# NURSING FUNDAMENTALS

## Caring & Clinical Decision Making

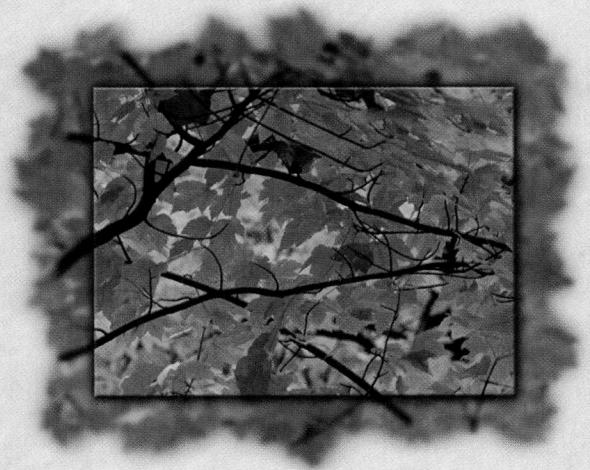

**Rick Daniels, RN, PhD**
*Oregon Health and Science University*
*Ashland, Oregon*

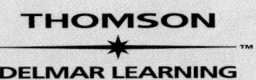

THOMSON

DELMAR LEARNING

Australia     Canada     Mexico     Singapore     Spain     United Kingdom     United States

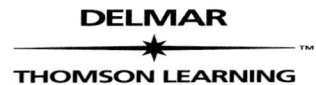

# DELMAR
## THOMSON LEARNING

**Nursing Fundamentals: Caring & Clinical Decision Making**
by Rick Daniels, RN, PhD

**Vice President, Health Care Business Unit:**
William Brottmiller

**Editorial Director:**
Cathy L. Esperti

**Acquisitions Editor:**
Matthew Filimonov

**Senior Developmental Editors:**
Marah Bellegarde, Elisabeth F. Williams

**Editorial Assistant:**
Patricia Osborn

**Marketing Director:**
Jennifer McAvey

**Marketing Channel Manager:**
Tamara Caruso

**Marketing Coordinator:**
Karen Summerlin

**Production Manager:**
Barbara A. Bullock

**Project Editor:**
Mary Ellen Cox

**Art/Design Specialist:**
Connie Lundberg-Watkins

**Production Coordinator:**
Kenneth McGrath

**Technology Director:**
Laurie K. Davis

**Technology Project Manager:**
Victoria Moore

**Technology Production Coordinator:**
Sherry Conners

Library of Congress Cataloging-in-Publication Data

Nursing fundamentals : caring & clinical decision making / Rick Daniels.
    p. ; cm.
    Includes bibliographical references.
    ISBN 0-7668-3836-6
    1. Nursing.  2. Nursing assessment.
    I. Daniels, Rick, RN.
    [DNLM: 1. Nursing Care.  2. Nursing.
    WY 100 N97324 2004]
    RT41.N873 2004
    610.73–dc22          2003055706

Asia (Including India):
Thomson Learning
60 Albert Street, #15-01
Albert Complex
Singapore 189969
Tel 65 336-6411
Fax 65 336-7411

Australia/New Zealand:
Nelson
102 Dodds Street
South Melbourne
Victoria 3205
Australia
Tel 61 (0)3 9685-4111
Fax 61 (0)3 9685-4199

Latin America:
Thomson Learning
Seneca 53
Colonia Polanco
11560 Mexico, D.F. Mexico
Tel (525) 281-2906
Fax (525) 281-2656

Canada:
Nelson
1120 Birchmount Road
Toronto, Ontario
Canada M1K 5G4
Tel (416) 752-9100
Fax (416) 752-8102

UK/Europe/Middle East/Africa:
Thomson Learning
Berkshire House
1680-173 High Holborn
London WC1V 7AA
United Kingdom
Tel 44 (0)20 497-1422
Fax 44 (0)20 497-1426

Spain (includes Portugal):
Paraninfo
Calle Magallanes 25
28015 Madrid
España
Tel 34 (0)91 446-3350
Fax 34 (0)91 445-6218

## NOTICE TO THE READER

I dedicate this textbook to Nancy, Luke, and Jennie, who are the best wife, son, and daughter a man could love, and to David Greer, who will always be an inspiration to me.

# CONTENTS

## Unit II
The Nursing Process
and Decision Making

## Chapter 10
Critical Thinking and the
Nursing Process

## Chapter 11
Assessment

## Chapter 12
Nursing Diagnosis

## Chapter 13
Outcome Identification
and Planning

## Chapter 14
Implementation

## Chapter 15
## Evaluation

## Chapter 16
## Documentation and Reporting

## Unit III
## Client Care Across the Life Span

## Chapter 17
## The Pediatric Client

## Chapter 18
## The Adult Client

## Chapter 19
## The Geriatric Client

## Unit IV
Arenas of Client Care

## Chapter 20
Acute Care

## Chapter 21
Restorative Care

## Chapter 22
Home Care

# Unit VI
## Concepts of Therapeutic Nursing

## Chapter 26
### Infection Control

## Chapter 27
### Health Assessment

## Chapter 28
### Client Education

# Section II
## Nursing of Human Function

## Unit VII
### Health Perception and Health Maintenance

### Chapter 32
### Health Maintenance, Health Promotion, and Wellness

### Chapter 33
### Safety and Hygiene

## Unit VIII
### Nutritional-Metabolic

### Chapter 34
### Fluid, Electrolyte, and Acid-Base Balance

# Unit IX
## Elimination

## Chapter 37
### Urinary and Bowel Elimination

# Unit X
## Activity-Exercise

## Chapter 38
### Mobility and Biomechanics

## Chapter 39
### Oxygenation

## Unit XIII
## Self-Perception/ Self-Concept

## Chapter 43
## Self-Concept

## Unit XIV
## Role-Relationship

## Chapter 44
## Family, Roles, Relationships, and Social Support

## Chapter 45
## Loss and Grief

## Unit XV
### Sexuality-Reproductive

### Chapter 46
#### Sexuality

## Unit XVI
### Coping-Stress Tolerance

### Chapter 47
#### Stress, Anxiety, Coping, and Adaptation

## Unit XVII
### Value-Belief

### Chapter 48
#### Spiritual Health

# CONTRIBUTORS AND REVIEWERS

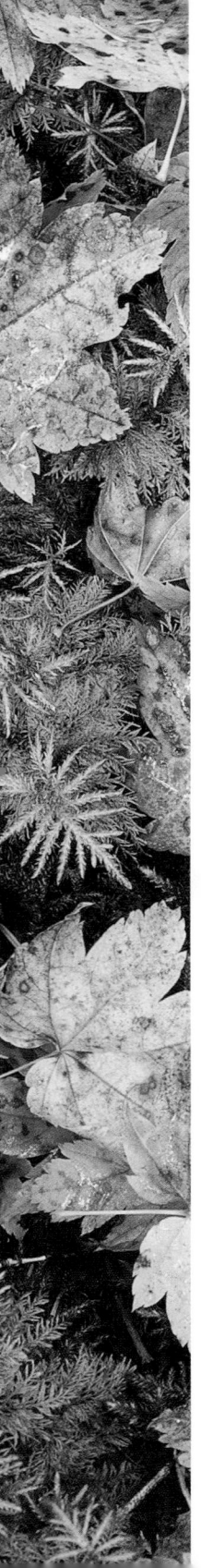

## Contributors

**Crisamar J. Anuncido, MS, FNP, RN, C**
Senior Specialist
Intermediate Care Unit
Sharp HealthCare
San Diego, California
*Chapter 29 Diagnostic Testing*

**Michael Brody, RN, BSN**
Wellness Coordinator—Center for Healthy Aging
Oregon Health and Science University
Portland, Oregon
*Chapter 4 The Nurse-Client Relationship*
*Chapter 14 Implementation*

**Kate Caelli, RN, RM, PhD**
Associate Professor of Nursing
University of Alberta
Alberta, Edmonton, Canada
*Chapter 6 Evidenced-Based Practice*
    *and Nursing Research*

**Carol Craig, PhD, FNP-C, RN**
Associate Professor
Oregon Health and Science University
Klamath Falls, Oregon
*Chapter 1 Evolution of Nursing Practice*
*Chapter 2 The Health Care Delivery System*
*Chapter 48 Spiritual Health*

**Annemarie Day, RN, MSN, FNP-C**
Family Nurse Practitioner
Medford, Oregon
*Chapter 38 Mobility and Biomechanics*
*Chapter 41 Sensation, Perception, and Cognition*

**Dorothy B. Doughty, MN, RN, FNP, CWOCN, FAAN**
Director
Wound Ostomy Continence Nursing
    Education Center
Emory University
Atlanta, Georgia
*Chapter 36 Skin Integrity and Wound Healing*

**Deborah L. Fell-Carson, BSN, RN, COHN-S, HEM**
Employee Health Coordinator/Safety Officer
Lebanon Community Hospital
Lebanon, Oregon
*and*
Lieutenant Colonel
Army Nurse Officer
Oregon Army National Guard
Monmouth, Oregon
*Chapter 25 Management and Policy*
*Chapter 33 Safety and Hygiene*

**Heather Freiheit, RN, BSN, EMT-P**
Clinical Manager
Emergency Services

Rogue Valley Medical Center
Medford, Oregon
*Chapter 15 Evaluation*

**Leonard H. Friedman, PhD, MPH**
Associate Professor of Public Health
Oregon State University
Corvallis, Oregon
*Chapter 24 Leadership, Delegation, and Collaboration*

**Ruth N. Grendell, DNSc, RN**
Professor Emerita
Point Loma Nazarene University
San Diego, California
*and*
Adjunct Professor
University of Phoenix
San Diego, California
*Chapter 7 Advanced Technology and Information Systems*
*Chapter 10 Critical Thinking and the Nursing Process*
*Chapter 12 Nursing Diagnosis*
*Chapter 13 Outcome Identification and Planning*
*Chapter 17 The Pediatric Client*
*Chapter 39 Oxygenation*
*Chapter 43 Self-Concept*
*Chapter 47 Stress, Anxiety, Coping, and Adaptation*

**Melissa Halas, RD, MA, CNSD**
Certified Nutrition Support Dietitian
Pasadena, California
*Chapter 35 Nutrition*

**Emily Wurster Hitchens, EdD, RN**
Associate Dean
School of Health Sciences
Lydia Green Nursing Program
Seattle Pacific University
Seattle, Washington
*Chapter 16 Documentation and Reporting*

**Sandra B. Holmes, RN, BSN, MA (C)**
Quality Improvement Analyst
Lebanon Community Hospital
Lebanon, Oregon
*Chapter 28 Client Education*
*Chapter 32 Health Maintenance, Health Promotion, and*
    *Wellness*

**Kathleen Lagana, RN, PhD**
Assistant Professor of Nursing
Oregon Health and Science University
Ashland, Oregon
*Chapter 44 Family Roles, Relationships, and Social Support*

**Katherine Moore, RN, PhD**
Assistant Professor of Nursing
University of Alberta
Alberta, Edmonton, Canada
*Chapter 6 Evidence-Based Practice and Nursing Research*
*Chapter 37 Urinary and Bowel Elimination*

**Larry A. Mullins, FACHE, CFAAMA**
President/CEO

Samaritan Health Services
Corvallis, Oregon
*Chapter 24 Leadership, Delegation, and Collaboration*

**Wendy Neander, MSN, RN**
Assistant Professor
Oregon Health and Science University
Ashland, Oregon
*Chapter 23 Community Care*
*Chapter 32 Health Maintenance, Health Promotion, and
   Wellness*

**Tina H. Olson, EdD, RN**
Professor, College of Health Sciences
Midwestern University
Glendale, Arizona
*and*
Senior Research Scientist
Mayo Clinic
Scottsdale, Arizona
*Chapter 9 Ethical Issues*
*Chapter 19 The Geriatric Client*

**Kathy Player, RN, EdD**
Chair, Division of Professional Studies
Grand Canyon University
Phoenix, Arizona
*Chapter 8 Legal Accountability and Responsibilities*

**Ellen Poole, DNSc (c), RN, CCRN, CPAN**
Associate Professor of Nursing
Grand Canyon University
Samaritan College of Nursing
Phoenix, Arizona
*Chapter 3 Framework of Nursing Practice*

**Marilyn Housel Poysky, RN, MSN, CS**
Assistant Professor
School of Health Sciences
Seattle Pacific University
Seattle, Washington
*Chapter 21 Restorative Care*
*Chapter 30 Medication Administration*

**Sharon M. Rayman, RN, MS, CPTC, CCTC**
Assistant Professor
Grand Canyon University
Samaritan College of Nursing
Phoenix, Arizona
*Chapter 11 Assessment*
*Chapter 27 Health Assessment*

**Diana Amaya Rodriquez, RN, PhD**
Associate Professor
Department of Nursing
Assistant Chair
Point Loma Nazarene University
San Diego, California
*Chapter 5 Culture and Ethnicity*

**Milena Segatore, RN, BscN, MscN, MNI-PG, CNRN**
Clinical Nurse Specialist—Neurosurgery/ Trauma
St. Michael's Hospital
30 Bond Street
Toronto, Ontario, Canada
*Chapter 20 Acute Care*
*Chapter 34 Fluid, Electrolyte, and Acid-Base Balance*

**Valerie Lindquist Stalsbroten, RN, MN**
Adjunct Faculty
School of Health Sciences
Seattle Pacific University
Seattle, Washington

*Chapter 18 The Adult Client*
*Chapter 22 Home Care*

**Debra L. Topham, PhD, RN, CNS, ACRN**
Assistant Professor
Oregon Health and Science University
Portland, Oregon
*Chapter 31 Alternative and Complementary Therapies*
*Chapter 40 Sleep and Rest*
*Chapter 42 Pain*
*Chapter 45 Loss and Grief*
*Chapter 46 Sexuality*

**Elizabeth Torrence, RN, MN, EdD**
Associate Professor
School of Health Sciences
Seattle Pacific University
Seattle, Washington
*Chapter 18 The Adult Client*

**Fred Wilkins, RN, MN (C)**
Nurse Manager
Roseburg Veterans Administration Hospital
Roseburg, Oregon
*Chapter 26: Infection Control*

## Additional Contributors

**Carma Andrus, MN, RN, CNS**
Dauterive Primary Care Clinic
St. Martinville, Louisiana

**Billie Barringer, RN, CS, APRN**
School of Nursing
Northeast Louisiana University
Monroe, Louisiana

**Barbara Brillhart, PhD, RN, CRRN, FNP-C**
College of Nursing
Arizona State University
Tempe, Arizona

**Ali Brown, MSN, RN**
Assistant Professor
College of Nursing
University of Tennessee
Knoxville, Tennessee

**Virginia Burggraf, MSN, RN, C**
Gerontological Nurse Consultant
Kensington, Maryland

**Beth Christensen, MN, RN, CCRN**
Touro Infirmary
New Orleans, Louisiana

**Jan Corder, DNS, RN**
Dean, School of Nursing
Northeast Louisiana University
Monroe, Louisiana

**Julie Coy, MS, RN, C**
Pain Consultation Service
The Children's Hospital
Denver, Colorado

**Sue C. DeLaune, MN, RN, C**
Adjunct Faculty
William Carey College
New Orleans, Louisiana
*and*
President, SDeLaune Consulting
Mandeville, Louisiana

**Mary Ellen Zator Estes, MSN, RN, CCRN**
Assistant Professor
School of Nursing
Marymount University
Arlington, Virginia

**Mary Frost, RN, BSN**
Covington, Louisiana

**Norma Fujise, MS, RN, C**
School of Nursing
University of Hawaii
Honolulu, Hawaii

**Mikel Gray, PhD, CURN, CCCN**
Nurse Practitioner/Clinical Investigator
Associate Professor
Department of Urology
University of Virginia Health Sciences Center
Charlottesville, Virginia
*and*
Adjunct Professor
Lancing School of Nursing
Bellarmine College
Louisville, Kentucky

**Janet Kula Harden, RN, MSN**
Faculty
Wayne State University
College of Nursing
Detroit, Michigan

**Lucille Joel, EdD, RN, FAAN**
**Professor**
College of Nursing
Rutgers—The State University of New Jersey
Newark, New Jersey

**Patricia K. Ladner, MS, MN, RN**
Consultant for Nursing Practice
Louisiana State Board of Nursing
New Orleans, Louisiana

**Claire Lincoln, MN, RN, CS**
Psychiatric Mental Health Clinical Nurse Specialist
Touro Infirmary
New Orleans, Louisiana

**Judy Martin, MS, RN, JD**
Nurse Attorney
Louisiana Department of Health and Hospitals
Health Standards Section
Baton Rouge, Louisiana

**Linda McCuistion, PhD, RN**
Assistant Professor
School of Nursing
Our Lady of Holy Cross College
New Orleans, Louisiana

**Elizabeth "Betty" Hauck Miller, MPH, BSN**
Director of Education
Meadowcrest Hospital, Gretna, Louisiana
*and*
JoEllen Smith Regional Medical Center,
New Orleans, Louisiana

**Mary Anne Modrcin-McCarthy, PhD, RN**
Associate Professor and Director of the Undergraduate
    Program
College of Nursing
University of Tennessee—Knoxville
Knoxville, Tennessee

**Barbara S. Moffett, PhD, RN**
Associate Professor of Nursing
School of Nursing
Southeastern Louisiana University
Hammond, Louisiana

**Brenda Owens, PhD, RN**
Associate Professor
School of Nursing
Louisiana State University Medical Center
New Orleans, Louisiana

**Demetrius Porche, DNS, RN, CCRN**
Associate Professor and Director
Bachelor of Science in Nursing Program
Nicholas State University
*and*
Adjunct Assistant Professor
Tulane University
School of Public Health and Topical Medicine
New Orleans, Louisiana

**Suzanne Riche, RN, C, MS**
Associate Professor
Charity School of Nursing
New Orleans, Louisiana

**Cheryl Taylor, PhD, RN**
Associate Professor of Nursing
North Carolina Agricultural and Technical
    State University
Greensboro, North Carolina

**Lorrie Wong, RN, MS**
School of Nursing
University of Hawaii
Honolulu, Hawaii

**Martha Yager, RN**
Assistant Director of Nurses
Bennington Health and Rehabilitation Center
Bennington, Vermont

**Rothlyn Zahourek, MS, RN, CS**
Certified Clinical Nurse Specialist
Amherst, Massachusetts

## Technical Writer and Reviewer

**Nancy Daniels, BSN, MEd**
Educator
Ashland School District and Southern Oregon
    University
Ashland, Oregon

## Reviewers

**Aris Andrews, RN, MS**
Assistant Professor of Nursing
Creighton University
Hastings, Nebraska

**Henrietta Bernal, RN, PhD**
Professor Emerita
School of Nursing
University of Connecticut
Storrs, Connecticut

**Diane Blanchard, RN, CNS, PhD**
Professor of Nursing
Alcorn University
Natchez, Mississippi

**Terre Bryan, RN, MSN, C, CFNP**
Assistant Professor of Nursing
Alcorn University
Natchez, Mississippi

**Beverly J. Bye, RN, MS Med, CS-FNR, FNE, CCES, CRNP**
Clinical Assistant Professor
Towson University
Towson, Maryland

**Joseann H. Dewitt, RN, MSN, C, CLNC**
Assistant Professor of Nursing
Alcorn State University
Natchez, Mississippi

**Lisa M. Fiorentino, RN, PhD**
Instructor of Nursing
University of Pittsburgh—Bradford
Bradford, Pennsylvania

**Mary Beth Gillis, RN, MS**
Assistant Professor of Nursing
Elmira College
Elmira, New York

**Marilyn Handley, RN, PhD**
Capstone College of Nursing
Professor of Nursing
University of Alabama
Tuscaloosa, Alabama

**Nicole Harder, MS**
Lecturer, Faculty of Nursing
University of Manitoba
Winnipeg, Manitoba, Canada

**Virginia Hedger, RN, BSN, MSN, PhD**
Assistant Professor of Nursing
Northern Kentucky University
Highland Heights, Kentucky

**Beth Hickey, BSN, MSN**
Instructor of Nursing
Northern Kentucky University
Highland Heights, Kentucky

**Alicia Horkan, RN, MSN, CNN**
Clinical Instructor of Nursing
Valdosta State University
Valdosta, Georgia

**Patricia Kaiser-McCloud, RN, MS**
Lecturer of Nursing
University of Michigan
Ann Arbor, Michigan

**Kathie M. Larke, RN, MEd, BC**
Nurse Educator
Middlesex Hospital
Portland, Oregon

**Sharon Little-Stoetzel, RN, MSN**
Instructor of Nursing
Graceland University
Independence, Missouri

**Cindy W. McCoy, RN, PhD**
Assistant Professor of Nursing
Troy State University
Troy, Alabama

**Nancy McGowan, RN, PhD**
Professor of Nursing
The University of Texas—Brownsville
Brownsville, Texas

**Lisa Oswalt, MSN, RN, BC**
Instructor of Nursing
Delta State University
Cleveland, Mississippi

**Carol A. Rafferty, RN, MSN, ANP**
Instructor of Nursing
Fox Valley Technical College
Appleton, Wisconsin

**Anita Reed, RN, MSN**
Instructor of Nursing
St. Elizabeth School of Nursing
Lafayette, Indiana

**Catherine Sikorski, MSN, APRN, BC**
Clinical Instructor of Nursing
Wayne State University
Detroit, Michigan

**Marilyn Stoner, RN, PhD**
Lecturer of Nursing
California State University
Long Beach, California

**Susan S. Sumner, RN, MS**
Instructor of Nursing
Holyoke Community College
Holyoke, Massachusetts

**Barbara Voshall, RN, MSN**
Assistant Professor of Nursing
Graceland University
Independence, Missouri

**Theresia Witt, MSN, RN-C**
Associate Professor of Nursing and
    Program Director
Alderson-Broaddus College
Philippi, West Virginia

**Michele Woodbeck, RN, MS**
Associate Professor of Nursing
Hudson Valley Community College
Troy, New York

# PREFACE

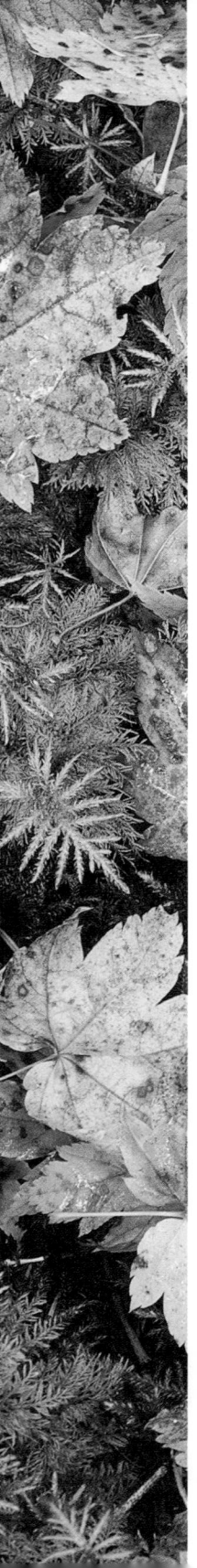

Nursing Fundamentals: Caring & Clinical Decision Making is a comprehensive text created for nursing students that addresses the fundamental topics that support nursing practice. It provides a learner-oriented, logically organized source of information to help students understand the knowledge required to become caring and responsible practitioners.

As the new century unfolds, the health care delivery system is more complex in many ways. Technological advancements are challenging and numerous, but just as challenging are the changing client situations to which nurses must adapt in order to provide their leadership in the system. Acute care stays have shortened, acuity levels have risen, and the percentages of clients in ambulatory, home care, and outpatient settings have grown. In addition, there are critical shortages of skilled nurse providers across all arenas of care. Nursing must embrace these challenges by preparing its students to be professionals who will not only provide the quality care that is needed but also exhibit leadership for the future.

## Conceptual Approach

The concept for Nursing Fundamentals arose from a need identified during the author's years of instruction to offer nursing students a thorough, organized, and practical approach to content delivery and skill mastery. Solid, accurate content is presented in a pedagogical framework that appeals to the various learning styles unique to each student learner. References to websites, cues to DVD nursing skills, and step-by-step procedures within the text are examples of methods of instruction that optimize learning for each reader. In addition, a wide variety of special features focusing on client education, research, and problem solving, among other things, fosters effective nursing practice and develops the critical thinking skills of the learner.

The client is the focus of the book, with a holistic perspective that encourages the nursing student to see each person with potential for health promotion and wellness, in addition to the needed focus on disease prevention and management across all levels of care. Case studies at the end of each chapter provide practical scenarios for application and synthesis of concepts. Full-color pages, a visually appealing design, boxes that emphasize essential points, and additional student tutorial references all engage the learner in a user-friendly approach. The information and learning processes, in collaboration with critical thinking skills of the active student-participant, foster the development of a caring, ethical, and responsible practicing professional nurse.

## Organization of the Text

Nursing Fundamentals consists of 48 chapters, which are organized under two global sections divided into 17 units. **Section I, Foundations of Nursing**, comprises Chapters 1 through 31 and provides the organization for the basic elements of nursing. **Section II, Nursing of Human Function**, includes Chapters 32 through 48 and uses Gordon's Functional Health Patterns as the organizing framework to focus on the implementation of the nursing process.

### Section I: Foundations of Nursing

**Unit I, Foundations of Nursing Practice** (Chapters 1 through 9), introduces the student to the basics of nursing and lays the foundation for learning about nursing. The first two chapters present a historical basis for the profession of nursing and an overview of the health care delivery system. Chapter 3 provides information describing the theoretical framework for nursing practice. Chapter 4 emphasizes the importance of the relationship between clients and nurses. Chapter 5 describes the implications of both the cultural and ethnic backgrounds of clients. Chapters 6 and 7 emphasize the value of evidence-based practice and the challenges and benefits of the information systems and technology of this era. Chapters 8 and 9 discuss invaluable legal and ethical issues relevant to nursing practice.

**Unit II, The Nursing Process and Decision Making** (Chapters 10 through 16), reviews decision making, the nursing process specific to the practice of nursing, and the necessary element of documentation/reporting in nursing practice.

**Unit III, Client Care Across the Life Span** (Chapters 17 through 19), covers the major nursing issues for the three broad categories of human development: pediatric, adult, and geriatric. Each of these chapters provides information explaining different considerations specific to the age of the client.

**Unit IV, Arenas of Client Care** (Chapters 20 through 23), includes individualized needs for the role of nurses in the different arenas of client care. Acute care (Chapter 20) is a traditional area of nursing care impacted heavily by advanced technology. Restorative care (Chapter 21) is emphasized due to the increasing numbers of aging clients. Chapters 22 and 23 focus on the increasing percentages of clients in home care settings and the continuing need for community nursing care.

**Unit V, Leadership in Nursing** (Chapters 24 and 25), offers information necessary for the increasing leadership roles of nurses (Chapter 24) in the health care delivery system. Nurses are intricately involved as managers and policy makers (Chapter 25) and continue to have greater responsibilities as leaders in the health care professions.

**Unit VI, Concepts of Therapeutic Nursing** (Chapters 26 through 31), explains various topics of interest pertinent to nursing practice. Chapter 26 provides the practice foundation of principles of infection control, Chapter 27 explores the techniques of health assessment, and Chapter 28 addresses the necessary element of client education in nursing practice. The importance and value of diagnostic testing is presented in Chapter 29. Chapter 30 describes the principles of medication administration, while Chapter 31 provides information regarding alternative and complementary therapies.

## Section II: Nursing of Human Function

**Unit VII, Health Perception and Health Maintenance** (Chapters 32 and 33), discusses the first functional health pattern which focuses on the importance of health maintenance and wellness (Chapter 32) and safety considerations (Chapter 33).

**Unit VIII, Nutritional-Metabolic** (Chapters 34 through 36), covers the important elements of the nutritional-metabolic pattern. Chapter 34 provides information on fluid and electrolyte implications and Chapter 35 focuses on nutrition as it impacts client care. Chapter 36 demonstrates the complications associated with skin integrity and wound healing care.

**Unit IX, Elimination** (Chapter 37), describes the elimination pattern, focusing on the impact of both bowel and urinary elimination to client care.

**Unit X, Activity-Exercise** (Chapters 38 and 39), explains the activity-exercise pattern. Chapter 38 presents important information regarding the principles of biomechanics and mobility issues for client care.

Chapter 39 adds the important nursing implications of oxygenation issues specific to respiratory and cardiovascular functioning.

**Unit XI, Sleep-Rest** (Chapter 40), addresses the sleep-rest pattern and its importance to client health.

**Unit XII, Cognitive-Perceptual** (Chapters 41 and 42), discusses the cognitive-perceptual pattern. Chapter 41 explores the elements of sensation, perception, and cognition involved in client conditions. Chapter 42 follows with specific information regarding the implications of pain and the associated nursing care directed towards client comfort.

**Unit XIII, Self-Perception/Self-Concept** (Chapter 43), describes the self-perception/self-control pattern and the nursing implications for clients with alterations in self-concept.

**Unit XIV, Role-Relationship** (Chapters 44 and 45), addresses the role-relationship pattern. Chapter 44 identifies the roles displayed by clients and explains the concept of social support in the context of nursing care. Chapter 45 examines loss and grief as related to clients and their conditions.

**Unit XV, Sexuality-Reproductive** (Chapter 46), discusses the sexuality health pattern. It describes the importance of human sexuality and the implications for nursing care in an open and sensitive manner.

**Unit XVI, Coping-Stress Tolerance** (Chapter 47), addresses the coping-stress tolerance pattern. The effects of stress and anxiety are emphasized, along with the role of nursing to assist clients in coping and adapting to their stressors.

**Unit XVII, Value-Belief** (Chapter 48), explores the value-belief pattern. The spirituality of clients is emphasized and the nursing implications for clients and their spiritual health are presented.

**Appendices:** Seven appendices augment *Nursing Fundamentals*. They include the NANDA nursing diagnoses, symbols and abbreviations, recommended dietary allowances, reference laboratory values, English/Spanish words and phrases, Standard Precautions, and concept mapping.

A detailed glossary is also included.

## Special Features

Enlightening features in *Nursing Fundamentals* stimulate critical thinking and self-reflection and assist the learner in synthesizing and applying the information provided in the text. These complements to the text information create a supportive learning environment as the student transitions to a practicing professional.

**Chapter Competencies** are placed at the beginning of each chapter to provide the main points within each chapter. They provide direction for study and give organization to the content.

**Key Terms** are printed in bold in the chapters to denote terms of particular importance to the reader. In addition, these terms are defined in the glossary for further reference.

**Case Studies/Nursing Care Plans** include sample client examples where pertinent history, physical assessment data, and laboratory findings emphasize the nursing role in the clinical setting. These examples engage the reader in making real and practical client care decisions.

**Stop and Think** boxes encourage critical thinking. They are clinical questions that stimulate problem solving and clinical decision making.

**Nursing Strategy** features are specific nursing interventions that offer a wide variety of hints, tips, and strategies for the provision of client care.

**Client Education** boxes present concise, relevant teaching interventions for clients, family, or support persons necessary to enhance or maintain health.

**Clinical Alerts** concisely indicate cautionary information for the nurse, including emergency findings and life-threatening situations.

**Client Reflections** are anecdotes that relate first-person experiences of clients in the health care system. Each example presents a brief client scenario, which includes quotes reflecting the client's feelings, questions, or concerns to humanize the client to the reader.

**Focus on Wellness** boxes include concepts of wellness and health promotion illustrating holistic nursing practices as well as the importance of disease prevention.

**Legal and Ethical Issues** highlights demonstrate legal implications or ethical issues that arise from a given area of nursing care.

**Life Span Considerations** highlight nursing implications of given developmental stages (e.g., pediatric, geriatric) in a brief narrative format that informs the reader of life span issues.

**Community/Home Care** boxes present relevant information about the nursing implications of care in the community or home setting.

**Research Focus** elements provide a cogent synopsis of research studies emphasizing evidence-based practice for the concepts fundamental to basic nursing practice. These refereed journal sources support the student in developing a knowledgeable base for learning.

**Procedures** present detailed step-by-step instructions on how to perform specific nursing skills. Many of these procedures have a video or DVD counterpart that accompanies the text as supplemental material.

**Key Concepts** highlight the primary points in the chapter and direct the reader in reviewing pertinent information.

**Review Questions and Activities** offer readers an opportunity to evaluate understanding of specific chapter content. Questions include recall, application, and synthesis formats to stimulate critical thinking skills.

**Multimedia Links** appear in some chapters to link them to video or DVD resources that support the chapter content. A complete list of these links is also included on page xxxiv.

**Web Resources** at the end of each chapter provide meaningful assistance to the reader in further research of a topic or with a clinical practice issue.

**References** at the end of each chapter document a current and varied theoretical basis for the content of the text.

# Teaching/Learning Package

The complete ancillary package was created to achieve two goals:

1. To assist students in learning the skills and information essential to securing a career in the profession of nursing;

2. To assist instructors in planning and implementing their programs for the most efficient use of time and other resources.

## Electronic Classroom Manager (ISBN 0-7668-3843-9)

The Electronic Classroom Manager is available to facilitate classroom preparations, presentation, and testing. Components include:

- **Computerized test bank** with approximately 1,800 questions geared to text chapters and following the NCLEX format
- **PowerPoint presentation** designed to support and facilitate lecture and classroom instruction
- **Electronic image library** containing files of hundreds of images from the text
- **Instructor's Manual** with strategies and answers to the Review Questions and Activities found in the text

## Online Companion (ISBN 0-7668-3844-7)

The Online Companion allows users of *Nursing Fundamentals* to access a wealth of information designed to enhance the book. Through the Delmar Learning site on the World Wide Web, this companion offers, by chapter, a content overview, thought-provoking questions with suggested responses, and useful Internet links.

## Procedures Checklist

(ISBN 1-4018-4045-0)

This teaching/learning tool contains key steps for every procedure in *Nursing Fundamentals*. The checklists may be used to help students evaluate their comprehension and execution of the procedures.

## Study Guide (ISBN 0-7668-3837-4)

The Study Guide offers a full array of study questions in varying formats (multiple choice, matching, fill in the blank) to facilitate and reinforce student learning.

## Multimedia Resources

A rich array of video and DVD resources is available to supplement and enhance text content. Icons are included in text procedures that have a video or DVD counterpart; a chapter-closing Multimedia Links element also highlights the tie to multimedia content. Available videos include:

Christensen *Core Concepts in Nursing Videos:*
- *Assessment and Diagnosis,* ISBN 0-7668-2553-1
- *Client Education,* ISBN 0-7668-2556-6
- *History of Nursing,* ISBN 0-7668-2557-4
- *Nursing Process,* ISBN 0-7668-2552-3
- *Nutrition and Diet Therapy,* ISBN 0-7668-2554-X
- *Planning and Intervention,* ISBN 0-7668-2555-8
- *Therapeutic Communication,* ISBN 0-7668-2559-0

Videos in the Altman and Morrison series include:
- *Delmar's Basic Nursing Care Skills Videos: Physical Assessment,* ISBN 1-4018-5098-7
- *Delmar's Basic Nursing Care Skills Videos: Vital Signs,* ISBN 1-4018-5100-2
- *Delmar's Basic Nursing Care Skills Videos: Basic Care I: Personal Care,* ISBN 1-4018-5101-0
- *Delmar's Basic Nursing Care Skills Videos: Basic Care II: Bed-Making,* ISBN 1-4018-5102-9
- *Delmar's Basic Nursing Care Skills Videos: Basic Care III: Infection Control and Bathing,* ISBN 1-4018-5103-7
- *Delmar's Basic Nursing Care Skills Videos: Basic Care IV: Aiding Client Movement I,* ISBN 1-4018-5104-5
- *Delmar's Basic Nursing Care Skills Videos: Basic Care V: Aiding Client Movement II,* ISBN 1-4018-5105-3
- *Delmar's Basic Nursing Care Skills Videos: Specimen Collection,* ISBN 1-4018-5106-1
- *Delmar's Intermediate Nursing Skills Videos: Nutrition and Elimination I,* ISBN 1-4018-5107-X
- *Delmar's Intermediate Nursing Skills Videos: Nutrition and Elimination II: Catheter Care,* ISBN 1-4018-5108-8
- *Delmar's Intermediate Nursing Skills Videos: Nutrition and Elimination III,* ISBN 1-4018-5109-6
- *Delmar's Intermediate Nursing Skills Videos: Wound Care,* ISBN 1-4018-5118-5
- *Delmar's Intermediate Nursing Skills Videos: Medication Administration I,* ISBN 1-4018-5110-X
- *Delmar's Intermediate Nursing Skills Videos: Medication Administration II: Routes of Administration,* ISBN 1-4018-5111-8
- *Delmar's Intermediate Nursing Skills Videos: Medication Administration III: Parenteral Medication,* ISBN 1-4018-5112-6
- *Delmar's Intermediate Nursing Skills Videos: Medication Administration IV: Intravenous Medication,* ISBN 1-4018-5113-4
- *Delmar's Advanced Nursing Care Skills Videos: Circulatory I: Venipuncture and Starting IV Therapy,* ISBN 1-4018-5114-2
- *Delmar's Advanced Nursing Care Skills Videos: Circulatory II: Maintaining IV Therapy,* ISBN 1-4018-5115-0
- *Delmar's Advanced Nursing Care Skills Videos: Circulatory III: Blood Transfusions,* ISBN 1-4018-5116-9
- *Delmar's Advanced Nursing Care Skills Videos: Oxygenation,* ISBN 1-4018-5117-7

Available Altman and Morrison DVDs include:
- *Delmar's Basic Nursing Skills DVD-ROM,* ISBN 1-4018-1071-3
- *Delmar's Intermediate Nursing Skills DVD-ROM,* ISBN 1-4018-1072-1
- *Delmar's Advanced Nursing Skills DVD-ROM,* ISBN 1-4018-1073-X

# ACKNOWLEDGMENTS

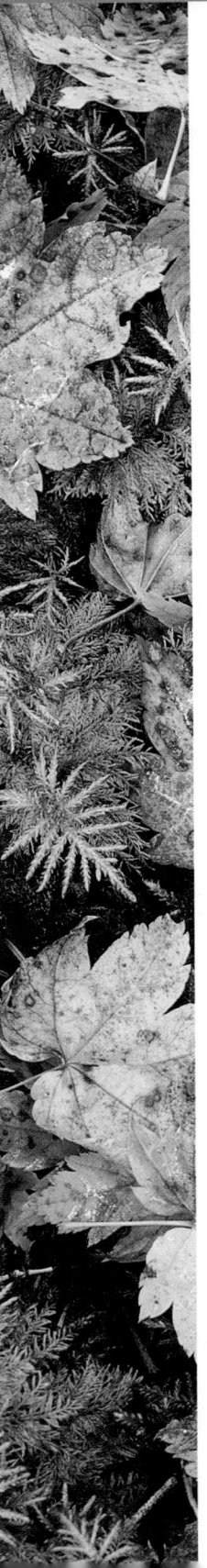

I would like to thank all the contributors to this comprehensive book for their time and effort in sharing their knowledge gained through the years. I also thank the reviewers for their time spent in critically reviewing the manuscripts and providing valuable comments that have been added to this text.

I would like to acknowledge and thank the members of the team at Delmar Learning who have worked with me in making this text a reality. Matthew Filimonov, acquisitions editor, and Marah Bellegarde and Elisabeth F. Williams, developmental editors, are incredible people whose knowledge and professional guidance assisted me with this project.

I particularly want to acknowledge my parents, "Corky" and Jennie, my brother Neil, and my grandparents. They raised me to love, to care, and to know that I could do whatever I wanted in life. From an early age they enveloped me with an attitude that was supportive of my being the best person I could become. I always knew if I needed anything, if it was in their power, they would be there for me.

Last, a very special thank-you to my immediate family: my adult children, Luke and Jennie, who are a constant joy to me; and my wife, Nancy, who acted as a technical writer and reviewer, and who helped me through every stage of this text. She is my constant and loving companion, with whom I am truly blessed. And I am most appreciative to the Lord for His direction in my life.

Rick Daniels obtained a bachelor of science in nursing from the University of Oregon Nursing School, Portland, Oregon, a master of science in nursing from the University of San Diego, California, and a PhD in nursing from the University of Texas in Austin.

He has taught nursing in associate, baccalaureate, and graduate schools of nursing, as well as in RN degree completion programs. Dr. Daniels has taught fundamentals of nursing, medical/surgical nursing, pharmacology, and research in a variety of programs. In addition, he teaches pathophysiology via distance learning and traditional classroom settings. He has also taught many adult health and illness topics at seminars and has presented posters for national organizations (e.g., Association of Operating Room Nurses, National League for Nurses, Educators Conference). Dr. Daniels administers clinical practicum courses in critical care and perioperative nursing arenas.

Dr. Daniels's clinical practice is kept current by practicing nursing as a colonel in the Oregon Army National Guard. He recently received an appointment as the Deputy State Commander of Oregon under the supervision of the Oregon State Surgeon.

Dr. Daniels' research is primarily associated with the concept of health promotion, and he has received three successive fundings with the Department of the Army to implement health promotion programs with National Guardsmen. In addition, Dr. Daniels publishes in nursing journals and authors nursing textbooks. He has membership in a number of professional nursing organizations, such as Sigma Theta Tau and the American Nurses Association.

Dr. Daniels is currently an associate professor with tenure at Oregon Health and Science University, School of Nursing.

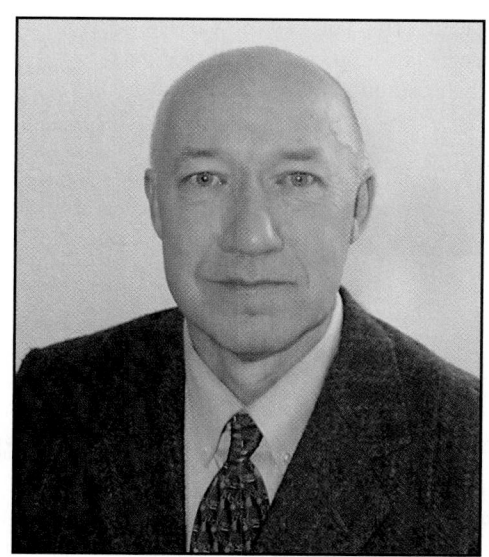

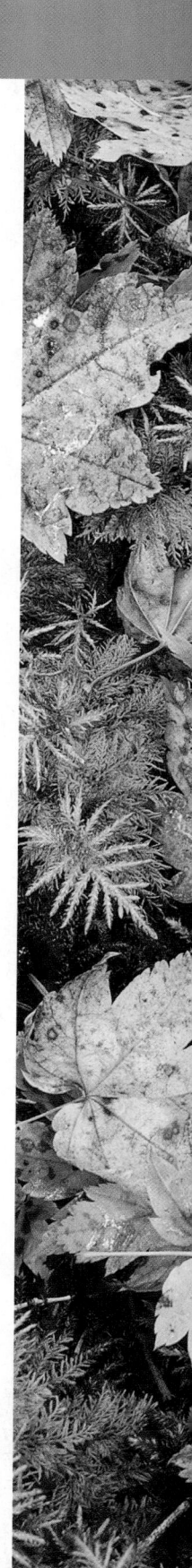

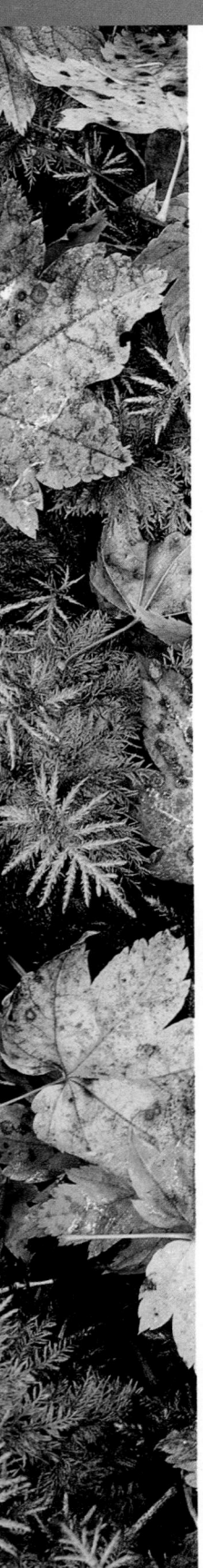

# HOW TO USE THIS TEXT

## STOP AND THINK

### What Is Cleanliness?

Cleanliness is highly valued by mainstream American society. However, in some cultures, a daily bath is not perceived as necessary or desirable. In fact, some cultures do not define natural body odors as offensive. It is important to consider the client in the context of cultural beliefs before labeling a client.

- Define the terms *dirty*, *unkempt*, and *foul-smelling*.

- Discuss how these value-laden terms can cloud the assessment process.

- Discuss how care can be affected by labeling a client as "dirty," "unkempt," or "foul-smelling."

## Stop and Think

Reading text materials does not always make you think critically. These boxes offer a client situation or topic that allows you to participate in decision making processes. Each example presents questions that stimulate you to think about chapter content and devise your individual answers.

## Nursing Strategy

In any profession there are many helpful hints that assist you in performing more efficiently. This is definitely true for nursing. These boxes list specific nursing interventions that offer you a wide variety of hints, tips, and strategies to help you as you work toward professional advancement. Share these ideas with your colleagues.

## NURSING STRATEGY

### Communicating Clearly in Nurses' Notes

[fol]lowing questions can assist the nurse in [do]cumentation:

[Are] exact times and dates for client assess-[me]nt and interventions noted?

[Is t]he purpose for client assessment and inter-[ven]tion indicated?

[Can] you identify what the nurse saw, smelled, [tou]ched, or heard?

[Is t]he client quoted directly? Is the client's [res]ponse noted?

5. Are the plans and expected client outcomes congruent with the observations?

Adapted from Carelock, J., & Innerarity, S. (2001). Critical incidents: Effective communication and documentation. *Critical Care Nursing, 23*(4), 59–66.

## CLIENT EDUCATION

### Preventing Skin Cancer

The following are preventive measures against developing skin cancer:

✓ Do not try to tan if your skin burns easily.
✓ Avoid unnecessary exposure to the sun.
✓ Avoid sunburn.
✓ Apply sunscreen of SPF 15 or higher when in the sun (note: cloudy days still produce dangerous ultraviolet rays). Sunscreens are rated in strength from 4 (lowest) to 50 (highest). The SPF indicates the solar protection factor, or how long a person can stay in the sun before getting burned.
✓ Wear protective clothing (broad-brimmed hat, long sleeves) if you are an at-risk individual.
✓ Use a lip balm that contains a sunscreen with the highest SPF number.

Adapted from American Cancer Society, 2003. Available: http://www.cancer.org

## Client Education

Clients benefit greatly from knowledge of self-care, and nurses presenting information in a collaborative manner promotes health. Therefore, these boxes present relevant teaching interventions for clients, family, or support persons necessary to enhance their health. Various instructions on how to equip clients with knowledge of well-being and preparing for procedures or outcomes is vital.

## CLINICAL ALERT

### Risk Factors for Skin Cancer

The following are people with risk factors for skin cancer:

- Fair-skinned, fair-haired, blue-eyed people
- People who sustain sunburn and do not tan
- People with longtime sun exposure (farmers, fisherman, construction workers)
- Adults who sunburn as frequently as children
- Elderly people and those with sun-damaged skin
- People exposed t⌐ (arsenic, nitrates⌐ oils and paraffins

Adapted from Schofield, J. R.
*really need to know about mol⌐*
Hopkins Press.

## Clinical Alerts

As a professional nurse, you will need to be able to react immediately in selected situations to ensure the health and safety of your clients. Pay careful attention to this feature as it will assist you in beginning to identify and respond to critical situations on your own, both efficiently and effectively.

## CLIENT REFLECTIONS

### Personalizing Nursing Interventions

Carlson is a 74-year-old client on your med⌐
⌐it. You are assessing her one morning when
⌐ys, "There's always so much going on here.
⌐imes I feel like you nurses forget you are
⌐all your procedures to real people. What if
⌐e your grandmother in this bed?" As her
⌐how would you respond to Mrs. Carlson?

## Client Reflections

The perspective of clients is extremely valuable, allowing you to empathize with their conditions. This box presents actual client scenarios with personal quotations, letting you determine the feelings and emotions that often accompany the client conditions. Use these examples to personalize your nursing care.

## FOCUS ON WELLNESS

### Illness Care versus Health Car⌐

Clients in hospital settings often feel that they⌐
receiving "illness care" rather than health⌐
While members of the health care team are⌐
implementing various interventions designe⌐
combat disease, the nurse can help the client f⌐
on those things the client can do to improve her
health. The specific steps vary depending on the
client's condition, but generally the client can
actively facilitate the healing process by getting
sufficient rest, movement, and nutrition; managing
her stress and pain; and maintaining a positive
attitude. By reminding the client of these simple
but important steps, and⌐
ly follow the plan of car⌐
client to implement es⌐
contribute to her wellne⌐

## Focus on Wellness

There are many clients with illnesses for which nurses do not consider the wellness and health promotion implications. These boxes include concepts of wellness and health promotion information in an attempt to make you realize that all clients can participate in health-oriented interventions.

## Legal and Ethical Issues

Our health care delivery system has many legal and ethical issues for the nurse to consider in the practice setting. These boxes describe client situations that make it easier for you to see the legal-ethical implications as you provide client care. Incorporate these insights into your professional growth and development as an ethical practitioner.

## LEGAL AND ETHICAL ISSUES

### Completeness in Charting

Is "If it wasn't charted, it wasn't done" just a⌐
⌐ince the purpose of the medical record is⌐
⌐ment the care administered to the client,⌐
⌐a practitioner convince a jury that care⌐
⌐ministered if it is not documented in the⌐
⌐record? Consider the following. A nurse,⌐
⌐t, always administers an intramuscular⌐
⌐in the ventrogluteal site (although both⌐
⌐rogluteal and dorsogluteal sites are within⌐
⌐pted guidelines of care). The nurse, how-⌐
⌐ils to chart the site on the medication⌐
⌐tration record (MAR). The client files a suit⌐
⌐ic nerve damage. Knowing that there is an⌐
⌐d greater risk factor for sciatic nerve injury⌐
⌐dorsogluteal site, do you think it would be
difficult to defend care given in this case?

## LIFE SPAN CONSIDERATIONS

### Blood Pressure Measurement

*Pediatric*

- Sma
  proc
  to h

- A cu

- It m
  arte

- BP v
  adol

- Take BP first before other anxiety or pain-
  producing procedures.

*Geriatric Variations*

- Elderly clients may have lost muscle mass and
  their upper arms may be quite thin. Be sure to
  adjust the cuff size to accommodate the
  client's arm.

- Many elderly clients have a history of hypertension and are taking antihypertensive
  medications.

## Life Span Considerations

It is important to recognize the specific implications for your care of clients at different developmental ages. You need to review such aspects as the physiological and psychological implications of different ages. This will assist you in delivering individualized nursing care.

## RESEARCH FOCUS

**Title of Study:** Infection control: New hand hygiene practices reduce drug-resistant germs in Washington, DC, hospital

**Study Purpose:** There is extremely poor compliance in health care workers using consistent handwashing techniques. This study's primary goal was to determine if staff could use alcohol-based hand-rubs (e.g., foam, gel, lotion), which are much less time-consuming than soap and water handwashing, and reduce nosocomial infection rates.

**Methods:** A 2-year study began at a VA medical center (an inner-city, tertiary-care teaching hospital with 167 acute and 120 long-term care beds). Five hundred alcohol-based dispensers were installed in all

## Research Focus

Evidence-Based Practice is essential to your development of knowledge and growth as a professional nurse. As you read these boxes, focus your attention on the elements of research that are presented and incorporate the application as appropriate in your nursing practice.

the study, the number of new cases of MRSA decreased by 21%, and the number of vancomycin-resistant enterococcus (VRE) decreased by 43%. The number of CD cases decreased about 22%. In addition
number of cases of new,
stant germs, the alcohol-
pular with the busy staff.
ture, there is the possibil-
rubs could take the place
. The new aseptic tech-
for staff, and ultimately
ct time for nurses and
infections.

## COMMUNITY/HOME CARE

### Taking Blood Press
in the Home

*Home Care Variations*

- Use the same cuff the client nor
  his home readings.

- Compare home readings to read
  cuff you know is properly calibra

- Assess the client's financial abili
  own sphygmomanometer.

- Consider use of an electronic BP cuff if the
  client has a hearing deficit.

*Long-Term Care Variations*

- Be aware of any injurie
  appliances that may co
  pressure reading at the

## Community/Home Care

Clients in the community and in their homes require specific care considerations. Many times these different settings require adaptation of techniques for delivering nursing care. As you read these examples, incorporate their principles into your practice and remember them for your own nursing practice.

**PROCEDURE 27-5    Taking Blood Pressure**

### EQUIPMENT NEEDED

- Stethoscope (Figure 27-27)
- Mercury sphygmomanometer with bladder
  and cuff
- Gloves if required
- Alcohol swabs

## Procedures

Procedure boxes are step-by-step instructions for performing basic clinical nursing skills. These features assist you as you practice in laboratory settings and then with clients in the clinical arenas. Use these procedures as a method of achieving competent behaviors in client care.

EMENTATION—ACTION/RATIONALE

### RATIONALE

achial Artery

most appropriate
ssure reading on an
one in which an

1. Reduces transmission of microorganisms.

2. Cuff inflation can temporarily interrupt blood
   flow and compromise circulation in an extremity
   already impaired or a vein receiving intravenous
   fluids.

# CASE STUDY/NURSING CARE PLAN

Mr. Wilkins, age 88, is hospitalized in the intensive care unit (ICU) with complications of diabetes mellitus type 1. Most recently, he is experiencing diabetic ketoacidosis (DKA) with a blood glucose of 340 mg/dL. In addition, he has coronary heart disease (CHD) from the microvascular complications of his diabetes (note: he has a pulmonary artery catheter to monitor his hemodynamic status). His primary clinical manifestations from the CHD ~~are~~ ... occasional arrhythmias. At present, his level of consciousness is ... espirations, his breath is acetone in nature, and he is extremely ... used in the careful documentation of his care, and charting takes ... places his vital signs, blood glucose, daily weights, and oxygen ... tion, there is a separate flow sheet for the ongoing neurological ... the medications he is receiving, including his titrated insulin, anti-

... ciated with type 1 diabetes mellitus. Specifically, he has a primary diagnosis of DKA (blood glucose = 340 mg/dL. In addition he has hypertension, atrial cardiac arrhythmias, and a decreased LOC. He is being monitored in an ICU.

## Nursing Diagnosis #1

*Deficient Fluid Volume* related to osmotic diuresis associated with hyperglycemia.

**NOC:** Electrolyte and Acid-Base Imbalance; Fluid Balance; Hydration; Nutritional Status; Food and Fluid Intake

**NIC:** Fluid Management; Hypovolemia Management; Shock Management: Volume

### Expected Outcomes
The client will:
1. Maintain a blood glucose level in the 150–180 mg/dL range within 72 hours.
2. Demonstrate no signs/symptoms of dehydration during his admission in the ICU.

---

## Case Study/Nursing Care Plan

These real-life scenarios present a client situation followed by nursing responsibilities outlined in a nursing process format.

---

## Review Questions and Activities

These activities stimulate your learning and allow you to synthesize and evaluate the knowledge gained when you study each section.

---

## Review Questions and Activities

1. Nate Jefferson, a nursing stude... his client's chart. The list of nursing diagnoses included in the chart seemed to describe the client well. However, something disturbed Jefferson about the list. The list he reviewed appears below. What is your response to this list? Identify the nursing diagnoses that seem to be problematic and the reasons for your conclusions.
   a. *Impaired Swallowing* as evidenced by stasis of food in oral cavity after chewing
   b. *Risk for Injury* as evidenced by weight and being dropped by staff
   c. *Impaired Skin Integrity* RT infrequent repositioning by staff
   d. *Chronic Confusion* as evidenced by Alzheimer's disease
   e. *Acute Pain* RT pain in right foot

2. Mr. Tyler is a 37-year-old client who limps into the clinic with pain in the right foot and swelling in the extremity. He is 5 feet 6 inches tall and weighs

---

## Multimedia Links

Refer to these links in selected chapters to learn what other sources are available for learning and practicing skills.

## Multimedia Links

Christensen *Core Concept Videos: Assessment and Diagnosis*

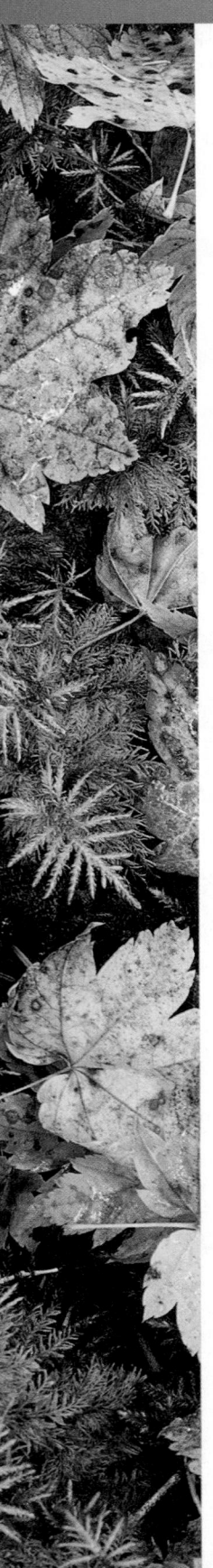

# MULTIMEDIA LINKS MATRIX

Many of the content areas and procedures in this book are designed to correlate with an accompanying video series. These videos show the step-by-step actions of the procedure, with an emphasis on new learners and correct practice. This matrix shows the correlation between the text content or procedure and the accompanying step-by-step video or DVD, which allows students to visualize the correct steps of the skill. The matrix below and the Multimedia Links listed at the end of chapters indicate the videos and DVDs where these content areas and procedures may be found.

## Key to Videos

Altman, *Basic Care*  Altman, Morrison: *Delmar's Fundamental and Advanced Nursing Skills Videos: Basic* (ISBN 1-4018-1079-9)

Altman, *Intermediate Care*  Altman, Morrison: *Delmar's Fundamental and Advanced Nursing Skills Videos: Intermediate* (ISBN 1-4018-1080-2)

Altman, *Advanced Care*  Altman, Morrison: *Delmar's Fundamental and Advanced Nursing Skills Videos: Advanced* (ISBN 1-4018-1081-0)

Christensen, *Core Concepts*  *Core Concepts in Nursing* Video Series (eight-tape set: ISBN 0-7768-2551-5)

## Key to DVD-ROMs

Altman, *Basic Care*  Altman, Morrison: *Delmar's Comprehensive Nursing Skills DVD-ROM: Basic* (ISBN 1-4018-1071-3)

Altman, *Intermediate Care*  Altman, Morrison: *Delmar's Comprehensive Nursing Skills DVD-ROM: Intermediate* (ISBN 1-4018-1072-1)

Altman, *Advanced Care*  Altman, Morrison: *Delmar's Comprehensive Nursing Skills DVD-ROM: Advanced* (ISBN 1-4018-1073-X)

| Chapter or Procedure Number | Content Area or Procedure Title | Video Link | DVD-ROM Link |
|---|---|---|---|
| 1 | History of Nursing | Christensen, *Core Concepts: History of Nursing* | — |
| 4 | The Nurse-Client Relationship | Christensen, *Core Concepts: Therapeutic Communication* | — |
| 11 | Assessment | Christensen, *Core Concepts: Nursing Process* | — |
| 12 | Nursing Diagnosis | Christensen, *Core Concepts: Assessment and Diagnosis* | — |
| 13 | Outcome Identification and Planning | Christensen, *Core Concepts: Planning and Intervention* | — |
| 14 | Implementation | Christensen, *Core Concepts: Planning and Intervention* | — |
| 16 | Documentation and Reporting | Christensen, *Core Concepts: Nursing Documentation* | — |
| 26-1 | Handwashing | Altman, *Basic Care III: Infection Control and Bathing* | Altman, *Basic Care: Handwashing* |
| 26-2 | Surgical Asepsis: Preparing and Maintaining a Sterile Field | — | Altman, *Basic Care: Preparing a Surgical Site* |
| 26-3 | Applying Sterile Gloves via the Open Method | — | Altman, *Basic Care: Applying Sterile Gloves via the Open Method* |
| 26-4 | Donning a Cap and Mask | — | Altman, *Basic Care: Donning and Removing Clean and Contaminated Gloves, Cap, and Mask* |
| 26-5 | Surgical Scrub | — | Altman, *Basic Care: Surgical Scrub* |
| 26-6 | Applying Sterile Gloves via the Closed Method | — | Altman, *Basic Care: Applying Sterile Gloves and Gown via the Closed Method* |
| 27-1 | Taking a Temperature | Altman, *Basic Care: Vital Signs* | Altman, *Basic Care: Taking a Temperature* |
| 27-2 | Taking a Pulse | Altman, *Basic Care: Vital Signs* | Altman, *Basic Care: Taking a Pulse* |
| 27-3 | Counting Respirations | Altman, *Basic Care: Vital Signs* | Altman, *Basic Care: Counting Respirations* |
| 27-4 | Administering Pulse Oximetry | — | Altman, *Advanced Care: Administering Pulse Oximetry* |
| 27-5 | Taking a Blood Pressure | Altman, *Basic Care: Vital Signs* | Altman, *Basic Care: Taking Blood Pressure* |
| 28 | Client Education | Christensen, *Core Concepts: Client Education* | — |

*(continues)*

| Chapter or Procedure Number | Content Area or Procedure Title | Video Link | DVD-ROM Link |
|---|---|---|---|
| 29-1 | Performing Venipuncture (Blood Drawing) | Altman, *Advanced Care: Circulatory I: Venipuncture and Starting IV Therapy* <br> Altman, *Basic Care: Specimen Collection* | Altman, *Advanced Care: Performing Venipuncture (Blood Drawing)* |
| 29-2 | Skin Puncture | Altman, *Basic Care: Specimen Collection* | Altman, *Basic Care: Performing a Skin Puncture* <br> Altman, *Intermediate Care: Obtaining an Arterial Blood Gas Specimen* <br> Altman, *Advanced Care: Assisting with Arteriography* |
| 29-3 | Obtaining a Residual Urine Specimen from an Indwelling Catheter | Altman, *Basic Care: Specimen Collection* <br> Altman, *Intermediate Care: Nutrition and Elimination II: Catheter Care* | Altman, *Basic Care: Collecting a Clean-Catch, Midstream Urine Specimen* <br> Altman, *Basic Care: Testing Urine for Specific Gravity, Ketones, and Occult Blood* <br> Altman, *Intermediate Care: Obtaining a Residual Urine Specimen from an Indwelling Catheter* |
| 29 | Blood Glucose Monitoring | — | Altman, *Basic Care: Measuring Blood Glucose Levels* |
| 29 | Collecting Nose, Throat, and Sputum Specimens | Altman, *Basic Care: Specimen Collection* | Altman, *Basic Care: Collecting Nose, Throat, and Sputum Specimens* |
| 29 | Testing Occult Blood | — | Altman, *Basic Care: Testing for Occult Blood with a Hemoccult Slide* |
| 29 | Wound Culturing | — | Altman, *Intermediate Care: Obtaining a Wound Drainage Specimen for Culturing* |
| 29 | ECG | — | Altman, *Advanced Care: Administering an Electrocardiogram* |
| 29 | MRI | — | Altman, *Advanced Care: Magnetic Resonance Imaging (MRI)* |
| 29 | CT Scan | — | Altman, *Advanced Care: Assisting with Computed Tomography (CT) Scanning* |
| 29 | Liver Biopsy | — | Altman, *Advanced Care: Assisting with a Liver Biopsy* |
| 29 | Thoracentesis | — | Altman, *Advanced Care: Assisting with a Thoracentesis* |
| 29 | Paracentesis | — | Altman, *Advanced Care: Assisting with an Abdominal Paracentesis* |
| 29 | Bone Marrow Biopsy and Aspiration | — | Altman, *Advanced Care: Assisting with a Bone Marrow Biopsy/Aspiration* |
| 29 | Lumbar Puncture | — | Altman, *Advanced Care: Assisting with a Lumbar Puncture* |
| 29 | Amniocentesis | — | Altman, *Advanced Care: Assisting with Amniocentesis* |

*(continues)*

| Chapter or Procedure Number | Content Area or Procedure Title | Video Link | DVD-ROM Link |
|---|---|---|---|
| 29 | Bronchoscopy | — | Altman, *Advanced Care: Assisting with Bronchoscopy* |
| 29 | Endoscopy | — | Altman, *Advanced Care: Assisting with a Gastrointestinal Endoscopy* |
| 29 | Proctosigmoidoscopy | — | Altman, *Advanced Care: Assisting with a Proctosigmoidoscopy* |
| 29 | PET Scanning | — | Altman, *Advanced Care: Positron-Emission Tomography Scanning* |
| 30-1 | Administering Oral, Sublingual, and Buccal Medications | Altman, *Intermediate Care: Medication Administration II: Routes of Administration* | Altman, *Intermediate Care: Administering Oral, Sublingual, and Buccal Medications* |
| 30-2 | Withdrawing Medication from an Ampoule | Altman, *Intermediate Care: Medication Administration III: Parenteral Medication* | Altman, *Intermediate Care: Withdrawing Medication from an Ampoule* |
| 30-3 | Withdrawing Medication from a Vial | Altman, *Intermediate Care: Medication Administration III: Parenteral Medication* | Altman, *Intermediate Care: Withdrawing Medication from a Vial* |
| 30-4 | Mixing Medications from Two Vials into One Syringe | Altman, *Intermediate Care: Medication Administration III: Parenteral Medication* | Altman, *Intermediate Care: Mixing Medications from Two Vials into One Syringe* |
| 30-5 | Administering an Intradermal Injection | Altman, *Intermediate Care: Medication Administration III: Parenteral Medication* | Altman, *Intermediate Care: Administering an Intradermal Injection* |
| 30-6 | Administering a Subcutaneous Injection | Altman, *Intermediate Care: Medication Administration III: Parenteral Medication* | Altman, *Intermediate Care: Administering a Subcutaneous Injection* |
| 30-7 | Administering an Intramuscular Injection | Altman, *Intermediate Care: Medication Administration III: Parenteral Medication* | Altman, *Intermediate Care: Administering an Intramuscular Injection* |
| 30-8 | Administering Medications via Secondary Administration Sets (Piggyback) | Altman, *Intermediate Care: Medication Administration IV: Intravenous Medication* | Altman, *Intermediate Care: Adding Medications to an IV Solution*<br>Altman, *Intermediate Care: Administering Medications via Secondary Administration Sets (Piggyback)*<br>Altman, *Intermediate Care: Administering Medications via IV Bolus or IV Push*<br>Altman, *Intermediate Care: Administering Medications via Volume Control Sets* |
| 30-9 | Administering Eye and Ear Medications | Altman, *Intermediate Care: Medication Administration II: Routes of Administration* | Altman, *Intermediate Care: Administering Ear and Eye Medications*<br>Altman, *Intermediate Care: Administering Skin/Topical Medications* |
| 30-10 | Administering Nasal Medications | Altman, *Intermediate Care: Medication Administration II: Routes of Administration* | Altman, *Intermediate Care: Administering Nasal Medications* |

*(continues)*

| Chapter or Procedure Number | Content Area or Procedure Title | Video Link | DVD-ROM Link |
|---|---|---|---|
| 30-11 | Teaching Self-Administration with a Metered Dose Inhaler | Altman, *Intermediate Care: Medication Administration II: Routes of Administration* | Altman, *Intermediate Care: Administering Nebulized Medications* |
| 30-12 | Administering Rectal Medications | Altman, *Intermediate Care: Medication Administration II: Routes of Administration* | Altman, *Intermediate Care: Administering Rectal Medications* |
| 30-13 | Administering Vaginal Medications | Altman, *Intermediate Care: Medication Administration II: Routes of Administration* | Altman, *Intermediate Care: Administering Vaginal Medications* |
| 30 | Z-track injection | Altman, *Intermediate Care: Medication Administration III: Parenteral Medication* | Altman, *Intermediate Care: Administering Medication via Z-Track Injection* |
| 30 | Controlled Substances | Altman, *Intermediate Care: Medication Administration I* | Altman, *Intermediate Care: Managing Controlled Substances* |
| 31-1 | Therapeutic Massage | — | Altman, *Basic Care: Therapeutic Massage* Altman, *Basic Care: Guided Imagery* Altman, *Basic Care: Progressive Muscle Relaxation* |
| 33-1 | Applying Restraints | Altman, *Basic Care: Basic Care II: Bed-Making* | Altman, *Basic Care: Applying Restraints* |
| 33-2 | Bathing a Client in Bed | Altman, *Basic Care: Basic Care III: Infection Control and Bathing* | Altman, *Basic Care: Bathing a Patient in Bed* Altman, *Basic Care: Warm Soaks and Sitz Baths* |
| 33-3 | Changing Linens in an Unoccupied Bed | Altman, *Basic Care: Basic Care II: Bed-Making* | Altman, *Basic Care: Changing Linens in an Unoccupied Bed* |
| 33-4 | Changing Linens in an Occupied Bed | Altman, *Basic Care: Basic Care II: Bed-Making* | Altman, *Basic Care: Changing Linens in an Occupied Bed* |
| 33-5 | Perineal and Genital Care | Altman, *Basic Care: Basic Care III: Infection Control and Bathing* | Altman, *Basic Care: Perineal and Genital Care* |
| 33-6 | Oral Care | Altman, *Basic Care: Basic Care I: Personal Care* | Altman, *Basic Care: Oral Care* |
| 33-7 | Eye Care | Altman, *Basic Care: Basic Care I: Personal Care* | Altman, *Basic Care: Eye Care* |
| 33 | Backrubs | Altman, *Basic Care: Basic Care III: Infection Control and Bathing* | Altman, *Basic Care: Giving a Backrub* |
| 33 | Hand and Foot Care | Altman, *Basic Care: Basic Care I: Personal Care* | Altman, *Basic Care: Hand and Foot Care* |
| 33 | Hair and Scalp Care | Altman, *Basic Care: Basic Care I: Personal Care* | Altman, *Basic Care: Hair and Scalp Care* |
| 33 | Shaving a Client | Altman, *Basic Care: Basic Care I: Personal Care* | Altman, *Basic Care: Shaving a Client* |
| 34-1 | Measuring Intake and Output | Altman, *Basic Care: Specimen Collection* | Altman, *Basic Care: Measuring Intake and Output* |

*(continues)*

| Chapter or Procedure Number | Content Area or Procedure Title | Video Link | DVD-ROM Link |
|---|---|---|---|
| 34-2 | Preparing an IV Solution | Altman, *Intermediate Care: Medication Administration IV: Intravenous Medication*<br>Altman, *Advanced Care: Circulatory I: Venipuncture and Starting IV Therapy*<br>Altman, *Advanced Care: Circulatory II: Maintaining IV Therapy* | Altman, *Intermediate Care: Preparing an IV Solution*<br>Altman, *Advanced Care: Starting an IV*<br>Altman, *Advanced Care: Inserting a Butterfly Needle*<br>Altman, *Advanced Care: Preparing the IV Bag and Tubing*<br>Altman, *Advanced Care: Setting the IV Flow Rate*<br>Altman, *Advanced Care: Changing the IV Solution* |
| 34-3 | Adding Medications to an IV Solution | Altman, *Intermediate Care: Medication Administration IV: Intravenous Medication* | Altman, *Intermediate Care: Adding Medications to an IV Solution* |
| 34-4 | Assessing and Maintaining an IV Insertion Site | Altman, *Advanced Care: Circulatory II: Maintaining IV Therapy* | Altman, *Advanced Care: Assessing and Maintaining an IV Insertion Site*<br>Altman, *Advanced Care: Discontinuing the IV and Changing to a Saline Lock* |
| 34-5 | Administering a Blood Transfusion | Altman, *Advanced Care: Circulatory III: Blood Transfusions* | Altman, *Advanced Care: Administering a Blood Transfusion*<br>Altman, *Advanced Care: Assessing and Responding to Transfusion Reactions* |
| 35-1 | Inserting and Maintaining a Nasogastric Tube | Altman, *Intermediate Care: Nutrition and Elimination I* | Altman, *Intermediate Care: Inserting and Maintaining a Nasogastric Tube* |
| 35-2 | Assessing Placement of a Large-Bore Feeding Tube | Altman, *Intermediate Care: Nutrition and Elimination I* | Altman, *Intermediate Care: Assessing Placement of a Large-Bore Feeding Tube*<br>Altman, *Intermediate Care: Assessing Placement of a Small-Bore Feeding Tube* |
| 35 | Nutrition | Christensen, *Core Concepts: Nutrition and Diet Therapy I, II, III* | — |
| 36-1 | Obtaining a Wound Drainage Specimen for Culturing | — | Altman, *Intermediate Care: Obtaining a Wound Drainage Specimen for Culturing* |
| 36-2 | Irrigating a Wound | — | Altman, *Intermediate Care: Irrigating a Wound* |
| 36-3 | Applying a Dry Dressing | — | Altman, *Intermediate Care: Applying a Dry Dressing* |
| 36-4 | Applying a Wet to Damp Dressing (Wet to Dry to Moist Dressing) | — | Altman, *Intermediate Care: Applying a Wet to Damp Dressing (Wet to Dry to Moist Dressing)* |
| 36 | Closed Wound Drainage System | Altman, *Intermediate Care: Wound Care* | Altman, *Intermediate Care: Maintaining a Closed Wound Drainage System* |

*(continues)*

| Chapter or Procedure Number | Content Area or Procedure Title | Video Link | DVD-ROM Link |
|---|---|---|---|
| 36 | Jackson-Pratt (JP) Drain Site | — | Altman, *Intermediate Care: Care of the Jackson-Pratt (JP) Drain Site and Emptying the Drain Bulb* |
| 36 | Preventing and Managing the Pressure Ulcer | Altman, *Basic Care: Basic Care IV: Aiding Client Movement* | Altman, *Basic Care: Preventing and Managing the Pressure Ulcer* |
| 36 | Wound Care | Altman, *Intermediate Care: Wound Care* | Altman, *Basic Care: Maintaining a Closed Wound Drainage System* |
| 36 | Applying Dry Heat | — | Altman, *Basic Care: Applying Dry Heat* |
| 36 | Applying Cold Treatment | — | Altman, *Basic Care: Applying Cold Treatment* |
| 37-1 | Assisting with a Bedpan or Urinal | — | Altman, *Basic Care: Assisting with a Bedpan or Urinal* |
| 37-2 | Applying a Condom Catheter | Altman, *Intermediate Care: Nutrition and Elimination II: Catheter Care* | Altman, *Intermediate Care: Applying a Condom Catheter* |
| 37-3 | Inserting an Indwelling Catheter: Male | Altman, *Intermediate Care: Nutrition and Elimination II: Catheter Care* | Altman, *Intermediate Care: Inserting an Indwelling Catheter: Male* |
| 37-4 | Inserting an Indwelling Catheter: Female | Altman, *Intermediate Care: Nutrition and Elimination II: Catheter Care* | Altman, *Intermediate Care: Inserting an Indwelling Catheter: Female* |
| 37-5 | Irrigating a Urinary Catheter | Altman, *Intermediate Care: Nutrition and Elimination II: Catheter Care* | Altman, *Intermediate Care: Irrigating a Urinary Catheter* |
| 37-6 | Irrigating the Bladder Using a Closed-System Catheter | — | Altman, *Intermediate Care: Irrigating the Bladder Using a Closed-System Catheter* |
| 37-7 | Administering an Enema | Altman, *Intermediate Care: Nutrition and Elimination III* | Altman, *Intermediate Care: Administering an Enema* |
| 37-8 | Changing a Bowel Diversion Ostomy Appliance: Pouching a Stoma | Altman, *Intermediate Care: Nutrition and Elimination III* | Altman, *Intermediate Care: Changing a Bowel Diversion Ostomy Appliance—Pouching a Stoma* |
| 38-1 | Proper Body Mechanics and Safe Lifting | — | Altman, *Basic Care: Proper Body Mechanics and Safe Lifting/ Transferring* |
| 38-2 | Turning and Positioning a Client | Altman, *Basic Care: Basic Care IV: Aiding Client Movement* | Altman, *Basic Care: Turning and Positioning a Client* |
| 38-3 | Administering Passive Range-of-Motion (ROM) Exercises | Altman, *Basic Care: Basic Care V: Aiding Client Movement* | Altman, *Basic Care: Administering Passive Range-of-Motion (ROM) Exercises* |
| 38-4 | Moving a Client in Bed | Altman, *Basic Care: Basic Care V: Aiding Client Movement* | Altman, *Basic Care: Moving a Client in Bed* |
| 38-6 | Assisting from Bed to Wheel-chair, Commode, or Chair | Altman, *Basic Care: Basic Care V: Aiding Client Movement* | Altman, *Basic Care: Assisting from Bed to Wheelchair, Commode, or Chair* |

(continues)

| Chapter or Procedure Number | Content Area or Procedure Title | Video Link | DVD-ROM Link |
|---|---|---|---|
| 38-7 | Assisting from Bed to Stretcher | Altman, *Basic Care: Basic Care V: Aiding Client Movement* | Altman, *Basic Care: Assisting from Bed to Stretcher* |
| 38-8 | Using a Hydraulic Lift | — | Altman, *Basic Care: Using a Hydraulic Lift* |
| 38-9 | Assisting with Ambulation and Safe Falling | — | Altman, *Basic Care: Assisting with Ambulation and Safe Falling* |
| 38 | Assisting from Bed to Walking | Altman, *Basic Care: Basic Care V: Aiding Client Movement* | Altman, *Basic Care: Assisting from Bed to Walking* |
| 38 | Applying Restraints | Altman, *Basic Care: Basic Care II: Bed-Making* | Altman, *Basic Care: Applying Restraints* |
| 39-1 | Maintaining and Cleaning the Tracheostomy Tube | — | Altman, *Advanced Care: Maintaining and Cleaning the Tracheostomy Tube* Altman, *Advanced Care: Maintaining a Double Cannula Tracheostomy Tube* Altman, *Advanced Care: Plugging the Tracheostomy Tube* |
| 39-2 | Suctioning Endotracheal and Tracheal Tubes | — | Altman, *Advanced Care: Suctioning Endotracheal and Tracheal Tubes* Altman, *Advanced Care: Maintaining and Cleaning Endotracheal Tubes* |
| 39-3 | Administering Oxygen Therapy | Altman, *Advanced Care: Oxygenation* | Altman, *Advanced Care: Administering Oxygen Therapy* Altman, *Advanced Care: Assisting a Client with Controlled Coughing and Deep Breathing* Altman, *Advanced Care: Assisting a Client with an Incentive Spirometer* Altman, *Advanced Care: Administering Pulmonary Therapy and Postural Drainage* Altman, *Advanced Care: Administering Pulse Oximetry* |
| 39-4 | Performing the Heimlich Maneuver | — | Altman, *Basic Care: Performing the Heimlich Maneuver* |
| 39-5 | Administering Cardiopulmonary Resuscitation (CPR) | — | Altman, *Basic Care: Administering Cardiopulmonary Resuscitation (CPR)* |
| 39 | Oxygenation | Christensen, *Core Concepts: Oxygenation* | — |
| 46 | Breast Exam | — | Altman, *Basic Care: Breast Examination* |

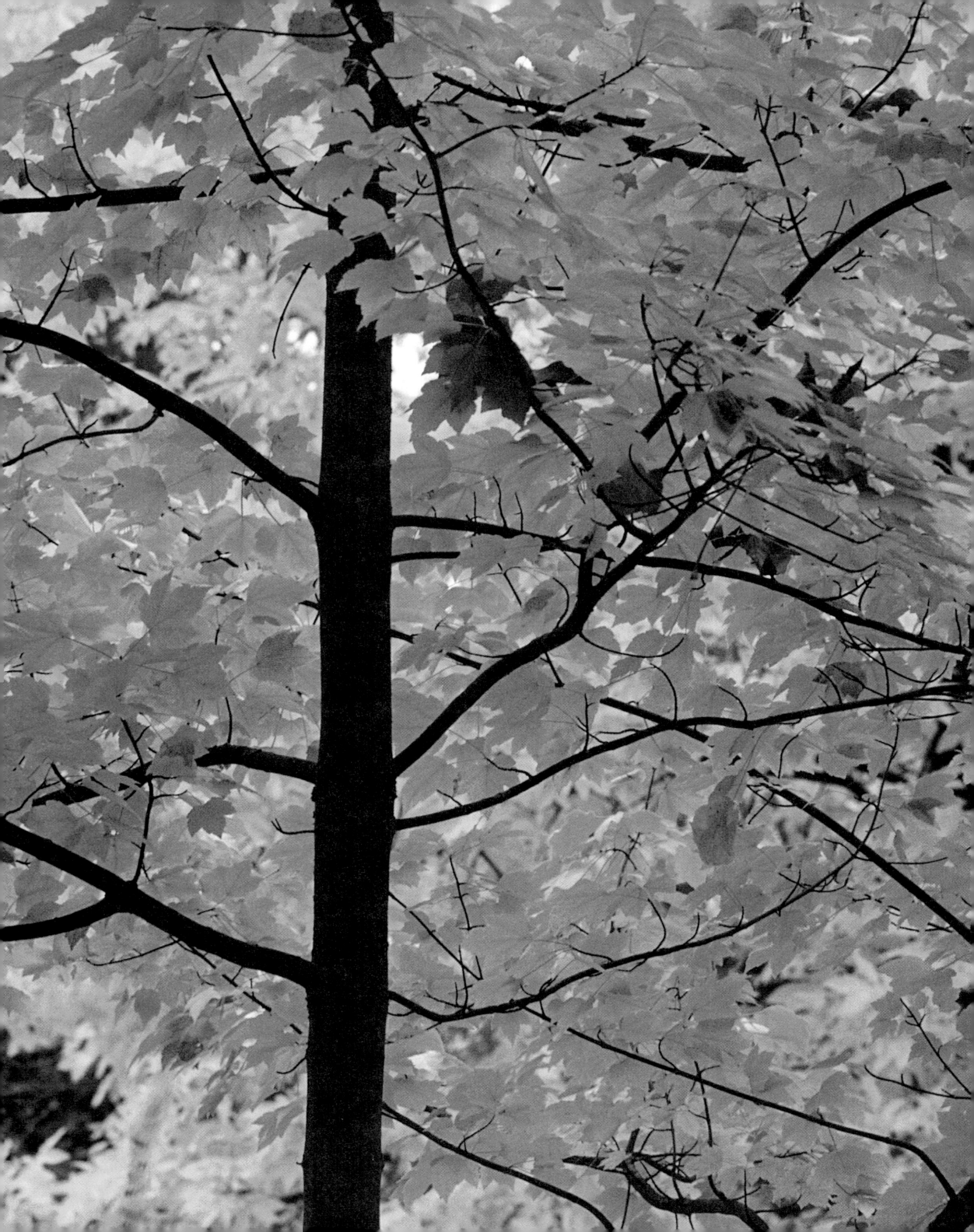

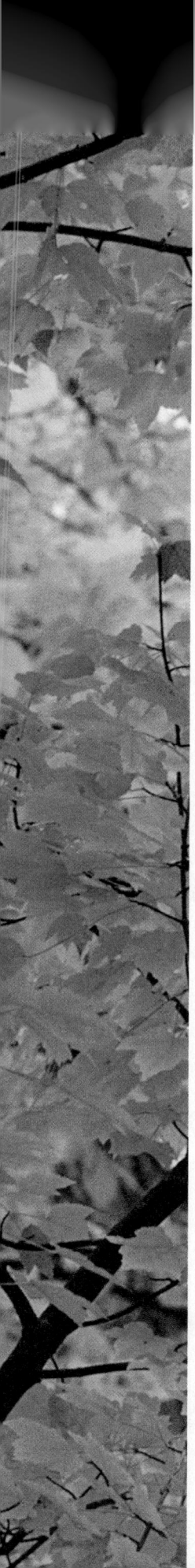

# Foundations of Nursing

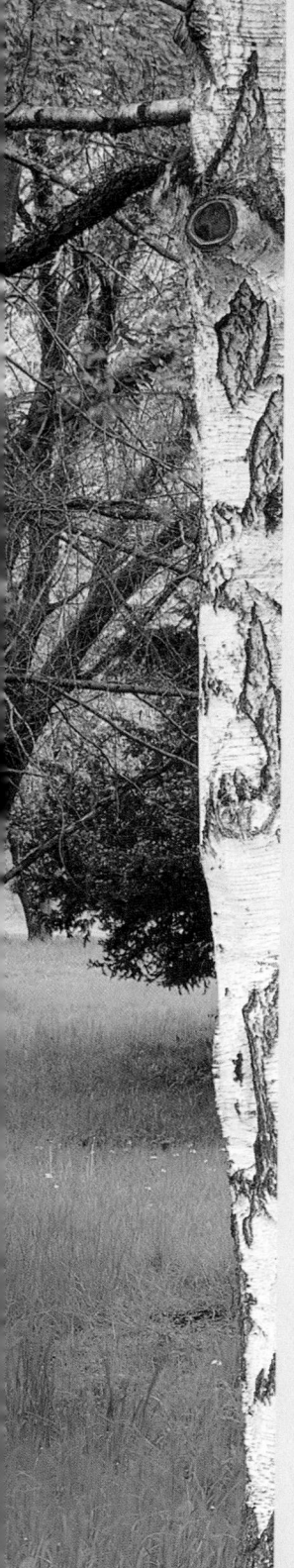

# UNIT

# Foundations of Nursing Practice

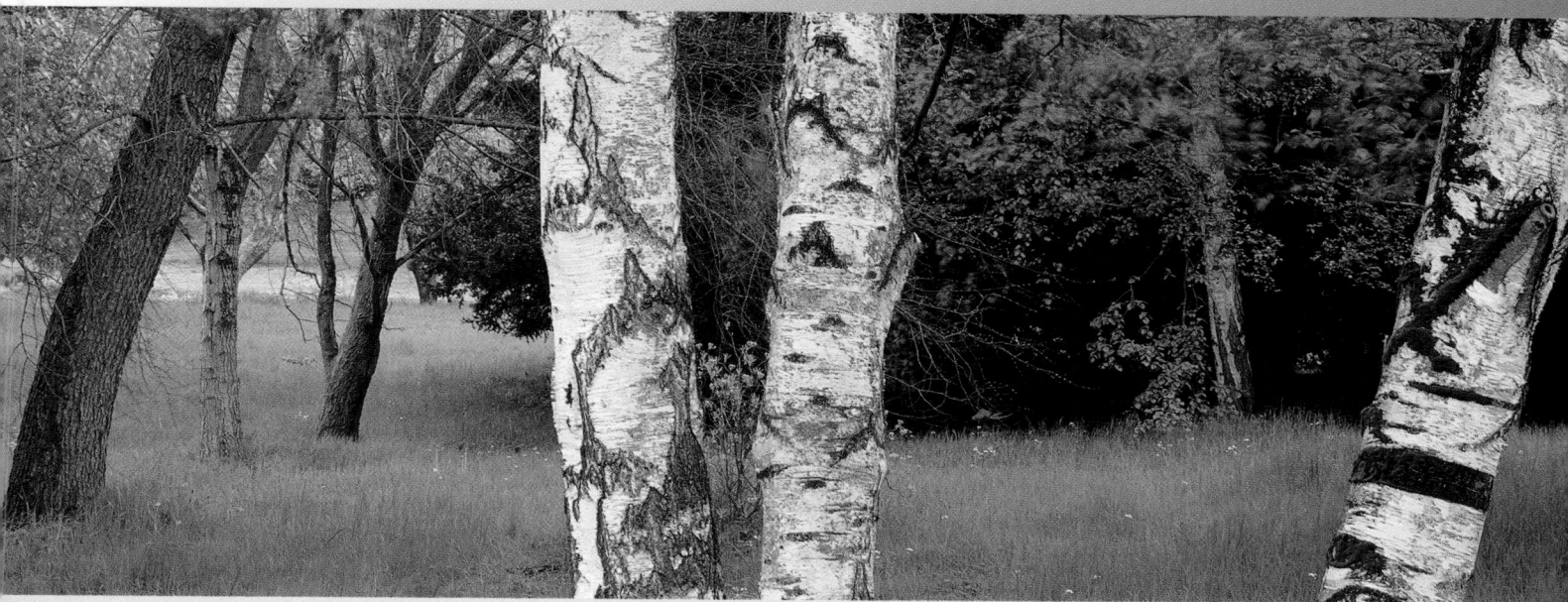

# Evolution of Nursing Practice

Carol Craig, PhD, FNP, RN
Rick Daniels, RN, PhD

*"History provides current nurses with the same intellectual and political tools that determined nursing pioneers applied to shape nursing values and beliefs to the social context of their times. Nursing history is not an ornament to be displayed on anniversary days, nor does it consist of only happy stories to be recalled and retold on special occasions. Nursing history is a vivid testimony, meant to incite, instruct and inspire today's nurses as they bravely tread the winding path of a reinvented health care system."*

*(American Association for the History of Nursing, 2002)*

# Chapter Competencies

## Upon completion of this chapter, the reader should be able to:

1. Evaluate nursing as both an art and a science.
2. Identify major historical and social events that have shaped current nursing practice.
3. Describe Florence Nightingale's impact on current nursing practice.
4. Discuss the contributions of early leaders in American nursing.
5. Evaluate the impact of selected landmark reports on nursing education and practice.
6. Relate the social forces of nursing's evolution to the current status of the professional nurse.
7. Anticipate the effect of the current nursing shortage on the health care system.

# Key Terms

autonomy
empowerment
evidence-based practice

health maintenance
  organization
history

nursing
primary health care

**N**ursing is an art and a science by which people are assisted in learning to care for themselves whenever possible and cared for by others when they are unable to meet their own needs.

Nursing has evolved from an unstructured method of caring for the ill to a scientific profession. The result has been movement from the mystical beliefs of primitive times to a "high-tech, high-touch" era. Nursing combines art and science. Using scientific knowledge in a humane manner, nursing combines critical thinking skills with caring behaviors.

Nursing requires a delicate balance of promoting clients' independence and dependence. Nursing focuses not on illness but rather on the client's *response* to illness.

Nursing promotes health and helps clients move to a higher level of wellness. This aspect of nursing also includes assisting a client with a terminal illness to maintain comfort and dignity in the final stage of life.

This chapter traces the evolution of nursing by exploring its rich heritage. Social forces that have affected the development of nursing are examined.

## Historical Overview

To understand the present status of nursing, it is necessary to have a base of historical knowledge about the profession. By studying nursing history, the nurse is better able to understand such issues as **autonomy** (being self-directed), unity within the profession, supply and demand, salary, education, and current practice. **History** is a study of the past that includes events, situations, and individuals (Figure 1-1). By learning from

historical role models, nurses can enhance their abilities to create positive change in the present and set a course for the future.

The study of nursing history offers another advantage—learning where the profession has been and its advancements. **Empowerment** is the process of enabling others to do for themselves. Only when nurses are empowered are they truly autonomous. Autonomy has historically been difficult for nurses to achieve. Nurses have had difficulty with empowerment and autonomy due to the discrimination that has existed toward the nursing profession. Nurses have had to overcome the inequity historically shown against women and men in nursing. The image of nursing has ranged from "servant to sex object," "angel to idiot." In addition, the media has not accurately portrayed nurses, and stereotypes continue to obscure the complex, holistic work that nurses perform. Empowerment and autonomy go together and are necessary for nursing to bring about positive changes in health care today (Figure 1-2). Power is not authority—authority is power.

Learning from the past is the major reason for studying history. Ignoring nursing's history can be detrimental to the future of the profession. By applying the lessons gained from a historical review, nurses will indeed be a vital force in the new millennium.

## Evolution of Nursing

Nursing has evolved with the development of civilization of mankind. Refer to Table 1-1 and the following for a discussion of nursing from early civilizations to the present era of advanced nursing practice and health care reform.

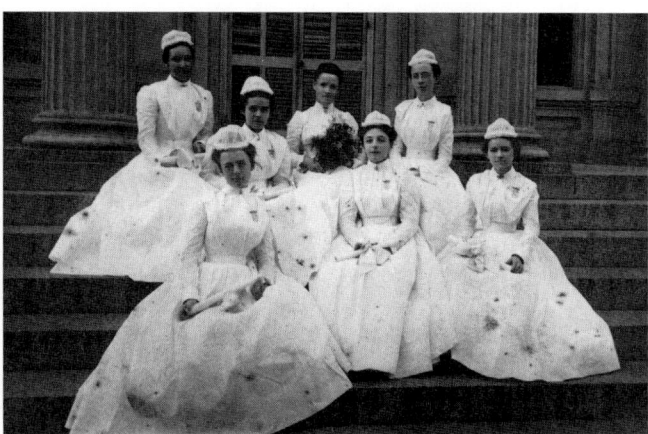

**Figure 1-1    Graduating class (1900) of Touro Infirmary Training School for Nurses.** *Photo courtesy of Touro Infirmary Archives, New Orleans, LA*

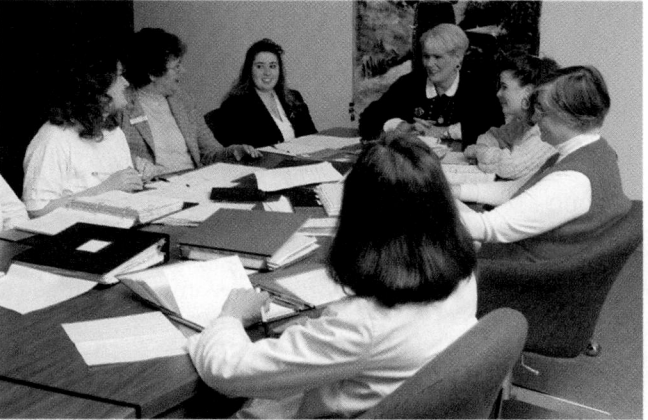

**Figure 1-2    Nurses collaborating with one another regarding client care leads to autonomy and empowerment.**

## STOP AND THINK

### The Value of Nursing History

- How has history changed the concept of empowerment and its relationship to nursing?

- What is the practical value of examining the history of nursing?

- Why should you familiarize yourself with the history of nursing and its leaders?

## Early Civilizations

The practice of nursing predates recorded history. Most human groups provided care for their sick and wounded. Prehistoric human remains show evidence of healed major fractures of the legs, arms, and skull, which attest to someone providing care so the person could heal. The recorded evolution of nursing dates back to 4000 BC, to primitive societies in which mother-nurses worked with priests. In 2000 BC, the use of wet nurses is recorded in Babylonia and Assyria.

## Ancient Greece

The ancient Greeks built temples to honor Hygeia, the goddess of health. These temples were more like health spas rather than hospitals in that they were religious institutions governed by priests. Priestesses (who were not nurses) attended to those housed in the temples. The nursing that was done by women was performed in the home.

## Roman Empire

Hospitals were first established in the Eastern Roman Empire (Byzantine Empire). St. Jerome was responsible, through one of his disciples, Fabiola, for introducing hospitals in the West. Western hospitals were primarily religious and charitable institutions housed in monasteries and convents. The caregivers had no formal training in therapeutic modalities and cared for the sick as a religious duty.

## Middle Ages

Military, religious, and lay orders of men continued to provide care throughout the Middle Ages. Some of the most famous were the Knights Hospitalers, the Teutonic Knights, the Teriaries, the Knights of St. Lazarus, the Order of the Holy Spirit, and the Hospital Brothers of St. Anthony (Kalisch & Kalisch, 1995).

Hospitals in large Byzantine cities were staffed primarily by paid male assistants and male nurses. During the medieval era, these hospitals were established primarily as almshouses, with care of the sick being secondary.

Medical practices in Western Europe remained basically unchanged until the 11th and 12th centuries, when formal medical education for physicians was required in a university setting. Although there were not enough physicians to care for all the sick, other caregivers were not required to receive any formal training. The dominant caregivers in the Byzantine setting were men; however, this was not true in the rural parts of the Eastern Roman Empire and in the West. In these societies, nursing was viewed as a natural nurturing job for women.

## Renaissance

During the Renaissance (AD 1400–1550), interest in the arts and sciences emerged. This was also the time of many geographic explorations by Europeans. As a result, the world literally expanded.

Because of renewed interest in science, universities were established, but no formal nursing schools were founded. Because of social status and customs, women were not encouraged to leave their homes; they continued to fulfill

## TABLE 1-1    HISTORICAL EVENTS INFLUENCING THE EVOLUTION OF NURSING

| Date | Event |
|---|---|
| 4000 BC | Primitive societies |
| 2000 BC | Babylonia and Assyria |
| 800–600 BC | Health religions of India |
| 700 BC | Greece: source of modern medical science |
| 460 BC | Hippocrates |
| 3 BC | Ireland: pre-Christian nursing |
| AD 390 | Fabiola founded first hospital |
| 390–407 | Early Christianity, deaconesses |
| 711 | Field hospital with nursing, Spain |
| 1100 | Ambulatory clinics, Spain (Moslems) |
| 1440 | First Chairs of Medicine, Oxford and Cambridge |
| 1522 | Military nursing orders |
| 1600–1752 | Deterioration of hospitals and nursing |
| 1633 | Founded: Daughters of Charity |
| 1820 | Florence Nightingale born |
| 1836 | Kaiserwerth deaconesses reestablished |
| 1837 | First American college for women, Mount Holyoke |
| 1841 | Founded: Nursing Sisters of the Holy Cross |
| 1848 | Women's Rights Convention, Seneca Falls, New York |
| 1854–1856 | Crimean War |
| 1859 | *Nightingale's Notes on Nursing* published in England |
| 1860 | First Nightingale School of Nursing, St. Thomas' Hospital, London |
| 1861–1865 | Civil War, United States: nursing nuns, untrained nurses provided care |
| 1863 | Charter granted to the New England Hospital for Women, Boston |
| 1871 | New York State Training School for Nurses, Brooklyn Maternity, Brooklyn, New York |
| 1872 | New England Hospital for Women: one-year program for nurses |
| 1873 | America's first trained nurse, Linda Richards |
|  | First three Nightingale schools in United States: Bellevue (New York City), Connecticut, and Massachusetts General |
|  | America's first trained African American nurse, Mary Eliza Mahoney |
| 1881 | Founded: American Red Cross |
| 1882 | Founded: American Association of University Women |
| 1888 | Founded: International Council of Women (ICW) |
|  | Founded: National Council of Women (NCW) |
| 1893 | First Nurses' Settlement House, New York City, founded by Lillian Wald and Mary Brewster |
|  | Founded: first American Nursing Society, American Society of Superintendents of Training Schools for Nurses (Superintendents' Society) |

*(continues)*

## TABLE 1-1    HISTORICAL EVENTS INFLUENCING THE EVOLUTION OF NURSING (*continued*)

| Date | Event |
|------|-------|
| 1896 | Founded: National Association of Colored Women |
| 1896–1911 | Founded: Nurses' Associated Alumnae of the United States and Canada (Associated Alumnae) |
| 1899 | Founded: International Council of Nurses (ICN) |
| | First postgraduate courses for nurses at Teachers College, Columbia University |
| 1900 | *American Journal of Nursing (AJN)* |
| 1901–1912 | Founded: American Federation of Nurses (Federation) |
| | Federation Joins NCW and ICW |
| 1903 | New York: efforts failed to pass a nurse licensing law |
| | North Carolina: passes first state nurse registration law |
| | Founded: Army Nurse Corps |
| 1905 | Federation withdraws from NCW and joins ICN |
| 1908 | National Association of Colored Graduate Nurses (NACGN) |
| | Founded: Navy Nurse Corps |
| 1909 | Founded: first 3-year diploma school in a university setting at University of Minnesota |
| 1910 | Flexner report |
| 1911 | Founded: American Nurses Association (ANA), formerly the Associated Alumnae |
| 1912 | Founded: National Organization of Public Health Nursing (NOPHN) |
| | Founded: National League of Nursing Education (NLN), formerly the Superintendents' Society |
| | ANA represents American nurses at ICN |
| | Nutting Report: Educational Status of Nursing |
| | Developments in preventive medicine |
| | Founded: Town and Country Rural Nursing Service |
| 1913 | Founded: National Women's Party |
| 1916 | Founded: National Association of Deans of Women |
| 1920 | Founded: National League for Women Voters |
| | Congress passes the federal suffrage amendment |
| 1920s | Depression: social programs and health insurance |
| | First prepaid medical plan, Pacific Northwest |
| | Founded: Bureaus of Medical Services |
| | Hospitals offered a prepaid plan |
| | Baylor Plan (prototype of Blue Cross) |
| | Goldmark report |
| 1921 | Women earn right to vote |
| | Founded: Sigma Theta Tau National Society for Nursing |
| 1922 | Studies of institutional nursing |

*(continues)*

## TABLE 1-1     HISTORICAL EVENTS INFLUENCING THE EVOLUTION OF NURSING (*continued*)

| Date | Event |
| --- | --- |
| 1923 | Studies of nursing education |
| | Goldmark report |
| | Founded: Yale University School of Nursing |
| 1926 | Burgess report |
| 1929 | Stock market crash begins the Great Depression |
| 1933 | American Hospital Association endorses Blue Cross |
| 1938 | American Medical Association endorses Blue Shield |
| | Economic Security Program for Nurses |
| 1940 | Cost studies of nursing education and service |
| 1943 | Founded: Federal Cadet Nurse Corps |
| 1948 | Brown report: *Future of Nursing* |
| 1952 | *Journal of Nursing Research* |
| 1953 | U.S. Public Health Services Studies in Nursing Education |
| 1955 | Practical Nursing (Title III) Health Amendment Act |
| 1956 | Hughes study: *20,000 Nurses Tell Their Stories* |
| 1960s | Created: Medicare and Medicaid |
| 1961 | Surgeon General's Consultant Group |
| 1964 | Nurse Training Act |
| 1965 | ANA position paper on entry into practice |
| 1966 | Educational opportunity grants for nurses |
| 1967 | First nurse practitioner program, pediatric |
| 1970 | Secretary's commission to study extended roles for nurses |
| 1973 | Health Maintenance Organization Act |
| 1977 | Rural Health Clinic Service Act |
| | National Commission for Manpower Policy Study |
| 1979 | U.S. Surgeon General Report *Healthy People* |
| 1980 | Omnibus Budget Reconciliation Act |
| 1982 | Budget cut to Health Maintenance Organization Act |
| | Tax Equity Fiscal Responsibility Act (TEFRA) |
| 1983 | Institute of Medicine Committee on Nursing and Nursing Education study |
| 1987 | Secretary's Commission on Nursing |
| 1990s | Health care reform |
| 1991 | U.S. Department of Health and Human Services Healthy People 2000 |
| 1997 | Agency for Health Care Policy and Research, now known as the Agency for Healthcare Research and Quality, established 12 evidence-based practice centers |
| 2000 | U.S. Department of Health and Human Services Healthy People 2010 |
| 2002 | Nursing shortage clearly identified as a crisis for health care delivery system |

the traditional role of nurturer and caregiver in the home. The Protestant Reformation (AD 1500–1700) dissolved Catholic hospitals in many European countries and the sick no longer had institutional care.

## Enlightenment and Industrial Revolution

The Industrial Revolution introduced technology that led to a proliferation of factories. Conditions for the factory workers were deplorable. Long hours, grueling work, and unsafe conditions prevailed in the workplace. The health status of laborers received little, if any, attention.

Medical schools were founded, including the Royal College of Surgeons in London in 1800. In France, men who were barbers also functioned as surgeons by performing procedures such as leeching, giving enemas, and extracting teeth.

At the end of the 18th century, there were no standards for nurses who worked in hospitals. In the early to mid-1800s, nursing was considered unseemly for women even though some hospitals (almshouses) relied on women to make beds, scrub floors, and bathe the poor. These women were frequently alcoholics and prostitutes who were sentenced to work in hospitals in lieu of jail time. Most nursing care was still performed in the home by female relatives of the ill.

## Religious Influences

The strong influence of religions on the development of nursing started in India (800–600 BC) and flourished in Greece and Ireland in 3 BC with male nurse-priests. In India, only men were considered "pure" enough to be nurses (Kalisch & Kalisch, 1995).

In 1836, Theodor Fleidner revived the Church Order of Deaconesses to care for those in a hospital he had founded. These deaconesses of Kaiserwerth became famous because they were the only ones formally trained in nursing. Pastor Fleidner had a profound influence on nursing because Florence Nightingale received her nurse's training at the Kaiserwerth Institute.

The Nursing Sisters of the Holy Cross was founded in LeMans, France, by Father Bassil Moreau in 1841. Father Sorin brought four sisters to Notre Dame in South Bend, Indiana, in 1841. In 1844, these sisters established St. Mary's Academy in Bertrand, Michigan. In 1855, the school was moved to Notre Dame and became known as Saint Mary's College, which became influential on the emerging role of women in nursing.

## Florence Nightingale

Florence Nightingale is considered the founder of modern nursing. She grew up in a wealthy upper-class family in England during the mid-1800s. Unlike other young women of her era, Nightingale received a thorough education including Greek, Latin, history, mathematics, and philosophy. She had always been interested in relieving suffering and caring for the sick. Social mores of the time made it impossible for her to consider caring for others, because she was not a member of a religious order. She became a nurse over the objections of society and her family.

After completing the 3-month course of study at Kaiserwerth Institute, Nightingale became active in reforming health care. The advent of Britain's war in the Crimea presented the stage for Nightingale to further develop the public's awareness of the need for educated nurses (Figure 1-3). The implementation of her principles in the areas of nursing practice and environmental modifications resulted in reduced morbidity and mortality rates during the war. In 6 months, mortality rates dropped from 42.7% to 2.2%.

Nightingale forged the future of nursing education as a result of her experiences in training nurses to care for British soldiers. She established the Nightingale Training School of Nurses at St. Thomas' Hospital in London. This was the first school for nurses that provided both theory-based knowledge and clinical skill building. She revolutionized not only the public's perception of nursing but also the method for educating nurses. Some of Nightingale's novel beliefs about nursing education were:

- A holistic framework inclusive of illness and health
- The need for a theoretical basis for nursing practice
- A liberal education as a foundation for nursing practice
- The importance of creating an environment that promotes healing
- The need for a body of nursing knowledge that was distinct from medical knowledge (Nightingale, 1969)

Nightingale introduced many other concepts that, though unique in her time, are still used today. She advocated: (1) having a systematic method of assessing clients,

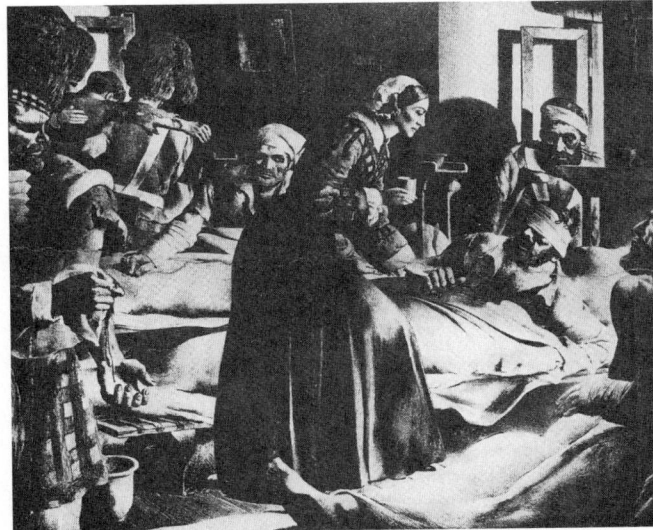

**Figure 1-3    Florence Nightingale.** *Photo courtesy of Parke-Davis, a division of Warner-Lambert Company*

## RESEARCH FOCUS

**Title of Study:** Religion, Gender, and Autonomy: A Comparison of Two Religious Women's Groups in Nursing and Hospitals in the Late Nineteenth and Early Twentieth Centuries

**Study Purpose:** This comparative study examines cases of Catholic nuns and Mormon women, and their effect on nursing in the American frontier in the 1800s and 1900s. The purpose of the study was to show how beliefs about religion and gender translated into power that women used to effectively administer health care services.

**Methods:** A comparative study of selected case studies was done to analyze the effect of Catholic nuns and Mormon women on the delivery of nursing care in the pioneer American West.

**Findings:** The two groups studied, Catholic nuns and Mormon women, lived in separate cultures on the frontier together. However, there are remarkable parallels in religious devotion, unique gender initiatives, autonomy, and the use of power. The numerous parallels include the following:

- The women in both groups were strong and capable in a society that promoted modesty and self-effacement of women.
- Women of both groups had a compelling sense of purpose ("mission") that empowered them to provide health care services.
- They received trust and support from male leaders because of their religious beliefs that broadened their roles in the community.
- The religious calling or mission did not interfere with or compromise professional competence of the women.
- Both groups of women had a privileged status and authority within their communities.

**Implications:** The role of religious groups in the American frontier has been largely ignored by modern historical research. This study is the beginning effort to focus importance on the experience of women as nurses and administrators of health care institutions.

Marshall, E. S., & Wall, B. M. (1999). Religion, gender, and autonomy: A comparison of two religious women's groups in nursing and hospitals in the late nineteenth and early twentieth centuries. *Advances in Nursing Science, 22*(1), 1–22.

## STOP AND THINK

### The Impact of Florence Nightingale

- What characteristics of Florence Nightingale would you incorporate into your practice?

- Based on the assertive example modeled by Nightingale, how would you teach other nurses to change their practice?

(2) individualizing care on the basis of the client's needs and preferences, and (3) maintaining confidentiality.

Nightingale also recognized the influence of environmental factors on health. She advocated that nurses provide clean surroundings with fresh air and light to improve the quality of care (Nightingale, 1859). Nightingale believed that nurses should be formally educated and should function as client advocates.

## Nursing and the Civil War

America's need for nurses increased dramatically during the Civil War (1861–1865). The sisters of the Holy Cross were the first to respond to the need for nurses during the Civil War. Answering a request of Indiana's governor, 12 sisters started caring for wounded soldiers. By the end of the war, 80 sisters had cared for soldiers in Illinois, Missouri, Kentucky, and Tennessee.

During the Civil War, nursing care was provided by the Sisters of Mercy, Daughters of Charity, Dominican Sisters, and the Franciscan Sisters of the Poor. The sisters were influenced by the roles assigned to women during the 19th century. Although they were submissive to authority, they were willing to take risks when human rights were threatened. Women volunteered to care for the soldiers of both the Union and Confederate armies (Figure 1-4). These women performed various duties, including the implementation of sanitary conditions in field hospitals.

Dorothea Dix, a New England schoolteacher, was appointed Superintendent of the Female Nurses of the Army in 1861; no woman had ever before been appointed to an administrative position by the federal government. As a result of her recruitment efforts, more than 2,000 women cared for the sick in the Union Army. After the Civil War, Dix concentrated her energies on reforming treatment of the mentally ill.

Realizing that "women played a special role in providing aid during times of crisis" (Frantz, 1998), Clara Barton began her efforts to establish an organization after the Civil War. Although nursing in America was not recognized as an acceptable career for women, Barton lobbied presidents and senators to allow nurses to form an organ-

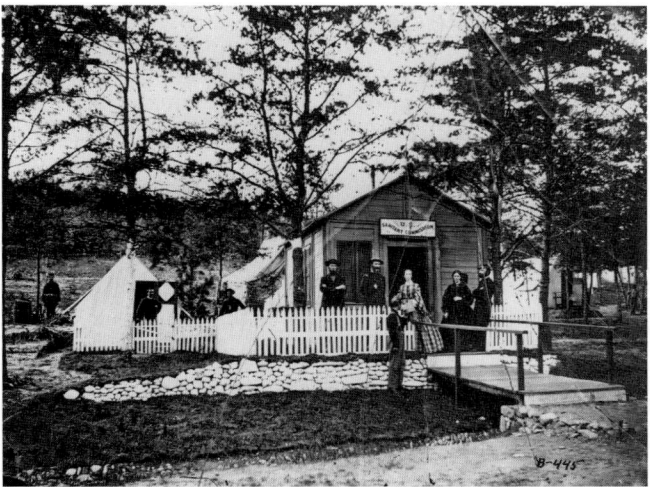

**Figure 1-4    During the Civil War, women were instrumental in the effort to minimize the risk of spreading contagious diseases among wounded soldiers.** *Photo courtesy of Corbis-Bettmann*

ization to provide war relief. Determined to provide aid in times of crisis, Barton, who was unsuccessful in her lobbying efforts to sponsor war relief, established the American Red Cross in 1881 to provide disaster relief. States rallied with support by creating their own branches of the American Red Cross. In 1898, Barton's knowledge from the Civil War allowed her and the State of Texas to effectively provide war relief to the Cuban citizens, and eventually to the American army during the Spanish-American War in Cuba (Frantz, 1998).

## The Women's Movement

In 1848, the Women's Rights Convention in Seneca Falls, New York, signaled the beginnings of social unrest. Women were not considered equal to men, society did not value education for women, and women did not have the right to vote. With suffrage, not only were the rights of women advocated but also the nursing profession itself advanced. By the mid-1900s, more women were being accepted into colleges and universities, even though only limited numbers of university-based nursing programs were available.

## Nursing Pioneers and Leaders

Modern nursing was forged by the contributions of many outstanding nurses through the years. The establishment of public health nursing, the provision of rural health care services, and the advancement of nursing education occurred as a result of the works of nurse pioneers, who are discussed below. Note that the term *trained nurse* was used historically as the predecessor of *registered nurse*. Information is presented in alphabetic, not chronological, order.

## Mary Breckinridge

In 1925, Mary Breckinridge introduced a system for delivering health care to rural America. She created a decentralized system for primary nursing care services in the Kentucky Appalachian Mountains. This system, the Frontier Nursing Service, lowered the childbirth mortality rate in Leslie County, Kentucky, from the highest in the nation to below the national average.

## Jane Delano

During World War I, Jane Delano (Figure 1-5), a graduate of Bellevue School of Nursing and former American Nurses Association (ANA) president, took one of the first stances that created a division among nursing leaders. In 1912, physicians wanted the Red Cross to put untrained nursing aides at their sides to assist with war casualties. Physicians, not nurses, would train the aides in caring for the sick.

Delano was opposed to the aide education plan because it violated the educational standards already established by nursing. This position pitted Delano against Annie Goodrich and Adelaide Nutting. The Red Cross recognized Delano's leadership abilities and dropped the aide plan. Delano was active in the Army Nurse Corps until she resigned her Army position in 1912 to work full time with the Red Cross. She died during wartime service in Europe.

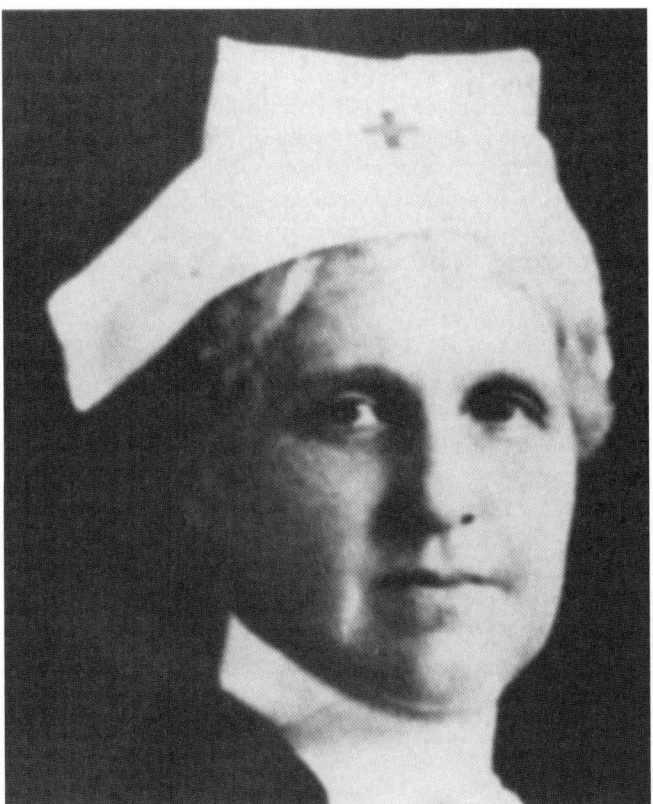

**Figure 1-5    Jane Delano.** *Photo courtesy of the American Nurses Association*

## Lavinia Dock

An influential leader in American nursing education was Lavinia Dock, who graduated from Bellevue Training School for Nurses in 1886. In her early nursing practice, she worked at the Henry Street Settlement House in New York City providing visiting nursing services to the indigent. She wrote one of the first nursing textbooks, *Materia Medica for Nurses*. Dock wrote many other books and was the first editor of the *American Journal of Nursing (AJN)*. Dock was a political activist who in 1914 encouraged nurses to unite when physicians objected to reforming labor laws to include nursing students.

## Martha Franklin

Martha Franklin was one of the first people to advocate racial equality in nursing. She was the only African American graduate of her class at Women's Hospital Training School for Nurses in Philadelphia. In 1908, Franklin organized the National Association of Colored Graduate Nurses (NACGN), which advocated that black nurses meet the same standards required of other nurses to prevent a double standard based on race. In 1951, the NACGN merged with the ANA.

## Annie Goodrich

Annie Goodrich (Figure 1-6) was influential in national and international nursing issues. During World War I, the supply of civilian nurses was greatly depleted because of the Army's need for trained nurses. Goodrich pushed for the establishment of an Army training school for nurses, which she envisioned as a model for other schools of nursing. She then was appointed dean of the Army School of Nursing. As an advocate of college-based educational nursing programs, Goodrich became the first dean of Yale University School of Nursing.

## Amelia Greenwald

Amelia Greenwald was a pioneer in public health nursing on the international scene. In 1908, she entered the Touro Infirmary Training School for Nurses in New Orleans, Louisiana. After graduation, Greenwald studied psychiatric and public health nursing. She served as chief nurse in several field hospitals during World War I. In 1923, she accepted the challenge of establishing a school of nursing in Poland. She received the Polish Golden Cross of Merit for her contributions to the welfare of the people. Greenwald was a catalyst for international public health nursing.

## Mamie Hale

In 1942, Mamie Hale (Figure 1-7) was hired by the Arkansas Health Department to upgrade the educational programs for midwives. Hale, a graduate of Tuskegee School of Nurse-Midwifery, gained the support of granny midwives, public health nurses, and obstetricians. Through education, Hale decreased superstition and illiteracy of those functioning as midwives. Hale's efforts resulted in improved mortality rates for both mothers and infants.

## Mary Mahoney

America's first African American professional nurse, Mary Mahoney (Figure 1-8), was a noted nursing leader who

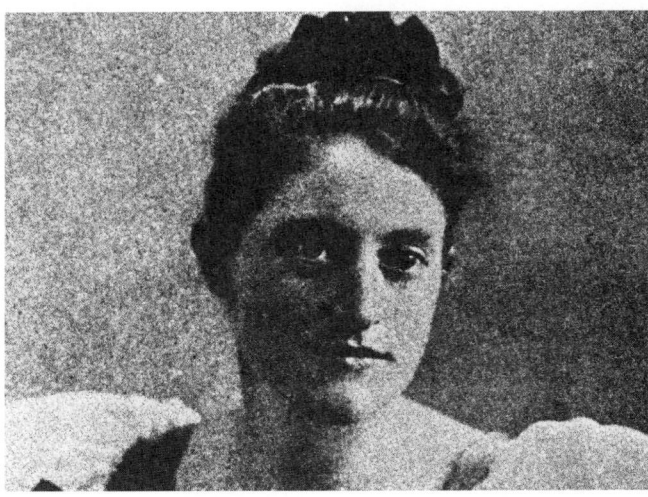

**Figure 1-6    Annie Goodrich.** *Photo courtesy of the American Nurses Association*

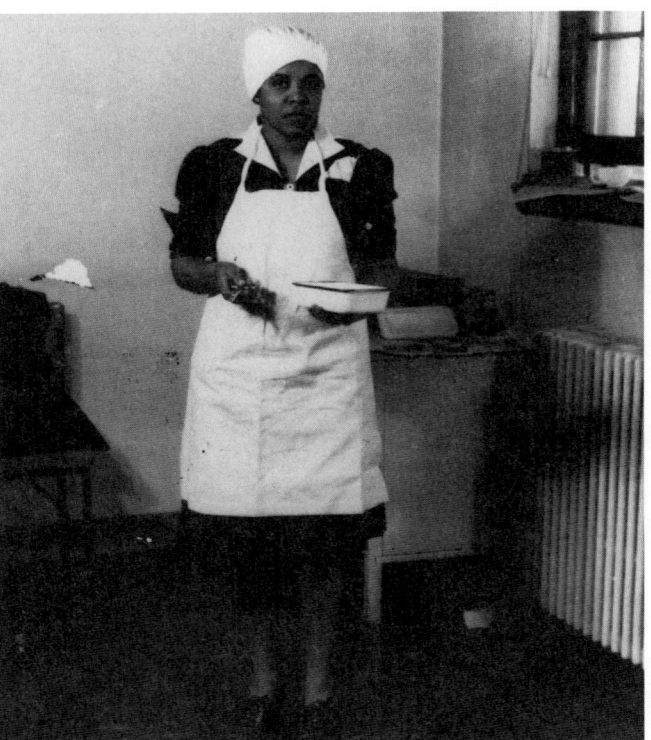

**Figure 1-7    Mamie Hale.** *Photo courtesy of the Historical Research Center, University of Arkansas for Medical Sciences Library, Little Rock, RG 515, Box 47*

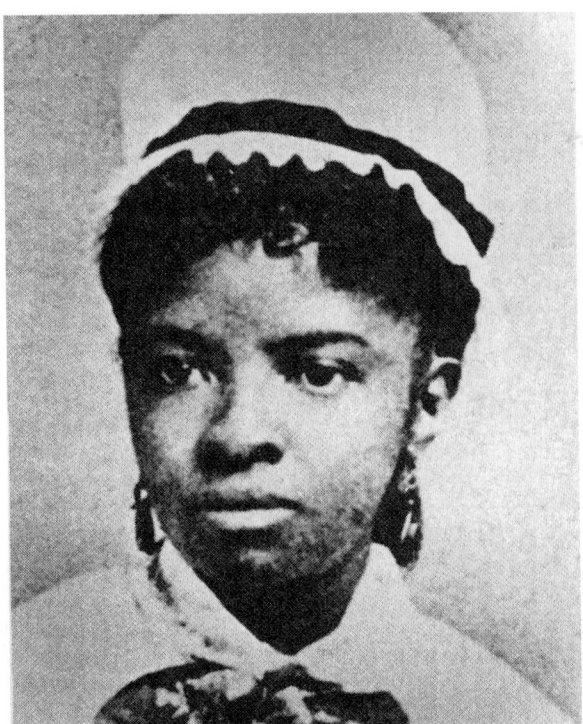

**Figure 1-8    Mary Mahoney.** *Photo courtesy of the American Nurses Association*

encouraged a respect for cultural diversity. Today, the ANA bestows the Mary Mahoney Award in recognition of individuals who make significant contributions toward improving relationships among multicultural groups.

## Adelaide Nutting

Adelaide Nutting was a nursing educator, historian, and scholar. She actively campaigned for nurses being educated in university settings and was the first nurse to be appointed to a university professorship. In 1910, Nutting was appointed to direct the newly established department of nursing and health at Teachers College, Columbia University, in New York City. This department was established to prepare nurses for teaching and supervision in nurse training schools, for administration in hospitals, and for work in preventive and social aspects of nursing.

## Harriet Neuton Phillips

Harriet Neuton Phillips was the first known graduate of the Women's Hospital of Philadelphia. A 6-month training course for nurses had been established by Dr. Ann Preston in 1861. Although no formal diplomas were awarded, the graduate nurses worked in the hospital and did private duty nursing in homes. Thus, Harriet Phillips can claim the title of the first American nurse to receive a training certificate. As a pioneer in community nursing, she worked with Chinese immigrants in San Francisco and with Native Americans in Wisconsin.

## Linda Richards

In 1873, the first diploma from an American training school for nurses was awarded to Linda Richards. Richards founded or reorganized 10 hospital-based training schools for nurses. She introduced the practice of keeping nurses' notes and physicians' orders as part of medical records. Also, Richards began the practice of nurses wearing uniforms. As the first Superintendent of Nurses at Massachusetts General Hospital, she demonstrated that trained nurses gave better care than those without formal nursing education.

## Isabel Hampton Robb

Isabel Hampton Robb (Figure 1-9) was responsible for founding several nursing organizations, namely the Superintendents' Society in 1893 and the Nurses' Associated Alumnae of the United States and Canada in 1896. She recognized the necessity of nurses participating in professional organizations to establish unity throughout nursing on positions and issues. She was instrumental in establishing both the American Nurses Association and the National League of Nursing Education. Robb was also an early supporter of the rights of nursing students. She called for shorter working hours and emphasized the role of the nursing student as learner instead of employee.

## Margaret Sanger

In 1912, Margaret Sanger (Figure 1-10), a nurse living in New York City, became concerned with women who had too many children to support. She coined the phrase

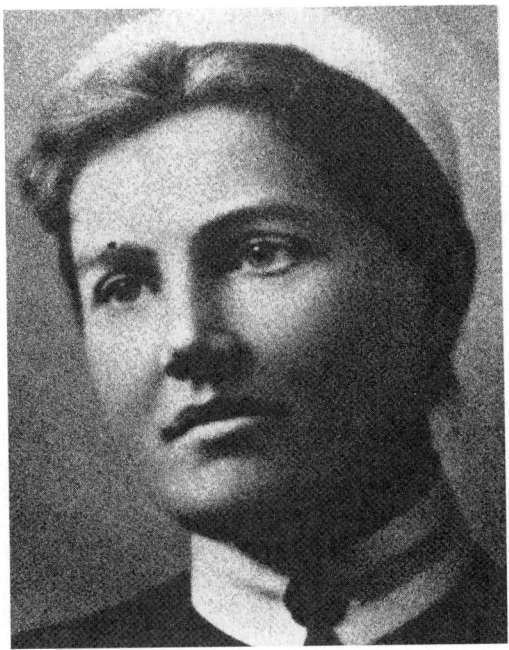

**Figure 1-9    Isabel Hampton Robb.** *Photo courtesy of the American Nurses Association*

"birth control" and began writing about contraceptive measures. Sanger fought to revise legislation that prohibited dissemination of information about contraception.

Sanger was not afraid of controversy and spent 1 month in jail for distributing information on birth control. As a true activist, Sanger made birth control an issue and fought for the rights of poor women. She understood the relationship between poverty, overpopulation, and high infant and maternal mortality rates. Sanger founded the American Birth Control League and was the first president of the International Planned Parenthood Federation.

## Adah Belle Thoms

Adah Belle Thoms was a crusader for improved relationships among persons of all races. In the early 1900s, she became acting director of nursing of the Lincoln School for Nurses in New York when African Americans rarely held high-level positions (Chinn, 1994). Thoms was one of the first to recognize public health as a field of nursing. She campaigned for equal rights for black nurses in the American Red Cross and the Army Nurse Corps.

## Shirley Titus

Shirley Titus received a diploma from St. Luke's Hospital School of Nursing in San Francisco in 1915. During her career, Titus served as dean of the School of Nursing at Vanderbilt University and in 1940 was the executive director of the California State Nurses' Association. She advocated improved economic security for nurses. Some of the many approaches to economic security for which she campaigned were malpractice insurance coverage, improved salaries and benefits, and collective bargaining.

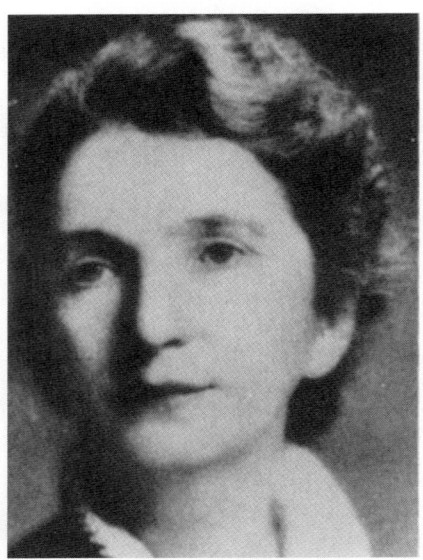

**Figure 1-10    Margaret Sanger.** *Photo courtesy of the American Nurses Association*

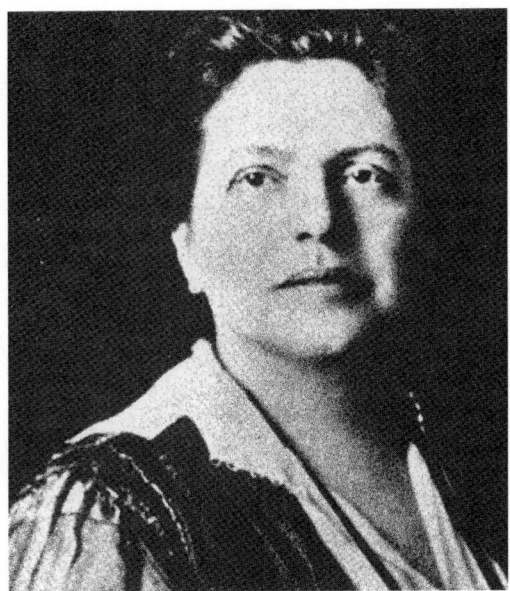

**Figure 1-11    Lillian Wald.** *Photo courtesy of the American Nurses Association*

## Lillian Wald

Lillian Wald (Figure 1-11) spent her life providing nursing care to the indigent population. In 1893, as the first community health nurse, she founded public health nursing with the establishment of the Henry Street Settlement Service (Figure 1-12) in New York City. Wald was a tireless reformer who:

- Improved housing conditions in tenement districts
- Supported education for the mentally challenged
- Advocated passage of more lenient immigration regulations
- Initiated change of child labor laws and founded the Children's Bureau of the U.S. Department of Labor

In addition to initiating public health nursing, Wald also established a school of nursing.

## Nursing in the 20th Century

The beginning of the 20th century brought about changes that have influenced contemporary nursing. Several landmark reports about medical and nursing education, as well as some contemporary reports, are discussed below. The establishment of visiting nurse associations and their use of protocols are also discussed.

## Flexner Report

In 1910, supported by a Carnegie grant, Abraham Flexner visited the 155 medical schools in the United States and Canada. The Flexner report was based on these findings, and its goal was to increase accountability in medical edu-

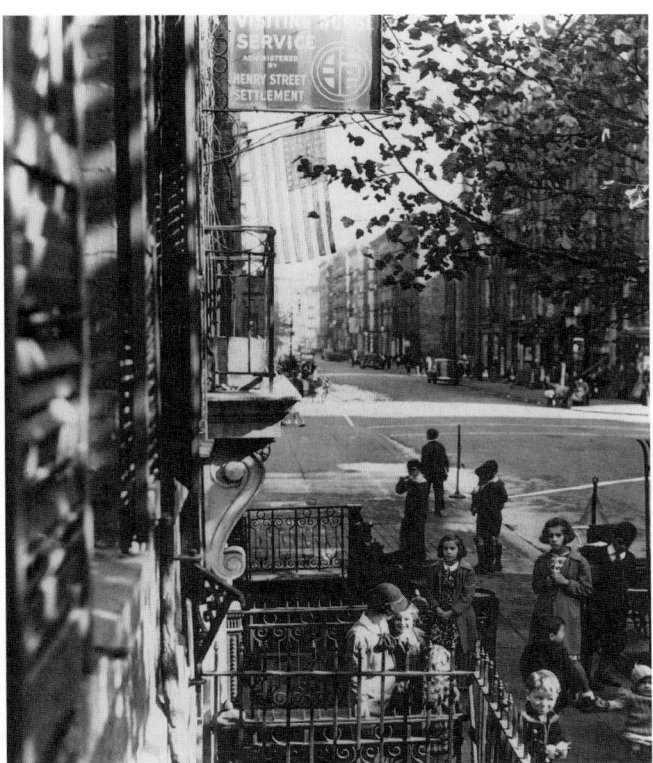

**Figure 1-12    Henry Street Settlement.** *Photo courtesy of Visiting Nurses Service of New York*

cation. The results of the study brought about the following changes: closure of inadequate medical schools, consolidation of schools with limited resources, creation of nonprofit status for remaining schools, and establishment of medical education in university settings based on standards and strong economic resources.

Adelaide Nutting saw the value and impact of the Flexner report on medical education and, in 1911, together with other colleagues of the Superintendents' Society, presented a proposal to the Carnegie Foundation to study nursing education. This foundation never allocated monies to study nursing education, but it supported educational studies in other disciplines such as law, dentistry, and teaching.

Although the efforts of Nutting and other nursing leaders went unheeded, in 1906 Richard Olding Beard successfully established a 3-year diploma school of nursing at the University of Minnesota under the College of Medicine.

## Early Insurance Plans

At the turn of the 20th century, there were more than 4,000 hospitals and 1,000 schools of nursing. During this time, the concepts of third-party payments and prepaid health insurance were instituted. Third-party payments refer to situations in which someone other than the recipient of health care (usually an insurance company) pays for the health care services provided. One of the earliest plans, involving teachers in Texas, provided 3 weeks of inpatient care, operating expenses, anesthesia, laboratory, and medication fees for 50 cents per month. Prepaid medical plans were started in Pacific Northwest lumber and mining camps, where employers contracted for and paid a monthly fee for medical services. This led to the establishment of the Bureau of Medical Services, where the employer contracted for medical services and the subscriber selected one of the physicians in the bureau.

Lillian Wald suggested the establishment of a national health insurance plan when she was the first president of the National Organization for Public Health Nursing.

### Blue Cross and Blue Shield

The Depression provided the main impetus for the growth of insurance plans. In addition, the American philosophy of health care for all contributed to the growth of insurance plans. In 1920, American hospitals offered a prepaid hospital plan that led to the "Baylor Plan," which eventually became the prototype of Blue Cross.

Blue Cross was the result of a joint venture between hospitals, physicians, and the general public. The American Hospital Association pioneered the development of an insurance company to provide benefits to subscribers who were hospitalized. Blue Shield was developed by the American Medical Association to provide reimbursement for medical services provided to subscribers. In 1933, the American Hospital Association endorsed Blue Cross, and in 1938 the American Medical Association endorsed Blue Shield.

## COMMUNITY/HOME CARE

### Community Care in an Urban Environment

The following story portrays a visit by a nurse to a home-based client:

Mrs. Corbett lives in a tenement building in a large urban setting. She has diabetes mellitus and suffers from peripheral vascular tissue destruction. Community care nurses need to visit Mrs. Corbett and assess her living situation as related to the disease process of diabetes. The nurse will need to assess Mrs. Corbett's level of knowledge about her disease and then develop a plan of care that addresses circulatory implications of her disease, as well as potential nutritional and activity related issues. It is interesting to reflect on the historical roots of community nurses (e.g., Lillian Wald) and their impact on current nursing practice in the community settings.

The federal government became more involved in health care delivery in 1935 with the passage of the Social Security Act, which provided for (among other things) benefits for the elderly, child welfare, and federal funding for training of health care personnel. Health insurance for all citizens was considered at this time but dropped after strong opposition from physicians (Kalisch & Kalisch, 1995). During World War II, the U.S. government extended the benefits for military services to include health care for veterans and their dependents.

### Visiting Nurses Associations

In 1901, at the suggestion of Lillian Wald, the Metropolitan Life Insurance Company, which provided visiting nursing services to its policyholders, entered into an agreement with the Henry Street Settlement. Wald worked with Metropolitan to expand the services of the Henry Street Settlement to other cities; thus, one form of managed care began.

Nurses providing care in the home environment experienced greater autonomy of practice than hospital-based nurses (Figure 1-13). This led to conflicts with some physicians about the scope of medical practice versus nursing practice parameters. Some physicians thought nurses were taking over their practice, whereas other physicians encouraged nurses to do whatever was necessary to care for the sick at home.

In 1912, in an effort to provide direction to home health staff nurses, the Chicago Visiting Nurse Association developed a list of standing orders for nurses to follow in providing home care. These orders were to direct the nursing care of clients when the nurse did not have specific orders from a physician. Thus, the groundwork for nursing protocols was established.

## Landmark Reports in Nursing Education

During the first half of the 20th century, a number of reports were issued concerning nursing education and practice. Three of them, the Goldmark, the Brown, and the Institute of Research and Service in Nursing Education reports, are discussed below.

### Goldmark Report

In 1918, Adelaide Nutting (relentless in her efforts to document the need for nursing education reform) approached the Rockefeller Foundation for support. Funding was provided, and, in 1919, the Committee for the Study of Nursing Education was established to investigate the training of public health nurses. E. A. Winslow, professor of public health, Yale University, chaired the committee, composed of ten physicians, two laypersons, and six nurses: Adelaide Nutting, Mary Beard, Lillian Clay, Annie Goodrich, Lillian Wald, and Helen Wood. Josephine Goldmark, a social worker, served as the secretary to the committee.

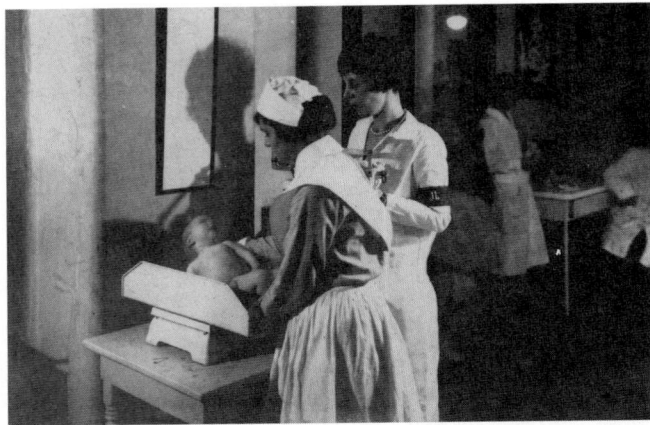

**Figure 1-13    A baby being weighed by a student nurse.** *Photo courtesy of Touro Infirmary Archives, New Orleans, LA*

As secretary, Goldmark developed the methodology of data collection and analysis for a small sampling of the 1,800 schools of nursing in existence. The study of 23 of the best nursing schools across the nation represented a cross-sample of schools—small and large, public and private.

The Goldmark report, entitled *Nursing and Nursing Education in the United States,* was published in 1923. Goldmark identified the major weakness of the hospital-based training programs as that of putting the needs of the institution (service delivery) before the needs of the student (education). Nursing tradition and the apprenticeship form of education reinforced putting the needs of the client before the learning needs of the student.

Some major inadequacies in nursing education identified by the study were limited resources, low admission standards, lack of supervision, poorly trained instructors, and failure to correlate clinical practice with theory. The report concluded that for nursing to be on equal footing with other disciplines, nursing education should occur in the university setting.

### Brown Report

In 1948, Esther Lucille Brown, a social anthropologist, published *Nursing for the Future and Nursing Reconsidered: A Study for Change.* Several recommendations were put forth in this study, including the need for nurses to demonstrate greater professional competence by moving nursing education from the hospital to the university setting.

Although published 20 years after the Goldmark report, the Brown report identified many of the same problems in diploma education—nursing students were still being used for service by the hospitals, and inadequate resources and authoritarianism in hospitals still prevailed in nursing education.

Brown recognized that nursing education in the university setting would provide the proper intellectual climate for the professional. Visionary nurse educators were securing necessary learning resources: libraries, laboratories, and clinical facilities. Professional endeavors such as research and publication were being implemented by nurse leaders.

### Institute of Research and Service in Nursing Education Report

During the 1950s, there was a deficit in the supply of nurses as the post–World War II demand for nursing services increased. Some contributing factors to the dearth of nurses were the low esteem of nursing as a profession, long hours with a heavy workload, and low salaries.

The Institute of Research and Service in Nursing Education report resulted in the establishment of practical nursing under Title III of the Health Amendment Act of 1955. There was a proliferation of associate degrees in nursing programs and practical nursing schools in the United States to increase the supply of nurses.

## Other Health Care Initiatives

In the 1960s, health care services were provided to the elderly and the indigent with the federal government's inception of Medicare and Medicaid.

This era also saw passage of the Nurse Training Act (1964), which provided federal funds to expand enrollments in schools of nursing. Federal funds were used to construct nursing schools, and student loans and scholarships were made available to nursing students.

### Selected Legislation

The Health Maintenance Organization Act of 1973 provided an alternative to the private health insurance industry. **Health maintenance organizations** (HMOs) are prepaid health plans that provide primary health care services for a predetermined fee (Kalisch & Kalisch, 1995). Because the fee is set in advance of services being rendered, HMOs provide cost-effective services. **Primary health care** refers to the client's point of entry into the health care system and includes assessment, diagnosis, treatment, coordination of care, preventive services, and education (Kalisch & Kalisch, 1995).

The National Commission for Manpower study, released in 1977, resulted in amendments to the House of Representatives 2504 of Title XVIII of the Social Security Act that provided payment for rural health clinic services. Through the efforts of Anne Zimmerman, former president of the ANA, the bill was amended to substitute the term *primary care providers* for *physician extenders* and therefore allowed nurse practitioners to be paid directly for their services. This was a major success for nursing.

The Rural Health Clinic Service Act of 1977 covered services rendered by nurse practitioners and nurse-midwives. The Omnibus Budget Reconciliation Act of 1980 mandated payment for nurse-midwife services to needy recipients (Kalisch & Kalisch, 1995). Nursing became an integral part in meeting the needs of vulnerable populations.

## Education and Practice: Contemporary Reports

During the 1980s, several important studies were commissioned to examine the areas of nursing education and practice.

## National Commission on Nursing

The National Commission on Nursing was created in 1980 by the American Hospital Association (AHA), the Hospital Research and Education Trust, and the American Hospital Supply Corporation to study nursing education and related issues in hospital management, nursing practice, and nursing education. The commission's conclusions addressed the need for:

- Adequate clinical education for students
- Baccalaureate education and educational mobility
- Involvement of nurses in collaborative institutional and clinical decision making
- Improved working conditions, specifically, salaries, flexible scheduling, and differentiated practice

As a result of the commission's study, attention was given to the need for physicians and nurses to enter into collaborative practice.

### Institute of Medicine

Concurrent with the National Commission on Nursing study, another study was initiated by Congress in 1979 and conducted by the Institute of Medicine (IOM). The study, *Nursing and Nursing Education: Public Policies and Private Actions*, focused on the need for continued federal funding to nursing education. The findings indicated that there was not a shortage of the general supply of nurses, but there was a serious shortage of nurses in research, teaching, administration, and advanced clinical practice. A significant nursing shortage existed in preventive and primary care for the disadvantaged and elderly in inner cities and rural areas.

### Secretary's Commission on Nursing

Although the IOM study indicated that there were sufficient numbers of staff nurses, based on supply and demand, hospitals continued to report severe shortages. As a response to hospitals' recruitment and retention challenges, Health and Human Services Secretary Otis R. Brown, MD, established the Secretary's Commission on Nursing, which made the following recommendations related to nursing practice:

- Nurse compensation
- Health care financing
- Nurse decision making

- Development, use, and maintenance of nursing resources (Secretary's Commission on Nursing, 1988)

This commission recognized that the federal government alone could not correct the problems facing nursing and health care but rather that the concerted efforts of health care organizations were needed for the implementation of the report's recommendations.

# Social Forces Affecting Nursing

From the earliest recordings of nursing, 4000 BC through the Christian era, women were allowed to perform the nurse role only in the home. Nursing's links with the church caused nursing to be viewed as a "service," not a profession such as medicine. The Crimean and Civil Wars had a significant impact on nursing's future by focusing on women as nurse providers and on the need for nurse training.

During the 20th century, the evolution of medical education as an established profession had far advanced that of nursing. The Flexner report carved the destiny for physicians. The Goldmark and Brown reports created havoc for nurses as they debated the issue of nursing education in the university setting.

The Depression and World War II brought social reform and created health and medical insurance that strengthened the organized power base of both physician and hospital. Nursing—almost exclusively a female profession—had little power and therefore did not exert much influence on the social forces at play. The greatest advances for nurses were seen in the realm of public health and preventive health care.

As physicians were released from military service after World War II, the era of specialized medicine began. Physicians used their veterans' educational entitlement benefits to take residency training in one or more specialty areas. By 1966, more than 70% of the physicians in practice were specialists.

The 1960s was a decade of growth and change. As technologic advances increased the scope of practice of medicine and nursing, other social forces were at play: access to health care services enhanced by Medicare and Medicaid, physician and nurse shortages, the feminist movement, the inception of nurse practitioners; and a focus on health maintenance.

The economic recession of the 1970s saw health care costs escalating along with unemployment. Professional autonomy was being debated, nursing theories were being developed, and nursing education was being integrated into the university setting. Nurses were becoming more politically astute in that they were working through professional organizations to affect health care legislation.

During the 1980s, nursing became more specialized and autonomous. The rapid technologic advances in medicine required more specialization in nursing. Nurse practitioners were being more widely accepted by the general public and other health care providers. Expanded roles of nurses were developing in response to greater demands for nursing services. One factor that led to an increased need for nursing was the proliferation of health maintenance organizations (HMOs) in the early 1980s.

During the 1990s, nurses were actively assuming more responsibilities for the delivery of health care. Evolving technology mandated nurses to continue to advance their knowledge base and skills. The aging of the population called for more nursing involvement with the elderly. Nurses, as individuals and as members of professional organizations, were involved in shaping policies for health care reform. Nursing was a stronger advocate for vulnerable populations: the elderly, those living in poverty, the homeless, and those with human immunodeficiency virus (HIV) and acquired immunodeficiency syndrome (AIDS).

## Healthy People Initiatives

Healthy People initiatives has become the nation's health agenda. This initiative began with a report entitled *Healthy People: The Surgeon General's Report on Health Promotion and Disease Prevention in 1979*. The report described the Healthy People as the nation's health agenda to guide policy on public health initiatives for health promotion and disease prevention activities during the decade 1980–1990. Five goals were identified to decrease the mortality rates for four distinct age groups (infants, children ages 1–14 years, adolescents and young adults up to age 34, adults ages 25–65) and to reduce the average number of days of illness among those over age 65 (U.S. Public Health Service, 1979). Also identified in the report were 15 strategies to achieve the goals; these strategies were studied by panels of experts and resulted in quantifiable objectives to implement the 15 strategies by governmental bodies and private sector agencies at the national, state, local, and community levels (U.S. Public Health Service, 1979). Achievement of the 226 objectives was measured and reported at 2-year increments by the National Center for Health Statistics. While positive changes were achieved for infants, children, and adults, the goals for adolescents and the elderly were not achieved by 1990 ("Results of the 1990 Objectives," 1992).

 **STOP AND THINK**

### The Women's Movement and Nursing

- How did the women's movement have an impact on nursing?

- What issues were created by the high percentage of women in the nursing profession?

The outcomes from the 1979 Healthy People initiative led to the development of the Healthy People 2000 Objectives. Coordinated by the U.S. Public Health Service, this program identified the following goals to be achieved from 1990 to 2000: increase the span of healthy life, reduce health disparities, and promote access to preventive services for all Americans (U.S. Department of Health and Human Services, 1991). The original 15 strategies were expanded to include 22 priority areas, and the total number of objectives was increased to 319. The objectives were classified into three major categories: health promotion, health protection, and preventive services. Wilson (1999) described the Healthy People 2000 Objectives as a challenge to the nation to move beyond merely saving lives, to decrease unnecessary suffering, illness, and disability, and to improve the quality of life. Although methodologies were similar to the first study regarding data collection and analysis, it is difficult to measure this program's success since many of the surveillance systems needed to measure outcomes were not in place at the onset of the study (Wilson, 1999).

The first draft of Healthy People 2010 initiatives appeared in the September 1997 issue of the *Federal Register*. Early work focused on identifying the 2000 objectives to be continued into the 2010 agenda. The Healthy People Consortium, an alliance that includes more than 350 national organizations and 270 state public health, mental health, substance abuse, and environmental agencies, launched in January 2000 the following Healthy People 2010 goals and objectives:

- Major goals
  1. Increase quality and years of healthy life.
  2. Eliminate health disparities.

- Enabling goals
  1. Promote healthy behaviors.
  2. Promote healthy and safe communities.
  3. Improve systems for personal and public health.
  4. Prevent and reduce diseases and disorders.

 **LIFE SPAN CONSIDERATIONS**

**Healthy People 2010 Goals and the Aged**

Often the elderly do not conceptualize goals to progress toward wellness behaviors. As the nurse, you are the most appropriate member of the health care team to increase the knowledge level of the elderly concerning wellness. You can use the Healthy People 2010 goals and objectives when working with the geriatric age group in achieving wellness (Hogstel, 2001).

 **CLIENT REFLECTIONS**

**Technology and Aging**

Mr. Abernathy is 65 years old and admitted to your coronary care unit. He says, "I feel like a lot of the nurses here are more interested in these machines I am hooked up to than they are in me." As his nurse, how would you respond to his statement?

An additional 26 focus areas, objectives, and developmental objectives were identified to support the achievement of the major and enabling goals.

Success of the Healthy People program requires the cooperative efforts of all health care disciplines to pool their resources and services in order to provide accessible, quality health care and preventive services for all Americans regardless of nationality, ethnicity, age, and economic status (Wilson, 1999).

## Alternative Methods of Health Care Delivery

As it has evolved over time, nursing is still focused on caring. Rapid technologic advances, the changing climate of financing health care, and the explosion of alternative delivery methods present challenges to nurses. How are nurses responding to these challenges?

- By shaping health care policies
- By collaborating with other health care providers
- By continuing to advance nursing education

Nursing in the new millennium will be vastly different from what it has been. Collaborative health care services and innovative settings for the delivery of health care are currently being developed by nurses.

### Costs and Quality Controls

During the 1970s, the cost-control systems of various federal government health programs were inadequate because of the rapid escalation of health care expenditures. Consequently, the Tax Equity Fiscal Responsibility Act (TEFRA) of 1982 was created in response to the $287 billion spent on health care in 1981. While the federal government, with TEFRA and prospective payment legislation, tried to control costs, there was also a heightened concern with the quality of health care.

Business and industry embraced quality control systems in the 1940s and 1950s. However, the health care industry failed to see the need for these types of controls until the 1980s. The Joint Commission on the Accreditation of Healthcare Organizations' (JCAHO) agenda for change in the late 1980s emphasized monitoring quality for outcomes rather than process, thus advocating change from a static quality assurance system to dynamic quality improvement. The JCAHO (1996) views quality of care as an ongoing process that continuously looks for ways to improve the care provided. See Chapter 25 for a discussion of the issue of quality management in nursing and health care.

## Health Care Reform

Health care access and costs were the focus of attention in the 1990s with an ever-increasing number (over 60 million) of Americans being uninsured or underinsured. Children remain at risk for having their health care neglected; one in five American children is not insured.

Nursing as a profession has made great strides in effecting federal and state health care legislation (Figure 1-14). The 1990s were filled with challenges as nurses were held accountable for quality nursing care amidst cutbacks in staffing patterns. Some of these challenges were settled by legislative outcomes such as determining nurse-client ratios in skilled nursing facilities and prohibiting acute care hospitals from assigning unlicensed personnel to perform nursing functions, in lieu of a registered nurse. Nurses worked in collaboration with other health care professionals in providing community-based services and in developing **evidence-based practice** among diverse health care settings. "Evidence-based practice is the application of the best available empirical evidence, including

recent research findings to clinical practice in order to aid clinical decision-making" (Taylor-Piliae, p. 30, 1998).

## The Nursing Shortage

The history of nursing is a cycle of nursing shortages and surpluses, and currently the supply of nurses is decreasing. The pressing nursing shortage may be a more permanent problem due to a number of important changes in our society. This is not only an aging society, but also an aging workforce. Each year, fewer students enroll in nursing, leading to a steadily aging population of nurses. As the baby-boom generation of nurses retire, fewer nurses are available to take open positions. In addition to recruitment, the job market demand for nurses has expanded. An older population requires more nursing care, and new nursing positions in community-based health services has increased the need for nurses.

Along with an aging workforce, job satisfaction in nursing is low. Physician behavior toward nurses, shift work, and flat salaries are among the problems nurses face. As staffing vacancies rise, mandatory overtime, understaffing, and increasing workloads follow. This chapter points out that nursing has been a predominantly female profession. As more opportunities are created for women, the nursing profession competes with other careers that perhaps offer better working conditions and higher salaries. Fewer prospective students see nursing as the best option for their career choice. To attract both men and women into nursing, reforms in employment conditions and job expectations need to occur (Bednash, 2000).

## The Future of Nursing

History is being made daily for nurses and other health care providers as the citizens of this country decide which way to move with health care reform initiatives. Pressing issues for nursing include developing evidence-based prac-

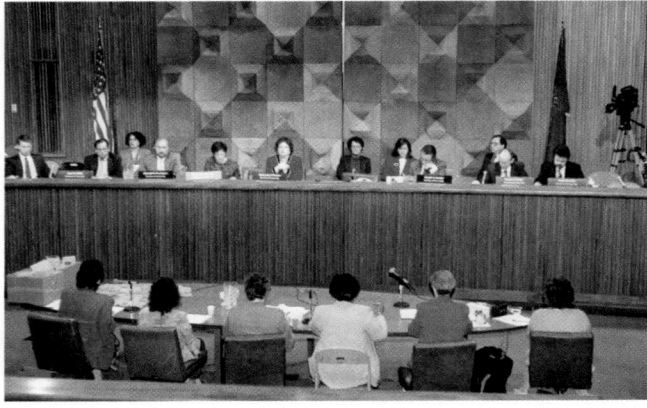

**Figure 1-14    Nurses making a presentation before a state legislature.** *Photo courtesy of the New York State Nurses Association*

## STOP AND THINK

### Distance Education

● If a nurse in Florida assists an online client in California, in which state is the nurse practicing?

● What do you think are some advantages and disadvantages of distance education for clients? For nursing students?

## NURSING STRATEGY

### Empowerment in Nursing

To increase the level of autonomy and increase the "power" in nursing:

● Participate in local, regional, and state specialty groups within nursing (e.g., Association of Operating Room Nursing, Critical Care Nursing, Clinical Nurse Specialist).

● Attend continuing education conferences and present information to those nurses you are associated with in your employment settings.

● Evaluate the contract agreements within your agency, attend business meetings, and join committees that represent nursing in your health care practice settings.

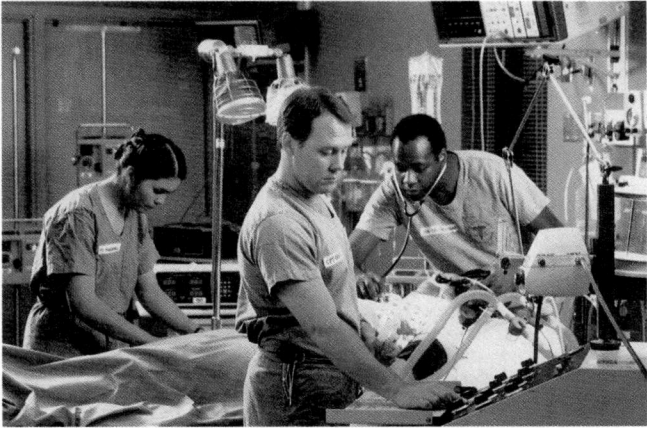

**Figure 1-15    Nurses in acute care setting.** *"Be All You Can Be," Courtesy of the U.S. Government, as represented by the Secretary of the Army*

tice that can be uniformly adopted in diverse nursing care settings; monitoring safe practice in a restructured health care environment; and designing systems that will enhance collaborative planning, and implement actions and policies to address the changes occurring in the nursing labor market. Nurses can make the most of this time of transformation, which is driven by societal needs. Nurses and nursing students need to stay abreast of current issues and be active with local nursing leaders to communicate nursing's position(s) on health care reform and alternative health care delivery models. Prominent new models of health care delivery will include distance technologies. Nurses are already delivering client education on the Internet (see Web Resources). Nursing degrees are offered entirely online. This new practice of distance education is increasing the need for changes in licensure (Schroeder & DePalma, 2001).

Nurses are being recognized as autonomous professionals and are involved in administrative and clinical decision making (Figure 1-15). Only when nurses are empowered are they truly autonomous.

## Key Concepts

• Nursing is an art and a science in which people are assisted in learning to care for themselves whenever possible and are cared for when they are unable to meet their own needs.

• Nurses will understand such issues as autonomy, unity within the profession, supply and demand, salary, education, and current practice and the empowerment of the profession by studying nursing's history.

• Nursing's early history was heavily influenced by religious organizations and the need for nurses to care for soldiers during wartime.

• Florence Nightingale forged the future of nursing practice and education as a result of her experiences in training nurses to care for soldiers.

• Nursing's early American leaders, professional organizations, and landmark reports have influenced the infrastructure of current nursing practice.

• Influential nursing leaders, such as Lillian Wald, Jane Delano, Isabel Hampton Robb, Annie Goodrich, Adelaide Nutting, and Lavinia Dock, were instrumental in the advancement of nursing education and practice.

• Other nursing pioneers, such as Amelia Greenwald, Mary Breckenridge, Mamie Hale, Mary Mahoney, Linda Richards, and Margaret Sanger, made important contributions to both nursing education and the fields of rural, public health, maternity, and multicultural nursing.

• In 1923, the Goldmark report concluded that for nursing to be on equal footing with other disciplines, nursing education should occur in the university setting.

• The Brown report (1948) addressed the need for nurses to demonstrate greater professional competence by moving nursing education to the university setting.

• The Health Maintenance Organization Act of 1973 provided an alternative to the private health insurance industry.

- Contemporary reports issued by the National Commission on Nursing, the Institute of Medicine, and the Secretary's Commission on Nursing focused on the areas of nursing education, practice, and nursing's role in health care financing policies.
- Developments such as alternative methods of health care delivery, evidence-based practice, and the efforts devoted to health care reform have led to diversified nursing roles.
- As the nursing profession continues to evolve and respond to the challenges within the health care system, nurses will remain responsive to societal needs.
- The current nursing shortage is critically affecting the entire health care delivery system.

## Review Questions and Activities

1. What does the phrase "using their own history" mean to nurses? After studying this chapter, list some major lessons nurses can derive from history.
2. Examine the history of your nursing school. Are the early leaders honored for their contributions?
3. Identify some contemporary nursing leaders. What are their contributions to the nursing profession?
4. Choose the correct answer. The major recommendation of both the Goldmark and Brown reports was to:
    a. recruit more people into the nursing profession
    b. compensate nurses with higher salaries and more comprehensive benefits
    c. place nursing education within institutions of higher learning
    d. increase the amount of clinical practice in nursing education programs
5. List some key legislative measures that have affected nursing's role in the delivery of health care in the United States.

## Multimedia Links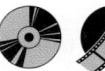

Christensen *Core Concept Videos: History of Nursing*

## Web Resources

Agency for Healthcare Research and Quality
    http://www.ahrq.gov
Ask the nurses
    http://www.med-help.com
American Association for the History of Nursing
    http://www.aahn.org
General health information provided by the government
    http://www.health.gov
Healthy People 2010
    HPWebsite@osophs.dhhs.gov

National Council of State Board of Nursing
    http://www.ncsbn.org
U.S. Department of Health and Human Services
    http://www.hhs.gov

## References

Bednash, G. (2000). The decreasing supply of registered nurses: Inevitable future or call to action. *Journal of the American Medical Association (JAMA), 283*(22), 2985–2993.

Brush, B. (1999). Has foreign nurse recruitment impeded African American access to nursing education and practice? *Nursing Outlook, 47*(4), 175–180.

Buerhaus, P. I. (2000). Implications of an aging registered nurse workforce. *Journal of the American Medical Association (JAMA), 283*(22), 2948–2953.

Chinn, P. L. (1994). *Developing the discipline: Critical studies in nursing history and professional issues.* Gaithersburg, MD: Aspen.

Cushing, A. (1995, Summer). An historical note on the relationship between nursing and nursing history. *International History Nursing Journal, 1*(1), 57–60.

Donahue, M. (1990). The past in the present. *Journal of Professional Nursing, 6*, 9.

Donahue, M. P. (1996). *Nursing: The finest art* (2nd ed.). St. Louis, MO: Mosby.

Dossey, B. (1995). Endnote: Florence Nightingale today. *Critical Care Nursing, 15*(4), 98.

Duncan, S., Leipert, B., & Mill, J. (1999). "Nurses as health evangelists?" Evolution of public health nursing in Canada, 1913–1939. *Advances in Nursing Science, 22*(1), 40–51.

Fairman, J., & Kagan, S. (1999). Creating critical care: The case of the Hospital of the University of Pennsylvania, 1950–1965. *Advances in Nursing Science, 22*(1), 63–77.

Frantz, A. (1998). Nursing Pride: Clara Barton in the Spanish-American War. *American Journal of Nursing, 98*(10), 39–40.

Freshwater, D. (2000). Crosscurrents: Against cultural narration in nursing. *Journal of Advances Nursing, 32*(2), 481–484.

Gordan, R. C. (1999). Linda Richards at the Kalamazoo State Hospital. *Journal of Psychosocial Nursing, 37*(11), 35–39.

Hall-Long, B. A. (1995, February-March). Nursing's past, present, and future political experience. *Nursing and Health Care Perspective Community, 16*(1), 24–28.

Hogstel, M. (2001). *Gerontology: Nursing care of the older adult.* Clifton Park, NY: Delmar Learning.

Institute of Medicine (1998). *Leading health indicators for healthy people 2010: Second interim report.* Washington, DC: National Academy Press.

Joint Commission on the Accreditation of Healthcare Organizations (1996). *Accreditation standards and scoring guidelines for hospital-based mental health.* Oak Brook Terrace, IL: Author.

Kalisch, P. A., & Kalisch, B. J. (1995). The Advance of American Nursing (3rd ed.). Philadelphia: Lippincott.

Kovner, C., & Harrington, C. (2000). Nursing counts. *American Journal of Nursing, 100*(9), 53–54.

Marshall, E. S., & Wall, B. M. (1999). Religion, gender, and autonomy: A comparison of two religious women's groups in nursing and hospitals in the late nineteenth and early twentieth centuries. *Advances in Nursing Science, 22*(1), 1–22.

Nightingale, F. (1969). *Nursing: What it is and what it is not.* New York: Dover Publications.

Olsen, T. (1995). Recreating past separations and the employment pattern of nurses, 1900–1940. *Nursing Outlook, 43*(5), 210–214.

Rafael, A. (1999). The politics of health promotion: Influences on public health promoting nursing practice in Ontario, Canada from Nightingale to the nineties. *Advances in Nursing Science, 22*(1), 23–29.

Results of the 1990 objectives for the nation (1992). *Journal of the American Medical Association, 268*(18).

The Robert Wood Johnson Foundation Anthology (1999). *To improve health and health care 2000.* San Francisco: Jossey-Bass Publishers.

Secretary's Commission on Nursing (1988). *Final report.* Washington, DC: Department of Health & Human Services.

Schroeder, B., & DePalma, N. (2001). As close as the phone: telemonitoring in home care. *Nurseweek, 9*(6) 23-26.

Stratton, T. D., Dunkin, J. W., & Juhl, N. (1995). Redefining the nursing shortage: A rural perspective. *Nursing Outlook, 43*(2), 71–77.

Taft, S. (2001). The nursing shortage: Introduction. *Online Journal of Issues in Nursing, 6*(1). http://www.nursingworld.org/ojin/topic14/tpc14ntr.htm

Taylor-Piliae, R. (1998). Establishing evidence-based practice: Issues and implications in critical care nursing. *Intensive Critical Care Nursing, 14*(1), 30–37.

Turkoski, B. B. (1995). Professionalism as ideology: A socio-historical analysis of the discourse of professionalism in nursing. *Nursing Inquiry, 2*(2), 83–89.

U.S. Department of Health and Human Services (1979). *Healthy people: The Surgeon General's report on health promotion and disease prevention.* (Publication No. PHS 79-55071.) Washington, DC: Department of Health, Education, and Welfare.

U.S. Department of Health and Human Services (1991). *National health promotion and disease prevention objectives for the nation.* Washington, DC: U.S. Public Health Services.

Wall, B. M. (1995). Courage to care: The Sisters of the Holy Cross in the Spanish American War. *Nursing Historical Review, 3*, 55–77.

Ward, S. F. (1995). Patient care has come full circle . . . faced with ever-changing patient care demands, hospitals are creating alternative care facilities—reverting to the days when the caregiver came to the patient. *Surgical Services Management, 1*(3), 6, 8–9.

Wieck, K. (2000). A vision for nursing: The future revisited. *Nursing Outlook, 48*(1), 7.

Wilson, L. M. (1999). Healthy people—A new millennium. *Journal of Nurse Attorney, 99*(1), 29–32.

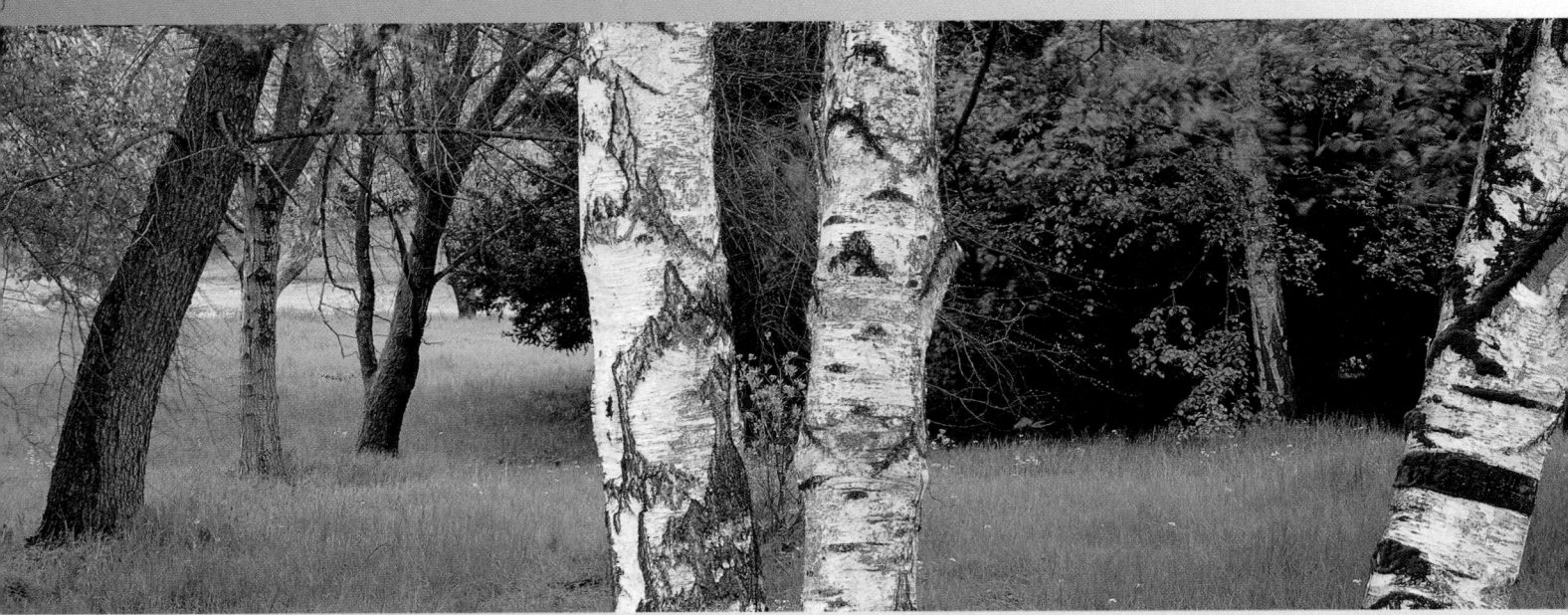

# The Health Care Delivery System

## Carol Craig, PhD, FNP, RN

*"The Twentieth Century will be remembered chiefly not as an age of political conflicts and technological inventions, but as an age in which human society dared to think of the health of the whole human race as a practical objective."*

(Arnold Toynbee, 1889–1975)

# Chapter Competencies

*Upon completion of this chapter, the reader should be able to:*

1. Describe the types of services of the U.S. health care delivery system.
2. Discuss the various health care settings through which health care services are delivered.
3. Identify the members of the health care team and their respective roles.
4. Describe the differences between the various financial programs for health care services and reimbursement.
5. Explain the factors that influence health care delivery.
6. Explore the challenges that exist within the health care system.
7. Discuss nursing's role in meeting the challenges within the health care system.
8. Describe the emerging trends and issues for the health care delivery system.

# Key Terms

advanced practice registered nurse
capitated rates
comorbidity
exclusive provider organization
fee-for-service

health care delivery system
health maintenance organization
managed care
medical model
preferred provider organization

prescriptive authority
primary care provider
primary health care
single-payer system
single point of entry
subacute care

A **health care delivery system** is a mechanism for providing services that meet the health-related needs of individuals. The U.S. health care delivery system is currently experiencing dramatic change. Health care institutions that once flourished economically are now searching for ways to survive. Health care providers are seeking cost-effective ways to deliver an ever-increasing range of services to consumers. Consumers are demanding greater accessibility to quality health care services that are affordable.

Nursing is a major component of the U.S. health care delivery system. Consequently, nurses must understand the changes occurring within this system, as well as their role in shaping the changes. This chapter discusses the types of health care services available, various settings in which these services are provided, and the members of the health care team. The economics of health care and the challenges within the health care delivery system are also discussed. Nursing's role in meeting these challenges is described.

Americans are becoming increasingly confused about the services and coverage offered by the health care system. This chapter examines some of the problems and possible solutions in health care delivery.

## Types of Health Care Services

Basically, health care services can be categorized into three levels: primary, secondary, and tertiary (Figure 2-1). The complexity of care varies according to the individual's need, provider's expertise, and delivery setting. Table 2-1 provides an overview of the types of care.

## Primary: Health Promotion and Illness Prevention

The major purposes of health care are to promote wellness and prevent illness or disability. Traditionally, the U.S. health care system focused on disease prevention rather than health promotion. However, within the past decade, society has begun to engage in health-promoting behaviors. Illness prevention activities are directed at the individual, the family, and/or the community.

Unfortunately, our entire system of health care delivery is not a *health* care system but rather an *illness* care system. Services are directed to caring for an individual after disease or disability has developed rather than emphasizing preventive aspects of care. Ideally, preventive care occurs in the community (e.g., homes, workplaces, schools) and emphasizes the development of healthy lifestyles.

## Secondary: Diagnosis and Treatment

Most services occur within this secondary type of health care. Diagnosis and treatment of most illnesses occurs in primary care clinics or provider's offices. Hospitals also do

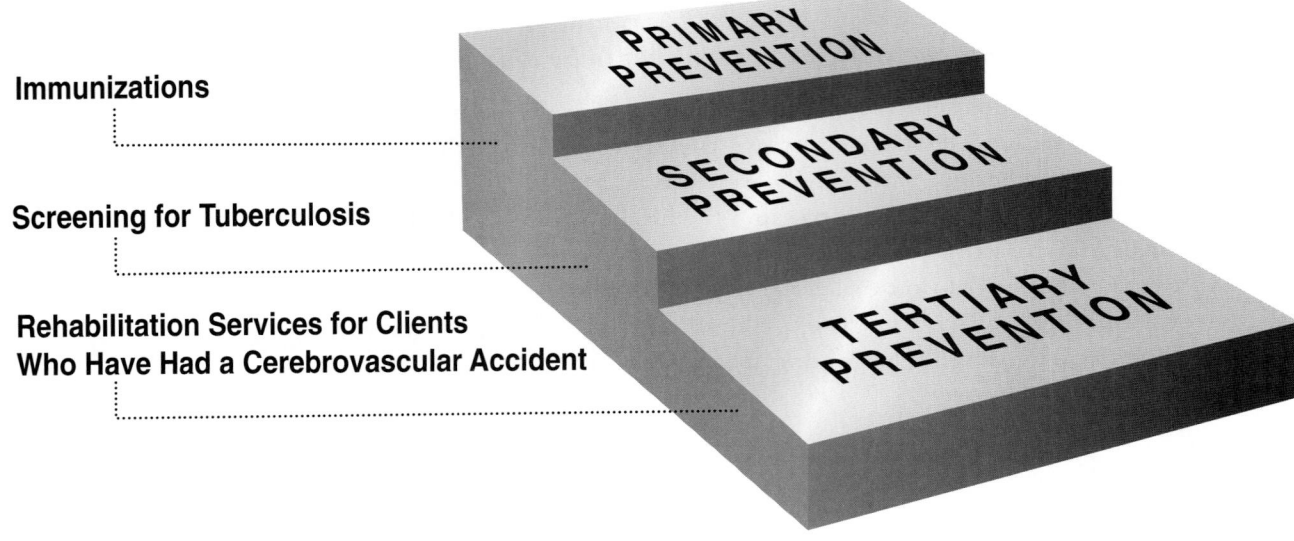

**Immunizations**

**Screening for Tuberculosis**

**Rehabilitation Services for Clients
Who Have Had a Cerebrovascular Accident**

**Figure 2-1    Three levels of prevention: examples**

| TABLE 2-1 | TYPES OF HEALTH CARE SERVICES | |
|---|---|---|
| Type of Care | Description | Examples |
| Primary | *Goal:* To decrease the risk to a client (individual or community) for disease or dysfunction | Teaching<br>Lifestyle modification for health (e.g., smoking cessation, nutritional counseling) |
| | *Explanation:*<br>General health promotion<br>Protection against specific illnesses | Referrals<br>Immunization<br>Promotion of a safe environment (e.g., sanitation, protection from toxic agents) |
| Secondary | *Goal:* Early detection and intervention to alleviate disease and prevent further disability | Screenings/diagnosis<br>Acute care<br>Surgery |
| | *Explanation*:<br>Early detection and intervention | |
| Tertiary | *Goal:* To minimize effects and permanent disability of chronic or irreversible condition | Education and retraining<br>Provision of direct care<br>Environmental modifications (e.g., advising on necessity of wheelchair accessibility for a person |
| | *Explanation*:<br>Restorative and rehabilitative activities to obtain optimal level of functioning | who has experienced a cardiovascular accident [stroke]) |

## STOP AND THINK

### Three Levels of Health Care Services

● Give examples of clients you have seen in each of the three levels of health care services.

● What types of services in your area meet the needs of the three levels of health care services?

secondary care, primarily through emergency departments. There is a growing movement to have diagnostic and therapeutic services provided in locations that are less expensive and more easily accessed by individuals. This trend is discussed later in this chapter.

## Tertiary: Rehabilitation

Restoring an individual to the state that existed before the development of an illness is the purpose of rehabilitative (or restorative) care. In situations in which the person is unable to regain previous functional abilities, the goal of rehabilitation is to help the client reach the optimal level of self-care. Restorative care is holistic, in that the entire person is cared for—physiological, psychological, social, and spiritual aspects.

## Health Care Settings

The U.S. health care delivery system is complex, involving myriad providers, consumers, and settings. Health care services in this country are delivered by both the public (including official and voluntary) and private sectors.

## Public Sector

Public agencies are financed with tax monies; thus, these agencies are accountable to the public. The public sector includes official (or governmental) agencies, voluntary agencies, and nonprofit agencies. Figure 2-2 shows the hierarchy of the public sector of health care delivery.

At the local level, services provided include immunizations, maternal-child care, and activities directed at control of chronic diseases. Each state varies in the provision of public health services. Generally, a state department of health coordinates the activities of local health units.

At the national level, the U.S. Department of Health and Human Services (DHHS) is administratively responsible for health care services delivered to the public. The Surgeon General is the chief officer of the U.S. Public Health Service (USPHS), the major agency that oversees the actual delivery of care services. Table 2-2 lists the USPHS agencies and their purposes.

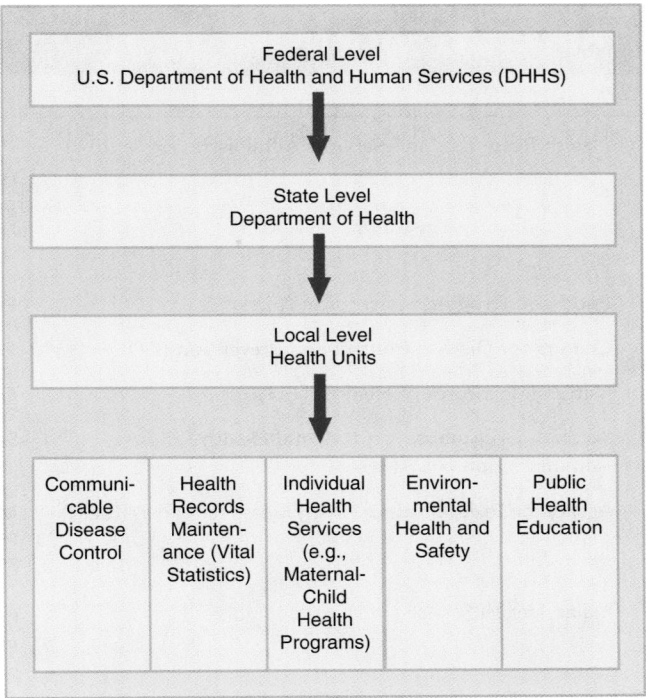

**Figure 2-2    The public sector of health care delivery**

An important part of the public sector of the health care delivery system is voluntary agencies. These not-for-profit agencies exert significant legislative influence (e.g., the American Nurses Association [ANA] and the American Medical Association [AMA]). Other voluntary agencies, such as the American Cancer Society and the American Heart Association, provide educational resources to the general public and to health care providers. Voluntary agencies are funded in a variety of ways, including individual contributions, corporate philanthropy, and membership dues.

## Private Sector

The private sector of the health care delivery system primarily comprises independent providers who are reimbursed on a **fee-for-service** basis (the recipient directly pays the provider for services as they are provided). The variety of settings in which health care is delivered and the roles of nurses in these settings are presented in Table 2-3. These practice settings are directly influenced by social and economic factors.

## The Health Care Team

Health care services are delivered by a multidisciplinary team. Table 2-4 provides a list of health care providers. Because nurses work with other care providers on an ongoing basis, it is necessary to understand the role of each provider. Nurses coordinate the care provided by other personnel (Figure 2-3).

## TABLE 2-2    AGENCIES OF THE U.S. PUBLIC HEALTH SERVICE

| Agency | Purpose |
| --- | --- |
| Health Resources and Services Administration (HRSA) | Provide health-related information<br>Administer programs concerned with health care for the homeless, people with human immunodeficiency virus (HIV) and acquired immunodeficiency syndrome (AIDS), organ transplants, rural health care, and employee occupational health |
| Food and Drug Administration (FDA) | Protect the public from unsafe drugs, food, and cosmetics |
| Centers for Disease Control and Prevention (CDC) | Prevent the transmission of communicable diseases |
| National Institutes of Health (NIH) | Conduct research and education related to specific illnesses |
| Alcohol, Drug Abuse, and Mental Health Administration (ADAMHA) | Serve as clearinghouse for information on substance abuse and mental health issues |
| Agency for Toxic Substances and Disease Registry (ATSDR) | Maintain registry of certain diseases<br>Provide information on toxic agents<br>Conduct mortality and morbidity studies on defined population groups |
| Indian Health Service (IHS) | Provide health care services to Native Americans, including health promotion, disease prevention, alcoholism prevention, substance abuse prevention, suicide prevention, nutrition, and maternal-child health |
| Agency for Healthcare Research and Quality (AHRQ) | Primary source of federal support for research related to quality of health care delivery |
| Administration for Children and Families (ACF) | Provide services and assistance to needy children and families<br>Provide funds to assist low-income families with child care<br>Support foster care and adoption services<br>Administer national child-support enforcement system |
| Administration on Aging (AOA) | Support a nationwide network to provide services to the elderly<br>Support meals-on-wheels, transportation, and at-home services<br>Provide policy leadership on aging |

## Nurse

What do nurses do? Nurses fulfill a variety of roles while assisting clients to meet their needs. Table 2-5 defines the most common roles of nurses. These roles are affected by changes in the health care environment. The percentage of nurses who work in hospitals is declining. The highest percentage was in 1984, when 66% of nurses worked in hospitals. This number has declined to 59% in 2000. The decline is due to the shift of more nurses working in the public health, community health, home health, and ambulatory care services (Health Resources and Services Administration, 2000). These "nonhospital" care arenas have greater numbers of clients because clients stay in the acute care settings for fewer days. Hospitals have discharged clients much more rapidly in the past 10 to 15 years due to the nature of the clients' care and to changes in third-party reimbursement. Nurses function in dependent, independent, and interdependent roles. The degree of autonomy nurses experience is related to client needs, expertise of the nurse, and practice setting.

## Economics of Health Care

Until recently, the reform movement in health care has been motivated primarily by health care costs. Denial of services has also become a major issue of debate in health care reform (Lens, 2002). Managed care was developed to cut cost while maintaining quality, but the evidence for its success is mixed (Fairfield, Hunter, Mechanic, & Rosleff, 1997). Rising costs slowed for a time, but now are rising at an annual rate of 7.3%, which outstrips the gross domestic product by 2.5% each year (Centers for Medicare and Medicaid Services, 2003). Control of costs has shifted from the health care providers to the insurers. As a result, there are increasing constraints on reimbursement. For years, the predominant method of covering health care costs was the fee-for-service method. There was little, if any, incentive for cost-effective delivery of care (Chamberlain, Chen, Osuna, & Yamamoto, 1995). All that is changing.

The U.S. health care system has a diverse financial base, composed of both private and public funding. As a result, administrative costs for health care reimbursement are

## TABLE 2-3   HEALTH CARE SETTINGS

| Setting | Services Provided | Nurse's Role |
|---|---|---|
| Hospitals | Diagnosis and treatment of illnesses (acute and chronic)<br>Acute inpatient services<br>Emergency care<br>Ambulatory care services<br>Critical (intensive) care<br>Rehabilitative care<br>Surgical interventions<br>Diagnostic procedures | Caregiver<br>Client educator<br>Provides ongoing assessment<br>Coordinates care and collaborates with other health care providers<br>Maintains client safety<br>Initiates discharge planning<br>Has a variety of areas in which to specialize:<br>  Cardiology      Oncology<br>  Critical care   Orthopedics<br>  Dialysis        Pediatrics<br>  Emergency    Psychiatry<br>  Geriatrics     Rehabilitation<br>  Infection control  Surgery<br>  Neurology |
| Extended care (long-term care) facilities (e.g., nursing homes, skilled nursing facilities) | Intermediate and long-term care for people with chronic illnesses or those who are unable to care for themselves<br>Restorative care until client is ready for discharge to home | Provides care directed at meeting basic needs (e.g., nutrition, hydration, comfort, elimination)<br>Provides teaching and counseling<br>Plans and coordinates care<br>Administers medications, treatments, and other therapeutic modalities |
| Home health agencies | Wide range of services, including curative and rehabilitative | Provides skilled nursing care<br>Coordinates health promotion activities (e.g., education) |
| Hospices | Care of individuals with terminal illnesses<br>Improving the quality of life until death | Promotes comfort measures<br>Provides pain control<br>Supports grieving families |
| Outpatient settings (clinics, health care practitioners' offices, ambulatory treatment centers) | Treatment of illness (acute and chronic)<br>Diagnostic testing<br>Simple surgical procedures | *Traditional Role:*<br>Checks vital signs<br>Assists with diagnostic tests<br>Prepares client for examination<br>*Expanded Role:*<br>Provides teaching and counseling<br>Performs physical (or mental status) examination<br>In some settings, advanced practice registered nurses (APRNs) are the primary care providers |
| Schools | School-based clinics (SBCs) are federally funded providers of physical and mental health services in middle and high schools. | Coordinates health promotion and disease prevention activities<br>Treats minor illnesses<br>Provides health education |
| Industrial clinics | Maintain health and safety of workers | Coordinates health promotion activities<br>Provides education for safety<br>Provides urgent care as needed<br>Maintains health records<br>Conducts ongoing screenings<br>Provides preventive services (e.g., tuberculosis testing) |
| Managed care organizations | Reimbursement for health care services | Serves as case manager<br>Uses triage to determine the most appropriate intervention for clients |
| Community nursing centers | Direct access to professional nursing services | Treats client's responses to health problems<br>Promotes health and wellness |
| Rural primary care hospitals (RPCHs) | Stabilize clients until they are physiologically able to be transferred to more skilled facilities | Performs assessments and provides emergency care |

## TABLE 2-4    HEALTH CARE PROVIDERS

| Professional | Function/Role |
| --- | --- |
| Nurse (RN) | Provides care to individuals who are unable to care for themselves; with a holistic approach, nurses assist clients to cope with illness or disability<br>Addresses the needs of the client (individual, family, community)<br>Emphasizes health promotion |
| Physician (MD) | Makes medical diagnoses and prescribes therapeutic modalities<br>Performs medical procedures (e.g., surgery)<br>May specialize in a variety of areas (e.g., gynecology/obstetrics, oncology, surgery) |
| Physician assistant (PA) | Provides medical services under the supervision of a health care practitioner |
| Advanced practice registered nurse | Diagnoses and manages common health problems<br>Performs medical procedures (e.g., suturing, casting) |
| Pharmacist (RPh) | Prepares and dispenses drugs for therapeutic use<br>Often involved in client education |
| Dentist (DDS) | Diagnoses and treats conditions affecting mouth, teeth, and gums<br>Performs preventive measures to promote dental health |
| Dental hygienist | Provides dental health education and prevention services |
| Dietitian (RD) | Plans diets to meet special needs of clients<br>Promotes health and prevents disease through education and counseling<br>May supervise preparation of meals |
| Social worker (SW) | Assists clients with psychosocial problems (e.g., financial, marital)<br>Conducts discharge planning<br>Makes referrals for placement |
| Respiratory therapist (RT) | Administers pulmonary function tests<br>Performs therapeutic measures to assist with respiration (e.g., oxygen administration, ventilators) |
| Physical therapist (PT) | Works with clients experiencing musculoskeletal problems<br>Assesses person's strength and mobility<br>Performs therapeutic measures (e.g., range of motion, massage, application of heat and cold)<br>Teaches new skills (e.g., walking with crutches)<br>Wound care |
| Occupational therapist (OT) | Works with clients with functional impairment to learn skills for activities of daily living |
| Chaplain | Assists in helping clients meet spiritual needs<br>Provides individual counseling<br>Provides support to families<br>Conducts religious services |
| Unlicensed assistive personnel (UAP) | Assists in provision of client care activities under the direction of the RN<br>May include certified nurses aide, personal care assistant, nursing assistant, orderly, and certified phlebotomist |

## TABLE 2-5    NURSING ROLES

| Role | Description |
| --- | --- |
| Caregiver | Traditional and most essential role<br>Functions as nurturer<br>Provides direct care<br>Is supportive<br>Demonstrates clinical proficiency<br>Promotes comfort of client |
| Teacher | Provides information<br>Serves as counselor<br>Seeks to empower clients for self-care<br>Encourages compliance with prescribed therapy<br>Promotes healthy lifestyles<br>Interprets information |
| Advocate | Protects the client<br>Provides explanations in client's language<br>Acts as change agent<br>Supports client's decisions |
| Manager | Makes decisions<br>Coordinates activities of others<br>Allocates resources<br>Evaluates care and personnel<br>Serves as a leader<br>Takes initiative |
| Expert | Advanced practice clinician<br>Conducts research<br>Teaches in schools of nursing<br>Develops theory<br>Contributes to professional literature<br>Provides testimony at governmental hearings and in courts |
| Case manager | Tracks client's progress through the health care system<br>Coordinates care to ensure continuity |
| Team member | Collaborates with others<br>Possesses highly skilled communication methods<br>Performs therapeutic measures to assist with respiration (e.g., oxygen administration, ventilators) |

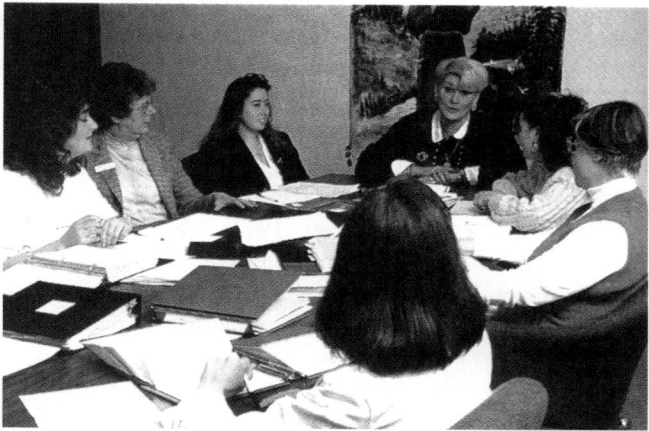

**Figure 2-3    Members of the health care team led by the nurse in brainstorming together for the benefit of the client.** *Photo courtesy of PhotoDisc*

higher in this country than in countries with a **single-payer system** (a model in which the government is the only entity to reimburse health care costs: e.g., Canada). The level of U.S. health care expenditures is higher than in any other nation, and previous cost-containment measures have been mixed. Despite the enormous expenditures of public funds, the United States has not found a way to provide adequate health care coverage for all citizens. About 39 million people had no health insurance in 1999, which is about 15% of the population (Nelson & Mills, 2001). Coverage varies by race and cultural background. Among Hispanic people, 33.4% have no health insurance; among African Americans, 21.2% lack coverage; while only 11% of Caucasians are without any coverage.

## Private Insurance

The system for financing health care services in the United States is based on the private insurance model. One of the largest sectors of the health care system is private insurance companies. Most private health insurance is an employment benefit, and employment-related health plans cover 64.1% of the population (U.S. Department of Commerce, 2001). Payment rates to health care providers vary among insurance companies.

Insured individuals are paying substantial monthly premiums and deductibles for health care services. These costs limit access for many Americans. In addition, insurers will no longer pay for services that they deem unnecessary. The quality of care provided is being monitored by providers, third-party payers, and, ever-increasingly, by consumers. Quality of care is also disputed, as quality within managed care systems continues to be suboptimal (Blumenthal, 1999).

## Managed Care

**Managed care** is a system of providing and monitoring care in which access, cost, and quality are controlled before or during delivery of services. The goal of managed care is the delivery of services in the most cost-efficient manner possible. Managed care seeks to control costs by monitoring delivery of services and restricting access to expensive procedures and providers.

Managed care was designed to provide coordinated services with an emphasis on prevention and primary care (American Nurses Association, 1995). The rationale for managed care is to give consumers preventive services delivered by a **primary care provider** (a health care provider whom a client sees first for health care) that, in turn, results in less expensive interventions.

Managed care has been in existence for years; however, only within the past few decades has it received national prominence. The Health Maintenance Organization Act (passed in 1973) implemented two mandates. First, federal grants and loans were made available to **health maintenance organizations** (HMOs) (prepaid health plans that provide primary health care services for a preset fee and focus on cost-effective treatment measures) that complied with strict federal regulations as opposed to the less restrictive state requirements. Second, the act required large employers to provide an HMO as an option for employees for health care coverage (Society for Ambulatory Care Professionals, 1994). From their inception, HMOs have been a viable alternative to the traditional fee-for-service system.

Managed care is not a place but rather an organizational structure with a few variations. One is represented by HMOs, which are both providers and insurers. Other variations are represented by **preferred provider organizations** (PPOs) (a type of managed care model in which member choice is limited to providers within the system) and **exclusive provider organizations** (EPOs) (organizations in which care must be delivered by the plan for clients to receive reimbursement). The latter creates a network of providers (such as physicians and hospitals) and offers the incentive of consumer services with little or no copayment if these providers are used exclusively. Table 2-6 provides a comparison of independent practice and managed care organizational structures.

The impact of managed care is that caregivers and institutions must change from providing as many services as possible under a fee-for-service payment approach to keeping the client well and providing fewer services so as to protect their financial interests. "In a fee-for-service system, the concern is that a client might receive too many or unnecessary services; in a prepaid system, the concern is that too few services might be given in order to save the provider and the managed care plan money" (Hitchcock, Schubert, & Thomas, 2003, p. 54).

## Health Maintenance Organizations

The HMOs often maintain primary health care sites and commonly employ provider professionals. They use **capitated rates** (a preset flat fee that is based on membership in, not services provided by, the HMO), assume the risk of

clients who are heavy users, and exert control on the use of services. HMOs have been noted for their use of advanced practice registered nurses (APRNs) as primary care providers, precertification programs to limit unnecessary hospitalization, and an emphasis on client education for health promotion and self-care.

Another common feature of HMOs is the practice of **single point of entry** (entry into the health care system is required through a point designated by the plan) through which primary care is delivered. **Primary health care** is the client's point of entry into the health care system and includes assessment, diagnosis, treatment, coordination of care, education, preventive services, and surveillance. It consists of the spectrum of services provided by a family practitioner (nurse or physician) in an ambulatory setting. Primary care providers (PCPs) serve as "gatekeepers" to the health care system in that they determine which, if any,

| TABLE 2-6 | COMPARISON OF INDEPENDENT PRACTICE WITH MANAGED CARE |
|---|---|
| Type | Description |
| Independent practice | Fee-for-service |
| | Functions within socially prescribed boundaries (professional ethics) |
| | Consumer choice of provider |
| | Disease-oriented philosophy |
| Health maintenance organizations (HMOs) | Provide services to a group of enrolled persons |
| | Fee is preset and prepaid |
| | Service provision is limited |
| Preferred provider organizations (PPOs) | Networks of providers that give discounts to sponsoring organization |
| | Members are not mandated to select a primary care health care practitioner but must use a health care practitioner in the network |
| Exclusive provider organizations (EPOs) | Plan pays no benefit if member is treated outside the network |
| | Are usually regulated by state insurance laws |

## RESEARCH FOCUS

**Title of Study:** Systematic Review of Whether Nurse Practitioners Working in Primary Care Can Provide Equivalent Care to Doctors

**Study Purpose:** To determine whether nurse practitioners can provide care at first point of contact equivalent to doctors in a primary care setting.

**Methods:** A systematic review of randomized, controlled trials and prospective observational studies was conducted. A total of 34 studies were analyzed. The study was conducted in England but reviewed studies from a number of countries.

**Findings:** People were more satisfied with care by a nurse practitioner than with care by a physician. No differences in health outcomes were found. Nurses spent more time with clients and ordered more tests than did physicians. No differences were found in prescriptions, return visits, or referrals. Quality of care in client education, communication, and documentation was better from nurses.

**Implications:** This meta-analysis of recent studies of nurse practitioners provides evidence for the effectiveness of nurse practitioner care. The analysis supports the utilization of nurse practitioners in primary care.

Horrocks, S., Anderson, E., & Salisbury, C. (2002). Systematic review of whether nurse practitioners working in primary care can provide equivalent care to doctors. *British Medical Journal, 324*, 819–823.

referrals to specialists are needed by the client. To reduce costs, direct access to specialists is limited. Extensive data collection proves that APRNs are exceptionally suited to these primary provider/gatekeeper roles (American Nurses Association, 1993a). Managed care plans assume a significant portion of the risk of providing health care and, consequently, encourage both prudent use by consumers and prescription by providers.

### Preferred Provider Organizations

The most common managed care systems are PPOs. A PPO is a contractual relationship between hospitals, providers, employers, and third-party payers to form a network in which providers negotiate with group purchasers to provide health services for a defined population at a predetermined price. Even though PPOs have been very popular with the American public, HMOs are gaining in market share among the American public and now enroll

78.5 million (28.3%) of the population (Centers for Disease Control, 2001). Medicare-sponsored HMOs are rapidly expanding, with 393 plans and 6.8 million people enrolled (Health Care Financing Administration, 1999).

The state of health care in the United States today is very confusing. Managed care was proposed in the 1990s as the solution to rising health care costs and lack of accessibility. In the early years of the new millennia, premium costs and the numbers of uninsured are rising.

## Federal Government Insurance Plans

The federal government became a third-party payer for health care services with the advent of Medicare and Medicaid in 1965. The Health Care Financing Administration (HCFA) is a federal agency that regulates Medicare and Medicaid expenditures. Public funding is used for 12% of the population under age 65 who are covered under the Medicaid program and 97% of the population over age 65 who are covered under the Medicare program (Health Care Financing Administration, 1999). The HCFA changed to the Centers for Medicare and Medicaid Services (CMS) on July 1, 2001, in compliance with Medicare funding issues. The CMS collects and analyzes statistics on health care spending, insurance coverage, and the cost of the U.S. health care system (Hitchcock, Schubert, & Thomas, 2003). There are myriad public programs for financing health care, with Medicare and Medicaid being the predominant ones. Medicare is the federally funded program that provides health care coverage for the elderly and the disabled. Medicaid is a jointly administered program between the federal and state governments that provides health care coverage for the economically disadvantaged.

The federal government created diagnosis-related groups (DRGs) to curtail spending for hospitalized Medicare recipients and to ensure that health care dollars would get to those who most need them. Through this system, an inclusive rate is established for each episode of hospitalization based on the client's age, principal diagnosis, and the presence or absence of surgery and **comorbidity** (existence of simultaneous disease processes within an individual). Hospitals are now reimbursed only for services that are determined to be medically necessary. An accelerating trend for the federal government is to give recipients of public monies the personal right to choose, through the use of vouchers, a managed care program in the private sector.

### Medicare

When Medicare was established in 1965, it was intended to protect individuals over the age of 65 from exorbitant costs of health care by providing public funds to cover the majority of health care services.

In 1972, Medicare was modified to include permanently disabled individuals and those with end-stage renal disease.

**LIFE SPAN CONSIDERATIONS**

### Changes in Health Insurance Coverage with Aging

Health insurance coverage can change as a person ages. The federal government provides health care insurance for all uninsured children through the State Children's Health Insurance Program, but this coverage stops once the child reaches adolescence or adulthood (programs vary from state to state). Medicare is a program for all people who are 65 years or older, but does not cover some basic health care needs such as long-term care, glasses, or hearing aids. Adults in the middle years are most at risk for not having health care insurance when they are employed in jobs that do not provide health care benefits. As the case scenario at the end of the chapter points out, when a person loses a job, health care concerns can lead to major medical and financial crises.

Centers for Medicare and Medicaid Services (2002). National Health Expenditures Projections: 2001–2011. Retrieved from www.hcfa.gov/stats/NHE-Proj/proj2001/default.htm

 **STOP AND THINK**

### Is Our Health Care System in Crisis?

- What health insurance problems does the United States face?

- Do you think the U.S. system provides adequate care? Why or why not?

- What changes would you suggest?

## Medicaid

Medicaid is a shared venture between the federal and state governments. Each state has latitude in determining who is "medically indigent," and thus qualifies for public monies. Minimal services covered by Medicaid are defined by the federal government and include inpatient and outpatient hospital services, physician services, laboratory services (including x-rays), and rural health clinic services. States may elect to cover other services, such as dental, vision, and prescription drugs.

## Canadian Health Insurance

Canada has a national health insurance program that covers each citizen for short- and long-term care. This mandatory program is financed with tax dollars. Each province runs its own health system in accordance with federal rules and with a fixed federal monetary contribution. Physicians are reimbursed on a prenegotiated fee-for-service basis.

Although some disagreement persists in the nursing community, the Canadian (or single-payer) model is not generally seen as the best choice for the United States. The Canadian system is more suited to a highly homogeneous population and the ethos of "the greatest good for the most people." The latter sounds like an incontestable truth, but it is a questionable fit with the American spirit, which is more aligned with the idea of equal opportunity

for all plus the availability of extra services for those who can afford them.

It is also appropriate to challenge the illusion of the Canadian health care system as a panacea. During the 1990s, the Canadian system suffered from shortages of physicians and nurses, which resulted in problems with acute care. Long waits for some diagnostic and therapeutic services such as hip replacement and radiotherapy are common (Inglehardt, 2000). Further, increasing costs are prompting a debate in Canada about which services are really affordable and whether copayment and deductibles will eventually be necessary. The Canadian government is implementing a plan that responds to the need for more nurses in all sectors of health care. In Canadian provinces that have additionally chosen to enrich the basic standard established at the national level, there is the possibility of cutbacks (Hirsch, 1999).

## Factors Influencing the Delivery of Health Care

Despite cost-containment efforts (such as DRGs established by the federal government and managed care by the insurers), the U.S. health care system still has problems with issues of cost, access, and quality.

### Cost

Why is consideration of cost so important? The very existence of the health care system depends on fiscal issues. Cost has been a driving force for change in the health care system, as evidenced by the strength and numbers of managed care plans, increased use of outpatient treatment, and shortened hospital stays. These market forces (to maximize profits by minimizing costs) are dominating the current changes in the health care system.

The U.S. government spends more on health care per person than any other country. In addition, U.S. health care values differ enormously from Canadian values, and those values drive political decisions. In the United States, leading values toward health care are a preference for pluralism and choice, ambivalence toward government management, confidence that innovation and new technology will solve health problems, and belief that competition is the best way to ensure services. The United States does not share values with countries that have universal access, such as Canada, which include health care as a right and public administration as an appropriate method to deliver health care. The increasing consumption of federal funds for health care in the U.S. means that resources are being moved from other areas of need, such as education, housing, and social services.

The cost of providing health care has risen dramatically during the past 20 years. By 2011, CMS predicts that the percentage of the gross domestic product will rise from 13.4% in 2000 to an estimated 17% in 2011 (Centers for Medicare and Medicaid Services, 2002).

The health care bureaucracy has become mammoth. The most cost-efficient programs in terms of administration are Medicare and Medicaid because of the number of people eligible for these benefits. In contrast, some private plans, particularly small business plans, use over 40 cents of each dollar for administration. The cost of health care has seriously compromised American business and industry for some time. For example, the chief executive officer of Ford Motor Company stated that the costs for health care coverage of employees exceeded the total expenditures on steel used in building cars (Grace & Brock, 1994). This policy has lead businesses to invest less money in growth and development, a decision that places the United States at risk in global markets. Over the last generation, the United States has moved rapidly toward becoming a service-dominated economy. Yet, a society's economic strength depends on its manufacturing and industry. This imbalance leaves few resources to return our industries to a position of world prominence. The cost of employee health care benefits is an expensive commitment for small businesses and is a serious factor when one considers that the economy of this country has survived—if not thrived—because of the contributions of small businesses.

Major factors that increase the cost of health care include: (1) an oversupply of specialized providers, (2) a surplus of hospital beds, (3) the passive role assumed by most consumers, (4) inequitable financing of services, and (5) very expensive technological advances in health care (Ginzberg, 1998). Other factors that contribute to the high cost of health care are the aging of the population, the increased number of people with chronic illnesses, the increase in health-related lawsuits that has resulted in the unnecessary use of services, and advanced technology that has allowed more people to survive disabling illnesses.

## Access

In addition to the issue of cost, access to health care services has a serious impact on the functioning of the health care

system. As a result of the cost, health care for many people is crisis-oriented and fragmented. A large number of Americans are unable to gain access to health care services owing to low income or lack of insurance, and, therefore, their illnesses progress to an acute stage before they seek intervention. Poverty often adversely affects an individual's access to health care services. For example, limited transportation (lack of an automobile or funding for public transit) interferes with the ability to travel to health care facilities. Services used by individuals during acute illnesses are typically those provided by emergency departments. Emergency room and acute care services are expensive when compared with early intervention and preventive measures.

Approximately 39 million Americans are uninsured (United States Census Bureau, 2001). Only a small portion of the medically indigent are covered by Medicare. In addition, many individuals are underinsured. These people are neither poor nor old, but middle-class unemployed Americans or those in jobs without adequate health care benefits.

In addition to poverty and unemployment, other factors impede a person's ability to obtain insurance. Refer to Box 2-1, which lists factors affecting access to health care services.

Other variables affecting access are the increase in the number of women employed outside the home and the number of single-parent families. These factors impair access to health care services because it is often difficult for parents to take time off from work to transport children to health care providers.

## Quality

It is estimated that 30% to 40% of diagnostic and medical procedures performed in this country are unnecessary (Lee, Soffel, & Luft, 1994). This inappropriate use of

---

**BOX 2-1    FACTORS LIMITING ACCESS TO HEALTH CARE SERVICES**

- No provision for insurance by an employer due to prohibitive costs
- Inability to obtain individual insurance due to high costs
- Difficulty for people with certain medical problems (preexisting conditions) to obtain insurance
- Cultural barriers
- Shortages of health care providers in some geographic areas (especially rural or inner city areas)
- Limited access to ancillary services (e.g., child care, transportation)

resources can be traced to several causative factors, including:

- The litigious environment creates the tendency toward defensive practice.
- Resource consumption is highly influenced by the widely held American belief that more is better.
- Lack of access to and continuity of services results in subsequent misuse of acute care services.

In an attempt to provide universal access to services in a cost-effective manner, quality does not have to be sacrificed. For example, hospitals that are reducing the numbers of registered nurses ("downsizing") risk endangering quality. Safety and quality are frequently compromised by inappropriate substitution of unqualified personnel for registered nurses in direct care of clients. The Economic Policy Institute (1999) released a study that indicates that as more tasks are delegated to unlicensed assistive personnel (UAP), the quality of data used in decision making diminishes. Studies of acute care inpatients found that with average acuity, the proportion of care delivered by registered nurses was inversely related to client outcomes.

A study conducted in 2002 revealed that 73% of nurses surveyed stated that the quality of care provided at their hospitals had deteriorated because of cost-containment measures. Rischer and Applebaum (2002) found that nurses' perception of the eroding quality in health care is directly attributed to the nursing shortage. Even more problematic, studies from 1988 to 1998 reveal that 30% of people in acute care received contraindicated care, and 28% of people in chronic care received contraindicated care (Schuster, McGlynn, & Brook, 1998). Cross-training of staff, increased use of unlicensed personnel, and reductions in full-time positions for nurses are affecting the type of care delivered in hospitals. In an attempt to be cost-effective, some hospitals have decreased the number of registered nurses, thereby creating unsafe situations for clients. Any movement toward reform must focus on providing quality nursing care to all consumers.

# Challenges within the Health Care System

The major challenges facing the U.S. health care delivery system include the nursing shortage, loss of control over health care decisions, decreased use of hospitals and the impact on quality of care, changing practice settings, ethical issues, and vulnerable populations.

## The Nursing Shortage

"The future of health care in the United States increasingly pivots on a sufficient supply of appropriately educated and skilled professional registered nurses" (Bednash, 2000, p. 2953). A shortage of nurses is here, and it is likely unique. The shortage has been created by fewer people entering the workforce than are leaving, and by an increasing demand for nursing services. Fewer people are entering the profession, because other career options appear less demanding and more remunerative. Women, who once had fewer career opportunities, are no longer choosing nursing as other careers are becoming more viable for them (Bednash, 2000). In addition, nurses, like the population at large, are aging. The average age for registered nurses is 51. When these nurses retire in 10 to 15 years, the shortage will worsen (Bednash, 2000). As technological and medical advances assist people to live longer with complex chronic illnesses, the need for skilled nursing care increases. By 2020, the workforce is forecast to be 20% below requirements (Buerhaus, Staiger, & Auerbach, 2000).

## Positive Perception of Nurses

Several studies verify the public's trust in nurses. The public sees nurses as part of the solution, not the problem, and believes that if nurses were allowed to use their skills, they would significantly enhance quality and reduce cost. Nurses are persistently seen as having the highest standards of honesty and ethics. Nursing was the highest ranking of all professions for ethics in a recent Gallup poll (Carlson, 2000). In the Gallup poll, nurses were rated as having "high" or "very high" standards by 79% of Americans. Only 63% of physicians were ranked as high. One survey inquired about consumer receptivity to nurses assuming expanded responsibilities. Respondents supported **prescriptive authority** (legal recognition of the ability to prescribe medications) for nurses and endorsed their role in performing physical examinations and managing minor acute illnesses. Nurses have limited their own vision of their roles owing to the roots of their education in the **medical model** (traditional approach to health care in which the focus is on treatment and cure of disease) and their socialization into the hierarchy that this model assumes.

## Loss of Control

Consumers express the sentiment of feeling terrorized by the health care delivery system. They feel they have lost personal control, and they do not trust the people who represent them. Many Americans stay in unsatisfying jobs because of their health care benefits and relinquish employment mobility due to a fear of being denied a new policy because of pre-existing conditions. Many American workers state that their greatest concern is the possible loss of health care coverage and shrinking health care benefits (American Nurses Association, 1999).

## Decreased Hospital Use

In the early 20th century, hospitals focused on providing care to those who had no caregivers in the family or community. The focus of these early institutions was care, not cure (Grace, 1994). The focus of hospitals changed in the mid-1940s as a result of technologic changes and the passage of the Hill-Burton Act by Congress in 1946, which provided funding for renovation and construction of hospitals. One unanticipated outcome of this act was a substantial oversupply of hospital beds. Health care costs escalated with the need to keep the hospital beds occupied.

From 1945 to 1982, the demand for hospital beds steadily increased. After 1982, a steady decline in the number of hospital admissions and the length of stay occurred (Grace, 1994). "As patient care services continue to move to outpatient settings, HCFA says that hospitals can expect to get only 30% of the nation's total expenditures by 2007—that's 5% less than in 1997" (Ventura, 1999, p. 14).

Currently, hospitals continue to be the nucleus of the health care delivery system in the United States. Hospitals account for the largest proportion of expenditures and employ the majority of health care workers. Hospitals have fewer clients today because of the trend toward rapid discharge and more procedures being performed in outpatient settings. The clients who are hospitalized require more nursing care because of the greater complexity of needs and severity of illness. Box 2-2 lists factors that have contributed to the decreased hospital population.

As a result of the changes in reimbursement practices, hospitals are restructuring (also referred to as redesigning and reengineering). Examples of restructuring activities include mergers with larger institutions; development of integrated systems that provide a full range of services focusing on continuity of care such as preadmission, outpatient, acute inpatient, long-term inpatient, and home care; and the substitution of multiskilled workers for nurses. Approximately 59.1% of registered nurses are employed by hospitals, which is down from a high of 66% in 1984 (Spratley, Johnson, Sochalski, Fritz, & Spencer, 2000). The majority of these nursing positions are direct care providers (staff nurses). In some institutions, restructuring includes replacing registered nurses with unlicensed personnel, which may lead to decreased quality of care. Nurses must ensure that cost-cutting efforts do not threaten client safety.

As the average lengths of stay in hospitals decline, the acuity level of clients increases. The presence of increasingly ill clients requires nurses who possess technical expertise, critical thinking skills, and interpersonal competence. Community-based services, such as home health, will need

to continue to expand to meet the increased needs of the steadily growing elderly population (Hull, 1994).

## Changing Practice Settings

Most nurses currently practice in hospitals and will continue to do so in the future but in a decreasing percentage (Spratley, Johnson, Sochalski, Fritz, & Spencer, 2000). However, there is an ever-increasing need for nurses in different areas of practice. Social and political changes are affecting nurses by creating the need for expanded services and settings. Because of these changes, demand for nursing care fluctuates. For example, nursing employment outside the hospital continues to increase rapidly. Health care expenditures for home care are rapidly increasing. It is predicted that 70% to 80% of care will be delivered in the home by the year 2010 (Conger et al., 1999). Since the advent of Medicare and Medicaid, home health care has grown rapidly (Figure 2-4).

More nurses will be needed in the future because:

- The growing elderly population will require more health care services.
- The number of people admitted to nursing homes is steadily growing.
- The number of homeless individuals, who are most often denied access to health care, is increasing.

As health care reform occurs, some nurses may be displaced from their current jobs. But overall, many more jobs will be created by the demand for greater access to health care services. Some examples of areas in which larger numbers of nurses will be required are primary care, public health, extended care facilities, and the home setting.

## Ethical Issues

The United States is struggling with a major ethical conflict of cost containment versus compassionate quality

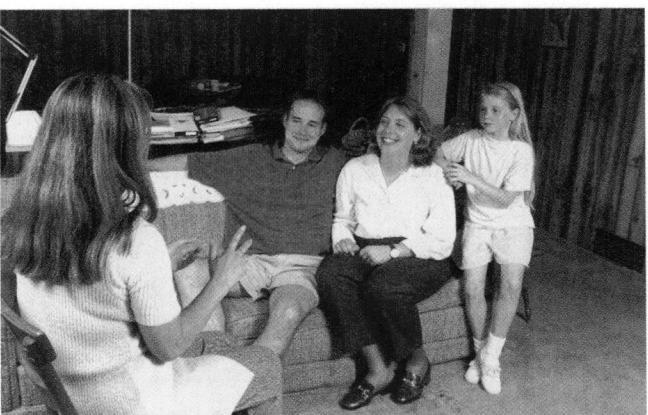

**Figure 2-4   The percentage of home health nurses is increasing in numbers, as health care reform places more nurses (such as this home health nurse) outside the acute care setting.**

**BOX 2-2   FACTORS INFLUENCING DECREASED HOSPITAL POPULATION**

- Shorter lengths of stay
- Technologic advances
- Greater availability of outpatient facilities
- More services available in outpatient settings
- Expectations/demands of third-party payers

## LEGAL AND ETHICAL ISSUES

### Should Health Care Be a Right of Citizenship?

The United States is one of only two industrialized nations that does NOT provide basic health care as a right of citizenship. We spend more than any other nation on health care, almost twice as much as the next most expensive country, Switzerland. Unlike Switzerland, however, we did not provide basic health care to all of our citizens. National health spending is accelerating once again (HCFA, 2000). Despite health care costs in excess of one trillion dollars, we do not have the highest longevity of any nation or the lowest maternal-child death rate (Inglehardt, 2000).

We do not have a mandate in the United States to provide health care insurance to every person. About 16% of our population are uninsured for health care (Inglehardt, 2000). Is it ethical to treat health care as a privilege? Why or why not? Should we tie health insurance for adults to employment? How would this affect small businesses? What should we do about those who are uninsured?

care. No country, regardless of how wealthy it is, can provide all citizens with every health care service they desire or need. Today, the U.S. health care delivery system is faced with the dilemma of citizens' needs being greater than available resources. Thus, some difficult choices must be made to determine which needs will be met and which will remain unmet.

The expectation that "everything must be done to save" a dying person has created an enormous drain on the health care resources of this country. As decisions are made about allocating scarce resources, there will be much debate about the ethics involved. The appropriateness of futile life-sustaining measures must be addressed (Rowe, 1996). Nurses must continue to strongly advocate for just and ethical distribution of resources as health care reform progresses.

## Vulnerable Populations

Meeting the health care needs of underserved populations is especially challenging. Groups that may be unable to gain access to health care services include children, the elderly, people with AIDS, the homeless, and others living in poverty. Approximately 39 million people in America had no health insurance in 2000 (U.S. Census Bureau, 2001), a slight decrease that reflects an increase in the number of children with health insurance.

Medicaid is no longer adequate to meet the needs of the medically indigent.

Our current health care system is trying to address the overall needs of children. Children are more likely than adults to be uninsured. One in five children lives in families with income below the poverty level. To respond to this problem, the State Children's Health Insurance Program was passed by Congress in 1997. The purpose of this program is to expand health insurance coverage to uninsured low-income children. Programs vary from state to state, but all states provide some coverage. Despite a slow start in implementation, the rate of uninsured children appears to be decreasing across the country (Rosenbach, Ellwood, Czajka, Irvin, Coupe, & Quinn, 2001). The number of uninsured children fell from 12.1% in 1997 to 9.2% in 2001 (Strunk & Cunningham, 2002).

Immunization rates increased from 65% in 1994 to 78% in 1999 (Mills, 2001). Inequities remain, however. Seventy-three percent of children in poverty are fully immunized, compared to 81% of higher income children (Mills, 2001). Preventive health care should be available to children of all ages, with an emphasis on early immunization. In addition, maternal-child health among select ethnic and racial minorities in certain geographic areas of this country is poorer than that in developing countries. The health of a country is often judged by its maternal-child health indicators (Author, 2001).

Over 300,000 Americans have been diagnosed with AIDS and approximately 800,000 Americans are infected with HIV (Centers for Disease Control and Prevention, 2001). The most rapid spread of the disease is occurring among women, children, and intravenous drug users and their sexual partners. Women who have AIDS have a higher mortality rate than men, and decreased access to health care may be one contributing factor to this higher mortality rate (CDC, 2001). Although the cost of the AIDS epidemic is unmeasurable in terms of human suffering, approximately $7.7 billion dollars was spent on care of people with AIDS in 2000 (CDC, 2001). This amount was sufficient to care for half of the people living with HIV (Levi & Kates, 2000). As people live longer, the total number of people who need HIV care is significantly increased. Not only will additional funding be necessary, but also outpatient care settings (such as hospices, home care, and clinics) must be expanded to care for those affected by this epidemic.

Traditionally, rural areas have always had few health care providers and facilities that were easily accessible. A large number of elderly people live in rural areas; 18% are rural, as opposed to 15% who live in urban areas (Rogers, 2000). Because people in rural areas tend to work for small businesses or are self-employed, many of them have no health insurance. Also, many hospitals in rural areas have been closed due to economic pressures.

Usually, adults in the United States who receive little assistance in health promotion maintain unhealthy lifestyles, which lead to the development of chronic illnesses. Older adults who have accumulated problems that could have been prevented are admitted to nursing homes, which are very costly (Rogers, 2000).

It is in the best interests of society to see that those who cannot afford the basic health services are not denied such services. The entire society's health is threatened when some sectors are denied basic care. As a group, nurses are concerned with the availability of health care services to everyone, regardless of their ability to pay.

# Nursing's Response to Health Care Challenges

As the United States continues to look for ways to address the issue of health care reform, the implications for nursing will continue to increase. Some nurses feel threatened by impending changes, whereas others are excited about the possibility of transforming the health care system into something better. The nursing profession has responded to the myriad challenges in health care delivery by proposing a plan for nursing's future.

## Nursing's Agenda for the Future

In response to the current nursing shortage and predictions of an unprecedented shortage in the near future, the ANA brought together a number of national nursing organizations and nursing leaders to create a strategic plan. The plan, Nursing's Agenda for the Future, focuses on strategies to improve professional conditions for nurses and quality of health care (American Nurses Association, 2002).

The plan is based on a vision statement for what nursing should be and should look like in the year 2010. The steering committee identified 10 focus areas to implement this statement. The 10 domains are:

| | |
|---|---|
| Leadership and planning | Economic value |
| Delivery systems | Work environment |
| Legislation/regulation/ policy | Public relations/ communication |
| Professional/nursing culture | Education |
| Recruitment/retention | Diversity |

Each focus area has objectives to make the vision statement a reality by 2010. Achieving these objectives will take large numbers of nurses from every sector of nursing practice, along with support from other health care professionals and organizations.

### Concept Mapping as a Method of Nursing Education's Addressing the Needs of the Future

Nursing education has consistently addressed the future needs of nursing by implementing new and innovative approaches to teaching nursing students. An example is **concept mapping**, which is a current method nurse edu-

cators are using to organize nursing care. Concept mapping is a process of analyzing the meaning of interrlationships among several concepts. A **concept map** is a graphic design that provides a visual "picture" of the analytical thinking process and interpretation of the information (Kathol, Geiger, & Hartig, 1998). Concept mapping includes the organization of client information within the phases of the nursing process that demonstrates the connections to the plan of care. Concept mapping enhances motivation and facilitates the learning process (Beitz, 1998). There are several examples of concept maps spread throughout this text, and specific information is referred to in Appendix A.

## Standards of Care

Another approach to the challenges experienced by the health care delivery system has been the move toward standardization of care. In December 1990, the Agency for Health Care Research and Quality (AHRQ), formerly known as the Agency for Health Care Policy and Research (AHCPR), was established with the specific charge of achieving consensus within the medical/health care community on the usual treatment of high-volume and expensive disease conditions that differ in their therapeutic management despite substantial research. More simply put, there is significant variation in the diagnosis and treatment of certain illnesses and diseases. The medical justification for such variance has been that every client is an individual and the choice of treatment is a private decision involving client and physician. The AHRQ aims to identify the standards of treatment for which the health care community can be held accountable. The AHRQ has developed a National Guidelines Clearinghouse (http://www.guideline.gov) for evidence-based health care guidelines. These guidelines have become the national standards for evidence-based practice and research.

When AHRQ was created, the ANA recognized the need to strengthen nursing practice standards. Three interdisciplinary panels chaired by nurses were created to propose standards for conditions that are highly responsive to nursing interventions. The 10 Nursing-Sensitive Quality Indicators are evaluation standards for acute health care settings (Box 2-3). Currently, AHRQ published guidelines are available to the public and should be integral to nursing practice.

## Advanced Practice

The advanced practice of nursing has evolved as nursing has become more complex and specialized. Since the late 1960s, nurse practitioners (NPs), clinical nurse specialists (CNS), certified nurse midwives (CNMs), certified registered nurse anesthetists (CRNA) (Figure 2-5), and other advanced practice registered nurses (APRNs) have provided primary health care services to individuals, many of whom would have had inadequate or no access to services. APRNs possess

## BOX 2-3     NURSING-SENSITIVE QUALITY INDICATORS

**Mix of RNs, LPNs, and Unlicensed Staff Caring for Patients**

*Recommended Definition:* The percent of registered nursing care hours as a total of all nursing care hours. This measure includes only staff on acute care units.

**Total Nursing Care Hours Provided per Patient Day**

*Recommended Definition:* Total number of productive hours worked by nursing staff with direct patient care responsibilities on acute care units per patient day.

**Pressure Ulcers**

*Recommended Definition:* Total number of patients with pressure ulcers divided by the number of patients in a prevalence study.

**Patient Falls**

*Recommended Definition:* Total number of patient falls leading to injury divided by the total number of patient days multiplied by 1,000.

**Patient Satisfaction with Pain Management**

*Recommended Definition:* Patient opinion of how well nursing staff managed patient's pain.

**Patient Satisfaction with Educational Information**

*Recommended Definition:* Patient opinion of nursing staff efforts to educate patient regarding patient's conditions and care requirements.

**Patient Satisfaction with Overall Care**

*Recommended Definition:* Patient perception of the hospital experience related to satisfaction with overall care.

**Patient Satisfaction with Nursing Care**

*Recommended Definition:* Patient opinion of care received from nursing staff during the hospital stay.

**Nosocomial Infection Rate**

*Recommended Definition:* Number of confirmed bacteremia associated with sites of central lines divided by 1,000 patient days per unit.

**Nurse Staff Satisfaction**

*Recommended Definition:* Job satisfaction expressed by nurses working in a hospital setting.

Needleman, J., Buerhaus, P. I., Mattke, S., Stewart, M., & Zelevinsky, K. (2001). *Nurse staffing and patient outcomes in hospitals.* Washington, DC: HRSA.

advanced skills and in-depth knowledge in specific areas of practice. Even though there are differences in various advanced practice roles, all APRNs are experts who work with clients to prevent disease and to promote health.

There are currently more than 200,000 APRNs in the United States (HRSA, 2000). It is predicted that there will be a 50% to 75% increase in the demand for APRNs in the next 10 years, with an accompanying decrease in demand for RNs without APRN preparation (Peterson, 1999). Nurses in advanced practice are also moving toward independent practice. Data suggest that APRNs can independently diagnose and resolve over 80% of the primary health care problems of the American public (ANA, 1997a). Nurses are preferable to other providers in terms of client compliance with a therapeutic regimen, consumer satisfaction, and client gains in functional ability and self-care. NPs facilitate access to and continuity of care and provide high-quality care (Horrocks, Anderson, & Salisbury, 2002). APRNs prescribe less-expensive diagnostic tests, the length of their visits is comparable to that of physicians, and they charge less for services because of the low cost of professional liability insurance. Despite repeated proof of the cost-efficiency and therapeutic effectiveness of APRNs, obstacles to this role for nurses persist. In a Division of Nursing report on APRNs, the singular most formidable obstacle to practice is the fact that most people are unaware of what APRNs offer.

For APRNs, direct access to clients is a necessity and requires direct reimbursement, prescriptive authority, sufficient professional liability insurance, autonomy in managed care plans, professional staff privileges in service systems, and adequate practice acts. As the social and economic barriers to advanced practice are removed, utilization of these nurse specialists will increase.

Recently, progress has been made on the access issues that constrain APRNs. Reimbursement is now available to some segments of the advanced practice community in every federal entitlement program. The Balanced Budget Act of 1997 gave nurse practitioners and clinical

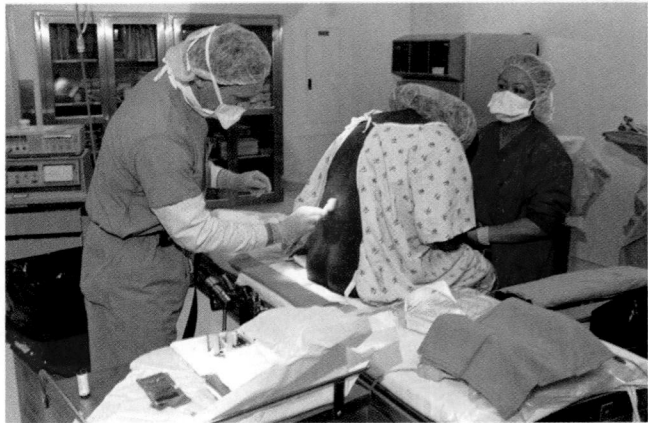

**Figure 2-5     A nurse anesthetist in an advanced practice role prepares a cesarean section client for spinal anesthesia.**

nurse specialists the right to be directly reimbursed by Medicare in all locations and specialties. The American Medical Association is still trying to limit APRN practice and reimbursement, and some state Medicare organizations don't understand the scope of practice for APRNs (Trossman, 2002). Nursing organizations continually join forces to oppose limitations to practice and reimbursement. Although insurance providers in the private sector are governed by state law and vary to the extent that they recognize advanced practice, APRNs report some form of reimbursement (in addition to that which is federally mandated) in every state and the District of Columbia (Pearson, 1996). Currently, every state and the District of Columbia award APRNs some type of prescriptive authority.

The ANA (through the Joint Commission on the Accreditation of Healthcare Organizations [JCAHO] and HCFA) began the groundwork for professional staff privileges for APRNs in its revision of the official definitions of professional staff that include a broad range of providers. The issue of institutional privileges is complicated given the fact that a facility may impose additional requirements on these privileges, including joint or collaborative practice with a physician (American Nurses Association, 1993b).

## Public versus Private Programs

The combination of public and private sector resources for health care seems to be comfortable for Americans. The competition between the two types of settings has encouraged quality and progress. Each setting provides benefits as well as drawbacks to health care recipients.

The nursing profession supports an integration of public and private sector programs and resources. Public dollars are required to help the poor and those who do not receive health care benefits through the workplace. Actual services should be available through a variety of public and private sources. To safeguard the health care system from becoming a two-tiered process based on personal resources, both the poor and nonpoor and the privileged and nonprivileged must be enrolled in the same programs.

Finally, the basic required package of services must be defined in the same way in each state and required as the minimum for both public and private sector programs. The persistence for national standards must be tempered with a respect for local needs and differences. In other words, set minimal national standards, but promote local planning and implementation. Local insights are particularly critical to the public health, meaning the health of a community as an aggregate of people, and not personal health services delivered in the community.

The states' rights philosophy prevailing in the United States creates an obstacle to national standards, which are necessary for several areas of assurance. Some coast-to-coast consistency in the cost of services is needed with local area adjustments. Further, a national standard to qualify for public entitlement is long overdue.

## Public Health

Public health includes services such as immunizations, prenatal care, environmental concerns, and analysis of the prevailing disease patterns in a community. Current public health problems include:

- Increase of sexually transmitted diseases that were once nearly eradicated (e.g., syphilis and gonorrhea)
- Appearance of new fatal diseases (e.g., AIDS and the Ebola virus)
- Emergence of drug-resistant strains of tuberculosis
- Underimmunization of infants and children
- Prevalence of overweight and inadequately nourished young people
- Presence of toxic environmental conditions

For today's needs, the medical model is insufficient. Table 2-7 presents a comparison of the medical model and the nursing model. In most instances, the nursing profession's approach to these issues transcends a health model and looks to a social model for response and assistance. Social models view areas of health, housing, education, and employment, in fact all social welfare concerns and programs, as an integrated whole. Education for healthy living is a good example. Healthy personal behaviors from adults are possible only if they have filtered down into the schools for the purposes of educating for health and influencing the peer systems that reinforce behaviors.

Nursing's strategic plan, as described in *Nursing's Agenda for Health Care Reform* (American Nurses Association, 1991), for achieving a better balance between illness and cure, and wellness and care, is only an interim step. Nursing must document its effectiveness in providing quality, cost-efficient services. Establishing joint ventures, procuring grant monies and other funding sources, and conducting research are avenues that nursing must pursue to achieve these objectives.

## Community Health

Community-oriented primary care combines elements of public health with primary care to provide solutions for

| TABLE 2-7 | MEDICAL MODEL VERSUS NURSING MODEL |
|---|---|
| **Medical Model** | **Nursing Model** |
| Focuses on disease and illness | Focuses on wellness |
| Cure oriented | Care oriented |
| Fragmented cases | Holistic perspective |

improving a community's health outcomes. Community-based care focuses on prevention and primary care. Community health nurses work in a variety of settings, including homes, clinics, workplaces, schools, church parishes, and organizations (Figure 2-6). They are skilled at providing services to populations at high risk for illness, homeless persons, aging populations, and those experiencing chronic illness. Regardless of the setting, fundamental principles of community care include the following (Hunt, 1998):

- Focusing on prevention
- Advocating client self-care
- Interactive nature between family, culture, and community
- Continuity of care
- Collaborative care

## School Nursing

The advent of school nursing was an extension of public health nursing in the early 1900s. Los Angeles became the first city to hire school nurses. The emphasis was on preventing the spread of communicable diseases. Early school

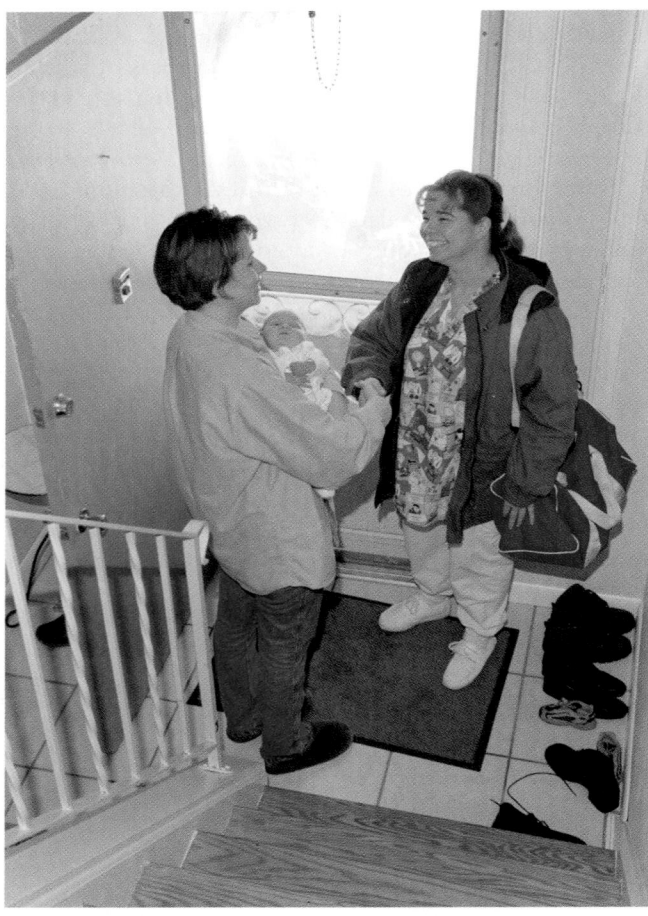

**Figure 2-6   A community health nurse introduces herself as she makes a home visit to a new mother and infant.**

nurses also provided health education to students and their families, performed physical assessments, and treated minor infections (Hitchcock, Schubert, & Thomas, 2003). Currently, services provided by school nurses have expanded to include maintaining a safe, healthy school environment, case finding, referral, and teaching other personnel how to care for children with special health care needs. Nursing has a rich heritage of providing community services. Thus, as nursing reclaims community-based practice as an integral part of its role, it is returning to its professional roots.

This scope and immediacy of health care services is extremely significant to school children. A generation ago, programs funded by the Robert Wood Johnson Foundation demonstrated that school nurse practitioners can identify over 90% of the health problems of school-age children and independently resolve over 80% of those problems. Despite these data, such services continue to be inaccessible to many children (Author, 2001).

## Long-Term Care

Nurses propose a community-personal partnership in addressing long-term care and support various financial plans that enable individuals to anticipate their long-term care needs; for example, long-term care insurance, long-term care individual retirement accounts (IRAs), and accessing the equity in property and life insurance policies to use for health care costs. Nurses are also aware that need will exceed resources for many chronically ill, frail, and disabled Americans. In those cases where there is catastrophic need, government dollars must be available.

Nurses also support the concept of **subacute care** (short-term aggressive care that emphasizes restorative interventions before the client's reentry into the community). The idea is not new but dates back to the Loeb Center of Montefiore Hospital in New York City in the 1960s (Joel & Kelly, 2003).

## Trends and Issues

As current trends continue in the millennium, the delivery of health care services will continue to change. Box 2-4 lists factors that will continue to shape reform of the health care delivery system.

The states and private sector will lead the way through a process to a product suited to the American character. The nursing profession has reached a point in time where there are few questions about the direction or process of health care reform. As health care reform occurs, some professions will experience opportunities while others will experience losses. The challenge is to improve the nation's delivery of health care services by positioning nursing to preserve its integrity and guarantee its preferred future. Nurses must continue to be in the forefront of change.

## BOX 2-4    TRENDS AFFECTING DELIVERY OF HEALTH CARE SERVICES

- The nursing shortage
- The aging of the U.S. population
- Increasing diversity in the U.S. population
- Increased number of single-parent families, with more children living in poverty
- Continued growth in outpatient settings with a greater demand for primary care providers
- Advances in technology with a resultant ability to perform more services in outpatient settings (including the home)
- More states using managed care models to deliver services to the medically indigent
- More emphasis on disease prevention and health promotion at the workplace
- Expectations of third-party payers and providers for clients to assume more personal responsibility for care
- Incentives for individuals who participate in preventive activities
- Federal funding of health care provider education focusing on service to underserved populations and areas
- The system as a union of both public and private sector resources and services
- Managed care dominating as the context for service delivery
- The right for individuals to enhance a basic package or expand their choices if they care to purchase that privilege
- Continuing focus on quality improvement

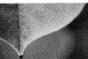

# CASE STUDY/NURSING CARE PLAN

Jim Knutson is a 58-year-old male who has just been hospitalized for diabetic ketoacidosis. Mr. Knutson was newly diagnosed with diabetes mellitus type 2 three months ago. One week before his admission to the hospital, he lost his job as a middle manager in a computer manufacturing plant. When he lost his job, he also lost his health insurance. Now he cannot afford his diabetes medications, which cost $450 per month without insurance copayments. Mr. Knutson also cannot afford to attend the diabetes education classes that were recommended when he was diagnosed. He lives with his wife, who is a homemaker.

### Assessment
On admission, Mr. Knutson has a blood glucose level of 570 mg/dL and is lethargic. His breath has a fruity odor. Mr. Knutson has the complication of diabetic ketoacidosis. His wife is anxious and tearful about both his condition and how they will pay for his hospitalization.

### Nursing Diagnosis #1
Ineffective coping related to the complexity of self-care regimens due to the complications of diabetic ketoacidosis.
**NOC:** Coping; Decision Making; Information Processing Knowledge: Diabetes Management
**NIC:** Coping Enhancement

### Expected Outcomes
The client will:
1. Resolve hyperglycemic condition by obtaining a blood glucose level within normal limits in 24 hours.
2. Learn the clinical manifestations of diabetic ketoacidosis and verbalize these symptoms within 24 to 72 hours.
3. Identify appropriate measures to keep diabetic complications from developing within 24 to 72 hours.

### Planning/Interventions/Rationales
1. Administer appropriate amounts of insulin per physician's order. *Decreases blood glucose levels to within normal limits.*

*(continues)*

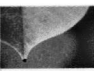

# CASE STUDY/NURSING CARE PLAN (continued)

2. Explore with the client and his wife their anxieties and knowledge about diabetes. *Common frustrations associated with diabetes stem from problems involving the disease, treatment regimes, and the health care system. Recognizing that these problems are common and can be managed increases confidence in the ability to cope. Provide client education regarding causes and management of diabetes.*

3. Assist the client and his wife to explore inexpensive options to manage blood glucose levels, such as diet, exercise, and educational materials (Web-based information and literature through public libraries, etc.) *Free information is easily accessible and will assist the family in finding new ways to cope with their problems.*

4. Refer the client to local diabetes support groups and to social services. *Social services can help the client to find pharmaceutical assistance, frequently through programs run by pharmacy companies. Support groups may provide opportunities for gaining mutual support and problem solving.*

## Evaluation

Client maintained a blood glucose level within 80–120 mg/dL within 24 hours.

## Nursing Diagnosis #2

Deficient knowledge related to pathophysiology of diabetes mellitus complications.
**NOC:** Knowledge: Diabetes Management; Information Processing
**NIC:** Learning Facilitation; Teaching: Individual

## Expected Outcomes

The client will:
1. Understand options for accessing the health care system to afford care for diabetes and verbalize those options to nurse within 1 week.
2. Verbalize an understanding of interventions for blood glucose levels within 1 week.

## Planning/Interventions/Rationales

1. Teach multiple levels of treatment options for diabetes mellitus. *To prevent diabetic complications.*
2. Refer client to social services within 1 week to discuss options for access to health care. *State health care insurance plans may be available to client if other resources are expended. Client and wife may need to seek other employment. Knowing options will allow client and wife to make realistic appraisal of their situation and plans for the future.*

## Evaluation

Client able to verbalize options to help him cope with diabetes and his treatment regimen within 5 days.

# Key Concepts

- The three levels of health care services can be categorized as primary, secondary, and tertiary levels.
- Health care services are delivered by both the public (official, voluntary, and nonprofit agencies) and private (hospitals, extended care facilities, home health agencies, hospices, outpatient settings, schools, industrial clinics, managed care organizations, community nursing centers, and rural hospitals) sectors.
- The health care team is composed of nurses, APRNs, physicians, physician assistants, pharmacists, dentists,

dental hygienists, dietitians, social workers, therapists, and chaplains.
- Health care in the United States is financed through a combination of both private and public funding.
- Managed care organizations seek to control health care costs by monitoring the delivery of services and restricting access to costly procedures and providers.
- Managed care plans include health maintenance organizations, preferred provider organizations, and exclusive provider organizations.
- The primary federal government insurance plans are Medicare, the program that provides health care coverage for the elderly and disabled, and Medicaid, the

jointly administered program that provides health care services for the poor.

- Health care reform must address the three critical issues of cost, access, and quality of health care services to achieve equity for all Americans.
- The cost of health care has been influenced by the oversupply of specialists, a surplus of hospital beds, the passive role assumed by most consumers, and the inequitable financing of health care services.
- The challenges that the health care delivery system need to overcome are the nursing shortage, the public's loss of control over health care decisions, the decreased use of hospitals and the related impact on quality of care, the change in practice settings, ethical issues, and the health care needs of vulnerable populations.
- *Nursing's Agenda for the Future*, written by the American Nurses Association, outlines nursing's proposals for easing the current problems in health care delivery.
- The Agency for Health Care Research and Quality aims to identify therapeutic standards for which the health care community can be held accountable.
- For advanced practice nurses to continue to provide access to high quality care, issues such as direct reimbursement for services, prescriptive authority, comprehensive professional liability insurance, autonomy in managed care plans, professional staff privileges in health care facilities, and adequate practice acts need to be resolved.
- A primary goal of the nursing profession within the areas of public health, community health, and long-term care is to provide health care services that emphasize prevention and primary health care to clients in these settings and thus help reduce the cost and increase the quality of health care.

## Review Questions and Activities

1. How does insurance influence health care?
2. What factors influence the nursing shortage?
3. What is the difference between the private and public sectors of health care?
4. What factors influence the delivery of health care?
5. How do Medicare and Medicaid differ?
6. How do primary, secondary, and tertiary care differ?
7. How do HMOs, PPOs, and private providers differ?
8. What are the different settings for health care delivery?

## Web Resources

Agency for Healthcare Research and Quality
   http://www.ahrq.gov
Agency for Health Care Policy and Research (AHRD)
   http://www.guideline.gov

American Association of Nurse Executives
   http://www.aone.org
American Nurses Association
   http://www.nursingworld.org
Centers for Disease Control and Prevention
   http://www.cdc.gov
Centers for Medicare & Medicaid Services
   http://www.cms.hhs.gov
Community Health Status Indicators Project
   http://www.communityhealth.hrsa.gov
Health Resources and Services Administration
   http://www.hrsa.gov
Healthcare Financing Administration
   http://www.hcfa.gov
Insure Kids Now
   http://www.insurekidsnow.gov
Medicare: The Official U.S. Government Site for Medicare Information
   http://www.medicare.gov
United States Census Bureau
   http://www.census.gov
United States Department of Commerce
   http://www.doc.gov
U.S. Department of Health & Human Services
   http://www.hhs.gov

## References

Agency for Health Care Policy and Research (AHRQ, 2003). http://www.guideline.gov

American Nurses Association (1997a). *Advanced practice nursing: A new age in health care.* Washington, DC: ANA.

American Nurses Association (1997b). *Implementing nursing's report card.* Washington, DC: ANA.

American Nurses Association (1999). *Nursing-sensitive quality indicators for acute care settings and ANA's safety and quality initiative.* Washington, DC: ANA.

American Nurses Association (1991). *Nursing's agenda for health care reform.* Kansas City, MO: Author.

American Nurses Association (1993a, September). Consumers willing to see a nurse for routine "doctoring" according to Gallup poll [news release]. Washington, DC: Author.

American Nurses Association (1993b, September). *States with some form of nurse privileging.* Washington, DC: Author.

American Nurses Association (1995). Managed care: Challenges and opportunities for nursing. *Nursing Facts* (Item PR-27). Washington, DC: Author.

American Nurses Association (2002). http://www. nursingworld.org

Author (2001). America's children: 2001. http://www.childstats.gov/americaschildren

Bednash, G. (2000). The decreasing supply of registered nurses: Inevitable future or call to action. *Journal of the American Medical Association, 283*(22), 2985–2953.

Beitz, J. (1998). Concept mapping: Navigating the learning process. *Nse Educ. 23*(5), 35–41.

Blumenthal, D. (1999). Health care reform at the close of the 20th century. *The New England Journal of Medicine, 340*(24), 1916-1920.

Buerhaus, P. I., Staiger, D. O., & Auerbach, D. I. (2000). Implications of an aging registered nurse workforce. *Journal of the American Medical Association, 283*(22), 2948-2954.

Carlson, D. K. (2000). Nurses remain at top of honesty and ethics poll. http://www.gallup.com/poll/releases/pr001127ii

Centers for Disease Control and Prevention (CDC) (2001). *HIV/AIDS Surveillance Report.* http://www.cdc.gov/hiv/stats/htm

Centers for Medicare and Medicaid Services, 2002. http://www.cms.hhs.gov

Centers for Medicare and Medicaid Services (2002). National Health Expenditures Projections: 2001-2011. http://www.hcfa.gov/stats/NHE-Proj/proj2001/default.htm

Chamberlain, P., Chen, Y., Osuna, E., & Yamamoto, C. (1995). Innovative culture shock prescribed for health care. *Nursing Outlook, 43*(5), 232-234.

Conger, C., Baldwin, J., Abegglen, J., & Callister, L. (1999). The shifting sands of health care delivery: Curriculum revision and integration of community health nursing. *Journal of Nursing Education, 38*(7), 304-311.

Economic Policy Institute (1999). *Sharing care: The changing nature of nursing.* Washington, DC: Author.

Fairfield, G., Hunter, D., Mechanic, D., & Rosleff, F. (1997). Managed care: Origins, principles, and evolution. *British Medical Journal, 314*(7097), 1823-1826.

Ginzberg, E. (1998). The changing U.S. health care agenda. *Journal of the American Medical Association, 279*(7), 501-504.

Grace, H. K. (1994). Can medical costs be contained? In J. C. McCloskey, & H. K. Grace (Eds.), *Current issues in nursing* (4th ed.). St. Louis: Mosby-Yearbook.

Grace, H. K., & Brock, R. M. (1994). Solving the health care dilemma: What will work? In J. C. McCloskey and H. K. Grace (Eds.), *Current issues in nursing* (4th ed.). St. Louis: Mosby-Yearbook.

Health Care Financing Administration (1999). *1999 Health Care Financing Administration Health Statistics.* http://www.hcfa.gov/stats

Health Care Financing Administration (2000). *Medicare 2000: 35 years of celebrating Americans' health and prosperity.* Washington, DC: Health Care Financing Administration.

Health Resources and Services Administration (2000). *The registered nurse population: Findings from the national sample survey of registered nurses.* Washington, DC: Health Resources and Services Administration.

Hirsch, D. (1999, Jan–Mar). Canadian government supports nurses. *Your Shift,* p. 4.

Hitchcock, J. E., Schubert, P. E., & Thomas, S. A. (2003). *Community health nursing: Caring in action* (2nd ed.). Clifton Park, NY.

Horrocks, S., Anderson, E., & Salisbury, C. (2002). Systematic review of whether nurse practitioners working in primary care can provide equivalent care to doctors. *British Medical Journal, 324,* 819–823.

Hull, K. (1994). Hospital trends. In C. Harrington and C. L. Estes (Eds.), *Health policy and nursing: Crisis and reform in the U.S. health care delivery system.* Boston: Jones & Bartlett.

Hunt, R. (1998). Community-based nursing: Philosophy or setting? *American Journal of Nursing, 98*(10), 44–47.

Inglehardt, J. R. (2000). The Canadian health care system. *The New England Journal of Medicine, 342*(26), 2007–2012.

Joel, L., & Kelly, L. (2003). *Kelly's Dimensions of professional nursing* (9th ed.). New York: McGraw-Hill.

Kathol, D. Geiger, M. & Hartig, J. (1998). Clinical correlation map: A tool for linking theory and practice. *Nse Educ. 23*(4), 31–34.

Lee, P. R., Soffel, D., & Luft, H. (1994). Costs and coverage: Pressures towards health care reform. In P. Lee, C. Estes, & N. Ramsay (Eds.), *The nation's health* (4th ed.). Boston: Jones & Bartlett.

Lens, V. (2002). Managed care and the judicial system. *Health and Social Work, 27*(1), 27–36.

Levi, J., & Kates, J. (2000). HIV: Challenging the health care delivery system. *American Journal of Public Health, 90*(7), 1033–1036.

Mills, R. J. (2001). *Health insurance coverage: 2000.* Washington, DC: U.S. Census Bureau.

Needleman, J., Buerhaus, P. I., Mattke, S., Stewart, M., & Zelevinsky, K. (2001). *Nurse staffing and patient outcomes in hospitals.* Washington, DC: Health Resources and Services Administration.

Nelson, C.T., & Mills, R. J. (2001). *The March CPS insurance verification question and its effect on estimates of the uninsured.* Washington, DC: U.S. Census Bureau.

Pearson, L. J. (1996). Annual update of how each state stands on legislative issues affecting advanced nursing practice. *Nurse Practitioner, 21*(1), 10–701.

Risher, P., & Applebaum, S. (2002). *Nurseweek/American Organization of Nurse Executives national survey of registered nurses.* Rochester, NY: Harris Heritage, Inc.

Rogers, C. C. (2000). *Changes in the older population and implications for rural areas.* Washington, DC: U.S. Department of Agriculture Economic Research Services.

Rosenbach, M., Ellwood, M., Czajka, J., Irvin, C., Coupe, W., & Quinn, B. (2001). *Implementation of the State Children's Health Insurance Program: Momentum is increasing after a modest start.* Washington, DC: Health Care Financing Administration.

Rowe, J. W. (1996). Health care myths at the end of life. *Bulletin of the American College of Surgeons, 81*(6), 11–18.

Schuster, M. A., McGlynn, E. A., & Brook, R. H. (1998). How good is health care in the United States? *Milbank Quarterly, 76*(4), 517–563.

Society for Ambulatory Care Professionals (1994). *Glossary of managed care terms: An issue briefing.* Chicago: American Hospital Association.

Spratley, E., Johnson, A., Sochalski, J., Fritz, M., & Spencer, W. (2000). *Findings from the National Sample Survey of Registered Nurses.* Washington, DC: Health Resources and Services Administration.

Strunk, B. C, & Cunningham, P. J. (2002). *Treading water: Americans' access to needed medical care.* 1997–2001. http://www.hschange.com

Toynbee, Arnold. (1916). A summary of Armenian history up to and including the year 1915. In Viscount Bryce, *The Treatment of Armenians in the Ottoman Empire 1915–16: Documents presented to Viscount Grey of Fallodon, Secretary of State for Foreign Affairs by Viscount Bryce* (pp. 637–653). New York and London: G. P. Putnam's Sons, for His Majesty's Stationary Office, London.

Trossman, S. (2002). APRNs fight for their right to practice. *American Journal of Nursing, 102*(1), 63, 65.

United States Census Bureau, 2001. http://www.census.gov

U.S. Department of Commerce (DOC) (2001). *More people have health insurance.* Washington, DC: U.S. Department of Commerce.

Ventura, M. J. (1999). Healthcare spending projected to double. *RN, 62*(1), 14.

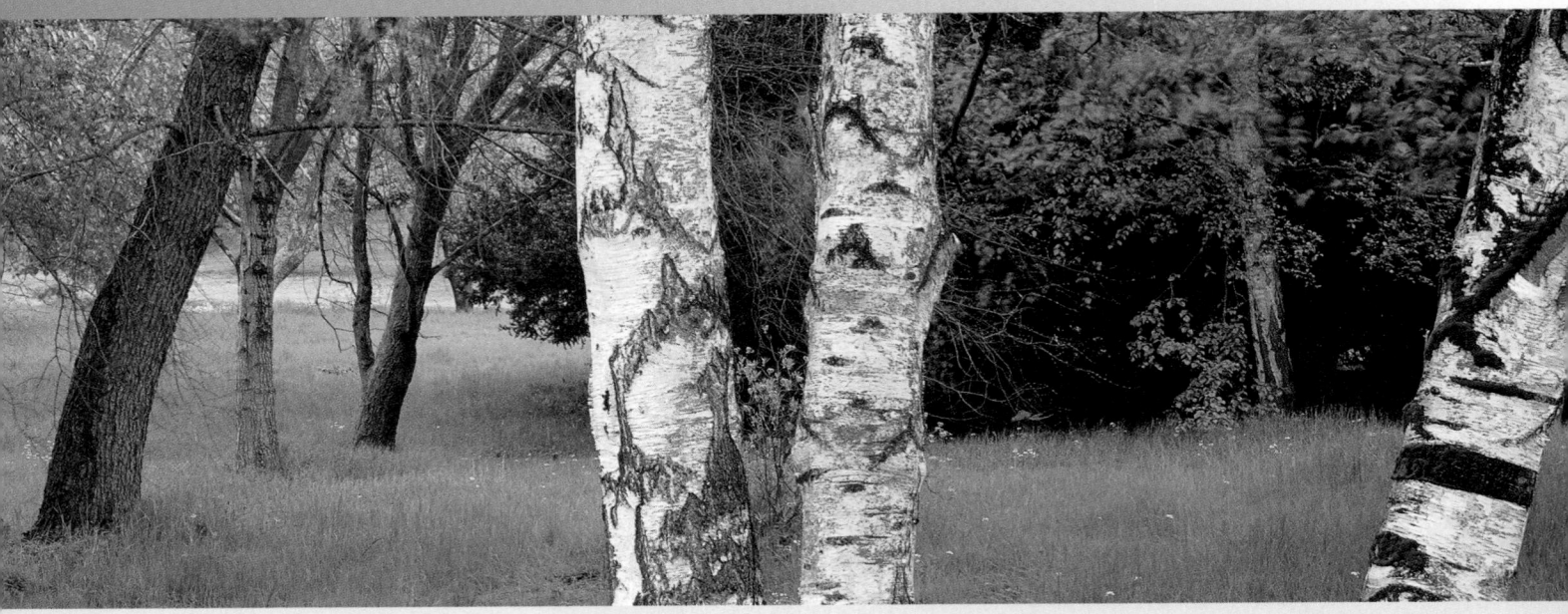

# 3 CHAPTER

# Framework of Nursing Practice

Ellen L. Poole, DNSc(c), RN, CCRN, CPAN

*"The art of nursing is not an indulgent nicety, but instead an essential activity grounded in practice and manifest in helping patients create coherence and meaning in lives threatened by transitions of many kinds."*

(LeVassuer, 1999)

# Chapter Competencies

*Upon completion of this chapter, the reader should be able to:*

1. Identify the purposes and essential elements of nursing theories.
2. Describe nonnursing theories and their role as related to nursing.
3. Recognize major nursing theories and their relevance to nursing practice.
4. Identify the major concepts within nursing theories.
5. Analyze the relationship between Nightingale's theoretical works and the early development of nursing theory.
6. Describe the knowledge development in nursing specific to metaparadigm and paradigm concepts.
7. Identify the main concepts of the early nursing theorists.
8. Describe the primary aspects of the contemporary nursing theories.
9. Analyze the theories of the new worldview of nursing.
10. Examine nursing theory and the standards of nursing practice.
11. Explain the relationship of functional health pattern typology to nursing theory.
12. Synthesize concepts of nursing theory developments as nursing moves into the 21st century.

# Key Terms

| | | |
|---|---|---|
| concept | grand theory | paradigm revolution |
| conceptual framework | health | paradigm shift |
| conceptual model | metaparadigm | person |
| discipline | middle-range theory | phenomenon |
| environment | nursing | proposition |
| existentialism | nursing research | self-care |
| functional health patterns | paradigm | theory |

Since the advent of modern nursing with Florence Nightingale over 150 years ago, nursing and nursing theory have evolved into a complex system that includes philosophy, grand theories, and middle-range theories. Nursing theory provides the theoretical foundation of the profession. In providing that foundation, nursing theory defines what nursing is, what it does, and the goals and outcomes of nursing care. Nursing is not guided or defined by one specific theory but is the synthesis of many theories. This synthesis of ideas is discussed in this chapter.

This chapter addresses the basic ideas and meanings of nursing theory and its relevance to the nursing profession. The purpose, use, and evolution of nursing are presented. A broad overview of selected nursing theories is described along with their specific applications to nursing practice. The chapter ends with an explanation of the use of functional health patterns in nursing practice.

## Components of the Theoretical Foundation

The basic elements that structure a nursing theory are concepts and propositions. In a theory, propositions represent how concepts affect each other.

### Concepts

A concept is the basic building block of a theory. A **concept** is a vehicle of thought. According to Chinn and Kramer (1999, p. 54), the term *concept* is a "complex mental formulation of . . . [our] perceptions of the world." A concept labels or names a **phenomenon**, an observable fact that can be perceived through the senses and explained. A concept assists in formulating a mental image about an object or situation. Concepts help to name things and occurrences in the world, and assist in communicating with each other about the world. Independence, self-care, and caring are just a few examples of concepts frequently encountered in health care. Theories are formulated by linking concepts together. A **conceptual framework** is a structure that links global concepts together and represents the unified whole of a larger reality. Whereas, a **conceptual model** is the "symbolic representation of empiric experience in words, pictorial or graphic diagram, mathematical notations, or physical material" (Chinn & Kramer, 1999, p. 255). The specifics about phenomena within the global whole are better explained by theory.

By its nature, a concept is a socially constructed label that may represent more than a single phenomenon. For example, upon hearing the word *plate*, a mental image that probably comes to mind is an item of dinnerware used for eating. The word *plate* could represent many different kinds of dinnerware for eating, such as a dinner plate, salad plate, or bread plate. Further, the word *plate* could also represent a print of a woodcut or a lithograph. The meaning of the word *plate* depends on the contextual usage.

In health care, the concept of *wandering* may be represented by meanings such as aimless and random movement, disorganized thought processes, and conversation that is difficult to follow. To be useful, the multiple meanings that often underlie a concept must be thoroughly understood and clearly defined within its context.

It is important to remember that the same concept may be used differently in various theories. For example, one nursing theory may use *health* to mean a dynamic state in a life cycle with continued goal attainment and adjustment to stressors through optimal use of resources. Another theory may use the concept of health to mean a dynamic state influenced by bio-psycho-social factors, without a focus on illness.

## Propositions

A **proposition** (another structural element of a theory) is a statement that proposes a relationship between concepts. An example of a nonnursing proposition is the statement "people seem to be happier in the sunshine." This proposition establishes a relationship between the concept of happiness and the type of day. A nursing propositional statement linking the concepts of futility, hopelessness, and powerlessness is stated as "futility may lead to a feeling of hopelessness, and hopelessness leads to a feeling of powerlessness." Propositional statements in a theory represent the theorist's view of which concepts fit together and in most theories, establish how concepts affect one another.

## Theories

A **theory** is a set of concepts and propositions that provide an orderly way to view phenomena. In scientific literature, *theory* may be defined in many different ways, with subtle nuances specific to the particular scientist's viewpoint.

These various explanations share a common notion of the theory's purpose, that being description, explanation, and prediction. "The purpose of a theory in scientific disciplines is to guide research to enhance the science by supporting existing knowledge or generating new knowledge" (Parse, 1987, p. 3). A theory not only helps to organize thoughts and ideas, but also may help direct in what to do and when and how to do it.

However, the use of the term *theory* is not restricted to the scientific world. It is often used in daily life and conversation. For example, a person telling a friend about a mystery novel may say, "I have a theory about who committed the crime." Or a track coach may say to his polevaulters, "I have a theory about how to improve your vault." The way in which *theory* is used in these statements provides a useful mechanism for thinking about its meaning.

# Theories from Other Disciplines

In addition to using theories specifically constructed to describe, explain, and predict the phenomena of concern to nursing, the nursing profession has long used theories from other disciplines. A **discipline** is a field of study. Theories from biologic, physical, and behavioral sciences are commonly used in the practice of nursing.

From psychology, Abraham Maslow's *Hierarchy of Human Needs* (1970) is frequently used to explain the progression of people's needs. Within this system, Maslow describes six levels of needs. Starting with basic physiological needs, an individual meets the lower needs before striving for the next level of needs (Figure 3-1).

Ludwig von Bartlaffny (1968) developed the General Systems Theory. Within this theory, Von Bartlaffny proposed that a system is greater than the sum of all of its parts. In general systems theory, all systems must be goal oriented. Each part may be acted upon separately, but it is interdependent with all the parts of the whole. There are implicit boundaries with human systems being open and dynamic. This theory reminds nurses that as they see a change in an individual's respiratory status (one system), it is interdependent with cardiac function; therefore, there is a change in cardiac function and the rest of the body.

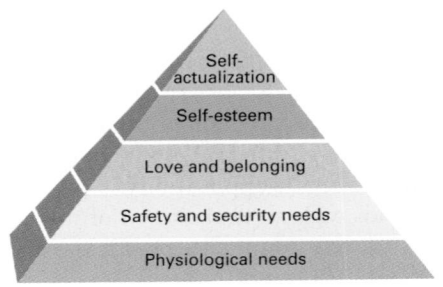

**Figure 3-1    Maslow's Hierarchy of Needs**

# Importance of Nursing Theories

Why do we have nursing theories? In the early part of nursing's history, knowledge was extremely limited and almost entirely task oriented. The knowledge explosion that occurred in health care in the 1950s produced the need to systematically organize the tremendous volume of new information being generated. From the very beginnings of nursing education, there was a need to categorize knowledge and to analyze client care situations in order to communicate in coherent and meaningful ways.

The literature about the relationship between theory and nursing care yields many interpretations in terms of the role each component plays in the health care environment. According to Barnum (1998, p. 1), "a theory is a construct that accounts for and organizes some phenomenon." Chinn and Kramer (1999, p. 51) define theory as a "creative and rigorous structure of ideas that projects a tentative purposeful and systematic view of phenomena." Meleis (1997, p. 12) stated that a theory is "a systematic depiction of aspects of reality that are discovered or invented for describing, explaining, predicting, or prescribing responses, events, situations, conditions, or relationships." Similarly, Fawcett (1999, p. 4) defined theory as a "set of relatively concrete and specific concepts and the propositions that describe or link those concepts."

Nursing theories provide a framework for thought in which to examine situations. As new situations are encountered, this framework provides a structure for organization, analysis, and decision making. In addition, nursing theories provide a structure for communicating with other nurses and with other members of the health care team. Nursing theories assist the discipline of nursing in clarifying beliefs, values, and goals. In addition, nursing theories help define the unique contribution of nursing, proclaim professional autonomy, and ultimately, control certain aspects of nursing practice.

In the broadest sense, nursing theory is necessary for the continued development and evolution of the discipline of nursing. As the world of health care changes daily, nursing must continue expanding its knowledge base to proactively respond to changes in societal needs. Knowledge for nursing practice is developed through nursing research, which in turn is used for either testing existing theories or generating new theories. **Nursing research** is the systematic application of formalized methods for generating valid and dependable information about the phenomena of concern to the discipline of nursing (Chinn & Kramer, 1999).

The relationship between nursing practice, theory, and research is depicted in Figure 3-2. These processes are so closely related that to consider one aspect without considering the other two aspects would be seeing only a part of the whole. Nursing practice is the focal point of the relationship between practice, theory, and research. Nursing practice provides the raw material for the ideas that are sys-

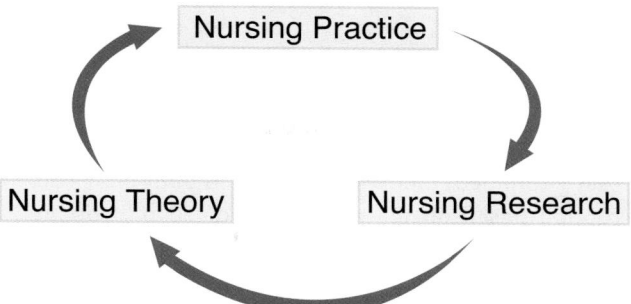

Figure 3-2   Process of knowledge development: Nursing practice, theory, and research are interdependent. Nursing theory development and nursing research activities are directed toward developing nursing practice guidelines.

tematically developed and organized in the form of nursing theory. The ideas proposed by nursing theory must be tested and validated through nursing research. In turn, new knowledge that results from nursing research is used to transform and inform nursing practice. Alternatively, nursing practice generates questions that serve as the basis for nursing research. Nursing research then influences the development of nursing theory, which in turn transforms nursing practice.

Myra Levine states that "exploring a variety of nursing theories ought to provide nurses with new insights into patient care, opening nursing options otherwise hidden, and stimulating innovative interventions" (1995, p. 13). Theoretical thinking enhances and strengthens the nurse's role and helps the nurse to actually *think* nursing. As nurses learn more about specific nursing theories, they may discover that they can relate more to one theory than another or that they appreciate ideas from several different theories. Nurses may use a specific nursing theory to help guide their practice or may choose a more eclectic approach and adopt ideas from several theories. Both approaches are valid. Furthermore, nurses may find particular theories more appropriate for certain situations. In that case, one theory can be used with a client in a home health care setting, whereas another theory may apply more to a client in an acute care environment. Regardless of the chosen approach, nurses will recognize the value and usefulness of nursing theory as a tool for effective nursing practice.

## Scope of Theories

"A theory is defined as one or more relatively concrete and specific concepts that are derived from a conceptual model, the propositions that narrowly describe these concepts, and the propositions that state relatively concrete and specific relations between two or more concepts" (Fawcett, 2000, p. 18). Essentially, two different categories relate to the scope of theories: grand theories and middle-range theories. This classification is applicable to both nursing and nonnursing theories.

## RESEARCH FOCUS

**Title of Study:** A grounded theory of reimaging

**Study Purpose:** This study proposed a conceptual (grounded) theory of adapting to body image disruption based on the experiences of 28 participants who had experienced an alteration in a physical appearance or function.

**Methods:** In this qualitative study, participants (n = 32) were recruited through newspaper advertisements and health professional referrals to clients. Purposive sampling ensured diversity in age and type of physical change. A total of 28 participants completed all aspects of the study. Within 3 months of a significant alteration in physical appearance or function, participants entered the study. Interviews were conducted at 3, 6, 12, and 18 months following the alteration. Coming from a wide range of socioeconomic backgrounds, participant ages ranged from 19 to 85 years. Participants were primarily Caucasian with one Native American, one African American, and one resident from India. Three-fourths (n = 21) were women. Physical changes causing body image disruptions were: significant weight change, loss or paralysis of body parts, ostomies, scarring from burns or trauma, or surgical reconstruction.

A constant comparative method of concurrent data collection analysis is used in grounded theory development. Using a broad interview guide, three investigators conducted interviews focused on participants' perceptions of themselves and experiences before and during the study, their thoughts, feelings, adaptive strategies, and perceptions of the responses of others. Investigators reviewed transcript copies and field notes, arrived at consensus, and generated areas for exploration in upcoming interviews.

**Findings:** Reimaging emerged as the basic social process that occurs in response to significant alterations in the physical appearance or functioning of the body. The process is comprised of three phases: (a) body image disruption, (b) wishing for restoration, return to former self, and (c) reimaging self, based on physical alteration. The phases are characterized by assimilation, accommodation, and interpretation. This process results in reconciliation, incorporation of new image, and normalization of lifestyle.

**Implications:** Recognition of the significance and meaning of behaviors and emotions of clients engaged in the process of reimaging enables the nurse to anticipate problems or needs, provide information and support, and develop alternative problem-solving strategies. Future research is needed to test relationships between influencing factors, action processes, and outcomes of the reimaging process.

Norris, J., Kunes-Connell, M., & Spelic, S. S. (1998). A grounded theory of reimaging. *Advances in Nursing Science, 20*(3), 1–12.

## Grand Theory

A **grand theory** is composed of concepts representing global and extremely complex phenomena. It is the broadest in scope, represents the most abstract level of development, and addresses the broad phenomena of concern within the discipline. Typically, a grand theory is not intended to provide guidance for the formation of specific nursing interventions, but rather it provides an overall framework for structuring broad, abstract ideas (Fawcett, 2000). An example of a grand theory is Margaret Newman's Theory of Health and Expanding Consciousness.

## Middle-Range Theory

A theory that addresses more concrete and more narrowly defined phenomena than does a grand theory is known as a **middle-range theory**. Descriptions, explanations, and predictions put forth in a middle-range theory are intended to answer questions about nursing phenomena, yet they do not cover the full range of phenomena of concern to the discipline. A middle-range theory provides a perspective from which to view complex situations and a direction for interventions (Fawcett, 2000). Currently, middle-range theory can be delineated into three levels of abstractness: high middle-range theory, middle middle-range theory, and low middle-range theory (McEwen & Wills, 2002). Another name for low middle-range theory is a practice theory that deals exclusively with one specific phenomena. Examples of middle-range theories are high middle-range, Patricia Benner's Model of Skills Acquisition in nursing (1984); middle middle-range theory, Theory of Resilience (Polk, 1997); and low middle-range, Ramona Mercer's Maternal Role Attainment Theory (1981).

## The Influence of Florence Nightingale on the Early Development of Nursing Theory

Prior to Nightingale (1859), nursing did not have a clear direction or identity. Nightingale, an educated English gentlewoman, was "called" to nursing. After she was called, she trained at Kaiserworth, Germany, for a brief 6 months.

Nightingale described nursing as both an art and a science. The art is the practice, the interaction between nurse and client, whereas the science speaks to the empirical, or scientific, knowledge of nursing. In addition, theory is identified as being necessary to guide practice, education, and research.

Nightingale did not develop a theory of nursing as theory is defined today; rather, she provided the nursing profession with the philosophical basis from which other theories have emerged and developed. Nightingale's ideas about nursing have guided both theoretical thought and actual nursing practice throughout the history of modern nursing. Her writings did not focus on the nature of the person, but did stress the importance of caring for the ill person rather than caring for the illness. In Nightingale's view, the person was a passive recipient of care, and nursing's primary focus was on the manipulation of the person's environment to maintain or achieve a state of health.

Despite the fact that Nightingale did not believe in the germ theory, her experiences in the Crimean War magnified her interest in the principles of sanitation and the relationship between environment and health. A person's health was the direct result of environmental influences, specifically cleanliness, light, pure air, pure water, and efficient drainage. Through manipulating the environment, nursing "aims to discover the laws of nature that would assist in putting the patient in the best possible condition so that nature can effect a cure" (Nightingale, 1859, p. 6). Nursing's main focus was health, and health was closely related to nursing. Nursing was concerned with the healthy as well as the sick (Nightingale, 1859).

Nightingale's principles regarding environment/ health/nursing were implemented in America at the turn of the 20th century. With the development of hospital-based schools of nursing, Nightingale's principles of sanitation were used to clean up the rat-infested, dirty hospitals of the day. As Nightingale's ideas were put in use, hospitals became a place for people to recover rather than a place to die. When, for a variety of reasons, hospitals did not hire their own nursing graduates, nurses applied Nightingale's principles in the community to the development of public health nursing. The Henry Street Settlement founded by Lillian Wald is an excellent example of Nightingale's theory in practice.

Private duty nursing and public health nursing remained the primary focus of nursing practice until World War II. At this time, a tremendous increase in scientific knowledge and technology was affecting health care. As the practice of medicine became more scientifically based, more clients were cared for in hospital settings. Nursing practice likewise became centered in the hospital rather than the home. With this development, it became clear that nursing did not have an adequate theory base to organize new knowledge and guide nursing practice. Nursing began to develop its knowledge base further by incorporating Nightingale's principles into modern nursing theory.

## The Evolution of Nursing Theory

The work of early nursing theorists in the 1950s focused on the tasks of nursing practice from a somewhat mechanistic (i.e., cause and effect) viewpoint. Because of this emphasis, much of the art of nursing—the value of caring, the relationship aspects of nursing, and the aesthetics of practice—was diminished. During the decades of the 1960s, 1970s, and 1980s, many nursing theorists struggled with making nursing practice, theory, and research fit into the prevailing view of science.

Reflecting changes in global awareness of health care needs, several contemporary nursing theorists have projected a new perspective for nursing that truly unifies nursing as both an art and a science. Noted nursing theorists such as Leininger, Watson, Rogers, Parse, and Newman have been urging the discipline of nursing to embrace this emerging view that is seen as more holistic, humanistic, client focused, and grounded in the notion of caring as the core of nursing.

Since the early 1950s, many nursing theories have been systematically developed to help describe, explain, and predict the phenomena of concern to nursing. Each of these established theories provides a unique perspective, and each is distinct and separate from other nursing theories in its particular view of nursing phenomena. An overview of several nursing theories is presented later in the chapter.

## Knowledge Development in Nursing

The knowledge in a particular discipline can be arranged in a hierarchical structure that ranges from abstract to concrete. Theories represent the most concrete component of a discipline. Several theories that share a common view of the world can be grouped together to form a paradigm. A **paradigm** is a particular viewpoint or perspective. Each discipline has a defined metaparadigm, which is the most abstract component of knowledge and can consist of more than one paradigm (Fawcett, 2000). A **metaparadigm** is

 **STOP AND THINK**

### Florence Nightingale and Modern Nursing

- Why is Florence Nightingale considered important to modern nursing?

- How does Florence Nightingale continue to influence nurses today?

the unifying force in a discipline that names the phenomena of concern to that discipline.

## The Metaparadigm of Nursing

What distinguishes nursing from any other discipline such as biology, sociology, or psychology? Each of the other disciplines is concerned with specific aspects of the human being. "Each discipline singles out certain phenomena with which it will deal in a unique manner" (Fawcett, 1989, p. 5). The field of biology (the study of living organisms) has defined limits and boundaries that do not extend into psychology. Similarly, psychology (which is concerned with the behavior of individuals) does not extend its concerns into the domain of sociology (which focuses mainly on the social behavior of human beings).

The broadly identified concerns of a discipline are defined in its metaparadigm, and most metaparadigms consist of several major concepts. The metaparadigm concepts provide the boundaries and limitations of a discipline.

Initial consensus on the metaparadigm concepts in nursing was achieved in 1984. According to Fawcett (1984), the major concepts that provide structure to the domain of nursing are *person, environment, health,* and *nursing*. **Person** refers to the individual, family, or group who are the interest of nursing. **Health** is the continuum of wellness to terminal illness of individuals. **Environment** is the place or community where care is provided; it also describes the world a person lives in and interacts with. **Nursing** is the actions and interactions of the nurse with the person. These metaparadigm elements name the overall areas of concern for the nursing discipline. Each nursing theory presents a slightly different view of the metaparadigm concepts. Refer to the section entitled "Contemporary Nursing Theories" for a discussion of how various theorists address and link the metaparadigm concepts.

Consider for a moment the practice of nursing by a home health nurse, a critical care nurse, and a nurse educator. What is the unifying thread among these various nurses? Although each nurse's practice is obviously different, they all consider their work as part of the nursing profession because they share the same major concerns. Regardless of the setting or the type of client involved, each nurse is concerned with person, environment, health, and nursing.

How is nursing's metaparadigm different from that of other helping professions? The metaparadigm of medicine focuses on the pathophysiology and curing of disease. Nursing's metaparadigm is broader and focuses on the person, health, and the environment. Consider a physician's view and a nurse's view of a client who is newly diagnosed with hypertension. The physician is concerned with reducing the client's abnormal blood pressure values to normal levels, if possible. The physician prescribes medications, an exercise regime, and nutritional counseling in an effort to control blood pressure levels. In dealing with the same client situation, the nurse is concerned with the impact of the diagnosis on all aspects of the client's life. Issues include the client's ability to cope with a chronic condition, the effect of the diagnosis on the client's family, and teaching about the need for changes in the client's daily living patterns. Although both health care providers are viewing the same client situation, each has a different perspective or focus. Each discipline's metaparadigm provides a viewpoint that leads to the development of knowledge as seen within that viewpoint.

Although person, health, environment, and nursing are generally accepted metaparadigm concepts in nursing, there is growing discontent with the limitation of these concepts. As dialogue continues and clarity emerges, the metaparadigm concepts will change to reflect contemporary thought and practice.

One example of this evolution in the discipline of nursing is the inclusion of caring as a basic core concept, central to the practice of nursing. Nurse scholars have urged a reconsideration of the identified metaparadigm elements. Watson (1985, p. 35) stated that "care is the essence of nursing and the most central and unifying focus for nursing practice." According to Watson (1990, p. 21), "human caring needs to be explicitly incorporated into nursing's metaparadigm."

## Paradigms in Nursing

The metaparadigm of a discipline identifies common areas of concern. A paradigm is a particular way of viewing the phenomena of concern that have been delineated by the metaparadigm of the discipline. The term *paradigm* stems from the work of Kuhn (1970), who referred to a paradigm as a "worldview" about the phenomena of concern in a discipline.

Two individuals with different paradigmatic views can look at precisely the same phenomenon and each will "see" the phenomenon differently. For example, consider the viewpoints of a mother and father who are watching their daughter at baseball practice. The mother looks at her daughter and "sees" a graceful, yet somewhat shy child who has shown improvement in her ability to make new friends. The father, on the other hand, "sees" a strong runner who needs help with batting drills. Each parent is operating from a different paradigm.

The prevailing paradigm in a particular discipline represents the dominant viewpoint of particular concepts. This viewpoint is supported by theories and research that address the concerns of the discipline. By consensus, the community of scholars in a discipline accepts and agrees on a particular viewpoint or worldview. When new theories and research surface that challenge the prevailing paradigm, a new paradigm emerges to compete with the prevailing worldview. The competition between the paradigms results in what Kuhn (1970) refers to as a paradigm revolution. A **paradigm revolution** is the turmoil and conflict that occur in a discipline when a competing paradigm gains acceptance over the dominant paradigm. If the competing paradigm answers more questions and solves more problems for the discipline than the prevailing paradigm does, then a paradigm shift occurs. A **paradigm shift** refers to the acceptance of the competing paradigm over the prevailing paradigm or a shifting away from one worldview toward another worldview. Again, by consensus the competing paradigm becomes the dominant paradigm and the process begins again (Kuhn, 1970).

The notion of paradigm revolution can be likened to a revolution that occurs in a country where the ruling government is overthrown by a competing group that proposed to have more and better solutions to the country's problems. In this situation, power shifts from one ruling body to another. In another example, a paradigm shift occurred when people began to view the world as round rather than flat. Once the community of scholars agreed that the world was round (now the prevailing paradigm), all other views about the world also changed. Paradigms can be mutually exclusive. Members of a discipline cannot subscribe to two competing paradigms at the same time. One cannot believe at the same time that the world is flat *and* that the world is round.

## Four Levels of Knowing

In 1978, Carper introduced "four patterns of knowing" to nursing knowledge. She identified and defined four levels of knowledge: (1) *empirical*—scientific knowledge that is descriptive, seeking to develop abstract theoretical meaning; (2) *aesthetics*—art of nursing, which is more than the technical skills and embodies the nurse's creative ability to individualize care; (3) *personal*—embodies the interpersonal interaction between nurse and client, recognizing the individual's unique humanness; and (4) *ethics*—embodies a specific moral code of right versus wrong from both the nurse and the client. White (1995) added sociopolitical knowledge from the contextual cultural location of nurse-client interaction as well as from the broader context where nursing and health care take place.

Debate, dialogue, discussion, theory development, and research continue within the discipline of nursing. Some nursing scholars argue about the structural elements of the discipline, some debate the value of competing paradigms, and some present alternative metaparadigm elements. Yet for all the uncertainty created by these questions and alternative ideas, the ongoing dialogue is a healthy sign of the development of the nursing profession.

## Early Nursing Theories

By its very nature, the development of nursing's theoretical base has progressed in a methodical and systematic, albeit slow, fashion. A variety of nursing theorists have emerged to create a foundation for contemporary nursing knowledge (Figure 3-3). The ongoing process of knowledge development is often influenced by driving forces outside the discipline of nursing. The early nurse theorists attempted to address the metaparadigm concepts because initial consensus on these had not yet been achieved and an agreed-upon definition for nursing did not exist.

## Hildegard Peplau

Hildegard Peplau, a psychiatric nurse instructor, combined her research and experience in the development of a theory of psychodynamic nursing, published in *Interpersonal Relations in Nursing* (1952). Drawing from her own knowledge and that from other disciplines, Peplau defined the concepts and stages involved in the development of the nurse-client relationship. From that relationship, she identified the roles of the nurse as stranger, resource person, teacher, leader, surrogate, and counselor. Peplau developed a middle-range theory with a focus on both nursing and the person, and she did not incorporate all aspects of the metaparadigm into her theory. Although other theories may view the nurse-client relationship differently, the primacy of this relationship in nursing has remained.

## Virginia Henderson

Virginia Henderson's definition of nursing, considered to be a classic, first appeared in 1955:

> The unique function of the nurse is to assist the individual, sick or well, in the performance of those activities contributing to health or its recovery (or to a peaceful death) that he would perform unaided if he had the necessary strength, will, or knowledge. And to do this in such a way as to help him gain independence as rapidly as possible (Henderson, 1966, p. 15).

Together with Bertha Harmer, Henderson attempted to identify those basic human needs viewed as the basis of nursing care. These needs include the need to maintain physiological balance, to adjust to the environment, to communicate and participate in social interaction, and to worship according to one's faith. Her 14 basic needs were published in the *Textbook of the Principles and Practice of Nursing* (1955), one of the first nursing textbooks. Henderson viewed the nursing role as helping the client from dependence to independence. As an early nursing theorist, Henderson did not intend to develop a theory of nursing; rather, she attempted to define the unique focus of nursing. Henderson's emphasis on basic human needs as the central focus of nursing practice has led to further theory development regarding the person's needs and how nursing can assist in meeting those needs.

## Faye Abdellah

Faye Abdellah (1960), acknowledging the influence of Henderson, expanded Henderson's 14 needs into 21 problems that she believed would serve as a knowledge base for nursing. Throughout her career, she strongly supported

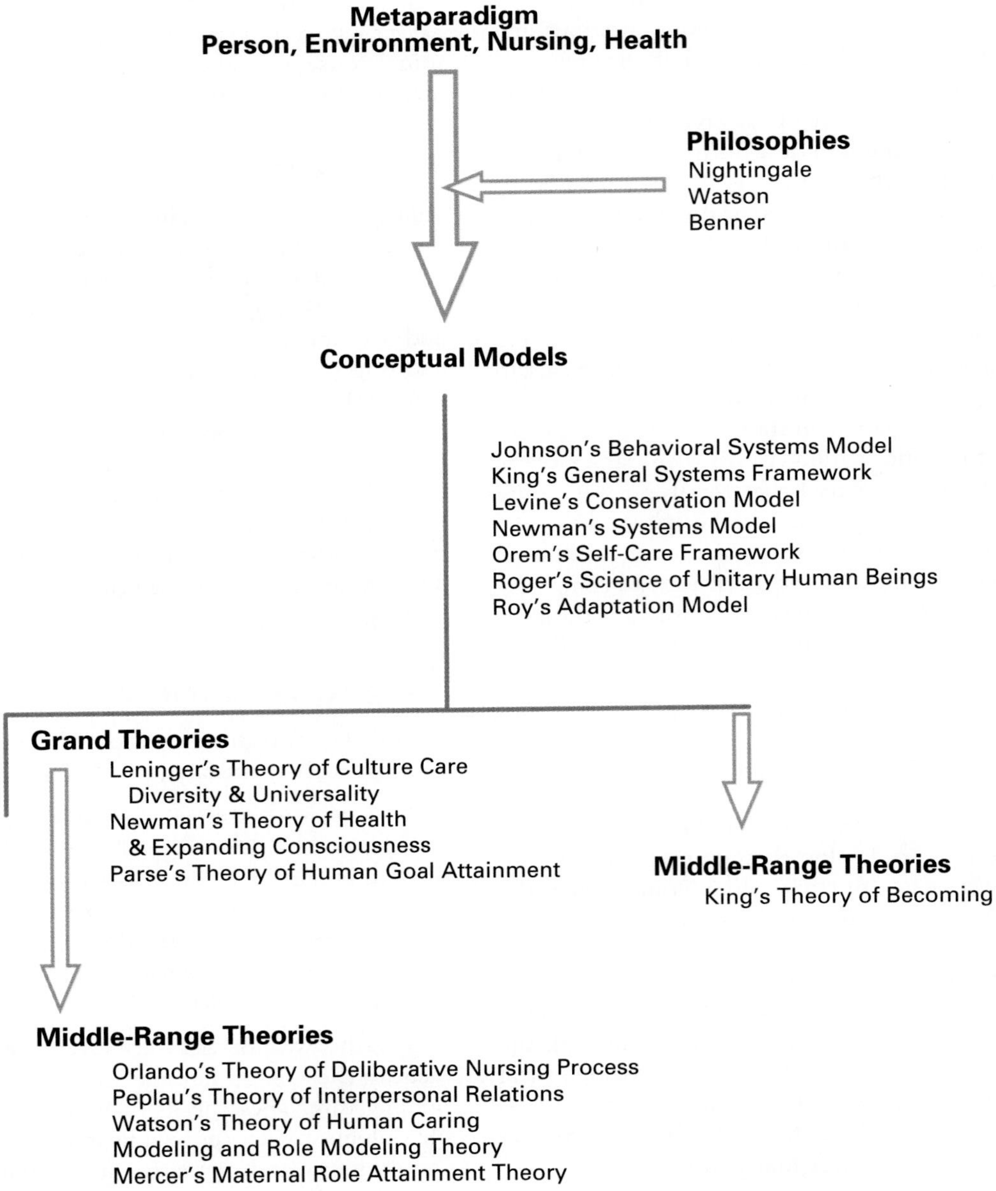

**Metaparadigm**
**Person, Environment, Nursing, Health**

**Philosophies**
Nightingale
Watson
Benner

**Conceptual Models**

Johnson's Behavioral Systems Model
King's General Systems Framework
Levine's Conservation Model
Newman's Systems Model
Orem's Self-Care Framework
Roger's Science of Unitary Human Beings
Roy's Adaptation Model

**Grand Theories**
Leninger's Theory of Culture Care
    Diversity & Universality
Newman's Theory of Health
    & Expanding Consciousness
Parse's Theory of Human Goal Attainment

**Middle-Range Theories**
King's Theory of Becoming

**Middle-Range Theories**
Orlando's Theory of Deliberative Nursing Process
Peplau's Theory of Interpersonal Relations
Watson's Theory of Human Caring
Modeling and Role Modeling Theory
Mercer's Maternal Role Attainment Theory

**Figure 3-3**    **Structural hierarchy of contemporary nursing knowledge components.** *Based on information from Meleis, A. I. (1997). Theoretical nursing: Development and progress (3rd ed.). Philadelphia: Lippincott*

the idea that nursing research would be the key factor in helping nursing to emerge as a true profession. The research done regarding these common needs and problems has served as a foundation for the development of what is now known as nursing diagnoses.

## Joyce Travelbee

Joyce Travelbee, an educator and psychiatric nurse, was influenced by the philosophy of **existentialism**, a movement centered on individual existence in an incomprehensible world and the role that free will plays in it, and she searched to find meaning in life's experiences. She extensively developed the ideas of sympathy, empathy, and rap-

port in which the nurse could begin to comprehend and relate to the uniqueness of others. Her work focused on the human-to-human relationship and on finding meaning in experiences such as pain, illness, and distress. Travelbee based most of her theory on her own experiences and readings and first published her work in *Interpersonal Aspects of Nursing* in 1966.

## Josephine Paterson and Loretta Zderad

The work of Josephine Paterson and Loretta Zderad was similar to that of Travelbee in that it emphasized the humanistic and existential basis of nursing practice.

## NURSING STRATEGY

### Applying Nursing Theories

To become comfortable with nursing theories, consider the following activities:

- Study the various nursing theorists, and find the one who most likely fits your philosophy of nursing.

- As you develop nursing interventions, assess their application from different nursing models.

- Several nursing theories have nursing societies or organizations. Attend a nursing conference sponsored by one of these societies.

Adapted from Meleis, A. I. (1997). *Theoretical nursing: Development and progress* (3rd ed.). Philadelphia: Lippincott.

## LIFE SPAN CONSIDERATIONS

### Nursing Theory and the Aged

Nursing theories cover clients of all age groups. For the pediatric client, caregivers are included in the theory, such as Mercer's Maternal Role Attainment Theory. Geriatric clients are adults; however, Levine's Conservation Model and Roy's Adaptation Model easily speak to the modifications necessary for the older adult.

---

According to Paterson and Zderad (1976), theory developed from the practice of nursing. Although the models proposed by Travelbee and Paterson and Zderad had some impact at the time of their initial introduction, they did not gain wide popularity and application in nursing. Current theorists, such as Watson, Rogers, Parse, Fitzpatrick, and Newman (who have an existential orientation), are rediscovering the merits of Travelbee and Paterson and Zderad.

## Contemporary Nursing Theories

Although early nursing theorists attempted to answer the question "What is nursing?", contemporary theorists addressed the metaparadigm concepts in more depth, focused more specifically on nursing actions, and tried to answer the question "When is nursing needed?" The work of contemporary theorists such as Myra Levine, Dorothea Orem, and Sister Callista Roy form the theoretical basis for many interventions in current nursing practice.

### Myra Levine

Myra Levine's Conservation Model is directly grounded in nursing practice. In her attempt to describe, explain, and predict phenomena of concern to nursing, Levine published the four conservation principles in 1969 in *Introduction to Clinical Nursing.* Conservation is derived from the Latin word "to keep together." Levine believed in the wholeness of the human being, and the primary focus of conservation is to maintain that wholeness. Levine viewed nursing as assisting clients with the conservation of their uniqueness by helping them to adapt appropriately. Conservation principles (Box 3-1) are universal princi-

ples designed to link concepts into a cohesive framework within which nursing practice can be performed in different environments (Levine, 1991).

According to Levine, the *person* is who the person knows himself or herself to be and the *environment* is the context in which the person lives his or her life. In Levine's view, *health* is socially defined and the goal of *nursing* is based on the four conservation principles. Levine did not operationally define and relate the metaparadigm concepts in her theory, because her original work was initially intended to be a medical-surgical nursing textbook and not a developed nursing theory. In reevaluating her theory 20 years later, Levine stated that she has "grown in [her] conviction that they [the conservation principles] continue to offer an approach to nursing that is scientific, research oriented, and above all suitable in daily practice in many environments" (Levine, 1989, p. 331).

A nurse who is involved in acute care situations such as an emergency room or intensive care unit often deals with clients who are exposed to severe threats to physiological integrity. The conservation of structural integrity is often the immediate priority in these acute care situations. For example, when a nurse in an emergency room is dealing with a client who has been in a severe motor vehicle accident, the client's structural integrity is at risk. When the client's structural integrity has been damaged, the client must put all available energy into healing the self. The nurse tries to provide care for that client so the client can conserve energy for the processes of healing. In addition to a threat to structural integrity, this client has other needs as well. The client has social relationships, which are also disrupted by the accident. The nurse is concerned with the client's significant other and family who are part of the social unit. Even in this time of crisis in the emergency room, the client's social integrity is of concern. Finally, the nurse is also concerned about the client's personal integrity because the traumatic experience and necessary treatment can be frightening and dehumanizing. As the nurse strives to maintain the client's structural, social, and personal integrity, the nurse recognizes that the client is a unique individual.

## BOX 3-1    LEVELS OF EVIDENCE

Levine's Four Principles of Conservation

1. **Conservation of energy:** "The individual requires a balance of energy and a constant renewal of energy to maintain life activities" (Levine, 1989, p. 197).

2. **Conservation of Structural Integrity:** "Structural integrity is concerned with the processes of healing . . . to restore wholeness and continuity after injury or illness" (Levine, 1989, p. 333).

3. **Conservation of Personal Integrity:** "Everyone seeks to defend his or her identity as a self, in both that hidden, intensely private person that dwells within and in the public faces assumed as individuals move through their relationships with others" (Levine, 1989, p. 334).

4. **Conservation of Social Integrity:** "No diagnosis should be made that does not include the other persons whose lives are entwined with that of the individual" (Levine, 1989, p. 336).

Adapted from Levine, M. E. (1989). The four conservation principles: 20 years later. In J. Riehl-Sisca (Ed.), *Conceptual models for nursing practice* (3rd ed.). Stamford, CT: Appleton & Lange.

Levine's four conservation principles can also be useful in a home setting in which the family rather than a single individual is the client. The nurse recognizes that energy within the family needs to be maintained to keep the family whole. In caring for the family, the nurse needs to maintain the structural, social, and personal integrity of the family and of each individual while dealing with the illness of a specific family member. Consider, for example, the nurse who makes a home health visit to see a child with cystic fibrosis. In this situation, the nurse's attention needs to be directed toward conservation of energy for the child. To help conserve the child's energy for breathing, exercises must be taught to and done by others. The nurse directs strategies toward conserving the child's structural integrity while recognizing that the child is both a unique individual and a member of a social group, the family. Conservation of social integrity would be accomplished through maintaining interest in and monitoring the family dynamics.

Levine is pragmatic, and the conservation principles can be applied to most nursing situations. Her theory is appropriate for use in situations where the nurse has had a long-term relationship with the client, yet it is also useful for short-term relationships.

## Dorothea Orem

In attempting to plan a nursing curriculum for licensed practical nurses, Dorothea Orem was searching for a pragmatic framework to organize nursing knowledge. She focused on the questions "What is nursing?" and "When do people need nursing care?", and from these questions she derived that people need nursing when they are unable to care for themselves. In 1971, she presented the Self-Care Deficit Theory of Nursing (S-CDTN) in the book *Nursing Concepts of Practice* and has continually revised and updated her theory.

Orem's theory incorporates the medical model rather than rejects it, centers on the individual, is problem oriented, and is easily adaptable in varied clinical situations. These attributes create its wide appeal for application in nursing practice. Meleis (1997, p. 400) stated that it has "the widest circle of all theories in practice." As a grand theory, the S-CDTN has three interconnecting theories: Theory of Self-Care, Theory of Self-Care Deficit, and Theory of Nursing Systems.

### Theory of Self-Care

According to this theory, **self-care** is a learned behavior and a deliberate action in response to a need. Orem identified three categories of self-care requisites: universal self-care requisites, developmental self-care requisites, and health-deviation self-care requisites. Universal self-care requisites are common to all human beings and include both physiological and social interaction needs. Developmental self-care requisites are the needs that arise as the individual grows and develops. Health-deviation self-care requisites result from the needs produced by disease or illness states. Self-care is performed by mature and maturing individuals. When someone else must perform a self-care need, it is termed dependent care.

### Theory of Self-Care Deficit

Orem's theory purports that nursing care is needed when people are affected by limitations that do not allow them to meet their self-care needs. The relationship between the nurse and the client is established when a self-care deficit is

    **STOP AND THINK**

### Applying Orem's Nursing Theory

Miss Taylor is a 25-year-old nursing assistant. She is currently hospitalized for problems with her diabetes. While answering questions in a nursing history, Miss Taylor states, "I have been unable to buy my insulin this month. I have no way of monitoring my sugar levels."

Why is Orem's theory a good theoretical model to guide you in responding to this client's needs?

present. Self-care deficits, not medical diagnosis, determine the need for nursing care. According to Orem, the only legitimate reasons for nursing care are self-care deficits.

## Theory of Nursing Systems

This is the unifying theory that subsumes the theory of self-care deficit and with it, the theory of self-care. The Theory of Nursing Systems attempts to answer the question "What do nurses do?" This was the original question that prompted the development of Orem's theory.

The nurse determines whether or not there is a legitimate need for nursing care. Is a person able to meet self-care needs? Does a deficit exist? If a deficit exists, then the nurse plans care that identifies what is to be done by whom: the nurse, the client, or other (family or significant other). Collectively, the actions of all these people are called the nursing system. Orem identified three types of nursing systems: wholly compensatory, partly compensatory, and supportive-educative.

In the wholly compensatory nursing system, the nurse supports and protects the client, compensates for the client's inability to care for self, and attempts to provide care for the client. The nurse would use the wholly compensatory nursing system when caring for a newborn or with a client recovering from surgery in a postanesthesia care unit. Both of these clients are completely unable to provide self-care.

In the partly compensatory nursing system, both the nurse and client perform care measures. For example, the nurse can assist the postoperative client to ambulate. The nurse may bring in a meal tray for the client who can feed his- or herself. The nurse compensates for what the client cannot do. The client can perform selected self-care activities, but also accepts care performed by the nurse for needs the client cannot meet independently.

In the supportive-educative nursing system, the nurse's actions are to help clients develop their own self-care abilities through knowledge, support, and encouragement. Clients must learn and perform their own self-care activities. The supportive-educative nursing system is being used when a nurse guides a new mother to breastfeed her baby. Counseling a psychiatric client on more adaptive coping strategies is another example of the use of the supportive-educative nursing system.

Orem focused primarily on the needs of the person and the action nursing takes to meet those needs. Lesser emphasis was given to defining health and the environment. The S-CDTN is useful in determining the kind of nursing assistance needed by the client and, therefore, has merit as a theory that guides nursing practice.

## Sister Callista Roy

Sister Callista Roy combined general systems theory with adaptation theory to produce the Roy Adaptation Model (Roy, 1976). Roy was greatly influenced by her teacher and mentor, Dorothy E. Johnson, a nursing theorist who developed the Behavioral Systems Model. Roy first published her model in 1976 and has continued to further refine and develop the theory. As a contemporary theorist, Roy worked with defining and relating the metaparadigm concepts.

Roy defines a person as "an adaptive system . . . a whole comprised of parts that function as a unity for some purpose" (Roy & Andrews, 1991, p. 4). The person is a biopsychosocial being in constant interaction with a changing internal and external environment. Nursing attempts to alter the environment when the person is not adapting well or has ineffective coping responses.

"The world around and within (the person as an adaptive system) is called the environment" and "includes all conditions, circumstances, and influences that surround and affect the development and behaviors of the person" (Roy & Andrews, 1991, p. 18). The *environmental stimuli* can be classified as either focal, residual, or contextual. *Focal stimuli* are immediately present in the person's environment. Focal stimuli are the objects or events that most attract one's attention. Most stimuli never become focal. *Residual stimuli* are attitudes developed during previous experiences in one's life whose effects on the current situation are unclear. *Contextual stimuli* are "all the other stimuli present in the situation that contribute to the effect of the focal stimulus" (Roy & Andrews, 1991, p. 9). Because stimuli are constantly changing, a stimulus that is focal one minute can become residual the next.

According to the Roy Adaptation Model, the person has coping mechanisms that are broadly categorized in either the regulator or cognator subsystem. Adaptation is accomplished through these coping mechanisms that are innate, "genetically determined . . . and automatic processes" (Roy & Andrews, 1991, p. 13). The *regulator subsystem* functions through the autonomic nervous system, which "responds automatically through neural, chemical, and endocrine coping process" (Roy & Andrews, 1991, p. 14). The *cognator subsystem* enables the person to respond to stimuli through processing stimuli, learning, judgment, and emotion. All input into the system (the person) is channeled through the regulator and cognator subsystems. If the regulator or cognator subsystem fails, there is ineffective adaptation.

Neither the regulator nor the cognator subsystem can be observed directly. Only their responses are observable. Roy categorized these responses into four adaptive modes: physiological, self-concept, role function, and interdependence. The *physiological mode* allows individuals to respond physiologically to their environment. The *self-concept mode* "focuses on psychologic and spiritual aspects of the person" (Roy & Andrews, 1991, p. 16). The basic underlying need of the self-concept mode is psychological integrity. The *role function mode* focuses on the need to know who one is at core. The emphasis of the *interdependence mode* is affectional adequacy or the feeling of security in nurturing relationships.

The purposes of adaptation are survival, growth, reproduction, and mastery. "Adaptive responses contribute to these goals, whereas ineffective responses may threaten the person's survival, growth, reproduction, or mastery" (Roy & Andrews, 1991).

The goal of nursing is "the promotion of adaptation in each of the four modes, thereby contributing to the person's health, quality of life, and dying with dignity" (Roy & Andrews, 1991, p. 20). Nursing care needs to be provided when a person has unusual stressors or when usual coping mechanisms are ineffective. Basically, the nurse attempts to manipulate stimuli in such a way as to allow the client to cope effectively. Roy defines health as "a state and a process of being and becoming an integrated and whole person" and says further that a "lack of integration represents lack of health" (Roy & Andrews, 1991, p. 419).

In Roy's view, the nurse must first assess how the client behaves in each adaptive mode and then determine what can be altered in that mode to produce more efficient and effective adaptive responses. The nurse either alters the environment directly or helps the person to alter the environment for better adaptive responses.

In the physiological mode, problems may arise in areas such as exercise, nutrition, elimination, fluid and electrolytes, temperature regulation, and oxygenation. For example, in caring for a client with a fever, the nurse helps the client to adapt by administering medications to lower the temperature, administering cool baths, and providing adequate fluids. Through these interventions, the nurse is attempting to alter both the internal and external environments of the person.

In the self-concept mode, the term *self-concept* refers to both the physical self and the personal self. The physical self is affected or threatened during invasive procedures such as surgery. Anxiety, guilt, and distress are responses within the personal self to physical or emotional stressors. For example, in caring for an obese person who feels guilty developing diabetes at an early age, a nurse can help reframe the client's thinking to work through the guilt and anxiety. Through the use of counseling tech-

niques, the nurse can teach the client how to adapt to the present situation and learn to cope with it in the future.

Within the framework of the role function mode, the nurse would help a woman disabled with arthritis to identify adaptive approaches to maintain the roles of wife and homemaker. Nursing actions might include referral to occupational therapy for needed adaptive devices that could assist the client in maintenance of roles.

In the interdependence mode, problems may include feelings of alienation, disengagement, loneliness, or disenfranchisement experienced in various relationships. Examples of clients with problems in interdependence may include a grieving widow or a person with an abusive spouse.

The Roy Adaptation Model has gained wide acceptance in nursing practice, research, and education and is part of the dominant worldview of nursing.

## Theories for the New Worldview of Nursing

Theories for the new worldview of nursing describe, explain, and predict the phenomena of concern to nursing from a unique, more holistic perspective. In the new worldview, the client has primacy and the client-environment interaction is of utmost importance. Theories by Jean Watson, Martha Rogers, and Rosemarie Parse exemplify the new worldview.

### Jean Watson

In the 1980s, Jean Watson developed the Theory of Human Caring, which focuses on the art and science of human caring. According to Watson (1985, p. 33), "caring is the essence of nursing and the most central and unifying focus of nursing practice." This theory offers a new way of conceptualizing and maximizing human-to-human transactions that occur daily in nursing practice. Watson's theory is influenced by Eastern philosophy and is "based on a metaphysical, spiritual-existential, and phenomenological orientation" (Fawcett, 1993, p. 220). These influences link Watson's theory to the work of early theorists such as Travelbee and Paterson and Zderad.

The Theory of Human Caring evolved from Watson's beliefs, values, and assumptions about caring. In Watson's view (1985), care and love comprise the primal universal psychic energy and are the basis for people's humanity. Watson noted that throughout its history nursing has been involved in caring and has actually evolved out of caring. Furthermore, she stated that caring will determine nursing's contribution to the humanization of the world.

Watson's theory is composed of ten carative factors, which are classified as nursing actions or processes. Watson's carative factors are listed in Box 3-2. The first three carative factors serve as the philosophical foundation for the science of caring. The remaining seven provide more specific direction for nursing actions.

Watson stated that "health refers to unity and harmony within the mind, body, and soul. Health is also associated with the degree of congruence between the self as perceived and the self as experienced" (Watson, 1985, p. 48). In Watson's view (1985, p. 49), the goal of nursing "is to help a person gain a higher degree of harmony with the mind, body, and soul." The nurse uses the above carative factors to accomplish the goal of nursing.

Although the concept of caring is being de-emphasized in today's health care environment because of exploding technology and cost-containment strategies, nursing must persevere in delivering care to clients. The challenge of nursing is to create moments of caring through human-to-human interaction in the face of the fast-paced world of health care.

## Martha Rogers

Martha Rogers, a visionary leader and pioneer in the development of nursing's unique knowledge base, developed the highly abstract theory of the Science of Unitary Human Beings. According to Rogers, "nursing is a learned profession: a science and an art. A science is an organized body of abstract knowledge. The art involved in nursing is the creative use of science for human betterment" (Rogers, 1990, p. 198). Rogers' contribution to the discipline of nursing was revolutionary and provided new directions for the practice of nursing. Rogers first presented her ideas in the book *An Introduction to the Theoretical Basis of Nursing* (1970). Her ideas regarding the person and the environment as energy fields were not considered to be consistent with the dominant paradigm of the 1970s.

According to Rogers (1990, p. 108), "the uniqueness of nursing is identified in the phenomena of concern. Nursing is the study of unitary, irreducible human beings and their respective environments." The unitary person is an irreducible pandimensional energy field characterized by pattern and expressing qualities that are unique to the whole and cannot be foreseen from knowledge of the parts (Rogers, 1990). Environment is defined as "an irreducible pandimensional energy field identified by pattern and integral with a given human field" (Rogers, 1990, p. 109).

Within the viewpoint of the Science of Unitary Human beings, the person is a unified whole and is seen as greater than the sum of the parts. The whole person cannot be known by examining any particular aspect or dimension of the person, because all aspects combine together to form an entity different from the collection of parts. It is the characterization of the person as a human energy field that unites all aspects of the person into a unified whole. The whole of the person's energy field interacts with the whole of the environmental energy field, which results in the process of life. There is a constant exchange of matter and energy between the person-environment unit, yet the uniqueness of each person is maintained through rhythmical patterns and relationships. In a worldview where person and environment are in a constant, dynamic, simultaneous process of change, the concept of homeostasis is obsolete.

Nursing identifies the patterns and organization of the person-environment unit and aims to repattern the rhythm and organization of these energy fields so that the person's integrity is heightened. "Maintenance and promotion of health, prevention of disease, nursing diagnosis, intervention, and rehabilitation encompass the scope of nursing's goals" (Rogers, 1970, p. 86).

## Rosemarie Parse

Rosemarie Parse synthesized Rogers' Science of Unitary Human Beings with existential-phenomenological

---

### BOX 3-2   WATSON'S CARATIVE FACTORS

1. Formation of a humanistic-altruistic system of values

2. Nurturing of faith-hope

3. Cultivation of sensitivity to one's self and to others

4. Developing a helping-trusting, human caring relationship

5. Promotion and acceptance of the expression of positive and negative feelings

6. Use of creative problem-solving method processes

7. Promotion of transpersonal teaching and learning

8. Provision for a supportive, protective, or corrective mental, physical, sociocultural, and spiritual environment

9. Assistance with gratification of human needs

10. Allowance for existential-phenomenological forces

Watson, J. (1985). *Nursing: Human science and human care, a theory of nursing.* East Norwalk, CT: Appleton-Century-Crofts.

## STOP AND THINK

### Choosing a Nursing Theory

● What nursing theory best describes your understanding of nursing practice?

● How do your standards of nursing practice relate to the various nursing theories?

philosophy and added emphasis on the meaning and values that influence a person's behavioral choices (Parse, 1981). Parse differs from Rogers in that she "does not view Man as an energy field, but rather as an open being who cocreates personal health" (Parse, 1987, p. 159). According to Leddy and Pepper (1993, p. 170), health is a "constantly changing process of becoming that incorporates values. Because it is not a state, health cannot be contrasted with disease." Parse (1987, p. 169) states that "the practice of nursing . . . is a subject-to-subject interrelationship, a loving, true presence with the other to promote health and quality of life." Parse provides a

practice methodology in which the nurse helps clients understand their own feelings and situation, find meaning within themselves and the situation, and plan for changes in the lived health patterns. In Parse's perspective, the nurse does things *with* people, as opposed to *for* them or *to* them.

## Nursing Theory and Standards of Practice

Standards of clinical practice (American Nurses Association, 1998) are developed out of nursing theories. Nursing research guided by nursing theory assists in identifying safe practices. Practice and standards are set by nursing organizations, such as American Nurses Association (ANA), American Association of Critical Care Nurses (AACN), and Association of Operating Room Nurses (AORN). The ANA Code of Ethics (2001) defines the ethical duties of nursing (see Chapter 9). Recently updated to reflect the changes in nursing and health care, the ANA Code of Ethics specifically addresses such issues as professional relationships, the nurse's primary commitment to the client, accountability, integrity, collaboration, and advancement of the profession.

### BOX 3-3    THE 11 FUNCTIONAL HEALTH PATTERNS

The following are the 11 functional health patterns:

1. **Health perception and health management:** What the individual perceives health to be, and how the person takes care of him- or herself

2. **Values/Beliefs:** What the individual values and believes, includes religious and ethnic practices

3. **Elimination:** Bodily functions of elimination

4. **Nutrition/Metabolic:** Assessment of energy needs and how those needs are supplied

5. **Activity/Exercise:** Mobility/ability of muscles to function

6. **Roles/Relationships:** Roles and relationships that each individual has

7. **Cognition/Perception:** Deals with both level of consciousness and sensory perceptions such as sight and hearing

8. **Sexuality/Reproduction:** Self-description of sexuality and reproductive function

9. **Self-perception/Self-concept:** How do the individuals see themselves; what is the individual's concept of self?

10. **Coping/Stress Tolerance:** Assesses the individual's ability to deal with stress; what mechanisms does the individual use—are they effective?

11. **Sleep/Rest:** Assessment of the individual's ability to sleep and provide enough rest to continue with routine functioning

Gordon, M. (2000). *Manual of Nursing Diagnosis*, 9th ed. St. Louis, MO: Mosby.

# Functional Health Patterns as a "Theory" That Guides Practice

From a practice standpoint, middle-range theories serve to explain and guide nursing care. The influence of Maslow's Hierarchy of Human Needs (1970) and Von Bartlaffny's General Systems Theory (1968) can be seen in Gordon's **Functional Health Patterns** (1994). The premise of Functional Health Patterns (FHP) is a systematic holistic approach to evaluate all areas of human needs, recognizing that the needs are interdependent. Gordon's FHP are integrated into this textbook as described in Section II with Chapters 32–48. The rationale for choosing Gordon's FHP is its nursing focus and practical nursing approach to client care. The 11 functional health patterns provide a very appropriate method for organizing the topics of client care necessary in this fundamentals nursing textbook. From the FHP assessment, the nurse is able to develop specific nursing diagnoses and a nursing plan of care. The 11 FHP incorporate physical and psychosocial assessments of the individuals, families, groups in both subjective and objective infor-

mation. Box 3-3 explains the FHP. A schematic of the FHP is found in Figure 3-4.

# Continuing Evolution of Nursing Theory

Current theorists are continually expanding and refining the work of theorists before them, and they are developing new ways of looking at the metaparadigm concepts of person, environment, health, and nursing. The nature of nursing is and always has been in a state of change. Although change is healthy and leads to growth, it is not always easy. Knowledge is not static, and what one learns today may be challenged by different thoughts tomorrow.

The world of health care changes on a daily basis. Client needs and problems often change on a minute-by-minute basis. Knowledge, information, and technology in both health care and nursing are growing at unprecedented rates. In the face of these advances, nursing strives to preserve *the notion of caring* in health care. Theories are needed to organize knowledge and to guide nursing practice and nursing research. More nursing research is needed

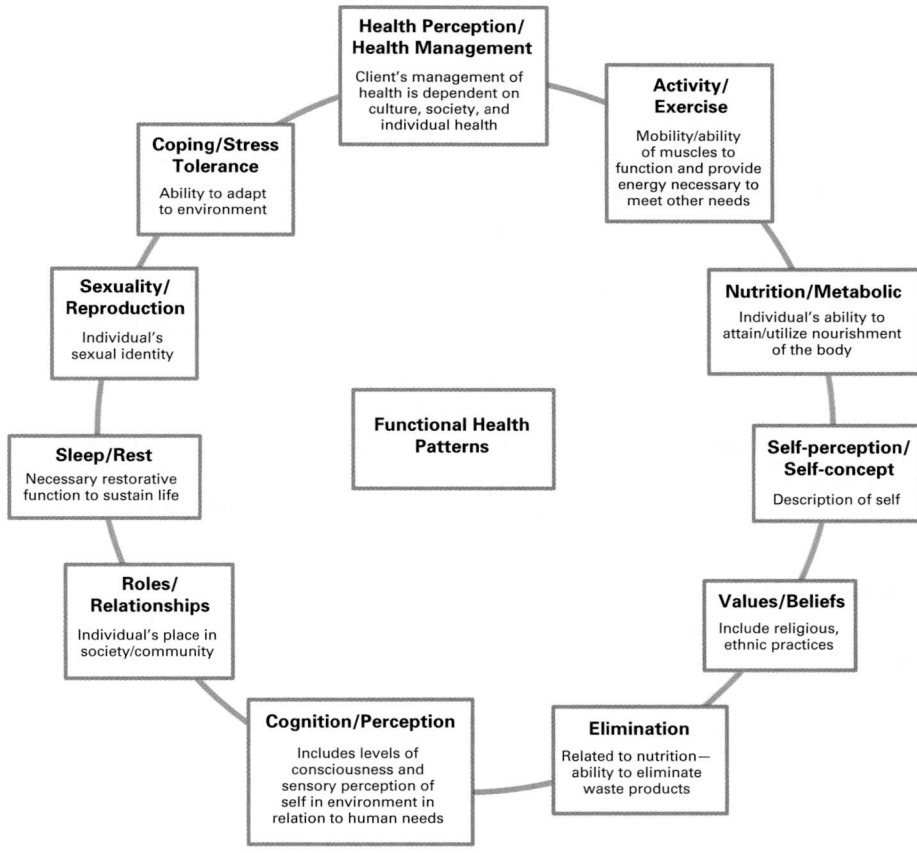

**Figure 3-4    Schematic of Functional Health Patterns.** *Based on information from Gordon, M. (2000). Manual of Nursing Diagnosis (9th ed.). St. Louis: Mosby.*

to confirm or refute theories. A strong theoretical foundation on which to base the practice of nursing is essential.

Nurses encounter a variety of clinical situations in which application of nursing theory is needed. In these occurrences, nurses may discover that specific theories will be more appropriate for certain clinical situations than others. Knowledge of specific theories should expand as nurses gain experience in nursing practice. Theories that are selected for application in practice should be congruent with the nurse's own beliefs and values.

With the advent of modern nursing under Florence Nightingale, nursing knowledge has expanded in multiple ways. Not only are there theories upon which to understand the profession, but there are theories to guide and direct nursing practice and research. Over the past 150 plus years, nursing leaders have consistently looked for ways to improve care for clients.

Nursing theory defines and guides the nursing profession. Starting with Nightingale, theory has been a continuum that reflects the times in which nursing is practiced. With the evolving changes in the 21st century, nursing theory will also change. Middle-range theories will be more fully developed to assist in the understanding of clinical practice. New theorists will come from a global perspective, and international nursing leaders will have great influence on nursing theory in the 21st century.

## FOCUS ON WELLNESS

### Functional Health Patterns and a Wellness Focus

Julie Wassersmith, RN, is preparing to talk to Mr. Sanchez regarding his discharge instructions after inguinal hernia surgery. Julie is interested in including a wellness focus during his discharge experience. Her instructions include diet, exercise, and return-to-work recommendations. Julie reviews Mr. Sanchez's FHP assessment and discovers that he visits the gym three times a week; eats three meals a day, including purchasing lunch in the workplace cafeteria; and is employed as a warehouse stocker, which requires lifting 50 or more pounds on a routine basis. With this information, Julie is able to assist Mr. Sanchez in making realistic plans for his gym work (gradual return to routine workout), diet (consider bringing a "healthy" lunch), and work expectations (avoid lifting more than 10 to 15 pounds for 3 to 6 weeks). Nurse Wassersmith evaluates her plan of care and concludes the wellness focus has been met.

# CASE STUDY/NURSING CARE PLAN

Mrs. Evans came to the emergency room complaining of chest pain unrelieved by nitroglycerin (NTG) and rest. She was admitted to the telemetry unit with congestive heart failure. During the physical exam, the nurse discovers that Mrs. Evans has a history of three previous heart attacks prior to triple bypass surgery 5 years ago. Over the past year, she has had an increase in shortness of breath, chest pain, and fatigue. She complains of being unable to socialize with family and friends or to complete her housework without several 10- to 20-minute rest periods. Her physical exam reveals bibasilar rales, pale skin, and capillary refill of >3 sec.

## Assessment
This client has a history of cardiac disease with an increase in chest pain, fatigue, and shortness of breath. The physical exam's results of rales in the lungs and pale skin with decreased capillary refill indicate problems with oxygenation and tissue perfusion. The client's expressed concern about social function and daily living activities indicate a need for conservation measures. Levine's Conservation Model will be a good fit as a plan of care is implemented.

## Nursing Diagnosis #1
Activity intolerance as related to imbalance between oxygen supply and demand, as evidenced by complaints of shortness of breath, chest pain, need for frequent rest periods during activities, and an inability to complete household activities
**NOC:** Endurance; Energy Conservation; Activity Tolerance; Self-Care Activities of Daily Living
**NIC:** Energy Management; Activity Therapy

## Expected Outcomes
The client will:
1. No longer complain of shortness of breath upon discharge to home

*(continues)*

# CASE STUDY/NURSING CARE PLAN (continued)

2. Have no episodes of chest pain upon discharge to home
3. Be able to complete household activities within 1 week of discharge

## Planning/Interventions/Rationales

1. Review therapeutic regimen with client (e.g., medications, activities, rest periods). Following therapeutic regimen, such as taking medications to improve cardiac function and to increase urinary output, decreases and eliminates shortness of breath and chest pain. *Preserves structural integrity.*
2. Assist client in planning rest periods during periods of physical activity, such as when carrying out household duties. *Allows for conservation of energy to complete activities with decreased stress and anxiety.*
3. Assess client's ability to employ household help, or refer to home health agencies for assistance with household activities that client is unable to complete. *Preserves personal integrity.*

## Evaluation

Client experienced no shortness of breath or chest pain and is following therapeutic regimen at home. Client took rest periods at least every 3 to 4 hours and was able to complete household chores within the first week of discharge home.

## Nursing Diagnosis #2

Fatigue as related to disease state (congestive heart failure) as evidenced by complaints of inability to complete household activities and an inability to maintain family and social functions
**NOC:** Endurance; Concentration; Nutritional Status; Energy; Energy Conservation
**NIC:** Energy Management

## Expected Outcomes

The client will:
1. State her energy levels are greater in 1 week and will be able to complete household activities within 1 week.
2. Allow family and friends to visit her at home and will make arrangements to socialize within 2 weeks of discharge.

## Planning/Interventions/Rationales

1. Teach energy-saving techniques for daily-living activities and household duties. *Conservation of energy allows client to complete activities with decreased anxiety and to consider other activities of life.*
2. Assess family and social support system (e.g., church groups, social groups), and plan activities that the client can participate in with decreased energy expenditure. *Preserves both personal and social integrity of the client.*

## Evaluation

Client completed daily-living activities and household duties within 1 week of discharge and states her energy level is higher than when first discharged home. Client went to church in first week and also invited family members to her home for dessert the second week of discharge.

# Key Concepts

- The components of theoretical foundations are concepts, propositions, and theories.
- Nonnursing theories such as Maslow's Hierarchy of Human Needs further define and clarify nursing theories and nursing practice.
- Multiple nursing theories define nursing practice. Grand theories, such as Orem's Self-Care Deficit Theory of Nursing, are applicable across multiple areas of nursing. Middle-range theories, such as Benner's Model of Skills Acquisition and Mercer's Maternal Role Attainment Theory, assist the nurse in planning client care.
- Four major concepts are defined within nursing theories: person, health, environment, and nursing.
- Florence Nightingale's concepts of nursing practice were very influential to nursing theory development.
- Knowledge development in nursing is founded on the impact of metaparadigm and paradigm concepts.
- The early nursing theorists are Peplau, Henderson, Abdellah, Travelbee, and Paterson and Zderad.
- The contemporary nursing theorists are Levine, Orem, and Roy.

- The new worldview nursing theorists are Watson, Rogers, and Parse.
- Functional health patterns make up a holistic system that can be utilized to assess an individual, family, group, or community.
- Nursing theory continues to evolve into the 21st century.

## Review Questions and Activities

1. Define concepts and propositions. How are concepts and propositions related to theory?
2. How have nonnursing theories influenced the development of nursing theories?
3. What is the purpose of nursing theory?
4. Describe the relationship between nursing theory, practice, and research.
5. Identify and define the four metaparadigm concepts in nursing.
6. How has Florence Nightingale influenced modern nursing theory?
7. How do nursing theories influence standards of nursing practice?
8. Define Functional Health Patterns as a middle-range theory.

## Web Resources

American Nurses Association
   http://www.nursingworld.org
Nursing Diagnosis (North American Nursing Diagnosis Association)
   http://www.nanda.org

## References

Abdellah, F. G. (1960). *Patient-centered approaches to nursing.* New York: Macmillan.

American Nurses Association (1998). *Standards of clinical practice* (2nd ed.). Washington, DC: Author.

Barnum, B. J. S. (1998). *Nursing theory: Analysis, application, evaluation.*(5th ed.). Philadelphia: Lippincott.

Benner, P. (1984). *From novice to expert: Excellence and power in clinical nursing practice.* Menlo Park, CA: Addison-Wesley.

Carper, B. (1978). Fundamental patterns of knowing. *Advances in Nursing Science, 1*(1), 13–23.

Chinn, R. L., & Kramer, M. K. (1999). *Theory and nursing: Integrated knowledge and development* (5th ed.). St. Louis, MO: Mosby.

DeLaune, S., & Ladner, P. (2002). *Fundamentals of Nursing* (2nd ed.). Clifton Park, NY: Delmar Learning.

Erickson, H., Tomlin, E., & Swain, M. (1983). *Modeling and role-modeling: A theory and paradigm for nursing.* Englewood Cliffs, NJ: Appleton & Lange.

Estes, M. (2002). *Health Assessment & Physical Examination* (2nd ed.). Clifton Park, NY: Delmar Learning.

Fawcett, J. (1984). The metaparadigm of nursing. Current status and future refinements. *Image: Journal of Nursing Scholarship, 16,* 84–87.

Fawcett, J. (1989). *Analysis and evaluation of conceptual models of nursing* (2nd ed.). Philadelphia: F. A. Davis.

Fawcett, J. (1993). *Analysis and evolution of nursing theories.* Philadelphia: F. A. Davis.

Fawcett, J. (1999). *The relationship of theory and research* (3rd ed.). Philadelphia: F. A. Davis.

Fawcett, J. (2000). *Analysis and evaluation of contemporary nursing knowledge: Nursing models and theories.* Philadelphia: F. A. Davis.

Fitzpatrick, J. J., & Whall, A. L. (1996). *Conceptual models of nursing: Analysis and application* (3rd ed.). Stamford, CT: Appleton & Lange.

Gordon, M. (1994). *Nursing diagnosis: Process and application* (3rd ed.). St. Louis, MO: Mosby.

Gordon, M. (2000). *Manual of Nursing Diagnosis,* 9th ed. St. Louis, MO: Mosby.

Hall, L.E. (1964). Nursing: What is it? *Canadian Nurse, 60,* 150–154.

Harmer, B., & Henderson, V. (1955). *Textbook of the principles and practice of nursing.* New York: Macmillan.

Henderson, V. (1966). *The nature of nursing: A definition and its implications for practice, research, and education.* New York: Macmillan.

Johnson, D. (1976). Behavioral systems and nursing.

King, I. (1971). *Toward a theory for nursing: General concepts of human behavior.* New York: John Wiley & Sons.

Kuhn, T. (1970). *The structure of scientific revolutions* (2nd ed.). Chicago: The University of Chicago Press.

Leddy, S., & Pepper, J. M. (1993). *Conceptual basis of professional nursing* (3rd ed.). Philadelphia: Lippincott Williams & Willkins.

Leininger, M. M. (1978). *Transcultural nursing: Concepts, theories, and practice.* New York: John Wiley & Sons.

Levine, M. E. (1969). *Introduction to clinical nursing.* Philadelphia: F. A. Davis.

Levine, M. E. (1989). The four conservation principles: 20 years later. In J. Riehl-Sisca (Ed.), *Conceptual models for nursing practice* (3rd ed.). Stamford, CT: Appleton & Lange.

Levine, M. E. (1991). The conservation model: A model for health. In K. M. Schaefer & J. B. Pond (Eds.), *The conservation model: A framework for nursing practice* (pp. 1–11). Philadelphia: F. A. Davis.

Levine, M. E. (1995). The rhetoric of nursing theory. *Image: Journal of Nursing Scholarship, 27,* 11–24.

Maslow, A. H. (1970). *Motivation and personality* (2nd ed.). New York: Harper & Row.

McEwen, M., & Wills, E. M. (2002). *Theoretical basis for nursing*. Philadelphia: Lippincott Williams & Wilkins.

Meleis, A. I. (1997). *Theoretical nursing: Development and progress* (3rd ed.). Philadelphia: Lippincott.

Mercer, R. T. (1981). A theoretical framework for studying factors that impact on the maternal role. *Nursing Research, 30*, 73–77.

Neuman, B. (1980). The Betty Neuman health-care systems model: A total person approach to patient problems. In J. P. Riehl & C. Roy (Eds.), *Conceptual models for nursing practice* (2nd ed., pp. 119–134). Norwalk, CT: Appleton-Century-Crofts.

Newman, M. A. (1979). *Theory development in nursing*. Philadelphia: F. A. Davis.

Nightingale, F. (1859). *Nursing: What it is and what it is not*. London: Harrison & Sons.

Norris, J., Kunes-Connell, M., & Spelic, S. S. (1998). A grounded theory of reimaging. *Advances in Nursing Science, 20*(3), 1–12.

Orem, D. E. (1971). *Nursing: Concepts of practice*. New York: McGraw-Hill.

Orlando, I. J. (1961). *The dynamic nurse-patient relationship: Function, process, and principles*. New York: G. P. Putnam.

Parse, R. R. (1981). *Man-Living-Health: A theory of nursing*. Clifton Park, NY: Delmar Learning.

Parse, R. R. (1987). *Nursing science: Major paradigms, theories, and critiques*. Philadelphia: Saunders.

Paterson, J. G., & Zderad, L. T. (1976). *Humanistic nursing*. New York: Wiley.

Peplau, H. E. (1952). *Interpersonal relations in nursing: A conceptual frame of reference for psychodynamic nursing*. New York: G. P. Putnam's Sons.

Polk, L. V. (1997). Towards a middle-range theory of resilience. *Advances in Nursing Science, 19*(3), 1–13.

Rogers, M. E. (1970). *An introduction to the theoretical basis of nursing*. Philadelphia: F. A. Davis.

Rogers, M. E. (1990). Nursing: Science of unitary, irreducible human beings: Update 1990. In E. Barrett (Ed.), *Visions of Rogers' science based nursing*. New York: National League for Nursing.

Roy, C. (1976). *Introduction to nursing: An adaptation model*. Englewood Cliffs, NJ: Prentice-Hall.

Roy, C., & Andrews, H. A. (1991). *The Roy adaptation model: The definitive statement*. Norwalk, CT: Appleton & Lange.

Travelbee, J. (1966). *Interpersonal aspects of nursing*. Philadelphia: F. A. Davis.

Von Bartlaffny, L. (1968). *General systems theory: Foundations development, application*. New York: George Brazeller.

Watson, J. (1985). *Nursing: Human science and human care, a theory of nursing*. East Norwalk, CT: Appleton-Century-Crofts.

Watson, J. (1990). Caring knowledge and informed moral passion. *Advances in Nursing Science, 13*(1), 15–24.

White, J. (1995). Patterns of knowing: Review, critique, and update. *Advances in Nursing Science, 17*(4), 73–86.

Wiedenback, R. (1964). *Clinical nursing: A helping art*. New York: Springer.

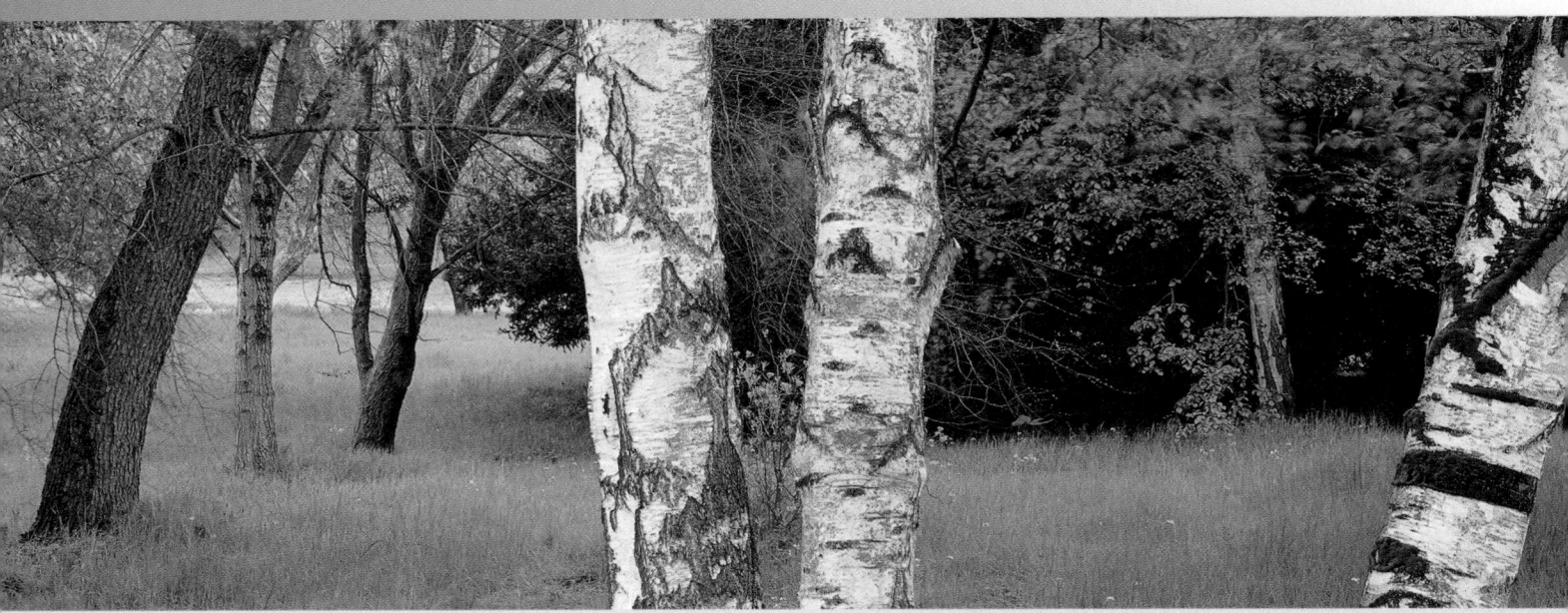

# 4 CHAPTER

# The Nurse-Client Relationship

Michael Brody, RN, BSN

*"People will forget what you say to them. They will never forget how you make them feel."*

*(Anonymous)*

# Chapter Competencies

*Upon completion of this chapter, the reader should be able to:*

1. Discuss the process of communication.
2. Identify and explain the components of the communication process.
3. Compare and contrast the different levels of communication.
4. Explain the various modes of communication.
5. Explore the role of therapeutic communication in the nurse-client relationship.
6. Identify the barriers to therapeutic communication.
7. Analyze the impact of communication in the nursing process.

# Key Terms

active listening
aphasia
artifact
auditory channel
channel
cohesiveness
communication
external stimuli
feedback

group communication
group dynamics
internal stimuli
interpersonal communication
intrapersonal communication
jargon
kinesthetic channel
message
nonverbal message

paraverbal cue
perception
receiver
sender
therapeutic communication
therapeutic relationship
verbal message
visual channel

Communication is not merely the sharing of facts; it is the essence of an innate quest to understand and be understood. People communicate in order to define themselves and find meaning in their interactions with the world around them. The nurse-client relationship depends on effective communication. Nurses must communicate effectively in order to perform their roles as educator, case manager, and active member of the health care team. As fundamental as communication is, it is rarely simple. It takes varied forms, occurs on many levels, and is vulnerable to multiple barriers. This chapter's goal is to discuss the process of communication and explore the ways in which nurses can use effective communication not only to improve their relationships with clients and thus improve outcomes of care, but also to improve the overall function of the entire health care team.

## The Communication Process

**Communication** is the exchange of thoughts, feelings, and other information. In a sense, it is impossible for people *not* to communicate (Figure 4-1). Humans are born with not only the capacity, but also the compulsion to self-express. From birth infants communicate with the world,

sending and receiving messages upon which their survival may depend. As infants grow, they develop increasingly complex forms of communication, enhancing their ability to understand and be understood. The extent to which infants communicate effectively helps determine their ability to form and maintain healthy relationships.

Nurses endeavor to understand and meet the many needs of a diverse client population. In order to do so, nurses must establish therapeutic relationships with their clients, and the quality of those relationships is directly related to the quality of communication between nurse and client (Desmond & Copeland, 2000).

## Components of the Communication Process

When seeking to understand a concept so complex as communication, it may be helpful initially to examine the whole as a sum of the parts that each play a role. In this conceptualization, the parts are sender, message, channel, receiver, and feedback (Figure 4-2). While not intended to encompass all the subtle intricacies of the communication process, the model that follows provides a framework for understanding the basics of how people communicate.

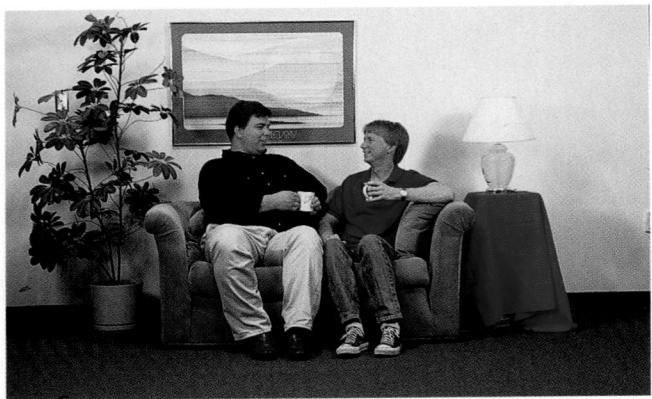

**Figure 4-1** Communication is the exchange of thoughts, feelings, and other information.

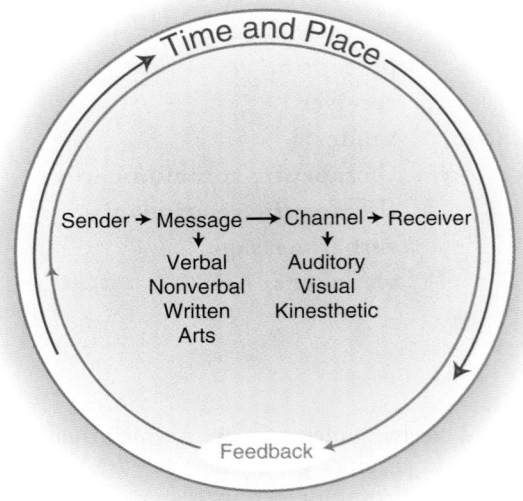

**Figure 4-2** A communication model

## Sender

As illustrated in Figure 4-2, the communication process is described as a line within a circle. Clearly the process is cyclical, and although a linear representation may oversimplify the process, it is helpful to consider communication as having a starting place. In the communication model, the starting place is the sender. The **sender** initiates the process of communication by generating a message. Messages emerge from people's need to relate to others and to create meaning from the world around and inside themselves.

## Message

The **message** derives from the sender's internal and external experiences. **External stimuli** include physical sensations, sights, sounds, touch, tastes, and smells. **Internal stimuli** include but are certainly not limited to hunger, fatigue, and cognitive experiences (e.g., thoughts, fantasies).

These internal and external stimuli generate messages that the sender then communicates to a receiver verbally, nonverbally, or in some other symbolic form (e.g., art). Verbal and nonverbal messages, as well as the influence of cognitive factors on communication, are discussed in detail later in this chapter.

## Channel

The **channel** is the medium through which the sender transmits the message. The three main communication channels are auditory, visual, and kinesthetic. The **visual channel** involves sight, which in turn allows for visual observation and perception. The **auditory channel** consists of spoken words and other verbal cues. The **kinesthetic channel** refers to physical sensations mediated by touch. Many people are aware of having a dominant channel—one that they subconsciously rely upon more than the others to send and receive messages—which influences the ways in which each individual communicates.

## Receiver

In addition to receiving the sender's message, the **receiver** interprets the message, infusing it with meaning specific to his personal experience. Different receivers may glean various meanings from the same message (see discussion on perception). Many factors influence each phase of the communication process, some of which are discussed in the following section. In terms of the receiver, physiological, psychological, and cognitive processes may have a significant impact. The physiological component involves the senses described above. For example, if the receiver's hearing is impaired, that person may not be able to hear spoken messages. If vision is affected, important visual cues may go unnoticed. Psychological processes exert a powerful influence on communication. In a mild stress response, for example, the receiver becomes acutely aware of her surroundings—able to perceive and interpret subtle messages rapidly and efficiently. If stress becomes severe or chronic, anxiety may seriously impede the receiver's ability to understand even the simplest messages. The cognitive processes, or thoughts, that occur within a receiver's mind help determine for each individual what the message exactly means (see section on intrapersonal communication for further discussion).

## Feedback

The receiver's reaction to the sender's message is labeled **feedback**. The function of feedback is to provide the sender with information about the receiver's perception of the interaction. This sometimes subtle and complicated process occurs constantly, shaping and reshaping the communication process. Feedback can either facilitate or impede effective communication. In the context of the nurse-client relationship, feedback must reflect and support the therapeutic nature of the communication process. Box 4-1 displays characteristics of effective feedback.

## BOX 4-1   CHARACTERISTICS OF EFFECTIVE FEEDBACK

- Specific rather than general
- Descriptive
- Provided in a supportive, nonthreatening manner
- Given in a timely manner
- Practical and appropriate for the individual client
- Clear and unambiguous
- Direct and honest

## Factors Influencing Communication

In terms of this model of communication, the sender, the message, the channel, and the receiver may all exert powerful influences on the process of communication. A discussion of other potentially influential factors includes perception, cultural context, space and distance, and time.

### Perception

**Perception** is an individual's subjective sense of the world around him. "Rather than hear a story, we construct a story about what we think we are hearing" (Greenhalgh & Hurwitz, 1998, p. xiii). It would be inaccurate to say there are as many different perceptions of the world as there are people. However, each individual, as a function of her social, cultural, family, and individual experience, perceives things in a unique and individual way. People often depend on presumed similarities between the way they see the world and the way they imagine others to see it; they assume commonality of meaning. This is especially true when people speak a common language. It is easy for the sender to assume that when he says "blue," "delicious," or "big," the receiver gets an image in mind similar to the sender. However, these assumptions can and often do lead people to misunderstand each other, as they attempt to fill inevitable gaps between intended meaning and perception.

### Cultural Context

Communication varies significantly from culture to culture. Not only may people from different cultures speak different languages, but they also may attach different meanings to other elements of communication, such as touch, personal space, and eye contact (Giger & Davidhizar, 1999). See Chapter 5 for a more in-depth discussion of cultural variations related to communication.

### Space and Distance

Each person has an invisible buffer zone, or personal space, which defines for that individual how close others should be when communicating with the individual (Figure 4-3). Table 4-1 describes the types of personal space. This boundary is culturally defined as well as particularly defined per the individual. An individual whose personal space has been invaded may experience discomfort, anxiety, and perhaps a strong desire to flee or defend himself (the fight-or-flight response). The nurse must consider and respect each client's right to personal space. This is especially important when the nurse is examining or touching the client. Before making contact, the nurse should explain the procedure and allow the client to ask questions. During the procedure, the nurse should communicate constantly with the client, explaining what she is doing and why.

### Time

Time is an increasingly challenging aspect of the nurse-client relationship. Today's nurses care for a greater number of clients with complex medical conditions than ever before. Nurses must learn to manage time effectively in order to complete the many and varied tasks that fall under their responsibility. By spending time with the client, the nurse allows the client to feel cared for, valued, and ideally, understood. When the busy nurse is unable to spend time with the client, that client may feel that he is not important and his needs may not be met. Finding ample time to avoid appearing rushed, to gather important diagnostic facts, to educate clients, and to establish therapeutic relationships remains a significant challenge for every nurse.

One important time-saving strategy is to take the time up front to do the job right the first time around. Many nurses may feel they don't have the time to communicate fully and effectively with a client during the initial assessment. However, studies indicate that the time invested in establishing rapport and listening to the

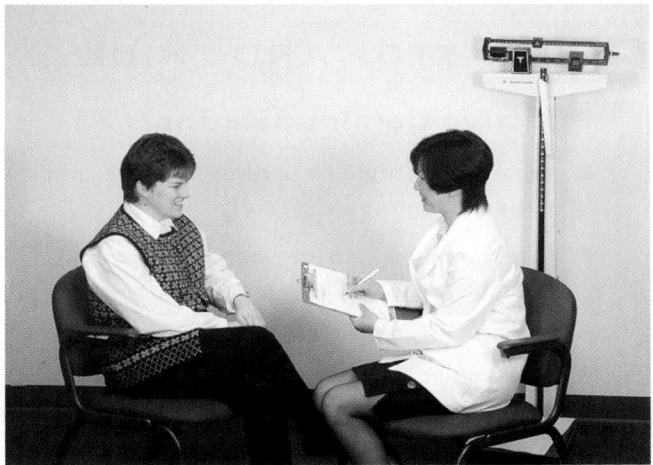

**Figure 4-3   Appropriate distance between the nurse and the client during an interview creates a more comfortable setting.**

## TABLE 4-1    TYPES OF PERSONAL SPACE

| Type | Description | Nursing Implications |
|---|---|---|
| Intimate distance (0 to 18 inches around the person's body) | • Reserved for people who feel close<br>• Vision is affected in that it is restricted to one portion of the other's body; may be distorted<br>• Tone of voice may seem louder<br>• Body smells are noticeable<br>• Increased sensation of body heat | • Nurses often must intrude on this space to provide care<br>• Explain intention to client<br>• Respect client's space as much as possible<br>• This space may be used for comforting and protecting<br>• Therapeutic examples:<br>—Rocking a toddler<br>—Administering a massage<br>—Checking vital signs (temperature, pulse, respiratory rate, and blood pressure) |
| Personal distance (zone extends 1.5 to 4 feet around the person's body) | • Usually maintained with friends<br>• Vision is clear since more of the other person is visible<br>• Tone of voice is moderate<br>• Sensations of body smells and heat are lessened | • Better able to read nonverbal communication at this distance<br>• Therapeutic examples:<br>—Conversation between client and nurse usually occurs in this zone<br>—One-to-one teaching<br>—Counseling |
| Social or public distance (zone extends from 4 feet and beyond) | • Generally used when conducting impersonal business<br>• Communication is more formal and less intense<br>• Sensory involvement is less intense<br>• Increased eye contact | • Therapeutic examples:<br>—Making rounds<br>—Leading a group<br>—Teaching a class |

Adapted from Giger, J. N., & Davidhizar, R. E. (1999). *Transcultural nursing: Assessment and intervention* (3rd ed.). St. Louis, MO: Mosby; Johnson, B. S. (2003). *Psychiatric-mental health nursing: Adaptation and growth* (5th ed.). Philadelphia: Lippincott.

client is invaluable. The nurse can avoid mistakes and complaints that arise later due to incomplete or inaccurate assessments and diagnoses. In addition, the nurse must establish a **therapeutic relationship** (i.e., a relationship that benefits the client's health status) with the client. A client who is fully informed is a more effective partner in the health care team (Hubert, 1998).

## Levels of Communication

Communication occurs at various levels, with each level influencing the others. Examples of different levels of communication include intrapersonal, interpersonal, group, and interdisciplinary, which are discussed below.

### Intrapersonal Level

**Intrapersonal communication**, also known as self-talk, is the deluge of thoughts, feelings, and information that circulate inside one's own mind. Everyone organizes,

## STOP AND THINK

### Effective Communication

● What words could be used to facilitate effective communication?

● How can nurses ensure, in the limited time available, that they have understood what a client intended to say?

● How can nurses determine whether a client has understood them?

● What potential harm might result from an even inadvertent misunderstanding?

interprets, and assigns meaning to every communication. Like perception, self-talk influences the way individuals understand the messages they receive from others. Figure 4-4 illustrates some of the elements involved in the process of self-talk. This process subtly but inevitably influences each individual's perception of a given message.

The speaker's intended message may vary dramatically from the message the receiver perceives, because of the intrapersonal communication process of the sender and receiver. For example, a client may determine in her self-talk process that she dislikes health care providers asking questions about her past. Then when the nurse asks questions in the interview process about the client's past, the client is negative toward the nurse's questions. At its worst, self-talk can interfere with attention to others and widen the gap between communicators during interpersonal exchanges. The more the nurse is aware of self-talk and the influence it may have on perception and the communication process as a whole, the more effectively the nurse can minimize the potentially disruptive nature of intrapersonal communication.

## Interpersonal Level

**Interpersonal communication** is the process that occurs between two individuals either in face-to-face encounters, over the telephone, or through other communication media. Interpersonal communication builds on the intrapersonal level in that each person communicates with himself in the process of communicating with others. Interpersonal communication represents an essential element in the development and maintenance of any interpersonal relationship, and without skillful interpersonal communication, the nurse-client relationship is in serious jeopardy.

## Group Communication Level

Communication between three or more individuals is defined as **group communication**. Because each member in a group engages in intrapersonal and interpersonal communication, the number of participants in the communication process is often directly related to increased complexity: the more communicators, the more challenges.

### NURSING STRATEGY

#### Spatial Arrangements of Group Members

In dealing with groups, the nurse should be aware of the nonverbal messages apparent in the spatial arrangement of group members. For example, the leader tends to sit at the end or head of the table. Timid or uninterested participants tend to sit at the back of the room. Seating clients in a circle rather than in rows promotes more egalitarian interaction, drawing group members closer together and facilitating group cohesion.

**Group dynamics** is the study of events that occurs in the context of group interaction. The dynamics of any group inevitably impact the productivity of the group. Nurses deal with groups constantly as they interact with families of clients, treatment teams, therapy groups, and committees within the health care setting. Groups represent potentially powerful therapeutic interventions, and nurses can participate not only by sharing professional insights, but also by listening actively and collaborating with multidisciplinary team members (e.g., social workers, clergy) to initiate the referral process.

**Cohesiveness** refers to bonding between and among members of a group (Figure 4-5). Groups often are formed around a common purpose or goal. Table 4-2 describes several different types of groups in which nurses are likely to participate. Nurses' participation in groups depends on educational background and professional licensing. According to the American Nurses Association (2000), nurse generalists, those prepared at the baccalaureate level or lower, may lead and colead all types of groups except for psychotherapy groups. Only nurse specialists with graduate degrees may lead psychotherapy groups.

### Interdisciplinary Communication

The health care team consists of the client (and family) and all health care personnel (e.g., social workers, physical therapists, occupational therapists) involved in providing care. Each member of the team performs important roles in the health care delivery system. It is essential that all health care team members communicate effectively with each other regarding assessment, intervention outcomes, and client status. The interdependent nature of the health care team requires especially skillful communication; breakdown of communication between team members could interfere with the client's treatment and ultimate outcomes.

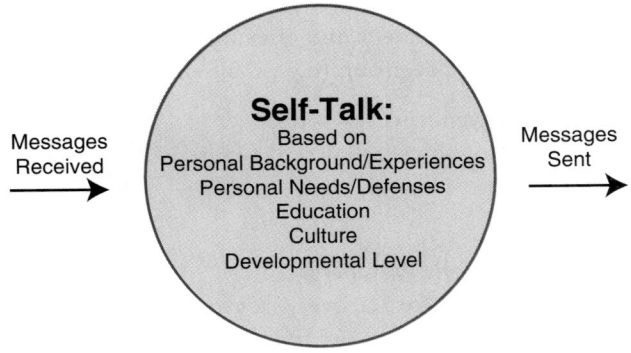

**Figure 4-4    Self-talk**

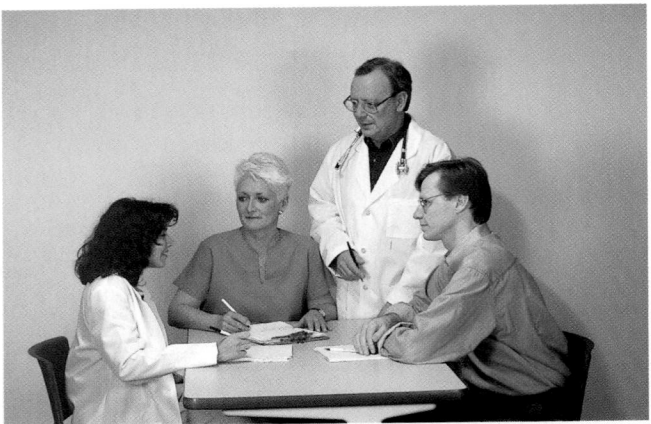

**Figure 4-5    Members of a group in a team conference**

# Modes of Communication

People communicate not only with verbal messages (words), but through nonverbal actions as well. Communication can therefore be categorized as either verbal or nonverbal.

## Verbal Messages

**Verbal messages** are communicated through words or language. Spoken and written language is comprised of verbal cues. Often **paraverbal** (or paralinguistic) **cues** accompany verbal messages. These cues include pitch and tone of voice; speed, inflection, and volume; grunts and other nonlanguage vocalizations. Paraverbal cues add meaning to verbal messages and can influence the listener as much as, if not more than, words do. Regardless of the words a person uses, concurrent paraverbal cues will likely

significantly impact the listener's understanding of what is said.

Cultural differences may lead to challenges in accurately interpreting verbal messages, most obviously because of difficulties understanding spoken language. No less confounding, however, are the culturally idiosyncratic paraverbal cues. Tone of voice, volume, and inflection varies from language to language and may easily be misinterpreted. On the other hand, other paraverbal messages like a friendly smile or tears during a period of grief seem practically universal and help to bridge the language gap.

The advent of Internet communication has given rise to a new set of challenges. Electronic mail (e-mail), for example, has become a pervasive form of modern communication technology. Though similar in some ways to traditional written communication (e.g., letters), certain elements of e-mail make it a unique form of communication with unique benefits as well as challenges. First, e-mail is immediate, allowing participants in an e-mail "conversation" to exchange information much more rapidly than would be possible using other forms of written communication. On the other hand, very much like a letter sent via traditional mail, the writer need not be immediately present to face the consequences of her message. Also like traditional mail, and seemingly incongruous in light of the speed of the Internet, e-mail confers upon the recipient of a message the advantage of time and forethought in drafting a response. A disadvantage is the lack of nonverbal communication and that the message may be more easily misinterpreted. For all its advantages and disadvantages, it seems clear that e-mail is here to stay. Nurses must therefore join other health care professionals in becoming proficient in using this technology and developing applications to benefit client care.

| TABLE 4-2 | TYPES OF GROUPS | |
| --- | --- | --- |
| Type | Description | Examples |
| Task group | Focuses on achievement of a specific goal<br>Emphasizes problem-solving and<br>    decision-making | Diabetes education group<br>Committee to study staffing issues<br>Student Nurses Association |
| Therapeutic group | Increases members' coping abilities<br>Offers support<br>Provides education and information | Stress management class<br>Bereavement and grieving<br>Exercise group (e.g., mall-walkers club) |
| Therapy group | Helps members learn about and change<br>    problematic behaviors<br>Focuses on emotional and behavioral<br>    disorders | Psychotherapy group<br>Cognitive-behavioral group |
| Self-help group | Focuses on a common experience of<br>    all members<br>Often led by nonprofessionals | Weight Watchers<br>Reach for Recovery (a group for women<br>    who have had mastectomies)<br>Alcoholics Anonymous |

## Nonverbal Messages

Just as paraverbal cues often confer more meaning than their accompanying words, so do nonverbal messages carry great meaning in human communication. People send **nonverbal messages** via body language rather than words, though the two very often coexist. Communication experts estimate that the majority of communication occurs through nonverbal messages. Nurses must pay close attention to nonverbal cues in order to accurately interpret changes in client behavior. Following is a brief discussion of specific types of nonverbal communication.

### Facial Expressions

The face is the ultimate conveyor of nonverbal messages (Figure 4-6). Unlike anywhere else in the body, the muscles of the face are connected directly to the skin, allowing for fine motor control of facial expressions to communicate the subtlest of messages. Facial expressions give clues that betray feelings and reactions not expressed in words. In addition, facial expressions support, contradict, or disguise the verbal message. Nurses attuned to changes in clients' facial expressions may be aware of emotional reactions and needs that a client might be reticent to express verbally, leading not only to better client care, but also to helping the client feel understood.

In addition to its central role in verbal communication, the mouth speaks volumes nonverbally as well. The lips smile (warmth, friendliness), frown (sadness, disapproval), quiver (fear, impending tears), and snarl or pout (malevolence, anger).

The eyes and surrounding structures (eyebrows and eyelashes) demonstrate interest, concern, sadness, dishonesty, or sincerity, and they are the windows into emotions such as anger, happiness, sadness, and fear. The French neurologist G. B. Duchenne discovered in his 19th century experiments that there are certain muscles that control movement of the facial structures surrounding the eyes and mouth that do not respond to conscious control, but rather are "only put into play by the sweet emotions of the soul," (Purves, Augustine, Fitzpatrick, Katz, LaMantia, McNamara, & Williams, 2001, p. 628).

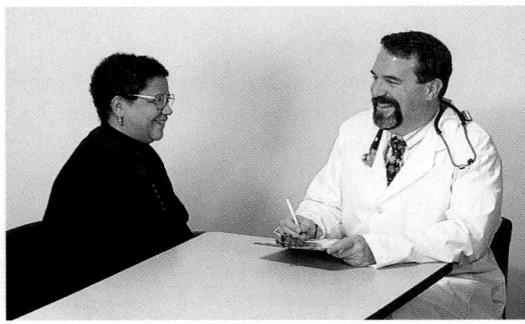

**Figure 4-6    A smile from the health care provider communicates positive caring to the client.**

### Posture

The nurse can learn much about the client and the client's family by observing and accurately interpreting posture. Posture may indicate anxiety, relaxation, and positive or negative self-image. Standing straight and tall usually indicates confidence, while slumping often indicates depressed, tired, or bored individuals. Leaning forward usually indicates interest; leaning backward might point to aversion, rejection, or a lack of engagement. On the other hand, a client who is very relaxed and self-assured might lean back during communication as well, illustrating the fact that just as verbal communication is subject to interpretation and vulnerable to inadvertent misunderstanding, so too is nonverbal communication potentially ambiguous.

### Gestures

Gestures like shrugging the shoulders, waving the hands, tapping the feet, and shaking the head all add to verbal communication. The nurse communicates openness and a willingness to listen by facing the client in a relaxed position. Crossed arms, for example, might indicate to the client that the nurse does not accept or has no interest in

## STOP AND THINK

### Nonverbal Cues

● Give an example of where your client is saying one thing while her facial expression, body language, or other nonverbal cues say something altogether different.

● How will you resolve this incongruence?

● What might you say to or ask your client in order to arrive at a more complete understanding?

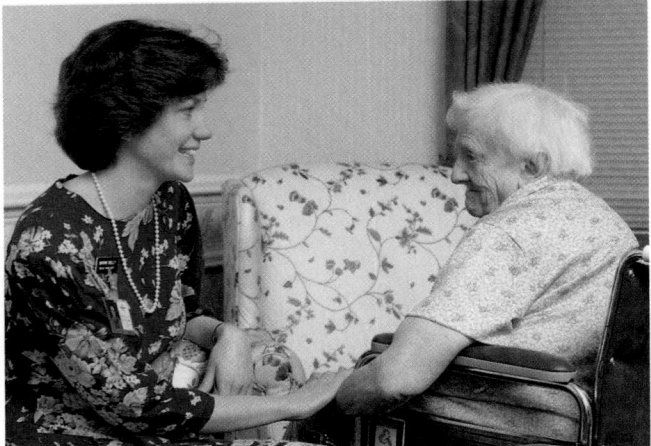

**Figure 4-7    Touch promotes bonding between the nurse and the client.**

what the client has to say. Looking repeatedly at a watch or clock tells the client the nurse does not have time to spend, regardless of what the nurse says.

### Touch

Touch is a powerful vehicle for communication, and is arguably underutilized in today's modern medical world, where machines and medications are the order of the day (Figure 4-7). Touch can be used to soothe, comfort, and establish rapport and a therapeutic bond between nurse and client. Touching someone is an age-old demonstration of caring, as in the case when a nurse holds a client's hand during a painful procedure or when delivering bad news.

Despite the nurse's best intentions, touch can also be perceived as intrusive or hostile. It is especially important to use touch cautiously with clients who are confused, suspicious, or aggressive, and with clients who have been victims of abuse. In addition, the nurse must understand the cultural significance of touch in order to prevent potential problems. See Chapter 5 for a discussion of various cultural perceptions of touch.

### Physical Appearance

Physical appearance and **artifacts** (items in the client's environment, grooming, clothing, jewelry) may convey important nonverbal messages. Uniforms can demonstrate professionalism and inspire confidence, but at the same time they may be perceived as symbols of superiority, hindering interpersonal connections. For this reason, nursing uniforms are not worn in certain areas, such as pediatrics, psychiatry, and some home health care settings.

## Therapeutic Communication

**Therapeutic communication**, using communication for the purpose of creating a beneficial outcome for the client, is the hallmark of the nurse-client relationship. Like touch, therapeutic communication may seem

almost trivial in the context of the modern medical miracles that technology makes possible for today's clients. However, while every client deserves and presumably desires to benefit from these technological advances, it is equally if not more important to every individual to feel cared for and understood; this is the goal of therapeutic communication. Brain scans, biochemistry, and other technology cannot replace dialogue; with its use nurses have a unique, demanding, and irreplaceable role in caring for clients. Table 4-3 presents the essential elements of therapeutic communication: empathy, trust, honesty, validation, caring, a nonjudgmental approach, and the use of active listening.

## Principles of Therapeutic Communication

Generally speaking, therapeutic communication is purposeful, in that it is directed toward a specific outcome. Most important, therapeutic communication is nonjudgmental and client-centered. While a therapeutic approach to communication may come somewhat naturally to many nurses, it behooves all nurses to practice techniques specifically designed to enhance the therapeutic value of communication. A discussion of basic principles for guiding therapeutic communication follows.

### Time and Place

Time and place are important to the elements of therapeutic communication. Not only the amount of time the nurse spends with each client, but also the timing of an interaction may have a significant impact on the outcome of the interaction. If the client is distracted by visitors or fatigued from a recently completed procedure or even a favorite television show, he may be too preoccupied to participate actively in the nurse-client interaction. Taking into consideration the timing of the interaction will also show the client that the nurse has the client's needs in mind.

The physical environment should be as comfortable and private as possible. The nurse can help ensure the client is comfortable by inquiring about the temperature, ventilation, and positioning of the client, and making any necessary adjustments. In addition, if pain is an issue, the nurse can intervene as appropriate. However, it should be noted that pain medication might have a sedative effect on the client and thereby render active participation by the client more difficult.

The client must be assured of confidentiality in order to feel safe in sharing information of a very private nature. This includes securing as private a location as possible for the interaction, as well as reiterating to the client that the conversation is confidential and information will be shared only with those directly involved in the client's care.

### Setting the Stage

Setting the stage for therapeutic communication is important. Having established an appropriate time and place, the nurse should introduce herself and clarify the purpose of the interaction and the expected duration. Setting the stage in this way allows the client to begin the interaction on a more equal footing with the nurse; each knows who the other is, as well as why and how long they will be there.

### Accepting the Client

Accepting the client "as is" is important to therapeutic communication. A judgmental approach to any interaction will limit the ability for mutual understanding. It is essential for every nurse to remain aware of his own biases and to approach each client from a perspective of acceptance. Often it is difficult for nurses to understand why clients behave in certain ways, especially when this behav-

ior endangers the client's health. While the nurse's feelings may stem from the best of intentions for the client's well-being, these feelings often drive a wedge between the nurse and client, rendering effective therapeutic communication nearly impossible. The nurse serves the client best by reserving judgment and trying to accept and understand the client as she is.

### Active Listening

Active listening is an important element to therapeutic communication. Thomas Gordon defines **active listening** as "a method of listening where you reflect back your understanding of what a person says to you." This is meant to confirm to the person that you understand his message, and to give him a chance to correct you if you don't. More important, however, active listening communicates your acceptance of the person's thoughts and emotions. Clearly understanding the client requires more than just hearing what she is saying. In addition to paying careful attention to what is said as well as what is not said (i.e.,

---

## COMMUNITY/HOME CARE

### Incorporating Family Members into Communication

It may be very challenging for the nurse to balance the need to include the client's family members with having to provide ample opportunity for private nurse-client interaction. The nurse should consult clients (privately) and ask how they want their family members involved in their care. The nurse can obtain a sense for a client's preference regarding how much the family is to be included in the nurse-client interactions. The nurse should ensure at least some one-to-one communication with the client.

---

## LEGAL AND ETHICAL ISSUES

### Confidentiality

One of the nurse's primary duties is to protect the client's right to confidentiality. However, should the client divulge information that indicates a real and present danger to the client or another individual, the nurse may be required by law to intervene by reporting this information to the appropriate authorities. *Tarasoff v. Regents of the University of California* describes a case in which a psychiatric patient shared with his therapist his intention to kill Tatiana Tarasoff, a young woman who had spurned the patient's affections. When the patient eventually followed through with his plan, Tatiana's parents sued the system for neglecting to better protect their daughter. The Tarasoff case has inspired two decades of debate regarding health care providers' obligations to the safety of third parties, and each state currently defines these obligations differently. Needless to say, it is essential that each nurse be aware of his state's regulations. While breaching client confidentiality may in rare situations be warranted or even required, nurses should never discuss clients casually or in settings or contexts outside the clients' direct care.

Trowbridge, B. (2002). "Law in Washington: Duty to Protect." Website: http://lawcrawler.findlaw.com/

## TABLE 4-3   THE ELEMENTS OF THERAPEUTIC COMMUNICATION

| Definition | Behaviors of the Nurse | Outcomes |
|---|---|---|
| **Empathy:** An emotional linkage between two or more people through which feelings are communicated; involves trying to imagine what it must be like to be in another person's situation | **Verbal comments:**<br>• "This must make you feel sad."<br>**Nonverbal actions:**<br>• A nod of the head to indicate understanding.<br>• Mirroring the client's facial expression in a genuine way. | • Promotes understanding of the client's feelings and condition.<br>• Enables the nurse and client to relate better.<br>• Provides the client with clues that the nurse is following and understanding what is being said. |
| **Trust:** The client's belief that the nurse will behave predictably and competently while respecting the client's needs | • Ensure confidentiality.<br>• Be consistent.<br>• Do exactly what you say you will do for the client.<br>• Arrive on time.<br>• End the session on time.<br>• Return when you say you will.<br>• Be consistently friendly, open, and honest. | • Provides the basis for progress during future encounters.<br>• Sets up the foundation of the therapeutic relationship.<br>• Makes the client feel comfortable with the nurse, rather than guarded or afraid. |
| **Honesty:** The ability to be truthful, frank, and sincere | • Provide realistic reassurance.<br>• Avoid false reassurance.<br>• Develop insight into the way your feelings and reactions affect the client.<br>• Accept yourself. | • Promotes the development of trust.<br>• Enables the nurse to gain personal insight. Consequently, behavior with the client can be modified as needed. |
| **Validation:** Listening to the client and responding congruently in order to be sure that the nurse and client have the same understanding of a problem or issue | **Verbal comments:**<br>• "So you are saying that . . ."<br>• "Let me be sure I understand what you are saying."<br>• "Tell me what you understand about what I just said." | • Clarifies communication.<br>• Helps the client to feel accepted, respected, and understood. |
| **Caring:** The level of emotional involvement between the nurse and the client | **Nonverbal actions:**<br>• Seeking the client out each day.<br>• Spending quality time with the client.<br>• Paying attention to the client's needs.<br>• Using tactile messages, such as a pat on the back, to show support. | • Makes the client feel accepted.<br>• Provides the client with the knowledge that the nurse is willing to help. |
| **Active listening:** Hearing and interpreting language, noticing nonverbal and paraverbal enhancements, and identifying underlying feelings | • Taking time to listen.<br>• Giving the client your undivided attention.<br>• Making eye contact.<br>• Responding to verbal and nonverbal leads, clues, and signals from the client.<br>• Analyzing and validating throughout the conversation.<br>• Suspending judgment.<br>• Listening between the lines.<br>• Understanding the feelings behind the facts.<br>• Noticing discrepancies between facts and feelings.<br>• Noticing things omitted such as topics that the client should be discussing but avoids.<br>• Using communication principles and techniques to be a sounding board. | • Promotes understanding of the client.<br>• Allows the client to express self more freely.<br>• Helps the client gain a better understanding of the problem(s).<br>• Promotes problem solving by the client.<br>• Enhances the client's self-esteem. |

Adapted from Johnson, B. S. (2003). *Psychiatric-mental health nursing: Adaptation and growth* (5th ed.). Philadelphia: Lippincott; Kneisl, C. R. (1996). Therapeutic communication. In H. S. Wilson & C. R. Kneisl, *Psychiatric nursing* (5th ed.). Menlo Park, CA: Addison-Wesley; Varcarolis, E., (2002). *Foundations of psychiatric mental health nursing* (4th ed.). Philadelphia: Saunders.

facial expressions, body language), nurses can encourage clients to engage in interaction by practicing the elements of active listening in Box 4-2.

Table 4-4 describes a number of specific techniques to enhance therapeutic communication. Every nurse should be aware of these techniques, but in the end each nurse must find a style of communication that fits his own unique personality.

# Barriers to Therapeutic Communication

Communication is challenging even under the most ideal circumstances. The situations in which nurses and clients must communicate often present obstacles, which the nurse and client must navigate in order to communicate effectively. Common barriers to effective communication are discussed below, followed by suggestions to help nurses overcome these barriers.

## Language

Even when two people speak the same language, it may be difficult for them to understand each other. In addition to linguistic barriers, such as discrepancies in sophistication of vocabulary, for example, intrusive self-talk, preconceptions, and individual differences in the use of certain words and expressions can render messages unintelligible despite a shared dialect. Imagine the potential barriers when two people do not speak the same language!

When English is the nurse or client's second language, the nurse can enhance the client's understanding by seeking common ground. Nurses can endeavor to learn some of the client's language. When this is not practical, nurses must bridge language gaps by thinking critically and creatively. Interpreters, foreign language dictionaries, pictures, and symbols are some potentially effective tools the nurse can use to enhance communication with a client who speaks a different language.

## Culture

Cultural differences in communication transcend spoken language. For example, while people from one culture may consider it perfectly appropriate to express thoughts and feelings with spontaneity and exuberance, people from another culture may value stoicism and reservation in verbal communication. Eye contact, physical proximity and contact, and the role of small talk are but a few examples of culturally idiosyncratic elements of communication. See Chapter 5 for a more in-depth discussion of cultural influence on communication.

## Gender

While it is certainly a generalization with many evident exceptions, men and women sometimes differ in their communication styles. Many people believe, for example, that women tend to be more adept at reading nonverbal cues and are more comfortable than men are with close physical proximity when communicating with another individual. Recent developments in brain imaging techniques indicate possible gender-based differences in the speech centers of men and women, and it will be interesting to follow this science as it develops (Williams, 2001). That said, as with any generalization, it is important to avoid relying on rigid preconceptions based on stereotypical gender-based differences.

## Health Status

The client who is in pain or is preoccupied with her condition may have difficulty communicating effectively.

---

**BOX 4-2   ELEMENTS OF ACTIVE LISTENING**

- **Let the client take the lead.** The nurse may need to gather important information in a short period of time, but it is essential to allow the client to initiate. This helps the client maintain some control in a situation (illness, hospitalization) that may have significantly attenuated his sense of control.

- **Seek clarification.** It can be very useful for the nurse to pause occasionally in order to verify that she has understood what the client has said. One very effective technique is reflection and restating (see Table 4-5). The nurse rephrases that which she believes the client has said. This not only allows the client to clarify his message, but hearing it in different words may also help the client to better understand and identify her own thought process. Not insignificantly, it also helps the nurse demonstrate to the client that she is fully engaged in the interaction.

- **When in doubt, listen.** Nurses' sincere desire to help clients can inadvertently sabotage the therapeutic communication process. By focusing on the myriad ways she can help, the nurse may forget to actually listen to the client. As tempting as it is to solve the client's problems, it is essential to hear the client out and, if possible, to guide him into playing a role in solving his own problems. This is the key to active listening.

## TABLE 4-4    TECHNIQUES OF THERAPEUTIC COMMUNICATION

| Technique | Description | Example |
|---|---|---|
| *Techniques that allow the client to set the pace* | | |
| Offering self | Nurse is available, physically and emotionally<br>Indicates nurse's willingness/intent to help<br>Nurse's presence is reassuring; may prompt client to continue<br>Indicates nurse's attention and interest | "I'll sit with you awhile."<br>"Go on."<br>"Uh-huh."<br>Head nodding |
| Broad openings | Encourages client to choose topic for discussion<br>Demonstrates respect for client's thoughts<br>Emphasizes importance of client's needs | "What do you want to talk about?"<br>"Can you tell me more about that?"<br>"How have things been going?" |
| Silence | Gives client time to reflect<br>Encourages client to express self<br>Indicates interest in what client has to say<br>Increases nurse's understanding of client's message<br>Helps to structure and pace the interaction<br>Conveys respect and acceptance | Sit quietly and observe client's behavior<br>Use appropriate eye contact<br>Employ attending behaviors<br>Control own discomfort during quiet periods or conversation lulls |
| *Techniques that encourage spontaneity* | | |
| Open-ended comments | Unfinished sentences that prompt client to continue<br>Questions that cannot be answered with a one-word answer<br>Allows client to decide what content is relevant | "Tell me about your pain?" instead of "Are you in pain?"<br>"Tell me about your family" rather than "How many children do you have?" |
| Reflection | Focuses on content of client's message and feelings<br>Repeating client's last words in order to prompt further expression<br>Communicates nurse's interest<br>Lets client know the nurse is actively listening | *Client:* "Do you think I should tell the doctor I stopped taking my medication?"<br>*Nurse:* "What do you think about that?"<br>*Client:* "I probably should. But the medicine makes me so tearful and agitated."<br>*Nurse:* "You sound a bit agitated now." |
| Restating | Repeating or paraphrasing client's main idea<br>Indicates nurse is listening to client<br>Encourages further dialogue<br>Gives client an opportunity to explain or elaborate | *Client:* "I told the doctor that I had problems with this medicine, but he just didn't listen to me!"<br>*Nurse:* "Sounds like you're pretty angry at him."<br>*Client:* "I don't sleep well anymore."<br>*Nurse:* "You're having problems sleeping?" |
| *Techniques that focus on the client by responding to verbal, paraverbal, and nonverbal cues* | | |
| Exploring | Attempts to develop in more detail a specific area of concern to client<br>Identifies patterns or themes | "Tell me more about how you feel when you do not take your medication."<br>"Could you tell me about one of those times when you felt so upset?" |
| Recognition | Nurse points out observed cues to client | "I notice that you became embarrassed when . . ."<br>"I see that you have some pictures of the new baby." |
| Focusing | Questions or statements that help client develop or expand an idea<br>Directs conversation toward key topics | "You mentioned that you are having a problem with . . ."<br>"You say you feel nauseous a lot." |

*(continues)*

## TABLE 4-4   TECHNIQUES OF THERAPEUTIC COMMUNICATION (*continued*)

| Technique | Description | Example |
|---|---|---|
| Directing | Comments that elicit specific information from the client<br>Is used to collect assessment data, not to satisfy nurse's curiosity | *Client:* "They told me I needed to see a specialist."<br>*Nurse:* "What made them say that to you?" or "When were you told this?" or "Where were you when they told you?" or "How do you feel about seeing another doctor?" |
| *Techniques that encourage expression of feelings* | | |
| Verbalizing the implied | An attempt to detect the true meaning of verbal messages | *Client:* "How much is this x-ray going to cost?"<br>*Nurse:* "You're worried about your medical bills?" |
| Making observations | Nurse calls attention to behavior indicative of feelings | "You seem sad today."<br>"You're limping as if your leg hurts." |
| Clarifying | Makes the meaning of client's message clear<br>Prevents nurse from making assumptions about client's message | *Client:* "Whenever I talk to my doctor, I feel upset."<br>*Nurse:* "Tell me what you mean by upset."<br>*Client:* "They said I could be discharged tomorrow."<br>*Nurse:* "Who told you this?" |
| *Techniques that encourage the client to make some changes* | | |
| Confronting | Nurse's verbal response to incongruence between client's words and actions<br>Encourages client to recognize potential areas for change | *Client:* "I am so angry at her" (stated while smiling).<br>*Nurse:* "You say you're angry, yet you're smiling."<br>*Client:* "I never know which of my symptoms to pay attention to. I think maybe I'm just a hypochondriac."<br>*Nurse:* "You say you're not sure which symptoms are important, yet you knew when to come to the clinic for help." |
| Limit setting | Stating expectations for appropriate behavior<br>Establishing behavioral parameters | *Nurse:* "It seems that you are feeling unsure of how to behave right now."<br>*Client:* "What do you mean?"<br>*Nurse:* "Well, you're asking me a lot of personal questions. The reason you're here is because you have some health problems. How can I help you tell me more clearly what brought you here to the clinic?" |

Adapted from Johnson, B. S. (2003). *Psychiatric-mental health nursing: Adaptation and growth* (4th ed.). Philadelphia: Lippincott; Kneisl, C. (1996). Therapeutic communication. In H. S. Wilson & C. R. Kneisl, *Psychiatric nursing* (5th ed.). Menlo Park, CA: Addison-Wesley; Stuart, G. W., & Laraia, M. T. (1998). *Principles and practice of psychiatric nursing* (7th ed.). St. Louis: Mosby; Sundeen, S. J., Stuart, G. W., Rankin, E. A., & Cohen, S. A. (1998). *Nurse-client interaction: Implementing the nursing process* (6th ed.). St. Louis: Mosby; Varcarolis, E. (2002). *Foundations of psychiatric mental health nursing* (4th ed.). Philadelphia: Saunders.

Similarly, confusion and perceptual alterations such as loss of hearing or vision may impact the communication process. See Table 4-5 for a description of techniques that may be helpful when communicating with clients whose physical and/or cognitive condition might potentially impede effective communication.

## Developmental Level

Failure to communicate at the client's individual developmental level can represent a significant roadblock to effec-

tive communication. Young children, for example, are generally incapable of abstract thought. Knowing this, the nurse will communicate with the child in relatively concrete terms. It is important that the nurse consider not only the age but also the developmental stage of the client, which may be affected by preexisting diseases.

## Emotions

In the health care setting, providers are sometimes guilty of treating the client as a curiosity, a problem, or a disease.

## TABLE 4-5    COMMUNICATING WITH VULNERABLE POPULATIONS

| | |
|---|---|
| Clients who are hearing impaired | Determine if the client reads lips. If so, face the client and reduce background noise to a minimum.<br>If client is using a hearing aid, check to see that it is in working order.<br>Always face the client.<br>Speak at a normal pace in a normal tone of voice.<br>Focus on nonverbal cues from the client.<br>Use gestures and facial expressions to reinforce verbal messages.<br>Provide pen and paper to facilitate communication if client is literate. |
| Clients who are visually impaired | When speaking to visually impaired clients, always face them as if they were sighted.<br>Follow the cues of the clients in order to allow as much independence as possible.<br>Look directly at the client.<br>Speak in a normal tone of voice; it is demeaning to yell.<br>Ask for permission before touching the client.<br>Orient the client to the immediate environment. |
| Clients who are aphasic | Assess the client's usual method of communication; adapt the interaction to accommodate the client's abilities.<br>Use a written interview format, letter boards, or yes/no cards.<br>Allow additional time for client's responses.<br>Do not answer for the client.<br>Use closed (one-word response) questions when possible.<br>Repeat or rephrase the comment if client does not understand.<br>Speak directly to the client, not to the intermediary.<br>To reinforce verbal messages, use facial expressions, gestures, and voice tone. |
| Unconscious clients | Assume the client can hear.<br>Talk to the client in a normal tone of voice.<br>Engage in normal conversational topics as with any client.<br>Speak to the client before touching.<br>Use touch to communicate a sense of presence.<br>Decrease environmental stimuli (especially auditory). |
| Confused clients | Maintain appropriate eye contact.<br>Keep background noises to a minimum.<br>Use simple, concrete words and sentences.<br>Use pictures and symbols.<br>Use closed rather than open-ended questions.<br>Give the client time to respond. |
| Angry clients | Use caution when communicating with a client who has a history of violent behavior or poor impulse control.<br>Do not turn your back on the client. Arrange the setting so that the client is not between you and the door to the room.<br>Focus on the client's body language.<br>Be alert for physical indicators of impending aggression: narrowed eyes, clenched jaw, clenched fist, or a loud tone of voice.<br>Model the expected behavior by lowering your tone of voice.<br>Stay within the client's line of vision.<br>Do not use touch. |

This stance may engender emotional distance, an unwillingness to "be there" with the client. Despite the need to focus on the client's alterations, the nurse must remember that the client is, first and foremost, a human being in need of empathy and understanding. Emotional distance precludes any modicum of therapeutic communication.

On the other hand, excessive emotional involvement on the part of the client or the nurse may prove equally disruptive to the communication process. The client may be so emotionally distraught that the nurse would do best to allow the client time to experience the emotions, without trying to intervene. In the interest of the client, the nurse, too, must maintain some control over his own emotions. A saying in hospice nursing goes, "It's OK to cry with the client, as long as you don't cry more than the client."

The role of emotions in the communication process, and in the overall nurse-client relationship, is complex. This complexity requires the nurse to remain conscious of her own emotional state as well as that of the client, and to ensure that neither emotional distance nor emotional excess derails the communication process.

## Using Health Care Jargon

Health care professionals often distance themselves from clients by using **jargon**, technical language that may be perfectly appropriate when communicating with other providers, but is confusing and potentially frightening to the client. Nurses should use language that is easily understood by the average layperson, explaining medical terminology in "plain English" at every opportunity. At the same time, nurses must avoid "talking down" to the client. Once again, review of basic therapeutic communication principles will help ensure that the nurse and client understand each other. In addition, nurses must also employ specific considerations when communicating with elderly clients (Figure 4-8).

## Communication Blocks

Certain responses that are acceptable in the context of social conversation may be inappropriate during therapeutic interaction. Communication roadblocks, some of which are described in Table 4-6, can stall the interview process and potentially confuse, intimidate, or even anger the client. Not only must nurses continuously monitor their communication with clients as well as other members of the health care team in order to identify potential roadblocks, but they also should strive to develop strategies and techniques to optimize the therapeutic value of their interactions.

# Communication, Critical Thinking, and the Nursing Process

In terms of effective communication, critical thinking refers to the vigilance nurses must use in their ongoing assessment of the communication between themselves, their clients, and their fellow health professionals. Thinking critically about communication helps the nurse to identify and

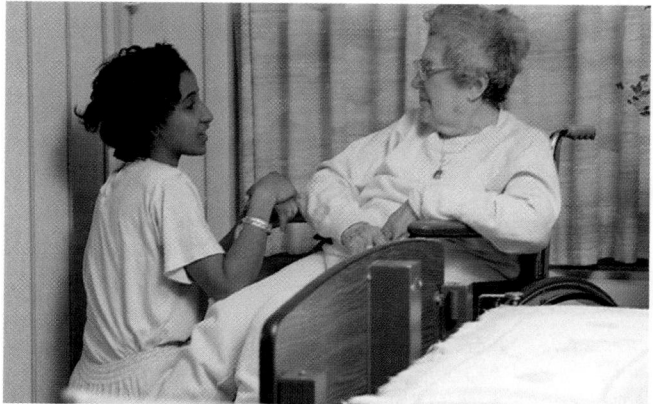

**Figure 4-8    A nurse communicating with an elderly client**

## LIFE SPAN CONSIDERATIONS

### Communicating with the Elderly

According to U.S. Census data (2001), the elderly population in the United States is expected to increase from 33.5 million in 1995 to 39.4 million in 2010, a 17% increase. From 2010 to 2030, the number of those aged 65 and over is expected to grow by 75% to over 69 million. Furthermore, the number of the oldest Americans (age 85 and over) is expected to grow by 46% from 2000 to 2010. One in three people over the age of 60, and half of those older than 85 years old, have hearing loss. Clearly, every nurse must develop skills in communicating effectively with elderly clients who have hearing loss. It may help to face the client directly, minimize distracting background noise, and if necessary, increase the volume of your voice—but do not yell.

In addition to adjusting the way you speak to an elderly client to ensure that she can hear you, it is essential to refrain from patronizing elderly clients by speaking to them as though they cannot understand. Every client, regardless of age, is an autonomous individual who deserves your compassion and your respect, which you can best demonstrate by communicating effectively. Refer to Table 4-6 for other suggestions to improve your skills in communicating with clients who are hearing impaired.

## TABLE 4-6    COMMUNICATION ROADBLOCKS

| Roadblock | Definition | Examples |
|---|---|---|
| Reassuring | Comments that indicate to the client that concerns or fears are unwarranted | • "Everything will be fine."<br>• "You will feel better soon." |
| Agreeing | Comments that indicate that the nurse's views are those of the client | • "I agree."<br>• "I think you are right." |
| Approving | Comments that indicate that the client's views, actions, needs, or wishes are "good" rather than "bad" | • "That's good."<br>• "I think you did the right thing." |
| Defending | Comments that are aimed at protecting the nurse, someone else, or something from verbal attack | • "I did not say that."<br>• "Doctor Jones is a good doctor."<br>• "I am sure your father meant nothing by that comment." |
| Using yes-or-no questions | Questions or comments that can be answered by the client with a Yes or No | • "Are you tired?"<br>• "Would you like some water?"<br>• "Could we talk now?"<br>• "Did you sleep well?" |
| Using stereotyped comments | "Pat" answers or clichés that indicate that the client's concerns are unimportant or insignificant | • "C'est la vie."<br>• "That's the way the ball bounces."<br>• "It will all come out in the wash." |
| Changing focus | Switching to a topic that is more comfortable to discuss | • *Client:* "I wish I were dead."<br>• *Nurse:* "Did your wife visit today?" |
| Judging | Comments or actions by the nurse that indicate pleasure or displeasure with what the client says | • A stern look<br>• Rolling the eyes<br>• "I like that."<br>• "I do not like that." |
| Blaming | Accusing the client of misconduct; undermines the client's need to be loved and accepted | • "You should know better than to talk like that."<br>• "If you had not moved, I would have been able to complete this venipuncture." |
| Belittling the client's feelings | Indicating to the client that feelings expressed are unwarranted or unimportant | • "Don't feel that way."<br>• "Be a big boy and stop crying." |
| Advising | Giving the client opinion or direction about solving a problem | • "If I were you, I would talk to your husband about this."<br>• "I think you should do something for yourself for a change." |
| Rejecting | Indicating to the client that certain topics are not open to discussion | • "Let's not talk about that right now." |
| Disapproving | Indicating displeasure about comments or behaviors and/or placing a value on them | • "That's bad." |
| Probing | Pressuring the client to discuss something before she is ready. | • "Why do you feel this way?"<br>• "Why did you come to the hospital?"<br>• "Why are you angry with your son?" |

Adapted from Johnson, B. S. (2003). *Psychiatric-mental health nursing: Adaptation and growth* (4th ed.). Philadelphia: Lippincott; Kneisl, C. R. (1996). Therapeutic communication. In H. S. Wilson & C. R. Kneisl. *Psychiatric nursing* (5th ed.). Menlo Park, CA: Addison-Wesley; Sundeen, S. J., Stuart, G. W., Rankin, E. A., & Cohen, S. A. (1998). *Nurse-client interaction: Implementing the nursing process* (6th ed.). St. Louis: Mosby; Varcarolis, E. (2002). *Foundations of psychiatric mental health nursing* (4th ed.). Philadelphia: Saunders.

successfully employ appropriate communication techniques. In addition, critical thinking can yield a deeper understanding of the client's experience and needs, ideally facilitating better outcomes.

## Assessment

The nurse theorist Hildegarde Peplau (1960) once said that, to encourage the client to participate in identifying and assessing his problems is to engage him as an active partner—an enterprise of great importance to him. Peplau's statement speaks to the importance of therapeutic communication in the quest to engage the client more fully in the healing process. Therapeutic communication is the vehicle for establishing a partnership between client and nurse. When assessing the client, the nurse seeks to understand the client by processing both verbal and nonverbal messages. When the client denies pain, for example, do her facial expression and body language support her words? Is there some incongruity between words and behavior? Refer to the Nursing Strategy box for guidelines that may be helpful in communicating with clients during the assessment process. Following these guidelines facilitates communication and thereby improves the accuracy and usefulness of assessment data.

## NURSING STRATEGY

### Communication Strategies

- Use open-ended questions to enhance the client's sense of control.

- Consider the client's age, developmental level, cultural background, and health status.

- Be mindful of the client's knowledge and literacy level, and speak neither down to the client nor over the client's head.

- Maintain a calm and caring demeanor, even if time is limited.

Ongoing assessment of the client's ability to communicate involves collecting information regarding both physical and psychological barriers. Several types of **aphasia**, impairment or absence of language function (Figure 4-9), are described in Table 4-7.

## Nursing Diagnosis

"Accurate diagnosis is an art of communication perfected by experience" (Hubert, 1998, p. 16). Accurate diagnosis derives from a therapeutic relationship with the client, one in which the client feels safe to express all relevant concerns. By paying meticulous attention to and correctly interpreting the client's verbal and nonverbal messages, nurses develop an understanding of the client's most compelling needs and can use this information to form their diagnostic judgments.

Whenever a client is unable to send, receive, or interpret messages accurately, the diagnosis of Impaired Verbal Communication is applicable. According to the North American Nursing Diagnosis Association (2003), the diagnosis of Impaired Verbal Communication is indicated when the client demonstrates a decreased, delayed, or absent ability to process, receive, or transmit meaning.

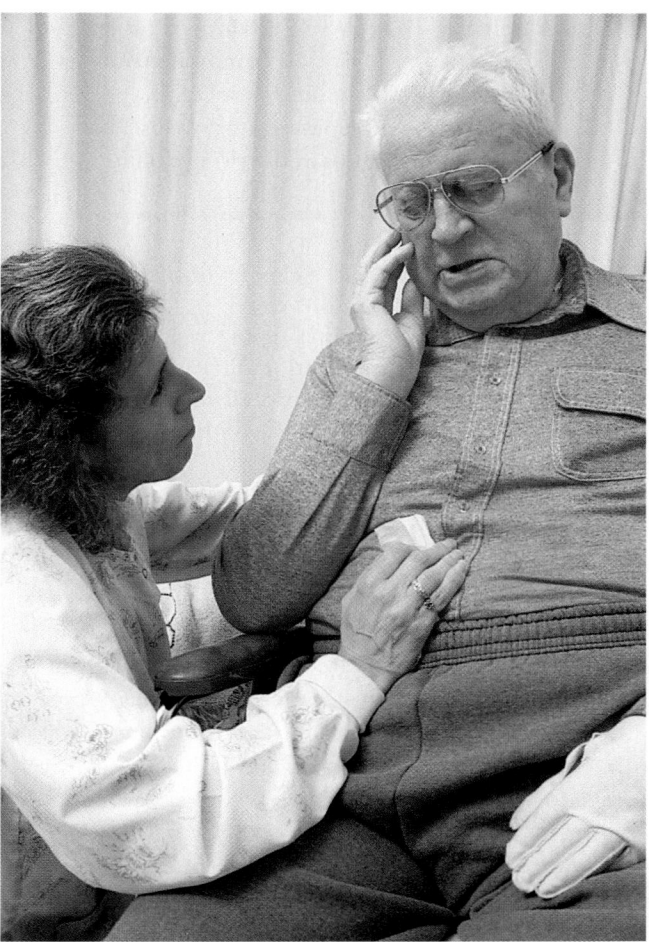

**Figure 4-9    A nurse comforts an elderly client who is depressed from his expressive aphasia condition.**

## TABLE 4-7    CLASSIFICATION OF APHASIAS

| | |
|---|---|
| Broca's aphasia | Slow, hesitant speech<br>Difficulty selecting and organizing words<br>Naming, word, and phrase repetition<br>Writing impaired<br>Slight comprehension defects |
| Wernicke's aphasia | Auditory comprehension impaired<br>Impaired speech content<br>Client unaware of deficits |
| Anomic aphasia | Unable to name objects or places<br>Comprehension and repetition of words and phrases intact |
| Conduction aphasia | Difficulty repeating words, substitutes incorrect sounds for another |
| Global aphasia | Severe impairment of oral and written comprehension<br>Impaired naming and repetition of words<br>Impaired writing ability |

Defining characteristics of the client with impaired verbal communication are shown in Box 4-3.

Other potentially relevant nursing diagnoses for the client experiencing communication difficulties include the following: (1) social isolation related to impaired verbal communication, (2) anxiety related to impaired verbal

## CLIENT REFLECTIONS

### Inability to Speak

Mr. Perez is recovering from a stroke and is unable to speak. You enter his room to find him agitated and making every effort to get you to take a piece of paper he has in his hand. In addition, he is making slurring noises, and you know he is trying to talk to you. On the paper he has written in shaky print, "I can't get anyone to take the time to listen to me. Please help!" What interventions can you suggest for yourself and other members of the health care team?

## BOX 4-3    CHARACTERISTICS OF IMPAIRED VERBAL COMMUNICATION

- Disorientation
- Inability or unwillingness to speak
- Difficulty speaking
- Difficulty expressing thoughts verbally
- Partial or total visual defect
- Stuttering or slurring of words
- Willful refusal to speak
- Unable to speak dominant language

communication, and (3) self-esteem disturbance related to impaired verbal communication.

## Planning and Outcome Identification

The nurse and client work together to develop goals and identify appropriate outcomes, a process that relies heavily on effective therapeutic communication. When impaired communication is an issue for the client, the nurse may employ any of the following approaches to overcome language barriers:

- Speak slowly in a normal tone of voice, enunciating clearly.
- Use gestures or pictures, when appropriate, to clarify meaning of words.
- Avoid clichés, medical jargon, and judgmental terms.
- Avoid body language that might appear defensive or frustrated.
- Consider the client's reading level when providing written material, and whenever possible, offer materials written in the client's native language.
- Ideally, use a professional interpreter fluent in medical terminology. Speak to the client rather than the interpreter.
- If possible, use the same interpreter for each interaction.

## Implementation

According to the National Institutes of Health (2001), it is estimated that communication disorders (including speech, language, and hearing disorders) affect 1 of every 10 people in the United States. Nurses inevitably interact with clients experiencing impaired communication, and these interactions can be very challenging.

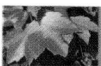

## RESEARCH FOCUS

**Title of Study:** Nursing the patient with severe communication impairment.

**Study Purpose:** In light of the currently scant research on nurses' experience caring for clients with severe communication impairment, this study provides descriptive information from interviews with 20 nurses who have cared for clients with severe communication impairment.

**Methods:** Initially, the authors conducted focus groups and a small pilot study designed to develop an interview protocol. Subsequently, the main study consisted of interviews with 20 nurses (17 women, 3 men) who had cared for at least 2 clients with significantly impaired communication in various in-patient hospital settings in the past 12 months. While one member of the research team conducted the 2-hour interview, another researcher entered responses into a portable computer. Following the interview, the interviewer checked the transcript for accuracy. Both descriptive and quantitative analyses were conducted to generate information regarding how often nurses used augmentative and alternative communication (AAC) strategies, and to explore general themes.

**Findings:** Not surprisingly, the interviews indicated that significant challenges are inherent in caring for clients with severe communication impairment. Many of these difficulties were attributed to a dearth of readily accessible support systems designed to aid in the nurse-client communication process.

**Implications:** This study indicates a need to educate nurses in the use of alternative modes of communication. Examples include sign language, gestures, alphabet boards, and electronic communication devices. In addition, nurses might benefit from a more collaborative working relationship with speech pathologists.

Hemsley, B., Sigafoos, J., Balandin, S., Forbes, R., Taylor, C., Green, V. A., & Parmenter, T. (2001). Nursing the patient with severe communication impairment. *Journal of Advanced Nursing*, 35(6), 827–835.

## Evaluation

Communication is an essential tool in evaluating the client's achievement of expected outcomes. This is especially true when evaluating the effectiveness of the nurse's efforts to educate the client regarding aspects of self-care. The nurse must pay careful attention to verbal and non-verbal cues and validate that these cues might indicate a need for further teaching. Generally speaking, nurses must ask themselves if communication is impeding this client's healing process, and if so, what interventions might resolve this problem.

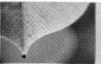

## CASE STUDY/NURSING CARE PLAN

Mrs. Sinclair brought her 16-year-old daughter to the emergency department (ED), distraught over Jennifer's plans to kill herself. Jennifer had become sullen and isolated, dropping out of school and refusing to talk to her mother except when they argued, which was daily at this point. Recently, the arguments often ended with Jennifer's promise to commit suicide, and tonight Mrs. Sinclair had found Jennifer alone in her room cutting her wrist with a pair of scissors. While the cuts were not serious, they frightened Mrs. Sinclair and convinced her that she had to seek help for her daughter. In the ED there were two distinct communicative approaches to this situation.

The nurse practitioner (NP), a longtime veteran of the ED, spoke mainly with Mrs. Sinclair to gather the history, engaging Jennifer only to admonish her for her selfishness. The NP spoke to Jennifer as if she could read the young woman's mind. She labeled character traits and thought patterns that she assumed Jennifer identified with. She also seemed to not register Jennifer's denials of feeling or thinking as the NP described. Jennifer and her mother became increasingly uncomfortable, and Mrs. Sinclair eventually asked if there might be someone else they could talk to. An inexperienced registered nurse (RN) approached the situation very differently, speaking directly to Jennifer in a comforting and sincere tone, asking her what she was experiencing and why she thought things had progressed to the point of suicide ideation. Jennifer gradually responded to this approach, eventually agreeing to spend the night in the hospital and to speak to a counselor the following day.

*(continues)*

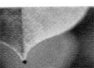

# CASE STUDY/NURSING CARE PLAN (continued)

### Assessment
Client demonstrates suicidal ideation. She presents with minor cuts on her wrists, saying that next time she will use a razor and "finish the job." She is initially reticent to discuss her situation, feeling as though no one understands. The NP does not use good principles of therapeutic communication, but the young RN communicates very appropriately.

### Nursing Diagnosis #1
High risk for self-directed violence
**NOC:** Cognitive Ability; Depression Control; Distorted Thought Control; Impulse Control; Suicide Self-Resistant
**NIC:** Anger Control Assistance; Anxiety Reduction; Coping Enhancement; Crisis Intervention; Suicide Prevention

### Expected Outcomes
The client will:
1. Reside in a safe setting to prevent self-harm while in facility.
2. Attend initial counseling session when scheduled.

### Planning/Interventions/Rationales
1. Admit client on inpatient basis, and place on 24-hour observation overnight. *Ensure client safety.*
2. Establish referral to counseling service provider. *Provide access to ongoing psychiatric care.*

### Evaluation
Verify that client is safe and that she has attended initial counseling session.

### Nursing Diagnosis #2
Impaired verbal communication related to depression
**NOC:** Communication Ability; Communication: Expressive Ability
**NIC:** Active Listening

### Expected Outcomes
The client will:
1. Receive counseling to address underlying issues within 24 hours.
2. Verbalize that she is being heard and understood by the end of session four.

### Planning/Interventions/Rationales
1. Employ active listening techniques. *Engage client in therapeutic communication process.*
2. Employ anxiety reduction techniques. *Allow client to process emotions from a calm and rational perspective.*

### Evaluation
Verify that the client feels she is being heard and understood.

## Key Concepts

- The communication process is fundamental to any human relationship.
- The components of the communication process include sender, message, channel, and receiver.
- There are several different levels in which persons communicate with one another, including intrapersonal, interpersonal, group, and interdisciplinary.
- Verbal and nonverbal messages are modes of communication that exist in the nurse-client relationship.
- Perception, culture, space, distance, and time influence communication.
- The goal of therapeutic communication is for all clients to feel that they are cared for and understood.
- Obstacles that must be considered in developing a therapeutic relationship are language, culture, gender,

health status, developmental levels, emotions, and use of health care jargon.

- The nursing process impacts communication in the nurse-client relationship.

## Review Questions and Activities

1. How is effective communication central to the nurse-client relationship?
2. In what ways might poor communication skills hinder the nurse's ability to work productively within the health care team?
3. What is therapeutic communication?
4. How might a nurse go about communicating with a client who just had a stroke that impaired the client's ability to speak?
5. In what ways can a nurse communicate with children in order to comfort them during a frightening clinical experience?

## Multimedia Links

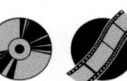 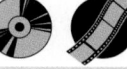

Christensen *Core Concept Videos: Therapeutic Communication*

## Web Resources

Administration on Aging
   http://www.aoa.gov
Center for the Advancement of Health
   http://www.cfah.org
Gordon Training International
   http://www.activelistening.com
National Institutes of Health
   http://www.nih.gov
National Institutes of Mental Health
   http://www.nimh.nih.gov

## References

DeLaune, S., & Ladner, P. (2002). *Fundamentals of Nursing* (2nd ed.). Clifton Park, NY: Delmar Learning.

Desmond, J., & Copeland, L. (2000). *Communicating with today's patient*. San Francisco: Jossey-Bass.

Giger, J. N., & Davidhizar, R. E. (1999). *Transcultural nursing: Assessment and intervention* (3rd ed., pp. 43–60). St. Louis: Mosby.

Greenhalgh, T., & Hurwitz, B. (1998). *Narrative Based Medicine: Dialogue and Discourse in Clinical Practice*. London: BMJ Books.

Hemsley, B., Sigafoos, J., Balandin, S., Forbes, R., Taylor, C., Green, V. & Parmenter, T. (2001). Nursing the patient with severe communication impairment. *Journal of Advanced Nursing, 35*(6), 827–835.

Hubert, P. M. (1998). Revealing patient concerns. *American Journal of Nursing, 98*(10), 16H-16L.

Johnson, B. S. (2003). *Psychiatric-mental health nursing: Adaptation and growth* (4th ed.). Philadelphia: Lippincott.

Kneisl, C. R. (1996). Therapeutic communication. In H. S. Wilson & C. R. Kneisl, *Psychiatric nursing* (5th ed.). Menlo Park, CA: Addison-Wesley.

North American Nursing Diagnosis Association (2001). *Nursing diagnoses: Definitions and classification: 2001–2002*. Philadelphia: Author.

Peplau, H. (1960). Talking with patients. *American Journal of Nursing, 60*(7), 964.

Purves, D., Augustine, G. J., Fitzpatrick, D., Katz, L. C., LaMantia, A., McNamara, J. O., & Williams, S. M. (2001). *Neuroscience* (2nd ed.). Sunderland: Sinauer Associates, Inc.

Stuart, G. W. & Laraia, M. T. (1998). *Principles and practice of psychiatric nursing* (7th ed.). St. Louis: Mosby.

Sundeen, S. J., Stuart, G. W., Rankin, E. A., & Cohen, S. A. (1998). *Nurse-client interaction: Implementing the nursing process* (6th ed.). St. Louis: Mosby.

Trowbridge, B. (2002). "Law in Washington: Duty to Protect." http://lawcrawler.findlaw.com/

Varcarolis, E. (2002). *Foundations of psychiatric mental health nursing* (4th ed.). Philadelphia: Saunders.

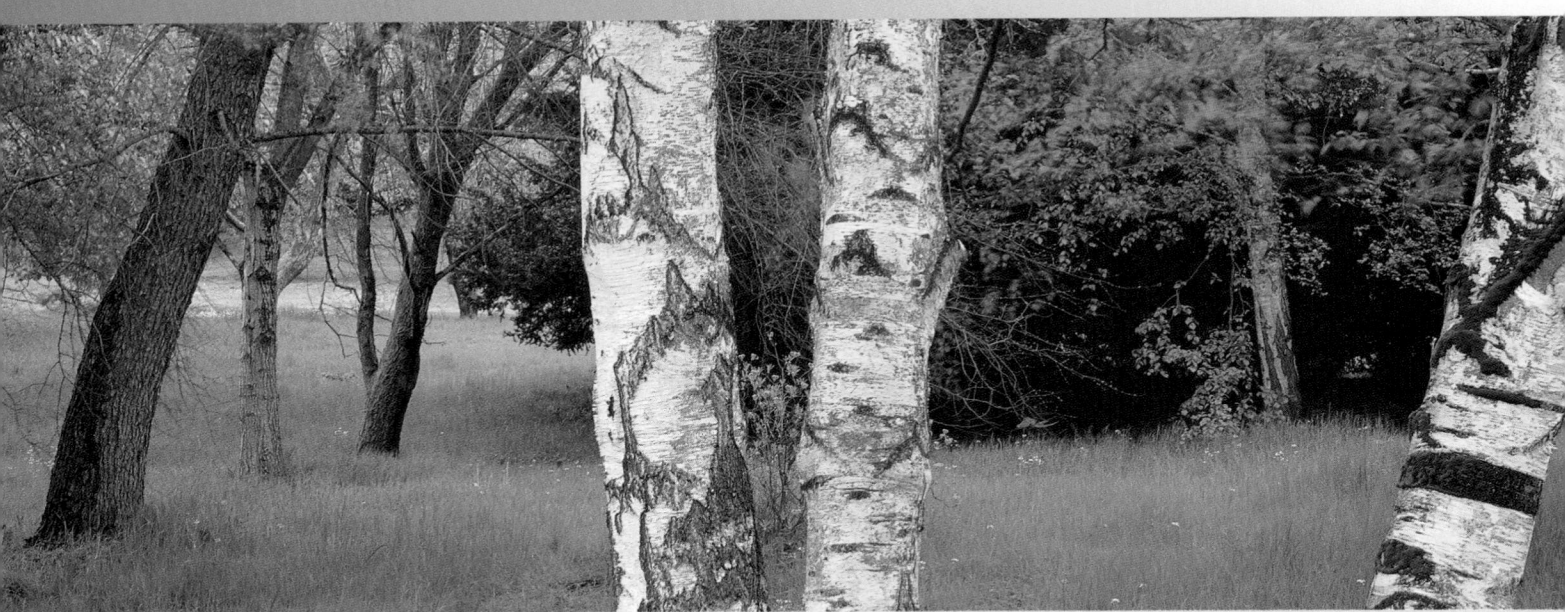

# Culture and Ethnicity

Diana Amaya Rodriguez, RN, PhD

*"If you can't see that your own culture has its own set of interests, emotions, and biases, how can you expect to deal successfully with someone else's culture?"*

(Anne Fadiman, 1997)

# Chapter Competencies

*Upon completion of this chapter, the reader should be able to:*

1. Identify the concepts of culture, ethnicity, race, ethnocentrism, and stereotyping.
2. Describe multiculturalism in the United States.
3. Discuss the organizing phenomena of culture.
4. Describe the process of transcultural nursing.
5. Evaluate how nurses maintain sensitivity to cultural diversity.
6. Discuss nursing strategies that ensure delivery of culturally sensitive care.

# Key Terms

| | | |
|---|---|---|
| acculturation | dominant culture | race |
| cultural assimilation | ethnicity | racism |
| cultural competence | ethnocentrism | stereotyping |
| cultural diversity | minority group | subculture |
| culture | oppression | transcultural nursing |

Every aspect of one's life (including attitudes, beliefs, and values) is influenced by one's culture. Behavior, including behavior affecting health, is culturally determined. As the population of the United States continues to diversify, recognition of cultural differences and their impact on health care becomes more critical. Nurses provide health care to culturally diverse client populations in a variety of settings. Knowledge of culturally relevant information is essential for delivery of competent nursing care. This chapter discusses the various concepts related to culture, the importance of diversity in American society, the influence of culture on health, and transcultural nursing.

## Concepts of Culture

Each individual is culturally unique. Behavior, self-perception, and judgment of others all depend on one's cultural perspective. This section discusses the concepts of culture, race, ethnicity, and stereotyping and provides an overview of the dominant cultural values in the United States. To provide holistic care, the nurse needs a thorough understanding of the following concepts.

### Culture

**Culture** refers to knowledge, beliefs, behaviors, ideas, attitudes, values, habits, customs, languages, symbols, rituals, ceremonies, and practices that are unique to a particular group of people. This structure of knowledge, behaviors, and values provides a group with a "blueprint" or a general design for living "that guide their worldview and decision-making" (Purnell & Paulanka, 1998, p. 4).

Culture is not static nor is it uniform among all members within cultural groups. Culture represents adaptive dynamic processes learned through life experiences. People have culturally predetermined values and beliefs that may change as new information is gained. There is much diversity among cultural groups. Such differences result from individual perspectives and practices. Consider for example how a family deals with a crisis. A crisis may cause some families to become closer, whereas the same situation may cause another family to withdraw and create distance among its members.

Cultural messages are transmitted in a variety of ways such as through schools and churches. The various media are also powerful transmitters and shapers of culture.

People learn about culture through traditions. When people state, "That's how we've always done it," they are describing cultural traditions. Cultural beliefs, values, customs, and behaviors are transmitted from one generation to another. Grandparents, other elders, and parents teach children cultural expectations and norms through role modeling, demonstration, and discussion (Figure 5-1).

### Characteristics of Culture

Differences exist among cultural groups and among individuals within a single culture. Despite these variances, all cultures exhibit the characteristics shown in Box 5-1.

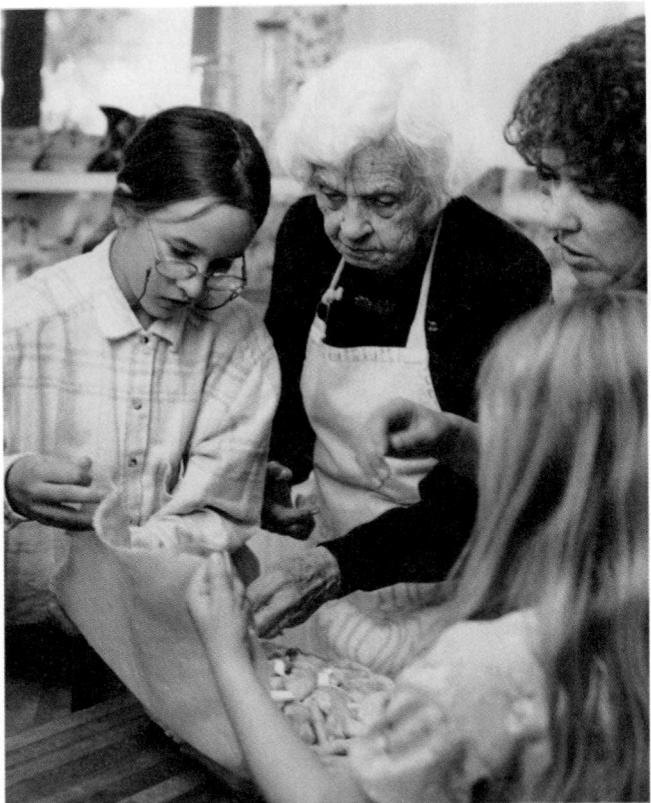

**Figure 5-1** Cultural expectations and traditions are shared through formal and informal activities.

## Ethnicity and Race

**Ethnicity** is a cultural group's perception of themselves (group identity). This self-perception influences how the group's members are perceived by others. Ethnicity is a sense of belongingness and a common social heritage that is passed from one generation to the next. Members of an ethnic group demonstrate their shared sense of identity in common customs and traits.

**Race** refers to a grouping of people based on biological similarities. Members of a racial group have similar physical characteristics such as blood group, facial features, and color of skin, hair, and eyes. There is often overlap between racial and ethnic groups because the cultural and biologic commonalities support one another (Giger & Davidhizar, 2004). The similarities of people in racial and ethnic groups reinforce a sense of commonality and cohesiveness. However, there may be differences with regard to individuals' perceptions of their racial backgrounds and their social relationships. The nurse must be careful to assess clients individually when considering race and ethnicity.

## Labeling and Stereotyping

Problems arise when differences across and within cultural groups are misunderstood. Misperception, confusion, and

---

**BOX 5-1    CHARACTERISTICS OF CULTURE**

- *Culture is learned and taught.* Cultural knowledge is transmitted from one generation to another. A person is not born with cultural concepts but instead learns them through socialization.

- *Culture is shared.* The sharing of common practices provides a group with part of its cultural identity.

- *Culture is social in nature.* Culture develops in and is communicated by groups of people.

- *Culture is dynamic, adaptive, and ever-changing.* Adaptation allows cultural groups to adjust to meet environmental changes. Cultural change occurs slowly and in response to the needs of the group. This dynamic and adaptable nature allows a culture to survive.

---

### 🌰 LIFE SPAN CONSIDERATIONS

#### Racial Background and Aging

Elderly persons of different racial backgrounds may have very different perspectives on the implications of their cultural heritage. For example, an older African American person raised in the southern United States may have experienced a great deal of discrimination and consequently is somewhat distrustful of white health care providers. The nurse may not realize the reasons for this perception and thus inaccurately assess the elderly person's attitude of distrust. The nurse must remember to consider age and experience as related to the client's racial background.

---

ignorance often accompany people's expectations of others. There are numerous ways in which people are different and, thus, classified by others (see Box 5-2).

Members of some cultural groups have historically and globally experienced oppression in the forms of racism, sexism, and classism. The basic underlying premise of these biases is that one way is assumed to be better or "right" and every other way is inferior. **Ethnocentrism** is the belief that one's own culture is superior to all others. According to the American Nurses Association (1998a):

| BOX 5-2 | WAYS IN WHICH PEOPLE DIFFER |
| --- | --- |

- Age
- Gender
- Educational level
- Language
- Occupation
- Residence (rural, urban, suburban)
- Socioeconomic status
- Religion
- Functional abilities
- Cognitive abilities
- Racial composition
- Nationality
- Family structure and ties
- Rituals (food, births, deaths, holidays)

This belief is common to all cultural groups; all groups regard their own culture as not only the best but also the correct, moral, and only way of life. This belief is pervasive, often unconscious, and is imposed on every aspect of day-to-day interaction and practices including health care. It is this attitude which creates problems between nurses and clients of diverse cultural groups. (p. 3)

Ethnocentrism results in oppression. **Oppression** occurs when the rules, modes, and ideals of one group are imposed on another group. Oppression is based on cultural biases, which stem from values, beliefs, traditions, and cultural expectations. **Racism**, a form of oppression, is defined as discrimination directed toward individuals who are misperceived to be inferior due to biologic differences.

**Stereotyping** is an expectation that all people within the same racial, ethnic, or cultural group act alike and share the same beliefs and attitudes. Stereotyping results in labeling people according to cultural preconceptions; therefore, an individual's unique identity is often ignored.

## Dominant Values in the United States

Cultural differences refer to values, practices, and rituals that vary from those of the dominant culture. The domi-nant culture of the United States is composed of white middle-class Protestants of European ancestry. A **dominant culture** is the group whose values prevail within a society. The European value orientation has had an important influence on U.S. culture, as illustrated by the following dominant beliefs:

- Achievement and success
- Individualism, independence, and self-reliance
- Activity, work, and ownership
- Efficiency, practicality, and reliance on technology
- Material comfort
- Competition and achievement
- Youth and beauty

Frequently, these dominant values (which may be blatant or subtle) conflict with the values of minority groups. Generally, a **minority group** can be composed of an ethnic, racial, or religious group that constitutes less than a numerical majority of the population. Because of their cultural or physical characteristics, such groups are labeled and treated differently from others in the society. Minority groups are usually considered to be less powerful than the dominant group (Giger & Davidhizar, 2004).

People assume the characteristics of the dominant culture through **acculturation** (process of learning norms, beliefs, and behavioral expectations of a group). Acculturation is encouraged through schools and the media. Assimilation is "cultural and structural blending into a dominant entity" (Kavanagh et al., 1999, p. 10). **Cultural assimilation** occurs when individuals from a minority group are absorbed by the dominant culture and take on the characteristics of the dominant culture.

## Multiculturalism in the United States

"The United States, already one of the most diverse societies in the world, is becoming increasingly multicultural and multilingual" (Lester, 1998, p. 26). The U.S. population is composed of many ethnic/racial subcultures. A **subculture** is a group of people "who have experiences different from those of the dominant culture by virtue of status, ethnic background, residence, religion, education, or other factors that functionally unify the group" (Purnell & Paulanka, 1998, p. 8). It is important to note that, even though a number of these subcultures possess less than their equal shares of money, influence, and prestige, these populations are increasing at a rapid rate. "By the year 2050, white Americans' share of the total population will decline from 75% to under 50%. In many localities so-called minorities are now, in fact, the majority" (American Nurses Association, 1998, p. 5). The numbers of immigrants and refugees entering the United States from non-European countries have added to this multicultural composition within the American universal culture.

## STOP AND THINK

### Culturally Competent Care

- Why is culturally competent care important when providing care to clients?

- Is there a group that should not be considered for culturally competent care?

- Why did you choose this group?

- What from your cultural background do you bring into the relationship with your clients?

- How do the beliefs of the dominant society compare with your personal beliefs?

Native Americans, African Americans, Asian Americans, and Hispanic Americans will be the most populous groups in the future. All four of these cultural groups have shown significant growth and are expected to increase. Within the next 50 years, the Asian population is expected to increase to 11%, the Black population to 16%, and the Hispanic population to 21% (Campinha-Bacote, 1999, p. 203). These growing minority groups increase the percentages of impoverished populations and have tremendous unmet health care needs. The result is a negative impact on the health care budget and adds to the health care spending deficit in the United States.

## Value of Diversity

**Cultural diversity** is the differences among people that result from ethnic, racial, and cultural variables. Cultural diversity refers to the differences between people based on a shared ideology and value set of beliefs, norms, customs, and meanings evidenced in a way of life (American Nurses Association, 1998b). The United States has a vast potential of human resources, which with divergent viewpoints and behaviors enriches the sociopolitical climate. New ideas, other viewpoints, increased problem-solving approaches, and increased tolerance are all outcomes of a diverse population. In addition to these advantages, there are also some disadvantages to living and working within such a culturally diverse environment. For example, the amount and types of variances can lead to splitting and ethnocentrism.

Cultural diversity presents special challenges for nurses who must provide care that is congruent with a person's expectations. Nurses caring for clients who are different from themselves must remember to determine the client's perception and significance (meaning) of the event (illness). The nurse honors each individual's differences while understanding that culture influences how clients are viewed and treated within health care settings.

# Organizing Phenomena of Culture

Cultural factors determine the worth of behaviors, whether behaviors are acceptable, and whether behaviors are incorporated into daily living. When these behavioral concepts are applied to health, they influence the individual's expectation of health care. Diversity of expectations among cultural groups influences health care. The nurse must be sensitive to the client's cultural context in order to provide care that meets individual needs. Each cultural group has the same basic organizational factors (see Box 5-3). Following is a discussion of the six organizing factors that must be considered when delivering culturally competent care.

## Communication

Communication is the vehicle for transmitting and preserving culture. To share complete and accurate information, nurses must be aware of the cultural variances related to communication. See Chapter 4 for a complete discussion of communication.

Nurses provide information to clients by using two types of communication: verbal and nonverbal. Verbal communication consists of words, both spoken and written. When cultural variances exist, communication problems may occur. The nurse must validate the meaning of and interpret words to ensure that clients receive the intended message.

Even when both client and nurse speak the same language, communication problems may occur because of varying cultural contexts in which words have different meanings to different people. Fear, compounded with illness, can affect the client's ability to hear what is being said, greatly interfering with communication.

When a nurse has a client who does not speak English, every effort should be made to obtain a qualified interpreter. For many reasons, using family members, hospital staff not hired for interpreting, or other clients or their

---

### BOX 5-3    ORGANIZING PHENOMENA OF CULTURE

- Communication

- Space

- Orientation to time

- Social organization

- Environmental control

- Biologic variations

families, results in less than optimal care for the client who does not speak English. First, just because someone is able to speak another language does not mean that person can adequately translate medical information. Second, using family members to translate has the potential to create a power imbalance within the family that may not be acceptable to them. Third, use of family members or others who are not interpreters may result in the interpreter not wanting to translate sensitive information to the client. The interpreter may even try to protect the client by changing the information. Conversely, the information could be misinterpreted because the family does not want the nurse to know everything—they may be overprotective of their family member. Finally, the use of someone who is not a qualified interpreter potentially violates client confidentiality by disclosing information without the consent of the client.

Nonverbal communication consists of body language (such as facial expressions, posture, and gestures); the use of silence; and paralinguistic cues (voice tone, pitch, and rate). An example of how nonverbal communication can be culturally misunderstood is the presence or absence of eye contact. For example, in Native American and Asian American cultures, eye contact may be considered intrusive and disrespectful. However, in the dominant U.S. cultural group, eye contact between individuals indicates trustworthiness.

## Space

An individual's personal space includes one's body, the surrounding environment, and objects and people within that environment. Culture determines the amount of social distance tolerated by a person. Members of British, German, and American cultures usually require more personal space than do people of Hispanic and French backgrounds (Giger & Davidhizar, 2004).

Nurses must be aware of the client's degree of comfort with closeness since diverse groups have varying norms for the use of touch. Touch may be perceived as invasive by clients from some cultures. Who can touch a person, when a person can be touched, and what forms of touch are appropriate are culturally determined. For example, members of the dominant U.S. culture often greet each other with handshakes, while it is commonly accepted in European cultures to greet others with a kiss on the cheek.

## Orientation to Time

Time orientation (being focused on the past, the present, or the future) varies according to cultural group. European Americans are future oriented as evidenced by their development of plans, such as retirement savings. Many Native Americans have a different concept of time in that they tend to live in the present moment (Giger & Davidhizar, 2004). For many Native Americans, watching the clock and timeliness/tardiness have little importance. Time is considered a circular, rather than a linear, process. Most health care providers value quickness and efficiency, which is interpreted by members of the Lakota tribe as insincerity and a lack of interest (Kavanagh et al., 1999). The nurse's nonverbal behavior can be changed to build interpersonal rapport by spending time, sitting down with clients, and demonstrating presence.

## Social Organization

Social organization refers to the ways in which groups determine rules of acceptable behavior and roles of individual members. Examples of social organizations include family and other kinship ties, religious groups, and ethnic groups.

### Family

Just as the nurse approaches the client with culturally competent care, the nurse must show the family the same cultural competency. Consideration of the family from a cultural perspective is important because culture profoundly affects the way that families respond to threats to a family member's health. Conclusions of how families are supposed to act, based on knowledge of their cultural background, can lead to erroneous assumptions.

---

## CLINICAL ALERT

### Assumptions and Communication

When the nurse assumes that the client understands the intended message and fails to confirm client understanding, cultural blindness can hamper the communication process.

---

## NURSING STRATEGY

### Consideration of Time Among Cultures

- In mainstream American culture, time is a valuable commodity (i.e., "Time is money!").

- Clients from diverse cultures may view time differently.

- When a client is late for an appointment, avoid jumping to the conclusion that the client is lazy or inconsiderate.

Degazon, C. (2000). Cultural diversity and community health nursing practice. In M. Stanhope & J. Lancaster (Eds.), *Community health nursing: Promoting health of aggregates, families, and individuals* (5th ed.). St. Louis: Mosby-Yearbook.

## BOX 5-4    TYPES OF FAMILY STRUCTURES

- *Nuclear*      Parents and children
- *Extended*     Parents, children, and other relatives (such as grandparents, cousins)
- *Attenuated*   Single parent with children
- *Incipient*    Married couple with no children
- *Blended*      Married couple and their children from previous unions; may indicate step-parents, step-siblings, half siblings.

The primary factors that lead to family differences within cultural groups are related to the family life cycle, the socioeconomic and social class status of the family, and the family's degree of acculturation. The various types of family structures are described in Box 5-4. It is vital for the nurse to know who will be involved in making decisions related to health care. Including the family according to their cultural expectations is a hallmark of quality nursing care. Family patterns usually are of one of three types: linear, collateral, or individualist. See Table 5-1 for an explanation of these types of family patterns.

In many cultures, the family assumes greater importance than the individual (Figure 5-2). For example, in most Native American tribes, the extended family is the basic family structure. The extended family is also extremely important in Hispanic American cultural groups. In some Hispanic groups, the family may include third and fourth cousins as well as close friends who are not related by ties of kinship.

Pickens (1998) identified the following attributes as necessary for nurses in order to collaborate with families:

- Nonjudgmental attitude (i.e., do not expect all families to be alike and behave similar to one's own)
- Self-awareness of own preconceptions about family members
- Respect for others' beliefs and values
- Recognition of families as significant providers of support
- Value the participation of families in caregiving

### Gender

Gender roles vary according to cultural context. For example, in families with a patriarchal structure (the man is the head of the household and chief authority figure), the husband/father is the dominant person. Such expectations are the cultural norm for Latino, Hispanic, and traditional Muslim families. The husband/father is the one

## TABLE 5-1    FAMILY PATTERNS

| Kinship Pattern | Explanation | Most Common Cultural Context |
|---|---|---|
| Linear | • Goals focus on needs of extended and hereditary family.<br>• Patriarchal structure is present.<br>• Enculturation of children is an important function.<br>• Elders are respected. | • Asian<br>• Middle Eastern<br>• Upper-class Euro-American |
| Collateral | • Individual member's goals are less important than those of the family.<br>• Nuclear family is present.<br>• Men are "head of household," yet women contribute to decision making (especially about childcare).<br>• Children are highly valued.<br>• Socialization revolves around family groups | • Hispanic<br>• Native American |
| Individualist | • Individual's goals take precedence over that of family.<br>• Emphasis is on individual accountability and self-responsibility.<br>• There is less respect for authority figures.<br>• Elders are not as honored.<br>• Family responsibilities are shared between men and women. | • Middle-class Euro-American<br>• Single-parent family<br>• Gay family |

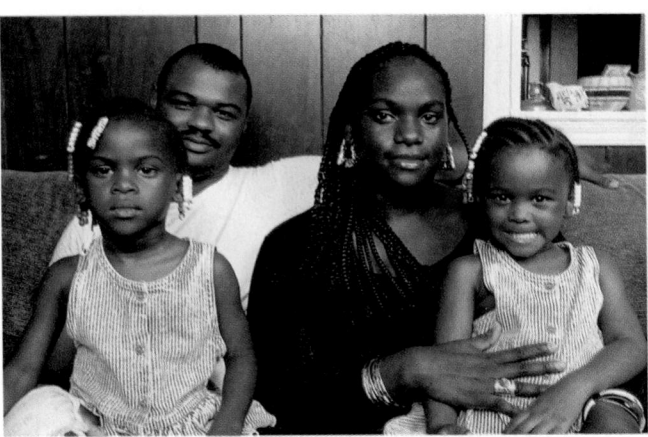

**Figure 5-2** Within this family, decisions about health care are made on a very personal level among the parents and children.

who makes decisions regarding health care for all family members. Also, in such cultures, the wife is responsible for child care and household maintenance, whereas the father's role is to protect and support the family members (Luckmann, 2000).

## Lifestyle

In addition to an increased heterogeneity of population groups in the United States, lifestyles are also becoming more diverse. Some examples of alternative lifestyles are homosexual couples, single-parent families, and communal groups. Figure 5-3 illustrates a variety of types of families. Nurses must demonstrate respect for clients' lifestyles even when they differ from those of the nurse.

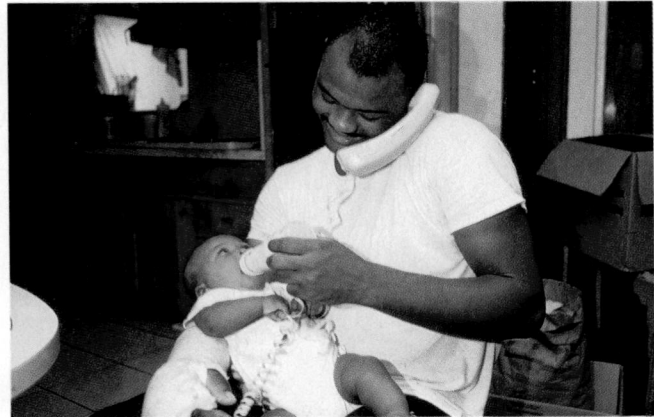

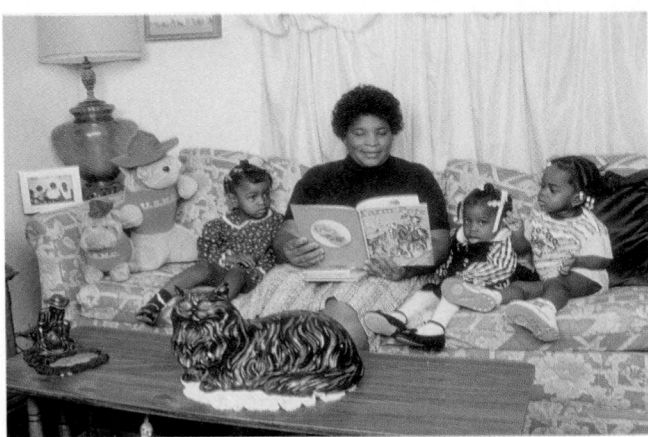

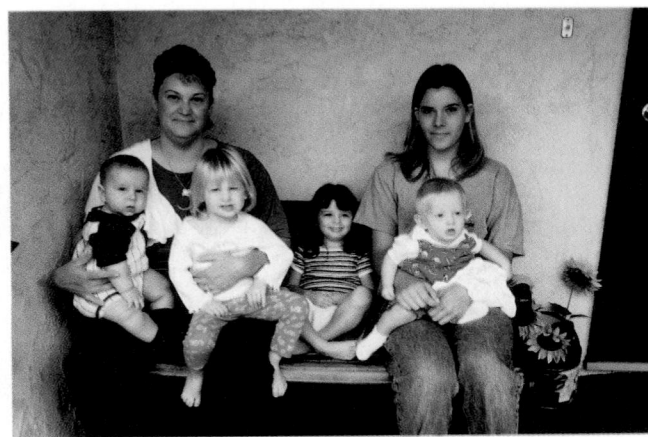

**Figure 5-3** There are diverse family structures and types, as shown in these photographs.

Some specific ways in which nurses can respect clients with differing lifestyles are:

- Be aware of own tendency to be ethnocentric.
- Be sensitive to client's needs, especially those expressed nonverbally.
- Use self-awareness to determine the impact of own beliefs and values.

Often the nurse and client are of different cultural backgrounds; see Figure 5-4. The nurse must be culturally

---

## FOCUS ON WELLNESS

### Prayer and Other Cultures

Different cultures emphasize the value and importance of prayer associated with their religious beliefs. The nurse should remember that clients with strong religious faiths may practice prayer regularly as part of their wellness practices. The nurse should create private times for the client to support the client's prayer times. In addition, the nurse should also remember that some cultures have identified persons (e.g., herbalist, rabbi, shaman) who are important to spiritual practices such as prayer.

Sherwood, G. D. (2000). The power of nurse-client encounters: Interpreting spiritual themes. *Journal of Holistic Nursing, 18*(2), 159–175.

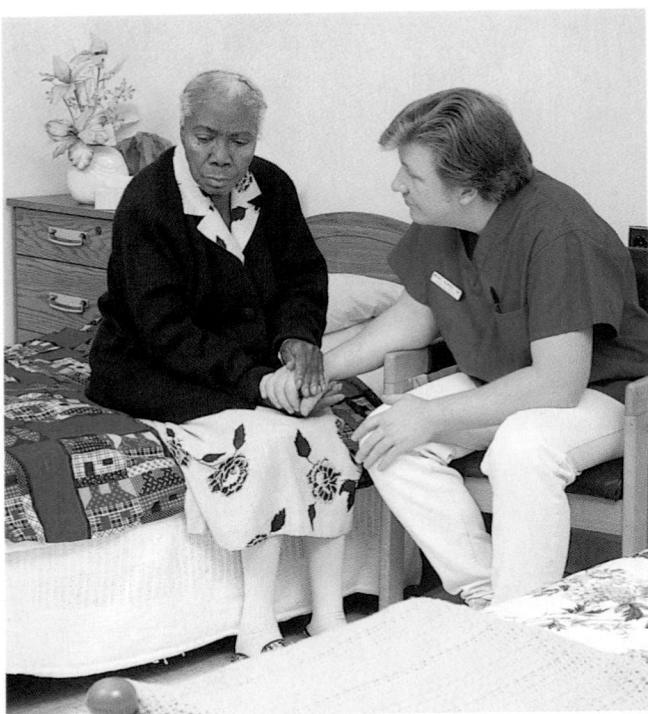

**Figure 5-4** Providing culturally sensitive care depends on establishment of a therapeutic nurse-client relationship.

sensitive in order to promote the development of a therapeutic nurse-client relationship.

## Religion

Religious beliefs influence a person's response to major life events such as birth, illness, and death. Religious practices are often a source of comfort during stressful life events and provide support during the healing process. Crises such as illness and treatment modalities are often the catalyst for increased spiritual needs; see Figure 5-5.

## Cultural Disparities in Health and Health Care Delivery

"Researchers suggest that cultural insensitivity can create more than mere discomfort. It can create real barriers to accessing health care" (Lester, 1998, p. 28). Language and other cultural differences often present barriers to necessary health care including:

- Appointment procedures
- Transportation
- Directions written in an unfamiliar language

There are disparities in the health of Americans. According to the American Nurses Association (ANA) (1998a), minorities experience some diseases at a much

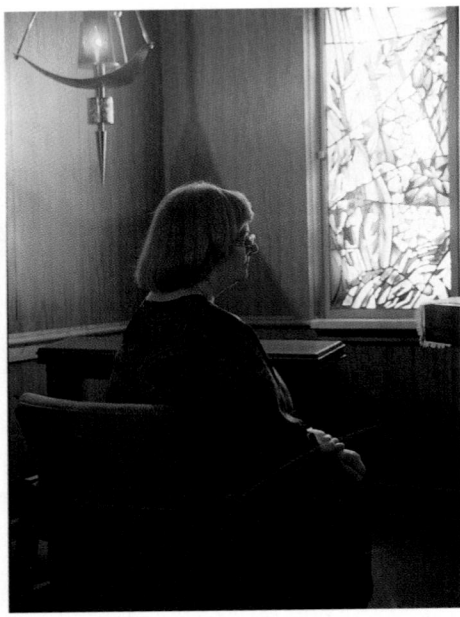

**Figure 5-5** Spiritual needs often become more important during times of stress such as illness.

higher rate than white Americans. The following examples are listed in the ANA's *Position Statement on Discrimination and Racism in Health Care* (1998b):

- Cancer is the leading cause of death for Chinese and Vietnamese individuals.
- Vietnamese women suffer from cervical cancer at nearly five times the rate of white American women.
- Compared with the general population, Hispanics have a higher incidence of cancer of the stomach, esophagus, pancreas, and cervix.
- African Americans have a life expectancy that is six years shorter than the life expectancy for white Americans.
- The Native American population has significant rates of diabetes, sudden infant death syndrome, and congenital malformations.

One of the major objectives established by the U.S. Office of Public Health in its *Healthy People 2010 Objectives* is the elimination of disparities in health status by providing equitable services for people of all groups (Chrvala & Bulger, 1999). Yet, while the objectives of *Healthy People 2010* call for providing equitable services for all groups of different backgrounds, the shift in health care toward a managed care model causes concern. The emphasis of a managed care model is cost-containment, which has the potential to place less priority in providing services that are culturally competent (Chinn, 2000). This is concerning because managed care organizations increasingly are serving more culturally diverse, undeserved populations since Medicaid recipients are enrolled into such services (Health Resources and Services Administration, 2001).

## LIFE SPAN CONSIDERATIONS

### Application of Developmental Theories

Application of child developmental theories to all children, regardless of their cultural or ethnic backgrounds, needs to be done with caution. Normative development has been defined according to Eurocentric standards, leaving little room for any other differences in the developing child. Five major sources of influence impact the developmental outcome of minority children, which include the effects of culture, health status, socioeconomic status, family structure, and biologic factors, all of which operate together but are difficult to isolate. Children from culturally or ethnically diverse backgrounds may not meet currently established milestones for various reasons. Consequently, a common child development assessment tool, the Denver Developmental II, which originally was developed from a Eurocentric perspective, underwent a major revision and restandardization to determine its usefulness with ethnic groups (Frankenburg, Dodds, Archer, Shapiro, & Bresnick, 1992). More recently, the Centers for Disease Control and Prevention updated the widely used growth charts, using government data from the last 30 years on children from all ethnic groups (CDC, 2003). The old chart, which was widely used prior to its updating, was developed utilizing data from a private study of formula-fed, primarily white children in Ohio.

## Vulnerable Populations

As a result of societal changes, more people are at risk for health problems. Groups that are especially susceptible for health-related problems include the poor, the homeless, migrant workers, abused individuals, the elderly, pregnant adolescents, and people with sexually transmitted diseases such as acquired immunodeficiency syndrome (AIDS).

The United States is currently facing many economic, social, and political challenges related to the delivery of health care services to vulnerable population groups (Edelman & Mandle, 2002). As a result, many vulnerable populations are underserved because of the high demand for services, lack of services, and limited availability and access to services.

### The Poor

Poverty affects health status and accessibility to health care services. According to the Centers for Disease

Control and Prevention (CDC) (1998), "increase in either income or education increases the likelihood of good health status. This relationship between socioeconomic status and health was observed for persons in every race and ethnic group examined" (p. 52). Living in poverty means being unable to meet the financial demands of basic living expenses, such as food, shelter, and clothing. Socioeconomic status is determined by family income, educational level, and occupation. "Childhood poverty has long-lasting negative effects on one's health. Children in low-income families fare less well than children in more affluent families. In 1999, 17% of American children lived in poverty" (U.S. Bureau of the Census, 2000). In 1999, a family of four with an annual income below $17,029 was below the federal poverty threshold. The poor population has more complex health problems, including a higher incidence of chronic illness (U.S. Bureau of the Census, 2000).

The CDC (1998) has identified the following as health risk factors that are related to lower income:

- Higher prevalence of cigarette smoking
- Greater incidence of obesity
- Elevated blood pressure
- Sedentary lifestyle
- Less likely to be covered by health insurance
- Less likely to receive preventive health care services

Increasing numbers of federally mandated health care initiatives are being implemented to address the historic racial and class disparities in health care. Entitlement programs imply that the government is legally mandated to provide services to the programs' eligible populations. Entitlement programs such as Medicare, Medicaid, and Women, Infants, and Children (WIC) were developed, in part, because of social and political pressures. WIC, a special supplemental food program for women, infants, and children, is a U.S. Public Health–sponsored program that targets low-income pregnant and breastfeeding mothers and their children age 5 years or younger. WIC links health care services, food supplements, and health education into a combined service package for eligible members. Medicaid is a program designed to provide access to health care for medically needy infants, children, and adults. Medicare is an entitlement program that finances health care services for individuals over the age of 65.

Poverty interferes with a child's ability to be housed, clothed, and fed adequately and can deprive the child of a safe (physical and psychological) environment. Children with access to health care have the possibility of getting necessary health care services. Children with health insurance (public or private) are much more likely than children without insurance to have a regular and accessible source of health care (U.S. Bureau of the Census, 2000). "There are many reasons why a child's parent(s) are uninsured . . . related to employment, limited health care benefits, and recent immigration" (Scott, 2000, p. 26).

## STOP AND THINK

### Factors That Correlate with Poverty

- How does cultural heritage correlate with factors that cause a person to be economically impoverished?

- Is poverty a result of socioeconomic political conditions, the individual's lack of initiative, or other factors?

- How do you feel about a person who cannot afford adequate health care services?

- Should the person be provided with access to health care?

## The Homeless

Even though it is difficult to determine the exact number of homeless people, it is estimated that 350,000 to 6 million people are homeless in the United States (Walker, 1998, p. 27). Societal factors that contribute to homelessness are:

- Lack of affordable housing
- Increasingly stringent criteria for public assistance
- Decreased availability of social services
- Inadequate or lack of employment
- A history of psychosocial trauma
- Deinstitutionalization of clients from mental health facilities *without* adequate community support (such as halfway houses and group homes)

Approximately 85% of homeless people are on the streets because they have some form of mental illness or are addicted to alcohol or other drugs (Walker, 1998). "We must confront the mistaken notion that hopelessness is a choice . . . It's important to understand the connection between hopelessness and chronic mental illness, for with understanding can come the sensitivity and compassion necessary to serve this population" (Walker, 1998, p. 27).

Those who are homeless are at greater risk for illness and injuries (Edelman & Mandle, 2002) (see Box 5-5). Hatton (1997) identified the following as major health care needs of homeless women: mental health, sexually transmitted diseases, and substance abuse. Access to basic health care services is limited because the homeless lack health insurance coverage. Those few facilities that do provide services to the homeless are not always accessible due to lack of transportation.

Children are especially vulnerable to the perils of homelessness. Presently, the federal government does not regularly collect data on the number of homeless children in the United States. However, 1998 statistics (U.S.

## BOX 5-5   COMMON HEALTH PROBLEMS EXPERIENCED BY THE HOMELESS

| Problem | Impact of Homelessness |
|---|---|
| Diabetes | • Lack of regularly scheduled nutritious meals<br>• Inadequate rest<br>• Insufficient exercise |
| AIDS | • Higher rate of sexual assault<br>• Intravenous drug use<br>• Lack of treatment or inadequate follow-up |
| Respiratory diseases (e.g., tuberculosis, pneumonia) | • Crowded living conditions<br>• Inadequate nutrition<br>• Limited or no access to treatment facilities |
| Cardiovascular diseases | • Impaired peripheral circulation as a result of extended time of walking on the streets and/or sleeping in upright, seated position<br>• Food served in many shelters has a high sodium content<br>• Consumption of alcohol and tobacco products |
| Parasitic infestations | • Shared personal items (clothing, bedding, hairbrushes)<br>• Close physical contact (as in shelters)<br>• Lack of facilities for bath, showers<br>• Inability to treat all those in contact with the affected person |

Data from Acquaviva, T., & Lancaster, J. (2000). Poverty and homelessness. In M. Stanhope & J. Lancaster (Eds.), *Community health nursing: Promoting health of aggregates, families, and individuals* (5th ed.). St. Louis: Mosby-Yearbook.

Bureau of the Census, 2000) show that 36% of U.S. households with children had housing problems, including physically inadequate housing and crowded housing. Adolescents who are homeless are at high risk for physical and mental health problems, including malnutrition, substance abuse, accidental pregnancy, and sexually transmitted disease.

The social and political reforms that are needed to create solutions to homelessness have just begun. There is great *urgency* to meet the immediate needs of the homeless and to provide health care that emphasizes both disease prevention and health promotion.

"Nonprofit nursing centers and clinics try to halt the epidemic of uninsured children" (Scott, 2000, p. 26). Listed below are a few examples of nursing's efforts in responding to the needs of vulnerable clients:

- Community Volunteers in Medicine is a nonprofit organization in which nurses, doctors, and dentists volunteer their time and services to treat uninsured people of all ages living in Chester County, Pennsylvania.
- Philadelphia-based Regional Nursing Centers Consortium (RNCC) sees approximately 250,000 clients annually. Up to 50% of these clients are uninsured.
- In 1999, LaSalle Neighborhood Nursing Center in Philadelphia identified 300 uninsured children and enrolled them in the Children's Health Insurance Program (CHIPs) or for medical assistance (Scott, 2000).

## Environmental Control

Environmental control refers to the relationships between people and nature and to a person's perceived ability to control activities of nature, such as factors causing illness.

A person's belief about the causation of disease will determine the type of treatment (if any) sought. According to Andrews and Boyle (1998), there are three types of health belief systems: magicoreligious, biomedical, and holistic. The magicoreligious belief system is based on the concept that health and illness are determined by supernatural forces (such as a higher power or the gods). The biomedical belief system states that illness is a result of an impairment in physical or biochemical processes. The holistic belief system views health as a result of harmony among the elements of nature; conversely, disease is caused by disharmony.

## Folk Medicine

Most cultures have preferences about health care, including:

- The type of care that is necessary and appropriate
- When care/treatment should be sought
- The appropriate caregiver

Because the presence of a folk medicine system (also referred to as alternative medicine) can present challenges to nurses caring for clients from diverse cultures, knowledge of basic beliefs about illness, factors contributing to illness, and home remedies is necessary. Nurses must realize that clients are often utilizing folk medicine or remedies at home but may be reluctant to disclose this information. It is important to try to obtain information about possible use of home remedies, because some home remedies may alter the function of some medical interventions. See Chapter 31 for a complete discussion of complementary/alternative treatment methods.

Folk healers are knowledgable about cultural norms and are usually familiar to the one seeking care (Edelman & Mandle, 2002). Table 5-2 presents the various healers within different cultures and describes common folk healing practices within these cultures. Nurses must be able to relate care and treatment to the client's cultural context to incorporate informal caregivers, healers, and other members of the clients' support system as allies in treatment. "The patient-centered orientation of nursing makes it imperative that nurses be able to respond to the unique cultural needs of different people. Nurses are challenged to provide effective caring and curing in varied cultural contexts" (Lester, 1998, p. 26).

## Biologic Variations

Biologic variations that distinguish one cultural group from another include enzymatic differences and susceptibility to disease (Andrews & Boyle, 2002; Giger & Davidhizar, 2004). Enzymatic differences account for diverse responses of some groups to dietary therapy and drugs (Table 5-3). Nutritional variations include food preferences that may contribute to health problems (Table 5-4).

## Transcultural Nursing

The ANA (1998) states that culture is a central concept of nursing. Acknowledgment and acceptance of cultural differences and understanding of culturally specific responses to illness are prerequisites for providing safe and effective care.

The conceptual framework for understanding cultural diversity and providing culturally competent care is based on Madeline Leininger's transcultural nursing theory. **Transcultural nursing**, according to Leininger (1978), focuses on the study and analysis of different cultures and subcultures with respect to cultural care, health beliefs, and health practices, with the goal of providing health care within the context of the client's culture.

A basic assumption of transcultural nursing is that when health care providers see problems from the client's cultural viewpoint, they are more open to understanding, appreciating, and working effectively with these clients (Figure 5-6). Other assumptions of transcultural nursing theory are:

- Every culture has some kind of system for health care that is based on values and behaviors.
- Cultures have certain methods for providing health care. These methods of care are often unknown to nurses from other cultures (Leininger, 1978).

Due to rapid globalization, every nurse must have an understanding of human conditions in diverse societies. Nurses do not need to travel to foreign countries to engage in international nursing. Nurses encounter cultural diversity everywhere—from inner-city hospitals to suburban

## TABLE 5-2    FOLK MEDICINE: HEALERS AND PRACTICES

| Cultural Group | Traditional Healers | Healing Practices |
|---|---|---|
| *African American* | • Elderly women healers<br>• "Community Mother" or "Granny"<br>• "Root doctor"<br>• Voodoo healer ("Mambo" or "oungan")<br>• Spiritualist | • Herbs, roots<br>• Poultices<br>• Oils<br>• Religious healing through rituals, (e.g., laying on of hands)<br>• Talismans are worn around the wrist or neck, or carried in a pouch to ward off disease |
| *Asian American* | • Herbalist<br>• Physician | • Use of hot and cold foods<br>• Herbs (e.g., ginseng root, which is used as a restorative potion)<br>• Soups<br>• Cupping, pinching, and rubbing<br>• Meditation<br>• Acupuncture (puncturing the skin at specified areas with metal needles)<br>• Acupressure (applying pressure with the fingertips to specified areas of the body)<br>• Application of tiger balm (a salve) to relieve muscular pains<br>• Energy to restore balance between yin and yang |
| *European American* | • Nurse<br>• Physician | • Exercise<br>• Medication (prescribed and over-the-counter)<br>• Modified diets<br>• Amulets<br>• Religious healing rituals |
| *Hispanic American* | • *Curandero*<br>• *Espiritualista*<br>• *Yerbero* (herbalist)<br>• *Brujo* (healer who uses witchcraft)<br>• *Sobadora*<br>• *Santiguadora* | • Hot and cold foods to treat some conditions<br>• Herbal teas, such as *Manzanilla*, used to treat gastrointestinal problems, insomnia, and menstrual cramps<br>• Prayers and religious medals<br>• Massage<br>• *Azabache*, a black stone worn as a necklace or bracelet to ward off the "evil eye"<br>• Some Haitian mothers practice the "three baths" ritual: they bathe for the first 3 postpartum days in water boiled with special leaves |
| *Native American* | • Shaman<br>• Medicine man/woman | • Use of plants and herbs<br>• Medicine bundle or bag filled with herbs that have been blessed by a medicine man/woman during a healing ceremony<br>• Sweet grass (herbs) burned to purify the ill person<br>• *Estafiate* (dried leaves) boiled to produce a tea for treating stomach disorders<br>• The *Blessingway* ceremony (a healing ritual conducted by the medicine man/woman)<br>• In some Navajo tribes, the medicine man/woman uses sand painting as a diagnostic method |

Data from Degazon, C. (2000). Cultural diversity and community health nursing practice. In M. Stanhope & J. Lancaster (Eds.), *Community health nursing: Promoting health of aggregates, families, and individuals* (5th ed.). St. Louis: Mosby-Yearbook; Giger, J. N., & Davidhizar, R. E. (2004). *Transcultural nursing: Assessment and intervention* (4th ed.). St. Louis: Mosby-Yearbook; Grossman, D. (1996). Cultural dimensions in home health nursing. *American Journal of Nursing, 96*(7), 33–36.

## TABLE 5-3    EFFECTS OF BIOLOGIC VARIATIONS ON SELECTED DRUGS

| Cultural Group | Effect of Biological Variance on Drugs |
|---|---|
| African American | • Isoniazid (drug used to treat tuberculosis) is rapidly metabolized, thus becoming inactive quickly; occurs in approximately 60% of population. <br>• An enzyme deficiency interferes with metabolism of primaquine (used to treat malaria); occurs in approximately 35% of population. <br>• Antihypertensive drugs (e.g., propranolol) need to be administered in higher doses to produce same effects as in European Americans. |
| Asian American | • Isoniazid (drug used to treat tuberculosis) is rapidly metabolized, thus becoming inactive quickly; occurs in approximately 85%-90% of population. <br>• Rapid metabolism of alcohol results in excessive facial flushing and other vasomotor symptoms. <br>• Chinese men need only about half as much propranolol (antihypertensive drug) as European American men. <br>• Asian people need smaller doses of alprazolam (antianxiety drug) to achieve same blood levels as their European American counterparts; the drug is also metabolized more slowly (remains in the bloodstream longer) in Asian men. |
| European American | • Due to liver enzyme differences, caffeine is metabolized and excreted faster than by people of other cultural groups. |
| Native American | • Isoniazid (drug used to treat tuberculosis) is rapidly metabolized, thus becoming inactive quickly; occurs in approximately 60%-90% of population. <br>• Rapid metabolism of alcohol results in excessive facial flushing and other vasomotor symptoms. |

Data from Andrews, M. M., & Boyle, J. S. (2002). *Transcultural concepts in nursing care* (4th ed.). Philadelphia: Lippincott; Giger, J. N., & Davidhizar, R. E. (2004). *Transcultural nursing: Assessment & intervention* (4th ed.). St. Louis: Mosby-Yearbook.

## TABLE 5-4    FOOD PREFERENCES AND RELATED EFFECTS ON HEALTH

| Cultural Group | Food Preferences | Nutritional Excess | Related Health Problem |
|---|---|---|---|
| African American | • Pork <br>• Greens <br>• Rice <br>• Fried foods | • Calories <br>• Cholesterol <br>• Carbohydrates <br>• Sodium | • Obesity <br>• Cardiovascular illnesses (hypertension, coronary heart disease) |
| Asian American | • Raw fish <br>• Rice <br>• Soy sauce | • Calories <br>• Cholesterol <br>• Carbohydrates <br>• Sodium | • Coronary heart disease <br>• Liver disease <br>• Stomach cancer <br>• Ulcers |
| Hispanic American | • Beans <br>• Fried foods <br>• Chili <br>• Carbonated beverages | • Calories <br>• Cholesterol <br>• Carbohydrates <br>• Sodium | • Obesity <br>• Coronary heart disease <br>• Diabetes |
| Native American | • Blue cornmeal <br>• Fish <br>• Game <br>• Fruits and berries | • Calories <br>• Carbohydrates | • Malnutrition <br>• Diabetes |

Data from Andrews, M. M., & Boyle, J. S. (2002). *Transcultural concepts in nursing care* (4th ed.). Philadelphia: Lippincott; Giger, J. N., & Davidhizar, R. E. (2004). *Transcultural nursing: Assessment & intervention* (4th ed.). St. Louis: Mosby-Yearbook.

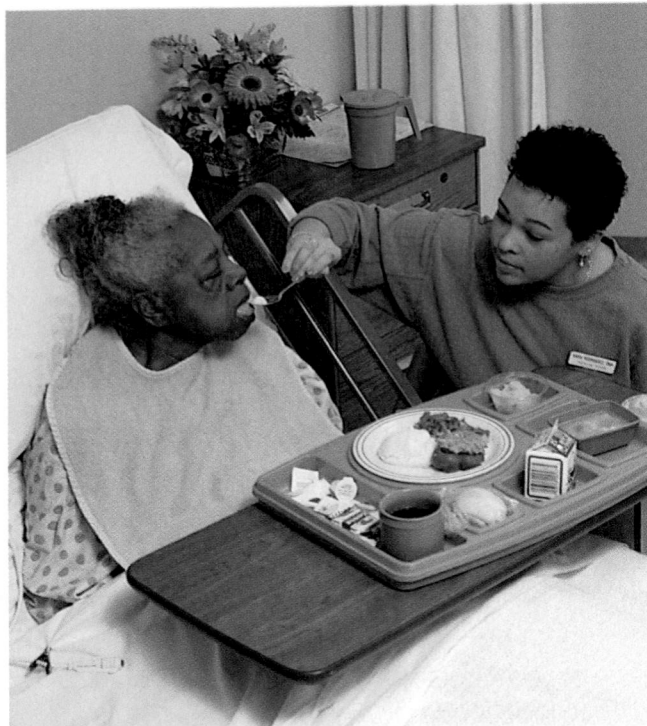

**Figure 5-6** The relationship between this nurse and client is based on a mutual acceptance of each other's cultural viewpoints.

| TABLE 5-5 | ELEMENTS OF CULTURAL COMPETENCE |
|---|---|
| **Element** | **Definition** |
| Cultural Awareness | A cognitive process in which the nurse becomes aware of and sensitive to the client's cultural values, beliefs, and practices |
| Cultural Knowledge | The nurse seeks a sound educational base about different cultures. |
| Cultural Skill | The nurse's ability to perform a culturally specific assessment (i.e., physical and psychosocial) |
| Cultural Encounters | The nurse interacts with clients from diverse cultural backgrounds. |
| Cultural Desire | The nurse's motivation ("want to") to become culturally competent |

Data from Campinha-Bacote, J. (1999). A model and instrument for addressing cultural competence in health care. *Journal of Nursing Education, 38*(5), 204–205.

clinics, from technologically sophisticated institutions to homes in rural, inner-city, and suburban areas.

## Cultural Competence

Community, social and kinship ties, religion, language, food, and cultural perceptions of illness are all areas that need to be considered by the nurse when working with culturally diverse clients. Cultural diversity challenges nurses to bridge cultural gaps with clients by providing culturally relevant care. An understanding of the client's cultural context permits nurses to become familiar with the client as a person instead of focusing only on the illness or problem.

**Cultural competence** is the process through which the nurse provides care that is appropriate to the client's cultural context. Culturally competent nurses are those who demonstrate knowledge and understanding of the client's culture; accept and respect cultural differences; and adapt care to be congruent with the client's culture (Purnell & Paulanka, 2003). Culturally competent nurses have knowledge about cultural values related to health and illness. Also, nurses who provide care in a culturally sensitive manner are flexible in their approaches and thinking. Campinha-Bacote (1999) defines five elements of cultural competence; see Table 5-5 for an explanation of each element.

## Cultural Competence and Nursing Process

Cultural sensitivity is requisite in every phase of the nursing process. The nurse's role in providing culturally competent care includes performing a cultural assessment, formulating nursing diagnoses, identifying expected client outcomes, planning care to assist clients in achieving the expected outcomes, intervening to address the client's nursing diagnoses, and evaluating the plan of care. In its *Guide to Nurses for Providing Culturally Sensitive Care*, the College of Nurses of Ontario (1991) identifies four elements of providing culturally sensitive care: self-reflection, facilitating client choice, gaining cultural knowledge, and effective communication. These four elements permeate the nursing process.

## Assessment

Caring for a client from a different culture can be challenging to the nurse. Using the client's strengths and respecting the client's values are essential components of effective nursing care. To begin providing culturally competent care, the nurse should use questions to gather infor-

## BOX 5-6 CULTURAL ASSESSMENT FACTORS

- Client's ethnic heritage
- Family role and function
- Religious practices
- Food preferences
- Native language
- Social networks
- Educational experiences (formal and informal)
- Health care beliefs
- Family patterns of health care

mation about the client's cultural background. The factors pertinent to cultural assessment are listed in Box 5-6.

The questions in the Cultural Assessment Interview Guide, shown in Figure 5-7, can either be incorporated into a general nursing assessment tool or used separately as a cultural assessment tool.

Understanding how a client explains and understands her illness is an important part of conducting a cultural assessment. When nurses are able to understand the client's perspective, they are better able to develop culturally appropriate plans of care that are inclusive of the client's thoughts, values, and perspectives about the illness. The Patient's Explanatory Model by Kleinman (Fadiman, 1997) is very useful for the nurse to explore the client's thoughts with some or all of the questions.

## Nursing Diagnosis

Diagnoses approved by the North American Nursing Diagnosis Association (NANDA, 2003) are used extensively by nurses. However, one stated disadvantage to NANDA diagnostic statements is that sometimes the diagnoses are worded in ways that result in cultural bias (Luckmann, 2000). Box 5-7 lists some diagnoses that may be culturally biased.

Consider the following examples of ways in which these diagnoses may be used in a culturally inappropriate manner:

- Applying the diagnosis *impaired verbal communication* to clients who speak a language different from the nurse
- Using the diagnosis *noncompliance* with a client who rejects a prescribed treatment method in order to adhere to culturally sanctioned folk healing methods

It may be more appropriate to use another term instead of *noncompliant*. Ward-Collins (1998) suggests "nonadherent" by stating that this term may present less of a stigma to clients than "noncompliant."

## RESEARCH FOCUS

**Title of Study:** Preparing Culturally Competent Practitioners

**Study Purpose:** To evaluate whether international student nursing clinical experiences could change student's ethnocentricism, cultural sensitivity, and cultural self-efficacy.

**Methods:** This exploratory study examined the relationship among cultural immersion, cultural self-efficacy, and cultural competence by using a triangulated research design. The study involved 10 different groups of students who volunteered to participate in international nursing experiences. The study was conducted during a 2-year time frame.

**Findings:** Quantitative analysis found statistically significant differences in the achievement of cultural self-efficacy for the students who completed international nursing clinical experiences as compared to the students who remained in the United States.

**Implications:** Short-term clinical cultural immersion experiences help move nursing students toward a greater understanding and achievement of cultural competence.

St. Clair, A., & McKenry, L. (1999). Preparing culturally competent practitioners. *Journal of Nursing Education, 39*(5), 228–234.

## BOX 5-7 NURSING DIAGNOSES THAT MAY BE CULTURALLY BIASED

- Noncompliance
- Impaired verbal communication
- Impaired social interaction
- Deficient knowledge
- Disturbed thought processes
- Powerlessness

# Cultural Assessment Interview Guide

Name: _____

Nickname or other names or special meaning attributed to your name: _____

Primary language:

        When speaking _____

        When writing _____

Date of birth: _____

Place of birth: _____

Educational level or specialized training: _____

To which ethnic group do you belong? _____

To what extent do you identify with your cultural group? _____

Who is the spokesperson for your family? _____

Describe some of the customs or beliefs that you have about the following:

        Health _____

        Life _____

        Illness _____

        Death _____

How do you learn information best?

    ☐ Reading

    ☐ Having someone explain verbally

    ☐ Having someone demonstrate

Describe some of your family's dietary habits and your personal food preferences. _____

_____

Are there any foods forbidden from your diet for religious or cultural reasons? _____

_____

Describe your religious affiliation. _____

What role do your religious beliefs and practices play in your life during times of good health and bad health? _____

_____

Whom do you rely on for health care services or healing and what type of cultural health practices have you been exposed to? _____

_____

Are there any sanctions or restrictions in your culture that the person taking care of you should know? _____

_____

Describe your current living arrangements. _____

How do members of your family communicate with each other? _____

Describe your strengths. _____

Who /what is your primary source of information about your health? _____

Is there anything else that is important about your cultural beliefs that you want to tell me? _____

**Figure 5-7    Cultural Assessment Interview Guide**

## NURSING STRATEGY

### Kleinman's Client Explanatory Model

Ask the client the following questions to explore the client's thoughts:

1. What do you call the problem?

2. What do you think has caused the problem?

3. Why do you think it started when it did?

4. What do you think the sickness does? How does it work?

5. How severe is the sickness? Will it have a short or long course?

6. What kind of treatment do you think you should receive? What are the most important results you hope to gain?

7. What are the chief problems the sickness has caused?

8. What do you fear most about the sickness?

Adapted from Fadiman, A. (1997). *The spirit catches you and you fall down*. New York: Noonday Press.

## CLIENT REFLECTIONS

### English Second Language Difficulties

Juan, age 32, is a Hispanic client who speaks broken English, and he has home health care three times per week for his new ostomy. He states, "Sometimes the nurses act like I am stupid because I speak English bad—and other times they [nurses] act like I am lazy. I think they [nurses] label me as lazy because they [nurses] think all Hispanics are lazy. I just can't speak English that good."

What would your care to this client involve?

## Planning and Outcome Identification

Cultural groups are not homogeneous; there are individual variations in personality, behavior, and expectations. It is important not to consider one member of a particular group to be like all the others of that same group.

In order to develop effective plans of care, nurses need to understand the following (American Nurses Association, 1998a):

• Cultural groups' perspectives on life processes (e.g, birth, death)
• Cultural definitions of health and illness
• How cultural groups maintain wellness
• Culture's perspectives on the causes of illness
• Use of healers in the cure and care of illness
• The influence of the nurse's cultural background on the delivery of care

It is also necessary to consider how the client's beliefs may impact the plan of care. Cultural beliefs greatly influence perceptions about health and, therefore, may create barriers to adhering to prescribed treatment plans. Culture influences the following:

• Perceptions of illness versus health
• Responses to illness

• Perceptions about the significance of symptoms
• The types of treatment approaches (i.e., alternative and/or conventional) (Muscari, 1998, p. 27)

## Implementation

Caring for culturally diverse clients requires three major nursing interventions: self-awareness, use of a nonjudgmental approach, and client education. Each of these aspects is discussed in the following section. The accompanying Community/Home Care box offers guidelines for providing culturally sensitive care for clients at home.

### Self-Awareness

In an increasingly diverse society, the nurse must be aware of the potential for bias or misunderstanding. Self-awareness can be used to help nurses recognize their own stereotypes, biases, and prejudgments about clients who are culturally different. Further experience, introspection, and study empower nurses to appreciate their own cultures and the strengths of other cultures.

### Nonjudgmental Approach

A nonjudgmental attitude is essential in the provision of culturally sensitive care. When caring in a manner sensitive to the client's cultural background, the nurse enables the client to offer open, honest feedback, to disagree, or to discuss real or perceived problems. A health care partnership is the outcome of this approach. "A key component of successful interactions with culturally diverse patients is to avoid using stereotypical, judgmental words" (Ward-Collins, 1998, p. 30).

### Client Education

Educating clients is an integral part of nursing practice. Education not only must be relevant to the client's needs but also must be provided in a culturally sensitive manner. Lester (1998) states, "You need to present the information in a way that the patient grabs onto what is important to her. We need to learn how to present teaching so that people can

## COMMUNITY/HOME CARE

### Providing Culturally Sensitive Nursing Care in the Home

- Remember that the setting for care is controlled by the client and family, not by the health care provider.

- The nurse is often viewed as a guest by the client and family. Social chatter may be necessary to facilitate rapport.

- The nurse must be nonjudgmental about the condition of the home (e.g., presence of clutter and disarray).

- Show respect and consideration for the client. For example:
  - Ask permission to use the sink or bathroom to wash your hands.
  - Wipe your feet before entering the home.
  - Ask permission before moving client's belongings, and replace items after you have finished the task.

- Take advantage of the home environment to assess cultural values and norms. Cultural clues may include:
  - Orderliness and decor of the home
  - Assignment of family roles and tasks
  - Types of interactions among family members
  - Value placed on privacy
  - Value placed on possessions

## NURSING STRATEGY

### Culturally Sensitive Teaching Guidelines

When caring for clients from diverse cultures, the nurse should consider the following guidelines for client teaching:

- Assess and incorporate family history of health care:
  - Fluency in English; obtain an interpreter if necessary
  - Extent of family support
  - Community resources
  - Level of education
  - Change of social status as a result of coming to this country

- Affirm client strengths.

- Recognize informal caregivers (family members and significant others) as an integral part of treatment.

- Evaluate the client's current knowledge base by asking the client to state what he knows about the specific topic.

- To ascertain the client's perception of need, ask the client and family what they need or want to learn.

- Observe the interaction between the client and family to determine family roles and authority figures. Include the dominant family member in your teaching.

- Use language easily understood by the client; avoid medical jargon.

- Clarify your verbal and nonverbal messages with the client.

- Have the client repeat the information learned, and if possible, demonstrate back what was taught.

- Inquire if the client has any further questions.

- Summarize at the end of teaching segment.

Luckmann, J. (2000). *Transcultural communication in nursing.* Clifton Park, NY: Delmar Learning; St. Clair, A., & McKenry, L. (1999). Preparing culturally competent practitioners. *Journal of Nursing Education, 39*(5), 228–234.

hear it. If people can't hear it, then we will not succeed in what we are trying to teach" (p. 29). See the Nursing Strategy box for culturally sensitive teaching guidelines.

## Evaluation

The final phase of the nursing process, evaluation, is extremely important in determining the client's achievement of expected outcomes and the efficacy of nursing interventions in delivery of culturally sensitive care.

Provision of culturally competent care requires that the nurse view the client as a partner of the health care team. It is important to demonstrate caring behaviors rather than just tolerating cultural variations in client's behavior. Awareness of cultural similarities and variations allow nurses to accept and appreciate the impact of culture on health care.

# CONCEPT MAPPING CASE STUDY

Mr. Ming Chang, a 68-year old Chinese gentleman, has been admitted to the short-term care unit for wound management of an ulcer on the plantar surface of his right foot. He was diagnosed with Non-Insulin Dependent Diabetes Mellitus (NIDDM), or type II diabetes, 5 years ago. His fasting blood glucose levels continue to fluctuate above 270 mg/dl, even though several months ago his physician prescribed exercise, an appropriate diet, and added tolazamide (Tolinase), a hypoglycemic medication, 100 mg daily. Mr. Chang complains of swelling and numbness in his feet and legs, but he does not have foot pain. The ulcerated area, near the metatarsal heads, has no drainage; the surrounding skin appears dry, cracked, and calloused; the pedal pulses are normal; the foot is warm to the touch; his toenails are long and thick.

Mr. Chang is a widower and lives with his daughter and her family. He understands some English, but cannot read it. He prefers that his daughter, Margaret, serve as his interpreter. She prepares his meals and administers his medications; however, he frequently will not submit to the finger sticks or scheduled blood draws for checking his glucose levels, and sometimes refuses the prescribed medication. (In addition to his diabetes, Mr. Chang has been diagnosed with hypertension and propranalol hydrochloride [Inderal] 40 mg b.i.d. was prescribed.) He prefers taking the Chinese herbal remedies that he feels are better for him. Margaret mentions that her father stopped his daily walks and Tai Chi exercises when the ulcer first appeared 4 months ago and he now spends most of his time watching television and smoking. He has given up one of his favorite pastimes, reading the Chinese newspapers, since he was recently diagnosed with a cataract. His appetite is good. In fact, he has gained some weight recently. Margaret is concerned about her father's health, but she feels helpless in trying to convince him to follow the plan of care.

The scenario has been designed to integrate cultural factors that can impact the plan of care. Create a concept map using the information that has been provided.

1. Refer to the concept map example in Appendix A for areas to include in your map. Add concepts from the case study into the areas where you believe they belong. (Some concepts may belong in more than one area.)
2. Have you placed the client in the center of the map?
3. Cluster related concepts together. Draw connecting lines to indicate relationships.
4. What are the risk factors related to culture and adherence to the plan of care?
5. Identify at least two nursing diagnoses related to Mr. Chang's health problem and his cultural beliefs.
6. Prioritize the client needs and list nursing interventions you would make to meet the needs.
7. What do you need to know about the Chinese culture to have appropriate interactions with Mr. Chang and his daughter/family?
8. Make a list of additional information that you would like to have in order to develop an appropriate plan of care for a client from a different culture.
9. What *optimal* client outcomes would you like to see?
10. Develop a basic teaching plan related to diabetes management and wound care. How will you need to adjust the teaching plan to minimize the cultural barriers to learning and application?
11. Compare your map with other students. How do they differ?
12. Discuss how cultural sensitivity is an essential component of safe and effective nursing care.

## Suggested References

Andrews, M., & Boyle, J. (2002). *Concepts in nursing care*. Philadelphia: Lippincott.

Leininger, M., & McFarland, M. (2002). *Transcultural nursing*. New York: McGraw-Hill.

Spector, R. (1999). *Cultural diversity in health & illness*. Upper Saddle River, N.J.: Prentice Hall.

Medical-Surgical texts for wound care and diabetes information.

Malarkey, L., & McMorrow, M. (2000). *Laboratory Tests and Diagnostic Procedures*. Philadelphia: W.B. Saunders.

Myers, B. (2003). *Wound management: principles and practice*. Upper Saddle River, N.J.: Prentice Hall.

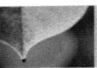

# CASE STUDY/NURSING CARE PLAN

Noah was a 35-year-old man who was brought to the emergency room by his brother. He had been having trouble sleeping, severe headaches, and episodes of blackouts. He was admitted to the hospital for a neurological workup of his symptoms. The doctor ordered some medications to relieve his pain, but Noah refused it. Morning reports from the night shift included that he continued to have trouble sleeping and that he had been crying. By the third day of admission, a mental health caseworker found that Noah was a refugee who had escaped from Sudan during the wars a year ago. While fleeing persecution, several of Noah's family members were killed, including his father. But Noah had to leave his father's body on the roadside, unburied. Noah believed that because his father was not buried, his spirit was angry with him and wandering the earth, causing Noah to be sick. A plan of care specific to Noah's ethnic and cultural background was to be implemented when Noah was discharged with follow-up home health nursing care.

## Assessment

Client is experiencing severe sleep disturbances and blackouts. He believes that his symptoms are caused by the angry spirit of his dead father because he was not buried after his death. Because Noah believes that his symptoms are due to a spiritual cause and not a physical one, he is refusing his medication.

## Nursing Diagnosis #1

Anxiety related to the unmet personal and cultural needs as evidenced by sleeplessness, headaches, and blackouts

**NOC:** Anxiety Control; Coping

**NIC:**   Anxiety Reduction; Presence; Calming Technique; Emotional Support

## Expected Outcomes

The client will:
1. Experience a relief of symptoms as evidenced by no further reports of headaches, sleeplessness, and blackouts within 1 week.
2. Attend culturally familiar activities (initiated by self) within 2 weeks.

## Planning/Interventions/Rationales

1. Seek out a community network of resources, such as the African Alliance organization, to explore ways to help Noah achieve peace about his father's death. *Encourages collaboration with a person familiar with Noah's cultural background and beliefs.*
2. Facilitate an opportunity for Noah to participate in a ritual that is acceptable to him so he may acquire peace. *Including Noah in the process will assure that he finds this intervention acceptable.*
3. Utilize nonpharmacological methods for pain relief, such as relaxation, distraction, massage, and a calm, quiet environment that promotes relaxation. *Provides client with options for pain relief that also respects his decision to not take medication for pain.*
4. Encourage creating an environment that is conducive to sleep, which includes such things as a quiet, darkened sleeping environment, and herbal teas acceptable to client. *Provides client with opportunities to sleep, which may help to alleviate some of his symptoms.*

## Evaluation

Client attended ritual 1 week after returning home. In the 2 weeks following discharge, Noah has only had two headaches, reports he is "sleeping better," and has had no blackouts.

## Key Concepts

- Every aspect of a person's life is influenced by one's culture.
- Behavior affecting health is culturally determined.
- Culture is a dynamic structure of behaviors, ideas, attitudes, values, habits, beliefs, customs, languages, rituals, ceremonies, and practices that are unique to a particular group of people. This structure of knowledge, behaviors, and values provides a group with a "blueprint" for behavior.
- Cultural norms are transmitted from one generation to another.

- Ethnicity is described as a sense of belongingness that is shared by other members of that same group. Ethnic groups are usually composed of people with the same racial composition.
- Race refers to a grouping of people based on biologic similarities. Members of a racial group have similar physical characteristics, such as blood type, facial features, and color of skin, hair, and eyes.
- Members of some racial and ethnic groups have experienced oppression in the forms of racism, sexism, and classism.
- The dominant values of the United States include achievement and success; individualism, independence, and self-reliance; activity, work, and ownership; efficiency, practicality, and reliance on technology; material comfort; competition and achievement; and youth and beauty.
- There is great value in cultural diversity, including a broader perspective of others, enhanced problem-solving ability and creativity, and improved productivity in the workplace.
- The six organizing phenomena of culture are communication, space, orientation to time, social organization, environmental control, and biologic variations.
- Transcultural nursing is based on the belief that when nurses view problems from the client's cultural viewpoint, they are more open to understanding and working more effectively with clients from other cultures.
- Understanding and accepting cultural differences and responses to illness are prerequisites for providing quality nursing care.
- The provision of culturally sensitive care is achieved through the use of approaches such as nonjudgmental attitudes and self-awareness and tools such as cultural assessment guides and client education strategies.

## Review Questions and Activities

1. Describe the difference between culture and ethnicity.
2. Identify the factors that contribute to the multiculturalism environment in the United States.
3. Explain the organizing phenomena of culture, and provide examples for each phenomenon.
4. Discuss how managed care has the potential to hinder culturally competent care.
5. What can a nurse do to provide culturally competent nursing care?
6. Why is it important to use caution when applying child developmental theories to children of diverse backgrounds?
7. What are several questions the nurse could ask to assess a client's cultural values?
8. What can a nurse do to achieve the best level of communication possible with a client whose primary language is not English?
9. Describe culturally sensitive teaching guidelines to use when teaching a client of a diverse background.

## Web Resources

American Nurses Association
    http://www.ana.org
American Psychiatric Nurses Association
    http://www.apna.org
The Cross-Cultural Health Care Program
    http://www.xculture.org
National Association of Hispanic Nurses
    http://www.thehispanicnurses.org
National Black Nurses' Association
    http://www.nbna.org
National Latino Children's Institute
    http://www.nlci.org
Owl Star, Native American News & Culture
    http://www.owlstar.com
Transcultural Nursing Society
    http://www.tcns.org

## References

Acquaviva, T., & Lancaster, J. (2000). Poverty and homelessness. In M. Stanhope & J. Lancaster (Eds.), Community health nursing: *Promoting health of aggregates, families, and individuals* (5th ed.). St. Louis: Mosby-Yearbook.

American Nurses Association (1998a). ANA addressing cultural diversity in the profession. *American Nurse, 30*(1), 25.

American Nurses Association (1998b). *Position statement on discrimination and racism in health care.* Washington, DC: Author.

Andrews, M. M., & Boyle, J. S. (2002). *Transcultural concepts in nursing care* (4th ed.). Philadelphia: Lippincott.

Campinha-Bacote, J. (1999). A model and instrument of addressing cultural competence in health care. *Journal of Nursing Education, 38*(5), 203–207.

Centers for Disease Control and Prevention (1998). Socioeconomic status and health chartbook. In *Health, United States, 1998*. (PHS)98-1232-1.

Chinn, J. L. (2000). Culturally competent health care. *Public Health Reports, 115,* 25–33.

Chrvala, C. A., & Bulger, R. J. (1999). *Leading health indicators for healthy people 2010: Final report,* Division of Health Promotion and Disease Prevention, Institute of Medicine. Washington, DC: National Academy Press.

College of Nurses of Ontario (1991). *A guide to nurses for providing culturally sensitive care.* Ontario: Author.

Degazon, C. (2000). Cultural diversity and community health nursing practice. In M. Stanhope & J. Lancaster (Eds.), *Community health nursing: Promoting health of aggregates, families, and individuals* (5th ed.). St. Louis: Mosby-Yearbook.

Edelman, C. L., & Mandle, C. L. (2002). *Health promotion throughout the life span* (5th ed.). St. Louis: Mosby-Yearbook.

Fadiman, A. (1997). *The spirit catches you and you fall down.* New York: Noonday Press.

Frankenburg, W. K., Dodds, J., Archer, P., Shapiro, H., & Bresnick, B. (1992). The Denver II: A major revision and restandardization of the Denver Developmental Screening Test. *Pediatric, 89*(1), 91–97.

Giger, J. N., & Davidhizar, R. E. (1998). *Canadian transcultural nursing: Assessment and intervention.* St. Louis: Mosby.

Giger, J. N., & Davidhizar, R. E. (2004). *Transcultural nursing: Assessment & intervention* (4th ed.). St. Louis: Mosby-Yearbook.

Hatton, D. C. (1997). Managing health problems among homeless women with children in a transitional shelter. *Image: The Journal of Nursing Scholarship, 29*(1), 33–37.

Health Resources and Services Administration (2001). *Cultural Competence Works,* 8-0372(P). Merrifield, VA: U.S. Department of Health and Human Services.

Kavanagh, K., Absalom, K., Beil, W., & Schliessmann, L. (1999). Connecting and becoming culturally competent: A Lakota example. *Advances in Nursing Science, 21*(3), 9–31.

Kleinman, A. (1988). *The Illness Narratives: Suffering, Healing and the Human Condition.* New York: Basic Books.

Leininger, A. M. (1998). *Culture care diversity and universality: A theory of nursing.* New York: National League for Nursing.

Leininger, M. (1978). *Transcultural nursing: Concepts, theories, and practice.* New York: Wiley.

Lester, N. (1998). Cultural competence: A nursing dialogue: Part I. *American Journal of Nursing, 98*(8), 26–34.

Luckmann, J. (2000). *Transcultural communication in nursing.* Clifton Park, NY: Delmar Learning.

Muscari, M. E. (1998). Rebels with a cause: When adolescents won't follow medical advice. *American Journal of Nursing, 98*(12), 26–30.

New pediatric growth charts. Centers for Disease Control, 2003. http://www.cdc.gov

North American Nursing Diagnosis Association. (2001). *Nursing diagnoses: Definitions and classification 2001–2002.* Philadelphia: Author.

Pickens, J. (1998). Formal and informal care of people with psychiatric disorders: Historical perspectives and current trends. *Journal of Psychosocial Nursing, 36*(1), 37–43.

Purnell, L. D., & Paulanka, B. J. (2003). *Transcultural health care: A culturally competent approach* (2nd ed.). Philadelphia: F. A. Davis.

Scott, A. (2000). Helping uninsured children. *Advance for Nurses: Special Edition Job Watch, 2000,* 25–26.

Sherwood, G. D. (2000). The power of nurse-client encounters: interpreting spiritual themes. *Journal of Holistic Nursing, 18*(2), 159–175.

St. Clair, A., & McKenry, L. (1999). Preparing culturally competent practitioners. *Journal of Nursing Education, 39*(5), 228–234.

Steward, M. (1998 Jan). Nurses need to strengthen cultural competence for the next century to ensure quality patient care. *American Nurse, 30*(1), 26–27.

U.S. Bureau of the Census (2000). Current population reports, Series P60-210, *Poverty in the United States: 1999.* Washington, DC: U.S. Government.

Walker, C. (1998). Homeless people and mental health: A nursing concern. *American Journal of Nursing, 98*(11), 26–32.

Ward-Collins, D. (1998). Noncompliant: Isn't there a better way to say it? *American Journal of Nursing, 98*(5), 27–31.

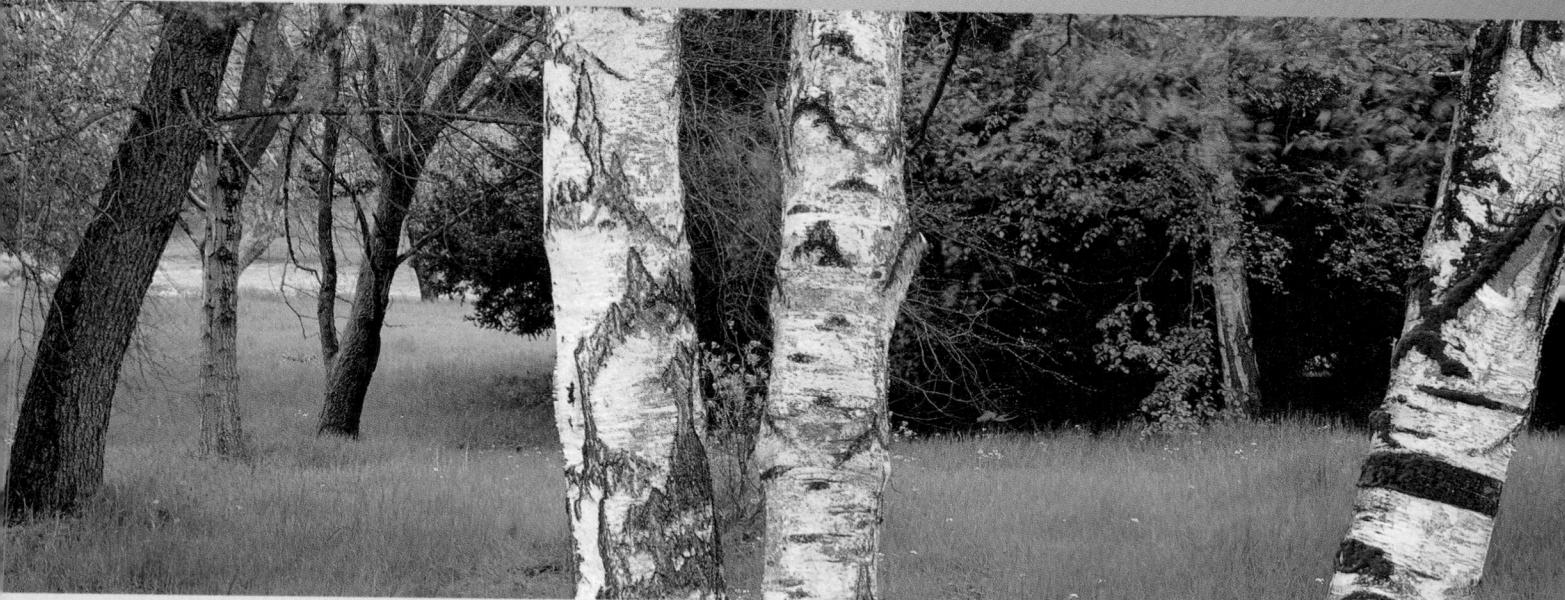

# CHAPTER 6

# Evidence-Based Practice and Nursing Research

Katherine Moore, RN, PhD
Kate Caelli, RN, RM, PhD

*"Scholarliness is a hallmark of the 1990s because research and theory help explicate major agreed-on nursing phenomena; because nursing is able to articulate its mission in theoretical terms and with scientific data."*

*(Meleis, 1997)*

# Chapter Competencies

*Upon completion of this chapter, the reader should be able to:*

1. Describe the historical development of nursing research.
2. Analyze how nursing knowledge is formulated.
3. Define evidence-based practice.
4. Compare and contrast research designs, methods, and methodologies.
5. Identify the parts of a research proposal.
6. Synthesize how to critically read a quantitative study and a qualitative study.
7. Explain the importance of writing and publishing a research study.
8. Analyze the implementation of research into nursing practice.
9. Evaluate potential directions for nursing research in the future.

# Key Terms

biographical method
case study method
correlational designs
cross-section studies
dependent variable
descriptive studies
ethnography
ethnomethodology

evidence-based practice
experimental designs
exploratory studies
grounded theory
historical research
independent variable
level of evidence
literature review

longitudinal studies
phenomenology
prospective studies
qualitative research design
quantitative research design
quasi-experimental designs
retrospective studies
survey method

Nursing research makes a difference in the care of clients, advances the discipline of nursing, and helps develop nursing knowledge. Although such research may be informed by theories developed by other disciplines, such as medicine, physiotherapy, and social work, nursing possesses a distinct body of knowledge with its own thought and philosophy. In this chapter, nursing research will be examined using specific examples of research challenges.

## The Historical Development of Nursing Research

Historically, research from the sciences and medicine influenced nursing practice. But nurses themselves have always had a voice, and since at least 1900, when the first issue of *American Journal of Nursing* was published, nurses have been publishing practice-related articles. The aim of the first issue's editors (and which continues today) was to "present month by month the most useful facts, the most progressive thought, and the latest news that the profession has to offer . . . such knowledge, gained through private work and in the hospital . . . cannot fail to make the

*Journal* not only interesting but of great educational value" (pp. 64–65). Educational projects and cost-effective practice issues were common during these early days of the 1900s. It was not until the 1970s that nurses began to independently investigate the effects of nursing care on their clients. Although by today's standards the designs of these early research studies were flawed, they formed the beginning of a nursing focus on the care of the person and were a significant move away from prevailing medical approaches. It was another 15 years before nursing research gained status among other health care disciplines (Table 6-1). In 1985, the National Center for Nursing Research (NCNR) was established, which became the first time federal tax dollars were dedicated to the study of nursing care. This happened because of an increasing sophistication in nursing and an overt recognition by the U.S. government and the medical field that nursing had significant research potential that was substantially more advanced than other disciplines. Then in 1993, the National Center for Nursing Research became the National Institute for Nursing Research (NINR), and the development of this organization continued to establish nursing as a research-based discipline. Nursing research studies have continued to expand greatly through the rest

## TABLE 6-1    LANDMARKS IN NURSING RESEARCH

**1900**    *American Journal of Nursing* first published.

**1936**    Sigma Theta Tau awards first research grant of $600 to Alice Crist Malone Ohio State University for the study "Measuring Achievement in Nursing Based Upon the Principles and Objectives Set Forth in the New Curriculum."

**1952**    *Nursing Research*, the official research journal of the American Nurses Association (ANA) is first published; chairman of the editorial board is Helen L. Bunge, Frances Payne Bolton School of Nursing, Case Western Reserve; the first editorial was written by Genevieve Knight Bixler, PhD, consultant in research at Case Western Reserve and former member of the board of directors of the National League of Nursing. The editorial was entitled "What is Research?"

**1955**    American Nurses Foundation (ANF) is formed as the research, education, and charitable affiliate of the ANA.

**1963**    Surgeon General's Consultant Group on nursing research.

**1965**    ANA sponsored the first of a series of research conferences to stimulate clinical studies focusing on quality of care.

**1972**    ANA Commission on Nursing Research established the Council of Nurse Researchers to be a forum to advance ideas, encourage research activities, and recognize excellence in research.

**1976**    ANA Commission on Nursing Research
Nursing research journals:
- *Advances in Nursing Science* (1978)
- *Research in Nursing and Health* (1977)
- *Western Journal of Nursing Research* (1978)

**1981**    ANA Commission on Nursing Research: Research Priorities for the 1980s (ANA. [1981]. *Research priorities for the 1980s. Generating a scientific base for nursing practice.* Publication #D-68. Kansas City, MO).

**1983**    The Institute of Medicine recognized the unique contributions of nurses to research, and encouraged separate funding. The result was the National Center for Nursing Research (NCNR) established in 1985 at the National Institute for Health. It was the first time federal tax dollars were dedicated to the study of nursing care. The purpose of the NCNR was the "conduct, support, and dissemination of information regarding basic clinical nursing research, training, and other programs in patient care research" (National Institute of Nursing Research, Undated).

**1985**    The ANA Cabinet on Nursing Research expanded its priorities for nursing research.

**1993**    The National Center for Nursing Research became the National Institute for Nursing Research (NINR). With the title change came an increased recognition of nursing as a research-based health profession.

**21st century**    Three major areas of nursing research funding are (1) health promotion/disease prevention, (2) acute and chronic illness, and (3) nursing system.

Adapted from Dempsey, P. A., & Dempsey, A. D. (2000). *Using nursing research: Process, critical evaluation, and utilization* (5th ed.). Baltimore: Lippincott Williams & Wilkins; Polit, D., Beck, S., & Hungler, B. (2001). *Essentials of nursing research: Methods, appraisal, & utilization* (5th ed.). Philadelphia: Lippincott.

of the 1990s. Now, in the 21st century the science of nursing produces tremendous research studies with great benefits to the health care system (Polit, Beck, & Hungler, 2001).

## Organizations That Support Nursing Research

Many organizations have been foundational in their support of the historical development of nursing research. Early on, a most important event for nursing was the American Nurses Association's (ANA) announcement in 1952 of the intention to devise new ways of improving nursing service based on research. In 1955, the American Nurses Foundation (ANF) was established as the research, education, and charitable affiliate of the ANA (American Nurses Association, 2002). The foundation continues to complement the work of the ANA, the largest nursing organization in America, by raising funds and by developing and managing grants to support advances in research, education, and clinical practice. In response to initiatives by the ANA and others, the first nursing journal dedicated to nursing research, *Nursing Research,* was established in 1952. The 1980s were outstanding in terms of nursing research, particularly in the field of urinary incontinence (UI). The National Institute for Aging (NIA) called specifically for incontinence studies, and several nursing leaders were successful in receiving grants in this area. Such a landmark achievement by nurses was unprecedented in the medically dominated research world, and it set the standard on which all other nursing research applications continue to be based.

### The National Institute of Nursing Research

The government authorized the creation of the National Center for Nursing Research (NCNR) at NIH in 1983. The NCNR became the National Institute of Nursing Research (NINR) in 1993. The impetus for establishing the NINR came from the findings of two federal studies: a 1983 report from the Institute of Medicine recommending that nursing research be included in the mainstream of biomedical and behavioral sciences, and a 1984 NIH Task Force study identifying nursing research activities relevant to the NIH mission (National Institute of Nursing Research, 2002). The NINR continues to be a tremendous asset for nursing research and is the fundamental organization for coordinating and supporting the research efforts within the nursing profession (NINR, 2002).

## Development of Nursing Knowledge

Nursing developed its distinctive body of knowledge and its own thoughts and philosophies about research via both traditional and nontraditional research approaches based on

changing understandings of what is meant by "knowledge." Nursing knowledge owes much to the experiences of nurses over time, gained through trial and error during the caregiving process. However, to "know" something in research terms means to be aware of the reality, truth, or actuality of that something. To know a phenomenon sometimes means that the knower must be able to perceive the particular phenomenon directly and be able to recognize and comprehend its real nature. Each discipline has certain aspects of professional knowing that make it unique. Nursing involves care and support based on well-established knowledge of nursing phenomena. For knowledge to be regarded as well established, it must be continually examined and tested to be sure that the "known" remains known in the face of variations, challenges, and distortions. To be truly known in a research sense in the context of the 21st century, nursing knowledge must be examined in the light of evidence.

## Evidence-Based Practice

**Evidence-based practice** is the integration of best research evidence with clinical expertise and patient values. When these three elements are integrated, clinicians and patients form a diagnostic and therapeutic alliance which optimizes clinical outcomes and quality of life. (Sackett, Stauss, Richardson, Rosenberg, & Haynes, 2000, p. 1).

Evidence-based practice may also be called research-based practice, best evidence, or best practice. Underlying this is the idea that opinion and usual care are not adequate reasons for justifying decision making and practice. The move toward supporting practice with evidence began in the mid-1980s, particularly with a group in Oxford, England, led by Dr. Archie Cochrane, a British medical researcher and epidemiologist. Cochrane's work led to the internationally known Cochrane Centres for Systematic Reviews. He challenged medical practice, noting that much of it was based on tradition rather than strong evidence. He asserted that health care resources were limited and would continue to be so, and therefore physicians had an obligation to provide care that had been shown, via randomized controlled trials, to provide reliable outcomes. Cochrane's emphasis on the importance of comprehensive literature analysis means that systematic reviews have become a very important method for disseminating the current state of evidence on a wide number of topics (The Cochrane Collaboration, 2001).

Taking research to the clinical area was the work of the archived Agency for Health Care Policy and Research (AHCPR), a U.S. government agency that developed many clinical practice guideline statements for nurses to choose from, ranging from wound care and pain control to benign prostatic hyperplasia. In 2002, with a significantly expanded mandate, the AHCPR has been renamed Agency for Healthcare Research and Quality. Among its responsibilities are (1) regular publishing of updated reviews of evidence, (2) publishing clinical practice guidelines, and (3) supporting nursing research.

Evidence-based practice in nursing has also been promoted by an Australian group, the Joanna Briggs Institute for Evidence-Based Nursing and Midwifery (2002). Through its Website (http://www.joannabriggs.edu.au), it provides Best Practice Information Sheets on a wide variety of topics specifically related to nursing, including catheter care, oral hygiene, total parental nutrition (TPN), resident safety, smoking, and preoperative teaching. All groups reviewing the evidence do their evaluations and draw conclusions based on the prescribed level of evidence.

## Level of Evidence

**Level of evidence** is the amount of research support generated to support a particular strategy in care. The four levels of evidence are described specifically in Box 6-1. For example, pelvic floor muscle exercises have been shown in randomized controlled studies to reduce urinary incontinence in women, so the level of evidence is 1. An example of level 2 evidence is research with radical prostatectomies, which are believed to control the progress of prostate cancer, and expert opinion and nonrandomized studies support the research. There are no

randomized studies, however, so the level of evidence is 2. With level 3 evidence, randomization has not been done, but the researchers have made attempts to control for subject differences. Level 4 evidence is supported by consensus opinion and intuition. For example, experts recommend that behavioral strategies for the treatment of urinary incontinence should be the first step, but little systematic study has been conducted in this area (Joanna Briggs Institute, 2002).

## Research Designs, Methods, and Methodologies in Nursing

A paradigm is a way of viewing something from a particular perspective—of seeing the world's phenomena in a certain way. Research is no different from any other way of perceiving and interpreting phenomena to determine how knowledge is acquired. The two main research paradigms in nursing are quantitative and qualitative.

## Quantitative Research Designs

**Quantitative research design** involves drawing conclusions about some procedure, usually under researcher-controlled conditions, and using statistical methods. Quantitative researchers use deductive reasoning, logic, and measurable aspects of experience to produce new knowledge. There are many ways to obtain research evidence, and researchers will often combine methods. Quantitative research methods include descriptive, exploratory, survey, historical review, cross-section, longitudinal, retrospective, prospective, correlational, quasi-experimental, and experimental studies (Polit, Beck, & Hungler, 2001).

### Descriptive Studies

**Descriptive studies** describe a phenomenon of interest, such as nurses' workloads during a 24-hour period. The study might include observations of their activities, or it might be based on interviews with nurses describing their workloads. Descriptive studies often are an important starting point for developing other studies by presenting information on the prevalence of a condition, such as asthma in community-dwelling seniors. Descriptive studies might also be called clinical observations and can lead to exploratory studies (Polit, Beck, & Hungler, 2001).

### Exploratory Studies

**Exploratory studies** describe in detail the nature of phenomena and try to identify contributing factors. Nurses in community care may have identified in a descriptive study that asthma in seniors was far more prevalent than they realized. The next step would be to explore the specifics of the problem such as triggers, risk factors, medication use, referrals, assessment, and prevention (The Cochrane Collaboration, 2001).

---

**BOX 6-1    LEVELS OF EVIDENCE**

- Level 1: Evidence obtained from a systematic review of all relevant randomized controlled trials (RCT)

- Level 2: Evidence obtained from at least one properly designed RCT

- Level 3A: Evidence obtained from well-designed controlled trials without randomization

- Level 3B: Evidence obtained from well-designed cohort or case control analytic studies, preferably from more than one center or research group

- Level 3C: Evidence obtained from multiple time series with or without the intervention; dramatic results in uncontrolled experiments

- Level 4: Opinion of respected authorities, based on clinical experience, descriptive studies, or reports of expert committees

Source: Joanna Briggs Institute for Evidence-Based Nursing and Midwifery. (2002). *Best practice information sheets.* Retrieved March 15, 2002, from http://www.joannabriggs.edu.au

## Survey Method

The **survey method** involves surveying a group of individuals for responses to certain questions. For example: *Do you smoke? How long have you smoked? Have you ever tried to quit? What does smoking mean to you?* In a survey, the research attempts to obtain information from a representative sample (Figure 6-1). For example, to determine the number of smokers in the population over age 16, researchers might survey every third person with a driver's license in the state of California and compare that with a similar survey in the state of Kentucky.

## Historical Research

**Historical research** is a specialized area in which data relating to past events is systematically collected and critically evaluated in the context of the past events (Dempsey

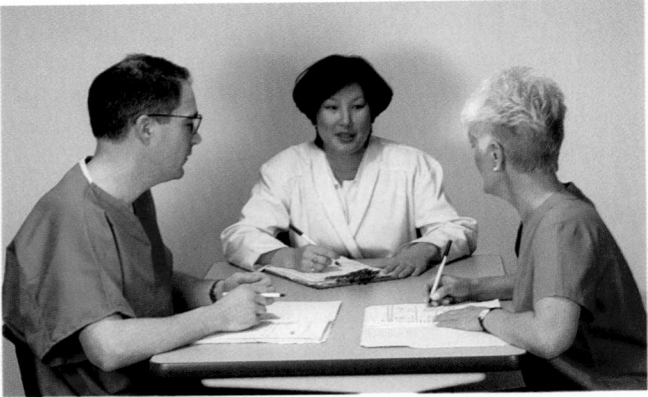

**Figure 6-1    A nurse researcher gives directions to research assistants whom she is training to implement her survey method of research.**

& Dempsey, 2000). Historical research has much greater implications than just "looking at the past." This type of research is extremely valuable for putting concepts in perspective, and is establishing parameters for continued research in a given area of focus.

## Cross-Section Studies

**Cross-section studies** involve data collected at one specific measurement point. The advantage of cross-sectional data is that it allows a relatively large number of individuals to be sampled in a short period of time. Researchers might collect cross-sectional data on the number and type of over-the-counter and herbal medications that people are using. The disadvantage of cross-sectional data is that it describes only a single event, rather than tracking events over a period of time. Longitudinal data collection provides a more comprehensive view of the sample.

## Longitudinal Studies

**Longitudinal studies** involve data collection over time in a particular research sample. It is extremely valuable to evaluate the effects of nursing interventions over periods of time. An example is a study on the effectiveness of diet change in obese people at risk of type II diabetes. Subjects can be surveyed on their HgA1c, diet record, and reported exercise every 3 months for 3 years. Longitudinal data can provide a better understanding of diet modification's impact on glycemic control in subjects at risk, and gives researchers a better understanding of the issues than would a single, cross-sectional survey, which only shows the effects on the subjects at one time period.

## Retrospective Studies

**Retrospective studies** involve reviewing existing data usually found in medical records or hospital charts. The limitations of retrospective reviews are significant and include missing data, missing subjects, missing charts, lack of follow-up, and poor subject recall. However, a carefully conducted retrospective review can provide the research questions for a prospective study. For example, a researcher might wish to know the urologic complications experienced by children who use intermittent catheterization. In a retrospective study, the researcher would review the medical records and attempt to contact the key players—such as parents, children, and the physicians—and confirm whether the data relating to the problems are complete. The nurse could then conduct a prospective, longitudinal study, in which children and their parents were followed over a prolonged period (e.g., 10 years).

## Prospective Studies

**Prospective studies** may evolve from a retrospective review. A prospective study actively follows subjects over the period of the study; it does not rely on data collected retrospectively, except as background information. A prospective study is more valid than a retrospective study because the researcher can control all information collected.

## Correlational Designs

**Correlational designs** investigate the correlation (relationship) of one variable to another. This study design is often used in clinical practice research studies, because of the large number of variables associated with "human research." The outcome of corrrelational research is that one cannot determine "cause and effect" with this type of analysis. Rather, there is simply a numerical value assigned to the degree of relationship that exists among variables. An example is shown in this question: Are scores on a quality of life scale correlated with either self-efficacy or self-esteem?

## Quasi-Experimental Designs

**Quasi-experimental designs** are modified experiments where control or randomization is not possible, so that all subjects have some exposure to the independent variable. This might include all subjects who have a certain procedure, and they would be tested in a pre-posttest design so that the subjects serve as their own controls. In a quasi-experimental design, though, one can never be certain whether some other variable than the independent variable caused a change or improvement of the condition. A quasi-experimental design is less robust than a true experimental design (Campbell & Stanley, 1966).

## Experimental Designs

**Experimental designs** involve an **independent variable**, such as pelvic floor muscle exercises, and are tested against a **dependent variable**, such as the number of incontinence episodes in a day. In other words, if a reduction in incontinence occurs, it "depends" on the treatment protocol of pelvic floor muscle exercises. The subjects are randomized to a treatment or control group. The objective outcome measures in such a study would be incontinence episodes before and after the therapy. The subjective measures could include the subjects' feelings about the pelvic floor therapy (e.g., Did they like it? Was it difficult to adhere to? Did they think it helped?). Experimental design is held up as the "gold standard" in research design.

## Qualitative Research Designs

**Qualitative research design** involves the systematic collection and consideration of data relating to humans' interactions in and with the world, and frequently involves interview data. Qualitative research uses a more holistic approach to data collection and is conducted in natural settings, generally where the participants live or conduct their lives. Many research texts refer to qualitative research reasoning as inductive rather than deductive.

Frequently, outlined under the title "qualitative research" in nursing texts, references to biographical

## STOP AND THINK

### Experimental Designs

● In an experimental study, why is it important to have subjects randomized to groups?

● If subjects are not randomized, what issues may arise with data interpretation?

● What is the purpose of a control group?

● What other considerations are important when choosing a group for a research study?

method, ethnography, grounded theory, phenomenology, and, more recently, case study method can be found. Ethnomethodology, or ethnoscience, and narrative analysis might also be found. Other research approaches, however, can be qualitative but frequently are not identified. These are critical theory, action research, critical ethnography, feminist research approaches, and postmodernism, poststructuralism, and deconstructionism (Caelli, 2000). Although it is important for students to recognize that there are many qualitative research approaches, only those most commonly found in nursing are addressed in this chapter (i.e., biographical method, case study method, ethnography, grounded theory, phenomenology).

## Biographical Method

The **biographical method** involves writing about people's lives (Smith, 1994). The sources of data in biographical research are diaries, letters, artifacts, personal stories of the person whose life is to be studied, contemporary accounts, membership in organizations or groups about which something is known, and historical facts that relate to the period. Data analysis is a process of sorting and relating all the gathered information in order to write about it. Biographical research is time-consuming and demanding work (Smith, 1994). Florence Nightingale performed biographical research by examining historical documents from her era.

## Case Study Method

The **case study method** may refer to a single case, a subject, a group, or an institution. The case study methodology in the qualitative genre differs somewhat from case studies in quantitative research because of the use of multiple sources of data and a variety of data collection strategies. Qualitative case studies take a multidimensional approach to research, which may encompass both quantitative and qualitative data, either alone or together (Yin, 1999).

In the case study approach that incorporates both quantitative and qualitative data, any theoretical positions

## RESEARCH FOCUS

**Title of Study:** Nurses' knowledge of wound irrigation and pressures generated during simulated wound irrigation

**Study Purpose:** To describe nurses' knowledge of wound irrigation and their ability to produce appropriate irrigation pressures established by the U.S. Agency for Healthcare Research and Quality (AHRQ) during simulated procedures.

**Methods:** This study was comprised of a convenience sample of 28 registered nurses and licensed practical nurses from a university medical center in the northwest United States. Participants were asked to complete a demographic data sheet and a questionnaire related to wound irrigation and to perform two simulated wound irrigations. The questionnaire developed for the study contained nine questions about general knowledge of wound irrigation and nine questions about wound irrigation technique. A device to measure the pressures generated by the participants during simulated wound irrigation was developed and calibrated using a transducer calibrated by the National Institute of Science and Technology.

**Findings:** Participants' scores were high on items querying general knowledge of wound irrigation, but lower on questions relating to irrigation technique. Thirteen participants achieved irrigation pressures within the guidelines established by the AHRQ, 14 fell below the guidelines, and 1 produced pressures exceeding the guidelines. The majority of nurses participating in this small study had some difficulty answering questions relating to wound irrigation technique. In addition, performance on simulated irrigation showed that the majority were not able to generate pressures in the recommended range.

**Implications:** Nursing professionals and educators should be aware of these knowledge and performance issues, and incorporate educational content and experiences in nursing programs designed to aid nurses in improving wound irrigation practice.

Campany, E., Johnson, R. W., & Whitney, J. D. (2000). Nurses' knowledge of wound irrigation and pressures generated during simulated wound irrigation. *Journal of Wound Ostomy and Continence Nursing, 27,* 296–303.

---

that exist and might be used to guide the data collection need to be considered during the design phase (Yin, 1994). These works may provide guidance about categories that may be important. Sampling is twofold and purposive in case study research. It relies on replication logic (searching for replication examples or disconfirming data) rather than sampling logic (Yin, 1994). Because the probabilities are unknown and unpredictable, the aim of sampling is not to achieve a representative, probability-based sample. Sampling is focused toward achieving data from multiple sources, gained from as many differing types of events, factors, and influences, and in as many different situations and contexts, as possible (Yin, 1994). Like ethnographic research, everything in the culture or subculture under study needs to be considered so that the case can be described comprehensively.

### Ethnography

Although there is considerable debate about its origins, from the early 20th century, it has generally been accepted that **ethnography** is the research approach of anthropology. The essential core of ethnography is the study of the meanings of actions and events to the people who are being studied (Spradley, 1980). Ethnography is descriptive research within a particular context. It seeks to describe the culture that is studied, as well as the behav-

## COMMUNITY/HOME CARE

### Qualitative Research in the Home Environment

Nurses involved in qualitative research may visit clients in their own homes. The nurse researcher always needs to be aware of personal safety. If a researcher was investigating substance abuse by inner-city residents, she may be advised to have a partner along, notify someone else of the visit, and carry a cell phone. For the most part, clients are very appreciative of the researcher taking the time to visit them in their homes. Visits can be very informative for the researcher as she views the client within the home setting rather than at the clinic. Home visits are very time-consuming and can be labor intensive, so researchers will need to account for the additional time involved in data collection. Moreover, techniques that are easy to do in a clinic setting (such as biofeedback for pelvic floor muscle exercises) can be far more challenging in the home.

iors that are observed within the context of the culture. The process of ethnography involves (1) intense periods of fieldwork in which everything in the culture is reviewed and described, (2) participant behavior is observed within the setting, (3) participants are interviewed about the meaning of the behaviors, and (4) artifacts that represent aspects of the culture are collected. Data sources are therefore the behaviors of the study group, their explanations of those behaviors, interviews, and artifacts that may help others to understand the culture (Roper & Shapira, 2000). Ethnographic research is longitudinal research and requires considerable periods of time to complete.

## Ethnomethodology

**Ethnomethodology** derives from the work of Garfinkel (1967) and is based in ethnography and the phenomenological work of Husserl (1931). Rather than a descriptive approach, the objective of ethnomethodology is to provide interpretive descriptions of what is happening in a particular social world. Ethnomethodology is concerned with how people make sense of their social world. There are no set methods for conducting an ethnomethodological study.

## Grounded Theory

**Grounded theory** is a form of field research used in nursing that seeks to explore and describe phenomena in naturalistic settings like hospitals, nursing homes, and outpatient clinics (Carpenter, 1999). Arising from symbolic interactionism in psychology, grounded theory is a qualitative research approach that is concerned with exploring social processes as they occur within human interactions. The aim of grounded theory is to provide explanation or beginning theory about how the social process works—for example, how clients make decisions about one particular type of treatment over another. First proposed in 1967 (Glaser & Strauss, 1967), there are now several differing approaches to grounded theory.

The process of grounded theory is complex, and there are multiple stages of data collection. Data sources include participant observations and in-depth interviews, which later become more targeted toward emerging categories of information. This latter process is known as theoretical sampling, and it continues until data saturation is reached. Data is saturated when the same categories or codes (types of information) keep recurring during theoretical sampling and no new information is forthcoming. Rather than just claiming that saturation has been reached, the research report should specify how, when, and under what circumstances it occurred (Hein, 2001).

## Phenomenology

**Phenomenology** differs from other qualitative research approaches in that it is a philosophy or a variety of distinctive yet related philosophies. In addition, phenomenology is also concerned with approaches to research and therefore, the methods used to conduct such research. As philosophers, phenomenologists hold differing views on epistemological questions (e.g., How do we know what we know?) and ontological questions (e.g., What does it mean to be or to exist?). Therefore, on-the-way phenomena may reveal themselves through the phenomenological process. The character of phenomenology is diverse, and the assumptions inherent in the various phenomenological approaches to understanding, and the methods they advocate, differ greatly. Eighteen different types of phenomenology were identified at the 1998 conference of the Society for Phenomenology and Existential Philosophy in Colorado. This means that researchers who plan to use phenomenological methodology must be very clear about the approach they are to use and must implement it consistently throughout the research.

Silverman (1987) asserts that American approaches to phenomenology are more concerned with extending the understanding of an issue as it has been initiated in the methodology. This means that the object of research is somewhat different between the two broad approaches, with traditional phenomenology focusing on the phenomenon, stripped as far as possible of its cultural overtones, while American phenomenology allows a focus on the issue involved, such as the experience itself. Furthermore, American phenomenological research generally does not insist on an objective scrutiny of the phenomenon under examination. American phenomenology does not require participants to reexamine their experience of the phenomena subsequent to describing it, or to ask themselves, "Is this what it was really like?" American phenomenology has been of particular value to nursing, because it allows an understanding of the behaviors in ways that were previously closed to nursing (Paley, 1997).

Phenomenology, in all its forms, begins in silence (Spiegelberg, 1982) or in profound reflection on the phenomenon to be studied; that way, researchers can come to know how they came to understand the phenomenon in the way that they do. Data sources in phenomenology may include texts, either biographical or fictional; diaries; photographs; images; and in-depth interviews. Phenomenological research involves intense reflection on the phenomenon so that its nature or meaning may be apprehended, interpreted, and described. Some forms of phenomenology are descriptive while others are interpretive, and the methods used to conduct the research differ depending on the methodology used.

## Literature Review

The **literature review** is the process by which published and unpublished materials are selected to develop support for the research project. A computerized literature search is the starting point for developing a research article or proposal. The well-known databases of CINAHL, Medline, ERIC, and PSYCH LIT should provide an initial comprehensive review. Many other sources of information such as abstract databases (e.g., nursing, dissertation, sociology, psychology) may have valuable studies not yet published. Sources of systematic reviews are York Database, Cochrane Trials Register, Evidence-Based Nursing, and Evidence-Based Practice. In addition, other sources of information are conference abstracts of relevant conferences such as the Wound, Ostomy and Continence Nurses; the Society of Urologic Nurses and Associates; and the Oncology Nurses Association. These and many of the official nursing organizations are extremely important sources of unpublished data, which may inform research questions. The reference lists of all retrieved sources are another extremely important source of potential studies. In addition, nurses must read resources very critically and differentiate among the various materials (Table 6-2).

## Developing a Research Proposal

The development of a research proposal is integral to the research process. When the researcher has chosen the question(s) to be explored and has clearly articulated a problem statement (Box 6-2), then the framework for answering the question is developed. The framework for the research proposal consists of sampling, measurement, data collection, data analysis, results, and application and implications for nursing.

## Writing and Publishing Research Studies

Upon completion of a research study, the researcher must be encouraged to publish the results in a referred journal. Publishing is an involved process and requires determination on the part of the author. The nurse researcher must first identify which journal is the most appropriate periodical for disseminating the study's results. Then the specific criteria for publication must be met, which usually begins with the author's submission of an abstract and manuscript of the study. As the process continues, the journal will notify the author of whether the new potential article is accepted "as is," "requires changes," or is denied acceptance. The end result is an accepted and then published article that assists in communicating the research results to other nurses and members of the health care team.

## Implementing Research into Nursing Practice

A published research report in a nursing journal sitting on a library shelf may not assist nursing practice. Research utilization has become a research priority and an area of research itself because of the gap between published studies and the use of the studies in clinical practice. Researchers have an obligation to present findings in user friendly language and to speak at conferences where practicing nurses will attend, or during research awareness days at the local hospital or health unit. In order for research findings to be implemented, they must clearly be better than the current practice (Polit, Beck, & Hungler, 2001). Finally, change in practice requires support from management. Change can be difficult if those at the administrative level do not encourage critical analysis of practice. Administrative attitudes should not be a reason to promote or not promote practice changes. Part of being a professional is also being a change agent. Characteristics of a change agent include the ability to take risks along with the ability to determine the risk and benefit of one's actions and then to decide to act; a commitment to the value of the change based on a full understanding of the study's findings and application; and a foundation in nursing knowledge that includes understanding research, basic science, communication, and interpersonal relations (Mauksch & Miller, 1981). In addition, nursing research in the clinical settings must be legal and ethical.

---

### BOX 6-2    PROBLEM STATEMENT

*Will lifestyle changes such as exercise and weight loss prevent people at risk from developing type 2 diabetes?*

---

 **STOP AND THINK**

#### Changes Based on Research in Practice

A nurse from another hospital tells you that the hospital has implemented a diabetes education program at their center that is reducing the anxiety and concerns of people who are newly diagnosed with type 2 diabetes. Before you approach the diabetes clinic in your hospital, what are some things you need to consider?

## TABLE 6-2    COMPARISON OF QUANTITATIVE AND QUALITATIVE WAYS OF READING A PUBLISHED ARTICLE

| Quantitative | Qualitative |
|---|---|
| • **Sample**<br>What is the target population?<br>What are the criteria for inclusion?<br>How is the sample selected?<br>What is the sample size?<br>Are these four elements of sample appropriate to this design?<br>Was an appropriate power analysis provided? | • **Participation**<br>What are the criteria for inclusion or exclusion?<br>Is the number of participants stated?<br>Is the number appropriate to the research approach?<br>Is the number of interviews with each participant stated?<br>Are these elements appropriately explained? |
| • **Methods**<br>What are the variables under study?<br>What methods were used to collect data for the study?<br>Were issues of reliability and validity of measurement adequately addressed?<br>Are the procedures adequately explained?<br>Are the methods the most appropriate ones that could have been selected? | • **Methods**<br>Is the methodology (i.e., the philosophical basis of the approach) adequately explained?<br>Is it appropriate to the question?<br>What methods were used to collect the data?<br>Are the methods appropriate to the methodology?<br>Are they the most appropriate methods that could have been selected?<br>Are the data collection steps explained? |
| • **Data Analysis**<br>Did the data analysis provide an answer to the research question?<br>Is there sufficient power to support statements made about the relationship(s) between or among independent and dependent variables?<br>Are the analysis techniques appropriate and properly conducted? | • **Data Analysis**<br>Was the data analysis in accord with the methodology?<br>If not, were the differences adequately explained?<br>Were the assumptions of the methodology explicitly taken into account when analyzing the data?<br>Does the discussion reflect the appropriate methodological assumptions and understanding?<br>Are the findings consistent with the intent of the methodology? |
| • **Internal Validity**<br>Could there be an alternative explanation for the relationships observed (or not observed) among the variables?<br>If so, what might these be? | • **Rigor**<br>Is the study credible—that is, faithful to human experience of the phenomenon? |
| • **External Validity**<br>Would the findings be applicable to other settings, times, people, and places? | • **Fittingness, Auditability, and Confirmability**<br>Do the findings fit into situations outside the study context?<br>Can you follow the decision trail of the researcher—that is, is the study auditable? Was any attempt made to confirm the findings with participants?<br>If not, was it clear why this was not appropriate? |

From Wood, M., & Caelli, K. (2000). *Comparison of quantitative and qualitative ways of reading a published article.* Unpublished course material, Faculty of Nursing, University of Alberta, Canada. Reprinted with permission.

# Legal Aspects of Research Exemplified in the Informed Consent

Protection of subjects in all research studies is mandatory. A primary method for ensuring that subjects are protected is the informed consent. The nurse researcher normally gives a written consent form that explains the purpose of the project, the time involved, the risks and benefits of the research, and how the project is confidential (Figure 6-2). For example, participants in a descriptive study need to know that their actions are being observed and recorded. The ANA and the U.S. government have published guidelines to ensure subjects' rights are protected in the informed consent (American Nurses Association, 2002). A subject's rights are protection from harm, full disclosure of information, ability to be free to participate or not, and to have all privacy and confidentiality respected. Additional steps must be taken to ensure no harm in the case of vulnerable subjects such as children, the mentally ill, the cognitively impaired, and the elderly. The informed consent is one method of protecting the clients involved in research. In addition, the Institutional Review Board (IRB) is another means of protecting the client during the research process. The IRB provides a structure for research to be implemented in both a legal and ethical environment. Normally, the IRB is the component of the institution that approves the informed consents, as well as the research projects in general.

## Nursing Research in the Year 2002 and Beyond

Basic nursing education does not prepare nurses to be researchers; that is the role of graduate school. But all nurses must be prepared to ask questions about practice, to be willing to explore the literature, and to bring issues back to the nursing unit. The most relevant questions for improving nursing care are generated by the nurse work-

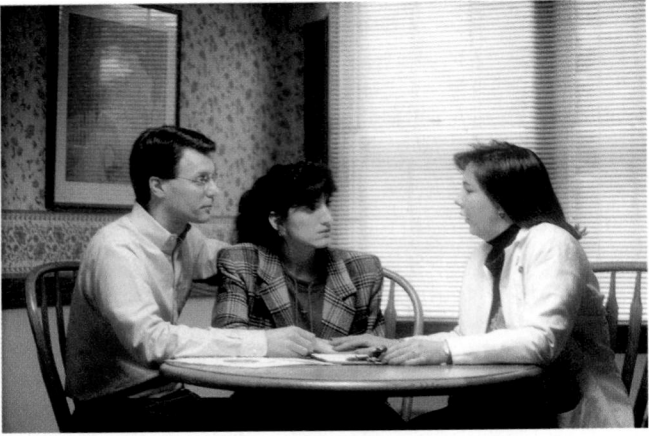

**Figure 6-2    The nurse plays an important role in a client's informed consent. Courtesy of Bellevue, The Women's Hospital, Niskayuna, NY.**

## LIFE SPAN CONSIDERATIONS

### Informed Consent for Vulnerable Clients

Individuals who cannot give consent for themselves are vulnerable and require protection. These groups include those with cognitive impairment such as confused elderly, unconscious clients, or underage clients. Typically, these populations are underrepresented in the research literature and pose a challenge to health care providers in obtaining consent for research studies. Family members or legal guardians must give consent for the research to be conducted, and many prefer that their loved one not be bothered. The researcher must give special consideration to the impact that their study may have on both the family and the potential subject. Consent must be obtained from a proxy, such as a legal guardian, parent, or spouse. A conflict may arise if a child wants to participate in a study but the parents do not wish the child to participate, or if the elderly person has given legal guardianship to his child but is still capable of making decisions for herself.

ing in the clinical area. The new nurse must use the library, understand online searches, and read research reports. Some of the professional responsibilities of the nurse are to remain current in the practice, be it home care or acute care, by attending conferences, reading journals, and sharing ideas. The use of distance learning technology (e.g., Internet, electronic mail) means that even in remote communities nurses can now share and collaborate with one another and with other members of the health care team (Polit, Beck, & Hungler, 2001).

In the past, nurses and other health care professionals worked alone on research studies and the studies reflected the clinical interest of the researchers. The present and future focus is on collaboration and development of teams of researchers who are skilled in several aspects of a discipline and who see health promotion and disease prevention as significant foci of research. A nurse interested in asthma, for example, could easily develop a team of collaborators interested in all aspects of the disease, from primary prevention to tertiary prevention. The team will include such individuals as a pharmacist, respiratory therapist, physician, physiologist, and social worker. Researchers need not be at one center; they may be located across the United States or have team members in Europe, Asia, or elsewhere. The ability of researchers to contact experts around the world is unsurpassed. Such collaboration will enhance the quality of research as well as help use it once it is completed.

## Key Concepts

- Nursing research began its development from the 1900s and has greatly expanded in the past two decades.
- Nursing knowledge is unique to its discipline and is based on nursing phenomena.
- Evidence-based practice involves client-focused research and has been promoted greatly in recent years in health care research.
- The two main research paradigms for nursing research designs are quantitative and qualitative methods. Quantitative design uses deductive reasoning, logic, and measurable aspects of experience. Qualitative design is a holistic approach to data collection and is often conducted in the client's natural setting.
- A research proposal consists of sampling, measurement techniques, data collection and analysis, results, and implications for nursing.
- Writing and publishing a research study is a complex process that begins with submitting an abstract and a manuscript.
- The implementation of nursing research into nursing practice involves research utilization, making changes in nursing practice, and applying legal and ethical principles in the research.
- The nursing profession's future depends on the continued advancement of research and its application in the practice arena. The use of distance learning technology and collaborative efforts among nurses in different locations are examples of future changes in nursing research.

## Review Questions and Activities

1. What are the historical roots of research in nursing?
2. What is the importance of nursing research as a way of knowing in nursing?
3. What implications for nursing research does evidence-based practice have?
4. What are several common methodologies used in nursing research? Explain each.
5. What are the primary elements in a research proposal?
6. What are the steps involved in publishing a research study?
7. What is involved in implementing research into nursing practice?
8. What changes are likely in the future of nursing research?

## Web Resources

American Nurses Association (ANA)
http://www.nursingworld.org

The Cochrane Collaboration
http://www.cochrane.org

Joanna Briggs Institute for Evidence-Based Nursing and Midwifery
http://www.joannabriggs.edu.au

National Institute of Nursing Research
http://www.nih.gov/ninr

## References

American Nurses Association (ANA) (2002). *About the American Nurses Foundation.* http://www.nursingworld.org

Caelli, K. (2000). The changing face of phenomenological research: Traditional and American phenomenology in nursing. *Qualitative Health Research 10*(3), 366–377.

Campany, E., Johnson, R.W., & Whitney, J.D. (2000). Nurses' knowledge of wound irrigation and pressures generated during simulated wound irrigation. *Journal of Wound Ostomy and Continence Nursing, 27,* 296–303.

Campbell, D. T., & Stanley, J. C. (1966). *Experimental and quasi-experimental designs for research.* Boston: Houghton Mifflin Company. (Reprinted from *Handbook of research on teaching*, by N. L. Gage [Ed.], 1963, Skokie, IL: Rand McNally & Company)

Carpenter, D. R. (1999). Grounded theory as method. In H. J. Streuber & D. R. Carpenter (Eds.), *Qualitative research in nursing: Advancing the humanistic imperative* (2nd ed., pp. 99–115). Philadelphia: Lippincott.

The Cochrane Collaboration (2001). *Cochrane brochure.* http://www.cochrane.org/cochrane

Dempsey, P. A., & Dempsey, A. D. (2000). *Using nursing research: Process, critical evaluation, and utilization* (5th ed.). Baltimore: Lippincott Williams & Wilkins.

Editorial (1900). The Editor. *American Journal of Nursing 1,* 64–65.

Garfinkel, H. (1967). *Studies in ethnomethodology.* Oxford: Polity Press.

Glaser, B., & Strauss, A. (1967). *The discovery of grounded theory.* New York: Aldine.

Hein, S. A. W. (2001). Empirical and hermeneutic approaches to phenomenological research in psychology: A comparison. *Psychological Methods 6*(1), 317.

Husserl, E. (1931). *Ideas: General introduction to pure phenomenology.* London: George Allen & Unwin.

Joanna Briggs Institute for Evidence-Based Nursing and Midwifery (2002). *Best practice information sheets.* http://www.joannabriggs.edu.au

Mauksch, I. G., & Miller, M. H. (1981). *Implementing change in nursing.* St. Louis: C. V. Mosby.

Meleis, A. (1997). *Theoretical Nursing: Development and Progress* (3rd ed.). Philadelphia: Lippincott.

National Institute of Nursing Research (NINR), 2002. *About NINR: A brief history of the NINR.* http://www.nih.gov/ninr

Paley, J. (1997). Husserl, phenomenology and nursing. *Journal of Advanced Nursing 26*(1), 193–197.

Polit, D., Beck, S., & Hungler, B. (2001). Essentials of Nursing Research: Methods, Appraisal, & Utilization (5th ed.). Philadelphia: Lippincott Co.

Roper, J., & Shapira, J. (2000). *Ethnography in nursing research*. Thousand Oaks: Sage Publications, Inc.

Sackett, D. L., Stauss, S. E., Richardson, W. S., Rosenberg, W., & Haynes, R. B. (2000). *Evidence-based medicine: How to practice and teach EBM*. New York: Churchill Livingstone.

Silverman, H. (1987). *Inscriptions: Between phenomenology and structuralism*. New York: Routledge & Kegan Paul.

Smith, L. M. (1994). Biographical method. In N. K. Denzin & Y. S. Lincoln (Eds.), *Handbook of qualitative research* (pp. 286–305). Thousand Oaks, CA: Sage Publications Inc.

Spiegelberg, H. (1982). *The phenomenological movement: A historical introduction* (3rd ed.). The Hague: Martinus Nijhoff.

Spradley, J. P. (1980). *Participant observation*. New York: Holt, Rinehart & Winston.

Wood, M., & Caelli, K. (2000). *Comparison of quantitative and qualitative ways of reading a published article*. Unpublished course material, University of Alberta, Canada.

Yin, R. K. (1994). *Case study research: Design and methods*. Newbury Park: Sage Publications Inc.

Yin, R. K. (1999). Enhancing the quality of case studies in health services research. *Health Services Research* 34(5 Pt 2), 1209–1224.

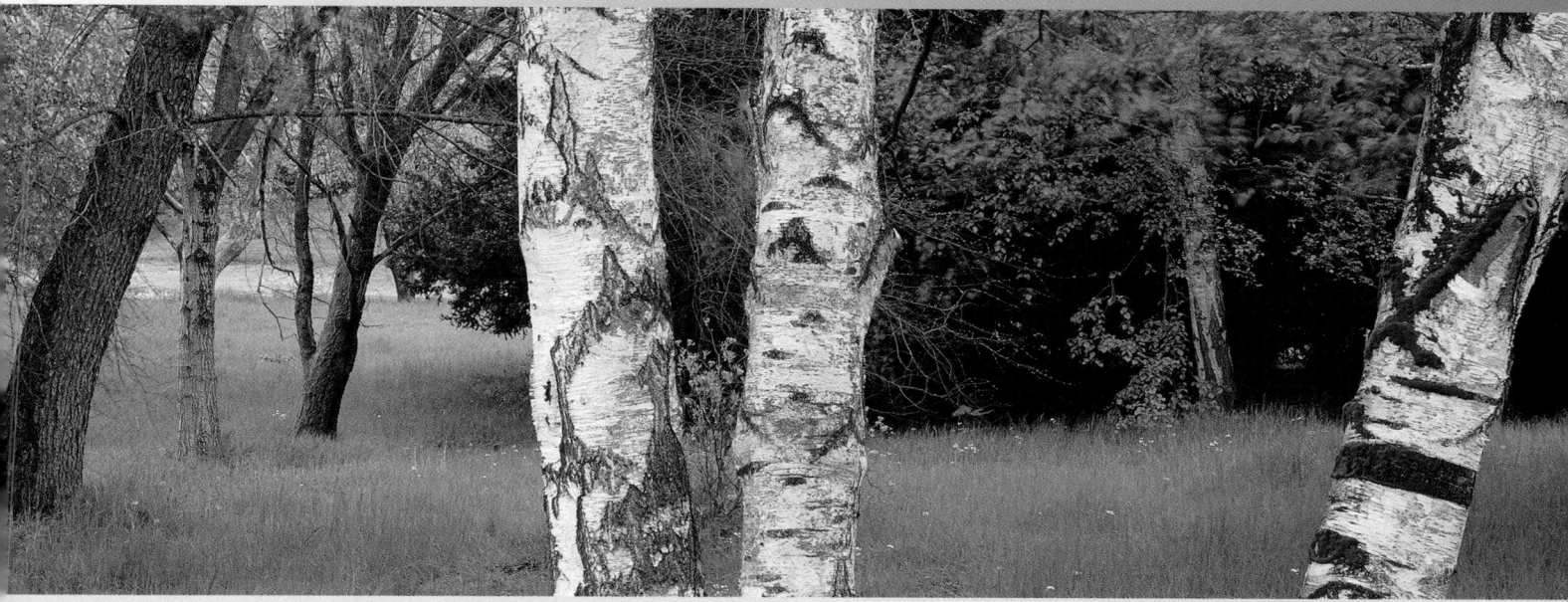

# Advanced Technology and Information Systems

Ruth N. Grendell, DNSc, RN

*"Nursing must be open to new information and ideas. More information is now available which creates a new decision-making process. Computers will be involved in almost every area of direct client care . . . Work can be accomplished more effectively and efficiently and the computer makes possible what we thought impossible."*

(Lindeman, 2000; Young, 2000)

# Chapter Competencies

*Upon completion of this chapter, the reader should be able to:*

1. Describe how information systems are used in health care and specifically in nursing.
2. Describe ethical issues embedded in the use of specific technologies.
3. Identify the variety of ways that technological advancements affect ambulatory care services.
4. Identify technological developments used in the home and the community.
5. Discuss the major effects of telehealth, telemedicine, and telenursing.
6. Identify technological advances and specific developments as used in biotechnology.
7. Describe the roles for nurses in the use of technology.
8. Describe the role of advanced technology in the research process.
9. Evaluate the technological classification systems developed for nursing language.
10. Discuss the concerns regarding a balance between the use of advanced technology and the caring aspects of nursing.

# Key Terms

ambulatory care
care map
community health information networks (CHINs)
distance learning
electronic health record (EHR)

electronic mail (e-mail)
expert systems
firewall
information technology
nursing informatics
personal digital assistants (PDA)

smart card
telehealth
telemedicine
telenursing
unified nursing language system (UNLS)

Information systems and advancements in technology have greatly changed the health care delivery system. For example, large databases are now accessible, thus creating new decision-making processes and improved client outcomes. The addition of **information technology** (the use of computers to gather, organize, process, and communicate information) is one of the highest priorities in health care organizations today (Young, 2000). It is imperative for nurses to use the latest equipment and computer resources as advancements in technology rapidly permeate every aspect of nursing and health care. The frequent addition of newer technology into the system will continue to impact the three principal areas of nursing: clinical practice, education, and research.

Access to computerized records, diagnostic reports, and other nursing care resources and the addition of programmed physiological monitoring systems have changed the way nurses practice at the hospital bedside, in outpatient services, in homes, and in the community. Educational institutions have embraced advanced technology in many ways to facilitate learning. The shift in emphasis from an illness episodic model to a holistic model requires skills in information management and communication. The impact of technology has led many nursing schools to reconfigure their curricula. For example, many schools have implemented **distance learning** (educational courses designed in formats that allow the educators and the students to be in different geographic locations) courses and have integrated the Internet and computers in the implementation of new delivery methods for their curricula (Figure 7-1) (Green, Esperat, Seale, Chalambaga, Smith, Walker, Ellison, Berg, & Robinson, 2001). Staff development programs in the clinical setting rely on information systems and the computer as teaching and assessment tools. Nurse managers and clinicians use advanced technology for administrative purposes such as creating staffing schedules and developing financial and other reports. Computer word processing software, graphic programs, and statistical programs are valuable resources to nurse researchers in conducting literature searches, analyzing statistics, and communicating their study findings.

Technology has brought many benefits to the health care system and its clients; these benefits are evident in the acute care setting, in ambulatory care, in the home and community, and in the arena of telehealth delivery. This chapter discusses many of the types and uses of technology in health care, and the standards, ethical issues, and future trends related to the discipline of nursing. The impact of technology as well as advances in biomedical technology on the nurse-client relationship is included. Brief discussions of advantages and disadvantages related to advanced technology are interspersed throughout the chapter.

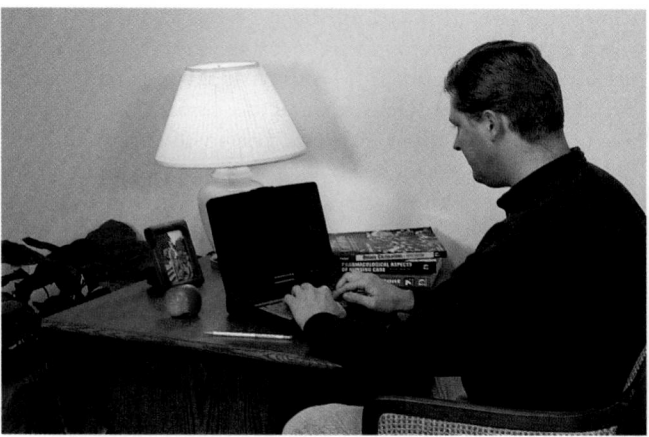

**Figure 7-1    A nurse working on the Internet for a distance learning, graduate-level nursing course.**

# Technological Advancements in Acute Care Clinical Practice

The acute care setting offers an arena for a wide variety of technological advancements. Hospitals have an incredible amount of equipment and advanced technology that is up-to-date and ever changing. Computerized infusion pumps monitor the flow rate of fluids (Figure 7-2) and medications as well as gastric tube feedings. Patient-controlled analgesia (PCA) machines can be programmed to deliver a predetermined amount of narcotic medication as the individual pushes a button (Figure 7-3). To avoid overdosage, a "lockout" device limits the amount of medication that can be delivered each time (Baker, 2001). Physiological monitoring of vital signs, oxygen saturation blood levels, cardiac perfusion, pulmonary artery pressure, and central venous pressure informs the nurse of changes and irregularities. In some cases, a microprocessing chip can regulate the equipment setting to correct client problems. In critical care specialty units, sophisticated computer-assisted equipment includes ventilators, pulmonary function monitoring systems, blood gas analyzers, and intracranial pressure monitors.

## Wireless Communication

A number of wireless systems allow nurses to communicate with one another in acute care settings. Paging systems allow nurses to be contacted regardless of their location. Wireless hospital telephone systems allow nurses' prompt attention to clients' needs and promote rapid communication with other personnel (Chaffee, 1999). Also, nurses can carry an electronic phone device (e.g., cell phone) that allows two-way communication from any location.

## Computers at the Bedside

Computer terminals at the bedside facilitate efficient recording of assessments and other activities, and allow other health care workers who are directly involved in the

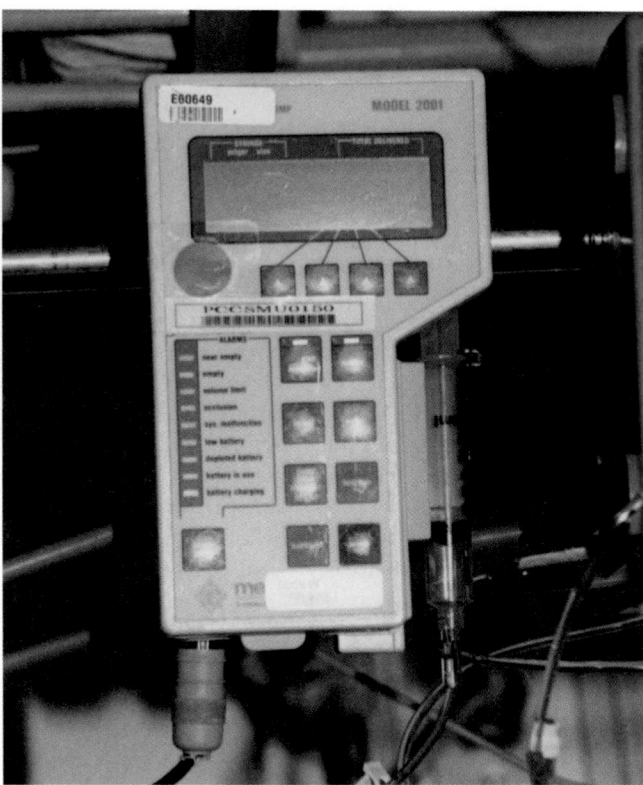

**Figure 7-2    An infusion pump used with a syringe to deliver an intravenous medication.**

client's care to review the most current information. The computer has also facilitated the development of standardized language classifications for documenting nursing actions (Gordon, 1998; Weston & Soloman, 1999). The classifications can serve as valuable tools for nurse researchers in gathering and analyzing data and reporting their findings. In some hospitals, nurses have access to handheld wireless computer devices, sometimes referred to as **personal digital assistants (PDA)**, for recording information and as reference sources (Benner, 2001). Newer versions that combine the handheld computer and cellular phone are entering the market (Grinsven, 2001).

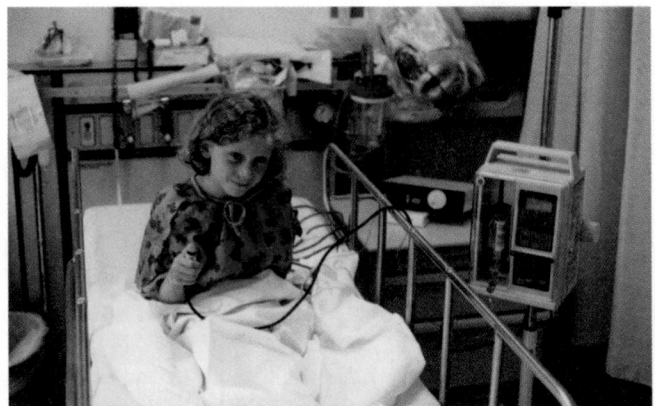

**Figure 7-3    This child is controlling her pain level with a PCA pump.**

## Electronic Health Record

Documentation in an **electronic health record (EHR)** (a method of documentation where all information related to the client is recorded electronically) is legible and more complete than the traditional handwritten form. EHR also offers more logical organization of content and less redundancy. All members of the health care team have access to a client's record in institutions with networking computer systems. Orders for multiple services (e.g., diagnostic studies, medications, and physical therapy) are entered at a unit computer terminal and received by the appropriate department. Laboratory results are posted directly into the client's record, appointments are scheduled, medications are ordered and the pharmacist can enter guidelines for medication administration, and nursing notes are entered more uniformly through answering a menu of preprogrammed statements. Printed discharge planning and teaching guides can be customized and shared with clients and their families. Home care nurses who have access to the hospital information system can obtain discharge summaries and referral orders. Access to the record can be made from any point of service within the institutional system (Allen & Englebright, 2000).

## Decision-Making Support Systems

**Expert systems**, or decision-making support systems, assist the nurse in many ways. They have been designed to alert the nurse to abnormal values on diagnostic tests, and to warn that certain medications are incompatible with other medications that are ordered. Medication administration programs can also alert the nurse when a specific assessment is needed related to a medication or when a medication is overdue. Other programs can generate an appropriate list of nursing diagnoses by analysis of a client's history and assessment data. Some programs also support the use of the nursing process by presenting a selected list of questions to answer regarding the client information, and then providing a set of suggested nursing diagnoses that pertain to the person's health problems. The programs can suggest options to modify a standard care plan in order to meet the unique needs of the client. The program prompts the nurse to complete all designated items before progressing to another area, thus assuring that each problem will be adequately addressed. Special purpose programs provide a wide array of information, including guidelines for performing procedures, infection control measures, client education, and discharge planning (Smith, 2000).

## Technological Advancements in Ambulatory Care Services

Advances in technology have made many treatments and procedures available that were not possible years ago. Health care providers use **ambulatory care** services (client care

delivered in institutional episodes of less than 24 hours), which encompass many short-term services, as an efficient method of care (Figure 7-4) (Warzynski, 2001). Many of the ambulatory care centers are satellites (branches) within a hospital network. Often, manufacturers will design or modify technical equipment specifically for use in an ambulatory care setting (e.g., clinic, physicians' office, surgical center, dialysis unit). Ambulatory care procedures that require advanced technology might include infusion therapy, endoscopic examination, elective surgery for minor and complex procedures, dialysis, radiation, and chemotherapy.

A networking information system within an institution allows access to a client's previous hospital and clinic electronic records and diagnostic reports by all the interdisciplinary team members. These information systems are also used to order prescriptions, schedule tests and future appointments or consultations, and record information related to the visit (Baker, 2001).

## Care Map

Advancements in technology have allowed ease of implementation of a **care map** (a plan of care based on standards that reflect optimal timing of sequential steps provided by all members of the health care team or managing chronic health problems) (Tyson, 2000). Some nurse-client contacts

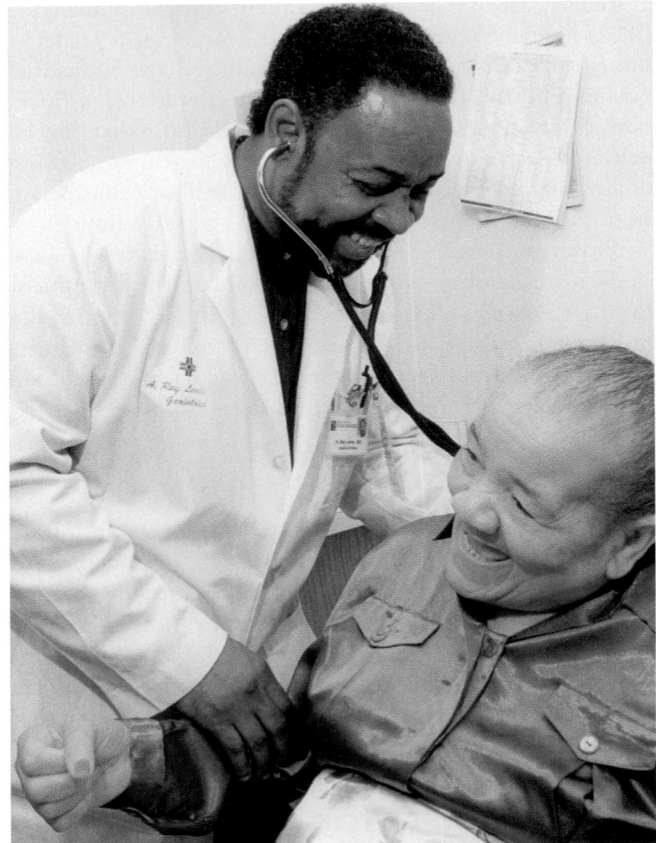

**Figure 7-4   A nurse assessing a client in an ambulatory care setting.**

may be through telephone and computer messages. The duration of contacts with health care providers is determined by the client's needs. Access to computer resources can help the client and family to understand and learn how to maintain the prescribed protocol (refer to Chapter 20 for further information on care maps, and note that several care maps are highlighted throughout this text).

## Advanced Technology

Advanced technology plays an important role in ambulatory care. For example, advanced technology equipment has facilitated development of freestanding birthing centers that have become very popular in the last decade. Other agencies that have benefited from the use of advanced technology include day care and rehabilitation centers and community-based nurse-managed centers (Figure 7-5). These agencies are often used as teaching/learning centers for student nurses to participate in care for clients across the life span. Computer and information technologies have been useful as resources for storing and retrieving important data as well as being communication tools between students and faculty. For example, some offices have computer terminals where clients can view educational materials. Teaching aids and brochures can be obtained from Internet resources for distribution to clients. Nurses in these areas frequently create their own demographic databases for documenting services, for follow-up care, and for annual reports to employers or school administrators (Benthein, 2001).

## Technological Advancements in the Home and the Community

Computers and advanced technology have produced benefits and positive changes in home health and community-based nursing practice. Nurses work more autonomously as care managers in the community, and their roles will con-

tinue to expand as they accept additional responsibilities. Computer access to client records, diagnostic information, and other resources enhances decision making and communication with others on the health care team. In some states, rural health care is provided through extensions of large urban networks. For example, nurses are often involved in telephone triage where they can answer (on the phone) health-related questions from clients in rural settings. Clients can also access the Internet for health care concerns (Schroeder & DePalma, 2001) (Figure 7-6).

Several new health care devices (e.g., mechanical ventilators, infusion pumps) have been modified for use in the home and community settings, thus permitting earlier discharge of clients from acute care settings who require continued short-term nursing care in the home. Home health care has also expanded to accommodate management of the long-term needs for the growing number of clients with chronic health problems. Progress reports are often communicated among the team members through **electronic mail (e-mail)** (method of transmitting data or text files from one computer to another over an intranet

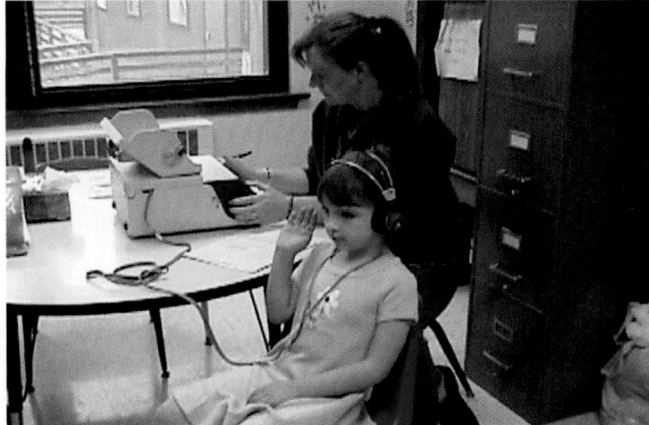

**Figure 7-5    This child is having an audiology test performed in a community-based nurse managed center.**

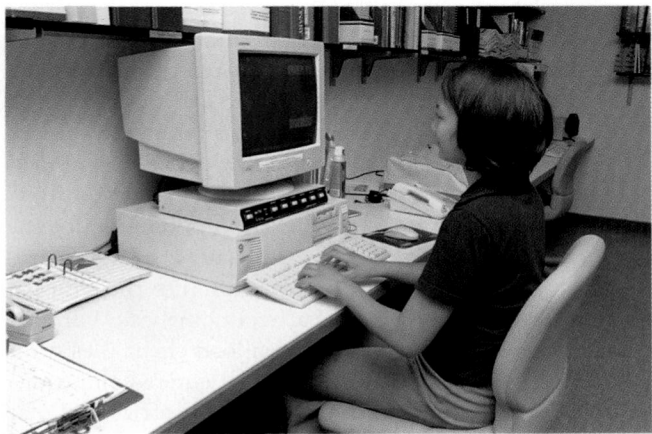

**Figure 7-6    This adolescent is "surfing the Net" (using the Internet) to find information about her newly diagnosed condition of juvenile onset diabetes.**

## COMMUNITY/HOME CARE

### Future Technology for Home Health Care

The home health care nurse can benefit tremendously from adapting care to include the use of advanced technological devices. Many software programs are available to assist the nurse in planning care, developing care outcome plans, and organizing the environment of the client. As more wireless devices are available, the home health nurse will have ready access to two-way audio/visual communication and the ability to access record keeping, information, and computer-assisted instruction aids in the home. For example, a wound could be photographed in the home setting and an enterostomal nurse specialist consulted over the fiber-optic networks. The technological advancements are quickly increasing the positive client management outcomes.

Baker, B. (2001). Home care's future is now. *AARP Bulletin*, 42(9), 7, 9.

or the Internet). Health education programs that promote compliance with the plan of care, and adjustment to lifestyle changes, assist individuals to live independently at home as long as possible (Schroeder & DePalma, 2001).

## Advanced Technology and Documentation

Regulations for reimbursement for community-based health care services set by the government and insurance agencies (third-party payers) necessitate a significant amount of documentation. Traditionally, client records are retained in the agency office and information is entered by the attending nurse at the end of the clinical day, or recorded on a tape recorder and submitted for typing. Documentation in client files is very time-consuming, and some information may be forgotten or omitted. Portable computers and handheld computers reduce the amount of paperwork and increase accuracy of the recording through direct entry of information into the required format during or immediately after a home visit. Portable computers can also be used to download client files prior to the home visit, and new data can be entered and transmitted to the host computer in the main office. Cellular phones have streamlined communication between nurses and their offices and other agencies. The phones have also been used effectively in emergency situations (Stricklin, Jones, & Niles, 2000).

## Home Care Monitoring Devices

Home care monitoring devices can alert health care providers about changes in a client's condition or be programmed to assist a client, and nonprofessional care provider, to adhere to the prescribed plan of care, such as maintaining a medication routine, monitoring blood sugar levels, or recording vital signs (Baker, 2001). Three such systems are discussed below.

### Cardiovascular System Monitoring Devices

The portable Holter® cardiac monitor and diagnostic tool records a continuous electrocardiogram tracing over a particular amount of time. Analysis of the data can determine a correlation between the symptoms and abnormal, or dysrhythmic, cardiac activity. The device is also useful in determining the effectiveness of a pacemaker and antiarrhythmic drugs (Daniels, 2003). Cardiac pacemakers can be monitored and regulated by a computerized telephone system. A special transmitter converts the electrical activity of the client's heart to frequency-modulated tones that are sent to an EKG (electrocardiogram) receiver. A tracing printout of the client's heart rate and pulse width is made for diagnostic purposes and for the client record.

### Maternal Child System Monitoring Devices

In the past, women who were diagnosed with high-risk pregnancies required hospitalization or were placed on bed rest at home with frequent evaluation visits by the home health care nurse. The introduction of home monitoring equipment has permitted evaluation of uterine activity and fetal heart rate via telephone and television hookup. When findings are outside the accepted range, the nurse can provide the mother with instructions by a follow-up phone call or by a home visit when necessary.

 **STOP AND THINK**

### Internet Resources for Home Health Clients

Select a consumer health information Website and determine if the information is appropriate for the public.

- How does it compare with the information in your nursing text?

- Could you use this information in developing a teaching plan? Discuss your opinions with some of your classmates.

## STOP AND THINK

### Availability of Computerized Equipment

● How might the cost of certain computerized records management systems influence an agency's decision to adopt an electronic system?

● What factors in addition to cost must be considered before implementing a computerized system into a community setting?

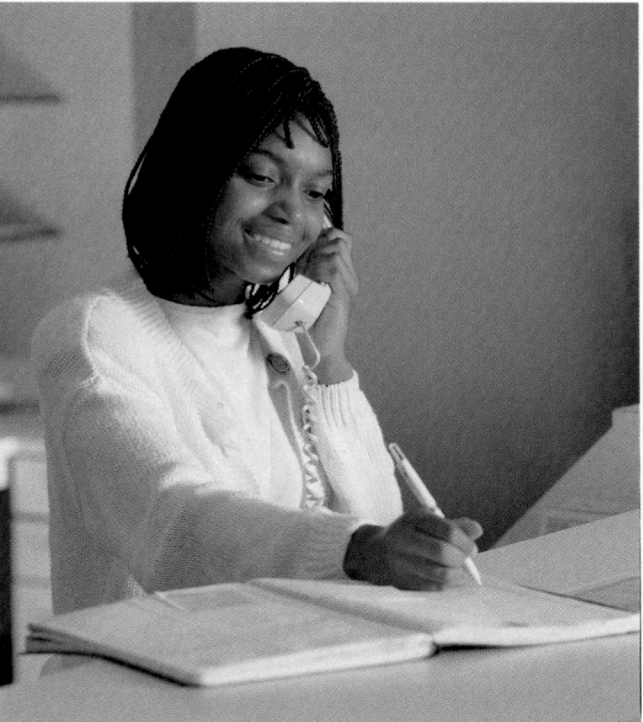

**Figure 7-7** **A nurse implementing a follow-up telephone call after a home visit.**

The home monitor provides a support system for the mother through a potentially difficult pregnancy or newborn care (Littleton & Engebretson, 2002) (Figure 7-7).

### Automated Telephone Monitoring System

Stricklin, Jones, and Niles (2000) reported the effectiveness of "Home Talk," an automated telephone monitoring system considered to be particularly useful in managing clients with chronic health problems. In response to telephone calls at designated times, the client answers a menu of "problem specific" questions by using a Touch-Tone phone. The scores are tallied immediately and rated according to a predetermined standard. When the responses indicate a negative change in condition, or if the person fails to answer a call, phone contact is made to determine if everything is all right (Box 7-1). The validity of the questions as indicators of a client's stable or deteriorating condition

was tested in a pilot study. There was 92% agreement in the findings between the client's responses and assessments conducted during a nurse's home visit within 1 hour after the scheduled phone contact.

Stricklin, Jones, and Niles (2000) mentioned that 50% of the home health care nurse's time is spent in teaching and providing information. "Healthy Talk," a health screening and health education program, was designed with a similar format to assist individuals to set healthy lifestyle goals. Thirty-seven clients diagnosed with hypertension or congestive heart failure participated in a second pilot study that included the telephone monitoring and health education programs. Eighteen participants were assigned to the experimental group and 19 received traditional home care management. At the end of a 60-day period, both groups were satisfied with their care and adhered to their prescribed therapy. Individuals in the experimental group were more likely to follow their diet, had increased awareness of their disease, and were more organized in reporting changes in their conditions. They also reported feeling more secure with the scheduled frequency of the telephone monitoring calls. There were no observable differences in lifestyle changes between the groups. However, higher costs were associated with the increased amount of time, travel expenses, and number of visits for the traditional (control) group. A final phase to the program is the addition of computerized standard care paths, or Healthy Steps, that will serve as guidelines for nurse education materials and assist clients to establish self-health promotion goals.

## CLIENT EDUCATION

### Holter® Monitoring

✓ Explain that the Holter® monitoring system evaluates the electrical activity of the heart on a continuous basis.

✓ Inform the client that the monitor will be worn for 24 to 48 hours in its carrying cover.

✓ Instruct the client to keep a diary for recording daily activity and any symptoms that may occur.

✓ Tell the client that there is a "marker button" on the machine that should be pushed when symptoms are felt (e.g., chest discomfort, faintness).

✓ Advise client to avoid tub bathing or showering while wearing the Holter® monitor.

Daniels, R. (2003). *Delmar's manual of laboratory and diagnostic tests.* Clifton Park, NY: Delmar Learning.

## BOX 7-1    TELEPHONE MONITORING

- Telephone calls are placed by the home health nurse at scheduled times. A specific menu of questions related to the client's health problem is given. Answers require a yes or no response.

  If yes, press 1. If no, press 2.

  If you need the question repeated, press 7.

- The client responds by Touch-Tone phone, pressing (1) for yes or (2) for no.

- Responses are scored immediately to a predetermined standard.

- The home health nurse is notified immediately if the results indicate a deviation from the standard range.

- The nurse telephones the client to obtain additional information.

- The nurse analyzes the information and may give instructions or make a home visit.

Examples of questions (in telephone monitoring) for a client with a chronic respiratory problem.

1. Is your breathing more rapid or more difficult at rest since your last nurse visit?
2. Have you used oxygen within the last 6 hours?
3. Do you feel better after using the oxygen?
4. Have you changed any routine in your medications?
5. Have you had any restlessness?
6. Do you feel anxious?

Adapted from Stricklin, M., Jones, S., & Niles, S. (2000). Home talk/healthy talk: Improving patient's health status with telephone technology. *Home Healthcare Nurse, 18*(1), 53.

Groups best served by telemonitoring are persons diagnosed with congestive heart failure (CHF), chronic obstructive pulmonary disease (COPD), diabetes mellitus, and chronic renal failure with continuous ambulatory peritoneal dialysis. Populations who benefit from telemonitoring include individuals who are noncompliant, frail and anxious, have a history of frequent hospitalizations or emergency room visits, or need frequent home visits without direct care (Schroeder & DePalma, 2001).

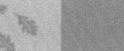

## CLIENT REFLECTIONS

### Home Monitoring of Newborn

Mrs. Cazares delivered her child two months ago and makes the following comments to her family nurse practitioner in the well-child clinic: "I really appreciated your calming me down throughout my pregnancy with your phone calls. Your idea for me to get a cell phone to keep in my purse made me know I could always call you and ask questions about my pregnancy. Rudy (Mrs. Cazares' new son) had so many times where I thought his heart was racing and then I would call you. You would monitor his heart rate, and reassure me that my son was just fine. I will always be grateful for your help and for those monitors used for Rudy's heart."

## Emergency Response Monitoring Systems

Emergency response systems are particularly helpful to elderly persons who prefer to live at home. The home telephone is equipped with a direct link to a monitoring agency that alerts the health care provider whenever a call for help comes through. Voice-activated systems are very beneficial to the person who cannot reach a phone. When the call comes into the health care agency, a designated neighbor can be called to check on the individual immediately and report back for instructions if needed. A home visit by a nurse may be indicated. Reminder services can be programmed to play on a daily, weekly, or other timed basis. A care partner in the home can have peace of mind knowing that professional help is available in case a person should fall, have a heart attack, or other health emergency (Schroeder & DePalma, 2001).

## Ethical Issues: Privacy and Confidentiality

One disadvantage of computerized systems is the danger of breeching confidentiality and privacy issues. To protect client privacy and confidentiality of information, certain precautions must be taken to preserve security for computer hardware and software (refer to Chapter 16 for more specific information on documentation). A **firewall**, a protective mechanism that establishes limited access into a computer system, can be programmed into the system. Limited access is also protected through assigning passwords or codes to personnel to enter only authorized documents and files. Preservation of information is ensured by making daily backup, or duplicate, files that are stored in a separate place. Physical placement of the computers in a secure area, use of closed-circuit television surveillance,

**STOP AND THINK**

### Privacy and Confidentiality When Using Computerized Documentation

- What precautions can you take to protect client privacy when documenting with computers?

- What can you say to your clients to reassure them that confidentiality is being maintained in their records?

and an automatic recording when any activity occurs can be used to discover the point of origin of altered, lost, or incorrectly used data (Smith, 2000).

## Telehealth, Telemedicine, and Telenursing

**Telehealth**, **telemedicine**, and **telenursing** (services that involve telecommunications in health care delivery, medicine, and nursing, respectively) had their beginnings in the 1950s. Now there is a renewed interest in their benefits to home health care. These services are conducted through video, audio, and computer systems in at least 20 states. Clients can test their blood pressure, oxygen levels, and blood sugar levels; send the results to their health care providers; and receive instructions. They can access online courses that teach them how to manage chronic conditions. "Virtual office visits" permit the client and physician, or nurse, to see each other and communicate via audio-video monitors. Clients and their providers can also communicate by e-mail. Clients are satisfied because the home-based technology provides a greater access to care, gives them the opportunity to participate in their own care, and the ability to stay at home as long as possible. Pilot studies indicated a reduction in hospitalization, clinic, and pharmacy costs (Baker, 2001).

### The Government's Role

The government has shown considerable interest in the benefits of telehealth programs. Several U.S. agencies, including the Department of Defense, are contributing significant resources to explore telehealth's uses. Military personnel around the world are often many miles from the care they need. Interest has been expressed in the role of telehealth applications to support emergency care for combat casualties, diagnostic studies, computerized client records, and links for aeromedical evacuation (Chaffee, 1999).

### Telehealth Distribution

Chaffee also reported on new projects of worldwide connections between health professionals and clients, and the

 **LEGAL AND ETHICAL ISSUES**

### Computerized Documentation

When documenting with computers, the nurse must still remember the principles for legal documentation. The nurse must first ensure that the right client and record are identified. This prevents the obvious legal challenge of an inaccurate recording. Then the date and time of each entry is needed so that an individual event can legally be placed in context of the chronology of the client's care. Next, the nurse must remember to "sign" the entry with the correct professional credentials required by the institution. This declares the legal rights and responsibilities of the nurse involved in the documentation. Errors are easy to "delete" on computerized systems, so . . . As in any charting system, the nurse must still remember to carefully review each entry for clarity, accuracy, and completeness.

Adapted from: Estes, M. (2002). *Health assessment and physical examination* (2nd ed.). Clifton Park, NY: Delmar Learning.

possibility of a mobile telehealth system to transmit client information from inside ambulances during transport. The telehealth system will present many opportunities to nurses, including giving care to clients at distant locations, designing telehealth programs, participating in research, and taking continuing education courses (Box 7-2).

### Finances and Telehealth

Many of the existing systems were initiated with start-up grants that are now expired. The high costs of the equipment and installation of sophisticated communication lines is prohibitive for many agencies. The reluctance by some physicians and other health care personnel, and clients themselves, to use the system is another factor. A major obstacle is obtaining reimbursement from private and governmental insurers (Shaffer & Sheets, 2000). Approximately one-third of travel time and expenses of in-person visits have been eliminated where the telehealth system has been in place (Carr, 2001). However, reimbursement and interstate licensure restrictions have limited widespread acceptance throughout the nation.

### Advances in Biotechnology

The advances in biotechnology have produced many diagnostic (Figure 7-8) and treatment instruments. Magnetic resonance imaging (MRI) and computed tomography (CT), sophisticated diagnostic tools that produce multidimensional images of organs, bones, muscles, soft tissues,

## FOCUS ON WELLNESS

### Wellness and Telenursing

Telenursing creates an open door to wellness because of the increased ability to communicate with the client in the home environment. In addition, the nurse can create health promotion programs without having to "travel" to the client's home, and communication can allow the nurse to evaluate the client's progress "from a distance." Nurses have to learn to think from a different perspective to desire to monitor wellness from a telecommunications paradigm.

Stricklin, M., Jones, S., & Niles, S. (2000). Home talk/healthy talk: Improving patient's health status with telephone technology. *Home Healthcare Nurse, 18*(1), 53.

### BOX 7-2    TELEHEALTH SERVICES

- Development of individualized care plan (clinical path)

- Ostomy care instructions

- Evening calls to augment regular hospice visits; video "check-in" contacts by the hospice nurse to answer questions and concerns of family caregivers

- Specialty services for the elderly—such as physical therapy needs, rehabilitation needs, and pre-dementia

- Programs for clients with spinal cord injury

- Coordination of care for a client population

- Monitoring high-risk pregnant women

- Support for families of high-risk newborns

- Pain management

- Health education programs

- International links

- Space programs

- Monitoring child abuse

American Nurses Association, 2003: Maddox, P. (2002). Ethics and the Brave New World of E-Health. Retrieved 5/1/03. http://www.nursingworld.org; Chaffee, M. (1999). A telehealth odyssey. *American Journal of Nursing, 99*(7), 27–29.

or a section of the body, have revolutionized medical diagnoses, treatments, and surgery. For example, an MRI can determine the size of a heart chamber, valvular function, beating of the heart, and blood flow through the great vessels, among other functions. Additional diagnostic instruments are the electromyography that measures electrical activity of muscles, and the arthroscope, a fiberoptic instrument that permits direct visualization of the interior of joints, which can assist during surgical procedures. The computerized microscope is a major contribution to microsurgical procedures, allowing greater magnification of minute structures. Images can be transmitted to a television monitor in the operating room and other viewing areas, and serve as a teaching method. Digital cameras are frequently used as adjunct equipment. Images can be downloaded to the computer and integrated into a presentation program, sent by e-mail for consultation purposes, or analyzed for medical applications (Nice & Gurevich, 2003). Other predictions describe further development of technology, computers and software, biosensors, implants, genetic therapies, imaging devices, and computer-assisted surgery (Holaday, 2000).

## Cost of Biotechnology

Evolvements in biotechnology information are expanding at a rapid pace. Frequent media reports of breakthroughs in scientific discoveries promote expectations of the public and the health care providers for more definitive diagnostic results and cure of diseases. There is a great incentive to allocate resources to purchase and implement the most recent technology to meet the demand for these therapeutic procedures (Figure 7-9). Possibly in some

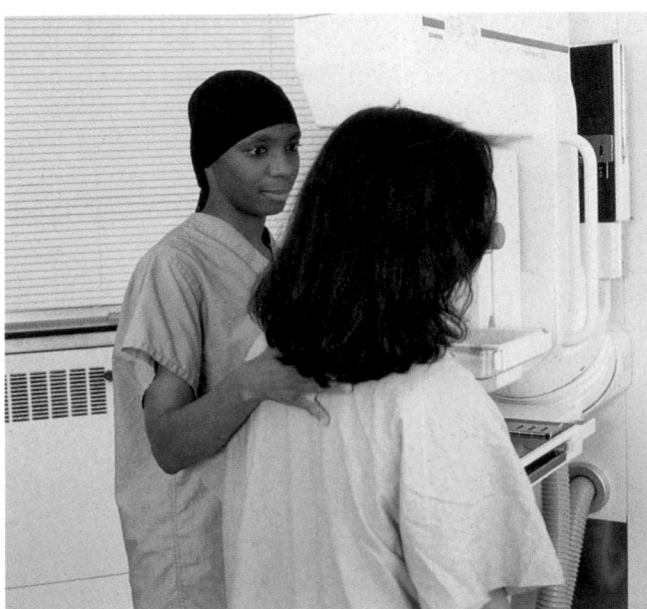

**Figure 7-8    Mammogram technology has become a common method for wellness promotion for women over the age of 40.**

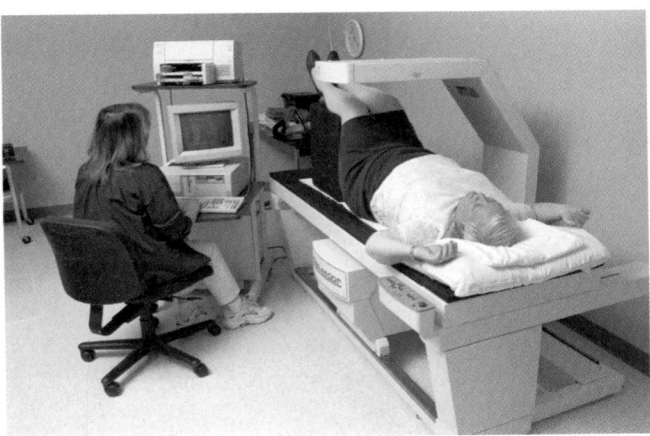

**Figure 7-9**    This bone density scan equipment is very expensive and requires adequate resource allocation for smaller health care agencies to afford its purchase.

## STOP AND THINK

### Advanced Technology for Everyone

● Only 41% of Americans have Internet access at home or at work. How does this disparity of access affect nursing?

● The cost of certain "high tech" health care initiatives is prohibitive to large portions of the population in need of these services. How would you reconfigure our health care system to be "fair" to a greater percentage of the population?

cases, overuse of technology further contributes to the rising cost of health care and raises new ethical issues concerns. Research and development costs can amount to more than $10 billion per year, thus leaving minimal funds for illness and disease prevention and health promotion measures. Some have questioned the value of extremely high-cost technology interventions that may not promote quality of life, as well as questioning who has access to these measures. The government and insurers have introduced cost control strategies to decrease these rising costs. Managed care that is designed to coordinate a broad range of health care services in the most efficient and least expensive manner has become the major reimbursement system in place at this time (Kerfoot, 2000).

## Types of Nursing Roles and the Use of Advanced Technology

A newer model of care includes the nurse as care manager, who coordinates the client's health care services over an extended period of time. Computer information systems are ideal in communicating client information among the various team members, and allow access to educational resources. An extended action plan can be developed and assist in decision making along the continuum of care. A central computer in one agency with data links to **Community Health Information Networks (CHINs)** permits access to a client's electronic health record by authorized personnel from various agencies within the community. Physicians, pharmacists, nurses, community hospitals, suppliers, and other agencies can also enter client care information to update the record. The central computer serves as a router for the various services. The **smart card** (a computer disk for carrying information), similar in size to a credit card carried by the client, is another method for supplying information regarding

insurance coverage, emergency care, and electronic address information to obtain access to the client's health care record. A medication profile listing all the drugs that a client takes can avoid duplications and detect drug interactions and potential adverse drug reactions. The care manager can also monitor the client's compliance with the plan of care. Specific criteria to measure outcomes can be entered into a database. Chronic disease management software can be linked with laboratories, pharmacies, and other service areas. Statistical packages readily aid in the analysis of findings, filing of reports, and decision making for future planning purposes (Warzynski, 2001) (Box 7-3).

## Advanced Technology Use by Nurse Administrators and Managers

Nurse administrators and managers in all areas of clinical practice need to be adept in all aspects of information management, including being proficient in word processing, use of spreadsheets for mathematical calculations, developing presentation graphic programs, and use of e-mail and Internet systems. The spreadsheet programs are powerful tools to manage a great deal of data and for predicting trends. Data from other programs can be imported and then statistically analyzed, organized, and prepared for reports, and be transferred to the presentation software if desired. Most nurse administrators hold graduate degrees in business or nursing administration and are frequently involved in data-based decisions and in developing strategic planning models for integrated health care delivery networks and to assure quality of care. Some nurses have specialty certificates in **Nursing Informatics** (information technologies used by nurses) (McPeck, 2001; Skiba & Cohen, 2000; Snyder-Halpern & Chervany, 2000). Administrators also use computer programs for monitoring care processes and improvements, and staff performance and compliance with standards; maintaining

## BOX 7-3    HOME MONITORING IN THE FUTURE

Thirteen percent of the U.S. population is over 65, and 76 million baby boomers are approaching retirement: the need for home-based care will increase. One solution under development is the "smart house." A smart house will monitor the health status of the house occupants and will serve as memory aids. Sensors will analyze the person's gait in walking up stairs and between rooms. If changes occur, a signal will be sent to designated relatives or friends. The occupants will wear badges that work via radio waves or infrared light. Cameras will view certain tasks to determine if interruptions prevent an individual from completing a task. Alarms will alert the person to take medications. Individuals can remain independent longer in their own living environments. Smart homes are expected to be on the market in 3 to 5 years. Costs will average $1,000 per room and $400 for the computer setup. Maintenance fees have not been determined.

Allen & Englebright (2000). Patient-centered document: An effective and efficient use of clinical information systems. *Journal of Nursing Administration, 30*(2), 90.

## STOP AND THINK

### A Virtual Reality Learning Environment

- What are advantages of a virtual reality learning environment? Visit the Belmont University Website (2001) for a virtual tour at http://www.belmont.edu

- What are some of the advantages and disadvantages of learning in this format?

personnel files and inventories; planning budgets; and communicating with other agency personnel. Computer access to agency information, including regulatory changes, is used in coordinating and facilitating the work of subordinates in order to meet the organizational goals (Allen & Englebright, 2000; Azzarello, 1999).

## Advanced Technology Use by Nurse Educators

Advanced technology is an integral part of nursing educational programs. Examples include computer-assisted instructional programs, audio-visual presentations, distance learning, and videoconferencing. Many nursing texts include computer disks and CD-ROMs to reinforce learning. Online courses and electronic products such as CDs and DVDs are also often available to enhance and augment the learning experience. Other uses of technology include "virtual learning labs" for monitoring of physiological data, charting, scheduling diagnostic studies and access to diagnostic reports, monitoring of medication administration, developing unique therapeutic regimens, and client education (McPeck, 2001).

Distance learning is probably the greatest change that technology has brought to the educational structure (Billings, 1999; Lindeman, 2000). The current student body consists of a diverse population with a variety of learning styles and needs. Many students continue to work while attending classes, some fulfill multiple roles, and others live great distances from educational institutions. The traditional school schedule does not meet their needs. Distance learning allows students to fit their learning experiences with their busy schedules and residence locations. Distance learning for advanced degrees is also beneficial to "travel nurses" who do not remain in a location for an extended period of time.

## Nursing Research and Advanced Technology

Advanced technology has greatly enhanced nursing research activities, which in turn have expanded the discipline's knowledge base. Efficient and comprehensive literature searches can be achieved by exploring the several computer databases, including international links. Prior to the development of nursing information systems, it was very difficult to gather data for comparison and analysis purposes. Documentation of nursing activities varied and did not necessarily describe what nursing actions actually were performed. Nursing activities were either based on medical diagnoses or by body system classifications.

Many dramatic changes have occurred in nursing research and education through advanced technology. In the near future, theses and dissertations of graduate students will be submitted electronically to their universities and will be available through digital libraries that will facilitate searches for studies related to research, education, or practice (Holaday, 2000).

Many health-related websites now exist; however, exploring for resources can be a very time-consuming and tedious process. Nurse researchers may not be aware of any ongoing local research or unpublished work. The Washington (D.C.) Area Nursing Research Resources (WANRR) Website was developed in 1997 as a directory of local nurse researchers; their areas of expertise, interests, and methodologies used in conducting research studies; and their e-mail addresses for communicating with each other. A news column was added for sharing information

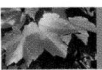

## RESEARCH FOCUS

**Title:** Evaluation of traditional classroom teaching methods versus course delivery via the World Wide Web.

**Study Purpose:** This study evaluated the perceptions of graduate nursing students toward traditional and computer-based portions of a course. The traditional seminar portion included lecture, video presentations, and group discussions.

**Methods:** Approximately one-fourth to one-third of the course was allocated to computer-based (WWW) learning modules. Following the course, a convenience sample of 96 students completed an eight-item survey related to the course content, participation, critical thinking, faculty preparation, and communication and technical skills. A Likert scale was used to tally the responses. Reliability and validity were established, and percentages of agreement and disagreement for each item for the two teaching methods were tabulated. In addition, three open-ended questions were asked regarding what the students liked or disliked about the course and how the course could be improved. The survey was repeated 2 weeks later.

**Findings:** There was a strong agreement that course content covered in the classroom involved more interaction and participation. The faculty's preparation and expertise was viewed as very important. Students expressed a need for better communication skills. The researchers evaluated the responses to the three open-ended questions independently, and themes were identified. Some responded that valuable time was wasted and some students monopolized conversation, while others participated only sporadically. Students believed the WWW portion improved their technical and writing skills, offered opportunities to network with other nurses, and encouraged them to independently search deeper for information. The convenience was a major benefit. Negative aspects included feeling disconnected from the class interaction and face-to-face contact with faculty. Some were unsure of the assignment, grading system, and instructions. Suggested improvements were to continue the combination of teaching methods, but to limit the number of modules on the WWW. Interviews with faculty indicated that careful planning is necessary in developing newer strategies. The faculty also indicated that expertise is required and workload was increased, but that the benefits outweighed the problems.

**Implications:** The use of both teaching methods provides a wider range of opportunities to accommodate diverse learning needs. More orientation sessions are needed prior to use of the computers. Availability of mentors to provide assistance for WWW modules may minimize feelings of isolation.

Ryan, M., Carlton, K., & Ali, N. (1999). Evaluation of traditional classroom teaching methods versus course delivery via the World Wide Web. *Journal of Nursing Education, 38*(6), 272–277.

about fellowship and research assistant opportunities, recent articles, new software, a calendar of research events in the area, and access to the five collaborating universities to check on available research courses. The Website is used to post recent doctoral dissertations. The Website also links regional, national, and international researchers, and as an example encourages collaboration among nurses and other disciplines.

## Classification Systems for Nursing Language

The widespread use of nursing diagnosis language increased the need for similar classification systems for the different nursing diagnoses. Perhaps the computer's greatest contributions to nursing are in facilitating development of a standardized language for documenting nurse-sensitive outcomes and client outcomes that reflect the quality and effectiveness of nursing interventions.

### Unified Nursing Language System

The **Unified Nursing Language System (UNLS)** developed by the American Nurses Association (ANA) in 1991 is a language system that encompasses common nursing terms from a variety of vocabularies that can be used interchangeably. Several criteria were established in order for classifications, or taxonomies, to be approved by the ANA. Currently, the ANA recognizes four classifications: The North American Nursing Diagnosis Association (NANDA), the Omaha Classification System (OCS), the Home Healthcare Classification (HHC), and the Nursing Interventions Classification (NIC). (Note: these are expanded upon in Chapter 12.) Selection criteria for classification schemes are (1) clinical usefulness for making diagnostic, intervention, and outcome decisions, (2) clear definition of terms, (3) test for reliability and validity, (4) documentation of systematic development, (5) process for periodic review and provision for revision, and (6) a unique identifier or code for each term in the classification (Young, 2000). Advanced technology has allowed for an easier use of these classifications systems by allowing the assimilation of large amounts of information.

# High-Tech, High-Touch Nursing

It is imperative that nurses balance "high-tech" (advanced technology) care with the caring aspect of nursing (Figure 7-10). Personal contact is still a very important part of nursing that technology cannot replace. The presence of the nurse is considered to influence client satisfaction and healing potential. The interpersonal nurse-client relationship aids in building trust and can empower the client and family (Skott, 2001; Godkin, 2001). For example, the nurse can touch the client's hand when first coming to the bedside, rather than initially examining the equipment and devices connected to the client. This reinforces to the client that the nurse is interested in his personal well-being and that the nurse cares for him. Another example of "high-touch" nursing is the caring tone of voice that the nurse can use when describing the care she is going to provide. The client will be comforted in recognizing that the nurse places a priority on caring for him, and will also realize that the nurse is providing "high-tech nursing care."

Nurses will need to be self-reliant, independent, and well equipped with "high-touch, high-tech" skills as related to critical thinking, decision making, and problem solving. As participants in the multidisciplinary team, nurses will need to develop skills in specialty areas of communication, leadership, information technology, research, and research utilization. Health promotion and client education; holistic care, including culturally sensitive care; and care of the geriatric population will be primary concerns. Technology will assist nurses in providing high-quality, cost-effective care. Nurses will be called upon to be leaders in replacing the traditional sick-care model and to be leaders in health promotion. Specific outcome criteria will be important in determining the quality of care and will become health care facilities' overriding concern in the future.

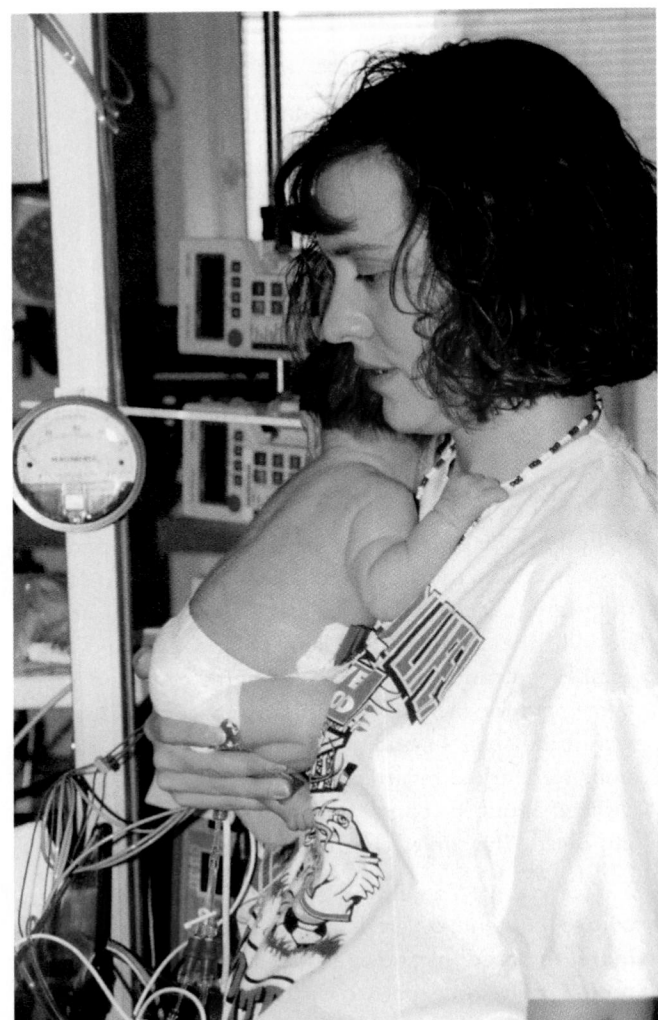

**Figure 7-10**   Neonate intensive care unit nurse practices caring while delivering high-tech nursing to infant.

# CASE STUDY/NURSING CARE PLAN

Frances Campbell, a 79-year-old woman diagnosed with cardiac insufficiency resulting from congestive heart failure and chronic obstructive lung disease, was admitted to your intensive care unit (ICU). She also has a history of hypertension. This is her fifth hospital admission during the past 10 months. Her symptoms include tachycardia, respiratory distress, coughing, wheezing, and rapid breathing. She appears cyanotic and tells you that she often uses her lounge chair at night because she has difficulty breathing in bed. She also says she has gained weight in the last few days, and you note that her feet and ankles are edematous and that it is difficult to feel her pedal pulses. In the ICU, Mrs. Campbell has the following technological devices applied as treatment modalities: pulmonary artery catheter, an arterial line, intra-aortic balloon pump, noninvasive blood pressure monitor, pulse oximetry, titrated medications to control her blood pressure, electrophysiology, and a mechanical ventilator.

*(continues)*

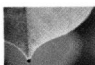

# CASE STUDY/NURSING CARE PLAN (continued)

## Assessment

Client is currently admitted to an acute care facility for the inability to compensate for cardiac insufficiency. She is experiencing a variety of acute clinical manifestations related to her inability to oxygenate adequately from a decreased cardiac output. Her blood pressure = 88/52; pulse = 112; R = 20/minute; oxygen saturation = 92%; cardiac output = 5 L/min. Her treatments involve a variety of advanced technological devices.

## Nursing Diagnosis #1

Decreased cardiac output related to left-sided heart failure and chronic obstructive pulmonary disease.
**NOC:** Cardiac Pump Effectiveness; Circulatory Status; Vital Signs Status
**NIC:** Cardiac Care; Cardiac Care: Acute; Circulatory Care

### Expected Outcomes

The client will:
1. Experience an increased oxygenation level of at least 95% within 48 hours
2. Demonstrate adequate cardiac output within 48 hours as evidenced by cardiac output below 4 L/min; blood pressure of at least 100 systolic and at least 60 diastolic; pulse below 100/minute; respirations unlabored; and lack of cyanosis

### Planning/Interventions/Rationales

1. Monitor for signs of decreased oxygenation and administer low-level oxygen as indicated. *Oxygen therapy increases circulating oxygen levels, and high flow rates increase $CO_2$ retention in persons with COPD (chronic obstructive pulmonary disease).*
2. Monitor for clinical manifestations of left-sided heart failure as manifested in vital signs, pulse oximetry, and cyanosis detection. *Assesses the effectiveness of the course of management.*

### Evaluation

Client continued to have tachycardia with pulse = 110/minute, blood pressure still hypotensive (88/54), high cardiac output (< 4 L/minute), and generalized cyanosis. In addition, her oxygen saturation levels have stayed at 92% or lower.

## Nursing Diagnosis #2

Ineffective tissue perfusion, (cardiopulmonary) related to disorders of COPD and left-sided heart failure.
**NOC:** Circulation Status; Cardiac Pump Effectiveness; Tissue Perfusion: Cardiac
**NIC:** Circulatory Care: Arterial Insufficiency

### Expected Outcomes

The client will:
1. Demonstrate improved tissue perfusion within 48 hours, as evidenced by decreased peripheral edema and fluid weight loss of at least 3 pounds.
2. Demonstrate within 48 hours bilateral pedal pulses that can be felt with palpation.

### Planning/Interventions/Rationales

1. Reduce or improve external venous compression by frequent changing of position, applying thromboembolic stockings, and measuring baseline circumference of lower extremities. *Provides ongoing assessment of client in regard to peripheral circulation, and decreases predisposition to thrombus and embolus production.*
2. Perform daily weights in the morning. *Assesses accurately the fluid status of the body and evaluates edema condition.*
3. Administer regular passive range-of-motion movements to client's extremities, being careful to monitor for clinical manifestations of deoxygenation during movements. *Encourages circulation at therapeutic levels.*

### Evaluation

Client gained 2 pounds in 48 hours and still had peripheral edema. Also, still unable to palpate pedal pulses within the 48 hours.

## Key Concepts

- Ambulatory care services use a tremendous variety of technological advancements.
- The use of computers in the health care delivery system involves many ethical and legal issues.
- Technological advancements and new health monitoring devices add much to nursing in ambulatory care services, the home, and the community.
- Telenursing methods are continuing to provide efficient methods of providing interventions to clients.
- Biotechnology has greatly improved diagnostic and treatment methods across the multitude of client health disorders and complications.
- Nurses benefit greatly by using advanced technology in decision making within the health care system.
- Nurse educators use distance learning strategies to implement new curricula across a greater variety of student populations.
- Nursing research uses new information systems and data analysis methods to proliferate the amount of evidence-based practice changes.
- The American Nurses Association has implemented four specific classification systems for the profession of nursing.
- The expansion of advanced technology has increased the need for nursing to focus on the human aspects of caring and interpersonal relationships.

## Review Questions and Activities

1. Describe several ways that the computer can help the nurse discover previous information and locate resources that will assist in planning and implementing care for Mrs. Campbell during her hospitalization.
2. How can the nurse use the computer to help Mrs. Campbell learn about healthy functional patterns after she is discharged from the hospital?
3. Discuss the computer communication methods in community-based nursing that can facilitate long-term health care management.
4. Describe the financial implications of using efficient technological advancements in the health care system.
5. Enumerate the technological advancements in acute care, ambulatory care, home care, and community care.
6. How does nursing research benefit from the use of high-tech in nursing?
7. What are the implications for the concept of caring as related to the technological advancements in nursing?

## Web Resources

American Nurses Association
http://nursingworld.org
Belmont University (2001). Virtual learning laboratory tour: http://www.belmont.edu
Caton, K. (1998). So you are a nurse, or nursing student: Why do you need to know anything about computers?: http://www.ohsu.edu (go to Library and Info services).
Goldsmith, C., & Rogers, J. (2000). High-tech in home care: More options, better services. (Part 1). http://www.nurseweek.com
Goldsmith, C., & Rogers, J. (2000). High-tech in home care: More options, better services. (Part 2). http://www.nurseweek.com
Nice, K., & Gurevich, G. (2003). How Digital Cameras Work http://www.howstuffworks.com

## References

Allen, J., & Englebright, J. (2000). Patient-centered document: An effective and efficient use of clinical information systems. *Journal of Nursing Administration, 30*(2), 90.

American Nurses Association, 2003: Maddox, P. (2002). Ethics and the Brave New World of E-Health. http://nursingworld.org

Azzarello, J. (1999). Nursing informatics: Could this specialty be for you? *Home Healthcare Nurse, 17*(10), 634.

Baker, B. (2001). Home care's future is now. *AARP Bulletin, 42*(9), 7, 9.

Belmont University (2001). Virtual learning laboratory tour. http://www.belmont.edu

Benner, J. (2001). In the palm of your hand: Buying a PDA. *Nursing, 31*(11), 55.

Benthein, J. (November 1, 2001). Personal interview with director of Point Loma Nazarene University Health Services. San Diego, CA.

Billings, D. (1999). The "next generation" distance education: Beyond access and convenience. *Journal of Nursing Education, 38*(6), 246–247.

Carr, E. (2001). Growing pains. *Nurseweek, 14*(22), 13–14.

Chaffee, M. (1999). A telehealth odyssey. *American Journal of Nursing, 99*(7), 27–29.

Daniels, R. (2003). *Delmar's manual of laboratory and diagnostic tests.* Clifton Park, NY: Delmar Learning.

Estes, M. E. (2002). *Health assessment: physical examination (2nd ed.).* Clifton Park, NY: Delmar Learning.

Godkin, J. (2001). Healing presence. *Journal of Holistic Nursing, 19*(1), 5–21.

Gordon, M. (1998). Nursing nomenclature and classification development. *Online Journal of Issues in Nursing.* Kent State University College of Nursing (pub.).

Green, A., Esperat, C., Seale, D., Chalambaga, M., Smith, S., Walker, G., Ellison, P., Berg, B., & Robinson, S. (2001). The evolution of a distance education initiative into a major telehealth project. *Nursing and Health Care Perspectives, 21*(2), 66–70.

Grinsven, L. (October 23, 2001). Handspring to top rivals with handheld's built-in phone. *Computer-link,* p. 12.

Hogstel, M. (2001). *Gerontology: Nursing care of the older adult.* Clifton Park, NY: Delmar Learning.

Holaday, B. (2000). Tapping into technology: The future of electronic theses and dissertations. *Excellence in Nursing Education, 1*(4), 1, 3.

Kerfoot, K. (2000). The health care organizations and patterns nursing care delivery. In J. Zerwekh and J. Claborn (Eds.), *Nursing Today.* Philadelphia: W. B. Saunders.

Lindeman, C. (2000). The future of nursing education. *Journal of Nursing Education, 39*(1), 5-12.

Littleton, L., & Engebretson, J. (2002). Maternal, neonatal, and women's health nursing. Clifton Park, NY: Delmar Learning.

McPeck, P. (October 8, 2001). The goalkeepers. *Nurseweek, 14*(12), 10–12.

Nice, K., & Gurevich, G. (2003). How Digital Cameras Work. www.howstuffworks.com

Ryan, M., Carlton, K., & Ali, N. (1999). Evaluation of traditional classroom teaching methods versus course delivery via the World Wide Web. *Journal of Nursing Education, 38*(6), 272–277.

Schroeder, B., & DePalma, N. (2001). As close as the phone: Telemonitoring in home care. *Nurseweek, 9*(6) 23–26.

Shaffer, F., & Sheets, V. (2000). Multi-state licensure: Opportunities for nurses to practice in new ways. *Nursing Administration Quarterly, 25*(2), 38.

Skiba, D., & Cohen. E. (2000). Case management and teaching: A necessary fit for the future. *Nursing Administration Quarterly, 25*(1), 132.

Skott, C. (2001). Caring narratives and the strategy of presence: Narrative communications in nursing practice. *Nursing Science Quarterly, 15*(3), 249–255.

Smith, L. (2000). Safe computer charting. *Nursing, 100*(9), 85.

Snyder-Halpern, R., & Chervany, N. (2000). A clinical information system strategic planning model for integrated health care delivery networks. *Journal of Nursing Administration, 30*(12), 583.

Stricklin, M., Jones, S., & Niles, S. (2000). Home talk/healthy talk: Improving patient's health status with telephone technology. *Home Healthcare Nurse, 18*(1), 53.

Tyson, T. (2000). The internet: Tomorrow's portal to non-traditional healthcare services. *Journal of Ambulatory Care, 23*(2), 1

Warzynski, D. (2001). Chronic care: How to achieve continuity across the continuum. *Nurseweek, 14*(14), 18–19.

Weston, B., & Soloman, D. (1999). Omaha system: Bridging homecare and technology. *On-line Journal of Nursing Informatics, 3*(1).

Winslow, E. (2001). Patient education materials. *American Journal of Nursing, 101*(10), 33–37.

Young, K. (2000). Nursing informatics. In J. Catalano (Ed.), *Nursing now: Today's issues, tomorrow's trends.* Philadelphia: F. A. Davis.

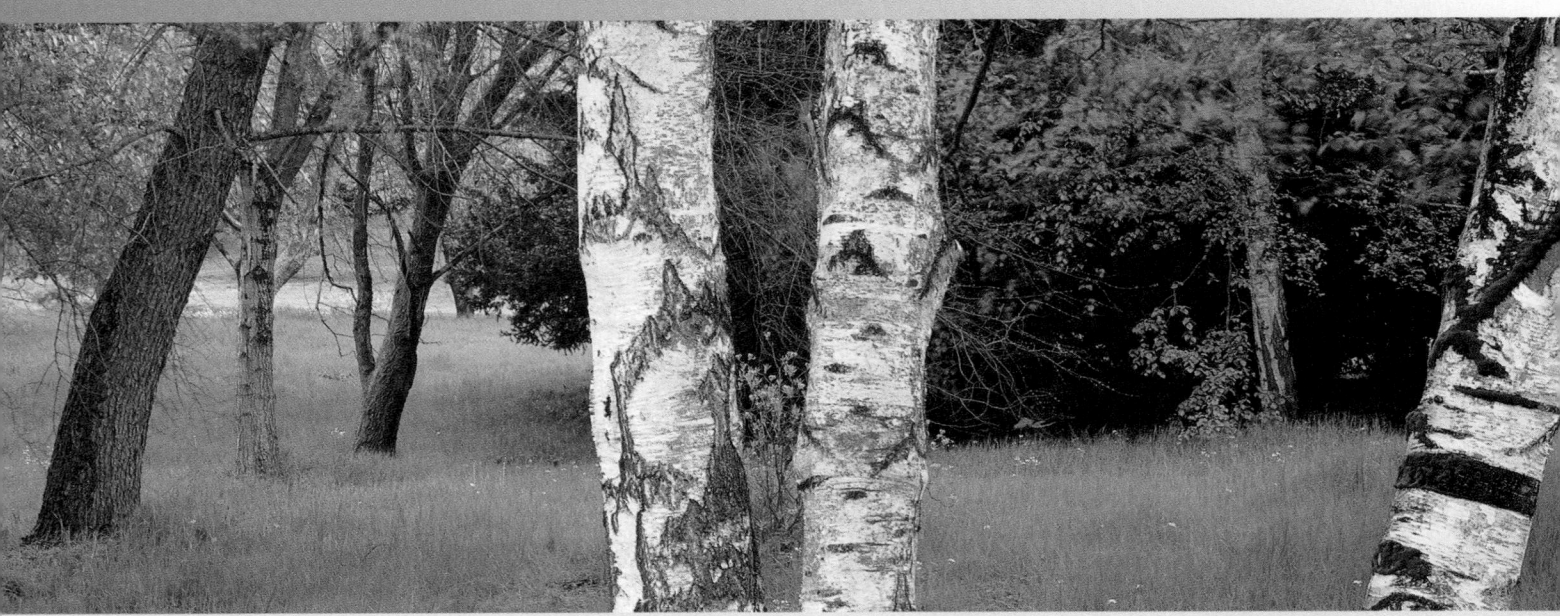

# 8 CHAPTER

# Legal Accountability and Responsibilities

Kathy Player, RN, EdD

*"I do not feel obligated to believe that the same God who has endowed us with sense, reason, and intellect has intended us to forgo their use."*

(Galileo Galilei)

# Chapter Competencies

*Upon completion of this chapter, the reader should be able to:*

1. Compare and contrast public law and civil law as they relate to nursing practice.
2. Define the two major areas of legal liability in nursing, and discuss how these relate to nursing practice.
3. Explain the four legal regulations and roles of professional nurses.
4. Define the legal responsibilities of nursing students.
5. Describe the legal safeguards that decrease the risk of liability in nursing practice.
6. List and explore the six major health care laws and regulations and how they affect nursing practice.
7. Describe the legal considerations for nurses involved in various client care situations.

# Key Terms

| | | |
|---|---|---|
| administrative law | euthanasia | liability |
| advance care medical directive | expert witness | living will |
| advance directive | expressed contract | malpractice |
| assault | false imprisonment | mandatory overtime |
| battery | felony | misdemeanor |
| causation | formal contract | negligence |
| civil law | fraud | plaintiff |
| consent | Good Samaritan acts | public law |
| constitution | impaired nurse | statutory law |
| contract law | implied contract | testimony |
| criminal law | informed consent | tort |
| defamation | injury | tort law |
| defendant | interstate nursing practice | understaffing |
| durable power of attorney | invasive | unprofessional conduct |
| duty | jurisprudence | whistle-blowing |
| equity | law | |

Law, like nursing, is responsive to the changing needs, roles, and relationships in society. As the nursing profession has continued to evolve, the scope of applicable law has enlarged considerably. This chapter discusses the laws affecting nursing practice and the legal responsibilities of nurses to clients.

## Legal Foundations of Nursing

The word **law** is derived from an Anglo-Saxon term meaning *that which is laid down or fixed*. The two types of law are **public law**, which deals with an individual's relationship to the state, and **civil law**, which deals with relations between individuals.

## Sources of Law

The three sources of public law at the federal and state levels are constitutional, administrative, and criminal. The three sources of civil law at the federal and state levels are contracts, torts, and protective/reporting laws.

### Public Law

As shown in Table 8-1, public law governs the legal aspects of constitutional, administrative, or criminal law. The law of the United States is set forth in the Constitution. A **constitution** is a set of basic laws that defines and limits the powers of government. Laws enacted by legislative bodies are referred to as **statutory law**. State boards and professional practice acts, such as nurse practice acts, are created and governed under statutory laws.

**TABLE 8-1   TYPES OF PUBLIC LAW**

| Constitutional Law | | Administrative Law | | Criminal Law | |
|---|---|---|---|---|---|
| *Federal* | *State* | *Federal* | *State* | *Federal* | *State* |
| U.S. Constitution Civil Rights Act | State Constitutions | Food, Drug, and Cosmetic Act Social Security Act National Labor Relations Act | Practice acts (e.g., nurse, medical, pharmacy) Worker's Compensation laws State Labor Relations Act Employment Security Act | Controlled Substance Act Kidnapping | Criminal codes (define murder, manslaughter, criminal negligence, rape, fraud, illegal possession of drugs, theft, assault, and battery) |

Data from Goldberg, K., Kaplan, H., & Shaw, M. (Eds.) (1996). *Nurse's legal handbook* (3rd ed.). Springhouse, PA: Springhouse.

**Administrative law** (regulatory law) is developed by groups who are appointed to governmental administrative agencies and who are entrusted with enforcing the statutory laws passed by the legislature. Under administrative law, state boards of nursing are given the power to further delineate the rules and regulations governing nursing as set forth in nurse practice acts. In these administrative rules, boards identify the specific processes for licensure, grounds for disciplinary proceedings, and the establishment of fees for the services and penalties rendered by the board.

The most common example of public law is **criminal law**, which refers to acts or offenses against the welfare or safety of the public. In criminal law there are two types of crimes: a **felony** (crime of a serious nature usually punishable by imprisonment in a state penitentiary at hard labor or by death, or a crime in violation of federal statute in which punishment is more than 1 year incarceration) and **misdemeanor** (an offense that is less serious than a felony and may be punished by a fine or sentence to a local prison for less than 1 year).

### Civil Law

Civil law deals with crimes against a person or persons in such legal matters as contracts, torts, and protective/reporting law (Table 8-2). Most cases of malpractice (professional liability) fall within the civil law of torts (Flight, 1997).

### Contract Law

**Contract law** is the enforcement of agreements among private individuals. A legal contract has three essential elements:

1. Promise(s) between two or more legally competent individuals stating what each individual must do or not do
2. Mutual understanding of the terms and obligations the contract imposes on each individual
3. Compensation for lawful actions performed

Contracts are recognized at the state level as shown in Table 8-2.

The terms of a contract may be agreed on orally or in writing; however, a written contract (**formal contract**) cannot be changed legally by an oral agreement. With an **expressed contract**, the conditions and terms of the contract are usually given in writing by the concerned parties. An **implied contract** recognizes a relationship between parties for services.

In accord with U.S. and Canadian contract law, the nurse is legally required to:

1. Adhere to the employer's policies and standards unless they are in conflict with federal or state law
2. Fulfill the terms of contracted service with the employer
3. Respect the rights and responsibilities of other health care providers, especially in areas that promote the continuity of client care

Accompanying these legal responsibilities are the nurse's rights to:

1. Expect adequate and qualified assistance in providing care
2. Receive reasonable and prudent conduct from the client
3. Expect from the employer compensation for services and provision of a safe environment with the necessary resources to perform the services
4. Be treated with prudent, reasonable behaviors from other health care providers

### Tort Law

**Tort law** is the enforcement of duties and rights among individuals independent of contractual agreements. **Tort** is a civil wrong committed on a person or property stemming from either a direct invasion of some legal right of the person, the infraction of some public duty, or the violation of some private obligation by which damages accrue to the person. Tort liability can be classified as unintentional (negligence and malpractice) and intentional (assault and battery, false imprisonment, invasion of privacy, defamation, and fraud). Intentional torts must prove that the defendant intended to commit the act. Examples of tort law are listed in Table 8-2 (Dempski & Killion, 2001).

## The Judicial Process

**Equity** acts in accordance with the spirit, not the letter, of the law. An outgrowth of English law, *equity allowed the king to hear an appeal when the application of the civil law became too harsh or when there was no adequate remedy in the common law*

## TABLE 8-2    TYPES OF CIVIL LAW

| Contract Law | | Torts | | Protective/Reporting Laws | |
| Federal | State | Federal | State | Federal | State |
| --- | --- | --- | --- | --- | --- |
| None | Employment contracts<br>Business contracts with clients<br>Contracts with allied groups<br>Uniform Commercial Code | Federal Torts Claims Act | State Torts Claims Act (to allow claims against the state)<br>Negligence (common law claim)<br>Malpractice statutes (professional liability)<br>Assault<br>Battery<br>False imprisonment<br>Invasion of privacy<br>Libel<br>Fraud | Child Abuse Prevention and Treatment Act<br>Privacy Act of 1974 | Age of Consent statutes (medical treatment, drugs, sexually transmitted disease)<br>Privileged Communication Statute<br>Abortion Statute<br>Good Samaritan Act<br>Abuse statutes (child, elderly, domestic violence)<br>Involuntary Hospitalization Statute<br>Living will legislation |

Data from Goldberg, K., Kaplan, H., & Shaw, M. (Eds.) (1996). *Nurse's legal handbook* (3rd ed.). Springhouse, PA: Springhouse.

*to satisfy the needs of the petitioner.* Therefore, the appeal was made to *conscience* (the king's innate sense of justice).

Equity evolved with its own set of principles, rules, and precedents, and when these clashed with their counterparts in the common law courts, equity prevailed. Equity continues to play an important role in the operation of the American judicial system (Brent, 1997).

### Judicial Law

Courts interpret a state's laws as they apply to everyday events. Once a court in the same jurisdiction, such as state or city, interprets a law in a certain manner, other courts tend to follow the same interpretation. This is often referred to as "setting a precedent."

Additionally, lower courts in the same jurisdiction must adhere to the interpretations of higher courts in the same region. Thus, all of a state's lower courts must adhere to the interpretations and procedures specified by that state's supreme or highest court and all courts in the United States must follow the rules established by the U.S. Supreme Court.

This body of judge-made law is referred to as **jurisprudence**. A well-known and controversial example of jurisprudence is the constitutional right to an abortion recognized by the Supreme Court that limits a state's ability to restrict a woman's access to an abortion.

## Legal Liability in Nursing

### Negligence and Malpractice

When the nurse fails to meet the legal expectations of care, the client can initiate action if harm or injury is incurred by the client. **Liability** is an obligation one has incurred or might incur through any act or failure to act. The term

**malpractice** refers to the behavior of a professional person's wrongful conduct, improper discharge of professional duties, or failure to meet the standards of acceptable care, which result in harm to another person (Zerwekh & Claborn, 2000). **Negligence** (breach of duty) is the failure of an individual to provide care that a reasonable person would ordinarily use in a similar circumstance. In other

 **LEGAL AND ETHICAL ISSUES**

### An Emergency Room Nurse Who Was Negligent for Failing to Do an EKG

The client had severe angina pain and called 911, believing she was having a heart attack. When she arrived at the emergency room, the triage nurse put her on oxygen, connected a heart monitor, and left her alone in an examination room with the curtain drawn.

An EKG machine was close by and not in use, but the nurse did not obtain an EKG strip. The client was not seen by a physician until almost an hour after she arrived. She survived the heart malfunction but had irreversible cardiac damage.

The jury found the emergency room nurse negligent for failing to do an EKG and for failing to summon the emergency room physician promptly.

Supreme Judicial Court of Massachusetts, 2001

Adapted from Snyder, E. (2002). *Legal eagle eye newsletter for the nursing profession, 10*(2), 2–7.

words, action that is contrary to the conduct of a reasonable person and results in harm is considered to be negligent behavior. When a nurse commits a negligent act that results in injury, it is known as malpractice.

Proof of liability depends on four elements:

1. **Duty** is an obligation created either by law or contract or by any voluntary action. It is the first element that must be proved for malpractice as it arises from the nurse-client relationship.
2. **Breach of duty** occurs when a nurse fails to act in accord with the standard of care. An act of commission or omission of the nurse may constitute a breach of the standard of care.
3. **Injury** (physical, financial, or emotional harm) must be demonstrated by the person making the claim to prove negligence. Damages is the money or other compensation awarded by the court to the **plaintiff** (the party who initiates a lawsuit that seeks damages or other relief).
4. **Causation** is the breach of duty that must be proved to have legally caused the injury. A cause-and-effect relationship must be clearly established.

To succeed in a malpractice suit, the plaintiff must first show that the **defendant** (the person being sued) owed him a duty. The plaintiff must then show that the defendant did not meet the duty and that this breach of duty caused harm, requiring compensation. Once the plaintiff files charges, the defendant must either refute the charges by demonstrating that, if a duty was owed, the duty was fulfilled or that, if a duty was breached, the breach was not

the cause of the plaintiff's complaint of injury. "Perhaps the most difficult concept in negligence is that of causation—proving that the negligent act was the cause of the injury" (Fiesta, 1997a, p. 24).

A person typically has no difficulty showing that a nurse owed a duty. All that needs to be demonstrated is that the nurse was working on the day of the injury and was responsible for the person's care as verified by the staffing schedules and assignment sheets. It is more difficult to prove that the duty owed was breached.

Courts usually apply the *reasonable person standard* that asks: "What would a reasonable nurse do in a similar situation?" To answer this question, courts look to the institution's policies and procedures to determine how client care is to be performed in that facility. When determining a breach of a duty, the actions of the nurse are also compared against the professional standards of nursing care. This is done by using published nursing standards of specialty nursing groups or by having another nurse testify as an expert witness. An **expert witness** is a person called by parties in a malpractice suit who is a member of the same profession as the party being sued and who is qualified to testify to the expected behaviors usually performed by members of the profession in a similar situation.

When a nurse is called to testify in a malpractice lawsuit either as the defendant or as an expert witness, the **testimony** (written or verbal evidence given by a qualified expert in an area) must be based on "facts." The jury and the court must form an opinion on their own; they are not interested in the witness's opinions on the matter in dispute.

Nurses are expected to administer client care based on both institutional policy and procedure and the professional standards of care. The nurse defendant would use the same methods to prove that a breach of duty did not occur: showing that the facility's policies and procedures were followed and that the actions followed accepted nursing standards. An expert witness is often asked to describe the relevant standards of care that will demonstrate that the client had the right to receive a *duty owed* from the nurse.

It is not sufficient to imply that the nurse breached a duty. The claimant must also show that this breach caused harm. A person cannot be compensated for a breach that caused no harm. Frequently, complaints against nurses are in one of the following categories: client falls, medication errors, failure to monitor a client in restraints, improper technique in giving treatment, failure to follow hospital procedures, and failure to supervise nonlicensed employees (Pozgar, 1999).

## NURSING STRATEGY

### Increasing Understanding and Comfort of Legal Responsibility

- Actively participate and network in local state nurses association.
- Attend nursing organizational meetings such as the Association of Legal Nurse Consultants.
- Familiarize yourself with the regulations of your State Board of Nursing, and call with any questions or concerns related to the parameters of your license.
- Attend continuing education conferences, and share new information with the colleagues in your work setting.
- Stay current in your knowledge of hospital policies and procedures.

American Association of Legal Nurse Consultants. (1997). *Legal nurse consulting: Principles and practice.* Washington, DC: CRC Press.

### Informed Consent

Laws regarding informed consent protect the client's right to self-determination. A client is able to make an informed decision about consenting to or refusing a treatment regime only if adequate information has been presented.

The law requires that clients or their representatives be given sufficient information regarding various treatment modalities so that the consent is an informed process. A

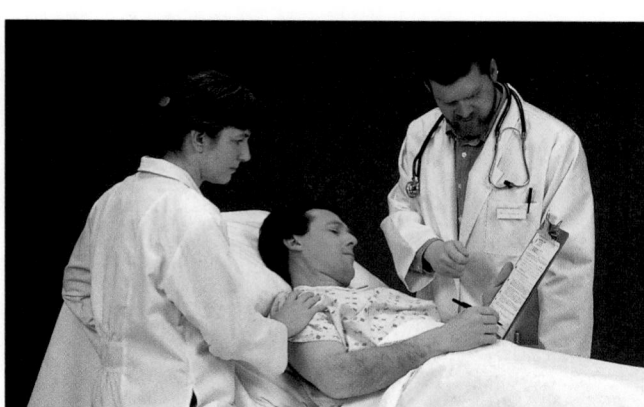

**Figure 8-1    This nurse is witnessing the signing of a consent form after the physician has fully informed the client about the proposed treatment. How does the nurse's compliance with the policy of informed consent lessen the nurse's liability in terms of this client's care?**

**consent** is a voluntary act by which a person agrees to allow someone else to do something. **Informed consent** means that the client understands the reason for the proposed intervention, and its benefits and risks, and agrees to the treatment by signing a consent form (Figure 8-1). Consent forms must be obtained for all **invasive** (accessing body tissues, organs, or cavities through some type of instrumentation) procedures.

Legally the client must be mentally competent to give consent for medical procedures. It is the legal responsibility of the health care provider performing the procedure to obtain the client's informed consent. Informed consent is a process consisting of information and consent, not merely the signing of a form. Obtaining the informed consent requires client teaching by the health care provider (Brent, 1997).

The health care provider may not coerce the client to sign the consent. The client has the right to refuse the information, waive the informed consent, and undergo treatment, but this decision must be documented in the medical record. The signing of an informed consent can also be waived for urgent medical and surgical intervention as long as institutional policy so indicates (Fiesta, 1999).

Parental or guardian consent should be obtained before treatment is initiated on a minor. There are three exceptions to this ruling: an emergency; situations where the consent of the minor is sufficient, such as treatment of a sexually transmitted disease; and when a court order or other legal authorization has been obtained. If a client is a minor and the parents or legal guardian deny the lifesaving treatment, the court may overrule the decision. Under the laws of most states and Canadian provinces, an emancipated minor (one who is married, pregnant, a parent, or financially independent) can give a valid consent to treatment. Most states legally mandate that a client's HIV status remain confidential (Cady, 1999). Therefore, nurses may be held liable for inappropriate disclosure, whether intentional or not, of information about a person's HIV status.

Switzer (1995) discusses how the courts have not always been clear in defining nursing responsibilities regarding informed consent. The general rules to keep in mind are:

1. The physician cannot delegate the responsibility for obtaining informed consents. However, a nurse could be held liable on a battery claim if the nurse knows the client has not given informed consent.
2. As directed by institutional policy, the nurse may witness a client's signing of a consent form or may be responsible for making sure the signed form is in the chart (Figure 8-2). As a witness to the client's signature, the nurse is confirming that the client was fully alert and aware of what was being signed.
3. When the nurse discovers circumstances that render a signed consent form invalid (such as a change in the client's condition), the nurse should notify the physician. If the client will not be harmed by a delay, the nurse is justified in refusing to assist with a procedure until the requirements for the informed consent are satisfied.

Although the law does not require staff nurses to obtain a formal informed consent for nursing procedures, the nurse has the responsibility of explaining to the client what to expect during the procedure.

### Assault and Battery

**Assault** is a stated intent to touch a person in an offensive, insulting, or physically intimidating manner. **Battery** is the touching of another person without the person's consent. The legal issues arising from assault and battery are usually based on whether the client consented to the touching that occurred.

Because assault and battery both deal with *acts of touching*, the client's cultural values, beliefs, and practices must be respected by the nurse. If the nurse should fail to recognize cultural differences, undesired outcomes may occur in the nurse–client relationship.

### False Imprisonment

**False imprisonment** occurs when clients are made to wrongfully believe they cannot leave a place. The most common example of this tort is telling a client not to leave the hospital until the bill is paid (Zerwekh & Claborn, 2000). Another example of false imprisonment is the misuse of physical or chemical restraints.

### Restraints or Seclusion

The Omnibus Budget Reconciliation Act (OBRA) of 1987 outlines the rights of the client and the responsibilities of health care providers regarding the use of both physical and chemical restraints. The nurse is to use safety measures, such as keeping the client's bed in a low position and checking on the client whenever the nurse or other caregivers pass the client's room, in an effort to avoid the use of restraints. Chemical restraints, primarily psychotropic medications (such as sedatives, hypnotics, antianxiety agents, and neuroleptics) are used to control hyperactive behavior of agitated clients.

---

**TULANE MEDICAL CENTER**
Hospital and Clinic
1415 Tulane Avenue
New Orleans, Louisiana  70112

Consent for medical procedure and acknowledgement
of receipt of information

Date_____

In keeping with the Louisiana State Law, you are being asked to sign a confirmation that we have discussed your contemplated operation or medical procedure. We have already discussed with you the common problems or risks. We wish to inform you as completely as possible. Please read the form carefully. Ask about anything that you do not understand and we will be pleased to explain it.

1.]  I hereby authorize and direct Dr._____ , with associates or assistants of his choice, to perform

upon_____ , the following surgical, diagnostic, or medical procedure

_____

_____

including any necessary or advisable anesthesia.

2.]  In general terms, the nature and purpose of this operation or medical procedure is:

_____

_____

3.]  This procedure has been explained to me. Alternate methods have also been explained to me, as have the advantages and disadvantages. I am advised that though good results are expected, the possibility and nature of complications cannot be accurately anticipated and that, therefore, there can be no guarantee as expressed or implied either as to the result of surgery or as to cure. The possible risks include death, brain damage, quadriplegia, paraplegia, loss of organ, loss of an arm or leg, or disfiguring scars.

4.]  I authorize the administration of a blood transfusion and such additional transfusion as may be deemed advisable in judgement of the attending physician, or his associates or assistants.
It has been fully explained that blood transfusions are not always successful in producing a desirable result and that there is a possibility of ill effects, such as the transmission of infectious hepatitis or other diseases or blood impairments. Also, it has been explained that emergencies may arise when it may not be possible to make adequate cross-matching tests, and that immediate need may make it necessary to use existing stocks of blood which may not include compatible blood types.

5.]  I further authorize the doctors to perform any other procedure that in their judgement is advisable for my well being. I hereby authorize and direct the above named physician and associates or assistants to provide such additional services as they may deem reasonable and necessary including, but not limited to, the administration of any anesthetic agent, or the services of the X-ray department or laboratories, and I hereby consent thereto.

6.]  I hereby state that I have read and understand this consent, all questions about the procedure or procedures have been answered in a satisfactory manner, and that all blanks were filled in prior to my signature.

Witness_____    Signature_____
                                                                                                (patient or person authorized to consent)

Witness_____    Relationship_____
(required only for telephone consent or consents signed with an X)

I certify that all blanks in this form were filled in prior to signature and that I explained them to the patient or his representative before requesting the patient or his representative to sign it.

                                                    Signature_____
                                                                        (above named physician to sign)

**CONSENT FOR MEDICAL PROCEDURE AND ACKNOWLEDGEMENT
OF  RECEIPT OF INFORMATION**

**Order by priority when consenting to medical/surgical procedure (except for care and treatment of mentally ill)**

1. Any competent adult, age 18 or older, for himself.
2. Any parent, whether an adult or minor, for his minor child.
3. Any married person, whether an adult or minor, for his/her spouse if spouse is unable to consent.
4. Any person temporarily standing in place of a parent whether formally served or not for the minor under his care and any guardian for his ward.

5. Any female regardless of age or marital status, for herself when given in connection with pregnancy or childbirth.
6. In the absence of a parent, any adult, for his minor brother or sister.
7. In the absence of a parent, any grandparent for his minor grandchild.

---

**Figure 8-2    Example of a consent form.** *Courtesy of Tulane University Hospital and Clinic, New Orleans, LA*

**LIFE SPAN CONSIDERATIONS**

### Legal Implications of an Impaired Elderly Client Signing an Informed Consent

An elderly individual may have difficulty hearing or be cognitively impaired. This would make the client unable to understand or conceptualize what the nurse is trying to explain in regards to a procedure (Figure 8-3). It is imperative not to rush the client into signing an informed consent without ensuring complete understanding. If the nurse has any doubt about the client's level of comprehension, the document should not be signed and the physician notified.

Adapted from Hogstel, M. (2001). *Gerontology: nursing care of the older adult*. Clifton Park, NY: Delmar Learning.

Restraints are legal only if they are necessary to protect the client or others from harm. If a competent client refuses to follow orders and the nurse uses restraints, the nurse can be charged with false imprisonment and/or assault and battery. In an emergency situation when a client becomes violent and is in imminent danger of harming self or others, the nurse may apply restraints and then immediately obtain an order from the physician. The law mandates that the use of restraints or seclusion must have a physician order. The nurse is legally accountable for the client in restraints or seclusion. Care of clients in restraints requires documentation as prescribed in specific agency policies.

### Privacy and Confidentiality

According to Badzek and Gross (1999), the concept of privacy includes the right to:

- Be left alone (i.e., freedom from intrusion)

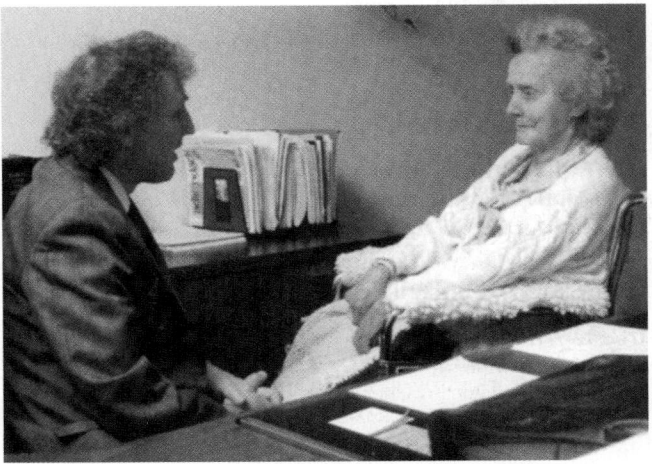

**Figure 8-3** **Nurse explaining procedure to an elderly client who is cognitively impaired.**

- Determine bodily integrity (to consent to or refuse treatment)
- Control how personal information is shared

Nurses are accountable for respecting the client's right to privacy. State laws guarantee that no one will reveal confidential information without the client's permission. Nurses must obtain the client's permission before disclosing any information regarding the client, going through the client's personal belongings, performing procedures, and photographing the client. An essential component of nursing practice is protecting the client's confidentiality and privacy. The American Nurses Association Code for Nurses (1985) identifies privacy and confidentiality as key elements in maintaining the integrity of the nursing profession.

The Canadian Nurses' Association (CNA) has developed its own Code of Ethics. CNA's Code of Ethics has involved nurses in all provinces and territories in Canada. Within the CNA's Code of Ethics, the value that applies to confidentiality states that the nurse is responsible to hold confidential all information about a client learned in health care settings. The nurse-client relationship is based on trust. Any violation of the client's privacy or breach of confidentiality may interfere with trust.

Nurses must ensure that clients understand their privacy rights including withholding information such as their diagnoses from the family. As another example, clients with sexually transmitted diseases or who are positive for the human immunodeficiency virus (HIV) may choose to withhold this information from their family. Most states recognize 18 years as the age at which adolescents are competent to make decisions regarding themselves. Nurses must be aware of the legislation in the state of practice since issues regarding health care of children varies from state to state (Muscari, 1999).

Privacy involves more than privilege doctrine. Nursing care should be delivered with a caring attitude that provides for privacy, such as keeping the door to the client's room

### COMMUNITY/HOME CARE

### Legal Implications of Potential Elder Abuse

Abuse of the elderly is an ever-growing issue and concern. Elderly parents cannot always afford assisted living environments, so as an alternative they live with family members. Nurses must be aware of the prevalent issue of elder abuse and note any suspicious bruises, cuts, or burns. If a nurse is not satisfied with the explanation of origin, these cases must be reported immediately to the authorities.

Fulmer, T. (2003). Elder abuse and neglect assessment. *Journal of Gerontological Nursing, 29*(1), 8–9.

closed, knocking before entering the client's room, closing the curtains around the bed before exposing the client, and draping the client appropriately for procedures (Figure 8-4).

A rapidly increasing problem that threatens privacy and confidentiality is access to electronic data. The technological proliferation of cellular phones, facsimile machines, and computerized medical records may jeopardize the privacy of information. In 1998, the American Nurses Association initiated a movement to regulate telecommunication technologies used in health care. "Confidentiality of client visits, client health records, and the integrity of information in our health care system is essential" (American Nurses Association, 1998, p. 4).

## Defamation

**Defamation** occurs when information is communicated to a third party that causes damage to someone else's reputation either in writing (libel) or verbally (slander). The most common examples of this tort are giving out inaccurate or inappropriate information from the medical record; discussing clients, families, or visitors in public areas; or speaking negatively about coworkers (Zerwekh & Claborn, 2000).

## Fraud

**Fraud** results from a deliberate deception intended to produce unlawful gain. Examples of fraudulent claims in health care are illegal billing and deceit in obtaining or attempting to obtain a nursing license (Flight, 1997). Fraudulent billing practices include overcharging for services and billing for services that were not provided. Other examples of fraud in health care include obtaining and using false credentials and falsifying medical records.

What should nurses do when they suspect fraud is occurring in the workplace? Nursing activities to deter fraud include the following:

* Documenting facts accurately
* Reporting illegal activities

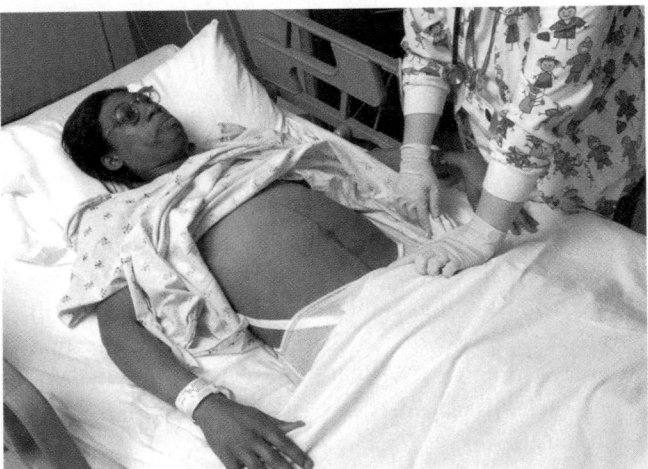

**Figure 8-4** Nurse examining the abdomen of a pregnant woman, while using appropriate techniques to maintain privacy.

 **LEGAL AND ETHICAL ISSUES**

### Nurse Reported Violence Threat: Suit Dismissed over Breach of Confidentiality

A college student was receiving mental health treatment at a mental health clinic and at a psychiatric center. His parents phoned the nurse who ran a parents' group at the psychiatric center and also spoke in the group about their son's statements that he might act out violently at the college's graduation ceremony. The nurse reported this to the local mental health authorities, who relayed the information to the local police. College officials questioned the young man, but let him participate in the graduation ceremony and nothing unusual happened.

The client claimed the nurse released confidential information from his mental health treatment records. That is not what happened. The client's parents talked to the nurse. The nurse called the county mental-health crisis team to report what the parents told her. The crisis team called the town police, who called the campus police. The decision was that there was no breach of medical confidentiality as the nurse did not disclose any information that was shared by the student during mental health visits.

New York Supreme Court, Appellate Division, 2001

Taken from Snyder, E. (2002). *Legal eagle eye newsletter for the nursing profession, 10*(2), 2–7.

* Educating peers and the public as to what constitutes fraud

The federal False Claims Act protects an employee who experiences any type of retaliation for reporting fraudulent practices (Kleiman, 1999).

## Unprofessional Conduct

Conduct that could adversely affect the health and welfare of the public constitutes **unprofessional conduct**. The following actions or omissions constitute unprofessional conduct: breach in client confidentiality; failure to use sufficient knowledge, skills, or nursing judgment when practicing nursing; physically or verbally abusing a client; assuming duties without sufficient preparation; knowingly delegating nursing tasks to unlicensed personnel that places the client at risk for injury; failure to accurately maintain a record for each client or falsifying a client's record; and leaving a nursing assignment without properly notifying appropriate personnel.

## CLIENT REFLECTIONS

### Confidential Information Shared with the Nurse

Mr. Wilson is a 64-year-old client admitted to your psychiatric unit. As his nurse, you have developed a therapeutic relationship with him, and he asks to speak confidentially to you. Mr. Wilson says, "I feel life has no purpose anymore, and I question my reason for living." He further adds, "Lately I have been having thoughts about ending my life."

As his nurse, what would you do with his confidential information?

---

### BOX 8-1 SUBSTANCE ABUSE INDICATORS

- Social isolation (e.g., requesting to work the night shift)
- Changes in personal appearance and mood
- Excessive work-related tardiness, absences, and accidents
- Excuses for being unavailable while on duty
- Resistance to change
- Defensive when questioned about client complaints and discrepancies in the narcotic control sheet
- Failure to meet schedules and deadlines
- Inaccurate and sloppy documentation

---

## Controlled Substances

The improper use of controlled substances may lead to criminal penalties in the United States and Canada under laws governing the distribution and use of controlled substances (narcotics, depressants, stimulants, and hallucinogens). Under law, agencies that distribute controlled substances must follow federal and state regulations regarding the security and access to these drugs. Title II of the Comprehensive Drug Abuse Prevention and Control Act of 1970 (Controlled Substances Act) requires accurate documentation of narcotic administration.

## The Impaired Nurse

If a nurse suspects a coworker is abusing chemicals, the nurse has a duty to report the individual to nursing administration in a confidential manner with the goal of treatment being the priority issue. Nursing administration should then notify the board of nursing regarding the nurse's behavior.

The ANA's *Code for Nurses* (1985) states that the nurse acts to safeguard the client and the public when health care and safety are affected by incompetent, unethical, or illegal practice of any person. Some boards of nursing will discipline a nurse for failing to report a fellow nurse who is abusing drugs. An **impaired nurse** is habitually intemperate or is addicted to the use of alcohol or habit-forming drugs. See Box 8-1 for indicators of substance abuse in nurses.

With the formation of the Task Force on Addiction and Psychological Disturbance by the ANA in 1981, many states have initiated programs to identify, treat, and assist impaired nurses. Intervention programs allow the nurse to seek and comply with a treatment regimen as an alternative to disciplinary action.

## Safety

The promotion of physical safety is one of the most important responsibilities of the nurse. There are four areas regarding client safety in which nurses are at legal risk:

(1) failure to monitor client status, (2) medication errors, (3) falls, and (4) use of restraints.

"Failure to monitor is a basis for liability that nurses must be particularly aware of" (Fiesta, 1997b, p. 16). The nurse must be aware of the client's condition. This calls for frequent assessment of all clients and adherence to policy guidelines regarding assessment of clients with special needs, such as those who are immobile, critically ill, or unconscious.

It is predicted that approximately 800,000 hospitalized clients will experience an adverse drug event each year. Almost 50% of adverse drug events are preventable (Fiesta, 1997b). Nurses play a major role in the prevention of adverse drug events by careful drug administration and client assessment.

A major area for potential liability is client falls (Figure 8-5). "Numerous lawsuits have demonstrated the importance of assessing patients for fall potential and taking necessary precautions in caring for patients who are likely to fall" (Eskreis, 1998, p. 34).

Another potential problem is the use of medical equipment. The nurse has the legal duty to use reasonable care when choosing and using medical equipment (Eskreis, 1998).

## Understaffing

**Understaffing** refers to the failure of a facility to provide a sufficient number of professional staff to meet client needs. Health care providers must have written staffing guidelines for each client population and setting to comply with the standards of the Joint Commission for the Accreditation of Healthcare Organizations. Usually staffing policies are in place to direct the decision making regarding increasing or downsizing staff numbers.

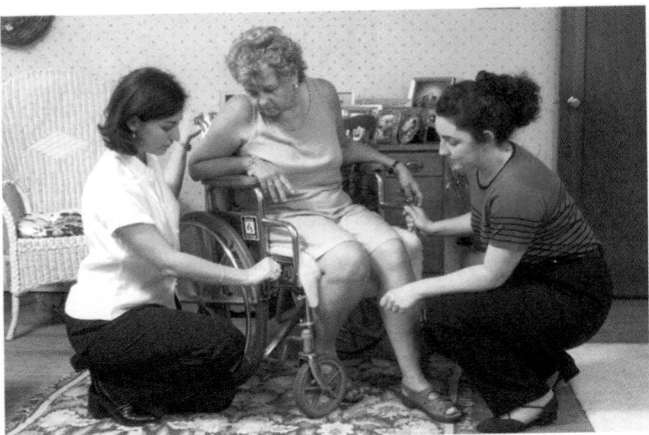

**Figure 8-5** A nurse explaining the correct method of sitting down in a wheelchair to avoid a fall.

## Mandatory Overtime

**Mandatory overtime** is defined as work hours imposed on an employee over an agreed-upon, predetermined work schedule. Across the country, nurses are reporting an increase in the use of mandatory overtime. As professionals, registered nurses are licensed by the state. It is through the process of licensure that the state protects the safety of the public. Once licensed, a nurse is declared to have met the minimal competency standards. This in turn provides the nurse with the authority to use professional judgment in all aspects of client care. The Nurse Practice Act provides the guidelines for professional practice, which are enforced by the Board of Nursing. When nurses are forced to work mandatory overtime, their professional judgment may be impaired or undermined as a result of fatigue. Nurses who challenge employers on this issue may in fact be terminated. Since nurses have few avenues to challenge mandatory overtime and can face licensure censure or revocation for providing less than adequate care because of stress, legislators must step in to protect the professional judgment of nurses and protect their clients' right to safe, quality care (American Nurses Association, 2002).

This issue is receiving much attention at both the local and national level. Legislators across the country are responding to the concern of nurses, as demonstrated by the fact that in 2001, 16 states introduced legislation to prohibit mandatory overtime.

## Reassignment

Questions are often raised by nurses in hospitals regarding the liabilities of "floating" (reassignment to work in an unfamiliar unit). This is an acceptable, legal practice used by hospitals to solve their understaffing problems. Legally, a nurse cannot refuse to float unless a union contract guarantees that nurses work only in a specified area or the nurse can prove the lack of knowledge for the performance of assigned tasks.

When reassignment occurs, nurses should set priorities and identify potential areas of harm to the client. Nursing

---

## FOCUS ON WELLNESS

### Ensuring a Safe Environment

Nurses have the responsibility to assess for and provide a safe client environment and anticipate areas of high risk (for both the client and the nurse). Client falls are one of the most prevalent reported injuries, and with proper assessment these incidents could be drastically reduced. Also, infection control measures need to be practiced on a consistent basis. Using basic critical thinking can prevent an injury or infection, as well as a lawsuit. Always assess a client's environment relative to the individual client, diagnosis, and administered medications. Reassess environment as needed. Remember: "An ounce of prevention is worth a pound of cure."

Adapted from Gershon, R., Karkashian, C., Grosch, J., Murphy, L., Escamilla-Cejudo, A., Flanagan, P., Bernacki, E., Kasting, C., Martin, L. (2000). Hospital safety climate and its relationship with safe work practices and workplace exposure incidents. *American Journal of Infection Control, 26*(3), 211–221.

---

experts recommend the practice of "nurses speaking out when they don't feel competent to take care of certain patients or perform certain procedures" (Trossman, 1999, p. 2). The nurse is legally mandated to be competent before performing procedures; inexperience is no legal excuse for errors. "When floating, it's especially important to ask questions of the regular staff" (Ahmed & Fecik, 1999, p. 12). All pertinent facts relating to client care problems and safety issues should be documented. Nurses who are required to "float" should receive orientation prior to reassignment.

## Executing Prescribed Orders

Medical practice acts of states and provinces usually define medicine as any act of diagnosis, prescription, surgery, or treatment. This definition allows for the initiation of written or verbal physician orders. In accord with nurse practice acts, nurses are obligated to follow the orders of a licensed physician or other designated health care provider *unless the orders would result in client harm.*

The nurse has a legal responsibility to the client to ensure that the order is clear and appropriate to the client's treatment. Ahmed and Fecik (1999) state "Questioning unclear orders testifies to a nurse's sense of responsibility" (p. 12). When the nurse questions a physician order, the physician should be contacted to obtain clarification. If, after physician clarification the nurse still questions the order, the nurse should institute agency policy; for example, notify the supervisor. Following the

## CLINICAL ALERT

### Medication Administration and Liability

Remember that the nurse remains liable for incorrectly administering a medication even if it is ordered incorrectly by a physician. "You're not exempt from liability because you were following a doctor's order" (Eskreis, 1998, p. 36).

agency's policy in this matter protects the nurse from employer disciplinary action.

Nurses are not encouraged to accept verbal orders from a physician because of the risks of error. See Chapter 16 for a complete discussion of how to document verbal orders.

## Legal Responsibilities and Roles of Professional Nurses

Nurses are legally responsible to practice nursing as set forth in nurse practice acts and professional standards of care. There are several roles performed by nurses related specifically to legal accountability.

### Provider of Service

The nurse is legally responsible to ensure that the client receives competent, safe, and holistic care. Nurses are expected to:

- Render care based on their education, experience, and circumstances (standards of a "reasonable, prudent person")
- Discuss with the client the associated risks and outcomes inherent in the plan of care as well as alternate treatment modalities
- Supervise and evaluate aspects of care that have been delegated to licensed and unlicensed caregivers
- Document the care the client receives and other significant events affecting the client
- Maintain clinical competency

The nurse is also responsible for the client's physical safety as discussed in this chapter in the section on safety.

### Expert Witness

To qualify as an expert witness, the nurse's education and experience are presented to the court to prove the nurse is knowledgeable about current standards and practice. The credentials of an expert witness have to match or exceed a defendant's qualifications. During the trial, the plaintiff's and the defendant's attorneys have the right to use the testimony of the expert witness for their respective cases.

## Forensic Specialist

A relatively new role for nurses is that of forensic nurse. In 1997, the American Nurses Association published *Scope and Standards of Forensic Nursing Practice*, which describes some of the responsibilities of forensic nurses as treating incarcerated clients, investigating trauma cases, and serving as expert witness in court. As violence continues to escalate in the United States, there will be an increased demand for forensic nurses.

## Reporting Responsibilities

Nurses should know which situations have to be reported because reporting statutes vary among the states and provinces; refer to Table 8-2 for protective/reporting laws. Criminal acts of rape and sexual assault must also be reported in most states and provinces.

## Legal Responsibilities of Students

Nursing students must act as reasonably prudent persons, equivalent with education and experience, when performing nursing duties. When employed as caregivers, nursing students must perform only those tasks that they are competent to perform, as stated in their job description.

## Legal Safeguards for Nursing Practice

There is a common set of actions a nurse can take to protect himself against ligation. Although each client encountered presents unique situations that can place the nurse at legal risk, certain general nursing care activities decrease this risk. Following the guidelines in the checklist should help protect nurses from lawsuits as well as provide defense in the event of a suit (Fiesta, 1998).

## CLIENT REFLECTIONS

### Blood Transfusion Controversy

Mary Jane Lucas is 10 years old and has just been admitted to the pediatric unit with a dangerously low hemoglobin level. Mary Jane's parents state, "We are Jehovah's Witnesses and will refuse any form of blood transfusion for our daughter. We both understand that Mary Jane may die without intervention and are willing to take that risk."

As Mary Jane's nurse, how would you proceed with this issue?

## Institutional Policies

All health care facilities have policies. Nursing students and registered nurses are obligated to know the policies and follow the procedures/protocols that flow from policy. Although policies are not laws, courts generally rule against nurses who violate policies.

## Whistle-Blowing in Health Care

The primary responsibility of nurses is to provide excellent health care. Nurses best serve the public when they can be candid and honest without reservation. Unfortunately, nurses do not always feel free to speak out about their quality-of-care concerns without fear of reprisal and retaliation. According to Fletcher, Sorrell, & Silva (1998), **whistle-blowing** is a warning issued by a member or former member of an organization to the public about a serious wrongdoing or danger created or concealed within the organization (Dempski & Killion, 2001). The ANA Guidelines on Reporting Incompetent, Unethical or Illegal Practices and the ANA Code of Ethics stipulate that a nurse who is aware of inappropriate or questionable practice in the provision of health care should express concern to the person carrying out the practice or to a responsible superior. In states without whistle-blower protection, nurses are faced with a choice between keeping quiet to keep their jobs or speaking out to improve client care.

Whistle-blowing is never a first choice; rather it is a last resort and indicates that the whistle-blower must have attempted, unsuccessfully, all other possible channels to right a wrong (Fletcher, Sorrell, & Silva, 1998). In other words, if a nurse finds working conditions to be unsafe, whether due to staffing levels, safety issues, or quality care, these instances should be reported to an administrator and be documented. There is much literature on the impact whistle-blowing has on a whistle-blower's life. Many have had to fight or leave the profession after reporting fraudulent workplace conduct and behavior. In an ethically responsible health care organization, whistle-blowing should not have to occur, because there would be

internal procedures to address staff concerns. If the concerns are addressed in a manner set forth by the organization, yet no action is taken, "whistle-blowing becomes a moral action of last resort, that under certain circumstances is not only appropriate but necessary" (Fletcher, Sorrell, & Silva, 1998, p. 3).

Some states have passed legislation protecting whistle-blowers from retaliation. Regardless, should an instance arise, a nurse should assess current whistle-blower protection in the state of employment and have documentation of incident(s) and attempts to resolve the situation internally before going outside an organization with charges.

## Professional Liability Insurance

Nurses should consider purchasing their own liability insurance for protection against malpractice lawsuits. Nurses may erroneously assume that they are protected by their employer's professional liability policies. When securing liability insurance, the nurse should validate the company's reputation. Most professional nursing organizations offer group liability insurance.

Usually when a nurse is sued, the employer is also sued for the nurse's actions or inaction. Even though this is the norm, nurses are encouraged to have their own malpractice insurance. For example, a suit may be filed for an incident that occurred in a facility where the nurse is no longer employed. Having one's own insurance also provides the nurse protection as an individual and allows the nurse to have an attorney who has only the nurse's interests in mind.

## Interstate Nursing Practice

Historically, regulation of the nursing practice has been a state-based function, whereby each state regulates the standards of practice within its geographic boundaries. Typically, nurses who hold more than one license have successfully passed the licensure exam in one state and applied for reciprocity in one or more other states (Silva & Ludwick, 1999). However, with the increased use of telecommunication (such as telehealth consultation), air transport nursing, or those nurses living on the border of two states, it can be understood how nursing practice is crossing state lines (Gaffney, 1999).

The National Council of State Boards of Nursing (NCSBN) (1997), a private association of state regulatory agencies, has proposed a solution known as the Nurse Licensure Compact. This legislation is an agreement among states to mutually recognize each other's licenses and allow for **interstate nursing practice** to occur. States that have adopted this legislation are referred to as *party* states, and states in which a nurse uses the multistate privilege are known as *remote* states. According to the terms of the compact proposed by the NCSBN, a nursing license would be issued by the state in which the nurse resides. Each nurse working within this compact agreement will be held accountable for complying with all laws governing

## STOP AND THINK

### Legal Implications for Nursing Students

When agency policy conflicts with the nurse practice act, what should you do? Remember that the state legislature empowers the board of nursing to define and monitor practice. If, as a nursing student, you willfully violate the state board's ruling, what future implication(s) could this have on your ability to apply for licensure?

## NURSING STRATEGY

### Actions to Decrease the Risk of Liability

- Communicate with your clients by keeping them informed and listening to what they say.

- Acknowledge unfortunate incidents and express concern about these events without either taking the blame, blaming others, or reacting defensively.

- Chart and time your observations immediately, while facts are still fresh in your mind.

- Take appropriate actions to meet the client's nursing needs.

- Follow the facility's policies and procedures for administering care and reporting incidents.

- Acknowledge and document the reason for any omission or deviation from agency policy, procedure, or standard.

- Maintain clinical competency and acknowledge your limitations. If you do not know how to do something, ask for help.

- Promptly report any concern regarding the quality of care, including the lack of resources with which to provide care, to a nursing administration representative.

- Use appropriate standards of care.

- Time and document changes in conditions requiring notification of the physician and include the response of the physician.

- Delegate client care based on the documented skills of licensed and unlicensed personnel.

- Treat all clients and their families with kindness and respect

nursing practice in the state in which the client is located. "Although the remote state (compact state) may discontinue the multistate privilege, the state of residence (home state) retains authority to take disciplinary action against the licensee" (Gaffney, 1999, p. 4).

This is a relatively new solution and approach to a growing concern. Over time the profession will have to assess issues ranging from confidentiality of information, to nonmaleficence (to do no harm), to autonomy of practice (what might be the standard of practice in one state may be taken away in another) among others.

## Risk Management Programs

Risk management is a method of identifying, evaluating, and decreasing the agency's risk of financial loss. Most health care facilities are required to have formal risk management programs in place by agencies such as the Department of Health and Human Services, accrediting bodies, and liability insurance carriers. These programs are based on systematic reporting of incidents or unusual occurrences, for example, client falls (Brown, Grigsby, Walsh, & Kaye, 2002).

## Incident Reports

In accord with the agency's policies, nurses are required to file incident reports when a situation arises that could or did cause client harm. When filing an incident report, the nurse should state only the *facts* surrounding the incident. The nurse's opinions or conclusions about the incident are not to be documented. Also, the client's medical record should not contain any reference to the filing of an incident report.

## Client Education

Safe nursing care requires that the client has a thorough understanding of the treatment plan. Although the physician has specific responsibilities regarding client education, the nurse must also provide client teaching and document the degree of learning.

## Legislation Affecting Nursing

There are legal, as well as ethical, implications inherent in nursing practice, which require nurses to know and comply with the specific existing health care laws and regulations in their state of licensure. The common legal liabilities in some nursing practice settings are discussed in the following section (Figure 8-6).

## Advance Directives

The Omnibus Reconciliation Act of 1990, called the Patient Self-Determination Act (PSDA), defines an **advance directive** as a written instruction that is recognized under state law and is related to the provision of such care when the individual is incapacitated (Cate & Gill, 1991). There are three types of legal instruments that comply with the act's definition:

1. A **living will** is a document prepared by a competent adult that provides direction regarding medical care in the event the person becomes unable to make decisions personally.

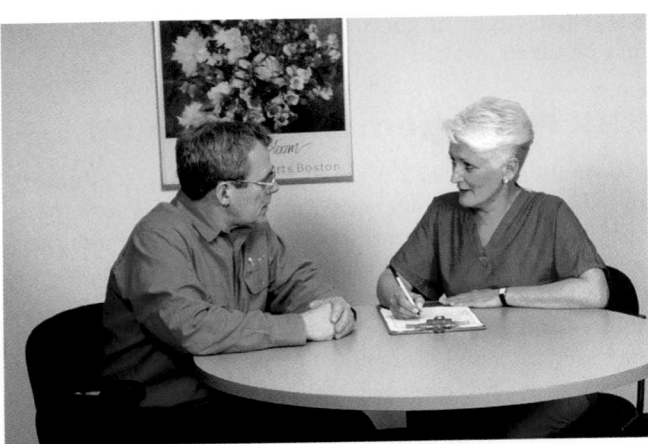

**Figure 8-6** A client and nurse discussing and completing advance directives.

2. **Durable power of attorney** (health care proxy) is an authorization that enables any competent individual to name someone to exercise decision-making authority, under specific circumstances, on the individual's behalf.
3. **Advance care medical directive** is a document in which an individual, in consultation with the physician, relatives, or other personal advisers, provides precise instructions for the type of care the client wants or does not want in a number of scenarios (Lieberson, 2002).

The living will is the most widely available instrument for recording future health care–related decisions. However, it is not an enacted statute in all 50 states. Figure 8-7 presents a sample document of a living will. All states provide for a general durable power of attorney.

American Health Consultants (1995) discussed the need to provide public education about initiation of advance directives in a non–health care setting in simple, easily understood language. Follow-up systems need to be put into place on a community level to ensure that citizens are aware of the purpose and provisions of advance directives and share these documents with their primary physician and family members.

As the total number of citizens in their eighties and nineties increases (Hogstel, 2001), the numbers of those who are not able to handle their own affairs and make decisions for themselves increases (Zronek, Daly, Rhee, 1999). This situation frequently requires the caregiver to become involved in legal affairs. Nurses who work with older clients should be aware of community resources to assist the elderly in legal matters. Local groups (e.g., the American Association of Retired Persons) are often able to refer people to agencies providing legal assistance for reasonable charges.

## Abortion

The 1973 Supreme Court decision of *Roe v. Wade* increased the safety and availability of abortions in the United States. Health care agencies and practitioners in various states may be required to report abortions performed as well as other information about the client, the procedure, and any resulting complications. Some states only require the reporting of abortions for minors.

Nurses may need to explore their own feelings or beliefs about abortion before assisting with these procedures. The nurse should also be aware of the client's feelings before the abortion so that the appropriate referral can be made for postprocedure care if necessary (Brent, 1997).

## The Americans with Disabilities Act

Passed by the U.S. Congress in 1990, The Americans with Disabilities Act (ADA) prohibits discrimination on the basis of disability in employment, public services, and public accommodations. The ADA defines a person with a disability as having a physical or mental impairment that substantially limits one or more of the major life activities. See Box 8-2 for disabilities that are covered by the ADA.

## Good Samaritan Acts

**Good Samaritan acts** are laws that provide protection to health care providers by ensuring immunity from civil liability when assistance is provided at the scene of an emergency and the caregiver does not intentionally or recklessly cause client injury. The caregiver will be evaluated by how a reasonable and prudent caregiver would have responded in a similar situation. Good Samaritan acts are examples of common and statutory laws as determined by the individual states. Although all 50 states and the District of Columbia have Good Samaritan acts, some of the Canadian provinces (e.g., Ontario and Quebec) do not have Good Samaritan acts.

Good Samaritan acts vary in coverage from state to state, and it is the responsibility of caregivers to know the law for their own jurisdictions. Keep in mind that some states only cover nurses licensed in that state and that these acts are amended periodically by legislation. Good Samaritan acts do not provide immunity to the nurse who is providing care as an employee (Zerwekh & Claborn, 2000).

 **STOP AND THINK**

### Coworker with Hearing Impairment

How would you feel about a nurse coworker who is hearing impaired and cannot hear heart, lung, and bowel sounds? What are your responsibilities in such a situation?

**Declaration**

Declaration made this _____ day of _____ (month, year).

I, _____, being of sound mind, willfully and voluntarily make known my desire that my dying shall not be artificially prolonged under the circumstances set forth below and do hereby declare:

If at any time I should either have a terminal and irreversible incurable injury, disease, or illness or be in continual profound comatose state with no reasonable chance of recovery, certified by two physicians who have personally examined me, one of whom shall be my attending physician, and the physicians have determined that my death will occur whether or not life-sustaining procedures are utilized and where the application of life-sustaining procedures would serve only to prolong artificially the dying process, I direct that such procedures be withheld or withdrawn and that I be permitted to die naturally with only the administration of medication or the performance of any medical procedure deemed necessary to provide me with comfort care.

In the absence of my ability to give directions regarding the use of such life-sustaining procedures, it is my intention that this declaration shall be honored by my family and physician(s) as the final expression of my legal right to refuse medical or surgical treatment and accept the consequences from such refusal.

I understand the full import of this declaration and I am emotionally and mentally competent to make this declaration.

Signed: _____

City, Parish, and State of Residence _____

The declarant has been personally known to me and I believe him or her to be of sound mind.

Witness: _____

Witness: _____

**Figure 8-7    Sample of a living will.** *Courtesy of Louisiana Hospital Association, Baton Rouge, LA*

## National Practitioner Data Bank

The Health Care Quality Improvement Act was enacted in 1986 to identify unsafe health care providers and restrict their unsafe practice. The major goal of this legislation was to deter incompetent practitioners from moving to a new state without having to report on problematic care delivery in previous states. There were two major components of this law: (1) to establish a National Practitioner Data Bank, which would serve as a clearinghouse for information on unsafe practitioners; and (2) to provide immunity for reporting incompetent peers.

## Occupational Safety and Health Act

In 1970, the Occupational Safety and Health Act (OSHA) was enacted to ensure safe work environments for Americans. The intent of the act was to decrease work-related injuries. The act was expanded in 1991 to develop standards for safety of those who may experience work-related exposure to blood-borne contaminants. Employers are fined if they violate OSHA rules and regulations.

## Legal Issues Related to Death

## Do Not Resuscitate Orders

Sudden death from a cardiac arrest requires the initiation of cardiopulmonary resuscitation (CPR) by competent persons. In health care settings, caregivers (often a nurse) perform CPR and other lifesaving measures according to agency policy unless the primary physician has written a *do not resuscitate* (DNR) order in the client's medical record.

## STOP AND THINK

### Good Samaritan Acts

If, as a nurse, you charge or accept a fee for the services rendered during an emergency situation, will you still be protected by a Good Samaritan act? What are the legal implications for accepting compensation for your professional services?

The physician's DNR order provides an exception to the universal standing order to resuscitate.

Health care agencies are required to have policies in place that provide a mechanism for reaching a DNR decision as well as for resolving conflicts in decision making. The principles of informed consent must be respected by the physician who writes a DNR order. When the client is either comatose or near death, there should be knowledgeable concurrence by the physician and the client's family or guardian about the actions to prolong the client's life. It is the responsibility of the nurse to know and follow the client's wishes relative to resuscitation and the application of life-support systems. This information must be documented in the client's medical record (Lieberson, 2002).

## Euthanasia

**Euthanasia** refers to an intentional action or lack of action causing the merciful death of someone suffering from a terminal illness or incurable condition. The issue of euthanasia is a difficult one for society, the courts, and health care facilities (Flight, 1997).

## Wills

The United States and Canada have laws regarding the legal requirements for written and oral wills. These laws define the format of wills, the number of witnesses needed, who can be a witness, what makes a will valid or invalid, how to invalidate a will, and how to contest a will (Goldberg, Kaplan, & Shaw, 1996). Nurses are usually required to notify the physician and nurse supervisor before acting as a witness and signing a will. Nurses should refrain from assisting the client with the wording of the will.

## Pronouncement of Death

Medicine has yet to agree on one acceptable definition of death. The various definitions are as follows: the absence of awareness of external stimuli, lack of movement or spontaneous breathing, absent reflexes, a flat brain wave repeated twice in 24 hours, and the Uniform Definition of Brain Death, which requires irreversible cessation of all functioning of the brain (Zerwekh & Claborn, 2000).

State regulatory boards have initiated laws to protect the public when dealing with issues of death. It is usually within the scope of practice of medicine to pronounce a client dead. However, some boards of nursing allow the nurse, in certain circumstances and with thorough documentation, to make a determination and pronouncement of death (Bosna, 1995; State of Alaska, 1994). Because state laws vary concerning this issue, it is important for the registered nurse to know the laws in the state(s) or province(s) of licensure.

## Care of the Deceased

When a client dies, the nurse is obligated to treat the deceased with respect and dignity. The nurse should prepare the body for removal to the morgue in accord with agency policies. The nurse is responsible for properly identifying the body. In *Lott v. State* (1962), a nurse mislabeled two bodies, causing a Roman Catholic to be prepared for an Orthodox Jewish burial, and an Orthodox Jew to be prepared for a Roman Catholic burial; the court found the nurse liable (Goldberg et al, 1996).

## RESEARCH FOCUS

**Title of Study:** Elderly patients' understanding of advance directives

**Study Purpose:** To determine client's beliefs and levels of understanding about advance directives (AD).

**Methods:** This was a descriptive study conducted by use of medical records reviews and client interviews. During the interviews, clients were read a questionnaire and the answers were recorded by an interviewer. The questions sought information about the type of AD completed, the client's source of information about ADs, and beliefs or communications regarding the completion of the AD.

**Findings:** A majority of clients interviewed were able to clearly state what an AD means. Ninety percent of respondents stated that they had discussed ADs with family members. Ninety-eight percent reported that they had discussed their feelings about life-sustaining treatment measures with potential surrogate decision makers. Many of those surveyed stated the belief that ADs facilitate client choice and decrease family suffering. Generally, clients believed ADs would "make a difference" for them at the end of their lives.

**Implications:** The clients in this study expressed a wish to simplify end-of-life decisions. They also stated a strong belief that ADs were useful in meeting this goal.

Zronek, S., Daly, B., & Lee, H. (1999). Elderly patients' understanding of advance directives. *JONA's Healthcare Law, Ethics, and Regulation, 1*(2), 23–28.

## Organ Donation

All 50 states have adopted the Uniform Anatomical Gift Act for cadaveric organ donation. In the United States and Canada, any person 18 or older may become an organ donor by written consent. In the absence of appropriate

## STOP AND THINK

### What Constitutes Death?

Considering the various definitions of death, is it absolutely clear when the moment of death occurs? Based on these definitions, when can the life-supporting machines be turned off? Although the right of the client to refuse treatment, which may lead to death, has been established, can you identify clinical circumstances where the client might be deprived of the right to die?

documentation, a family member or legal guardian may authorize donation of the organs. Nurses and other caregivers are expected to approach families for organ donation in the absence of documentation of the client's wishes. Consent for an organ donation requires the collaborative efforts of the nurse with physicians, social workers, and clergy to ensure timely removal of the organ(s) (Aiken, 2000).

## Autopsies

An autopsy is performed to determine the *cause of death*. Autopsy results are used in cases of suspicious death or the presence of communicable disease. The cause of death also has implications regarding payment from insurance policies and worker's compensation.

Autopsy cases are the most frequent cause of litigation involving dead bodies and hospitals. A few states require the consent in writing, whereas other states accept telegrams or documented telephone conversations. Regardless of how the consent is obtained, the physician must document that the consent was obtained and identify in the client's record who authorized the autopsy. In some states, the consent for an autopsy is not required in unwitnessed deaths because this situation requires a mandatory autopsy. The nurse has the responsibility for ensuring that all documentation is in place before releasing the body for autopsy (Brent, 1997).

## CASE STUDY/NURSING CARE PLAN

Sam Kelsey is a 48-year-old male admitted to the psychiatric unit for depression with suicidal ideation. He admitted that his wife left him 2 weeks ago, taking their 5-year-old son with her because of Sam's "jealous outbursts." Sam admitted to having difficulty managing his anger at times but did not see it as a major problem. He denied any recent violent altercations with his wife, but confessed to having been abusive in the past. Sam stated to the nurse that it had been about "1 year since I hit her." When asked about his alcohol intake, he stated that he had a history of drinking one to two cans of beer at night after work, but his drinking has increased to five to six cans of beer per night since his marital separation. Sam mentioned that

*(continues)*

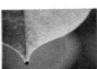 **CASE STUDY/NURSING CARE PLAN** (continued)

over the past week he called in sick to work on three occasions because he was just "too tired" to deal with things. He describes feelings of hopelessness and helplessness, yet expresses fierce anger at his wife for "wrecking his life."

After 48 hours in the psychiatric unit, Sam states to his doctor that he no longer is having thoughts of hurting himself. A discharge order is written. Later that shift, the nurse working on his discharge overhears the client make the statement, "My wife will regret what she has done to me. I swear I will get even with her if it's the last thing I do," and then give an inappropriate laugh. The nurse continues to monitor the client's affect and further evaluates his appropriateness for discharge.

### Assessment
The assessment reveals a 48-year-old Caucasian male who recently experienced a marital separation. Upon further clinical assessment for depression with suicidal ideation, it is revealed that the client has a history of domestic violence and regular alcohol intake. The client's age, race, gender, alcohol intake, and crisis situation make him a higher than average risk for suicide and violence toward others. As the time for discharge is approaching, the client is becoming increasingly agitated and stressed.

### Nursing Diagnosis #1
Risk for other-directed violence related to catastrophic personal events in life.
**NOC:** Abusive Behavior Self-Control; Aggression Control; Impulse Control; Risk Detection
**NIC:** Anger Control Assistance; Environmental Management: Violence Prevention

### Expected Outcomes
The client will:
1. Attend regularly scheduled counseling meetings within 1 week of discharge.
2. State practical methods for controlling his anger within first two counseling sessions.
3. Verbalize the necessity to stop alcohol consumption and attend Alcoholics Anonymous support group during first counseling session with health care provider.

### Planning/Interventions/Rationales
1. Attend biweekly counseling sessions for anger management with health care provider. *Anger is treatable with short-term, structured management programs.*
2. Allow client to ventilate and express his emotions when anger first develops, and encourage client to identify practical methods for controlling his anger. *Clearly identifying emotions assists client in developing coping strategies for anger management.*
3. Encourage client to cease alcohol consumption and attend Alcoholics Anonymous support group. *Alcohol consumption decreases personal control and decreases rationale decision-making processes.*

### Evaluation
By the second week of counseling sessions, the client began to verbally express his feeling related to anger instead of acting out on impulses. He also began attending Alcoholics Anonymous within 1 week of discharge.

## Key Concepts

- Laws define and limit relationships among individuals and the government.
- The three sources of public law at the federal and state levels are constitutional law, administrative law, and criminal law.
- Administrative law empowers state boards of nursing to protect the public by regulating the scope of nursing practice.
- The three sources of civil law at the federal and state levels are contract law, tort law, and protective/reporting laws.
- A nurse employed by a health care facility is legally responsible for the terms of an implied contract.
- The two types of tort law at the state level are unintentional torts, which include negligence and malpractice, and intentional torts, which include assault and battery, false imprisonment, invasion of privacy, defamation, and fraud.

- Protective/reporting laws such as The Americans with Disabilities Act and Good Samaritan acts protect a designated group of individuals.
- Even when working mandated overtime hours, nurses assume complete responsibility for any nursing errors.
- The legal responsibilities of the nurse, defined in practice acts and standards of care, include elements such as providing services to clients and acting as expert witnesses in malpractice suits.
- Incident reports are filed by the nurse when a situation arises that could or did cause client harm.
- To prevent incurring liability due to the policy of "floating," nurses should set priorities and identify potential areas of harm to the client, receive orientation and cross-training before reassignment, and document all pertinent information about client care problems and safety issues.
- The ANA Code of Ethics stipulates that a nurse who is aware of inappropriate or questionable practice in the provision of health care should express concern to the person carrying out the practice or to a responsible manager.
- Legal instruments such as informed consent and advance directives uphold the right of all people to control decisions relating to their own health care.
- Nurse Licensure Compact is an agreement among states to mutually recognize each other's licenses and allow for interstate nursing practice to occur.
- Nurses may witness the signing of a consent form by a client as permitted by institutional policies; however, if the nurse discovers circumstances that render a signed consent form invalid, the nurse should notify the physician and, if necessary, the nurse manager.
- In terms of specific client care issues such as abortion, pronouncement of death, do not resuscitate orders, euthanasia, care of the deceased, wills, organ donation, and autopsies, nurses must know and comply with the existing laws and regulations that pertain to these areas in their individual states and provinces of licensure.

## Review Questions and Activities

1. Provide an example of a:
   a. Public law
   b. Civil law
2. Explain each type of law:
   a. Constitutional
   b. Administrative
   c. Criminal
   d. Protective/reporting
3. List the three essential elements of a legal contract.
4. Identify the types of intentional torts.
5. What are the four elements that must be proven by the plaintiff in a malpractice case?
6. Discuss the relationship of the reasonable person standard in relation to professional standards of practice.
7. Identify common acts of commission and omission that lead to nursing malpractice complaints.

## Web Resources

American Association of Colleges of Nursing
   http://www.aacn.nche.edu
American Association of Legal Nurse Consultants
   http://www.aalnc.org
American Association of Nurse Attorneys
   http://www.taana.org
American Nurses Association
   http://www.ana.org
National Center on Elder Abuse
   http://www.elderabusecenter.org
Nursing World
   http://www.nursingworld.org

## References

Ahmed, D. S., & Fecik, S. (1999). Med errors: Floating faux pas. *American Journal of Nursing, 99*(7), 12.

Aiken, T. (2000). *Legal issues in nursing* (2nd ed.). Philadelphia: F. A. Davis.

American Association of Legal Nurse Consultants (1997). *Legal nurse consulting: Principles and practice.* Washington, DC: CRC Press.

American Health Consultants (1995). Registry aims to solve case of the missing directive. *Medical Ethics Advisor, 11*(8), 105–107.

American Nurses Association (1985). *Code for nurses with interpretative statements.* Kansas City: Author.

American Nurses Association (1998). *Core principles on telehealth.* (Publication No. 9901TH.) Washington, DC: Author.

American Nurses Association (2002). *ANA position paper on mandatory overtime.* Washington, DC: Author.

Badzek, L., & Gross, L. (1999). Confidentiality and privacy: At the forefront for nurses. *American Journal of Nursing, 99*(6), 52–54.

Bosna, M. (1995). Legal questions. *Nursing 95, 25*(7), 71–73.

Brent, N. J. (1997). *Nurses and the law: A guide to principles and applications.* Chicago: Saunders.

Brown, B. B., Grigsby, J., Walsh, A. C., & Kaye, K. (2002). *Mental capacity: Legal and medical aspects of assessment and treatment* (2nd ed.). New York: Clark.

Cady, R. F. (1999). The legal forum. *Journal of Nursing Administration, 1*(2), 8–11.

Cate, F. H., & Gill, B. A. (1991). *The Patient Self-Determination Act.* Northwestern University: The Annenberg Washington Program.

Dempski, K. M., & Killion, S. W. (2001). *Legal and ethical issues in nursing.* Thorofare, NJ: SLACK, Inc.

Eskreis, T. R. (1998). Seven common legal pitfalls in nursing. *American Journal of Nursing, 98*(4), 34–40.

Fiesta, J. (1997a). Legal update—1996, Part 3. *Nursing Management, 28*(7), 24–26.

Fiesta, J. (1997b). Legal update—1996, Part 2. *Nursing Management, 28*(6), 16–17, 19.

Fiesta, J. (1998). *Law and liability: A guide for nurses.* New York: Wiley.

Fiesta, J. (1999). Informed consent: What health care professionals need to know, Part 2. *Nursing Management, 30*(7), 6–7.

Fletcher, J., Sorrell, J., & Silva, M. (1998). Whistleblowing as a failure of organizational ethics. *Online Journal of Issues in Nursing.* http://nursingworld.org

Flight, M. (1997). *Law, liability, and ethics* (3rd ed.). Clifton Park, NY: Delmar Learning.

Fulmer, T. (2003). Elder abuse and neglect assessment. *Journal of Gerontological Nursing, 29*(1), 8–9.

Gaffney, T. (1999). The regulatory dilemma surrounding interstate practice. *Online Journal of Issues in Nursing.* http://www.nursingworld.org

Gershon, R., Karkashian, C., Grosch, J., Murphy, L., Escamilla-Cejudo, A., Flanagan, P., Bernacki, E., Kasting, C., Martin, L. (2000). Hospital safety climate and its relationship with safe work practices and workplace exposure incidents. *American Journal of Infection Control, 26*(3), 211–221.

Goldberg, K., Kaplan, H., & Shaw, M. (Eds.). (1996). *Nurse's legal handbook* (3rd ed.). Springhouse, PA: Springhouse.

Hogstel, M. O. (2001). *Gerontology: Nursing care of the older adult.* Clifton Park, NY: Delmar Learning.

Hutcherson, C. (2001). Legal considerations for nurses practicing in a telehealth setting. *Online Journal of Issues in Nursing.* http://www.nursingworld.org

Kleiman, M. A. (1999). The false claims act. *JONA's Healthcare Law, Ethics, and Regulations, 1*(2), 17–22.

Lieberson, A. D. (2002). *Advance medical directives.* New York: Clark.

Muscari, M. E. (1999). When can an adolescent give consent? *American Journal of Nursing, 98*(5), 18–19.

National Council of State Boards of Nursing (1997). Quarterly Reports, July 1996–June 1997. New Jersey: The Chauncy Group.

Pozgar, G. D. (1999). *Legal aspects of health care administration* (7th ed.). Gaithersburg, MD: Aspen Publishers.

Silva, M., & Ludwick, R. (1999). Interstate nursing practice and regulation: Ethical issues for the 21st century. *Online Journal of Issues in Nursing.* http://www.nursingworld.org/ojin/ethicol/ethics_1.htm

Snyder, E. (2002). *Legal eagle eye newsletter for the nursing profession, 10*(2), 2–7.

State of Alaska (1994). *Alaska Statutes.* Published in the Alaska Administrative Code.

Switzer, H. (1995). The legal side. *American Journal of Nursing, 95*(6), 66-67.

Trossman, S. (1999, January/February). Staffing smart: A difficult proposition. *The American Nurse,* 1–2.

Zerwekh, J., & Claborn, J. C. (2000). *Nursing today: Transition and trends* (3rd ed.). Philadelphia: Saunders.

Zronek, S., Daly, B., & Lee, H. (1999). Elderly patients' understanding of advance directives. *JONA's Healthcare Law, Ethics, and Regulation, 1*(2), 23–28.

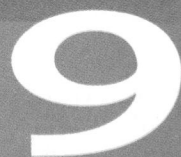

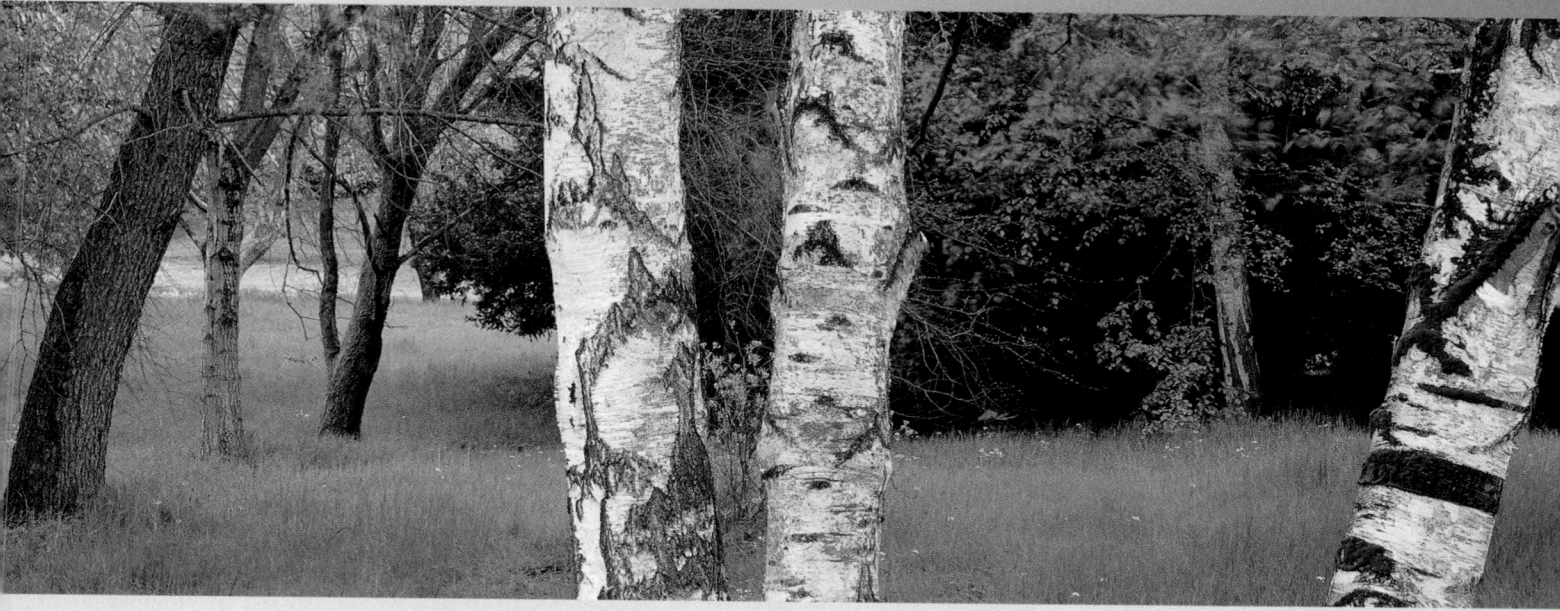

# CHAPTER 9

# Ethical Issues

Tina H. Olson, EdD, RN

*"Do and dare what is right, not swayed by the whim of the moment."*

(Dietrich Bonhoeffer, 1955)

# Chapter Competencies

*Upon completion of this chapter, the reader should be able to:*

1. Explain the relationship between ethics and law.
2. Discuss the ethical theories of teleology and deontology.
3. Describe the major ethical principles that affect health care.
4. Explain the link between ethics and values.
5. Relate the ethical codes developed by the International Council of Nurses, the American Nurses Association, and the Canadian Nurses Association to daily nursing practice.
6. Identify the rights of the client as established by the American Hospital Association.
7. Apply the steps identified in the framework for ethical decision making to issues such as euthanasia, refusal of treatment, and use of scarce resources.

# Key Terms

| | | |
|---|---|---|
| active euthanasia | ethical principles | nonmaleficence |
| assisted suicide | ethical reasoning | passive euthanasia |
| autonomy | ethics | paternalism |
| beneficence | euthanasia | teleology |
| bioethics | fidelity | utility |
| categorical imperative | justice | values |
| client advocate | material principle of justice | values clarification |
| deontology | morality | veracity |
| ethical dilemma | | |

Every day, nurses encounter situations in which they must make decisions based on the determination of right and wrong. How do they make such decisions? Which values determine the rightness of an action?

The delivery of ethical health care is becoming an increasingly difficult issue in contemporary society. Nurses are committed to maintaining clients' rights in terms of the provision of information about health care and treatment. This desire to maintain clients' rights, however, often conflicts with professional duties and institutional policies. It is important to balance these two perspectives so that the primary objective, delivery of quality care, is achieved (White, Coyne, Patel, 2001).

In considering the situations presented throughout this chapter, realize that there are no absolute right answers. Dealing with the gray areas (ambiguities) causes discomfort for some nurses. Ethical rules are impossible to prove (Burkhardt & Nathaniel, 1998, p. 25). Because clients and nurses are humans, no two situations can ever be exactly alike. This chapter explores the concept of ethics, ethical theories and principles, values and ethics,

ethical codes, ethical decision making, and the application of ethical guidelines to nursing practice.

## Concept of Ethics

**Ethics** is the branch of philosophy that examines the differences between right and wrong. Simply put, ethics is the study of the rightness of conduct. Ethics deals with one's responsibilities (duties and obligations) as defined by logical argument. Ethics looks at human behavior—what people do under what type of circumstances. But ethics is not merely a philosophical discussion; ethical persons put their beliefs into action.

Often the term *morals* is mistakenly used when ethics is meant. **Morality** is behavior in accordance with custom or tradition and usually reflects personal or religious beliefs. An example of a moral belief is a person's desire to maintain her right to die. Ethics is the free, rational, and publicly stated assessment of alternative actions in relation to theories, principles, and rules. Ethics is rooted in the legal system and reflects the political values of our society. An example of an ethical belief is the practice of parents' teaching their children the importance of telling the truth.

## Relationship Between Legal and Ethical Concepts

There is a connection between acts that are legal and acts that are ethical. Sometimes, it is difficult to separate legalities from ethics (see Chapter 8 for discussion about the legal responsibilities of nurses). Some legal acts are considered to be unethical and vice versa. According to Burkhardt and Nathaniel (1998), the following contribute to the occasional discrepancies between law and ethics:

- Ethical opinions reflect individual differences.
- Human behavior and motivation are too complex to be accurately reflected in law.
- The legal system judges action rather than intention.
- Laws change according to social and political influences.

Professional nursing actions are both legal and ethical.

## Ethics in Health Care

The application of general ethical principles to health care is referred to as **bioethics**. Ethics affects every area of health care, including direct care of clients, allocation of finances, and utilization of staff. Ethics does not provide easy answers, but it can help provide structure by raising questions that ultimately lead to answers (Newell, 2002).

Ethics is exerting an ever-increasing influence on health care today. Several factors contribute to an increased need to provide health care in an ethical manner. Some of these factors are:

1. An increasingly technological society. The nature of advanced technology creates situations involving complicated issues that never had to be considered before.

As a result of technological advances:
- Many newborns are surviving at earlier gestational ages, and many of them have serious health problems (Lea & Thomas-Lawson, 2001).
- People are living much longer than ever before.
- Organ transplants and the use of bionic body parts are becoming more common.

2. The changing fabric of society. Family structure is moving from extended families to nuclear families, single-parent families, and nonrelated groups living together as families.
3. Clients are becoming more knowledgeable about their health and health-related interventions. As consumer demand for information increases, health care providers must adapt quickly. The result is an increased focus on the consumer-driven system.
4. The proportion of total federal funds allocated for health care is continually decreasing (Figure 9-1).

Nurses face situations in which they must make decisions that transcend technical and professional concerns. These situations may or may not be life-threatening. "Too often, the 'smaller,' more common conflicts, such as how to determine whether a patient's refusal of treatment is informed or how to effectively advocate on a patient's behalf, get less attention" (Kennedy-Schwarz, 2000, p. 71) than the life-or-death issues revolving around imminent death. Such situations raise complex problems that cannot be answered completely with technical knowledge and professional expertise. Technological advances have created unprecedented choices, not only for society at large, but specifically for clients and nurses. For example, the Human Genome Project has tremendous implications for society, and particularly clients and nursing.

There is emphasis on ethical issues involving life-or-death situations. However, nurses daily encounter challenges about what *ought* to be done, even in the most ordinary circumstances. The way in which nurses relate to

 **STOP AND THINK**

### Legal and Ethical Concepts

Which of the following behaviors is (or are) ethical and illegal? Legal and unethical? Illegal and unethical? Legal and ethical?

- Working in a clinic that performs abortions

- Honoring a terminally ill client's request to have "no heroic" actions taken

- Discontinuing a comatose client's life support at the request of the family

- Diverting medications from a client for your own use

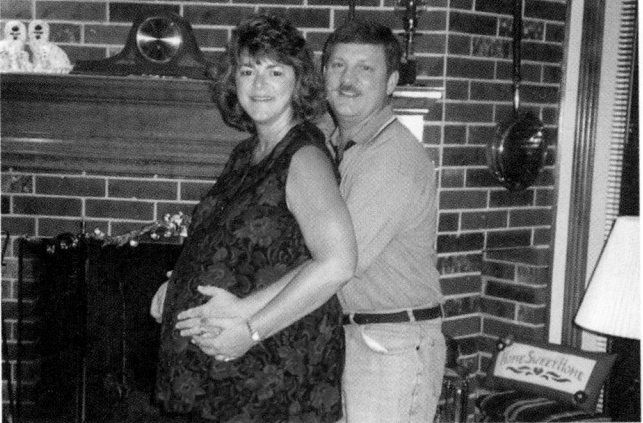

**Figure 9-1** This couple is planning a home birth because the husband recently lost his job and they do not have health insurance. Scarce resources create the ethical dilemma exemplified in the question, "Should health care benefits be provided for everyone in society?"

## LEGAL AND ETHICAL ISSUES

### Human Genome Project

The Human Genome Project completed in 2001 has been compared to the Manhattan Project, which produced the atomic bomb, and the Apollo project, which put man on the moon, in terms of scope, scientific discovery, and costs. The world now has a "map" of the human genome, which may enable scientists to ultimately develop new organs to: make a better spine to protect one from back strain, regenerate hands from cuts and injury, create stomach enzymes to digest cellulose so people can eat more foods like grasses, and engineer in the qualities of flies' eyes or sonar from whales to improve vision and hearing. How will the ethical principles of autonomy, nonmaleficence, beneficence, justice, veracity, and fidelity come into play for involved health professionals?

Lea, D. H, & Thomas-Lawson, M. (2001). Bringing genetics into the classroom: A practice-based approach. *Nursing and Health Care Perspectives, 22*(23), 147–151.

clients, families, and other health care providers is the true demonstration of ethical behavior.

## Ethical Theories

Ethical theories were debated by ancient philosophers such as Plato and Aristotle, and the debate continues today. No theory in and of itself can provide the "correct" answer to any single ethical conflict. Ethical theories can be used as a way to analyze ethical problems.

## Teleology

**Teleology** is the ethical theory stating that the value of a situation is determined by its consequences. Thus, the outcome of an action—not the action itself—is the criterion for determining the goodness of that action. This theory (also called the consequentialist theory) was advocated by the philosopher John Stuart Mill. The principle of **utility** is a basic concept of teleology; utility states that an act must result in the greatest amount of good for the greatest number of people involved in a situation. "Good" refers to positive benefit. Any act can be ethical if it delivers "good" results. Every alternative is assessed for its potential outcomes, both positive and negative. The selected action is the one that results in the most benefits and the least amount of harm for all those involved.

## Deontology

**Deontology** is the ethical theory that considers the intrinsic significance of the act itself as the criterion for determination of good. That is, in determining the ethics of a situation, a person must consider the motives of the actor, not the consequences of the act.

This theory (also called formalism) was postulated by the philosopher Immanuel Kant. Kant established the concept of the **categorical imperative**, which states that one should act only if the action is based on a principle that is universal (everyone would act in the same way in a similar situation). The categorical imperative also mandates that a person should never be treated as a means to an end. Adherence to this concept may pose an ethical concern to health care researchers, who sometimes may risk the well-being of a person participating in an experimental procedure for the sake of finding a drug that will save many from suffering.

## Ethical Principles

**Ethical principles** are tenets that direct or govern actions. They are widely accepted and generally are based on the humane aspects of society. Ethical decisions are principled; that is, they reflect what is best for the client and society. Table 9-1 summarizes the major ethical principles. Each principle is discussed in detail in the following paragraphs.

By applying ethical principles, nurses become more systematic in solving ethical conflicts. Ethical principles can be used as guidelines in analyzing dilemmas; they can also

| TABLE 9-1 | OVERVIEW OF ETHICAL PRINCIPLES |
| --- | --- |
| **Principle** | **Explanation** |
| Autonomy | Respect for an individual's right to self-determination; respect for individual liberty |
| Nonmaleficence | Obligation to do or cause no harm to another |
| Beneficence | Duty to do good to others and to maintain a balance between benefits and harms |
| Justice | Equitable distribution of potential benefits and risks |
| Veracity | Obligation to tell the truth |
| Fidelity | Duty to do what one has promised |

serve as a justification (rationale) for the resolution of ethical problems. Remember that these principles are not absolute; there can be exceptions to each principle in any given situation.

## Autonomy

The principle of **autonomy** refers to the individual's right to choose and the ability to act on that choice. The individuality of each person is respected when autonomy is maintained. This respect for personal liberty is a dominant value in American society.

Nurses should respect a client's right to decide and protect those clients who are unable to decide for themselves. The ethical principle of autonomy reflects the belief that every competent person has the right to determine her own course of action. The right to free choice rests on the client's competency to decide.

Informed consent is based on the clients' right to decide for themselves. Upholding autonomy means that the nurse accepts the client's choices, even when the nurse believes those choices are not in the client's best interests. Following are examples of clients' autonomous behavior that can impair recovery or treatment:

- Smoking after a diagnosis of emphysema or lung cancer
- Refusing to take medication
- Continuing to drink alcohol when one has cirrhosis
- Refusing to receive a blood transfusion because of religious beliefs

The Patient Self-Determination Act of 1990 was legislated to ensure that clients have the right to make their own health care decisions. Based on the principle of autonomy, this act requires that every person admitted to a health care facility be informed of the right to self-determination. The client's directives then need to be communicated, documented, and executed.

## Nonmaleficence

**Nonmaleficence** is the duty to cause no harm to others. Harm can take many forms: physiological, psychological, social, spiritual. Nonmaleficence refers to both actual harm and the risk of harm. The principle of nonmaleficence helps guide decisions about treatment approaches; the relevant question is "Will this treatment modality cause more harm or more good to the client?" Determining whether technology is harmful to the client is not always a clear-cut decision. Factors to consider include:

- The treatment must offer a reasonable prospect of benefit.
- It must not involve excessive expense, pain, or other inconvenience.
- The client is fully informed about side effects, consequences, and costs.

Nonmaleficence requires that the nurse act thoughtfully and carefully, weighing the potential risks and benefits of research or treatment. Sometimes it is easier to weigh the risk than to measure the benefit. It is possible to violate this principle without acting maliciously and without ever being aware of the harm.

Nonmaleficence is considered a fundamental duty of health care providers. Both the Nightingale Pledge and the Hippocratic Oath state that providers are to cause no harm to clients. Some clinical examples of nonmaleficence are:

- Preventing medication errors (including drug interactions)
- Being aware of potential risks of treatment modalities
- Removing hazards (e.g., obstructions that might cause a fall)
- Preventing the loss of autonomy

When upholding the principle of nonmaleficence, the nurse practices according to professional and legal standards of care. The question most frequently asked in court of a nurse is "Did you cause any harm?"

---

## CLIENT REFLECTIONS

### Informed Consent

Mr. Tippins is having you, a home health nurse, change his ostomy after a colostomy surgery. In reminiscing about his surgery, Mr. Tippins tells you, "I felt like the nurse who had me sign the consent form really didn't want to take time to answer my questions about the surgery. I kind of thought she (the nurse) was in a hurry and just wanted my signature on the paper. So I signed it, but I really had a lot of questions that weren't answered."

What would you say to this client?

---

## STOP AND THINK

### Nonmaleficence

Weighing the potential benefit and harm of treatment approaches is value-laden. At what point does pain, inconvenience, or expense become excessive? Who determines excessiveness? Is the result of a therapy that will prolong the client's life a benefit or a burden? Who determines what is an acceptable and what is an unacceptable quality of life?

## STOP AND THINK

### Paternalism

Listen to the messages communicated to clients by health care professionals. What comments can you think of that would be considered paternalistic? Would you consider the following comments to be paternalistic? Why?

● "Just follow the doctor's orders and everything will be OK."

● "We know what's best for you, trust us."

● "This is for your own good."

## Beneficence

**Beneficence** is the ethical principle that means the duty to promote good and to prevent harm. There are two elements of beneficence: (1) providing benefit, and (2) balancing benefits and harm.

One undesirable outcome of beneficence is **paternalism**, an occurrence in which health care providers decide what is "best" for clients and then attempt to coerce (or "encourage") them to act against their own choices. Paternalistic health care providers treat competent adults as if they are children who need protection.

Paternalism is usually not considered an ethical approach. However, in some situations paternalism may be advisable. For example, when prevention of harm overrides the loss of individual freedom and when an individual's ability to choose is limited by incompetency, paternalism may be justified.

## Justice

The principle of **justice** is based on the concept of fairness. The major health-related issues of justice involve fair treatment of individuals and allocation of resource distribution. Justice considers action from the point of view of the least fortunate in society. With equal and similar treatment of people, benefits and burdens are distributed equally.

The ethical principle of justice requires that all people be treated equally unless there is a justification for unequal treatment. The **material principle of justice** is the rationale for determining when there can be unequal allocation of scarce resources. This concept specifies that resources should be allocated:

• Equally
• According to need
• According to individual effort
• According to the individual's merit (ability)
• According to the individual's contribution to society

An application of the material principle of justice is the Department of Veteran Affairs (VA). Individuals who gave to their country by serving in the military are eligible to receive health care through the VA in ambulatory, acute care, and psychiatric facilities.

According to the American Nurses Association (ANA)(1991), three types of actions are considered to be unjust:

1. Discrimination or arbitrarily unequal treatment in enforcing policies/rules
2. Exploiting (taking unfair advantage of) another
3. Making unfair (false or derogatory) remarks about others

In health care institutions, the principle of justice is being strenuously tested on the issue of allocation of one important resource: nursing personnel. Many institutions and agencies are downsizing their professional staff as a cost-containment measure. As a result, some health care facilities are so poorly staffed or have such a high ratio of underqualified personnel providing care that quality care is being sacrificed. "Some 72% of the respondents report that the quality of care at their hospital has deteriorated over the past year because of cost-containment decisions" (Wolfe, 1999, p. 28).

The principles of justice and beneficence often conflict. For example, should federal funds be spent on a costly transplant that will benefit only one Medicaid recipient, or should the funds be spent on less expensive measures that would prevent disease in many (e.g., immunizations)?

## Veracity

**Veracity** means truthfulness, neither lying nor deceiving others. Deception can take many forms: intentional lying, nondisclosure of information, or partial disclosure of information. Veracity often is difficult to achieve. It may not be hard to tell the truth, but it can be very hard to decide how much truth to tell.

## STOP AND THINK

### Client Advocate

A 15-year-old girl visits a family planning clinic because she suspects she is pregnant. Her suspicion is confirmed after an examination. She informs the nurse practitioner that she wants an abortion, and she refuses to tell her parents about this situation. In considering this dilemma, keep in mind that the client is a minor. What are the ethical obligations of the nurse practitioner? Do the ethical obligations coincide or conflict with the legal responsibilities? How would you resolve this conflict?

## Fidelity

The concept of **fidelity** (which is the ethical foundation of nurse-client relationships) means faithfulness and keeping promises (Gastmans, 2002).

Clients have an ethical right to expect nurses to act in their best interests. As nurses function in the role of **client advocate** (a person who speaks up for or acts on behalf of the client), they are upholding the principle of fidelity. Fidelity is demonstrated when nurses:

- Represent the client's viewpoint to other members of the health care team
- Avoid letting their own personal values influence their advocacy for clients
- Support the client's decision even when it conflicts with the nurse's preferences or choices

# Values and Ethics

The close relationship between ethics and values both illuminates and complicates the nurse's approach toward balancing the principles of health care delivery with those of the client. Nurses need to examine their own value systems in order to determine the best approach in managing the care of clients whose values differ. In order to practice ethically, nurses must understand the impact of their own values. **Values** influence the development of beliefs and attitudes and thus affect behaviors indirectly. Almost nothing in life is value-free, even though individuals often fail to consider the impact of values on decisions and resultant behaviors. Values are similar to breathing; people don't think about it until there's a problem.

Nurses often care for clients whose value systems conflict with theirs. Determining what is meaningful to the client is based on an understanding of the client's value system. The nurse's values can become problematic when they conflict with the values of clients (Killen, 2002).

## Values Clarification

Through values clarification, a nurse can increase self-awareness and become better able to care for people with different values. **Values clarification** is the process of analyzing one's own values to better understand what is truly important. In their classic work *Values and Teaching*, Raths, Harmin, and Simon (1978, p. 47) formulated a theory of values clarification and proposed a three-step process of valuing as follows:

1. *Choosing:* Beliefs are selected freely (that is, without coercion) from among alternatives. The choosing step involves analysis of the consequences of various alternatives.
2. *Prizing:* The beliefs that are selected are cherished (prized).
3. *Acting:* The selected beliefs are demonstrated consistently through behavior.

Values are individual rather than universal; therefore, nurses should not impose their own values on clients. The provision of ethical nursing care is directly related to one's values. For example, the nurse who strongly values the sanctity of life may experience an ethical conflict when caring for a terminally ill client who refuses treatment that may extend life for a short time.

# Ethical Codes

One hallmark of a profession is the determination of ethical behavior for its members. According to Sills (2000):

> . . . the profession has certain obligations to the society: to do no harm, to be proficient in one's work, to behave and reason with high moral and ethical standards, to control the entrance of a person to the professional ranks, to discipline professionals who fail to meet acceptable standards, and to use its knowledge to treat people in need and to teach the public what it needs to know for self-care. (p. 30)

Several nursing organizations have developed codes as guidelines for ethical conduct. In its 1973 Code for Nurses, the International Council of Nurses (ICN) states: "The nurse, in providing care, promotes an environment in which the values, customs, and spiritual beliefs of the individual are respected" (ICN, 1973).

The ANA has also established a code for ethical conduct. The ANA Code of Ethics spells out the nurse's obligations to clients and society at large. "A code of ethics indicates a profession's acceptance of the responsibility and trust with which it has been invested by society" (American Nurses Association, 1985, p. 1). The ethical code, which provides broad principles for determining and evaluating nursing care, is not legally binding for registered nurses. In most states, however, the Board of Nursing has authority to reprimand nurses for unprofessional conduct that results from violation of the ethical code.

The Canadian Nurses Association (CNA) developed a code of ethics in 1980 and revised it in 1991. The CNA code serves as a guide for professional nursing actions.

# Clients' Rights

The concept of rights is often misused, overused, and abused. American society tends to take rights for granted; rights and obligations are culturally defined. The dominant American society has an ethnocentric perspective in believing that its rights and values are shared globally.

Clients have certain rights including, but not limited to, the right to:

- Make decisions regarding their care
- Be actively involved in the treatment process
- Be treated with dignity and respect

These rights apply to all clients regardless of the setting for delivery of care. For example, during the initial assessment, the home health nurse discusses these rights with the client.

When clients are admitted to short-term acute care agencies or extended care facilities, they are also entitled to certain rights. In 1972, the American Hospital Association (AHA) established a *Patient's Bill of Rights*, which includes the rights and responsibilities of clients receiving care in hospitals. This document was revised in 1992. The *Patient's Bill of Rights* increases health care providers' awareness of the need to treat clients in an ethical manner and encourages all health care providers to protect the rights of clients. Congress is currently debating a national patients' [clients'] "Bill of Rights" (January 2003).

## Ethical Dilemmas

An **ethical dilemma** occurs when there is a conflict between two or more ethical principles (see Box 9-1). The most beneficial decision depends on the circumstances. When an ethical dilemma occurs, the nurse chooses between two alternatives. Ethical analysis is not an exact science. In some cases, even after a dilemma seems to have been resolved, questions remain. This ambiguity may make it emotionally painful for the persons involved. The emotional discomfort is often a result of the nurse trying to second-guess the decision and may lead to such self-messages as "If only I had done this" or "Maybe I should have . . ."

## Ethical Decision Making

Nurses must understand the basis on which they make their decisions. **Ethical reasoning** is the process of thinking through what one ought to do in an orderly, systematic manner to provide justification of actions based on principles. Ethical decision making is used in situations where the right decision is not clear or where rights and duties conflict. A framework for resolving ethical dilemmas follows.

## Framework for Ethical Decision Making

Once an ethical dilemma is identified, the nurse must determine the relevant parts of the conflict in order to resolve it. When making an ethical decision, the nurse must consider the following relevant parts:

- Which theories are involved?
- Which principles are involved?
- Who will be affected?
- What will be the consequences of the alternatives (ethical options)?
- What does the client desire?

To resolve ethical dilemmas, the nurse must be able to make decisions in a systematic fashion. Figure 9-2 illustrates a method for making ethical judgments that uses steps similar to those of the nursing process.

The first step of ethical analysis is to gather relevant data in order to identify the problem. Determine what type of ethical problem exists: Do principles conflict with principles? Do actions conflict with actions? Do actions conflict with principles?

Next, consider all the people involved. What are their rights, responsibilities, duties, and decision-making abilities? Who is the most appropriate person to make the decision? It is important to identify several possible alternatives and predict the outcome of each. Then, and only then, select a course of action—one that, it is hoped, ends in resolution of the problem. The final step of ethical decision making is evaluation of the resolution process. Consider the following two issues: euthanasia and refusal of treatment.

---

| BOX 9-1 | FREQUENTLY OCCURRING ETHICAL DILEMMAS |
|---|---|

- Informed consent
- Refusal of treatment
- Use of scarce resources
- Cost-containment initiatives that negatively affect client well-being
- Incompetent health care providers

Adapted from Gastmans, C. (2002). A fundamental ethical approach to nursing; some proposals for ethics education. *Nursing Ethics, 9*(5), 494–507.

---

 **STOP AND THINK**

### Ethical Conflicts

As a nurse, you will often be caught in a dilemma involving what you *ought* to do (on the basis of one ethical principle) and what you *ought not* to do (on the basis of another principle). For example, should you tell a client who has been diagnosed as having breast cancer the complete truth about the diagnosis, or should you soft-pedal the bad news because it might result in loss of hope? The dilemma is a conflict between the principles of veracity and nonmaleficence. Also, the principle of autonomy is violated. Not telling the client denies that person the right to make an informed choice.

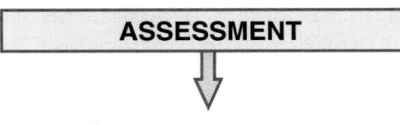

Determination of claims and parties

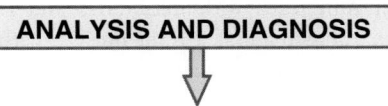

Problem identification: Statement of the ethical dilemma

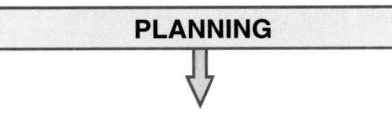

Consideration of priorities of claims,
generation of alternatives for resolving the dilemma,
consideration of the consequences of alternatives

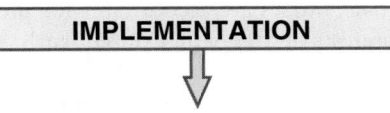

Carrying out selected moral actions

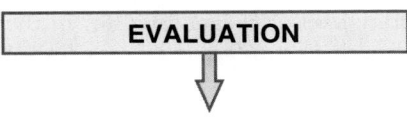

Assessing the outcome of moral actions;
"Were the actions ethical?"
"What were the consequences?"

**Figure 9-2    Ethical decision-making model**

## Euthanasia

Most people hope to experience a peaceful, gentle death when their "time comes." The word **euthanasia** comes from the Greek word *euthanatos*, which literally means "good, or gentle, death." In current times, *euthanasia* refers to mercy killing (deliberate ending of life as a humane action) (Tucker, 2002).

**Active euthanasia** refers to taking deliberate action that will hasten the client's death. In contrast, **passive euthanasia** means cooperating with the client's dying process. Passive euthanasia is the omission of an action that would prolong dying, such as the discontinuation of tube feedings.

**Assisted suicide** is a form of active euthanasia in which a health care professional provides a client with the means to end his own life. Recently, physician-assisted suicide has been the topic of much controversy. Nurses have differing opinions regarding assisted suicide. Some view it as a violation of the ethical principles upon which the practice of nursing is based: autonomy, nonmaleficence, beneficence, justice, veracity, and fidelity. Other nurses view assisted suicide as a humane act. Regardless of a nurse's personal viewpoint, assisted suicide is still illegal except in Oregon, the

**STOP AND THINK**

**Ethical Debate: Euthanasia**

What does the phrase "good death" mean to you? For some people, it means:

● Dying with dignity

● Being pain-free

● Dying in the company of loved ones and friends

To others, dying a good death means:

● Being at home

● Determining when death will occur (maintaining control)

only state that has designated assisted suicide as a legal action. Other nurses may see assisted suicide as an ethical dilemma; they agree that it violates some ethical principles but question whether it violates others. For example, does assisted suicide violate the principle of autonomy? From one standpoint, it is *refusal* to assist a suicide that violates a client's autonomy. In its *Position Statement on Active Euthanasia*, the ANA (1994) states that participation in active euthanasia violates nursing's ethical code. However, some states are debating this position.

## Refusal of Treatment

The client's right to refuse treatment is based on the principle of autonomy. In fairness, the client can refuse only after the treatment methods and their consequences have been explained. A client's right to refuse treatment and the right to die challenge the values of some health care providers (Cameron, 2002).

Consider the use of ventilators. Medical technology makes it possible for clients to continue breathing as long as they are connected to a machine; without the machine, these clients would die. But what are the costs—emotional, physical, psychological, and fiscal? And what is the quality of a life prolonged by technology?

## Scarce Resources

With the current emphasis on containing health care costs, the use of expensive services is being examined closely. The use of specialists, organ transplants, and distribution of services is being influenced by social and political forces. For example, the length of stay in a hospital and the number of office visits allowable for individual clients are already predetermined by many third-party payers. In addition to economics, the availability of goods (such as organs) is contributing to a scarcity of resources. In many situations, clients experience extended waiting periods

## STOP AND THINK

### Allocation of Scarce Resources

The following two people are in desperate need of a liver transplant:

- A 62-year-old alcoholic who is destitute and has no family

- A 24-year-old mother of three young children

One liver is available. In your opinion, who should get the liver? What influenced your decision?

before receiving a donated organ. The allocation of scarce resources is emerging as a major ethical dilemma in today's health care environment. "When nursing care is viewed as a kind of commodity or resource, it must be dis-

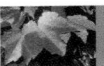

## RESEARCH FOCUS

**Title of Study:** Confirming older adult patients' views of who they are and would like to be

**Study Purpose:** To investigate the ethical nursing care of older adults in geriatric units.

**Methods:** Semi-structured qualitative interviews with 12 cognitively intact older adults from 70 to 91 years of age. They had been hospitalized in geriatric units from 10 to 15 days and discharged to their homes. Purposeful sampling strategy was used to select participants. The survey instrument was developed based upon 10 categories of integrity by Kihlgren and Thorsen asking such questions as "What was your experience in the hospital"? Many of the subjects provided rich and detailed experiences about their hospitalizations. Their narrative stories were analyzed phenomenologically.

**Findings:** The clients' basic needs for ethical care were not met. Nursing staff did not see these older adults as unique individuals who could make their own decisions. In order to cope with this lack of ethical care, the clients played the role of "old cognitively impaired clients." In this role, they obtained some needed nursing care.

**Implications:** Ethical care is dependent on a caregiver's ability to respect and confirm each client for who they are and would like to be.

Randers, I., Olson, T. H., & Mattiasson, A. C. (2002). Confirming older adult patients' views of who they are and would like to be. *Nursing Ethics, 9*(4), 416–431.

tributed fairly and equitably to meet the needs of a population group" (American Nurses Association, 1991, p. 2).

Our population is living longer, giving rise to increases in the demand for services. As improvements in health care technologies lead to further declines in mortality, the number of Americans with disabilities and functional restrictions will increase, as will the number with chronic, irremediable conditions. As costs increase, so too will the demand to contain costs. . . . We are spending more on health care than any other industrialized country but providing less coverage for our citizens. (Koloroutis & Thorstenson, 1999, p. 9–10)

As the above quotation illustrates, health care reform will be needed to ensure services to all citizens.

## Ethics and Nursing

As professionals, nurses are accountable for protecting the rights and interests of the client. Consequently, sound nursing practice involves making ethical decisions. Ethics affects nurses in most health care settings, and each practice setting presents the nurse with its own set of ethical concerns. For example, consider home health nursing. With the increased acuity level of clients cared for in the home setting, home health nurses face ever-increasing ethical challenges of continuing to provide quality care under federally mandated cost-containment initiatives (Gastmans, 2002).

Whatever the setting, nurses need to balance their ethical responsibilities to each client with their professional obligations. Often there is an inherent conflict. The Nursing Strategy box provides guidelines for promoting ethical care.

## NURSING STRATEGY

### Providing Ethical Care

- Initiate dialogue concerning the client's wishes. Do more listening than talking. (For example, the following is a question you might ask to help determine the client's wishes: "If your heart stopped, would you want us to try to start it again?")

- Assess the client's understanding of the illness and available treatment options

- Allow time for the client to explore values and to communicate

- Facilitate communication of the client's desires to family and other health care providers

- Facilitate development of advance directive resources

## Ethics Committees

The provision of ethical health care usually requires self-examination of the care provider and the opportunity for dialogue with other health care providers. Many health care agencies now recognize the need for a systematic manner to discuss ethical concerns. Formation of multidisciplinary committees (also referred to as Institutional Ethics Committees) is one approach for facilitating dialogue regarding ethical dilemmas. In addition to serving as a forum where ethical issues are discussed, ethics committees can lead to the establishment of policies and procedures for prevention and resolution of dilemmas.

## Nurse as Client Advocate

When acting as a client advocate, the nurse's first step is to develop a meaningful relationship with the client. The primary ethical responsibility is to protect clients' rights to make their own decisions. The nurse who functions as a client advocate is adhering to the ANA Code of Ethics. Specific examples of advocacy behaviors include empower-

## LIFE SPAN CONSIDERATIONS

### Standardized Forms

Many hospitals now offer admitted clients standardized forms to complete for medical power of attorney or advance directives. The focus is often on geriatric clients. Often these clients are nervous, anxious, severely ill, in pain, and medicated. How should nurses in the outpatient setting prepare elderly clients for this paperwork, and how can nurses in the inpatient setting improve this type of policy?

ment of clients through education, providing support, actively listening to client's concerns, and acting as a liaison between client and other health care providers. Elderly clients often require nurses to fulfill the client advocate role in a proactive manner and in ways that other groups of clients might not need.

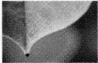

## CASE STUDY/NURSING CARE PLAN

Clyde Oster is an 86-year-old Latino male who has been hospitalized for 6 weeks with severe and irreversible congestive heart failure. His physical and mental state have continued to decline, requiring increasing doses of diuretics, narcotics, Digoxin, and oxygen by mask. Mr. Oster's mental state is "comatose" in the progress notes. He is on IV hydration and has a urinary catheter. Mr. Oster's family physician of 30 years, primary care nurse, and 22 family members have a meeting in the conference room at the hospital to discuss his prognosis. Mr. Oster's physician tells the family that Mr. Oster is in a "persistent vegetative state" and death is imminent. Mr. Oster's wife, Polly, who is a competent, 80-year-old woman, has medical power of attorney. She states that her husband did not want a mechanical ventilator or CPR in the event that he had a cardiac arrest. She and her husband had agreed that it was best for "the Lord to take him when his time had come." The family was in agreement, as was the physician. Legal documents were signed, dated, and witnessed, and DNR (do not resuscitate) orders were written.

During the night, a medical intern was on call as part of the house staff, and Mr. Oster had a cardiac arrest. Somehow in the confusion, the intern ordered CPR and Mr. Oster was put on a ventilator. When the primary care nurse came on at 7:00 A.M., she called the family. The family arrived at the hospital and were shocked that their wishes, which had been documented by the physician in the medical chart, were not executed.

### Assessment

The assessment reveals an 86-year-old male in a "persistent vegetative state" due to congestive heart failure. Client has diminished vital signs, irregular EKG, flat EEG, and fails to respond to stimuli. The spouse, who is competent, has medical power of attorney and signs legal document for "no heroic measures including CPR and mechanical ventilation." Physician agrees and documents DNR orders in medical record. Primary care nurse communicates this to nursing staff. Client arrests during the middle of the night, and medical intern institutes CPR and mechanical ventilation.

### Nursing Diagnosis #1

Spiritual distress related to the professional staff not implementing the family's desires concerning the DNR orders of the family physician and the family.

**NOC:** Hope; Spiritual Well-Being

**NIC:** Spiritual Support; Coping Enhancement; Emotional Support

*(continues)*

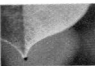

# CASE STUDY/NURSING CARE PLAN (continued)

## Expected Outcomes

The client and family will:

1. Identify alternative medical treatments by physician, nursing staff, and family within 8 hours of finding client on mechanical ventilator.
2. Verbalize feelings regarding problem immediately after finding family member on mechanical ventilator.
3. Have decisions communicated clearly and effectively from the medical and nursing staff as they are made.

## Planning/Interventions/Rationales

1. Offer family conference room to discuss in private options for client care and feelings regarding finding family member on mechanical ventilator. *Preserves autonomy.*
2. Support family and physician's decision to reduce oxygen level of ventilator to room air, which will allow Mr. Oster to die slowly. *Supports beneficent endeavors.*
3. Tell family about how long it may take Mr. Oster to die with room air only. *Encourages veracity.*
4. Allow family to be with Mr. Oster during this time; around the clock if necessary. Inform the family that they can call their physician and nurses at any time before treatments will be employed. *Provides justice and promotes fidelity.*

## Evaluation

Mr. Oster died 28 minutes after the physician turned the oxygen level to room air. The family grieved openly and left the hospital feeling that although their initial autonomy had been compromised, their loved one "was now in Heaven and not suffering anymore."

## Key Concepts

- Ethics is the study of the rightness of conduct.
- Ethics examines human behavior—what people do under what circumstances.
- Morality is not the same as ethics. Morality is behavior in accordance with custom or tradition and usually reflects personal or religious beliefs.
- There is a connection between acts that are legal and acts that are ethical. Professional nursing actions are both legal and ethical.
- Teleology is an ethical theory that states that the moral nature of a situation is determined by its consequences.
- Deontology is an ethical theory that considers the intrinsic moral significance of the act itself as the criterion for determination of good.
- Ethical decisions are based on principles such as autonomy, nonmaleficence, beneficence, justice, veracity, and fidelity.
- Because ethics and values are closely associated with each other, nurses need to explore their own values in order to acknowledge the different value systems possessed by their clients.
- Values clarification is a process through which nurses can gain knowledge of their values and apply that understanding to the care of clients.
- Ethical codes that have been developed by nursing organizations such as the International Council of Nurses, the American Nurses Association, and the Canadian Nurses Association establish guidelines for the ethical conduct of nurses with clients, coworkers, society, and the nursing profession.
- The *Patient's Bill of Rights* is designed to guarantee ethical care of clients in terms of their decision making about treatment choices and other aspects of their care.
- Nurses must apply the process of ethical reasoning to resolve ethical dilemmas in which conflict exists between principles and duties.
- The framework for ethical decision making consists of five steps: assessment, analysis and diagnosis, planning, implementation, and evaluation.

## Review Questions and Activities

1. Apply the ethical analysis framework to each of the following case situations.

Case Example 1:

Mary Washington delivers a baby with multiple congenital defects. The prognosis is poor; the infant is not expected to live longer than 12 months at most. Mary says, "We can't afford to pay for the baby's care." Who should determine the degree of intervention? Should the cost of care be the foremost basis for the decision?

Case Example 2:

An 80-year-old woman is in a persistent vegetative state as a result of a cardiovascular accident. She has always talked about "someday" signing a living will requesting that heroic measures not be taken. But her family wants "everything to be done that can be done." Whose wishes should prevail? Can her undocumented statements be legally honored?

2.  Read the following situation and determine the ethical ramifications of each scenario. How do your values influence your decisions?
    A married couple seek an abortion:
    •   Because the wife was raped by a stranger
    •   As a birth control measure
    •   Because the woman has been told by her doctor that going through another pregnancy will threaten her life
    •   To select a female baby because they already have a son

3.  Assumption: *The client's right to privacy and confidentiality must always be upheld by the nurse.* Do you agree? Think about a young sexually active female who is diagnosed as HIV-positive. Your conflict is the client's right to privacy versus the public's right to safety. What do you do?

4.  Clients have a right to self-determination, even when their decisions result in self-harm.
    •   Do you agree with this statement?
    •   How will you support a client's right to refuse treatment?
    •   How do you respond to a client's decision to continue self-harmful practices?

5.  A person's responses to clients are based on personal values. How do your feelings toward people with AIDS (acquired immunodeficiency syndrome) change in the context of values? For example, will your response be the same for all of these clients?
    •   A child infected through a contaminated blood transfusion
    •   A homosexual male who was infected by a promiscuous partner
    •   A female prostitute who became infected by sharing needles with other drug users

6.  What impact does the following information have on your provision of professional care?
    •   The client is a convicted rapist.
    •   The client is homeless.
    •   The client is a member of a very wealthy and influential family.
    •   The client is a nurse.
    •   The client is a physician.

## Web Resources

Biomedical Ethics Resources
    http://www.nova.edu
Ethics of Reproductive Technology
    http://www.acusd.edu
The Hastings Center for Bioethics
    http://www.thehastingscenter.org

Kennedy Institute of Ethics
    http://www.georgetown.edu

## References

American Hospital Association (1992). *A patient's bill of rights.* Chicago: Author.

American Nurses Association (1985). *Code for nurses, with interpretive statements.* Kansas City: Author.

American Nurses Association (1991). *Position statement: Ethics and human rights.* Washington, DC: Author.

American Nurses Association (1994). *Position statement: Active euthanasia.* Washington, DC: Author.

Burkhardt, M. A., & Nathaniel, A. K. (1998). *Ethics and issues in contemporary nursing.* Clifton Park, NY: Delmar Learning.

Cameron, M. E. (2002). Older persons' ethical problems involving their health. *Nursing Ethics, 9*(5), 537–556.

Canadian Nurses Association (1991). *Code of ethics for nursing.* Ottawa: Author.

Gastmans, C. (2002). A fundamental ethical approach to nursing. Some proposals for ethics education. *Nursing Ethics, 9*(5), 494–507.

International Council of Nurses (1973). *ICN code for nurses: Ethical concepts applied to nursing.* Geneva: Imprimeries Populaires.

Kennedy-Schwarz, J. (2000). The "ethics" of instinct. *American Journal of Nursing, 100*(4), 71–73.

Killen, A. R. (2002). Stories from the operating room: moral dilemmas for nurses. *Nursing Ethics, 9*(4), 405–415.

Koloroutis, M., & Thorstenson, T. (1999). An ethics framework for organizational change. *Nursing Administration Quarterly, 23*(2), 9–18.

Lea, D. H., Thomas-Lawson, M. (2001). Bringing genetics into the classroom: A practice-based approach. *Nursing and Health Care Perspectives, 22*(23), 147–151.

Newell, C. (2002). Individual actions or social issues? Toward ethical biotech futures in a civil society. *Nursing Ethics, 9*(5), 459–460.

Randers, I., Olson, T. H., Mattiasson, A. C. (2002). Confirming older adult patients' views of who they are and would like to be. *Nursing Ethics, 9*(4), 416–431.

Raths, L., Harmin, M., & Simon, S. (1978). *Values and teaching* (2nd ed.). Columbus, OH: Merrill.

Sills, G. M. (2000). Peplau and professionalism: The emergence of the paradigm of professionalization. *Journal of the American Psychiatric Nurses Association, 6*(1), 29–34.

Tucker, E. H. (2002). The importance of end-of-life treatment preferences among older adults. *Nursing Ethics, 9*(5), 561–562.

White, K. R., Coyne, P., and Patel, U. (2001). Can Nurses Adequately be Prepared for End-of-Life Care? *Journal of Nursing Scholarship 33*(2), 147–152.

Wolfe, S. (1999). Quality vs. cost. *RN, 62*(1), 28–34.

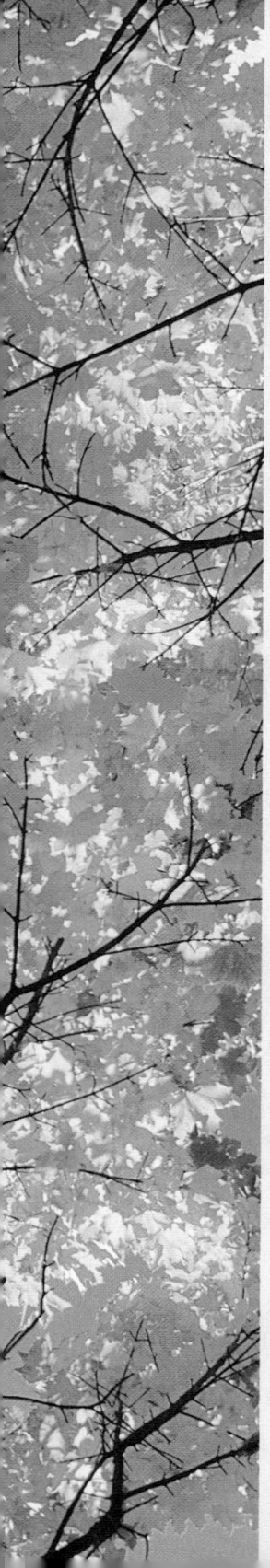

# II UNIT

# The Nursing Process and Decision Making

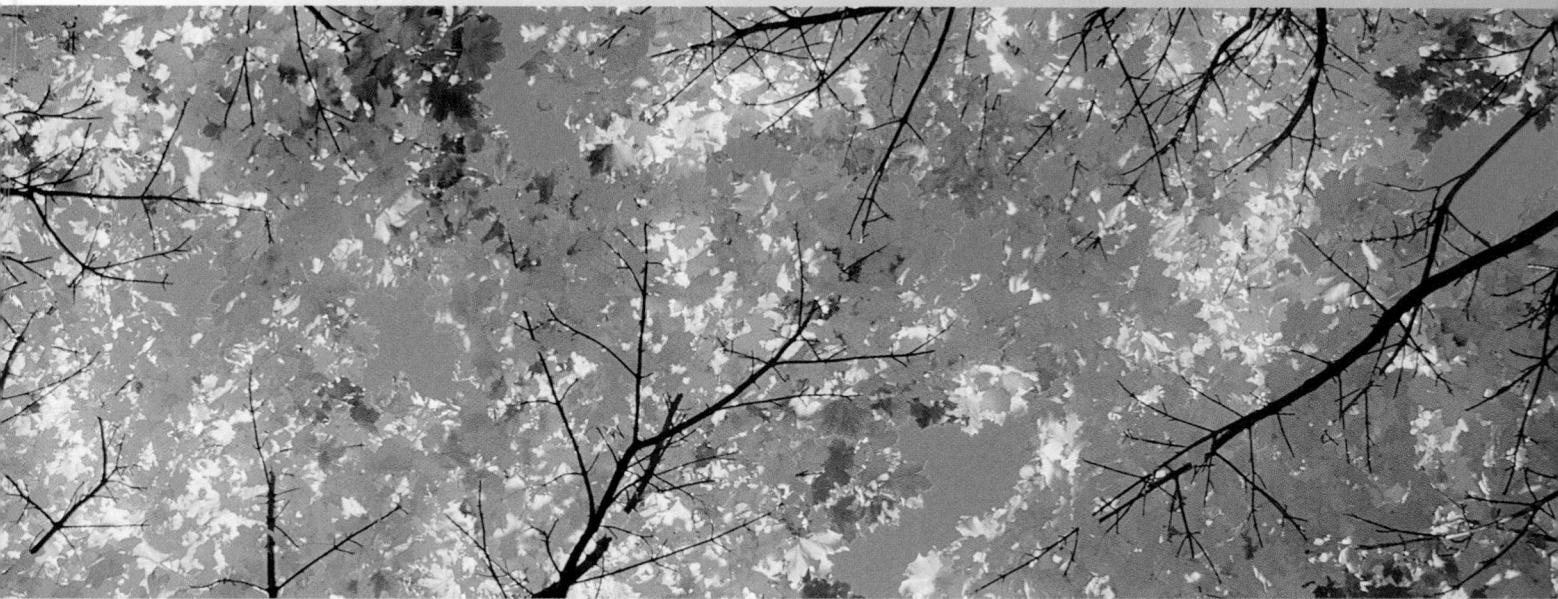

# CHAPTER 10

# Critical Thinking and the Nursing Process

Ruth N. Grendell, DNSc, RN

*"There is nothing, however, that requires more insight, acumen, skill, and cooperation on the part of persons concerned with the treatment, care, and guidance of the patient [client] than the working out of an effective and flexible plan of care."*

(Virginia Henderson, 1944)

# Chapter Competencies

*Upon completion of this chapter, the reader should be able to:*

1. Identify the components of critical thinking.
2. Describe how critical thinking relates to problem solving and decision making.
3. Relate critical thinking to the nursing process.
4. Describe the components of the assessment step of the nursing process.
5. List the tasks involved in the outcome identification and planning step of the nursing process.
6. Discuss the types of skills that nurses must possess in order to perform the nursing interventions during the implementation step of the nursing process.
7. Identify factors that may influence evaluation.
8. Relate the nursing process to the problem-solving method.

# Key Terms

| | | |
|---|---|---|
| actual nursing diagnosis | goal | possible nursing diagnosis |
| analysis | groupthink | primary source |
| assessment | implementation | process |
| collaborative problems | nursing diagnosis | risk nursing diagnosis |
| critical thinking | nursing intervention | secondary source |
| decision making | nursing process | subjective data |
| evaluation | objective data | synthesis |
| expected outcome | planning | wellness nursing diagnosis |

Nurses fulfill many roles that require critical-thinking, problem-solving, and decision-making skills, whether as direct care providers, coordinators of care, managers, educators, or client advocates. "One of the most important responsibilities that nurses have is to make correct and safe decisions in a variety of client care situations" (Catalano, 2000, p. 95). This chapter presents information about the relationships between critical thinking, decision making, and the nursing process (Figure 10-1). "**Critical thinking** is based on reason and reflection, knowledge, and instinct derived from experience" (Catalano, 2000, p. 95). The nursing process, a problem-solving method, is used to guide nursing practice in providing holistic care for individuals, groups, and communities, and can be used for clients across the life span in a variety of settings. The chapter also discusses applying critical thinking to the nursing process, thus enhancing the role of critical thinking as a powerful problem-solving tool for a wide range of client health needs.

## Critical Thinking

Baker (2001, p. 203) states, "Critical thinking is an intellectual skill based on theories and principles guided by logic and sound judgment to allow for the provision of safe quality nursing." Critical thinking is a highly desirable skill that can be learned, and has been identified by the National League of Nursing (NLN) (and supported by the American Association of Colleges in Nursing) as a criterion outcome of the nursing education curriculum. Students entering an educational program have a wide range of thinking styles and critical-thinking abilities that have been influenced by different educational backgrounds and the degree of cognitive maturity. "The purpose of higher education is to increase students' reasoning skills" (Redding, 1999).

Knowing how one thinks helps the nurse work collaboratively with other health care providers (Rubenfeld & Scheffer, 1999). Critical thinkers are people who know how to think. They possess intellectual autonomy, in that they refuse to accept conclusions without evaluating the evidence (facts and reasons) for themselves. Critical thinkers have the ability to think beyond the obvious and make connections between ideas.

## Characteristics of Critical Thinking

Critical thinking is a multifaceted and complex concept that is best explained by the characteristics and attitudes of

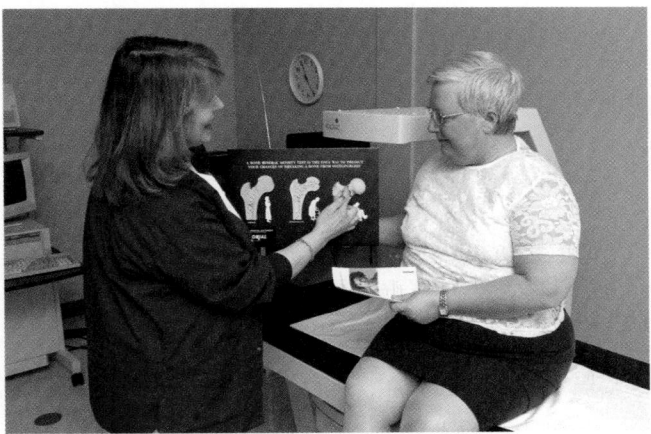

**Figure 10-1   A nurse using the nursing process with a client to make a critical decision about treatments for osteoporosis during menopause.**

people who use the critical-thinking processes when making decisions. Critical thinking enhances the ability to modify and expand existing knowledge and its application to new situations. "The ability to see the whole of any situation allows for looking at how the present situation is connected to or affected by other situations, thus offering more possibilities and opportunities from which to select when decisions need to be made" (Bower, 2000, p. 37). Redding (1999) identifies five cognitive skills of clinical judgment that rely on the application of critical-thinking skills:

1. A systematic approach to problem solving
2. Caring: Sensitivity to client information as supportive evidence of a problem or need
3. Unbiased inquiry and creative analysis of cause and effect: Alternative perspectives are reviewed and incorporated into the final conclusion
4. Intuition: Decision is based on values and assumptions gleaned from internal and external sources. There is trust in one's reasoning processes. (This is more evident and more accurate in the experienced nurse who has repeated exposure to similar situations.)
5. Reflection in action (evaluation): Valid conclusions are based on logical consistency. This process involves a

reciprocal relationship between nursing domain-specific knowledge and action. (This process may be the best example of critical thinking in nursing. Changes in a plan of care and choices for new actions are based on the client's adverse responses and a realignment of the nurse's knowledge of the situation.)

Critical thinking is considered to be the basis of self-reliance and functioning as a professional (Catalano, 2000). Professional nurses are accountable for actions and draw from a distinct body of knowledge. See the characteristics of critical thinking proposed by several theorists in Box 10-1.

## Development of Critical-Thinking Skills

The development of critical-thinking skills is a gradual process related to the individual's maturity, because maturity enhances the ability to suspend judgment until the data have been collected. It takes time to break habitual ways of thinking and doing.

Listed below are some specific strategies that promote the development and application of critical thinking:

- Identify goals.
- Determine what knowledge is required.
- Assess the margin for error.
- Determine the amount of time available for decision making.
- Identify available resources.
- Recognize factors (i.e., biases, fatigue) that may influence decision making (Alfaro-LeFevre, 2004).

Table 10-1 lists skills necessary for critical thinking to occur.

## Critical Thinking and Creativity

Creative thinking is the foundation for individualizing client care, in that the nurse identifies unique needs of each client and develops interventions specific to those needs. Without creative thinking, nursing care would become routine and habitual.

There is a strong link between critical and creative thinking. In order to develop creative solutions to problems, the nurse needs to use critical intellect. Also, to be an excellent critical thinker, the nurse exercises creative thinking (Le Storti, Cullen, Hanzlik, Michiels, Piano, Rya, & Johnson, 1999).

## Barriers to Creative Thinking

Factors affecting decision making include internal and external factors. An individual's perception can be influenced by physical and emotional states, and personal characteristics (i.e., values, past experiences, interests, and knowledge). External factors include environmental conditions and time. Unpredictable events and uncertainty in clinical settings can influence the availability of

## LEGAL AND ETHICAL ISSUES

### Legal Implications of Critical Thinking

Critical-thinking skills are extremely important to sound nursing practice. Nurses must familiarize themselves with the critical-thinking concepts in their decision-making processes, particularly when it comes to client safety issues. Critical thinking may decrease the possibility of malpractice and enhance optimal nursing care and interventions.

## BOX 10-1    CHARACTERISTICS OF CRITICAL THINKING

- Creativity: explores new ideas and alternative ways to reach a conclusion

- Logical, rational, reflective processes: bases decisions on rationale and facts

- Prudent, inquisitive, cautious, truth-seeking, self-confident, systematic, mature

- Self-regulating judgment: uses reflective thought to analyze decisions

- Intellectual humility: sensitive to one's own strengths, weaknesses, and biases; open to input from other sources

- Independent thinking: autonomous, not influenced by bias

- Challenges rituals and habits: willing to take risks, comfortable with ambiguity

- Action-orientation: directed toward goal or resolution of a problem

- Expertise based on experience and knowledge: able to perceive a situation holistically rather than in parts, recognizes patterns in phenomena

- Clear thinking thought processes are orderly, focused, and persistent

- Ability to see multiple meanings in a situation: blends logic and intuitive feelings (based on experience)

- Anticipates events, takes initiative, examines strategies to use, recognizes consequences of each strategy, and makes a decision

- Ability to work collaboratively in reaching a decision: respects perspectives of others

Bower, F. (2000). *Nurses taking the lead: Personal qualities of effective leadership.* Philadelphia: W. B. Saunders.

## CLINICAL ALERT

### The Element of Time in Critical Thinking

The nurse will learn with experience that prioritizing critical-thinking skills in a timely manner is essential in providing care. For example, when a client is having respiratory difficulties, the nurse needs to decide what to do quickly in order to give safe and efficient care.

intellectual courage to think something new and different from one's peers, and then act on those thoughts. Independent thinking is a hallmark of persons who think critically and creatively.

Lachman (1999) reported that unresolved conflicts among team members pose barriers to problem solving. These conflicts can be due to different levels of critical-thinking skills in the group, which include stereotyping that limits reflective thinking and exploration of new ideas, conformity to rules, decreased independent thought, and concern with maintaining group harmony. Group decisions may not be made based on scientific principles, and flaws in judgment may be undetected. Conflict resolution requires critical-thinking skills in applying assertiveness, negotiation, and other decision-making strategies. There are a variety of barriers to critical-thinking skills that are listed in Box 10-2.

## TABLE 10-1    CRITICAL THINKING SKILLS

| Interpretation | Categorize, decode sentences, clarify meanings |
|---|---|
| Analysis | Examine ideas, identify and analyze arguments |
| Inference | Query evidence, conjecture alternatives, draw conclusions |
| Explanation | State results, justify procedures, present arguments |
| Evaluation | Assess claims, assess arguments |
| Self-regulation | Self-examination, self-correction (if necessary) |

Data from Pesut, D. J., & Herman, J. (1999). *Clinical reasoning: The art and science of critical and creative thinking.* Clifton Park, NY: Delmar Learning.

data. Agency policies often dictate a standard format that blocks creative thinking. Traditional methods of problem solving include trial and error, experimentation, habit, and "wait and see" approaches (Welch, 1999).

Another major block to creativity is **groupthink** (going along with the majority opinion while personally having another viewpoint). Nurses who engage in groupthink generally wish to avoid interpersonal conflict. It takes

# Critical Thinking and Problem Solving

Critical thinking includes problem-solving and decision-making processes. People use problem solving in their daily lives. With the problem-solving method, problems are identified, information is gathered, a specific problem is named, a plan for solving the problem is developed, the plan is put into action, and results of the plan are evaluated. However, this kind of problem solving is frequently based on incomplete data, and plans are sometimes based on guesses. Conversely, the nurse uses the **nursing process** to identify and to make decisions about client needs. It is a systematic and scientifically based process that requires the use of many cognitive and psychomotor skills.

Critical thinkers avoid the pitfalls listed above by clearly defining the problem, analyzing the data, understanding the causes, and creating new ideas that will lead to problem resolution.

# Critical Thinking and Decision Making

When making a clinical decision, the nurse determines action that will help move the client toward achievement of the expected outcomes. Thus, **decision making** is defined as considering and selecting interventions from a repertoire of actions that facilitate the achievement of a desired outcome (Pesut, 1999). Nurses exercise clinical judgment by making sound decisions; clinical judgment can be viewed as critical thinking applied in clinical situations. Nursing judgments are formed after collecting

## BOX 10-2    BARRIERS TO CREATIVE THINKING

The following is a list of barriers to creative thinking:

- Rigid mind-set
- Practice guided by tradition, habit, routines, or rituals
- Stereotypical perception of client-care is not individualized
- Unwilling to take risks or look for alternative strategies
- Resistant to change, comfortable with status quo
- Hasty decision making without sufficient data
- Decisions are not supported by rationale
- Failure to evaluate effectiveness of nursing actions
- Fear of making mistakes

## NURSING STRATEGY

### Problem-Solving and Decision-Making Strategies

- Gather additional information from a variety of sources that will support an action or argue against the action.
- Consult with others regarding their approaches to resolving problem situations. (Peer thinking is a valuable resource. Comparing notes is the beginning of lifelong collaboration.)
- Conduct literature review. Examine effective strategies used by others.
- Seek alternative methods, and try new approaches to resolving problems.

Adapted from Welch, R. (1999). Problem solving and decision making. In P. Yoder-Wise, *Leading and managing in nursing* (pp. 91–106). St. Louis: C.V. Mosby.

## COMMUNITY/HOME CARE

### Adapting to the Home Environment

Often nurses must adapt to the home care environment when delivering nursing care. Nurses are used to having "easy access" to equipment and supplies, but these are often not available in the home setting. For example, when a nurse performs a dressing change for a client at home in the bedroom, a sink and trash containers may not be available nearby. The nurse must remember to bring (1) handwash gels with disposable wipes and (2) trashbags with ties to take the place of unavailable equipment.

Hitchcock, J., Schubert, P., & Thomas, S. (2003). *Community health nursing: Caring in action.* Clifton Park, NY: Delmar Learning.

assessment data and examining the relationships among those data. Since nursing judgments form the basis of client care, they occur in every phase of the nursing process (Rubenfeld & Scheffer, 1999).

It is important that nursing decisions be the best decisions possible, be based on reliable information, and be made with as much critical thought as possible. The nursing process is the specific problem-solving method used by nurses to arrive at the point at which decisions about client care can be made.

A comparison of problem solving and the nursing process is presented later in this chapter.

## The Nursing Process

The **nursing process** is the systematic framework for providing professional, quality nursing care. It directs nursing activities for health promotion, health protection, and disease prevention, and is used by nurses in every practice setting and specialty. "The cognitive pieces of critical thinking (assumptions, inferences, and arguments) interface with the steps of the nursing process (assessing, planning, intervening, and evaluating)" (Baker, 2001).

### Historical Perspective

The term *nursing process* was mentioned by Hildegarde Peplau (1952), Lydia Hall (1955), Dorothy Johnson (1959), Ida Jean Orlando (1961), and Ernestine Wiedenbach (1963). At that time, the nursing process involved only three steps: (1) assessment, (2) planning, and (3) evaluation. The process was formally introduced as a tool for nursing practice in 1967. In their classic book *The Nursing Process*, Yura and Walsh (1967) identified four steps in the nursing process: (1) assessing, (2) planning, (3) implementing, and (4) evaluating.

The *Standards of Practice*, first published in 1973 by the American Nurses Association (ANA), included eight standards. These standards identified each of the steps, including nursing diagnosis, that are now included in the nursing process.

Fry (1953) first used the term *nursing diagnosis*, but it was not until 1974, after the first meeting of the group now called the North American Nursing Diagnosis Association (NANDA), that Gebbie and Lavin added nursing diagnosis as a separate and distinct step in the nursing process. Prior to this, nursing diagnosis had been included as a natural conclusion to the first step, assessment.

Following publication of the ANA standards, the nurse practice acts of many states were revised to include the steps of the nursing process specifically. The ANA made revisions to the standards in 1991 to include outcome identification as a specific part of the planning phase. Currently, the steps in the nursing process are:

1. Assessment
2. Diagnosis
3. Outcome identification and planning
4. Implementation
5. Evaluation

The ANA practice standards address each step of the nursing process.

The nursing process is now included in the conceptual framework of all nursing curricula (Doenges & Moorhouse, 2002). Definitions of the nursing process and its component steps have undergone revisions over the years and now include emphasis on professional accountability, multiculturalism, and aging issues (Atkinson & Murray, 2000). In essence, the nursing process is an organizing framework that guides what nurses do in practice. It is derived from the scientific method of problem solving.

## Overview of the Nursing Process

A process is a series of steps or acts that lead to accomplishment of some goal or purpose. The purpose of the nursing process is to provide care for clients that is individualized, holistic, effective, and efficient. The steps of the nursing process build upon each other, but they are not linear. There is overlap of each step with the previous and subsequent steps (Figure 10-2).

The nursing process is dynamic and requires creativity for its application. The steps remain the same, but the application and results will be different in each client situation. The nursing process is designed to be used with clients throughout the life span and in any setting in which a nurse provides care for clients. It is also a basic organizing system for the National Council Licensure Examination for Registered Nurses (NCLEX-RN). The benefits of the nursing process for the nurse include self-confidence, job satisfaction, and professional growth. Benefits for the client are the potential for greater participation in their own care and continuity of quality care.

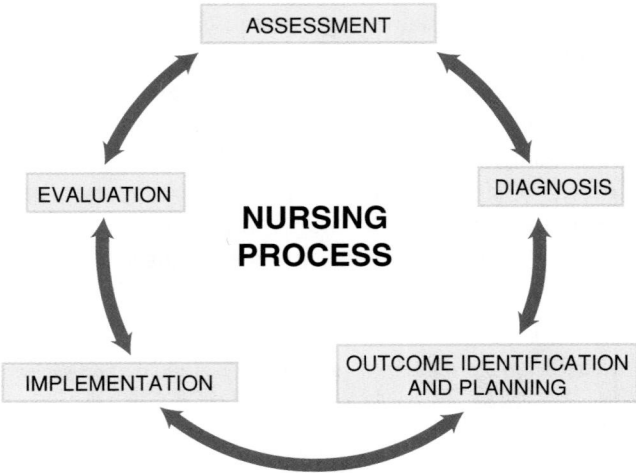

**Figure 10-2   Components of the nursing process**

## Assessment

Assessment is the first step in the nursing process and includes collection, verification, organization, interpretation, and documentation of data. The completeness and correctness of the information obtained during assessment are directly related to the accuracy of the steps that follow. Assessment involves several steps:

- Collecting data from a variety of sources
- Validating the data
- Organizing data
- Categorizing or identifying patterns in the data
- Making initial inferences or impressions
- Recording or reporting data

Data are collected from a variety of sources; however, the client should be considered the **primary source** of data (the major provider of information about self). As much information as possible should be gathered from the client, using both interview techniques and physical examination skills. Sources of data other than the client are considered **secondary sources** and include family members, other health care providers, and medical records and diagnostic reports.

Assessment provides information that will form the client database. Two types of information are collected through the assessment component: subjective and objective.

**Subjective data** are data from the client's point of view and include feelings, perceptions, and concerns. The method of collecting subjective information is primarily the interview. Using therapeutic interviewing techniques,

the nurse collects data that will begin to build the client database. Examples of subjective information include such statements as:

- "I drink only coffee for breakfast."
- "I have had pains in my legs for three days now."
- "I go to sleep easily each night, but I wake up about two hours later and cannot go back to sleep until it is time to get up in the morning."

**Objective data** are observable and measurable data that are obtained through both standard assessment techniques performed during the physical examination and diagnostic tests. The primary method of collecting objective information is the physical examination, which provides information about the function of body systems (Figure 10-3). Examples of objective information include:

- T 98.6°F, P 100, R 12, B/P 130/76
- Bowel sounds auscultated in all four quadrants
- Gait slow, shuffling, and unsteady

This objective information may add to or validate subjective information. Validation is a critical step in data collection to avoid omissions, prevent misunderstandings, and avoid incorrect inferences and conclusions.

Collected data must be organized to be useful to the health care professional collecting the data as well as others involved with the client's care. Clustering similar cues

---

### STOP AND THINK

#### Cultural Influences

You are collecting data from a 35-year-old Asian American woman while her parents and older brother are in the room. Family is very important to this client, whose parents consistently interrupt her while she is answering your questions. If you ask the family to leave the room while you complete the interview, you risk offending the client and her family and creating barriers to your communication process. If you allow the family to remain in the room, the parents may influence the client's responses so that you are unable to make a complete assessment.

- How do you respect family dynamics while ensuring that the client receives the most appropriate care?

- What do you say to the family?

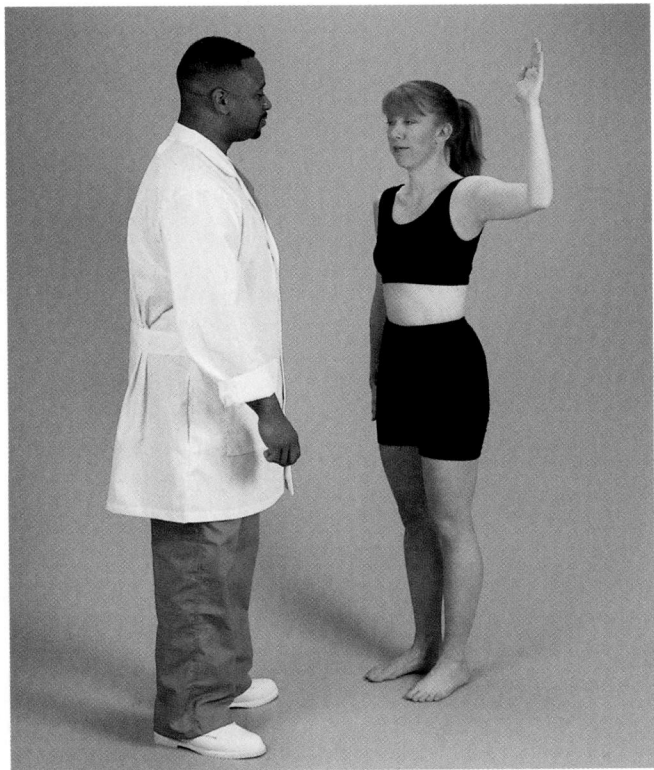

**Figure 10-3**    **This nurse is gathering objective data through assessment of the client's ability to perform ROM activity.**

or pieces of information assists the nurse in constructing a picture of the client's problems and strengths. There are a number of organizing frameworks for collection of data—for example, Gordon's Functional Health Patterns. Many health care agencies use an admission assessment format, which assists the nurse in collecting data in specific categories of functioning.

Critical thinking is used in determining the significance of data collected. Once data are organized into categories, the data are clustered into groups of related pieces. Placing data into clusters helps the nurse to recognize patterns of response or behavior. When data are placed into clusters, the nurse can:

- Distinguish between relevant and irrelevant data
- Determine if and where there are gaps in the data
- Identify patterns of cause and effect

With this information, the nurse, through critical thinking, can begin to develop impressions or inferences about what the data mean.

Assessment data must be recorded and reported. The nurse must make a judgment about which data are to be reported immediately and which data need only to be recorded at that time. Data that reflect a significant deviation from the normal (for example, rapid heart rate with irregular rhythm, severe difficulty in breathing, or high levels of anxiety) would need to be reported as well as recorded. Often the elderly deviate significantly from other age ranges in their physical assessment data. Examples of data that need only to be recorded at the time include a report that prescribed medication has relieved a headache and a determination that an abdominal dressing is dry and intact.

Assessment does not end with the initial interview and physical examination. Assessment is dynamic and continues with each nurse-client interaction (Alfaro-LeFevre, 1998; Wilkinson, 1998).

## Diagnosis

The second step in the nursing process involves further **analysis** (breaking the whole down into parts that can be examined) and **synthesis** (putting data together in a new way) of the data that have been collected. Formulation of the list of nursing diagnoses is the outcome of this process. According to the North American Nursing Diagnosis Association (NANDA, 2002) a **nursing diagnosis**

> is a clinical judgment about individual, family, or community responses to actual or potential health problems/life processes.

The nursing diagnoses developed during this phase of the nursing process provide the basis for client care delivered through the remaining steps.

Client problems are labeled by both medical and nursing diagnoses. Clients receive both medical and nursing diagnoses. Table 10-2 compares the two categories of diagnoses (Ackley & Ladwig, 2002; Carpenito, 2002).

See the Nursing Strategy box for a nursing intervention of applying critical thinking when determining nursing diagnoses.

## Types of Nursing Diagnoses

Analysis of the collected data leads the nurse to make a diagnosis in one of the following categories:

---

### LIFE SPAN CONSIDERATIONS

## Elderly Deviations in Physical Assessment Data

The elderly often present with a wide variety of differences in their physical assessment "norms." The nurse must be aware of these differences when making assessments. For example, just in the cardiovascular system, the elderly often have (1) more systolic and diastolic murmurs, (2) decreased vascular integrity from the fibrosis that occurs with aging, (3) decreased efficiency of venous return, (4) a variety of electrophysiological changes correlated with aging, and (5) an increased tendency toward left- or right-sided heart failure from atherosclerosis associated with aging.

Estes, M. (2002). *Health assessment & physical examination* (2nd ed.). Clifton Park, NY: Delmar Learning.

---

| TABLE 10-2 | COMPARISON OF MEDICAL DIAGNOSES AND NURSING DIAGNOSES | |
| --- | --- | --- |
| **Medical Diagnosis** | **Nursing Diagnosis** |
| Focuses on the illness, injury, or disease process. | Focuses on the responses to actual or potential health problems or life processes. |
| Remains constant until a cure is effected. | Changes as the client's response and/or the health problem changes. |
| Identifies conditions the health care practitioner is licensed and qualified to treat. | Identifies situations in which the nurse is licensed and qualified to intervene. |

## NURSING STRATEGY

### Using Critical-Thinking and Decision-Making Skills

The nurse uses critical-thinking and decision-making skills in developing nursing diagnoses. This process is facilitated by asking questions such as:

- Are there problems here?

- If so, what are the specific problems?

- What are some possible causes for the problems?

- Is there a situation involving risk factors?

- What are the risk factors?

- Is there a situation in which a problem can develop if preventive measures are not taken?

- Has the client indicated a desire for a higher level of wellness in a particular area of function?

- What are the client's strengths?

- What data are available to answer these questions?

- Are more data needed to answer the questions?

- If so, what are some possible sources of the data that are needed?

### TABLE 10-3   TYPES OF NURSING DIAGNOSES

| Nursing Diagnosis | Example |
|---|---|
| Actual diagnosis | *Deficient Fluid Volume* related to nausea and vomiting as manifested by dry skin and mucous membranes and decreased oral intake of fluids |
| Risk diagnosis | *Risk for Infection* related to presence of invasive lines (intravenous line and indwelling bladder catheter) |
| Possible diagnosis | *Possible Imbalanced Nutrition: Less Than Body Requirements* related to insufficient oral intake |
| Wellness diagnosis | *Readiness for Enhanced Spiritual Well-Being* |
| Collaborative problem | *Potential Complication* (PC): *Increased Intracranial Pressure* |

- Actual problems
- Potential problems (including those where risk factors exist and there are possible problems)
- Wellness conditions
- Collaborative problems

Examples of the various types of diagnoses are shown in Table 10-3.

An **actual nursing diagnosis** indicates that a problem exists, and is composed of the diagnostic label, related factors, and signs and symptoms. An example of an actual diagnosis is *Impaired Skin Integrity* related to prolonged pressure on bony prominence as manifested by (AMB) Stage II pressure ulcer over coccyx, 3 cm in diameter.

A **risk nursing diagnosis** (potential problem) indicates that a problem does not yet exist, but special risk factors are present. A risk diagnosis is composed of the diagnostic label preceded by the phrase "risk for," with the specific risk factors listed. An example of a risk diagnosis is *Risk for Impaired Skin Integrity* related to inability to turn self from side to side in bed.

A **possible nursing diagnosis** indicates a situation in which a problem could arise unless preventive action is taken. In addition, a possible diagnosis may state a "hunch" or intuition by the nurse that cannot be confirmed or eliminated until more data have been collected. A possible diagnosis is composed of the diagnostic label and related factors. An example of a possible diagnosis is *Possible Self-Esteem Disturbance* related to recent retirement and relocation. The nurse may not yet have enough data to confirm this diagnosis or a more specific one. However, this diagnosis will alert other nurses to collect data that will either confirm this or another diagnosis, verify a risk diagnosis, or rule out the existence of a problem.

A **wellness nursing diagnosis** indicates the client's expression of a desire to attain a higher level of wellness in some area of function. It is composed of the diagnostic label preceded by the phrase "potential for enhanced." For example, a client who is neither overweight nor underweight tells the nurse that she knows she could improve her diet in some ways. She states that she eats only a small number of vegetables and fruits and thinks that the fat content of her diet is probably high. She expresses a desire to know more about how to improve her diet. The nurse would make a wellness diagnosis of *Potential for Enhanced Nutrition*.

Carpenito introduced the bifocal clinical practice model that includes nursing diagnoses and collaborative problems. **Collaborative problems** are defined as physiological complications monitored by nurses to assess changes in client

## FOCUS ON WELLNESS

### When Writing Nursing Diagnoses

Nurses often focus on illness and forget they can focus on the concept of wellness when applying the nursing process. For example, a client who normally participates in aerobic activities (e.g., jogging, swimming) but is currently recovering from an appendectomy, can likely have a nursing diagnosis of potential for effective activity and exercise. Another example is the client who has a positive outlook on life and is being treated for stable angina. This client can have a wellness-oriented nursing diagnosis labeled "potential positive self-esteem."

Pender, J., Murdaugh, C., & Parsons, M. A. (2002). *Health promotion in nursing practice* (4th ed.). Upper Saddle River, NJ: Prentice-Hall.

status. Collaborative problems are managed through the use of interventions prescribed by other health care practitioners and/or nurses (Carpenito, 2002). Collaborative problems include those conditions in which the nurse seeks medical input for treatment of potential medical problems. Usually, collaborative problems involve alterations in organ and/or system function or structure (e.g., myocardial infarction, duodenal ulcer). Collaborative problems begin with the label *Potential Complication* (PC) followed by the situation—for example, *Potential Complication: Hemorrhage*.

Analysis of the data also assists the nurse in identifying strengths of the client. For example, the client's strong family support system would be identified as a strength. These areas of positive functioning will be reinforced and used as a basis for planning care for those areas where functioning is less than optimal.

After it is formulated, the list of diagnoses is presented to the client for confirmation if possible. If that is not

## NURSING STRATEGY

### A Continuous Process

Remember that the nursing process is not linear but involves overlapping steps. The steps are explained one after the other for ease of understanding. In actual practice, there may not be a definite beginning or end to each step. Work in one step may begin before work in the preceding step is completed.

possible, family members may be able to confirm the diagnoses. Finally, the list of nursing diagnoses is recorded on the client's record. Once this list is developed and recorded, the remainder of the client's plan of care can be completed. The list of nursing diagnoses is not static. It is dynamic, changing as more data are collected and as client goals and client responses to interventions are evaluated.

### Outcome Identification and Planning

**Planning** is the third step of the nursing process and includes the formulation of guidelines that establish the proposed course of nursing action in the resolution of nursing diagnoses and the development of the client's plan of care. Once the nursing diagnoses have been developed and client strengths have been identified, planning can begin. The planning phase involves several tasks:

- The list of nursing diagnoses is prioritized.
- Client-centered long- and short-term goals and outcomes are identified and written.
- Specific interventions are developed.
- The entire plan of care is recorded in the client's record.

Once the list of nursing diagnoses has been developed from the data, decisions must be made about priority. Critical thinking enables the nurse to make decisions about which diagnoses are the most important and need attention first. A number of frameworks are used to prioritize nursing diagnoses; however, those diagnoses involving life-threatening situations are given the highest priority. For example, the following nursing diagnoses would be stated in this order of priority:

- *Ineffective Airway Clearance* related to excessive and thick secretions and pain secondary to surgery and inability to cough effectively; respirations: 25, shallow, wheezing
- *Risk for Injury* (falls) related to unsteady gait
- *Imbalanced Nutrition: Less Than Body Requirements* related to nausea and vomiting

Client-centered goals are established in collaboration with the client whenever possible. A **goal** is an aim, intent, or end. Goals are broad statements that describe the intended or desired change in the client's behavior. Goal statements refer to the diagnostic label (or problem statement) of the nursing diagnosis. If the client or significant others are unable to participate in goal development, the nurse assumes that responsibility until the client is able to participate. Client-centered goals assure that nursing care is individualized and focused on the client.

**Expected outcomes** are specific objectives related to the goals and are used to evaluate the nursing interventions. They must be measurable, have a time limit, and be realistic. Once goals and expected outcomes have been established, nursing interventions are planned that enable the client to reach the goals.

A **nursing intervention** is the activity that the nurse will execute for and with the client to enable accomplishment of the goals. Nursing interventions refer directly to the related factors in the actual nursing diagnoses and the risk factors in risk nursing diagnoses. If the nursing interventions can remove or reduce the related factors and the risk factors, the problem can be resolved or prevented. Nursing interventions also refer to the diagnostic label for possible diagnoses and focus on data needed to confirm or eliminate the diagnosis.

For each nursing diagnosis, there may be a number of nursing interventions. Nursing interventions are individualized and are stated in specific terms. Examples of nursing interventions are:

- Turn, cough, and deep breathe q 2 h beginning at 0800, 2/10.
- Teach "nipple care when breastfeeding" at 1000, 2/11.
- Weigh client at each visit.

Once the interventions have been determined for each diagnosis, the interventions are recorded on the client's plan of care. As is true with other steps in the nursing process, the list of interventions is not static. As the nurse interacts with the client, assesses responses to interventions, and evaluates those responses, interventions may change.

### Implementation

The fourth step in the nursing process is implementation. **Implementation** involves the execution of the nursing plan of care derived during the planning phase. It consists of performing nursing activities that have been planned to meet the goals set with the client. Nurses may delegate some of the nursing interventions to other persons assigned to care for the client—for example, the licensed practical nurses and unlicensed assistive personnel.

Implementation involves many skills. The nurse must continue to assess the client's condition before, during, and after the nursing intervention. Assessment prior to the intervention provides the nurse with baseline data (Figure 10-4). Assessment during and after the intervention allows the nurse to detect positive or negative responses the client may have to the intervention. If negative responses occur during the procedure, the nurse must take appropriate action. If positive responses occur, the nurse adds this information to the database for use in evaluating the efficacy of the intervention. The nurse must also possess psychomotor skills, interpersonal skills, and critical-thinking skills to perform the nursing interventions that have been planned. The nurse uses psychomotor skills when performing procedures such as giving injections, changing dressings, and helping the client perform range-of-motion (ROM) exercises. Interpersonal skills are necessary as the nurse interacts with the client and the family to collect data, provide information in teaching sessions, and offer support in times of anxiety.

## RESEARCH FOCUS

**Title of Study:** Intuition: An important tool in the practice of nursing.

**Study Purpose:** This study examines the various definitions of intuition and the perceived benefits derived from using intuition when used in making decisions.

**Methods:** This qualitative study used comparative analysis of focus group interviews to create questions for a Delphi survey, which was distributed to nurses who had used intuition in their practice.

**Findings:** Intuition is a synergy of experience, expertise and knowledge, the existing environment, personality of the decision maker, and personal acceptance of intuition as a valid tool. These interactions are dependent and reciprocal—providing a "gestalt," or total picture of the situation involved. Respondents believed that acting on intuitive feelings was "the right thing to do," and that the use of intuition can change client outcomes. Inexperienced nurses were perceived to be reluctant to risk acting on their intuitive feelings.

**Implications:** This study continues to add to the knowledge related to the concept of intuition. There is a correlation between nurses using intuition and positive effects on client outcomes. In the future, studies on the influence of intuition in evidenced-based practice can prove to be very useful.

McCutcheon, H., & Pincombe, J. (2001). Intuition: An important tool in the practice of nursing. *Journal of Advanced Nursing, 35*(3), 342–348.

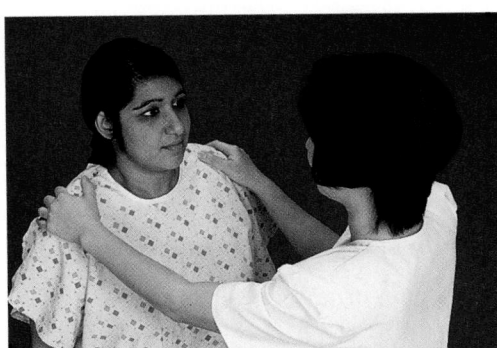

**Figure 10-4    A nurse applying assessment skills (i.e., assessment of cranial nerve XI) during the implementation phase of the nursing process.**

## TABLE 10-4    EXAMPLES OF CRITICAL-THINKING QUESTIONS FOR USE WITH THE NURSING PROCESS

| Nursing Process Step | Critical-Thinking Question |
|---|---|
| Assessment | Are the data complete? What other data do I need? What are some possible sources of those data? What assumptions or biases do I have in this situation? What is the client's point of view? Are there other points of view? |
| Diagnosis | What do these data mean? What else could be happening? Are there any gaps in the data? How are these data similar and how are they different? What assumptions or biases do I have in this situation? Have my assumptions affected my interpretation of the data? If so, in what way? |
| Outcome identification and planning | What are the goals for this client? What do I want to accomplish? How are my goals related to what the client wants to accomplish? What are the expected outcomes for this client? What interventions are to be used? Who is the best-qualified person to perform these interventions? How much involvement can the client and family or significant others have at this time? How much involvement does the client wish to have at this time? |
| Implementation | What is the client's current status? What are the most critical steps in this intervention? How must I alter the intervention to best meet this client's needs and maintain principles of safety? What is the client's response during and after the intervention? Is there a need to alter the intervention in any way? If so, why and how? |
| Evaluation | Were the interventions successful in assisting the client to achieve the desired goals? How could things have been done differently? What data do I need to make new decisions? Where will I get the data? Were there assumptions, biases, or points of view that I missed that affected the outcomes? What can be done about these assumptions, biases, or points of view? |

## TABLE 10-5    COMPARISON OF PROBLEM SOLVING AND NURSING PROCESS

| Problem Solving | Nursing Process |
|---|---|
| Encountering problem | Assessing |
| Collecting data | Assessing |
| Identifying exact nature of problem | Formulating nursing diagnosis |
| Determining plan of action | Planning |
| Carrying out plan | Implementing |
| Evaluating plan in new situation | Evaluating |

Adapted from Pesut, D. J., & Herman, J. (1999). *Clinical reasoning: The art and science of critical and creative thinking.* Clifton Park, NY: Delmar Learning.

Critical-thinking skills enable the nurse to think through the situation, ask the appropriate questions, and make decisions about what needs to be done.

The implementation step also involves reporting and documentation. Data to be recorded include the client condition prior to the intervention, the specific intervention performed, the client response to the intervention, and client outcomes.

### Evaluation

**Evaluation**, the fifth step in the nursing process, involves determining whether the client goals have been met, partially met, or not met. If the goal has been met, the nurse must then decide whether nursing activities will cease or continue in order for status to be maintained. If the goal has been partially met or not been met, the nurse must reassess the situation. Data are collected to determine why the goal has not been achieved and what modifications to the plan of care are necessary. There are a number of possible reasons that goals are not met or are only partially met, including:

- The initial assessment data were incomplete.
- The goals and expected outcomes were not realistic.

## TABLE 10-6 APPLICATION OF CRITICAL THINKING TO NURSING PROCESS

| Assessment | Diagnosis | Outcome Identification | Implementation | Evaluation and Planning |
|---|---|---|---|---|
| • Gather pertinent data<br>• Interpret data<br>• Keep an open mind by questioning assumptions about data<br>• Think about what information to collect<br>• Determine the significance of data<br>• Make conclusions based on the data | • Develop well-thought-out conclusions<br>• Seek reasons and principles that justify nursing judgments<br>• Test conclusions against criteria<br>• Suspend judgment when data is insufficient<br>• Differentiate essential and trivial data | • Explore alternative actions<br>• Collaborate with others<br>• Examine assumptions<br>• Reframe problems in order to generate solutions<br>• Generate ideas and possible solutions | • Communicate with others to solve complex problems<br>• Accurately report data and clues<br>• Action is based on sound rationale | • Establish standards (criteria) based on logic rather than assumptions<br>• Analyze course of action<br>• Critique outcomes<br>• Evaluate the soundness of conclusions |

• The time frame was too optimistic.
• The goals and/or the nursing interventions planned were not appropriate for the client.

Evaluation is an ongoing process. Nurses continually evaluate data in order to make informed decisions during other phases of the nursing process.

## Critical Thinking Applied in Nursing

Critical thinking is a skill that can be learned just as other skills are learned. The skill of critical thinking is important and useful in all aspects of a person's life. However, it is a vital tool for the nurse in using the nursing process. Critical thinkers develop a questioning attitude and delve into situations in order to seek possible explanations for what is happening. Examples of questions the nurse as a critical thinker might ask at each step in the nursing process are listed in Table 10-4.

There are many similarities between the nursing process and the problem-solving process, as shown in Table 10-5.

Nurses use critical-thinking skills in each step of the nursing process. "Everything nurses do requires high-level thinking; no action is performed without critical thinking" (Rubenfeld & Scheffer, 1999, p. 3). Table 10-6 provides examples of how critical thinking is used in each phase of the nursing process.

"Because the conclusions and decisions we as nurses make affect people's lives, our thinking must be guided by sound reasoning—precise, disciplined thinking that promotes accuracy and depth of data collection, and seeks to clearly identify the issues at hand" (Alfaro-LeFevre, 1998, p. 64).

# CASE STUDY/NURSING CARE PLAN

Mr. Boswick is a 70-year-old client who was admitted to your orthopedic unit 2 days ago with a fractured left hip. He had an ORIF (open reduction and internal fixation) on the day of admission. He is currently recovering, with his primary problem being acute pain that is restricting his ability to ambulate. He was injured while climbing on a ladder at home. He is widowed and recently retired from an administrative position with a large company in Florida. He has two children, who both live within 3 hours' driving time. Mr. Boswick lives alone in a two-bedroom condominium that is located about two blocks from your hospital. Mr. Boswick will be discharged from the acute care setting within 1 to 2 days and is being referred to either (1) a convalescent facility, or (2) home health agency for follow-up care.

*(continues)*

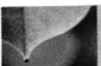

# CASE STUDY/NURSING CARE PLAN (continued)

## Assessment

Mr. Boswick has had a successful repair of a fractured hip and is recovering, with the problem of acute pain. He is awaiting discharge and needs client education in this regard. Mr. Boswick will need direction as to whether he is able to go home with home health nursing supervision and assistance or if he will need to be admitted to a convalescent setting.

## Nursing Diagnosis #1

Acute pain related to recent repair of a fractured left hip.
**NOC:** Pain Level; Pain Control; Comfort Level; Pain: Disruptive Effects
**NIC:**  Pain Management; Analgesic Administration; Patient-Controlled Analgesia

## Expected Outcomes

The client will:
1. State he has a decreased level of pain (on a pain scale of 1 to 10) within 48 hours.
2. Verbalize successful measures that improve his comfort level before discharge.

## Planning/Interventions/Rationales

1. Collaborate with client in determining what methods can be used to reduce the pain level. *Increases the self-efficacy of the client in pain-relief methods.*
2. Premedicate the client 30 to 60 minutes prior to ambulating. *Prevents pain level from increasing beyond the pain threshold.*

## Evaluation

Client states that his pain level has decreased from 6 to a 3 on the pain management scale of 1 to 10 and that he is able to ambulate with less discomfort.

## Nursing Diagnosis #2

Ineffective health maintenance from recent surgery, as related to impending discharge.
**NOC:** Health Beliefs: Perceived Resources; Health-Promoting Behavior; Health-Seeking Behavior
**NIC:**  Health System Guidance; Support System Enhancement; Health Education

## Expected Outcomes

The client will:
1. Identify barriers to health maintenance in whichever environment he is discharged to, within 3 days of relocating.
2. Engage in health maintenance behaviors, such as personal hygiene, within 3 days of relocating.

## Planning/Interventions/Rationales

1. Client will assess for barriers to health maintenance. *Encourages client to discover methods for improving his state of health.*
2. Assist the client in identifying health behaviors that are compatible with his lifestyle after the surgical repair of his left hip. *Allows a realistic plan for client to adapt to his limitations created from the recent surgery.*

## Evaluation

Client identified the health barriers of his recent surgery and developed a plan for overcoming those deficiencies.

# Key Concepts

- Critical thinking, problem-solving, and decision-making skills are important for use in the nursing process.
- Critical thinkers ask questions, evaluate evidence, identify assumptions, examine alternatives, and seek to understand various points of view.
- The nursing process is an organized method of planning and delivering nursing care.

- The nursing process is composed of five steps: assessment, diagnosis, outcome identification and planning, implementation, and evaluation.
- Assessment is the first step in the nursing process and involves collecting, validating, organizing, categorizing, and recording data.
- Both subjective data (information given by the client) and objective data (information collected by the health

care provider using the senses) are collected during the assessment process.

- The second step in the nursing process involves further analysis and synthesis of the data and results in a list of nursing diagnoses.
- Types of nursing diagnoses include actual, potential (including risk and possible), and wellness.
- Planning, the third step in the nursing process, involves prioritizing nursing diagnoses, identifying and writing goals and client outcomes, developing nursing interventions, and recording the plan of care in the client's record.
- Implementation, the fourth step in the nursing process, involves performing or delegating nursing activities.
- The nurse uses psychomotor skills, interpersonal skills, and cognitive skills when performing nursing activities.
- Evaluation, the fifth step in the nursing process, involves deciding whether the client goals have been met, been partially met, or not been met.
- The steps in the nursing process are similar to those in the problem-solving method in that problems are identified, information is gathered, a specific problem is named, a plan for solving the problem is developed, the plan is put into action, and the results of the plan are evaluated.

## Review Questions and Activities

1. Think of all the ways you can use your senses when assessing clients. What type of information can you gather through vision, hearing, smell, and touch?
2. Mrs. Rose was admitted to your unit 2 hours ago. The following data are recorded on her chart. Which data are objective? Which data are subjective? Use "S" and "O" to indicate your response.

   | | |
   |---|---|
   | __ Temperature 102°F | __ Pulse 98, irregular |
   | __ "My head hurts." | __ Red maculopapular rash |
   | __ Nausea | __ Vomiting for 3 days |
   | __ Grimaces when blinds open | __ Skin flushed, hot |

3. Match the steps in the nursing process (Column B) with the activities listed in Column A. Use the letters to indicate your answers.

   | COLUMN A | COLUMN B |
   |---|---|
   | 1.__ Examine the data for pattern. | a. Assessment |
   | 2.__ Write client outcomes. | b. Diagnosis |
   | 3.__ Take the client's blood pressure. | c. Outcome identification and planning |
   | 4.__ Take the health history, using interviewing techniques. | d. Implementation |

   | | |
   |---|---|
   | 5.__ Select appropriate nursing actions. | e. Evaluation |
   | 6.__ Document client response to walking. | |
   | 7.__ Conduct a physical assessment. | |
   | 8.__ Measure results of nursing interventions. | |
   | 9.__ Identify client strengths. | |
   | 10.__ Prioritize nursing diagnoses. | |

4. What is the advantage of using the nursing process when you provide nursing care to your clients?
5. What do you believe about how people react when they are in pain? How do you and the people you know respond when in pain? Your beliefs form the basis for assumptions about pain response. How could these assumptions influence your interpretation of client responses to pain?

## Web Resources

American Nurses Association
   http://www.nursingworld.org
AMI Care Map
   http://www.hsc.mb.ca
Critical Thinking Consortium
   http://www.criticalthinking.org

## References

Ackley, B. J., & Ladwig, G. B. (2002). *Nursing diagnosis handbook: A guide to planning care* (5th ed.). St. Louis: Mosby.

Alfaro-LeFevre, R. (2004). *Critical thinking in nursing: A practical approach* (3rd ed.). Philadelphia: Saunders.

Alfaro-LeFevre, R. (1999). *Applying nursing process* (4th ed.). Philadelphia: Lippincott.

American Nurses Association (1998). *Standards of clinical nursing practice.* Kansas City, MO: Author.

Atkinson, L., & Murray, M. (2000). *Understanding the nursing process in a changing care environment.* New York.: McGraw-Hill.

Baker, D. (2001). Nursing reasoning model. *Nursing Educator, 26*(5), 203–204.

Bower, F. (2000). *Nurses taking the lead: Personal qualities of effective leadership.* Philadelphia: W. B. Saunders.

Carpenito, L. (2002). *Nursing diagnosis: Application to clinical practice* (8th ed.). Philadelphia: J. B. Lippincott.

Catalano, J. (2000). *Nursing now: Today's issues, tomorrow's trends.* Philadelphia: F. A. Davis.

Doenges, M., Moorhouse, M., & Geissler-Murr, A. (2002). *Nurse's pocket guide: Diagnoses, interventions, and rationales* (8th ed.). Philadelphia: F. A. Davis.

Estes, M. E. Z. (2002). *Health assessment & physical examination* (2nd ed.). Clifton Park, NY: Delmar Learning.

Fry, V. S. (1953). The creative approach to nursing. *American Journal of Nursing, 53*(3), 301–302.

Gebbie, K. M., & Lavin, M. A. (1974). Classifying nursing diagnoses. *American Journal of Nursing, 74,* 250–253.

Hall, L. (1955, February). *Quality of nursing care.* Address at meeting of Department of Baccalaureate and Higher Degree Programs, New Jersey League for Nursing, Seton Hall University, Newark, NJ.

Harmer, B., & Henderson, V. (1944). *Textbook of the principles and practice of nursing.* New York: Macmillan Co.

Hitchcock, J., Schubert, P., & Thomas, S. (2003). *Community health nursing: Caring in action.* Clifton Park, NY: Delmar Learning.

Johnson, D. (1959). A philosophy for nursing diagnosis. *Nursing Outlook, 7,* 198–200.

Lachman, V. (1999). Breaking the quality barrier: Critical thinking and conflict resolution. *Nursing Care Management, 4*(5), 224–227.

Le Storti, A. J., Cullen, P. A., Hanzlik, E. M., Michiels, J. M., Piano, L. A., Rya, P. L., & Johnson, W. (1999). Creative thinking in nursing education: Preparing for tomorrow's challenges. *Nursing Outlook, 47*(2), 62–66.

McCutcheon, H., & Pincombe, J. (2001). Intuition: An important tool in the practice of nursing. *Journal of Advanced Nursing, 35*(3), 342–348.

National League for Nursing (1997). *Interpretive guidelines for standards and criteria 1997: Baccalaureate and higher degree.* New York: National League for Nursing Accrediting Commission.

Nicoteri, J. A. (1998). Critical thinking skills: Applying theory to real-life patient care. *American Journal of Nursing, 98*(10), 62–66.

North America Nursing Diagnosis Association (2002). *A vision for nursing. Trends in RN Education programs: White Paper.* http://www.nanda.org

Nunnery, R. (1997). *Advancing your career: Concepts of professional nursing.* Philadelphia: F. A. Davis.

Orlando, I. (1961). *The dynamic nurse-patient relationship.* New York: G.P. Putnam & Sons.

Pender, J., Murdaugh, C., & Parsons, M.A. (2002). *Health promotion in nursing practice* (4th ed.). Upper Saddle River, NJ: Prentice-Hall.

Peplau, H. (1952). *Interpersonal relations in nursing.* New York: Putnam.

Pesut, D. J., & Herman, J. (1999). *Clinical reasoning: The art and science of critical and creative thinking.* Clifton Park, NY: Delmar Learning.

Redding, D. (1999). Development of critical thinking among students in baccalaureate nursing education. *Holistic Nursing Practice, 15*(4), 57–65.

Rubenfeld, M. G., & Scheffer, B. K. (1999). *Critical thinking in nursing: An interactive approach* (2nd ed.). Philadelphia: Lippincott.

Welch, R. (1999). Problem solving and decision making. In P. Yoder-Wise, *Leading and managing in nursing.* St. Louis: C.V. Mosby, pp. 91–106.

Wiedenbach, E. (1963). The helping art of nursing. *American Journal of Nursing, 63*(11), 54–57.

Wilkinson, J. M. (1998). *Nursing process in action: A critical thinking approach* (2nd ed.). Redwood City, CA: Addison-Wesley Nursing.

Yura, H., & Walsh, M. B. (1967). *The nursing process.* Washington, DC: The Catholic University of America Press.

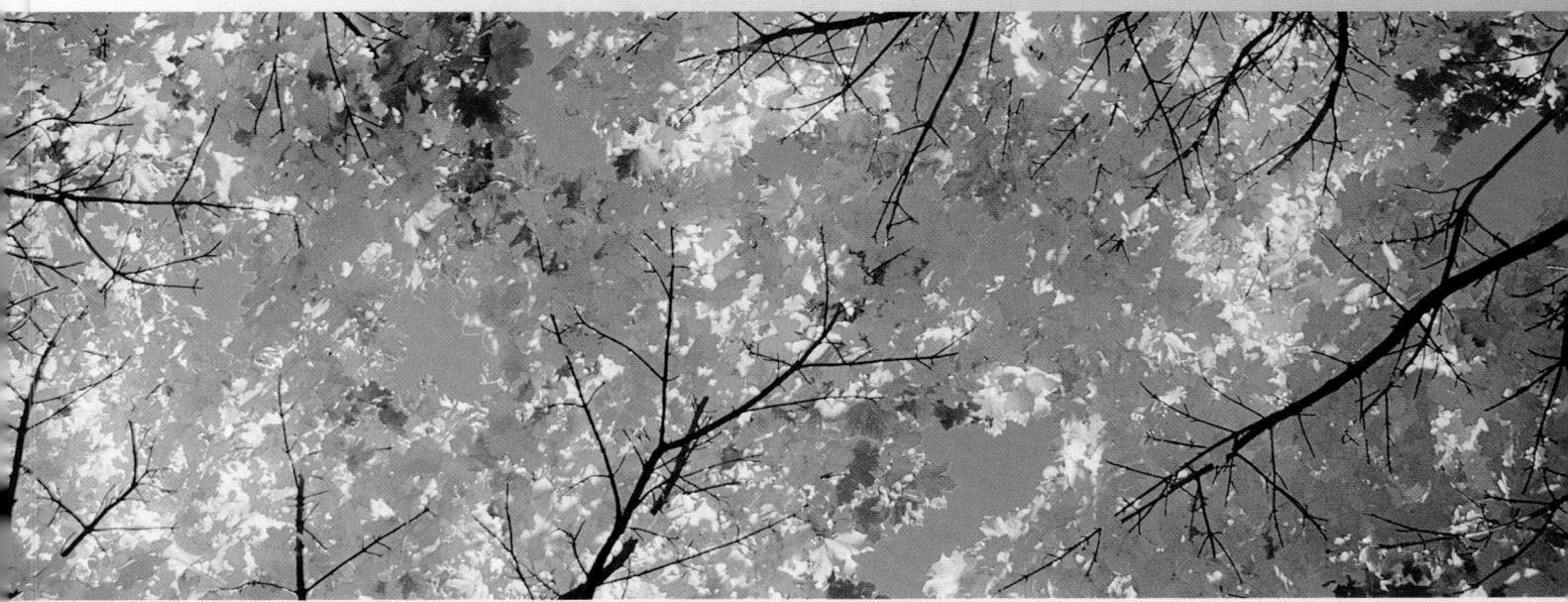

# CHAPTER 11

# Assessment

Sharon M. Rayman, RN, MS, CPTC, CCTC

*"The most important practical lesson that can be given to nurses is to teach them what to observe—how to observe—what symptoms indicate improvement—what the reverse—which are of importance—which are of none—which are the evidence of neglect—and of what kind of neglect. All this is what ought to make part, and an essential part, of the training of every nurse."*

(Florence Nightingale, Notes on Nursing, 1860/1969)

# Chapter Competencies

*Upon completion of this chapter, the reader should be able to:*

1. Describe the primary purpose of the assessment process.
2. Explain the types of assessment.
3. Identify five essential elements of the assessment process.
4. Explain the types of information that may be exchanged between the nurse and client during the assessment process.
5. Describe four types of assessment databases.
6. Differentiate subjective data from objective data.
7. Describe five methods involved in data collection.
8. Describe the process of data verification.
9. Identify examples of nursing and nonnursing models used in collecting and organizing data.
10. Discuss the use of data clustering in organizing the information obtained about the client.
11. Identify four types of formats for documentation of assessment data.

# Key Terms

assessment
assessment model
auscultation
closed-ended questions
comprehensive assessment
data clustering
data interpretation
data verification

emergency assessment
focused assessment
focused questions
health history
inspection
interview
objective data
observation

ongoing assessment
open-ended questions
palpation
percussion
primary source
review of systems
secondary source
subjective data

Assessment is the first step in the nursing process and includes systematic collection, verification, organization, interpretation, and documentation of data for use by health care professionals. Nursing assessments focus upon the client's response to health problems, perceived health needs, and health practices and values. Box 11-1 presents the essential elements of the assessment process. Effective planning of client care depends on a complete database and accurate interpretation of information. Incomplete or inadequate assessment may result in inaccurate conclusions and incorrect nursing interventions. Proper collection of assessment data directs decision-making activities of professional nurses.

The goal of assessment is the collection and analysis of data that are used in formulating nursing diagnoses, identifying outcomes and planning care, and developing nursing interventions. This chapter discusses the purpose of assessment, types of assessment, and the use of data in the assessment process.

## Purpose of Assessment

The purpose of assessment is to establish a database about a client's physical and emotional well-being, intellectual

---

**BOX 11-1    ELEMENTS OF THE ASSESSMENT PROCESS**

- Data collection
- Data verification
- Data organization
- Data interpretation
- Data documentation

functioning, social relationships, and spiritual condition. This information is used to identify health-promoting behaviors as well as actual and/or potential health problems. The American Nurses Association (ANA), in its *Standards of Clinical Nursing Practice* (1998), supports the use of the nursing process and outlines the essential components of assessment in this process. The data must be relevant to client needs, collected from a variety of valid sources, obtained using appropriate techniques and in a systematic manner, and documented in a usable format. Through assessment, the nurse determines the client's functional abilities and the absence or presence of dysfunction. The client's normal routine for activities of daily living and lifestyle patterns are also assessed. Identification of the client's strengths provides the nurse and other members of the treatment team information about the skills, abilities, and behaviors the client has available to promote the treatment and recovery process. Some examples of client strengths are family support, intelligence, spiritual beliefs, and coping skills (how previous problems have been solved). The assessment phase also offers an opportunity for the nurse to form a therapeutic interpersonal relationship with the client. During assessment, the client is provided an opportunity to discuss health care concerns and goals with the nurse (Alfaro-LeFevre, 2002).

## Types of Assessment

The type and scope of information needed for assessment are usually determined by the health care setting and needs of the client (Figure 11-1). Four types of assessment databases are comprehensive, focused, ongoing, and emergency. Although a comprehensive assessment is most desirable in initially determining a client's need for nursing care, time limitations or special circumstances may dictate the need for abbreviated data collection, as represented by the focused assessment. The assessment database can then be expanded after the initial focused assessment, and data should be updated through the ongoing assessment process.

## Comprehensive Assessment

A **comprehensive assessment** is usually completed upon admission to a health care agency and includes a complete health history to determine current needs of the client. This database provides a baseline against which changes in the client's health status can be measured and should include assessment of physical and psychosocial aspects of the client's health, the client's perception of health, the presence of health risk factors, and the client's coping patterns.

## Focused Assessment

A **focused assessment** is an assessment that is limited in scope in order to focus on a particular need or health care problem or potential health care risks. Focused assessments are not as detailed as comprehensive assessments and are often used in health care agencies in which short stays are anticipated (e.g., outpatient surgery centers and emergency departments), in specialty areas such as labor and delivery, and in mental health settings or for purposes of screening for specific problems or risk factors (e.g., well-child clinics). See the Nursing Strategy box for sample questions used to assess a client experiencing labor.

## Ongoing Assessment

Systematic follow-up is required when problems are identified during a comprehensive or focused assessment. An **ongoing assessment** is an assessment that includes systematic monitoring and observation related to specific problems. This type of assessment allows the nurse to broaden the database or to confirm the validity of the data obtained during the initial assessment. Ongoing

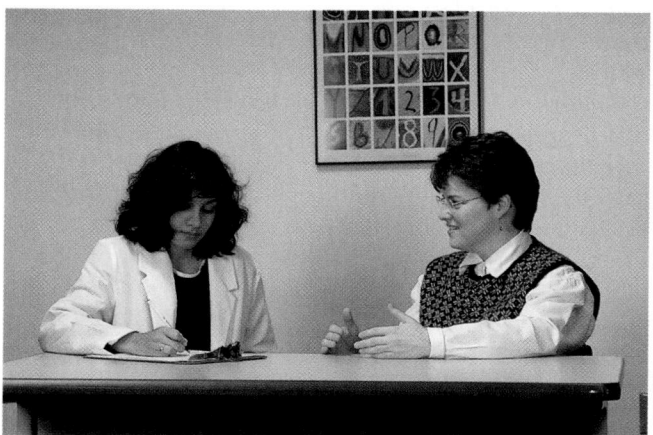

**Figure 11-1** In this focused assessment, the nurse is collecting data about the client prior to elective surgery.

### NURSING STRATEGY

#### Sample Focused Assessment: The Woman Experiencing Labor

Following are examples of questions that focus on essential information for the nurse caring for a woman during labor:

- When did your contractions begin?
- How far apart are the contractions?
- Are they getting stronger?
- When did your water break?

## NURSING STRATEGY

### Sample Ongoing Assessment: The Woman Experiencing Labor

- What led up to your most recent hospitalization?

- What medications were prescribed for you during that time?

- What kind of diet were you on?

- What type of activities did you do while you were in the hospital?

- While in the hospital, what did you learn about . . . ?

- What adaptations for your comfort and care have you and your family made since your return home?

## NURSING STRATEGY

### Sample Emergency Assessment: Potential of Suicide

The following are questions for the nurse to ask the client who is considering suicide:

- Have you lost interest in things or activities that you usually have found enjoyable?

- Have you thought about harming yourself?

- If you were to hurt yourself, how would you do it?

- Describe the items you need to carry out your plan.

- Are the resources to carry out your plan available?

- What has kept you from harming yourself?

assessment is particularly important when problems have been identified and a plan of care has been implemented to address these problems. Systematic monitoring and observations allow the nurse to determine the response to nursing interventions and to identify any emerging problems.

The nurse delivering care to a client at home uses ongoing assessment. In the home, the nurse often has to direct the client to provide information relevant to the current problem, as the client may have a tendency to spend a lot of time telling stories of past medical problems and treat-

## LEGAL AND ETHICAL ISSUES

### Legal Implications of Emergency Care

If the assessment of a client takes place "in the field" (primary setting), the nurse must remember that both Good Samaritan and abandonment laws apply. That is, the nurse must begin to give whatever emergency care is within the nurse's clinical practice, and the nurse must stay with the client until relieved by other qualified health care providers (e.g., paramedics). If the nurse did not begin to give care or left the scene prior to adequate care being established, that nurse would be liable.

Adapted from Gastmans, C. (2002). A fundamental ethical approach to nursing; some proposals for ethics education. *Nursing Ethics, 9*(5), 494–507.

ment, as opposed to providing information relevant to the situation at hand (Humphrey, 1998). Use of specific questions will be most helpful in eliciting specific information.

## Emergency Assessment

An **emergency assessment** involves a rapid assessment of a client who is experiencing a life-threatening problem or crisis. This problem can be of a physiological and/or psychological and sociological nature. In the event of a cardiac arrest, the nurse will ask few questions but will immediately focus on airway patency, breathing status, and circulation status. Whereas with clients who present with emotional crises, the nurse will focus on immediate safety and coping abilities and strategies.

Risk for suicide among older adults is a growing problem in today's society. Suicide by older adults accounts for 20% of all suicides, but only 12% of the population (Salvatore, 2000). In assessing clients for potential suicide, it is helpful to have a series of questions. The basic components of suicide assessment to evaluate are suicidal thoughts; prior attempts; suicide plan; lethality of plan; availability of resources to implement plan; coexisting health, social, emotional problems; and the extent of feelings of hopelessness or worthlessness (Hogstel & Weeks, 2000). Specific questions to assess the potential for suicide are in the accompanying Nursing Strategy box.

## Data Collection

The nurse must possess strong cognitive, interpersonal, and technical skills in order to elicit appropriate information and make relevant observations during the data collection process. This process often begins prior to initial contact between the nurse and the client, primarily through the nurse's review of biographical data and medical records. Upon meeting the client, the nurse continues data collection through interview, observation, and examination. A variety of sources and methods are used in compiling a comprehensive database

## Types of Data

Client data include information that the client communicates concerning perceptions of her own health status, as well as specific observations made by the nurse. These two types of information are referred to as subjective and objective data. **Subjective data** are data from the client's point of view and include feelings, perceptions, and concerns. The data (also referred to as symptoms) are obtained through interviews with the client. They are called subjective because they rely on the feelings or opinions of the person experiencing them and cannot be readily observed by another.

**Objective data** are observable and measurable (quantitative) data that are obtained through observation, standard assessment techniques performed during the physical examination, and laboratory and diagnostic testing. These data (also called signs) can be seen, heard, or felt by someone other than the person experiencing them. Assessments that are comprehensive and accurate include both subjective and objective data (Estes, 2002). A sample application for types of data appears in Box 11-2.

## Sources of Data

A comprehensive database should include data from every possible source (see Box 11-3). The client is always the **primary source** of data and, if possible, should always be consulted. However, other sources of data should not be overlooked. Data from sources other than the client are considered **secondary sources** of information. The client's family and significant others can also provide useful information, especially if the client is unable to verbalize or relate information. In addition, other health care professionals who have cared for the client may contribute valuable information. Medical records should also be reviewed, including the medical history and physical examination; results of laboratory and diagnostic tests and various health care professionals should also be consulted.

Pertinent literature should be investigated in order to pursue relevant information and plan appropriate nursing interventions. Written standards are valuable sources of data for comparison—for example, a standard table of infant growth to determine if an infant's weight and height are within normal growth range. Another valuable source of data is knowledge about the client's normal parameters of functioning. The nurse's knowledge based on experience is another important source of data.

---

**BOX 11-2 SAMPLE APPLICATION: TYPES OF DATA**

| Data | Types of Data |
|---|---|
| Charlene Rhodes, age 47, has come to the clinic after "passing out" twice in the last 2 days. She tells the nurse that she becomes "lightheaded" after almost any type of activity. She has experienced some nausea since yesterday and vomited after eating breakfast this morning. She also tells the nurse that she is very nervous about these occurrences because she remembers her mother having similar symptoms when the mother suffered from a brain disorder. The nurse observes that the client's gait is unsteady and her skin is pale. The client also has large bruises on her right arm and the right side of her face, which she says occurred when she fell. | **Subjective (Symptoms)** Report of fainting Complaint of dizziness Nausea Verbalization of anxiety Self-reported fall  **Objective (Signs)** Vomiting Unsteady gait Pale skin Bruises on right side of face and right arm |

---

**BOX 11-3 SOURCES OF DATA**

Primary

- Client

Secondary

- Family/significant other

- Other health care professionals

- Medical records

- Interdisciplinary conferences, rounds, and consultations

- Results of diagnostic tests

- Relevant literature

- Nurse's knowledge and experience

Adapted from Estes, M. (2002). *Health assessment & physical examination* (2nd ed.). Clifton Park, NY: Delmar Learning.

## LIFE SPAN CONSIDERATIONS

### A Comprehensive Database

Molly, age 2, with a history of a seizure disorder, was admitted to the pediatric intensive care unit following a near-drowning incident. She is responsive to verbal instructions. She has not had any seizures since admission. Her care is managed by a pediatric clinical nurse specialist. Molly's parents are at the bedside. Her pediatrician has admitting privileges to the hospital. You are the bedside nurse assigned to collect a comprehensive assessment database. You need to assess the primary data source, which is Molly herself. Your focus with Molly is to provide emotional support specific to a 2-year-old and to provide information that Molly can understand. In addition, you need to assess the secondary data sources, which include Molly's parents, other medical records as they are applicable, and the documentation provided by other members of the health care team.

Adapted from Potts, N., & Mandleco, B. (2002). *Pediatric nursing: Caring for children and their families.* Clifton Park, NY: Delmar Learning.

## COMMUNITY/HOME CARE

### Observation Skills in the Home Setting

The home health nurse must learn to carefully assess the total environment, and not just the client's condition alone, when admitting a client in the home care setting. A much greater variety of items need consideration in the home care arena. For example, if the client is going to self-administer parenteral antibiotics, he will need to set up his equipment in an environment that is relatively easy to keep clean and close to a sink for washing hands. The nurse would need to assess the home for a location that addresses these needs. Overall, observation in the home setting requires advanced, critical decision-making skills for the nurse.

Hogstel, M. (2001). *Gerontology: Nursing care of the older adult.* Clifton Park, NY: Delmar Learning; Humphrey, C. J. (1998). *Home care nursing handbook* (3rd ed.). Gaithersburg, MD: Aspen.

## Methods of Data Collection

The nurse collects information through the following methods: observation, interview, health history, symptom analysis, physical examination, and laboratory and diagnostic data. These approaches require systematic use of assessment skills that are discussed below.

## Observation

The nurse uses the skill of **observation** to carefully and attentively note the general appearance and behavior of the client. These observations occur whenever there is contact with the client and include factors such as client mood, interactions with others, physical and emotional responses, and any safety considerations. Observation helps the nurse determine the client's status, both physical and mental. By carefully watching the client, the nurse can detect nonverbal cues that indicate a variety of feelings, including presence of pain, anxiety, and anger. Observational skills are essential in detecting the early warning signs of physical changes (e.g., pallor and sweating). Additional skills are required in the home setting.

## Interview

An **interview** is a therapeutic interaction that has a specific purpose The purpose of the assessment interview is to collect information about the client's health history and current status in order to make determinations about

the client's health needs. Effective interviewing depends on the nurse's knowledge and ability to skillfully elicit information from the client using appropriate techniques of communication. Observation of nonverbal behavior during the interview is also essential to effective data collection (Figure 11-2).

### Interview Preparation

The interview is more productive if the nurse has an opportunity to prepare for the interaction. Such preparation includes review of the client's medical records, conversations with other health care team members (e.g., personnel in emergency departments or long-term care facilities), and research of the presenting medical diagnosis. This information can be useful in obtaining the

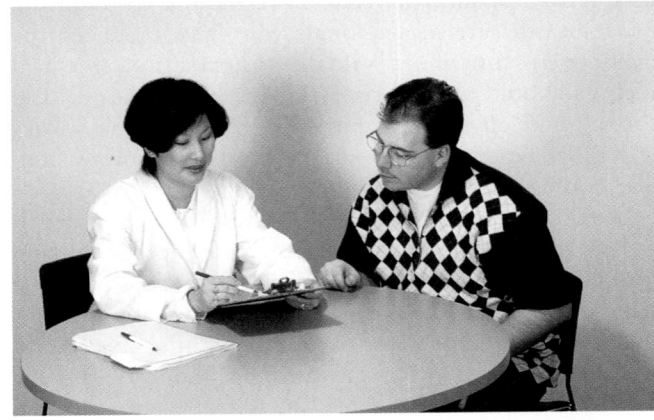

**Figure 11-2    A nurse gathering data by interviewing a client.**

client's relevant history and formulating a current needs assessment.

The client is more likely to respond freely if the interview environment provides comfort and privacy and if rapport exists between the client and the nurse. The nurse should sit (if possible), establish eye contact with the client, and listen attentively. It is the nurse's responsibility to note nonverbal messages that can indicate that the client is uncomfortable, tired, or preoccupied with other matters. If this situation occurs, it might be necessary to complete the interview at a later time. For example, if the client is guarding an incision and verbalizing discomfort or is extremely anxious about an impending procedure, only essential data are collected and the comprehensive interview is postponed until immediate needs have been met.

The Nursing Strategy box provides guidelines to prepare the environment for the interview.

### Interview Stages

Since the assessment interview often occurs at the beginning of a nurse-client relationship, it is helpful to begin the process with an orientation phase. During this period introductions are made, rapport is established, and roles are defined. The nurse interviews for a variety of reasons throughout the nurse-client relationship, including data collection, teaching, exploration of the client's feelings or concerns, and provision of support. The first few minutes of the nurse-client meeting may give an indication of the type of interviewing needed, so it is important that the nurse exhibit good listening skills as the relationship leads into the interview process. There are three stages to an interview: introduction, working, and closure.

**Introduction** The introduction stage of the interview establishes the goals for the interaction. The primary goal of the assessment interview is the collection of data about the client. In this phase of the interview, the purpose and use of the data collection should be discussed. For exam-

ple, the nurse might state, "I need to ask you a few questions and talk to you for a few minutes about your health so that we can better plan your care." Adequate time and privacy should be allowed for the interview so that the client feels free to share any information that may be relevant. The nurse should also inform the client about the approximate duration of the interview.

**Working** The working stage of the interview focuses on the details of data collection. The scope of the assessment interview depends on the type of assessment to be conducted (e.g., comprehensive or focused). The interview may be structured and formal (used in situations when a large amount of information needs to be obtained) or unstructured and informal (used in interactions that focus on a specific area of concern to the client). The nurse should be familiar with the specific assessment format used by the health care agency so that attention can be focused toward the client rather than the form itself.

The interview generally begins with questions about biographical and other nonthreatening information. The client's reason for seeking health care is also addressed early in the working phase. The depth of the majority of questions that the nurse will ask the client depends on the data collection model used by the health care agency. Information is usually gathered from the general to the specific, with details about intimate or potentially embarrassing topics reserved until later in the interview.

Techniques used during the interview are determined by the setting and purpose of the interview. A comprehensive interview that seeks to identify problems and concerns is facilitated by open-ended questions, while an interview that focuses on specific details about a presenting problem is facilitated by direct, closed-ended questions. For example, an emergency setting would likely employ more direct, closed-ended questions, while admission to a long-term care facility might require greater use of open-ended questions.

**Closed-ended questions** are questions that can be answered briefly or with one-word responses. For example, the question "Have you been in the hospital before?" is a closed-ended question that can easily be answered by a one-word response. Questions about the dates of and reasons for the hospitalizations are also closed questions that require brief answers.

**Open-ended questions** are questions that encourage the client to elaborate about a particular concern or problem. For example, the question "What led to your coming here today?" is open-ended and allows the client flexibility in response. Both closed-ended and open-ended questions can be effective in collecting information.

**Focused questions** are asked to obtain information that is more specific about a problem or condition (Desmond & Copeland, 2000). Focused questions allow the client to provide a response that is more than a yes or no response. This type of question usually begins with words such as *describe, explain, tell*—for example, "Describe the pain in your chest,"

---

## NURSING STRATEGY

### Prepare Environment for Interview

- Assure adequate lighting.
- Maintain comfortable room temperature.
- Control for noise and distractions.
- Maintain client privacy.
- Establish time guidelines for interview.
- Promote client comfort.

Estes, M. (2002). *Health assessment & physical examination* (2nd ed.). Clifton Park, NY: Delmar Learning.

## STOP AND THINK

### Interview Techniques

Formulate a closed-ended question, open-ended question, and focused question to elicit information from a client about the following areas: diet, activity and exercise, and support system(s).

- Which questions do you think will elicit the most useful and complete information from the client?

- Under which assessment database would each type of question be best used?

## NURSING STRATEGY

### Guidelines for Promoting a Caring Interview

Establish rapport.

- Provide time for introductions.
- Explain your purpose.

Listen attentively.

- Listen for feelings.
- Observe body language.

Gather information.

- Ask open-ended questions.
- Ask closed-ended questions.
- Ask focused questions.

Observe.

- Use your senses.
- Notice interaction patterns.

Provide closure.

- Summarize.
- Ask for validation.
- Offer resources or follow-up.
- End with a positive statement.

or "Tell me about the activities your child was involved with prior to the fainting spells."

**Closure**    Closure is established in the introduction phase when approximate time parameters are set. As the interview session concludes, the nurse should indicate closure by stating that almost all the information needed has been obtained or that the time for the interview is almost over. This action allows the client an opportunity to present any other relevant information, and it avoids surprises when the interview terminates. During the closure phase, the nurse summarizes what was covered or accomplished during the interview and requests validation of perceptions with the client. If the nurse or the client feels that additional time is needed for further exploration of specific points discussed during this session, plans can be made for future interviews.

### Health History

A primary focus of the data collection interview is the health history. The **health history** is a review of the client's functional health patterns prior to the current contact with a health care agency. While the medical history concentrates on symptoms and the progression of disease, the nursing health history focuses on the client's functional health patterns, responses to changes in health status, and alterations in lifestyle. The health history is also used in developing the plan of care and formulating nursing interventions.

### Demographic Information

Personal data including name, address, date of birth, gender, religion, race and ethnic origin, occupation, and type of health plan and insurance should be included. This information may be useful in helping to foster understanding of a client's perspective.

### Reason for Seeking Health Care

The client's reason for seeking health care should be described in the client's own words. For example, the

statement "fell off 4-foot ladder and landed on right shoulder; unable to move right arm" is the client's actual report of the event that precipitated her need for health care. The client's perspective is important because it explains what is significant about the event from the client's point of view. It is also important to determine the time of the onset of symptoms as well as a complete symptom analysis.

### Perception of Health Status

Perception of health status refers to the client's opinion of his general health. It may be useful to ask clients to rate their health on a scale of 1 to 10 (with 10 being ideal and 1 being poor), together with the clients' rationale for their rating score. For example, the nurse may record a statement such as the following to represent the client's perception of health: "Rates health a 7 on a scale of 1 (poor) to 10 (ideal) because he must take medication regularly in

## CLINICAL ALERT

### Clients Who Are Adopted

Keep in mind that clients who are adopted will have varying degrees of knowledge about their biologic parents. Sensitivity to this issue is critical in gaining client trust during the interview process.

order to maintain mobility, but the medication sometimes upsets his stomach."

### Previous Illnesses, Hospitalizations, and Surgeries

The history and timing of any previous experiences with illness, surgery, or hospitalization are helpful in order to assess recurrent conditions and to anticipate responses to illness, since prior experiences often have an impact on current responses.

### Client/Family Medical History

The nurse needs to determine any family history of acute and chronic illnesses that tend to be familial. Health history forms will frequently include checklists of various illnesses that the nurse can use as the basis for questions about this aspect. The client should be instructed that family history refers to blood relatives. It is also helpful to indicate *who* the relative is in relation to the client (e.g., mother, father, sister).

### Immunizations/Exposure to Communicable Disease

Any history of childhood or other communicable diseases should also be noted. In addition, a record of current immunizations should be obtained. This is particularly important with children; however, records of immunizations for tetanus, influenza, and hepatitis B can also be important for adults. If the client has traveled out of the country, the time frame should be indicated in order to determine incubation periods for relevant diseases. The client should also be asked about potential exposure to communicable diseases such as tuberculosis, or to human immunodeficiency virus (HIV).

### Allergies

Any drug, food, or environmental allergies should be noted in the health history. In addition to the name of the allergen, the type of reaction to the substance should also be noted. For example, a client may report that she developed a rash or became short of breath. This reaction should be recorded. Clients may report an "allergy" to a medication because they developed an upset stomach after ingesting it, which the nurse will recognize as a side effect that would not necessarily preclude administration of the drug in the future.

## CLINICAL ALERT

### Assessment for Allergies

It is essential that the nurse explore possible allergies prior to administering any medications. Allergic reactions can be life-threatening and can occur even with very low dosages of medications. A client's sensitivity to a drug can also change over time, resulting in severe reactions even though the client has successfully taken the drug during prior illnesses or experienced only mild reactions to the drug in the past.

### Current Medications

All medications currently taken, both prescription and over-the-counter, are to be recorded by name, frequency, and dosage. Remind clients that this information should include medications such as birth control pills, laxatives, and non-prescription pain relief medications. Ask which, if any, herbal preparations the client uses. Patterns related to caffeine and alcohol intake and use of tobacco or recreational drugs should also be explored. Use of alternative/complementary treatment methods, including herbals, is often not shared by health care consumers. Some clients fear rejection or ridicule when divulging such information with health care providers. The nurse uses a sensitive, nonjudgmental approach when assessing for the client's use of all healing practices.

### Developmental Level

Knowledge of developmental level is essential for considering appropriate norms of behavior and for appraising the achievement of relevant developmental tasks. Any recognized theory of growth and development can be applied in order to determine if clients are functioning within the parameters expected for their age group. For example, if the nurse uses Erikson's stages of psychosocial development, an adult client's attainment of the developmental task of generativity versus stagnation can be validated by the nurse's statement, such as "client prefers to spend time with his family; very involved in children's school activities."

### Psychosocial History

Psychosocial history refers to assessment of dimensions such as self-concept and self-esteem, as well as usual sources of stress and the client's ability to cope. Sources of support for clients in crisis, such as family, significant others, religion, or support groups, should be explored.

### Value and Belief System

It is important to identify the client's values and beliefs about life, death, health, illness, and spirituality. The value and belief system is the basis of a person's philosophy of life.

The client's cultural and ethnic background and spiritual dimensions influence views about health and illness. The degree to which traditional ethnic values are maintained may affect health care practices, health-related decisions, and behaviors in life-threatening situations.

## Sociocultural History

In exploring the client's sociocultural history, it is important to inquire about the home environment, family situation, and client's role in the family. For example, the client could be the parent of three children and the sole provider in a single-parent family. The responsibilities of the client are important data through which the nurse can determine the impact of changes in health status and thus plan the most beneficial care for the client.

## Activities of Daily Living

The activities of daily living is a description of the client's lifestyle and capacity for self-care and is useful both as baseline information and as a source of insight into usual health behaviors. This database should include the following areas:

- *Nutrition:* Includes type of diet and foods eaten and fluids consumed regularly, food preparation, the size of portions, and the number of meals per day. Food preferences and dislikes, as well as the client's need for assistance in food preparation or eating, should also be determined.
- *Elimination:* Includes both urinary and bowel elimination frequency and patterns. Any recent changes or problems in these patterns should be noted.
- *Rest/sleep:* Includes the usual number of hours of sleep, number of hours of sleep needed to feel rested, sleep aids used, and the time within the day or night when sleep usually occurs. Any bedtime rituals (especially with children) should also be noted.

---

## FOCUS ON WELLNESS

### Incorporating Wellness Into a Client Assessment

The nurse must remember to assess the wellness activities of the client. It is important to remember to ask the client what types of health promotive behaviors he engages in (e.g., walking, eating low-fat substances, quitting smoking). These wellness activities "balance" the negative consequences of illness and also allow the nurse to have a more complete assessment of the client's health status.

Adapted from Pender, J., Murdaugh, C., & Parsons, M. A. (2002). *Health promotion in nursing practice* (4th ed.). Upper Saddle River, NJ: Prentice-Hall.

---

- *Activity/exercise:* Includes types of exercise and patterns in a typical day or week. If assistance is needed with activities such as walking, standing, or meeting hygienic needs, this information should be noted.

## Review of Systems

The **review of systems** (ROS) is a brief account from the client of any recent signs or symptoms associated with any of the body systems. This allows the client an opportunity to communicate any deviations from normal that have not been otherwise identified. The review of systems relies on subjective information provided by the client rather than on the nurse's own physical examination. When a symptom is encountered, either while eliciting the health histo-

---

 ## LIFE SPAN CONSIDERATIONS

### Age and the Assessment Interview

The age of the client being interviewed affects the way the interview is conducted.

#### Children
A child's age, verbal communication skills, and attention span will determine the degree to which a child can participate in an interview. Toddlers have short attention spans and may have difficulty with the interview. School-age children may respond more to play and visual activities. Adolescents may be more willing to share information without the presence of a parent. The following communication guidelines may assist with interviewing children: (1) identify the child's age and developmental stage, (2) establish rapport, and (3) observe family interactions.

#### Elderly Client
The nursing health history for the aged client must include functional, cognitive, affective, and social well-being. Additionally, a life history filled with people, places, and events demands adaptations in interviewing styles and techniques. Adaptations (such as the following) that reflect a sensitivity toward the elderly client will enhance the interview process: (1) establish rapport—demonstrate respect, (2) evaluate sensory alterations—hearing and visual acuity, (3) allow adequate time—rest periods, and (4) allow for time to reminisce about past memories.

Adapted from Estes, M. (2002). *Health assessment & physical examination* (2nd ed.). Clifton Park, NY: Delmar Learning; Leukenotte, A. G. (2000). Gerontologic assessment. In A. G. Leukenotte (Ed.). *Gerontologic nursing* (2nd ed.). St. Louis: Mosby.

ry or during the physical examination of the client, the nurse should obtain as much information as possible about the symptom. Relevant data include:

- *Location:* The area of the body in which the symptom (such as pain) can either be pointed to or described in detail.
- *Character:* The quality of the feeling or sensation (e.g., sharp, dull, stabbing).
- *Intensity:* The severity or quantity of the feeling or sensation and its interference with functional abilities. The sensation can be rated on a scale of 1 (very little) to 10 (very intense).
- *Timing:* The onset, duration, frequency, and precipitating factors of the symptom.
- *Aggravating/alleviating factors:* The activities or actions that make the symptom worse or better (see Box 11-4).

## Physical Examination

The purpose of the physical examination is to make direct observations of any deviations from normal and to validate subjective data gathered through the interview. Baseline measurements are obtained, and physical examination techniques are used to gather objective data.

## Baseline Data

Baseline data collection is the systematic organization of observations obtained during the physical examination that forms the basis for comparison and evaluation to establish the status of a client at a given point in time. Measurement of height, weight, and vital signs (temperature, pulse, respirations, and blood pressure) is important for comparison with future measurements in order to judge the significance of any changes (progress or regression) over time.

## Assessment Techniques

The physical examination incorporates the use of visual, auditory, tactile, and olfactory senses and the use of systematic assessment techniques. The use of visual, auditory, and tactile senses will be described with each of the specific assessment techniques. In addition, olfaction (sense of smell) is helpful in detecting characteristic odors as well as those associated with altered health states. For example, presence of infection is sometimes first detected by the change in the characteristic odor of body fluids or drainage. The four assessment techniques used in physical examination are inspection, palpation, percussion, and auscultation (Estes, 2002).

**Inspection    Inspection** involves careful visual observation. The client is observed first from a general point of view and then with specific attention to detail. For example, the nurse first observes for patterns of skin lesions and then focuses on the specific characteristics of individual lesions. Instruments such as a penlight and otoscope are often used to enhance visualization. Effective inspection requires adequate lighting and exposure of the body parts being observed. Beginning nurses often feel

---

### BOX 11-4    ELEMENTS OF THE HEALTH HISTORY

- Demographic information: name, age, gender, marital status
- Reason for seeking health care: concern that initiated visit
- Perception of health status: client's view of health
- Previous illnesses, hospitalizations, and surgeries: any chronic illness or acute episodes that led to hospitalization or surgery
- Client/family medical history: illness or cause of deaths in blood relatives
- Immunizations/exposure to communicable disease: childhood immunizations or relevant immunizations of adulthood; any known exposure to communicable disease
- Allergies: prior allergic reactions to medications, food, or environmental substances
- Current medications: prescription or over-the-counter medications, including laxatives, birth control pills, pain medications
- Developmental level: evidence of accomplishing developmental tasks for age group
- Psychosocial history: sources of stress, coping mechanisms, self-concept
- Values and belief system: cultural and ethnic background, spiritual beliefs, participation in religious activities, personal and cultural remedies
- Sociocultural history: role in family, relationships, occupational history
- Activities of daily living: patterns of nutrition, elimination, rest/sleep, and activity/exercise
- Review of systems: recent signs and symptoms associated with body systems

---

self-conscious or embarrassed using the technique of inspection; however, most become comfortable with the technique over time. Nurses must also be sensitive to the client's feelings of embarrassment with the use of inspection and respond to this situation by discussing the technique with the client and using measures such as draping in order to increase the client's comfort level.

## CLINICAL ALERT

### Palpation

Deep palpation is a technique requiring expertise and should not be employed by beginning nursing students without supervision.

**Palpation**    **Palpation** uses the sense of touch to assess texture, temperature, moisture, organ location and size, vibrations and pulsations, swelling, masses, and tenderness. Palpation requires a calm, gentle approach and is used systematically, with light palpation preceding deep palpation and palpation of tender areas performed last.

The technique of palpation uses the hands and fingers in different ways for assessment of:

- *Temperature:* Best detected using the dorsal (back) surface of the hand
- *Texture, pulses, and swelling:* Best detected using fingertips
- *Vibration:* Best detected with the base of the fingers
- *Shape and consistency of organs or masses:* Best detected by grasping organ or mass between fingertips

**Percussion**    **Percussion** uses short, tapping strokes on the surface of the skin to create vibrations of underlying organs. It is used for assessing the density of structures or determining the location and the size of organs in the body. Structures with relatively more air (such as the lungs) produce louder, deeper, and longer sounds with percussion than more dense, solid structures (such as the liver), which produce softer, higher, and shorter sounds (Figure 11-3).

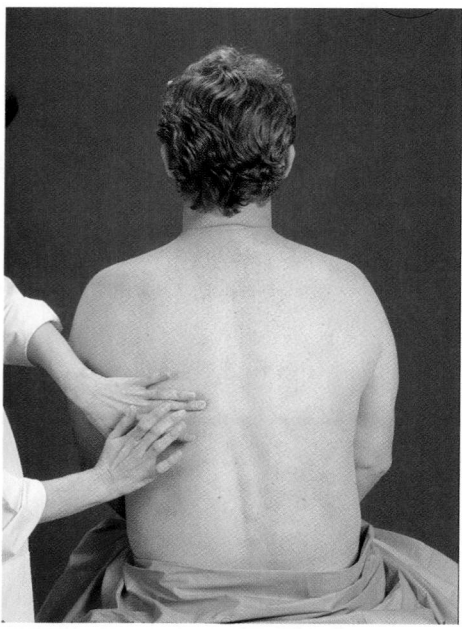

**Figure 11-3    A nurse using percussion to assess the posterior thorax of a client.**

**Auscultation**    **Auscultation** involves listening to sounds in the body that are created by movement of air or fluid. Areas most often auscultated include the lungs, heart, abdomen, and blood vessels. Although direct auscultation is sometimes possible, a stethoscope is usually employed in order to channel the sound.

### Laboratory and Diagnostic Data

Results of laboratory and diagnostic tests can be useful objective data as these values often serve as defining characteristics for various altered health states; these can also be helpful in ruling out certain suspected problems. For example, diabetic clients who are poorly controlled on diet, medication, or both will usually have an elevated blood glucose level. The pattern of these types of variations is useful in determining a plan of care. In addition, the effectiveness of nursing and medical interventions and progress toward health restoration are often monitored through laboratory and diagnostic test data.

## Data Verification

**Data verification** is the process through which data are validated as being complete and accurate. Once the nurse completes the initial data collection, the data are reviewed for inconsistencies or omissions. This process is particularly important if data sources are considered unreliable. For example, if a client is confused or unable to communicate, or if two sources provide conflicting data, it is necessary for the nurse to seek further information or clarification. Data verification is done by examining the congruence between subjective and objective data. For example, a client might exhibit nonverbal expressions of pain (e.g., guarding a part of the body, facial grimacing) but verbally deny feeling pain. The nurse would need to consider possible reasons for this discrepancy in findings and collect more information before formulating conclusions or planning care. Findings should also be compared with norms. Any grossly abnormal findings should be rechecked and confirmed (Ackley & Ladwig, 2002).

## Data Organization

After data collection is completed and information is validated, the nurse organizes, or clusters, the information together in order to identify areas of strength and weakness. This process is known as **data clustering.** How data are organized depends on the assessment model used.

### Assessment Models

An **assessment model** is a framework that provides a systematic method for organizing data. The use of a model helps to ensure comprehensive and organized data collection. A guiding framework also provides direction for decision making about nursing diagnoses. A number of nursing and nonnursing models are used to assist with organization of data. This section describes only a few of the many assessment models available to nurses.

## Nursing Models

Nursing models have been developed to focus on a wide range of human responses to alterations in health status. These models typically include psychosocial, sociocultural, and behavioral data as well as biophysical data. Nursing models may offer the advantage of organizing information in a mode that more easily allows transition from data collection to nursing diagnoses.

### Functional Health Patterns

Marjory Gordon's Human Functional Health Patterns (Gordon, 1997) is not based on a particular theory of nursing but does provide a systematic framework for data collection that focuses on 11 functional health patterns. These patterns can be used in assessment of individuals, families, and communities.

These functional health pattern areas allow gathering and clustering of information about a client's usual patterns and any recent changes in order to determine if the client's response is functional or dysfunctional. For example, the activity-exercise pattern is assessed for a client who recently experienced a stroke. Data collection would be focused on mobility and exercise patterns prior to the stroke, current muscle strength and joint mobility, and the effect of any changes on the client's lifestyle and functional ability.

### Human Response Patterns

The North American Nursing Diagnosis Association (NANDA), in an effort to standardize terminology related to client problems, has developed a taxonomy of nursing diagnoses (North American Nursing Diagnosis Association, 2003). The first taxonomy was completed in 1973 and consisted of 31 diagnostic categories. This taxonomy has developed into over 100 diagnostic categories arranged in a hierarchical structure that is organized according to nine human response patterns. This framework suggests that a person's health status is evidenced by observable phenomena that can be classified into one of these response patterns. These human response patterns can then be used as a model for organizing data collection.

### Theory of Self-Care

The theory of self-care, developed by Orem (1995), is based on a client's ability to perform self-care activities. Self-care is a learned behavior and a deliberate action in response to a need. It includes activities that an individual performs to maintain health. A major focus of this theory is the appraisal of the client's ability to meet self-care needs and the identification of existing self-care deficits. Since this theory focuses on deficits in care, it primarily addresses illness states.

### Roy Adaptation Model

The Roy Adaptation Model is organized around adaptive behaviors (Andrews & Roy, 1991). The individual is con-

sidered a product of biologic, psychological, and sociological influences and is in constant interaction with the environment. The ability of the person to cope with internal and external stressors determines the health status of the individual. Assessment is focused toward an individual's response to stimuli in the environment in the areas of physiological status, self-concept, role function, and interdependence.

### Leininger Sunrise Model

Madeline Leininger (2001), a well-known nurse anthropologist, postulates that caring is the essence of nursing and that human caring, although culturally derived, varies among cultures in its expressions, processes, and patterns. In the early 1990s, she developed the Sunrise Model to depict cultural care diversity and universality. This model provides a framework for areas of concern. The Sunrise Model emphasizes that health and care are influenced by elements of the social structure, such as technology, religious and philosophical factors, kinship and social systems, cultural values, political and legal factors, economic factors, and educational factors. These social factors are addressed within environmental contexts, language expressions, and ethnohistory. Each of these systems is part of any society's social structure; health care expressions, patterns, and practices are also integral parts of these social factors (Leininger, 1993). A culturally relevant assessment starts with the client's reality. By letting the clients tell their story and asking reflective questions to ensure understanding, the nurse learns to make sense of the cultural context of the health care needs, client behaviors, social roles, values and beliefs, and economic and educational factors.

## Nonnursing Models

Nursing, of course, neither exists nor functions in a vacuum. Nursing uses related health concepts from other disciplines, some of which are discussed next.

### Body Systems Model

Approaching data collection by examining body systems is sometimes referred to as the "medical model," since it is frequently used by physicians to investigate presence or absence of disease. This method organizes data collection according to the organ and tissue function in various body systems (e.g., cardiovascular, respiratory, gastrointestinal). Although nurses often use this method as well, the body systems model does not facilitate the formulation of nursing diagnoses. In addition, psychosocial aspects of the client's status are often neglected with resultant fragmentation of care.

### Hierarchy of Needs

Abraham Maslow's hierarchy (1970) of needs proposes that an individual's basic needs (physiological) must be met before progressing to higher-level needs. Maslow's framework can be used to prioritize needs. Use of a hierarchy of needs model requires initial assessment of all

## RESEARCH FOCUS

**Title of Study:** Factors associated with adherence to treatment regimens after lung transplantation

**Study Purpose:** This study was designed to examine the demographic and psychological factors associated with compliance in clients who have had lung transplants.

**Methods:** Eighteen women and 13 men, an average of 24 months post-transplant, completed a demographic form, a self-report compliance measure, a social support questionnaire, and the Multidimensional Health Locus of Control Scale. A significant other or family member and the post-transplant nurse coordinator also assessed the client's compliance with the post-transplant regimen.

**Findings:** Five findings are of note:
- Although clients rated themselves as being compliant with aspects of their self-care, on more subtle measures of compliance their self-reported compliance was not as impressive.
- Clients with more recent transplants appeared more compliant.
- Clients with cystic fibrosis used their spirometer more often than clients with other lung diseases.
- Family support significantly correlated with self-reported compliance.
- Clients' and family members' ratings were significantly correlated across a variety of compliance measures, while clients' and transplant coordinators' compliance rates were not as consistently correlated.

**Implications:** How researchers ask clients about treatment adherence may influence clients' perceptions of compliance. Clients may become less compliant the longer it has been since their transplant, which may imply the need for periodic reassessment of educational and self-care needs. Longitudinal studies are needed to assess the degree to which compliance affects the number of rejection and febrile episodes as well as client mortality after lung transplant.

Teichman, B. J., Burker, E. J., Weiner, M., & Egan, T. M. (2000). Factors associated with adherence to treatment regimens after lung transplantation. *Progress in Transplantation, 10*(2), 113–121.

## STOP AND THINK

### Assessment Models

Consider the following client data:

- Breathing is rapid and labored.
- Client states "nervous about what might be wrong."
- Unable to eat or sleep for last 3 days.
- Becomes short of breath with minimal activity.
- Unable to work for 3 days. Client is afraid will not be able to return to work.

Where would each observation be included using the various models described? Which of these models do you feel most comfortable using? Why?

physiological needs, followed by assessment of higher-level needs. Using Maslow's theory, a person's needs should be addressed in the following order:

First: Physiological needs—the basic survival needs, such as food, water, and oxygen

Second: Safety and security needs—both physical (e.g., protection from bodily harm) and psychological (e.g., security and stability) needs

Third: Need for love and belonging—humans have an innate need to be a part of a group and to feel accepted by others

Fourth: Self-esteem needs—individuals need to feel they are valued and worthwhile

Fifth: Self-actualization needs—the need to function at one's optimal level and to be personally fulfilled.

## Data Interpretation and Documentation

Data clustering facilitates recognition of patterns and determination of further data that are needed. **Data interpretation** is necessary for identification of nursing diagnoses.

Accurate and complete recording of assessment data are essential for communicating information to other health care team members. In addition, documentation is the basis for determining quality of care and should include appropriate data to support identified problems (Figures 11-4 through 11-7).

### Types of Assessment Formats

Health care agencies may choose from a variety of assessment forms for documentation depending on the type of

**Application:  Assessment in the Industrial Clinic**

The following is an example of an occupational health history used in industrial settings.

I.    **Current Job:**

A.  What is your current job title? _____

B.  How long have you had this job?_____

C.  What are specific tasks you perform on the job?_____

_____

_____

D.  Are you exposed to any of the following on your present job?

___Chemicals          ___Infectious agents          ___Stress

___Dusts              ___Loud noise                ___Vapors, gases

___Extreme            ___Radiation                 ___Vibrations
temperature
changes

E.  Do you think you have any work-related health problems?

If so, describe:_____

F.  How would you describe your satisfaction with your job?

___Very satisfied  ___Satisfied  ___Somewhat satisfied  ___Dissatisfied  ___Very Dissatisfied

G.  Have there been any recent changes in your job or work hours?

H.  Do you use protective equipment/clothing on your job?

If so, list items used:_____

II.    **Past Work Experience:**

Please provide the following information, starting with your first job:

| Job Title | Dates Held | Brief description of job | Exposures | Injuries/Illnesses |
|-----------|-----------|--------------------------|-----------|--------------------|
|           |           |                          |           |                    |

**Figure 11-4    Application: assessment in the industrial clinic**

**HEALTH HISTORY**

Name_____     Date_____ Time_____

**Demographic Data:** Date of birth_____     Gender_____ _____     Marital status_____

**Reason for Seeking Health Care:**_____
_____

**Perception of Health Status:**_____
_____

**Previous Illness/Hospitalization/Surgeries:**_____
_____

**Client/Family Medical History:**
Addiction(drugs/alcohol)_____     Diabetes_____     Mental disorders_____
Arthritis_____     Heart disease_____     Sickle cell anemia_____
Cancer_____     Hypertension_____     Stroke_____
Chronic lung disease_____     Kidney disease_____     Other_____

**Immunizations/Exposure to Communicable Disease:**_____
_____

**Allergies:**_____
_____

**Home Medications:**_____
_____

**Developmental Level:**_____
_____

**Psychosocial History:**
Alcohol use:_____
Tobacco use:_____
Drug use:_____
Caffeine intake:_____

**Self-perception/Self-concept:**_____
_____

**Sociocultural History:**
Family structure_____
Role in family_____
Cultural/ethnic group_____
Occupation/work role_____
Relationships with others_____

**Activities of Daily Living:**
*Nutrition:* Type of diet_____     Usual weight_____
Eating patterns_____
Types of snacks_____
Food likes/dislikes_____
Fluid intake: Type_____     Amount_____
*Elimination (usual patterns):* Urinary_____     Bowel_____
*Sleep/Rest:*
Usual sleep patterns_____
Relaxation techniques/patterns_____
*Activity/Exercise:*
Usual exercise patterns_____
Ability to perform self-care activities_____

**Review of Systems:**
**Respiratory**_____
**Circulatory**_____
**Integumentary**_____
**Musculoskeletal**_____
**Neurosensory**_____
**Reproductive/Sexuality**_____

**Health Maintenance Activities:**
Usual source of health care_____
Date of last exam (physical, dental, eye)_____
Other health maintenance activities_____

**Figure 11-5    Sample assessment form: open-ended**

# NORTH OAKS MEDICAL CENTER
## Initial Nursing Patient Assessment

| Admission Date | Room | Time |
|---|---|---|
| | | ___ AM ___ PM |

How admitted: ☐ Ambulatory ☐ Wheelchair ☐ Stretcher ☐ Ambulance ☐ Other: ___

Accompanied by: ☐ Family ☐ Friend ☐ Other: ___

| VITAL SIGNS | | ORIENTATION | | |
|---|---|---|---|---|
| Temperature | Height | Call Light/Bed Control ☐ | Visitation Rules ☐ | Bed locked ☐ |
| Pulse | Weight (Actual)) lbs. | Television ☐ | Phone ☐ | |
| Respiration | | Educational Channels ☐ | Bathroom/Emergency Light ☐ | |
| B/P | | Lights ☐ | ID Band On ☐ | |

### PERSONAL ESSENTIALS LIST / TRANSFER INFORMATION

| Valuables to Safe ☐ No ☐ Yes (list on valuables envelope only) ☐ Sent Home | Date/Room | Date/Room | Date/Room | Date/Room |
|---|---|---|---|---|
| Essentials at bedside: (check only those that apply) Rings: ☐ Plain yellow metal ☐ Yellow metal with stone ☐ Plain white metal ☐ White metal with stone | | | | |
| Watch – Describe | | | | |
| Hearing Aid ☐ Left ☐ Right | | | | |
| ☐ Eyeglasses ☐ Contacts ☐ Right ☐ Left | | | | |
| Dentures Full: ☐ Upper ☐ Lower Partial: ☐ Upper ☐ Lower | | | | |
| Other (wheelchair, prosthesis, cane, etc.) | Admission | Sending RN | Sending RN | Sending RN |
| | | Receiving RN | Receiving RN | Receiving RN |

### ALLERGIES

☐ No Known Allergies ☐ Yes

Allergy: ___ Type of Reaction: ___

| HEALTH PERCEPTION/HEALTH MANAGEMENT PATTERN (May be completed by RN or LPN) | Nursing Diagnosis (Must be completed by RN) |
|---|---|
| 1. Informant: ☐ Patient ☐ Family Member ☐ Friend ☐ Unable to Obtain | ☐ Health Maintenance. Altered |
| 2. Present Illness/Current Complaint/Reason for Hospitalization: | ☐ Noncompliance (Specify) |
| 3. Date last admitted to North Oaks Medical Center ☐ Never admitted | ☐ Infection, Potential for |
| 4. Previous Hospitalization/Surgical Procedures: | ☐ Injury, Potential for ☐ Other (Specify) |

5. Medical History: ☐ Diabetes ☐ Respiratory Disease ☐ Cancer ☐ Kidney Disease ☐ Mental Illness ☐ Hypertension ☐ Hepatitis ☐ GI Disease ☐ Thyroid Disease ☐ Arthritis ☐ Heart Disease ☐ Vision Disorder ☐ Sickle Cell ☐ Neuro-Muscular Disorders ☐ Sexually Transmitted Disease ☐ Tuberculosis ☐ Seizure Disorder ☐ Blood Disorder ☐ Problems with Anesthesia ☐ Other:

6. Medications: Including OTC Drugs/Treatment Used at Home
☐ See Emergency Department Medication Review Sheet ☐ List below if Patient not seen in Emergency Room

| Name | Dose/Frequency | Time Last Dose |
|---|---|---|
| | | |
| | | |
| | | |

Insulins:
Transdermals:

7. Do you take your medications as ordered? ☐ Yes ☐ No Why? ___

8. Disposition of Medications: ☐ Not Brought with Patient ☐ Sent Home with Family ☐ Sent to Pharmacy

9. Use of: ☐ Alcohol ☐ Tobacco ☐ Recreational Drugs ☐ Alcohol ☐ Tobacco ☐ Recreational Drugs
How Much ___ How Long ___

*(continues)*

**Figure 11-6** Sample assessment form: checklist. *Reprinted with permission of North Oaks Medical Center, Hammond, LA*

| SYSTEMS ASSESSMENT | (May be completed by RN or LPN) | Nursing Diagnosis (Must be completed by RN) |
|---|---|---|

**Cardiovascular**

☐ Chest Pain  Rhythm: ☐ Regular  Radial ☐ Palpable  Dorsalis ☐ Palpable  Edema: ☐ Present
☐ Orthopnea  ☐ Irregular  Pulses: ☐ Non-palpable  Pedis: ☐ Non-palpable  ☐ Pitting
☐ Hypertension  Type: ☐ Pounding  ☐ Other  ☐ Other  ☐ Non-pitting
☐ Pacemaker  ☐ Thready  ☐ Absent
☐ Apical Pulse  ☐ Weak

**Respiratory**

☐ Cough  Chest ☐ Symmetrical  Breath ☐ Labored  Breath ☐ Clear all lobes
☐ Productive  Appearance: ☐ Asymmetrical  Pattern: ☐ Non-labored  Sounds: ☐ Equal & Bilateral
☐ Non-productive  ☐ Crackles
☐ Dyspnea  ☐ Rhonchi
☐ Orthopnea  ☐ Wheezes

**Cardiopulmonary**

** 1. Mobility Status: ☐ Ambulatory ☐ Ambulatory with Assist ☐ Bedrest ☐ Transfer with Assist ☐ Walker
2. Assistive Devices: ☐ None ☐ Cane ☐ Wheelchair ☐ Crutches ☐ Prosthesis ☐ Pillows #_____
☐ Other _____
3. Limitations ☐ None ☐ Weakness ☐ Fatigue ☐ Other _____
_____
4. Do you have enough energy for desired activity? ☐ Yes ☐ No  Describe _____
5. Activities of Daily Living: I=Independent  A=Assist  D=Dependent
___ Feeding ___ Bathing ___ Grooming  Describe _____
___ Toileting ___ Dressing ___ Other

Nursing Diagnosis column:
☐ Activity Intolerance
☐ Airway Clearance. Ineffective
☐ Breathing Pattern. Ineffective
☐ Decreased Cardiac Output
☐ Activity Intolerance. Potential
☐ Gas Exchange Impaired
☐ Home Maintenance Management. Impaired
☐ Physical Mobility. Impaired
☐ Self-Care Deficit (Specify)
☐ Other (Specify)

**Musculoskeletal**

** ☐ Pain  ☐ Cramping  Muscle strength: (S=Strong  W=Weak  N=None)
☐ Joint Stiffness  ☐ Spasms  Grips: ☐ Right ☐ Left
☐ Swelling  ☐ Tremors  Pushes: ☐ Right ☐ Left

**Neurological**

** ☐ Headache/Pain  Pupil Size: ☐ PERL  Level of ☐ Alert  Oriented to: ☐ Person
☐ Motor Disturbances  ☐ Other  Consciousness: ☐ Stuporous  ☐ Place
☐ Seizures  Right _____  ☐ Semicomatose  ☐ Time
☐ Numbness  Left _____  ☐ Comatose  ☐ Event
☐ Tingling  ☐ Combative
☐ Anxious
☐ Confused

** 1. Visual Impairment ☐ None ☐ Wears Glasses   4. Communication/Language Barrier: ☐ Yes ☐ No
☐ Contacts   5. Level of Education:
☐ Blind _____ Right _____ Left   Grade _____
2. Hearing Impairment ☐ None ☐ Hard of Hearing   6. Pain/Discomfort:
☐ Deaf _____ Right _____ Left   Describe: _____
☐ Uses Hearing Aid _____ Right _____ Left   A. Precipitating Factors:
3. Speech Impairment   Describe: _____
☐ None ☐ Cannot Express   _____
☐ Slurring ☐ Cannot Understand   B. How is pain controlled?
☐ Mute ☐ Tracheostomy   Describe: _____
☐ Stutters ☐ Laryngectomy

Nursing Diagnosis column:
☐ Pain
☐ Pain Chronic
☐ Communication. Impaired Verbal
☐ Knowledge Deficit (Specify)
☐ Injury. Potential for
☐ Sensory/Perception. Altered (Specify)
☐ Thought Processes. Altered
☐ Unilateral Neglect
☐ Other (Specify) _____

**Integumentary**

☐ Normal  Temperature: ☐ Hot  Describe: ☐ Decubitus ☐ Bruises
☐ Pale  ☐ Warm  ☐ Rashes ☐ Scars
☐ Flushed  ☐ Cool  ☐ Wounds ☐ None Visible
☐ Cyanotic  Turgor: ☐ Good  ☐ Lesions ☐ Other
☐ Jaundiced  ☐ Fair
☐ Other  ☐ Poor
☐ Skin Intact

(body figures illustration)  cm  1  2  3  4  5

**Nutritional / Metabolic**

1. Special Diet: ☐ Yes ☐ No
Describe: _____
2. Frequency of Meals: _____
Describe: _____
3. Recent Changes in Appetite / Eating / Patterns? ☐ Yes ☐ No
Describe: _____
_____
4. Have you experienced ☐ Indigestion ☐ Vomiting ☐ Difficulty Chewing ☐ Choking with Meals
current/recent ☐ Nausea ☐ Sore Mouth ☐ Difficulty Swallowing ☐ Full Feeling in Throat
Describe: _____
5. Recent Weight Loss/Gain? ☐ Yes ☐ No
Describe: _____

Nursing Diagnosis column:
☐ Body Temperature. Potential Altered
☐ Fluid Volume Deficit
☐ Fluid Volume Excess
☐ Swallowing Impaired
☐ Infection. Potential for
☐ Nutrition. Less than Body Requirements. Altered
☐ Nutrition. More than Body Requirements. Altered
☐ Oral Mucous Membrane. Altered
☐ Skin Integrity. Impaired
☐ Skin Integrity. Potential Impaired
☐ Other (Specify)

| HEALTH PATTERNS ASSESSMENT | (May be completed by RN or LPN) | |
|---|---|---|

**Gastrointestinal**

General ☐ Well Nourished  Oral ☐ Dry  Bowel ☐ Present  ☐ Ostomies
Appearance: ☐ Malnourished  Mucosa: ☐ Moist  Sounds: ☐ Absent  ☐ Gastrostomy
☐ Obese  ☐ Nasogastric
☐ Jejunostomy

**Figure 11-6**   *(continued)*

## Patients At Risk to Develop Pressure Sores  (May be completed by an LPN)

Identify any patient at risk to develop pressure sores by assessing the seven clinical condition parameters and assigning a score. Patients with intact skin, but scoring 8 or greater, should have the Nursing Diagnosis "Potential Impairment of Skin Integrity." Directions: Choose the number which best describes the patient's status. Total the seven numbers.

| Clinical Condition Parameters | Score | Clinical Condition Parameters | Score | Clinical Condition Parameters | Score |
|---|---|---|---|---|---|
| **General physical condition (health problem)**<br>Good (minor) — 0<br>Fair (major but stable) — 1<br>Poor (chronic/serious not stable) — 2 | | **Mobility (extremities)**<br>Full active range — 0<br>Limited movement with assistance — 2<br>Move only with assistance — 4<br>Immobile — 6 | | **Skin/Tissue Status**<br>Good (well nourished/skin intact) — 0<br>Fair (poorly nourished/skin intact) — 1<br>Poor (skin not intact) — 2 | |
| **Level of Conciousness (to commands)**<br>Alert (responds readily) — 0<br>Lethargic (slow to respond) — 1<br>Semi-Comatose (responds only to verbal or painful stimuli) — 2<br>Comatose (no response to stimuli) — 3 | | **Incontinence (bowel and/or bladder)**<br>None — 0<br>Occasional (less than 2x in 24 hours) — 2<br>Usually (more than 2x in 24 hours) — 4<br>No Control — 6 | | **Nutrition (for age and size)**<br>Good (eats/drinks adequately—3/4 of meal) — 0<br>Fair (eats/drinks inadequately – at least 1/2 meal) — 1<br>Poor (unable/refuses to eat/drink – less then 1/2 meal) — 2 | |
| **Activity**<br>Ambulant without assistance — 0<br>Ambulant with assistance — 2<br>Chairfast — 4<br>Bedfast — 6 | | | | Total | |

### HEALTH PATTERNS ASSESSMENT                    (May be completed by RN or LPN) cont.

**Nursing Diagnosis** (Must be completed by RN)

**Genito-urinary**

Description per _____ Nurse _____ Patient

Urine Color:  ☐ Clear  ☐ Hematuria  ☐ Bladder Distention  ☐ Suprapubic Catheter
☐ Dark  ☐ Cloudy  ☐ Foley Catheter  ☐ Urostomy
☐ Other  ☐ Dialysis Access _____

**Elimination**

Description per _____ Nurse _____ Patient

1. Bowel:  ☐ No Problems  ☐ Diarrhea  ☐ Pain  ☐ Blood in stool
☐ Constipation  ☐ Incontinence  ☐ Hemorrhoids  ☐ Other
Describe: _____

2. Bladder:  ☐ No Problems  ☐ Incontinence  ☐ Frequency  ☐ Burning  ☐ Nocturia
☐ Retention  ☐ Dribbling  ☐ Dysuna  ☐ Urgency  ☐ Other
Describe: _____

3. Interventions:  ☐ None  ☐ Laxatives  ☐ Suppositories  ☐ Enemas  ☐ Other
Describe: _____

*Nursing Diagnosis:*
☐ Constipation
☐ Diarrhea
☐ Incontinence. Bowel
☐ Incontinence. Functional
☐ Incontinence. Total
☐ Urinary Elimination. Altered
☐ Urinary Retention
☐ Other (Specify)
_____

**Reproductive**

*Male*
☐ Penile Discharge  ☐ Pain  ☐ Inguinal Mass  ☐ Penile Implant  ☐ Other
☐ Tenderness  ☐ Scrotal Mass  ☐ Breast Lumps  ☐ STD's (Sexual Transmitted Diseases)

*Female*
LMP _____    Last Pap Smear _____    Pain with:    Pregnant
Para _____   ☐ Itching     ☐ Breast Lumps   ☐ Menstruation   ☐ Yes
Gravada _____   ☐ Abnormal Bleeding   ☐ PMS   ☐ Intercourse   ☐ No
☐ Contraceptive   ☐ Discharge     ☐ Other

*Nursing Diagnosis:*
☐ Role Performance. Altered
☐ Sexual Dysfunction
☐ Sexuality Patterns. Altered
☐ Rape Trauma Syndrome
☐ Body Image Disturbance
☐ Other (Specify)

**Role Relationship**

1. Home Environment:  ☐ Lives with Spouse  ☐ Lives Alone  ☐ Lives with Family  ☐ Lives with Friend
2. Who do you rely on for emotional support?  ☐ Spouse  ☐ Family  ☐ Friend  ☐ Self  ☐ Other
Describe: _____
3. How does your illness/hospitalization affect your family/significant others?
Describe: _____

*Nursing Diagnosis:*
☐ Communication Impaired
☐ Verbal
☐ Family Processes. Altered
☐ Grieving, Anticipatory
☐ Parenting. Altered
☐ Social Interaction Impaired
☐ Social Isolation

**Coping/Stress**

1. Have you had any recent changes in your life (job, move, divorce, death, major surgeries, recent abuse)?
☐ Yes  ☐ No  Describe: _____
2. Do you feel you are dealing successfully with stresses associated with this change?
Describe: _____

*Nursing Diagnosis:*
☐ Violence. Potential for self-directed or directed toward others
☐ Role Performance. Altered
☐ Fear
☐ Other (Specify)

**Sleep/Rest**

1. Sleep: ☐ No problem  ☐ Difficulty falling asleep  ☐ Difficulty staying asleep  ☐ Does not feel rested after sleep
Other _____
2. What helps you sleep?

*Nursing Diagnosis:*
☐ Sleep Pattern Disturbance
☐ Other (Specify)

**Self-Perception**

1. What concerns you most about your illness/hospitalization?
Describe: _____
2. Does your illness and/or hospitalization affect your sexuality/body image?  ☐ Yes  ☐ No

*Nursing Diagnosis:*
☐ Anxiety
☐ Fear
☐ Powerlessness
☐ Self-Esteem Disturbance
☐ Other (Specify)

**Values Beliefs**

1. Is religion important in your life?  ☐ Yes  ☐ No  ☐ Religion/Faith _____
2. Do you have special religious request during this hospitalization?  ☐ Yes  ☐ No  ☐ Notify Volunteer Services for Clergy
Describe: _____

*Nursing Diagnosis:*
☐ Spiritual Distress
☐ Other (Specify)

**Safety**

1. All areas with ** should be considered for FPP.
2. FPP should automatically be instituted for pts. who have/are:  A) fallen previously
B) confused, disoriented or combative
C) chemical or physical restraints required

**Figure 11-6**  *(continued)*

# ADMISSION ASSESSMENT

Date_____ Time_____

Admitted from: Home____ER____Other____

Allergies_____

Baseline Data:  Ht____Wt____T____P____R____BP____

Mode of Transport:  Stretcher____W/C____Amb____

Home Meds:    _____    _____
              _____    _____
              _____    _____

| Mental Status | | | Comment |
|---|---|---|---|
| Alert/Oriented | Yes | No | _____ |
| Confused | Yes | No | _____ |
| Anxious | Yes | No | _____ |
| Comatose | Yes | No | _____ |
| Combative | Yes | No | _____ |

Other_____

| Communication | | | Comment |
|---|---|---|---|
| Speaks English | Yes | No | _____ |
| Aphasic | Yes | No | _____ |
| Speech Impediment | Yes | No | _____ |

| Sensory | | | Comment |
|---|---|---|---|
| Hearing Impaired | Yes | No | _____ |
| Visually Impaired | Yes | No | _____ |
| Amputation | Yes | No | _____ |
| Hemiplegia | Yes | No | _____ |
| Paraplegia | Yes | No | _____ |

## Diet/Nutrition

Diet at Home_____

Likes/Dislikes_____

Appetite_____

| Skin | | | Location |
|---|---|---|---|
| Warm/Dry | Yes | No | _____ |
| Abrasions/Bruises | Yes | No | _____ |
| Laceration/Scar | Yes | No | _____ |
| Reddened Areas | Yes | No | _____ |
| Decubitus Ulcers | Yes | No | _____ |
| Burns | Yes | No | _____ |
| Rash/Scaling | Yes | No | _____ |
| Diaphoretic | Yes | No | _____ |

Other_____

Color:        Pale    Normal    Cyanotic

**Treatments in Progress**_____
_____
_____

| Elimination | | | Comment |
|---|---|---|---|
| GI: Constipation | Yes | No | _____ |
| Frequency | Yes | No | _____ |
| Laxatives | Yes | No | _____ |

Other_____

| GU: Frequency | Yes | No | _____ |
|---|---|---|---|
| Burning | Yes | No | _____ |
| Incontinent | Yes | No | _____ |

Other_____

| Sleeping | | | Comment |
|---|---|---|---|
| Unable to fall asleep | Yes | No | _____ |
| Awakens frequently | Yes | No | _____ |
| Sleep meds | Yes | No | _____ |
| Naps | Yes | No | _____ |

| ADL | | | Comment |
|---|---|---|---|

Assistance needed for:

| Ambulation | Yes | No | _____ |
|---|---|---|---|
| Eating | Yes | No | _____ |
| Bathing | Yes | No | _____ |
| Dressing | Yes | No | _____ |
| Eliminating | Yes | No | _____ |
| Turning | Yes | No | _____ |

Other_____

| **Denture** | Yes | No | _____ |
|---|---|---|---|
| **Glasses** | Yes | No | _____ |
| **Contact Lenses** | Yes | No | _____ |

**Personal Habits:**

| Tobacco use | Yes | No | _____ |
|---|---|---|---|
| | | | (quantity) |
| Alcohol use | Yes | No | _____ |
| | | | (quantity) |

**Chief Complaint:**_____
_____
_____

**Other Assessment Data:**_____
_____

**Figure 11-7    Sample assessment form: combination**

agency, the population served by the facility, and the primary reasons for documentation. For example, clients seeking health care in a clinic or physician's office might be asked to complete a brief self-questionnaire, while a client admitted to an acute-care facility for labor and delivery might be asked to provide only information directly related to pregnancy and child care needs. Four types of documentation formats include open-ended, checklist, combination, and specialty. See Figure 11-4 for an example of a form used in occupational nursing.

### Open-Ended Formats

The open-ended format for documentation allows the nurse to write a narrative description of observations (Figure 11-5). This format is more time-consuming for the nurse but allows flexibility in recording findings.

### Checklist Formats

Formats that include checklists facilitate documentation by summarizing findings in an abbreviated form (Figure 11-6). They also provide more consistency in the recording of information and reduce the likelihood of omitting relevant information. However, checklists may discourage nurses from obtaining elaboration about observations from clients that require further explanation. For example, if a checklist indicates that mobility is impaired, further explanation is required in order to determine the extent of the impairment and thus plan the necessary interventions.

### Combination Formats

Combination formats often allow the convenience of a checklist together with space to document a complete narrative description of any significant or abnormal findings (Figure 11-7). Some agencies provide cues on the form to alert personnel when further information is needed. This format provides for some consistency in recording data while allowing flexibility for documenting specific information.

### Specialty Formats

Specialty areas such as outpatient surgery, labor and delivery, and psychiatric facilities may use abbreviated formats focused directly on assessment needs for the particular service provided. In addition, specialty assessment forms may be included together with comprehensive assessment forms for clients at particular risk for various conditions (e.g., falls, impaired skin integrity).

Documentation of assessment data is essential as a means of communication among health care team members to assure accurate problem identification, determination of appropriate client outcomes, and continuity of care.

### The MDS Medicare Prospective Payment System Assessment Form (MPAF)

The Minimum Data Set (MDS) was developed by the Health Care Financing Administration (HCFA) (currently Centers for Medicare and Medicaid Services [CMS]) to perform clinical assessments to facilitate the development of a comprehensive care plan for every resident of Medicare/Medicaid certified nursing homes. As such, the MDS is a standardized assessment instrument used in all skilled and long-term care facilities that are funded by CMS. This comprehensive assessment instrument is designed to collect data on the following client characteristics (Centers for Medicare and Medicade Services, 2003):

- Sensory, cognitive, and communication patterns
- Mood and behavior patterns
- Activities of daily living
- Physical functioning and structural problems
- Medical conditions, medications and treatments, and procedures and therapies
- Discharge potential

## CASE STUDY/NURSING CARE PLAN

Mrs. Juarez, a fashionably dressed and groomed female, 60 years of age, arrived at her gynecologist's office for her scheduled annual appointment. Mrs. Juarez has had an annual gynecological evaluation for the past 10 years. She is married and has three adult children. She does not drink alcohol or smoke. She exercises three times per week at the local health club. She has just retired from working at the local police department as an administrative assistant for 40 years. She is active in her local church group and with the civic women's club. Mrs. Juarez reported that for the past 2 weeks she has had to "go to the bathroom a lot and it burns when I pass my water" and that her urine "smells strong and is a dark orange." When asked how much fluid she consumes daily, Mrs. Juarez responded, "I drink one big cup of coffee in the morning, one can of diet soda at lunch, one glass of milk at dinner, and maybe one glass of water at bedtime." She also stated that "my skin feels very dry and my lower back hurts."

Vital signs revealed a temperature of 100°F, pulse 100, lying blood pressure of 140/78, and a standing blood pressure of 110/70. Height is 5 feet 4 inches; weight, 135 pounds. A urine specimen for urinalysis and for culture

*(continues)*

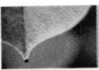
# CASE STUDY/NURSING CARE PLAN (continued)

and sensitivity were ordered by the physician. The nurse observed that Mrs. Juarez's urine was foul-smelling, dark amber, cloudy, and thick. Her skin turgor revealed tenting with the shape remaining for 15 seconds. Her fluid intake for the past 24 hours was 960 cc. The urinalysis revealed a specific gravity >1.030, and the culture and sensitivity report disclosed the presence of *Escherichia coli* with a sensitivity to all penicillins. Her hemoglobin was 14, hematocrit was 45%, and white blood cell count was 12,000. In addition, Mrs. Juarez guards her lower back upon movement.

## Assessment
Client is a 60-year-old female with a urinary tract infection that has existed for the past 2 weeks. She is febrile, has subjective complaints of pain from the infection, and her urine is concentrated, dark colored, and foul smelling.

## Nursing Diagnosis #1
*Impaired Urinary Elimination* related to irritation to bladder secondary to infection as evidenced by foul-smelling, dark amber, cloudy, thick urine; oral temperature 100°F; urine culture reveals *Escherichia coli*.
**NOC:** Urinary Elimination; Urinary Continence
**NIC:**  Urinary Elimination Management

## Expected Outcomes
The client will:
1. Experience no urinary urgency as evidenced by voiding 240 to 400 cc every 6 to 8 hours within 3 days of initiating treatment.
2. Report no pain or burning upon urination within 24 hours of initiating treatment.
3. Be free of infection as evidenced by clear, non-foul-smelling urine; pain-free urination; white blood count between 5,000 and 10,000 within 3 days of initiating treatment.

## Planning/Interventions/Rationales
1. Evaluate previous patterns of voiding. *Voiding patterns are unique to each client and can vary. Urinary tract infection can cause retention but is more likely to cause frequency.*
2. Assess the balance between intake and output. *Intake greater than output may indicate retention.*
3. Monitor results of urinalysis, urine culture, and sensitivity. *Retention of urine can predispose the client to urinary tract infections.*
4. Assess client description of pain: quality, nature, and severity using a pain rating scale every 4 hours. *Urinary tract infections are described as burning on urination; if renal involvement, client may experience back or flank pain.*
5. Encourage fluids by offering fluids of choice every 2 hours. *Fluid intake should be 1,500 cc per 24 hours to promote renal blood flow and flush bacteria from urinary tract.*

## Evaluation
Client's urine is clear and non-foul-smelling, and white blood cell count is between 5,000 and 10,000 within 3 days of initiating treatment. The client is free of urinary urgency and voids 240 to 400 cc every 6 to 8 hours within 3 days of initiating treatment. In addition, the client rates the severity of burning upon urination as a 0 on a severity rating scale of 0 to 5 (with 0 being no burning and 5 severe burning upon urination) within 24 hours of initiating treatment.

## Nursing Diagnosis #2
*Deficient Knowledge* related to lack of information about causes for urinary tract infections and not seeking health care treatment.
**NOC:** Knowledge: Disease Process; Health Behaviors; Health Resources; Infection Control; Treatment Procedures; Treatment Regimen
**NIC:**  Teaching: Disease Process; Teaching: Individual

*(continues)*

**CASE STUDY/NURSING CARE PLAN** *(continued)*

### Expected Outcomes

The client will:

1. Accurately verbalize measures to prevent or reduce risk of reinfection by eliminating beverages with caffeine, consuming liquids or products that acidify urine, and drinking at least 1,500 cc of fluids per 24 hours within 7 days of initiation of treatment and at the follow-up appointment visit.
2. Implement measures that will reduce the risk for introduction of pathogens into the urethra.

### Planning/Interventions/Rationales

1. Assess knowledge of nature of urinary tract infections. *To identify client's knowledge and understanding of the risk factors for urinary tract infections.*
2. Teach client the importance of adequate fluid intake. *Keeps tissues hydrated and decreases bladder irritation.*
3. Teach client to consume products and liquids that acidify urine (e.g., cranberry juice). *Bacteria grow poorly in acidic environment.*
4. Teach client to avoid or reduce caffeine intake. *Caffeine is a diuretic, which may lead to dehydration.*

### Evaluation

Client verbalizes measures to prevent or reduce risk of reinfection by eliminating beverages with caffeine, drinking fluids that acidify urine, and drinking at least 1,500 cc of fluids per 24 hours within 7 days of initiation of treatment and at the follow-up appointment visit. In addition, the client verbalizes that showering, wiping from front to back after voiding, and voiding immediately after sexual intercourse decreases the concentration of pathogens that may enter the urethra.

## Key Concepts

- Assessment includes collection, verification, organization, interpretation, and documentation of data.
- The nurse uses the process of assessment to establish a database about the client, to form an interpersonal relationship with the client, and to provide the client with an opportunity to discuss health care concerns.
- Assessment can be comprehensive, focused, ongoing, or emergency, depending on the health care setting and needs of the client.
- The two types of data collected during the assessment process are subjective (data from the client's point of view) and objective (observable and measurable data that are obtained through both the physical examination and laboratory and diagnostic tests).
- Although a variety of sources should be used in data collection, the client is the primary source of information.
- Assessment models such as Gordon's functional health patterns, NANDA's human response patterns, Orem's theory of self-care model, Roy's adaptation model, Leininger's Sunrise Model, the body systems model, and Maslow's hierarchy of needs model ensure comprehensive data collection and organization.
- Data are collected through the interview, health history, symptom analysis, physical examination, and laboratory and diagnostic tests.
- The three stages of assessment interview are the introduction, working, and closure phases.
- A comprehensive health history is useful in determining the client's functional health patterns, responses to changes in health status, and alterations in lifestyle.
- The elements of the health history are demographic information; reason for seeking health care; perception of health status; previous illnesses, hospitalizations, and surgeries; client/family medical history; immunizations/exposure to communicable disease; allergies; current medications; developmental level; psychosocial history; values/beliefs; sociocultural history; activities of daily living; and review of systems.
- The purposes of the physical examination are to gather baseline data, confirm data obtained in the interview and health history, and evaluate progress toward established goals. The examination includes the techniques of inspection, palpation, percussion, and auscultation.
- Accurate and complete documentation of assessment findings is essential for communication to other health care team members and may be recorded on a variety of assessment tools, such as open-ended, checklist, combination, and specialty formats.

## Review Questions and Activities

1. Write *S* in the blank if the data listed is subjective and *O* if the data is objective:

   \_\_Temperature 103.2  \_\_Right upper quadrant pain
   \_\_Nausea  \_\_Swelling in ankles
   \_\_Hematocrit 33%  \_\_Itching

2. Change each of the following closed-ended questions to open-ended questions:
   a. Are you able to take care of yourself at home?
   b. Is your cough productive?
   c. Are you satisfied with your health status?
   d. Is your chest pain sharp or dull?
3. Millie Jones is a new employee in the corporation in which you are employed as a nurse. What categories of information would you need to include for a complete health history of Ms. Jones?
4. List the four assessment techniques, and give an example of how each is used in a physical examination.
5. In reviewing data collected from Mr. Robbins, a client admitted to the adult acute care unit, you note his statement that he takes his blood pressure medication as prescribed. His blood pressure is very high (190/110). His wife does not remember the prescription being filled for over 2 months. What would you say to Mr. Robbins to clarify this incongruence?
6. Mr. Larsen, age 72, is visiting the clinic with a complaint of difficulty urinating. What type of assessment is most appropriate for this situation?
7. Identify the stage of assessment interview for each of the following statements made by the nurse. Write *IP* for interview preparation, *I* for introduction, *W* for working, and *C* for closure.
   ___ "I need about 10 minutes to ask you questions about your health practices."
   ___ "I reviewed your record prior to your visit."
   ___ "What would you like to talk about?"
   ___ "Our time together is almost over; you expressed your concerns about how to manage your care following discharge from the clinic."

## Multimedia Links

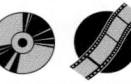

Christensen *Core Concept Videos: Nursing Process*

## Web Resources

American Nurses Association
   http://www.nursingworld.org
Centers for Medicare and Medicaid Services
   http://www.cms.gov
North American Nursing Diagnosis Association
   http://www.nanda.org

## References

Ackley, B. J., & Ladwig, G. B. (2002) *Nursing diagnosis handbook: A guide to planning care* (5th ed.). St. Louis: Mosby.

Alfaro-LeFevre, R. (2002). *Applying nursing process: Promoting collaborative care* (5th ed.). Philadelphia: Lippincott.

American Nurses Association (1998). *Standards of clinical nursing practice* (2nd ed.). Washington, DC: Author.

Andrews, H. & Roy, C. (1991). *The Roy Adaptation Model: The definitive statement.* Norwalk, CT: Appelton & Lange.

Desmond, J., & Copeland, L. (2000). *Communicating with today's patient.* San Francisco: Jossey–Bass.

Estes, M. (2002). *Health assessment and physical examination* (2nd ed.). Clifton Park, NY: Delmar Learning.

Gastmans, C. (2002). A fundamental ethical approach to nursing; some proposals for ethics education. *Nursing Ethics, 9*(5), 494–507.

Gordon, M. (1997). *Manual of nursing diagnosis, 1997–1998 edition.* St. Louis: Mosby.

Health Care Financing Administration (n.d.). *MDS 2.0 manual and forms.* http://www.hcfa.gov/medicaid/mds20/man-form.htm

Hogstel, M. O. (2001). *Gerontology: Nursing care of the older adult.* Clifton Park, NY: Delmar Learning.

Hogstel, M. O., & Weeks, S. M. (2000). Mental health. In A.G. Leukenotte (Ed.). *Gerontologic nursing* (2nd ed). St. Louis: Mosby.

Humphrey, C. J. (1998). *Home care nursing handbook* (3rd ed.). Gaithersburg, MD: Aspen.

Leininger, M. M. (Ed.). (2001). *Culture care diversity and universality: A theory of nursing.* New York: National League for Nursing/Jones and Bartlett Publishers: Pub. No. 15-2402.

Leininger, M. M. (1993, Winter). Towards conceptualization of transcultural health care systems: Concepts and a model. *Journal of Transcultural Nursing, 4,* 32–40.

Leukenotte, A. G. (2000). Gerontologic Assessment. In A.G. Leukenotte (Ed.). *Gerontologic nursing* (2nd ed). St. Louis: Mosby

Maslow, A. H. (1970). *Motivation and personality* (2nd ed.). New York: Harper & Row.

Nightingale, Florence. (1969). *Notes on nursing.* New York: Dover Publications, Inc. (Original work published 1860.)

North American Nursing Diagnosis Association (2003). *Nursing diagnoses: Definitions and classification, 2003–2004.* Philadelphia: Author.

Orem, D. E. (1995). *Nursing: Concepts of practice* (5th ed.). St. Louis: Mosby.

Pender, J., Murdaugh, C., & Parsons, M. A. (2002). *Health promotion in nursing practice* (4th ed.). Upper Saddle River, NJ: Prentice-Hall.

Potts, N., & Mandleco, B. (2002). *Pediatric nursing: Caring for children and their families.* Clifton Park, NY: Delmar Learning.

Salvatore, T. (2000). Elder suicide: A gatekeeper strategy for home care. *Home Healthcare Nurse, 18*(3), 180–186.

Teichman, B. J., Burker, E. J., Weiner, M., & Egan, T. M. (2000). Factors associated with adherence to treatment regimens after lung transplantation. *Progress in transplantation, 10*(2), 113–121.

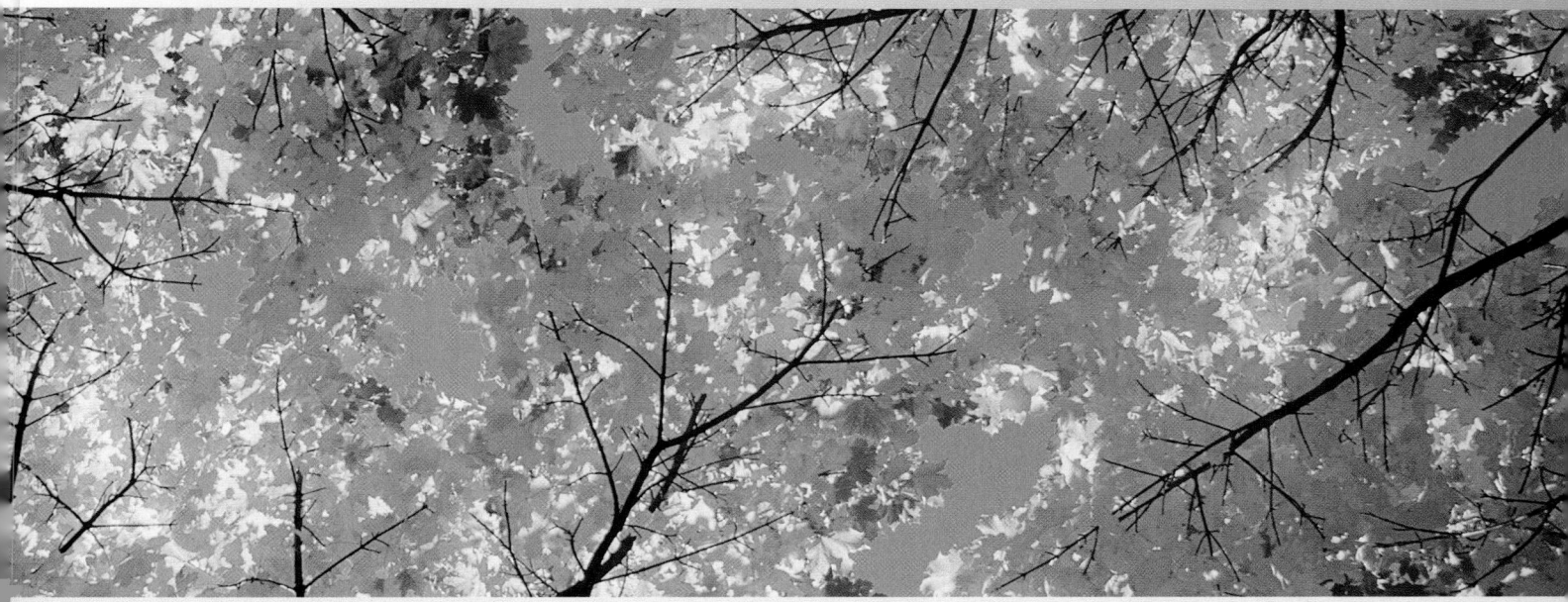

# CHAPTER 12

# Nursing Diagnosis

## Ruth N. Grendell, DNSc, RN

*A true understanding of a behavior requires knowledge about the person (past experiences, present attitudes, and strengths or capabilities) and also, knowledge of the immediate situation from that person's perspective.*

*(Adapted from M. Deutsch, 1968)*

# Chapter Competencies

*Upon completion of this chapter, the reader should be able to:*

1. Define nursing diagnosis as a nursing function, and compare and contrast with medical diagnosis.
2. Identify the historical perspective of the construct of the nursing diagnosis.
3. Explain the purposes of nursing diagnoses.
4. List the components of a nursing diagnosis.
5. Explore characteristics of the nursing diagnosis taxonomy.
6. Describe the process of developing a nursing diagnosis.
7. Identify errors that can occur in the development of a nursing diagnosis.
8. Discuss the limitations of a nursing diagnosis.
9. Explore barriers that can affect the use of a nursing diagnosis.
10. Describe strategies to overcome the barriers to using nursing diagnosis.
11. Describe how a nursing diagnosis enables the delivery of holistic or comprehensive nursing care.
12. Explain how a nursing diagnosis enhances accountability and empowerment in the nursing profession.

# Key Terms

| | | |
|---|---|---|
| cluster | diagnosis | nursing diagnosis |
| cues | etiology | taxonomy of nursing |
| defining characteristics | medical diagnosis | diagnoses |

The **nursing diagnosis** is both a pivotal step in the nursing process and a diagnostic reasoning process. As the second step in the nursing process, it is a professional clinical judgment about individual, family, or community (aggregate) *responses* to actual or at-risk health problems, to wellness states, or to life process events. As a diagnostic reasoning process, nursing diagnosis includes the nurse's critical thinking and interpretation of the meaning and significance of evidence, or cues, derived from assessment data. The purpose of a nursing diagnosis is to effectively communicate the health care needs of individuals and aggregates among members of the health care team and within the health care delivery system. When a nursing diagnosis is a part of the client's plan of care, the nurse is able to communicate the client's needs to other professionals involved in that care. These needs encompass physiological, role function, self-concept, interdependence, and spiritual dimensions. In order to determine individualized therapeutic nursing interventions, the nurse must first collect and organize assessment data before developing appropriate nursing diagnoses.

This chapter describes the nature of a nursing diagnosis, its purposes, and the components of a nursing diagnostic statement. It also discusses the process involved in developing a nursing diagnosis and methods through which nurses can avoid errors in the formulation of nursing diagnoses. This chapter concludes with strategies for overcoming barriers to the use of a nursing diagnosis in the clinical setting (Figure 12-1).

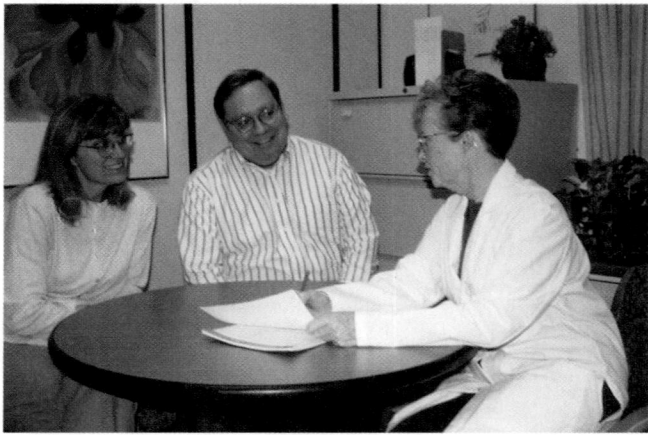

**Figure 12-1    A nurse gathering information from the parents of a pediatric client to develop accurate nursing diagnoses.**

# Definition of Nursing Diagnosis

**Diagnosis** is the science and art of identifying problems or conditions. Members in a variety of professions, including physicians, lawyers, nurses, social workers, psychologists, and educators, use this process. The diagnostic process aids in defining problems and conditions related to the specific professional area of expertise. The process consists of collecting data, critically analyzing the data, forming the data into categories or clusters, validating the data, and identifying the problem or condition. Each nursing diagnosis requires an identified outcome in order to predict expected goals of care. Nursing diagnoses and nursing interventions aid in defining the scope of nursing practice (Figure 12-2).

Many definitions of nursing diagnosis have evolved over the past decades. At the 12th North American Nursing Diagnosis Association (NANDA) conference, the following working definition of nursing diagnosis was approved:

> A clinical judgment about individual, family or community responses to actual and potential health problems/life processes. Nursing diagnoses provide the basis for selection of nursing interventions to achieve outcomes for which the nurse is accountable (North American Nursing Diagnosis Association [NANDA], 1996, p. 8).

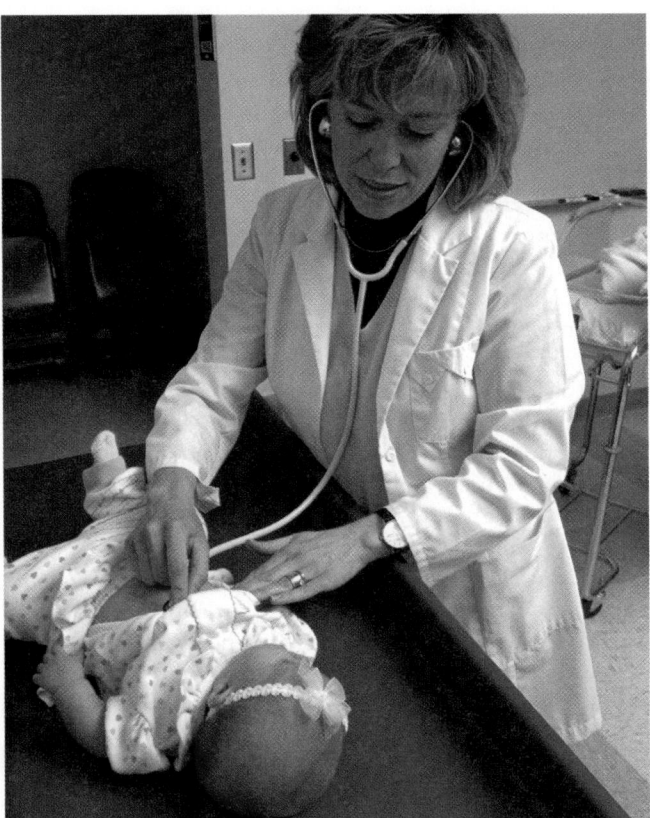

**Figure 12-2  Evaluating heart sounds is essential when a nursing diagnosis involves a decreasing cardiac output.**

Additional definitions of nursing diagnosis abound in the nursing literature. It is clear that although all definitions are not exactly alike, there are similar attributes among them, such as a focus on client-centered problems; the promotion of nursing accountability; an awareness of the human response to health problems; the formation of clinical judgments about individuals, families, or communities; and the development of nursing interventions that a nurse is licensed to enact. Following are selected descriptions of nursing diagnoses that reflect the historical evolution of the concept:

- "A creative approach to nursing involves a nursing diagnosis and the design and means for carrying out a plan for the care of an individual person. There are five areas of patients' needs on which the nursing diagnosis is based . . . treatment and medication, personal hygiene, environmental, guidance and teaching and human or self-needs" (Fry, 1953, p. 301).
- "Use of the term *diagnosis* is gaining acceptance as the logical end product of nursing assessment" (Gebbie & Lavin, 1974, p. 250).
- "A nursing diagnosis is a statement that describes the human response (health state or actual/potential altered interaction pattern) of an individual or group which the nurse can legally identify and for which the nurse can order the definitive interventions to maintain the health state or to reduce, eliminate, or prevent alterations" (Carpenito, 1989, p. 5).
- "Nursing diagnosis is defined in the Roy Adaptation Model as a judgment process resulting in a statement conveying the person's adaptation status" (Roy & Andrews, 1991, p. 37).
- "Nursing diagnosis provides the basis for selection of nursing interventions to achieve outcomes for which the nurse is accountable" (NANDA, 1996, p. 8).
- "Nursing diagnosis deals with identifying the individual's ability to meet human needs with or without assistance, taking into account that person's strength, will and knowledge," Virginia Henderson, pioneer nursing leader and theorist (cited in Anderson, 2000).
- "Nursing diagnosis is a process whereby nurses interpret assessment data and apply standardized labels to health-related phenomena that they identify and anticipate treating" (Berger & Williams, 1999, p. 444).

## Comparison of Nursing and Medical Diagnoses

It is important to have a clear understanding of the nature of a nursing diagnosis as compared to a medical diagnosis. Clarification of this point is necessary to distinguish between the nursing and medical professions and the potential legal ramifications.

Nursing diagnoses assist nurses in defining their scope of practice just as medical diagnoses assist physicians in defining their scope of practice. In addition, the use of diagnoses in nursing and medicine enables clarification of the legal boundaries for practice.

Medicine uses the term *medical diagnosis* and nursing uses the term *nursing diagnosis* to identify problems relating to a client's health status:

- **Medical diagnosis** is the terminology used for a clinical judgment by the physician that identifies or determines a specific disease, condition, or pathologic state.
- **Nursing diagnosis** is the terminology used for a clinical judgment by the professional nurse that identifies the client's or aggregate's actual risk, wellness, or syndrome responses to a health state, problem, or condition.

The philosophy of nursing is holistic in nature, not only indicating a concern for restoring a client to optimal health, but also placing a focus on preventing illness and disease and maintaining health, or relieving pain and discomfort when a return to health is not possible (Doenges, Moorehouse, & Geissler-Murr, 2000). The client is the primary recipient of nursing care and the term *client* can refer to a single individual, small groups, or a collective of individuals in the community. As the understanding of human nature has developed, the client is considered to be more than a person who needs restorative care due to illness or disease. The client is now viewed as a complex entity influenced by interrelationships between the mind, spirit, and body and other individuals, and the environment. This is one of the clearest distinctions between medical models and nursing models. Medical models are restrictive and are almost exclusively devoted to curing diseases and to restoring health (Doenges et al., 2002).

See Box 12-1 for a comparison of nursing and medical diagnoses.

The term *nursing diagnosis* is used in three different contexts: (1) as a data analysis and decision-making process, (2) as a product or diagnostic label, and (3) as an organized classification system, or taxonomy (Berger & Williams, 1999). Taxonomy is a classification system in which the nursing diagnoses are organized according to client responses to specific conditions.

The interdisciplinary relationship between nursing and medicine has implications for both. This relationship also extends to members of other disciplines who have contact with the individual client and family. Data are exchanged, ideas are shared, and plans of care are developed. Clients, as well as the family and significant other(s), are included as much as possible in the process. Although nurses work within the medical and psychosocial domains, nursing's phenomena of concern are the patterns of human response, *not* disease processes (Doenges et al., 2002). Nursing diagnoses and the nursing plan of care involve independent and collaborative nursing actions rather than mimicking medical and psychiatric diagnoses (Ackley & Ladwig, 2002).

Medical and nursing diagnoses have both similarities and differences. The similarities include using the com-

| BOX 12-1 | COMPARISON OF SELECTED NURSING AND MEDICAL DIAGNOSES |
|---|---|
| **Nursing** | **Medicine** |
| *Ineffective Breathing Pattern* | • Chronic Obstructive Pulmonary Disease |
| *Activity Intolerance* | • Cerebrovascular Accident |
| *Acute Pain* | • Appendectomy |
| *Body Image Disturbance* | • Amputation |
| *Risk for Altered Body Temperature* | • Strep Throat |

prehensive diagnostic process in making a clinical judgment (diagnosis), and determining expected outcomes. The diagnosis is the basis for interventions and treatment within the legal dimensions and standards of the respective profession (Ackley & Ladwig, 2002; Berger & Williams, 1999; Doenges et al., 2002). An example of these similarities can be illustrated by considering Alan Brown, a client who has a medical diagnosis of asthma. The physician and nurse would both collect assessment data on respiratory status. The physician would use this information to treat the disease of asthma and the nurse would use this information to focus on Mr. Brown's response to the disease, which would result in a nursing diagnosis of *Ineffective Breathing Pattern*.

Nursing diagnoses are different from medical diagnoses in (1) purpose, (2) goals, and (3) therapeutic interventions. The *purpose* of a nursing diagnosis is to focus on the human response or responses of the individual family or community to identified problems or conditions, including life processes. Medical diagnoses center on the disease state or pathological condition. For example, if the medical diagnosis for Sheila Barrington is breast cancer, appropriate nursing diagnoses may include *Fear*, *Deficient Knowledge* related to treatment measures, *Anticipatory Grieving*, *Body Image Disturbance*, *Powerlessness*, and *Ineffective Coping*. In addition, the *goals* (aims, intent, or ends) that accompany these nursing diagnoses differ, as do the specific, individualized therapeutic nursing *interventions* (nursing actions to promote or restore health and enhance general well-being).

## Historical Perspective

The term *nursing diagnosis* has been in the literature since the early 1950s. Fry (1953) identified that nursing diagnosis is integral to the plan of nursing care and is an important tool for individualizing client care. However, these ideas were slow to gain momentum despite the interests of several nurse theorists and the focus on client-centered problems in the 1960s and the 1970s. In 1973, the First National Conference for the Classification of Nursing Diagnoses convened in St. Louis, Missouri. Nurses met at that time and "began the formal effort to identify, develop, and classify nursing diagnoses" (NANDA, 1996, p. 107). In 1982, at the fifth national conference, the organization was renamed the North American Nursing Diagnosis Association (NANDA). Since its inception, NANDA continues to hold conference meetings every 2 years (NANDA, 2003). At the seventh NANDA national conference in 1986, the Taxonomy I classification was adopted. This classification places nursing diagnoses into nine human response patterns, a categorical order that is applicable to computerization. The definitions of the nine patterns were expanded in 1990. Expanded definitions of the response patterns are discussed later in the chapter. Taxonomy II was adopted at the 14th national conference in 2000 (NANDA, 2001). Refer to Table 12-1 for listings of the two classifications.

Additional endorsement for nursing diagnosis came from the American Nurses Association (ANA) in 1973 in the publication entitled *Standards of Nursing Practice* (American Nurses Association [ANA], 1973). Ongoing discussions occurred in the nursing literature, with increasing support evident by the 1980s for nursing diagnosis and the diagnostic process. The ANA continued to support nursing diagnosis as the second step of the nursing process through publication of *Nursing: A Social Policy Statement* (ANA, 1995) and *Standards of Clinical Nursing Practice* (ANA, 1998). See Box 12-2 for the standard of care related to nursing diagnosis. At the 13th conference in 1998, NANDA developed 21 new nursing diagnoses and revised 37 nursing diagnoses by clarifying existing diagnoses and their definitions, defining their characteristics, and related factors. Following the biennial conference in April 1994, the Taxonomy Committee identified the need to revise the structure of Taxonomy I. During the 14th biennial conference in April 2000, NANDA adopted the taxonomy, Taxonomy II. "Taxonomy II was designed to be multiaxial in its form, thereby substantially improving the flexibility of the nomenclature and allowing for easy additions and modifications" (NANDA, 2001, p. 212). With the publication of these standards, the nurse has both a professional and legal obligation to practice as defined by the professional organization for nurses.

## Nursing Diagnoses

The 1995 ANA Social Policy Statement outlines a framework for development and classification of nursing diagnoses, and to help ensure a discipline-specific perspective for interventions provided by professional nurses. The policy statement defines nursing as the: "attention to a

---

### BOX 12-2 DIAGNOSIS AS A STANDARD COMPONENT OF CARE: ANA STANDARDS

**Standard II. Diagnosis**

The nurse analyzes the assessment in determining diagnoses. Guidelines: Diagnoses must be:

- Based on data collected during assessment of client

- Validated with client, significant others, and health care providers

- Documented so that they can be used in further development of expected outcomes and plan of care

Data from American Nurses Association. (1998). *Standards of clinical nursing practice.* (2nd ed.). Washington, DC: Author.

---

full range of human experiences and responses to health/illness without restriction to a problem-focused orientation (ANA, 2002). This statement supports the use of wellness nursing diagnoses. "The most essential and distinguishing feature of any nursing diagnosis is that it describes a *human condition or response* that can be resolved or enhanced (in the case of wellness diagnoses) primarily by nursing interventions or therapies." (NANDA & ANA statements, cited in Berger & Williams, 1999). A wellness nursing diagnosis identifies a human response that indicates a potential for enhancement to a higher level of wellness. Examples include *family coping: readiness for enhanced growth, health seeking behaviors*, and *effective breast feeding*.

Diagnoses approved and accepted by NANDA have been refined to the point for clinical use and testing. Currently, there are 155 NANDA–approved diagnoses. Seven new diagnoses were added at the 14th conference in 2000 (NANDA, 2003). Refer to Table 12-1 for a comparison of Taxonomy I and II.

Use of the nursing process and development of a taxonomy of nursing diagnoses have assisted in identifying trends related to client problems and the nursing care provided. NANDA continues to refine, test, and update nursing diagnoses through a system of clinical expert review. Nursing diagnoses are easily linked to the standardized language of the Nursing Interventions Classification (NIC) and Nursing Outcomes Classification (NOC) systems, including computerized documentation systems that will be discussed later in this chapter. All of these systems have improved data collection and the nursing process by standardizing the data through a set of common definitions (Nursing Practice FAQs Sheet, 1999).

## TABLE 12-1    NANDA–APPROVED NURSING DIAGNOSES: TAXONOMY I TO TAXONOMY II

| Taxonomy I Nursing Diagnosis | Taxonomy II Nursing Diagnosis |
| --- | --- |
| *Exchanging* | |
| Altered nutrition: More than body requirements | Imbalanced nutrition: More than body requirements |
| Altered nutrition: Less than body requirements | Imbalanced nutrition: Less than body requirements |
| Altered nutrition: Risk for more than body requirements | Risk for imbalanced nutrition: More than body requirements |
| Risk for infection | Risk for infection |
| Risk for altered body temperature | Risk for imbalanced body temperature |
| Hypothermia | Hypothermia |
| Hyperthermia | Hyperthermia |
| Ineffective thermoregulation | Ineffective thermoregulation |
| Dysreflexia | Autonomic dysreflexia |
| Risk for autonomic dysreflexia | Risk for autonomic dysreflexia |
| Constipation | Constipation |
| Perceived constipation | Perceived constipation |
| Diarrhea | Diarrhea |
| Bowel incontinence | Bowel incontinence |
| Risk for constipation | Risk for constipation |
| Altered urinary elimination | Impaired urinary elimination |
| Stress incontinence | Stress urinary incontinence |
| Reflex urinary incontinence | Reflex urinary incontinence |
| Urge incontinence | Urge urinary incontinence |
| Functional urinary incontinence | Functional urinary incontinence |
| Total incontinence | Total urinary incontinence |
| Risk for urinary urge incontinence | Risk for urge urinary incontinence |
| Urinary retention | Urinary retention |
| Altered tissue perfusion (specify type: renal, cerebral, cardiopulmonary, gastrointestinal, peripheral) | Ineffective tissue perfusion (specify type: renal, cerebral, cardiopulmonary, gastrointestinal, peripheral) |
| Risk for fluid volume imbalance | Risk for imbalanced fluid volume |
| Fluid volume excess | Excess fluid volume |
| Fluid volume deficit | Deficient fluid volume |
| Risk for fluid volume deficit | Risk for deficient fluid volume |
| Decreased cardiac output | Decreased cardiac output |
| Impaired gas exchange | Impaired gas exchange |
| Ineffective airway clearance | Ineffective airway clearance |
| Ineffective breathing pattern | Ineffective breathing pattern |
| Inability to sustain spontaneous ventilation | Impaired spontaneous ventilation |
| Dysfunctional ventilatory weaning response | Dysfunctional ventilatory weaning response |
| Risk for injury | Risk for injury |
| Risk for suffocation | Risk for suffocation |
| Risk for poisoning | Risk for poisoning |
| Risk for trauma | Risk for trauma |

*(continues)*

## TABLE 12-1    NANDA–APPROVED NURSING DIAGNOSES: TAXONOMY I TO TAXONOMY II (*continued*)

| Taxonomy I Nursing Diagnosis | Taxonomy II Nursing Diagnosis |
| --- | --- |
| **Exchanging (*continued*)** | |
| Risk for aspiration | Risk for aspiration |
| Risk for disuse syndrome | Risk for disuse syndrome |
| Latex allergy response | Latex allergy response |
| Risk for latex allergy response | Risk for latex allergy response |
| Altered protection | Ineffective protection |
| Impaired tissue integrity | Impaired tissue integrity |
| Altered oral mucous membrane | Impaired oral mucous membrane |
| Impaired skin integrity | Impaired skin integrity |
| Risk for impaired skin integrity | Risk for impaired skin integrity |
| Altered dentition | Impaired dentition |
| Decreased adaptive capacity: Intracranial | Decreased intracranial adaptive capacity |
| Energy field disturbance | Disturbed energy field |
| **Communicating** | |
| Impaired verbal communication | Impaired verbal communication |
| **Relating** | |
| Impaired social interaction | Impaired social interaction |
| Social isolation | Social isolation |
| Risk for loneliness | Risk for loneliness |
| Altered role performance | Ineffective role performance |
| Altered role performance | Ineffective role performance |
| Altered parenting | Impaired parenting |
| Risk for altered parenting | Risk for impaired parenting |
| Risk for altered parent/infant/child attachment | Risk for impaired parent/infant/child attachment |
| Sexual dysfunction | Sexual dysfunction |
| Altered family processes | Interrupted family processes |
| Caregiver role strain | Caregiver role strain |
| Risk for caregiver role strain | Risk for caregiver role strain |
| Altered family processes: Alcoholism | Dysfunctional family processes: Alcoholism |
| Parental role conflict | Parental role conflict |
| Altered sexuality patterns | Ineffective sexuality patterns |
| **Valuing** | |
| Spiritual distress (distress of the human spirit) | Spiritual distress |
| Risk for spiritual distress | Risk for spiritual distress |
| Potential for enhanced spiritual well-being | Readiness for enhanced spiritual well-being |

*(continues)*

## TABLE 12-1    NANDA–APPROVED NURSING DIAGNOSES: TAXONOMY I TO TAXONOMY II (*continued*)

| Taxonomy I Nursing Diagnosis | Taxonomy II Nursing Diagnosis |
| --- | --- |
| *Choosing* | |
| Ineffective individual coping | Ineffective coping |
| Impaired adjustment | Impaired adjustment |
| Defensive coping | Defensive coping |
| Ineffective denial | Ineffective denial |
| Ineffective family coping: Disabling | Disabled family coping |
| Ineffective family coping: Compromised | Compromised family coping |
| Family coping: Potential for growth | Readiness for enhanced family coping |
| Potential for enhanced community coping | Readiness for enhanced community coping |
| Ineffective community coping | Ineffective community coping |
| Ineffective management of therapeutic regimen: Individual | Ineffective therapeutic regimen management |
| Noncompliance (specify) | Noncompliance (specify) |
| Ineffective management of therapeutic regimen: Families | Ineffective family therapeutic regimen management |
| Ineffective management of therapeutic regimen: Community | Ineffective community therapeutic regimen management |
| Effective management of therapeutic regimen: Individual | Effective therapeutic regimen management |
| Decisional conflict (specify) | Decisional conflict (specify) |
| Health-seeking behaviors (specify) | Health-seeking behaviors (specify) |
| *Moving* | |
| Impaired physical mobility | Impaired physical mobility |
| Risk for peripheral neurovascular dysfunction | Risk for peripheral neurovascular dysfunction |
| Risk for perioperative-positioning injury | Risk for perioperative-positioning injury |
| Impaired walking | Impaired walking |
| Impaired wheelchair mobility | Impaired wheelchair mobility |
| Impaired transfer ability | Impaired transfer ability |
| Impaired bed mobility | Impaired bed mobility |
| Activity intolerance | Activity intolerance |
| Fatigue | Fatigue |
| Risk for activity intolerance | Risk for activity intolerance |
| Sleep pattern disturbance | Disturbed sleep pattern |
| Sleep deprivation | Sleep deprivation |
| Diversional activity deficit | Deficient diversional activity |
| Impaired home maintenance management | Impaired home maintenance |
| Altered health maintenance | Ineffective health maintenance |
| Delayed surgical recovery | Delayed surgical recovery |
| Adult failure to thrive | Adult failure to thrive |
| Feeding self-care deficit | Feeding self-care deficit |
| Impaired swallowing | Impaired swallowing |
| Ineffective breastfeeding | Ineffective breastfeeding |

*(continues)*

## TABLE 12-1    NANDA–APPROVED NURSING DIAGNOSES: TAXONOMY I TO TAXONOMY II (*continued*)

| Taxonomy I Nursing Diagnosis | Taxonomy II Nursing Diagnosis |
| --- | --- |
| *Moving (continued)* | |
| Interrupted breastfeeding | Interrupted breastfeeding |
| Effective breastfeeding | Effective breastfeeding |
| Ineffective infant feeding pattern | Ineffective infant feeding pattern |
| Bathing/hygiene self-care deficit | Bathing/hygiene self-care deficit |
| Dressing/grooming self-care deficit | Dressing/grooming self-care deficit |
| Toileting self-care deficit | Toileting self-care deficit |
| Altered growth and development | Delayed growth and development |
| Risk for altered development | Risk for delayed development |
| Risk for altered growth | Risk for disproportionate growth |
| Relocation stress syndrome | Relocation stress syndrome |
| Risk for disorganized infant behavior | Risk for disorganized infant behavior |
| Disorganized infant behavior | Disorganized infant behavior |
| Potential for enhanced organized infant behavior | Readiness for enhanced organized infant behavior |
| *Perceiving* | |
| Body image disturbance | Disturbed body image |
| Chronic low self-esteem | Chronic low self-esteem |
| Situational low self-esteem | Situational low self-esteem |
| Personal identity disturbance | Disturbed personal identity |
| Sensory/perceptual alterations (specify: visual, auditory, kinesthetic, gustatory, tactile, olfactory) | Disturbed sensory perception (specify: visual, auditory, kinesthetic, gustatory, tactile, olfactory) |
| Unilateral neglect | Unilateral neglect |
| Hopelessness | Hopelessness |
| Powerlessness | Powerlessness |
| *Knowing* | |
| Knowledge deficit (specify) | Deficient knowledge (specify) |
| Impaired environmental-interpretation syndrome | Impaired environmental interpretation syndrome |
| Acute confusion | Acute confusion |
| Chronic confusion | Chronic confusion |
| Altered thought processes | Disturbed thought processes |
| Impaired memory | Impaired memory |
| *Feeling* | |
| Pain | Acute pain |
| Chronic pain | Chronic pain |
| Nausea | Nausea |
| Dysfunctional grieving | Dysfunctional grieving |
| Anticipatory grieving | Anticipatory grieving |

(continues)

## TABLE 12-1   NANDA–APPROVED NURSING DIAGNOSES: TAXONOMY I TO TAXONOMY II (*continued*)

| Taxonomy I Nursing Diagnosis | Taxonomy II Nursing Diagnosis |
| --- | --- |
| *Feeling (continued)* | |
| Chronic sorrow | Chronic sorrow |
| Risk for violence: Directed at others | Risk for other-directed violence |
| Risk for self-mutilation | Risk for self-mutilation |
| Risk for violence: Self-directed | Risk for self-directed violence |
| Post-trauma syndrome | Post-trauma syndrome |
| Rape-trauma syndrome | Rape-trauma syndrome |
| Rape-trauma syndrome: Compound reaction | Rape-trauma syndrome: Compound reaction |
| Rape-trauma syndrome: Silent reaction | Rape-trauma syndrome: Silent reaction |
| Risk for post-trauma syndrome | Risk for post-trauma syndrome |
| Anxiety | Anxiety |
| Death anxiety | Death anxiety |
| Fear | Fear |
| | **New to Taxonomy II** |
| | Risk for falls |
| | Risk for powerlessness |
| | Risk for relocation stress syndrome |
| | Risk for situational low self-esteem |
| | Self-mutilation |
| | Risk for suicide |
| | Wandering |

Used with permission from North American Diagnosis Association. (2003). *Nursing diagnoses: Definitions and classification 2003–2004.* Philadelphia: Author.

## Research

With the inception of the first conference on nursing diagnoses, NANDA supported research endeavors on the development of a nursing diagnosis classification system. The first type of research conducted was identification studies, where the clinician repeatedly observed a condition in order to label nursing diagnoses. At the sixth conference in 1986, Fehring identified the need for two standardized research methodologies for data collection: (1) diagnostic content validity (DCV), retrospective evidence from experts on the characteristics of a given label; and (2) clinical diagnostic validity (CDV), prospective evidence on the characteristics from a clinical perspective (Whitley, 1999). In 1989, NANDA sponsored an invitational conference on research methodologies for generating and validating existing diagnoses and to develop new methodologies to direct future studies. Although there is an abundance of DCV studies, only a few clinical studies have been conducted because the CDV model is more complicated to execute. *Nursing Diagnosis: The Journal of Nursing Language &*

*Classification* is the official publication of NANDA. The journal was first published in 1989 to promote the development, refinement, and use of nursing language and classification.

Carlson-Catalano et al. (1998) conducted a clinical validation study on three respiratory diagnoses: *Ineffective Breathing Pattern (IBP), Ineffective Airway Clearance (IAC),* and *Impaired Gas Exchange (IGE).* The diagnoses were added to the NANDA list in 1980 and are among the most frequently used diagnoses; however, there were no reported clinical validation studies of the defining characteristics.

Recent validation studies have been conducted on the nursing diagnoses of *Relocation Stress Syndrome (RSS), Fatigue,* and *Impaired Swallowing.* Study findings have contributed to the refinement and modification of nursing diagnoses and interventions. Mallick and Whipple (2000) suggest that *RSS* may not be a valid diagnosis for group moves. The defining characteristics of dependency, confusion, anxiety, depression, and withdrawal symptoms commonly associated with *RSS* were not evident for a group of

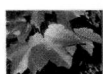

## RESEARCH FOCUS

**Title of Study:** Clinical validation of ineffective breathing pattern, ineffective airway clearance, and impaired gas exchange

**Study Purpose:** To conduct a clinical validation of etiologies and defining characteristics of the three respiratory diagnoses, and to determine the most important interventions for each diagnosis

**Methods:** A literature-based concept analysis revealed 37 possible characteristics (including those defined by NANDA) associated with the three diagnoses. The investigators developed an instrument to determine the presence or absence of these characteristics, their importance in making a diagnosis, etiologies or contributing factors, and the importance of specific nursing interventions. Subjective cues suggested by the literature analysis, but not included in NANDA definitions, were included in the instrument. Expert nurses were prepared to evaluate 76 clients selected for the study with a variety of medical-surgical problems.

**Findings:** The majority of the clients experienced *Impaired Breathing Pattern* or *Ineffective Airway Clearance.* *Impaired Gas Exchange* was present only in combination with one or both of the other diagnoses. Many different etiologies associated with the variety of acute and chronic medical-surgical problems were identified. The percentages of defining characteristics were also varied with this population; many did not meet the criterion of 50%. Subjective expressions of fatigue and anxiety were accepted as defining characteristics in this study, representing a "whole-person response." Fatigue was represented in 86.9% of the sample. High percentages of the importance of nursing interventions support the NANDA approval of these human responses as "nursing" diagnoses.

**Implications:** The findings suggest that NANDA-approved defining characteristics for each of the diagnoses should be reconsidered. Fewer cues may be needed, thus increasing efficiency in making these diagnoses. Clinical experts identified the importance of teaching interventions and a need for teaching expertise at the bedside. The authors suggested replication of the study with other populations, further longitudinal studies with follow-up, and determination of which interventions more likely will be associated with positive outcomes for each diagnosis.

Carlson-Catalano, J., Lunney, M., Paradiso, C., Bruno, J., Luise, B., Martin, T., Massoni, M., & Pachter, S. (1998). Clinical validation of ineffective breathing pattern, ineffective airway clearance, and impaired gas exchange. *Image: Journal of Nursing Scholarship, 30*(3), 243–248.

long-term residents who were relocated en masse to a new extended care facility.

Acute or chronic fatigue is associated with numerous physical and psychological health problems. Self-reports of the severity and effects of fatigue have formed the basis for several definitions and measurement tools of this complex human response. Depression and a sense of powerlessness were prevalent findings in two recent studies by Dzurec, Hoover, & Fields (2002) and Aaronson et al. (1999). The researchers suggest that the client's subjective rating of severity, distress, and impact of fatigue on daily living would aid in assessment and measures of fatigue. However, no single measure can adequately address the complexity of the fatigue phenomenon.

Difficulty in swallowing is a significant problem for persons with neurological disorders associated with dysphagia and aspiration, and others are at risk, including the elderly and clients following extubation. Yet feeding is often one of the first tasks nurses delegate to less-skilled personnel. McHale, Phipps, Horvath, & Schemlz (1998) examined the methods used by expert nurses to assess and feed clients. The study findings support the monitoring and feeding interventions listed in the NIC. There is, also, an overlap with the nursing diagnoses of *High Risk for Aspiration* and *Impaired Swallowing.*

Whitley (1999) suggests the development of a "research agenda" to promote research in a coordinated fashion, since interest about nursing diagnoses has spread in the international community, at a time when a common nursing language is needed to strengthen nursing's bases for practice. In 1998, the NANDA Board instituted an ad hoc research committee to coordinate nursing diagnosis research and funding and to develop a "research agenda."

## Purposes of Nursing Diagnosis

Prior to the 1980 ANA Social Policy Statement, the medical model served as the basis for nursing practice, and there was no clear definition of nursing (Schall & Flannery, 2000). The nursing process quickly became recognized as the organizational framework for professional nursing practice, thus permitting nurses to assess, diagnose, and plan interventions within a nursing perspective (Carrol-Johnson, 2001). The emphasis of the 1995 ANA Social Policy Statement was on health promotion, as the nation's health care system required increased professional accountability for cost-effective quality care and efficient use of resources. The document also supports a professional knowledge base derived from nursing science, philosophy, and ethics, and physical, economic, biomedical, behavioral, and social sciences (ANA, 1995; Schall & Flannery, 2000).

The thrust of NANDA's work continues to meet the need for establishing a standardized language, or vocabulary, that reflects treatment modalities of the nursing discipline (Berger & Williams, 1999). For evaluation of nursing services and for reimbursement purposes, standardized ways of communicating are viewed as critical indicators of good nursing practices (*Minnesota Nursing Accent*, 1999). In addition, communication about nursing diagnoses is possible through computer search. The *Cumulative Index to Nursing and Allied Health Literature* (CINAHL), NANDA, and links to related sources and other nursing organizations (NursingCenter.com and Nursing World.com) provide a wealth of research-based information. Box 12-3 further illustrates the purposes of nursing diagnosis.

Nursing diagnosis also provides a means for effective communication. It is generally agreed among nurses, health care practitioners, and other health care professionals that there is a need for a common language within the health care sector. A mutual vocabulary that can be used for describing practice, research, and education benefits both the profession and the consumer. With this language, collaboration and international exchanges regarding nursing and health care are possible.

Holistic client, family, and community-focused care are facilitated with the use of nursing diagnosis. The list of

NANDA–approved nursing diagnoses (NANDA, 2003) for clinical use provides assistance for the nurse in individualizing care and developing comprehensive therapeutic nursing interventions. Quality care and continuity of care are enhanced with identified nursing diagnoses as part of the client's plan of nursing care. Box 12-4 illustrates the value of applying nursing diagnosis to a home health care situation.

In summary, nursing diagnosis allows for empowerment of the profession of nursing, facilitates effective communication, and provides a means to individualize nursing care. Nursing diagnosis is essential to clinical practice and education, and pivotal for theory development and research.

## Nursing Diagnoses and Diagnostic-Related Groups

Payment for services was shifted from the number of days in a hospital to the individual's medical diagnosis, with the purpose of controlling delivery of care and reducing Medicare costs. Prospective payment financing designates an amount of money for each DRG and only that amount is paid. "There are no set codes for nursing diagnosis or care, in spite of growing evidence that nursing care directly affects length of stay and [client] outcomes" (*Michigan Nurse,* 2000).

The development of nursing's standardized languages has provided a mechanism to recognize the contributions made by nurses (Clingerman, 1999). For more than a

---

**BOX 12-3 PURPOSES OF NURSING DIAGNOSIS**

- Identifies areas that nurses can resolve or enhance

- Demonstrates professional judgment

- Organizes decision making as part of the nursing process

- Promotes use of standardized language and process

- Defines the scope of nursing practice

- Clarifies the nursing profession's services to society

- Promotes accountability of the nurse

- Provides communication among nurses and other health care professionals

- Promotes collaboration with others and clients

- Decreases costs

- Provides a mechanism for conducting nursing research

- Aids building of a scientific body of knowledge for the nursing profession

---

**BOX 12-4 HOME HEALTH CARE**

Individualizing care of the home health client is an important function of nursing diagnosis. For example, the following questions can be used as a guide in developing nursing interventions in response to the nursing diagnosis of *Compromised Family Coping*— related to a caregiver appearing to be unable to assist a client with management of a health problem:

- Is the client experiencing difficulty with the caregiver's response about the type and level of care needed?

- Has the caregiver expressed concern or anxiety about performing certain functions for the client?

- Does the care performed by the caregiver for the client yield satisfactory results in terms of alleviation of symptoms?

- What changes have occurred within the family situation that have altered the dynamics between the client and caregiver?

decade, research at the University of Iowa has focused largely on identifying and categorizing nursing interventions and their effects on client outcomes. The development of the NIC and the NOC linked with NANDA diagnoses has aided nurses in documenting, retrieving, and comparing discrete nursing contributions (McCloskey & Bulecheck, 2000) (see Box 12-5 and Box 12-6).

Each item in the classifications has been defined, labeled, and numerically coded. Each intervention is accompanied by a selection of nursing activities to facilitate an individualized plan of care; each outcome has a set of observable and measurable indicators that are rated on a scale of 1 (least desirable client status) to 5 (most desirable client status). Since an outcome can vary and change over time, it can be monitored across a life span and in a variety of environmental settings. The classifications are continually reviewed and updated, and have been translated into several international languages (McCloskey & Bulecheck, 2000; Clingerman, 1999; Nursing Practice FAQs Sheet, 1999). NANDA now works closely with the National Library of Medicine, the International Council of Nursing, and the American Nurses Association toward a unified nursing language system.

The NIC and NOC classifications have been linked with the standardized languages used by NANDA, the Omaha System, Home Health Care System, and Nursing Home Resident Assessment Protocols, and both NIC and NOC classifications are recognized by the ANA. The classifications and other standard languages are included in the unified medical language (UML) and CINAHL. The NIC/NOC classifications have also been accepted by the Joint Commission of Accreditation of Healthcare Organizations (JCAHO) as one system to meet standards on uniform care. An alliance formed by NANDA, NIC, and NOC will participate in collaborative research.

Standardized languages and computerization have enhanced the visibility of nursing contributions. The coding of data identifies specific information and "captures" the most efficient and effective interventions. NIC and NOC also facilitate the development of critical and clinical pathways (interdisciplinary care plans) standards of care, and serve as the basis for research activities (Clingerman, 1999; Nursing Practice FAQs Sheet, 1999).

Nurses need a working knowledge of health care reimbursement and the language of health economists, accountants, administrators, and lawmakers for nursing to have an impact on the health care system. Management of health care dollars will continue to change and be affected by population demographics, the economy, advances in technology, laws, and resources of third-party payers (*Michigan Nurse*, 2000).

# Components of a Nursing Diagnosis

Several formats have been used to structure nursing diagnosis statements. Two formats that are frequently seen in the nursing literature are the two- and three-part statements. The two-part statement is NANDA-approved and is used by most experienced nurses, in large part because of its brief and precise format. The three-part statement is preferred by those nurses desiring to strengthen the diagnostic statement by including specific manifestations, an attribute that is not possible through the use of the two-part format.

## The Two-Part Statement

The components of a nursing diagnosis typically consist of two parts. The first component is a problem statement

---

**BOX 12-5  EXAMPLE OF NURSING OUTCOMES CLASSIFICATION (NOC)**

**Cardiac Output Status**

*Definition*

Cardiac output (CO), cardiac index (CI), pulmonary artery pressure (PAP), pulmonary artery wedge pressure (PAWP) within expected range for the individual

| Scale: | Extreme Deviation from Expected Range | Substantial Deviation from Expected Range | Moderate Deviation from Expected Range | Mild Deviation from Expected Range | No Deviation from Expected Range |
|---|---|---|---|---|---|
| **Indicators:** | | | | | |
| CO | 1 | 2 | 3 | 4 | 5 |
| PAP | 1 | 2 | 3 | 4 | 5 |
| PAWP | 1 | 2 | 3 | 4 | 5 |
| CI | 1 | 2 | 3 | 4 | 5 |

## BOX 12-6    EXAMPLE OF NURSING-INITIATED NURSING INTERVENTION (NIC)

### Dressing

**Definition**

Selecting, putting on, and removing clothes for a person who cannot do so independently

**Activities**

- Dress client after personal hygiene implemented.

- Encourage participation in selection of clothing.

- Dress in nonrestrictive clothing, as appropriate.

- Dress in personal clothing, as appropriate.

- Select shoes or slippers conducive to ambulation.

or diagnostic label that describes the client's response to an actual, possible, and risk health problem or a wellness condition. Table 12-1 presents the list of NANDA-approved nursing diagnoses. (Note the addition of new diagnoses in Taxonomy II.)

The second component of a two-part nursing diagnosis is the etiology. The **etiology** is the related cause or contributor to the problem. The diagnostic label and etiology are linked by the term *related to* (RT). Examples of nursing diagnoses are *Disturbed Body Image* RT loss of left lower extremity and *Activity Intolerance* RT decreased oxygen-carrying capacity of cells. Descriptive words or terms may be added to clarify specific nursing diagnoses. These descriptive words are called qualifiers and include *Acute, Chronic, Decreased, Deficient, Depleted, Disturbed, Dysfunctional, Enhanced, Excessive, Impaired, Increased, Ineffective, Intermittent, Potential for,* and *Risk.* These terms specify a degree of qualification for the identified nursing diagnosis and are placed (used) before the problem statement.

## The Three-Part Statement

The nursing diagnosis can also be expressed as a three-part statement. As in the two-part statement, the first two components are the diagnostic label and the etiology. The third component consists of **defining characteristics** (collected data that are also known as signs and symptoms, subjective and objective data, or clinical manifestations). In the three-part nursing diagnosis format, the third part is joined to the first two components with the connecting phrase "as evidenced by" (AEB). Defining characteristics list the relevant clinical manifestations, such as signs or symptoms for the identified client problem and the related etiology. Defining characteristics are identified for each NANDA–approved diagnosis. These characteristics continue to evolve as they are reviewed and updated at the biennial conference. It is important to emphasize that defining characteristics may assist the nurse in identifying client goals, measurable client outcome criteria, and relevant nursing interventions.

Some nurses believe that the three-part statement strengthens the diagnostic process. However, other nurses prefer the two-part statement and refer to the defining characteristics as part of the original database. Table 12-2 depicts the components and relationship of the three versions of the diagnosis statement. Although the most commonly used format is the two-part statement, it is beneficial for the nurse to be knowledgeable about the use of the three-part statement for development of a nursing diagnosis. See Table 12-3 for a comparison of selected approved NANDA diagnoses in the two- and three-part statements.

## Categories of Nursing Diagnoses

Nursing diagnoses may be classified into three categories: actual, risk, and wellness. The most common nursing diagnoses used are actual and risk diagnoses. Wellness diagnoses were adopted by NANDA 1996, and Carpenito (2004) described possible nursing diagnoses.

- *Actual diagnoses* are those problems identified by the nurse that are already in existence. Actual diagnoses may include *Excess Fluid Volume* related to (RT) intra-

## TABLE 12-2    COMPARISON OF ONE-, TWO-, AND THREE-PART NURSING DIAGNOSIS STATEMENTS

| One-Part Statement | Two-Part Statement | Three-Part Statement |
|---|---|---|
| Part 1: Wellness condition/state to be enhanced (no related to, no etiology, and no defining characteristics) | Part 1: Problem Related to<br>Part 2: Etiology (no defining characteristics) | Part 1: Problem Related to<br>Part 2: Etiology<br>Part 3: Defining Characteristics |

## TABLE 12-3    EXAMPLES OF NURSING DIAGNOSES EXPRESSED IN TWO- AND THREE-PART STATEMENTS

| Nursing Diagnosis | Two-Part Statement | Three-Part Statement |
|---|---|---|
| *Feeding Self-Care Deficit* | *Feeding Self-Care Deficit* RT decreased strength and endurance | *Feeding Self-Care Deficit* RT decreased strength and endurance AEB inability to maintain fork in hand from plate to mouth |
| *Ineffective Airway Clearance* | *Ineffective Airway Clearance* RT fatigue | *Ineffective Airway Clearance* RT fatigue AEB dyspnea at rest |
| *Anxiety* | *Anxiety* RT change in role functioning | *Anxiety* RT change in role functioning AEB insomnia, poor eye contact, and quivering voice |
| *Deficient Knowledge* | *Deficient Knowledge* RT misinterpretation of information | *Deficient Knowledge* RT misinterpretation of information AEB inaccurate return demonstration of self-injection |
| *Spiritual Distress* | *Spiritual Distress* RT separation from religious ties | *Spiritual Distress* RT separation from religious ties AEB crying and withdrawal |

Data from North American Nursing Diagnosis Association (NANDA) (2003). *Nursing diagnoses: Definitions and classification 2003–2004.* Philadelphia: Author.

venous infusion therapy overload and *Anxiety* RT unknown results of breast biopsy.

- *Risk diagnoses* are identified by the nurse in situations in which problems might occur but are not currently in existence. Examples of risk diagnoses may include *Risk for Poisoning* RT increased mobility of infant and failure to have house child-proofed and *Risk for Deficient Fluid Volume* RT excessive number of stools.
- *Wellness diagnoses* identify the individual or aggregate condition or state that may be enhanced by health-promoting activities. These consist of a one-part statement (no "related to" phrase) that uses the label "Readiness for Enhanced" followed by the state the nurse desires to enhance. Examples of wellness diagnoses may include *Readiness for Enhanced Community Coping* and *Readiness for Enhanced Spiritual Well-Being.*

## Taxonomy of Nursing Diagnosis

The **taxonomy of nursing diagnoses** is the type of classification under which the diagnostic label is grouped based on which human response the client is demonstrating to the actual or perceived stressor. Rather than consult the alphabetical listing of NANDA diagnoses, some nurses might find it more helpful to review the NANDA listing by pattern of human response. This listing is called the NANDA Taxonomy II and organizes the NANDA-approved nursing diagnoses under the corresponding human response category. The NANDA nursing diagnosis taxonomy is composed of nine patterns of human response:

- Exchanging
- Communicating
- Relating
- Valuing
- Choosing
- Moving
- Perceiving
- Knowing
- Feeling

Refer to Box 12-7 for expanded definitions.

Although the word *taxonomy* may be somewhat overwhelming for the beginning practitioner, remember it is only an organizational framework and one should not be intimidated by it. Rather, view this approach as another way to find appropriate nursing diagnoses for clients on the basis of the classification of human response.

## Developing a Nursing Diagnosis

The development of a nursing diagnosis is a systematic process in which certain activities need to be executed. Box 12-8 illustrates the steps in the development of nursing diagnoses.

## Critical Thinking in Nursing Diagnosis

Contemporary nursing practice, with its focus on nursing diagnoses, interventions, and outcomes, requires critical thinking (Pesut & Herman, 1999). Interpreting data cues is one example of critical thinking that the nurse must use on a daily basis when working with clients. Specifically, the synthesis of information that takes place when interpreting data cues demonstrates how essential it is for the nurse to think critically. Interpreting Mr. Zachary's cues (see Stop and Think box) is pivotal for

## BOX 12-7    EXPANDED DEFINITIONS OF HUMAN RESPONSE PATTERNS

- **Exchanging:** To relinquish or lose something while receiving something in return; a mutual giving and receiving

- **Communicating:** Sending messages—transmission of thoughts, feelings, or information—internally or externally, verbally or nonverbally

- **Relating:** Establishing a link; to connect; to be in some association to another thing, person, or place

- **Valuing:** Being concerned about or assigning relative worth or usefulness; to equate importance

- **Choosing:** Selection of alternatives; to exercise preference of one matter over another

- **Moving:** Activity; to change the place or position of a body or part of the body; to take action; to cause an excretion or discharge

- **Perceiving:** Reception of information; to become aware through the senses

- **Knowing:** To recognize meaning associated with information; to be knowledgeable about factual information and principles; to understand

- **Feeling:** Subjective or conscious awareness of information; to be emotionally affected by the experience.

Adapted from Doenges, M., Moorehouse, M., & Geissler-Murr, A. (2002). *Nurse's pocket guide: Diagnosis, interventions and rationales* (8th ed.) Philadelphia: F. A. Davis.

## BOX 12-8    STEPS IN DEVELOPING A NURSING DIAGNOSIS

1. Data cues are collected from the assessment phase.

2. Data cues are validated and examined.

3. Data cues are interpreted and assigned a meaning through the use of critical thinking.

4. Data are grouped into clusters.

5. The NANDA list is consulted.

6. The first part of the nursing diagnosis statement is written.

7. Related to (RT) factors are identified.

8. Phrases from steps 6 and 7 are combined to form a two-part nursing diagnosis.

9. Defining characteristics (AEB) are identified.

10. Phrases from steps 6, 7, 8, and 9 are combined to form a three-part nursing diagnosis.

Data from American Nurses Association. (1998). *Standards of clinical nursing practice* [2nd ed.] (p. 9). Washington, DC: Author.

output, and complaint of thirst. The expert nurse immediately processes these cues and determines a nursing diagnosis, plans client outcomes, and implements therapeutic nursing interventions. The novice nurse must proceed more cautiously and use additional time to process these data cues.

correctly diagnosing his actual or at-risk problem, or wellness state. The accompanying display provides questions that are helpful in developing appropriate diagnoses.

## Assessing Database

In the assessment phase, the nurse collects data cues from the client. **Cues** are small amounts of data that are applied to the decision-making process. Nurses should be attentive to the cues gathered from the interview, health history, symptom analysis, physical examination, and laboratory and diagnostic data, since they increase the index of suspicion and stimulate further observation of additional sets of cues. Examples of cues might be poor skin turgor, parched lips, dry skin, decreased urine

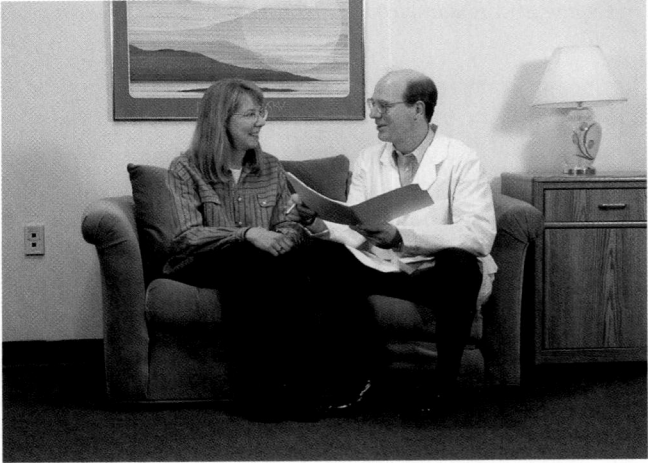

**Figure 12-3    This nurse is validating the cues collected from this client during the assessment phase.**

## STOP AND THINK

### Identifying Data Cues

What relevant data cues can be gathered from the following assessment data for Peter Zachary, age 44?

**Subjective Data**

- "I am the father of two boys."

- "I paint houses for a living."

- "I go to church every Sunday."

- "I always seem to be hungry, and I eat five or six times a day."

- "I've gained 12 pounds this year."

**Objective Data**

- Client is 5 feet 10 inches and weighs 204 pounds.

- Protruding abdomen over belt and waist of pants

- Double chin

- Fleshy loose upper arms

- Dimpling of buttocks

- One bowel movement every other day

- Vital signs: HR 92; BP 130/80; R 17; T 98.9°F

- Red scaly patches on skin

- Nonproductive cough

- Birthmark right upper hip

## STOP AND THINK

### Development of a Nursing Diagnosis

The following questions should be considered by the nurse in the development of a nursing diagnosis:

- Do I have enough data to formulate a nursing diagnosis?

- Are any data missing?

- Is there any information on my database that seems incomplete or uncertain?

- Should I talk to the client and family again?

- What data fit together or have something in common?

- What specific cues from the client made me form this conclusion?

- What elements of this situation, condition, or problem are able to be enhanced or resolved by therapeutic nursing interventions?

- What elements need to be referred to another discipline (e.g., medicine, social services, dietary)?

data cues. In order to interpret Mr. Zachary's subjective and objective data cues, the nurse should ask the following questions:

- What is this information telling me?
- Is there a pattern?
- Can this information be put together?
- Is the information falling into a logical arrangement?
- Is the information forming natural groupings?

## Validating Cues

After reviewing the data cues, the nurse validates that information and examines it carefully (Figure 12-3). In the example of Mr. Zachary, the nurse determines if the information is accurate and complete. This process involves verifying subjective and objective data. Verification can be done by interviewing Mr. Zachary again and reassessing data cues—for example, weighing him and measuring abdominal girth.

## Interpreting Cues

Through interpretation of data cues and use of critical-thinking strategies, the nurse assigns a meaning to the

## Clustering Cues

Once the cues have been collected, validated, and interpreted, the data are then grouped into clusters. A **cluster** is a set of data cues in which relationships between and among cues are established to identify a specific health state or condition. Related pieces of information about the client are grouped together. Conclusions are drawn from the data cues. One piece of information by itself can be misleading. This idea is analogous to the assembly of a jigsaw puzzle. One puzzle piece by itself does not give an accurate idea of the picture. In the same way, one data cue (or piece of assessment data) does not have much relevance by itself. When more pieces of the puzzle are put together or when more data assessment cues are put together, the nurse may have a beginning idea of what the puzzle picture or the client's health looks like.

In Mr. Zachary's situation, data cues that can be clustered together include

Subjective: "I always seem to be hungry and I eat five or six times a day," and "I've gained 12 pounds in the past year."

Objective: weight 204 pounds, protruding abdomen, double chin, fleshy loose upper arms, and dimpling of buttocks.

## Consulting NANDA List of Nursing Diagnoses

After the data have been organized into clusters, the nurse needs to consult the NANDA list to ascertain similarities and differences between the clusters and NANDA diagnoses. The clustered data are then matched with a particular NANDA diagnosis. In Mr. Zachary's case, the NANDA–approved diagnosis is *Imbalanced Nutrition: More Than Body Requirements.*

## Writing the Nursing Diagnosis Statement

The nursing diagnosis selected from the NANDA list becomes the diagnostic label, the first part of the diagnosis statement. Etiologies are also identified from the NANDA list. The appropriate etiology is selected and joined to the first part of the statement with the "related to" phrase. Because the NANDA list of nursing diagnoses is constantly evolving, there may be times when no etiology is provided. In such cases, the nurse should attempt to describe likely contributing factors to the client's condition. In a two-part statement, the nursing diagnosis for Mr. Zachary would be *Imbalanced Nutrition: More Than Body Requirements* RT excessive food intake. The three-part statement would be *Imbalanced Nutrition: More Than Body Requirements* AEB weight gain, increased appetite, excess adipose tissue, and increased abdominal girth.

## Avoiding Errors in Developing a Nursing Diagnosis

The holistic view of nursing supports the collection of a large amount of health history data, which is time-consuming but provides a wealth of information regarding the client's ability to function in a variety of settings. Errors can occur during the diagnostic process, such as incomplete and inaccurate data collection, or misinterpretation of data and placement into inappropriate categories (clusters). Access to the client's subjective data may be restricted due to the client's inability to provide information. The nurse may fail to validate data with the client or other sources, or record a nursing diagnosis incorrectly. Errors related to physical assessment, observation, personal bias, and interpretation of diagnostics can also lead to missed or incorrect diagnoses. The following is a discussion of guidelines to help avoid these common errors in developing nursing diagnoses.

### Accurate and Complete Collection of Data

Errors in judgment can occur from insufficient data collection and insufficient data analysis. The inexperience of the novice nurse and lack of understanding for the scope of the client's health concerns often lead to premature closure of the data collection and to hasty decisions. The experienced nurse may rely heavily on knowledge from past experiences, stereotype client health concerns, and neglect to fully analyze the data (Berger & Williams, 1999). In either case, important cues can be overlooked or misinterpreted.

The accuracy and completeness of the health history reported by the client provides important information; however, several factors may prevent an in-depth assessment. Ideally, data should be collected in one time frame. This may not be practical in an acute care setting, and the nurse collects data that is pertinent to the immediate situation. Therefore, it is important to learn how to modify the procedure and gather a complete database over time, and to be alert to subtle cues that may arise.

A large amount of data must be placed within an organizational, or topical, framework in order to understand its meaning and interrelationships. An accurate assessment requires the nurse to be cognizant of both physical and psychosocial normal parameters before being able to recognize abnormal findings. The quality and amount of collected data are affected by the nurse's interview and assessment skills, as well as sensitivity to the uniqueness of the client. A mutual sharing of information between nurse and client increases the validity of the diagnosis (Berger & Williams, 1999).

The initial, or working, diagnosis is subject to change and ongoing revision. As additional data become available or as the client's condition changes, alternative explanations may confirm or rule out the original diagnosis. Data may also support more than one diagnosis. The diagnoses then need to be prioritized to determine which diagnosis needs immediate intervention.

Some diagnoses such as fatigue, fear, and deficient knowledge require a qualifying statement to make the diagnosis more specific to the client situation. Examples include (1) fatigue: altered sleep patterns due to changing work shifts or increased demands in family caregiving role; (2) fear: postoperative pain; and (3) deficient knowledge: self-administration of medications.

An organized, or structured, format facilitates a complete and accurate collection of data. The interview and physical assessment findings are documented in the client's record according to the specific agency protocol. The format may consist of narrative outline or checklist with provision for comments. Agency-approved abbreviations and terminology facilitate communication among the various health care team members.

## Use of Resources

When a client cannot provide the necessary information, the family can be a valuable resource regarding the health history and cultural beliefs and practices related to the client's health care needs. An interpreter can be used to overcome a language barrier when necessary. Additional resources are nursing diagnosis and intervention texts that provide accurate definitions of diagnostic labels, which help clarify the relationship of a diagnosis, its etiology, and its defining characteristics. As an example, the definition listed for *Impaired Skin Integrity* is a "state in which the individual's skin is adversely altered" (Doenges et al., 2002). Rationales for decisions are often included as well.

## Validation of Data

Previously collected data, such as an admission blood pressure reading, should be validated by comparison with more recent results to avoid premature conclusions. The diagnostic process involves ongoing data collection and examination of the meanings of cue clusters of subjective and objective symptoms. Some symptoms may present themselves as "red flags," indicating risk factors or a serious change in the client's condition. As an example, a recent large weight gain accompanied by excessive thirst, edema, and low urine output are not normally related directly to overeating, and indicate that further assessment is required. Including specific etiology and defining characteristics in the statement supports the nursing diagnosis.

It is important to validate the meaning, or inference, of data clusters through consultation with authoritative sources such as experienced personnel, textbooks, and published research, and by sharing conclusions with the client or family. In many instances, certain defining characteristics must be present for a diagnosis to be made, and are absent when the diagnosis is absent. Reexamination of the cues and clusters may indicate another diagnosis. Data cues that did not seem to fit into one of the original clusters can suggest the basis for a new data cluster and a new nursing diagnosis. A careful analysis of the client's profile, including history, lifestyle, culture, and values and beliefs,

## NURSING STRATEGY

### Summary Statements for Avoiding Common Diagnostic Errors

The nurse must be competent in interviewing and assessment skills, sensitive to the uniqueness of the client, and knowledgeable of normal physical and psychosocial parameters. The following strategies help to avoid making common diagnostic errors:

- Collect a sufficient amount of subjective and objective data.

- Thoroughly analyze all data.

- Use an organizational framework for clustering data cues.

- Avoid personal bias in interpreting data and grouping into clusters.

- Recognize that an initial diagnosis is subject to change and ongoing revision.

- Continue to collect and analyze data for use in revision process.

- Prioritize diagnoses if more than one diagnosis is evident in order to meet client's immediate need(s).

- Validate conclusions with authoritative sources, client, and/or family.

- Document findings and conclusions in client record according to agency protocol.

- State diagnosis as a client response or client need.

- State expected client-oriented outcomes in desirable and measurable terms.

- Write a diagnostic statement in standard format indicating (1) nursing diagnosis, (2) etiology, and (3) defining characteristics.

- Remember that etiology is often the focus for planning nursing interventions.

- State the diagnosis to reflect conditions that nurses are able to treat.

is a major resource for identifying cue clusters as well as risk factors. The analysis is also helpful in determining healthy functional patterns or dysfunctional ones, and aids in developing and planning nursing interventions

(Ackley & Ladwig, 2002; Berger & Williams, 1999). The nursing diagnosis must be developed from the cues presented by the client data assessment.

One or more expected client outcomes may be identified for each nursing diagnosis. These outcomes represent client progress and are stated in desirable and measurable terms related to the client's physiological, psychosocial, and spiritual health status, and acquisition of knowledge or skills.

## Incorrect Writing of the Nursing Diagnosis Statement

Errors in writing a nursing diagnosis include the use of a symptom as the diagnosis, or repeating the diagnostic label as the etiology. For example: *Deficient Knowledge* RT lack of information does not truly explain the etiology of the diagnosis. A correct statement is *Deficient Knowledge: self-management of medications* RT lack of exposure to information (the etiology is often the main focus for treatment because eliminating the causative factors may resolve the diagnosis). Another error is the misuse of a medical diagnosis that is not amenable to treatment by nurses (Berger & Williams, 1999). The accompanying Nursing Strategy box summarizes strategies for avoiding common diagnostic errors.

In conclusion, the health assessment and diagnosis steps are ongoing processes that can be done formally or informally. A client's condition can change rapidly; the nurse must focus on the mental as well as physical status of the client. Diagnoses may need to be revised in light of analysis and interpretation of new assessment data, as well as a selection of appropriate interventions to meet the client's needs. A primary goal of the nursing process is to develop an individualized plan of care rather than one based on standards or norms (Carrol-Johnson, 2001).

## Limitations of Nursing Diagnosis

A number of limitations and professional concerns are associated with nursing diagnosis. The primary concern is directed toward the lack of consensus among nurses regarding the NANDA–approved nursing diagnosis list. Criticisms about the list include disagreement over specific labels in the classification system and the perception that the list is confining, incomplete, acute care oriented, and confusing. Some nurses feel that the diagnosis classifications detract from humanistic care, and state a label stigmatizes clients (Pesut, 2002). However, the list is not meant to be inclusive. Development and refinement of diagnoses continue to be the focus of NANDA conferences.

Nurses in home health care and outpatient settings consider the Omaha and Home Health Care classifica-

## LIFE SPAN CONSIDERATIONS

### Planning Appropriate Care for the Elderly

Many times in acute care settings, the elderly client will be awaiting discharge without having practical considerations in the nursing care plan for the home care setting. The nurse must remember to do a thorough health history that includes the home environment and how the client's lifestyle is impacted at home. The nurse also needs to include the spouse and family members in regard to applying the nursing process at home.

tions to be more appropriate. Nurses in other specialties have been encouraged to contribute diagnoses that are specific to their areas. Pesut (2002) suggests that those who are skeptical about the use of nursing diagnosis should suspend their judgment until they familiarize themselves with the more than 30 years of research and application projects.

Collaboration between NANDA, ANA, the Iowa Project (NIC and NOC), and other groups will facilitate the integration of the nursing languages and health care databases. The purpose of NANDA is to increase the visibility of nursing's contribution to client care. NANDA is also recognized as a major contributor to the development of nursing knowledge through identifying, using, and refining concepts that are the building blocks of nursing science (NANDA, 2003).

Novice nurses need to know nursing diagnosis and nursing process in order to understand how the discipline of nursing intersects with the other health care providers. NANDA (1999) recognizes that health care is moving into an interdisciplinary, client-focused care environment that requires standardization of languages across disciplines. Many acute care facilities use an interdisciplinary care plan such as care maps and/or critical pathways to monitor

client outcomes. All health care providers use the same care plan to document the client's response to specific interventions. Common "client problems" listed on a critical pathway are written as nursing diagnoses, such as *Risk for Infection* or *Risk for Injury*.

There are also legal considerations concerning the use of nursing diagnoses. Nurses are accountable for their actions and must document their interventions. If a nursing diagnosis is inappropriate or a nursing diagnosis list is incomplete and as a result the interventions are inappropriate or lacking, the nurse is liable for these errors in clinical judgment. These errors can be avoided by collecting comprehensive assessment data and by critically analyzing these data.

## Overcoming Barriers to Nursing Diagnosis

NANDA's language is still relatively new (approximately 25 years) compared to modern medical language that has existed for several hundred years. Some nurses would rather wait until the NANDA listing is complete before

## STOP AND THINK

### Nursing Diagnosis: A Standard Language

- How do you think nursing diagnoses assist nurses with communication among themselves?

- How do nursing diagnoses influence communication among nurses and other health care professionals?

## NURSING STRATEGY

### Strategies for Optimizing the Use of Nursing Diagnosis

Nurses should implement the following strategies when working with nursing diagnoses:

- Agree on a common language.

- Acknowledge and embrace the fluid nature of the language of nursing diagnosis.

- Discuss the purpose and value of nursing diagnosis with administrators and medical staff.

- Support colleagues when they use nursing diagnosis language.

- Adopt a positive attitude toward the principles and taxonomy of nursing diagnosis.

- Be willing to add to the existing body of knowledge by describing unusual nursing phenomena.

- Participate in conferences, workshops, and other educational activities that advance and promote nursing diagnosis.

- Continue communicating with other nurses about nursing diagnosis

they use it. However, it is unrealistic to think that a system such as NANDA should not be used until it is completed. The ever-changing health care scene dictates that nurses participate in evolving methods to communicate within the health care industry.

Familiarity with this language empowers the nurse to communicate more effectively with other nurses and health care team members. Effective communication, in turn, improves the accuracy in nursing diagnoses. Ultimately, the quality of care should improve and the costs associated with that care should decrease. Because many acute-care facilities are asking nurses to do more with fewer resources, nurses are challenged to learn more efficient ways of performing their duties. Nurses' time is spent more efficiently if less time is spent deciphering meanings of words.

When a nurse encounters client situations that do not readily fit the nursing diagnosis language, every attempt should be made to describe the phenomena. The nurse may be on the threshold of documenting the need for a new, as-yet-undiscovered nursing diagnosis.

As nurses collaborate on the refinement of nursing diagnoses, it may be possible to agree on certain aspects of the language. The achievement of this goal will end the use of multiple approaches and will make choices less complicated. Enhanced communication among nurses in everyday settings and among professionals who convene nationally and internationally to exchange ideas about nursing diagnoses is essential.

Most nursing educational programs now offer standardized content related to nursing diagnoses. In addition, experienced nurses need opportunities to review principles of nursing diagnoses, especially since so many are working in settings that tend to favor medical diagnoses and focus on achievement of tasks by the nurse.

Professional advantages of nursing diagnosis include the focus on prescribing nursing interventions that are diagnosis-specific, which should enhance the effectiveness of nursing care. The diagnostic process supports specific rationales for client care based on nursing assessment, and helps create comprehensive and individualized client care. Diagnosis also facilitates evaluation of nursing interventions, and assists in defining the discipline of nursing. The standardized vocabulary aids in communication with other health care disciplines, and provides a framework for developing a system for nursing service reimbursement (Berger & Williams, 1999).

# CASE STUDY/NURSING CARE PLAN

Mr. Lowder is a 62-year-old male who was admitted last night through the emergency room because of difficulty breathing. He was also experiencing some difficulty voiding. His lower extremities are very swollen. History reveals he smokes one pack of cigarettes a day and has done this for the past 45 years. His vital signs are P 112; R 30; BP 172/96; T 101.1°F. He has an eighth-grade education, attends church every week, is estranged from his daughter, and says, "I hate hospitals because my mother died in one."

The nurse takes the necessary amount of time to develop the nursing care plan, which has not yet been added to Mr. Lowder's record of care.

## Assessment
This is a 62-year-old male with dyspnea (respiratory rate, 30/minute), oxygen saturation at 93%, and urination difficulties. He is hypertensive (172/96), and he has tachycardia (pulse, 112/minute). In addition, he has dependent edema and is nervous about being in the acute care setting.

## Nursing Diagnosis #1
*Ineffective Breathing Pattern* as evidenced by hyperventilation
**NOC:** Respiratory Status: Ventilation, Vital Signs Status; Respiratory Status: Airway Patency
**NIC:** Airway Management; Respiratory Monitoring; Vital Signs Monitoring

## Expected Outcomes
The client will:
1. Maintain an effective respiratory rate of below 18/minute within 24 hours
2. Identify and relate the causative factors, if known, to the adaptive ways of coping with them

## Planning/Interventions/Rationales
1. Administer oxygen per physician's order, and monitor oxygen saturation levels and signs or symptoms of respiratory system. *Assesses effective cellular oxygenation.*
2. Reassure client that measures are being taken to ensure the maintenance of adequate cellular oxygenation. *Reinforces decreased anxiety, which assists in the control of the hyperventilatory state.*

*(continues)*

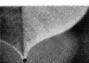

# CASE STUDY/NURSING CARE PLAN (continued)

3. Slow the client's breathing pattern by role-modeling a slower rate of breathing and educating the client as to the need to slow his respiratory rate. *Assists in voluntary control of respiratory rate.*

## Evaluation
Client will be monitored for effective oxygenation by monitoring respiratory rate, oxygen saturation levels, and effective oxygenation.

## Nursing Diagnosis #2
*Ineffective Tissue Perfusion* as demonstrated by inability to void and peripheral edema
**NOC:** Circulation Status; Cardiac Pump Effectiveness; Tissue Perfusion: Cardiac
**NIC:**   Circulatory Care: Arterial Insufficiency

## Expected Outcomes
The client will:
1. Improve renal tissue perfusion as demonstrated by return of renal function.
2. Demonstate a decreasing blood pressure, peripheral edema, and pulse rate within 24 to 48 hours.

## Planning/Interventions/Rationales
1. Measure blood pressure and renal output every 2 hours. *Provides accurate assessment of renal function.*
2. Restrict fluids, decrease sodium intake, and measure daily weight. *Decreases peripheral edema, lowers blood pressure, and evaluates edema.*
3. Promote factors that improve venous return, such as keeping lower extremities elevated. *Decreases peripheral edema.*

## Evaluation
Blood pressure monitored every 2 hours and client is still hypertensive (166/94). Renal output measured every 2 hours and is averaging 80 cc/hr. Legs are slightly less in circumference in 24 hours, and overall weight is decreased by 1 pound.

# Key Concepts

- Nursing diagnosis is the second step in the nursing process and is the clinical judgment about individual, family, or community (aggregates) responses to actual or risk problems, wellness states, or syndromes.
- Through the efforts of NANDA and ANA, the identification and validation of nursing diagnosis as the second step of the nursing process has been substantiated and forms the basis for professional accountability.
- Nursing diagnosis has a label or title, and etiology. A three-part statement also includes defining characteristics.
- Nursing diagnosis contributes to a clearer conceptualization of knowledge unique to nursing, improved communication among nurses and other health care professionals, promotion of individualized client care, and support for theory development and nursing research.
- Nursing diagnoses can be written as either two-part statements (diagnostic label and etiology) or three-part statements (diagnostic label, etiology, and defining characteristics).
- The NANDA nursing diagnosis taxonomy is composed of nine human response patterns: exchanging, communicating, relating, valuing, choosing, moving, perceiving, knowing, and feeling.

- The process of developing a nursing diagnosis includes analysis of assessment cues, validation of cues, interpretation of cues, clustering of data, consulting NANDA's list of approved nursing diagnoses, and writing the nursing diagnosis statement.
- When the nurse is knowledgeable about the components of the nursing diagnosis process and is equipped to develop the diagnostic statement, the nurse is able to make appropriate decisions regarding therapeutic nursing interventions.
- To avoid committing errors in the nursing diagnostic process, the nurse should ensure that the data collection is complete, that the interpretation of the data is accurate and based upon the nursing and not the medical diagnosis, and that the client's response to a health problem is amenable to therapeutic nursing interventions.
- The barriers that have been identified as preventing the use of nursing diagnosis in a more universal manner are the constraints on the time nurses can devote to client care, the continuing organization of health care according to medical diagnosis, the constantly evolving refinement of the nursing diagnosis language, and the availability of numerous approaches for formulation and application of nursing diagnoses.

- Although barriers to the use of nursing diagnosis may be present, they may be overcome by employing specific strategies such as agreeing on a common language, supporting colleagues' attempts to use nursing diagnoses, adopting a nonjudgmental attitude, and continuing to communicate with other nurses at national and international levels.
- Nursing Interventions Classification (NIC) is a standardized language of treatments, activities, and interventions performed by nurses on behalf of clients. The classification consists of more than 486 intervention labels covering both direct and indirect care. NIC has been field tested, can be used in computer documentation systems, and is linked to NANDA nursing diagnoses. (NIC/NOC Center, University of Iowa, 2002; Nursing Practice FAQs Sheet, 1999).
- Nursing Outcomes Classification (NOC) is a comprehensive standardized language to describe client outcomes that are sensitive to nursing intervention in all settings and all specialties. Currently, there are over 260 outcomes. Each outcome contains a list of indicators with a five-point scale that can be used to measure the effectiveness of interventions. NOC is linked to nursing diagnosis and is used with NIC. (Ackley & Ladwig, 2002; Nursing Practice FAQs Sheet, 1999).
- Client outcomes are client behaviors or perceptions that are responsive to nursing intervention.

## Review Questions and Activities

1. Nate Jefferson, a nursing student, was reviewing his client's chart. The list of nursing diagnoses included in the chart seemed to describe the client well. However, something disturbed Jefferson about the list. The list he reviewed appears below. What is your response to this list? Identify the nursing diagnoses that seem to be problematic and the reasons for your conclusions.
   a. *Impaired Swallowing* as evidenced by stasis of food in oral cavity after chewing
   b. *Risk for Injury* as evidenced by weight and being dropped by staff
   c. *Impaired Skin Integrity* RT infrequent repositioning by staff
   d. *Chronic Confusion* as evidenced by Alzheimer's disease
   e. *Acute Pain* RT pain in right foot
2. Mr. Tyler is a 37-year-old client who limps into the clinic with pain in the right foot and swelling in the extremity. He is 5 feet 6 inches tall and weighs 275 pounds. While consulting the approved NANDA list of diagnoses, develop initial nursing diagnoses based on these data.

3. Alison Jones, RN, performs the nursing assessment and physical exam on Mr. Evans, a newly admitted client. Due to an emergency at home, Ms. Jones must leave, and Dolores Smythe, RN, is assigned to care for Mr. Evans. Discuss possible sources of errors and ways to avoid them in planning Mr. Evans's care.
4. *Impaired Physical Mobility* is an approved NANDA diagnosis. List several etiologies that are appropriate for this diagnosis. Develop a two-part nursing diagnostic statement.
5. Select one strategy to overcome barriers to using nursing diagnoses. Describe how you would use this strategy in your clinical setting.
6. John Babcock, RN, asks: "What's all the fuss about nursing diagnoses?" What would your response to him be?
7. Nursing diagnoses empower the nursing profession. Money is usually associated with power. Discuss how the use of nursing diagnoses affects both power and reimbursement in the nursing profession.

## Multimedia Links

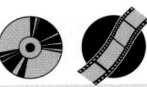

Christensen *Core Concept Videos:* Assessment and Diagnosis

## Web Resources

North American Nursing Diagnosis Association (NANDA)
   http://www.nanda.org
Nursing Net
   http://www.nursingnet.org
Nursing World
   http://www.nursingworld.org

## References

Aaronson, L., Teel, C., Cassmeyer, V., Neuberger, G., Pallikkathayil, L., Pierce, J., Press, A.,Williams, P., and Wingate, A. (1999). Defining and measuring fatigue. *Image: Journal of Nursing Scholarship, 31*(1), 45–50.

Ackley, B., & Ladwig, G. (2002). *Nursing diagnosis handbook: A guide to planning care* (5th ed.). St. Louis: Mosby.

American Nurses Association (1973). *Standards of nursing practice.* Kansas City, MO: Author.

American Nurses Association (1995). *Nursing: A social policy statement.* Kansas City, MO: Author.

American Nurses Association (1998). *Standards of clinical nursing practice.* Washington, DC: Author.

American Nurses Association (2001). *Nursing diagnoses: Reflections and classifications 2001–2002.* Philadelphia: Author.

American Nurses Association (2003). *Standards of clinical practice*. Philadelphia: Author.

Anderson, M. (2000). Virginia Avenel Henderson: A modern legend. *Wyoming Nurse, 12*(1), 9–10.

Berger, K., & Williams, M. (1999). *Fundamentals of nursing: Collaborating for optimal health*. Stamford, CT: Appleton & Lange.

Carpenito, L. (1989). *Nursing diagnosis: Application to clinical practice* (3rd ed.). Philadelphia: J. B. Lippincott.

Carpenito, L. (1995). *Nursing diagnosis: Application to clinical practice* (6th ed.). Philadelphia: J. B. Lippincott.

Carpenito, L. (2002). *Nursing diagnosis: Application to clinical practice* (8th ed.). Philadelphia: J. B. Lippincott.

Carpenito, L. (2004). *Nursing diagnosis: Application to clinical practice* (10th ed). Philadelphia: J. B. Lippincott.

Carrol-Johnson, R. (2001). Learning to think. *Nursing Diagnosis, 12*(2), 43–44.

Carlson-Catalano, J., Lunney, M., Paradiso, C., Bruno, J., Luise, B., Martin, T., Massoni, M., & Pachter, S. (1998). Clinical validation of ineffective breathing pattern, ineffective airway clearance, and impaired gas exchange. *Image: Journal of Nursing Scholarship, 30*(3), 243–248.

Clingerman, E. (1999). Recognizing nursing's contributions to patient care. *Michigan Nurse, 72*(5), 7–8.

Deutsch, M. (1968). Field theory in social psychology. In G. Lindzey & E. Aronson (Eds.). *The handbook of social psychology*. Reading, MA: Addison-Wesley.

Doenges, M., Moorehouse, M., & Geissler-Murr, A. (2002). *Nurse's pocket guide: Diagnoses, interventions, and rationales* (8th ed.). Philadelphia: F. A. Davis.

Doenges, M., Moorehouse, M., & Burley, J. (2000). *Application of nursing process and nursing diagnosis* (3rd ed.). Philadelphia: F. A. Davis.

Dzurec, L., Hoover, P., & Fields, J. (2002). Acknowledging unexplained fatigue of tired women. *Journal of Nursing Scholarship, 34*(1), 41–46.

Fry, V. (1953). The creative approach to nursing. *American Journal of Nursing, 53*, 301–302.

Gebbie, K., & Lavin, M. (1974). Classifying nursing diagnoses. *American Journal of Nursing, 74*(2), 250–253.

Mallick, M., & Whipple, T. (2000). Validity of the nursing diagnosis of relocation stress syndrome. *Nursing Research, 49*(2), 97–100.

McCloskey, J., & Bulecheck, G. (2000). *Nursing interventions classifications (NIC)* (3rd ed.). St. Louis: Mosby Year Book.

McHale, J., Phipps, M., Horvath, K., & Schmelz, J. (1998). Expert nursing knowledge in the care of patients at risk of impaired swallowing. *Image: Journal of Nursing Scholarship, 30*(2), 137–141.

*Michigan Nurse* (2000). Reimbursement for nursing activities. http://www.minurses.org

*Minnesota Nursing Accent* (1999). Communication through standardized language. http://www.roch.edu/Library

North American Nursing Diagnosis Association (1996). *Nursing diagnoses: Definitions and classification, 1995–1996*. Philadelphia: Author.

North American Nursing Diagnosis Association (1999). *Nursing diagnoses: Definitions and classification, 1999–2000*. Philadelphia: Author.

North American Nursing Diagnosis Association (2001). *Nursing diagnoses: Definitions and classification, 2001–2002*. Philadelphia: Author.

North American Nursing Diagnosis Association (2003). *Nursing diagnoses: Definitions and classification, 2003–2004*. Philadelphia: Author.

Nursing practice FAQs sheet no. 5 (1999). Standardized nursing language. *Minnesota Nursing Accent, 71*(6), 9–10.

Pesut, D., & Herman, J. (1999). *Clinical reasoning: The art and science of critical and creative thinking*. Clifton Park, NY: Delmar Learning.

Pesut, D. J. (2002). Education, Nursing Nomenclatures, and Eye-Roll Anxiety Control. *Journal of Professional Nursing, 18*(1), 3–4.

Roy, C., & Andrews, H. (1991). *The Roy Adaptation Model: The definitive statement*. Norwalk, CT: Appleton & Lange.

Schall, M., & Flannery, J. (2000). Directions for curricular change: The 1980 and 1995 American Nurses Association's policy statements. *Nurse Educator, 25*(1), 17–18.

Whitley, G. (1999). Processes and methodologies for research validation of nursing diagnoses. *Nursing Diagnosis, 10*(1), 5–13.

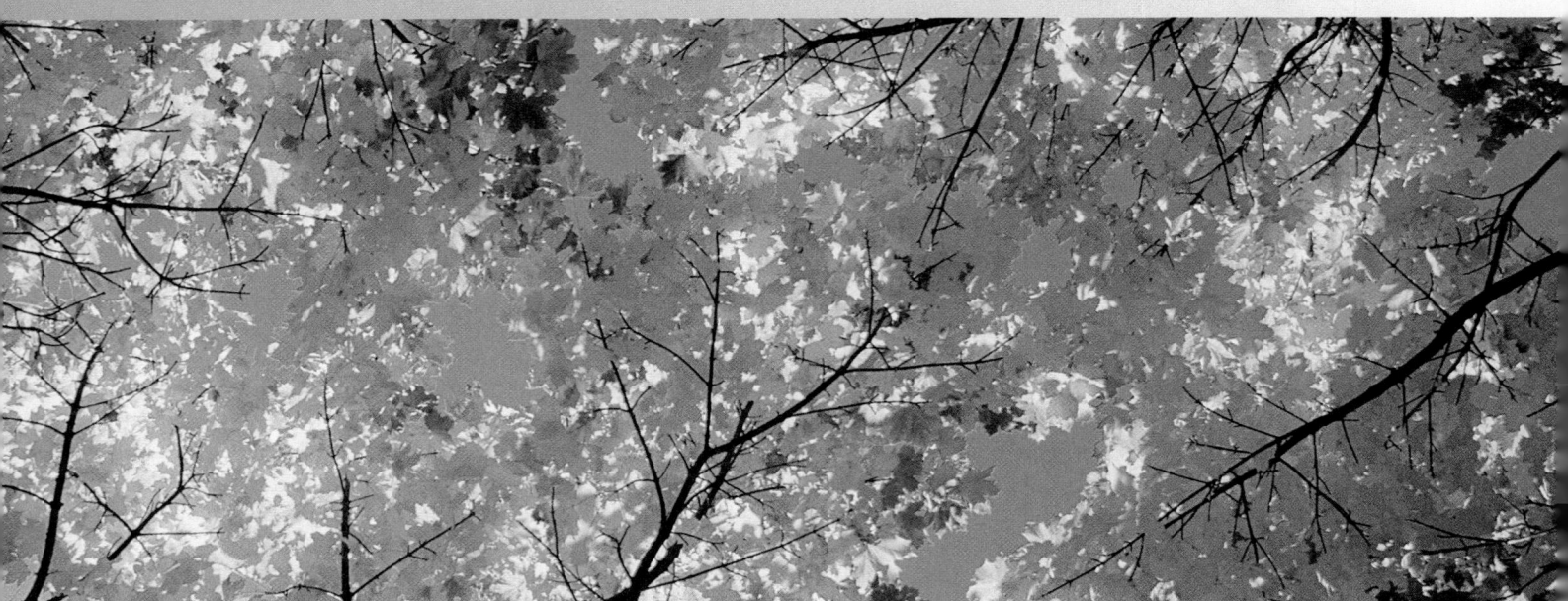

# Outcome Identification and Planning

Ruth N. Grendell, DNSc, RN

*"As a profession, I want nurses to develop expertise in clinical reasoning. To do so, there needs to be a shift in thinking from problems to OUTCOMES."*

*(Daniel Pesut, 2000)*

# *Chapter Competencies*

*Upon completion of this chapter, the reader should be able to:*

1. Explain the purposes of outcome identification and planning.
2. Describe the four elements of the process of outcome identification and planning.
3. Describe the characteristics of expected outcomes.
4. Discuss the components in the construction of expected outcomes.
5. Identify nursing strategies in planning nursing care.
6. Evaluate the nursing outcome classifications.
7. Describe the use of the care plan in the outcome identification and planning step of the nursing process.
8. Discuss strategies for overcoming barriers to effective planning of nursing care.

# *Key Terms*

collaboration

consultation

criteria

dependent nursing intervention

evidence-based nursing

expected outcome

independent nursing intervention

interdependent nursing intervention

long-term outcome

nursing intervention

nursing order

nursing sensitive outcome

plan of care

planning

rationale

short-term outcome

The third step of the nursing process encompasses outcome identification and planning. After a nurse thoroughly assesses a client and determines the client's unique nursing diagnoses, or health problems, a plan of action is developed. Client-specific outcomes are established to resolve the diagnoses that are measurable within a time frame for attainment. A "preferred outcome" statement describes (1) the expected client status (behavior or function) when a problem-focused nursing diagnosis has been resolved, (2) the modification of a condition that places the client at risk for a diagnosis, or (3) a client's positive adaptation that has been enhanced, as with a wellness diagnosis (Berger & Williams, 1999). "Desired outcomes encompass biologic, psychological, sociocultural and spiritual aspects of health, or related knowledge and skills" (Fortinash, 2000; Wilkinson, 1998).

The major components of planning are:

- Establishing diagnosis priorities
- Developing expected client outcomes and establishing outcome criteria
- Planning nursing strategies (with collaboration and consultation as needed)
- Writing the nursing care plan and nursing orders

The components of a client care plan are:

- Diagnostic statement(s)
- Desired client outcome statement(s)
- Description of nursing interventions
- Evaluation criteria

This chapter explains the planning component of the nursing process. The purpose, as well as the entire process, of the planning concept is illustrated with theory and examples. Strategies for effective planning of quality nursing care are described together with problems frequently encountered in this stage of the nursing process. The role of critical thinking in planning and outcome identification is emphasized.

## Purposes of Outcome Identification and Planning

The American Nurses Association (1998), in its *Standards of Clinical Nursing Practice*, identifies outcome identification and planning as essential principles for ensuring the delivery of competent nursing care and outlines these components in terms of their significance within the nursing process (see Box 13-1). Although the overall purpose of a client's plan of care should be to maintain or improve health at an optimal level, planning is a framework on which to base scientific nursing practice. Therefore, the purposes of the planning component of the nursing process are to provide adequate direction to ensure quality nursing care for individual clients, families, groups, and communities; to present a vehicle to improve

## BOX 13-1    OUTCOME IDENTIFICATION AND PLANNING AS A STANDARD COMPONENT OF CARE: ANA STANDARDS

### Standard III. Outcome Identification

The nurse identifies expected outcomes individualized to the client.

*Guidelines*

Outcomes should be:

- Based on diagnoses
- Documented in measurable terms
- Developed with the client and health care providers
- Realistic and achievable

### Standard IV. Planning

The nurse develops a plan of care that prescribes interventions to attain expected outcomes.

*Guidelines*

Planning should:

- Be individualized to the client's needs and status
- Be developed with the client, significant others, and health care providers
- Be documented
- Promote continuity of care

Used with permission from American Nurses Association. (1998). *Standards of Clinical Nursing Practice.* (2nd ed.). Washington, DC: Author.

communication with health care personnel; and to provide continuity in the delivery of individualized, quality nursing care to all clients.

The 1995 American Nurses Association (ANA) policy statement emphasized health promotion as a primary focus of nurses and nursing care. Nursing interventions are related to human experiences and responses to birth, health, illness, and death within the context of individuals, families, groups, and communities (Schall & Flannery, 2000).

Therefore, the purposes of the nursing process's planning component are to provide adequate direction to ensure quality nursing care for clients across the continuum of care, to present a mechanism for communication among health care personnel, and to provide continuity of quality nursing care that is unique to each client (Oermann & Huber, 1999; Wilkinson, 1998).

# Process of Outcome Identification and Planning

The five steps of the nursing process are at the very core in using scientific reasoning for the delivery of individualized, quality nursing care in any setting. The ability to make appropriate decisions based on a strong knowledge base and problem-solving strategies is an expected behavior of the professional nurse (Rubenfeld & Scheffer, 1999).

## Critical Thinking

The development and evaluation of a plan for individualized client care is a professional responsibility of all nurses. Nurses must have a strong foundation of nursing knowledge and a clear understanding of the nursing process, be skilled in assessment, and make decisions based on problem-solving skills and critical thinking (Berger & Williams, 1999).

The nursing process is not always an orderly process. Each step of the nursing process has feedback loops that influence the assessment and interpretation of data. The nursing process steps are also intertwined, thus changes in one step will affect the others (Rubenfeld & Scheffer, 1999). The most critical component of the planning process is the identification of appropriate nursing diagnoses and their priority rank (Singer, 2000). Environmental factors, changes in client condition, and new assessment feedback can suggest:

1. A change in the client's diagnosis
2. Overlapping diagnoses
3. New diagnoses in order to meet the expected outcome

Planning is sequential, dynamic, and future-oriented. Planning includes establishing priorities, identifying goals and expected outcomes, developing nursing interventions, and documenting the client's plan of care. Appropriate guidelines are used to prioritize urgent needs. The client's nursing diagnoses are determined and then ranked by mutual agreement of the nurse and client or significant others. The planning component continues with thorough examination of this prioritized list of nursing diagnoses and determination of the client's goals and desired expected outcomes. After a clear picture is obtained regarding the diagnoses and goals, the nursing interventions can be planned to achieve the desired outcomes.

In the planning phase, the nurse organizes "thought processes for clinical decision making" (Doenges, Moorehouse, & Geissler-Murr, 2002). To think critically is to examine an issue purposefully from a goal-directed perspective. Critical thinking "is based on principles of science and scientific method" (Alfaro-LeFevre, 2004). Skills needed by today's nurses include the ability to understand the process of care provision across the continuum, and the ability to analyze that care in terms of cost and benefit and make ethical decisions. Nurses must also have strong assessment and collaborative skills as well as be the client advocate (Kersbergen, 2000). Therefore, critical thinking is a useful procedure in the development of objectives and in the formulation of a blueprint to achieve those objectives. The formulation of objectives is accomplished by using valid and reliable data previously gathered during the assessment component of the nursing process.

## Establishing Priorities

The establishment of priorities is the first element of planning. In establishing priorities, the nurse examines the client's nursing diagnoses and ranks them in order of physiological or psychological importance. This method organizes a client's nursing diagnoses into an operational format for the planning of nursing care. These diagnoses should be mutually ranked by the nurse and client or family and significant others. Involving the client in shared decision-making power helps motivate the client and gives the client a feeling of control, which inspires successful achievement of each goal (Doenges et al., 2002). Determining priorities is a complex process that enhances quality and efficiency of care. Priorities do not remain constant but change with the client's condition or when diagnoses are resolved. In some instances, several problems may be ranked simultaneously as priority (Berger & Williams, 1999).

When an individual client has more than one diagnosis, the nurse and client need to establish priorities to identify which nursing diagnosis will be addressed initially in the plan of care (Carpenito, 2004) (Figure 13-1). By communicating this decision-making process to other members of the health care team, the nurse encourages an orderly approach to the achievement of optimal health for each client.

Various guidelines are used in the establishment of priorities for determining which nursing diagnosis will be addressed initially. The client's basic needs, safety, and desires, as well as anticipation of future diagnoses, must be

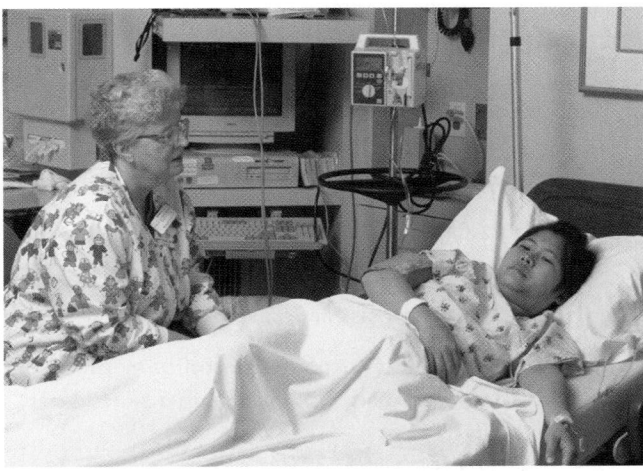

**Figure 13-1    Nurses working with clients in the acute care setting must set priorities while identifying multiple nursing diagnoses.**

## STOP AND THINK

### Prioritizing Nursing Diagnoses

Mr. Clyde Morrison, an elderly homeless client, was admitted to the hospital with a medical diagnosis of malnutrition. Identified nursing diagnoses include *Imbalanced Nutrition, Less Than Body Requirements* related to inability to procure appropriate food; *Constipation* related to inadequate fluid intake; and *Disturbed Body Image* related to feelings of inadequacy and inability to live up to identified standards. What should the priority ranking of this client's nursing diagnoses be?

considered. One of the most common methods of selecting priorities is the consideration of Maslow's hierarchy of needs, which requires that a life-threatening diagnosis be given more urgency than a non-life-threatening diagnosis. Once the basic physiological needs (e.g., respiration, nutrition, hydration, elimination) are met to some degree, the nurse may consider needs on the next level of the hierarchy (e.g., safe environment, stable living condition) and so on up the hierarchy until all the client's nursing diagnoses have been prioritized. Establishing priorities is a complex process that enhances quality and efficiency of care (Atkinson & Murray, 2000).

A useful guide for the beginning nursing student would be to examine each nursing diagnosis, determine its level of need, and rank the need in order of priority. Table 13-1 illustrates this process.

Another consideration in the designation of priorities is client preferences. If at all possible, the client should always be involved in the decision-making process of establishing priorities. If the nurse and the client do not mutually set priorities, there may be a contradictory course of direction and motivation, which may lead to noncompliance and nonresolution of the client's nursing

| TABLE 13-1 | RANKING NURSING DIAGNOSES | |
|---|---|---|
| Nursing Diagnosis | Maslow's Hierarchy of Needs | Rank |
| *Anxiety* related to hospitalization | Safety and security | Moderate |
| *Ineffective Coping* | Self-esteem | Low |
| *Ineffective Airway Clearance* related to excessive secretions | Physiological | High |

diagnoses. The client must participate in the identification of priorities so that the nature of the problem, as well as the client's values, is reflected in the selected course of action (Atkinson & Murray, 2000).

An additional point regarding the establishment of priorities is the anticipation of future diagnoses. Nursing diagnoses of low and moderate priorities often involve the prevention of anticipated potential or risk diagnoses. Although potential nursing diagnoses may not be a current threat to the client, their seriousness may require that the nurse consider the development of nursing interventions directed toward prevention of the problem. For example, a client in the Postanesthesia Care Unit may have a high-priority nursing diagnosis of *Ineffective Breathing Pattern* related to the anesthesia and sedative drugs. Despite the fact that the client currently has no problem in this area, this diagnosis is indeed the basis for the Postanesthesia Care Unit protocol of monitoring the client closely.

Establishing priorities does not mean that one diagnosis must be totally resolved before giving attention to another diagnosis. Nursing interventions for several diagnoses may be carried out simultaneously. However, at times, it is crucial that the nurse and client correctly identify the order of priority of the client's nursing diagnoses so that maximum effort can be directed toward resolution of the most urgent diagnosis. Table 13-2 illustrates this process.

| TABLE 13-2 | PRIORITIZING NURSING DIAGNOSES WITH ACCOMPANYING NURSING IMPLICATIONS | |
|---|---|---|
| Priority | Diagnosis | Nursing Implications |
| High | *Ineffective Breathing Pattern* | • Assess breath sounds.<br>• Auscultate lungs.<br>• Monitor vital signs.<br>• Reposition client. |
| Moderate | *Risk for Impaired Skin Integrity* | • Perform comprehensive skin assessment.<br>• Keep skin clean and dry.<br>• Provide turning schedule. |
| Low | *Ineffective Coping* | • Assist to identify problem.<br>• Encourage keeping daily journal.<br>• Teach client strategies for expressing feelings. |

## Identifying Expected Outcomes

After assessing the client, formulating nursing diagnoses, and establishing priorities, the nurse identifies and establishes expected outcomes for each nursing diagnosis. The purposes of setting expected outcomes are to provide guidelines for individualized nursing interventions and to establish evaluation criteria to measure the effectiveness of the nursing care plan.

Although the terms *goals, objectives,* and *outcomes* traditionally have been used interchangeably in many health care settings, *expected outcomes* is the preferred term. This term reflects terminology used in quality assurance, quality improvement, and case management protocols. "An **expected (or desired) outcome** is a description of the favorable client status that is achieved when a problem-focused nursing diagnosis has been resolved or positive adaptation has been enhanced" (Berger & Williams, 1999). Clearly written outcome statements stipulate the client's expected behavior or function within a specified time frame, rather than what the nursing interventions will accomplish. Some outcome statements require qualifiers, or the conditions involved with the client's activity. Examples are "with the help of a walker," "in a wheelchair," or "while on a specific diet." Desired outcome statements serve as the basis for selecting nursing interventions to assist the client in outcome attainment (Berger & Williams, 1999).

Each desired outcome statement is related to only one nursing diagnosis; however, one diagnosis may require more than one outcome statement (Box 13-2). Combining outcome statements that are related to more than one nursing diagnosis is confusing, as each diagnosis may have a different etiology and require different nursing interventions and evaluation measures. Although *Activity Intolerance* and *Ineffective Breathing Pattern* can be present concurrently, the outcome and the nursing interventions to resolve the two diagnoses should not appear in one outcome statement. Nursing interventions and related statements are discussed later in the chapter.

### STOP AND THINK

**Expected Outcomes**

(Refer to Table 13-2)

● What expected outcomes accompany the nursing diagnosis *Ineffective Breathing Pattern*?

● What expected outcomes accompany the nursing diagnosis *Risk for Impaired Skin Integrity*?

● What expected outcomes accompany the nursing diagnosis *Ineffective Coping*?

## BOX 13-2    SHORT-TERM AND LONG-TERM OUTCOMES

*Nursing Diagnosis: Chronic pain related to rheumatoid arthritis*

The basic structure of the outcome statement contains a subject (the client), a verb (task/action), and an object, or client outcome criteria (behavior/function).

*Short-term (focused on etiology, within hours/days)*

The client:

- Uses pain rating scale to identify current level of pain intensity

- Demonstrates ability to pace self, taking rest periods before they are needed

- Describes plan for pain relief (drug and non-drug therapies)

*Long-Term (focused on problem, within a longer time frame)*

The client:

- Functions on an acceptable ability level with minimal interference from pain and medication side effects

Adapted from Ackley & Ladwig, 2002; Atkinson & Murray, 2000.

of time, usually over weeks or months. See Box 13-2 for examples of short-term and long-term outcomes.

In the current managed care environment and due to shorter hospital stays, most long-term outcomes cannot be met; however, several short-term outcomes can be used as incremental progress steps in meeting a long-term outcome. Long-term outcomes may require direct nursing interventions (preserving skin integrity for a client on bed rest) or outcomes that are met by a series of short-term outcomes (e.g., the client loses a specific amount of weight within designated times until the outcome is reached) (Atkinson & Murray, 2000; Berger & Williams, 1999).

Another consideration in writing outcomes is the accuracy in identifying the etiology of the problem. If the etiology of the problem is incorrectly identified, the client may meet the short-term outcome without resolving the problem. Thus, it is important to correctly identify the etiology of the problem.

Setting long-term outcomes is important in successful discharge planning. Ideally discharge planning begins soon after the client is admitted to the acute care setting. It helps in coordinating all health care team members to accomplish the same overall purpose, that is, client discharge. Coordination promotes continuity of care into settings such as restorative care or home health.

### Expected Outcomes

Given the client's unique situation and resources, expected outcomes are constructed to be:

- Realistic
- Mutually desired by the client and nurse
- Attainable within a defined time period

## Writing Outcomes

Written outcomes need to be constructed clearly. Clear, precise terminology improves the chances that outcomes will be achieved. When outcomes are clearly written, their establishment provides direction for the nursing plan of care and for determination of effectiveness in the evaluation of nursing interventions. A guideline is provided for the desired change in the client, and the client has a clear idea of the direction needed to resolve each nursing diagnosis. Expected outcomes establish appropriate evaluation criteria to measure the effectiveness of planned nursing interventions to resolve the client's individual nursing diagnoses.

Outcomes should be established to meet the immediate, as well as long-term prevention and rehabilitation, needs of the client. A **short-term outcome** is a statement written in objective format demonstrating an expectation to be achieved in resolution of the nursing diagnosis in a short period of time, usually in a few hours or days. A **long-term outcome** is a statement written in objective format demonstrating an expectation to be achieved in resolution of the nursing diagnosis over a longer period

## LIFE SPAN CONSIDERATIONS

### Elderly and Expected Outcomes

There are a variety of nursing strategies to consider for elderly clients when developing expected outcomes:

- Allow an older client extra time to meet expected outcomes.

- Include families and support persons in the planning processes. They can provide valuable information about the client's abilities and lifestyle.

- Carefully assess the client's environment before establishing mutual goals.

- Perform a thorough holistic assessment to create realistic expected outcomes.

## Home Care and Expected Outcomes

Rosa Martinez has been recovering from orthopedic back surgery in a restorative care facility. She is discharged home, and her home health nurse identifies the following nursing diagnosis: *Risk for Disuse Syndrome* related to immobilization due to skeletal traction. The following factors need to be considered as the home health nurse writes the short-term and long-term outcomes for this client:

● Immediate needs: maintenance of elimination patterns, promotion of skin integrity, preservation of effective breathing patterns, and minimization of long-term immobility

● Rehabilitative needs: resumption of normal musculoskeletal function, ability to use assistive devices correctly, increase in activity tolerance, and enhancement of self-esteem and well-being

The short-term outcomes should focus on the maintenance of physiological patterns involving elimination, skin integrity, respiration, and mobility. The long-term outcomes should concentrate on the client's return to maximal functional capability and independence (Alexander & Kraposki, 1999) (Figure 13-2).

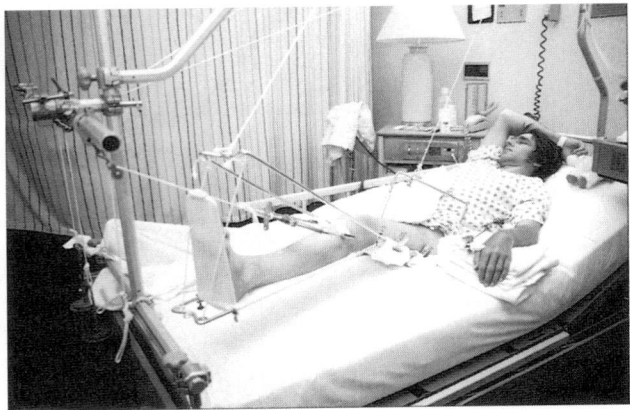

**Figure 13-2   It is often necessary to establish many long-term outcomes for clients with rehabilitative needs, such as for this orthopedic client.**

defining characteristics (symptoms). The absence of these characteristics indicates the problem has been resolved (Berger & Williams, 1999).

Each component of an appropriately written outcome is discussed in the following paragraphs. For clarity of each concept, examples are provided with related discussion. The examples are designed with the intent of developing skills in the construction of expected outcomes.

### Subject

The component to be considered initially in writing an outcome is the subject. The subject identifies the person who will perform the desired behavior or meet the outcome. In a client-centered plan of nursing care, the client is the person who needs to achieve a desired change in behavior. See the Nursing Strategy box for an application of the subject component.

Because nursing care is based on a holistic approach, expected outcomes may be written in the spiritual, emotional, physiological, developmental, and social dimensions. An expected outcome depicts measurable behavioral change or evidence of change in the client when the outcome has been met. Expected outcomes are used in the evaluation process by providing a standard for comparison to determine if the client successfully accomplished the outcome.

In the construction of expected outcome objectives, essential components include subject, task statement, criteria, the conditions (if necessary), and time frame (Doenges et al., 2002). When outcome statements are written clearly, the nurse can select nursing interventions to ensure that the client's baseline data are thoroughly assessed, individual client needs are identified, and appropriate approaches are used in the plan of care.

Each nursing diagnosis has one expected outcome that may have several measurable evaluation criteria, or evidence, that the outcome has been achieved. The nurse decides upon a nursing diagnosis based on the presence of

### Examples of Documentation of Expected Outcomes

1. By Saturday, the client will ambulate the entire length of the hallway three times a day.

2. The client will demonstrate the technique for self-administration of insulin by Friday.

3. The client will take own radial pulse and obtain the same results as the nurse by Saturday.

4. By Friday, the client will plan a low-salt diet for 24 hours in accordance with the diet plan left by the dietitian.

Note how each example reflects the client as the subject performing an action.

## NURSING STRATEGY

### Examples of Criteria Application

1. By Saturday, the client will ambulate the entire length of the hallway three times a day.

2. The client will demonstrate the technique for self-administration of insulin by Friday.

3. The client will take own radial pulse and obtain the same results as the nurse by Saturday.

4. By Friday, the client will plan a low-salt diet for 24 hours in accordance with the diet plan left by the dietitian.

The examples indicate the standards used to evaluate whether the behavior demonstrated by the client indicates that the goal has been reached.

Example 1 includes criteria of a time limit and amount of activity.

Example 2 demonstrates important characteristics of performance accuracy by stating "with aseptic technique."

Example 3 sets standards of performance accuracy and includes a time limit.

Example 4 includes a time limit and a sample plan to be followed.

### Task Statement

The next component in writing outcomes is the task statement or the action verb. This component describes what the client (or subject) will do to obtain an expected change in behavior. The task statement enables the evaluator to determine achievement of observable behavior. When the actual behavior is stated as a task statement that can be clearly and directly measured, the nurse can determine whether the client is demonstrating achievement of the expected outcome.

Only one task statement should be used for each outcome. It is clearer to write separate outcomes than to try to accurately measure a combination of tasks—for instance, "ambulate the entire length of the hallway" from number 1 in the Nursing Strategy box.

### Criteria

The next essential component is the criteria of an outcome. **Criteria** are standards used to evaluate whether the demonstrated behavior indicates accomplishment of the outcome. Criteria may be written in a variety of ways. Criteria may include:

- A time limit
- Amount of activity

- Important characteristics of accurate performance
- Description of the performance to be followed

The nurse should specify the precise performance to be considered acceptable in accomplishment of the outcome.

It is not always possible to specify a criterion with as much detail as one would like; however, the nurse should continue to communicate precise criteria as explicitly as possible. To provide better direction to the client, the nurse considers how well the client, family member, or significant other should perform the task. See the Nursing Strategy box on the following page for an application of criteria.

### Conditions

The next component to be included in writing proper outcomes is the conditions under which the client should perform or demonstrate mastery of the task. Although this component is optional in terms of writing outcomes, conditions may provide clarity and assist the client in demonstrating the expected behavior. The conditions may include the experiences that the client is expected to have before performing the task. Example 1 in the Nursing Strategy box states the condition with which the activity must be performed (i.e., "with the use of a walker"). Example 4 cites the condition by which the activity must be performed (i.e., "in accordance with the diet plan left by the dietitian").

### Time Frame

The last component to be included in writing outcomes appropriately is the time frame in which the client should perform or demonstrate mastery of the task.

## Strategies for Well-Written Expected Outcome Statements

Nursing students and inexperienced nurses are often reluctant to develop unique, or individualized, care plans, and may rely heavily on standard and textbook-created plans. Clients should be included in the decision and planning processes. The expected outcome and plan of care must be realistic, as well as congruent with and supportive of other therapies. See the Nursing Strategy box on the following page for helpful guidelines in writing effective expected outcome statements.

## Planning Nursing Interventions

Once the outcomes have been mutually agreed on by the nurse and client, the nurse should use a decision-making process to select appropriate nursing interventions. A **nursing intervention** is an action performed by a nurse that helps the client to achieve the results specified by the expected outcome. These terms are based on scientific principles and knowledge from behavioral and physical sciences. Usually, several nursing interventions are developed for each of the outcomes identified for the client (Berger & Williams, 1999). It is important to identify as

## NURSING STRATEGY

### Guidelines for Effective Expected Outcome Statements

- State the outcomes in terms of client outcomes, not nursing actions.

- Clearly describe the client's behavior or function that demonstrates reduction or resolution of a problem-focused nursing diagnosis, and positive adaptation with a wellness (health promotion) diagnosis.

- Use positive terms. State what client behavior you would realistically want to observe. Outcomes should be observable and measurable.

- Specify the expected time frame for the client to achieve the expected outcome.

- Relate each desired outcome to one specific nursing diagnosis. Each diagnosis should have an adequate number of outcomes.

- Determine whether the client and family or support system value the outcome.

- Collaborate with the client as a partner in the planning process to promote a mutual understanding of the situation. Shared decision making empowers the client, enhances trust, and implies consent.

- Start with short-term outcomes. This allows for frequent evaluation of the client's progress and permits a timely modification of the plan of care if necessary.

- Outcomes must be compatible with the total therapeutic plan. Outcomes should be included in the overall plan of care. Sharing information with all health care team members provides the client with the benefit of the collective expertise.

- Outcomes are stated based on professional knowledge, resources, and research, and are compatible with standards of care. Refer to the Evidenced-Based Practice and the Nursing Outcomes Classification (NOC) that are discussed later in the chapter

Ackley, B. & Ladwig, G. (2002). *Nursing diagnosis handbook: A guide to planning care.* St. Louis: Mosby; Atkinson, L. & Murray, M. (2002). *Understanding the nursing process in a changing care environment.* New York: McGraw-Hill.

many nursing interventions as possible so that if one proves to be unsuitable, others are readily available. The interventions are prioritized according to the order in which they will be implemented.

With the inclusion of scientific problem solving and critical thinking, the delivery of quality, individualized nursing care is greatly enhanced. Through critical thinking, sound conclusions are reached in the selection of nursing interventions to prevent, reduce, or eliminate the nursing diagnoses or problems. The nurse studies the entire issue thoroughly in the planning component of the nursing process by examining the assessment data and nursing diagnoses, analyzing the client's outcomes and expected outcomes, and selecting which nursing interventions should be used from a multitude of possibilities to ensure the delivery of quality nursing care for each client.

Several factors can assist the nurse in selecting nursing interventions. Just as the client's outcomes can be derived from the nursing diagnosis, the nursing interventions can be developed from the etiology of each nursing diagnosis. The effective nurse plans interventions that are directed toward the cause of the client's nursing diagnosis or problem. For example, for a client with angina who may have the nursing diagnosis of *Pain* related to myocardial ischemia, an appropriate nursing intervention would be to help the client conserve energy (i.e., bed rest).

The nurse may use various guidelines in selecting appropriate nursing interventions. These guidelines include the individual nurse practice acts, state boards of nursing standards, and the Joint Commission on Accreditation of Healthcare Organizations (JCAHO) standards for nursing care (2000). Other determining factors of appropriate nursing interventions include whether an action is realistic in terms of the abilities of the client and nurse, and if it is compatible with available resources, the client's values and beliefs, and other therapies planned for the client.

In determining which nursing interventions to use, the nurse should critically consider the consequences and risks of each intervention. After considering these factors, the nurse selects those that are most likely to be effective with the minimum of risk. Table 13-3 applies the guidelines for selection of appropriate nursing interventions for a specific nursing diagnosis.

After setting the outcomes and planning the appropriate nursing interventions, the nurse writes nursing orders to communicate the exact nursing interventions that are to be implemented for the client. A **nursing order** is a statement written by the nurse that is within the realm of nursing practice to plan and initiate. These statements specify direction and individualize the client's plan of care. For example, a health care practitioner's order to force fluids must be specified in the nursing order as the number of milliliters per hour or per shift (e.g., 100 ml/h or Day shift = 800 ml; Evening shift = 800 ml; Night shift = 400 ml).

Ensuring that nursing orders are well written requires several essential elements. These elements include the nursing order date, action verb, detailed description, time

## TABLE 13-3   NURSING INTERVENTIONS: SELECTION GUIDELINES

| Nursing Diagnosis: Acute Pain related to myocardial ischemia | Nursing Interventions: |
|---|---|
| | • Assess pain characteristics such as location, quality, severity, duration, onset, relief. |
| **Expected Outcome:** Client will verbalize relief of pain. | • At first signs of pain, instruct client to relax and discontinue activity. |
| | • Instruct client to take sublingual nitroglycerin. |
| | • If pain continues after repeating doses every 5 minutes for a total of three pills, notify the health care practitioner or nurse practitioner. |
| | • Administer oxygen as prescribed. |
| | • Note time interval between episodes of pain. |
| | • Maintain bed rest and quiet environment to decrease oxygen demands. |
| | • Give analgesic medications as prescribed. |
| | • Offer assurance and emotional support by explaining all treatments and procedures and by encouraging questions. |

## TABLE 13-4   ELEMENTS OF NURSING ORDERS

| | |
|---|---|
| • Date: | The date on which the order is written. This information is updated to reflect review and revision. |
| • Action verb: | Directs the nurse's action. Examples of action verbs are *explain*, *demonstrate*, and *auscultate*. |
| • Detailed description: | Precisely clarifies what the nurse's action will be. This phrase explains *what, when, where*, and *how*. |
| • Time frame: | Describes *when, how often*, and *how long* the nursing order is to be performed. |
| • Signature: | Indicates the nurse who writes the order. This element implies legal and ethical accountability. |

frame, and signature (Wilkinson, 1998). See Table 13-4 for a summary of the elements of a nursing order.

The type of nursing order written is determined by the client problem. The nurse is responsible for writing nursing orders that involve health promotion, observation, prevention, and treatment (Wilkinson, 1998). Table 13-5 gives examples of types of nursing orders.

## Categories of Nursing Interventions

Nursing interventions are classified according to three categories: independent, interdependent, and dependent. **Independent nursing interventions** are nursing actions initiated by the nurse that do not require direction or an order from another health care professional. These interventions are sanctioned by professional nurse practice acts derived from licensure laws. In many states, the nurse practice acts allow independent nursing interventions regarding activities of daily living, health education, health promotion, and counseling. An example of an independent nursing intervention is the nurse's action to elevate a client's edematous extremity.

**Interdependent nursing interventions** are those actions that are implemented in a collaborative manner by the nurse with other health care professionals. **Collaboration** is a partnership in which all parties are valued for their contribution. Collaboration is used to gather data, plan, implement, evaluate, and gain objectivity by examining another's viewpoint. Interdependent nursing interventions allow the client's nursing diagnoses to be resolved on the basis of recommendations of an interdisciplinary health care team approach. For example, a client care conference or a discharge planning committee uses an interdisciplinary approach that includes health care members such as a nursing supervisor, a home health care nurse, a dietitian, a social worker, a physical therapist, and occasionally a physician. The nurse assumes the responsibility of being both the primary coordinator of the client's plan of nursing care and intermediary of interdepartmental collaboration (Doenges et al., 2002).

In addition to collaboration, the planning of interdependent nursing interventions may also include consultation. **Consultation** is a method of soliciting help from a specialist in order to resolve nursing diagnoses. The need for consultation arises when an individual nurse identifies a problem that cannot be solved using his own knowledge, skills, or resources. In the management of the client's plan

## TABLE 13-5 TYPES OF NURSING ORDERS

| Type | Description | Example |
|------|-------------|---------|
| Health promotion | Nursing orders that encourage behaviors leading to a higher level of wellness | Teach the importance of a daily exercise regimen. |
| Observation | Nursing orders that include observations regarding potential complications as well as observations of client's current responses | Auscultate lungs q4h. |
| Prevention | Nursing orders that direct nursing care in the reduction of risk factors or the prevention of complications | Turn, cough, and deep breathe q2h. |
| Treatment | Nursing orders that include teaching, referrals, or physical care necessary in the treatment of an existing problem | Refer client to occupational therapist for assistance with skills for activities of daily living. |

of care, nurses may consult with other health care personnel including health care practitioners, clinical nurse specialists, nutritionists, physical therapists, and social workers. Nurses frequently consult to verify assessment data or to obtain clinical advice—for example, discussing with an oncology clinical nurse specialist the effects of chemotherapy on a client's self-esteem.

Consultation can be informal or formal. An informal consultation may simply involve another health care practitioner's ideas regarding a nursing problem. Some agencies have a formal protocol for the consultation of a health professional and may require that certain forms be completed. Steps in formal consultation reflect a logical sequence and include:

- Identifying the problem
- Collecting all relevant data
- Selecting a suitable consultant
- Communicating unbiased data regarding the problem
- Discussing recommendations with the consultant
- Incorporating the recommendations into the client's plan of care

The consultation process often generates new approaches to the client's individualized plan of care. Acquiring supplementary knowledge may help in ensuring that the best conceivable plan of care is being developed. In addition,

nurses who have sought the help of a consultant are presented with an opportunity to learn from the recommendations for future situations.

**Dependent nursing interventions** are those actions that require an order from another health care professional. An example of a dependent intervention is administration of a medication. Although this intervention requires specific nursing knowledge and responsibilities, it is not within the realm of legal nursing practice in many states to prescribe medications. The nurse may not order medications but, when administering them, the nurse is responsible for knowing the classification, the pharmacological action, normal dosage, adverse effects, contraindications, and nursing implications of the drugs. Therefore, dependent nursing interventions must always be guided by appropriate knowledge and judgment. It should be noted that many state nurse practice acts sanction advanced practice registered nurses to prescribe medications. In those states, prescriptive authority is an independent intervention for nurses in advanced practice. Figure 13-3 illustrates the three categories of nursing interventions.

All nursing interventions require critical thinking in making appropriate nursing judgments. Alfaro-LeFevre (2004) states that the development of critical reasoning skills by nurses is a progressive process that requires a dedication to examining common health problems, participating in diverse clinical experiences, and preparing for delivery of care in clinical settings. Given the emphasis on critical thinking in the planning step of the nursing process, the nurse does not automatically carry out a health care practitioner's order without due consideration. All requested orders are given consideration for their appropriateness. An in-depth knowledge base is necessary to recognize an error and seek clarification. The use of rationales helps the nurse practice decision making and substantiate judgments. The rationales should accompany the nursing intervention or nursing order statement on the written plan of nursing care. A **rationale** is an explanation based on theories and scientific principles of natural and behavioral sciences and the humanities.

## Evaluating Care

Evaluating care involves determining the client's progress toward achievement of expected outcomes. Effective planning is essential if evaluation is to be effective. In other words, the planned outcomes are the yardsticks by which effectiveness of therapies are evaluated. If there is no stated expectation of care (i.e., client outcome), how can progress be measured?

## Nursing Outcomes Classification (NOC)

Measuring outcomes in nursing began with Nightingale, who relied on mortality statistics as an indicator of quality of care for British soldiers in the Crimean War.

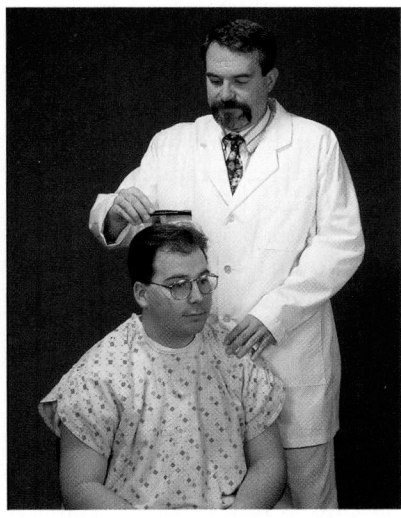
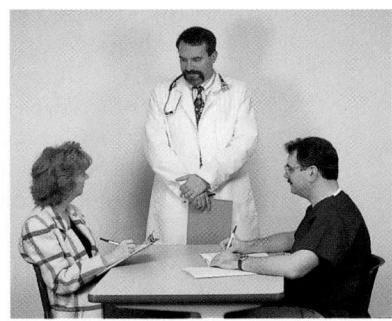
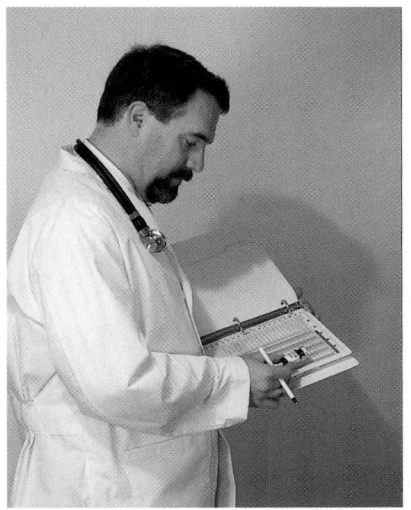

**Figure 13-3**   Examples of types of nursing interventions: (A) independent, (B) interdependent, (C) dependent.

Nightingale proved that the mortality rate for soldiers declined as a result of improved sanitation (Oermann & Huber, 1999). Recently, there has been increased emphasis by the nursing community on evaluating outcomes. There has been scant research or documentation to support the unique role of the nurse with the integration of multidisciplinary care (Schall & Flannery, 2000). The American Nurses Association (ANA) initiated a Quality Indicators Study in 1994 to answer the questions about what nurses do and the impact of nursing interventions on client outcomes. Clinical research activities have increased to provide answers to these questions (Spilsbury & Meyer, 2001). A **nursing-sensitive outcome** has been defined as "changes in client health status that reflect direct influence of nursing interventions" (Urden, 2001). (See Box 13-3 for outcome indicators for acute care and additional suggested outcomes related to nursing interventions.)

Nurse researchers (Maas & Johnson, 2000) at the University of Iowa have developed classifications of client outcomes, the Nursing Outcomes Classification (NOC). The NOC provides a standardized language that can be used to measure the effects of nursing practice on client outcomes. Just as the North American Nursing Diagnosis Association (NANDA) and the Nursing Interventions Classification (NIC) are continuing to develop standardized nursing language relative to diagnosis and intervention, NOC is striving toward a similar outcome of standardized language for classifying nursing interventions. An outcome classification system can be used to enhance decision making in clinical practice and research.

"**Evidence-Based Nursing** (EBN) is a decision-making approach based on integrating clinical expertise with the best available evidence from systematic research" (Kim, 2000). Several nursing interventions have been identified through clinical research to serve as guidelines for planning client care. Examples include the NIC, the Home Health Care Classification (HHCC) System, and the OMAHA Classification System (OCS) that are linked with the NANDA diagnosis taxonomy. Selection of any of these

interventions is always conditional upon the client's unique situation, needs, and capabilities (Ackley & Ladwig, 2002).

Linking nursing interventions to improved client outcomes through scientific research is important. Nurse researchers who are observing, measuring, and studying client outcomes believe that outcomes indicate the quality or effectiveness of the nursing interventions provided. Porter-O'Grady (1999) states that nurses need to provide empirical evidence of the "insights and intuition of their practice"(p. 7). Strengthening the links between nursing interventions and client outcomes will benefit not only clients, but nursing as well. Having solid research evidence that documents the effectiveness of nursing care on client outcomes will influence political and financial decisions relative to nursing. "By measuring patient outcomes, nurses can answer two pivotal questions: Do our patients benefit from our care? And if so, how?" (Oermann & Huber, 1999, p. 41).

The NOC taxonomy focuses on function, physiology, psychosocial aspects, health knowledge and behavior, and perceived self-health and family health. The NOC system, which defines over 190 client outcomes that are sensitive to nursing interventions, allows nurses to evaluate client status over time. Outcomes are to be evaluated along the continuum of care. Outcomes may be stated as short- or long-term. Time of measurement is important and should be as close to the intervention as possible (Urden, 2001).

## Plan of Care

The **plan of care** is a written guide that organizes data about a client's care into a formal statement of the strategies that will be implemented to help the client achieve optimal health. Nursing care plans usually include components such as assessment, nursing diagnoses, expected outcomes, nursing interventions, and evaluations. The nurse begins the nursing care plan on the day of admission and

## BOX 13-3    ANA OUTCOME INDICATORS FOR ACUTE CARE

A standardized list of outcome indicators for acute care developed by the ANA include:

- Nosocomial infection rate (measured by urinary tract infection after 72 hours of hospitalization)

- Client injury rate (measured by number of confirmed cases of bacteremia associated with central lines)

- Client falls and client satisfaction with nursing care (as measured by responses to surveys)

Typical indicators for measuring a client's ambulation include the ability to bear weight, effectiveness of gait, and distance walked.

Process indicators (such as pressure ulcers) evaluate the methods and amount of care that nurses provide.

Structure indicators examine the skill mix of registered nurses, licensed practical and vocational nurses, and unlicensed care providers.

Additional outcomes related to nursing interventions include client hygiene and self-care, nutrition and hydration, pain control, client education, rehospitalization, and medication errors.

Long-term outcomes in the home and community include physiological and psychosocial functions such as family function and home maintenance, family caregiver satisfaction, morbidity changes, maternal-child care, immunizations, education, health promotion, nutrition and hydration, and health care costs.

Adapted from Urden, L. (2001). Outcome evaluation: An essential component of clinical nurse specialist practice. *Clinical Nurse Specialist, 15*(6), 260–268; Alexander, J., & Kraposki, M. (1999). Outcomes for community health nursing practice. *Journal of Nursing Administration, 29*(5), 49–56; Oermann, M. H., & Huber, D. (1999). Patient outcomes: A measure of nursing's value. *American Journal of Nursing, 99*(9), 40–47.

continually updates and individualizes the client's plan of care until discharge.

The plan of care directs the efforts of the entire health care team regarding each client. This plan promotes the health care team's delivery of quality, holistic, individualized, and outcome-oriented care to the client. Attention to a comprehensive assessment of the entire person allows for a holistic approach. Individualization is enhanced by continuous reviewing and updating of the plan of care. A carefully formulated written plan of care prioritizes problems and addresses short- and long-term needs of the client. JCAHO standards state that each client will be assessed and reassessed according to the health care facility policy (JCAHO, 2000). The written plan of care authenticates activities of assessment by maintaining written records and providing evidence of nursing interventions, the client's response to nursing interventions, and changes in the client's condition.

Although plans of care differ in various institutions from handwritten to computerized forms, they all have the same basic elements in common. The plan of care is realistically designed and customized to each individual client's health status and is the final result of the planning component of the nursing process. The nursing plan of care documents health care needs, coordinates nursing care, promotes continuity of care, encourages communication within the health care team, and promotes quality nursing care.

There are several types of care plans. These different types include student-oriented, standardized, institutional, and computerized care plans. The student-oriented care plan promotes learning of problem-solving skills, the nursing process, verbal and written communication skills, and organizational skills. This comprehensive care plan has great depth for teaching the process of planning care. Educational programs vary, but usually the student-oriented care plan begins with assessment and proceeds in a sequential manner until it concludes with the plan of care evaluation.

The standardized care plan is a preplanned, preprinted guide for the nursing care of client groups with common needs. This type of care plan generally follows the nursing process format (i.e., problem, outcomes, nursing orders, and evaluation). The nurse may use standardized care plans when a client has predictable, commonly occurring problems. Individualization may be accomplished by the inclusion of additional handwritten notes on unusual problems.

Institutional nursing care plans are concise documents that become a part of the client's medical record after discharge. The Kardex nursing care plan is an example of this type of care plan and is frequently used. The institutional nursing care plan may simply include the problem, outcome, and nursing action. In addition, the Kardex nursing care plan may be expanded to include assessment, nursing diagnosis, outcome, implementation, and evaluation. Figure 13-4 provides an example of an institutional care plan.

Computers are used for creating and storing nursing care plans and can generate both standardized and individualized nursing care plans. The nurse selects appropriate diagnoses from a menu suggested by the computer, which then lists possible outcomes and nursing interventions. The nurse has the option of reading the client's plan of care from the computer screen or printing out an updated working copy. Figure 13-5 presents an example of a computerized nursing care plan.

| NURSING DIAGNOSIS | NURSING INTERVENTIONS | EVALUATION |
|---|---|---|
| Ineffective breathing pattern R/T operative site/incisional pain. | 1. Auscultate breath sounds q 4h. & PRN. 2. Assist pt. to TCDB q 2h while awake. | 1. Lungs clear on auscultation. 2. "It doesn't hurt as much to cough today." |
| Potential for infection R/T surgical incision & indwelling catheter | Assess for S/S of infection q 4h. | T-100.2°, incision site warm & pink, non-edematous. "It really hurts under the bandage." |
| Altered bowel elimination R/T abdominal surgery. | 1. Restart oral fluids gradually. Offer clear liquids frequently. 2. Observe for abd. distension & evaluate tolerance when pt. begins taking fluid/foods. | Unable to tolerate oral fluids — nauseated p taking ice chips. |
| | | |
| | | |
| | | |
| | | |

**Figure 13-4   Handwritten institutional care plan.**

# Strategies for Effective Care Planning

In planning quality nursing care for each client, the nurse assumes responsibility for the coordination of total nursing care. The nurse coordinates the participation of various health care team members to implement their recommendations into the delivery of quality nursing care. Critical thinking assists the nurse in establishing collaborative relationships with other members of the health care team and managing complex nursing systems.

An important strategy for effective planning is clear communication of the client's plan of care to other health care personnel. Hansten and Washburn (2001) suggested a model focused on attention to client outcomes and the influence of nursing interventions on the outcomes. The model incorporates reporting short- and long-term outcomes to other health care team members during daily reports. Continuity of care is assured as team members describe their roles and provide updates on the client's status.

 **STOP AND THINK**

## Coordination of Care

Mr. Eduardo Rodriquez has been admitted with arthritis. His left knee is extremely edematous, and the health care practitioner has ordered heat application of 100°F to the left knee four times a day for 2 hours. In considering the appropriateness of this order, the nurse detects an error regarding the time frame because heat produces maximum vasodilation in 20 to 30 minutes to dissipate the edema; further application of heat may lead to a rebound phenomenon of tissue congestion and vessel constriction, as well as potential burns. At this point, the nurse needs to seek clarification of the order from the health care practitioner. What would be appropriate methods of handling this situation?

## PLAN OF CARE

PC: ABDOMINAL SURGERY

PB: TD:____/____Ineffective breathing pattern r/t: op site/incision pain.

EO: Respiratory rate & effort WNL with good chest expansion.

  1: Ausculate breath sounds Q4H & PRN. Note diminished/absent sounds, rales wheezing, crackles, rhonchi. DOCUMENT IN NURSES' NOTES.

  2: Assist pt to TCDB Q2H while awake. Support incision. DOCUMENT RESPONSE & EFFORT.

PB: TD:____/____Potential for infection r/t surgical incision/indwelling cath.

EO: Surgical incision healing w/out s/s of infection.

  1: Assess for s/s of infection Q4H: (fever, chills, swelling, redness, pain, drainage, increased WBC, etc) DOCUMENT IN NURSE'S NOTES.

PB: TD:____/____Pain r/t_____ surgical incision/operative site.

EO: Pt reports pain relieved/ controlled.

  1: Implement Patient Controlled Analgesia (PCA) Protocol and PCA Teaching Protocol.

PB: TD:____/____Altered bowel elimination r/t_____surgery.

EO: Pt' bowel elimination is normal within limits of surgical procedure.

  1: Restart oral fluids gradually. Offer clear liquids frequently.

  2: Observe for abdominal distention & evaluate tolerance when Pt begins taking fluid/foods post-op. DOCUMENT IN NURSES' NOTES.

INT    SIGNATURE

**Figure 13-5   Computerized institutional care plan.** *Courtesy of St. Tammany Parish Hospital, Covington, LA*

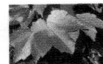

## RESEARCH FOCUS

**Title of Study:** Through the eyes of beholder: Multiple perspectives on quality in women's health care.

**Study Purpose:** To describe "quality of care" as an outcome indicator as perceived by clients, physicians, nurses, and third-party payers associated with a hospital-based health care service line for women.

**Methods:** A qualitative study was used to compare and contrast the various definitions of "quality of care." Data was collected via interviews, focus groups, and survey methods.

**Findings:** Eight key outcomes were identified from the analysis of assessment data. These are a caring environment and professional attitude of caregivers, professional competence, sensitivity to meeting needs in a timely manner, congenial relationships among professionals and clients, scope of services provided, clean and safe environment, and supportive systems within the organization.

**Implications:** The several definitions and different meanings of "quality of care" are ellusive. However, the study did reveal several factors that the nurse can use to improve client care (e.g., timeliness, caring environment, professional attitude).

Stickler, J., & Weiss, M. (2001). "Through the eyes of beholder: Multiple perspectives on quality in women's health care." *Journal of Nursing Care Quality, 15*(3), 59–74.

The nurse must always communicate the plan of care in clear, precise terms. Avoid using vague terminology such as *improved, adequate,* and *normal.*

Another strategy for effective planning is to establish a realistic nursing plan of care, because this will avoid setting an outcome that is too difficult or impossible to achieve. If an outcome is too ambitious or is unattainable, the client and nurse may become discouraged or apathetic about the resolution of nursing diagnoses. In addition, outcomes should be measurable. Quantitative terms assist in the determination of measurement. Finally, the outcomes should be future-oriented. Because an outcome is an aim or a desired achievement, outcomes should be written in future tense format.

Once appropriate nursing diagnoses are individualized to the client, the plan of care has a stable framework on which an optimum level of wellness for the client can be reached. Although some clients may not achieve complete resolution of all nursing diagnoses, the individualized nursing plan of care can improve health to the client's optimal level.

# CASE STUDY/NURSING CARE PLAN

Mr. Ballenger, age 64, is recovering from a chronic occlusive arterial disorder of both lower extremities in his home setting. He was recently hospitalized for 2 days and was given intravenous anticoagulants during the acute care admission. He is continuing to take 5 mg of Coumadin (anticoagulant) daily. Upon an initial assessment by his home health nurse, he states that his "biggest problem is that he has not been sleeping well." In addition, Mr. Ballenger says that his feet are still a little cool. The nurse explains that she will examine Mr. Ballenger's peripheral pulses with a Doppler listening device and she will visit him once a week until his condition "stabilizes." The nurse then assesses his lower extremities and asks specific questions about his coagulation status.

## Assessment

Mr. Ballenger has experienced a recent hospitalization for chronic arterial occlusions of his legs. He was admitted to the acute care setting for 2 days and is now at home with a home health nurse visiting weekly. His primary problems are continuing intermittent claudication and the inability to sleep well.

## Nursing Diagnosis #1

Ineffective Tissue Perfusion: Peripheral related to chronic arterial occlusive disease
**NOC:** Circulation Status; Tissue Perfusion: Peripheral
**NIC:** Circulatory Care: Arterial Insufficiency

## Expected Outcomes

The client will:
1. Demonstrate palpable peripheral pulses in 1 week.
2. Identify changes in lifestyle that are needed to increase tissue perfusion.

## Planning/Interventions/Rationales

1. Assess client for clinical manifestations of poor coagulation by checking peripheral pulses at each visit. *Provides ongoing assessment of client's circulatory status.*
2. Wear protective footwear when ambulating. *Decreases the likelihood of skin breakdown and potential bleeding tendencies.*

## Evaluation

Client's peripheral pulses are palpable and bilateral within 48 hours and lower extremities developed warmth to the touch within 48 hours. Client wearing slippers at all times and did not have any skin deterioration on feet.

## Nursing Diagnosis #2

*Disturbed Sleep Pattern* related to chronic arterial occlusive disease.
**NOC:** Sleep; Rest; Well-Being
**NIC:** Sleep Enhancement

## Expected Outcomes

The client will:
1. Sleep uninterrupted for 6 hours.
2. Wake up less frequently during the night.
3. Verbalize plan to implement bedtime routines.

## Planning/Interventions/Rationales

1. Provide client with quiet, dark environment in which to sleep. *Enhances potential for uninterrupted sleep.*
2. Encourage client to listen to soothing music or read a book just prior to sleeping. *Creates a restful environment just before sleeping.*
3. Participation in stress management activities while recovering at home. *Enhances potential for successful sleeping pattern.*

## Evaluation

Client reported fewer interruptions in sleep times and verbalized being more rested on a daily basis.

## Key Concepts

- The outcome identification and planning component of the nursing process is a sequential, orderly method of using problem-solving skills and critical thinking to formulate a nursing plan of care to resolve nursing diagnoses.
- The planning component of the nursing process includes establishing priorities, developing expected outcomes, selecting nursing interventions, and documenting the plan of care.
- The purposes of outcome identification and planning are to provide direction for nursing care, to improve communication among health care providers, and to provide continuity of nursing care.
- The establishment of priorities may be guided by such factors as endangerment of well-being, Maslow's hierarchy of needs, client preferences, and anticipation of future diagnoses.
- Establishing expected outcomes provides guidelines for directing nursing interventions and establishes evaluation criteria by deciding on outcome statements that illustrate a desired change in the client's behavior.
- Expected outcome objectives include the components of subject, task statement, criteria, conditions, and time frame.
- Two common problems frequently encountered in planning with regard to outcomes are the improper format and unrealistic and nonmeasurable qualities of this component.
- In planning nursing care, the nurse uses an expansive scientific knowledge base and critical thinking to select independent, interdependent, and dependent nursing interventions guided by local and federal standards of care.
- The plan of care documents health care needs, coordinates nursing care, promotes continuity of care, encourages communication within the health care team, and promotes quality nursing care.
- Strategies for effective care planning include communication of the client's plan of care within the health care team, establishment of a realistic plan of care, and formulation of measurable and future-oriented outcomes.

## Review Questions and Activities

1. Decide whether the following statements are client-centered, and place a mark in front of all client-centered outcomes.

    _____ 1. The nursing assistant will ambulate client in the hall three times a day by Saturday.

    _____ 2. Will teach the client to plan a low-fat diet for 24 hours.

    _____ 3. The client will describe two purposes of a low-fat diet by Wednesday.

    _____ 4. Will encourage the client to walk the entire length of hallway two times a day by Thursday.

2. Decide whether the following statements have action verbs for their task assignment, and place a mark in front of all outcomes with action verbs.

    _____ 1. The client will know five reasons for proper nutrition.

    _____ 2. The client will be able to state where diabetic injection equipment may be purchased after discharge.

    _____ 3. The client will explain the purpose of maintaining asepsis in daily dressing changes by Wednesday.

    _____ 4. The client will understand how to change dressings on abdomen.

3. Indicate whether the following statements have criteria, and place a mark in front of all outcomes with criteria.

    _____ 1. The client will describe two purposes of the low-salt diet by Friday.

    _____ 2. The client will know the cause of low blood sugar.

    _____ 3. The client will understand the importance of returning for follow-up visits to the health care practitioner.

    _____ 4. The client will demonstrate crutch walking the entire length of the hallway twice a day.

4. Decide whether the following statements have conditions, and place a mark in front of all outcomes with conditions.

    _____ 1. The client will describe two purposes of the low-salt diet by Friday.

    _____ 2. The client will know the cause of low blood sugar.

    _____ 3. The client will understand the importance of returning for follow-up visits to the health care practitioner.

    _____ 4. The client will demonstrate crutch walking.

5. Decide whether the following statements have time frames, and place a mark in front of all outcomes with time frames.

    _____ 1. The client will describe two purposes of the low-salt diet by Friday.

    _____ 2. The client will know the cause of low blood sugar.

    _____ 3. The client will understand the importance of returning for follow-up visits to the health care practitioner.

    _____ 4. The client will demonstrate crutch walking.

6. The plan of nursing care includes:
   a. Client assessment data, medical treatment regime and rationales, and diagnostic test results and significance
   b. Doctor's orders, demographic data, and medication administration and rationales
   c. Collected documentation of all team members providing care for your client
   d. Client's nursing diagnoses, expected outcome objectives, and nursing interventions
7. When establishing priorities of a client's plan of nursing care, the nurse should rank the highest priorities to life-threatening diagnoses and the lowest priorities to:
   a. Safety-related needs
   b. The client's social, love, and belonging needs
   c. Needs of family members and friends who are involved in plan of care
   d. Needs of client regarding referral agencies
8. What is the main purpose of the expected outcome?
   a. To describe the education plans to be taught to the client
   b. To describe the behavior the client is expected to achieve as a result of nursing interventions
   c. To provide a standard for evaluating the quality of health care delivered to the client during the hospital stay
   d. To make sure that the client's treatment does not extend beyond the time allowed under the diagnosis-related group system
9. What are the essential components of an expected outcome?
   a. Nursing diagnosis, interventions, and expected client behavior
   b. Target date, nursing action, measurement criteria, and desired client behavior
   c. Nursing action, client behavior, target date, and conditions under which the behavior occurs
   d. Client behavior, measurement criteria, conditions under which the behavior occurs, and target date
10. Which guideline is most appropriate when developing nursing interventions?
   a. Choose actions that a nurse can perform without leaving the unit or consulting with medical staff.
   b. Make intervention statements specific to ensure continuity of care.
   c. Write interventions in general terms to allow maximum flexibility and creativity in delivering nursing care.
   d. Make sure that nursing care activities receive priority over other aspects of the treatment regime.

## Multimedia Links

Christensen *Core Concept Videos: Planning and Intervention*

## Web Resources

Agency for Healthcare Research and Quality (EBN)
   http://www.ahcpr.gov
American Nurses Association
   http://www.nursingworld.org
Nursing Interventions Classification (NIC)
   http://www.nursinguiowa.edu
Outcomes data links:
   http://www.nurseweek.com

## References

Ackley, B., & Ladwig, G. (2002). *Nursing diagnosis handbook: A guide to planning care.* St. Louis: Mosby.

Alexander, J., & Kraposki, M. (1999). Outcomes for community health nursing practice. *Journal of Nursing Administration, 29*(5), 49–56. (special issue devoted to research in nursing administration)

Alfaro-LeFevre, R. (2004). *Critical thinking in nursing: A practical approach* (3rd ed.). Philadelphia: Saunders.

American Nurses Association (1998). *Standards of clinical nursing practice* (2nd ed.). Washington, DC: Author.

Atkinson, L., & Murray, M. (2000). *Understanding the nursing process in a changing care environment.* New York: McGraw Hill.

Berger, K., & Williams, M. (1999). *Fundamentals of nursing: Collaborating for optimal health.* Stamford, CT: Appelton & Lange.

Carpenito, L. J. (2004). *Handbook of nursing diagnosis* (10th ed.). Philadelphia: Lippincott.

Doenges, M. E., Moorehouse, M. F., & Geissler, A. C. (2002). *Nursing care plans: Guidelines for individualizing patient care* (6th ed.). Philadelphia: Davis.

Fortinash, K. (2000). The nursing process. In K. Fortinash & Holoday-Worret (Eds.). *Psychiatric mental health nursing* (pp. 122–147). St. Louis: Mosby.

Hansten, R., & Washburn, M. (2001). Outcomes-based care delivery (hospital extra). *American Journal of Nursing, 101*(2), 24A–24D.

Joint Commission of Healthcare Organizations (2000). *Comprehensive accreditation manual for hospitals: The official handbook (CAMH) 2000 update.* Chicago: Author.

Kersbergen, A. (2000). Managed care shifts health care from an altruistic model to a business framework. *Nursing and Health Care Perspectives, 21*(2), 81–83. (National League of Nursing, Pub.)

Kim, M. (2000). Evidence-based nursing: Connecting knowledge to practice. *Nursing, 97*(9), 1, 4–6.

Maas, M. L., & Johnson, M. (Eds.). (2000). *Nursing outcomes classification (NOC): Iowa outcomes project.* St. Louis: Mosby.

McCloskey-Dochterman, J., & Bulechek, G. (2000). *Nursing interventions classification (NIC).* St. Louis: Mosby Year Book.

Oermann, M. H., & Huber, D. (1999). Patient outcomes: A measure of nursing's value. *American Journal of Nursing, 99*(9), 40–47.

Pesut, D., & Herman, J. (1999). *Clinical reasoning: The art and science of critical and creative thinking.* Clifton Park, NY: Delmar Learning.

Porter-O'Grady, T. (1999). Making the case for nursing. *Nursing Management, 39*(3), 7.

Rubenfeld, M., & Scheffer, B. (1999). *Critical thinking in nursing: An interactive approach.* Philadelphia: J. B. Lippincott.

Schall, M., & Flannery, J. (2000). Directions for curricular change: The 1980 and 1995 American Nurses Association's policy statements. *Nurse Educator, 25*(1), 17–18.

Singer, C. (2000). Challenges of nursing management. In J. Zerwekh & J. Claborn (Eds.). *Nursing today: Transitions and trends* (pp. 109–130). Philadelphia: W. B. Saunders.

Spilsbury, K., & Meyer, J. (2001). Defining the nursing contributions to patient outcomes: Lessons from a review of the literature examining nursing outcomes, skill mix, and changing roles. *Journal of Clinical Nursing, 10*(1), 3–14.

Stickler, J., & Weiss, M. (2001). Through the eyes of beholder: Multiple perspectives on quality in women's health care. *Journal of Nursing Care Quality, 15*(3), 59–74.

Urden, L. (2001). Outcome evaluation: An essential component of clinical nurse specialist practice. *Clinical Nurse Specialist, 15*(6), 260–268.

Wilkinson, J. M. (1998). *Nursing process in action: A critical thinking approach* (2nd ed.). Redwood City, CA: Addison-Wesley Nursing.

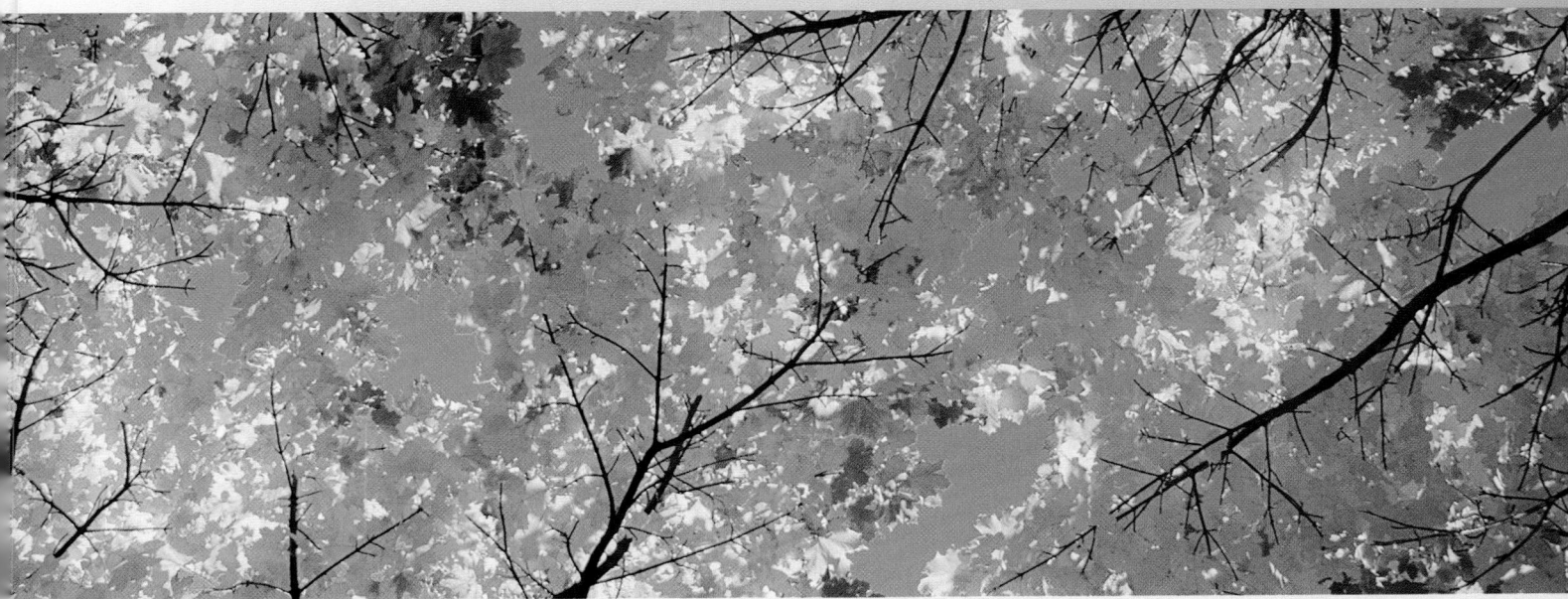

# CHAPTER 14

# Implementation

Michael Brody, RN, BSN

*"Knowing is not enough; we must apply. Willing is not enough; we must do."*

(Johann von Goethe, 1832)

# Chapter Competencies

## Upon completion of this chapter, the reader should be able to:

1. Describe the purposes of the implementation step of the nursing process.
2. Explore the types of skills required for effective implementation.
3. Discuss various implementation activities that nurses execute as directed by the nursing plan of care.
4. Explain the nurse's roles and responsibilities in the delegation of care to assistive personnel and its impact on implementation.
5. Identify the specific types of nursing interventions that are implemented by the nurse and the characteristics of each type.
6. Discuss the importance of documentation in the implementation process.

# Key Terms

delegation

discharge planning

implementation

nursing intervention

protocol

rationale

standing order

**I**mplementation is the fourth step in the nursing process and involves the execution of the nursing plan of care formulated during the planning phase of the nursing process. In the implementation phase, the nurse and other members of the health care team put the care plan into action. Nursing is a dynamic process, and every nurse must continually incorporate new assessment and diagnostic information into the implementation of the care plan (Frisch & Kelly, 2002). Nurses must therefore draw from a broad base of clinical knowledge, careful planning, critical thinking and analysis, and judgment.

This chapter explores the various elements that comprise the implementation process, the role of implementation in the general scope of the nursing process, and the skills each nurse must develop to successfully implement the plan of care. Although identified as the fourth step of the nursing process, the implementation phase begins with assessment and continually interacts with the other steps in the process to reflect the changing needs of the client and the response of the nurse to those needs.

## Purposes of Implementation

The complexity of the implementation process derives from the many and varied needs of each client. In implementing the plan of care, the skilled nurse considers all aspects of the presenting illness as well as the environmental, personal, and cultural elements that make each client a unique individual. In addition, the nurse is responsible for delegating appropriate tasks to staff members and ancillary personnel, and documenting the entire process, including what the nurse does and how the client responds.

The American Nursing Association (1998), in its *Standards of Clinical Nursing Practice*, describes the standards applicable to implementation in terms of both a standard of care and standards of professional performance. Adherence to these standards requires that the nurse have a current knowledge base, be proficient with technical and communication skills, and use sound judgment in determining safe and efficient use of personnel and materials.

## Requirements for Effective Implementation

The implementation phase of the nursing process requires cognitive (intellectual), psychomotor (technical), and interpersonal skills. These basic competencies serve as a foundation for effective nursing care.

 **STOP AND THINK**

### Implementation Activities

- When you think of the activities performed by nurses on a daily basis, what specific actions come to mind?

- How would you categorize the level of skill that is required for each activity?

- How comfortable would you feel executing all of these activities yourself?

## CLIENT EDUCATION

### Keeping the Client Informed

When implementing the plan of care, it is essential that the nurse make every effort to keep the client informed of the process, rationale, and expected outcomes. This includes:

✓ Explaining specifically what the intervention involves
✓ Describing what the client can expect to experience (pain, pressure, dizziness, etc.)
✓ Providing the rationale for the intervention
✓ Inviting the client to ask any questions in order to improve her understanding

## NURSING STRATEGY

### Assessing for Pain

Take the following steps to accurately assess a client's pain:

● Consider any developmental factors and sensory or cognitive impairments that might impact the client's ability to effectively use a given form of pain scale.

● Based on this assessment, use an appropriate pain scale (numeric, analog, color, etc.).

● Ensure that the client clearly understands the scale.

● Assess for level of pain, verifying your understanding of the client's rating.

● Carefully document the pain assessment in order to provide for subsequent comparative analysis.

Cognitive skills enable nurses to make appropriate observations, understand the rationale for the activities performed, and appreciate the differences among individuals and how they influence nursing care. Critical thinking is an important element within the cognitive domain because it helps nurses to analyze data, organize observations, and apply prior knowledge and experiences to current client situations.

Psychomotor skills enable the nurse to safely and effectively perform nursing activities. Nurses must be able to handle medical equipment with a high degree of competency and to perform skills such as administering medications and assisting clients with mobility needs (e.g., positioning and ambulating).

The use of interpersonal skills involves communication with clients and families as well as with other health care professionals. Effective implementation depends upon therapeutic communication with the client and family, as well as effective communication between members of the care team. Cognitive, psychomotor, and communication skills are essential aspects of the implementation process.

## Implementation Activities

Nursing implementation activities include:

• Ongoing assessment
• Establishment of priorities
• Allocation of resources
• Initiation of nursing interventions
• Documentation of interventions and client response

These activities are interactive, and each is discussed in further detail.

## Ongoing Assessment

The nursing plan of care is based on the initial assessment data collected by the nurse and the nursing diagnoses

derived from those data (Powers, 2002). Because a client's condition can change rapidly, or new data may become available through interaction with the client, ongoing assessment is necessary to validate the relevance of proposed interventions. Goals, expected outcomes, and interventions may change as new data emerge and the client status evolves. The nurse completes a focused assessment during the initial interaction with a client. The nurse continuously observes the client during the implementation process, adjusting the plan of care accordingly to better meet the changing needs of each individual client.

It is not unusual for nursing diagnoses to change or to be resolved in a short period of time. For example, the nursing care plan for Mrs. Cline, a preoperative client, might include an intervention to teach her about the use of a patient-controlled analgesia (PCA) pump. As she demonstrates proper use of the PCA, the nurse observes that Mrs. Cline is unable to depress the button easily with the fingers of her right hand. Mrs. Cline informs the nurse that she forgot to mention that her joints swell occasionally and she has very little strength in her hand during these times. This information is essential for both developing a nursing diagnosis concerning Mrs. Cline's impaired physical mobility and determining appropriate teaching methods for use of the PCA pump.

Ongoing assessment demands attention to verbal and nonverbal cues from the client and requires knowledge of expected responses to specific interventions. If nurses observe that responses are different from those expected, this assessment data can lead to a change in expected outcomes and accompanying interventions.

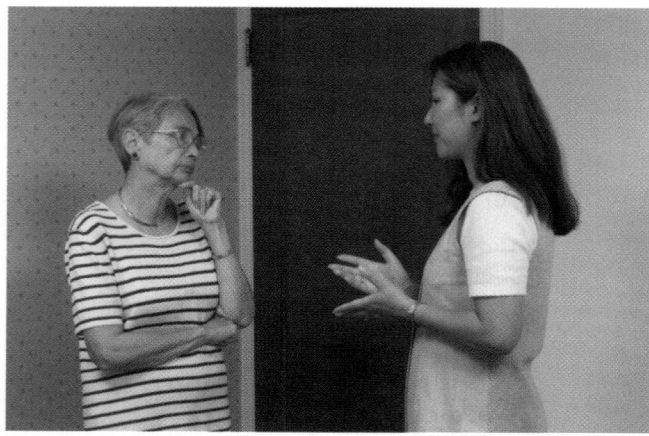

**Figure 14-1    A home health nurse assesses a client by gathering data while communicating with a client.**

Ongoing assessment is of equal importance in home health care or extended care settings when contact with skilled health care providers might occur less frequently and the length of time that the care is required varies. The nurse's assessment and clinical judgment often determine whether the client needs continued care or referral to other health care providers (Figure 14-1).

## Establishing Priorities

Based on the information derived from ongoing assessment and review of the problem list, the nurse establishes priorities for implementing the plan of care. Priorities are based on:

- Which problems are deemed most important by the nurse, the client, and family or significant others
- Activities previously scheduled by other departments (e.g., surgery, diagnostic testing)
- Available resources

The change-of-shift report can also be a valuable tool in determining priorities. A client's condition and variables in the clinical setting can change quickly and frequently—especially in acute care settings—requiring that the nurse exercise sound clinical judgment and maintain flexibility in organizing care. For example, the nursing care plan for Mr. Jenkins, who had hip replacement surgery, might reflect a priority nursing diagnosis of *Impaired Physical Mobility* with interventions focused toward learning to ambulate. When the nurse listens to Mr. Jenkins' breath sounds on a particular morning, it is noted that his breathing is more labored and crackles are present in the lung bases. This assessment is noted on the change-of-shift report, and the priorities of interventions change to focus on this new development.

Time management is important whether the nurse is caring for one client or a group of clients. It is helpful to make a list of tasks that need to be accomplished throughout the day and to create a worksheet outlining a target time for these activities. Those activities with specified times for

## LIFE SPAN CONSIDERATIONS

### Assessing Elderly for Falls

An important element in the ongoing assessment of elderly clients is the appraisal for the risk of falls. The following questions can help the nurse determine the seriousness of this risk:

- Which medications are currently prescribed for the client, and what are their effects on the central nervous system?

- Are there elimination problems, such as incontinence?

- Has the mental status of the client recently changed in terms of orientation to time and place?

- Does the client's level of mobility require ambulatory assistance devices such as a cane, walker, or wheelchair?

- If the client has previously experienced a fall, what were the conditions under which it occurred?

completion should be scheduled first. For example, medications usually allow a narrow time frame for administration and must be scheduled at specific times on the worksheet. An example of a worksheet that outlines a plan for activities is shown in Table 14-1. The time allotted for activities depends on the complexity of the task and the amount of assistance required by the client. An example of a worksheet for a group of clients is presented in Table 14-2.

## Allocating Resources

Before implementing the nursing plan of care, the nurse reviews proposed interventions to determine the level of knowledge and the types of skills required for safe and effective implementation. The assessment provides data for determining if an activity can be performed independently by the client, can be completed with assistance from family, or requires assistance of health care personnel.

## Delegating Tasks

The registered nurse is legally responsible for all nursing care given. Each member of the health care team, based on his individual educational background, professional experience, and licensure, brings essential knowledge and skills for effective implementation of the care plan. The nurse must identify and perform those interventions that require the specific knowledge and skills of a registered

## TABLE 14-1    SAMPLE WORKSHEET OF NURSING ACTIVITIES (ONE CLIENT)

| Time | Activity |
|---|---|
| 6:45 A.M. | Listen to change-of-shift report. |
| 7:00 | Perform head-to-toe assessment of client, including vital signs. |
| 7:10 | Check routine medication times. |
| 7:30 | Chart assessment findings. |
| 8:00 | Serve breakfast. While client eats breakfast, review chart for new laboratory test data. |
| 8:30 | Record I&O after breakfast; remove breakfast tray. |
| 8:40 | Gather supplies for hygiene. Assist with A.M. care. |
| 9:15 | Assist up to chair. Show films about diabetic skin care. |
| 10:00 | Document interventions and observations on chart. |
| 10:15 | Review care plan for any needed revisions. |
| 10:30 | Report status of client to charge nurse. Attend inservice on IV care. |
| 11:45 | Take and record vital signs. |

nurse, and at the same time, recognize that nonnursing personnel may be more appropriate to complete other aspects of the plan of care. **Delegation** is the process of transferring a selected nursing task in a situation to an individual who is competent to perform that specific task. However, while the nurse can effectively and appropriately assign some activities to other health care personnel, the registered nurse remains accountable for appropriate delegation and supervision of the care provided by these individuals. In general, registered nurses are authorized by law to both provide nursing care to clients directly and supervise and instruct others to deliver this care. Further, the registered nurse is empowered to delegate selected tasks to either licensed or unlicensed nursing personnel (Figure 14-2).

Decisions about delegation are guided by the needs of the client, the number and type of available personnel, and the nursing management system of the unit or agency. In performing delegated tasks, nursing students must determine if the intervention is either one that they have performed with supervision and can safely accomplish independently or is one for which assistance is needed.

The first consideration in determining the most appropriate nursing personnel to administer care is client safety. Nurse practice acts dictate to some extent which tasks can be legally delegated. For example, administration of blood or blood products is not an act that can be legally delegated to licensed practical nurses or unlicensed assistive personnel in most states. Other activities, such as assisting clients with activities of daily living (ADL, those activities performed by a person usually on a daily basis), ordering supplies, or transcribing orders, can often be safely delegated to other personnel.

If delegation of a particular activity is legally allowed, the nurse should validate the knowledge and skill level of personnel before delegation. If uncertain about the level of an

## TABLE 14-2    SAMPLE WORKSHEET OF NURSING ACTIVITIES (GROUP OF CLIENTS)

| | 7 A.M. | 8 A.M. | 9 A.M. | 10 A.M. | 11 A.M. | NOON |
|---|---|---|---|---|---|---|
| 351 Hughes | V/S assess | | Meds | Assist to chair | V/S Meds | Meds |
| 352 Parsons | V/S assess | Breakfast | To PT | D/C plan | V/S | Telem. strip |
| 353 Crowson | V/S assess | Ck. PTT results | Meds; Amb. in hall | Show video | BP sit/stand Meds | Telem. strip |
| 354 Robinson | V/S assess | q2h I/O | Meds | q2h I/O | | q2h I/O |
| 355 Temple | Pre-op OR on call | | Meds | | | |
| 356 Anderson | V/S assess | NPO | Meds | V/S Gastro | | Meds |

Abbreviations: Amb., ambulate; BP, blood pressure; D/C, discharge; I/O, input/output; NPO, nothing by mouth; OR, operation room; PT, physical therapy; PTT, partial thromboplastin time; telem., telemetry; V/S, vital signs

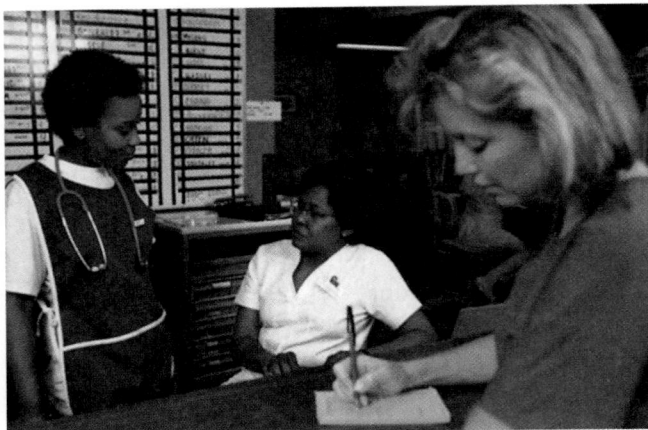

**Figure 14-2**    The registered nurse is responsible for delegating nursing tasks to other members of the health care team.

individual's competence to perform an activity, the nurse should not delegate the task even though it might be legally performed by that level of personnel. The registered nurse is held accountable to delegate only such care that can safely be done by the other individual and would be performed with the same level of competency and respect for state laws and regulations as would be evident in the nurse's performance of this care.

## Types of Management Systems

Once the nurse determines that he can safely delegate a task to another member of the care team, the nurse must consider cost. In the interest of wise and efficient use of finite resources, nurses delegate tasks to the most cost-effective level of personnel who can safely, legally, and proficiently perform the activity. The nursing management system often determines the numbers and types of personnel available. Changes in health care delivery in

### LEGAL AND ETHICAL ISSUES

#### Delegating in an Ethical and Legal Manner

In acute care settings, the nurse is often "time challenged"; that is, there is not enough time to do everything the nurse wants to do. Therefore, it is tempting to delegate many of the nurse responsibilities to other nonprofessional care providers (i.e., patient care assistants [PCA]). For example, the nurse might ask the PCA to "go see if my IV bag needs to be changed." While the PCA can likely perform this task, medication delivery is not in the PCA's legal practice. The nurse must be the care provider to perform this function.

### STOP AND THINK

#### Delegation

Your employer, a large acute care hospital, has hired consultants to examine the cost of care expended in the facility and to recommend a more cost-effective system. These consultants recommend decreasing the number of both registered nurses and licensed practical/vocational nurses and increasing the responsibilities of unlicensed assistive personnel. As a registered nurse in charge of the care of medical-surgical clients, what questions would you ask regarding this proposal? In what ways do you think your responsibilities would increase because of this situation? Do you think your responsibilities would decrease significantly? What impact would this proposal have on the ethical delivery of care to clients, specifically the nurse's need to cause no harm and promote good?

recent years have resulted in an increasing emphasis on cost containment and have subsequently created several unique management models. The redesign of the workplace in many health care agencies has included cross-training of employees, with nurses frequently assuming responsibilities formerly assigned to other health care providers. For example, nurses might draw blood for laboratory tests, perform electrocardiograms, or administer respiratory treatments, as care is focused around the client rather than the various departments in the agency. Nurses in community health settings have traditionally exercised a variety of roles in their practice. As health care delivery continues to evolve in this country, a variety of innovative approaches will emerge to better meet the needs of clients. The most common management systems currently used include functional nursing, team nursing, primary nursing, total client care, modular nursing, and case management.

### Functional Nursing

The functional nursing approach divides care into tasks to be completed and uses various levels of personnel depending on the complexity of the assignment. Each member of the staff performs her assigned task for each client. For example, one nurse may assess each client and document findings, and another may give all medications and treatments. Another nurse may be assigned to complete client teaching or **discharge planning** (process that enables the client to resume self-care activities before leaving the health care environment). One nursing assistant might serve all trays and collect intake and output records for each client, while another is responsible for giving baths or making beds.

## CLINICAL ALERT

### Unsafe Delegation Practices

Delegation is an important aspect of nursing care, as it allows the skilled nurse to effectively and efficiently engage other members of the health care team in the implementation of the client's care plan. The nurse is responsible to ensure that the delegation process has resulted in the ancillary provider having learned to safely implement the procedure in question. If the nurse is not completely confident in the abilities of the nonnursing personnel to perform the specific procedure in any given situation, the nurse should not delegate that responsibility.

## STOP AND THINK

### Management Styles

- What management style is used in the acute care facilities where you have practiced?

- What are the advantages and disadvantages to your facility's management style?

- How would you attempt to change this facility's management style to another style? What would you use as your rationale for the change?

Ideally, this system enables a relatively small number of personnel to care for a large number of clients. In addition, it allows the use of less skilled (and less expensive) personnel for some tasks and allows personnel to be used in areas for which they have special knowledge or skill. However, this system can also result in fragmented and depersonalized care and may invite omissions in care because no *one* person is responsible for the total care of the client.

### Team Nursing

The team nursing approach uses a variety of personnel (professional, technical, and unlicensed assistants) in the delivery of nursing care. The registered nurse is leader of the team and is responsible for supervision of the team, as well as planning and evaluating the results of caregiving activities. This management system uses professional nurses for skilled observations and interventions and provision of direct care to acutely ill clients, while licensed practical nurses care for less acutely ill clients, and nursing assistants are responsible for serving trays, making beds, and assisting the nurses with other tasks. This management system is frequently used because it is cost-effective and provides more individualized care than the functional approach.

### Primary Nursing

In the primary nursing management system, the professional nurse assumes full responsibility for total client care for a small number of clients. Although care may be delegated to nurse associates for shifts when the primary nurse is not in attendance, the primary nurse maintains responsibility for total client care 24 hours a day. The primary nurse sets health care goals with the client and plans care to meet those goals. The principal advantage of this approach is the continuity of care inherent in the system. Primary nursing is most effective with a total staff of registered nurses, which makes this system expensive to maintain.

### Total Client Care and Modular Nursing

Total client care and modular nursing are variations of primary nursing. Although these systems imply that one nurse is responsible for all the care administered to a client, responsibility for the client actually changes from shift to shift with the assigned caregiver. This system uses both registered nurses and licensed practical nurses; the registered nurses are assigned to more complex client situations. A unit manager or charge nurse typically coordinates activities on the unit. Modular nursing attempts to assign caregivers to a small segment or "module" of a nursing unit, ensuring that clients are cared for by the same personnel on a regular basis.

### Case Management

In the case management system, the nurse assumes responsibility for planning, implementing, coordinating, and evaluating care for a given client, regardless of the client's location at any given time. This approach is often used when care is complex and a number of health care team members are involved in providing care. Generally, a case management plan, or critical pathway, is developed (based on the norm or typical course of the condition), and the nurse evaluates the progress of the client in relation to what is expected, investigating and following up on any variance in the time required or the amount of improvement noted. Although the case load for the individual nurse might be smaller (thus making this approach expensive), continuity of care and collaboration are enhanced.

## Nursing Interventions

After reviewing the client's current condition, verifying priorities, and examining resources, the nurse should be ready to initiate nursing interventions. A **nursing intervention** is an action that the nurse performs to help the client achieve the results specified by the expected outcomes of the plan of care. All interventions must conform to standards of care. Nurses should understand the reason for any intervention, the expected effect, and any potential problems that may result. Understanding the reason for a nursing intervention is the hallmark of a professional nurse, in that the nurse is using logic and scientific reasoning as the basis of practice. Nursing interventions are a blend of science (rational acts) and art (intuitive actions). It is important for novice nurses to identify the **rationale** (an explanation based on the theories and scientific principles of natural and behavioral sciences and the humanities) for each intervention in order to effectively implement the plan of care. Prior to implementation, the nurse must determine exactly:

- What is to be done
- How it is to be done
- When it should be done
- Who will do it
- How long it should be done

The nurse considers the root cause of the client's problem, as well as other factors contributing to the nursing diagnosis, in an effort to determine which interventions are most likely to result in a positive outcome. Clients with similar nursing diagnoses may require different interventions, depending on the various characteristics of the individual client, which the nurse discovers through ongoing assessment. The nurse must consider the client's stated preferences, the developmental level of the client, and availability of resources. In addition, the health care practitioner's orders often have an impact on nursing interventions by imposing restrictions on factors such as diet or activity.

## Types of Nursing Interventions

Nurses may write nursing interventions as orders in the plan of care for each client. These orders may also derive from other health care providers or as a result of a collaborative effort between nurses and other health care professionals. Depending on the authority required to implement a given activity, the intervention may be categorized as independent, dependent, or interdependent.

Interventions can be implemented on the basis of standing orders or protocols. A **standing order** is a standardized intervention written, approved, and signed by a

## CLIENT REFLECTIONS

### Personalizing Nursing Interventions

Mrs. Carlson is a 74-year-old client on your medical unit. You are assessing her one morning when she says, "There's always so much going on here. Sometimes I feel like you nurses forget you are doing all your procedures to real people. What if it were your grandmother in this bed?" As her nurse, how would you respond to Mrs. Carlson?

## FOCUS ON WELLNESS

### Illness Care versus Health Care

Clients in hospital settings often feel that they are receiving "illness care" rather than health care. While members of the health care team are busy implementing various interventions designed to combat disease, the nurse can help the client focus on those things the client can do to improve her health. The specific steps vary depending on the client's condition, but generally the client can actively facilitate the healing process by getting sufficient rest, movement, and nutrition; managing her stress and pain; and maintaining a positive attitude. By reminding the client of these simple but important steps, and encouraging her to closely follow the plan of care, the nurse empowers the client to implement essential interventions that contribute to her wellness.

health care practitioner and kept on file where it remains available to the health care team to guide treatment interventions. Nurses can implement standing orders in these situations after they have assessed the client and identified the primary or emerging problem. For example, nurses in an ambulatory clinic or home health care agency may have standing orders for administering certain medications or ordering laboratory tests when indicated, or a health care practitioner may establish standing orders on an inpatient unit that specify certain medications that can be administered for common complaints such as a headache. Table 14-3 provides an example of standing orders used for client preparation for a barium enema.

A **protocol** is a series of standing orders or procedures that should be followed under certain specific conditions. They define what interventions are permissible and under what circumstances the nurse is allowed to implement the measures. Health care agencies or individual health care practitioners frequently have standing orders or protocols for client preparation for diagnostic tests or for immediate interventions in life-threatening circumstances. These protocols prevent needless duplication of writing the same orders repeatedly for different clients and often save valuable time in critical situations.

## Nursing Interventions Classification

The Iowa Intervention Project has developed a taxonomy of nursing interventions that includes both direct and indirect activities directed toward health promotion and illness management (Iowa Intervention Project, 1993). This taxonomy, the Nursing Interventions Classification (NIC), is a

## TABLE 14-3    EXAMPLE OF STANDING ORDERS

| Date | Physician's Orders |
|------|--------------------|
| 8/1  | Standing Orders for Barium Enema |
|      | *Prior to test:* |
|      | Clear liquid supper evening prior to test |
|      | 16 oz citrate of magnesia 6 P.M. |
|      | Ducolax tabs iii at 8 P.M. |
|      | NPO after midnight |
|      | Enemas until clear A.M. of test |
|      | *Following test:* |
|      | Milk of magnesia 30 ml PO |

standardized language system that describes nursing interventions performed in all practice settings. NIC is a method for linking nursing interventions to diagnoses and client outcomes (McCloskey, Bulechek, & Eoyang, 1999).

The format for each intervention is as follows: label name, definition, a list of activities that a nurse performs to carry out the intervention, and a list of background readings (see Table 14-4). NIC offers standardized language for research on nursing interventions and is a promising tool for determining reimbursement for nursing services.

### Nursing Intervention Activities

Nursing interventions are widely varied and yet individualized to the specific client. In general, nursing intervention categories include assisting with activities of daily living, delivering therapeutic interventions, monitoring and surveillance of the client's responses, client education, discharge planning, and supervising or coordinating nursing personnel. In the process of implementing the plan of care, the nurse must constantly consider the client's rights, as well as the ethical and legal implications associated with providing care.

Clients have the right to refuse any intervention. However, the nurse must explain the rationale for the intervention and possible consequences associated with refusing treatment. If the intervention refused was health-care-practitioner-initiated, the health care practitioner should be informed of the refusal of care. Ethical standards require that clients be afforded privacy and confidentiality. Matters related to a client's condition and care should be discussed only with individuals directly involved with the client's care, and any discussion should be held in a location where information cannot be overheard by visitors or bystanders. From a legal standpoint, the nurse must ensure that the authority for prescribing any intervention has been satisfied and that applicable standards of

care are maintained during implementation of all nursing interventions.

### Activities of Daily Living

Clients frequently need assistance with ADL such as bathing, grooming, ambulating, eating, and eliminating. The goal for most clients is to return to self-care or to regain as much autonomy as possible. The nurse's role is to determine the extent of assistance needed and to provide support for ADL while at the same time fostering independence. Ongoing assessment is important for determining the appropriate balance between ensuring safety and promoting independence. For example, ambulating may be an important activity for a client recovering from surgery. The nurse must determine, based on assessment findings as well as agency protocol or health practitioner orders, the extent to which the client may ambulate independently without putting himself at unnecessary risk. If the nurse assigns to other personnel the task of assisting the client to ambulate, the nurse must provide adequate training and supervision to ensure that the client is safe.

### Therapeutic Interventions

Therapeutic nursing interventions are those measures directed toward resolution of a current problem and include activities such as administrating medications and treatments, performing skilled procedures, and providing physical and psychological comfort. Written orders must be verified before implementing interventions requiring prescriptive authority. Reassessment of the client is also needed to determine if the intervention remains appropriate. In addition, a nurse must also understand the rationale, expected effects, and possible complications that could result from any intervention.

### Monitoring and Surveillance

Observation of the client's response to treatment is an integral part of the implementation of any intervention. Monitoring and surveillance of the client's progress or lack of progress are essential in determining the effectiveness of the plan of care and for detection of potential complications. Specific interventions require specific monitoring activities; however, typical monitoring activities include observations such as vital signs measurement, cardiac monitoring, and recording of intake and output.

### Client Education

A key element in health promotion and illness management is the education of clients to help them modify their behaviors in response to potential health risks and actual health alterations. As part of this teaching process, nurses must also discuss the rationales for the interventions that are included in the nursing plan of care.

Numerous opportunities arise every day for informal teaching related to client care. For example, teaching clients about the medications they are taking and possible side effects should occur routinely as medications are administered. Similarly, as nurses perform assessment activities, the sharing of observations with the client can

## TABLE 14-4 NURSING INTERVENTIONS CLASSIFICATION (NIC) TAXONOMY

| | Domain 1 | Domain 2 | Domain 3 | Domain 4 | Domain 5 | Domain 6 |
|---|---|---|---|---|---|---|
| LEVEL 1: DOMAINS | 1. Physiological: Basic Care that supports physical functioning | 2. Physiological: Complex Care that supports homeostatic regulation | 3. Behavioral Care that supports psychosocial functioning and facilitates lifestyle changes | 4. Safety Care that supports protection against harm | 5. Family Care that supports the family unit | 6. Health System Care that supports effective use of the health care delivery system |
| LEVEL 2: CLASSES | A Activity and Exercise Management: Interventions to organize or assist with physical activity and energy conservation and expenditure | G Electrolyte and Acid-Base Management: Interventions to regulate electrolyte/acid-base balance and prevent complications | O Behavior Therapy: Interventions to reinforce or promote desirable behaviors or alter undesirable behaviors | U Crisis Management: Interventions to provide immediate short-term help in both psychological and physiological crises | W Childbearing Care: Interventions to assist in understanding and coping with the psychological and physiological changes during the childbearing period | Y Health System Medication: Interventions to facilitate the interface between client/family and the health care system |
| | B Elimination Management: Interventions to establish and maintain regular bowel and urinary elimination patterns and manage complications due to altered patterns | H Drug Management: Interventions to facilitate desired effects of pharmacologic agents | P Cognitive Therapy: Interventions to reinforce or promote desirable cognitive functioning or alter undesirable cognitive functioning | V Risk Management: Interventions to initiate risk-education activities and continue monitoring risks over time | X Life Span Care: Interventions to facilitate family unit functioning and promote the health and welfare of family members throughout the life span | a Health System Management: Interventions to provide and enhance support services for the delivery of care |
| | C Immobility Management: Interventions to manage restricted body movement and the sequelae | I Neurologic Management: Interventions to optimize neurologic functions | Q Communication Enhancement: Interventions to facilitate delivering and receiving verbal and nonverbal messages | | | b Information Management: Interventions to facilitate communications among health care provider |
| | | J Perioperative Management: Interventions to provide care before, during, and immediately after surgery | | | | |

*(continues)*

## TABLE 14-4    NURSING INTERVENTIONS CLASSIFICATION (NIC) TAXONOMY (continued)

| Domain 1 | Domain 2 | Domain 3 | Domain 4 | Domain 5 | Domain 6 |
|---|---|---|---|---|---|
| *D Nutrition Support:* Interventions to modify or maintain nutritional status | *K Respiratory Management:* Interventions to promote airway patency and gas exchange | *R Coping Assistance:* Interventions to assist another to build on own strengths, to adapt to a change in function, or to achieve a higher level of function | | | |
| *E Physical Comfort Promotion:* Interventions to promote comfort using physical techniques | *L Skin/Wound Management:* Interventions to maintain or restore tissue integrity | *S Client Education:* Interventions to facilitate learning | | | |
| *F Self-Care Facilitation:* Interventions to provide or assist with routine activities of daily living | *M Thermoregulation:* Interventions to maintain body temperature within a normal range | *T Psychological Comfort Promotion:* Interventions to promote comfort using psychological techniques | | | |
| | *N Tissue Perfusion Management:* Interventions to optimize circulation of blood and fluids to the tissue | | | | |

Reprinted from *Nursing interventions classification (NIC): Iowa intervention project* (3rd ed.). McCloskey, J. C., & Bulechek, G. M. (1999). With permission from Elsevier.

If nurses have never performed a specific procedure or feel unsure about their ability to safely perform the skill, they must always secure assistance before implementation.

be informative in terms of what characteristics are desirable and what observations are sources of concern. This knowledge can be valuable to a client when self-monitoring (Figure 14-3).

Effective teaching requires insight into the client's knowledge base and readiness to learn. Only by seeking to understand the client's particular situation, including the family's impact and role, can the nurse help to establish realistic teaching goals and learning outcomes. The nurse can further facilitate learning by ensuring that the environment is conducive to the learning process. Limiting potentially threatening or disruptive environmental stimuli, avoiding unnecessarily technical vocabulary, and taking into consideration the client's individuality are examples of steps each nurse should take to support the client's learning.

### Discharge Planning

Preparation for discharge begins at the time of admission to a health care facility. As the average length of stay in acute care settings continues to decrease, early discharge planning becomes imperative. Expected outcomes dictate the type of planning required and the interventions necessary to attain the desired outcomes. Interventions directed toward discharge planning include activities such as teaching and consultation with other agencies (e.g., home health, rehabilitation facilities, nursing homes, social services) concerning follow-up care. The nurse must provide any teaching required to prepare the client for transition

to home or another health care facility. For example, changes in the client's diet, medications, or lifestyle may require instruction. In addition, the nurse should make every effort to anticipate potential barriers or problems

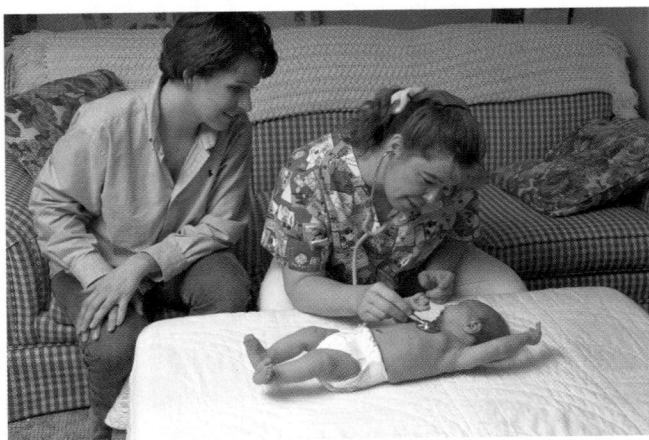

**Figure 14-3    A maternal-child nurse is assessing an infant with the mother and educating the mother in the various considerations for the new child.**

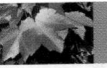

## RESEARCH FOCUS

**Title of Study:** Facilitating day-to-day decision making in palliative care

**Study Purpose:** To investigate the ways nurses support or restrict clients' participation in their care

**Methods:** Researchers evaluated field notes derived from observations of clients and their caregivers in two hospital-based palliative care units and from 23 transcripts of interviews with participating nurses and clients.

**Findings:**
- Nurses in the study subscribed to the values of client-centered care and the importance of developing close relationships with clients and their families. They asserted their commitment to provide opportunities for client decision-making and to respect the choices that clients made.
- The process of getting to know the client is critical to facilitating client choice, because it allows nurses to determine the role clients want to play in decisions about their care, the individual capacities of clients for choice, and the choices that are likely to be meaningful to each individual. Moreover, it allows nurses to tailor opportunities for client choice that maximize levels of participation without overburdening clients and without forcing participation on clients who are reluctant to make choices and wish to relinquish control to others.
- Notwithstanding the positive ramifications of this commitment for clients, knowing the client at this level increases the complexity of nursing care and raises the potential of moral distress for nurses. In the current research, nurses sometimes found it difficult to support client choices that conflicted with their own knowledge or experience (e.g., related to client comfort and safety).

**Implications:** Getting to know the client enables the nurse to better understand, anticipate, and meet that client's needs. In implementing the plan of care, nurses and clients benefit from the nurse's efforts to get to know the client.

Bottorff, J. L., Steele, R., Davies, B., Porterfield, P., Garossino, C., Shaw, M. (2000). Facilitating day-to-day decision making in palliative care. *Cancer Nursing, 23*(2):141–50.

## COMMUNITY/HOME CARE

### Involving Family in Interventions

Mrs. Chang has recently returned home from the hospital. Her cancer has not responded to treatment, and she is now under hospice care. Her family is unsure of how to cope with the concept of her dying, and is equally unprepared for the everyday logistics of caring for Mrs. Chang as she is dying. In addition to implementing the appropriate nursing interventions to keep Mrs. Chang comfortable, the hospice nurse must begin immediately to educate the family. The education process includes helping family members understand the predictable changes that will occur as Mrs. Chang proceeds through the dying process and what interventions they can perform to help her, as well as the things they should avoid doing. Many times, family members feel more comfortable when they develop basic skills that contribute to the client's care. By educating them in this way, the hospice nurse enlists the family, as well as Mrs. Chang, as active members of the health care team.

the client might encounter in the home environment, and to resolve these issues prior to discharge. Some agencies employ personnel whose primary responsibility is to provide discharge planning for groups of clients; however, the nurse who is caring for the individual client is also responsible for ensuring that all appropriate interventions have been implemented before discharge.

### Supervision and Coordination of Personnel

The management style and type of facility, as well as the needs of the client, determine the scope of interventions associated with supervision and coordination of client care. In a health care facility in which nurses are assigned clients within a total client care management system, responsibilities for supervision might be minimal, whereas facilities that use a variety of ancillary personnel for certain client activities might require a large percentage of time devoted to supervision of care. In home health care, for example, the primary role of the professional nurse might be supervision of personnel who provide assistance with ADL. Although a nurse might delegate certain tasks to other personnel, it is still the nurse's responsibility to ensure that the task was completed according to standards of care and to note the response of the client in order to evaluate progress toward expected outcomes.

Regardless of management style or type of facility, coordination of client activities among various health care providers remains the nurse's responsibility. For example, in acute care settings, the nurse needs to coordinate client activities around the schedule of diagnostic tests or physical therapy. Scheduling of procedures, therapy, treatments, and medications for a number of clients often requires considerable organizational skills, creativity, and resourcefulness.

## Evaluating Interventions

In order to provide the highest quality of care, the implementation process must include careful evaluation of each intervention. One approach to determining the efficacy of nursing interventions is by evaluating clients' achievement of expected outcomes. The NIC, previously described in this chapter, provides a systematic method for linking nursing activities to client outcomes. When treatment can be shown to directly improve client outcomes, both nursing and health care consumers benefit.

Another taxonomy, the Nursing Outcomes Classification (NOC) has been specifically designed to evaluate nursing interventions. NOC provides a common language for measuring client responses to nursing interventions.

## Documentation of Interventions

The nurse is responsible for both written documentation of the implementation process as well as verbal communication with other care providers, especially when responsibility for the client's care is transferred from one provider to another. The nurse is legally required to record all interventions and observations related to the client's response to treatment. This not only provides a legal record but also provides the basis for effective communication with other health care team members, thus enhancing continuity of care. In addition, written documentation becomes essential in the reimbursement process, as well as in the ongoing effort to track indicators for continuous quality improvement.

Checklists, flow sheets, and narrative summaries are examples of different forms of written documentation. However, in the event of any unexpected or significant changes in the client's status, the nurse must provide a complete written description, regardless of the form of documentation being used.

Effective verbal communication among members of the health care team is a prerequisite for quality care. Nurses who delegate any aspect of client care must elicit accurate feedback from the assistive personnel regarding the activities performed and the client's response to those interventions. In addition, assistive personnel should know which data might be meaningful in regard to client status, in order to more effectively inform the nurse responsible for that client's care, as well as other members of the health care team. For example, if a nursing assistant observes that Mrs. Robbins, hospitalized with a deep vein thrombosis of the left leg, is having difficulty swallowing and has eaten very little, this information should be reported to the nurse. This is especially important if the behavior is a new occurrence and not a part of the established problem list, because the nurse might not otherwise seek this information.

Communication between nurses generally occurs at the change of shift, when the responsibility for care changes from one nurse to another. Nursing students must communicate relevant information to the nurse responsible for their clients when they leave the unit. Information that should be shared in the verbal report includes:

- Activities completed and those remaining to be completed
- Status of current relevant problems
- Any abnormalities or changes in assessment
- Results of treatments (i.e., client response)
- Diagnostic tests scheduled or completed (and results)

All communication—written and verbal—must be objective, descriptive, and complete. The communication includes observations rather than opinions and is stated or written so that an accurate picture of the client is conveyed. For example, if it is noted that a client is less alert today than yesterday, the *behavior* that led to that conclusion should be documented. This observation can be objectively and descriptively communicated by the statement: "Does not respond unless firmly touched; quickly returns to sleep." This description results in a more complete picture of the client than simply stating: "Less alert today." Thorough and detailed communication of implementation activities is fundamental to ensuring that client care and progress toward goals can be adequately evaluated.

# CASE STUDY/NURSING CARE PLAN

Mr. Thomson presented to the emergency department (ED) with his wife, who had driven him to the hospital and now had to physically help him through the doors. A new nurse is working in the ED and is learning to triage clients, a process that consists of making a brief assessment to determine the acuity of the client's condition. Mr. Thomson is grimacing with pain and short of breath. He is diaphoretic. He denies chest pain, and as the new nurse begins the assessment process, the charge nurse takes one look at him and immediately helps him back to an exam room. On the way past the new nurse, the charge nurse says two words: "Kidney stone." The charge nurse then states that the first priorities for nursing implementation procedures are monitoring his shortness of breath, positioning Mr. Thomson in as comfortable a position as possible, taking his vital signs, and requesting an analgesic for pain.

## Assessment
A brief history, urinalysis, and finally radiography confirmed the charge nurse's assessment. Mr. Thomson had a stone blocking his left ureter. He was in excruciating pain and very nauseated.

## Nursing Diagnosis #1
*Acute Pain* related to urinary tract obstruction
**NOC:** Comfort Level; Pain Control
**NIC:**  Analgesic Administration; Pain Management

## Expected Outcome
Client will experience pain relief by stating pain is at a 3 within 24 hours.

## Planning/Interventions/Rationales
1. Assess level of pain using a scale from 1 to 10. *Provides quantitative baseline assessment of client's pain and allows for subsequent assessment of effectiveness of pain control interventions.*
2. Administer analgesics as prescribed. *Provides treatment for the pain.*
3. Report increased pain to physician. *May indicate change in condition that could necessitate revised intervention strategy.*

## Evaluation
Pain level reported as a 2 within 24 hours. Client taking analgesics every 4 hours.

## Nursing Diagnosis #2
*Deficient Knowledge* related to diagnostic and treatment procedures.
**NOC:** Knowledge: Treatment Procedures
**NIC:**  Teaching: Procedure/Treatment

*(continues)*

# CASE STUDY/NURSING CARE PLAN *(continued)*

### Expected Outcome
Client will develop understanding of procedures at the time of explanation and have relevant questions answered to the best of the nurse's ability.

### Planning/Interventions/Rationales
1. Assess client's current level of understanding of diagnostic tests and treatment procedures. *Informs nurse of specific knowledge gaps.*
2. Describe procedures in simple language, and assess client's understanding of explanations. *Client is in pain and likely anxious about his situation, making it more difficult for him to comprehend explanations and instructions.*
3. Provide opportunities for client to ask questions before, during, and after procedures. *Reinforces education and minimizes likelihood of further knowledge gap.*

### Evaluation
Client verbalizes an understanding of diagnostic and treatment procedures as they are taught. Client asked two questions after a procedure was explained.

## Key Concepts

- During the implementation phase of the nursing process, the nurse applies assessment and diagnostic information to carry out the plan of care. Implementation might require the nurse to provide direct client care, to delegate tasks to other members of the health care team, or to do both. In either case, the nurse must carefully document each activity involved in the implementation process.
- Implementation requires cognitive, psychomotor, and intellectual skills to accomplish goals and make progress toward expected outcomes.
- Implementation activities include ongoing assessment, establishment of priorities, allocation of resources, initiation of specific nursing interventions, and documentation of interventions and client responses.
- In order to determine the extent to which interventions have been effective and to discover emerging problems, the nurse must include ongoing assessment in the implementation of the care plan.
- Changing variables in clients and the environment demands clinical judgment and flexibility in organizing care.
- Time management skills are essential in implementing client care.
- The nurse maintains responsibility for care delegated to other health care personnel.
- The most common management systems currently used include functional nursing, team nursing, primary nursing, total client care, modular nursing, and case management.
- Interventions can be nurse-initiated, health-care-practitioner-initiated, or collaborative in origin, and thus are considered dependent, independent, or interdependent.

- Nursing Interventions Classification (NIC) is a system for sorting, labeling, and describing nursing interventions.
- Nursing interventions include assisting with activities of daily living, skilled therapeutic interventions, monitoring and surveillance of response to care, teaching, discharge planning, and supervision and coordination of nursing personnel.
- Communication concerning interventions should be provided verbally and in writing.

## Review Questions and Activities

1. Label each of the following nursing interventions as dependent (dep.), independent (ind.), or interdependent (int.).

    _____ **a.** Applying a heating pad to a shoulder for 20 minutes

    _____ **b.** Administering a pain medication as needed following surgery

    _____ **c.** Turning a client with impaired mobility every 2 hours

    _____ **d.** Teaching a client about side effects of a medication

    _____ **e.** Assisting a client with oral care

    _____ **f.** Sending an order for a diagnostic laboratory test

    _____ **g.** Reviewing and conveying abnormal lab test results

    _____ **h.** Starting intravenous fluids

2. List five implementation activities, and give an example of each.

3. List two reasons for documentation of client care.

4. *Situation:* Mary Long, age 42, has come to the clinic because of recurrent chest pains (although symptom-free at this time). Although there is a strong family history of heart disease, she has no personal history of heart problems. She is approximately 60 lb overweight, and you determine that her lifestyle is rather sedentary and her diet high in fat content. She lives at home with her husband. Her children no longer live at home. Although she works part-time as a receptionist, her favorite activity is cooking.

   Her health care practitioner mentions diet, exercise, and weight control as long-term activities, orders a series of tests to be done as an outpatient, and gives her a prescription for nitroglycerin tablets for chest pain.

   What interventions do you think will be necessary and appropriate for Mrs. Long? How would you organize priorities for Mrs. Long?

5. Consider your most recent clinical experience. How could you have organized your time more effectively? Apply these same time management principles to your study time. How could you arrange your time more efficiently?

6. The next time you are in a clinical agency, examine your client's record for the previous 8 hours. Does it provide a vivid and accurate description of the client? How could the written documentation be improved?

7. Ask a nurse what activities occupy most of his or her time. What activities does the nurse most enjoy? What does the nurse least enjoy? Compare this nurse's perceptions with your own ideas.

8. How does the nurse practice act in your state address delegation? Does the definition specifically address the registered nurse's role in supervising other nursing personnel? Licensed practical nurse's role? Delegation of nursing care to others? Has the board of nursing in your state established rules on delegation? If so, what do these rules allow? If not, how is the issue of delegation of nursing care addressed?

9. You are caring for Mr. Sims, who has had a stroke. The care plan includes the following activities and interventions:

   - Up in chair at bedside three times a day for at least 30 minutes
   - Assist bed bath/assist with eating
   - CT of head at 10:00 A.M.
   - Strengthening exercises per physical therapy at 9:00 A.M.
   - Routine medications at 9:00 A.M. and 1:00 P.M.

   You are responsible for total client care for Mr. Sims. Write a plan of your activities with Mr. Sims.

10. If you were a client in a hospital, which nursing management system would you prefer? Why?

## Multimedia Links

Christensen *Core Concept Videos: Planning and Intervention*

## Web Resources

Agency for Healthcare Research and Quality
    http://www.ahcpr.gov
American Nurses Association
    http://www.nursingworld.org
National Institute of Nursing Research
    http://www.nih.gov/ninr
North American Nursing Diagnosis Association
    http://www.nanda.org

## References

American Nurses Association (1998). *Standards of Clinical Nursing Practice* (2nd ed.). Washington, DC: Author.

Bezon, J., Echevarria, K. H., & Smith, G. B. (1999). Nursing outcome indicator: Preventing falls for elderly people. *Outcomes Management for Nursing Practice, 3*(2), 112–117.

Bottorff, J. L., Steele, R., Davies, B., Porterfield, P., Garossino, C., Shaw, M. (2000). Facilitating day-to-day decision making in palliative care. *Cancer Nursing, 23*(2),141–50.

Chitty, K. K. (2000). *Professional nursing: Concepts and challenges.* (2nd ed.). Philadelphia: Saunders.

Frisch, N. C., & Kelly, J. H. (2002). Nursing diagnosis and nursing theory: exploration of factors inhibiting and supporting simultaneous use. *Nursing Diagnosis,* 13(2), 53–61.

Iowa Intervention Project (1993). The NIC taxonomy structure. *Image: Journal of Nursing Scholarship,* 25(3), 187–192.

Johnson, M., Maas, M., & Dochterman, J. M. (2000). *Nursing diagnoses, outcomes, and interventions: NANDA, NOC and NIC linkages.* St. Louis: Mosby.

McCloskey, J. C., Bulechek, G. M., & Eoyang, T. (Eds.). (1999). *Nursing interventions: Effective nursing treatments* (3rd ed.). Philadelphia: Saunders.

McCloskey, J. C., & Bulechek, G. M. (1999). *Nursing interventions classification (NIC): Iowa intervention project* (3rd ed.). St. Louis: Mosby.

Powers, P. (2002). A discourse analysis of nursing diagnosis. *Qualitative Health Research,* 12(7), 945–965.

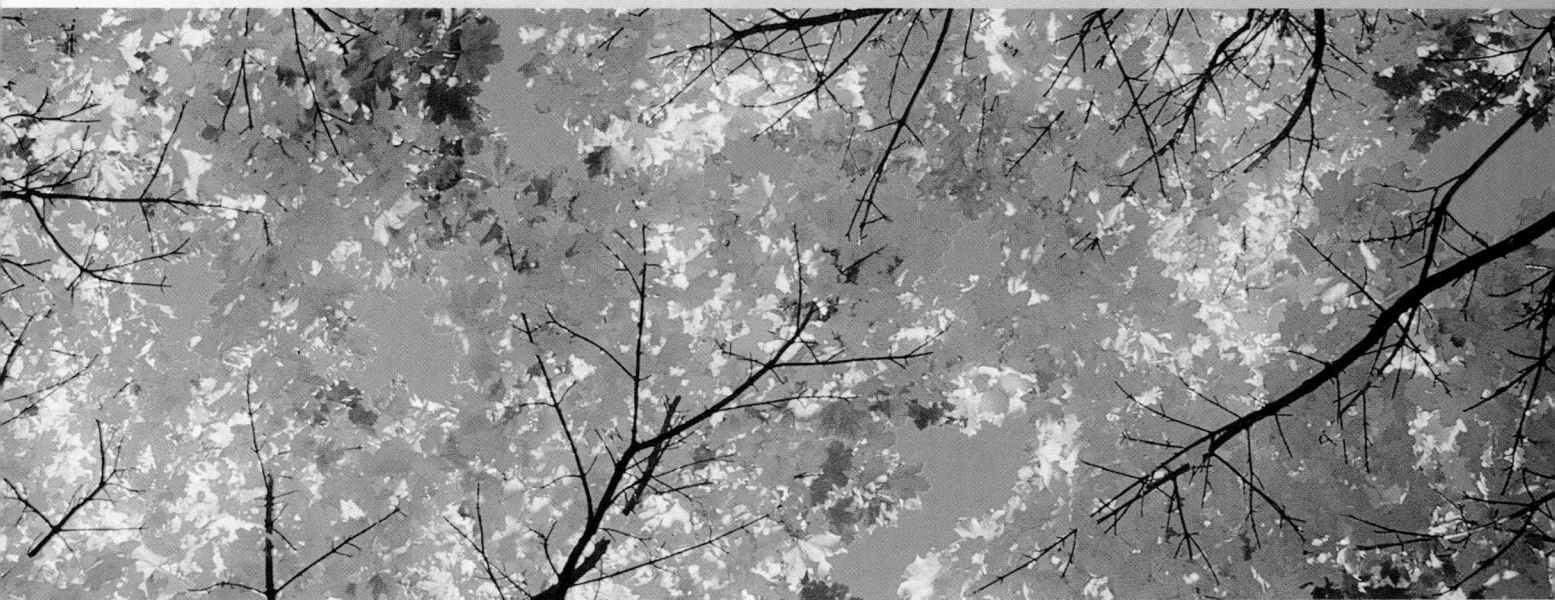

# CHAPTER 15

# Evaluation

Heather Freiheit, RN, BSN, EMT-P

*"We don't know who we are until we see what we can do."*

*(Martha Grimes, 2001)*

# Chapter Competencies

## Upon completion of this chapter, the reader should be able to:

1. Explain the evaluation phase of the nursing process.
2. List the components of evaluation.
3. Describe the methods of evaluation.
4. Relate how the quality of client care is affected by the evaluation phase.
5. Show how accountability interfaces with evaluation.
6. Explain why client evaluation must be a multidisciplinary action.

# Key Terms

accountability

evaluation

nursing audit

outcome evaluation

peer evaluation

process evaluation

structure evaluation

**E**valuation is the fifth step in the nursing process and involves determining whether the client goals have been met, have been partially met, or have not been met. Even though it is the final phase of the nursing process, evaluation is an ongoing part of daily nursing activities. Ongoing evaluation can determine if the client has achieved the expected outcomes or if care needs to be modified to help achieve these outcomes. Also, it is an integral process in determining the quality of health care delivered.

This chapter discusses the purposes, components, and methods of evaluation. The relationship between evaluation and quality of care is also examined.

## Evaluation of Client Care

Evaluation is the measurement of the degree to which objectives are achieved. Therefore, evaluating the care provided to clients is an essential part of professional nursing. Evaluation is a systematic process that measures the health of the client against the desired expected outcomes. The American Nurses Association (1998), in its *Standards of Clinical Nursing Practice*, designates evaluation as a fundamental component of the nursing process. The purposes of evaluation include:

- To determine the client's progress or lack of progress toward achievement of expected outcomes
- To determine the effectiveness of nursing care in helping clients achieve the expected outcomes
- To determine the overall quality of care provided
- To promote nursing accountability (discussed later in this chapter)

Evaluation is done primarily to determine whether a client is progressing—that is, experiencing an improvement in health status. Not an end to the nursing process, evaluation is rather an ongoing mechanism that assures quality and effective interventions. Evaluation is performed continuously, not just prior to termination of the client's care (Box 15-1). Evaluation is closely related to each of the other stages of the nursing process. The client's plan of care may be modified during any phase of the nursing process as determined through evaluation. Client goals and expected outcomes provide the criteria for evaluation of care (Figure 15-1).

## Components of Evaluation

Evaluation is a fluid process that is dependent on all the other components of the nursing process. As shown in Figure 15-2, evaluation affects, and is affected by, assessment, diagnosis, outcome identification and planning, and implementation of nursing care (Fitzpatrick, 2002). Ongoing evaluation is essential if the nursing process is to be implemented appropriately. As Alfaro-LeFevre (2004) states:

> When we evaluate early, checking whether our information is accurate, complete, and up-to-date, we're able to make corrections *early*. We avoid making decisions based on outdated, inaccurate, or incomplete information. Early evaluation enhances our ability to act safely and effectively. It improves our *efficiency* by helping us stay focused on priorities and avoid wasting time continuing useless actions.

There are specific criteria to be used in the process of evaluation. The evaluation criteria must be planned, goal-

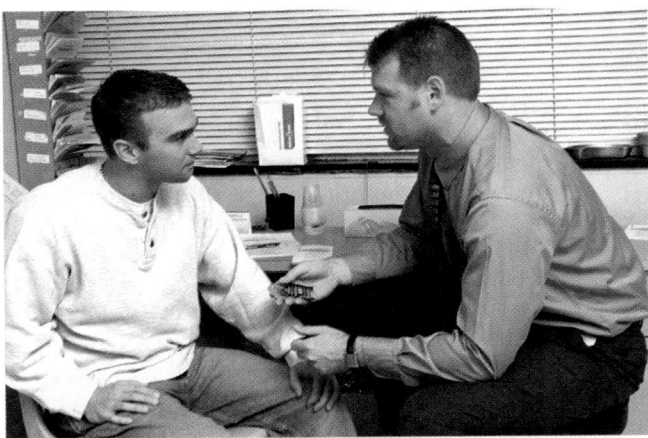

**Figure 15-1   A nurse involved in a follow-up evaluation to set goals with an adolescent in a wellness clinic.**

directed, objective, verifiable, and specific (that is, strengths, weaknesses, achievements, and deficits must be considered).

## Techniques

Effective evaluation results primarily from the nurse's accurate use of communication and observation skills. Both verbal and nonverbal communication between the nurse and the client can yield important information about the accuracy of the goals and expected planned outcomes and the nursing interventions that have been executed for resolution of the client's problems. The nurse needs to be sensitive to clients' willingness or hesitation to discuss their responses to nursing actions, and must use the techniques of therapeutic communication to collect all necessary data.

The nurse must be sensitive to changes in the client's physiological condition, emotional status, and behavior. Because these changes are often subtle, they require astute observational skills on the part of the nurse. What the nurse sees, hears, smells, and feels when touching the client all provide clues to the client's current health status (Figure 15-3).

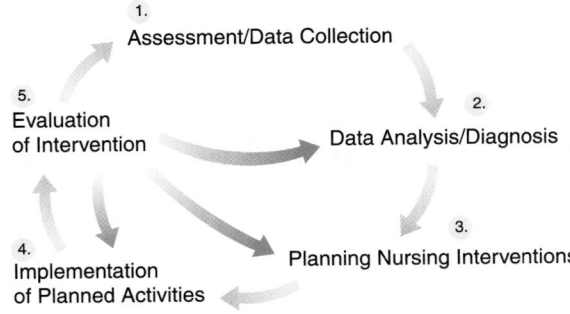

**Figure 15-2   Relationship of evaluation to the nursing process**

> ### BOX 15-1   EVALUATION AS A STANDARD COMPONENT OF CARE: ANA STANDARDS
>
> #### Standard VI: Evaluation
> The nurse evaluates the client's progress toward attainment of outcomes.
>
> #### Guidelines
> Evaluation must:
>
> - Be performed as a systemic process
> - Occur on an ongoing basis
> - Lead to revision of the plan of care when needed
> - Involve the client, significant others, and other members of the health care team
> - Be documented
>
> From American Nurses Association. (1998). *Standards of clinical nursing practice* (2nd ed.). Washington, DC: Author. Reprinted with permission of the author.

## Sources of Data

Evaluation is a mutual process occurring among the nurse, client, family, and other health care providers. Both subjective and objective data are used in evaluating the client's status. Asking clients to describe feelings results in subjective data. Objective data consist of observable facts, such as laboratory values and the client's behavior. When a nurse communicates an assessment of a client's response to an actual or potential health problem, clients and families are empowered to discuss their concerns and questions. When feedback is given, the nurse must avoid being defensive or judgmental, because that attitude may cause clients or families to avoid being open and honest. As a result, they may say only what they think the nurse wants to hear or they may completely refuse to participate in the evaluation process. The nurse's verbal and nonverbal communication establishes the atmosphere in which clients and families freely share their comments, both positive and negative.

## Goals and Expected Outcomes

The effectiveness of nursing interventions is evaluated by examination of goals and expected outcomes. Goals provide direction for the plan of care and serve as measurements for the client's progress or lack of progress toward resolution of a problem.

Realistic goals are necessary for effective evaluation. These goals must take into consideration the client's

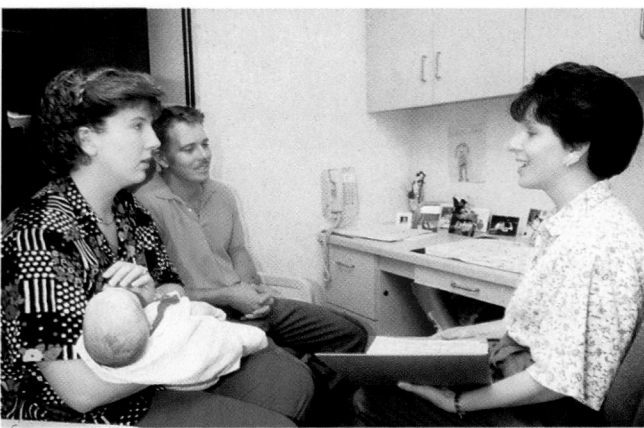

**Figure 15-3    A nurse using therapeutic communication techniques in evaluating postpartum care with two parents.**

## STOP AND THINK

### Evaluation Scenarios

- How would you evaluate a hearing impaired client, who communicates with American Sign Language, for mental confusion after a diagnosis of a cerebrovascular accident?

- What subjective and objective data would you use to evaluate the effectiveness of a pain medication administered to a two-year-old?

- What criteria would you use to evaluate the diet of a diabetic client who is resistive to diabetic teaching?

strengths, limitations, resources, and the time frame for achievement of the objectives. Examples of client strengths are educational background, family support, and financial resources (for instance, money to purchase medications and foods that support the prescribed interventions). Examples of client limitations are delayed developmental level, poverty, and unwillingness to change.

## Methods of Evaluation

The nurse who successfully evaluates nursing care uses a systematic approach that ensures thorough, comprehensive collection of data. Evaluation is an orderly process consisting of eight steps.

### Establishing Standards

Specific criteria are used to determine whether the demonstrated behavior indicates goal achievement. Standards are established before nursing action is implemented. Evaluation of criteria examines the presence of any changes, direction of change (positive or negative), and whether the changes are expected or unexpected.

### Collecting Data

Assessment skills are used to gather data pertinent to goals and expected outcomes. The nurse must be proficient in assessment skills for effective, comprehensive evaluation to occur. Evaluation data are collected to answer the following question: Were the treatment goals and expected outcomes achieved?

### Determining Goal Achievement

Data are analyzed to determine whether client behaviors indicate goal achievement. This process is validated through analysis of the client's response to the specific nursing interventions that are developed in the plan of

care. For example, these data can take the form of either physiological responses (such as the client's being able to cough productively in order to promote effective breathing patterns) or psychosocial responses (such as the client's being able to verbalize concerns about an impending surgical procedure in order to alleviate anxiety) (Cocchairella, 2000).

### Relating Nursing Actions to Client Status

Nursing interventions are examined to determine their relevance to the client's needs and nursing diagnoses. Efficient nursing actions are those that address pertinent client needs and are proven to be primary factors in helping clients appropriately resolve actual or potential problems (McInnes, Duff, Fennessey, Seers, & Clark, 2001).

### Judging the Value of Nursing Interventions

Critical-thinking skills are used to determine the degree to which nursing actions have contributed to the client's improved status. Critical thinking enables the nurse to apply an analytical focus to the client's responses to the nursing interventions, thereby evaluating the benefits of those interventions and identifying additional opportunities for revision.

### Reassessing the Client's Status

The client's health status is reevaluated through use of assessment and observation skills. Evaluation focuses on the client's health status and compares it with baseline data collected during the initial assessment. Omissions or incomplete data within the database are identified so that an accurate picture of the client's health status is obtained.

## Modifying the Plan of Care

If the evaluation data indicate a lack of progress toward goal achievement, the plan of care is modified. These revisions are developed through the following process: reassessment of the client, formulation of more appropriate nursing diagnoses, development of new or revised goals and expected outcomes, and implementation of different nursing actions or repetition of specific actions to maximize their effectiveness (for instance, client teaching).

Evaluation is performed by every nurse, regardless of the practice setting. For example, the home health nurse evaluates the care provided regularly throughout the client's relationship with the agency. Evaluation of the home care client is carried out in order to determine whether the care was delivered in an effective and efficient manner, to modify the plan of care as needed, and to decide when the client is ready for discontinuation of home care services. The accompanying Nursing Strategies box provides guidelines to analyze the nursing intervention.

## Critical Thinking and Evaluation

Evaluation is a critical thinking activity. It is a deliberate mechanism used to analyze and make judgments. Nurses need to remain objective when evaluating client care in order to modify care based on reason rather than emotion. One critical-thinking strategy, juxtaposing, is described as "putting the present state condition next to the outcome state in a side-by-side contrast" (Pesut & Herman, 1999, p. 93). Nurses use juxtaposing throughout evaluative activities by comparing client responses to expected behaviors. They make conclusions about whether expected outcomes have been met. In order to make such conclusions, assessment data is needed to determine client progress toward achievement of objectives. Evaluation involves analysis and is much more complex than merely answering questions.

### NURSING STRATEGY

**Application of Nursing Process**

The following guidelines demonstrate the nurse's application of the nursing process with the client:

- Assessment was thorough and accurate.

- Nursing diagnoses were relevant.

- Client and family participated in goal setting.

- Goals were specific, measurable, and realistic.

- Nursing action addressed client's problems.

- Client and family participated in evaluation.

- Evaluation was ongoing and resulted in a revised plan of care as the client's status changed.

- Plan of care was revised according to the client's needs.

- Documentation reflected the client's status, including responses to nursing interventions.

### COMMUNITY/HOME CARE

**Plan of Care Evaluation**

The home health care nurse evaluates the plan of care through the following questions to examine client achievement of expectant outcomes:

1. Were the goals realistic in terms of the client's abilities and time frame?

2. Were there external variables that prevented goal achievement (e.g., housing problems, impaired family dynamics)?

3. Did the family have the resources to assist in meeting the goals (e.g., transportation)?

4. Was the care coordinated with other providers to facilitate efficient delivery of care (e.g., occupational therapy)?

# Evaluation and Quality of Care

Evaluation is performed at the individual and institutional levels. For example, individual evaluation focuses on the client's achievement of goals and also on the individual nurse's delivery of care (King & Lipsky, 2000). Quality and evaluation are closely related. This section examines the role of evaluation in assuring the delivery of quality health care. Because it is the mechanism used by nurses in determining the need for improvement, evaluation assists in the provision of quality care. The aspects that need to be evaluated to determine the quality of health care are:

- Appropriateness (the care provided adhered to standards and resulted in achievement of goals)
- Clinical outcomes
- Client satisfaction
- Cost-effectiveness
- Access to care
- Availability of resources

Quality management involves constant, ongoing evaluation (monitoring of activities).

## Elements in Evaluating the Quality of Care

Organizational evaluation examines the agency's overall ability to deliver quality care. Evaluation can be classified according to what is being evaluated: the structure, the process, or the outcome. Table 15-1 provides an overview of the types of evaluation. Figure 15-4 illustrates the variables to be assessed in each type of evaluation.

### Structure Evaluation

**Structure evaluation** is a determination of the health care agency's ability to provide the services offered to its client population. This type of evaluation focuses on assessing the systems by which nursing care is delivered (Barnum & Kerfoot, 1995). Structure evaluation examines the physical facilities, resources, equipment, staffing patterns, organizational patterns, and the agency's qualifications for staff. The majority of problems with providing effective health care stems from problems in the structural area. The purpose of structure evaluation is to identify any system errors, which can then be corrected.

Structure evaluation involves determining whether client care meets legal and professional standards. A frequently used method to evaluate whether the agency provides care within legal parameters is a review of policy and procedure manuals to check for compliance with regulations.

### Process Evaluation

**Process evaluation** is the measurement of nursing actions by examination of each phase of the nursing process. This type of evaluation is done to determine whether nursing care was effective and efficient. Nursing

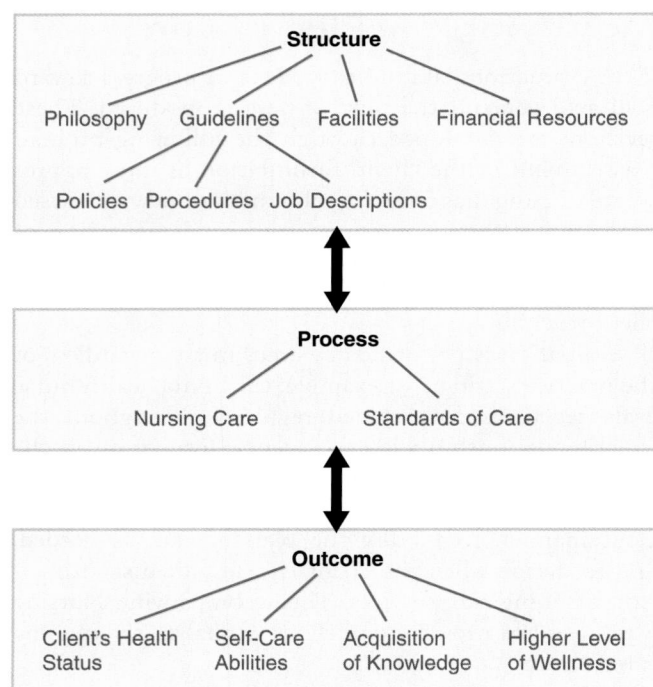

**Figure 15-4    Elements within each type of evaluation**

interventions are judged to be effective when use of the action results in the desired outcome. A nursing intervention is determined to be efficient through analysis of the intervention's cost-benefit ratio. Process evaluation determines the nurse's ability to establish an environment that promotes the client's health. See Table 15-1 for sample questions used during process evaluation.

### Outcome Evaluation

**Outcome evaluation** is the process of comparing the client's current status with the expected outcomes. This type of evaluation examines all direct care activities that affect the client's health status. Outcome evaluation, though challenging, is the most meaningful way to judge the effectiveness of nursing interventions.

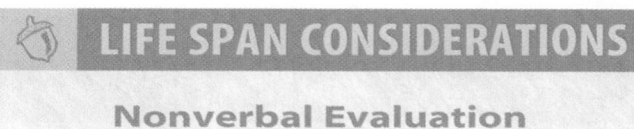

## LIFE SPAN CONSIDERATIONS

### Nonverbal Evaluation of Pediatric Clients

In contrast to working with adults, evaluating the pediatric population can be challenging. Pediatric clients can be nonverbal or have difficulty expressing their symptoms. As a nurse you may have only objective data to help you determine if the intervention achieved the desired outcome.

Potts, N., & Mandleco, B. (2002). *Pediatric nursing: Caring for children and their families.* Clifton Park, NY: Delmar Learning.

## TABLE 15-1    TYPES OF EVALUATION

| Purpose | Data Sources | Sample Evaluation Questions |
|---|---|---|
| *Structure Evaluation* | | |
| Measures the adequacy of facility to meet needs of clients | Policy and procedure manuals<br><br>Job descriptions (including qualifications)<br><br>Staffing patterns<br><br>Credentials of staff<br><br>Written care plans<br><br>Orientation programs | Does the orientation program provide nurses with information relevant to the needs of their assigned areas?<br><br>Do the nursing policies adhere to legal requirements?<br><br>Are nursing policies easily accessed by staff?<br><br>Do staffing patterns reflect ability to meet acuity needs of clients? |
| *Process Evaluation* | | |
| Measures the adequacy of nursing activities in implementing the nursing process | Client interviews<br><br>Demonstration of client's skills and knowledge<br><br>Documentation in client's record of nursing actions performed | Is every client assessed by a nurse upon admission to the agency?<br><br>Is the plan of care individualized for each client?<br><br>Is the nursing care based on identified client needs?<br><br>Is the client's response to the nursing actions documented? |
| *Outcome Evaluation* | | |
| Compares client's progress to expected outcomes | Observation of client<br><br>Client interview<br><br>Chart audits<br><br>Written discharge plans | Does the client demonstrate new knowledge or skills?<br><br>Is there documented evidence of client progress toward achievement of expected outcomes?<br><br>Is there documentation of the client's abilities to cope with the problem after discharge? |

Data from Barnum, B. S., & Kerfoot, K. M. (1995). *The nurse as executive* (4th ed., pp. 236–248). Gaithersburg, MD: Aspen; Gillies, D. A. (1994). *Nursing management: A systems approach* (3rd ed., pp. 511–535). Philadelphia: Saunders; Kenney, J. W. (1995). Evaluation. In P. J. Christensen & J. W. Kenney (Eds.), *Nursing process: Application of conceptual models* (4th ed., pp. 195–207). St. Louis: Mosby.

Outcome evaluation focuses on changes in the client's health status. A basic question to ask when evaluating the outcome is, Has the expected change occurred? Such changes may include modifications of symptoms, signs, knowledge, attitudes, satisfaction, skill, and compliance with treatment regimen. Another variable assessed during outcome evaluation is the client's self-care ability. Has the client demonstrated an improved ability to care for self? Does the client verbalize knowledge related to self-care needs? See Table 15-1 for suggested approaches to performing outcome evaluation. In addition, there need to be varied approaches to evaluating the outcomes of different age ranges.

## Nursing Audit

A **nursing audit** is the process of collecting and analyzing data to evaluate the effectiveness of nursing interventions. A nursing audit can focus on implementation of

## CLIENT REFLECTIONS

### Evaluation of Pain

"How is your pain level now, Mr. Jones?" questioned the nurse.

"Thank you for asking; it is well controlled at a 2," replied Mr. Jones. "Initially I could not figure out why all my nurses kept asking me to rate my pain. After you explained to me that this was a way to assess how my pain medication was working, it all made sense. I appreciate your dedication and concern."

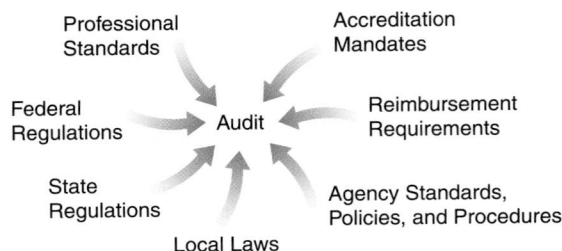

Figure 15-5    Influences affecting the nursing audit

the nursing process, client outcomes, or both in order to evaluate the quality of care provided. Nursing audits examine data related to:

- Safety measures
- Treatment interventions and client responses to the interventions
- Preestablished outcomes used as basis for interventions
- Discharge planning
- Client teaching
- Adequacy of staffing patterns

Audits are based on components such as institutional policies; federal, state, and local regulations; accreditation standards; and professional standards (Figure 15-5). Audits assist in identifying strengths and weaknesses that, in turn, provide direction for areas needing revision. Corrective action plans are developed in accordance with the audit results (Stone, Bakken, & Curran, 2002).

## Peer Evaluation

Another method of evaluating quality of care is **peer evaluation** (also referred to as *peer review*), the process by which professionals provide to their peers critical performance appraisal and feedback that are geared toward corrective action. According to the ANA (1988):

## RESEARCH FOCUS

**Title of Study:** Managing the outcome of infection: Nosocomial infection initiative

**Study Purpose:** To demonstrate that the incidence of nosocomial pneumonia can be reduced by changing clinical practice

**Methods:** This study was conducted on clients who had cardiovascular surgery. A tool was designed to identify clients who were at high risk for developing pneumonia. Clients scoring higher than the cutoff rate on the scoring tool were placed on a newly designed protocol for pneumonia prevention. Two clinical practices, hand washing and suctioning techniques, were selected as the variables for evaluating (by use of a checklist) clinicians' skills.

**Findings:** Within 1 year following implementation of the protocol, the pneumonia rate for cardiovascular surgery clients decreased by 37%.

**Implications:** This study demonstrates that changing clinical practice may affect client outcomes. Evaluation of other nursing interventions could be considered for future study.

Houston, S. (1999). Managing the outcome of infection: Nosocomial infection initiative. *Outcomes Management for Nursing Practice, 3*(2), 73–77.

Peer review in nursing is the process by which practicing Registered Nurses systematically assess, monitor, and make judgments about the quality of nursing care provided by peers, as measured against professional standards of practice. (p. 3)

In 1984, Lucille Joel postulated that peer review is the basis of nursing's autonomy and self-governance (Joel, 1984). This perspective is still very relevant in today's health care climate. By evaluating itself, nursing is demonstrating an essential criterion by which professions are recognized. Peer evaluation promotes both professional and individual accountability.

The quality of nursing care is strongly evident to coworkers and nurses who are expected to assess the work of their peers. "Peer review is an essential mechanism for evaluating the judgment and performance of clinical providers" (Wakefield, Helms, & Helms, 1995, p. 11).

Such judgment may result in one of the following outcomes:

- Destructive: complaints and attacks that undermine morale and cohesiveness
- Constructive: positive feedback that improves the quality of care

## NURSING STRATEGY

### Principles of Effective Peer Evaluation

Effective peer evaluation

- Improves the quality of client care

- Promotes professional growth

- Is timely, frequent, and ongoing

- May be formal or informal, verbal or written

- Is not anonymous

- Is objective—that is, addresses specific behavior

- Is not linked to financial rewards (salary raises) or promotional opportunities

- Needs to be documented

Data from Cohen, B., Berube, R., & Turrentine, B. (1996). A peer review program for professional nurses. *Journal of Nursing Staff Development, 12*(1), 13.

Peer evaluation can be destructive if the parties involved begin to personalize the process, misunderstand the purpose, or deliver feedback in an unfeeling and nonobjective manner. Peer evaluation can be threatening when guidelines have not been established for the process and when the assessment focuses on emotions and personalities instead of on behaviors. Conversely, peer evaluation is con-

## STOP AND THINK

### Peer Evaluation and Friendship

Your coworker is also a close friend. You are assigned to perform a peer evaluation with her. Before the process begins, she asks you to be especially lenient when evaluating her performance. When collecting information about the quality of her work, you discover that she is often hurried and unorganized, a practice that results in her providing only mediocre care. You know that if the evaluation is not above average, your friend will likely experience disciplinary action from her supervisor. In view of your friendship, what do you do in this situation?

structive when the focus remains on quality improvement and encourages the continued growth and learning of all the parties involved. The accompanying Nursing Strategy box provides principles that promote the use of objective, nonbiased peer evaluation.

## Evaluation and Accountability

**Accountability** means assuming responsibility for one's actions. Evaluation enhances nursing accountability by providing a mechanism for assisting the nurse to define, explain, and measure the results of nursing actions. Accountability is increased by ongoing evaluation; nurses are continually checking their own progress against predetermined standards.

Accountability is an integral part of professional nursing practice and is an important method through which commitment to quality client care can be demonstrated. Nurses are accountable for designing effective care plans, implementing appropriate nursing actions, and judging the effectiveness of their nursing interventions. In other words, nurses are accountable for their judgments, decisions, and actions to:

- Clients, families, and significant others
- Colleagues
- Employers
- The general public (society)
- The nursing profession
- Themselves

Nurses demonstrate their commitment in a variety of ways, including:

- Maintaining expertise in skills
- Participating in continuing education programs
- Achieving and maintaining certification
- Participating in peer evaluation

## Multidisciplinary Collaboration in Evaluation

Evaluating the quality of care provided is a responsibility shared among members of the health care team. In addition to those directly involved (the health care providers, clients, and families), others interested in the outcomes of evaluation include the community and third-party payers (both public and private reimbursement organizations).

An ongoing monitoring process is implemented to evaluate quality of care. Ideally, every discipline monitors its own quality efforts. No single discipline is responsible for all-inclusive evaluation of client care. However, in most health care agencies, nurses are actively involved in monitoring evaluation activities. Many agencies have nurses on

## CLINICAL ALERT

### Professional Accountability

A component of evaluation includes taking professional accountability by notifying the primary health care provider when you discover critical changes in a client's status.

staff who function either as quality management coordinators, utilization review evaluators, or both.

When health care providers from all the relevant disciplines are involved in evaluation, the result is decreased fragmentation of care. The team approach mandates active involvement of all care providers in the evaluation of quality care. Multidisciplinary evaluation helps promote a continuum of care for the client, from the preadmission phase to discharge planning and follow-up care.

# CASE STUDY/NURSING CARE PLAN

Mr. Carver, age 68, was admitted yesterday through the emergency room with right-sided weakness. He was treated for a medical diagnosis of cerebral vascular accident (CVA) after confirmation with a CT (computed tomography) scan. He was then admitted to the medical unit for follow-up care. Mr. Carver's assessment shows that he is normally right-handed and now has difficulty holding a fork. In addition, he is weak in his right leg movements and his verbalizations are slightly slurred. His history reveals that he resides alone in the house on his farm where he and his wife lived for 40 years, as she died last year.

## Assessment
- "I can't handle this milk carton with only one hand."
- "I do not like to use that walker. It gets in my way."
- Gait unsteady and shuffling
- Asymmetrical strength in arms and legs
- Unable to hold fork in right hand

## Nursing Diagnosis #1
*Feeding Self-Care Deficit* related to weakness in right hand and inability to hold fork
**NOC:** Nutritional Status; Nutritional Status: Food and Fluid Intake
**NIC:** Nutrition Management; Nutritional Counseling

## Expected Outcomes
The client will:
1. Attend a teaching session on feeding himself with his left hand at 1000, on 2/12.
2. Practice using adaptive spoon at 1400 on 2/12.
3. Use adaptive spoon for meals beginning with breakfast on 2/13.

## Planning/Interventions/Rationales
1. Present a teaching session "Feeding oneself with the nondominant hand" at 1000, on 2/12. *For clients recovering from illness and/or injury, information about adapting to limitations fosters independence.*
2. Provide the client with four foods of differing textures, adaptive spoons, and apron for a practice session at 1400, on 2/12. *Providing practice time reinforces skills learned and fosters an improved confidence level in the learner.*
3. Notify the dietary department to include a left-hand adaptive spoon with breakfast tray on 2/13. *Using adaptive devices provides safety and promotes independence.*
4. Encourage client to feed self independently at each meal, beginning 2/13. *Recognizing and commending success promotes positive self-esteem.*
5. Assist client with food preparation and feeding as needed at each meal, beginning 2/12. *Assistance preserves strength and avoids tiring the client, promotes safety, and decreases frustration as the client strives for independence.*

## Evaluation
1. Mr. Carver attended teaching session on 2/12, asked questions, and participated in the practice session.

*(continues)*

# CASE STUDY/NURSING CARE PLAN (continued)

2. Goal partially met. Mr. Carver practiced using a spoon in his left hand to feed himself oatmeal, soup, ice cream, and canned peaches on 2/12. Successful self-feeding with all foods except soup. Continue practice, reevaluate 2/19.

3. Goal partially met. On 2/13, fed self 75% of each meal, using adaptive spoon. Continue. Reevaluate on 2/15.

## Nursing Diagnosis #2

*Risk for Injury:* Falls related to unsteady, shuffling gait

**NOC:** Risk Control; Safety Behavior: Home Environment; Safety Behavior: Personal; Safety Status: Falls Occurrence; Safety Status: Physical Injury

**NIC:** Health Education; Behavior Modification

## Expected Outcomes

The client will:

1. Participate in physical therapy evaluation of mobility strengths and weaknesses on 2/11 at 1100.

2. Attend a muscle-strengthening class on 2/12 at 1600.

3. Perform all strengthening exercises prescribed BID at 1000 and 1600, beginning 2/13.

## Planning/Interventions/Rationales

1. Request physical therapy consultation for appropriate assistive devices, strengthening exercises, and gait training on 2/11. *Collaboration with other health care providers provides the best care for the client.*

2. Escort client to muscle-strengthening class on 2/12 at 1600. *Provides safety and support as the client begins to learn new skills.*

3. Assigned caregiver will record each exercise, number of repetitions, and client response BID. *Documenting client progress toward the achievement of goals aids in outcome attainment and evaluation of care.*

## Evaluation

1. Goal not met. Appointment not kept on 2/11. Dental emergency. Continue. Reevaluate 2/15.

2. Goal not met. Unable to evaluate on 2/12. Continue. Reevaluate on 2/15.

3. 2/15: Goal met. Client attended muscle-strengthening class and has performed exercises as prescribed two times each day.

## Key Concepts

- Evaluation, the fifth step in the nursing process, involves determining whether the client goals have been met, have been partially met, or have not been met.

- The purposes of evaluation are to determine the client's progress or lack of progress toward achievement of client objectives, to judge the value of nursing actions in helping clients to achieve objectives, to determine the health care agency's overall ability to deliver care in an effective and efficient manner, and to promote nursing accountability.

- Evaluation is based primarily on the skills of communication and observation.

- Evaluation is a mutual, ongoing process occurring among the nurse, client, family, and other health care providers.

- The effectiveness of nursing interventions is evaluated by examination of goals and expected outcomes that provide direction for the plan of care and serve as standards by which the client's progress is measured.

- Evaluation is an orderly process consisting of seven steps: establishing standards, collecting data related to the goals and expected outcomes, determining goal achievement, relating nursing actions to client status, judging the value of nursing interventions in assisting clients to achieve goals and objectives, reassessing the client's status, and modifying the plan of care if necessary.

- There is a relationship between quality management and evaluation. Evaluation is necessary in the provision of quality care because it is the mechanism used by nurses in determining how to improve care.

- Structure evaluation judges a health care agency's ability to provide the services offered to its client population.

- Process evaluation measures nursing actions by examining each phase of the nursing process to determine the effectiveness of the actions in helping clients meet expected outcomes and goals.

- Outcome evaluation compares the client's current status with the expected outcomes and examines all direct care activities that affect the client's status.

- A nursing audit can focus on implementation of the nursing process, client outcomes, or both in order to evaluate the quality of care provided.
- Peer evaluation (peer review) is the process by which professionals provide to their peers performance appraisal feedback geared toward corrective action.
- Evaluation enhances professional nursing accountability by providing a mechanism for assisting the nurse to define, explain, and measure the results of nursing actions.
- Evaluating the quality of care is a shared responsibility among members of the health care team.

## Review Questions and Activities

1. When does evaluation of nursing care occur?
2. Describe the three types of evaluation, and compare them in terms of purpose and methodology.
3. How does evaluation promote the individual nurse's accountability?
4. State specific ways in which a nurse can perform process evaluation.
5. What are the advantages of peer evaluation?
6. Develop criteria for conducting a nursing audit related to client safety in an extended-care facility.

## Web Resources

American Nurses Association
http://www.nursingworld.org
Joint Commission on Accreditation of Healthcare Organizations
http://www.jcaho.org
National Committee for Quality Assurance
http://www.ncqa.org

## References

Alfaro-LeFevre, R. (2004). *Critical thinking in nursing: A practical approach* (3rd ed.). Philadelphia: Saunders.

American Nurses Association (1988). *Peer review guidelines*. Kansas City: Author.

American Nurses Association (1998). *Standards of clinical nursing practice* (2nd ed.). Washington, DC: Author.

Barnum, B. S., & Kerfoot, K. M. (1995). *The nurse as executive* (4th ed.). Gaithersburg, MD: Aspen.

Carpenito, L. J. (2002). *Nursing diagnosis: Application to clinical practice* (8th ed.). New York: Lippincott.

Cocchairella, L. (2000). *Guides to the evaluation of permanent impairment*. American Medical Association.

Cohen, B., Berube, R., & Turrentine, B. (1996). A peer review program for professional nurses. *Journal of Nursing Staff Development, 12*(1), 13–18.

Fitzpatrick, J. (2002). The nursing shortage revisited: Focus on patient outcomes. *Applied Nursing Research, 15*(3), 117.

Gillies, D. A. (1994). *Nursing management: A systems approach* (3rd ed.). Philadelphia: Saunders.

Grimes, M. (2001). *The Blue Last*. New York: Viking Press.

Grindel, C. G., Peterson, K., Kinneman, M., & Turner, T. L. (1996). The practice environment project: A process for outcome evaluation. *Journal of Nursing Administration, 26*(5), 43–51.

Hill, M. (1999). Outcomes measurement requires nursing to shift to outcome-based practice. *Nursing Administration Quarterly, 24*(1), 1–16.

Houston, S. (1999). Managing the outcome of infection: Nosocomial infection initiative. *Outcomes Management for Nursing Practice, 3*(2), 73–77.

Jennings, B. M. & Staggers, N. (1999). A provocative look at performance measurement. *Nursing Administration Quarterly, 24*(1), 17–30.

Joel, L. (1984). Self-regulation protects nursing's growing edge. *The American Nurse, 16*(2), 4, 22.

Johnson, M., & Maas, M. (Eds.). (1999). *Nursing outcomes classification (NOC): Iowa outcome project*. St. Louis: Mosby.

Kenney, J. W. (1995). Evaluation. In P. J. Christensen & J. W. Kenney (Eds.). *Nursing process: Application of conceptual models* (4th ed.). St. Louis: Mosby.

King, M., & Lipsky, M. (2000). Evaluation of nursing home patients: A systematic approach can improve care. *Postgraduate Medicine, 107*(2), 201–215.

McCloskey, J., & Bulechek, G. (1995). Validating and coding of the NIC taxonomy structures: Iowa intervention project. *Image: Journal of Nursing Scholarship, 27*(1), 43–49.

McInnes, E., Duff, H., Fennessey, G., Seers, K., & Clark, E. (2001). Implementing evidence based practice in clinical situations. *Nursing Standard, 15*(41), 40–44.

Murrary, R. B., & Zentner, J. P. (2000). *Nursing assessment and health promotion: Strategies through the life span* (7th ed.). New Jersey: Prentice Hall.

Pesut, D. J., & Herman, J. (1999). *Clinical reasoning: The art and science of critical and creative thinking*. Clifton Park, NY: Delmar Learning.

Potts, N., & Mandleco, B. (2002). *Pediatric nursing: Caring for children and their families*. Clifton Park, NY: Delmar Learning.

Stone, P., Bakken, S., & Curran, C. (2002). Evaluations of studies of health economics. *Evidence Based Nursing, 5*(4), 100–104.

Wakefield, D. S., Helms, C. M., & Helms, L. (1995). The peer review process: The art of judgment. *Journal of Healthcare Quality, 17*(3), 11–15.

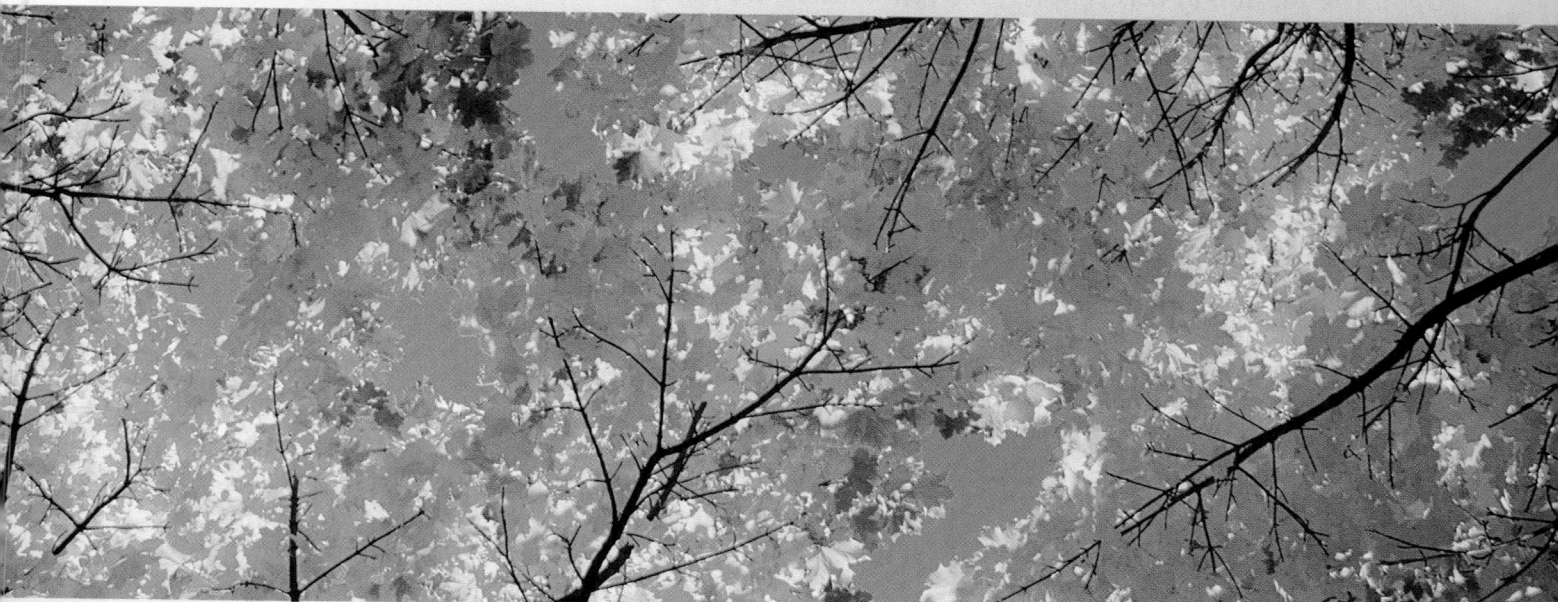

# CHAPTER 16

# Documentation and Reporting

Emily Wurster Hitchens, EdD, RN

*"Of all the patient's [client's] medical attendants the nurse is with him most constantly. For this reason the quality of her observations and reports, written and oral, are of the utmost importance."*

(Harmer & Henderson, 1955)

# Chapter Competencies

*Upon completion of this chapter, the reader should be able to:*

1. Explain the purposes of documentation in health care.
2. Discuss the principles of effective documentation.
3. Compare and contrast the various methods of documentation.
4. Identify various types of documentation records.
5. Evaluate the latest trends in documentation.
6. Describe the variety of reporting methods used in nursing.

# Key Terms

advance directive
case management
charting by exception (CBE)
communication
critical pathway
documentation
durable power of attorney
focus charting
incident report

informed consent
Kardex
narrative charting
nursing interventions
    classification (NIC)
nursing minimum data set
    (NMDS)
point-of-care charting

problem, intervention,
    evaluation (PIE) charting
problem-oriented medical
    record (POMR)
SOAP charting
source-oriented (S.O.) charting
variations
walking rounds

Throughout the development of modern nursing, a variety of documentation systems have emerged in response to changes inherent in health care delivery. Changes in consumer and legal expectations, federal and state regulations, accreditation standards, and research findings direct provider accountability for the documentation of services. Systems of recording and reporting data pertinent to the care of clients have evolved primarily in response to the demand for health care practitioners to be held accountable to societal norms, professional standards of practice, legal and regulatory standards, and institutional policies and standards.

As with all facets of health care, advanced technology has affected the expectations for documentation. Benchmarking activities in quality improvement and cost containment have also increased the demands on health care practitioners to create efficient documentation systems. Efficiency is measured in terms of time, thoroughness, and the quality of the observations being recorded. The documentation systems in use today reflect the specific needs and preferences of the numerous health care agencies. Selected systems and their ramifications are discussed in this chapter.

## Documentation as Communication

**Communication** is a dynamic, continuous, and multidimensional process for sharing information. Reporting and recording are the major communication techniques used by health care providers to direct client-based decision making and continuity of care. The medical record serves as a legal document for recording all client activities assessed and initiated by health care practitioners (Figure 16-1).

## Documentation Defined

**Documentation** is defined as written evidence of:

1. The interactions between and among health professionals, clients, their families, and health care organizations
2. The administration of tests, procedures, treatments, and client education
3. The results or client's response to these diagnostic tests and interventions

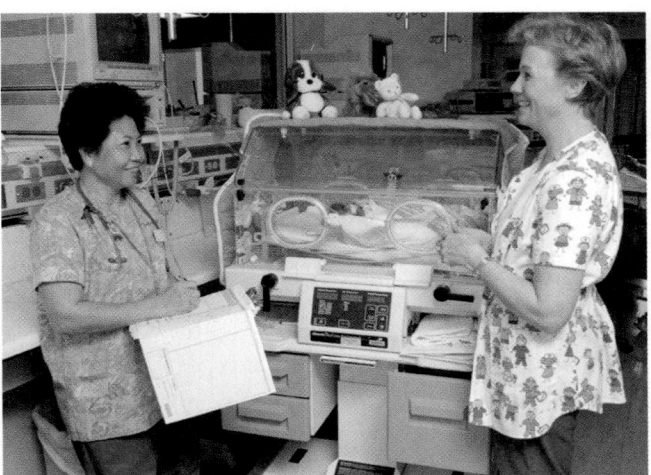

**Figure 16-1    Documentation is a responsibility of the entire interdisciplinary care team.**

Documentation provides written records that reflect client care provided on the basis of assessment data and the client's response to interventions.

Nurses rely on documentation tools that support the implementation of the nursing process. These tools are the charting records and systems that facilitate a logical sequencing of events. All the tools used by nurses to record their nursing care should form a system. Systematic documentation is critical because it presents the care administered by nurses in a logical fashion, as follows (Carelock & Innerarity, 2001):

1. Assessment data (obtained by interviewing, observing, and inspecting) identifies the client's specific alterations and provides the foundation of the nursing care plan.
2. The risk factors, the identified alteration in the functional health pattern, or both direct the formulation of a nursing diagnosis.
3. Identifying the nursing diagnosis promotes the development of the client's short-term goals, long-term goals, and expected outcomes, and also triggers the nursing interventions. These activities occur during the planning and implementation phases of the nursing process.
4. The plan of care identifies the actions necessary to resolve the nursing diagnosis.
5. Implementation is evidenced by actions the nurse performs to assist the client in achieving the expected outcomes.

The effectiveness of the nursing interventions in achieving the client's expected outcomes becomes the criterion for evaluation that determines the need for subsequent reassessment and revision of the plan of care.

The system becomes a vehicle for expressing each phase of the nursing process. Nurses rely on systems that provide thorough, accurate charting reflective of the nurse's decision-making ability and the client's plan of care. The nurse's

critical-thinking skills, judgments, and evaluation must be clearly communicated through proper documentation.

## Purposes of Health Care Documentation

Professional responsibility and accountability are two primary reasons practitioners document. Other reasons to document include communication, education, research, meeting legal and practice standards, and reimbursement. Documentation is the professional responsibility of all health care practitioners. It provides written evidence of the practitioner's accountability to the client, the institution, the profession, and society.

### Communication

Recording is a method of communication that validates the care provided to the client. It should clearly communicate all important information regarding the client (Calloway, 2001). Thorough documentation provides:

- Accurate data needed to plan the client's care in order to ensure the continuity of care
- A method of communication among the health care team members responsible for the client's care
- Written evidence of what was done for the client, the client's response, and any revisions made in the plan of care
- Compliance with professional practice standards (e.g., American Nurses Association)
- Compliance with accreditation criteria (e.g., the Joint Commission on Accreditation of Healthcare Organization [JCAHO])
- A resource for review, audit, reimbursement, education, and research
- A written legal record to protect the client, institution, and practitioner

The client's medical record contains documents for record keeping. The type of document that constitutes the medical record is determined by the health care institution. References will be made to the various types of medical record documents throughout this chapter; refer to Table 16-1 for an explanation of these documents.

### Education

The documentation contained within the client's medical record can be used for the purpose of education. Health care students use the medical record as a tool to learn about disease processes, complications, medical and nursing diagnoses, and interventions. The results of physical examination and laboratory and diagnostic testing provide valuable information regarding specific diagnoses and interventions (Estes, 2002).

Nursing students can enhance their critical-thinking skills by examining the records in chronological order, analyzing the results, and following the health care team's

## TABLE 16-1 MEDICAL RECORD DOCUMENTS

| Document | Information |
| --- | --- |
| Face sheet | Biographical data: name, date of birth, address, phone number, Social Security number, marital status, employment, race, gender, religion, closest relative; insurance coverage; allergies; attending physician; admitting medical diagnosis; assigned diagnosis-related group; statement of whether the client has an advance directive. |
| Consent form | *Admit:* Gives the institution and physician the right to treat. |
| | *Surgery:* Explains the reason for the operation in lay terms, the risks for complications, and the client's level of understanding. |
| | *Blood transfusion:* Permission to administer blood or blood products. |
| Medical history and physical examination | Results of the client's initial history and physical assessment as performed by the health care provider. |
| Prescriber order sheet | Medical orders to admit and the treatment plan. |
| Progress notes | Evaluation of the client's response to treatment; may contain the progress recording of interdisciplinary practitioners (e.g., dietary or social services). |
| Consultation sheet | Initiated by the physician to request the evaluation or services of other practitioners. |
| Diagnostic results | Contains the results from laboratory and diagnostic tests (e.g., X-ray, hematology). |
| Nursing admit assessment | Recording of data obtained from the interview and physical assessment conducted by the RN. |
| Nursing plan of care | Contains the treatment plan (e.g., nursing diagnosis or a problem list, initiation of standards of care, or protocols). |
| Graphic sheet | Data recording regarding vital signs and weight. |
| Flow sheet | Contains all routine interventions that can be noted with a check mark or other simple code; allows for a quick comparison of measurement. |
| Nurses' progress notes | Additional data that do not duplicate information on the flow sheet (e.g., client's achievement of expected outcome or revision of the plan of care). |
| Medication administration record (MAR) | Contains all medication information for routine and prn drugs: date, time, dose, route, site (for injections). |
| Patient education record | Recording of the nurses' teaching of the client, family, or other caregiver and the learner's response. |
| Health care team record | Treatment and progress record for nonmedical and nonnursing practitioners, when the physician's progress notes are not used by other practitioners (e.g., respiratory, physical therapy, dietary). |
| Clinical pathway | A multidisciplinary form for each day of anticipated hospitalization that identifies the interventions and achievement of client outcomes; the practitioner's initial implementation and variances from the norm are explained in the progress notes. |
| Discharge plan and summary | A multidisciplinary form used before discharge from a health care facility containing a brief summary of care rendered and discharge instructions (e.g., food-drug interactions, referrals or follow-up appointments). |
| Advance directive or living will | Federal law requires that health care providers discuss with clients the use of advance directives, commonly known as the living will or durable power of attorney. Most states recognize the living will as a legal document. If the client has advance directives, they are reviewed at the time of admission and placed in the medical record. |

## NURSING STRATEGY

### Communicating Clearly in Nurses' Notes

The following questions can assist the nurse in good documentation:

1. Are exact times and dates for client assessment and interventions noted?
2. Is the purpose for client assessment and intervention indicated?
3. Can you identify what the nurse saw, smelled, touched, or heard?
4. Is the client quoted directly? Is the client's response noted?
5. Are the plans and expected client outcomes congruent with the observations?

Adapted from Carelock, J., & Innerarity, S. (2001). Critical incidents: Effective communication and documentation. *Critical Care Nursing, 23*(4), 59–66.

## CLINICAL ALERT

### The Importance of Communication

Important information obtained from an assessment that warrants immediate intervention should not only be documented in the medical record but also communicated orally to the other practitioners. The element of time must direct decision making when critical information is obtained.

plan of care in terms of how the plan was developed, implemented, and evaluated. Students and all health care professionals need to be aware of confidentiality issues before reading any client's chart; these are discussed later in the chapter.

Clinical rounds and case conferences, which rely heavily on information contained in the medical record, have also proven to be effective teaching tools. These learning experiences usually involve several disciplines that contribute to the review and discussion of client outcomes.

Student nurses need to learn the "flow" of documenting clinical data according to institutional policy in a legible, descriptive, and time-sequenced fashion. A good way to learn the "flow" is to review the client's condition as presented in the chart before hearing the report. The data obtained from chart review should direct the assessment of signs and symptoms on rounds.

### Research

Researchers rely heavily on clients' medical records as a clinical data source to determine if clients meet the research criteria of a study. Documentation also can validate the need for research. For example, if documentation demonstrates an increased infection rate with intravenous catheters, researchers can identify and study the variables that may be associated with the increased infection rate.

### Legal and Practice Standards

Failure to document appropriately is a key factor in clinical mishaps and a pivotal issue in many malpractice cases, because the client's medical record is a legal document, and in the case of a lawsuit the record serves as the descrip-

tion of exactly what happened to a client. In 80% to 85% of malpractice lawsuits involving client care, the medical record is the determining factor in providing proof of significant events (Iyer & Camp, 1999). The legal issues of documentation require:

- Legible and neat writing
- Proper use of spelling and grammar
- Use of authorized abbreviations
- Factual and time-sequenced descriptive notations
- No omissions, blanks, or unused spaces

These elements of effective documentation are discussed later in this chapter.

Nurses are responsible for the care the client receives and can be held liable if appropriate interventions are not implemented in a timely manner when information is available that would dictate otherwise. The nurse is responsible for documenting on the chart when a "physician was notified" along with what significant information was orally communicated. If the nurse does not get a

## LEGAL AND ETHICAL ISSUES

### Completeness in Charting

Is "If it wasn't charted, it wasn't done" just a cliché? Since the purpose of the medical record is to document the care administered to the client, how can a practitioner convince a jury that care was administered if it is not documented in the medical record? Consider the following. A nurse, by habit, always administers an intramuscular injection in the ventrogluteal site (although both the ventrogluteal and dorsogluteal sites are within the accepted guidelines of care). The nurse, however, fails to chart the site on the medication administration record (MAR). The client files a suit for sciatic nerve damage. Knowing that there is an identified greater risk factor for sciatic nerve injury with the dorsogluteal site, do you think it would be difficult to defend care given in this case?

response from the physician that recognizes the urgency of the information, the nurse must document the physician's response and notify the supervisor of the situation. The better the communication between the caregivers and the client, the less likelihood of lawsuits or claims.

## Informed Consent

**Informed consent** means that the client understands the reason for and the risks of the proposed intervention and agrees to the treatment by signing a consent form. Legally, the client must be mentally competent, and the physician who is to perform the procedure is responsible for obtaining the client's informed consent (refer to Chapter 14).

In order to assist the physician with proper documentation of teaching, many facilities have preprinted informed consent documents that explain procedures in lay terms and identify the risk factors and possible complications. These documents are usually duplicate copies: the original goes in the medical record, and a copy is given to the client. This procedure provides the client with a written copy of the information that can be reviewed at a later time in a more relaxed environment.

Nurses are responsible for ensuring that the client understands the procedure or intervention and has signed the informed consent. The best way to assess a client's knowledge of an intervention is to ask him to explain, in his own words, what is going to be done and the common risks and possible complications. If the informed consent has not been signed or if the nurse assesses a lack of understanding on the client's part, the physician should be notified and the client should not be allowed to undergo the procedure. If the intervention is a surgical procedure, the nurse should notify the operating room at the time the physician is notified (Killion & Dempski, 2001).

Although most informed consents deal with medical interventions, nurses are sometimes responsible for implementing the interventions: for example, administering blood or blood products requires informed consent. It is also the responsibility of the nurse to obtain oral consent for certain nursing interventions, such as initiating intravenous therapy or inserting a nasogastric tube or urinary catheter. Consents require client education with an explanation of outcomes and documentation of the client's understanding of the procedure.

Once the client has been educated by the physician and nurse of the intervention, the informed consent needs to be signed by the client and witnessed. Witnessing the signing of the consent confirms that the person who signs the consent is in fact the client and *is competent, alert, and aware of all actions at that point in time.*

## Advance Directives

An **advance directive** is a statement made by clients that defines care they deem acceptable if they become incapacitated. It effectively allows clients, while competent, to participate in end-of-life decisions and to choose the types of life-sustaining procedures they will permit if they become unable to make their own decisions at a later time. A **durable power of attorney** allows the client to appoint a person to make health-related decisions when the client is incapable of making them. The Patient Self-Determination Act of 1990 requires health care facilities (hospitals, skilled-nursing facilities, and home health agencies) to inform adult clients of their rights regarding advance directives and to document in the medical record whether the client has such a directive (Lieberson, 2002).

## American Nurses Association (ANA) Standards of Care

Standards of documentation are established by professional organizations. ANA's *Standards of Clinical Nursing Practice* serve as a guideline for determining safe, quality nursing care and practice. The nursing process gives structure to the standards of care, with specific measurement criteria for each phase in the process. For each of the six standards (assessment, diagnosis, outcome identification, planning, implementation, and evaluation) there is a measurement criterion that states "are documented." ANA standards make explicit the role of data collection and documentation in nursing practice and specify that data collection be systematic and continuous and that data are accessible, communicated, and recorded (American Nurses Association [ANA], 2001).

## State Nurse Practice Acts

In an attempt to recognize and control the practice of nursing, nurse practice acts, on a state-by-state basis, have established guidelines to ensure safe practice and to demonstrate accountability to society. The standards of care, as set forth in the practice acts, are based on the phases of the nursing process and require evidence of compliance by documentation. Nurses should be familiar with the practice acts and rules of the state in which they work (Alternative Link Systems, Inc., 2001).

## Joint Commission on Accreditation of Healthcare Organizations (JCAHO)

The JCAHO surveys health care facilities to measure compliance with its standards for safe health care provision.

---

### CLINICAL ALERT

#### Consent from Sedated Clients

Sedated clients should never be requested or allowed to sign an informed consent. The client may not be capable of understanding the nature of and risks associated with the procedure, so the consent will be invalid, and the nurse and institution will be at legal risk. Wait instead for the client to be competent and free of sedation, or have a legally acceptable family member brought into the decision.

Although facilities voluntarily submit to this accreditation process, reimbursement eligibility for Medicare, Medicaid, and private funding is dependent upon JCAHO accreditation.

The JCAHO no longer requires that health care organizations have traditional nursing care plans, but documentation of an individualized plan of care must be evident for each client. JCAHO's standards require:

- The involvement of the client or family in the development of the plan, which must be documented in the medical record
- Interdisciplinary planning and implementation of all aspects of care

The use of interdisciplinary tools has proven to be an effective approach to documenting client and family education for agencies not yet using critical pathways (discussed later in the chapter) or care mapping. Compliance with JCAHO's client and family teaching standards through the use of an interdisciplinary record improved education documentation from 30% to 84% in one medical center studied (Tucker, 1995).

During the accreditation survey, the reviewer looks for evidence of an organized and systematic method of monitoring and evaluating client care that is reflected through documentation in the medical record. Documenting the steps of the nursing process ensures compliance with JCAHO's plan of care requirements.

## Reimbursement

Peer review organizations (PROs), consisting of physicians and nurses, are required by the federal government to monitor and evaluate the quality and appropriateness of care given. Medical record documentation is the mechanism for the PRO review, which evaluates the intensity of services and the severity of illness on the basis of a comparison of sample medical records from different facilities against specific screening criteria.

The federal enactment of the diagnosis-related group (DRG) classification system changed the health care provider reimbursement process from a cost-per-case formula to a prospective payment system (PPS). With PPS, the medical record must provide documentation that supports the DRG and the appropriateness of care. Nursing documentation must also show evidence of client and family education and discharge planning.

From a hospital's perspective, when information in the medical record demonstrates compliance with Medicare and Medicaid standards, the reimbursement is maximized. If nurses fail to document the equipment or procedures used daily (e.g., feeding pump; daily weight, intake and output; intravenous therapy; drug additives), reimbursement to the facility can be denied.

Another federal law, the Consolidated Omnibus Budget Reconciliation Act of 1986 (COBRA) allows employees to temporarily carry their employer-provided health insurance benefits for a period of time varying with

## STOP AND THINK

### Meeting COBRA Laws

Why would an emergency room want to transfer a COBRA client who has insurance? Do you think these clients are considered high risk? Suppose a pregnant client in the seventh month of gestation comes to the emergency room in labor. The client is assessed by the physician and nurse. Labor is in progress, but delivery is not imminent, and the client's blood pressure is 210/124. Treatment is initiated; however, the blood pressure remains high (190/110). Can this client be transferred? If not, why not? Why would this health care provider want to stabilize and transfer the client before delivery?

the qualifying event of termination, reduction in work hours, or retirement. The law requires that for any COBRA client receiving care in an emergency room, the client's condition must be stabilized before the client can be transferred to another facility. If the client's condition is not stable, then the institution cannot initiate a transfer.

Facilities in violation of COBRA laws are fined and stand to lose their eligibility for Medicare and Medicaid funding. Compliance with this law is evaluated through medical record review. The documentation concerning client transfers must include:

- Chronology of the event
- Measures taken or treatment implemented
- Client's response to treatment
- Results of measures taken to prevent the client's condition from deteriorating

## COMMUNITY/HOME CARE

### Documentation in Home Health Care

Home health agencies also keep documents: physician orders, history and physical forms, home care team records, and nursing records (initial assessment form, plan of care, problem list for daily progress notes, client teaching activities, and discharge summary). Home health care providers are required to comply with state and federal regulations that affect health care, documentation, and reimbursement.

# Principles of Effective Documentation

Documentation requirements will differ depending on the health care facility (hospital, nursing home, home health agency) and the setting within the facility (e.g., emergency room, perioperative, medical-surgical unit) and with specific client populations (e.g., obstetrics, pediatrics, geriatrics). Regardless of what client care is administered, the documentation of that care must reflect the nursing process. General documentation guidelines are listed in Table 16-2.

Nursing notes must be logical, focused, and relevant to care, and must represent each phase in the nursing process (Iyer & Camp, 1999). Nursing documentation based on the nursing process facilitates effective care because client needs can be traced from assessment, through the identification of the problems, to the care plan, implementation, and evaluation. A brief reminder of the elements of the nursing process follows:

- *Assessment:* Summarize, without duplication, assessment data that are related to an actual or potential health care need. With reassessment, highlight any new findings or any changes in the client's condition (e.g., increased pain). Table 16-3 outlines some assessment-specific documentation guidelines.
- *Diagnosis:* Identify the client's problem or need using NANDA terminology.
- *Outcome identification and planning:* Discuss with the client and communicate to members of the multidisciplinary team the expected outcomes or goals of client care.
- *Implementation:* After the intervention has been performed, document on the flow sheet and progress notes observations, treatments, teaching, and related clinical judgments. Client teaching should include learning needs, teaching plan content, methods of teaching, who was taught, and the client's response.
- *Evaluation:* Evaluate and document the effectiveness of the interventions in terms of the expected outcomes: progress toward goals; client response to tests, treatments, and nursing interventions; client and family response to teaching and significant events; questions, statements, or complaints voiced by the client or family.
- *Revisions of planned care:* Document the reasons for the revisions with the supporting evidence and client and family agreement.

Charting in accordance with the nursing process ensures thorough documentation in compliance with ANA's standards of care, practice acts, and reimbursement and accreditation criteria.

## Elements of Effective Documentation

Effective documentation requires:

- Use of a common vocabulary
- Legibility and neatness

## TABLE 16-2    GENERAL DOCUMENTATION GUIDELINES

- Ensure that you have the correct client record or chart and that the client's name and identifying information are on every page of the record.
- Document as soon as the client encounter is concluded to ensure accurate recall of data (follow institutional guidelines on frequency of charting).
- Date and time each entry.
- Sign each entry with your full legal name and with your professional credentials, or per your institutional policy.
- Do not leave space between entries.
- If an error is made while documenting, use a single line to cross out the error, then date, time, and sign the correction (check institutional policy); avoid erasing, crossing out, or using correction fluid.
- Never change another person's entry, even if it is incorrect.
- Use quotation marks to indicate direct client responses (e.g., "I feel lousy").
- Document in chronological order (if chronological order is not used, state why).
- Write legibly.
- Use a permanent-ink pen (black is usually preferable because of its ability to photocopy well).
- Document in a complete but concise manner by using phrases and abbreviations as appropriate and as approved by the institution.
- Document all telephone calls you make or receive that are related to a client's case.

Adapted from Estes, M. E. Z. (2002). *Health assessment & physical examination* (2nd ed.). Clifton Park, NY: Delmar Learning.

- Use of only authorized abbreviations and symbols
- Factual and time-sequenced organization
- Accurate inclusion of any errors that occurred

The following discussion of effective charting refers to all nursing documents, such as flow sheet, progress notes, and so on. Add to the nursing documents when:

## TABLE 16-3   ASSESSMENT-SPECIFIC DOCUMENTATION GUIDELINES

- Record all data that contribute directly to the assessment (e.g., positive assessment findings and pertinent negatives).

- Document any parts of the assessment that are omitted or refused by the client.

- Avoid using judgmental language such as "good," "poor," "bad," "normal," "abnormal," "decreased," "appears to be," and "seems."

- Avoid evaluative statements (e.g., "client is uncooperative," "client is lazy"); cite instead specific statements or actions that you observe (e.g., "client said 'I hate this place' and kicked trash can").

- State time intervals precisely (e.g., "every 4 hours," "bid," instead of "seldom," "occasionally").

- Do not make relative statements about findings (e.g., "mass the size of an egg"); use specific measurements (e.g., "mass 3 cm × 5 cm").

- Draw pictures when appropriate (e.g., location of scar, masses, skin lesion, decubitus, deep tendon reflex, etc.).

- Refer to findings using anatomical landmarks (e.g., left upper quadrant [of abdomen], left lower lobe [of lung], midclavicular line, etc.).

- Use the face of the clock to describe findings that are in a circular pattern (e.g., breast, tympanic membrane, rectum, vagina).

- Document any change in the client's condition during a visit or from previous visits.

- Describe what you observed, not what you did.

Adapted from Estes, M. E. Z. (2002). *Health assessment & physical examination* (2nd ed.). Clifton Park, NY: Delmar Learning.

## NURSING STRATEGY

### Using Common Vocabulary in Documentation

- Create reference list with examples of vocabulary, which is to be kept with other texts (e.g., laboratory books, medication texts).

- Place NANDA list of nursing diagnoses and texts with nursing care plans where nurses can access them easily.

- Include medical dictionary (e.g., Taber's) in reference texts.

- Schedule continuing education programs with quality improvement personnel reviewing documentation wording seen in chart audits.

Adapted from Estes, M. E. Z. (2002). *Health assessment & physical examination* (2nd ed.). Clifton Park, NY: Delmar Learning.

One reason these inadequacies exist is that the documented clinical data cannot be correlated without a common vocabulary for addressing client outcomes for specific nursing interventions. Nursing practice reflects the use of multiple terms for nursing interventions, preventing cross-institutional comparisons of nursing care. The current efforts under way to establish a taxonomy for nursing interventions determined by specific nursing diagnoses will enhance the quality of documentation and support the efforts of researchers. Use of common vocabulary will also improve intrateam communication and lessen the chance of misunderstandings.

### Legibility

Whatever is charted must be easily readable, without any chance of error. If your handwriting is not readable, print. If you make a mistake, do not erase or obliterate it; draw one line through the erroneous entry and state the reason for the error, then sign and date the correction, as shown in Figure 16-2.

### Abbreviations and Symbols

Facilities usually have a list of acceptable abbreviations and symbols, approved by the Medical Records Committee, to be used when documenting information in the client's record. Always refer to the facility's approved listing. Avoid abbreviations that can be misunderstood.

### Organization

Start every entry with the date and time. Chart in a chronological order, assessment data, observation, intervention, and evaluation (Figure 16-3). Comply with the time frame indicated in the facility's guidelines for documentation: for

- A change occurs in the client's condition
- Measuring the client's response to an intervention or expected outcome
- The client or family voices a complaint

### Use of Common Vocabulary

During the last decade, nurse researchers have observed inadequacies in the clinical record that prevent data collection and comparison among large groups of clients.

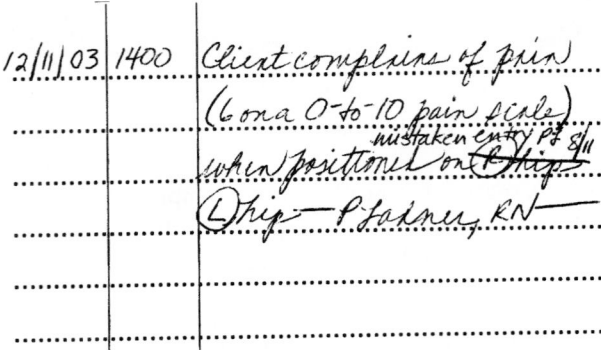

**Figure 16-2    Correcting a documentation error**

example, the frequency of charting observations for a client with restraints or the time frame within which the admit assessment must be completed.

Chart in a timely fashion to avoid the omission of pertinent data; it is not a good practice to wait until the end of the shift to chart on all the clients. Chart medications immediately after administration to avoid errors. Sign your name after each entry.

When the nurse forgets to document significant data, it is appropriate and advisable to include these data at a later date. There are several reasons a late entry might have to be made:

- The chart was not available (e.g., the chart was with the client in special procedures lab).
- Entries had to be added after notes were completed.
- Information was documented on the wrong record.

As with other aspects of documentation, follow the facility's policy for charting a late entry. Common practice is to enter the date and time and label "Late entry" to indicate that it is out of sequence. Then record the date and time it should have been charted in the body of the entry as shown in Figure 16-4.

## LEGAL AND ETHICAL ISSUES

### Use of Abbreviations

When using abbreviations, be certain that the meaning is not open to interpretation. For example, the abbreviation *PT* could be interpreted as *patient, part-time, physical therapy,* or *prothrombin time.* Legally, documenting with abbreviations requires the nurse to ascertain what the facility defines the abbreviation to mean. Incorrect use could change the meaning of a written statement and consequently make the documentation incorrect and therefore open to malpractice.

Adapted from Killion, S. W., & Dempski, K. M. (2001). *Quick look nursing: Legal and ethical Issues.* Clifton Park, NY: Delmar Learning.

## Nurses Progress Record

| Date | Hour | Progress Notes |
|---|---|---|
| 12/11/03 | 1730 | Client complains of a burning pain (5 on a 0-to-10 pain scale) in URQ, leaning forward; burning pain R/T gastric secretion reflux; admin. Mylanta 30 cc po PRN as ordered; head of bed elevated 45° — P Fodner, RN |
| 12/11/03 | 1815 | client states burning pain ↓ 2, P Fodner, RN |

**Figure 16-3    Charting a prn medication**

### Accuracy

Accuracy and objective data are crucial if the documentation is to be useful either clinically or for research. Use factual, descriptive terms to chart exactly what was observed or done—for example:

| INCORRECT | CORRECT |
|---|---|
| "Wound appears the same." | "Wound is 2.5 cm by 1.0 cm." |
| "Large amount of drainage." | "Foul-smelling, yellowish drainage completely saturated two 4 × 4s." |

Use correct spelling and grammar, and write complete sentences.

Differentiate who does what—for example, "Dr. Smith inserted a triple-lumen, 20-gauge catheter into the right subclavian vein." Read the notes recorded by nurses on previous shifts, and make further comments on their findings to maintain the continuity of care.

### Documenting a Medication Error

Facilities require nurses to report medication errors on incident reports (discussed later in this chapter). This

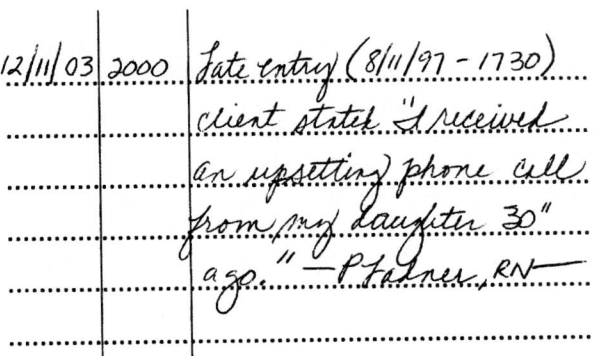

**Figure 16-4    Charting a late entry**

information should also appear on the medication administration record (MAR) with a notation in the nurses' progress notes. Remember, the purpose of the medical record is to report any care or treatment the client receives.

When a medication error occurs, the following should be charted:

1. Chart the medication on the MAR to prevent other caregivers from giving the client additional doses of the drug, similar drugs, or drugs that may be contraindicated.
2. Document the error in the nurses' notes as follows: name and dosage of the medication, time it was given, client's response to the medication, name of the practitioner who was notified of the error, time of the notification, nursing interventions or medical treatment to counteract the error, and client's response to treatment.

### Confidentiality

Nurses are bound by ethical codes and laws to treat all client information in a confidential and professional manner; this includes the client's record. The written documentation contained in the client's chart is a legal record

of care, and it should be available only to members of that client's health care team. The client's significant others, insurance companies, or other parties not directly involved in the care provided by the health care team may not have access to clients' records; it is the nurse's responsibility to protect the privacy and confidentiality of client interactions, assessments, and care. Even clients themselves must submit a written request to have their information released, and then they must specify exactly what information is to be released and to whom. In many institutions, particularly teaching hospitals, client records may be used for educational or research purposes. Members of these educational and research teams are held to the same standards of privacy protection and may not legitimately use client information for any purposes other than education or research or in any manner that would identify specific clients in any way (Killion & Dempski, 2001).

## Methods of Documentation

Documentation must reflect the complexity of care, and it must embody accuracy, completeness, and evidence of professional practice with efficient and cost-effective systems. The clinical standards (structure, outcome, process, and evaluation) are used to develop a system that complies with legal, accreditation, and professional practice requirements of documentation.

There are many methods used for documentation, including:

- Narrative charting
- Source-oriented charting
- Problem-oriented charting
- PIE charting
- Focus charting
- Charting by exception (CBE)
- Computerized documentation
- Case management with critical paths

### Narrative Charting

**Narrative charting**, the traditional method of nursing documentation, is a story format that describes the client's status, interventions, treatments, and response to treatments. Before the advent of flow sheets, this was the only method for documenting care. About 30% of nurses' time, during an 8-hour shift, was spent on narrative charting (Miller & Pastorino, 1990).

Narrative documentation is easy to use in emergency situations, in which a simple, chronological order is needed. However, in this type of documentation it is often difficult to avoid being subjective, and there is normally a lack of analysis and critical decision making on the part of the nurse. Narrative charting is now being replaced by other formats because:

- The flow of care is disorganized. It is difficult to show a relationship between data and critical-thinking skills.

---

### CLINICAL ALERT

#### Tips for Avoiding Medication Errors

The nurse must refrain from documenting medications before they are given. The nurse may be tempted to chart the medications in the MAR when the medications are obtained, and then go give the medications. This activity may lend itself to documenting medications that are not given, for whatever reason. In addition, the nurse must remember to double-check those medications that have severe consequences when misadministered (e.g., heparin, insulin).

Adapted from Reiss, B., Evans, M., & Broyles, B. (2002). *Pharmacological aspects of nursing care* (6th ed.). Clifton Park, NY: Delmar Learning.

- Each nurse writes with a unique style, making continuity of care difficult to identify.
- It fails to reflect the nursing process. The focus is on tasks without emphasis on assessment data or progress toward achievement of outcomes.
- It is time-consuming. The paragraphs are free-flowing, so it takes more time to record accurate data and for others to read it.
- The information is difficult to retrieve. The same problems may not be addressed from shift to shift, so it is difficult to track the client's progress. Auditors often disallow charges for equipment and supplies because consistent usage cannot be identified.

## Source-Oriented Charting

**Source-oriented (S.O.) charting** is described as a narrative recording by each member (source) of the health care team on separate records. Because each discipline has a separate record, care is often fragmented and communication between disciplines becomes time-consuming. S.O. charting has similar advantages and disadvantages to narrative charting since nurses use an unstructured approach when documenting in the progress notes.

## Problem-Oriented Charting

**Problem-oriented medical record (POMR)** was introduced in 1969 by Lawrence Weed, a physician at Case Western Reserve University. The focus of POMR documentation is on the client's problem, with a structured, logical format to narrative charting called **SOAP**:

- *S*: subjective data (what the client or family states)
- *O*: objective data (what is observed/inspected)
- *A*: assessment (conclusion reached on the basis of data formulated as client problems or nursing diagnoses)
- *P*: plan (actions to be taken to relieve client's problem)

SOAPIE and SOAPIER refer to formats that add:

- *I*: intervention (measures to achieve an expected outcome)
- *E*: evaluation (effectiveness of interventions)
- *R*: revision (changes from the original plan of care)

Figure 16-5 shows a sample of SOAPIE charting.

The POMR system was modified by nonmedical caregivers and is referred to as problem-oriented record (POR). The system is used by hospitals, nursing homes, and home care agencies (Souther, 2001).

There are four critical components of POMR/POR:

- Database: Assessment data, representative of all disciplines (history, physical, nursing admit assessment, laboratory findings, educational and discharge needs), which become the basis for a problem list evaluation of the client's condition.
- Problem list: Derived from the database; a listing of the client's problems as identified, with each problem

numbered and labeled as acute, chronic, active, or inactive. Nurses use NANDA terminology in writing client problems as nursing diagnoses; the list is revised as new problems arise and others are resolved.
- Initial plan: Based on problem identification; the starting point for care plan development with client participation in setting goals, expected outcomes, and learning needs.
- Progress notes: Charting based on the SOAP, SOAPIE, or SOAPIER format.

The POR system uses flow sheets to record routine care and a discharge summary that addresses each problem on the list and notes whether it was resolved. SOAP entries are usually made every 24 hours on any unresolved problem or whenever the client's condition changes.

## PIE Charting

After SOAP charting gained in popularity, the **problem, intervention, evaluation (PIE)** charting system was instituted at Craven Regional Medical Center in 1984 to streamline documentation. Whereas SOAP was developed on a medical model, PIE charting has a nursing origin. PIE is an acronym for *problem, intervention, and evaluation* of nursing care. The key components of this system are assessment flow sheets and nurses' progress notes with an integrated plan of care that eliminates the need for a separate care plan. Each client problem is labeled and numbered for easy reference. When interventions are implemented to manage the client's problem, the problem number is identified, as shown in Figure 16-6. This system eliminates the traditional care plan by incorporating an ongoing plan of care into the daily documentation.

## Focus Charting

**Focus charting** is a method of identifying and organizing the narrative documentation of client concerns to include data, action, and response. This method is not limited to client "problems" but allows for the identification of all "concerns" such as a significant event (e.g., results of a diagnostic test). Focus charting was created in 1981 at Eitel Hospital in Minneapolis, when the results from a SOAP audit revealed weaknesses in writing care plans (18% compliance) and charting the client's response to care (12% compliance) (Iyer & Camp, 1999). Focus charting uses a columnar format within the progress notes to distinguish the entry from other recordings in the narrative notes.

## Charting by Exception

**Charting by exception (CBE)** is a charting method that requires the nurse to document only deviations from preestablished norms per agency guidelines. When charting by exception is used, a thorough baseline assessment must be documented so that exceptions are discernible. Exceptions should have detailed descriptions; deficits

| Nurses Progress Record | | |
|---|---|---|
| Date | Hour | Progress Notes |

**12/11/03** — **0730**

Problem #2 Ketoacidosis

**S:** Client states "I feel sick all over." Client claims difficulty in breathing, abdominal pain + nausea.

**O:** Lungs clear, R 28/min, labored. Abdomen distended, bowel sounds underactive all 4 quadrants. 5+ abdominal pain.

**A:** Alteration in nutrition + comfort r/t ketoacidosis. Blood glucose 458 mg/dl. Ketones strongly positive. pH < 7.3.

**P:** Maintain IV infusion of 0.9% NS c̄ regular insulin as ordered. NPO. Oral hygiene hrly. Maintain accurate I + O. Assess for rales, hypotension, cardiac dysrhythmias. Monitor blood glucose + electrolytes. — P Fadner RN

should be noted as well. Otherwise, the client's medical record does will appear to not accurately reflect the client's current status and thus other clinicians will not be alerted to potential problems or complications (Helm, 2002). CBE was instituted in 1983 by St. Luke Medical Center in Milwaukee to overcome the recurring problem of lengthy, repetitive notes and to enable the identification of trends in client status. The CBE system has three key components:

1. Flow sheets: Highlight significant findings and define assessment parameters and findings.
2. Reference documentation: Is related to the standards of nursing practice. (All standards are met unless otherwise documented.)
3. Bedside accessibility: Is related to the documentation forms. CBE requires the nurse to document significant findings or exceptions to predefined norms.

**12/11/03** — **0730**

**I:** Called Dr Smith, blood glucose 458 mg/dl IV bolus regular insulin given as ordered. 1000 ml 0.9% N.S. infusing c̄ 17/H central line #1 via infusion pump. 50u regular insulin in 500 ml NS infusing c̄ 50 ml/H, central line #2 via infusion pump. EKG taken, placed on telemetry.

**12/11/03** — **0835**

**E:** Lungs clear, R 24/min, non-labored. NSR. 3+ abdominal pain. Urinary output 750 ml/hr. Blood glucose 360 mg/dl. — P Fadner RN

**Figure 16-5    Sample SOAPIE charting**

## Nurses Progress Record

| Date | Hour | Progress Notes |
|---|---|---|
| 12/11/03 | 0730 | P#4: nutrition R/T ketoacidosis. Blood glucose 458 mg/dl ketones strongly positive, pH 7.2. I#4: called Dr Smith, blood glucose 458 mg/dl IV bolus regular insulin given as ordered. 1000ml 0.9% NS infusing C 17/H central line #1 via infusion pump. 50 u regular insulin in 500 ml N.S. infusing C 50ml/H, central line #2 via infusion pump. EKG taken, placed on telemetry. |
| 12/11/03 | 0835 | E#4: Lungs clear, R/Thin non-labored. NSR. 3+ abdominal pain. Urinary output 750 ml. H (0730-0830) Blood sugar 360 mg/dl. — P. Jadner, RN — |

Figure 16-6    Sample PIE charting—the client problem is "Imbalanced Nutrition R/T Ketoacidosis";
once the problem is stated, the problem is referred
to by its number only (#4) in subsequent entries.

## Computerized Documentation

The contemporary health care system has directed nurse leaders to develop computerized records in response to the large demand for clinical, administrative, and regulatory information.

Nursing information systems (NIS) are being developed that will complement existing hospital information systems (HIS) (Larrabee et al., 2001). The NIS will collect, store, process, retrieve, display, and communicate timely information that supports:

- Administration of nursing services and resources
- Management of standardized client care information
- Linkage of research resources and educational applications to nursing practice

Health care facilities work in collaboration with producers of computer software to design medical record documents that complement existing documentation systems.

Computerized documentation has several advantages (Stangl, 2002). It enhances the systematic approach to client care through standardized protocols, teaching documents, data management, and communication. Computers are cost-effective and increase the quality of documentation. The practical advantages to staff nurses are:

- Saves documentation time: Data entry needs to be done only once; the system avoids duplication of effort. For example, a physician's medication order goes immediately to the pharmacy, eliminating the need to transcribe and transmit orders; the pharmacy receives the order (at preestablished computer-acceptable doses and routes), and the client's MAR is immediately updated. This system increases job satisfaction and saves more than 30% of nurses' time spent on charting.
- Increases legibility and accuracy: A computer printout is easy to read. Accuracy is achieved through standardized documents that prompt the nurse for information, making the charting more complete, thorough, concise, and organized. For example, the fall-prevention standard is automatically initiated for all high-risk clients. Bedside terminals allow for client care data to be entered in a timely fashion.
- Provides clear, decisive, and concise keywords: Standardized nursing terminology provides for usage of consistent keywords (e.g., *alert*) and avoids ambiguous phraseology (e.g., "appears to be"). Nurses can select nursing choices on a screen that automatically builds a comprehensive record of an event.
- Facilitates statistical analysis of data.
- Enhances implementation of the nursing process: Uses documentation tools that provide an individualized plan of care: admission and nursing history data, diagnosis, goals, measurable outcomes, and interventions, inclusive of client teaching. Improved documentation of interventions has improved the PRO reimbursement.
- Enhances critical thinking and decision making: Provides access to other data, such as laboratory results,

that can be correlated with the nurses' assessment data. If a trend is developing (e.g., decreasing levels of oxygenation), the nurse will recognize it quickly.

- Supports multidisciplinary networking: Information is quickly coordinated and integrated by other departments; all departments have access to the data.

Many of the disadvantages of computerized documentation are inherent in the computer and software itself: cost of installation, which limits the number of terminals at nursing stations; slow processing speed at peak usage times; and downtime (time for routine servicing or sudden unexpected failure). Practitioners are also often reluctant to change from the comfortable "pen-and-paper" methods to a high-tech electronic system.

A series of legal issues has developed from computerized documentation: problems in protecting client confidentiality, sharing of access codes (passwords), and determining who should have access to the clinical database and how it should be used. Computerized software can be designed to record all transactions, thus permitting the identification of all staff members who request sensitive information. In addition to the legal issues of computerized documentation, there are potential ethical ramifications.

### Point-of-Care System

**Point-of-care charting** allows health care providers to gain immediate access to client information. The system allows for inputting and retrieving client data at the bedside through a handheld portable computer. At the beginning of the shift, the nurse receives a client assignment and report with all client data downloaded from the main computer into the handheld portable computer. The nurse enters data (e.g., assessment, interventions, client's response, and evaluation) into the computer at the bedside. The information is enhanced at the bedside by interfacing the new data with other data to clarify options. At the end of the shift, or when the client's condition changes, the data from the handheld computer are downloaded back into the main computer.

The advantages of point-of-care charting are based on the efficiency of the computer system. Since health care providers can record client data at the point of care, it:

- Controls operating costs
- Complements existing information systems
- Eliminates redundant data entry
- Allows the provider more one-on-one time for client care
- Provides crucial client information to all health care providers in a timely fashion

Point-of-care computerized documentation also facilitates the transition to a managed-care system (an integrated health care team) by focusing on the continuum of care. The focus is to provide each health care practitioner with all pertinent client data to ensure continuity of care without duplication. Because the client's status can be reviewed at the bedside, practitioners have more time for interactions with their clients.

Based on focus and outcome, the point-of-care documentation system should promote quality of care, decrease the length of stay, and foster compliance with accreditation and regulatory standards.

## Case Management Process

**Case management** is defined as a methodology for organizing client care through an episode of illness so that specific clinical and financial outcomes are achieved within an allotted time frame. The outcome of this process is a DRG-specific case management plan that contains daily notes on assessment documentation, care plan, outcome-oriented multidisciplinary interventions, teaching, and discharge planning (Sheehan, 2002).

At admission, the nurse case manager and the admitting practitioner individualize the case management plan (called a critical pathway) to meet the client's specific needs. A **critical pathway** (or critical path) is an abbreviated summary of key indicators from the case management plan. The pathway is used by all health care providers as a monitoring and documentation tool to ensure that interventions are performed on time and that client outcomes are achieved on time. Health care providers must remember that critical pathways serve as care guidelines; when the actual status of the client changes, the provider may make other clinical judgment decisions. A critical pathway is not a substitute for critical thinking (Sheehan, 2002).

**Variations**, sometimes referred to as a variance, are goals not met or interventions not performed within the

---

 **LEGAL AND ETHICAL ISSUES**

### Computerized Documentation Methods

Computerized documentation methods create a wide variety of potential ethical problems. For example, the nurse may "feel" that documenting via this method violates the privacy of the client because information is put into a system that may be "hacked" (broken into). Another ethical situation created by computerized documentation is the temptation of one health care worker to use another health care worker's password in the interest of saving time. The problem this can create—in addition to risk of termination of employment for the perpetrator—is creating an inaccurate "paper trail" for the true writer of the documented material.

Chamrorro, T. (2001). Computer-based patient records. *Seminars in Oncology Nursing, 17*(1), 24–33.

time frame. The nurse documents on the back of the critical pathway the unexpected event (e.g., hospital-acquired decubiti), actions taken in response to the event, and appropriate discharge planning.

The advantages of case management are that it makes efficient use of time and increases the quality of care, with the expected outcomes identified on the plan. It also promotes collaboration, communication, and teamwork, which work to the advantage of the client and the facility, with discharge occurring in a timely manner. Case management also has several limitations; mainly, it is useful for clients with only one or two diagnoses. When clients have more than two diagnoses or variations, documentation becomes complicated because of limited space. This situation requires additional documentation forms to complement the pathway, such as intervention flow sheets and nurses' notes.

## Forms for Recording Data

Several types of forms are used in record keeping: Kardex, flow sheets, nurses' progress notes, and discharge summaries. All of these forms are designed to facilitate record keeping, reduce duplicate activity, and ensure quick and easy access to information.

### Kardex

A **Kardex** (client profile and client summary sheets) is a summary worksheet reference of basic client care information that traditionally is not part of the medical record. The Kardex, a concise client data source, is used as a reference throughout the shift and during change-of-shift reports. Kardexes come in various sizes, shapes, and types (and they may also be computer-generated). The Kardex is designed to complement the care delivery setting. For example, a home health Kardex would contain information related to family contacts, practitioners (physician), other services, and emergency referrals. The Kardex usually contains the following information:

- Client data: Name, age, marital status, religious preference
- Medical diagnoses: Listed by priority
- Nursing diagnoses: Listed by priority
- Medical orders: Diet, medications, IV therapy, treatments, diagnostic tests and procedures (inclusive of dates and results), and consultations
- Activities permitted: Functional limitations, assistance needed in activities of daily living, and safety precautions

### Flow Sheets

Flow sheets have vertical or horizontal columns for recording dates and times to show assessment and interventions, making it easy to track changes in the client's condition. Client teaching, use of special equipment, and IV therapy

are other aspects of the flow sheet. Because the flow sheets have small spaces for recording, these forms usually contain legends that identify the approved abbreviations for charting data. It is important to fill out flow sheets completely because blank spaces imply that an intervention was not completed, attempted, or recognized.

The information on the flow sheet can be formatted to meet the specific needs of client populations (special needs, activity, and measurement and intervention). For example, recording assessment data may be different in pediatric clinics and pediatric hospital units than in facilities for adults. Flow sheets in critical care settings are more comprehensive than are those on a medical-surgical unit (Carelock & Innerarity, 2001) (Figure 16-7). Flow sheets can also complement other types of records of specific interventions (e.g., MAR, IV therapy).

Flow sheets are used as supplements to most documentation systems because they decrease the redundancy of charting in the nurses' progress notes. But they do not replace the progress notes. Nurses still need to document observations, client responses and teaching, detailed interventions, and other significant data in the progress notes.

## Nurses' Progress Notes

The nurses' progress notes are used to document the client's condition, problems, and complaints; interventions; response to interventions; and achievement of outcomes. Progress notes include the following forms: nurses' notes, medication administration record (MAR), personal care flow sheets, teaching records, intake and output forms, vital sign records, and specialty forms (e.g., diabetic flow sheet and neurologic assessment form). The progress notes can be completely narrative or incorporated into a standardized flow sheet to complement SOAP(IER), PIE, focus charting, and other documentation systems.

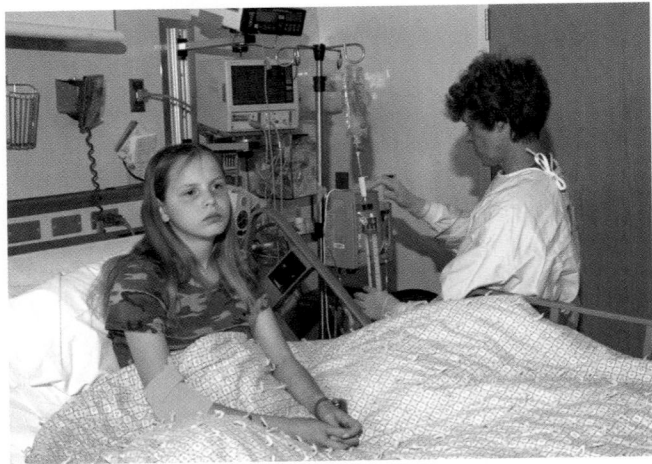

**Figure 16-7** Flow sheets used in critical care settings allow specific documentation in a complex setting.

## RESEARCH FOCUS

**Title of Study:** Evaluation of documentation before and after implementation of a nursing information system in an acute care hospital

**Study Purpose:** The purpose of the study is to evaluate documentation before and after implementation of a nursing information system in an acute care hospital.

**Methods:** The study site was a 100-bed acute care hospital in which three units implemented the nursing information system (NIS). It is a quasi-experimental study using a natural experiment. Nursing assessments of client outcomes (NASSESS), achievement of client outcomes (NGOAL), and nurse perceived quality (NQUAL) are measured using a nursing care plan, data collection instrument. Nurses volunteered as data collectors and were instructed in how to use the instrument, and acceptable inter-rater reliability is demonstrated prior to and during the study. Chart reviews averaged 2 hours per chart.

Eighteen months prior to implementation of the information system, the project team customized a module in an integrated information system. Before the system was implemented, all nurses were given an 8-hour training session provided by the vendor. During the week of implementation, the project team was available 24 hours a day for consultation on using the system. Data for the study was obtained using a retrospective chart review of 90 records three times before implementation and two times after implementation of the information system. Prior to the third chart review, a quality improvement retraining intervention was done with the nurses.

**Findings:** The nursing assessment scores (NASSESS) varied significantly between the three time frames. Units one and two, but not three, also varied significantly for the nursing goals score (NGOAL) and the nursing quality score (NQUAL). The retraining between the second and third times had a significant effect on the assessment, goal, and quality scores. For the assessment and quality scores, the time unit also was significant. All the scores improved, except the nursing quality score, by the third time measure. Since this Nursing Information System (NIS) did not mandate that all the variables be documented, one unit did not record some variables.

**Implications:** A more extensive educational program is needed to implement a nursing information system. Eight hours of education and consultation was not enough to ensure understanding and use of the information system. Just because the documentation is computerized, it is not correct to assume that documentation is complete. Differing characteristics of units and nurses may influence the recording of variables, so the NIS needs to address these differences. Agencies need to continue to periodically review the completeness of documentation and improve the system or the nurse's use of it.

Larrabee, J. H., Boldreghini, S., Elder-Sorrells, K., Turner, Z., Wender, R. G., Hart, J. M., & Lenzi, P. S. (2001). Evaluation of documentation before and after implementation of a nursing information system in an acute care hospital. *Computers in nursing, 19*(2), 56–65.

## Discharge Summary

Discharge summaries highlight the client's illness and course of care. When a narrative discharge summary is entered into the progress notes, it includes:

- The client's status at admission and discharge
- A brief summary of the client's care
- Intervention and education outcomes
- Resolved problems and continuing care needs for unresolved problems, inclusive of referrals
- Client instructions regarding medications, diet, food-drug interactions, activity, treatments, follow-up instructions, and other special needs

Many facilities have a documentation form that itemizes discharge and client instructions. The form has a duplicate copy for the client; the original goes in the medical record. Figure 16-8 shows the common elements of this tool.

## Trends in Documentation

"Health care is increasingly driven by information, and consequently, patient care will demand effective management of information" (Travis & Brennan, p. 162, 1998). In the 21st century with complex clinical practice, nurses face escalating information challenges inherent in processing and communicating computerized information.

Computerized nursing documentation requires the skills of technically competent nurses to improve client care and change the delivery of health care; however, technical competence includes not only equipment competence but also skill in the efficient use of information (Travis & Brennan, 1998). "To harness innovative technologies, nurses must recognize them and know what to do with them" (Brennan, 1999, p. 128).

# Tulane
## UNIVERSITY
### Medical Center

## COORDINATION OF DISCHARGE CARE

### DISCHARGE ASSESSMENT

| DESCRIPTION | | | COMMENT | DESCRIPTION | | | COMMENT | DESCRIPTION | | | | COMMENT |
|---|---|---|---|---|---|---|---|---|---|---|---|---|
| LOC | NL | AB | | respiration quality | NL | AB | | Foley removed/voided | N | Y | NA | |
| pupils | NL | AB | | lung auscultation | NL | AB | | bladder habit problems | N | Y | | |
| range of motion | NL | AB | | heart sounds | NL | AB | | sleep problems | N | Y | UTO | |
| extremity strength | NL | AB | | telemetry removed | N | Y | NA | IV removed and intact | N | Y | NA | |
| appetite | NL | AB | UTO | peripheral pulses | NL | AB | | break in skin integrity | N | | | |
| swallowing difficulty | N | Y | UTO | bowel sounds | NL | AB | | discomfort/pain | N | Y | UTO | |
| feeds self | N | Y | | bowel habit problems | N | Y | Date Last BM | | | | | |

Signature                    RN                        Date                    Time

### DISCHARGE MEDICATIONS

| ☐ None | Medication | Dosage | Route | Schedule | Special Instructions ▼medication instruction sheets given    food/drug interaction sheet given▲ | RX given |
|---|---|---|---|---|---|---|
| | | | | | ☐    ☐ | ☐ |
| | | | | | ☐    ☐ | ☐ |
| | | | | | ☐    ☐ | ☐ |
| | | | | | ☐    ☐ | ☐ |
| | | | | | ☐    ☐ | ☐ |
| | | | | | ☐    ☐ | ☐ |
| | | | | | ☐    ☐ | ☐ |

### HOME ROUTINE

**Activity:** ☐ As tolerated  ☐ Restrictions_____    **Physical Therapy** ☐ Exercise Program    ☐ Equipment

**Diet:** ☐ Regular  ☐ Modified    ☐ Gait Instruction                    *(SIGNATURE)*

**Special Instructions:** (document discharge sheet given to patient)    **Occupational Therapy:**

_____

_____                                    *(SIGNATURE)*

_____    **Nutrition Care:**

_____

_____

_____

_____                                    *(SIGNATURE)*

_____    **Other Services:**

**Social Services:**

                    *(SIGNATURE)*                                    *(SIGNATURE)*

### FOLLOW-UP CARE

Your MD is:            To Contact Call:            In An Emergency Call:

☐ No Appointment    ☐ Appointment(s) made:

| Name | clinic/floor | date/time | phone # |
|---|---|---|---|
| Name | clinic/floor | date/time | phone # |

Appointment(s) not made:

| Call | phone # ext. | for an appointment in | days/weeks with | MD |
|---|---|---|---|---|
| Call | phone # ext. | for an appointment in | days/weeks with | MD |

I understand the above instructions.

_____    _____    _____
Patient or Guardian's Signature    Date    Time of Discharge    Nurse's Signature & Title

**Figure 16-8    Common elements of an interdisciplinary discharge tool.** *Courtesy of Tulane University Medical Center, New Orleans, LA*

With the transition to managed care and the introduction of capitation by insurers, computerized charting is now prevalent in hospitals and is one of the strongest trends in documentation with home health agencies. In order for computerized nursing documentation to demonstrate the quality, effectiveness, and value of the services that nurses provide, standardized databases have to be developed to ensure accuracy and precision in nursing information systems.

## Nursing Minimum Data Set (NMDS)

In 1985, Werley and Lang convened an invitational working conference at the University of Wisconsin–Milwaukee to identify the elements that should be included in a **nursing minimum data set (NMDS)**; these are the elements that should be contained in clinical records and abstracted for studies on the effectiveness and costs of nursing care (Werley & Lang, 1988). Sixteen elements, grouped into three categories, were identified:

1. Demographics: personal identification, date of birth, gender, race and ethnicity, and residence
2. Service: unique facility or service agency number, episode admission or encounter date, discharge or termination date, disposition of client, expected payer, unique health record number of client,* and unique number of principal registered nurse provider*
3. Nursing care: nursing diagnosis,* nursing intervention,* nursing outcome,* and intensity of nursing care* (Werley & Lang, 1988)

Several challenges are inherent in the development of the four nursing care categories: diagnoses, interventions, outcomes, and intensity. Automated information systems must be capable of supporting cost-effective nursing practice through efficient, comprehensive documentation. Basic to standardizing databases is the consistent use of a taxonomy that promotes validity and reliability. NMDS, however, does not specify taxonomy for any of the four elements—for example, NANDA (2003) diagnoses, the Omaha System, Nursing Interventions Classification (NIC) (1995), and acuity ratings. Nursing needs to achieve consensus of terminology for clinical data to be included in nursing care elements of an NMDS.

## Nursing Diagnoses

A nursing diagnosis is a clinical judgment about individual, family, or community responses to actual or potential health problems or life processes (NANDA, 2003). The ANA endorsed NANDA to develop a classification for nursing diagnoses, and in 1992 the NANDA terms were accepted into the Unified Medical Language System

(Ozbolt, Fruchtnight & Hayden, 1994). Most recently, NANDA has revised its system to include a Taxonomy II, which incorporates improved statements of the nursing diagnoses and its organizing framework (Ackley & Ladwig, 2002). (Refer to Chapter 12 for a complete discussion of nursing diagnoses.)

## Nursing Interventions Classification (NIC)

The **nursing interventions classification (NIC)** is a comprehensive standardized language for nursing interventions organized in a three-level taxonomy (McCloskey & Bulechek, 1995). Initiated by a research team (Iowa Intervention Project) at the University of Iowa in 1987, the three-level taxonomy contains 6 domains, 26 classes, and 366 interventions. Each nursing intervention has a label, a definition, and a set of activities to carry out the interventions. *Activities are not interventions and should not be labeled as such in nursing information systems* (NIC, 1995).

The six domains are physiological: basic; complex; behavioral; family; health system; and safety. Within each domain is a set of classes (groups). An example of a class is perioperative care, which contains the nursing interventions (e.g., Teaching Preoperative) that contain sets of activities to carry out a specific intervention. Refer to Chapter 12 for additional discussion of NIC.

NIC interventions have been incorporated into health care data sets and the computerized client medical record. NIC has been recognized by the ANA as one of the first nursing languages to be included in the National Library of Medicine's Metathesaurus for the Unified Medical Language System (McCloskey & Bulechek, 1995).

Grobe and colleagues at the University of Texas at Austin have been developing a lexicon and taxonomy of nursing interventions taken from home care records. Omaha Visiting Nurses Association have developed and used intervention statements to direct client care (Gulanick & Myers, 2003).

## Nursing Outcomes Classification (NOC)

The **nursing outcomes classification (NOC)** is a "taxonomy of patient outcomes that are sensitive to nursing interventions" (Gulanick & Myers, 2003, p. 2). NOC allow nurses to work efficiently with managed care organizations, to decrease health care costs, and to improve quality of care. Well-written NOC allow nurses to quantify their interventions and measure client outcomes with more accuracy. In addition, the NOC improve documentation standards and ultimately improve client care. The new Taxonomy II organizing framework has evolved to improve both the NIC and the NOC of the NANDA system.

---

*Elements not included in the Uniform Hospital Discharge Data Set.

# Reporting

Reporting is the verbal communication of data regarding the client's health status, needs, treatments, outcomes, and responses. When a report is given, it needs to summarize the current critical information that facilitates clinical decision making and continuity of care. As with recording, reporting is based on the nursing process, standards of care, and legal and ethical principles. The nursing process provides structure for an organized report, a challenge inherent in verbal communications (Estes, 2002). In order to verbally communicate an efficient and well-organized report, the nurse must consider

- What needs to be said
- Why it needs to be said
- How to say it
- What the expected outcomes are

Considering these aspects of reporting before the communication will provide for a concise, organized report.

Another critical element in reporting is listening (refer to Chapter 4). Reports require participation from everyone present. When receiving a report, the nurse focuses behaviors to enhance listening skills: the nurse eliminates distractions, puts thoughts and concerns aside, concentrates on what is being said, and does not anticipate what the presenter will say next. The reporting process is an integral component of developing effective interpersonal and intrapersonal relationships that promote continuity of client care. Regardless of the type of communication, planned presentation of client data is a key to accurate, concise, effective reporting. Summary reports, walking rounds, telephone communication, and incident reports are all types of reporting.

## Summary Reports

Summary reports summarize pertinent client information that focuses on the client's needs as identified by the nursing process for the new caregiver. Summary reports commonly occur at the change of shift and when the client is transferred to another area.

A summary, or end-of-shift, report should be presented as follows:

- Background data obtained from client interactions and assessment of the functional health patterns
- Primary medical and nursing diagnoses and priority problems
- Identification of client risk problems
- Recent changes in condition or in treatments (e.g., new medications, elevated temperature)
- Effective interventions or treatments of priority problems, inclusive of laboratory and diagnostic results (e.g., client's response to pain medication)
- Progress toward expected outcomes: priority problems, teaching or discharge planning
- Adjustments in the plan of care
- Client or family complaints

This format will provide structure and organization to the data that are both logical and time-sequenced since the format follows the nursing process. The new caregiver needs to receive an accurate, concise report about what has happened during the previous shift in order to provide continuity of care. Client and family complaints should be addressed last for each client because these situations usually generate questions and discussion.

## Walking Rounds

Walking rounds can be either nursing rounds, physician-nurse rounds, or interdisciplinary rounds. **Walking rounds** is a reporting method used when the members of the care team walk to each client's room and discuss care and progress with each other and with the client.

Nursing rounds are used most frequently by charge nurses as their method of report. During the rounds, the on-coming nurse is introduced to the client and the off-going nurse discusses with the client and the on-coming nurse changes in the plan of care. Rounds are more time-consuming than the end-of-shift report but give the nurses and the client the opportunity to evaluate the effectiveness of care together (Figure 16-9).

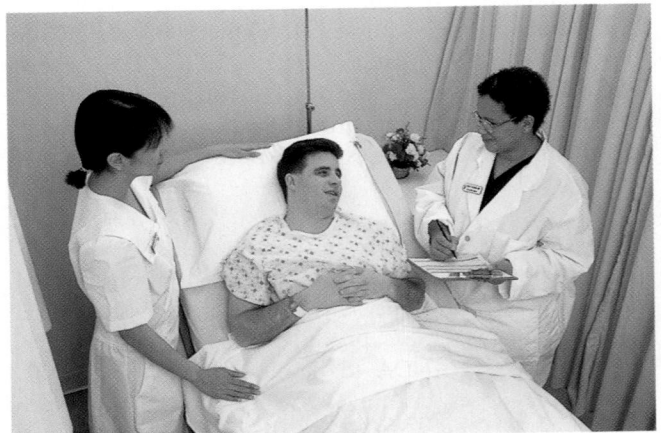

**Figure 16-9   Nursing rounds: What are some advantages of nursing rounds compared to traditional end-of-shift reports?**

## STOP AND THINK

### Recording and Reporting

How do recording and reporting data differ? Both serve as a method of communicating information about the client's care and other significant data. What would happen in a change-of-shift report if the two were identical?

## STOP AND THINK

### Nursing Rounds

Can nursing rounds foster team building among the nurses from different shifts? Do you think nursing rounds promote client satisfaction? If your critical analysis identifies that nursing rounds have the potential for fostering team building and client satisfaction, why do you think this method of reporting is not used by all charge nurses?

Nursing rounds are also used as a teaching method. The instructor introduces the client to the student, and together they discuss the client's care. The instructor can also use this time to appraise the student's observation, communication, and decision-making skills.

Nurse-physician rounds can involve either the staff nurse or the charge nurse with the physician. These rounds usually occur daily and provide the nurse, physician, and client the opportunity to evaluate the effectiveness of care.

Interdisciplinary rounds, in which many disciplines are involved, usually occur less frequently than the other types of rounds. Continuity of care, client satisfaction, and decreased costs are often the outcomes of daily interdisciplinary rounds (Curley, McEachern, & Speroff, 1998). The interdisciplinary concept recognizes that health care providers do not work independently of one another, but address clients' needs within the context of all team members. Interdisciplinary rounds are done most commonly in place of or to supplement case conferences and to discuss discharge planning. Interdisciplinary rounds support the concept of critical pathways and are seen most frequently in teaching hospitals.

## Telephone Communication

Telephone communications are another way nurses report transfers, communicate referrals, obtain client data, solve problems, and inform a physician and client's family members regarding a change in the client's condition. Nurses are expected to demonstrate phone courtesy and professionalism when initiating and receiving telephone reports and orders.

When initiating a phone call, organize the information to be reported or received. For example:

1. Make sure all lab results are back; if they are not, identify in advance which ones are missing and phone the lab or check the computer to determine if other results are available. Write down which tests have been per-

formed and the results. Spell the client's name and provide the client's medical record number to avoid the error of getting the results on the wrong client.

2. Review your notes and have your assessment data readily available, especially any significant client data that are related to the call. If you have not assessed the client, do an assessment before telephoning the practitioner; otherwise, the practitioner might ask you questions that you will not be able to answer.

3. Let the charge nurse or someone else at the nurses' station know that you are placing the call so that you will not be interrupted while on the phone.

When you place the call, state the reason you are calling: for example, "I am calling Dr. Smith regarding the blood sugar results for Mrs. White." Be brief and listen carefully. Repeat the test results and any orders the physician gives over the phone.

Record accurately in the medical record the date and time the phone call was placed, the client data you reported on the phone, the name of the person you spoke with, and whether an order was obtained. Do not chart "physician notified, no orders obtained." Rather, chart "Dr. Smith notified by phone, blood sugar 260 mg (drawn by the lab at 1300), orders received and recorded on the physician order sheet." Charting telephone orders and documentation in the nurses' progress notes should be done as soon as possible after the phone call to prevent an entry by another caregiver before you chart the telephone report.

Figure 16-10 demonstrates how to write a telephone order onto the physician order sheet: date and time the entry; record the order as given by the physician; then sign the order beginning with *t.o.* (telephone order), write the physician's name, and sign your name. If another nurse witnesses the phone order, that nurse's signature should go after yours.

The physician needs to countersign the order within a time frame as specified by the facility's policy. Fax machines have decreased the need for lengthy or complicated telephone orders, both saving time and avoiding error. To confirm the physician's identity as the initiator of the fax orders, telephone the physician. The physician

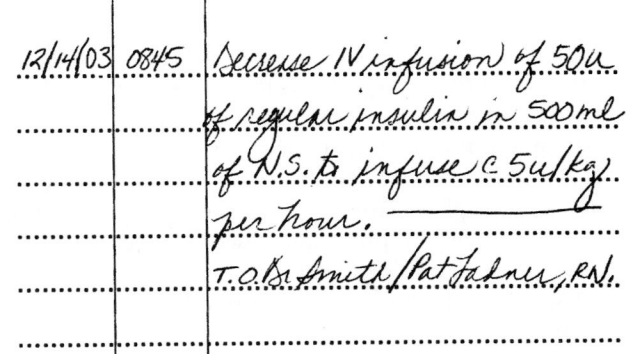

**Figure 16-10    Documenting a telephone order**

needs to countersign the fax orders according to agency policy.

## Incident Reports

**Incident reports**, or occurrence reports, are used to document any unusual occurrence or accident in the delivery of client care, such as falls or medication errors. The *Code for Nurses* (ANA, 2001) states that nurses are expected "to protect the client when safety is affected." Ethical practice requires that nurses file an incident report to protect the client, not to punish the caregiver.

The filing of incident reports is not only an internal device for the facility but is also a requirement by federal, national, and state accrediting agencies. Nurses are often advised not to document the filing of an incident report in the nurses' notes for legal reasons, but, as previously discussed, documenting medication errors requires an incident report and documentation in the nurses' notes to ensure that the client receives safe care.

The incident report serves two functions:

1. It informs the facility's administration of the incident, so risk management personnel can consider changes that might prevent similar occurrences in the future.
2. It alerts the facility's insurance company to a potential claim and the need for further investigation.

Litigation can be avoided if the facility takes prompt action by investigating an occurrence. The incident report is not part of the medical record, but it may be used later in litigation.

Each person with firsthand knowledge of the occurrence should fill out and sign a separate report. Although the incident report format varies from one facility to another, some key elements must be addressed when filing a report:

- Record the date, exact time, and place you discovered the occurrence.
- Identify the person(s) involved in the occurrence, including witnesses.
- Document accurately and objectively the exact occurrences that you witnessed or first saw after the incident; for example, record "found the client sitting on the floor" rather than "client fell."
- Record the exact details, in time sequence, what happened, and the consequences for the persons involved.
- Record your actions to provide care and results of your assessment for injuries or client complaints.
- Notify the supervisor on duty and record the time and name of the physician notified; if telephone orders were received from the physician, document as previously discussed and implement the orders.
- Do not record your opinions, judgments, conclusions, or assumptions about what occurred, point blame, or suggest how to prevent occurrence of a similar incident.
- Forward the incident report to the designated person as defined in the facility's policy.

Iyer and Camp (1999) suggest an additional safeguard for the nurse: write a brief, accurate description of the incident and keep it at home. In the description, include the details of the incident and the names of the people who were involved, especially if they can substantiate your information. Lawsuits may take several years from the time of an incident until the case goes to court; your personal notes will help you with accurate recall of the incident. Use the same elements described above in filing an incident report, because your personal notes may be read by the plaintiff's attorney.

Special attention should be given to documenting falls, because current research shows that client falls constitute a large percentage of the incident reports written in acute care settings. Client falls are the main reason nurses are sued (Iyer & Camp, 1999). (Refer to Chapter 33 for information on how to prevent client falls and their legal ramifications.)

---

## NURSING STRATEGY

### Documentation of Client Fall

*Assessment*

- Check for bruises, lacerations, or abrasions.
- Check blood pressure, pulse, and respirations.
- Perform a neurologic assessment (slurred speech, weakness, mental status).
- Check for incontinency (urinary or fecal).
- Note any pain or deformity in the extremities (arm, lumbar spine, hip, or leg).

*Interview the Client*

- Were there any symptoms prior to the fall (lightheadedness, impaired vision, dizziness, weakness, palpitations, shortness of breath, chest pain)?
- What were your actions prior to the fall (movements, muscle jerks, breathing pattern)?
- How did the fall occur (getting out of bed, while walking in the room)?
- Did anyone witness the fall?

Be sure to chart what you observe ("Client prone on floor"), not what you conclude ("Client fell out of bed"). Document all data in the nurses' progress notes and on the incident report.

# CASE STUDY/NURSING CARE PLAN

Mr. Wilkins, age 88, is hospitalized in the intensive care unit (ICU) with complications of diabetes mellitus type 1. Most recently, he is experiencing diabetic ketoacidosis (DKA) with a blood glucose of 340 mg/dL. In addition, he has coronary heart disease (CHD) from the microvascular complications of his diabetes (note: he has a pulmonary artery catheter to monitor his hemodynamic status). His primary clinical manifestations from the CHD are: hypertension, tachycardia, and occasional arrhythmias. At present, his level of consciousness is impaired, he is breathing with Kussmaul respirations, his breath is acetone in nature, and he is extremely fatigued. A variety of flow sheets are being used in the careful documentation of his care, and charting takes place more frequently than hourly. The nurse places his vital signs, blood glucose, daily weights, and oxygen saturation levels on one flow sheet. In addition, there is a separate flow sheet for the ongoing neurological assessment. There is also an MAR for all of the medications he is receiving, including his titrated insulin, anti-hypertensives, and antiarrhythmics.

## Assessment

An 88-year-old male with complications associated with type 1 diabetes mellitus. Specifically, he has a primary diagnosis of DKA (blood glucose = 340 mg/dL. In addition he has hypertension, atrial cardiac arrhythmias, and a decreased LOC. He is being monitored in an ICU.

## Nursing Diagnosis #1

*Deficient Fluid Volume* related to osmotic diuresis associated with hyperglycemia.

**NOC:** Electrolyte and Acid-Base Imbalance; Fluid Balance; Hydration; Nutritional Status; Food and Fluid Intake

**NIC:** Fluid Management; Hypovolemia Management; Shock Management: Volume

## Expected Outcomes

The client will:

1. Maintain a blood glucose level in the 150–180 mg/dL range within 72 hours.
2. Demonstrate no signs/symptoms of dehydration during his admission in the ICU.
3. Maintain a cardiac output in the normal range of 4–6 L/min during his admission to the ICU.

## Planning/Interventions/Rationales

1. Measure blood glucose levels Q 1 hour, and administer insulin per sliding scale orders. *Blood glucose levels are at a crisis level, and close monitoring prevents further complications of DKA.*
2. Evaluate cardiac output by assessing cardiac system with vital signs, hemodynamic monitor (pulmonary artery catheter), and electrophysiology. *Allows for close cardiac monitoring, which is necessary for the client's critical condition.*
3. Assess hydration status Q 1 hour by monitoring: urine specific gravity, intake/output (hourly urine output), skin turgor, and vital signs. *Frequent assessment detects subtle changes in hydration status during the critical complication of DKA.*

## Evaluation

The client has a blood glucose within a controlled range, stable hemodynamic readings of the pulmonary artery catheter, and no clinical manifestations of dehydration during his admission to the ICU.

## Nursing Diagnosis #2

*Ineffective Breathing Pattern of Kussmaul Respirations* related to metabolic acidosis associated with DKA.

**NOC:** Respiratory Status: Ventilation; Vital Signs Status; Respiratory Status; Airway Patency

**NIC:** Airway Management; Respiratory Monitoring

## Expected Outcomes

The client will:

1. Demonstrate an effective respiratory rate of 12 to 16 breaths/minute with an oxygen saturation level of at least 94% within 24 hours.

*(continues)*

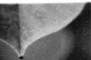

# CASE STUDY/NURSING CARE PLAN *(continued)*

2. Progressively regain level of consciousness within 24 to 48 hours.
3. Decrease sense of energy and experience less generalized fatigue within 24 to 48 hours.

## Planning/Interventions/Rationales

1. Monitor oxygen saturation levels and assess depth/rhythm of respirations Q 1 hour. *Detects respiratory compensation during a time of the respiratory crisis of Kussmaul breathing (caused by the DKA).*
2. Assess level of consciousness by evaluating neurological responses and client's ability to effectively answer questions Q 1 hour. *Provides constant monitoring of neurological status.*
3. Ask client questions regarding his level of energy, and ask client to quantify from 1 to 10 the level of his fatigue Q 1 hour. *Evaluates fatigue levels on constant basis.*

## Evaluation

The client has a progressive decrease in the Kussmaul breathing pattern, an increasing level of consciousness, and an increasing level of energy.

## Key Concepts

- Documentation provides a system of written records that reflect client care provided on the basis of assessment data and the client's response to interventions.
- The medical record can be used by health care students as a teaching tool and is a main source of data for clinical research.
- Nurses are responsible for assessing and documenting that the client has an understanding of the treatment prior to the intervention.
- Competent adult clients have the right, through an advance directive, to make decisions regarding life-sustaining interventions when they become incapacitated or terminally ill.
- Standards of care, as set forth by State Boards of Nursing and the American Nurses Association, require nurses to use the nursing process in their documentation.
- Accreditation and reimbursement agencies require accurate and thorough documentation of the nursing care rendered and the client's response to interventions.
- Effective documentation requires clear, concise, accurate recording of all client care and other significant events in an organized and chronological fashion, representative of each phase of the nursing process.
- Client safety requires appropriate reporting and recording of medication errors and other occurrences in compliance with the facility's policy.
- Computerized documentation saves time, increases legibility and accuracy, provides standardized nursing terminology, enhances the nursing process and decision-making skills, and supports continuity of care.
- Computerized documentation has both legal and ethical considerations unique to its method, as contrasted with other forms of documentation.
- The discharge summary is used to highlight the client's illness, course of care, and aftercare instructions.

- Incident reports are used to document any unusual occurrence in the delivery of client care.

## Review Questions and Activities

1. During your clinical laboratory, review the documentation tools:
   Do they form a system?
   Is the nursing process evident?
   Do you have to chart the same data on more than one form?
2. Read a client's medical record. Can you identify what was done for the client and the client's responses? If you cannot, what significant data are missing?
3. When planning the care for your clients, identify the critical elements of assessment that you will need to document. Analyze these data in relation to the documentation system of your assigned clinical facility and the types of forms for charting.
4. What information must be documented in the nurses' progress notes when using an assessment and intervention flow sheet?
5. Label each of the following statements, which describe the acronym components of problem-oriented charting (SOAP):
   ____ Abdomen distended; on auscultation, bowel sounds absent in all 4 quadrants
   ____ Imbalanced nutrition: less than body requirements related to inability to digest or absorb nutrients; first day postop. Risk for deficient fluid volume.
   ____ "I'm nauseated, I think I'm going to vomit."
   ____ Notified Dr. James of symptoms and client's

complaints. Placed NPO; increase intravenous fluids of normal saline to 150 ml/hr; measure I&O; keep environment quiet; reassure client.

**6.** Describe the format for focus charting.

**7.** What are legal and ethical issues specific to computerized documentation?

## Multimedia Links

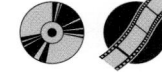

Christensen *Core Concept Videos: Nursing Documentation*

## Web Resources

American Association of Legal Nurse Consultants
http://www.aalnc.org
American Health Information Management Association
http://www.ahima.org
American Nurses Association
http://www.nursingworld.org
Healthcare Information and Management Systems Society
http://www.himss.org
Information Technology in Nursing
http://www.bcnsg.org.uk
Nursing Informatics Working Group of the American Medical Informatics Association
http://www.amia-niwg.org

## References

Ackley, B., & Ladwig, G. (2002). *Nursing diagnosis handbook: A guide to planning care* (5th ed.). St. Louis: Mosby.

Alternative Link Systems, Inc. (2001). *The state legal guide to nursing.* Clifton Park, NY: Delmar Learning.

American Nurses Association (ANA) (2001). *Code for nurses with interpretive statements.* Kansas City: Author.

American Nurses Association (ANA) (1997). *Standards of clinical nursing practice.* Kansas City: Author.

Brennan, P. F. (1999). Harnessing innovative technologies: What can you do with a shoe? *Nursing Outlook, 47*(3), 128–132.

Calloway, W. D. (2001). Preventing communication breakdown. *RN, 64*(1), 71–74.

Carelock, J., & Innerarity, S. (2001). Critical incidents: Effective communication and documentation. *Critical Care Nursing, 23*(4), 59–66.

Chamrorro, T. (2001). Computer-based patient records. *Seminars in Oncology Nursing, 17*(1), 24–33.

Curley, C., McEachern, J. E., & Speroff, T. (1998). Interdisciplinary rounds reduced hospital stay and costs and improved staff satisfaction. *Medical Care, 36*(5), 4–12.

Estes, M. (2002). *Health assessment & physical examination* (2nd ed.). Clifton Park, NY: Delmar Learning.

Gulanick, M., & Myers, J. (2003). *Nursing care plans: Nursing diagnosis and intervention* (5th ed.). St. Louis: Mosby.

Harmer, B., & Henderson, V. (1955). *Textbook of the principles and practice of nursing* (5th ed.). New York: The MacMillan Company, p. 259.

Helm, A. (2002). Charting by exception. *CNSO Risk Advisor, 2*(1), 3.

Iyer, P. W., & Camp, N. H. (1999). *Nursing documentation: A nursing process approach* (3rd ed.). St. Louis: Mosby Yearbook.

Killion, S. W., & Dempski, K. M. (2001). *Quick look nursing: Legal and ethical issues.* Clifton Park, NY: Delmar Learning.

Larrabee, J. H., Boldreghini, S., Elder-Sorrells, K., Turner, Z., Wender, R. G., Hart, J. M., & Lenzi, P. S. (2001). Evaluation of documentation before and after implementation of a nursing information system in an acute care hospital. *Computers in nursing, 19*(2), 56–65.

Lieberson, A. D. (2002). *Advance Medical Directives.* New York: Clark.

McCloskey, J. C., & Bulechek, G. M. (1995). Validation and coding of the NIC taxonomy structure. *Image: Journal of Nursing Scholarship, 27*(1), 43–49.

Miller, P., & Pastorino, C. (1990). Daily nursing documentation can be quick and thorough! *Nursing Management, 21*(11), 47–49.

North American Nursing Diagnosis Association (2003). *NANDA Nursing diagnoses: Definitions and classification: 2003–2004.* St. Louis: Author.

Nursing Intervention Classification (NIC) (1995). *The NIC letter, 3*(1), 4.

Ozbolt, J. G., Fruchtnight, J. N., & Hayden, J. R. (1994). Toward data standards for clinical nursing information. *Journal of the American Medical Informatics Association, 1*(2), 175–185.

Reiss, B., Evans, M., & Broyles, B. (2002). *Pharmacological aspects of nursing care* (6th ed.). Clifton Park, NY: Delmar Learning.

Sheehan, J. P. (2002). A liability checklist for clinical pathways. *Nursing Management, 33*(2), 23–25.

Souther, E. (2001). Implementation of the electronic medical record: The team approach. *Computers in Nursing, 19*(2), 47–55.

Stangl, R. (2002). Learning to love computerized charting. *Nursing, 32*(9), 12.

Travis, L., & Brennan, P. F. (1998). Information science for the future: An innovative nursing informatics curriculum. *Journal of Nursing Education, 37*(4), 162–168.

Tucker, J. L. (1995). Interdisciplinary record improves documentation. *Patient Education Management, 2*(3), 45–47.

Werley, H. H., & Lang, N. M. (1988). The consensually derived nursing minimum data set: Elements and definitions. In H. H. Werley & N. M. Lang (Eds.). *Identification of the nursing minimum data set* (pp. 402–411). New York: Springer.

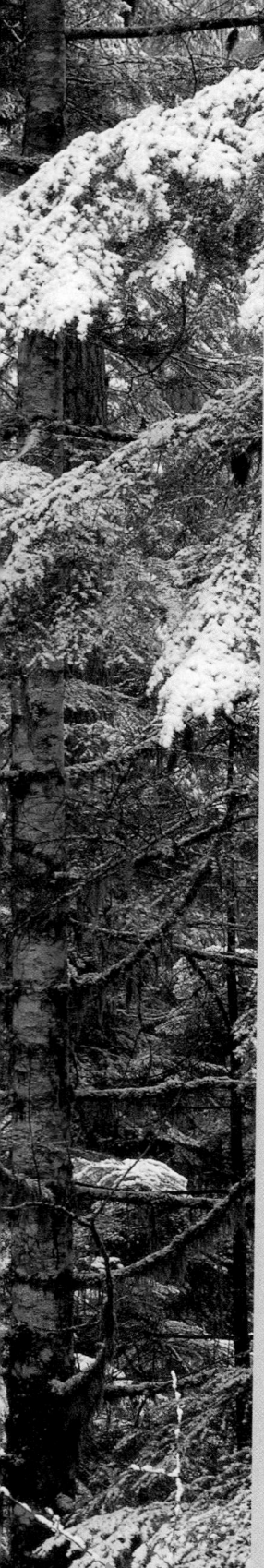

# III UNIT

# Client Care Across the Life Span

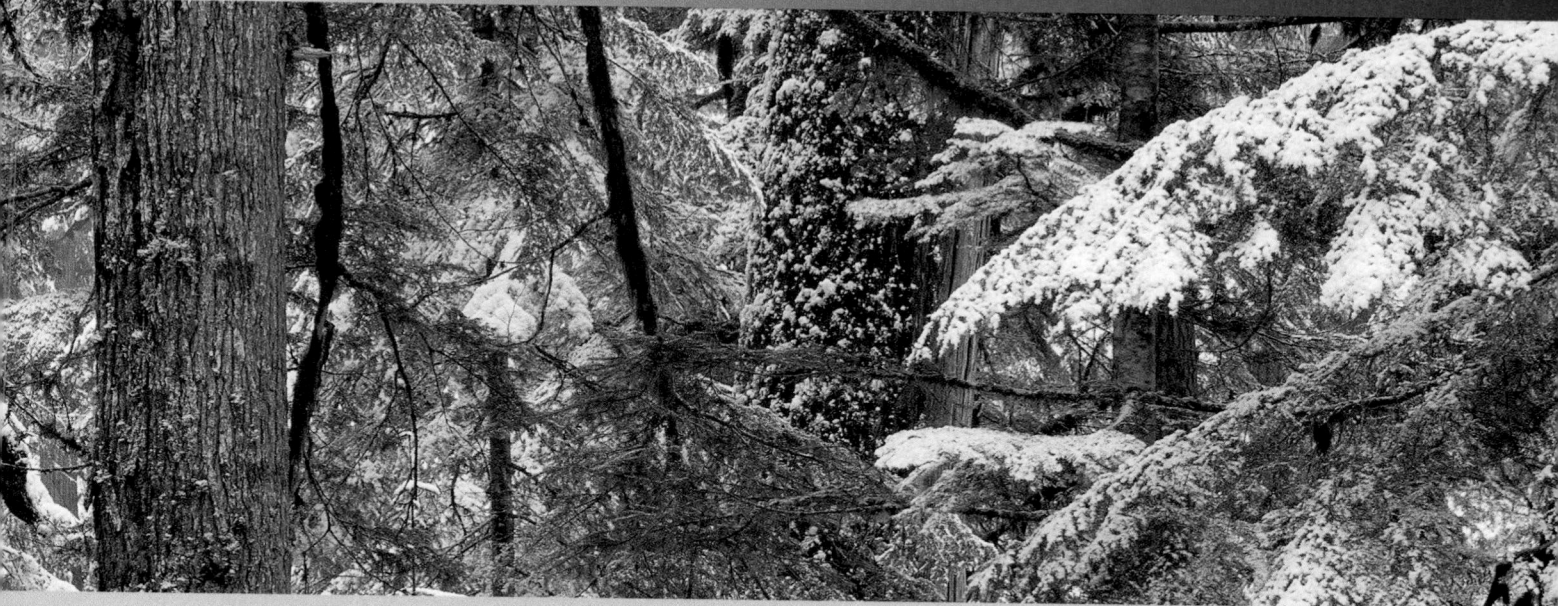

# CHAPTER 17

# The Pediatric Client

## Ruth N. Grendell, DNSc, RN

*"An adult may see human wisdom manifested in its highest form by watching a child's boundless capacity for making the most of today."*

(Anonymous)

# Chapter Competencies

*Upon completion of this chapter, the reader should be able to:*

1. Discuss the basic principles of growth and development.
2. Describe the theoretical foundations for growth and development.
3. Discuss the importance of development as a holistic framework for nursing.
4. Identify the stages of the life cycle.
5. Describe the nursing implications that are relevant to each stage of the life cycle from prenatal development through adolescence.

# Key Terms

accommodation
adaptation
adolescence
anorexia nervosa
assimilation
bonding
bulimia
critical period
development
developmental tasks
embryonic stage

fetal alcohol syndrome
fetal stage
germinal stage
growth
infancy
intrapsychic theory
learning
maturation
menarche
moral maturity
neonatal period

obesity
phenylketonuria (PKU)
preadolescence
prenatal period
preschool stage
puberty
school-age period
self-concept
spirituality
teratogenic substance
toddler

From conception to death, individuals are constantly changing. Physical, psychological, emotional, cognitive, moral, and spiritual development continues throughout life. Health status and developmental stages influence each other. A thorough understanding of developmental concepts and their relationship to health status is essential for professional nursing practice.

This chapter provides an overview of the information related to the various stages of growth and development from conception through adolescence. This time of life is best labeled as "childhood," and is commonly represented by the sequential stages of the prenatal period, the neonate (birth to 4 weeks of age), the infant (1 to 12 months), the toddler (1 to 3 years), the preschooler (3 to 5 years), the school-aged child (5 to 12 years), and the adolescent (12 to 18 or 20 years). Emphasis is on health promotion as well as the influence of common health problems within each developmental stage.

Major growth and developmental theories are presented and the application of age-specific theoretical concepts is addressed within the discussion of each childhood stage. The framework used is a holistic nursing perspective that includes the family as partner in promoting healthy growth and developmental patterns.

# Fundamental Concepts of Growth and Development

**Growth** is the quantitative (measurable) changes in physical size of the body and its parts, such as increases in cells, tissues, structures, and systems. Examples of growth are physical changes in height, weight, bone density, and dental structure. Even though growth is not a steady process through the life cycle, growth patterns can be predicted. Variations in growth, such as rapid increases contrasted with slower rates of physical change, occur with each individual. Rapid growth is most common in the prenatal, infant, and adolescent stages. An individual's growth depends on both genetic traits and environmental factors that promote consistent growth. Most physical growth is reached by late adolescence. Environmental factors that inhibit growth include malnutrition and trauma imposed by a nonnurturing or disruptive and changing environment (Martin, 2002; Berger & Williams, 1999).

**Development** is a qualitative term that refers to behavioral changes and increasing competency in functional abilities and skills. **Maturation** is another qualitative term that is closely related to development. "Development describes a change or expansion of a person's capabilities;

maturation describes a differentiation or increasing complexity of those capabilities that may come with age" (Berger & Williams, 1999, p. 238). Maturation depends on biologic growth, functional changes, and **learning** (assimilation of information with a resultant change in behavior). During each developmental stage of the life cycle, certain goals (**developmental tasks**) must be achieved. These developmental tasks set the stage for future learning and adaption.

The **critical period** is the time of the most rapid growth or development in a particular stage of the life cycle. During these critical periods, an individual is most vulnerable to stressors of any type.

Growth, development, maturation, and learning are interdependent processes. For learning to occur, the individual must be mature enough to grasp the concepts and make required behavioral changes. Cognitive maturation precedes learning. Physical growth is also a prerequisite for many types of learning; for example, a child must have the physical ability to control the anal sphincter before toilet training skills are learned.

## Principles of Growth and Development

All persons have individual talents and abilities that contribute to their development as unique entities. *There are no absolute rules in predicting the exact rate of development for an individual.* However, some general principles relate to the growth and development of all humans (Table 17-1).

The sequence of development is predictable even though the emergence of specific skills varies with each person. For example, not all infants roll over at the same age, but most roll over before they crawl (Ball & Bindler, 2003, Berger & Williams, 1979).

## Factors Influencing Growth and Development

Multiple factors such as heredity, life experiences, health status, and cultural expectations influence a child's growth and development. The interaction of these factors greatly influences how the individual responds to everyday situations; the choices a child makes regarding health behaviors are also greatly determined by these factors.

### Heredity

A complex series of processes transmits genetic information from parents to children. The genetic composition of an individual determines physical characteristics such as skin color, hair texture, facial features, and body structure, as well as a predisposition to certain diseases. Heredity is a genetic blueprint from which an individual grows and develops; it determines to a great extent the rate of physical and mental development.

## STOP AND THINK

### Nature or Nurture?

What determines a person's behavior—heredity or environment? This "nature versus nurture" issue remains a controversy today. What do you think is most important in determining a person's behavior: an individual's genetic predisposition or the response of other people and socialization? This question has no simple answers. As you continue to develop in your professional role, keep an open mind regarding the factors influencing behavior.

Many genetic or hereditary disorders are present from birth. Some of these abnormalities are serious and others are not. For example, autosomal recessive disorders such as Tay-Sachs disease can lead to serious consequences. Tay-Sachs results in neuromuscular and brain deterioration with death commonly occurring before the age of 5. The nurse must work closely with the family, and psychological and genetic counseling need to be incorporated into the plan of care (*Taber's Cyclopedic Medical Dictionary,* 2001).

### Life Experiences

A child's experiences can also influence the rate of growth and development. For example, contrast the differences in physical growth rates between a child whose family can afford food, shelter, and health care and a child whose family has little, if any, resources. The child who is poor has a higher risk of experiencing physical and mental lags in growth and development.

### Health Status

Children experiencing wellness are progressing normally along the life cycle. However, illness or disability can interfere with the achievement of developmental milestones. Individuals with chronic conditions will often meet developmental milestones but with a time delay. For example, children who are physically ill may not be able to progress through normal developmental tasks in the "normal time frame" for a given developmental stage.

### Cultural Expectations

Society expects people to master certain skills in each developmental period. The age at which an individual masters a particular task is determined in part by culture. For example, the time for mastery of toilet training is greatly influenced by cultural norms.

The following are examples of how societal expectations can either promote or hinder one's growth and development (Potts & Mandleco, 2002):

## TABLE 17-1   PRINCIPLES OF GROWTH AND DEVELOPMENT

| Principle | Example/Description |
| --- | --- |
| Development occurs in cephalocaudal (head-to-toe) direction. | An infant raises his head before sitting up. |
| Development occurs in a proximodistal manner. | The infant is able to move his arms before picking up objects with hands and fingers. Functions closer to the midline (proximal) of the body develop before functions farther away from the body's midline (distal). |
| Development occurs in an orderly manner from simple to complex and from the general to the specific. | An infant crawls before walking. A child holds a crayon with the entire hand before being able to grasp it between thumb and finger. Gross motor control is achieved before fine motor coordination. |
| The pattern of growth and development is continuous, orderly, and predictable. However, growth and development do not proceed at a consistent rate. | Periods of rapid growth (similar to growth spurts of adolescence) alternate with periods of slower growth. |
| Every person proceeds through stages of growth and development at an individual rate. | One adolescent boy may reach his full height by age 14, while another may continue to grow until age 20. |
| Every stage of development has specific characteristics. | An infant is dependent on others for physical and emotional survival. Adolescence is characterized by a search for identity. |
| Growth and development may temporarily be stalled or regress during critical periods. | A toddler may revert to infant behaviors when a new baby enters the family. |
| Each stage of development has certain tasks to be achieved or acquired during that specific time. Tasks of one developmental stage become the foundation for tasks in subsequent stages. | An infant must master the psychological task of developing trust in order to mature as an adolescent who can establish a separate identity. |
| Some stages of growth and development are more critical than others. | The first trimester of pregnancy is a critical time for fetal development. During this critical phase, the developing human is most vulnerable to damage from toxins (e.g., drugs, chemicals, viruses). |

- A child who grows up in an economically deprived home may receive inadequate food, shelter, emotional nurturing, or intellectual stimulation with resultant impairments in physical, psychosocial, and cognitive development.
- A child who is raised in a single-parent family may have a different sense of self-esteem in a culture that supports a nuclear family consisting of both mother and father (Figure 17-1).
- Other children and their parents may label the child who is homeschooled as lacking in social interpersonal skills.
- Cultural child-rearing practices (i.e., attitudes toward touching) may differ from the traditional social practices, leading to misunderstanding and isolation from interactions within the mainstream social structure.
- Cultural foods can have an influence on health.
- Swaddling infants and carrying infants on boards (as in the Native American practice) can delay walking.
- Hip dysplasia is rarely seen in children who are carried by straddling the mother's hips. (Note: dysplasia is caused by abducted position for prolonged period of time.)
- Social roles of men and women within a certain culture often influence the child's school activities and choice of careers.

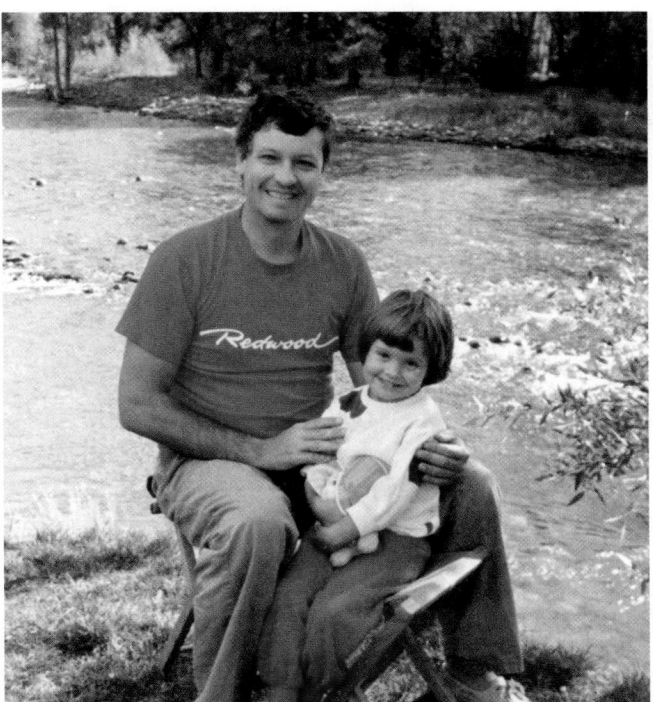

**FIGURE 17-1   All children will develop a sense of self-esteem stemming in part from their family.**

# Theoretical Perspectives of Human Development

Nurses must have a thorough understanding of human growth and development in order to provide individualized care. Remember that chronological age and developmental age are not synonymous. An overview of the major developmental theories is presented below. These theories are discussed more fully in the specific sections about each developmental period.

## Physiological Dimension

Physiological growth (physical size and functioning) of a child is influenced primarily by interaction of genetic predisposition, the central nervous system (CNS), the endocrine system, and maturation. The role of heredity in human development is complex and not yet fully understood. Genetics is the foundation for achievement of specific tasks. Factors such as the psychosocial environment and health status help children live up to their genetic potential.

## Psychosocial Dimension

The psychosocial dimension of growth and development consists of subjective feelings and interpersonal relationships. A favorable **self-concept** (view of one's self, including body image, self-esteem, and ideal self) is likely the

most important key to a person's success and happiness. Following are characteristics of an individual with a positive self-concept:

- Self-confidence
- Willingness to take risks
- Ability to receive criticism without defensiveness
- Ability to adapt effectively to stressors
- Innovative problem-solving skills

Self-esteem fluctuates as the child progresses through the various life stages. The patterns are usually established by the age of 3 or 4, but the process actually begins in infancy. Parental involvement and demonstration of love are critical. The child may see temporary setbacks as permanent. The parent can redirect the "I can't" and "I'm no good" expressions of failure to "I'll keep trying until I succeed" attitudes. Praising and rewarding the child's effort toward completion of a task rather than focusing on the outcome can redirect the child's inaccurate beliefs (Rutherford, Dowshen, & Mesinger, 2001).

People with a healthy self-concept believe in themselves; as a result, they set goals that can be achieved. The goal achievement reinforces the positive belief about one's self. Figure 17-2 illustrates this positive cycle of self-fulfilling beliefs and actions.

A person with a positive self-concept is likely to engage in health-promoting activities. For example, an adolescent who values self is more likely to avoid unhealthy habits, such as binge eating, smoking, or experimenting with drugs. Many different psychosocial theories explain the development of self-concept. This chapter presents the intrapsychic and interpersonal models of personality development.

## Intrapsychic Theory

**Intrapsychic theory** (also called psychodynamic) focuses on an individual's unconscious processes. Feelings, needs, conflicts, and drives are considered to be motivators of behavior, learning, and development. Sigmund Freud and Erik Erikson are two major intrapsychic theorists.

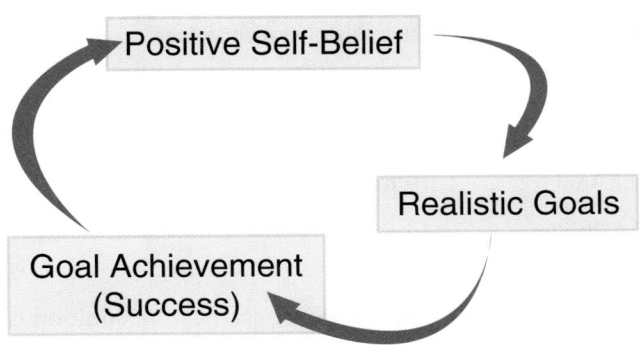

**Figure 17-2   Self-fulfilling cycle in positive self-concept**

## NURSING STRATEGY

### Touch Points

T. Berry Brazelton, pediatrician and author, describes critical periods as "touch points." The care giver must assess for:

- Regressive behaviors that are common just before a new development stage; many times, the behavior is part of the struggle for autonomy.

- Sibling rivalry, where the child may exhibit frequent crying, tantrums, waking at night; become "emotionally stuck"; be fearful; cling to parents; or revert to bedwetting.

- Self-calming habitual activities (i.e., pulling own hair and nail biting). These times can be opportunities to reassure the child regarding her unique place in the family, and to help reorganize the child's behavior in preparation for the new development tasks.

Brazelton, T. B., & Sparrow, J. (2001). *Touchpoints three to six.* Cambridge, MA: Perseus.

"According to Freud's early theory all behavior is motivated by a desire to satisfy biological needs and release of tension" (Oran, 2000, p. 179). Freud (1856–1939) believed that gratification behavior is expressed primarily through different body zones (oral, anal, genital) at certain ages during the course of personality development. "The goal of development is maximizing need gratification while minimizing punishment and guilt, using defenses to control anxiety" (Oran, 2000, p. 179). Freud's theory stated "Unresolved gratification at a certain stage leads to a fix-

ation of development at that stage" (Ball & Bindler, 2003). The personality was viewed as a three-part structure: the id (basic sexual energy), the ego (the realistic part of the person), and the superego (the moral system that contains a set of values and conscience). Freud believed the personality development was completed in the final stages of adolescence. He labeled the ages from 6 to 12 years as the "latency" period when the child expresses little interest in sexuality. This was disputed by recent studies indicating that children are sexual from birth and express sexual feelings in diverse behaviors as they develop (Kelly, 2001). Table 17-2 depicts Freud's stages of psychosexual development.

Erikson (1902–1994) expanded Freud's concept of developmental stages by theorizing that psychosocial development is a lifelong process that does not end with the cessation of adolescence. Just as physical growth patterns can be predicted, certain psychosocial tasks must be mastered in each developmental stage. Erikson's model (1968) proposes that psychosocial development is a series of conflicts that can have favorable or unfavorable outcomes. These conflicts occur in eight developmental stages of life as described in Table 17-3.

Havighurst (1972) theorized that there are six developmental stages of life, each with essential tasks to be achieved. Mastery of a task in one developmental stage is essential for mastery of tasks in subsequent stages. When a task in one stage is mastered, it is learned for life, independent of subsequent neurological change (which may occur with disease or injury). Table 17-4 presents Havighurst's developmental stages with the associated tasks.

### Interpersonal Theory

Harry Stack Sullivan (1953) theorized that relationships with others influence how one's personality develops. Approval and disapproval from significant others influence the formation of one's personality. To form satisfying relationships with others, an individual must complete six stages of development, which are shown in Table 17-5.

| TABLE 17-2 | FREUD'S STAGES OF PSYCHOSEXUAL DEVELOPMENT | |
| --- | --- | --- |
| Stage | Age | Description |
| Oral | Birth to 18 months | Pleasure is derived primarily through sucking and eating |
| Anal | 18 months to 3 years | Control of muscles, especially those controlling urination and defecation |
| Phallic ("Oedipal") | 3 to 6 years | Awareness of sex and genitalia |
| Latency | 6 to 12 years | Exhibition of latent sexual development and energy |
| Genital | 12 years to adulthood | Emergence of sexual interests and development of relationships with potential sexual partners |

Data from Freud, S. (1961). *Civilization and its discontents.* New York: Norton.

## TABLE 17-3    ERIKSON'S STAGES OF PSYCHOSOCIAL DEVELOPMENT

| Stage | Age | Task to Be Achieved | Implications |
|---|---|---|---|
| Trust vs. Mistrust | Birth to 18 months | Develop a sense of trust in others | Consistent, affectionate care promotes successful mastery. Inadequate, inconsistent care produces an unfavorable outcome at this stage. |
| Autonomy vs. Shame and Doubt | 18 months to 3 years | Learn self-control | The child needs support, praise, and encouragement to use newly acquired skills of independence. Shaming or insulting the child will lead to unnecessary dependence. |
| Initiative vs. Guilt | 3 to 6 years | Initiate spontaneous activities | Give clear explanations for events and encourage creative activities. Threatening punishment or labeling behavior as "bad" leads to development of guilt and fears of doing wrong. |
| Industry vs. Inferiority | 6 to 12 years | Develop necessary social skills | To build confidence, recognize the child's accomplishments. Unrealistic expectation or excessively harsh criticism leads to a sense of inadequacy. |
| Identity vs. Role Diffusion | 12 to 20 years | Integrate childhood experiences into a personal identity | Help the adolescent make decisions. Encourage active participation in home events. Assist with planning for the future. |
| Intimacy vs. Isolation | 18 to 25 years | Develop commitments to others and to a life work (career) | Teach the young adult to establish realistic goals. Avoid ridiculing romances or job choices. |
| Generativity vs. Stagnation | 21 to 45 years | Establish a family and become productive | Provide emotional support. Recognize individual accomplishments and provide appropriate praise. |
| Integrity vs. Despair | 45+ years | View one's life as meaningful and fulfilling | Explore positive aspects of one's life. Review contributions made by the individual. |

Data from Erikson, E. (1963). *Childhood and society*. New York: Norton; Varcarolis, E., & Rader, I. (2002). *Foundations of psychiatric mental health nursing* (4th ed.). Philadelphia: Saunders.

## Cognitive Dimension

The cognitive dimension is characterized by the intellectual process of knowing, which includes perception, memory, and judgment, and develops as an individual progresses through the life span. Intelligence is an adaptive process. Individuals use intelligence to adapt by changing the environment to meet their needs and by altering their responses to environmental stressors. The ability to change behavior in response to the demands of an ever-changing environment is characteristic of intelligent beings.

Jean Piaget (1963) studied the differences between children's thinking patterns at different ages and how intelligence is used to solve problems and answer questions. He theorized that children learn to think by playing (Figure 17-3).

Piaget and Inhelder (1969) categorized intellectual development into four phases: sensorimotor, preoperational, concrete operations, and formal operations. Table 17-6 provides a description of each phase. Each phase is

## TABLE 17-4     HAVIGHURST'S DEVELOPMENTAL STAGES AND TASKS

| Developmental Stage | Developmental Task |
|---|---|
| Infancy and Early Childhood | Eat solid foods<br>Walk<br>Talk<br>Control elimination of wastes<br>Relate emotionally to others<br>Distinguish right from wrong through development of a conscience<br>Learn sex differences and sexual modesty<br>Achieve psychological stability<br>Form simple concepts of social and physical reality |
| Middle Childhood | Learn physical skills required for games<br>Build healthy attitudes toward oneself<br>Learn to socialize with peers<br>Learn appropriate masculine or feminine role<br>Gain basic reading, writing, and mathematical skills<br>Develop concepts necessary for everyday living<br>Formulate a conscience based on a value system<br>Achieve personal independence<br>Develop attitudes toward social groups and institutions |
| Adolescence | Establish more mature relationships with same-age individuals of both sexes<br>Achieve a masculine or feminine social role<br>Accept own body<br>Establish emotional independence from parents<br>Achieve assurance of economic independence<br>Prepare for an occupation<br>Prepare for marriage and establishment of a family<br>Acquire skills necessary to fulfill civic responsibilities<br>Develop a set of values that guides behavior |
| Early Adulthood | Select a partner<br>Learn to live with a partner<br>Start a family<br>Manage a home<br>Establish self in a career/occupation<br>Assume civic responsibility<br>Become a part of a social group |
| Middle Adulthood | Fulfill civic and social responsibilities<br>Maintain an economic standard of living<br>Assist adolescent children to become responsible, happy adults<br>Relate to one's partner<br>Adjust to physiological changes<br>Adjust to aging parents |
| Later Maturity | Adjust to physiological changes and alterations in health status<br>Adjust to retirement and altered income<br>Adjust to death of spouse<br>Develop affiliation with one's age group<br>Meet civic and social responsibilities<br>Establish satisfactory living arrangements |

Data from Havighurst, R. J. (1972). *Developmental tasks and education.* New York: Longman.

## TABLE 17-5    SULLIVAN'S INTERPERSONAL MODEL OF PERSONALITY DEVELOPMENT

| Stage | Age | Description |
|---|---|---|
| Infancy | Birth to 18 months | Infant learns to rely on caregivers to meet needs and desires. |
| Childhood | 18 months to 6 years | Child begins learning to delay immediate need for gratification of needs and desires. |
| Juvenile | 6 to 9 years | Child forms fulfilling peer relationships. |
| Preadolescence | 9 to 12 years | Child relates successfully to same-sex peers. |
| Early Adolescence | 12 to 14 years | Adolescent learns to be independent and forms relationships with members of opposite sex. |
| Late Adolescence | 14 to 21 years | Person establishes an intimate, long-lasting relationship with someone of the opposite sex. |

Data from Sullivan, H. S. (1953). *Interpersonal theory of psychiatry.* New York: Norton.

characterized by the ways in which the child interprets and uses the environment. Approximate ages are indicated for each phase, but there is great variation among individuals.

The individual learns by interacting with others and the environment through three processes: assimilation, accommodation, and adaptation. **Assimilation** is the process of taking in new experiences or information. **Accommodation** allows for readjustment of the cognitive structure (mindset) to take in the new information; thus, understanding is increased. **Adaptation** refers to the changes that occur as a result of assimilation and accommodation (Murray & Zentner, 2000; Oran, 2000).

## Moral Dimension

The moral dimension consists of a person's value system that helps in differentiating right and wrong. **Moral maturity** (the ability to independently decide for oneself what is "right") is closely related to emotional and cognitive development.

Piaget and Lawrence Kohlberg (1977) are among the main theorists who have studied the development of moral judgment. Piaget, who was more interested in the process of development than in time frames, theorized that children are *amoral* until the age of 7 when they move to the stage of *moral realism.* At this stage, actions are judged in concrete terms as totally right or totally wrong, based on the consequences of the action. In the stage of *autonomous morality,* during middle childhood or early adolescence, children are able to consider the intentions behind the action and the consequences. Later, in the formal operation stage, children are able to analyze a situation from different moral viewpoints (Oran, 2000). "Although Piaget's work is considered a major achievement, recent research suggests that he underestimated children's abilities" (Berger & Williams, 1999).

Lawrence Kohlberg (1977) established a framework for understanding how individuals determine a moral code to guide their behavior. Kohlberg's model states that a person's ability to make moral judgments and behave in a morally correct manner develops over a period of time.

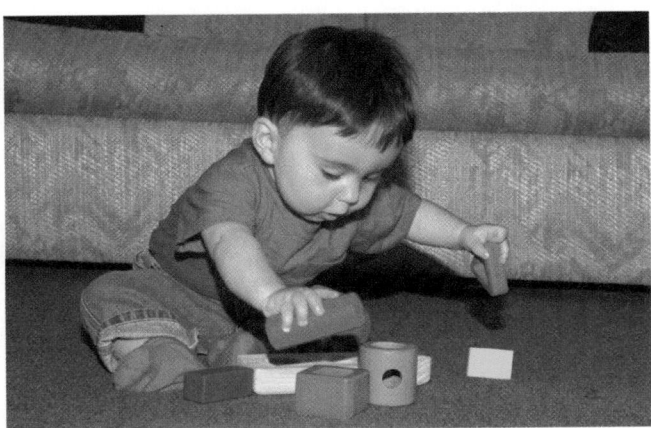

**Figure 17-3    A child's play is an important part of cognitive development.**

### CLINICAL ALERT

#### Therapeutic Play

Therapeutic play is specially designed play activities that help children express fears, conflicts, and feelings. This technique is especially useful with younger children who have not developed language skills to express feelings that commonly accompany illness, hospitalization, or traumatic situations.

Berger, K., & Williams, M. (1999). *Fundamentals of nursing: Collaborating for optimal health.* Stamford, CT: Appleton & Lange.

## TABLE 17-6   PIAGET'S PHASES OF COGNITIVE DEVELOPMENT

| Phase | Age | Description |
|---|---|---|
| **Sensorimotor** | **Birth to 2 years** | **Sensory organs and muscles become more functional** |
| Stage 1: Use of reflexes | Birth to 1 month | Movements are primarily reflexive |
| Stage 2: Primary circular reaction | 1 to 4 months | Perceptions center around one's body<br>Objects are perceived as extensions of the self |
| Stage 3: Secondary circular reaction | 4 to 8 months | Becomes aware of external environment<br>Initiates acts to change the environment |
| Stage 4: Coordination of secondary schemata | 8 to 12 months | Differentiates goals and goal-directed activities |
| Stage 5: Tertiary circular reaction | 12 to 18 months | Experiments with methods to reach goals<br>Develops rituals that become significant |
| Stage 6: Invention of new means | 18 to 24 months | Uses mental imagery to understand the environment<br>Uses fantasy ("make-believe") |
| **Preoperational** | **2 to 7 years** | **Emerging ability to think** |
| Preconceptual stage | 2 to 4 years | Thinking tends to be egocentric<br><br>Exhibits use of symbolism |
| Intuitive stage | 4 to 7 years | Unable to break down a whole into separate parts<br>Able to classify objects according to one trait |
| **Concrete Operations** | **7 to 11 years** | **Learns to reason about events in the here and now** |
| **Formal Operations** | **11+ years** | **Able to see relationships and to reason in the abstract** |

Data from Piaget, J. (1963). *The origins of intelligence in children.* New York: Norton.

Kohlberg identified three levels of morality: a preconventional level, based on obedience or punishment; a conventional level, or good-boy/nice-girl orientation; and a postconventional level when reasoning begins to focus on more abstract principles of right or wrong rather than on established moral rules. Within each level are various stages of development. Individuals move through five stages in a sequential fashion; however, not everyone reaches or goes beyond stage five, which is in the postconventional level (Oran, 2000). The levels and stages are summarized in Table 17-7.

## Spiritual Dimension

The spiritual dimension is characterized by a sense of personal meaning. **Spirituality** refers to relationships with one's self, with others, and with a higher power or divine source. Spirituality does not refer to a specific religious affiliation; rather, it can be defined as the core of a person. Development of spirituality is an ongoing, lifelong process.

Fowler's theory of spiritual development was influenced by the works of Erikson, Piaget, and Kohlberg. Fowler's theory is composed of a pre-stage and six distinct stages of faith development (Fowler, 1981). Even though

 **STOP AND THINK**

### Spiritual Awareness

The term *spirit* is derived from the Latin word meaning breath, air, and wind. Thus, *spirit* refers to whatever gives life to a person. What animates you? What is the core of your spirituality (life force)? The answers to these questions are truly individual. Remember that each client has a personalized definition of the spiritual self, even though some clients seem to be unaware of their spiritual nature.

## TABLE 17-7   KOHLBERG'S STAGES OF MORAL DEVELOPMENT

| Level and Stage | Description |
| --- | --- |
| **Level I: Preconventional** | **Authority figures are obeyed** (self-centered orientation) |
| Age 4 to 10 years | Misbehavior is viewed in terms of damage done. |
| *Stage 1:* Punishment and obedience orientation | A deed is perceived as "wrong" if one is punished; the activity is "right" if one is not punished. |
| *Stage 2:* Hedonistic and instrumental orientation | "Right" is defined as that which is acceptable to and approved by the self. When actions satisfy one's needs, they are "right." |
| **Level II: Conventional** | **Cordial interpersonal relationships are maintained.** (able to see victim's perspective) |
| Age 10 to 13, but can go into adolescence | Approval of others is sought through one's actions. |
| *Stage 3:* Good boy/girl orientation | Authority is respected. |
| *Stage 4:* Law-and-order orientation | Individual feels "duty-bound" to maintain social order. Behavior is "right" when it conforms to the rules. |
| **Level III: Postconventional** | **Individual understands the morality of having democratically established laws.** (underlying ethical principles are considered that include societal needs) |
| Adolescence and beyond | |
| *Stage 5:* Social contract orientation | It is "wrong" to violate others' rights. |
| *Stage 6:* Hierarchy of principles orientation | Judgments based on principles of justice, respect for dignity of human beings as individuals—Do to others as you would have them do to you. |

Adapted from Kohlberg, L. (1977). *Recent research in moral development.* New York: Holt Rinehart & Winston; Oran, D. (2000). Children and adolescents. In K. Fortinash & P. Holoday-Worret (Eds.). *Psychiatric mental health nursing* (2nd ed.). St. Louis: C.V. Mosby.

the ages at which individuals experience each stage will vary, the sequence of stages remains the same. Table 17-8 describes Fowler's theory.

Table 17-9 provides a comparison of the major concepts of the developmental theories.

# Holistic Framework for Nursing

Basic concepts of holistic professional nursing include consideration of the "wholeness" of individuals and supporting them in assuming responsibility for self-care. Growth and development patterns are predictable dynamic processes throughout life, yet remain uniquely different among individuals. Developmental progress, or lack of progress, in one aspect affects all other dimensions of life. The interacting dimensions of the holistic nature of individuals are depicted in Figure 17-4. Knowledge of growth and development concepts is essential in anticipating common health needs during specific stages of development, in understanding human responses to health problems and their effects on development, and in planning involvement of children and their families in making

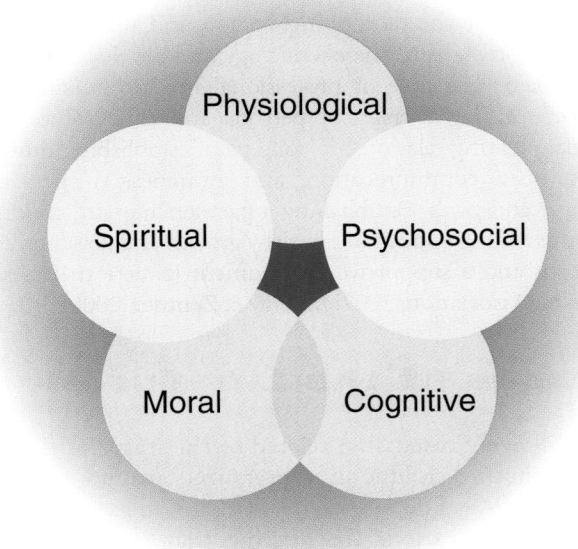

**Figure 17-4   Holistic nature of human beings**

## TABLE 17-8    FOWLER'S STAGES OF FAITH

| Stage | Age | Characteristics |
|---|---|---|
| Pre-Stage: *Undifferentiated faith* | Infant | Trust, hope, and love compete with environmental inconsistencies or threats of abandonment |
| Stage 1: *Intuitive-projective faith* | Toddler-preschooler | Imitates parental behaviors and attitudes about religion and spirituality |
| | | Has no real understanding of spiritual concepts |
| Stage 2: *Mythical-literal faith* | School-aged child | Accepts existence of a deity |
| | | Religious and moral beliefs are symbolized by stories |
| | | Appreciates others' viewpoints |
| | | Accepts concept of reciprocal fairness |
| Stage 3: *Synthetic-conventional faith* | Adolescent | Questions values and religious beliefs in an attempt to form own identity |
| Stage 4: *Individuative-reflective faith* | Late adolescent and young adult | Assumes responsibility for own attitudes and beliefs |
| Stage 5: *Conjunctive faith* | Adult | Integrates other perspectives about faith into own definition of truth |
| Stage 6: *Universalizing faith* | Adult | Makes concepts of love and justice tangible |

Data from Fowler, J. W. (1981). *Stages of faith: The psychology of human development and the quest for meaning.* New York: Harper & Row; Mohr, W. (2002). *Johnson's psychiatric-mental health nursing* (5th ed.). Philadelphia: Lippincott.

health care decisions. This knowledge also provides the basis for client education and nursing interventions to support healthy behaviors. Additional critical aspects of holistic nursing include considering the family as the basic unit for the developing person and tailoring communication skills to the client's age and development.

A major principle of professional holistic nursing is a respect for the diversity of persons and their values and beliefs. A caring relationship consists of establishing mutual trust, open communication, and awareness of personal motives and goals. Establishing a partnership with children and their families facilitates healthy growth and development patterns and a supportive environment (American Holistic Nursing Association, 2002; Murray & Zentner, 2000).

## Stages of the Life Cycle

The following discussion related to the stages of the life cycle denoting childhood is organized around the relevant growth and development information for each stage and the implications for nursing that include assessment, wellness promotion, safety precautions, the individual's responses to common health problems, and client education.

## Prenatal Period

The **prenatal period** (the developmental stage beginning with conception and ending with birth) is a critical time in a human being's development and consists of three developmental phases: the germinal, embryonic, and fetal stages. The **germinal stage** begins with conception and lasts approximately 10 to 14 days. This stage is characterized by rapid cell division and implantation of the fertilized egg in the uterine wall. In this very early stage, the CNS is already beginning to form.

## CLINICAL ALERT

### Media Health Information

The nurse must be keenly aware of the media health information that is available to the public. Some of the information, particularly on the Internet, may be misleading yet readily accepted as factual.

Potts, N., & Mandleco, B. (2002). *Pediatric nursing: Caring for children and their families.* Clifton Park, NY: Delmar Learning.

## TABLE 17-9    COMPARISON OF MAJOR CONCEPTS OF DEVELOPMENTAL THEORIES RELATED TO CHILDHOOD

| Theories | Freud Psychosexual Development | Erikson Psychosocial Development | Havighurst Developmental Stages and Tasks | Sullivan Personality Development | Piaget Cognitive Development | Kohlberg Moral Development | Fowler Stages of Faith |
|---|---|---|---|---|---|---|---|
| **Development Stage** | **Oral Stage** *Id* | **Trust vs. Mistrust** | **(Infant to early childhood)** | Infancy | **Sensiomotor stages 1–6 (Birth to 2 yrs.)** | **Preconventional (Birth to 9 yrs.)** | **Pre-stage Undifferentiated faith** |
| Birth to 18 Months | Oral activities provide major pleasures. Selfish: Unable to delay gratification of needs. | Develops sense of trust in others. A sense of self begins to develop. Separation anxiety occurs at approximately 6 months. | Crawl, walk, talk, eat solid foods. | Interpersonal relationships. Relies on caregivers to meet needs and desires. | Develops function of sensory organs and muscles. Develops rituals that become significant. | Level 1: Misbehavior is viewed in terms of damage done. Deed is wrong if child receives punishment; activity is right if one is not punished. | Trust/hope/love compete with environmental inconsistencies or threats of abandonment. |
| 18 months to 3 yrs. | **Anal Stage** *Ego* Gains control over elimination. | **Autonomy vs. Shame/Doubt** Learns self-control. | Progress in earlier tasks. Control of elimination needs. Relates emotionally to others. | **(Childhood to 18 months to 6 yrs.)** Learns to delay gratification of immediate needs. Identifies "Good Me" "Bad Me" "Not Me." | Uses mental imagery to understand the environment. Uses fantasy/make-believe. | **Preconventional** Level 2: Something is right if it satisfies personal needs. | **Stage 1: Intuitive-Projective Faith** Imitates parents. No real understanding of spiritual concepts. |

*(continues)*

## TABLE 17-9 COMPARISON OF MAJOR CONCEPTS OF DEVELOPMENTAL THEORIES RELATED TO CHILDHOOD (continued)

| Theories | Freud Psychosexual Development | Erikson Psychosocial Development | Havighurst Developmental Stages and Tasks | Sullivan Personality Development | Piaget Cognitive Development | Kohlberg Moral Development | Fowler Stages of Faith |
|---|---|---|---|---|---|---|---|
| 3 to 6 yrs. | **Phallic Stage** (Oedipal/Electra complex) *Superego* Learns values and rules from parents. Development of self-esteem. Awareness of gender and genitalia. | **Initiative vs. Guilt** Initiates spontaneous activities. | Development of conscience. Learns sex differences and gender modesty. Forms simple concepts of social and physical reality. | Progress in developmental tasks. | **Pre-operational** (2 to 7 yrs.) Thinking tends to be egocentric. Exhibits use of symbolism. | Level 2 (cont'd.) Progress in development of skills. | Stage 1 (cont'd) Progress in development of beliefs. |
| Development Stage | Latency | **Industry vs. Inferiority** | **(Middle Childhood)** | **Juvenile (6–9) Preadolescent (9 to 12 yrs.)** | **Concrete Operations (7 to 11 yrs.)** | **Level 2 Conventional** | **Mythical-literal faith** |
| 6 to 12 yrs. | Lack of sexual development and energy. (This has been disputed by later research noting sexuality is expressed throughout life.) | Develop necessary social skills. | Learns physical skills and healthy self-identity. Learns to socialize with peers. Learns appropriate male and female roles. Reads, writes. Develops conscience and value system. | Forms fulfilling peer relationships. Relates successfully to same-sex peers. | Progress in development. Learns to reason about current happenings/events. | Seeks approval and respect. Authority is respected. Obeys rules. | Accepts existence of a deity. Religious and moral beliefs symbolized by stories. Appreciates others' viewpoints. |

(continues)

## TABLE 17-9   COMPARISON OF MAJOR CONCEPTS OF DEVELOPMENTAL THEORIES RELATED TO CHILDHOOD (continued)

| Theories | Freud Psychosexual Development | Erikson Psychosocial Development | Havighurst Developmental Stages and Tasks | Sullivan Personality Development | Piaget Cognitive Development | Kohlberg Moral Development | Fowler Stages of Faith |
|---|---|---|---|---|---|---|---|
| 12 to 18 or 20 yrs. | Genital Stage (12 yrs. to adulthood)<br><br>Mastery of learning. Emergence of sex interests. Develops relationships with potential sex partners. | Identity vs. Role Differentiation (12 to 20 yrs.)<br><br>Integrates childhood experiences into personal identity. | Adolescence<br><br>More mature relationships. Develops gender identity. Becoming independent from parents. Preparation for occupation and adult roles. Has a set of values. | Early/Late Adolescence (12 to 14 yrs. and 14 to 21 yrs.)<br><br>Independent relationships with members of opposite sex. Establishes intimate, long-lasting relationship with someone of opposite sex. | Formal Operational Stage<br><br>Able to see relationships and reason abstractly. | Post-Conventional Stage<br><br>Understands morality of established laws. | Individual-Reflective Faith<br><br>Assumes responsibility for own attitudes and beliefs. |

**BOX 17-1    HEALTHY PEOPLE 2010 REPORT**

Statistical indicators of a healthy population include:

- Physical activity
- Overweight/obesity
- Tobacco use
- Substance abuse
- Responsible sexual behavior
- Mental health
- Injury and violence
- Environmental quality
- Immunizations

The nurse plays a primary role in health promotion and education. Consider these indicators as you learn about the stages of childhood. During which developmental stage is a child most vulnerable to specific indicators?

U.S. Department of Health and Human Services (2000). *Healthy People 2010 Report*. Washington, DC: Author.

The **embryonic stage** (the first 2 to 8 weeks after fertilization of an egg by a sperm) is characterized by rapid cellular differentiation, growth, and development of the body systems. This critical period is when the embryo is most vulnerable to noxious stimuli, which may lead to a spontaneous abortion (miscarriage) (Murray & Zentner, 2000).

The **fetal stage** (the intrauterine developmental period from 8 weeks to birth) is characterized by rapid growth and differentiation of body systems and parts. Table 17-10 provides an overview of fetal development.

## Nursing Implications

Common health problems during the prenatal period are related to the mother's lifestyle choices, physical and emotional health, nutritional status, and use of prenatal care (Littleton & Engebretson, 2002). The pregnant woman needs to have physical examinations and screenings during the entire pregnancy. Early prenatal care is essential for a positive pregnancy outcome.

Learning that one is pregnant may stimulate several emotions: happiness, fear, sadness, excitement, and anxiety. Emotions lead to alterations in biochemicals; therefore, the mother's emotional state can bring about biochemical changes in the fetus. By teaching pregnant women how to relax, the nurse can promote a supportive environment for the developing embryo and fetus.

### Wellness Promotion

The uterus is the primary environment affecting prenatal growth and development. Ideally, this environment nurtures positive growth of the embryo and fetus.

An ample supply of nutrients must be provided by the gestating woman. Women who consume insufficient amounts of protein during pregnancy have a high rate of giving birth to premature and low birth-weight infants. Such infants are at risk for developmental alterations.

When teaching the pregnant woman about nutrition, the nurse must emphasize that vitamin supplements are *not* to be substituted for adequate intake of food. Other nursing interventions that promote prenatal health include:

- Screening (blood pressure measurement, urine sugar analysis)
- Teaching (nutritional guidelines)
- Counseling (e.g., guidance about bonding with the child and incorporating a child into a family unit)
- Promoting the use of complementary/alternative modalities to reduce stress
- Working with economically disadvantaged clients to obtain prenatal care

(See the annotated listing of Websites at the end of the chapter for an excellent educational video program on prenatal development that is appropriate for the professional and the public.)

### Safety Considerations

The fetus is especially vulnerable to substances consumed by the mother during the first trimester. In addition to providing the fetus with wholesome nutrients, maternal blood can also transport toxins.

Cigarettes contain several toxic substances, such as nicotine, that cross the placental barrier and interfere with the transport of oxygen to the fetus. Such toxins often result in increased risk of premature birth, retarded growth, learning difficulties, and fetal death.

Use of alcohol during pregnancy can result in **fetal alcohol syndrome (FAS)**, a condition in which fetal development is impaired and is manifested in the infant by characteristic physical attributes and intellectual problems. Typically, FAS infants are small, have facial abnormalities (such as thin upper lips and short, upturned noses), and may have some degree of brain damage. Alcohol consumption is most dangerous during the first 3 months of pregnancy when the embryo's brain and other vital organs are developing. The effects of alcohol on the fetus are permanent. FAS is considered to be the leading cause of mental retardation among infants, and the incidence continues to increase (Hockenberry, 2003) (Figure 17-5).

In addition to nicotine and alcohol, there are many other teratogenic substances. A **teratogenic substance** is any substance that can cross the placental barrier and impair normal growth and development.

## TABLE 17-10    EMBRYO AND FETUS: GROWTH AND DEVELOPMENT

| Age | Characteristics |
| --- | --- |
| Weeks 1 to 3 | Rapid cell differentiation<br>Heart starts to pulsate<br>CNS formation<br>Presence of all organs |
| Week 4 | Beginnings of respiratory system<br>Basic structures for eyes and ears<br>Limb buds distinguishable |
| Week 5 | Embryo has a C-shaped body with a tail and large head<br>Each body system present in at least a rudimentary form<br>Umbilical cord developed<br>Brain vesicles developed<br>Nerve tissues more fully developed |
| Week 6 | Establishment of circulatory pathway (including heart with septa)<br>Limbs distinguishable as arms and legs<br>Intestine elongating<br>Lungs formed, with bronchi beginning to branch out<br>Liver begins production of blood cells |
| Week 9 | Fingers, toes, eyelids, nose, and jaw evident |
| Week 12 | Body growth speeds up while growth of head slows |
| Week 16 | Ossification of skeleton begins<br>Fingers and toes separated |
| Week 20 | Fetal movement felt by mother<br>Wake and sleep cycles evident<br>Formation of small amounts of body fat |
| Week 24 | Circulation of blood in vessels is visible<br>Accelerated weight gain<br>Ovaries/testes developed<br>Kidney tubules branch out<br>Brain grows rapidly |
| Week 28 | Eyes open and close<br>Thick hair on head<br>Lanugo (thick coating of body hair) is present<br>Rhythmic breathing patterns begin to be established |
| Week 32 | Maturation of respiratory system and temperature-regulating mechanism<br>Fat deposited in arms and legs<br>Fingernails and toenails present |
| Week 36 | Protrusion of mammary glands in both sexes<br>Lack of melanin leads to white skin in all fetuses at this stage |
| Week 40 | Completion of fetal development<br>Fetus is ready for extrauterine environment<br>Optimal time for birth |

Data from Guyton, A. C., & Hall, J. (2001). *Textbook of medical physiology* (10th ed.). Philadelphia: Saunders; Hockenberry, M., Wilson, D., Winkelstein, M., & Kline, N. (2003). *Wong's nursing care of infants and children* (7th ed.). St. Louis: Mosby-Yearbook.

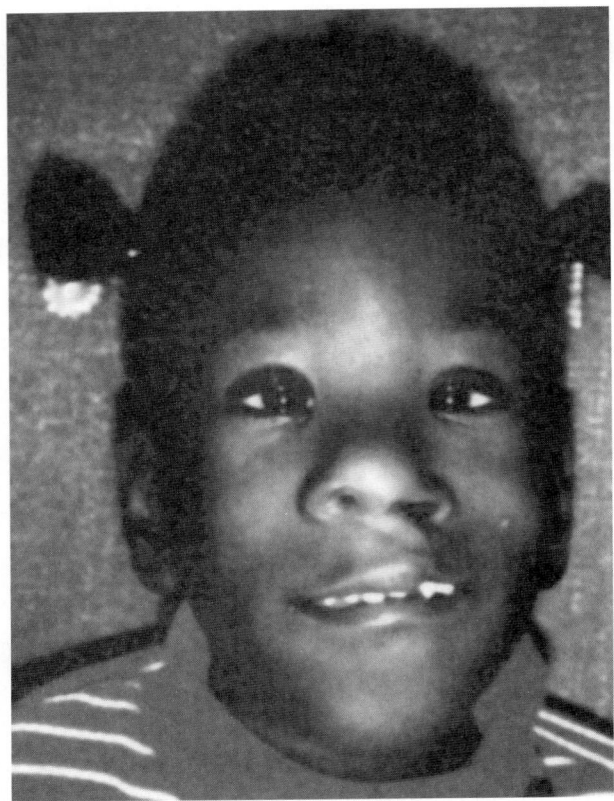

**Figure 17-5 Young girl with fetal alcohol syndrome—in this case the mother drank heavily from the onset of conception**

Client education consists of teaching pregnant women to check labels of *all* medicines for information about potential effects on the fetus. The Food and Drug Administration requires that all manufactured drugs list their potential for causing birth defects. The use of illegal drugs by pregnant women presents a very serious threat to the unborn. Substance abuse prevention programs can be effective in preventing or reducing this risk.

## Neonate

The **neonatal period** (the first 28 days of life following birth) is a time of major adjustment to extrauterine life. The energies of the neonate (newborn) are focused on achieving equilibrium through stabilization of major body systems. Table 17-11 describes neonatal development.

### CLINICAL ALERT

### Tobacco and Alcohol Use During Pregnancy

Total abstinence from cigarette smoking is advised during pregnancy. Because there has been no determination of "safe" amounts of alcohol consumption, caution all pregnant women to avoid drinking alcohol.

The neonate's activities, which are reflexive in nature, consist primarily of sucking, crying, eliminating, and sleeping (Figure 17-6). The neonate blinks in response to bright lights and demonstrates the startle reflex in response to loud noises. Neonatal reflexes play a major role in the ability to survive. Table 17-12 lists the reflexive activities of the neonate.

During the first month of life, the neonate progresses developmentally from a mass of reflexes to behavior that is more goal directed (purposeful). In addition to the major physiological adjustments necessitated by extrauterine life, the neonate also undergoes psychological adaptation.

The major psychological task of neonates is to adjust to the parental figures. **Bonding**, the formation of attachment between parent and child, begins at birth when the neonate and parent make initial eye contact. The quality of parent-neonate bonding lays the foundation for trust that is necessary for the development of future interpersonal relationships. Figure 17-7 shows bonding between neonate and parent.

### Nursing Implications

Common health problems for the neonate that may or may not affect growth and development include colic, diaper rash, and regurgitation. Responses to illness may include irritability and changes in feeding, sleep patterns, and elimination.

A complete and thorough assessment of the neonate, which is performed immediately after delivery, includes evaluation of the neonate's reflexes. In addition to focusing on the reflexes, the assessment also evaluates respiratory and cardiac functioning. Table 17-13 shows the Apgar assessment tool that is performed by the nurse at 1 minute and again at 5 minutes after birth.

In the first few hours after birth, encourage the parents to cuddle the newborn. Explain the neonate's interactive abilities. Encourage mutual eye contact between neonate and parents by showing parents how to hold the child face to face. In addition, the neonate must be evaluated for any abnormalities, such as thrush.

### Wellness Promotion

Teaching is one of the most important nursing activities promoting neonatal wellness. First-time parents need information about basic newborn needs (to be held, rocked, and talked to), nutrition, infection control (especially hand washing and hygienic diaper changing practices), care of the umbilicus, and incorporating the newborn into the family unit. Knowledge of growth and development milestones is necessary for parents to provide appropriate neonatal stimulation and have realistic expectations.

Other nursing interventions that promote neonatal wellness are listed below:

• Continually assessing the neonate's physiological status
• Providing a warm environment (neonates breathe more easily when they are warm)

**TABLE 17-11    NEONATE: GROWTH AND DEVELOPMENT**

| Dimension | Characteristics | Nursing Implications |
|---|---|---|
| *Physiological* | Circulatory function shifts from the umbilical cord to heart. | Accurately assess neonate's cardiovascular status. |
| | Gas exchange (oxygen and carbon dioxide) is transferred from placenta to lungs. Seconds after birth, respiratory reflexes are activated. | Immediately after birth, hold the neonate with head lower than body to allow for drainage of fluids that may block respiratory passages.<br><br>If spontaneous respirations do not occur, resuscitate immediately. |
| | Weak neck and shoulder muscles. | Carefully support the neonate's head. |
| | Immature temperature-regulating mechanism. | To conserve heat:<br>• Dry neonate immediately after birth and place in a warmed bassinet.<br>• Place a stockinette cap on neonate's head. |
| | Incomplete ossification (process of cartilage changing to bone). | Protect the anterior fontanelle on neonate's skull. |
| | Poor visual acuity; visual focus is generally rigid. | Instruct parents to be directly in front of the neonate (about 9 to 12 inches away from child's face) when communicating. |
| *Motor* | Reflexes direct the majority of movement. | |
| | The full-term neonate has some limited ability to hold the head erect. | Support neck and head when lifting. |
| | Able to lift head slightly when lying prone. | |
| *Psychosocial* | Crying is the neonate's method of communication. There is a reason for the cry. | Teach parents about the dynamics of crying to avoid having the neonate labeled as "fussy" or the parents developing the misconception that they are inadequate caregivers.<br><br>Encourage parents to learn to discriminate crying patterns. |
| | The bonding process begins shortly after birth. | Teach parents the importance of interacting with the neonate during every contact (feeding, bathing, changing, cuddling). |
| *Cognitive* | Neonates learn through sensory experiences. | To promote learning, encourage parents to provide frequent sensory stimuli (touching, talking, looking the neonate in the eyes). |
| | Learning is enhanced by an environment that provides stimuli without bombarding the neonate. | |
| | Learning occurs by repeated exposure to stimuli. | |

Data from Fuller, J., & Schaller-Ayers, J. (1999). *Health assessment: A nursing approach* (3rd ed.). Philadelphia: Lippincott; Murray, R. B., & Zentner, J. P. (2000). *Nursing assessment and health promotion through the lifespan* (7th ed.). New Jersey: Prentice Hall; Hockenberry, M., et al. (2003). *Wong's nursing care of infants and children* (7th ed.). St. Louis: Mosby-Yearbook.

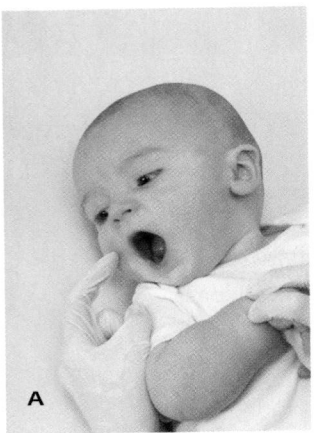
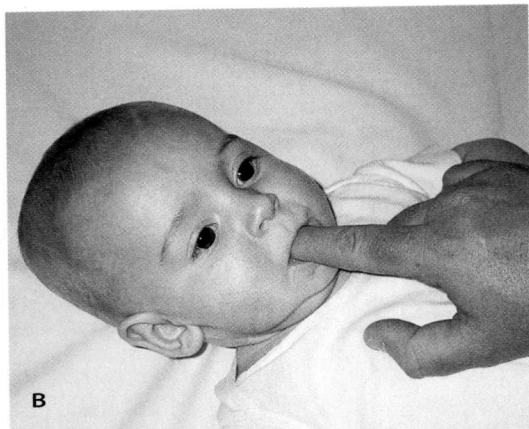
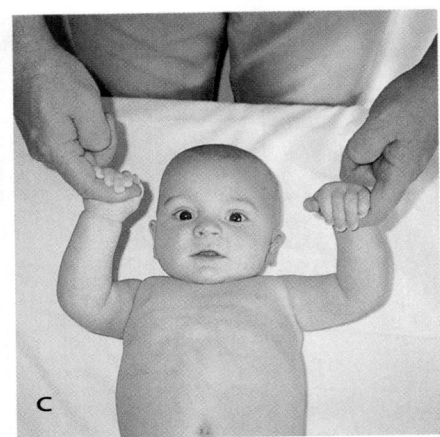
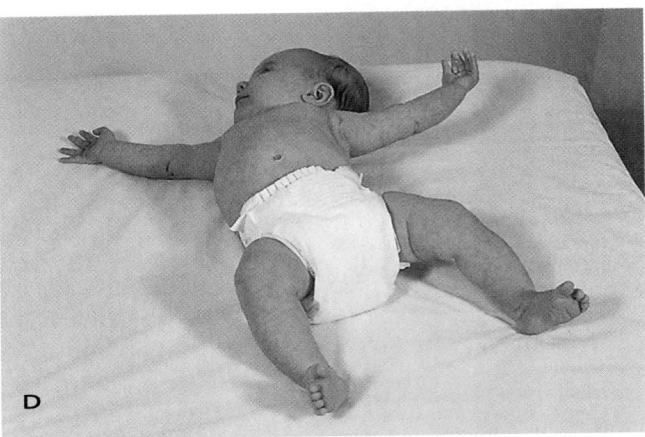
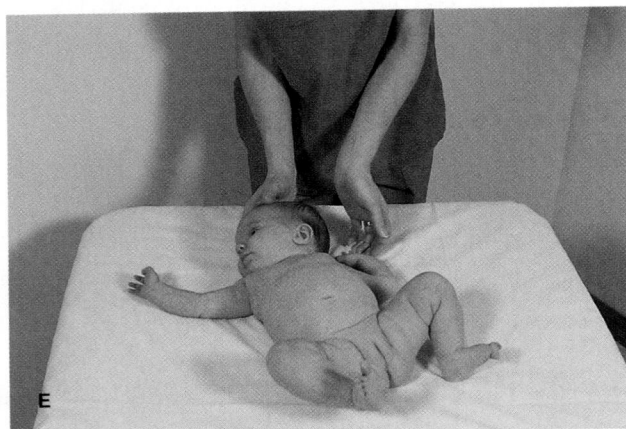

**Figure 17-6    Selected neonatal reflexes: A, rooting; B, sucking; C, grasp; D, Moro; E, tonic neck**

- Monitoring nutritional status. It is normal for neonates to lose weight (up to 10% of birth weight) during the first week of life.
- Providing a clean environment to protect neonates from infection, and teaching parents that neonates need a clean environment, not a sterile one
- Conducting screening tests; for example, the blood test for **phenylketonuria (PKU)**, a genetic disorder that, if untreated, can lead to impaired intellectual functioning
- Promoting *early* parent-neonate interaction

Selection of a feeding method for the neonate is a major decision for parents. Breastfeeding is one option. Commercially prepared formula is also available. For a comparison of feeding methods, see the discussion about nutrition for the infant.

## Safety Considerations

Safety is of primary concern when caring for neonates because neonates are totally dependent on others to meet their needs. Accidents are the primary cause of neonatal mortality (Fuller & Schaller-Ayers, 1999).

One of the most important neonatal accident prevention methods is to teach parents about the use of infant car seats. Under current federal law, neonates and infants must be secured in an approved infant car seat *every* time the child travels in a car. The infant car seat must be placed in the back seat facing the rear of the car, and be correctly fastened by the vehicle's seat belt.

In addition to accidents, infections pose a serious health risk to the neonate. Newborns should not be in contact with anyone experiencing an infectious disease. The skin is the body's major defense against invasion by disease-producing microorganisms; therefore, it is essential that the neonate's skin integrity be maintained. Parents must be taught the importance of skin cleanliness. Diaper rash is a common skin problem for newborns and infants because of the ammonia from urine in wet diapers. The ammonia burns and irritates the skin, resulting in localized irritation, blisters, or fissures. In addition to prompt changing of wet diapers, bathing and use of pro-

### CLINICAL ALERT

#### Neonatal Reflexes

A complete assessment of neonatal reflexes should be performed immediately after birth or as soon as the neonate is physiologically stable (Table 17-12).

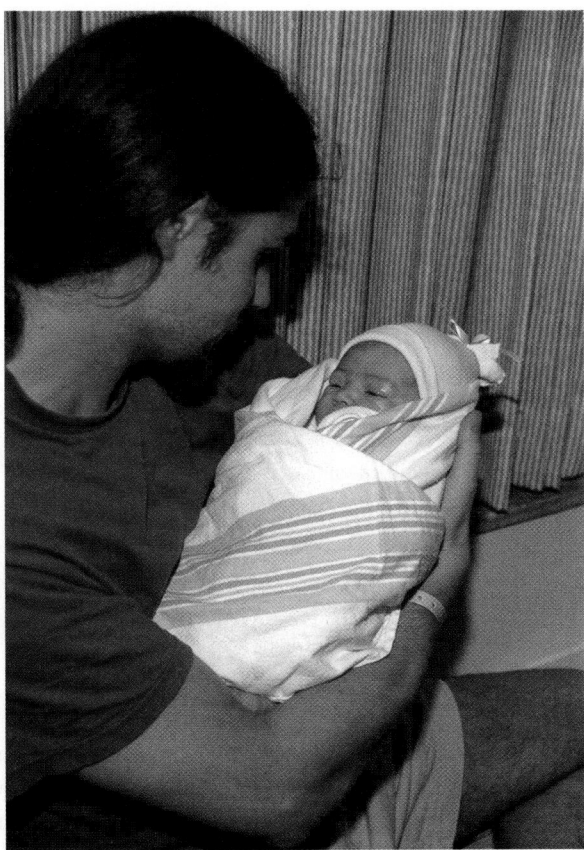

**Figure 17-7** Bonding between a parent and neonate; consider the factors that may have an impact on the early attachment between this father and daughter.

tective creams are useful in preventing skin breakdown. See Chapter 26 for a complete discussion of safety considerations and infections control practices.

## Infant

**Infancy** (the developmental stage from the first month to the first year of life) is a time of continued adaptation. During this stage, the infant experiences rapid physiologic growth and psychosocial development (Figure 17-8). Table 17-14 provides an overview of infant development in the physical, motor, psychosocial, cognitive, moral, and spiritual dimensions.

### Nursing Implications

The nurse caring for an infant must focus on safety, prevention of infection, and teaching parents about incorporating the child into the family. Teaching parents and other caregivers about developmental milestones is essential. Nursing care involves the provision of support, reassurance, and information to the parents.

Common health problems for infants include low birth weight, lack of prenatal care, poverty, infections, and accidents. Infants express their needs by crying and fussing; they may change their feeding and activity levels, be more

| TABLE 17-12 | MAJOR NEONATAL REFLEXES |
|---|---|
| Reflex | Description |
| Rooting | Turning the mouth and nose in the direction of any facial touch |
| Sucking | Using the tongue and mouth to take in liquid or food |
| Swallowing | Movement of throat muscles to push food from mouth to esophagus |
| Grasp | Firm contraction of hand muscles around an object |
| Babinski | When foot stroked, toes fan upward and outward |
| Moro | When startled, arms and legs swing quickly out, then immediately back and neonate curls up into a ball |
| Smiling | Turning lips upward; neonate looks "happy" |
| Blinking | Rapid closing and opening of eyelids |
| Sneezing | A violent, spasmodic, sudden expiration of breath |
| Coughing | Explosively expelling air from the lungs |
| Crying | Making a loud, wailing sound |
| Tonic neck | When head is turned to side, arm and leg on same side are extended in a fencing posture |
| Extrusion | Tongue pushes outward when touched by an object at the tip |
| Head turning | Moving face to one side or the other when airway is blocked by a surface, such as a bed or pillow |

"fussy" when they have an elevated temperature and may "splint" (hold or protect) a body part that is painful (Berger & Williams, 1999).

### Wellness Promotion

Nurses promote infant wellness by teaching growth and development concepts to parents and other caregivers. Knowledge of the type of behavior to expect at certain times during infancy serves as both guidance and reassurance for parents. Three specific areas in which parents need guidance

## TABLE 17-13    APGAR ASSESSMENT TOOL

| Sign | Value 0 | 1 | 2 |
|---|---|---|---|
| Heart rate | Absent | Less than 100 beats per minute | Over 100 beats per minute |
| Respiratory effort | Absent | Slow and irregular | Crying |
| Muscle tone | Flaccid | Some flexion of extremities | Active movement |
| Reflex irritability | No response | Weak cry or grimace | Vigorous cry |
| Color | Blue or pale | Pink body, cyanotic extremities | Entire body is pink |

The neonate is rated in each of the above categories. The rating for each category is totaled. A score of 7–10 indicates normal function; a score of 4–6 indicates that neonate needs special assistance; and a score of less than 4 indicates the neonate's need for *immediate* life-sustaining measures.

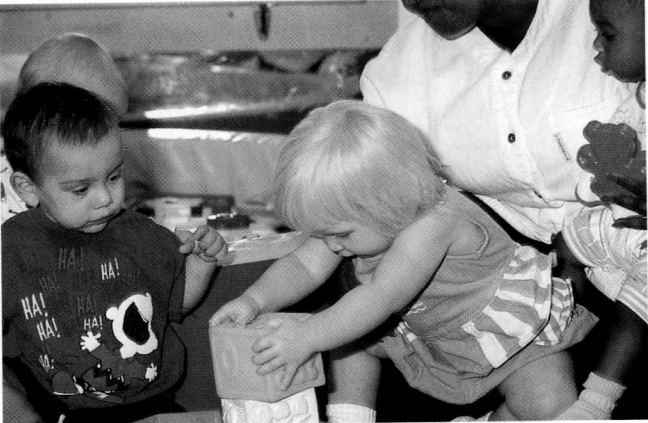

**Figure 17-8** These children are exploring their world and demonstrating mastery of both the physiological and cognitive dimensions of their development.

from the nurse in caring for their infants are nutrition, protection from infection, and promotion of sleep.

A major factor influencing health maintenance of the infant is the provision of adequate nutrients delivered in a loving, consistent manner. Caregivers should be taught that the nutrients must be germ free and provide the recommended amounts of carbohydrates, protein, calcium, iron, and vitamins. The American Academy of Pediatrics recommends that infants be breastfed for the first 6 to 12 months (Murray & Zentner, 2000). The act of breastfeeding promotes maternal-infant bonding (Hockenberry et al., 2003).

Breastmilk has several benefits over commercially prepared formulas, including:

- Offers immunologic benefits (e.g., contains immunoglobulins, lymphocytes, and other bacteria growth retardants)
- Is more easily digested because of smaller curds than those in cow's milk and formula

### CLINICAL ALERT

#### Shaken-Baby Syndrome

Crying is a form of communication by the neonate and infant. Incessant crying can be very frustrating to new parents or those who are unable to meet an infant's needs. Shaking an infant can cause brain damage, blindness, mental retardation, or death. Teaching positive parenting skills and stress management is an essential factor in prevention of shaken-baby syndrome. A careful screening of child-care providers is also necessary (McPeck, 2002).

### NURSING STRATEGY

#### Infant Dermatitis

Diaper dermatitis is the most common contact dermatitis in infants from 4 to 12 months of age, and can lead to secondary fungal and bacterial infections. Teach parents to avoid using baby wipes for infants with diaper dermatitis. The alcohol content in the wipes can exacerbate the condition. Diapers should be changed as soon as the infant is wet or at least every 2 hours during the day and once during the night. Avoid use of tight diapers and waterproof pants. Protect skin with A & D ointment, zinc oxide, or other approved products. When using cornstarch or other powders, keep them away from the infant's face. Place infant on absorbable pad, and expose the diaper area to air from time to time to aid in healing.

Potts, N., & Mandleco, B. (2002). *Pediatric nursing: Caring for children and their families.* Clifton Park, NY: Delmar Learning.

## TABLE 17-14   INFANT: GROWTH AND DEVELOPMENT

| Dimension | Characteristics | Nursing Implications |
|---|---|---|
| Physiological | Physical growth is rapid. Birth weight usually triples by end of first year. Height increases by approximately 50%. | Inform parents of the developmental norms. |
| | Progressive maturation of all body systems | Encourage parents to have "well-baby checkups" as recommended. |
| | Body temperature stabilizes. | |
| | Heart rate slows (approximately 80 to 130 beats per minute). | |
| | Blood pressure rises. | |
| | At approximately 4 to 6 months, eruption of teeth begins. | |
| | Rapid growth of brain (reaches about half the adult size) | |
| | Posterior fontanel closes at approximately 2 months. | Protect infant's skull. |
| | Eyes begin to focus. | |
| Motor | Physical maturation allows for development of motor skills. | Teach parents anticipated ages for motor skill development. |
| | Primitive reflexes are replaced by movement that is more voluntary and goal directed. | |
| | Motor skills develop rapidly:<br>    6 months: rolls over voluntarily<br>    6 to 7 months: crawls<br>    8 months: sits alone | |
| | Grasping objects is reflexive for first 2 to 3 months and gradually becomes voluntary. | |
| Psychosocial | *Freud:* Oral stage | Seeks immediate gratification of needs; receives pleasure and comfort through mouth, lips, and tongue. |
| | *Erikson:* Trust vs. mistrust | Encourage parents to feed in a prompt, consistent manner (feed on demand rather than a fixed schedule). |
| | A sense of self begins to develop. | |
| | Responds to caregiver's voice | Other activities that promote trust are providing warmth, diapering, and comforting. |
| | Separation anxiety occurs at approximately 6 months. | |
| | *Havighurst:*<br>Learns to eat solid food, crawl, walk, and talk | Teach parents approximate ages that developmental milestones are expected to occur. |
| Cognitive | *Piaget:* Sensorimotor stage | Encourage parents to provide a variety of sensory stimuli: visual, sensory, auditory, and tactile (e.g., colorful mobiles; musical toys; soft plush animals; rubbing, patting, stroking the infant's skin) |
| | Infant learns by interacting with the environment. | |
| | Language development includes babbling, repetition, and imitation. | Caregivers need to talk to infant often. |
| | | Encourage caregivers to name objects that are the focus of the infant's attention. |
| Moral | *Kohlberg:* Preconventional stage | Teach parents that now is the time to start teaching (by role modeling) the difference between "right" and "wrong." |
| Spiritual | *Fowler:* Stage of undifferentiated faith | Encourage caregivers to model the values they want the infant to learn. |

Data from Murray, R. B., & Zentner, J. P. (2000). *Health promotion strategies through the life span* (7th ed.). New Jersey: Prentice Hall; Hockenberry, M., et al. (2003). *Wong's nursing care of infants and children* (7th ed.). St. Louis: Mosby-Yearbook.

## CLINICAL ALERT

### Cow's Milk

Whole cow's milk is not recommended for infants under age 1 year. Human milk and commercially prepared formula are more easily digested.

- Enhances absorption of fat and calcium
- Is readily available and economical

Nurses must be aware that there are some cultural sanctions against breastfeeding, and some cultures view bottle-feeding as a status symbol.

Normal growth and development can occur without breastfeeding. Special formulas are available for infants who are hypersensitive to protein, who have PKU, and who experience fat malabsorption. Soy-based formulas have been developed for the infant with lactose deficiency or who is allergic to regular formula. Infants who are formula fed generally have greater deposits of subcutaneous fat (Murray & Zentner, 2000). The Client Education box provides teaching strategies for parents of bottle-fed infants.

It is important that the nurse provide accurate information about the types of feeding available and support the parents' decision about the method chosen.

Solid foods are usually introduced at 4 to 6 months of age. Rice cereal is the first solid food of choice because it has the fewest allergic responses (Murray & Zentner, 2000).

Infants are especially vulnerable to developing infections. Because the immune system is not fully matured, infections pose a great threat. Immunizations are of utmost importance in preventing infections. Nurses should confirm that infants receive all necessary immu-

nizations. Figure 17-9 provides a recommended schedule for childhood immunization; this is updated annually.

Parents often need information about normal sleep patterns of infants and how the patterns change with maturation. Activities that promote sleep include:

- Providing a quiet room for the infant
- Scheduling feedings and other care activities during periods of wakefulness instead of drowsy times
- Developing sensitivity to the unique sleep and rest periods established by the infant
- Providing comfort and security measures (e.g., rocking, singing)
- Establishing routine times for sleep

### Safety Considerations

The majority of infant injuries and deaths are related to motor vehicle accidents. Therefore, the consistent and proper use of infant car seats is one of the most effective measures parents can take to ensure their infant's safety.

## Toddler

The **toddler** period begins at 12 to 18 months of age, when a child begins to walk alone, and ends at approximately age 3. The family is very important to the toddler in that the family promotes language development and teaches toileting skills. During this stage, the child becomes more independent. Frequently, when attempts to demonstrate autonomy are prevented, the child will have a temper tantrum; thus, this stage is often referred to as

## CLINICAL ALERT

### Handwashing and Infant Care

Handwashing is the most useful action to prevent the transmission of microorganisms.

## CLIENT EDUCATION

### Bottle-Feeding

 The baby should be in a semi-reclining position cradled close to the mother's body with the mother in a comfortable position. Never prop a bottle in the baby's mouth, because choking may result.

 Use care if heating bottles. Do not warm bottles in the microwave, because the hot liquid can cause esophageal and oropharyngeal burns.

✓ Avoid using the bottle as a pacifier, because this action may result in tooth decay and set the stage for future obesity.

## CLINICAL ALERT

### Infants and Secondhand Smoke

A review of 10 studies in international health care settings revealed positive associations between infant exposure to tobacco smoke and gastro-esophageal reflux, colic, sudden infant death syndrome, lower respiratory tract infections, and other infant morbidities. Maternal smoking was a significant predictor of infant health outcomes. The prevalence of smoking in women in developed countries is currently 24%.

Gaffney, K. (2001). Infant exposure to environmental tobacco smoke. *Journal of Nursing Scholarship, 33*(4), 343–347.

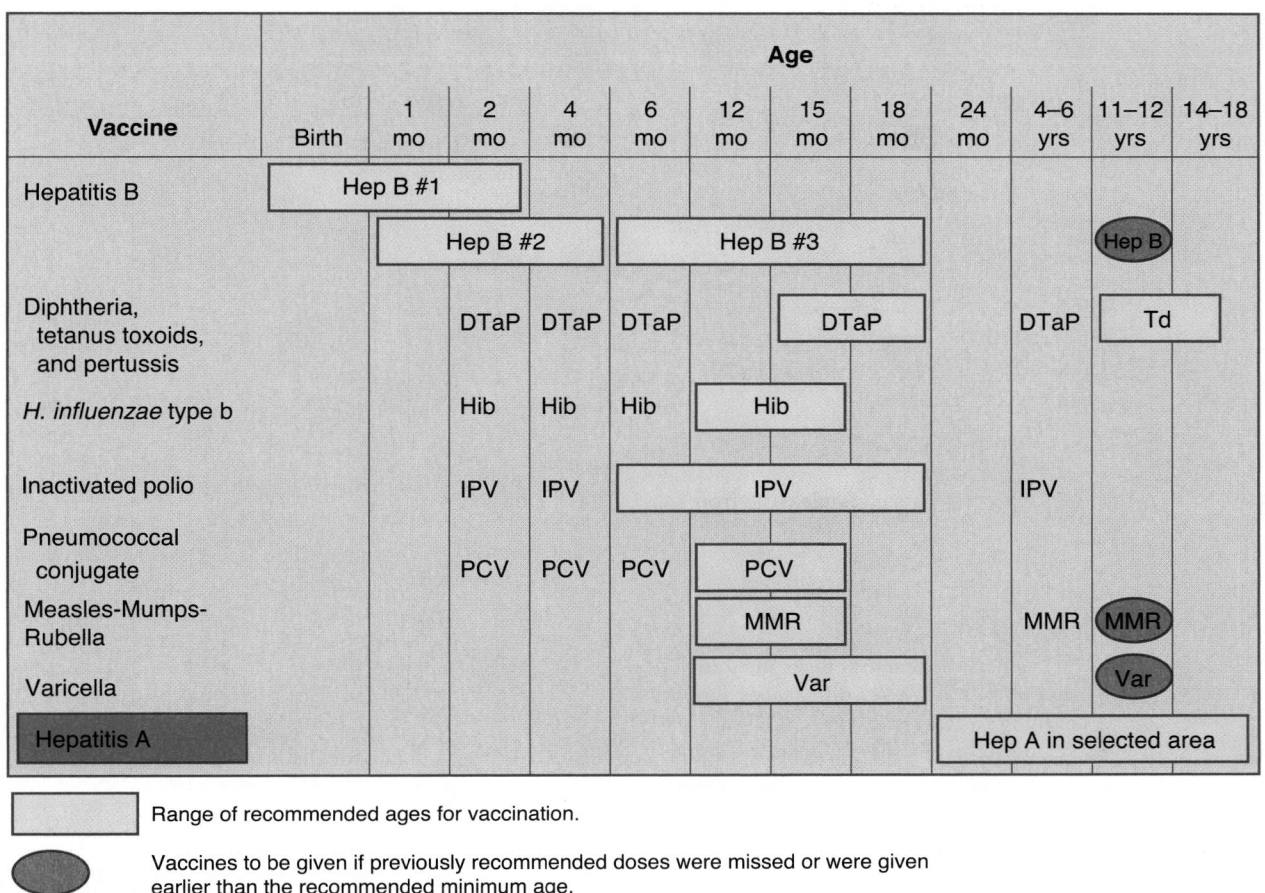

**Figure 17-9   Recommended childhood immunization schedule.** *From Centers for Disease Control and Prevention; recommended childhood immunization schedule—United States, January–December 2002). Available: http://www.cdc.gov/nip/recs/child-schedule.pdf.*

"the terrible twos." Parents must understand that the toddler's frequent use of the word "no" is an expression of developing autonomy.

Nurses can greatly influence the quality of parent-child interaction by teaching parents about developmental concepts. This information helps parents form *realistic* expectations of the toddler's behavior. The use of firm limits set in a consistent manner helps the toddler learn and provides parameters for safe and socially acceptable behavior. Table 17-15 describes the toddler's growth and development in the physiological, motor, psychosocial, cognitive, moral, and spiritual dimensions.

## Nursing Implications

Common health problems for toddlers that may affect growth and development are related to their increasing mobility and curiosity, their inability to make judgments, and their immature immune system. Toddlers may display negative behavior, and refuse medication or treatments. Separation anxiety, or the need to be with a parent, is particularly noticed during illness (Figure 17-10). Toddlers'

responses to illness are greatly influenced by parents' reactions (Rutherford, Dowshen, & Mesinger, 2001).

Nurses who work with toddlers must be sensitive to the fact that children of this age are likely to be anxious and fearful in the presence of strangers. The establishment of rapport with the child will help alleviate this stranger anxiety. Play is an effective tool for building rapport with toddlers.

When toddlers are hospitalized (for an extended time or only a day), fear and anxiety can make the experience a negative one. The major stressor resulting from hospitalization is the toddler's separation from parents. An unfamiliar environment also results in stress for the toddler. Nurses can help reduce stress in the hospitalized toddler by teaching both the child and parents about procedures.

Toddlers need to have regular health examinations, and immunizations remain an essential part of health care. Encourage parents to be involved during the examination and immunizations. Parents can alleviate the toddler's stress by holding the child and talking in a calm manner when in the presence of the health care provider.

## TABLE 17-15    TODDLER: GROWTH AND DEVELOPMENT

| Dimension | Characteristics | Nursing Implications |
|---|---|---|
| Physiological | Overall rate of growth slows. By 24 months, the toddler usually weighs four times more than at birth. | Instruct parents on need for vitamin D, calcium, and phosphorus. |
| | Rapid growth of brain | |
| | Bones in extremities grow in length. | Recognize that "growing pains" are normal. |
| | Physiological readiness for bowel and bladder training develops. | Instruct parents of timing for toilet training and need for consistency and patience. |
| Motor | Walks and runs | Assess home environment for safety as toddler becomes more mobile. |
| | Becomes more coordinated | |
| Psychosocial | *Freud:* Anal stage (receives pleasure from contraction and relaxation of sphincter muscles) | Instruct parents to avoid overemphasis on toilet training. |
| | *Erikson:* Autonomy vs. Shame and Doubt | Teach parents to encourage toddler's attempts at independence (e.g., trying to feed and dress self). |
| | *Havighurst:* Developmental tasks include: <br> • Beginning to learn sex differences <br> • Learning to talk | Explain that sexual curiosity is normal. <br> Encourage parents to talk to child frequently. |
| | Engages in parallel play (playing near other children but not necessarily interacting with them) | Provide opportunities for child to socialize with peers. |
| | A reemergence of separation anxiety often occurs. | Reassure child that parents will return. |
| | By age 3, most toddlers are able to tolerate being left with strangers. | |
| Cognitive | *Piaget:* Preoperational stage | |
| | Can follow simple directions | Instruct parents to give only one direction at a time. |
| | Concrete thought processes | |
| | Is able to anticipate future events | Use a calendar to show today's date and the number of days until a significant event. |
| | Short attention span | |
| | Comprehends self as a separate entity | Teach caregivers importance of calling child by name. |
| | *Language:* At approximately 1 year, can make two syllable sounds (e.g., ma-ma, da-da) | Talk to child frequently, avoiding use of "baby talk." |
| | At approximately 2 years, can form short sentences | |
| | Has a vocabulary of approximately 900 words | |
| Moral | *Kohlberg:* Preconventional stage | Parents need to be consistent in setting limits. |
| | Learns to distinguish right from wrong | Understand the significance of role modeling desired behavior to child. |
| Spiritual | *Fowler:* Intuitive-projective stage of faith | Instruct parents to provide simple answers to questions related to religion. |
| | | Instruct on importance of incorporating religious rituals and ceremonies into daily life. |

Data from Murray, R. B., & Zentner, J. P. (2000). *Health promotion strategies through the life span* (7th ed.). New Jersey: Prentice Hall; Hockenberry, M., et al. (2003). *Wong's nursing care of infants and children* (7th ed.). St. Louis: Mosby-Yearbook.

## RESEARCH FOCUS

**Title of Study:** Effects of home visits to vulnerable young families

**Study Purpose:** To determine the long-term effects of home visits by nurses on parenting skills and child development

**Methods:** Analysis of 20 experimental and quasi-experimental published studies of home visits to new parents identified with social risk factors, such as poverty and premature infants

**Findings:** Increased parenting skills and development of cognitive skills were supported in several studies, particularly for premature infants who were followed over a one-year period. Parent and infant interaction was enhanced. Maternal well-being (less depression, less anxiety, and a perceived mastery of parental skills) was noted in several studies. However, the visits did not increase health promotion activities such as immunizations and well-child clinic visits.

**Implications:** There is a need to promote safety precautions against infectious diseases, injuries, and other environmental dangers. The trusting relationship that developed over a period of time provides an excellent venue for introducing additional child-care information.

Kearney, M., York, R., & Deatrick, J. (2000). Effects of home visits to vulnerable young families. *Journal of Nursing Scholarship, 32*(4), 369–376.

## NURSING STRATEGY

### Preventing Infant Accidents

- To avoid vehicular accidents: use infant seats and keep the infant out of the paths of automobiles and other vehicles. Many infants can crawl very quickly!

- To prevent burns: keep infant away from open heaters, furnaces, fireplaces, hot stoves, and matches.

- To protect from falls: keep crib rails up at all times, never leave the infant lying unattended on furniture, and use protective gates and barriers to block stairways.

- To prevent drowning: never leave the infant unattended near water (bathtubs, buckets, swimming pools).

- To prevent electrocution: as the infant begins to crawl, use plastic safety plugs to cover all electrical outlets and keep electrical cords out of infant's reach.

- To prevent choking: closely monitor the infant who is exploring the environment. During this oral phase of development, infants tend to test out their environment and seek pleasure through the mouth. Aspiration accidents are common with infants who choke on objects such as buttons, coins, and food. The Heimlich maneuver is *not* used with infants, because it may force the foreign object further down the trachea. Figure 17-11 illustrates the proper technique of back blows and chest thrusts to use with an infant who is choking.

Some specific nursing approaches to use with toddlers include:

- Explain what is being done in a calm tone of voice.
- Use therapeutic play to alleviate anxiety (e.g., have the child examine a teddy bear or doll).
- Give short, simple directions.
- After a painful procedure, comfort the child (cuddling, rocking).
- Encourage parents' active participation in the care.

### Wellness Promotion

Teaching is done with both toddlers and their parents. Play can be used to establish an effective relationship with the child. Play is a valuable process for toddlers in that it is the primary mechanism for learning and socialization. To facilitate teaching, approach toddlers at eye level and use terminology that they can understand.

Respiratory infections are common health threats to the toddler. Parasitic diseases are also fairly common. Teaching parents preventive measures becomes the focus of wellness promotion.

Nutritional needs change during the toddler period as the rate of growth slows. The need for calories decreases from the requirements for infants. The required amount of protein is also lower than that of the infant; however, toddlers still need more protein than do older children. The toddler needs fewer fluids than the infant (Hockenberry et al., 2003). Because most toddlers become selective ("picky") with the foods they enjoy, it is sometimes difficult to provide increased intake of calcium and iron due to the toddler's food habits. The toddler should consume an average of 2 to 3 cups of milk a day to ensure adequate calcium intake. The toddler who drinks more than a quart of milk per day is at increased risk of developing anemia because the high milk consumption limits the amount of other nutrients taken in (Hockenberry et al., 2003).

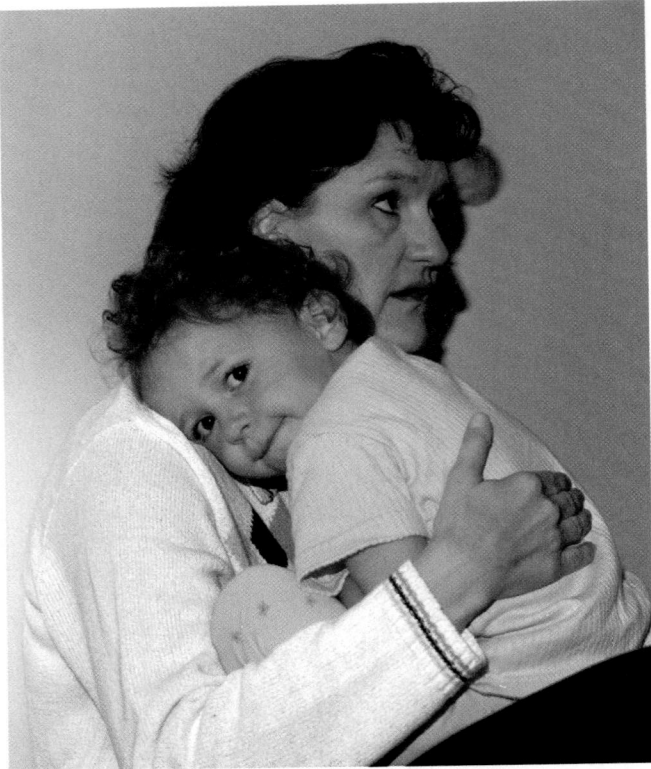

**Figure 17-10** **Stress due to illness often leads to separation anxiety.**

Nurses can play a key role in the toddler's nutritional counseling. The following points should be shared with parents about dietary practices:

- Avoid using food as a reward, because this may encourage overeating.
- Do not serve large helpings, because the child may be overwhelmed and refuse to eat.

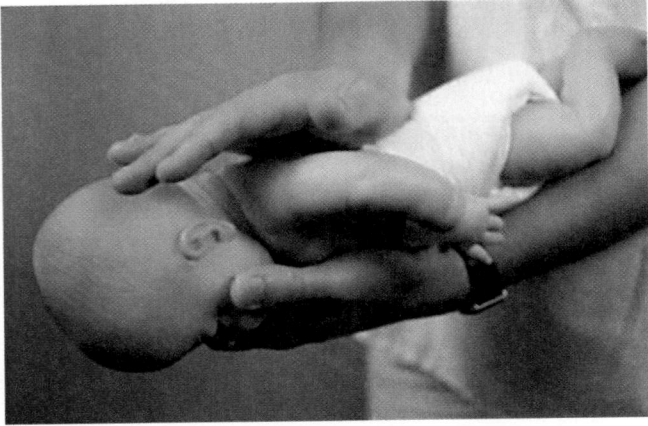

**Figure 17-11** **Intervention for a choking infant. Emergency care for an infant who is choking consists of a series of four blows to the back between the shoulder blades, followed by four thrusts midline on the chest approximately 1 inch below the nipple line.**

> ### CLINICAL ALERT
> ## Medications and Children
>
> Medications must be formalized in concentrations that the infant and child can tolerate. Scheduling of doses should be appropriate to the child's age, liver maturity, and kidney function to allow adequate excretion of drugs and toxic substances.
>
> Reiss, B., Evans, M., & Broyles, B. (2002). *Pharmacological aspects of nursing care.* Clifton Park, NY: Delmar Learning.

- Expect sporadic eating patterns (e.g., toddler eats a lot one day and very little the next; enjoys one food for several days, then suddenly will not eat it).
- Avoid power struggles related to meals. Trying to force a child to eat is counterproductive to establishing healthy eating habits.
- Establish a mealtime routine and follow it (rituals are comforting to toddlers).
- Provide nutritional snacks to meet dietary requirements.

### Safety Considerations

Accidents (especially those involving automobiles) are the most frequent cause of disability and death in toddlers (Edelman & Mandle, 2000; Murray & Zentner, 2000). Toddlers, about one year or older and over 20 pounds, should ride in the back seat buckled into an approved child safety seat. Children should not be left unattended in a motor vehicle for any reason.

Another common type of accident occurring with toddlers involves toys. Parents need to be taught to inspect toys for:

- Age appropriateness
- Sharp objects
- Small parts that can be swallowed
- Flammable or toxic materials (e.g., lead-based paint)

As children gain new skills, parents should be taught to reassess the safety of toys and of the home environment.

Toddlers, with their increased mobility and curiosity, are especially prone to accidental poisonings. Parents should be informed of the need for careful observation of the toddler and child-proofing the home. In addition, parents must be very careful when administering medications to children.

## Preschooler

The developmental stage from the ages of 3 to 6 is called the **preschool stage**. During this stage, physical growth slows and psychosocial and cognitive development are accelerated. Table 17-16 describes preschool development in detail.

## TABLE 17-16   PRESCHOOLER: GROWTH AND DEVELOPMENT

| Dimension | Characteristics | Nursing Implications |
|---|---|---|
| Physiological | Physical growth slows; average weight at age 5 is 45 pounds. | |
| | Size of head is approximate adult size. | |
| | Has a full set of deciduous teeth; these "baby teeth" start to fall out and be replaced by permanent teeth | Can eat larger meals and a variety of foods. |
| Motor | Development of fine motor skills, (e.g., ability to skip, throw a ball overhand, use scissors, tie shoelaces) | Provide a safe environment for play and exploration. Praise attempted independent activities. |
| Psychosocial | *Freud:* Phallic stage | |
| | Oedipal conflict leads to development of superego (conscience) | |
| | *Erikson:* Initiative vs. Guilt | Inform parents that preschoolers learn self-control through interacting with others. |
| | *Havighurst:* Developmental tasks include: <br>• Learning sex differences and modesty | Inform parents to provide sex education information at the child's comprehension level. |
| | • Language development and basic ability to formulate concepts | |
| | • Developing reading readiness | Encourage parents to read to child. |
| | • Distinguishing right from wrong | |
| Cognitive | *Piaget:* Preoperational stage | |
| | Improved ability to use reason and logic and increased curiosity result in frequent use of questioning. | Parents need to know that children of this age learn through frequent use of the word *why.* |
| | Play becomes more reality based. | |
| | As a result of increased ability to communicate, there is greater socialization with peers. | |
| Moral | *Kohlberg:* Preconventional stage | |
| | A conscience begins to develop. | |
| | Child fears wrongdoing. | Teach child basic values, ideally by role modeling. |
| | Child seeks parental approval. | Provide consistent praise and acceptance of child. |
| Spiritual | *Fowler:* Intuitive-projective stage of faith | |
| | Not yet able to understand spiritual concepts | |
| | Imitates parental behaviors | Remind parents that teaching by example is the best approach for a child this age. |

Data from Murray, R. B., & Zentner, J. P. (2000). *Health promotion strategies through the life span* (7th ed.). New Jersey: Prentice Hall; Hockenberry, M., et al. (2003). *Wong's nursing care of infants and children* (7th ed.). St. Louis: Mosby-Yearbook.

During this period of childhood, curiosity becomes pronounced and the child is better able to communicate. When teaching the parents, let them know that the child's frequent use of the word *why* is necessary for normal cognitive and psychosocial development.

The child's world begins to expand outside the immediate home environment. Play is the mechanism used by the preschooler to learn about and develop relationships.

Common health problems for preschoolers that may affect growth and development include injuries and susceptibility to infections of the ear, nose, throat, skin, or urinary tract. This is a period of slower growth, so preschoolers have small appetites and may not eat a balanced diet. Excess intake of fruit juices contributes to obesity. Preschoolers can be easily frightened, have difficulty coping with fears, and experience separation anxiety when exposed to health care environments (Berger & Williams, 1999).

### Nursing Implications

Play is a tool that can be used by nurses with preschoolers to help reduce fear and anxiety. Through the use of play, preschoolers learn about the environment, incorporate socially defined expectations for behavior, and reduce tension (Figure 17-12).

### Wellness Promotion

When working with a preschooler, it is important for the nurse to communicate at the child's level of comprehension without talking down to the child. Include the child in activities and decisions as much as possible. The preschool years are the optimum time for the child to begin showing interest in health. The astute nurse capitalizes on this by making health education fun to promote the development of lifelong health-promoting lifestyles.

A major wellness intervention for preschoolers is immunization. Teach parents about and encourage them to adhere to the recommended schedules. Each state in the United States has immunization requirements as prerequisites for school admission. The nurse should encourage parents to have children immunized and to keep the immunization records current. All states offer exemptions for children who have medical problems such as severe illness, immunocompromised status, or allergies to vaccine constituents (CDC, 2000).

### Safety Considerations

Accidents are the leading cause of death in young children. Eagerness to explore the environment and cognitive immaturity lead to the preschooler's risk for accidents. Children in this stage often act impulsively and cannot be expected to remember and follow all safety rules. Parents must understand the importance of teaching young children the meaning of "no" to prevent accidents.

Common accidents that involve preschoolers are automobile accidents, burns, falls, drowning, animal bites, and ingestion of poisonous substances.

It is important for the nurse to emphasize education about protection from potential hazards. The safety practices that are developed by the preschooler will tend to be lifelong. Adults can best teach preschoolers about accident prevention through role modeling. For example, parents who buckle their seat belts every time they get into a car are not only protecting themselves but are also teaching their children an important accident-prevention measure.

## School-Age Child

During the **school-age period** (developmental stage from the ages of 6 to 12 years), physical changes occur in a slow, even, continuous pace. Table 17-17 gives an overview of growth and development of the school-age child.

The school-age child's world expands greatly. Participation in school activities, team sports, and play contributes to an enlarging social network. As children continue to mature, their playtime becomes more structured and less spontaneous. Communication increases and vocabulary expands greatly to accommodate the expression of needs, thoughts, and feelings.

As the school-age child's cognitive abilities expand, creativity is expressed in a variety of unique ways. Involvement in academics, sports, and social activities stimulates the development of creativity and provides outlets for its expression.

### Nursing Implications

Common health problems seen in school-age children that may affect growth and development include: nutritional needs, obesity, dental caries and other dental prob-

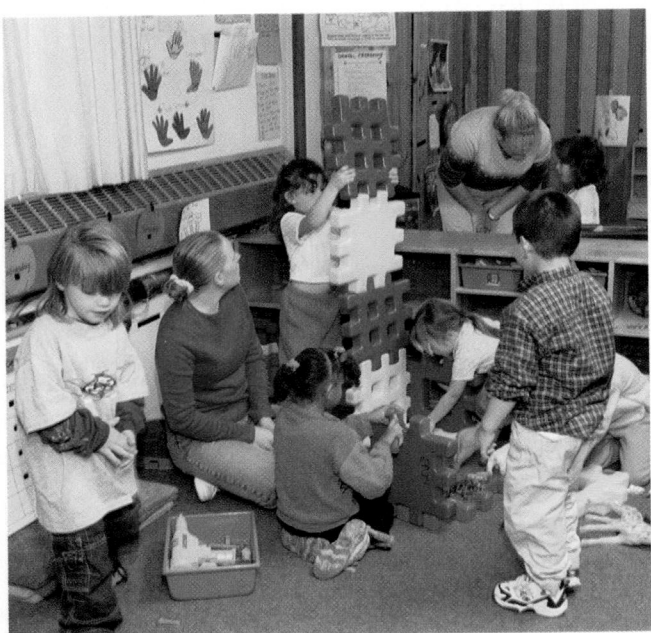

**Figure 17-12     Play is an important tool for socializing among preschoolers.**

## CLIENT REFLECTIONS

### A Hospitalized Child

Tony's mother: "I was so frightened when I first saw Tony after surgery. He was surrounded with technical equipment. I wanted to hold him and tell him that Mommy would make everything better, but of course I couldn't. Thank goodness, Mary, the nurse, sensed my concerns and told me what would be happening during the next few days. She even included me in planning Tony's care by asking me about Tony's likes and dislikes in food, about his daily habits, his favorite hobbies, and his reaction to pain. All the nurses involved me in Tony's care as much as possible and brought books for me to read to him. They also helped prepare me to care for Tony when he comes home."

Tony: "The nurses showed me some funny faces to use to let them know how much pain I was feeling. Mary always helped me get ready for the treatments. Sometimes the treatments hurt real bad, but I was glad that my Mom could stay and hug me or hold my hand."

What would you say to Tony's mother and to Tony?

## COMMUNITY/HOME CARE

### Difficulties for Children Experiencing Home Care

The family should be an integral part of the care plan for the hospitalized child, in discharge planning and in the care provided in the home. Frequently, parents must learn how to use specialized equipment such as intravenous lines, administer oxygen, monitor vital signs and blood sugar levels, perform physical and rehabilitative procedures, and be able to identify symptoms of distress and know when to report them. Nurses have an important role in preparing the child and family for home care. Early discharge planning includes assessment of the family's ability to provide care, consultation with the health care team, educating the family care provider, and assuring a smooth transition to the home. The community nurse verifies that the family uses the equipment correctly and follows the educational instructions. Nurses can also assist parents by acting as case managers to coordinate the child's overall care. They can plan an individualized education program with teachers and work with other service providers required for home care. Some communities have workshops for parents who manage the complex care of children with chronic illnesses or long-term care following an injury.

Hitchcock, J., Schubert, P., & Thomas, S. (2003). *Community health nursing: Caring in action* (2nd ed.). Clifton Park, NY: Delmar Learning.

lems, unintentional injury, vision and hearing deficits, learning disorders, and infectious diseases. Chronic conditions such as diabetes mellitus, asthma, and cystic fibrosis can affect 10–15% of this group of children. An illness may intensify fears in school-age children, and they may not view their situation logically (Berger & Williams, 1999). Furthermore, hospitalized children and their caregivers have difficulty with fears related to the acute care setting and have many specialized needs in that environment. In addition, children with illnesses who require home care have very special needs, and the nurses must work closely with the care providers in the administration of their home care.

### Wellness Promotion

Lifestyles begin to be established during childhood; nurses can intervene to promote the development of healthy lifestyles with children in schools. Schools are an area in which health promotion behaviors can be taught in a cost-effective manner. Nurses can promote wellness in the school-age child by teaching parents to:

- Encourage healthy lifestyles (nonsedentary activities, nutritious meals)
- Have children immunized
- Provide nutritious meals
- Teach children appropriate hygienic measures

- Schedule regular checkups with the primary health care provider
- Schedule dental checkups and encourage daily brushing and flossing
- Establish sleep patterns alternating with periods of activity
- Report any symptoms of illness immediately to the health care provider
- Teach safety precautions

### Safety Considerations

Many accidents experienced by school-age children occur during play. Injuries related to the use of skates, skateboards, in-line skates, and bicycles are common. Children should be taught safety rules for use of such toys (e.g., use of protective equipment; Figure 17-13). Parents must frequently remind children of the danger of playing near traffic (Figure 17-14). Children in this developmental stage

## TABLE 17-17    SCHOOL-AGE CHILD: GROWTH AND DEVELOPMENT

| Dimension | Characteristics | Nursing Implications |
|---|---|---|
| Physiological | Physical growth is steady (approximately 3 to 6 pounds and 2 to 3 inches per year). | Emphasize with parents the need for a balanced diet to sustain growth requirements. |
| | Due to changes in amount and distribution of fat, body has an overall slimmer shape. | |
| | Maturation of CNS is nearly completed. | |
| | By age 12, all permanent teeth are present (except second and third molars). | Teach parents need for dental hygiene (daily brushing and flossing) and regularly scheduled visits to dentist. |
| | | Instruct to change toothbrushes every 3 months. |
| Motor | Continued development of motor control. | Encourage participation in physical activities. |
| | Becomes less dependent on parents for activities of daily living. | Provide praise for independent activities. |
| Psychosocial | *Freud:* Latency stage | To develop a sense of confidence, encourage child to: |
| | Same-gender companions preferred. | • Participate in both group and individual activities |
| | | • Become involved in a variety of activities |
| | *Erikson:* Industry vs. Inferiority | |
| | Develops initiative and high self-esteem as shown in school and sports. | Encourage parents to praise child's efforts. |
| | Exhibits less dependency on family. | |
| | *Havighurst:* Developmental tasks include: | |
| | • Ability to perform more-complex motor functions (e.g., ride a bicycle, catch a ball) | |
| Cognitive | *Piaget:* Concrete operations stage | |
| | Ability to cooperate with others and begins to be able to see the other's point of view, which leads to more meaningful communication | Encourage child to engage in group activities. |
| | Reasoning ability moves from intuitive to logical and rational. | |
| | Ability to think in the abstract is not fully developed. | Communicate at child's level of comprehension. |
| | Develops the concept of time: | |
| | • Knows difference between past and present | |
| | • Begins to learn to tell time | |
| | • Better able to understand the process of aging | |
| | Able to order, categorize, and classify groups of objects as evidenced in increased interest in collections (coins, stamps, rocks) | |
| | Sees relationships between objects | |
| Moral | *Kohlberg:* Conventional stage | Provide consistent limits. |
| | Can understand what society deems as unacceptable behavior but cannot always choose between right and wrong without assistance | Role-model appropriate behavior. |
| | | Provide praise for appropriate behavior. |
| Spiritual | *Fowler:* Mythical-literal stage of faith | Encourage parents to discuss their beliefs. |
| | Accepts existence of a deity | Storytelling and use of parables can reinforce understanding of spiritual concepts. |
| | Beliefs are symbolized through stories. | |

Data from Edelman, C. L., & Mandle, C. L. (2000). *Health promotion throughout the life span* (4th ed.). St. Louis: Mosby-Yearbook; Murray, R. B., & Zentner, J. P. (2000). *Health promotion strategies through the life span* (7th ed.). New Jersey: Prentice Hall.

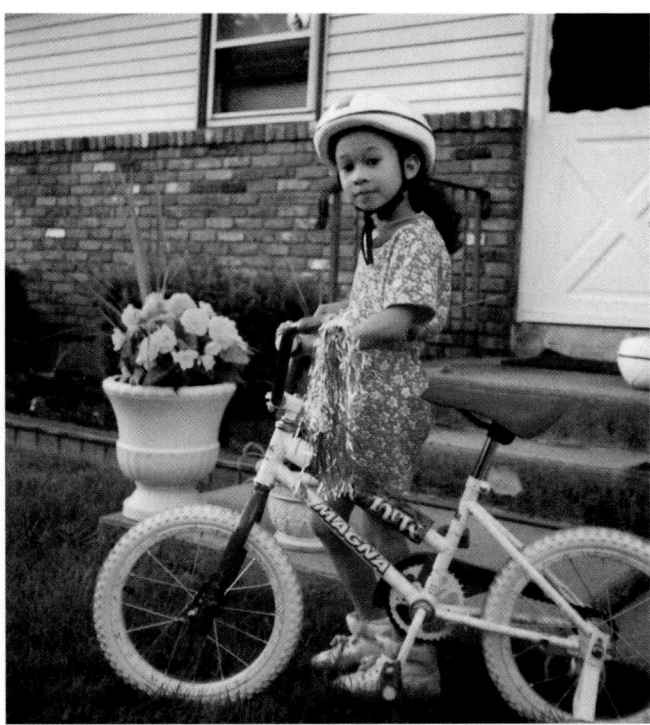

**Figure 17-13    The use of equipment such as safety helmets helps to protect school-age children from injury.**

must also be taught to use caution with strangers because of the possibility of abductions.

## Preadolescent

The later school-age years from 10 to 12 are frequently referred to as **preadolescence** or prepuberty. This stage is marked by rapid physiological changes with accompanying psychological, emotional, and social implications.

The child is beginning to experience hormonal changes that will result in the onset of **puberty** (appearance of secondary sex characteristics). There is a marked variation among individuals during this transition peri-

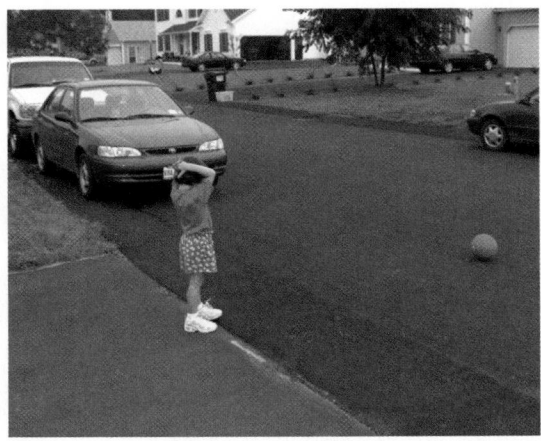

**Figure 17-14    Parents must teach children to use caution while playing near traffic.**

od. Girls generally experience preadolescence at a younger age than boys—approximately age 9 to 10 for girls and age 10 to 11 for boys (Edelman & Mandle, 2000). Table 17-18 provides an overview of preadolescent development.

In girls, breast development begins between the ages of 10 and 11. Further breast development is stimulated by the release of estrogen that occurs during puberty. The pattern of female breast development is described in Table 17-19. Other aspects of female sexual development are described in Table 17-20.

Approximately 2 years after the appearance of breast buds, **menarche** (onset of the first menstrual period) occurs. The first menstrual periods are usually irregular, scant, and may or may not be accompanied by ovulation. The average age of menarche in the United States is 12.8 years, which has gradually declined over the past century. This is probably due to improved general health status, particularly nutrition and sanitation (Hockenberry et al., 2003).

The menstrual cycle is a complex blend of physiological and psychological changes that occur approximately every month. After approximately the first 6 to 12 months, a girl's cycle will become established in a regular pattern. Some girls may have received inadequate or incorrect information regarding the onset of menstruation. Client teaching should include information about the physiological changes, emotional changes, and hygienic practices. Teaching should emphasize that the cyclical hormone-induced changes are normal.

One menstrual problem experienced by many females is premenstrual syndrome (PMS). PMS is a complex condition characterized by a variety of symptoms including headache, backache, fatigue, irritability, weight gain, and crying spells. Females need information about PMS to receive early intervention if needed.

In preadolescent boys, the first signs of puberty are:

- Testicular enlargement
- Penile enlargement
- The scrotum becoming thinner and redder
- Pubic hair growth

Table 17-21 illustrates the physiological changes in boys during sexual development of male genitalia.

### Nursing Implications

Common health problems for the preadolescent that may affect growth and development include sports injuries, exposure to violence, tobacco and substance abuse, unsafe sexual practices, excessive or insufficient food intake and eating "junk food," dental problems, and self-image disturbances related to body changes. Although preadolescents show increased maturity, they may lack judgment in decisions and participate in risky behaviors. "Children with chronic illnesses are at greater risk for other problems such as infectious diseases, injury, or developmental delay" (Ball & Bindler, 2003).

Sensitivity is essential for the nurse working with the preadolescent child. To increase one's sensitivity, the nurse

## TABLE 17-18    PREADOLESCENT AND ADOLESCENT: GROWTH AND DEVELOPMENT

| Dimension | Characteristics | Nursing Implications |
|---|---|---|
| Physiological | *Physiological Changes:*<br>Accelerated physical growth with changes in body proportion. Extremities grow first, then trunk and hips. Growth in skull and facial bones results in changes in physical appearance | Teach the child and parents about expected growth spurts.<br><br>Provide reassurance that it is not uncommon for facial appearance to change in only a few months. |
| | *Reproductive/Sexual Changes:*<br>Hypothalamus stimulates secretion of pituitary gonadotropins, leading to reproductive maturity. | Provide support and information about emerging sexual changes. |
| | Development of both primary and secondary sex characteristics. | Remember that the physiological changes are accompanied by psychological and social alterations. |
| | Beginning of puberty is evidenced in girls by:<br>• Breast development<br>• Pubic and axillary hair growth<br>• Menarche (onset of menses)<br>• Increases in height | |
| | Beginning of puberty is evidenced in boys by:<br>• Genital development<br>• Growth of facial, pubic, and axillary hair<br>• Nocturnal ejaculations<br>• Height increases<br>• Voice changes | |
| | *Musculoskeletal Changes:*<br>• Ossification of bones<br>• Increased muscle mass and strength | Encourage physical activities and intake of adequate amounts of calcium. |
| | *Cardiovascular Changes:*<br>• Heart increases in size and strength.<br>• Heart rate decreases to adult norms.<br>• Increased blood volume and blood pressure | |
| | *Respiratory Changes:*<br>• Rate decreases to an average of 15 to 20 respirations per minute<br>• Increased respiratory volume and vital capacity<br>• Growth of larynx, laryngeal cartilage, and vocal cords, and voice pitch deepens | Instruct about anticipated changes. |
| | *Gastrointestinal and Genitourinary Changes:*<br>• Spleen, liver, kidneys, and digestive tract enlarge but experience no functional changes. | |
| | *Dental Changes:*<br>• Eruption of last four molars | Emphasize importance of continued dental hygiene. |
| | *Integumentary Changes:*<br>• Skin becomes thicker and tougher.<br>• Activation of sebaceous glands leads to possibility of acne.<br>• Appearance of pubic hair | Teach proper skin care:<br>• Wash two to three times daily with soap and water.<br>• Avoid vigorous scrubbing.<br>• Females should avoid cosmetics with a fat or grease base.<br>• Use sunscreen and avoid prolonged exposure to sunlight.<br>• Provide support to children experiencing acne. |
| Motor | • Able to be completely independent with self-care activities | |

*(continues)*

## TABLE 17-18    PREADOLESCENT AND ADOLESCENT: GROWTH AND DEVELOPMENT (*continued*)

| Dimension | Characteristics | Nursing Implications |
|---|---|---|
| Psychosocial | *Freud:* Genital stage | |
| | *Erikson:* Identity vs. Role diffusion | Offer support. |
| | Major task: develop a sense of identity | |
| | Develops a new body image | |
| | Establishes intimacy with members of opposite gender | Provide sex education. |
| | Peer group is the primary mechanism of support | |
| | Rebels against adult authority | Inform parents that rebellion is a normal developmental experience. |
| | *Havighurst:* | |
| | Achieves personal independence | Encourage attempts to achieve independence while providing assistance and support as needed. |
| | Establishes more mature relationships with others | |
| Cognitive | *Piaget:* Formal operations stage | Teach parents expected developmental changes in thinking patterns. |
| | Logical, organized, consistent approach to thinking | |
| | Thinks in terms of cause and effect | |
| | **Note:** Not all adolescents achieve this level of cognitive development. Some are capable of flights from reality. | |
| | Tends to be extremely idealistic | |
| | Egocentric (self-centered) thinking is common with a view of oneself as omnipotent. | |
| | Sees self as exceptional, special, and unique, and possesses a belief that one is immune to problems | A false sense of immunity ("It can't happen to me" attitude) has an impact on health behaviors. |
| | | Teach safety issues to children:<br>• Safe sex practices<br>• Avoid driving and use of alcohol |
| Moral | *Kohlberg:* Postconventional stage | |
| | Tends to support the morality of law and order to determine right from wrong | Teach parents that questioning of values is normal. |
| | Begins to question status quo and discards and chooses different values | |
| | Moral maturity varies in context of the situation and the relationship. | |
| | Peer pressure may override the adolescent's own moral reasoning. | Teach child assertiveness skills to use in communicating with peers. |
| Spiritual | *Fowler:* Synthetic-conventional stage of faith | Inform parents that curiosity about other religious beliefs is normal. |
| | Questions values and beliefs | |

Data from Edelman, C. L., & Mandle, C. L. (2000). *Health promotion throughout the life span* (4th ed.). St. Louis: Mosby-Yearbook; Varcarolis, E., & Rader, I. (2002). *Foundations of mental health psychiatric nursing* (4th ed.). Philadelphia: Saunders.

## TABLE 17-19    SEXUAL MATURITY RATING FOR FEMALE BREAST DEVELOPMENT

**Developmental Stage**

1. Preadolescent stage (before age 10). Nipple is small, slightly raised.

2. Breast bud stage (after age 10). Nipple and breast form a small mound. Areola enlarges. Height spurt begins.

3. Adolescent stage (10–14 years). Nipple is flush with breast shape. Breast and areola enlarge. Menses begin. Height spurt peaks.

4. Late adolescent stage (10–14 years). Nipple and areola form a secondary mound over the breast. Height spurt ends.

5. Adult stage. Nipple protrudes; areola is flush with the breast shape.

Data from Estes, M. E. (2002). *Health assessment & physical examination* (2nd ed.). Clifton Park, NY: Delmar Learning.

uses a nonjudgmental approach and attends to the child's body language. It is imperative that the nurse establish a trusting relationship with the preadolescent in order to encourage the child to ask questions about any health-related concerns.

## Wellness Promotion

The preadolescent needs information about nutrition, rest and activity, and the physiological changes that are occurring. The child must learn about the growth spurt, sexual changes, and psychosocial changes. By preparing the

## TABLE 17-20    SEXUAL MATURITY RATING FOR FEMALE GENITALIA

| Developmental stage | Description |
|---|---|
| Stage 1 | No pubic hair, only body hair (vellus hair) |
| Stage 2 | Sparse growth of long, slightly dark, fine pubic hair, slightly curly and located along the labia (ages 11 to 12) |
| Stage 3 | Pubic hair becomes darker, curlier, and spreads over the symphysis (ages 12 to 13) |
| Stage 4 | Texture and curl of pubic hair are similar to those of an adult but not spread to thighs (ages 13 to 15) |
| Stage 5 | Adult appearance in quality and quantity of pubic hair; growth is spread to inner aspect of thighs and abdomen |

Data from Estes, M. E. (2002). *Health assessment & physical examination* (2nd ed.). Clifton Park, NY: Delmar Learning.

## LEGAL AND ETHICAL ISSUES

### Children with Disabilities

Several laws regarding the education of children with disabilities have been passed in recent years. The Individuals with Disabilities Education Act (IDEA) authorized by Congress in 1997 ensures that children ages 3 through 11 years with complex health problems will receive free and appropriate education in school settings in the least restrictive educational environment. The legislation greatly impacts the role of the school nurse and requires advanced clinical, communication, and decision-making skills in collaborating with parents, teachers, and other school personnel.

Potts, N., & Mandleco, B. (2002). *Pediatric nursing: Caring for children and their families.* Clifton Park, NY: Delmar Learning.

preadolescent for upcoming changes, the nurse is promoting physical and emotional health.

### Safety Considerations

The preadolescent is at risk for injury from sports and play activities. Another major health risk posed to many preadolescents is violence both in and away from the home. Education is a major preventive approach to violence; it is the tool for helping break the intergenerational cycle of child abuse.

Other topics for promoting preadolescent safety are: substance abuse prevention, sex education, and development of healthy lifestyles.

## Adolescent

Adolescence is the developmental stage that ranges from the onset of puberty to the ages of 18 to 20. (The earlier discussion of the preadolescent stage is frequently included in some texts as part of the discussion on adolescence.) The adolescent must adapt to the rapid body changes and emotional feelings over several years (Ball & Bindler, 2003). Furthermore, children with disabilities have special needs that health care providers must consider.

During adolescence, the individual undergoes the major transition from child to adult. Numerous physiological changes and rapid physical growth occur during this stage. The rapid changes that occur during adolescence are not only physical. Many psychosocial adjustments must be made by the adolescent. Establishing a sense of personal identity uses a great amount of the adolescent's psychic energy. Questions such as "Who am I?" and "What is *really* important?" are common for adolescents to consider. See Table 17-18 for an overview of adolescent development.

## CLIENT EDUCATION

### Preventing Eating Disorders

✓ Encourage a balance between exercise and food consumption.

✓ Promote an increased sense of self-esteem.

✓ Emphasize the importance of a healthy lifestyle rather than physical appearance.

✓ Avoid pressuring children to seek perfection or to strive for unrealistic goals.

✓ Recognize the indicators of eating disorders.

## LEGAL AND ETHICAL ISSUES

### Informed Consent

Parents and legal guardians are legally responsible for giving *informed* consent for care provided to minor children that includes invasive procedures or research participation. The physician must provide detailed explanation of a treatment, the potential benefits and risks involved, possible alternative treatments, and the right to refuse treatment on behalf of the child. Children can also actively participate in decision making when given age-appropriate information. In some states, 14- to 15-year-old adolescents who understand treatment risks can give consent for treatment or refuse treatment.

Potts, N., & Mandleco, B. (2002). *Pediatric nursing: Caring for children and their families.* Clifton Park, NY: Delmar Learning.

Most adolescents are greatly concerned about their appearance. This emphasis on physical attractiveness sometimes results in eating disorders, such as **anorexia nervosa** (a self-imposed starvation that results in a 15% loss of body weight). Approximately 1% to 2% of female adolescents are affected by anorexia; the rate in males is much lower—about 5% to 10% of the anorectic population is male (Stuart & Laraia, 2001). Other types of eating disorders common in adolescents are **bulimia nervosa** (episodic binge eating followed by purging) and **obesity** (weight that is 20% or more above the ideal body weight).

### Nursing Implications

Common health problems that occur during adolescence include injuries (motor vehicles and guns), tobacco, alcohol and substance abuse, nutritional and dental problems, pregnancy, and sexually transmitted diseases. Most adolescents may delay reporting their symptoms due to fear of losing control (Oran, 2000). Mental health problems (i.e., depression, anxiety disorders, and suicidal thoughts) may also occur (Lucas & Ferguson, 2000).

The nurse can support adolescents by providing information about the numerous body changes. Adolescents should be encouraged to share their health concerns with parents. However, the nurse must honor the adolescent's choice to withhold sensitive information from parents. The use of a nonjudgmental attitude is essential to the establishment of rapport when working with adolescents. Adolescents should be treated in a respectful, dignified manner. Avoid using a condescending attitude when communicating with them. Nurses are also responsible for providing client education to children and adolescents. This information has to be presented in language that is easily understood and care must be taken to include the caregivers throughout this sharing of information.

### Wellness Promotion

The nurse promotes the adolescent's wellness primarily through teaching. Areas to be emphasized in health education of adolescents include hygiene, nutrition, sex education, developmental changes, and substance abuse prevention.

Adolescents need education about the physical changes they are undergoing. Health teaching is often done by school nurses, and the establishment of nurse-managed clinics in schools is one avenue for promoting wellness among adolescents. School-based clinics are rapidly increasing. *Nursing's Agenda for Health Care Reform* (American Nurses Association, 1990) calls for the delivery of primary health care services to individuals in convenient, familiar places. What better place to teach adolescents about health care than in the schools?

### Safety Considerations

Unhealthy behaviors contribute to the three major causes of adolescent death: accidents, homicide, and suicide. The

## CLINICAL ALERT

### Late Onset of Menarche

Late onset of menarche can be the result of several factors. If you encounter a client who has not experienced the onset of menstruation by age 16 to 18, evaluate her for the following:

1. Inadequate nutrition
2. Presence of eating disorders
3. Chronic diseases (e.g., Crohn's disease, hypothyroidism)
4. Environmental stressors
5. Use of steroids or opiates

## TABLE 17-21    SEXUAL MATURITY RATING FOR MALE GENITALIA

| DEVELOPMENTAL STAGE | PUBIC HAIR | PENIS | SCROTUM |
|---|---|---|---|
| 1. | No pubic hair, only fine body hair (vellus hair) | Preadolescent; childhood size and proportion | Preadolescent; childhood size and proportion |
| 2. | Sparse growth of long, slightly dark, straight hair | Slight or no growth | Growth in testes and scrotum; scrotum reddens and changes texture |
| 3. | Becomes darker and coarser; slightly curled and spreads over symphysis | Growth, especially in length | Further growth |
| 4. | Texture and curl of pubic hair are similar to an adult's but hair not spread to thighs | Further growth in length; diameter increases; development of glans | Further growth; scrotum darkens |
| 5. | Adult appearance in quality and quantity of pubic hair; growth is spread to medial surface of thighs | Adult size and shape | Adult size and shape |

Data from Estes, M. E. (2002). *Health assessment & physical examination* (2nd ed.). Clifton Park, NY: Delmar Learning.

following developmental factors increase the adolescent's risk for accidents:

- Impulsive behavior
- Sense of being invulnerable to accidents (a feeling that "It can never happen to me!")
- Testing limits
- Rebelling against adult advice

As a result, many adolescents engage in unhealthy behaviors such as smoking, consuming alcohol and other drugs, reckless driving, violence, and unprotected sexual activity.

Many health problems in adolescents are related to sexual behaviors including acquired immunodeficiency syndrome, sexually transmitted diseases (STDs), and unplanned pregnancy.

## NURSING STRATEGY

### Therapeutic Approaches with the Adolescent Client

- Treat the adolescent as an active participant in health care to form a collaborative partnership.

- Answer all questions honestly.

- Be especially sensitive to nonverbal clues. Adolescents are often too embarrassed to initiate discussion of their health-related concerns.

- Remember that the peer group is of major importance to adolescents, and use group settings whenever possible to provide health education.

- Demonstrate acceptance of the adolescent even when limits need to be established to intervene with unhealthy or inappropriate behaviors.

- Questioning adult authority is a normal part of adolescent rebelliousness. Do not personalize testing behaviors. Nurses who personalize the behavior become defensive and lose their interpersonal effectiveness and credibility with adolescents.

## CLINICAL ALERT

### Legal Mandate to Report STDs

Laws concerning the dissemination of information about STDs vary among states and provinces. However, most have legislation that requires nurses to report the names of clients with certain STDs to the state/provincial health department. You must know the requirements for your state or province.

## FOCUS ON WELLNESS

### Adolescent Health Screening

Recommended health screening for adolescents (12 to 18 years) to identify early physical, emotional, and behavioral problems and to promote healthy lifestyles include:

- Recommendation of a health guidance visit with parent and child during early and middle adolescence related to parenting, development, diet and physical activity, healthy lifestyle, and prevention of injury.

- A screening history for eating disorders, sexual activity, tobacco, alcohol and other drug use, abuse, school performance, depression, and risk for suicide. Obtain health history and immunization schedule.

- Comprehensive physical exam, blood pressure, and body mass index during early, middle, and late adolescence.

- Diagnostic tests: (1) cholesterol (test if there is a family history of cardiovascular disease or hyperlipidemia); (2) hepatitis B (administer vaccine to children not previously vaccinated); (3) varicella vaccine should be given if there is no reliable history of chicken pox); (4) hepatitis A (vaccinate if at risk for infection); (5) measles/mumps/rubella (do not give vaccine if administered in last 5 years).

Adapted from Potts, N., & Mandleco, B. (2002). *Pediatric nursing: Caring for children and their families*. Clifton Park, NY: Delmar Learning.

The effect of teen pregnancy on families and communities is great. Social programs that provide resources for meeting the special needs of pregnant adolescents are decreasing. Many pregnant teens become trapped in a cycle of school failure (or dropout), limited employment opportunities, and poverty. Adolescents who become pregnant experience developmental difficulties in that they must make adult decisions before they are adults. Infants born to adolescent mothers are likely to experience health-related problems such as prematurity and low birth weight.

The pregnant adolescent needs expert prenatal care, a supportive environment, and information. Client teaching must emphasize the prevention of STDs because the pregnancy itself is evidence of high-risk (unprotected) sexual activity.

Sexually transmitted diseases present a serious health threat for adolescents. Shared sexual activity among

## CLINICAL ALERT

### Violence and Children

Physical or sexual abuse, neglect, or witnessing violence produces many problems during childhood and adolescence. Recently, the rates of physical aggression and antisocial acts by victims of child abuse has increased significantly. In addition, delinquency, acts of violence, running away, substance abuse, and teen pregnancy may occur.

Lucas, R., & Ferguson, M. (2000). Disorders of childhood and adolescence. In K. Fortinash & P. Holoday-Worret (Eds.). *Psychiatric mental health nursing.* St. Louis: C. V. Mosby.

## STOP AND THINK

### Values Clarification

As a nurse, you will often encounter clients whose value systems conflict with your own beliefs. How will you provide care to sexually active adolescents if you think their behavior is immoral or "wrong"? Is it ethical for you to try to change the adolescent's values to be congruent with yours? Should you change your values to be congruent with those of the client?

teenagers is on the rise. Three million adolescents are infected with a sexually transmitted disease (STD) (human immunodeficiency virus, genital herpes, Chlamydia, syphilis, gonorrhea) each year (Kelly, 2000). As male adolescents become increasingly sexually active, their use of condoms declines and they rely more on the female partner's method of birth control. This leads to vulnerability of both partners contracting an STD.

Nurses must educate adolescents about methods for preventing the spread of STDs. Preventive education should include the following topics:

- Methods of transmission
- Incubation period
- Clinical manifestations
- Treatment methods
- Consequences of lack of or inadequate treatment
- Notification of sexual partner(s)

Nurses who teach adolescent clients about safe sex practices need to be especially sensitive to cultural influences on sexual activity.

Another major health problem during adolescence is the high risk of suicide. Often, suicide is perceived by the adolescent as the only alternative to an overwhelming situation. Low self-esteem, lack of maturity, and impulsive behaviors may increase the risk of suicidal behavior. The rate of suicide is higher among adolescent males than females.

When assessing for suicidal potential, the nurse should always directly question the adolescent about any plans for harming or killing self. Box 17-2 lists signs indicative of suicide risk in adolescents.

When teaching suicide prevention, inform people to *immediately* contact a health care professional if someone is exhibiting any of the indicators of suicide risk. Many communities have a special telephone suicide-cope line available.

Another significant health problem for many adolescents is substance abuse. Using alcohol or other drugs is a

common maladaptive attempt to cope with the stressors of adolescence. Box 17-3 lists indicators of substance abuse in adolescents.

Nurses can play a vital role in substance abuse prevention with adolescents through primary, secondary, or tertiary prevention. Goals of primary prevention are to prevent nonusers from starting use of psychoactive substances, to prevent progression from experimentation to chronic use, and to prevent expansion to other substances.

## BOX 17-2   SIGNS OF SUICIDAL RISK IN ADOLESCENTS

- Anorexia
- Writing suicide notes
- Talking about suicide
- Aggressive behavior
- Substance abuse
- Running away from home
- Preoccupation with death
- Neglecting personal hygiene
- Giving away treasured objects
- Sudden changes in behavior
- Verbal cues (e.g., "You won't have to worry about me much longer")
- Fatigue
- Social withdrawal

## BOX 17-3    INDICATORS OF ADOLESCENT SUBSTANCE ABUSE

- Decline in academic performance
- Mood swings
- Changes in personality (such as confusion, euphoria, belligerence, withdrawal)
- Fatigue
- Drowsiness
- Behaviors indicative of depression (such as appetite changes, insomnia, weight loss, apathy)

(Legal substances, such as tobacco and alcohol, are considered "gateway drugs" leading to the use of other drugs.) An education program focuses on explaining the hazards of substance abuse and modification of risk factors. Goals of secondary prevention are early interventions and treatment before irreversible pathological changes occur. Nurses can prepare the family to be partners with professionals in the intervention process. A combination of treatment modalities that is geared to individual problems are usually more effective than a single mode. Tertiary prevention focuses on preventing a relapse into former substance abuse behaviors. Emotional support and encouragement, elimination of stressors, reinforcement of the individual's motivation to abstain from drug use, and support groups are helpful resources (Clark, 1999).

By providing such information, nurses can help adolescents make responsible, informed decisions before experimentation with drugs begins.

# CASE STUDY/NURSING CARE PLAN

Tony is a 7-year-old boy who was admitted to the emergency department as the result of an accident while inline skating. He was brought to the hospital by ambulance and had emergency surgery for the removal of his spleen and an open reduction and internal fixation (ORIF) of his left femur. Currently, Tony has been in the post-surgical unit for about 12 hours. His vital signs are stable (B.P. = 114/68, P = 86, R = 20, T = 37.4°C). His left femur is "pinned," is in traction, and has a hemovac for drainage. He has a dry dressing over his spleen area surgical incision, an IV of Lactated Ringers at 40 cc/hr, and he has other minor lacerations on his face and extremities.

Tony is recovering in a stable manner 12 hours post-op from orthopedic surgery of his left femur and the removal of his spleen. Several nursing diagnoses may apply to the case scenario, which may also be associated with growth and development. The client care plan that follows consists of selected areas of importance.

### Assessment
Pediatric client is recovering in stable manner after an ORIF of the left femur. His CMS (circulation, movement, sensation) checks are good, he is afebrile, his traction is in place, and his hemovac has a moderate amount of serosanguineous drainage.

### Nursing Diagnosis #1
*Acute Pain* related to the recent trauma and surgical interventions.
**NOC:** Pain Level; Pain Control; Comfort Level
**NIC:** Pain Management; Analgesic Administration

### Expected Outcomes
1. Reports pain level at a 3 (scale 1 to 10) within 24 hours.
2. Client will report pain and need for analgesics throughout hospitalization.

### Planning/Interventions/Rationales
1. Ongoing assessment of pain scale. *Allows for constant monitoring of subjective response to pain.*
2. Administer analgesics in timely fashion and determine specific medication most appropriate to pain level. *Most efficiently keeps acceptable pain level.*
3. Maintain proper positioning of traction and repaired femur. *Maintains child's body alignment.*

*(continues)*

# CASE STUDY/NURSING CARE PLAN (continued)

### Evaluation
Pain level at a 2 within 24 hours; traction and body kept in good alignment.

### Nursing Diagnosis #2
*Anxiety* related to recent trauma and uncertain outcome.
**NOC:** Anxiety Control; Aggression Control; Coping
**NIC:**  Anxiety Reduction

### Expected Outcomes
1. Client demonstrates improved concentration and accuracy of thoughts within 24 hours.

### Planning/Interventions/Rationales
1. Assist client in identifying precipitants to anxiety. *Provides method of "measuring level of anxiety."*
2. Involve Tony's parents in his care. *Assists in controlling his anxiety level, which contributes to pain level.*

### Evaluation
Tony has normal verbalizations in answering questions, and Tony's parents assisted with activities of daily living and communicated openly with their son.

# CONCEPT MAPPING CASE STUDY

Andrew (Drew) Peters, age 9, has been diagnosed with asthma, a chronic reactive airway disorder. He has been treated in the physician's office and the emergency department several times during the past 5 years for acute respiratory episodes, or "asthma attacks." The primary causes for these episodes were infections and exposure to allergens. He has been hospitalized twice during the past 2 years. He is currently admitted to the hospital for an acute respiratory infection. His temperature is 102.6°F, respirations are labored and rapid (30 to 40 per minute), pulse is 110, he has a productive cough of copious thick mucus, and expiratory wheezing is noted. Nasal flaring and intercostals retractions are noticed upon inspiration. The physical assessment indicates that Andrew is small for his age, his chest is slightly "barrel shaped," and he appears fatigued and anxious. His skin color is pale, lips and nailbeds are cyanotic, and his breath sounds are diminished. The physician orders pulmonary function tests, pulse oximetry, and a sputum culture. Additional orders include humidified oxygen via mask, respiratory therapy, and an intravenous line to be available for fluids and medications if needed. Medications include an aerosol bronchodilator, a systemic anti-inflammatory, and acetaminophen.

Drew's parents appear very anxious. His father leaves the room to smoke a cigarette. He promises Drew he will be right back. Mrs. Peters strokes Drew's arm and speaks softly to him. She mentions that he is worried about missing the school play in which he has a part tomorrow. She is also concerned regarding child care for his younger sister, Stephanie.

In this scenario, the family is your client. Refer back to the sample concept map for assistance in designing a map for Drew's case study. Add concepts where you believe they belong. (Some concepts may belong in more than one area.)

### Suggested References
Ball, J., & Bindler, R. (2003). *Pediatric nursing: Caring for children* (3rd ed.). Reading, MA: Pearson Education; current nurses drug guide or pharmacology text

*(continues)*

# CONCEPT MAPPING CASE STUDY (continued)

1. Why do you think the physician did not order an antibiotic for Drew at this time? (What additional information would you like to have?)
2. How would you evaluate the effectiveness of each of his medications? Discuss the nurse's role in monitoring Drew for drug-drug interactions.
3. List the nursing interventions you would use to:
   a. Facilitate easier breathing
   b. Promote decrease in Drew's temperature
   c. Assure adequate fluid balance
4. Identify the psychological needs of the family.
5. How would you cluster Drew's symptoms and needs for the nursing diagnoses of *Impaired Gas Exchange* and *Ineffective Airway Clearance*?
6. Select at least two additional nursing diagnoses. What clusters of information in the case study will you use to support your selected diagnoses?
7. How would you evaluate the family's knowledge in using an incentive spirometer?
8. Prioritize the items to include in home care instructions for Drew and his family.
9. Describe how you would communicate with the parents regarding stimuli, or triggers, in the environment that initiate Drew's asthmatic episodes.
10. What would you include in an individual school health management plan for Drew? (What measures would help to enhance Drew's self-image?)

## Key Concepts

- Growth is the quantitative changes in physical size of the body and its parts.
- Development is a qualitative term that refers to behavior changes and increasing competency in functional abilities and skills.
- Maturation, a qualitative term, describes a differentiation or increasing complexity of development capabilities that comes with age.
- During each developmental stage, certain developmental tasks must be achieved for normal development to occur.
- Growth and development of an individual are influenced by a combination of factors, including heredity, life experiences, health status, and cultural expectations.
- According to Freud, certain developmental tasks must be achieved at each of five psychosexual development stages from birth through adolescence. Failure to achieve, or a delay in achieving, the developmental task results in a fixation at a previous stage.
- Erikson stated that psychosocial development is a series of conflicts that occur during eight stages of life.
- Sullivan stated that personality development is strongly influenced by interpersonal relationships.
- Piaget's cognitive development theory states that there are four phases: sensorimotor, preoperational, concrete operations, and formal operations. Each phase is characterized by the ways in which the child interprets and uses the environment.
- Kohlberg's theory describes six progressive stages of moral development that determine an individual's moral code to guide personal behavior.
- Havighurst described the physical and behavioral developmental tasks for each developmental stage throughout the life span.
- Fowler's stages of faith theory states that there are six distinct stages of faith development and even though individuals vary in the age at which they experience each stage, the sequence of stages remains the same.
- Basic concepts of holistic professional nursing include consideration of the "wholeness" of individuals and supporting them in assuming responsibility for self-care.
- A major principle of professional holistic nursing is a respect for the diversity of persons and their values and beliefs.
- Nurses have important roles in promoting the health and safety of children and their families. Considering the family as "the client" is integral to providing comprehensive care.
- The stages of childhood include the prenatal, neonate, infant, toddler, preschooler, school-age child, the preadolescent, and adolescent.

## Review Questions and Activities

1. State three ways that Erikson's developmental theory relates to the nursing care of the toddler.

**2.** You are assigned to care for a 4-year-old girl. What games and toys would be appropriate for her?

**3.** What are several considerations the nurse should remember when performing client education with a 9-year-old boy?

**4.** You are a nurse in a clinic setting providing teaching to an adolescent male who has tested positive for Chlamydia (STD). What information will you discuss with him?

**5.** How does Erikson's concept of trust and mistrust relate to Fowler's theory stages of faith (undifferentiated faith)?

## Web Resources

Centers for Disease Control and Prevention
  http://www.cdc.gov
Healthfinder is maintained by the U.S. Department of Health and Human Services. It provides unbiased information, and links to many sites are listed.
  http://www.healthfinder.gov
Mental health information for children. A variety of topics are presented.
  http://www.mentalhelp.net
The National Association for Sport and Physical Education
  http://www.aahperd.org/naspe
National Health Information Center
  http://www.health.gov/nhic
The National Youth Sports Safety Foundation
  http://www.nyssf.org
Nemours Foundation (established by philanthropist Alfred duPont)
  http://www.kidshealth.org
Prenatal development from conception to time of birth
  http://www.visembryo.com
Parents' guide to childhood immunizations
  http://www.cdc.gov/nip

## References

Ackley, B., & Ladwig, G. (2002). *Nursing diagnosis handbook: A guide for planning care* (5th ed.). St. Louis: Mosby.

American Holistic Nursing Association (2002). Philosophy of organization. http://www.AHNA.org

American Nurses Association (1990). *Nursing's agenda for health care reform.* Washington, DC: Author.

Ball, J., & Bindler, R. (2003). *Pediatric nursing: Caring for children* (3rd ed.). Reading, MA: Pearson Education.

Berger, K., & Williams, M. (1999). Fundamentals of nursing: Collaborating for optimal Health. Stamford, CT: Appleton & Lange.

Black, J., Hawks, J., & Keene, A. (2001). *Medical-surgical nursing: Clinical management for positive outcomes.* Philadelphia: W. B. Saunders.

Brazelton, T. B., & Sparrow, J. (2001). *Touchpoints three to six.* Cambridge, MA: Perseus.

Centers for Disease Control and Prevention (2002). Parents' guide to childhood immunizations. www.cdc.gov/nip/publications/parents.guide/textreaderversion.htm

Clark, M. J. (1999). *Nursing in the community: Dimensions of community health nursing.* Stamford, CT: Appleton & Lange.

Edelman, C. L., & Mandle, C. L. (2001). *Health promotion throughout the life span* (5th ed.). St. Louis: Mosby-Yearbook.

Erikson, E. (1963). *Childhood and society.* New York: Norton.

Estes, M. E. (2002). *Health assessment & physical examination* (2nd ed.). Clifton Park, NY: Delmar Learning.

Fowler, J. W. (1981). *Stages of faith: The psychology of human development and the quest for meaning.* New York: Harper & Row.

Freud, S. (1961). *Civilization and its discontents.* New York: Norton.

Fuller, J., & Schaller-Ayers, J. (1999). *Health assessment: A nursing approach* (3rd ed.). Philadelphia: Lippincott.

Gaffney, K. (2001). Infant exposure to environmental tobacco smoke. *Journal of Nursing Scholarship, 33*(4), 343–347.

Guyton, A. C., & Hall, J. (2001). *Textbook of medical physiology* (10th ed.). Philadelphia: Saunders.

Havighurst, R. J. (1972). *Developmental tasks and education.* New York: Longman.

Herrmann, N. (1990). *The creative brain* (2nd ed.). Lake Lure, NC: The Ned Herrmann Group.

Hitchcock, J., Schubert, P., & Thomas, S. (2003). *Community health nursing: Caring in action* (2nd ed.). Clifton Park, NY: Delmar Learning.

Hockenberry, M., Wilson, D., Winkelstein, M., & Kline, N. (2003). *Wong's nursing care of infants and children* (7th ed.). St. Louis: Mosby-Yearbook.

Jean-Murat, C. (1999). *Menopause made easy.* Carlsbad, CA: Hay House.

Kearney, M., York, R., & Deatrick, J. (2000). Effects of home visits to vulnerable young families. *Journal of Nursing Scholarship, 32*(4), 369–376.

Kelly, G. (2001). *Sexuality today: The human perspective.* New York: McGraw-Hill.

Kohlberg, L. (1977). *Recent research in moral development.* New York: Holt, Rinehart, & Winston.

Kohlberg, L. (1983). The development of children's orientation toward a moral order. In W. Damon (Ed.), *Social and personality development essays on the growth of the child.* New York: W. W. Norton.

Littleton, L., & Engebretson, J. (2002). *Maternal, neonatal, and women's health nursing.* Clifton Park, NY: Delmar Learning.

Lucas, R., & Ferguson, M. (2000). Disorders of childhood and adolescence. In K. Fortinash & P. Holoday-Worret (Eds.), *Psychiatric mental health nursing.* St. Louis: C. V. Mosby.

Martin, S. (2002). Children exposed to domestic violence: Psychiatric considerations for health care practitioners. *Holistic Nursing Practice, 16*(3), 7–15.

McPeck, P. (2002). For Kieria's sake: Shaken Baby Syndrome. *NurseWeek Newsletter.* http://www.NurseWeek.com

Mohr, W. (2002). *Johnson's psychiatric-mental health nursing* (5th ed.). Philadelphia: Lippincott.

Murray, R., & Zentner, J. (2000). *Nursing assessment and health promotion strategies through the life span* (7th ed.). New Jersey: Prentice Hall.

Oran, D. (2000). Children and adolescents. In K. Fortinash & P. Holoday-Worret (Eds.), *Psychiatric mental health nursing* (2nd ed.). St. Louis: C. V. Mosby.

Piaget, J. (1963). *The origins of intelligence in children.* New York: Norton.

Piaget, J., & Inhelder, B. (1969). *The psychology of the child.* New York: Basic Books.

Potts, N., & Mandleco, B. (2002). *Pediatric nursing: Caring for children and their families.* Clifton Park, NY: Delmar Learning.

Reiss, B., Evans, M., & Broyles, B. (2002). *Pharmacological aspects of nursing care.* Clifton Park, NY: Delmar Learning.

Rutherford, K., Dowshen, S., & Mesinger, B. (2001). *Developing a child's self-esteem.* Nemours Foundation at: http://www.kidshealth.org

Sullivan, H. S. (1953). *Interpersonal theory of psychiatry.* New York: Norton.

*Taber's cyclopedic medical dictionary* (19th ed.) (2001). Sickle cell anemia; Tay-Sachs disease; Phenylketonuria. Author: Philadelphia: F. A. Davis.

U.S. Department of Health and Human Services (2000). *Healthy People 2010 Report.* Washington, DC: Author.

Varcarolis, E., & Rader, I. (2002). *Foundations of psychiatric mental health nursing* (4th ed.). Philadelphia: Saunders.

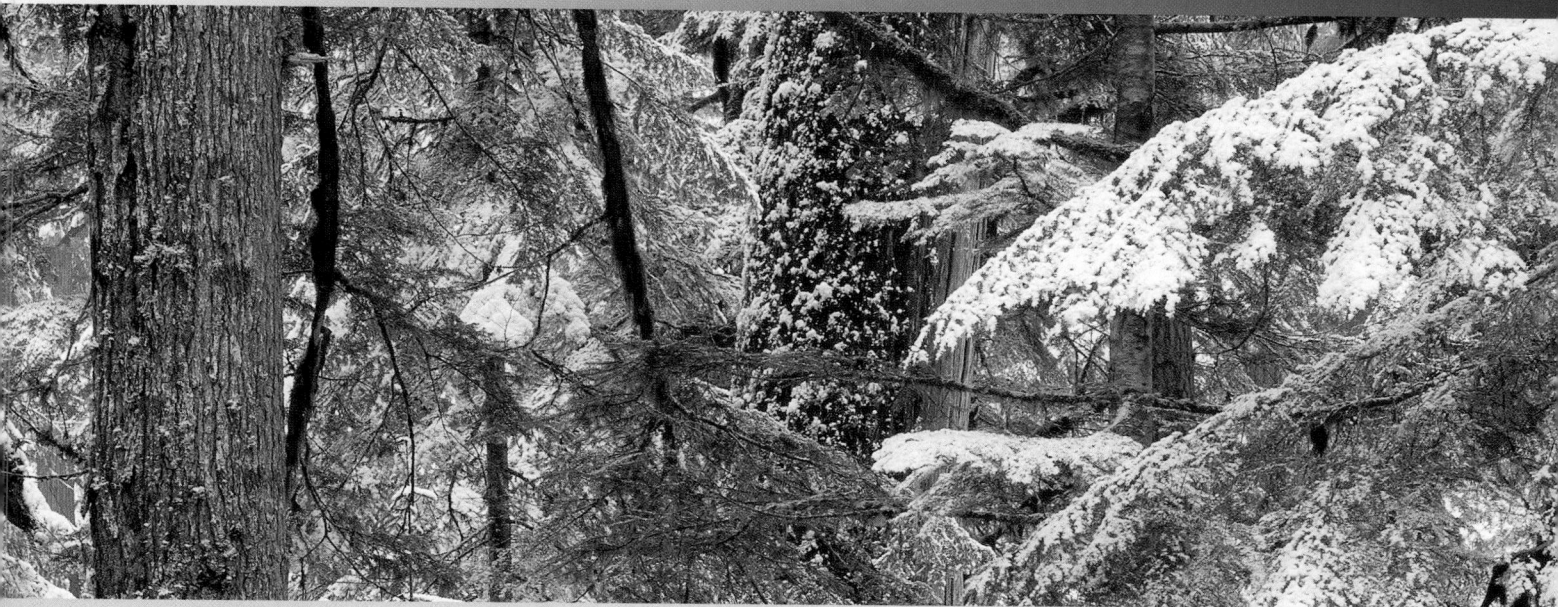

# CHAPTER 18

# The Adult Client

## Valerie Lindquist Stalsbroten, RN, MN
## Elizabeth Torrence, RN, MN, EdD

*"You are truly the generation in the middle! You have at once aging parents as well as maturing children to cope with, and you are not granted the deference accorded age, or the indulgence given the young."*

(H. Arnstein, 1978)

# Chapter Competencies

*Upon completion of this chapter, the reader should be able to:*

1. Identify the developmental context in which adulthood occurs.
2. Discuss young adulthood and the critical nature of this developmental stage in life.
3. Describe the issues in middle adulthood and the developmental implications of this age.
4. Integrate the nursing role into the health care issues experienced in young and middle adulthood.

# Key Terms

adherence

generativity

hardiness

middle adulthood

presbyopia

stagnation

young adulthood

This chapter discusses the growth and developmental issues that span the period from the end of adolescence through middle adulthood. Although physical growth is complete by adulthood, certain health-related changes continue to occur throughout adulthood. Often the physical and health changes associated with living have been called the effects of aging. In this section, the attribution of the changes through every age will be referred to as the effects of living.

## Passage Through Adulthood

The changes facing adults are very different from those of the infant, the child, and the adolescent. As a person leaves the *Sturm und Drang* (storm and stress) of the adolescent period and enters adult life, healthy independence and adult relationships become the focus. Relationships include family of origin relationships, selecting a life partner or choosing to remain single, marriage and family relations, connections with children, involvement with fellow workers and colleagues, spiritual and religious connections, and general formations in community life. These relationships are strongly influenced by the experiences of childhood and adolescence. Healthy independence is reflected in a lifestyle that selects health promotion activities and both short-term and long-term illness prevention strategies (Siegler, 2000).

### The Adult in Society

To describe the "average" adult in today's world is difficult. A description can be accurate in stereotype yet imprecise in relation to the individual person. The nurse must assess each person as an individual and apply what is known about the physiology, psychology, spirituality, and moral and cognitive development of adults to how the individual presents. The nurse must use a disciplined and reflective approach to assess each person's presentation (Rook, 2000).

## Ending Adolescence and Beginning Adulthood

Just as the adolescent struggles with developing identity, the individual in the late adolescent–early adulthood period continues with parallel issues. Continuity and change are present in developmental transitions in late adolescence, early adulthood, and adulthood. In late adolescence–early adulthood, the struggles of autonomy versus attachment to parents are reaching resolution and maturity. Peer pressure diminishes as the complexity of individual identity becomes clearer and is achieved. This transitional period from adolescence to adulthood is variously represented as a period that is as short as 2 years and as long as 8 to 10 years (Klein, Allan, Elster, Stevens, Cox, Hedberg, & Goodman, 2001).

Often the parameters that mark the transition from adolescence are financial independence and independent decision making (e.g., living on one's own). An indication of the transition into early adulthood is full-time employment and residence outside of the parental home. This takes place after either high school or college. Because of financial considerations, full-time employment can occur while in high school and hence the distinction of residing outside the parental home. The young adult establishes a relationship with the parent(s) as an independent person able to make decisions based on his own set of values and beliefs. During this time, the individual assumes responsibility for his own actions and behaviors (Scal, Evans, Blozis, Okinow, & Blum, 1999).

# Young Adulthood

The **young adulthood** period, often identified as between ages 18 and 30 (note: some sources use the ages 21 to 40), is as critical a precursor of future well-being and development as are the previous periods. Plans, behaviors, and decisions made during this time profoundly affect both the quality and length of one's current and future life (Potts & Mandleco, 2002).

## A Critical Period of Life

Young adults experience the true weight of adult decision making in issues such as choosing lifestyles, developing a diet and eating behaviors, selecting an appropriate exercise routine, using illicit drugs, consuming alcohol, developing a healthy sexuality, selecting a career and employment, establishing adult relationships, falling in love, becoming intimate, choosing a marriage partner or significant other, staying single or becoming divorced, and becoming a parent (Figure 18-1). The path of adulthood is filled with changes and decisions that have long-term effects (Klein et al., 2001) (Table 18-1).

## Health Issues and Implications for Nursing

Health issues during young adulthood are varied. Many times young adulthood is a healthy period in a person's life. However, healthy responses to the stressors of this period become an important objective. Some health issues continue from adolescence and constitute chronic illness. Transitional care programs are necessary to provide quality continuing care to the adolescent with a chronic illness who is converting to adult-oriented health care. Transition from pediatric to adult health care services depends on external financial funding sources and access (Scal et al., 1999). Nurses are invaluable resources to young adults in the areas of health promotion, teaching, and counseling.

### Pregnancy

Pregnancy is a time of transition and lifestyle adjustment that is experienced by many women in young adulthood (Potts & Mandleco, 2002). Table 18-2 lists a few of the changes commonly experienced by women during pregnancy (Figure 18-2). Throughout pregnancy, women experience changes in self-concept and may need reassurance that such changes are normal.

### Acute Problems

Statistically the young adult has a greater chance of dying in an accident or from suicide than from any other cause. Sexually transmitted diseases are problematic in the young adult and require knowledge and practice of sexually responsible behavior. HIV infection and AIDS have had a profound effect on sexual behavior and the need for safe

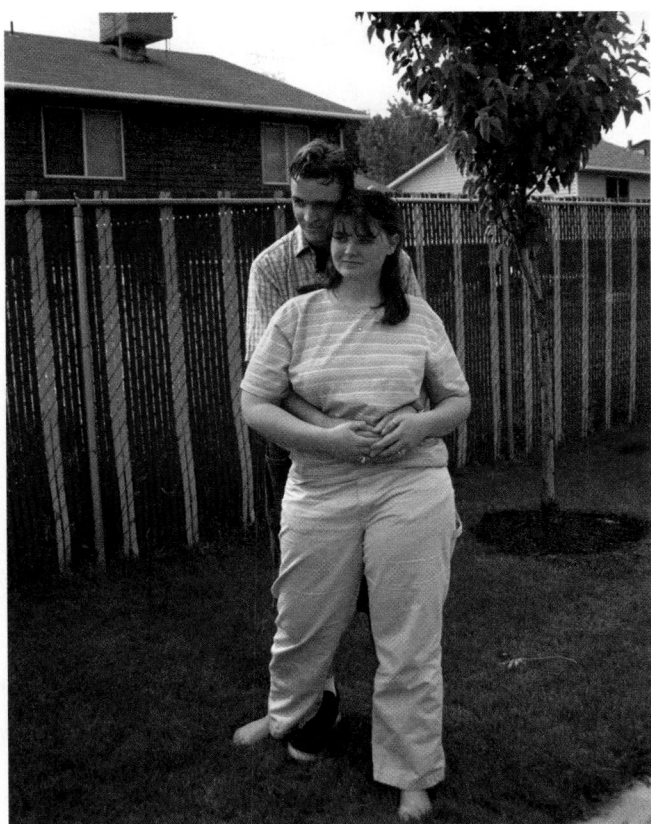

**Figure 18-1    Young adulthood brings a continuing drive to develop a healthy sexuality and to develop intimate relationships.**

## NURSING STRATEGY

### Assessment for Substance Abuse

The following are items you can ask about in assessing for substance abuse:

- Past and recurrent use of the substance
- Age when first began
- When was the substance last used
- Preferred method of use of the substance
- Amount of substance used
- Effect of the substance
- Circumstances associated with use of the substance
- How the substance is obtained
- Number of attempts to cease or decrease use

Adapted from Alcoholics Anonymous, 2003. Available: www.alcoholics-anonymous.org

## TABLE 18-1 YOUNG ADULT: GROWTH AND DEVELOPMENT

| Dimension | Characteristics | Nursing Implications |
|---|---|---|
| Physiological | *Physiological Changes:*<br>Physical growth stabilizes.<br><br>Physical functioning is optimum.<br><br>Maturation of body systems is complete.<br><br>*Cardiovascular Changes:*<br>Men are more likely to have increased cholesterol levels than women.<br><br>*Gastrointestinal Changes:*<br>After age 30, digestive juices decrease.<br><br>*Dental Changes:*<br>By mid-20s, dental maturity is achieved with emergence of last four molars ("wisdom teeth").<br><br>*Musculoskeletal Changes:*<br>At approximately age 25, skeletal growth is complete.<br><br>*Reproductive/Sexual Changes:*<br>System is completely matured.<br><br>*Women:*<br>Ages 20 to 30 are optimal years for reproduction.<br><br>*Men:*<br>Beginning at about age 24, male hormones slowly decrease; does not affect ability to reproduce. | The person is at physical peak and therefore less likely to be concerned with own health.<br>Teach importance of health promotion behaviors.<br><br>Encourage development of healthy lifestyles. |
| Psychosocial | *Erikson:* Intimacy vs. Isolation<br>Engages in productive work<br>Develops intimate relationships<br><br>*Havighurst:*<br>Becomes part of a social group<br>Selects a partner<br>Assumes civic responsibility | Emphasize need for social support as the person assumes new roles.<br>Teach time management skills.<br><br>Provide sex education information, including prevention of STDs. |
| Cognitive | *Piaget:* Formal operations stage<br>Problem-solving abilities are realistic.<br>Less egocentricism is demonstrated.<br>Many young adults are engaged in formal educational activities. | Encourage the development and use of appropriate judgment. |
| Moral | *Kohlberg:* Postconventional stage<br>Right and wrong is defined in terms of personal beliefs and principles.<br><br>*Gilligan:* Women consider morality to be based on caring for others and avoiding hurt. | Assess the person's value system and respect beliefs. |
| Spiritual | *Fowler:* Individuative-reflective faith<br>Assumes responsibility for own beliefs | Encourage client to use spiritual support system. |

Adapted from Beare, P. G., & Myers, J. L. (1998). *Adult health nursing.* (3rd ed.). St. Louis: Mosby-Yearbook; Edelman, C. L., & Mandle, C. L. (2002). *Health promotion throughout the life span* (5th ed.). St. Louis: Mosby-Yearbook.

## TABLE 18-2    CHANGES EXPERIENCED DURING PREGNANCY

| Physiological | Psychological |
| --- | --- |
| *First Trimester* | *First Trimester* |
| Fatigue | Emotional detachment as thoughts begin to focus on developing child |
| Nausea and vomiting | |
| Urinary frequency | Labile (rapidly changing) mood |
| Constipation | Ambivalence about the pregnancy |
| Breast tenderness and enlargement | Increased dependency on others |
| | Interest in learning about physical changes |
| *Second Trimester* | *Second Trimester* |
| Perception of fetal movement | Doubts and fears about ability to care for an infant |
| Fetal heart tone can be detected with fetoscope | Bond with mate either strengthened or threatened |
| Increased libido | Excited by fetal movement |
| | Initial attachment with fetus strengthened |
| *Third Trimester* | *Third Trimester* |
| Backache | Feels less attractive |
| Stretch marks on abdomen or breasts | Increased irritability |
| Urinary frequency | Insomnia |
| Heartburn | Anticipation of birth |
| Shortness of breath | Plans for incorporating child into family unit |
| Varicose veins on legs | |

Adapted from Edelman, C. L., & Mandle, C. L. (2002). *Health promotion throughout the life span* (5th ed.). St. Louis: Mosby-Yearbook; Fuller, J., & Schaller-Ayers, J. (1999). *Health assessment: A nursing approach* (3rd ed.). Philadelphia: Lippincott.

sex practices. Even so, AIDS is a leading cause of death in persons ages 25 to 44 (Joslin & Harrison, 2002).

Young adults seek intervention from health care providers for acute episodic short-term illnesses. The pattern of developing health-seeking and illness-preventing behaviors must begin either in the parental home or in

high school (Klein et al., 2001). Nurses in the college environment collaborate with counseling departments in providing programs to assist the late adolescent or young adult with support for these issues. Education has been found to be a strong predictor of healthy lifestyle choices; nurses can play a pivotal role by providing health education and guidance to the young adult.

### Health Promotion and Wellness

Health promotion and wellness for the young adult will typically focus on avoidance of accident, injury, and violence, and development of health promoting lifestyle behaviors. Nurses can share information regarding sexually transmitted diseases, prevention of unwanted pregnancy, and good health practices. Young adulthood is a critical time for nurses to teach: (1) men and women to perform monthly breast self-examinations (BSE), and (2) men to perform testicular self-examinations (TSE) (see Chapter 46 for more information on BSE and TSE). Nurses can also teach clients in regard to safety issues, such as "drinking and driving" and avoiding risk factors for skin cancer (e.g., overexposure to sun, tanning salons) (Schofield & Robinson, 2000).

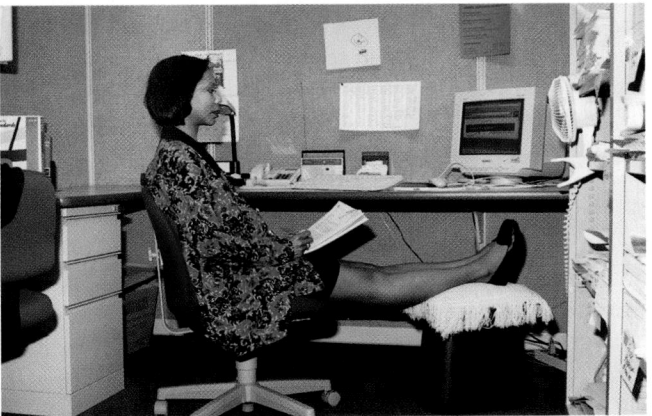

**Figure 18-2    Swollen lower extremities is just one of the common changes occurring during pregnancy.**

# Middle Adulthood

**Middle adulthood** is typically defined as the period between age 30 and 55; however, this age range is not fixed (note: some sources state 40 to 65 years). The percentage of individuals falling within this age range is increasing, as is the expected life span, so the years referred to as "middle age" are also occurring later (Hackler, 2001). Maintaining health and wellness during middle adulthood can be more challenging, as lifestyle choices, heredity, and environment play a large role in an adult's ability to remain healthy.

## Health Issues and Implications for Nursing

Just as behavior and choice affected the health of the young adult, so the continued behavior, choices, and consequences over time affect the health of the middle-aged adult. Stress and illness become strongly associated. Worry about one's health often begins or intensifies during the middle years. Psychological stress and distress cause neurohormonal changes that negatively impact the autonomic nervous system, the immune system, and the endocrine system. Cardiovascular disease, cancer, and obesity become a major cause of morbidity and mortality in the middle and later adult years. Automobile accidents, especially those involving the use of alcohol, are a serious health problem for middle-aged adults. Another significant problem is occupational health hazards such as expo-

## CLINICAL ALERT

### Risk Factors for Skin Cancer

The following are people with risk factors for skin cancer:

- Fair-skinned, fair-haired, blue-eyed people

- People who sustain sunburn and do not tan

- People with longtime sun exposure (farmers, fisherman, construction workers)

- Adults who sunburn as frequently as children

- Elderly people and those with sun-damaged skin

- People exposed to chemical pollutants (arsenic, nitrates, coal, tar and pitch, and oils and paraffins)

Adapted from Schofield, J. R., & Robinson, W. (2000). *What you really need to know about moles and melanoma*. Baltimore: Johns Hopkins Press.

## CLIENT EDUCATION

### Preventing Skin Cancer

The following are preventive measures against developing skin cancer:

✓ Do not try to tan if your skin burns easily.

✓ Avoid unnecessary exposure to the sun.

✓ Avoid sunburn.

✓ Apply sunscreen of SPF 15 or higher when in the sun (note: cloudy days still produce dangerous ultraviolet rays). Sunscreens are rated in strength from 4 (lowest) to 50 (highest). The SPF indicates the solar protection factor, or how long a person can stay in the sun before getting burned.

✓ Wear protective clothing (broad-brimmed hat, long sleeves) if you are an at-risk individual.

✓ Use a lip balm that contains a sunscreen with the highest SPF number.

Adapted from American Cancer Society, 2003. Available: http://www.cancer.org

sure to environmental toxins. Middle adulthood is also the time when a lifelong accumulation of unhealthy lifestyle practices, such as smoking, sedentary habits, inadequate nutrition, and overuse of alcohol may begin to exert adverse effects (Siegler, Bastian, & Bosworth, 2000).

## Developmental Considerations

Many developmental changes occur in middle adulthood (Table 18-3). The primary development task of middle-aged persons revolves around the conflict of **generativity** (a sense that one is making a contribution to society) versus **stagnation** (a sense of nonmeaning in one's life) (Figure 18-3). When an individual successfully resolves this developmental conflict, acceptance of age-related changes occurs. Achievement of the developmental task is indicated by the following: (1) demonstrating creativity, (2) guiding the next generation, (3) establishing lasting relationships, and (4) evaluating goals in terms of achievement. The evaluation of goals often leads to a midlife crisis, especially if individuals feel they have accomplished little or not lived up to earlier self-expectations (Erikson, 1968).

## Physiological Changes

Peak physical performance is attained in the late twenties and then begins to decline. Physical stamina begins to diminish as normal cardiovascular and respiratory changes occur.

In middle age, sensory changes may also occur. **Presbyopia**, or the inability of the visual lens to change shape, causes the farsightedness common in the middle years. Hearing begins to diminish, especially for high-

## TABLE 18-3 MIDDLE ADULT: GROWTH AND DEVELOPMENT

| Dimension | Characteristics | Nursing Implications |
|---|---|---|
| *Physiological* | *Cardiovascular Changes:*<br>Decreased functional aerobic capacity results in decreased cardiac output.<br>Blood vessels become thicker and lose elasticity. | Decreased capacity for physical activity.<br>Instruct client about necessity of remaining physically active. Predisposition for hypertension (high blood pressure), coronary artery disease, cerebral vascular accidents ("strokes").<br>Teach client about lifestyle modifications related to cardiovascular health:<br>• Smoking cessation<br>• Avoid secondary tobacco smoke<br>• Nutrition (low fat, low cholesterol)<br>• Engage in physical activity |
| | *Neurological Changes:*<br>Cellular changes (regulation, repair, and atrophy) occur gradually.<br>A gradual loss in efficiency of nerve conduction leads to impaired sensation of heat and cold. | Explain age-related changes.<br>Provide support and reassurance.<br>Teach safety precautions regarding:<br>• Exposure to sunlight<br>• Sensitivity to heatstroke<br>• Sensitivity to frostbite |
| | *Gastrointestinal Changes:*<br>Slower gastrointestinal motility results in constipation. | Teach client about:<br>• Nutrition (high-fiber food intake; adequate amounts of fluid)<br>• Maintaining physical activity |
| | *Genitourinary Changes:*<br>Nephron units diminish in number and size; diminished blood supply to kidneys.<br><br>Decreased glomerular filtration rate leads to decrease in urinary output with resultant dehydration. | Teach normal age-related changes.<br><br>Teach signs indicative of dehydration.<br>Inform client of need to maintain adequate fluid intake. |
| | *Integumentary Changes:*<br>Decreased moisture and turgor of skin and loss of subcutaneous fat leads to development of wrinkles.<br>Hair thins and turns gray. | Instruct client about effects of sun and cigarette smoking on the skin.<br>Assess client for body image alterations.<br>Use nonjudgmental listening.<br>Provide support. |
| | *Musculoskeletal Changes:*<br>Decreased bone mass and density.<br>Slight (from 1 to 4 inches) loss of height may occur.<br><br>Thinning of intervertebral disks.<br><br>Generalized decrease in muscle tone; "flabby" appearance and less agility. | Instruct client about:<br>• Need for calcium intake<br>• Importance of decreasing caffeine and alcohol consumption<br>• Effects of sedentary versus active lifestyle on osteoporosis<br>Increased risk of injury. Instruct client of need for proper posture (especially sitting), exercise, and adequate fluid intake.<br>Instruct client on need for adequate physical activity. |
| | *Endocrine Changes:*<br>Decreased metabolism results in reduced production of enzymes and increased hydrochloric acid.<br>Lead to acid indigestion and belching. | Instruct client to:<br>• Eat foods that are not spicy or fried<br>• Avoid eating within 2 hours before bedtime |

*(continues)*

## TABLE 18-3     MIDDLE ADULT: GROWTH AND DEVELOPMENT (*continued*)

| Dimension | Characteristics | Nursing Implications |
|---|---|---|
|  | *Reproductive/Sexual Changes—Women:*<br>Cessation of estrogen and progesterone production during menopause<br>Regression of secondary sex characteristics (decreased breast size, loss of pubic hair)<br>Decreased vaginal secretions<br>Note: With no pregnancy risk, some postmenopausal women enjoy sexual activity more. | Teach clients about age-related sexual/reproductive changes.<br>Encourage responsible sexual behavior.<br>Teach about prevention of sexually transmitted diseases. |
|  | *Reproductive/Sexual Changes—Men:*<br>Decreased levels of testosterone<br>Reduced amount of viable sperm<br>Decline in sexual energy; takes longer to achieve an erection; erection is sustained longer<br>Adaptation to developing chronic diseases and sexual problems may diminish self-esteem |  |
| Psychosocial | *Erikson:* Generativity vs. Stagnation<br>Adults who have achieved generativity feel good about their lives and are comfortable with themselves.<br>Become more involved in altruistic acts (e.g., community activities, volunteer work)<br>Usually experience changing family roles (e.g., caregiver to aging parents, grandparent) | Provide support as the client deals with aging.<br>Encourage to become involved in community activities.<br>Teach leisure skills.<br>Instruct in the need to care for self while caring for others. |
|  | *Havighurst:*<br>Fulfill social and civic responsibilities<br>Assist children to become independent<br>Adult children leaving home may lead to happiness or depression ("empty nest syndrome")<br>Maintain relationship with one's partner |  |
| Cognitive | *Piaget:*<br>Will use all stages, depending on the task (e.g., can move between formal operations, concrete operations, and problem solving as needed)<br>Able to reflect on the past and anticipate the future<br>Reaction time diminishes during late middle age.<br>Memory is unimpaired.<br>Learning ability remains intact if person is motivated and material is meaningful. | Encourage middle-age clients who are anticipating returning to school or engaging in other intellectually stimulating activities. |
| Moral | *Kohlberg:* Postconventional stage | Use nonjudgmental approach when client discusses values. |
|  | *Gilligan:*<br>Women tend to judge morality of issues according to a sense of fairness and avoiding hurt to others.<br>Establishes moral beliefs that are independent of what others think | Respect personal differences by individualizing care. |
| Spiritual | *Fowler:* Conjunctive faith<br>Is able to appreciate others' belief systems<br>Becomes less dogmatic with own beliefs<br>Religion is usually a source of comfort. | Encourage use of spiritual support.<br>Refer to clergy if desired by client. |

Adapted from Beare, P. B., & Myers, J. L. (1998). *Adult health nursing* (3rd ed.). St. Louis: Mosby-Yearbook; Edelman, C. L., & Mandle, C. L. (2002). *Health promotion throughout the life span* (5th ed.). St. Louis: Mosby-Yearbook; Fuller, J., & Schaller-Ayers, J. (1999). *Health assessment: A nursing approach* (3rd ed.). Philadelphia: Lippincott.

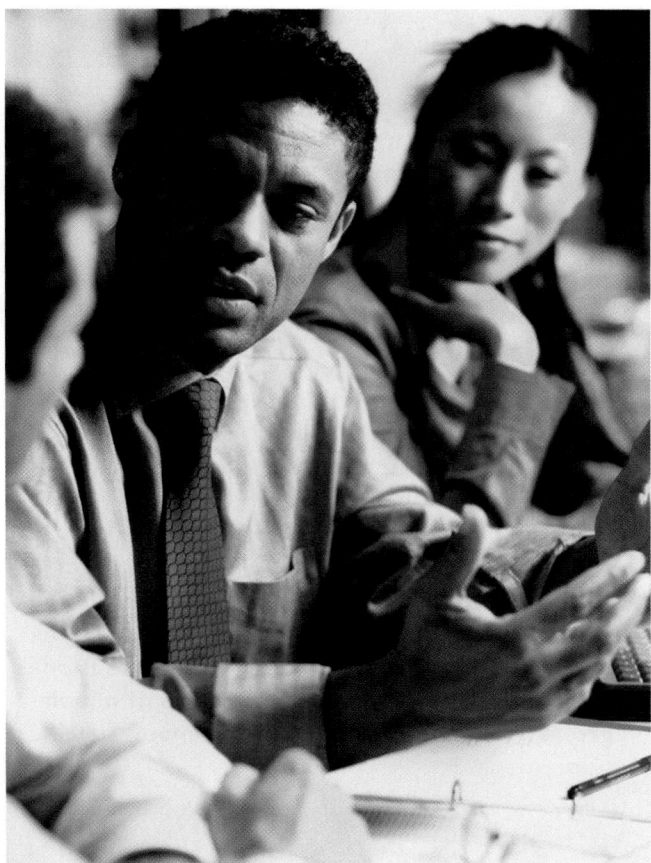

**Figure 18-3    A primary developmental task in middle adulthood is attaining success, which is often reflected in obtaining professional status.** *Courtesy of Photodisc*

frequency sound. Muscle tone begins to moderate and body fat begins to increase. Hair begins to gray, hair loss may occur, and subcutaneous fascia diminishes, causing skin wrinkles to appear. Menopause occurs in women due to a decrease in hormones. The loss of calcium from the bone increases the incidence of osteoporosis among postmenopausal women and some men (Hogstel, 2001).

## Stress Management

An adult in today's society may experience stress in all areas of life: work and professional life, personal and family life, and even in recreational activities. Psychosocial stressors of middle age may include increasingly dependent aging parents, relationships with adult children, and changes in professional or personal status. Stress can contribute to cardiovascular disability and disease, gastrointestinal disorders, alcohol-related problems, violence, vehicular deaths and injury, and psychiatric disorders from depression to suicide.

Of all predictors of health, stress is one of the most significant factors (Thomas, 1997). Stress can alter many aspects of a client's life (Chiriboga, 1997). Therefore, stress reduction and relaxation techniques should be fundamental to a nurse's practice. Maddi and Hightower

# STOP AND THINK

## Nurses Helping Clients Make Healthy Choices

- Why do you think many middle-aged clients do not participate in healthy lifestyles?

- What can nurses do to encourage clients to participate in healthy activities?

(1999) described the personality characteristic of **hardiness** (the ability to survive stress). Individuals who were hardy (i.e., who were generally resourceful and had a sense that problems were challenges and not threats) were generally healthier than those who did not display this characteristic. Adults who face these dilemmas need assistance in sorting out how to manage their increased responsibilities.

## Health Promotion and Wellness

The nurse plays an important role in helping individuals manage the changes in their lives by providing them with ways to practice personal wellness (Edwards & Ung, 2002; Gottlieb & Wolfe, 2002; Joslin & Harrison, 2002; McCarty & Drebing, 2002). A healthy lifestyle and preventive health care are keys to personal wellness. The middle-aged adult should have regular health checkups, eat a well-balanced diet, have a regular exercise program, and maintain body weight appropriate to body size (Institute of Medicine, 2002).

Nurses can encourage middle-aged adults to assume more responsibility for their own health (Figure 18-4) (see Research Focus box). Wellness promotion must also be a focus for community settings. Self-care education topics appropriate for middle-aged adults are shown in the Focus on Wellness box.

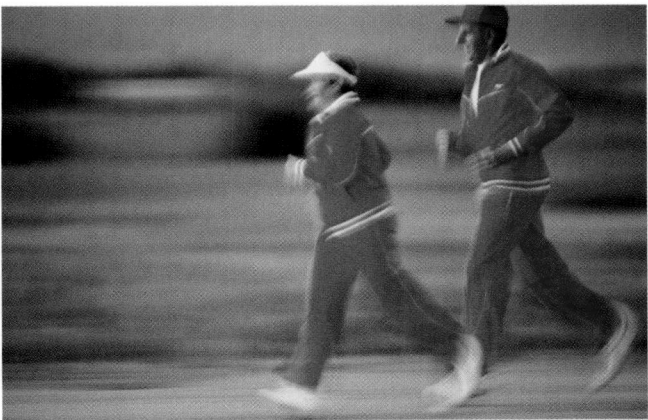

**Figure 18-4    Through activities such as running, these middle-aged adults have taken responsibility for their health and are learning to cope with the physiological changes that occur during this stage.**

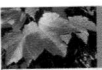

## RESEARCH FOCUS

**Title of Study:** Does adherence make a difference?: Results from a community-based aquatic exercise program

**Study Purpose:** An intervention research project that identifies the characteristics and outcomes for adult participants who adhere to a community-based aquatic exercise program.

**Methods:** Two hundred and forty-nine adults with osteoarthritis were recruited from Washington State for randomization to a 20-week Arthritis Foundation aquatic exercise program (n-125) or a wait-list control group (n-124). Adherers were defined as those attending at least two classes per week for 16 of 20 weeks. The measures included: Quality of Well-Being Scale, Health Assessment Questionnaire, Center for Epidemiological Studies-Depression Scale, and a single arthritis quality of life rating-item.

**Findings:** The baseline to postintervention change scores revealed that treatment-group adherers reported improved quality of well-being, physical function, and change in arthritis quality of life compared to the control group. When comparing treatment-group adherers to treatment-group nonadherers, the quality of well-being and depressed mood improved for adherers, but not for nonadherers.

**Implications:** When analyzed for level of participation, aquatic exercise benefits adults with osteoarthritis. Consistent participation in exercise programs results in better outcomes. Nurses can assist in improving the methods for enhancing adherence to exercise and assessing the intrinsic factors that increase adherence (e.g., self-esteem, self-efficacy).

Belza, B., Topolski, T., Kinne, S., Patrick, D., & Ramsey, S. (2002). Does adherence make a difference?: Results from a community-based aquatic exercise program. *Nursing Research, 51*(5), 285–291.

### Nurses and Illness Prevention

Understanding the health care needs of the middle-aged population is essential. Not only should the nurse have knowledge and information about particular illnesses or diseases that affect adults, but the nurse also needs to understand how these illnesses can be prevented (Figure 18-5). For example, insulin-dependent diabetics may not control their exercise regimen and be intermittent in their

## COMMUNITY/HOME CARE

### Addressing the Community Wellness Needs of the Middle-Aged Adult

Often the general health needs of the middle-aged adult community are not easily addressed. People of this age group usually only visit health care providers when they are ill. Consequently, disseminating pertinent information regarding specific changes in community health needs is most often addressed in the media and is usually illness oriented. This may not be the best approach to increasing the healthy status of middle-aged adults. Nurses must stay vigilant in their pursuit of providing wellness information, such as teaching preventive care and encouraging routine exams, to the adult community by whatever means possible. Implementing Healthy People 2010 activities is one means of increasing the wellness status of middle-aged adults (see Chapter 32 for more specific information).

Healthy People 2010, 2003. http://www.healthypeople.gov

## FOCUS ON WELLNESS

### Self-Care Education Topics for the Middle-Aged Adult

- Acceptance of aging
- Nutrition
- Exercise and weight control
- Substance abuse prevention
- Stress management
- Recommendations for health screening (cholesterol screening, prostate examination, mammogram, Papanicolaou [Pap] test)

Pender, J., Murdaugh, C., & Parsons, M. A. (2002). *Health promotion in nursing practice* (4th ed.). Upper Saddle River, NJ: Prentice-Hall.

## LEGAL AND ETHICAL ISSUES

### Nonjudgmental Attitude Toward Clients Who Do Not Adhere to Their Therapeutic Regimen

A difficult ethical issue for many nurses is how to accept clients who purposefully and knowingly do not adhere to their therapeutic regimen. It can be very frustrating for the nurse to see a client participate in unhealthy behaviors after a good teaching plan has been presented. The nurse must remember that nonadherence is not a personal attack by the client. In addition, there are many variables related to **adherence** (i.e., remaining faithful to a program of instruction or activity) (see Box 18-1). The nurse must remember to remain professional, exercise patience, and to "rise above" the emotional nature of the situation by seeking the reason for the noncompliance and by incorporating alternate teaching methods to encourage client cooperation.

O'Halloran, V. E. (1997). Defining educational settings to improve client health teaching. *MEDSURG Nursing, 6*(3), 130–136.

### BOX 18-1   VARIABLES THAT AFFECT THE DEGREE OF ADHERENCE TO A THERAPEUTIC REGIMEN

The following are some of the variables that affect a person's adherence to a therapeutic regimen:

- Illness variables, such as the severity of the illness and the type of clinical manifestations during the illness

- Demographic variables, such as age, gender, ethnic origin, education, and socioeconomic status

- Financial variables, particularly if the cost of the management program is above the client's budget process

- Treatment variables that are difficult to follow and hard to understand

- Presence and availability of an effective support system for the client

Adapted from Tierney, A. J., Worth, A., & Watson, N. (2000). Meeting patients' information needs before and after discharge from hospital, *Journal of Clinical Nursing, 9*(6), 14–19.

activities. The nurse needs to explain that blood glucose levels may vary within different exercise patterns, which changes the amount of insulin the body needs to maintain an adequate blood glucose level. Controlled exercise prevents diabetic complications, such as diabetic ketoacidosis, which is important for the nurse to teach to the client with diabetes. In addition, nurses must be professional when caring for clients who are noncompliant with their management regimen.

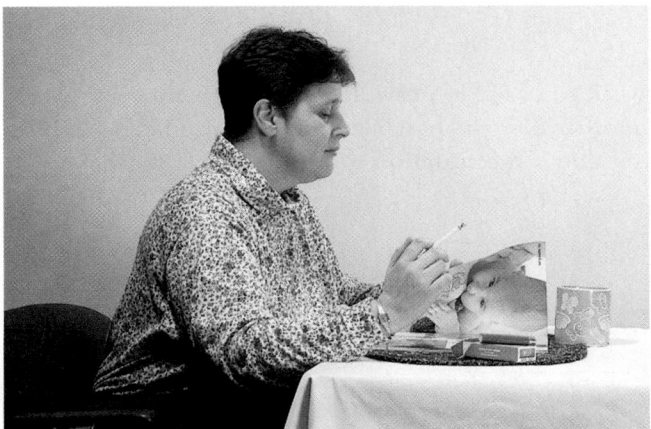

**Figure 18-5   This client is continuing to smoke, even though she knows that lung cancer is the leading cause of cancer death in women.**

### Resources for Wellness

The Agency for Health Care Research and Quality (AHRQ) sponsors and conducts research that provides clinicians with evidence-based information on health care outcomes. This agency sponsors the United States Preventive Services Task Force (USPSTF) (2003), which is responsible for evaluating and publishing the services that should routinely be incorporated into primary preventive health care (http://www.ahrq.gov).

The federal government has other programs available to nurses that provide useful information in the cause of health promotion and illness prevention. The Healthy People 2010 (2003) initiative is available at http://www.healthypeople.gov. This site's purpose is to ensure that good health, as well as long life, is enjoyed by all. Healthy People 2010 includes 10 leading health indicators. The indicators have resources for individuals to access related to each area (see Chapter 32).

The American Cancer Society (2003) is organized to eliminate cancer as a major health problem. It has proposed goals and objectives for the nation to be reached by 2015; these can be reviewed at http://www.cancer.org.

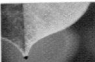

# CASE STUDY/NURSING CARE PLAN

Mrs. Mona Centurion has come into your urgent care center with complaints of mild headaches, stress, and fatigue. Mrs. Centurion is a 48-year-old professional stockbroker with two children ages 13 and 9. Her husband is a software engineer who works for a petroleum company and frequently travels. Mona's mother is a widow and has recently been diagnosed with Alzheimer's disease. She has been residing in an assisted living center for 4 years. One day, Mrs. Centurion received a phone call from the nursing director of the assisted living center, reporting that Mona's mother had assaulted another resident. The nursing director told Mona that her mother was no longer an appropriate resident for this living situation. She informed Mrs. Centurion that she had 30 days to find another placement for her mother. Mrs. Centurion could not find a care facility, took a temporary leave from work, and is caring for her mother in her own home.

## Assessment

Client is a 48-year-old professional who is just recently responsible for providing and coordinating the care of her mother. The mother has Alzheimer's disease, has been evicted from her resident living facility, and is now living in Mrs. Centurion's home. Mrs. Centurion is stressed over the circumstances, has mild hypertension (BP = 136/92, P = 86/minute), and is overweight (height = 5 feet 6 inches, weight = 148 pounds). In addition, Mrs. Centurion lives a sedentary lifestyle, prior to leave of absence normally worked 50 to 60 hours per week, and "eats when she is stressed." Mrs. Centurion is also very concerned for the financial implications related to her mother's care situation.

## Nursing Diagnosis #1

*Caregiver Strain* due to the sudden role change of caring for her mother in her home.

**NOC:** Caregiver Emotional Health; Caregiver Endurance Potential; Caregiver Lifestyle Disruption; Caregiver Performance: Direct Care; Caregiver Physical Health; Caregiver Stressors; Caregiver Well-Being

**NIC:** Caregiver Support

## Expected Outcomes

The client will:
1. Identify one source of support by her second appointment at the urgent care center.
2. Identify two changes that, if made, would improve her daily life within 2 weeks.

## Planning/Interventions/Rationales

1. Develop a plan of care for her mother that includes tasks that another person (e.g., home health aide) could provide. *Delegates caregiving tasks to decrease the client's stress.*
2. Allow spouse and children to watch the mother while client takes a half-hour walk each evening. *Decreases stress and encourages healthy behavior.*
3. Engage the family (separate from the caregiver) in appraisal of situation; potentially explore another caregiving facility. *Broadens the base of support for client.*

## Evaluation

Client hired a home health aide to visit three times per week to assist in providing care to the mother with Alzheimer's disease. The children and husband watch the mother every night while Mrs. Centurion takes a 30-minute walk. In 2 weeks, client stated she was feeling better about the situation of caring for her mother.

## Nursing Diagnosis #2

*Ineffective Health Maintenance* related to increased stress from caregiver strain.

**NOC:** Health Beliefs: Perceived Resources; Health-Promoting Behavior, Health-Seeking Behavior

**NIC:** Health System Guidance; Support System Enhancement; Health Education

## Expected Outcomes

The client will:
1. Decrease her blood pressure by 10% within 2 weeks.
2. Develop a balanced diet plan within 2 weeks and adhere to the diet on a daily basis.

*(continues)*

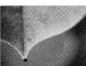

# CASE STUDY/NURSING CARE PLAN (continued)

3. Identify a goal weight to obtain, and lose 2 pounds per week for 4 weeks (and then progressively work toward maintaining her goal weight).

### Planning/Interventions/Rationales

1. Takes blood pressure daily. *Monitors blood pressure patterns.*
2. Eats a well-balanced diet that is normal in caloric intake for client, low in fat, and low in sodium. *Decrease mild hypertension by reducing cardiovascular risk factors associated with incorrect diet.*
3. Attends a social group that focuses on weight loss and maintaining a healthy lifestyle. *Increases the likelihood of success in losing weight and developing a wellness lifestyle.*

### Evaluation

Client took blood pressure every day and her blood pressure readings dropped an average of 8% within 2 weeks. In addition, she reports "eating healthy," attending Weight Watchers, and losing 5 pounds in 2 weeks.

## Key Concepts

- Specific developmental processes take place in adulthood as a person transitions from adolescence to young and middle adulthood.
- Young adulthood is a critical period in life where many important decisions are made (e.g., career choice, selection of marriage partner or significant other, becoming a parent).
- Generativity versus stagnation are developmental considerations seen in middle adulthood.
- Nurses are valuable resources for middle-age adult clients in the areas of health promotion, teaching, and counseling.

## Review Questions and Activities

1. What conceptual issues are involved in the transition from adolescence to young adulthood?
2. How would you describe the critical factors during young adulthood?
3. What interventions could you suggest to a client to avoid skin cancer from sun exposure?
4. What developmental considerations exist in your middle-aged family members?
5. How would you describe the physiological changes of middle adulthood?

## Web Resources

Alcoholics Anonymous
    http://www.alcoholics-anonymous.org
American Cancer Society
    http://www.cancer.org
Healthy People 2010
    http://www.healthypeople.gov

United States Preventive Services Task Force (USPSTF)
    http://www.ahrq.gov

## References

Alcoholics Anonymous, 2003: www.alcoholics-anonymous.org

American Cancer Society, 2003: www.cancer.org

Arnstein, H. (1978). *What to tell your child.* New York: Condor.

Beare, P. G., & Myers, J. L. (1998). *Adult health nursing* (3rd ed.). St. Louis: Mosby-Yearbook.

Chiriboga, D. A. (1997). Crisis, challenge, and stability in the middle years. In S. H. Qualls and N. Abeles (Eds.), *Psychology and the aging revolutions: How we adapt to longer life* (293–322). Washington, DC: American Psychological Association.

Edelman, C. L., & Mandle, C. L. (2002). *Health promotion throughout the life span* (5th ed.). St. Louis: Mosby-Yearbook.

Edwards, B., & Ung, L. (2002). Quality of life instruments for caregivers of patients with cancer: A review of their psychometric properties. *Cancer Nursing, 25*(5), 342–349.

Erikson, E. (1968). *Childhood and society.* New York: Norton.

Fuller, J., & Schaller-Ayers, J. (1999). *Health assessment: A nursing approach* (3rd ed.). Philadelphia: Lippincott.

Goodrick, G., Poston, II, W. S. C., & Kimball, K. T. (1998). Nondieting versus treatment for overweight binge-eating women. *Journal of Consulting Clinical Psychology, 66*(4), 363–368.

Gottlieb, B. H. & Wolfe, J. (2002). Coping with family caregiving to persons with dementia: A critical review. *Aging and Mental Health, 6*(4), 325–342.

Hackler, C. (2001). Troubling implications of doubling the human life span. *Generations, 25*(4), 15–19.

Healthy People 2010, 2003:
    http://www.healthypeople.gov/

Hogstel, M. (2001). *Gerontology: Nursing care of the older adult.* Clifton Park, NY: Delmar Learning.

Institute of Medicine (2002). *Dietary reference intakes for energy, carbohydrate, fiber, fat, fatty acids, cholesterol, protein, and amino acids, Part 1.* National Academies Press, http://www4.nas.edu/news.nsf

Joslin, D., & Harrison, R. (2002). Self-reported physical health among older surrogate parents to children orphaned and affected by HIV disease. *AIDS Care, 14*(5), 619–624.

Klein, J. D., Allan, M. J., Elster, A. B., Stevens, D., Cox, C., Hedberg, V. A., Goodman, R. A. (2001). *Improving adolescent preventive care in community health centers. Pediatrics 107*(2), 316–327.

Maddi, S. R., & Hightower, M. (1999). Hardiness and optimism as expressed in coping patterns. *Consulting Psychology Journal, 51,* 95–105.

McCarty, E. F., & Drebing, C. (2002). Burden and professional caregivers: Tracking the impact. *Journal for Nurses in Staff Development, 18*(5), 250–257.

O'Halloran, V. E. (1997). Defining educational settings to improve client health teaching. *MEDSURG Nursing, 6*(3), 130–136.

Pender, J., Murdaugh, C., & Parsons, M.A. (2002). *Health promotion in nursing practice* (4th ed.). Upper Saddle River, NJ: Prentice-Hall.

Potts, N., & Mandleco, B. (2002). *Pediatric nursing: Caring for children and their families.* Clifton Park, NY: Delmar Learning.

Rook, K. S. (2000). The evolution of social relationships in later adulthood. In S. H. Qualls and N. Abeles (Eds.), *Psychology and the aging revolutions: How we adapt to longer life,* 173–191. Washington, DC: American Psychological Association.

Scal, P., Evans, T., Blozis, S., Okinow, N., & Blum, R. (1999). Trends in transition from pediatric to adult health care services for young adults with chronic conditions. *Journal of Adolescent Health, 24*(4), 259–264.

Schofield, J. R., & Robinson, W. (2000). *What you really need to know about moles and melanoma.* Baltimore: Johns Hopkins Press.

Siegler, I. C. (2000). Aging research and health: A status report. In S. H. Qualls and N. Abeles (Eds.), *Psychology and the aging revolutions: How we adapt to longer life,* 207–218. Washington, DC: American Psychological Association.

Siegler, I. C., Bastian, L. A., & Bosworth, H. B. (2000). Health, behavior and aging. In A. Baum, T. A. Revenson, & J. E. Singer (Eds.), *Handbook of health psychology,* 469–476. Mahwah, NJ: Erlbaum.

Thomas, S. P. (1997). Psychosocial correlates of women's self-rated physical health in middle adulthood. In M. E. Lachman and J. B. James (Eds.), *Multiple paths of midlife development,* 257–291. Chicago: The University of Chicago Press.

Tierney, A. J., Worth, A., & Watson, N. (2000). Meeting patients' information needs before and after discharge from hospital, *Journal of Clinical Nursing, 9*(6), 14–19.

United States Preventive Services Task Force (USPSTF), 2003: http://www.ahrq.gov

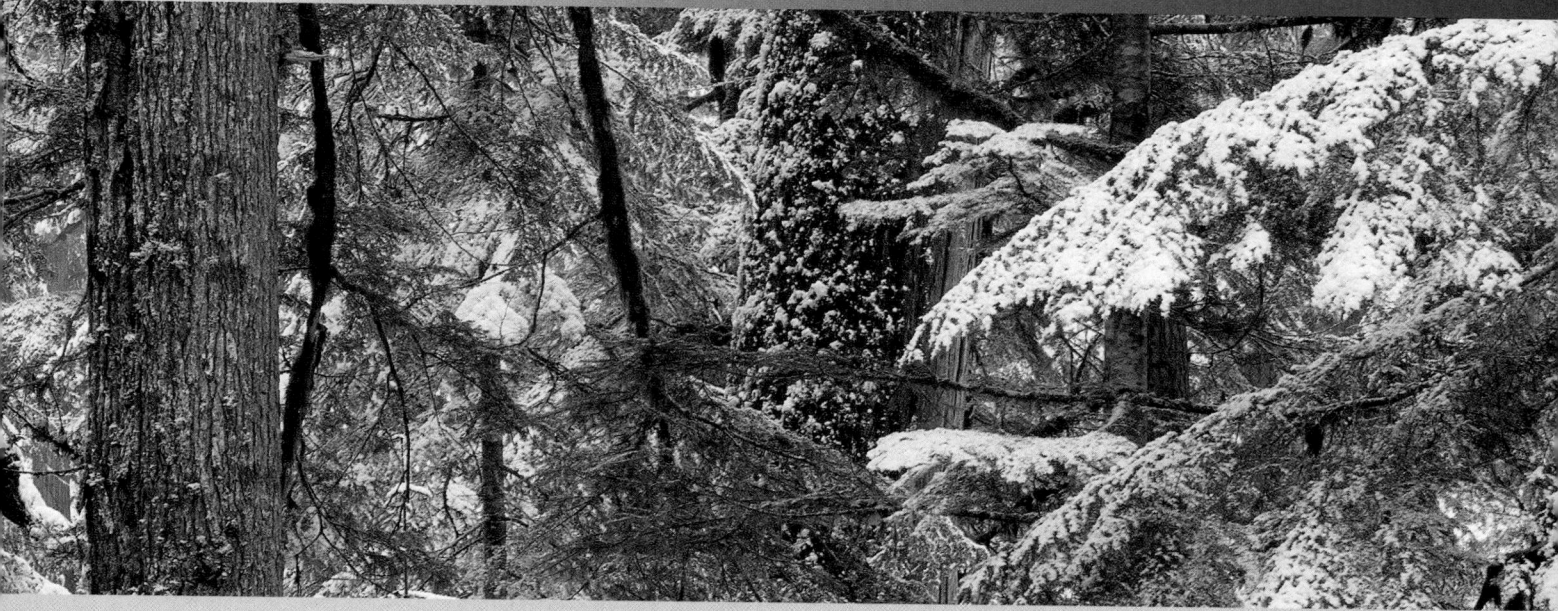

# CHAPTER 19

# The Geriatric Client

Tina H. Olson, EdD, RN

*"If aging is not your issue, it will be."*

*(Anonymous)*

# Chapter Competencies

*Upon completion of this chapter, the reader should be able to:*

1. Define selected demographics of the aging population in the United States and worldwide.
2. Evaluate the multiple physical changes associated with aging and the impact these may have on an older adult's ability to function and to perform activities of daily living.
3. Define polypharmacy and its significance in older clients.
4. Identify physical and psychological signs of neglect and abuse in older adults.
5. Discuss the impact of the Human Genome Project on aging.
6. Discuss the use of the nursing process with older clients.

# Key Terms

ageism
chronological age
genome

Human Genome Project
lentigo senilis
polypharmacy

presbycusis
restorative nursing care

What defines older adults? Some think older adulthood starts when individuals begin receiving their Social Security checks. Certain movie theaters and restaurants have "senior discounts" for people over age 55 on special days of the week or at special times of the day. A person can become a member of the American Association of Retired Persons at age 50. Is menopause women's rite of passage into older adulthood? For 5,000 years, people were considered "old" when they lived to the age of 50. Consider the commentary by the scientist who wrote about the "Iceman," who lived sometime between 3350 and 3100 BC. The Iceman was found frozen in the Italian Alps in 1991. The Iceman discovery is unique because he was not mummified or buried but clothed in his daily attire when he died, and then was frozen in glacier ice for 5,000 years. (Note: a museum in Bolzano, Italy, is dedicated to the Iceman, where his body, clothing, and personal items as well as a reproduction can be studied.)

> From the beginning, the question of the Iceman's age was raised. The fact that the teeth were so worn down and the erosion of the spine, knee, and ankle joints all indicate advanced age. The signs of age-related disintegration and changes of the bone structure which could be seen on the x-ray had to be taken into account. On the basis of these examinations, the scientist established a minimum age of 40 and a maximum age of 53. The average of various mathematical calculations result in an age of 46 which was an advanced age by Neolithic standards (Flecker and Steiner, 1998).

## Definition of Older Adults and U.S. Demographics

In 1900, the average life expectancy for people in the United States was just 47 years old—about the same age as the Iceman. Just one hundred years later, in 2000, the average life expectancy is over 75 years due to abundant clean water and food, and advances in medical technology, including immunizations and antibiotics. The statistics in Figure 19-1 confirm the increase of aged persons during the 1900s.

The older population as defined by the U.S. Census Bureau is persons 65 years and older with three subcategories of older adults: 65 to 74, 75 to 84, and 85 and over. The following statistics demonstrate that even older adults as a group are getting older. If the three groups are compared in 1900 and again in 1999, the results are as shown in Box 19-1.

There were about 35 million older adults in 1999, which represented 12.7% of the U.S. population or about one in every eight Americans. The majority are women with a gender ratio of 141 women to 100 men. The ratio increases as the population ages, with women continuing to live longer than men. The older population will continue to grow significantly with the aging baby boomers (born between 1946 and 1964) turning age 65. There are expected to be about 70 million older persons in 2030—more than twice their number in 1999! Though older adults represent about 13% of the U.S. population in the year 2000, they will represent about 20% of the population

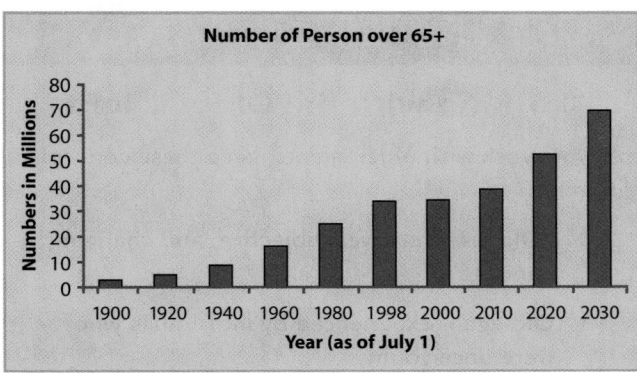

**Figure 19-1    Number of persons 65+, 1900–2030.** *Source: United States Bureau of the Census [1999]. Population and family characteristics:* Population estimates and projections. *Washington, DC: Author*

by 2030 (AARP, 2002). In 2000, over 50,000 centenarians (individuals who have reached age 100) were living in the United States. Belle Boon Beard conducted several thousand interviews with centenarians during a 40-year study. Some interesting characteristics of centenarians have been outlined in Box 19-2.

This data has profound implications for nurses and the health professions not only in the United States but worldwide. Global aging is a phenomenon particularly noted in developed countries that participated in World War II, in which the baby boomers were conceived. Not only do nurses need to prepare for this growing segment of the population in terms of numbers of professionals, but also they need to learn how to better care for older adults, as it is a global issue in countries that have clean water and ample food, and where communicable diseases have been eradicated.

## BOX 19-1    OLDER ADULTS INCREASING IN THE 1900s

Older adults are getting older when comparing statistics of 1900 to the present time:

- 65 to 74 years of age group (18.2 million) is 8 times larger than in 1900.

- 75 to 84 years of age group (12.1 million) is 16 times larger than in 1900.

- 85 or more years of age group (4.2 million) is 34 times larger than in 1900.

Hackler C. (Winter 2001). Troubling implications of doubling the human life span. *Generations,* 25(4): 15–19.

## BOX 19-2    CHARACTERISTICS OF CENTENARIANS

- Think they are healthy and practice good health habits

- Generally optimistic about life

- Eat a varied diet and drink coffee, tea, and alcohol in moderation

- Have lifelong habits of mental and physical activity, enthusiastically enjoy walking

- Regardless of educational level, most have good memories and continue to learn

- Over 90% say that religion was important to them, though they are tolerant and not dogmatic

- Tend to see the positive aspect of situations, are respectful of others, and content with own life situation

- Continue to have work to do; highly value work and doing things for others

- Have broad social contacts and interests

- Show tolerance for others and forgiveness of self

- Demonstrate integrity and independence

Summarized from Beard, B. B., *Centenarians: The new generation.* (N. K. Wilson & A. J. F. Wilson, Eds.). Westport, CT: Greenwood Press.

## Theories of Aging

Aging is a complex process of biologic, psychosocial, cultural, and experiential changes. No one theory on aging completely embraces and explains all the many facets of change. Following is a discussion of several biologic and psychosocial theories on aging that provide a frame of reference for providing nursing care to elderly clients.

### Biologic Theories

Biologic theories of aging are vast and may be derived from fields of genetics, microbiology, biochemistry, and sociology. Developing and testing aging theories is one of the newer scientific fields in the United States, which is beginning to receive more federal, state, and private research money to support this work. Stochastic theories hypothesize that aging occurs randomly and persistently with time. Nonstochastic theories suggest that aging is predetermined.

## STOP AND THINK

### Personal Views on Aging

Consider your own beliefs about aging. Do you feel that one of these theories best represents the older adult population? Would you classify your opinion of older adults as basically positive or basically negative? On what information have you based your views?

## NURSING STRATEGY

### Working with the Older Client

As you work with older clients, keep these concepts in mind:

- "Old" is a relative, subjective, and changing concept.

- Old age is experienced by individuals who were once young.

- Older persons are individuals; many of their attributes have nothing to do with their age.

- Ageism is unacceptable in the care and treatment of older persons.

- Older persons are entitled to the same high quality of health care as younger persons.

## Psychosocial Theories

Psychosocial theories on aging present the position that many factors in addition to genetics contribute to the aging process. The *disengagement theory* posits that as individuals age, they inevitably withdraw from society and society withdraws from them in a mutual dance of separation. The *continuity theory* suggests that an individual's values and personality develop over a lifetime and that goals and individual characteristics will remain constant throughout life. An individual thus learns to adapt to changes and will tend to repeat those reactions and behaviors that brought success in the past. The *activity theory* proposes that an individual's satisfaction with life depends on involvement in new interests, hobbies, roles, and relationships. Volunteering is one way many retirees stay connected to the community. In addition to providing social connection, volunteer activities provide a daily routine, a way to make a contribution, and a sense of being needed.

## Myths and Stereotypes of Aging

In our youth-driven society, old age often has a negative connotation. In many cultures, older people are accorded a position of respect, and young people feel a moral and familial responsibility to care for parents and older relatives. In American culture, misconceptions about older adults abound. Older adults are often stereotyped as being ill, bald, hard of hearing, forgetful, rigid, grumpy, or boring simply on the basis of their age and regardless of their competencies and individual characteristics. Many younger Americans also believe that all older people live in nursing homes, and fail to consider the independence of the older generation and their contributions to society. These types of attitudes are known as **ageism** (the process of stereotyping and discriminating against people because of their age).

To many, aging is synonymous with death; these individuals have a negative view of the aging process, which usually results from fear, lack of exposure to older individuals, and a lack of understanding of how varied experiences can enhance the overall quality of life. Surprisingly, many older adults have negative attitudes toward other older adults; these often result from fear of stereotypes and social stigmas, or a sense of anxiety over "guilt by association." Nurses need to be aware of these myths and stereotypes and to separate them from the realities of the aging process in order to provide sensitive and appropriate care to older clients.

## Quality of Life Among Older Adults

Quality of life is gaining more emphasis in today's aging society. Sadler (2000) states that the United States is experiencing a *longevity revolution*, in that many people are living twice as long as previously expected. In 18th-century America, the average life span was barely 40. In the 21st century, the average American life span is nearly 85. The increasing life span has both positive and negative outcomes. For example, Medicare beneficiaries (people aged 65 and over) spent an average of $2,810.00 each (19% of their income) for health care services in 2001 (AARP, 2002).

One of the greatest fears associated with advancing age is poor health. Everyone wants to live a long life, as long as it is a long *healthy* life, but the reality is that the elderly have more health problems than the general population. Fortunately, the trend is in fact for people to live longer *and healthier* lives. Many Americans over 65 live in relative financial comfort, able to continue working or start enjoying their retirement years. Good nutrition, proper exercise, continued work, travel, recreation, hobbies, and companionship are just a few of the healthy lifestyle choices many older people now have the means to afford.

Outlook and adaptation contribute to the high quality of life enjoyed by many older adults today. Although

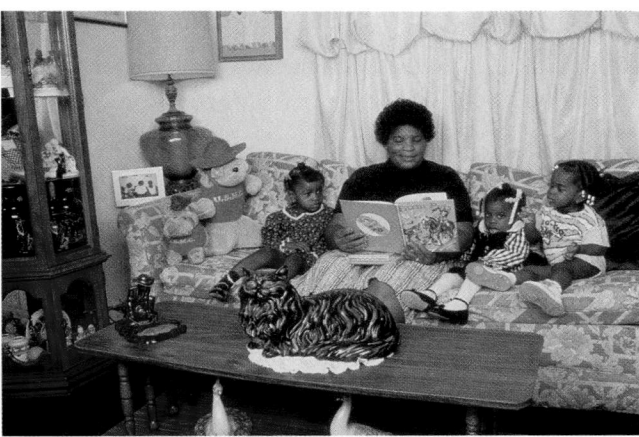

**Figure 19-2**  Older adults often assume new roles, such as grandparent, as they mature. They can gain immense pleasure in spending time with family and sharing wisdom and ideas with the younger generation.

many people over 65 have some kind of chronic health problem, most have found ways to keep their illnesses from lowering their enjoyment of life. Most older people accept a certain amount of declining health as a normal, expected part of aging, but do not allow health issues to interfere with the vigorous pursuit of enjoyment (Figure 19-2).

# Biopsychosocial Changes Associated with Aging

Change is an ongoing part of life. Changes of aging can be viewed as developmental, physiological, or psychosocial in nature.

## Developmental Changes

At every stage of life, including old age, new developmental challenges constantly arise. Like developmental challenges faced earlier in life, these occasions are opportunities for success or failure. Older people may experience feelings of satisfaction or success over completing certain developmental tasks associated with aging, such as:

- Gaining insight or wisdom, even if physical powers are in decline
- Developing better social skills, with more same-sex friendships
- Becoming more open-minded and tolerant
- Finding an unexpectedly active and pleasurable sexual dimension
- Seeing children transform into responsible, successful adults
- Becoming a grandparent
- Holding civic and community positions of responsibility
- Achieving mastery of one's occupation or skills
- Developing new skills, hobbies, and interests

- Renewing and deepening one's relationship with one's spouse, significant others, or friends
- Gaining new knowledge and experiences
- Accepting and adjusting to physical changes associated with aging
- Coping with aging parents, spouses, and friends

On the other hand, any older person would be challenged to find successful ways to cope with other developmental tasks of aging, such as:

- Adjusting to the death of a spouse
- Adapting to major declines in health or physical ability
- Adjusting to the loss of social role, prestige, occupation, income, or sense of usefulness
- Getting accustomed to loss of independent living
- Adjusting to any kind of loneliness or loss without boredom or depression
- Accepting a fixed income

It is important for the nurse to assess the nature of any developmental challenges a client may be experiencing, because a client's adaptation to changes can have a profound effect on health status.

## Physiological Changes

From the moment of birth, the human body begins the aging process. As a unique individual, each person ages differently; the rate of age-related changes varies from one individual to the next. However, some generalized physiological changes occur with the aging process, including:

- A decrease in the rate of cell mitosis
- A deterioration of specialized nondividing cells (such as neurons)
- Decreased elasticity and increased rigidity of connective tissue
- Decreased functional capacity

Some of the physical changes of aging, such as graying of the hair and decreased visual acuity, are readily apparent. Other changes are more subtle and may go undetected until a problem occurs.

The rate of aging is influenced by:

- Genetic composition
- Lifestyle (e.g., dietary and exercise patterns)
- Previous experience (e.g., adaptive responses to stressors)
- Presence of chronic illnesses
- Environmental influences (e.g., air quality)

### Neurological Changes

Aging brings about several changes in the nervous system that alter sensory and perceptual responses, as shown in Box 19-3. As a result of these changes, reaction time is usually slowed, which may affect driving ability. The generalized slower response to environmental changes leads to increased risk for falls, burns, and other injuries.

## BOX 19-3 AGE-RELATED NEUROLOGICAL CHANGES

- Fewer neurons

- Transmission of nerve impulses slowed

- The number of neurotransmitters (chemical messengers of the central nervous system) decreased

- Sensory threshold decreased (affects pain and tactile sensations)

From Murray, R. B., & Zentner, J. P. (2000). *Nursing assessment and health promotion: Strategies through the life span* (7th ed.). Norwalk, CT: Appleton & Lange

It is important that the nurse allow older clients time to respond to questions and instructions. Teaching safety measures is a preventive aspect of nursing when dealing with older clients.

## Sensory and Perceptual Changes

Sensory changes are progressive and usually cause some limitations in later years. The resultant changes may impair the individual's ability to enjoy life to the fullest, as well as present related health problems.

## Vision

The aging process causes some visual changes. For example, pupils decrease in size and are less responsive to light. Usually a loss of visual acuity occurs because of degenerative changes related to aging. By the age of approximately 42, the lens cortex becomes thicker, impairing its ability to change shape and focus. This condition, presbyopia, causes farsightedness and is corrected by the use of bifocals.

Cataracts, glaucoma, and age-related macular degeneration are the most common pathological visual problems experienced by older adults. Cataracts (or opacity of the lens) can be surgically corrected. If untreated, glaucoma can result in blindness; thus, annual screening is recommended for all individuals over age 40. Age-related macular degeneration is the loss of central vision; magnification must be used to compensate for the changes. Diabetes, hypertension, and other systemic diseases will exacerbate macular degeneration. Fewer tears are produced by the lacrimal glands so the cornea is likely to become irritated. Most elderly people experience a decreased ability to see colors; pastels fade, and monotones, blacks, and whites are difficult to see. These changes normally occur with aging.

The nurse caring for older clients must be aware of the client's increased sensitivity to glare and allow time for the eyes to accommodate changes in lighting. The use of eyedrops or artificial tears may also be beneficial. Brighter colors compensate for the decline in color discrimination.

## CLIENT REFLECTIONS

### Misperceptions of Older Adults Who Are Hard of Hearing

Mr. Devin, age 83, is somewhat hard of hearing but has no cognitive impairment. In addition, he is a retired university English professor. He is hospitalized for a colon resection and makes the following comments: "I am always amazed at the inept caregivers who assume that my difficulty in hearing is (falsely) accompanied with a lack of intelligence. Invariably, the nurse or nursing assistant will approach me with shouts of simplistic "commands" as though speaking to a 7-year-old. I usually don't get angry and try to be patient with their lack of accuracy in my abilities."

### Hearing

Generally, hearing is diminished with age. There is a drying and wrinkling of the auricle with a noticeable increase of hair in the auditory canal. Cerumen becomes drier and can cause impaction, which blocks transmission of sounds. The hearing loss associated with aging is called **presbycusis**. In the middle ear, bony joints show some degeneration. However, the major changes occur in the inner ear, where degeneration of the vestibular system and simultaneous atrophy of the cochlea and the organ of Corti produce deficits in equilibrium and hearing.

Nurses need to be very patient in their approach to the older client. With anticipated changes in sensory perception, it is important that nurses face their clients, speak slowly and clearly, and protect them from injury. It is important when teaching clients that nurses ask for feedback and evaluate comprehension.

### Taste and Smell

With aging, taste perception declines and salivation is diminished. Many older clients prefer more highly seasoned foods, with more salt and sugar to compensate for a

## STOP AND THINK

### Food Preferences

When you think about eating and preparing food for others, what are some of the things you consider? Think of a favorite meal and what you like most about it. Do you have preferences involving color, aroma, texture? Older people may experience gradual loss of taste and smell. What do you do to your food to enhance its taste appeal?

decreased sensation of taste. Increased loss of appetite often occurs and may be medication-related in some individuals. It may be helpful for older adults to eat small portions frequently throughout the day. The nurse should strive to make food visually appealing and know the client's food preferences. It is important to teach clients about healthy eating patterns.

Olfactory nerve cells decrease in number. The nurse should instruct family members and other caregivers to be alert for safety hazards associated with decreased sense of smell, such as the inability to detect smoke, leaking gas, or spoiled food.

### Pain Perception

More research in loss of pain perception is needed, as caregivers have observed that some older adults seem to lack specific responses to pain. Clients may have a silent myocardial infarction, appendicitis, or delayed responses to cold or heat. This poses challenges for the nurse in geriatrics who needs to be mindful of hot drinks like coffee, heating pads, iced items, or air temperatures that may be too hot or cold for the aging person.

### Cardiovascular Changes

As a result of aging, functioning of the cardiovascular system becomes less efficient. Reduced elasticity of the heart muscle and arteries causes a subsequent increase in systolic blood pressure. Increased fat deposits in the blood vessels lead to a reduced supply of oxygen. The arterial diameter decreases as a result of arteriosclerosis. Thickening of venous walls leads to decreased elasticity. Thickening of aortic and mitral valves leads to incomplete closure; murmurs may occur in some older people. Both arteries and veins become fibrotic and the endothelial cell variation increases. Of particular importance has been the recent research in cardiac syndrome X, a phenomena found primarily in postmenopausal women. The medical profile of clients presenting with this diagnosis as reported in the literature is typified in Box 19-4.

In the last 10 years, about 20 clinical sites worldwide have reported research in the assessment, diagnosis, treatment, or prognosis of coronary endothelial dysfunction, a syndrome found primarily in middle-age women. Despite the cost and morbidity of this syndrome, relatively little research has been conducted in the effective treatment of this international and increasingly recognized medical problem. Though the incidence of syndrome X is unknown, approximately 20% of angiograms in women with chest pain have no occlusions in the major coronary arteries. Thus, this will be important research to follow in relation to the health of aging women.

In the peripheral circulation, the vascular system is more stiff and rigid, losing its elasticity. Pooling of the blood increases the venous pressure, contributing to hypertension. Hypertension is defined as a systolic pressure at or above 140 mm Hg and diastolic pressure at or above 90 mm Hg. Cardiovascular disease is a major cause of morbidity and mortality in people age 65 and over.

## RESEARCH FOCUS

**Title of Study:** Quality of life of elderly patients after treatment in the ICU

**Study Purpose:** The purpose of this study was to determine the impact of intensive care unit (ICU) treatment on quality of life (QOL) outcomes for critically ill elderly clients 4 to 6 months after ICU discharge.

**Methods:** Sample site was a 250-bed Midwestern hospital. Surviving sample from two ICUs was n = 164. Telephone consent was obtained, and QOL questionnaires were mailed approximately 4 to 6 months after discharge. Several other scales were used to measure perceived health and impact of illness. Medical chart reviews of target sample were also reviewed to obtain pertinent hospitalization data.

**Findings:** A mean score of 21.4 (SD = 0.63) was obtained with the Quality of Life Index (Ferrans & Powers, 1985) indicating that all the ICU survivors in the sample reported good QOL, and were satisfied with areas of life that were important to them, and had higher levels of social support.

**Implications:** Clients in ICUs where nurses provide greater social support and there is better perceived health status, and clients who are there for fewer days of hospitalization received higher QOL scores.

Kleinpell, R. M., & Ferrans, C. E. (2000). Quality of life of elderly patients after treatment in the ICU. *Research in Nursing and Health, 25:* 212–221.

Hypertension increases the risk of cardiac disease. With the pooling of blood in the peripheral circulation, the development of varicose veins is common. As a result of decreased cardiac output, many older adults experience a decreased capacity for physical activity. A diminished cardiac output is problematic when the older person becomes physically, mentally, or emotional impaired (Ebersole, Hess, & Luggen, 2004).

### Respiratory Changes

Most older adults experience a decreased functional respiratory reserve capacity, with a generalized decreased elasticity and tone of muscles, including the muscles necessary for respiration. Physical changes in the lungs include fewer functioning alveoli and a decreased number of cilia. Therefore, ineffective clearing of the respiratory system occurs. Calcification of the chest wall and rib cage causes the lungs to remain hyperinflated on exhalation, thereby decreasing vital capacity. Factors contributing to respiratory problems are shown in Box 19-5.

## BOX 19-4   CLIENT PROFILE OF CLIENTS WITH CARDIAC SYNDROME X

- Female predominance

- Average age is 48 years old (range 40 to 65 years of age)

- Severe, disabling symptoms both at rest and with exercise

- Clients report angina-like chest pain

- EKG demonstrates ischemic-appearing ST-segment depression during exercise

- Normal epicardial coronary angiogram on negative stress echo or nuclear imaging study

- Inconsistent responses to conventional anti-ischemic therapy

Beers, H. M, & Berkow, R. (2000). *The Merck manual of geriatrics* (3rd ed.). Merck Research Laboratories, Merck, Inc.: Whitehouse Station, New Jersey.

## FOCUS ON WELLNESS

### Proper Amounts of Activity, Rest, and Sleep in Older Clients

The nurse should offer information to the client about the importance of remaining physically active and the need to balance activity with adequate rest and sleep. Older clients also need education on lifestyle modifications that promote cardiovascular health. Such instruction could include the following:

- Avoid smoking and use of other forms of tobacco

- Avoid secondary tobacco smoke and other forms of air pollution

- Eat a healthy diet that is low in fat, sugar, and salt, and high in protein, fruits, vegetables, and water

- Exercise for at least 30 minutes three times a week—for example, walking, leg lifting and arm raising while sitting, low-impact water aerobics

- Express emotions (e.g., anger) in an appropriate manner

- Avoid obesity

Thompson, B., Sierpina, V. S., & Sierpina, M. (Winter 2001). What is healthy aging? Family physicians look at conventional and alternative approaches. *Generations, 25*(4): 49–53.

Pneumonias are among the leading causes of death in older adults, with pneumococcal pneumonias being the most common bacterial respiratory infection. Other less common bacterial pneumonias are staphylococcus, streptococcus, Haemophilus influenzae, and Klebsiella. Older adults who are at risk are those who are sedated, have swallowing or breathing difficulties, or have an endotracheal tube. Chronic obstructive pulmonary disease (COPD) includes bronchiectasis, bronchitis, asthma, and emphysema (Beers & Berkow, 2000).

To manage respiratory changes, the nurse teaches the client how to breathe deeply and cough effectively. The client needs to establish a balance between exercise and activity to conserve respiratory effort while at the same time improving vital capacity. Because physical exercise increases lung capacity, nurses encourage clients to walk.

### Gastrointestinal Changes

Aging brings about several alterations in gastrointestinal functioning. The major changes are described in the following section.

### Mouth

Many older people lose their teeth for a variety of reasons, including years of inadequate dental hygiene and extended use of medication (e.g., anticonvulsant drugs). Other physiological changes include atrophy of oral mucosa, loss of elasticity in connective tissue, and a decreased number of nerve cells that control chewing, swallowing, and taste. Saliva production is decreased, and saliva becomes more alkaline. The older person's ability to chew food is often impaired by loss of teeth, gum recession, and degeneration of the mandible. The nurse should instruct the client and caregivers to have available foods that are easily chewed and swallowed. Frequent oral hygiene is beneficial.

### Gastrointestinal Tract

Peristaltic action decreases with a relaxation of the lower esophageal sphincter. This causes a decreased emptying of the esophagus and stomach. Intestinal motility is slowed. Shrinkage of gastric mucosa leads to changes in the levels of hydrochloric acid, the reason for many older persons' complaints of heartburn. Older adults have an inability to tolerate large amounts of foods containing fat.

Elimination is often impaired in older clients. As a result, absorption of nutrients decreases. Some loss of sphincter control may be noted. Nurses should instruct older clients about the importance of adequate nutrition, especially fluids and high fiber foods. Keep clients well hydrated by instructing them to drink at least 8 glasses of fluid daily. Other methods to prevent constipation are physical activity and a regular time for toileting.

## BOX 19-5 FACTORS CONTRIBUTING TO RESPIRATORY DISEASES

- *Smoking*—the major contributing factor to respiratory problems; workload of the lungs is increased due to decreased oxygenation level.

- *Impaired functioning of immune system*—increases the risk of respiratory infections.

- *Impaired mobility*—lung expansion is decreased; secretions pool in lungs and provide a medium for growth of microorganisms; increased risk of pneumonia.

- *Obesity*—leads to decreased lung expansion and volume.

- *Surgery*—most anesthetic agents cause decreased respiratory rate and decreased tidal volume and lead to hypoventilation

From Johnson, A. P. (1999). The pulmonary system and its problems in the elderly. In M. Stanley & P. G. Beare (Eds.), *Gerontological nursing* (2nd ed.). Philadelphia: Davis.

## Genitourinary Changes

Major changes in the structure and function of the urinary system are associated with aging. The kidneys, bladder, and ureters are all affected by the aging process.

The loss of some muscle tone in the bladder and urethra can result in incomplete emptying of the bladder. Residual urine can lead to bladder infection. Decreased bladder capacity may cause subsequent nocturia (nighttime elimination) and polyuria (excessive urination).

Renal function is the major determinant of an individual's fluid and electrolyte balance. In older adults, renal function is often affected by diminished blood flow to the kidneys as a result of arteriosclerosis, hypertension, and other cardiovascular disorders. The glomerular filtration rate slows and there are fewer functioning nephrons.

The risk of renal failure increases with age, as does fluid retention. Dehydration is a very real threat for many older adults. The aging body loses some of its functional ability to adapt to changes in total body water, which is essential for metabolism. The composition of body water declines from 60% to about 40% of an older adult's total body weight.

Nursing measures address the underlying problems that result in a fluid and electrolyte imbalance. For example, if clients are dehydrated, they should be instructed to drink 2,000 ml (10 glasses) of liquid a day. Note that the fluid intake should be limited 2 hours before bedtime to decrease the likelihood of nocturia.

## Endocrine Changes

During the aging process, the following changes occur in the endocrine system:

- Slowing of metabolism
- Alteration in pancreatic activity
- Decreased blood levels of growth hormone, estrogen, and testosterone

As a person ages, the number of hormonal receptors in the adrenal and thyroid glands decreases. Thus, the person's ability to respond effectively to stress is diminished. Aging is associated with altered functioning of the pancreas; levels of insulin and circulating glucose increase.

The major changes affecting men are enlargement of the prostate gland (benign hypertrophy) and decreased reserves of testosterone. The age-related changes for women include a loss of elasticity in breast tissue with resultant sagging of the breasts, decreased size of uterus and fallopian tubes, and decreased motility of fallopian tubes.

The nurse must provide information about the normal changes associated with aging and listen in a nonjudgmental manner when clients discuss their concerns about the physical changes.

## Reproductive/Sexual Changes

To promote discussion of sexuality, it is important for the nurse to have an understanding and accepting attitude. Sensitivity to verbal and nonverbal cues will also promote the client's expression of concerns. The nurse must not assume that the older client is heterosexual, sexually inactive, or uninterested in sex (Figure 19-3). "Sexual function is not normally lost with age, yet attitudes and expectations seem to imply that older adults are not interested in or capable of sex" (Eliopoulos, 1999, p. 405). It is important to recognize older adults as sexual beings and to provide privacy to promote intimacy. See Table 19-1 for a listing of sexual responses in older adults.

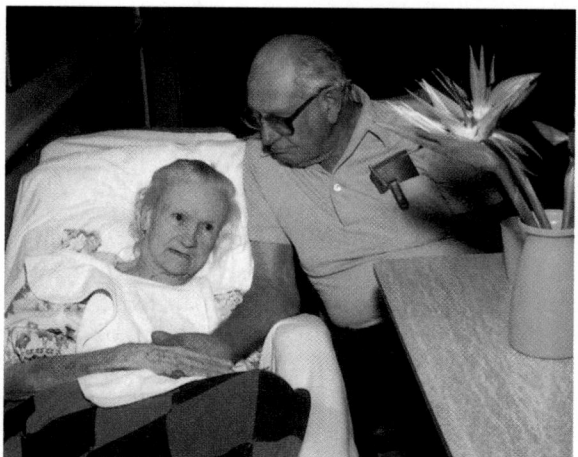

**Figure 19-3** **Older adults need companionship, as intimacy and sexuality remain important throughout the entire life span.**

## TABLE 19-1     AGE-RELATED CHANGES IN SEXUAL RESPONSES

| Women | Men |
|---|---|
| • Nipple erections during sexual excitement may last several hours postorgasm. | • It takes longer to achieve an erection. |
| • Orgasms are usually unchanged, except that vaginal contractions may be of shorter duration. | • More direct physical stimulation is required for erection. |
| • Vaginal lubrication is decreased. | • Erection is more readily lost after interruption. |
| • Urinary frequency and urgency occur after intercourse. | • There is an increased ability to prolong time before ejaculation. |
| • Clitoral response to stimulation is the same as in youth. | • Ejaculation may be less forceful or may not occur. |
| • Skin is less flushed due to superficial vasocongestive skin response. | • Orgasm is similar to that experienced in youth. |
| | • Less flushing of skin occurs. |

From Eliopoulos, C. (1999). *Manual of gerontologic nursing* (2nd ed.). St. Louis: Mosby.

Older adults who are sexually active may need education about sexually transmitted diseases (STDs), including AIDS. This is one health education topic that is frequently overlooked in health promotion for the elderly.

When caring for clients of either gender, the nurse should teach about the effects of aging on reproduction and sexuality and should use a nonjudgmental approach when clients discuss sexual issues.

### Changes in Men

As men age, the testes become softer and smaller as a result of decreased concentration of testosterone in the bloodstream. The production of sperm is inhibited or decreased, and ejaculations are less forceful. Sexual dysfunction increases in prevalence with aging.

Sexual dysfunction in men may be related to erection, ejaculation, orgasm, or partner-related issues. Erectile dysfunction (ED) is more commonly reported in contemporary society. The prevalence is about 52% among men ages 40 to 70 and is nearly 95% among men over the age of 70. ED or impotence is defined as "the inability to develop and sustain an erection sufficient for satisfactory sexual intercourse in 50% or more attempts at intercourse" (Beers & Berkow, 2000, p. 1166). Causes of erectile dysfunction may have multiple etiology and are shown in Box 19-6.

Vascular disorders are the most common etiology among older men, especially those who have hypercholesterolemia, diabetes, peripheral vascular disease, hypertension, or alcohol abuse, or those who smoke (Beers & Berkow, 2000, p. 1166). When taking a history, nurses can make men feel comfortable by explaining that erectile dysfunction is common and effective treatments are available such as pharmacotherapy, constriction rings, tumescent devices, penile prostheses, penile implants, revascularization surgery, and psychological counseling.

### Changes in Women

The older woman experiences a decline in the serum levels of estrogen. As a result, the vaginal walls thin and vaginal secretions decrease. The vulva, external genitalia, and breasts shrink because of loss of subcutaneous body fat. Other changes may include bone demineralization, as in osteoporosis; sleep disturbances; emotional symptoms; hot flashes or flushes; and diaphoresis. Postmenopausal changes, such as vaginal dryness, may cause the woman to experience pain during intercourse in which estrogen-based lubricants may help.

For many women, estrogen-replacement therapy diminishes the signs and symptoms of ovarian follicle failure. The many different kinds of preparations include estrogen patches, oral estrogen, estrogen injections, and vaginal creams. Significant contraindications include carcinoma of the breast and endometrium, and thromboembolic disease.

Libido, or sexual desire, seems to be testosterone-dependent in both women and men. Since ovarian hor-

### BOX 19-6     CAUSES OF ERECTILE DYSFUNCTION

● Vascular, neurologic and endocrine disorders

● Structural abnormalities of the penis

● Adverse effect of drugs

● Psychological disorders

Sadovsky, R. (1999). Management of erectile dysfunction. *CNS, Special Edition, 1*(1), 79–83.

mones and adrenal androgens begin to decrease prior to menopause, a decrease in libido, decreased sense of well-being, loss of energy, and loss of bone mass may result. The use of alcohol or drugs may also affect sexuality in women. Literature on the effect of drugs on libido is sparse, but anticonvulsants, anticancer drugs, and antidepressants may also inhibit libido, arousal, and orgasm (Beers & Berkow, 2000). Though decreased libido may benefit from androgen therapy if baseline testosterone levels are low, there are reported increased cardiovascular risks and virilization.

## Musculoskeletal Changes

Many people experience a decrease in height as they age. Long bones take on a disproportionate size, and many aged people assume a stooped posture. These postural changes occur primarily as a result of calcium loss from bone, creating osteoporosis and kyphosis. These conditions are more common in women than in men and are implicated in estrogen loss that occurs with aging.

Ligaments, tendons, and joints are also affected by age. They show results of collagen loss and become hardened, more rigid, less flexible, and predisposed to tears. Cartilage wears down around the joints, making flexion painful. Walking and a consistent exercise pattern can promote function and prevent the disabling effects of many of these changes (Ebersole et al., 2004).

The nurse should instruct women about the importance of calcium consumption and calcium supplements. Foods with a high calcium content include dairy products and green leafy vegetables. Encourage exercise, especially walking, to promote flexibility and perform passive range of motion exercises for those who need it. It is essential that the nurse teach safety measures, including fall prevention measures, to clients and caregivers.

## Integumentary Changes

Older adults frequently experience dry, wrinkled, flaccid skin. This is an expected condition that occurs with aging because the skin loses many of the properties that help make it appear youthful. It takes approximately 20 days for epidermal cells to be replaced in a young person, whereas in the older adult, this process takes about 30 days. Therefore, it takes longer for an elderly client's wounds to heal. Because of collagen loss, the skin of an older person loses its ability to stretch, and thus tears more easily. Loss of subcutaneous fat, moisture content of the skin, and elastic fibers causes the older person's skin to wrinkle, dry, and sag, leading to the development of elongated ears, jowls, and double chin. If the client has had years of sun exposure, skin drying is accelerated. "Photoaging" of the skin is the result of chronic UV radiation from sunlight and occurs most often on exposed skin areas such as the face and arms. Photoaging differs clinically, histologically, and physiologically from intrinsic aging. Some geriatric skin diseases like skin cancer occur primarily due to photoaged skin. "The use of sunscreens

with a sun protection factor (SPF) of at least 15 or greater should be used liberally when outdoors or swimming" (Beers & Berkow, 2000, p. 1237). For the aging smoker, dehydration of the skin is exacerbated even more.

The development of **lentigo senilis** (brown pigmented areas on the face, hands, and arms of older people) can cause the person concern over his appearance. Sometimes called liver spots or age spots, these colorations are benign. Some cosmetic agents may lighten or almost eliminate these spots.

Skin appendages (hair and nails) also undergo changes associated with aging. Hair loses its original color as the production of melanin decreases, turning it gray, and eventually, white. Hair also tends to thin, both on the head and elsewhere on the body. Nails thicken and become more brittle. Care of the toenails often becomes a problem for many older people because they may not have the flexibility to reach their feet easily. The nurse must take special care to assess the skin and its appendages. Referrals to a podiatrist may be necessary for an older person to receive adequate care of the toenails.

As a person ages, the number of sweat glands decreases; this decrease can result in heat exhaustion. The decreased amount of subcutaneous fat may also lead to increased susceptibility to cold. Other functional skin losses are provided in Box 19-7.

The accompanying Client Education box provides guidelines for dealing with integumentary changes. Some elderly clients will have body image changes as a result of these visible signs of aging. The nurse must assess for body image alterations. If the client has an altered body image, it may be appropriate to:

- Assist with grooming as necessary.
- Use photographs of client to help adjust to changing appearance.
- Use touch to help clarify body boundaries.

## Alterations in Mental Status

Alterations in mental status that occur with aging can be mild and have little impact on a client's functioning, or they can be severe and require the older adult to have assistance in managing psychosocial and physical needs. The nurse must understand the types of cognitive deficits experienced by older adults and what each one means to the client's health status.

*Acute confusion* is a state of diminished awareness and attention of typically short duration (hours to weeks). The level of confusion often varies according to the time of day, worsening at night; this may cause sleep pattern disturbances. The individual is usually unaware of the setting, time of day, or day of the week and needs frequent reorientation to reality.

An individual with *dementia* experiences chronic confusion, usually of a long duration (months to years), that impedes functioning. Individuals with dementia will exhibit personality changes, difficulty with sequential

## BOX 19-7   SKIN LOSSES THAT OCCUR WITH AGING

- Barrier function
- Cell replacement
- DNA repair
- Elasticity
- Immunologic responsiveness
- Inflammatory responsiveness
- Mechanical protection
- Sensory protection
- Sweating and sebum production
- Thermoregulation
- Vitamin D production
- Wound healing

Beers, H. M., & Berkow, R. (2000). *The Merck manual of geriatrics* (3rd ed.). Whitehouse Station, NJ: Merck Research Laboratories, Merck, Inc.

## CLIENT EDUCATION

### Responding to the Older Adult's Integumentary Alterations

1. Instruct client to avoid excessive use of soap, hot water, and brisk rubbing when bathing.
2. Teach client to pat skin dry instead of briskly rubbing.
3. Inform client of the need to use tepid bathwater.
4. Use lotion for itching and dryness.
5. Use a humidifier to help reduce dryness.
6. Avoid prolonged pressure on bony prominences.
7. Protect the skin from temperature extremes.
8. Protect skin from sun exposure (wear protective clothing, hats, sunglasses, and use sunblock with a high SPF factor).
9. Soak nails in water before trimming.
10. Dress appropriately for weather and climate.

speech and thoughts, and possibly a lack of orientation to reality. *Alzheimer's disease* is a type of dementia that causes numerous deficits, including diminished intellectual abilities, confusion, and impaired judgment.

*Depression* is an altered state of mood that lasts at least 6 weeks. Individuals suffering from depression typically are alert and oriented to their environment but are characterized by exaggerated sadness, apathy, and preoccupation with negative thoughts. Table 19-2 offers guidelines for distinguishing among acute confusion, dementia, delirium, and depression in the elderly. Many people believe that it is normal for older adults to become sad and withdrawn; this is a false assumption, which leads to lack of diagnosis and treatment of a serious health problem. Late-life depression can be successfully treated if it is not dismissed as an inevitable part of the aging process. Nursing intervention includes supportive therapy and psychiatric referral.

## Psychosocial Changes

The multitude of physical changes that occur with aging are accompanied by numerous psychosocial changes. As adults age, the nature of their daily lives changes along with their bodies. Major life events such as retirement, changes in social relationships and roles, changes in living arrangements, and dealing with loss are usually experienced during the later years of life and can affect an individual's health status and outlook on life.

### Retirement

An individual's view of retirement is a product of many factors, including overall life attitude, support of significant others, and personal expectations. For individuals who, during their adult years, defined themselves and their success according to their work contributions, retirement may produce feelings of uneasiness and anxiety. An individual who views retirement as the end of the productive years may dread the change in life pattern and social status and may fear being a burden to others, both socially and financially.

Many adults, though, look forward to retirement as their reward for years of hard work and contributions and fill their newly freed days with activities, travel, new skills or hobbies, and interests that time constraints had prohibited them from pursuing during their earlier years. These individuals typically led more balanced lives during their working years, viewing their value as a combination of many factors, including work, family, and community involvement; they adjust more easily to the loss of employment status by balancing this change with other positive aspects of their lives. Also, individuals who have planned for retirement and made arrangements (financial, housing, social) ahead of time tend to adjust more readily to this change in work status.

### Social Relationships and Roles

Relationships and roles change over time as an individual grows and develops. For the older adult, these changes may take on even more meaning because activities and involvement in other areas of life may change or diminish. Changes in relationships and roles typically occur in con-

## TABLE 19-2    DISTINGUISHING ACUTE CONFUSION, DELIRIUM, DEMENTIA, AND DEPRESSION

| Parameter | Acute Confusion | Delirium | Dementia | Depression |
|---|---|---|---|---|
| Definition | Inability to think with usual clarity, speed, and coherence | Perceptual disorder characterized by heightened awareness, hallucinations, vivid dreams, and intense emotional outbursts | Deterioration of all cognitive functions with little or no disturbance of consciousness or perception | Altered emotional state characterized by feelings of intense sadness, helplessness, and hopelessness |
| Onset | Variable | Sudden | Gradual | Variable |
| Duration | Reversible | Reversible | Irreversible | Reversible |
| Pathophysiology | Metabolic disorders Toxic substances Cerebrovascular accident (CVA) Trauma Febrile states | Drug intoxications Withdrawal from alcohol and other drugs Encephalitis Trauma Febrile states Hypoxia Fluid and electrolyte imbalance | Alzheimer's disease Metabolic disorders CVA Head injury | Neurochemical abnormalities Significant loss Parkinson's disease Alzheimer's disease CVA Medications |
| Attention | Impaired: dulled | Impaired: heightened or dull | Impaired | Intact |
| Memory | Short term: impaired Long term: may be impaired | Short term: impaired Long term: intact | Short term: impaired first Long term: intact until disease progresses to later stages | Variable because of concentration ability |
| Judgment | Impaired | Grossly impaired Impulsive Volatile | Impaired | Impaired |
| Insight | Impaired | Impaired | Impaired | Impaired if in bipolar (manic) phase |
| Spatial perception | May be impaired | Intact | Impaired | Intact |
| Thought process and content | Impaired, incoherent | Impaired, hallucinations | Impaired | Intact but may demonstrate flight of ideas (jumping rapidly from one unrelated topic to another) |

From Estes, M. E. Z. (2002). *Health assessment & physical examination* (2nd ed.). Clifton Park, NY: Delmar Learning.

junction with major life events, such as marriage, divorce, birth, death, relocation, and change in employment status. For instance, the older adult who has been a husband for 40 years will find his life and his roles greatly changed when he becomes a widower. The birth of his children's children will bring him new status as a grandparent, and his retirement will remove him from the full-time workforce and present opportunities for the development of relationships with new friends.

A key to successful aging is staying connected to others. Volz (2000) cites a definite link between social support and health: older people "do better if they continue to engage with life and maintain close relationships" (p. 27).

One type of relationship that many older adults experience is grandparenthood. This relationship may be a source of pride and happiness, or it can become a negative stressor. For many older Americans, grandparenting has become a full-time responsibility, as they are the sole caretakers of grandchildren. Over 2.4 million families in the United States were maintained by grandparents in 1998. This is a 19% increase since 1990 (Davidhizar, Bechtel, & Woodring, 2000). The changing role of grandparenthood "causes caregiver stress, adversely affects child health, and ultimately diminishes family functioning" (Davidhizar et al., 2000, p. 24). However, not all grandparents are overwhelmed by the role of child-rearing for a second generation; many find it rewarding (Davidhizar et al., 2000).

Listed below are some of the factors that have contributed to the increasing numbers of grandparents who are raising their grandchildren on a full-time basis:

- Divorce
- Unemployment
- Teen pregnancy
- Death of a grandchild's parent
- Abuse and/or neglect of the child
- Substance abuse
- Incarceration

## LEGAL AND ETHICAL ISSUES

### Grandparenting and Parenting at the Same Time

Sometimes grandparents find themselves making difficult decisions regarding their children's neglect of their grandchildren. The first ethical dilemma is when the grandparent is put in the awkward position of "taking over" and "stepping in" as the substitute parent. The next ethical dilemma is deciding how to let a grandchild learn through her mistakes and yet be sure to fulfill the child's need for a "good home." The nurse must be prepared to offer unbiased counseling or make a referral to family counseling.

Nurses should be knowledgeable about potential areas of stress imposed by the additional responsibilities of the new grandparenthood role. Also, knowledge of community resources is essential for appropriate referral. Some grandparents may also need information about current childhood problems that were not as prevalent during their years of parenting their own offspring (e.g., cyberporn, school violence).

## Living Arrangements

Advancing age often brings with it changes in living arrangements. The older client has many living options depending on income, health status, activity level, level of independence, and family or other support systems (Figure 19-4). A change in living arrangements is a significant event for any individual, but for older adults, this change may mean leaving family, friends, neighbors, and routines that have been a part of life for decades. Most older adults prefer to remain in their homes or dwellings, in a familiar environment and with familiar routines. In some cases, older adults may move in with their grown children and their families or have the grown children move in with them. The degree of physical, psychological, and financial independence of the older adult, and the status of the relationship with the children, will likely determine the success of this arrangement. Larsen (1998) reports:

> One of the most pressing community challenges we face is the care of elderly persons with a chronic illness. Home care for this population is provided primarily by family members who report chronic fatigue, anger, depression, stress, family conflicts, and excessive financial costs. (p. 8)

Older adults needing assistance to remain in their homes may take advantage of home care services, which provide assistance in the tasks of daily living, or day care services, which provide limited health and rehabilitation intervention. Assisted living facilities (ALFs) are quickly becoming the transition between living independently at home and residing in a nursing home (Kaas & Lewis, 1999). Nursing homes and ALFs are the most common types of residential treatment services used by the older adult. Other options include foster care, group living arrangements, and hospice (Fleming, 2000). "Although only 5% of the older population reside in nursing homes at any one time, about 43% of all people eventually spend

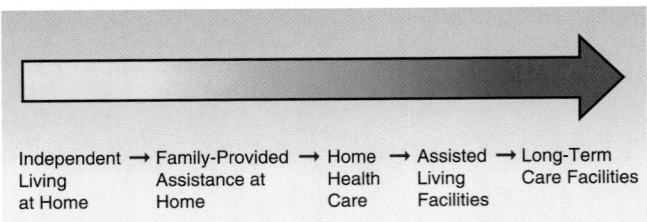

**Figure 19-4  Continuum of living arrangements for the elderly**

some time in such a facility" (National Institute of Aging, 2000). "Multilevel" living facilities may incorporate up to four levels of assistance for adults as depicted in Box 19-8.

Nurses should assist families with the selection of the appropriate setting for declining older adults who cannot stay in their own home. Social workers and case managers are excellent resources to include in these planning discussions. Families may ask about the certification or quality of various institutions. Some of the most common deficiencies in nursing homes are revealed in the statistics of citations of nursing homes noted by Harrington (Beers & Berkow, 2000). Nurses can recommend that families contact the appropriate board in their state to determine certification citations and recommendations of extended care facilities.

When health needs necessitate extensive or full-time supervision and care, a long-term care facility such as a nursing home may be the best living option. Nursing homes offer a variety of services to support the medical, personal, and psychosocial needs of the aging client. Older adults who are able to participate in the decision regarding their living arrangements generally adapt better to the change than those who are unable to participate or who are not involved in their care decisions.

## Coping with Loss

Loss is an inevitable part of life, and the longer a client lives, the more losses will be experienced. Losing a lifetime partner is one of the most stressful loss experiences an individual can face, and many older clients will face loss through death of a spouse at some point in their lives. As the years pass, deaths of children and friends may leave older adults grieving and feeling as if everyone they have known and loved has died before them. Feelings of isolation and hopelessness may arise; these can be compounded if the individual suffers multiple losses at once or within a short period of time. Losses are magnified in older adults who are socially isolated. Fleming (2000) states:

> We need to move away from making old people invisible. We need to care for them. We're the longest-living people planet Earth has ever seen. It's no wonder we never planned for it. We don't know how to live this long. (p. 2)

Helping older adults stay connected with others in the community is an effective intervention for those who are

## NURSING STRATEGY

### Monitoring Drug Use by the Older Adult

Watch for nonspecific side effects, such as appetite disturbance, altered behavior, and falls. Many side effects of medication use are subtle and, therefore, not detected.

---

## BOX 19-8   FOUR LEVELS OF ASSISTANCE FOR ADULTS IN "MULTILEVEL" LIVING FACILITIES

*Level 1*  Living independently in an apartment with a kitchen, a bathroom, and one's own furniture; may elect to take meals in a group setting with a common dining or prepare meals in own room

*Level 2*  Same as number one but services can be purchased such as medication administration and monitoring by staff nurse, assistance with bathing, grocery shopping, clothes washing, and housekeeping

*Level 3*  Living less dependently in a private or double room with usually a bed, chair, closet, and dresser; may share room with roommate; no kitchen; shared bathroom with support bars; may need wheelchair or walker assistance; meals brought to room or taken in common dining room; services in level 2 are available in level 3

*Level 4*  Extensive care usually for severely disoriented or physically disabled older adults; may be fed meals if needed or served in bed; therapies may be needed such as speech, occupational, physical; nurse practitioner, physician assistant, or physician may make rounds on regular basis; intravenous nutrition and urethral catheters utilized; advance directives, living wills, and/or do-not-resuscitate orders may be discussed and documented. Some level 4 units have a philosophy of supporting a quiet, comfortable dying experience to those older adults in whom death is imminent; others have a policy of sending clients to the hospital if they are at near death.

Adapted from Mathieson, K. M., Jacobs Kronenfeld, J., & Keith, V. M. (February 2002). Maintaining functional independence in elderly adults: The roles of health status and financial resources in predicting home modifications and use of mobility equipment. *The Gerontologist, 42*(1): 24–31.

---

experiencing loss and resultant depression. Some avenues for helping elders develop a social support system are churches, senior citizen centers, neighborhood/apartment associations, and community support groups. Often, loss will lead older clients to reflect on their lives and their relationships and to review their successes and shortcomings.

## STOP AND THINK

### Understanding the Meaning of Loss

Consider the perspective of an older client who has experienced the loss of loved ones, such as a spouse of 50 years, or a child. How many losses of this magnitude have you experienced? Do you feel you will be able to relate to and show empathy to an older adult whose life experiences may differ dramatically from your own? What steps can you take to ensure that you treat these clients with dignity, respect, and compassion?

Individuals who feel isolated and abandoned often feel angry and hopeless. Nursing actions that promote a sense of hope in older adults include making time to be sure that the client is included in the discussion and asking about daily plans. Recalling the stages of grief by Dr. Kübler-Ross (1975) can be helpful to nurses' understanding of older adults' emotional responses to losses of loved ones, home, personal belongings, friends, livelihood, and physical capabilities (see Chapter 45).

## Medications and the Older Adult

### Adverse Drug Reaction

The physiological changes of aging can complicate drug therapy in the older adult. The normal effects of aging alter how the body metabolizes and excretes drugs. Therefore, older adults are more sensitive to both the toxic and therapeutic effects of medications. Another factor affecting older adult's drug use is **polypharmacy** (the concurrent use of several medications). Older adults may take more medicine than those who are young and as a result, they are at greater risk for adverse drug reactions (ADR). In addition to increased risk of an ADR, other problems associated with polypharmacy are:

- Medication errors
- Inappropriate prescribing
- Excessive drug costs
- Noncompliance

The presence of multiple diseases and the use of several medications place the elderly person at risk. The effectiveness of drug therapy in the older individual depends on the properties of the particular drug and the impact of age-related changes. As reported by Aparasu (1999), one in 20 prescriptions written for older outpatients may be for medications that should not be used by older clients.

## CLINICAL ALERT

### Use of NSAIDs by the Elderly

Older adults should take nonsteroidal anti-inflammatory drugs (NSAIDs) with caution. NSAIDs can contribute to renal disease. Older adults have renal changes that may exacerbate renal problems.

"Inappropriate prescribing is the primary cause of adverse drug effects in the geriatric population" (Aparasu, 1999, p. 438).

The symptoms of many ADRs are subtle and often are confused with the changes of aging or chronic illnesses. For example, confusion, constipation, fatigue, and dizziness are nonspecific symptoms of many conditions, including ADRs.

The older client's response to drugs is highly individualized. Therefore, the nurse must accurately monitor the client for therapeutic effectiveness and signs of adverse drug reactions.

### Compliance

In addition to assessing the client's responses to medications, the nurse also must assess the client's knowledge of medications being used. Knowledge about the medication, its intended effects, possible side effects, and how to reduce the side effects can increase the client's compliance with the medication regimen. Factors that may negatively affect medication compliance are as follows:

- Complicated dosing schedules and regimens
- Multiple dosing throughout the day
- Use of several medications concurrently (polypharmacy)
- Cost of drugs
- Limited mobility and range of motion (e.g., the client with arthritis who is unable to open childproof containers)
- Impaired memory (e.g., omission—i.e., the client forgets to take the medication; overdosing as a result of not remembering whether the medicine was taken)
- Clients who need assistance and live alone
- Small-print medication labels

Educating elderly clients and caregivers about medication, self-administration, and ways to increase compliance is a major nursing intervention.

### Mistreatment of the Older Adult

Mistreatment of older adults (also referred to as elder abuse) is a serious and ever-increasing problem and disturbing trend. It is estimated that annually 1 million or

## NURSING STRATEGY

### Improving Medication Compliance

1. Provide easily understood information about the medications.
2. Schedule administration of the medication around certain activities of daily living as a reminder to the client.
3. Provide the client with a name and telephone number of a person to contact when questions arise.
4. Assess how the medications are stored and arranged in the client's home. Make sure they are accessible.
5. Perform a complete drug history to determine *all* medications being taken. Instruct the client or caregiver to provide this information to the prescribing practitioner.
6. Encourage client and caregiver to discuss any concerns regarding the medication.
7. Assist with making large-print chart of medications.

## BOX 19-9    SIGNS OF PHYSICAL MISTREATMENT IN THE ELDERLY

- Contusions
- Abrasions
- Sprains
- Burns
- Bruising
- Human bite marks
- Sexual molestation
- Untreated but previously treated conditions
- Misuse of medications
- Freezing
- Depression
- Erratic hair loss from hair pulling
- Lacerations
- Fractures
- Dislocations
- Oversedation
- Over- or undermedication
- Welts
- Scratches
- Decubiti
- Dehydration
- Malnutrition
- Poor hygiene
- Head and face injuries (especially orbital fracture, black eyes, broken teeth)

From Pierce, A. G., Fulmer, T. T., & Edelman, C. L. (2002). Older adult. In C. L. Edelman & C. L. Mandle (Eds.), *Health promotion throughout the life span* (5th ed.). St. Louis: Mosby; Stuart, G. W., & Laraia, M. T. (2001). *Principles and practice of psychiatric nursing* (7th ed.). St. Louis: Mosby.

more older Americans are victims of some form of abuse. There are many forms of elder abuse, including:

- *Physical abuse*—willful infliction of injury
- *Neglect*—withholding goods or services (such as food, attention) to the detriment of the elder's physical or mental health
- *Psychological abuse*—withholding affection or imposing social isolation
- *Exploitation*—dishonest or inappropriate use of the older person's property, money, or other resources

Nurses in the home, clinic, hospital emergency department, and long-term care setting are often the first to identify signs of mistreatment in older people; see Box 19-9 for signs of physical abuse. Abused older adults may either cling to or act in a very guarded manner toward the abuser. Another indicator of possible abuse is vague explanations offered for the cause of the injuries. Psychosocial indicators of abuse may be anger and rage, depression, anxiety, and conflictual interactions between the older adult and the abuser.

When assessing for mistreatment, the nurse must be nonjudgmental and avoid any signs of disapproval that may evoke further feelings of anger and shame in the older client. A private setting should be used for interviewing to promote sharing; also, if the older victim thinks the perpetrator is able to hear the interview, the victim may withhold information or refuse to talk. It is essential that the interview findings be documented and reported in an accurate and unbiased manner.

Nursing interventions for the abused elder are primary, secondary, and tertiary. Primary intervention strategies emphasize prevention. Secondary nursing interventions consist of early identification and prompt treatment to minimize the long-term effects of the abuse. Tertiary interventions occur after the abuse and promote recovery and rehabilitation. Tertiary interventions are restorative in nature.

If the nurse suspects abuse or neglect, this concern should first be addressed with the client. Many abused older adults may not admit to abuse because of embarrassment and fear of reprisal. Most states and many local governments have an Adult Protective Services program. Nurses are responsible for knowing the local statues on mandatory reporting of elder abuse, as these laws may vary. Psychological counseling and support therapy in groups may be beneficial to the victim.

## Advances in Quality of Life and the Human Genome Project

In 2001, scientists in the United States and England completed the blueprint of the human **genome** (the DNA contained in an organism or a cell, which includes both the chromosomes within the nucleus and the DNA in mitochondria). This scientific discovery has been compared to the Apollo Project in outer space and the Manhattan project, which produced the atomic bomb, in terms of scope and costs. The goals of the **Human Genome Project** (an international research project to map each human gene and to completely sequence human DNA) are shown in Box 19-10.

Ultimately, scientists wanted to improve the early diagnosis and prevention of disease and to identify more diseases that could be treated. Currently, medical scientists are searching for heredity markers for alcoholism, depression, intelligence, criminality, sexual orientation, Alzheimer's, as well as aging. Brian Stableford states in McGee's (1997) text *The Perfect Baby* that there is a "new quest for better human beings" and "we will be masters of evolution" from cloning human organs to removing heritable pathologies to cure and prevent disease. Will these advances impact the aging process? Already there is research in "cell therapy" to replace tissues in Parkinson's, injured spinal cords, stroke, diseased heart muscle, liver cells, kidney cells, and skin cells for burn clients. It is an exciting time in the field of aging as new discoveries will impact the aging population's quality of life.

# Nursing Process and the Older Adult

Due to the changing demographics in the United States, older adults are currently the most frequent consumers of health care services (Sheffler, 1998). Thus, an ever-increasing number of nurses will provide care to the older client. "With advancing age, health-promoting interventions along with the management of chronic health problems become essential elements for maintaining independent living and minimizing use of costly health care services" (Tanner & Lethbridge, 1998, p. 354). Nurses are the ideal health care providers to help people change their behavior in order to take advantage of increased longevity.

According to Kamimoto, Easton, Maurice, Husten, & Macera (1999), older Americans could do more to improve their health and quality of life. Listed below are areas in which older adults need to develop health-promoting behaviors:

- Nutrition: More than 60% of older adults are not eating at least five fruits and vegetables daily.
- Exercise: Approximately 33% of those aged 55 to 74 are physically inactive; 46% of those over age 74 are not physically active.
- Use of preventive health services: Fewer than 60% of those over age 65 have received the pneumonococcal vaccine.
- Use of health screenings: (1) breast cancer screening decreases with age; (2) fewer than 33% of people aged 55 years and older had received a screening test for colorectal cancer (Kamimoto et al., 1999).

Increasing numbers of gerontological nurses are needed to provide quality of care. As stated by the American Nurses Association (2001):

Gerontological nursing is one of the profession's most challenging practice areas. Gerontological nurses will continue to work with populations at risk for health care problems as they recognize the needs of specific groups, including frail elders over age 85, minorities, the socially and financially impoverished, the homeless, and the institutionalized. (p. 7)

Professional standards for gerontological nurses were developed by the ANA in 1995; these standards are addressed in the next section.

## Assessment

The data-gathering phase of assessment begins with the first encounter with the older client. Overall appearance, dress, gait, presentation, and general behavior can be noted when a client first enters the room. Assessment of the older client can be a time-consuming yet rewarding process when the nurse works thoughtfully and sensitively with the client to discover strengths, resources, and limitations.

When interviewing the older client in the home, it is important to also include the client's caregivers in the assessment. The home care nurse assesses:

- Family interactions
- Caregiver motivation to participate in the rehabilitation process
- The motivational impact of the caregivers on the older person to accept some control over own care
- Feelings of caregivers toward their role (e.g., level of satisfaction or burnout)

## Health History

Older adults are individuals not only of age and wisdom, but also individuals with a long history that deserves telling. The nurse's role in conducting a health history with the older client is to draw facts and interpretations from the client that will shed light on current health status and health concerns. Eliciting these data requires time and patience on the part of both nurse and client, but it can be a rewarding and interesting process. To gather pertinent health data, the nurse may interview the client and the client's significant others to determine the client's past coping strategies, strengths, and health habits. A holistic approach will include discussion of physical, emotional, psychological, spiritual, and sociocultural aspects that contribute to the client's overall health.

Older clients often feel a loss of control over their lives when decisions, including health care decisions, are made by others. The nurse respects the client's dignity and independence during the interview process by facing the client, speaking directly to the client in a clear manner, and reacting appropriately to client concerns and needs.

## Physical Examination

The nurse must be knowledgeable about the normal physical changes of aging in order to conduct an efficient and informative physical examination of the older client. The physical changes must be noted: the impact these changes have on the client's quality of life and activities of daily living must also be determined. The assessment tools will need to be adjusted to the older person's abilities and limitations. For instance, the physical examination may need to be performed in more than one session to prevent client fatigue. Client positioning may need to be adjusted according to client comfort. The client may need assistance with disrobing or position changes, and the nurse must always be alert to protect the client from potential injury, such as falls. For an explanation of special considerations necessary in assessment of elderly clients, see Table 19-3.

## Nursing Diagnosis

Nursing diagnoses developed from the assessment of the older client will be as varied as the clients themselves. According to the ANA (2001), gerontological nurses are expected to analyze the assessment data in determining diagnosis.

Nurses must keep in mind that older clients may present with many needs, both physical and psychosocial, and that the nursing diagnoses will need to be prioritized. Client status may change frequently, so reevaluation of nursing diagnoses on a regular basis is warranted. Selected nursing diagnoses (North American Nursing Diagnosis Association [NANDA], 2003) that are frequently seen in older clients include:

- Physical
  - *Impaired Physical Mobility* related to intolerance to activity/decreased strength and endurance; pain/discomfort; perceptual/cognitive impairment; neuromuscular impairment; musculoskeletal impairment; depression/severe anxiety
  - *Activity Intolerance* related to bed rest/immobility; generalized weakness; sedentary lifestyle
  - *Self-Care Deficit* related to intolerance to activity; decreased strength and endurance; physical, perceptual, or cognitive impairment

- Psychosocial
  - *Social Isolation* related to absence of supportive significant others; alterations in physical appearance; alterations in mental status; inadequate personal resources
  - *Risk for Loneliness*: risk factors include affectional deprivation; physical isolation; social isolation
  - *Ineffective Role Performance* related to change in self-perception of role; change in physical capacity to resume role; change in usual patterns of responsibility
  - *Impaired Home Maintenance* related to disease or injury; insufficient finances; impaired cognitive or emotional functioning; inadequate support systems
  - *Acute Confusion* related to age; dementia; alcohol abuse; drug abuse; delirium

## Outcome Identification and Planning

Outcomes identified in the plan of care must be developed in partnership with the older client and the client's support system. See Box 19-11 for the ANA gerontological standards related to outcome identification and planning.

Outcomes should be realistic for the client's current status and desired goals and should be targeted to maintaining a certain level of health or restoring the client to a former state of health. Support systems, friends, and colleagues should be involved as agreeable with the client to assist in meeting health care needs. See the Nursing Strategy box for a discussion of a teaching plan for an older client.

## Implementation

Nursing interventions for the older client will typically focus on the areas of maintaining physical health, supporting psychosocial well-being, promoting safety, and providing restorative care. The ANA directs gerontological nurses to implement the interventions identified in the care plan.

Three major interventions used effectively with older clients are education, communication, and life review. The Nursing Strategy box provides information on communicating effectively with older adults.

Life review (also referred to as reminiscence therapy) is a structured intervention in which the nurse guides the client through remembrance of life, stage by stage. This intervention is especially therapeutic for clients who feel alienated and depressed, as it helps people develop a sense

## TABLE 19-3    SPECIAL CONSIDERATIONS FOR ASSESSING OLDER CLIENTS

| Assessment Area | Essential Points |
| --- | --- |
| Fluid balance | Older adults are more sensitive to fluid and electrolyte imbalances. <br> Older adults can become dehydrated quickly due to deficient volumes. <br> Monitor closely the amount of fluid administered (including oral ingestion, IV fluids, blood products). <br> Maintain accurate fluid intake and output record. |
| Body temperature | Decreased body tissue, diminished thermoregulation, and peripheral vascular changes place older adults at risk for hypothermia. <br> Watch closely for signs of chilling (e.g., shivering). <br> Assess environmental temperature. |
| Neurologic | Assess mental status. <br> Assess for underlying causes of confusion and memory loss, if necessary. |
| Sensory | Assess vision. <br> Assess hearing. <br> Determine level of orientation. |
| Cardiovascular | Assessment of peripheral pulses may be difficult because of atherosclerosis. <br> Monitor for baseline values (i.e., signs of hypoxia, hypovolemia, acidosis). <br> Reassess frequently. |
| Pulmonary | Monitor respiratory rate and characteristics. <br> Assess ability to cough productively. <br> Reassess frequently to detect early indicators of deterioration. |
| Musculoskeletal | Evaluate ability to ambulate (immobility contributes to risk of pulmonary embolism and deep vein thrombosis). <br> Determine amount of assistance needed for performing activities of daily living. |
| Integumentary | Less elastic, thin skin abrades easily and is vulnerable to pressure. <br> Assess for any reddened areas or fissures. <br> Check skin turgor. |

From Walhout, M. F., Tubergen, C. R., & Cook, K. J. (November 1998). Multiple accident victims: All elderly. *Nursing98, 59.*

### BOX 19-11    STANDARDS OF CLINICAL GERONTOLOGICAL NURSING CARE: OUTCOME IDENTIFICATION AND PLANNING

The gerontological nurse:

- Identifies expected outcomes individualized to each client

- Develops a plan of care that prescribes interventions to attain expected outcomes

From American Nurses Association (1995). *Scope and standards of gerontological nursing practice.* Washington, DC: Author.

of meaning and promotes achievement of the sense of integrity identified by Erikson (1968). Brady (1999) discusses the "power and efficacy of reminiscence and life review for the elderly" (p. 178). See Box 19-12 for some of the therapeutic outcomes of reminiscence.

### Maintain Physical Health

During the assessment phase, the nurse will identify which physical changes are the result of normal aging and which have underlying pathology. Clients will need to be educated as to what these changes mean, what impact they may have on their daily activities, and what strategies they can use to meet their needs given their new or changing abilities. It is critical to emphasize clients' assets and abilities, instead of focusing on limitations, to maintain a

## NURSING STRATEGY

### Outcome Identification and Planning

When developing client outcomes and a teaching plan:

1. Plan for a quiet, private environment that is conducive to learning.
2. Assess the client's readiness to learn as well as previous knowledge.
3. Treat the client as a partner whose input is valuable in the planning and outcome identification process.
4. Assess sensory status, especially sight and hearing, and adjust actions according to client needs.
5. Use language that is clear and easy to understand.
6. Encourage clients to ask questions and verbalize their understanding of what is being taught. For instance, state, "I want you to feel free to ask questions; all your questions are important."
7. Plan to include the family and significant others in the teaching session, not as a substitute for the client, but for support and reinforcement.
8. Plan for active learning experiences (e.g., use examples, simulations, games, and audiovisuals when appropriate).
9. Pace the learning. Do not give too much information at one time, and progress at the individual's learning pace. Stop if you see that the client is distracted or fatigued.
10. Plan to summarize and reinforce what has been taught.

## BOX 19-12 BENEFITS OF REMINISCENCE

- Enhances problem solving
- Provides an outlet for catharsis ("getting things off one's chest")
- Assists in resolving conflicts
- Maximizes long-term memory when short-term memory is impaired
- Maintains identity and self-esteem
- Promotes ability to attain perspective and find meaning

From Brady, E. M. (1999). Stories at the hour of our death. *Home Healthcare Nurse, 17*(3), 176–180; Eliopoulos, C. (1999). *Manual of gerontologic nursing* (2nd ed.). St. Louis: Mosby.

or lie down when fatigued, avoid carrying heavy parcels when ambulating).

### Support Psychosocial Well-Being

An older client's psychosocial health is as equally important as physical well-being. The use of touch and therapeutic communication helps the client overcome feelings of isolation and enhances a positive self-concept. Encouraging the older adult to be active in social groups, leisure activities, and hobbies supports a higher level of

healthy self-concept and to show clients how much independence they still maintain.

Specific interventions related to the physical changes of aging will depend on the nature of the alterations. For instance, skin changes such as dryness, wrinkling, or flaccidity can be partially overcome through the use of oils, moisturizers, and a humidifier. If deteriorating eyesight is a prominent complaint, nurses should instruct the client to avoid reading when fatigued, to use large-print materials, and to ensure that the reading environment is well lit with an overhead and desk lamp that does not create glare. If cardiovascular changes result in fatigue and shortness of breath on exertion, nurses should help the client learn the signs indicating his activity tolerance level and to adjust activity accordingly (e.g., plan for frequent rest periods, sit

## NURSING STRATEGY

### Communicating with Older Clients

1. Get the client's attention before you speak.
2. Minimize extraneous stimuli (e.g., background noises).
3. Sit directly facing the client, keep your mouth visible, and maintain eye contact.
4. Speak slowly and clearly. Use short, simple sentences. Give the client time to respond.
5. Speak loudly enough for the client to hear you, but avoid yelling.
6. Use repetition often.
7. Summarize frequently the most important elements of your message.

From Tips on overcoming communication breakdown with elderly patients (February 1999). *Home Healthcare Nurse, 17*(2), 78.

## COMMUNITY/HOME CARE

### Promoting a Safe Environment

- Provide adequate nonglare lighting.

- Place nightlights in bedroom, bathroom, and hallway.

- Secure loose rugs or do not use them.

- Keep electrical cords out of throughways.

- Install smoke alarms.

- Place a plastic chair in tub or shower.

- Install grab bars in tub or shower and next to toilet.

- Install high toilet lids.

- Have handrails next to stairs and long hallways.

- Use sturdy chairs with armrests.

- Purchase shoes that have flat rubber soles.

- Fix leaks in kitchen or bathroom plumbing.

- Have list of emergency phone numbers in large print next to phone.

- Observe client's behavior to know if cooking with electricity or gas is safe.

- Check safety features on winter floor heaters.

- Have vision checked annually for new eyeglass prescriptions.

- Purchase coffeemakers and irons with automatic turnoff.

self-esteem and pleasure with life and helps the client to focus on positive traits and abilities.

The client's family or significant others can have a significant impact on maintaining the client's psychosocial functioning. They can assist the client in maintaining a relatively independent lifestyle and may even be able to help the client sustain activities of daily living outside of an institutional environment. For clients without support systems, teaching how to cope with alterations in mental status (e.g., using calendars to orient to reality, reading the daily paper to keep aware of current events) and how to work within those parameters can help clients maintain a sense of independence and dignity. Referrals to community services may be beneficial.

### Promote a Safe Environment

Ongoing assessment includes observing the client's immediate environment for safety. This is especially critical for clients who will be remaining in their own homes or in a home situation where they, not the health care staff, are responsible for maintaining a safe environment. Family members and significant others should be included in the efforts to create a safe environment for the elderly client (Figure 19-5). See Chapter 33 for additional information on safety and preventing falls.

Falls are a major safety issue with many older adults. Box 19-13 lists some age-related factors that contribute to falls.

In order to promote a safe home environment for the older client, the nurse may suggest safety actions.

Each year, approximately 2 million older Americans are victims of crime. Older people are often easy targets for car theft, robbery, and burglary. For suggestions on preventing victimization, see Table 19-4.

### Restorative Care

**Restorative nursing care** (also referred to as rehabilitative care) seeks to assist the client in regaining maximal functional ability. Restorative care that is provided to clients who have residual impairment as a result of disease or injury seeks to increase the client's independence and ability to perform self-care. Nurses providing restorative care understand that sometimes the impairment in functional ability will remain. In such cases, the goal is to help the client function at the maximal level possible. Nurses constantly balance the client's need for dependence with the need for independence. In other words, nurses provide care as needed while encouraging the client to do for self as much as possible. Restorative care is provided in home health, assisted-living facilities, and long-term care facilities (e.g., nursing homes).

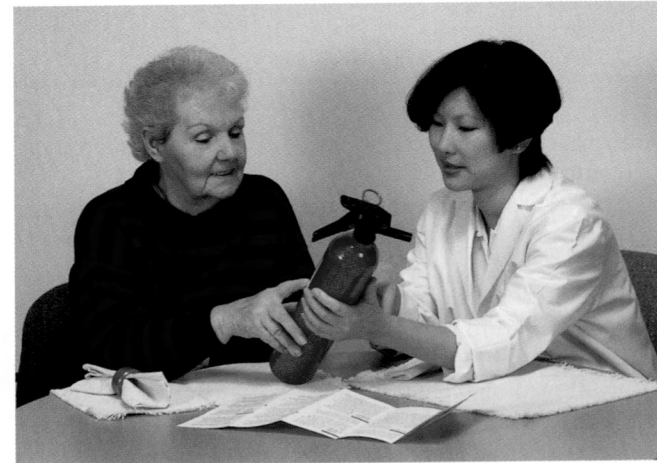

**Figure 19-5** **Educating the older client about safety, particularly in the home, is an essential nursing function that is facilitated by the use of clear step-by-step instructions.**

## BOX 19-13    AGE-RELATED FACTORS CONTRIBUTING TO FALLS

- Decreased visual acuity
- Poor vision in dimly lit areas
- Less foot and toe lift when walking
- Altered center of gravity
- Slower reflexes
- Impaired muscle control
- Orthostatic hypotension (blood pressure related to posture)
- Urinary frequency

From Ebersole, P., Hess P., & Luggen, A. (2004). *Toward healthy aging: Human needs and nursing response* (5th ed.). St. Louis: Mosby; Eliopoulos, C. (1999). *Manual of gerontologic nursing* (2nd ed.). St. Louis: Mosby.

## NURSING STRATEGY

### Guidelines for Providing Restorative Care

1. Encourage independence.
2. Use a positive, reassuring approach.
3. Be alert to limitations and client-expressed need for help.
4. Encourage client decision making.
5. Communicate with words easily understood by the client. Ask client to repeat directions in order to assess their comprehension.
6. Provide positive reinforcement often.
7. Use repetition through words and actions (i.e., demonstration).
8. Provide rest periods as needed.
9. Ensure client safety by safeguarding against injury at all times.

## TABLE 19-4    SUGGESTIONS FOR DECREASING THE RISK OF ELDER VICTIMIZATION

| | |
|---|---|
| In the home | Lock doors and windows. |
| | Be sure locks cannot be easily broken. |
| | Install an alarm system. |
| | Identify the caller before opening the door. |
| | Take photographs of valuable items; mark items with an identification number. |
| | Keep police phone number by phone. |
| | Tell phone solicitors to take you off list. |
| On the street | Always be vigilant. |
| | Avoid dark alleys and dark parking areas. |
| | Walk with others instead of alone. |
| | Have monthly income checks sent to the bank via direct deposit. |
| | Vary the time you go to the bank. |
| | Avoid using isolated ATM machines. |
| | Avoid keeping a lot of cash on hand, but if threatened by an assailant, hand over all cash. |
| Consumer fraud | Don't take money if a stranger tells you to do so. |
| | Avoid giving credit card or bank account numbers over the phone. |
| | Beware of deals that sound "too good to be true"; check with the local Better Business Bureau. |
| | Be alert to "miracle cures" for health problems. |

From National Institute on Aging (1996). *Age page: Crime and older people*. Gaithersburg, MD: Author.

Clients who might benefit from restorative care are those who:

- Are incontinent
- Have an indwelling catheter
- Are nonambulatory
- Have pressure sores (decubitus ulcers)
- Require partial or complete assistance with activities of daily living

See the Nursing Strategy box for interventions most useful in providing restorative care.

## Evaluation

Evaluation is an important function of all nurses working with the elderly. The ANA standard for gerontology requires nurses to evaluate the older person's progress toward attainment of expected outcomes. Evaluation is a major determinant of the need for continuing care of the older client. The nurse must decide whether the original assessment is still pertinent and if its accompanying diagnoses have been resolved. New diagnoses need to be established on the basis of client progress and changing needs, and new goals must be developed with the client and significant others that will foster maximum health status based on the client's abilities and capabilities. In terms of providing for continuity of care, the nurse should consider the ongoing needs of the client and offer resources or make referrals to ensure that the health and well-being of the client will continue to be monitored and enhanced.

 # CASE STUDY/NURSING CARE PLAN

Winston Evans, an 82-year-old man, is a retired grocer who was widowed 6 years ago. Until last year, Mr. Evans lived alone in a small home, was involved with his family, went to church regularly, and enjoyed socializing with peers at the community senior center. He now lives in his daughter's home. His daughter brings him to the clinic today stating, "We can't go on like this! Last night he walked out of the house and was missing for hours. The policeman brought him home while we were looking for him." This was Mr. Evans' fourth episode of wandering within the past 3 months. The daughter also stated that Mr. Evans was unable to take care of himself. "I have to feed and bathe him every day." Mr. Evans was unable to state the date, day of week, month, or year. He also did not know where he was, even though he had been treated by the nurse practitioner (NP) for several years at the clinic. He could not remember the names of his family except for his daughter. He was observed by the NP to be restless, and his speech was rambling and confused. Mr. Evans tells the NP, "Get away from me. No one's gonna hurt me." His medical diagnosis is severe arthritis, glaucoma, and congestive heart failure. He weighs 115 pounds (a weight loss of 24 pounds over the past 4 months), he "picks at his food," is constipated, sleeps most of the day, and is usually loud and restless at night. During the assessment, Mr. Evans is agitated and cries out several times, "Help me, help me!"

## Assessment

Client is disoriented to time and place, but is able to state his name. He is somewhat uncooperative and does not stay focused to the questions being asked. When answering questions, he cannot remember things that he says in the conversation. His facial expressions reflect a lack of sleep and his general color is slightly pale. Mr. Evans' lung sounds are clear and his breathing is unlabored. His vital signs are B/P = 146/74, P = 86, R = 18, T = 37.2. The client has evidence of arthritis in his hands.

## Nursing Diagnosis #1

*Noncompliance* of client with a therapeutic plan that will keep him free of injury, related to his confused mental status.

**NOC:** Adherence Behavior; Compliance Behavior; Knowledge: Treatment Regimen; Health Care Decisions
**NIC:** Behavior Modifications; Decision-Making Support; Patient Contracting; Health Education

## Expected Outcomes

The client will:

1. Be free of injury to self and others.
2. Have his activities monitored closely on constant basis.

*(continues)*

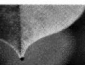

# CASE STUDY/NURSING CARE PLAN (*continued*)

## Planning/Interventions/Rationales

1. Approach in a calm, nonthreatening manner. *Decreases anxiety level, which further impairs mental status.*
2. Determine the presence of personal or environmental risk factors. *Identification of safety hazards is the first step in minimizing such hazards.*
3. Orient Mr. Evans regularly to his environment. *To decrease client's frustration level and better understand client needs.*
4. Closely supervise Mr. Evans at night to assess safety. *To determine which risk factors are present and what safety measures should be implemented.*
5. Set limits on self-destructive behavior. *To promote safety of client and others.*
6. Monitor judgment, decision-making ability, and impulse control. *Impaired judgment and impulsivity increase the likelihood of unsafe behaviors.*
7. Minimize specific hazards in the home (e.g., remove stove knobs, store cleaning products and medications in a locked area, clear floor and hallway of obstacles). *To make the home environment safer.*
8. Provide an ID bracelet for Mr. Evans to wear at home, and participate in local police registry if available. *To increase possibility of client's quick return to home if he wanders away.*
9. Keep nightlights on at night. *Decreases the potential for falls.*
10. Instruct family to install an alarm system on all exit doors. *To minimize the possibility of wandering.*

## Evaluation

Goal met. Mr. Evans remains free from physical injury and does not injure anyone else. He has not wandered off alone in the past week.

## Nursing Diagnosis #2

*Disturbed Sleep Pattern* related to altered mental status.
**NOC:** Anxiety Control; Sleep
**NIC:** Sleep Enhancement

## Expected Outcomes

The client will:

1. Sleep uninterrupted for periods of at least 4 consecutive hours, and sleep for at least 8 hours each night (beginning immediately).
2. Display affect that is not indicative of sleeplessness, and improve current generalized skin pallor within 72 hours.

## Planning/Interventions/Rationales

1. Monitor and keep a record of sleep patterns. *To determine a baseline for future evaluation of progress or lack of progress.*
2. Minimize daytime napping. *Older adults need less sleep, so daytime napping only subtracts from amount of sleep required at night.*
3. Schedule exercise 2 hours prior to scheduled bedtime. *To provide relaxation.*
4. Teach client and family simple relaxation techniques. *Keeping instructions simple helps the client who is confused to better absorb the information. Relaxation techniques can be used to promote sleep.*
5. Limit caffeine intake. *Caffeine can interfere with sleep.*
6. Ensure quiet environment with a soft nightlight. *Promotes relaxation and a sense of comfort.*
7. Provide comfort measures and teach such measures to family. *The use of back rubs and rearranging linens can promote comfort and relaxation.*

## Evaluation

Goal partially met. Family reports that Mr. Evans is sleeping every night in approximately 3-hour intervals, and skin pallor has improved.

# CONCEPT MAPPING CASE STUDY

Jason Rutherford, aged 81, is a retired schoolteacher. He is widowed and lives alone in the home that he and his wife shared for 43 years. His two adult sons and their wives live in the city, and they visit him at least once each week. His two grandchildren attend college in another state. A cleaning woman comes to his home every 2 weeks. Mr. Rutherford enjoys his independence, still drives his car, attends his church regularly, and likes to garden. He manages the routine cooking and household tasks rather well. He also belongs to a group of retired teachers who have breakfast meetings once a month.

Mr. Rutherford has hypertension and is taking daily doses of lisinopril 40 mg, an ACE-inhibitor medication; pravastatin 10 mg, an antilipemic medication; and low-dose (81 mg) aspirin. He takes Tylenol (OTC) for arthritis pain. He is scheduled for cataract surgery next month.

Yesterday, he tripped and fell when he was retrieving his mail from the mailbox by his driveway. He felt a sharp pain in his right hip and leg and was unable to get up. His next-door neighbor heard his shouts for help and ran out to assist him. She notified Mr. Rutherford's son and called 911. After being examined in the emergency department, he was diagnosed with a femoral neck fracture. He was transferred to the orthopedic unit and was scheduled for a total hip replacement (arthroplasty).

Postoperative orders include thigh-high support hose, an indwelling catheter (for 2 to 3 days), legs must remain abducted, and Mr. Rutherford cannot be turned. Assess the wound dressing and hemovac drainage. He has an intravenous fluid running. Intake and output are to be measured. Narcotic analgesics will be administered via a patient controlled analgesia device (PCA) for the first 2 days with transition to oral analgesics the third day if needed. Heparin is to be administered intravenously as a prophylactic measure against thrombophlebitis. Vital signs and neurovascular status of the lower extremities are to be evaluated on a routine basis.

**Note:** There is a current trend for using clinical pathways for managing the interdisciplinary care for total hip replacement. Clients can usually return to their regular presurgical diet on the second postoperative day. Hospitalization for this type of surgery is 4 to 5 days. The client is usually discharged to a rehabilitation facility for a period of time. Physical and occupational therapies and education related to transferring techniques, weight-bearing exercises, modifications in the home, and so on begins early in the postoperative treatment time. The nurse is also involved in education and monitoring the client's progress. The recovery period is approximately 4 to 6 weeks. As you respond to the discussion questions for this case study, consider the special needs of the geriatric client as they relate to the holistic mental, physical, spiritual, environmental, and safety needs. Refer to the sample concept map for assistance in designing a map for Mr. Rutherford. Add concepts where you believe they belong (note: some concepts may belong in more than one area).

## Suggested References
Current nurses drug guide or pharmacology text
Current medical/surgical nursing text
Current NANDA (nursing diagnosis) text

1. Describe the potential complications due to immobility. What are the nursing actions to prevent these complications?
2. What precautions should be taken when transferring Mr. Rutherford from the bed to a chair?
3. What clinical manifestations (respiratory, gastrointestinal, mental, etc.) would alert you to the adverse side effects of the narcotic medications?
4. Describe discharge instructions that you would provide for Mr. Rutherford.
5. If you were assigned to evaluate Mr. Rutherford's home, what safety precautions and adaptations would you suggest to minimize falls and promote his progress toward independent living?

## Key Concepts

- Persons in the late adulthood years are often classified as "young old" (those between 65 and 75), "middle old" (those between 75 and 85), and the "old" (those 85 and older).
- Biologic theories of aging state that the physical changes of aging are universal.
- Psychosocial theories of aging consider factors other than genetics when describing the aging process.
- Numerous myths about aging can be viewed as ageism, which is stereotyping and discrimination based on age.
- Advances in medicine and technology have greatly improved life expectancy as well as the quality of life for older adults.
- Developmental tasks of older adults include enhancing skills, gaining and sharing wisdom, renewing relationships, expanding knowledge, and adjusting to losses and change.
- The multiple physical changes associated with aging can have a profound impact on an older adult's ability to function and to perform activities of daily living.
- Retirement, changes in social relationships, changes in living arrangements, and loss may affect an older client's self-esteem, self-concept, impression of self-worth, and feelings of isolation.
- Individuals who have had a positive outlook on the aging process over the years tend to adapt better to retirement and the many other life changes that occur in late adulthood than do individuals who fear or do not understand the aging process.
- Physical assessment of the older client will need to be tailored to the client's functional level and activity tolerance.
- Including family and significant others in planning and implementing care for older clients enhances the chance for successful outcomes.
- Restorative nursing care (also referred to as rehabilitative care) seeks to assist the client in regaining maximal functional ability. Restorative care is provided to clients who have residual impairment as a result of disease or injury and aims to increase the client's independence and ability to perform self-care.
- Safety is a primary concern when caring for older clients; this can be addressed through thorough assessment and client and family teaching.

## Review Questions and Activities

1. Explain "old age" in terms of theories and misconceptions about aging.
2. What are the multiple physiological changes associated with aging and the impact these may have on an older adult's ability to function and to perform activities of daily living?
3. Discuss the psychosocial impact that retirement, changes in social relationships, changes in living arrangements, and loss may have on the older adult.
4. Define polypharmacy and its significance for nurses caring for older clients.
5. What are the physical and psychological signs of elder abuse?
6. What safety considerations for the elderly living at home should the nurse and caregivers evaluate?
7. Develop guidelines for teaching the older client.
8. As the nurse manager of a nursing home, you want to establish a program to encourage clients to engage in life review. You decide to conduct a weekly class for interested residents who want to share their life experiences. How would you prepare for the class? What agenda would you establish? How would you evaluate the effectiveness of the class?

## Web Resources

Administration on Aging
    http://www.aoa.dhhs.gov
American Association of Retired People
    http://www.aarp.org
American Society on Aging
    http://www.asaging.org
Healthcare Ethics
    http://www.Ascensionhealth.org
National Conference of Gerontological
    Nurse Practitioners
    http://www.ncgnp.org
National Council on Aging
    http://www.ncoa.org
National Institute on Aging
    http://www.nih.gov/nia
South Tyrol Museum of Archeology
    http://www.archaeologiemuseum.it

## References

AARP (2002). *A profile of older Americans.* Washington, DC: Author.

American Nurses Association. (2001). *Scope and standards of nursing practice.* Washington, DC: Author.

American Nurses Association. (1995). *Scope and standards of gerontological nursing practice.* Washington, DC: Author.

Aparasu, R. R. (1999). Inappropriate prescribing for elderly outpatients. *American Journal of Health Systems Pharmacy, 56,* 433–439.

Beard, B. B. (1991). Centenarians: The new generation (N. K. Wilson & A. J. F. Wilson, Eds.). Westport, CT: Greenwood Press.

Beers, H. M., & Berkow, R. (2000). *The Merck manual of geriatrics* (3rd ed.). Whitehouse Station, NJ: Merck Research Laboratories, Merck, Inc.

Brady, E. M. (1999). Stories at the hour of our death. *Home Healthcare Nurse, 17*(3), 176–180.

Davidhizar, R., Bechtel, G. A., & Woodring, B. C. (2000). The changing role of grandparenthood. *Journal of Gerontological Nursing, 26*(1), 24–29.

Ebersole, P., Hess, P., & Luggen, A. (2004). *Toward healthy aging: Human needs and nursing response* (6th ed.). St. Louis: Mosby.

Eliopoulos, C. (1999). *Manual of gerontologic nursing* (2nd ed.). St. Louis: Mosby.

Erikson, E. (1968). *Childhood and society.* New York: Norton.

Estes, M. E. Z. (2002). *Health assessment & physical examination* (2nd ed.). Clifton Park, NY: Delmar Learning.

Ferrans, C., & Powers, M. (1985). Quality of Life Index: Development and psychometric properties. *Advances in Nursing Science, 8,* 15–24.

Flecker, A., & Steiner, H. (1998). *The fascination of the neolithic age: The iceman.* Folio Verlag, Bolzano, Vienna and South Tyrol Museum of Archeology.

Fleming, K. C. (February 2000). Mayo clinic office visit: The ins and outs of long-term care. *Mayo Clinic Women's Healthsource Supplement, 3.*

Hackler, C. (Winter 2001). Troubling implications of doubling the human life span. *Generations, 25*(4), 15–19.

Johnson, A. P. (1999). The pulmonary system and its problems in the elderly. In M. Stanley & P. G. Beare (Eds.), *Gerontological nursing* (2nd ed.). Philadelphia: Davis.

Kaas, M. J., & Lewis, M. L. (1999). Cognitive behavioral group therapy for residents in assisted-living facilities. *Journal of Psychosocial Nursing, 37*(10), 9–15.

Kamimoto, L. A., Easton, A. N., Maurice, E., Husten, C. G., & Macera, C. A. (December 17, 1999). Surveillance for five health risks among older adults—United States, 1993–1997. *Morbidity & mortality report CDC surveillance summary, 48*(18): 51–88.

Kleinpell, R. M., & Ferrans, C. E. (2002). Quality of life of elderly patients after treatment in the ICU. *Research in Nursing and Health, 25,* 212–221.

Kübler-Ross, E. (1975). *Death: The final stage of growth.* Englewood Cliffs, NJ: Prentice Hall.

Larsen, L. S. (1998). Effectiveness of a counseling intervention to assist family caregivers of chronically ill relatives. *Journal of Psychosocial Nursing, 36*(8), 26–32.

Mathieson, K. M., Jacobs Kronenfeld, J., & Keith, V. M. (February 2002). Maintaining functional independence in elderly adults: The roles of health status and financial resources in predicting home modifications and use of mobility equipment. *The Gerontologist, 42*(1), 24–31.

McGee, G. (1997). *The perfect baby.* Lanham, MD: Rowman & Littlefield Publishers, Inc.

Murray, R. B., & Zentner, J. P. (2000). *Nursing assessment and health promotion: Strategies through the life span* (7th ed.). Norwalk, CT: Appleton & Lange.

National Institute on Aging (2000). *Working with your older patient: A clinician's handbook.* http://www.nih.gov/nia/pubs/clinicians-handbook

National Institute on Aging (1996). *Age page: Crime and older people.* Gaithersburg, MD: Author.

North American Nursing Diagnosis Association (2003). *Nursing diagnoses: Definitions and classification, 2003–2004.* Philadelphia: Author.

Pierce, A. G., Fulmer, T. T., & Edelman, C. L. (2002). Older adult. In C. L. Edelman & C. L. Mandle (Eds.), *Health promotion throughout the life span* (5th ed.). St. Louis: Mosby.

Sadler, W. (2000). *The third age: Six principles of growth and renewal after forty.* New York: Perseus Books.

Sadovsky, R. (1999). Management of erectile dysfunction. *CNS Special Edition, 1*(1), 79–83.

Sheffler, S. J. (1998). Clinical placement and correlates affecting student attitudes toward the elderly. *Journal of Nursing Education, 37*(5), 216–219.

Stuart, G. W., & Laraia, M. T. (2001). *Principles and practice of psychiatric nursing* (7th ed.). St. Louis: Mosby.

Tanner, E. K. W., & Lethbridge, D. J. (1998). Educational implications of "real-life" community health care delivery to underserved elders by RN baccalaureate nursing students. *Journal of Nursing Education, 37*(8), 354–357.

Thompson, B., Sierpina, V. S., & Sierpina, M. (Winter 2001) What is healthy aging? Family physicians look at conventional and alternative approaches. *Generations, 25*(4), 49–53.

Tips on overcoming communication breakdown with elderly patients (February 1999). *Home Healthcare Nurse, 17*(2), 78.w

United States Bureau of the Census. (1999). *Population and family characteristics: Population estimates and projections.* Washington, DC: Author.

Volz, F. (2000). Successful aging: The second 50. *Monitor on Psychology, 31*(1), 24–28.

Walhout, M. F., Tubergen, C. R., & Cook, K. J. (November 1998). Multiple accident victims: All elderly. *Nursing98,* 59.

# Arenas of Client Care

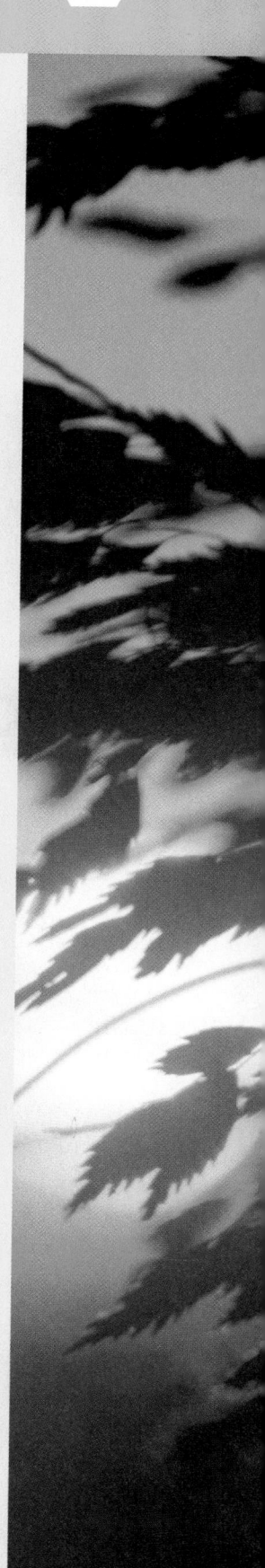

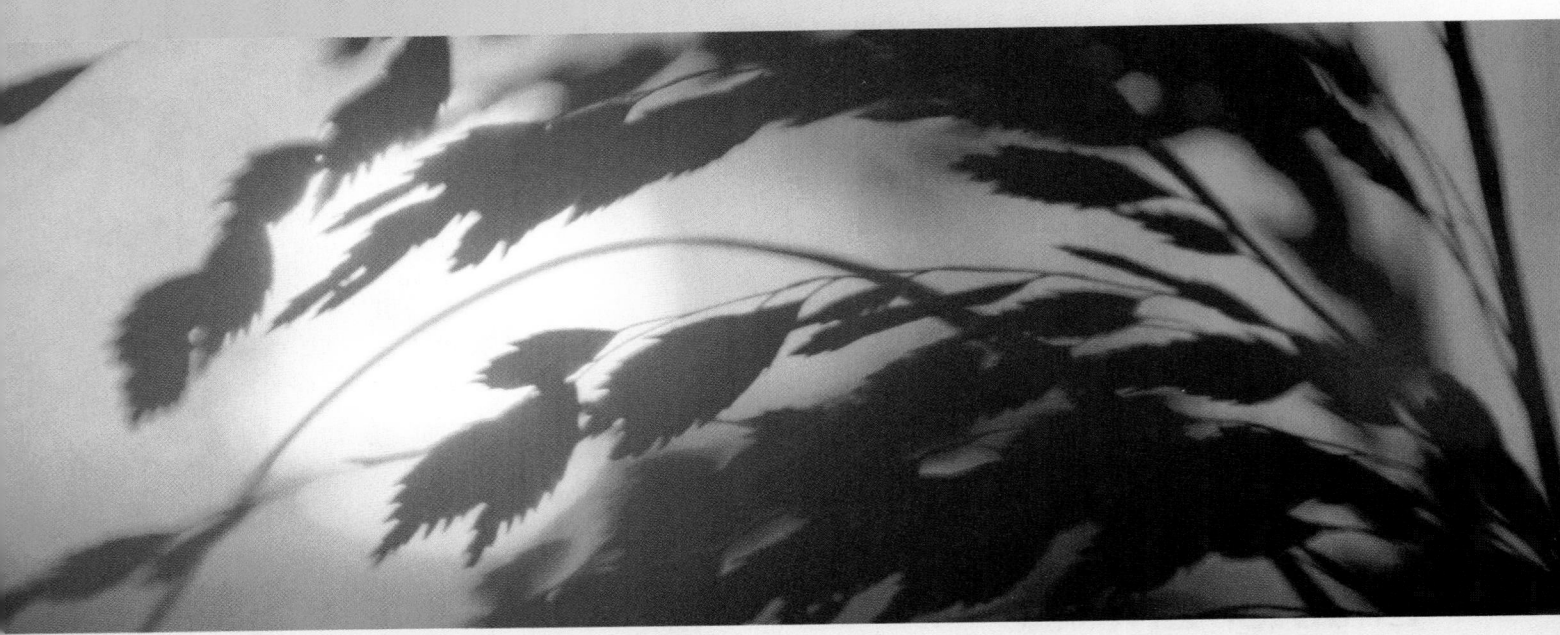

# Acute Care

Milena Segatore, RN, BscN, MscN, MNI-PG, CNRN

*"I will do all in my power to maintain and elevate the standard of my profession . . ."*

(Nightingale Pledge, 1859)

# Chapter Competencies

**Upon completion of this chapter, the reader should be able to:**

1. Define acute care nursing.
2. Differentiate acute care from other arenas of care delivery.
3. Describe various health care provider roles in the acute care setting.
4. Evaluate the role of critical thinking in acute care nursing.
5. Compare and contrast the various regulatory bodies associated with acute care nursing.
6. Identify the agencies that evaluate the standards of nursing in the acute care setting.
7. Discuss the importance of Evidence-Based Practice in acute care nursing.
8. Describe the role of values orientation in acute care nursing.
9. Evaluate the effects of capitalism on acute care practice.
10. Discuss contemporary societal influences that are shaping the structure and delivery of health care in the acute care setting.
11. Evaluate current issues in acute care nursing.

# Key Terms

| | | |
|---|---|---|
| acute care | clinical guidelines | managed care |
| advanced practice nurse | critical pathways | |
| care maps | long-term acute care | |

This chapter is about acute care nursing. It is unlikely that a clear consensus definition of "acute care" exists. It can be argued that the definition of acute care depends upon who defines it. Common themes in acute care include such concepts as "time limited" and "hospital care delivery." An accepted definition for acute care is "short-term hospital care provided to clients with conditions of short duration requiring stays of, on average, less than 30 days" (O'Brien-Pallas & Baumann, 2001). Funding and regulatory agency expectations of what should occur in acute care, staffing requirements, the aggregation of specific services, and the skill sets of involved professionals are appropriate indicators for acute care. Acute care is the most expensive of settings in which health care is delivered with regard to the required intensity of labor, sophistication of technology, service delivery, and nursing skill mix. The acute care arena is also at the heart of many current controversies in health care. Acute care is a place of breathtaking advances but also is the site of strife, angst, and controversy, regardless of if the system of care delivery is privately or publicly funded or a combination of the two. Acute care is at the crossroads of where tensions of access, cost containment, and quality intersect.

The right to provide nursing care is a privilege conferred in trust to practitioners by the public. On a daily basis, the acute care nurse fulfills a historic responsibility to care for, and render comfort to, the sick and injured. As such, nurses function at the highest levels to deliver safe and efficient care, and collaborate with others who control the use of resources to deliver efficient, effective, and where possible, evidence-based care. In addition, nursing care is provided from a foundation of compassion. Nurses as citizens also consume, shape, and participate in the reconfiguration of health care services. Nursing possesses a distinctive perspective and opportunity to contribute to the study and reshaping of health care public policy as related to acute care.

## Definition of Acute Care

Acute care is a descriptor for a type of nursing, as well as, more concretely, the place or venue for the delivery of nursing care. It is contrasted with restorative, community, and home arenas of care. The purpose of acute care nursing services is to support the restoration of normal life processes and functions (White & Duncan, 2002). Acute care embraces all age groups from preconception to care of older clients. Acute care also includes the full range of physical and mental alterations that may afflict an individual. The objectives of acute care can be diverse, from saving life, to prolonging it, to palliation of suffering. For example, the care in perioperative cardiovascular surgery, transplant, or multiple trauma is a high intensity activity and calls for a broad range of human skills and sophisticated technological support. The care of premature infants (Figure 20-1) and their families in neonatal intensive care units (NICU) over extended periods of time represents another high-resource, high-intensity environment where the locus of care expands to explicitly involve the family. In contrast, acute care palliative nursing uses medical, surgical, and pharmacological interventions to bring relief to individuals in the last stage of terminal illness or injury. The mix of expertise and technologies in this setting is a different, but no less intense, example of acute care with a greater orientation to skills of spiritual care and pain relief. The variable intensity or complexity of health problems in turn creates a range of demands for resource-intensive settings and skill sets. Acute care nursing requires nurses to care for stable clients with single-system problems that can be met easily with little technological support, and acute care nursing requires nurses to care for physiologically unstable clients with life threatening illnesses or injuries.

The etymology of the word *acute* sheds further light on the business of acute care. By definition, *acute* historically refers to arriving at a crossroad—of "coming sharply to a crisis; severe, not chronic" (Allen, 2000, p. 13). That is, acute problems may appear precipitously, striking a totally unsuspecting victim. Nurses must quickly detect changes in clients in the acute care setting. On the other hand, acute care clients can have problems that arise out of the background of a chronic illness. For

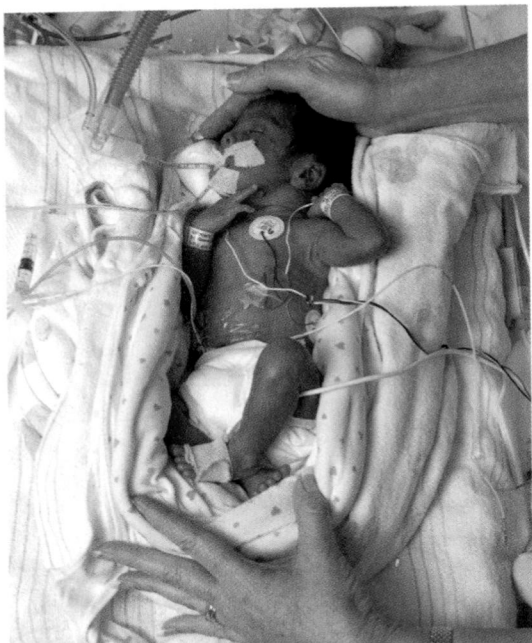

**Figure 20-1** Care for this preterm infant in the neonatal intensive care unit (NICU) requires extensive acute care skills and resources. It is a high-intensity environment in which the client and family receive acute care.

## CLINICAL ALERT

### Detecting Changes in the Acute Care Setting

The nurse must always be aware of changes that are detected in acute care clients. Many times, "warning signals" of physical crises occur prior to the event and the nurse must be aware of those clinical manifestations. For example, clients with diabetes may experience light-headedness, tremors, or diaphoresis just prior to a glycemic complication. The nurse might be able to prevent the diabetic complication if management therapies are implemented as soon as the changes are detected.

example, an acute myocardial infarction (MI) or stroke can cripple an apparently healthy individual without warning, or be the endpoint in a long history of cardiovascular disease. The MI is dramatic, and possibly a defining event in a client with a family history of vasculopathy and a personal history of poorly managed hypertension and smoking (risk factors). In both acute and chronic conditions, the MI represents a dramatic failure of prevention. Similarly, an individual with a history of chronic alcohol abuse, admitted to the intensive care unit (ICU) with acute hepatic failure or torrential gastrointestinal hemorrhage, punctuates a long trajectory of illness with an episode of high acuity.

## The Focus of Acute Care Nursing

The emphasis in acute care may include case finding and disease prevention prior to the appearance of first signs or symptoms (primary prevention). More commonly, however, acute care activities address the challenges of conditions associated with failures of secondary and tertiary prevention. Acute care is aimed at disease detection in a presymptomatic stage (secondary prevention), or preventing complications in clients with symptomatic chronic disease. Although acute care is designed to manage crisis, there is an ever-increasing focus on chronic illness management. Chronic disease care is increasing due to the technological advances and revolutions in disease management that are prolonging life and increasing morbidity, and the demographics that document an aging population. Chronic illness management is the epidemic of the 21st century. It is becoming increasingly evident that isolated management of acute illness episodes without a view to comprehensive disease management is short-sighted and increasingly inadequate for managing chronic disease (Ayanian, Weissman, Schneider, Ginsberg, & Zaslavsky, 2000). Acute care, displaced from its prior

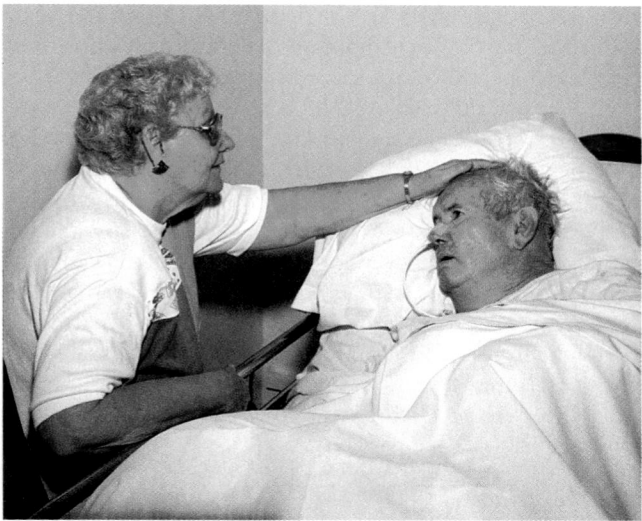

**Figure 20-2    A spouse is visiting her husband in a long-term acute care unit.**

prominence, is now poised at a more dynamic interface with many new participants in care delivery.

## Arenas of Acute Care

Just as the acuity of client conditions varies across a continuum, so, too, do the acute care delivery settings. Acute care venues can be proprietary or not-for-profit, general (e.g., St. Michaels' Hospital, Johns Hopkins, Duke Medical Center) or specialized (University of Texas M. D. Anderson Cancer Center, Midwest Children's Hospital). Becoming more common are **long-term acute care** (LTAC) facilities, which are designed to care for the survivors of acute ICU interventions. These institutions provide specialized acute hospital care for medically complex clients who are critically ill, have multisystem complications and/or failures, and require hospitalization averaging 25 days (Figure 20-2). Acute problems that require hospitalization often require the resources of specialty or tertiary care facilities, and within them, not uncommonly, the intensive care unit. Locale and cost of care are correlated positively with the use of more complex and technologically sophisticated technologies used in diagnosis and management. Nurses who possess familiarity with sophisticated physiological monitoring systems and complex interventions are needed. Thus, costs often parallel acuity and client location. Generally, an "ICU bed"—that is, intensive care setting—is considerably more expensive than a "ward bed" because of the complexity of care involved in the ICU arena. The consumers of acute care bring a range of demands that are met in multilayered environments that provide a different intensity of technological nursing. It should be noted that many systems of health care delivery are placing, within a

single physical environment, different venues of care. Commonly, post-acute rehabilitation or subacute services are linked to traditional acute care settings. These are accredited with reference to different standards by the Commission on Accreditation of Rehabilitation Facilities (CARF) and the Joint Commission on Accreditation of Healthcare Organizations (JCAHO) (Sochalski & Patrician, 1999).

## Providers of Acute Care Nursing

A wide range of nursing personnel, licensed and unlicensed, provide acute care nursing services. They bring to their work a variety of levels of preparation, from formal to informal methods of education and training (see Chapter 2). Providers of acute nursing care include (unlicensed) clinical assistants, nursing assistants, licensed practical (vocational) nurses, and registered nurses with one or more levels (e.g., associate, diploma, baccalaureate, graduate) of preparation. In addition to having a range of basic-level skills, nurses can also be certified or credentialed at an advanced or post-basic level in one or more specialties. This subgroup of practitioners, having received basic licensure to practice, has also usually satisfied additional educational and practice requirements in the form of university courses, continuing education credits, examinations at higher levels, or on-the-job advanced training through staff development departments. Nurses prepared at the master's and doctoral levels also participate in education, management, research, and client care consultation in the acute care setting. Four general categories of **advanced practice nurses** in acute care settings also contribute to nursing care. They include (1) clinical nurse specialists (CNS), (2) nurse practitioners (NP), (3) nurse midwives, and (4) nurse anesthetists. The growth has particularly increased for nurse practitioners, as the demand in the primary care sector has grown. Their practices are statutorily defined by each state, as well as are institutionally characterized. For example, in California, an NP is a "registered nurse who possesses additional preparation and skills in physical diagnosis, psychosocial assessment, and management of health-illness needs in primary health care, and who has been prepared in a program that conforms to board standards as specified in section 1484" (California Code of Regulations, 2001, Article 8, 1480, Definitions). The growth of new categories of personnel participating in direct client care and the emergence of clinical specialists and nurse practitioners have magnified the complexity of care delivery in acute care.

## The Importance of Critical Thinking in Acute Care Nursing

Familiarity with and the ability to use the nursing process is a necessary but not sufficient prerequisite for the delivery of acute care nursing. Nurses must not only acquire the ability to think critically, but also master the facts and concepts concerning the common problems that they encounter. That is, the nursing process is useful only when it is used with the general and specific content knowledge areas referable to specific acute problems. This body of knowledge consists of the content of nursing science, as well as of the foundation sciences of nursing: biomedical, pharmacological, sociological, psychological, and cultural and spiritual bodies of knowledge. The scientific foundations of acute care nursing can be seen as derivative, to the degree that many of the concepts and interventions flow from organized bodies of more traditional basic and applied sciences. The content of the discipline and the nursing process are applied against a tapestry of ethical expectations (see Box 20-1); acute care nursing is delivered within a macro environment involving employers, regulatory agencies, consumer groups, and government bodies. Even the philosophies of sponsoring bodies affect the quality and scope of acute care services offered to clients. For example, in networks sponsored by the Catholic faith, specific reproductive health policies limit service provision to women of childbearing age. The acute care nurse is challenged to apply principles of critical decision making in this complex environment (Figure 20-3).

## Aggregates of Clients in Acute Care

The organization of modern acute care nursing is increasingly marked by attempts to match the needs of the client to the skill sets of the nurses and other providers. In some centers, often depending upon the resources available and the size and complexity of specific populations, the trend is to physically aggregate clients with common problems

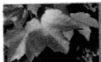

## RESEARCH FOCUS

**Title of Study:** Clinical decision-making process in perioperative nursing

**Study Purpose:** The purpose of this phenomenological study was to reveal the processes of clinical decision making by expert perioperative nurses.

**Methods:** Six expert nurses from five different hospitals in a large Southern metropolitan area participated in the study. Expert nurses were defined as having worked a minimum of 5 years and considered themselves to be expert circulating nurses in the operating room. Based on an interview guide, the participants were asked to describe any perioperative clinical situations in which they intervened on the client's behalf and affected the client's outcome by doing so. The interviews were transcribed verbatim; data were loaded into a software program to be categorized, sorted, and managed.

**Findings:** The predominant pattern contributing to the clinical decision-making process among the expert nurses was "seeing the big picture: engendered through caring." Multiple decisions were identified within each nurse's practice, and within each decision, certain characteristics were identified and categorized into themes. Data analysis identified three themes as requisite for expert clinical decision making: connecting with clients, advocating for clients, and embodied knowing.

**Implications:** This study demonstrates that positive client outcomes depend on the ability of the perioperative nurse to integrate all nursing knowledge, make rapid decisions, and constantly advocate for the client. These data also suggest that nurses and nursing students would both benefit if personal care experiences were shared so that the knowledge of clinical practice that was taken for granted could be examined, and caring practices could be made explicit.

Parker, C., Minick, P., & Kee, C. (1999). Clinical decision-making process in perioperative nursing. *AORN Journal, 70*(1), 45–62.

in units staffed by specially trained nurses (e.g., myocardial infarction clients in a coronary care unit, cancer clients in an oncology unit).

It is clear that the basic and applied sciences that form part of the foundation of acute care nursing are growing exponentially. Scientific knowledge is exploding and the technologies burgeoning. Time from discovery to application is shortening, whereas specialization in acute care is growing. In many acute care settings, nurses no longer

## BOX 20-1    ETHICAL CONCEPTS DEFINED FOR NURSING SERVICE

We are called to:

- Service of the poor—Generosity of spirit, especially for persons most in need

- Reverence—Respect and compassion for the dignity and diversity of life.

- Integrity—Inspiring trust through personal leadership

- Wisdom—Integrating excellence and stewardship.

- Creativity—Courageous innovation

- Dedication—Affirming the hope and joy of our ministry

Available: http://www.Ascensionhealth.org

---

have the opportunity to engage in generalist practice. Even so-called general medical-surgical units care for aggregated specialty populations with special needs. How has acute care nursing remained current with the growth of knowledge, basic and applied, that is shaping and reshaping the delivery of care? In large measure, acute care nurses have done so by becoming familiar with the state of the sciences relevant to their practice arenas.

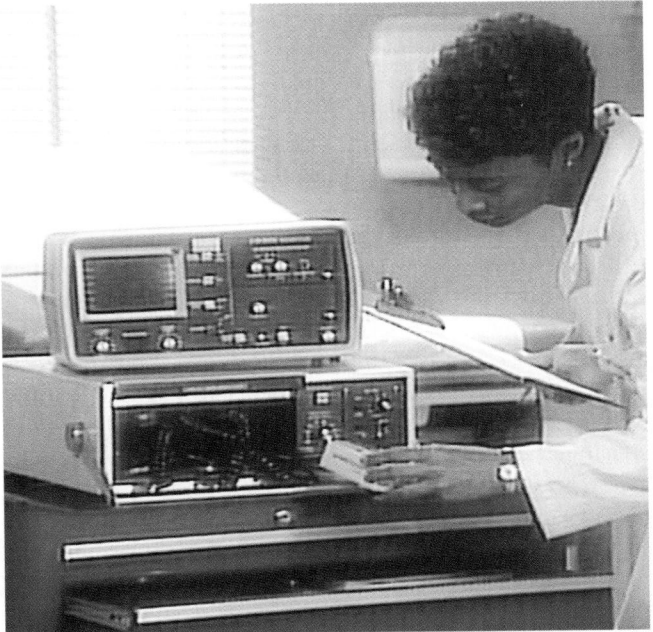

**Figure 20-3    A nurse making critical decisions when working with a "crash cart"**

# Regulatory Organizations for Acute Care Nursing Practice

Nurses have long recognized an ethical duty to maintain their competency in the face of scientific advancements (ICN Code of Ethics, 2000, p. 3). Nursing professional organizations worldwide have responded to the growth of the foundation sciences by certifying specialty content expertise that reflect and complement the medical specialty growth. For example, the American Nurses Association (ANA) recognizes numerous specialty organizations; the Canadian Nurses Association (CNA) recognizes and oversees certification examinations in 10 specialties. Many of those specialty organizations have developed specialty-specific core curricula, which summarize the scientific basis of their specialty practice (e.g., *Core Curriculum for Neonatal Intensive Care Nursing*, 2nd ed., 1999; *Core Curriculum for Oncology Nursing*, 3rd ed., 1998). One of the best known and most widely used specialty organizations in acute care is the *Core Curriculum for Critical Care Nursing* by the American Association of Critical Care Nurses (AACN). The value of a curriculum and related documents can extend far beyond just being educational. Notable in this regard is the output of the Intravenous Nurses Society (INS). The recent *Policies and Procedures for Infusion Nursing*, published by the INS Clinical Practice Committee, can serve as the definitive policy and procedure reference for infusion practice nationally, if not internationally. It is consistent with the Infusion Nursing Standards of Practice, also recently revised. It provides the opportunity for facilities that lack local resources to design practice and deliver care at the national standard. Other acute care nursing specialty groups are also developing specialized content summaries that capture their specialty practice areas, and are developing or have in place mechanisms for periodic updating and review. For example, the American Association of Neuroscience Nurses (AANN) has published and revised over time a number of guidelines. Consistent with and complementary to the literature on ischemic stroke is the *AANN Clinical Guideline Series Document*, which provides recommendations for nursing management of stroke clients (Beers & Berkow, 2000). More circumscribed guidelines include documents outlining seizure assessment, and technologically oriented documents addressed intracranial pressure monitoring and lumbar drain management. These guidelines seek to standardize care, reduce practice variation, and simultaneously reflect the highest standards of neuroscience nursing practice.

## Allied Disciplines and Acute Care Nursing

Nursing specialization is enriched by the parallel and complementary evolution of the allied disciplines. Using stroke or neurological care as an example, occupational and physical therapists can both sit for specialty certification: The

American Occupational Therapy Association (AOTA) offers board certification in neurorehabilitation, and the American Physical Therapy Association (APTA) offers specialist certification in neurology. In addition, medical technologists are responsible for the laboratory diagnostics that augment the information necessary for acute care clients. These and other disciplines work side by side to enrich the nursing care of specific populations across all venues of care.

In the past two decades, many medical specialty organizations have codified the scientific bases of their practice. That is, many societies have developed **clinical guidelines** regarding specific areas of specialty practice. These can be defined as "consensus statements that are systematically developed to assist practitioners in making [client] management decisions related to special clinical circumstances" (Every, Hochman, Becker, Kopecky, & Cannon, 2000, p. 1). Across specialties, the consensus statements, or the position papers, and their accompanying technical reviews are often available free of charge to interested readers. Regardless of individual physical proximity to a major academic medical center, libraries, or experts, summary or state-of-the science documents are accessible. These documents, which review the empirical bases of practice, are not intended to be narrowly prescriptive. They—along with ethical, intuitive, and aesthetic factors—are to be considered the "art" of the specialty.

## Regulatory Agencies for Cardiovascular Clients in Acute Care

Notable for the maturity and scope of its efforts is the American Heart Association (American Heart Association, 2003). Not only has it codified the science around the management of myocardial ischemia/infarction and congestive heart failure, as well as numerous other cardiovascular health topics, but it has also addressed the topic of cerebrovascular disease. The Stroke Council of the AHA has developed a body of literature over the past 10 years related to the management of ischemic and hemorrhagic strokes. The individual documents not only summarize the science upon which that practice is based, but evaluate the quality of the evidence and the strength of the recommendations found within. It has revised and updated the guidelines to reflect growth in the understanding, and as such, is an invaluable repository for every clinician who cares for the client with ischemic stroke. These documents are available in Web-based format (see Box 20-2).

## Standards for Care in Acute Care Nursing

Clinical guidelines have also served as valuable resources for establishing standards in acute care for both clients and professionals. The standards in turn have helped to

---

> ### BOX 20-2    SELECTED AMERICAN HEART ASSOCIATION GUIDELINE TOPICS (ON THE WEB) RELATED TO ISCHEMIC STROKE
>
> - ACC/AHA guidelines for the clinical application of echocardiography (1997)
> - Supplement to the guidelines for the management of transient ischemic attacks (1999)
> - Practice guidelines for the use of imaging in transient ischemic attacks and acute stroke (1997)
> - Guidelines for thrombolytic therapy for acute stroke; a supplement to the guidelines for the management of patients with acute ischemic stroke (1996)
> - Guidelines for the management of patients with acute ischemic stroke (1996)
>
> American Heart Association, 2003; Available: History of AHA, http://americanheart.org

---

create explicit expectations for providers and clients. Guidelines are also being used to develop different instruments that streamline and rationalize care planning, resource allocation, and program marketing, and facilitate cooperation across communities in the delivery of care for individuals with stroke. For example, nurses and others have used the documents to develop flow sheets (Figure 20-4), physician order sets, outcome systems, care plans, and databases specific to specific acute care populations. All of the instruments or tools are designed to streamline, organize, and elevate the quality of practice. Clinical guidelines have lent scientific rigor to common diagnoses with well-developed scientific understanding.

**Care maps** (Figure 20-5), also referred to as clinical or critical pathways, have grown in popularity as another means of reducing variations in care, reducing resource utilization, and improving client outcomes. Anchored in the relevant clinical guidelines or summary documents, **critical pathways** are defined as instruments or tools that "detail processes of care and highlight inefficiencies regardless of whether there is evidence to warrant changes in those processes" (Every et al., 2000, p. 1). Nurses are sharing these instruments across organizational boundaries, and different specialty organizations have made compilations available free of charge to interested parties. At this time, unfortunately, their explosive growth has not been matched by rigor in evaluation (Every et al., 2000, p. 2). In addition, one outcome of organized care is better client education. One type of client education material is material available on the Internet.

**THROMBOLYTIC THERAPY FOR
ACUTE STROKE PROTOCOL**

White - Medical Records
Yellow - Outcomes Based Care Mangement

| History: Time of stroke onset must be determined precisely to consider t-PA. | | | | | | | |
|---|---|---|---|---|---|---|---|
| | Age (18-77) | | Stroke Onset: Date | | ED Arrival: Date | | Transport to ED |
| | Sex | | Stroke Onset: Time | | ED Arrival: Time | | Weight: |

| Inclusion Criteria by History: Both must be "YES" to consider t-PA. | YES | NO |
|---|---|---|
| Is the initial clinical impression "Acute Ischemic Stroke?" (Language abnormality, focal neurological deficit/motor abnormality, facial droop) | | |
| Can evaluation be completed and treatment begun within 3 hours of stroke onset? NOTE: Tests take 1 hr. | | |

☐ **Call attending physician and neurologist**  ☐ **Alert Lab**  ☐ **Establish 2 peripheral IV lines**
☐ **Alert CT of potential stat CT Head**  (Coag Dept. x2232)  ☐ **O₂ 2L per nasal cannula or** _____

| Exclusion Criteria by History: All must be "NO" to consider t-PA | Time M.D. Assessment: | YES | NO |
|---|---|---|---|
| Illness/treatment predisposing to an increased risk of bleeding. | | | |
| Ongoing anticoagulant therapy (Heparin, Coumadin, etc.) See back for anticoagulant reference. | | | |
| Known brain tumor, arteriovenous (arteriovascular) malformation or aneurysm. | | | |
| Prior stroke or traumatic brain injury in the previous 3 months. | | | |
| Major surgery or serious trauma within the preceding 14 days. | | | |
| GI or GU bleeding in past 3 weeks. | | | |
| Recent MI or post MI pericarditis. | | | |
| Seizure at stroke onset. | | | |
| Pregnancy. | | | |
| Lumbar puncture or arterial puncture in past week. | | | |
| History of intracranial hemorrhage. | | | |
| NIH Stroke Scale Score greater than **22 or** any one or more of the following exist: ☐ Stupor  ☐ Flaccid hemiplegia  ☐ NIH Score _____  ☐ Gaze deviation  ☐ Severe global aphasia  (use of scale optional) | | | |

| Inclusion and Exclusion Criteria all met → stat evaluation for t-PA treatment. | |
|---|---|
| 1. Obtain stat: CT (non-contrast) | Time Ordered: |
| 2. Obtain stat - CBC c̄ platelets, electrolytes, BUN, blood glucose, creatinine, PTT, INR, type/screen | |
| 3. Obtain stat: 12 lead EKG. | |
| 4. Alert Pharmacy of potential candidate t-PA for CVA. | |

| Inclusion Criteria by Exam: Both must be "YES" before using t-PA. | Baseline BP: | YES | NO |
|---|---|---|---|
| Pre-t-PA therapy BP <185/110* (See Physician Order Set for optional BP treatment algorithm). | | | |
| Measurable and significant neurologic deficit. | | | |

| Exclusion Criteria by Exam: t-PA contraindicated if any "YES". | YES | NO |
|---|---|---|
| Active bleeding. | | |
| Sustained BP >185/110 after medication to reduce. | | |
| Rapidly improving neurological signs or isolated mild neurological deficits. | | |

| Exclusion Criteria by Lab and/or CT results: t-PA contraindicated if any "YES". | YES | NO |
|---|---|---|
| Glucose <50 or >400mg%. | | |
| Platelet count <100,000/mm³ | | |
| INR greater than 1.7, elevated PTT (greater than upper limit of normal for lab) | | |
| CT scan indicates hemorrhage or onset >3 hours (cerebral edema) or any major structural abnormality. | | |
| Time CT Read: | Time Decision to Treat: | |

| Risks benefits, alternatives and complications explained to patient related to procedure. | |
|---|---|
| If all criteria met and informed consent obtained, proceed with t-PA protocol for stroke. | |

| Neurology Consulted Time: | Dr.: | Total t-PA Dose: | Time Started: |
|---|---|---|---|

Triage RN _____  RN _____  Physician _____

St JOSEPH'S
HOSPITAL
5000 W. Chambers St. · Milwaukee, WI 53210-1688
A MEMBER OF *Covenant* HEALTHCARE
St. Joseph's Hospital is Sponsored by the Wheaton Franciscan-Sisters

THROMBOLYTIC THERAPY FOR
ACUTE STROKE PROTOCOL

PATIENT LABELS MUST BE PLACED HERE ON ALL
PAGES (PARTS) - SIDES - OR FOLD-OUT (PANELS) THAT
THIS BOX APPEARS ON.

Form 51864 10/98 ©1998

**Figure 20-4** St. Joseph's flow sheet used in the diagnostics and treatment for thrombolytic therapy for stroke clients. *Courtesy of St. Joseph's Regional Medical Center*

ST. JOSEPH'S HOSPITAL
E.D. DIAGNOSTIC & TREATMENT PROCESS FOR THROMBOLYTIC THERAPY FOR STROKE PATIENTS

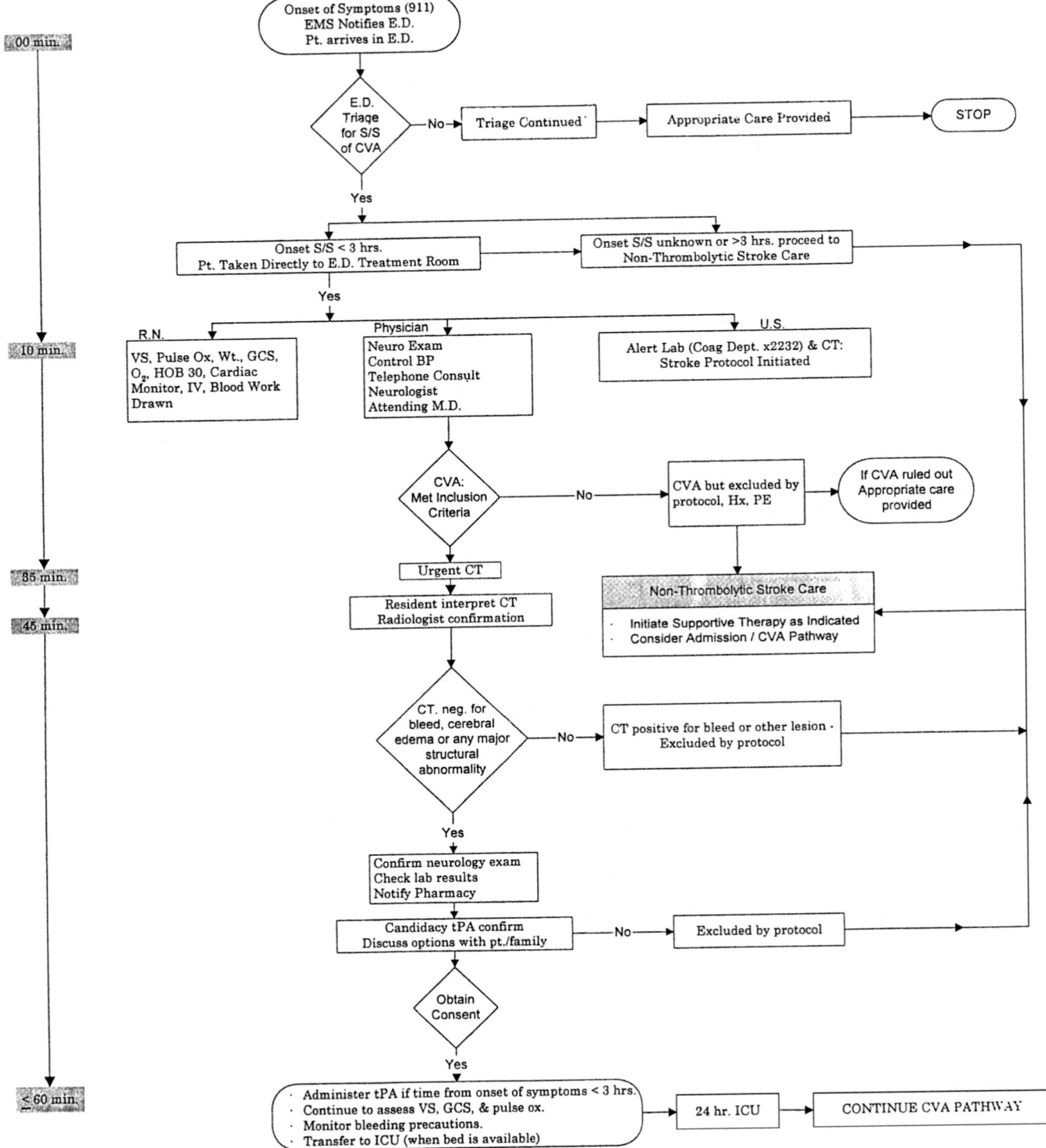

**Figure 20-5**    An example of a care map used for acute stroke protocol by St. Joseph's Hospital. *Courtesy of St. Joseph's Regional Medical Center*

## Evaluation of Acute Care Nursing

In response to the profusion of studies, and expansion and sophistication of the literature, a variety of organizations have emerged with mandates to systematically review topics of interest to acute care providers and other clinicians. These resources for critically examining and summarizing evidence are growing in number, with sophisticated information system infrastructures and analytical resources at their command. For example, the Agency of Healthcare Research and Quality (AHRQ, 2003), formerly the Agency for Health Care Policy and Research (AHCPR), is an agency of the federal government's Department of Health and Human Services and creatively addresses the relationships among care delivery, cost, and clinical outcomes. When the questions that arise out of daily clinical practice turn to outcomes and effectiveness, the interested party can access its services and resources. For example, the National Guideline Clearinghouse™ is a vast database of evidence-based clinical practice guidelines and their supporting documents. Nongovernmental agencies are also participating in information management. The Cochrane Collaboration (2001) produces reviews that are collated in the Cochrane Database of Systematic Reviews. These documents are the products of international expert review groups, which provide systematic, up-to-date reviews of all relevant randomized clinical trials (RCT) of health care. The Cochrane Injuries Group has posted 11 reviews related to the management of severe brain injury; they complement the Brain Trauma Foundation (BTF) guidelines. Informal national and local networks are also emerging for health care workers to share experiences and successes.

---

### CLIENT EDUCATION

#### Teaching Materials for Client Education on the Internet

Client education can consist of such things as:

1. References from national organizations (e.g., American Cancer Society, www.cancer.org; American Heart Association, http://www.americanheart.org)
2. Audio/visual aids developed for particular teaching needs, such as nutritional suggestions from the American Diabetic Association, http://www.diabetes.org
3. Health promotion and wellness materials from federal organizations, such as the Department of the Army's health promotion and wellness website, http://chppm-www.apgea.army.mil

---

For example, a "Best Practice Network" offers a forum for health care professionals to share ideas, collaborate, exchange ideas, and share best practice. Original participants had a strong representation from nursing.

## Quality Control Agencies for Acute Care

The acute care environment is an ever changing, complex arena of client care. Consequently, evaluation and quality control of the delivery of acute care is essential. A variety of agencies (i.e., hospitals, JCAHO, federal agencies) provide quality control in acute care settings and are addressed in this section.

### Hospitals

The hospital is the primary agency in acute care, and very specific agencies are responsible for quality control. For example, hospitals answer for safety to the Occupational Safety and Health Administration (OSHA); for laboratory quality to Clinical Laboratory Improvement Amendments (CLIA). Practice and billing/accounting structures are carefully scrutinized and can be audited by granting agencies (Centers for Medicare and Medicaid Services [CMS]), managed care organizations, and internal quality committees. Hospitals establish processes designed to identify and resolve problems and track outcomes. Hospital sector management is generally costly and rigid. Hospitals are increasingly stressed financially in providing even emergency services. Unionized settings add yet another layer of complexity. Individual classes of practitioners are held to their professional and ethical standards within this venue of care.

### Joint Commission on Accreditation of Healthcare Organizations (JCAHO)

Perhaps the best-known bureaucracy that impacts the acute care setting and day-to-day practice of acute care nursing is the Joint Commission on Accreditation of Healthcare Organizations (JCAHO) (see Chapter 2). Its mission is to "continuously improve the safety and quality of care provided to the public" (JCAHO, 2001). JCAHO operates nationwide, and through common standards and regular on-site visits, attempts to ensure high standards of care. It has been a strong voice in the movement to quality in health care. In 1986 JCAHO defined quality assurance as a "planned, systematic process for monitoring and evaluating the appropriateness of care, evaluating the quality of service, and resolving existing problems." JCAHO's role is also educational and supportive; in 1997, it integrated outcomes and other performance measures into the process of accreditation. This mission is complementary not only to the mission of all professional groups, including nursing, but to consumers as well.

## Federal Agencies

The federal government has organized an approach to combat provider and user fraud in the National Committee for Quality Assurance (NCQA). Where internal self-regulatory mechanisms have failed to address public concerns regarding safety and quality, state and federal resources have been created to assist the consumer seeking redress if mistreated, and adjudicate treatment decisions, such as denials of care. For example, some states have appointed ombudsmen to oversee complaints. The California Department of Managed Health Care, the first-in-the-nation consumer rights project, was implemented to help Californians resolve problems with HMOs as well as ensure a better, more solvent, and stable managed health care system. Massachusetts has an Ombudsman for the Managed Care consumer advisory board. There has been a growing political participation of invested consumers to ensure that their voices are heard on fund allocation and public policy (Kohn, Corrigan, & Donaldson, 1999). For example, organizations such as the Center for Responsive Politics, a nonprofit research group that tracks the flow and influence of money in politics, publishes papers relevant to health care issues (e.g., *Managed Care*). A Patient Bill of Rights was adopted by the AHA in 1973, with member hospitals encouraged to modify and adapt to better serve their clients. Lobbyists are numerous, representing every interest. For example, groups may be demographically defined (e.g., AARP), disease-related (e.g., American Parkinson's Disease Association), or more directly tied to specific industries (e.g., pharmaceutical).

## Institute of Medicine of the National Academy of Sciences

Acute care is a setting where the acuity is rising and where multiple caregivers struggle under extraordinary pressures to cut cost and control financial outcomes. Consequently, mistakes are made and errors in acute care are costly in human terms. Mistakes can result in death and dismemberment in extreme circumstances. Perhaps the most influential document to energize current thinking about safety is the recent report *To Err Is Human* (Kohn et al., 1999). A product of the Institute of Medicine of the National Academy of Sciences, which was formed to advise the government on scientific and technical matters, the report focuses on the improvement of client safety. It discusses error incidence, detection, analysis, and prevention and recommends a four-tiered approach to improve safety in health care.

## Evidence-Based Practice in Acute Care Nursing

In the face of ever changing and ever more complexity in the empiric foundations of acute care health delivery, every clinician finds it difficult to remain current with the science and art of his or her specialty. A movement that is growing to meet the need is Evidence-Based Practice, which requires close collaboration among information technology experts, clinicians, researchers, and policy makers (see Chapter 6). Its recent popularity in acute care settings has arisen from four pressing realities: 1) the need for rapidly available, valid information; 2) the realization that traditional sources may be limited, wrong, or hard to access; 3) that great disparity across knowledge and clinical judgment; and 4) the personal time required to update is shrinking proportional to the growth of knowledge. Evidence-Based Practice is conscientious, explicit, and judicious use of current best evidence in making decisions about the care of individual clients, and there is growing evidence that this can be accomplished on the front line of client care by busy clinicians who devote their scarce reading time to selective, efficient, client-driven searching, appraisal, and incorporation of the best available evidence (Goldman, Ganju, Drake, Gorman, Hogan, Hyde, & Morgan, 2001).

## Outcomes Research in Acute Care Practice

In addition, a quality practice must also involve measured outcomes (see Chapter 13). The range of outcomes available in the acute care setting is as diverse as the interests of participants in acute care, including consumers, practitioners, policy makers, and corporate interests. The range of the outcomes is as diverse as the client problems and the care delivery bureaucracies that they concern. By linking care delivery with the outcomes achieved, outcomes research has become a powerful means of monitoring and improving the quality of care in the acute care setting.

> Outcomes are the outputs or results of the program or the activities of the provider . . . Process/outcome evaluation is a decision-making process by which one examines the manner in which a program or provider delivers services or their outputs and makes judgments about what is done or how well objectives are met. Evaluation of . . . outcomes can be expected to lead to suggestions for action to improve effectiveness and efficiency. (Waltz, Strickland, & Lenz, 1991, p. 438–439.)

The Clinical Value compass is one of many models that propose a range of outcomes that must be addressed in the quest to improve quality of acute care (Nelson, Mohr, Batalden, & Plume, 1996). The outcomes can be diagrammed as four points of a directional compass, and include 1) functional status, risk status, and well-being; 2) costs; 3) satisfaction with health care and perceived benefit; and 4) clinical outcomes. In any given circumstance, the selection of particular outcomes reflects professional, economic, and societal values and priorities. Given the range, and the temptation to sample from all domains, "outcomes selected must be meaningful and salient to the focus of the investigation" (Waltz et al., 1991, p. 441).

## Mastery of Knowledge in Acute Care Nursing

Mastery of a broad knowledge base is a necessity for every acute care nurse. One recent client assignment on a busy medical-surgical unit shared by one nurse and one clinical assistant included the following clients: A 38-year-old unilingual Cambodian female awaiting surgery for an arteriovenous malformation in the brain; a 49-year-old black male with severe pancreatitis, receiving total parental nutrition (TPN) through a peripherally inserted central line (PICC) and medicated using a system of patient controlled analgesia (PCA); a 78-year-old white female with large dominant hemisphere stroke, and problems with swallowing, language, and mobility; and a 79-year-old gentleman recovering from a gastrointestinal hemorrhage linked to aspirin use. The knowledge base required to manage this small group encompassed a wide range of pathologies, all with different laboratory and radiological correlates. For example, the pharmacological management alone requires familiarity with multiple drug classes, as well as agents available to manage possible treatment complications (e.g., Narcan for overmedication with narcotics). It also clearly demanded a broad range of assessment skills related to every body system, as well as familiarity with cultural and age-related concepts. The prescribed medical treatments in turn created the demand that caregivers be familiar with common diagnostic and complication-related signs and symptoms (e.g., aspiration risk in acute stroke). The range of interventions was related to communication, dietary management and feeding, hygiene, pain management and positioning, as well as psychosocial support (e.g., related to the experience of uncertainty and fear). Technical demands included a facility with infusion devices, including those used for opiate and TPN administration, maintenance of infusion catheters, including PICC and peripheral lines, nasogastric tubes, indwelling bladder catheters, and splint care. Effective and efficient client management also required extensive communication within the nurse–clini-

### STOP AND THINK

**Where Does the Novice Turn for Knowledge?**

- Where would you go to learn about the pathologies of the disorders listed above?

- Who could you ask for information regarding diseases and treatments about which you lack knowledge?

- What would you say to a client when you are asked a question related to a disease and you do not have knowledge about that specific disease?

cal assistant dyad, as well as collaboration with representatives from multiple disciplines, including pharmacists, therapists, and an interpreter. The case mix may seem atypical. However, the level of acuity within acute care has risen dramatically, as many services have relocated to less expensive venues, such as clinics, laboratories, and outpatient procedure settings. That is, less acutely ill clients who were formerly admitted to in-patient venues are being served elsewhere, leaving only the sickest clients behind.

## Value Orientation and Acute Care Nursing

The arena of acute care nursing is replete with difficult ethical dilemmas and thus value orientation is an essential

### CLIENT REFLECTIONS

**Medication Use**

Mr. Clark is discussing with his acute care nurse his concerns regarding his medications. Mr. Clark states, "My doctor prescribed so many medications that I don't know what they all do. I have medications for my high blood pressure, high cholesterol, arthritis, and allergies. I am worried that they don't work well together or that one medication reacts with some of my other medications."

What would you say to Mr. Clark, and what resources would you use to answer Mr. Clark?

### LEGAL AND ETHICAL ISSUES

**Ethical Dilemmas in Acute Care**

Every acute care nurse has seen physiological function prolonged at the expense of quality of life. The tension between distributive and utilitarian perspectives is real, and confronts the health care system more and more frequently. On any given day, a nurse may also confront multiple dilemmas, arising from the relative superiority of individual over community or aggregate interest. With an increasingly tight supply of beds and other resources, nurses are being trained to participate in discussions and justify their decisions that allocate resources.

Burkhardt, M., & Nathaniel, A. (2002). *Ethics & issues in contemporary nursing* (2nd ed.). Clifton Park, NY: Delmar Learning.

## STOP AND THINK

### Values and Resource Utilization in Acute Care

- Does a society and a health care profession accept in specific circumstances a higher mortality for lower morbidity?

- How does our health care system make decisions about who gets health care?

- Do we expend resources on those most likely to recover and contribute to the public life, or salvage the most injured or diseased with the least probability of survival?

- Should resources be redirected from high technology, high-cost heroic "last ditch" interventions to primary prevention and disease management?

- Do we ask the wealthy to pay proportionally more for health care?

component to consider. The questions that arise in the acute care arena may be difficult to solve and are powerful in nature. Discussions about what ought to be valued, and how resource expenditure decisions are complex yet necessary, are important conversations in acute care. In addition, acute care nursing has many difficult ethical dilemmas. Every decision is accompanied by potentially serious consequences: people may die sooner than they might otherwise; clients may be exposed to undue risk and possible harm, and nurses and others may be liable when client needs are not matched to the appropriate skill level in a particular environment. More and more commonly, nurses find themselves accountable for justifying the promotion of one good over the other and for articulating justifiable reasons for limiting the provision of good in specific situations.

## Capitalism and Acute Care Nursing

The effect of capitalism on the acute care portion of the gross national product in the U.S. economy is mammoth. In the United States between 1970 and 1995, expenditures exploded from 73.2 to 988.5 billion dollars, reflecting an increase from 7.1% to 13.6% of the economy devoted to health care. Public sector (federal, state, and local) contributions increased during the same time period from 37.8% to 46.2%, reflecting increases in Medicare, Medicaid, and other spending (Sochalski & Patrician, 1999). The largest health care system in the United States is the federally owned and operated Veterans Health Administration of the Department of Veterans Affairs.

Research and development costs in the acute care setting are staggering, the regulatory maze is daunting, and the money to be made and lost is almost incalculable. Technology is exploding and is driven by advances in such areas as diagnostic testing (Figure 20-6), genetic sciences, and other basic sciences. New sophistication and increasing cost pressures are leading to relocation of specially trained clinicians and many diagnostic and therapeutic interventions to out-of-hospital settings (Blatchford, 2001). New pharmaceuticals are not only revolutionizing disease management, allowing control of numerous chronic illnesses (e.g., heart disease, AIDS), but are doing so at a price unimaginable 20 years ago. Computerization and information technology are transforming systems of care delivery, such as diagnostics, scheduling, billing, budgeting, disease surveillance, and outcome tracking. Within the health care sector, different interests compete for finite resources as well. Drug manufacturers, citizen coalitions, and managed care organizations may all be motivated by competing interests. The hospital sector is represented by the American Hospital Association (AHA), which is dedicated to a mission of leadership in public policy, representation and advocacy, and services.

## Philosophy of Capitalism and Health Care

Whereas Canada and many Western European nations have a public policy of universal access, the United States does not. This fact suggests that the American value orientation may be substantively different. De Tocqueville's mid-19th-century journey through America produced his book *Democracy in America* (2002), which describes an outsider's view of "typical" U.S. values: the society was perceived as individualist, egalitarian, decentralized, religious, and materialistic, with an antigovernment distrust or bias.

These seminal values tend to celebrate individual over aggregate good, pay less heed to the reality of resource scarcity and the inevitability of mortality, and celebrate the

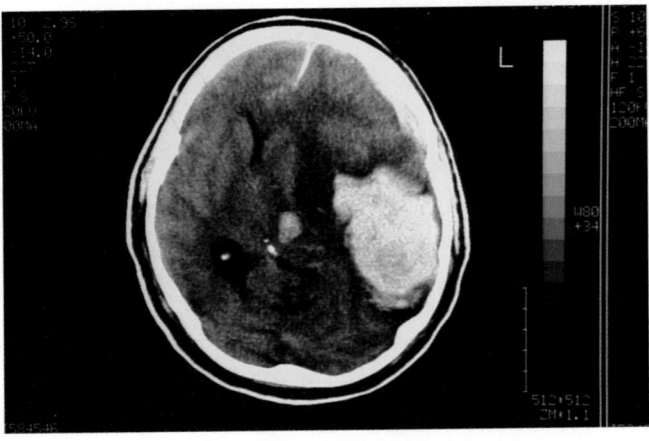

**Figure 20-6    Diagnostic advances like this CT scan of a subdural hematoma have greatly changed the management of critical clients in the acute care setting.**

expectation of a "quick fix." The legislative output affirms the importance of personal freedoms. For the most part, American health care is considered and treated more as a market commodity to be bought and sold rather than a right. And health care, particularly acute care, is only one of many competing economic or market sectors and is engaged in a continuous battle with competing initiatives (e.g., defense, education, environment, homeland security, infrastructure development). Like all those competing interests, there is infinite demand for finite resources.

## Managed Care Concepts in Acute Care

**Managed care** can be defined as health care financing and delivery arrangement designed to provide appropriate, effective, and efficient health care through organized relationships with health care providers. Physicians feel some enmity toward managed care, which has been seen, and continues to be by many, as a direct challenge to client and provider autonomy, infringing on the doctor-client relationship, and freedom to make a profit.

Physician and nursing groups, trial and malpractice litigators, legislators from both sides of the aisle, lobbyists, and others also bring vested interests to health care policy decision making. The complexity is staggering and in turn elicits responses. Nurses have formed the American Association of Managed Care Nurses (AAMCN), a nonprofit organization whose mission is to be recognized as the "expert and resource in managed care nursing." Cross competition is often fierce. For example, in response to the growth of managed care, a physician-owned-and-operated management company was formed to provide managed care management services to the specialty physician community, as well as needed systems and management to handle managed care effectively. Ironically, groups that may appear to be working at cross-purposes are often complementary and philosophically synergistic. For example, as sound business practice, managed care organizations track outcomes and tangibly reward improved outcomes (clinical and cost) with business. Many managed care institutions are strong allies with any and every group interested in quality health care. These managed care organizations demand that acute care service providers develop systems for tracking outcomes to improve their efficiencies.

## Social Issues Influencing Acute Care Nursing

The acute care setting exists within the larger society and the health care delivery system. This means that many societal issues impact acute care nursing. Examples of social issues currently affecting acute care nursing are human genome mapping, aging trends, and the third-party payment systems of insurance. Culture and ethnicity also heavily influence acute care nursing and are addressed in Chapter 5.

## Human Genome Mapping and Acute Care Nursing

Acute care will also be greatly affected by what is probably the best example of dynamism in health care—the ever growing impact of the mapping of the human genome. The Human Genome Project (HGP), cosponsored by the U.S. Department of Energy (DOE) and the National Institutes of Health (NIH), will likely stand as the seminal event in 21st-century medicine. Sequencing of the DNA in the human genome is shifting the focus of diagnostics and therapeutics to genetic and molecular levels. Along the way, it is generating a spate of new technologies, which carry important and far-reaching social implications. The National Human Genome Research Institute (NHGRI), which administers the HGP for the NIH, allocates 5% of the budget to ethical, legal, and social implications (Human Genome Research, 2001). Fundamental issues to be addressed include how the knowledge affects the acutely ill, and whether insurance will cover illness in the acute care setting if a "predisposition" for a particular disease is discovered.

## Aging and Acute Care

The growing number of older clients has tremendous consequences for acute care nursing. The need for and value of formal training that equips acute care practitioners to address salient issues dominating geriatric care, such as pharmacological principles and managing dementia and associated behavioral problems, are obvious (Panneton, 1998) (see Chapter 19). There is even a national institute for aging that has materials specific to caring for the aged. The generational shift is also catalyzing discussions about the appropriate use of technology and other health care resources, as well as legitimizing discussion about setting limits and other sensitive issues. Every acute care nurse who admits an older individual with a functionally devastating event, such as severe stroke, confronts this problem directly or indirectly. Every acute care nurse has consoled and advised a family regarding life-transforming treatment and resuscitation decisions. Not infrequently, it is the acute care nurse who provides the support and guidance to do so with equanimity, due deliberation, and sensitivity.

## Insurance and Acute Care

The lack of insurance ultimately causes many persons to require acute care. The number of uninsured persons, often the working poor, is significant and has been growing since the late 1980s. The number of uninsured, nonelderly individuals increased from 17.3% to 18.4% (by 4.2 million) between 1994 and 1998. The increase has been largely attributed to reductions in Medicaid and other public and private coverage (Holahan & Kim, 2000). The U.S. Census Bureau estimated in 2001 that 42.6 million Americans lack health insurance. The Health Insurance Association of America estimated the number at 43.5 million in 1998, and projected an increase of 10

## LIFE SPAN CONSIDERATIONS

### Neurological Assessment of the Acutely Ill Older Client

The neurological assessment of the acutely ill geriatric client is complex. Possible influences include the impact of underlying dementia or depression, with or without an overlying delirium attributable to the proximate cause of the acute illness. Focal neurological findings attributable to common neurological diseases of the elderly, including stroke or Parkinson's disease, may coexist. The nursing assessment must include a careful history, with attention to preadmission functional, behavioral, and socioemotional status. The mental status exam, with emphasis on attention, clarity of thinking, and psychomotor function, is often the key to recognizing delirium; the remainder of the neurological exam—cranial nerve, sensorimotor, and cerebellar assessments—may reveal focal deficits that suggest a discrete insult.

Adapted from Estes, M. (2002). *Health assessment & physical examination* (2nd ed.). Clifton Park, NY: Delmar Learning.

million by 2007. Additionally, a growing number of individuals may be losing traditional sources of access to care, notably doctors' offices (Moy, Bartman, Clancy, & Cornelius, 1998). The fact is that clients with identified risk factors for debilitating disease who cannot afford to see a health care provider often lack preventive services, which would be far less expensive to provide than the expensive emergency acute care services. The uninsured often experience major decompensation as a result of lack of attention to what were originally quite manageable problems. One study reported that over one-quarter of clients with known hypertension and diabetes mellitus, major risk factors for stroke and myocardial infarction, and blindness and end-stage renal failure necessitating dialysis, had not had a checkup from a health care provider in 2 years (Ayanian et al., 2000). Research has shown that day-to-day disease management in many cases can delay or prevent major deterioration and impose far lighter burdens on the client.

## Current Issues in Nursing and the Effect on Acute Care Nursing

Many issues within nursing affect acute care nursing. Several of these issues have been addressed in other chapters (e.g., nursing shortage in Chapter 2, critical decision making in Chapter 10). However, additional information is included in this section on the following issues: entry into practice, use of variably trained caregivers, and critical thinking in the acute care setting.

## Entry into Practice Issues and Acute Care

If increased interpersonal complexity weren't enough, the exponential growth of the sciences is also underscoring the necessity for lifelong learning, and compelling every nurse to address the issue of continuing education much more seriously. Although the ethical injunction to remain current is clear, continuing education is not mandated in every jurisdiction. Debate over who should bear the cost continues. Furthermore, in acute care, a practice context where new knowledge, new products (e.g., pharmaceuticals), and technologies are being introduced almost daily, failure to remain current can pose potential safety risks to clients. The qualification profile of practicing nurses raises a troubling question, which is at least as worrisome as the demographic graying of the nursing workforce: Is the education capable of addressing the complexity of care demands imposed on nurses? As of 1996, 58.4% of the employed nurses had less than a baccalaureate degree as their highest nursing credential, 31.8% had a bachelor's, and 6.3% were qualified in one of four categories as advanced practice nurses. Not all were nationally credentialed (Spratley, Johnson, Soohalski, Fritz, & Spencer, 2002). The related debate concerning the level of entry to practice is boiling, with the suggestion that by 2010, two-thirds of registered nurses in the United States be minimally baccalaureate prepared.

## Nonstandardized Care Providers in Acute Care

With about 60% of nurses employed in the hospital sector, acute care settings are definitely impacted by the nursing shortage (Figure 20-7). The increasing challenge is to pro-

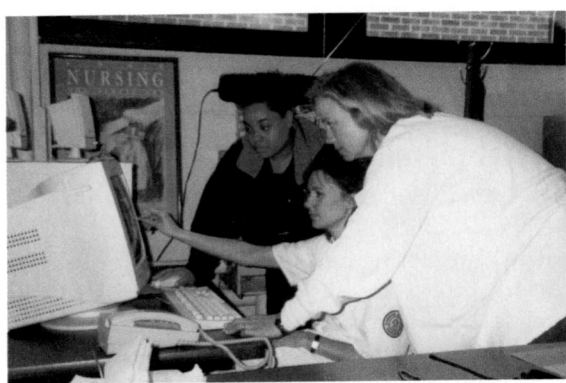

**Figure 20-7    A nurse is taking time to explain the assignments of her shift to two patient care assistants.**

vide quality care in an acute care environment with fewer and fewer nurses. One solution that emerges during this nursing shortage is the use of variably prepared caregivers (e.g., patient care assistants, nursing assistants). These persons often have education that is not standardized and roles that are not clearly defined. Ultimately the nurse is solely responsible for defining the capabilities of these individuals, which adds to the problem created by the shortage. Nurses must take additional time from already busy sched-

ules to outline the responsibilities of the ancillary care providers and ensure that these persons can perform their assignments and tasks. It has become increasingly difficult to define practice boundaries, negotiate delegation, and determine accountability. Individuals, institutions, and professional and regulatory organizations are being compelled by circumstance to address this lack of clarity and the consequences of the increasing interdependency (Frketich, 2001).

 # CASE STUDY/NURSING CARE PLAN

A 44-year-old male, James Carter, presented to the emergency department (ED) after a witnessed grand mal seizure on a nearby street corner. On arrival in the ED, the client was found drowsy but able to provide a history and answer questions. Mr. Carter had no focal neurological findings, and the toxicology screen was positive for cocaine and ethanol. The old chart revealed the client was well-known to the medical service, with a long history of poorly controlled hypertension and multisubstance abuse. The client was admitted for blood pressure control and neurological observation.

Upon arrival to the neurology unit, vital signs were notable for a blood pressure (BP) of 203/120 mm Hg. Mr. Carter was drowsy, opened his eyes to voice, was able to answer questions, and obeyed commands with all extremities. He was able to move himself from the stretcher to the bed. Pupils were 3 mm bilaterally and reacted to light. Approximately 30 minutes later, a passing registered nurse noted loud stertorous breathing from the client's room. On entering she noted that the respiratory rate was 25 and irregular, oxygen saturation was 92%, BP = 186/98, P = 90. Neurologically, Mr. Carter opened his eyes to painful stimulus and uttered incomprehensible sounds to pain. There was abnormal flexion of both upper extremities, and extensor rigidity of the lower limbs (decorticate). Right upper and lower limbs appeared to be weak, the upper more so than the lower. Pupils were noted to be asymmetric. The right was 3 mm and reactive; the left was 5 mm and sluggishly reactive to light.

## Assessment
Mr. Carter is a known hypertensive, post-ictal cocaine user with new onset respiratory abnormalities. He is experiencing focal neurological deficits, extreme hypertension, and a decreased level of consciousness.

## Nursing Diagnosis #1
*Impaired Gas Exchange* related to a focal neurological event.
**NOC:** Respiratory Status: Gas Exchange; Respiratory Status: Ventilation; Tissue Perfusion: Pulmonary
**NIC:** Airway Management; Oxygen Therapy; Respiratory Monitoring

## Expected Outcomes
The client will:
1. Demonstrate adequate respiratory function as measured by oxygen saturation levels returning to 95% or higher within 48 hours.
2. Maintain patent airway throughout hospitalization.

## Planning/Interventions/Rationales
1. Insert nasopharyngeal or oral airway. *Ensures airway functioning.*
2. Position head of bed to 30 degrees; neutral body position. *Encourages orthopneic position to increase oxygenation.*
3. Consider advising the placement of a nasogastric tube. *Decompresses stomach during time of decreased level of consciousness.*
4. Continuous monitoring of $O_2$ saturation. *Assesses accurate cellular oxygenation.*

## Evaluation
Oxygen saturation levels were maintained at 94%, and airway was patent without deterioration of breathing status.

*(continues)*

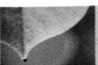

# CASE STUDY/NURSING CARE PLAN (continued)

## Nursing Diagnosis #2

*Impaired Cerebral Tissue Perfusion* related to ischemic event related to underlying hypertension or cocaine ingestion.

**NOC:** Circulation Status; Cardiac Pump Effectiveness: Tissue Perfusion: Cerebral

**NIC:**  Circulatory Care: Arterial Insufficiency

### Expected Outcome

The client will:

1. Demonstrate adequate cerebral perfusion as measured by stability in Glascow Coma Scale (GCS) with a score greater than 10.

### Planning/Interventions/Rationales

1. Monitor neurological status Q 5 to 10 minutes (e.g., Glasgow Coma Scale Score), pupillary size and reactivity, and respiratory rhythmicity. *Evaluates and assesses continuing neurological status.*
2. If there are sedatives prescribed, hold sedatives and contact physician. *Prevents potential negative consequences of decreasing cerebral function if the sedatives are administered.*

### Evaluation

Client has continuing stable GCS at a score of 10 or higher and a cerebral partial pressure ≥ 60 mm Hg.

## Key Concepts

- Nurses who practice in acute care settings are an integral part of one of the fastest growing applied sciences, benefiting and adapting to explosive growth in bench and clinical foundation sciences.
- Acute care is practiced by a wide variety of practitioners and is evaluated by the outcomes effected on the clients.
- Many organizations regulate nursing practice in the acute care settings and establish standards of care.
- Nurses share with their colleagues across the disciplines the obligation to maintain a current knowledge and skill base in order to support safe and evidence-based practice.
- Growing emphasis on the ability to demonstrate favorable client, provider, and organizational outcomes is shaping acute nursing care delivery.
- Nurses are active and compassionate participants in many of the ethical decisions that confront consumers and providers of health care.
- Societal priorities and public (government), capitalism, and private competing interests all shape the delivery of acute health care.
- Tenacity and courage are required to meet the challenges facing the nature and scope of acute care nursing in the 21st century.
- Entry into practice issues, and nonstandardized care providers influence current acute care nursing.

## Review Questions and Activities

1. Describe the typical arenas of acute care.
2. What are typical categories of advanced practice nurses seen in acute care nursing?

3. Describe several regulatory organizations used in monitoring acute care nursing practice.
4. Discuss clinical guidelines that are used as resources for establishing standards in acute care.
5. Describe the role of quality control in acute care.
6. Why do societal issues impact acute care nursing, and what is an example of such an issue?

## Web Resources

Agency of Healthcare Research and Quality
    http://www.ahrq.gov
American Cancer Society
    http://www.cancer.org
American Diabetic Association
    http://www.diabetes.org
American Heart Association History of the AHA
    http://www.americanheart.org
American Occupational Therapy Association (AOTA)
    http://www.aota.org
California Code of Regulations
    http://www.rn.ca.gov
Cochrane Collaboration
    http://www.campbell-reviews.com
Department of the Army's health promotion and wellness Website, http://chppm-www.apgea.army.mil
History of the American Hospital Association
    http://www.aha.org
Human Genome Research
    http://www.ornl.gov
International Council of Nursing
    http://www.icn.ch

Panneton K., 1998. Aging population pushes need for geriatric training http://albany.bcentral.com

Sochalski, J., & Patrician, P., 1999. *An overview of health care spending patterns in the United States: Using national data sources to explore trends in nursing services* http://www.nursingworld.org

# References

Agency of Healthcare Research and Quality, 2003 retrieved Feb 2, 2003 from www.ahrq.gov

Allen, R. E. (Ed.) (2000). *The concise oxford dictionary of current English.* Oxford: Clarendon Press.

American Cancer Society, 2003, www.cancer.org

American Diabetic Association, 2003, http://www.diabetes.org

American Heart Association, 2003: History of the AHA, http://www.aha.org/

American Occupational Therapy Association (AOTA), 2003, http://www.aota.org

Ayanian, J. Z., Weissman, J. S., Schneider, E. C., Ginsberg, J. A., Zaslavsky, A. M. (2000). Unmet health needs of uninsured adults in the United States. *Journal of the American Medical Association 284*(16), 2016–2019.

Beers, H. M., & Berkow, R. (2000). *The Merck manual of geriatrics* (3rd ed.). Whitehouse Station, NJ: Merck Research Laboratories, Merck, Inc.

Blatchford, C. (2001). In the ER pit. Emergency services in crisis. *National Post,* Saturday, June 9, Page B1.

Burkhardt, M., & Nathaniel, A. (2002). *Ethics & issues in contemporary nursing* (2nd ed.). Clifton Park, NY: Delmar Learning.

California Code of Regulations, 2001, http://www.rn.ca.gov

*Cochrane Collaboration* (2001), http://www.campbell-reviews.com/ccweb/cochrane.

Department of the Army's health promotion and wellness Website, 2003, http://chppm-www.apgea.army.mil/dhpw

De Tocqueville, A. (2002). *Democracy in America.* Canada: Penguin Books.

Estes, M. (2002). *Health assessment & physical examination* (2nd ed.). Clifton Park, NY: Delmar Learning.

Every, N., Hochman, J., Becker, R., Kopecky, S., & Cannon, C. P. (2000). Critical pathways. AHA scientific statement. *Circulation 101,* 461.

Frketich, J. (2001). Home care in chaos. Report cites lack of money, staff. *Hamilton Spectator, 12*(1).

Goldman, H. H., Ganju, V., Drake, R. E., Gorman, P., Hogan, M., Hyde, P. S., Morgan, O. (2001). Policy implications for implementing evidence-based practice. *Psychiatric Services, 52*(12), pp. 1591–1597.

History of the American Hospital Association, 2001, http://www.aha.org

Holahan, J., & Kim, J. (2000). Why does the number of uninsured Americans continue to grow? *Health Affairs 19*(4), 188–196.

Human Genome Research, 2001, http://www.ornl.gov

International Council of Nursing, 2000, http://www.icn.ch

Joint Commission on Accreditation of Healthcare Organizations (JCAHO, 2001).

Kohn, L., Corrigan, J., Donaldson, M. (Eds.) (1999). *To Err Is Human: Building a Safer Health System.* Committee on Quality of Health Care in America, Institute of Medicine. Washington, DC: National Academy Press.

Moy, E., Bartman, B. A., Clancy, & Cornelius, L. J. (1998). Changes in usual sources of medical care between 1987 and 1992. *Journal of Health Care for the Poor and Underserved 9*(2),126–138.

Nelson, E., Mohr, J., Batalden, P., & Plume, S. (1996). Improving health care, Part I: The clinical value compass. *The Joint Commission Journal of Quality Improvement, 22*(4), 112–115.

Nightingale, F. (1859). *Notes on Nursing. What it is, and what it is not.* London: Harrison & Sons.

O'Brien-Pallas, L. L., & Baumann, A. (2001). *Commitment and care: the benefits of a healthy workplace for nurses, their patients and the system. Executive Summary,* http://www.chsrf.ca/english/document-library/psescomcare_e.html

Panneton, K. (1998). Aging population pushes need for geriatric training , http://albany.bcentral.com

Parker, C., Minick, P., & Kee, C. (1999). Clinical decision-making process in perioperative nursing. *AORN Journal, 70*(1), 45–62.

Pender, J., Murdaugh, C., & Parsons, M. A. (2002). *Health promotion in nursing practice* (4th ed.). Upper Saddle River, NJ: Prentice-Hall.

Sochalski, J., & Patrician, P. (1999). *An overview of health care spending patterns in the United States: Using national data sources to explore trends in nursing services,* http://www.nursingworld.org

Spratley, E., Johnson, A., Sochalski, J., Fritz, M., & Spencer, W. (2002). *Findings from the National Sample Survey of Registered Nurses.* Washington, DC: Health Resources and Services Administration.

Waltz, C. F., Strickland, O. L., & Lenz, E. R. (1991). *Measurement in nursing research* (2nd ed.) Philadelphia: F. A. Davis.

White, L., & Duncan, G. (2002). *Medical-surgical nursing: An integrated approach* (2nd ed.). Clifton Park, NY: Delmar Learning.

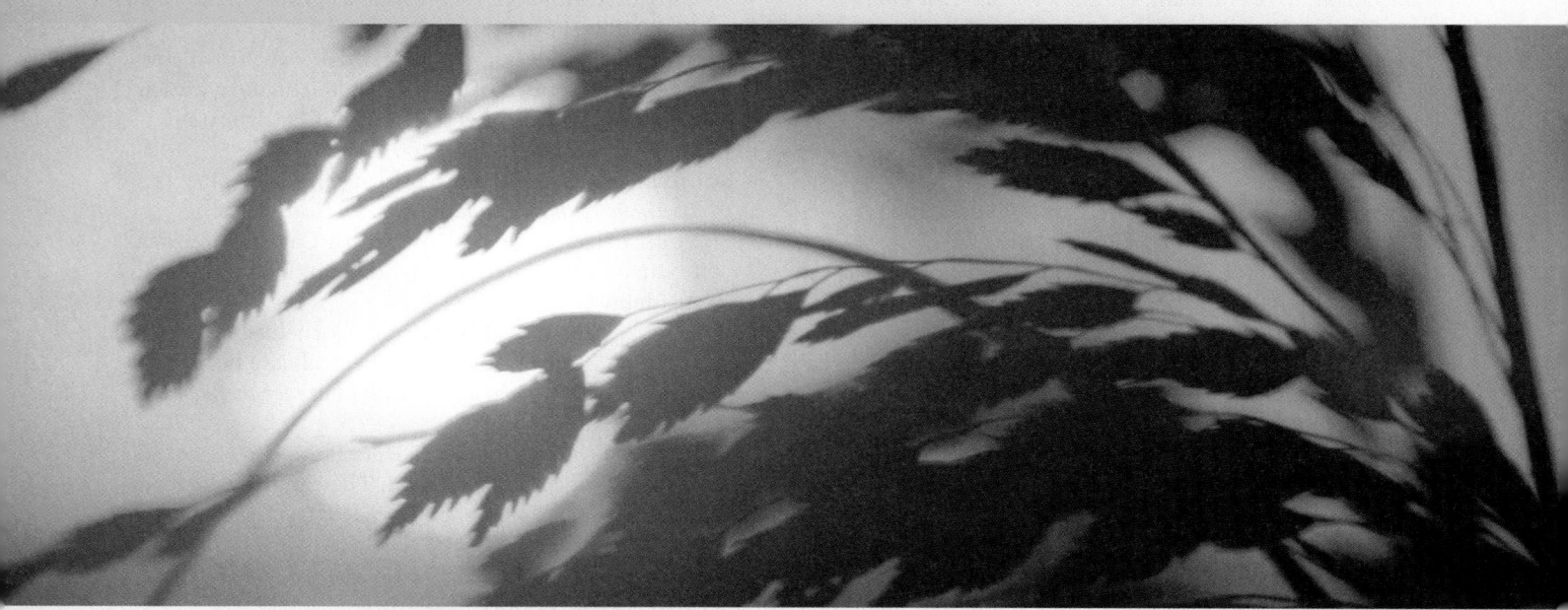

# Restorative Care

Marilyn Housel Poysky, RN, MSN, CS

*"The rehabilitation nurse helps clients and their families weave their lives back together and return to the community and to their roles as productive members of society."*

(Chin, Finocchiaro, Rosebrough, 1998)

# Chapter Competencies

*Upon completion of this chapter, the reader should be able to:*

1. Discuss the definition of restorative nursing.
2. Identify the types of settings in which restorative nursing care is given.
3. Discuss the philosophy and principles of restorative nursing care.
4. Discuss the life-span considerations in relation to restorative care.
5. Describe the roles of the restorative nurse on the interdisciplinary team.
6. Discuss the nursing role in discharge planning for the transition between acute, subacute, and home care, including assessment of the home setting.
7. Discuss quality improvement issues related to restorative care.
8. Discuss the historical, current, and future trends in restorative care.
9. Discuss the application of the nursing process in restorative care including assessing functional ability.
10. Compare nursing diagnoses, client outcomes, and restorative nursing interventions that are frequently used in restorative care.

# Key Terms

activities of daily living (ADL)

acuity

Barthel Index

Case management

comorbidity

disability

functional ability

Functional Independence Measurement (FIM)

handicap

impairment

rehabilitate

Relocation Stress Syndrome

restorative

Restorative care takes place in many types of health care settings, including acute care, outpatient clinics, long-term care facilities, and in-home health care. The focus of the restorative care nurse is on optimal health function and quality of life for the client. Disease, trauma, or congenital conditions can leave the client with decreased functional ability, interrupting daily living, lifestyle, and family or work roles. Restorative nursing interventions help the client return to normal functional ability or to adapt activities and lifestyle to resume family and work roles. Restorative care places the client at the center of the health care team. The purpose of the team is to teach, empower, and encourage the client to be in charge of his health care and to be as independent as possible.

In this chapter the philosophy, principles, and selected interventions of restorative nursing will be discussed with illustrations of how they are utilized in different settings and with varying client needs, from simple to complex. The role of the nurse and the interdisciplinary team, the use of the nursing process in longer-term situations, and the discharge planning required to accomplish the restorative process will be illustrated. Finally, the historical, current, and future trends in restorative nursing care will be described to provide perspective on its importance on quality health care.

# Definition of Restorative Care

Webster (Neufeldt, 2001) defines the term **restorative** as "to bring back into a former, normal, or unimpaired state or condition" (p. 1144). The term **rehabilitate** is defined by Webster (Neufeldt, 2001) as "to restore to a normal or optimal state of health and constructive activity by medical, physical, and psychological therapy . . . to prepare a disabled or disadvantaged person for employment by vocational counseling or training" (p. 1131). The term *rehabilitation* has been used in medical and nursing literature for over 60 years. Philosophically, some professionals believe the term *restorative* creates less stigma and labeling of disabled persons than does the term *rehabilitative*. However, the terms continue to be used interchangeably in current literature.

In 1988, two professional nursing organizations defined rehabilitation nursing as "the diagnosis and treatment of human responses of individuals and groups to actual or potential health problems stemming from altered functional ability and altered lifestyle" (American Nurses Association & Association of Rehabilitation Nurses, 1988, p. 4). The emphasis is on **functional ability** and the changes or adaptations a client needs to make in daily lifestyle. Functional ability is composed of the physical, cognitive, and emotional skills required to perform **activities of daily living (ADL)** related to self-care, such as grooming, as well as those activities required by the individual's family and work roles.

Using a broader perspective, Hickey defines *rehabilitation* "as a dynamic process in which the person is aided in achieving optimum physical, emotional, psychosocial, and vocational potential in order to maintain dignity and self-respect in a life that is as self-fulfilling as possible" (Derstine & Hargrove, 2001, p. 7). Rehabilitation is a process that is multifaceted and occurs over a period of time, often many months or years (Figure 21-1). It is a planned, orderly, and dynamic process that is individualized to each client's needs (Chin, Finocchiaro, & Rosebrough, 1998).

In the Omnibus Budget Act of 1987 (OBRA 87), restorative nursing was defined as "including exercises, transfer training, and carrying out of restorative or reha-

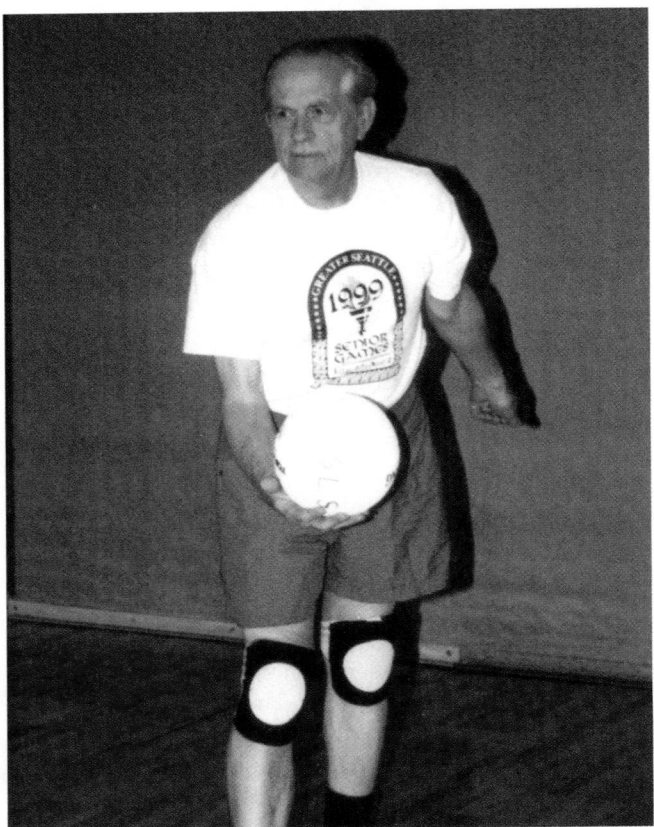

**Figure 21-1    A client in a rehabilitation program**

bilitative programs ordered by a physician" (Derstine & Hargrove, 2001, p. 72). It describes specific interventions that a restorative care nurse may teach the client or caregiver to do in ADL such as grooming, dressing, and eating. This legislation was particularly directed toward residents in long-term care facilities to ensure they attained and maintained their highest physical, mental, and psychosocial well-being (Resnick, 2000). The legislation had an enormous impact on long-term care in the last 12 years, changing it from a custodial philosophy to a restorative philosophy (Bonder & Wagner, 2001).

## Historical Trends in Restorative Care

Florence Nightingale in her *Notes on Nursing* (1859, p. 22) first stressed that "whatever a patient can do for himself, it is better and less anxiety for him to do for himself." She understood the importance of the client being an active participant in self-care, which is an underlying principle in restorative care.

The word *rehabilitation* first appeared in medical literature during World War I when thousands of war veterans returned home with amputations and other wounds. During this time, the government and the medical community recognized the importance of helping disabled veterans readapt their lives in their communities and to be vocationally productive. After the war, the Social Security Act of 1935 was the first legislation to give restorative services to the American public. However, at this point the physician was seen as the only specialist in the process. During the 1930s and 1940s, epidemics of poliomyelitis, which struck children and young adults in particular, stimulated study on how restorative care could be accomplished for this population. In 1941, the Australian nurse Sister Kenney changed the method of treating polio in the United States, instituting the use of muscle manipulation and hot packs (Chin et al., 1998).

World War II brought an even bigger increase of wounded veterans who had survived war wounds due to better field methods of medicine and the advent of antibiotics. But they now needed long-term rehabilitation to return to their communities. Howard Rusk, head of the Air Force Convalescent Training Program, was a leader in the establishment of separate centers for the rehabilitation of the veterans. He also established the first civilian rehabilitation program in 1948 in New York City. He especially emphasized the importance of good nursing care in the client's recovery (Chin et al., 1998). Examples of early rehabilitation nursing interventions at this time were the use of footboards to prevent foot drop, extra pillows for good positioning of the body, and frequent voiding programs to prevent incontinence.

By the 1960s, the polio epidemic was stopped, but an increase in head injuries stemming from motor vehicle and recreational accidents led to research exploring how rehabilitation could be applied to neurological impairment due to strokes or multiple sclerosis. In addition, new research was being conducted showing the benefits of cardiac rehabilitation.

In 1965, the American Nurses Association published its *Guidelines for the practice of nursing on the rehabilitation team: An answer to a growing need* because it was recognized that rehabilitation nursing was a specialization. The Association of Rehabilitation Nurses (ARN) was established in 1974 to further define issues important to rehabilitation nursing and to provide continuing education. Ten years later the ARN began certifying nurses who met the standards of the credentialing exam. The Association of Rehabilitation Nurses published their standards of care and standards of professional practice for rehabilitation nursing in 1994 and for advanced practice in rehabilitation nursing in 1996.

The Rehabilitation Act of 1973 was extremely important because the goal of the Act was to return clients to the community and to increase their control of their health care and life. It especially emphasized that rehabilitation services should be available in all communities. Equally important was the Americans with Disabilities Act of 1990, which mandated that all physical barriers and discrimination be removed in the areas of transportation, work, and education. Thus the disabled had the right to guide dogs in all public places, transportation systems that accommodated wheelchairs, access for those with hearing or visual impairments, and classrooms and restrooms that are accessible to wheelchairs (Figure 21-2).

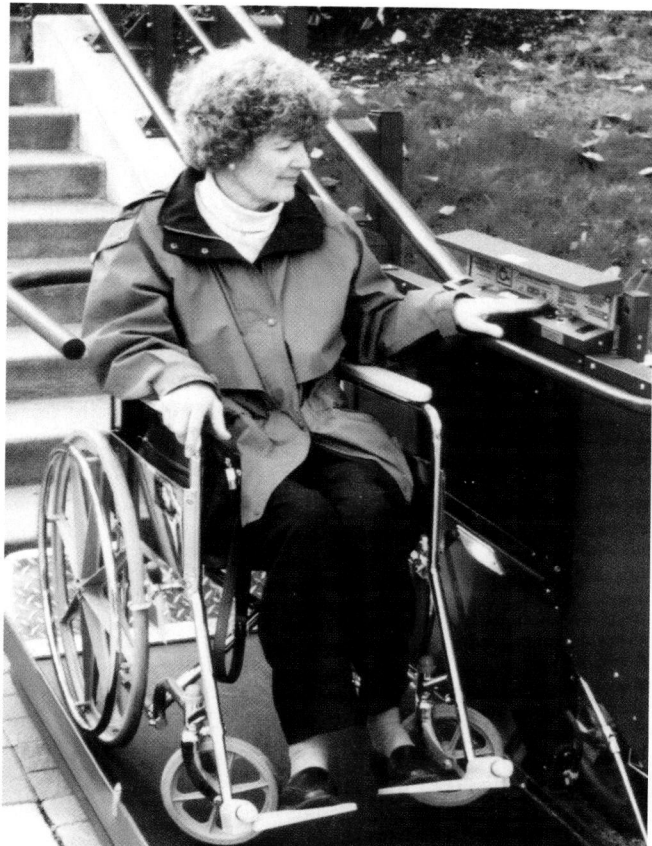

**Figure 21-2    A client using a wheelchair lift**

## Classification of Terms

Often the terms **disability**, **impairment**, and **handicap** are used interchangeably without distinguishing their meanings. The World Health Organization (WHO) defined these terms for scientific and clinical application to the rehabilitation process. Table 21-1 summarizes the WHO Classification, which is used worldwide. However, in the United States some health professionals believe the term *handicap* carries too great of a stigma. They have adopted an alternative model by Nagy, which uses the term *functional limitation* for loss of the ability to perform a

specific activity and the term *disability* for the loss of a role (Table 21-1). With either definition the goal of rehabilitation is to prevent further deterioration or complications and to aid the client in recovering functional ability and resuming his life roles.

## Types of Restorative Care Settings

The early rehabilitation centers in the 1950s through the 1970s delivered intensive, comprehensive rehabilitation for many types of clients. Goals were set with a long length

| TABLE 21-1 | CLASSIFICATION OF TERMS BY WHO AND NAGY | |
|---|---|---|
| **WHO Term** | **Definition** | **Nagy's Term** |
| Impairment | Loss of function at the organ level | Impairment |
| Disability | Restriction or lack of ability to perform an activity a normal person can perform | Functional limitation |
| Handicap | Inability to perform life roles due to disability | Disability |

Adapted from Hoeman, S. (2002). *Rehabilitation nursing: Process, applications, & outcomes* (3rd ed.). Philadelphia, Pennsylvania: W. B. Saunders Co.

of stay allowed for their accomplishment. However, in the last 10 years, due to managed care incentives to contain health care costs, most clients are assigned to subacute units, ambulatory care clinics, or home health care to accomplish their rehabilitation. In the changing state of health care today, many partnerships and alliances are occurring between types of facilities to provide restorative care in as cost-effective a way as possible. The following are examples of types of settings used for restorative nursing care in today's health care.

## Inpatient Rehabilitation Centers

Many large medical centers have inpatient rehabilitation units that offer intensive therapy, commonly called acute rehabilitation, for 4 to 6 hours a day. Also, some free-standing rehabilitation centers offer all phases of rehabilitation, including inpatient. Nursing staff have responsibility for teaching the client complex rehabilitation interventions and helping the client integrate the skills into everyday use. The nurse also coordinates services of a large interdisciplinary health care team. This type of setting is generally for the client with extensive rehabilitation needs who has the stamina required for the extended hours of therapy. In addition, these units benefit clients who live in a rural area with few community rehabilitation resources. Today, the length of stay averages 3 to 6 weeks.

## Acute Care Hospitals

If the client is hospitalized with acute care needs, restorative interventions are begun in the hospital by nurses, physical therapists, and others to prevent complications and to recover muscle strength. Examples of restorative interventions begun in acute care are range of motion exercises, analysis of feeding and caloric problems, use of splints to support joints, and increasing sitting balance and strength. The client may go to the physical therapy department for 30 to 60 minutes a day. Often these clients have experienced severe illness with complications. They fatigue very easily and cannot yet tolerate more intensive restorative interventions. Many are clients who have been ill for a long time waiting for an organ transplant or clients who have experienced Acute Respiratory Distress Syndrome (ARDS) or other complications following a routine surgery.

## Transition Hospitals

Currently about 120 hospitals fit in this classification in the United States (Tellis-Nayak, 1998). Often these hospitals receive clients directly from the intensive care unit (ICU). They provide long-term care for the client who has extensive needs for skilled nursing care, such as those paralyzed by a traumatic motor vehicle or recreational accident. The hospitals have a full range of rehabilitation services.

## Subacute Units

These units may be within an acute care hospital, as a free-standing facility, or within a long-term care facility. They care for clients who are convalescing from a surgery or illness and need more time for rehabilitation and strengthening before returning home. Clients have short-term needs with specific goals and a short time frame to meet them. A typical length of stay would be 10 to 14 days.

## Skilled Nursing Long-Term Unit

Traditionally these units are in nursing homes, but some are also in acute care facilities. Their clients have long-term needs with sufficient complexity to require some skilled nursing care 24 hours a day. Some units are specialty units, such as those for spinal cord injuries or Alzheimer's clients, whereas others have a general focus. Many have a majority of geriatric clients.

## Ambulatory Clinics

Restorative care clinics can offer nursing assessment and physical, occupational, and speech therapy to clients who are able to come daily to the setting. This is cost-effective and beneficial to the client who prefers living at home. However, the client needs a caregiver who can deliver the complexity of the nursing care required by the client. In addition, the client needs suitable daily transportation to the ambulatory setting and should not tire too much during the transportation time.

## Home Health Care

Neal (1999) states that "both rehabilitation nursing and home health nursing espouse the same primary goals of maximal patient independence and self-care" (p. 115). In home health care, the client's knowledge deficits are evaluated by the nurse, and the goals, interventions, and community resources are mutually chosen by the nurse and client. Physical therapists and other members of the health care team make home visits. The client should be sufficiently independent to be alone or have a caregiver who can manage the complexity of nursing care needed (Figure 21-3). Home health care is very cost-effective. However, both managed care and Medicare set a strict limitation on the number of visits allowed to accomplish the restorative goals.

# Life Span Considerations in Restorative Care

All age groups experience a wide variety of acute or chronic conditions that may require restorative nursing care. Nurses must have a clear understanding of the growth and development needs of these groups in order to deliver effective, compassionate care. A presentation of the con-

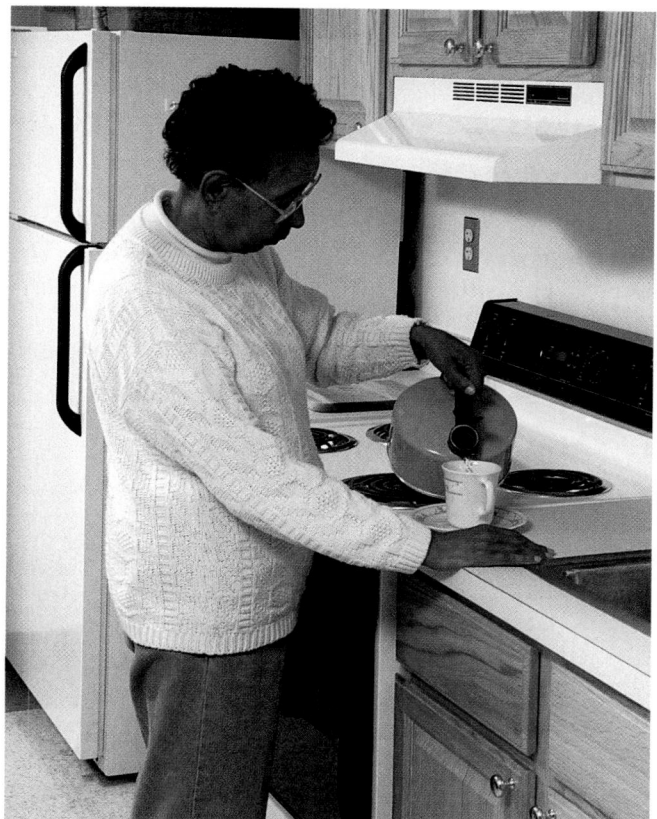

**Figure 21-3    Clients who are able to manage certain tasks independently or with minimal assistance are good candidates for home care.**

siderations for children, young adults and middle-age adults, and late middle-age and older adults follows in this section.

## Children

Newborns may be born with congenital conditions needing surgical correction and intensive rehabilitation. An example is an infant born with a congenital hip, which needs surgery and casting for a number of months, and

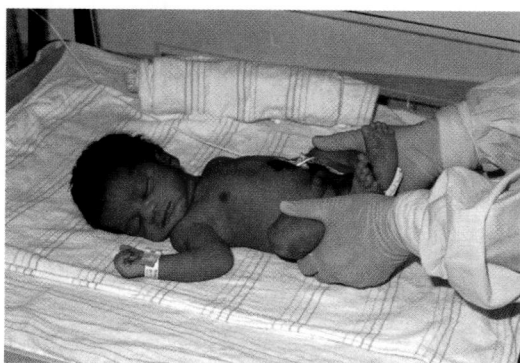

**Figure 21-4    Examination for congenital hip abnormality**

then physical therapy and strengthening of the hip muscles in preparation for learning to walk (Figure 21-4). Cerebral palsy is a birth injury that has long-term consequences requiring lifelong rehabilitation and restorative nursing interventions for many clients. In addition, children and adolescents may experience sports injuries, falls, or accidents that result in fractures, brain injuries, or spinal cord damage requiring restorative nursing care.

## Young Adults and Middle Age

Motor vehicle or recreational accidents, war injuries, and work-related injuries are a few causes of impairment and disability in young and middle-age adults. Rehabilitation involves recovering functional ability or adapting to functional limitations in ADL. It also involves family and work role adaptations, because most clients in this age group carry the heavy responsibilities of providing income for their families and raising children.

## Late Middle Age and Older Adults

The term *restorative care* has been broadened in recent years to also include a variety of other health conditions found in late middle-aged and older adults. Cardiac rehabilitation has proven beneficial for clients with myocardial infarctions or after cardiac surgery. Restorative care also

## COMMUNITY/HOME CARE

### Efficacy of Outpatient Infusion Units

Heart failure and the resulting decline of functional capacity take an enormous toll in health care costs, not to mention a decline in the individual's quality of life. A study by Warner compared the cost-effectiveness of an inotropic infusion outpatient unit to traditional hospitalization for heart failure treatment. Also incorporated into the study were a restorative care pathway, case management, telemanagement, and home inotropic infusion for palliative treatment. There was a 0% readmission rate and a 50% decrease in health care costs for clients using the outpatient infusion unit. There were numerous examples of increased activity levels and quality of life for clients using the unit compared to their health status before using the unit.

Warner, P. M., & Hutchinson, C. (1999). Heart failure management. *Journal of Nursing Administration, 29*(7/8), 28–37.

encompasses ambulatory infusion clinics for those older clients with heart failure (Warner & Hutchinson, 1999). Pulmonary rehabilitation is critical for persons with asthma or chronic obstructive lung disease. They are taught breathing exercises, strengthening exercises for walking tolerance, and other ways to adapt to their disease so that they can function at a higher level with less fatigue. Restorative care also encompasses ambulatory infusion clinics for those elderly with heart failure (Warner & Hutchinson, 1999). Restorative nursing care interventions are increasingly used with clients with cancer, including those in hospice or palliative treatment. Interventions with these clients help to extend their functional ability to care for themselves during the dying process. In addition, family members can be taught how to give care and support, enabling the client to remain at home until death (Michael, 2001). Box 21-1 is a partial list of conditions that frequently require restorative care.

The elderly population experiences falls and trauma accidents as well. They also have a high incidence of arthritis, which can lead to joint destruction and joint replacement surgery, necessitating restorative nursing care. Older clients may require restorative nursing because of failure to use their current physical abilities. For example, older clients frequently lack adequate exercise even if they do not have any physical limitation. In addition, they may experience fear of falling and depression, which keeps them less mobile. The immobility creates shortening of muscles,

stiffness, and loss of strength and balance, putting them at an even higher risk for falls.

## Acuity Level of Restorative Care Clients

Clients have a wide variation in the amount and complexity of restorative nursing care needed. **Acuity** is a term that classifies where the client is on the care contin-

---

 **LIFE SPAN CONSIDERATIONS**

### Physiological Changes and Conditions of Older Adults That Complicate or Prolong Restorative Care

- Decreased immune response—heal more slowly, contract infections more easily

- Less cardiac and respiratory reserve—fatigue easily, shortness of breath with exercise

- Cognitively process information more slowly—need more time to learn new mental or physical skills and adapt to changes

- Decreased visual acuity and hearing—difficulty hearing or reading instructions

- Experience increased anxiety and fear with change or the potential for change

Hogstel, M. (2001). *Gerontology: Nursing care of the older adult.* Clifton Park, NY: Delmar Learning.

---

### BOX 21-1    CONDITIONS FREQUENTLY NEEDING RESTORATIVE NURSING INTERVENTIONS

| | |
|---|---|
| Brain injury: trauma, aneurism, stroke, tumor | Guillain-Barre syndrome |
| Spinal cord injury: trauma, tumor | Postpolio syndrome |
| Amyotrophic lateral sclerosis (Lou Gehrig's disease) | Multiple sclerosis |
| Limb amputation | Joint replacement |
| Arthritis | Burns |
| Cardiac surgery | Heart failure |
| Chronic obstructive pulmonary disease | Myocardial infarction |
| Cancer | Organ transplantation |
| Alzheimer's and other dementias | AIDS |

---

### FOCUS ON WELLNESS

### Exercise and Older Adults

Two-thirds of persons over 65 do not exercise regularly. A major focus of restorative nursing is to find strategies to motivate this age group to exercise consistently for at least 20 minutes three or more times a week. In a research study using group exercises for women in a retirement setting, the most useful method was large group exercises twice a week, using a videotape and a nurse leading the group. The women refused small group exercise, peer leaders, or more frequent weekly exercise.

Grove, N. C., & Spier, B. E. (1999). Motivating the well elderly to exercise. *Journal of Community Health Nursing, 16*(3), 179–188.

uum from being highly dependent on complex nursing care to being independent in self-care at the other end of the continuum (Figure 21-5). The care continuum for restorative care clients can be visualized as having two components. One component is the amount of nursing assistance needed to physically accomplish ADL and mobility. The other component is the amount of education in self-care activities that the client and family need to assume the care themselves.

A low acuity client with hip joint replacement surgery may have simple teaching needs. The client will need some assistance with ADLs for 1 to 3 weeks, education in hip precautions, use of an assistive device for walking, and exercises for strengthening the joint muscles. A client injured in an accident resulting in a brain injury and partial T 10 spinal injury will be a high acuity client. He will have a high dependence on assistance in ADL and mobility, as well as need extensive education on skin, bowel, and bladder care. The education may require more time than usual due to the client's brain injury.

## High Technology Advancements and Acuity Level

The acuity level of clients is increasing due to several factors. One factor is the increased ability of emergency rescue teams to stabilize critically injured people in the field until they are transported to ICUs. A related factor is the increased knowledge and use of technology in the ICU to manage not only the injury but also the severe life-threatening complications, such as disseminated intravascular coagulopathy and acute respiratory distress syndrome, which may accompany it.

## Aging and Acuity Level

Another factor increasing the acuity of restorative care clients is the growing number of people who are aged 85 and over. This population group is expected to double from 3.3 million to 7.6 million by the year 2020 (Black, 1999). These people often have two or more **comorbidi-**

**ties**, which complicate and slow their return to their previous level of function. A comorbidity is a condition, usually a chronic disease, that the client had prior to the current condition requiring restorative nursing care. For example, if an older man falls and breaks his hip, returning to his baseline of functional ability is made more difficult if he also has chronic obstructive pulmonary disease that makes him short of breath with exertion. Box 21-2 shows examples of frequently occurring comorbidities in older clients. Arthritis is the most frequently occurring chronic disease in those over 65 years (Derstine & Hargrove, 2001).

## Nursing Theory and Restorative Care

Rehabilitation as an interdisciplinary field of practice is influenced by theories from the disciplines of nursing, psychology, education, and sociology. Theories from other disciplines include the disability theories of Dembo, Goffman, and Wright; the motivational theories of Abram Maslow and Dunn; theories of family and aging; and cognitive and social learning theories such as Piaget's (Hoeman, 2002). Although it is important to gain a deeper understanding of these theories from other disciplines, the nursing theories are most applicable in day-to-day restorative nursing care. One such example is illustrated in Dorothy Orem's self-care model (1995). Orem's model was developed in the 1950s and has had an important influence in rehabilitation nursing. It is based on the concept of self-care that Orem defined as "the practice of activities that individuals initiate and perform on their own behalf in maintaining life, health, and well-being" (Derstine & Hargrove, 2001, p. 14). The individual is in need of nursing care when the client's need exceeds ability, creating a self-care deficit. Nursing is viewed as a service helping the client and family to become capable of self-care. Restorative nurses recognize the emphasis on self-care, overcoming deficits, independence, self-esteem, worth of the client, and the importance of client education in Orem's model.

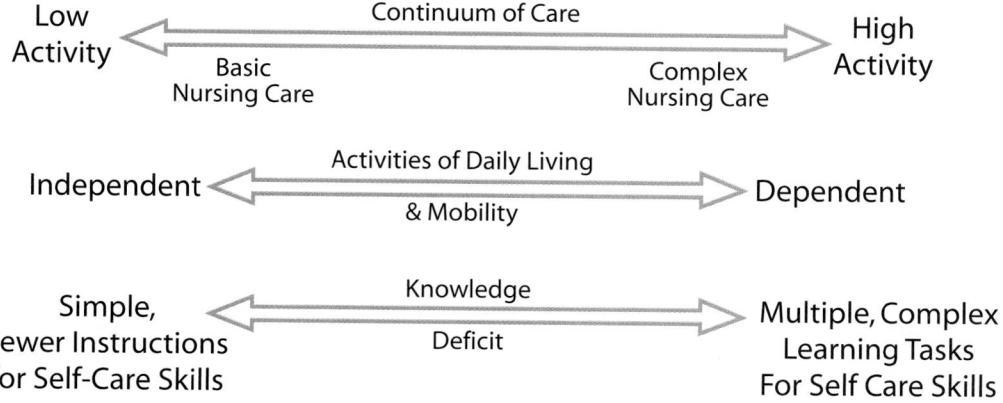

**Figure 21-5    Acuity continuum of care**

## BOX 21-2    FREQUENT COMORBIDITIES IN OLDER CLIENTS

| | |
|---|---|
| Chronic obstructive pulmonary disease | Stroke |
| | Diabetes |
| Heart failure | Arthritis |
| Alzheimer's | |
| Renal insufficiency | |

It is cautioned that nursing theories have not been thoroughly researched in the rehabilitation setting. It may be most useful to eventually develop an eclectic model for restorative care (Hoeman, 2002).

## Philosophy and Principles of Restorative Care

Restorative nursing care has a unique philosophy that focuses on self-care and independence of the client. The client is given the right to become the expert in her own health care. This is accomplished through client education and the development of self-care skills (Chin et al., 1998). It requires time and careful coordination of services with a perspective that views the client holistically, including her physical, psychological, emotional, spiritual, social, and vocational needs. The Commission on Accreditation of Rehabilitation Facilities (CARF) defines rehabilitation as "the process of providing in a coordinated manner, those comprehensive services deemed appropriate to the needs of a person with a disability in a program designed to achieve the objectives of improved health, welfare, and the realization of the person's maximal physical, social, psychological, and vocational potential for useful and productive activity" (Derstine, 2001, p. 7). Following are some of the principles that are basic to the philosophy of restorative nursing.

### Prevent Deterioration and Complications

First and foremost in restorative care is to institute interventions to prevent worsening of functional ability or complications that would impair it. This would include preventing the risks inherent in immobility such as joint contractures, muscle atrophy, blood clots, skin ulcers, and pneumonia. Stryker, an early pioneer in rehabilitation nursing, emphasized the need to begin restorative care as soon as the client first encounters disease or trauma (Chin et al., 1998). Restorative measures that are begun early can shorten and simplify the rehabilitation process later.

### Promote Optimum Functional Ability

The restorative care nurse seeks to increase or restore the client's functional ability. This involves careful assessment of the skills needed for self-care and identifying factors such as cognition that influence the client's performance. Through interventions such as exercises, splint, assistive aids, and tasks broken down into smaller steps, the client can recover or adapt to the change.

### Include Client and Family on the Team

Central to the philosophy is involvement of the client and family as part of the health care team, including being part of the decision making. Making the client a member of the team conveys not only respect for him as a person, but it allows the client to communicate and express personal viewpoints. The goal is to establish good communication and to foster understanding between health care providers and the client.

### Teach Client Rationale of Self-Care Skills

Teaching the rationale of self-care skills gives the client the knowledge base to do them correctly. In addition, it helps the client make informed decisions of how to incorporate the skills into her lifestyle and to make adjustments without causing harm. For example, doing pressure relief activities is extremely important to a wheelchair-bound client to prevent the development of skin ulcers.

Understanding the reason for the activities can help the client decide how to incorporate them into the work schedule or when traveling. Teaching goals need to take into account not only the client's physical capacity but also the cognitive ability. If the client has suffered brain injury, goals would need to be adjusted to compensate for it.

### View the Client Holistically

The client must be considered not only from a standpoint of functional ability, but also in light of the client's psychological, spiritual, social, and financial resources. Social, family, and work roles must be understood in order for the rehabilitation process to successfully help the client adapt to his roles and community setting. Clients with extensive functional limitations, such as children born with cerebral palsy or adults with brain injuries, need years of follow-up.

### Integrate Client into the Community

The focus of restorative care is to help prepare the client to live as independently as possible. The goal is a return to

## CLIENT REFLECTIONS

### Quality of Life

Ted, a survivor of a motorcycle accident, states, "After my accident I used to think I'd rather die than be unable to walk, climb mountains, run races. I couldn't imagine being useful again. But now, even though I am in a wheelchair, I realize how far I've come in putting my life back together again, piece by piece. And I really appreciate life itself much more than I did before the accident."

What would be your response to this client?

the family by creating a support system in the community. This does not happen unless there is extensive preparation and planning from the beginning of the illness or trauma episode (Chin et al., 1998). In the last 20 years, community reentry is viewed as a right by many who advocate for the disabled. American society has become much more accepting of the integration of persons with disabilities into schools, workplaces, and leisure activities.

## Advocate for Quality of Life

Ultimately, each person defines what "quality of life" means to them personally. It often must be redefined when a client encounters severe injury or impairment, even when restorative care interventions have been instituted. Complete functional recovery is not always possible. However, quality of life involves having a sense of purpose in life, dignity and self-respect, and some capacity of independence. The restorative care nurse is guided overall by attempting to provide optimal quality of life for the client.

## The Interdisciplinary Team

A client's need for restorative nursing care may be simple or complex. For example, a client with a joint replacement who has no postsurgical complications or comorbidities will need only the orthopedic surgeon, a nurse, and a physical therapist on the health care team. When restorative care is complex, it is important for it to be managed by a larger interdisciplinary team. The Joint Commission on Accreditation of Healthcare Organizations (JCAHO) requirements for a minimum interdisciplinary team are a physician, rehabilitation nurse, physical therapist, occupational therapist, speech therapist, and social worker. The Commission on Accreditation of Rehabilitative Facilities (CARF) requirements add a psychologist and a recreational therapist. A physician with a specialty in rehabilitation medicine is called a physiatrist and is often the team leader, although the nurse case manager also may be the leader.

Additional team members may be added, depending on client needs. For example, a client with 50% burns to his body may need not only a physical therapist, but also the skin graft surgeon, a nutritionist to determine calorie needs for healing, a pain management specialist from medicine or nursing, and a social worker to collaborate with community resources for long-term rehabilitation. Table 21-2 lists examples of interdisciplinary team members and their roles.

Besides the advantages of an increased knowledge base from each of the disciplines represented, an interdisciplinary team offers a more holistic view of the client, giving attention to the emotional, psychological, and financial needs. Continuity of care from the acute care center through rehabilitation and into the community setting must be provided by team members with expertise in community resources such as funding, availability of outpatient clinics, vocational retraining, and legoethical issues.

Generally, the interdisciplinary team meets on a regular basis to evaluate the client's progress and the current plan of care, obtain feedback from the client, family, and other team members, and to make revisions in the plan of care.

## LEGAL AND ETHICAL ISSUES

### Conflicts Between the Health Care Team and the Client

Sometimes clients make requests or choices that are not congruent with the health team's values or what they believe is the best health choice. Two examples:

- The paraplegic client who insists on going home even though he lives alone and has been admitted twice in the last 6 months with stage 4 decubiti on his buttocks.

- The client has suffered a severe stroke affecting her ability to swallow and paralyzing her right side. She has been sustained by tube feedings through a percutaneous endoscopic gastrostomy (PEG) tube. She insists the tube feedings be stopped.

When a conflict of health care decisions occurs, the health care team generally discusses the implications with the client and family, has outside consultation, and refers the case to the facility's ethics committee. The committee usually doesn't make a decision but advocates that all sides be considered. In the end, the client's decision must be respected.

Chin, P. S., Finocchiaro, D., & Rosebrough, A. (1998). *Rehabilitation nursing practice.* New York: McGraw-Hill.

## TABLE 21-2     INTERDISCIPLINARY HEALTH TEAM ROLES

| Team Member | Role |
| --- | --- |
| Nurse | See text for description of roles |
| Physician or physiatrist | Prescribe medical and pharmacological treatment |
| Physical therapist | Muscle and joint training |
| Occupational therapist | Fine muscle training, self-care skills |
| Nutritionist | Assess for caloric intake |
| Speech therapist | Swallow evaluations, speech retraining |
| Psychologist | Testing for cognitive, emotional, and psychological function; counseling grief, loss, depression |
| Social worker | Evaluate need for financial resources, community resources; counseling family issues |
| Visiting nurse | Evaluation of home setting; assess, teach, and coordinate home care |
| Vocational counselor | Vocational retraining, adaptation of work setting |
| Recreational therapist | Provides socialization opportunities; teaches how to adapt to community |
| Respiratory Therapist | Treatment of respiratory or ventilatory equipment problems |
| Clergy | Spiritual counseling |
| Clinical nurse specialist | Case management |

The meetings may be daily during the initial assessment and planning phase, then once or twice weekly after the care plan is initiated.

## Roles of the Restorative Nurse

The restorative care nurse is essential regardless of how the team is structured for the setting. The nurse knows the client best and can present the nursing concerns and advocate for the client's concerns. Consequently, the restorative nurse assumes several roles: educator, caregiver, counselor, coordinator, client advocate, researcher, and life care planner.

### Educator

Based on the principles of restorative care, one of the most important roles of the nurse is educator. In order for the client to become independent and manage her own care, the client must be taught the physiological basis of the problem and the specific skills and rationale for relief of the problem and prevention of complications. Without this information, the client would not be able to make wise decisions about her health care in the future when she is more independent and returns to the community.

### Caregiver

The restorative care nurse may be in a primary position responsible for the hands-on care. While doing the care,

the nurse can demonstrate and explain the rationale of what is being done. The restorative care nurse must have an extensive knowledge base to provide the appropriate nursing interventions for a wide variety of client needs.

### Counselor

The restorative nurse is often called on to act as a counselor. Because clients often have critical injuries with a long protracted recovery, there is an opportunity to form close nurse-patient relationships that give the nurse opportunity to listen to the client's concerns. The nurse can provide assistance in meeting psychological and emotional concerns about the recovery and rehabilitative process.

### Coordinator

A key role is that of coordinator of the plan of care. Whether in the role of primary nurse with hands-on care or that of a case manager for a number of clients, coordination of the many services both within the institution and in the community is extremely important. The nurse needs good communication and problem-solving skills when working with the client, family, varying disciplines, and departments to coordinate services and meet the goals of the care plan.

### Client Advocate

As in all types of nursing, being a client advocate is extremely important. Because the nurse often sees the client and the family the most, the nurse must be listening for questions, apprehensions, and misunderstandings and interpret these to the other team members. The client or family may feel very overwhelmed, too intimidated to speak up, or unable to verbalize their concerns themselves. It is very important for the nurse to always advocate the client's position as a member of the health care team and for the client's quality of life issues.

### Researcher

The restorative care nurse has two additional roles. One is that of researcher (Chin et al., 1998). It is extremely important that additional research be done to provide evidence that the restorative care interventions are both effective and cost-beneficial. Being able to apply nursing research to clinical practice and to aid in designing research are skills restorative care nurses should learn (Thorne, 2000).

### Life Care Planner

A life care planner is an expert witness for certain clients. The restorative care nurse applies nursing expertise and knowledge in projecting both current and future health care needs for those with very severe injuries (Chin et al., 1998).

# The Nursing Process in Restorative Care

The nursing process is the cornerstone of restorative nursing care. The nursing process is an organized, systematic process that is continual and ongoing throughout the rehabilitation process as the client adapts and functional ability changes. There are some differences in how the process is applied to rehabilitation clients. One difference is the longer period of time, often months or years, that is required for goals to be met. Comorbidities may complicate or slow progress. Goals must often be defined in small steps to show progress. Reevaluation must be done periodically to keep the care plan relevant to client needs.

## Assessment

The restorative nurse begins the nursing process with a thorough assessment of the client upon admission to the setting. This includes a complete physical exam to identify current physical problems that may be related to the primary injury or disease, to comorbidities, or to complications during recovery (Figure 21-6). Problems such as skin breakdown, abnormal lung sounds, and peripheral edema can be detected. The restorative nurse does a very specific assessment of the client's functional ability, identifying both the abilities and limitations of self-care activities and mobility, the two areas most basic for restorative care.

A number of tests and scales can be used to formally assess functional ability. The value of using formal tests is the data is more consistent and reliable compared to data

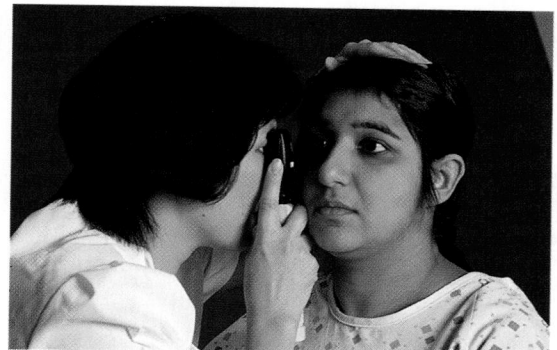

**Figure 21-6** Physical examination: the beginning of restorative care

from clinical observation. The two most widely used are the **Functional Independence Measurement (FIM)** and the **Barthel Index**. The FIM is a formal tool that evaluates an individual's ability to safely and independently perform ADL specific to self-care, sphincter control, transfers, locomotion, communication, and social cognition. The Barthel Index measures the ability of the client to perform in 10 domains of motor function for ADL (see Box 21-3).

## Nursing Diagnosis

The restorative care nurse analyzes the data and identifies nursing diagnoses. The nursing diagnosis names the client's actual or potential problem and identifies the causative factor or the risk factors. An example would be *Self-Care Deficit: Dressing/Grooming,* related to left hemiplegia, or *Walking, Impaired,* related to arthritis of the knee

---

**BOX 21-3 DOMAINS OF BARTHEL INDEX OF ACTIVITIES OF DAILY LIVING**

Feeding

Moving from wheelchair to bed and return

Personal grooming (wash face, comb hair, shave, brush teeth)

Bathing self

Dressing

Walking on level surface

Ascending and descending stairs

Controlling bowels

Controlling bladder

Adapted from Hoeman, S. (2002). *Rehabilitation nursing: Process, applications, & outcomes* (3rd ed.). Philadelphia, Pennsylvania: W. B. Saunders Co.

## LIFE SPAN CONSIDERATIONS

### Pediatric Assessment

Assessment of the child must be based on the principles of physical growth and human development. Development of skills is sequential and evaluation of developmental milestones is important when assessing a child's functional ability.

Estes, M. (2002). *Health assessment & physical examination* (2nd ed.). Clifton Park, NY: Delmar Learning.

## STOP AND THINK

### Functional and Cognitive Skills

- What functional skills does the client need to prepare a meal?

- What cognitive skills does the client need to safely move from a bed to a wheelchair?

- If your client wants to return to his work as an accountant, what functional and/or cognitive skills would he need?

joints (Figure 21-7). Box 21-4 lists examples of NANDA nursing diagnoses often used in restorative care (Ackley & Ladwig, 2002).

## Outcomes Identification

The restorative nurse can identify client goals from the nursing diagnoses. Accomplishment of the outcomes validates and quantifies the work of restorative nursing care. In addition, funding sources such as Medicare are now requiring documentation and evaluation of these outcomes (Gunderson, 2000). Generally the goals and outcomes for rehabilitation should be broken down into smaller steps so that a goal does not seem so overwhelming and progress can be better measured and appreciated.

## Plan of Care

Nursing interventions are selected that will enable the client to meet the outcomes of the plan. These include nursing actions of direct care as well as teaching and guiding the client and family in self-care. The plan of care is written so that the entire team, including the client and family, know the plan. Some institutions are using restorative care pathways that are specific to a common condi-

## RESEARCH FOCUS

**Title:** Functional performance and exercise of older adults in long-term care settings

**Study Purpose:** This study explored the variables that influence the functional performance and exercise activity in a group of nursing home residents.

**Methods:** This was a descriptive study with a convenience sample. Methods used included chart reviews; one-to-one interviews with residents, including pain scale; mini-mental-status exam; evaluation of functional performance using the Barthel Index with direct observation of the resident; and a self-efficacy test. Self-efficacy is an individual's belief in self-ability to perform a course of action to attain a desired outcome.

**Findings:** This group of residents was quite impaired functionally. Only 20% participated in a regular exercise program. There was no statistical correlation between medical condition and exercise or functional performance. Married women exercised more than widowed or single women. Pain if present was significant. In a regressive model, only self-efficacy and outcome expectations were statistically significant predictors of exercise behavior in the residents. There was a statistically significant relationship between perceived health status and functional performance and exercise behavior. Those who perceived themselves in better health were more likely to perform functional activities and to exercise regularly.

**Implications:** Interventions should be incorporated into a restorative nursing care program that focuses on strengthening self-efficacy and outcome expectations to ensure a successful program. It is important to teach residents and families the benefits of exercise and performing functional tasks. Nurses should identify specific goals for each resident, give verbal encouragement and positive reinforcement, and seek to decrease pain and fatigue barriers.

Resnick, B. (2000). Functional performance and exercise of older adults in long-term care settings. *Journal of Gerontological Nursing, 26*(3), 7–16.

tion, such as hip joint replacement. The interventions of all the disciplines are integrated. This helps keep the health care team focused on the time frame for client outcomes, which helps contain costs (Pearson, 2001; Cervizzi & Edwards, 1999). However, the pathway can be individualized to each client as needed.

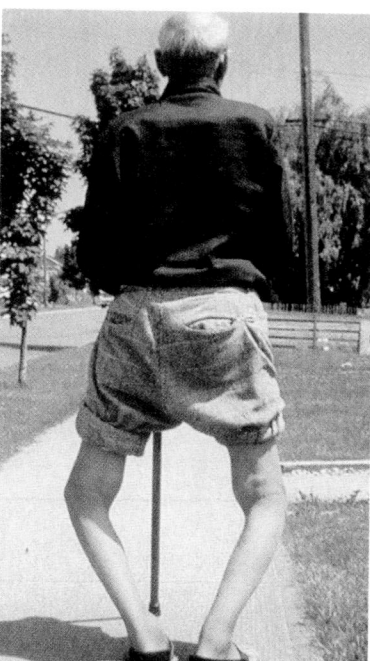

**Figure 21-7   A client with impaired walking related to arthritis of the knee joints**

## NURSING STRATEGY

### Client Independence

Too often nurses do "for the client." The goal of restorative nursing is to help the client be as independent as possible.

- Stryker described the importance of the nurse being "slow geared," meaning the nurse needs to be patient, allowing the client the time needed to accomplish the tasks himself (Chin et al., 1998).

- "Cueing" is used to teach the client the steps of a task. For example, in helping a client learn to safely transfer from the bed to a chair, cue the client by telling her: "Move to the edge of the bed, so that your feet are on the floor," "Grasp your walker and stand up," "Pivot on your left foot," "Place your hands on the chair arms," and "Lower yourself into the chair."

## Interventions

Numerous nursing interventions can be defined as restorative. Some are used daily with clients in all settings from ICU to home health care. Others are more specialized nursing

## BOX 21-4   NANDA DIAGNOSES FREQUENTLY USED IN RESTORATIVE CARE

Activity Intolerance

Disturbed Body Image

Disturbed Sensory Perception: Auditory or Visual

Caregiver Role Strain

Ineffective Coping

Bowel Incontinence

Impaired Physical Mobility

Impaired Urinary Elimination

Deficient Knowledge

Ineffective Therapeutic Regimen Management

Acute Pain

Chronic Pain

Self-Care Deficit

Situational Low Self-Esteem

Risk for Impaired Skin Integrity

Anticipatory Grieving

Spiritual Distress

Impaired Swallowing

Disturbed Thought Processes

Adapted from Ackley, B. J., & Ladwig, G. B. (2002). *Nursing diagnosis handbook: A guide to planning care.* (5th ed.). St. Louis: Mosby.

interventions in which the nurse may need additional training to apply them in complex client situations. Box 21-5 summarizes a partial list of the restorative nursing interventions. All of the nursing interventions and rationales can be taught to the client and caregiver.

Many interventions use assistive devices to help clients with their activities of daily living. For example, using a "reacher" or "pick-upper," a client can pick up items on the floor or from shelves that are beyond his reach (Figure 21-8). Other devices include Velcro instead of hooks or buttons on clothing and shoes, and tools for guiding the foot into a sock or shoe (Figure 21-9). Foam or Velcro grips can be put on toothbrushes or silverware to aid the client in holding the utensil, and plate guards can be attached to help keep food on the plate. There are shower sprays on long extensions so a client can sit while in the

## BOX 21-5    EXAMPLES OF RESTORATIVE NURSING INTERVENTIONS

Bowel and bladder training

Self-catheterization

Progressive mobility: safety issues, sitting balance, turning self in bed, transferring to chair or toilet, use of assistive aids

Assistive cough

Use of assistive devices for dressing, grooming, and eating

Skin checks and pressure relief activities

Self-administration of medications

Body positioning and support using pillows, splints

Safety issues and precautions for hip replacement surgery, prevention of aspiration, or sternum or spinal precautions

Sine, R., Liss, S. E., Roush, R. E., Holcomb, J. D., & Wilson, G. (2000). *Basic rehabilitation techniques* (4th ed.). Gaithersburg, MD: Aspen.

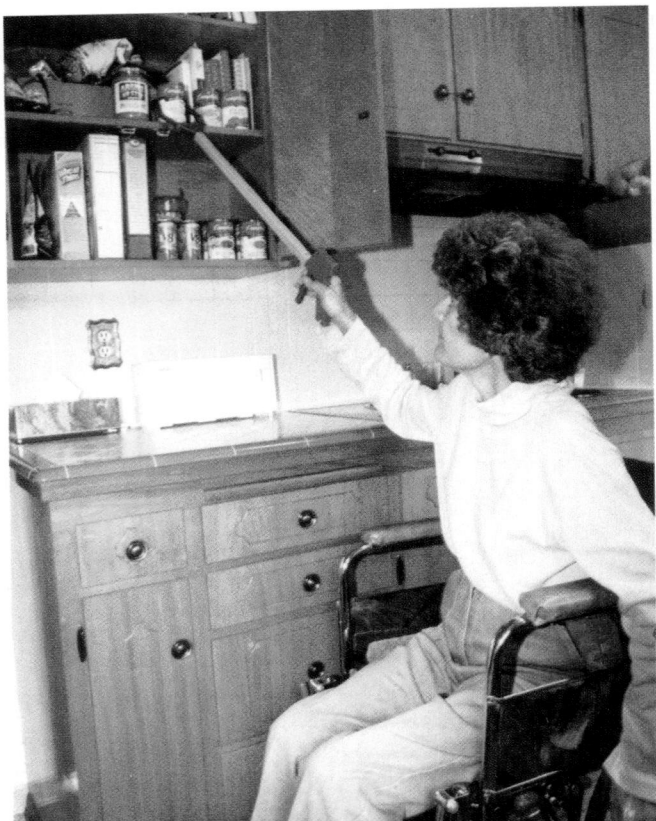

**Figure 21-8    The use of an assistive aid for out-of-reach items**

shower, bath and shower seats, safety bars that can be installed, and sliding boards used in transfers between the bed and wheelchair. Several kinds of walkers and canes help clients maintain balance.

## Documentation

Computer-generated charting systems are being designed for restorative care, using nursing diagnoses and outcomes that focus on the functional skills of the client (Cervizzi, 1999). The Minimum Data Set—Post Acute Care (MDS-PAC) is an eight-page form required by Medicare that evaluates the client's functional ability on days 4, 11, 31, and 61. It includes documentation of interventions and achievement of outcomes in detail (Bianchi, 2001).

## Evaluation and Revision of the Plan of Care

Because progress of the restorative care client is slower, evaluation and revision of the plan of care may be done only every 3 to 7 days. Ideally, the entire interdisciplinary team should evaluate the care plan and the client's progress together. The client and family should also be included. A weekly care conference enables everyone to hear information and feedback from each team member

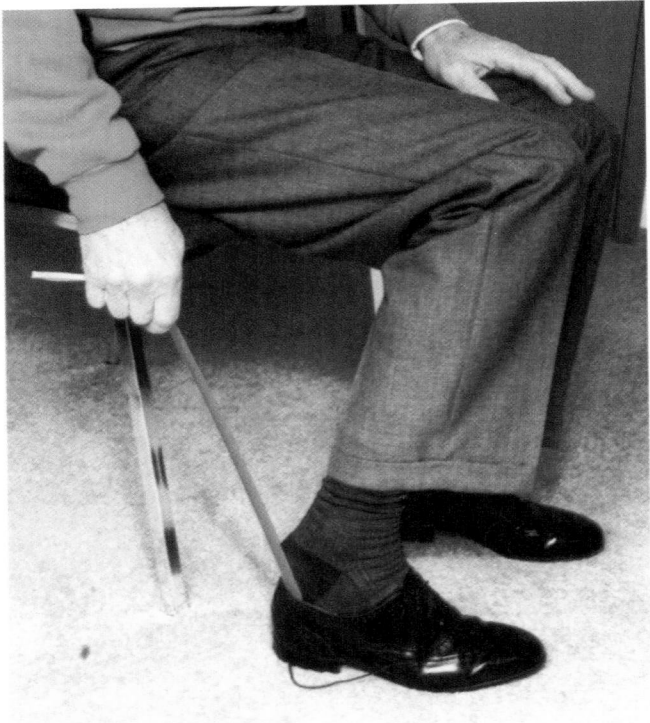

**Figure 21-9    Assistive aid for dressing**

## CLINICAL ALERT

### Unilateral Neglect

The client who has experienced a stroke with hemiplegia may have unilateral neglect, meaning he is unaware of the paralyzed limb. He may lie on it or bang it against a side rail, developing bruises or skin pressure areas. The client must be taught to support the arm and position it correctly. When up out of bed, the client must learn to put the arm in a sling to prevent subluxation of the arm from the shoulder joint.

and the client. Questions can be readily addressed, and changes to the goals and plan can be mutually agreed on.

## Transitions Between Care Settings: Discharge Planning

Ultimately, the entire interdisciplinary team focuses on discharge planning, but the social worker and the nurse have the greatest share of the responsibility. The social worker has an extensive knowledge of facilities and services available in the community. The nurse has an intimate knowledge of the client's functional ability, cognitive and perceptual skills, and her understanding of the rationale for self-care skills. Working together with the client and family, the nurse and social worker do the majority of the assessment and planning for the transition to either a care facility or the home setting.

When planning for a client's discharge to another care facility, the nurse needs to prepare a written care plan that is sent with the client. But it is also helpful to discuss the plan by phone with the nurse in the new setting. The client's current functional abilities in relation to transfers, fatigue level, knowledge and performance of self-care skills, and judgment and safety issues are important information needed by the nurse in the new setting. Further information about family members or issues, and areas needing further instruction, is also important.

## Preparation of the Client and Family

Regardless of what type of setting the client is transitioning to, the client and family experience a marked increase in anxiety. This is true even if the transition is done because the client has significantly improved. A transition to a new setting means loss of relationships with the current health team members and loss of a familiar routine. Uncertainty about the new environment

and what is required and learning to trust the new health team members may be issues. Concerns about the ultimate prognosis for recovery may add to the stress. The transition is even more difficult for those who are cognitively impaired or have an altered level of consciousness. Many older clients experience heightened confusion with a change of surroundings. This increased anxiety and confusion during transition is termed **Relocation Stress Syndrome**.

### Caregiver Strain

Careful discharge planning must be done when the restorative client is returning home. One of the problems causing unsuccessful transition to home occurs when a family member is unprepared or unwilling to be the caregiver. Another problem can be poor adaptation of the restorative skills to everyday life in the home setting (Alexander, Hiduke, & Stevens, 1999). Both the client and caregiver family members may feel very overwhelmed by the responsibility for safe, competent care. The nursing diagnosis *Risk for Caregiver Role Strain* is an important issue when planning a discharge home (Ackley & Ladwig, 2002). When the client is decreased significantly in functional ability and requires assistance in a multitude of ADL, the caregiver may experience signs and symptoms of strain. These include apprehension, fatigue, isolation, frustration, and depression. This is compounded even more in the elderly caregiver who often has a number of his own health issues and functional limitations. The impact of the disease and the anxiety of the transition may impair the memory and learning skills of both client and family. Medications may further impact the memory and learning skills of the client.

## Home Health Nursing and Restorative Care

Home health nursing care is extremely important for many clients to have a successful transition from facility to home. The home health nurse often comes to the inpatient setting to do an initial assessment. If this is not the case, the client's current nurse needs to do a careful written referral. Often this is followed by a phone call discussing issues in greater detail. The inpatient nurse must teach the client and caregiver the medication schedule, self-care skills such as transfers, and nursing care such as dressing changes. The inpatient nurse must be sure the client and caregiver understand the skills correctly and have the opportunity to practice and redemonstrate the skill. Planning for assistive equipment such as a hospital bed, walkers, raised toilet seats, and other assistive equipment is best done before discharge so that the equipment is available the first day home. In addition, important factors to assess are potential physical barriers to entry, wheelchair barriers, need for assistive devices, and safety issues.

## CLIENT EDUCATION

### PEG Feeding Instructions to Present to the Client for Intermittent Gravity Feeding

✓ Check for residual by pulling back on catheter-tip syringe.

✓ If 50 cc or less residual, pour 500 cc feeding solution into the feeding bag and administer by gravity at approximately 80 drops per minute over 15 to 20 minutes. Be sure you are sitting up at a 30-degree angle or higher during the feeding.

✓ As soon as feeding solution is done, flush PEG tube with 30 cc cool tap water and clamp tube. Remain with head up at 30 degrees or more for 30 minutes. Rinse feeding bag in soapy water and thoroughly rinse. Hang open to dry until next feeding.

✓ Clean PEG tube skin site each day with hydrogen peroxide diluted half and half with tap water, rinse with water, and pat dry. A dry dressing may be applied if you wish.

✓ If drainage or skin redness appear at the site, contact your home health nurse.

Alexander, T. T., Hiduke, R. J., & Stevens, K. A. (1999). *Rehabilitation nursing procedures manual* (2nd ed.). New York: McGraw-Hill.

## Case Management and Restorative Care

Continuity of care for the restorative client is a nursing goal in all types of settings. One of the most effective ways of accomplishing this is through **case management**. Case management as defined by Mullahy is "a collaborative process which assesses, plans, implements, coordinates, monitors, and evaluates the options and services to meet an individual's health needs, using communication and available resources to promote quality, cost-effective outcomes" (Mullahy, 1995, p. 5). Case management particularly lends itself to rehabilitation clients with complex long-term needs. The case management role is usually done by a certified rehabilitation nurse (CRRN) or by an advanced practice rehabilitation nurse. The role may be within one institution, coordinating various levels of care from ICU to acute care through a referral to a subacute facility. Case management may also be an external role across multiple health care settings. A case example would be a client injured in a motor vehicle accident resulting in L 2 paraplegia. The case manager could begin with the

## BOX 21-6    CURRENT AND FUTURE TRENDS IN RESTORATIVE NURSING

1. The biggest current challenge to restorative care is the impact of managed care and decreased coverage by third-party payers and Medicare.

2. Restorative care teams are challenged to give cost-effective yet individualized high-quality care and education to clients and their families.

3. Residents in long-term care facilities are greatly impacted by the fact that Medicare changed the way payment is done for restorative care in long-term care facilities.

4. Beginning in April, 2001, Medicare also changed the financing of intensive inpatient rehabilitation to a prospective payment service (PPS) system.

5. The current changes in funding for restorative care by Medicare is partly in anticipation of the huge demographic change in the elderly population, with the large baby-boomer population rapidly reaching age.

6. Therefore, restorative nurses need to design evidence-based nursing studies that prove restorative care nursing produces quality outcomes (Thorne, 2000). Furthermore, there is a need to design innovative models of care that can meet the demand for quality of care and cost-effectiveness (Dean-Barr, 1998).

7. Another challenge for restorative care is the increasing shortage of nurses, especially those with strong rehabilitation nursing skills.

8. Also, there is high turnover and low staffing levels of unlicensed nursing aides especially in subacute and long-term care.

9. Restorative care can benefit from the use of electronic-health through the Web by both clients and by nurses. Also, LISTSERV discussions by e-mail can help clients who share common problems (Buhrer, 2001).

client's admission to ICU and the stabilization of the spinal cord injury. The case manager would help in the transition of the client to a medical unit in acute care and the transfer to an intensive rehabilitation setting in the community. Finally, the case manager will coordinate the community services and equipment needed for the client to return home.

## Quality Improvement Issues in Restorative Care

Quality improvement as related to nursing care is evaluated by professional standards of care published by the Association of Rehabilitation Nurses. Nursing care is also evaluated by whether it is based on the scientific knowledge and principles outlined in current nursing texts and journals, whether the client meets the outcomes stated in the care plan, and client satisfaction. Quality improvement in today's health care environment must also incorporate cost-effectiveness. Cost-effectiveness is defined as outcomes that are met at a reasonable cost (Tappen, 2001). The cost for restorative care has multiplied many times in the last 10 years, especially as the number of older adults has increased. Both Medicare and third-party payers are demanding evidence that restorative nursing makes a difference (see Box 21-6). To contain costs, most providers have moved to an increased emphasis on patient outcomes as measures of treatment effectiveness (Gunderson, 2000).

# CASE STUDY/NURSING CARE PLAN

Mrs. Abernathy, a 79-year-old woman, was admitted to the ICU following an automobile accident. Her injuries upon admission included a pneumothorax and fractured right hip. She was confused at times. She was quickly stabilized with a chest tube and was taken to surgery the next day for an open reduction and internal fixation of her fractured hip. After surgery, she was admitted to the postsurgical nursing unit where her chest tube was removed and her lung fully expanded. Six days post surgery, she was transferred to a rehabilitation unit. Her hip incision was healing and physical therapy was attempting to teach her hip precautions and gait training using a walker. However, she was periodically confused with a short-term memory deficit, making it difficult for her to remember instructions. Prior to the accident, she had no history of confusion or memory loss.

Discharge planning had begun the day of surgery. Mrs. Abernathy lived with her husband, who was 83 years old and had a history of stroke with left-sided hemiplegia. Their home was single story with four steps to gain entry. Neither Mr. or Mrs. Abernathy drove any longer. Because clients with this type of surgery need continued physical therapy and because Mrs. Abernathy was frail and tired easily, it was evident that the first transition needed to be to a subacute facility that could meet her needs for convalescence and physical therapy. On admission to the subacute facility, the nurse followed the nursing process to establish a plan of care.

### Assessment
Mrs. Abernathy was fully recovered from the pneumothorax with normal breath sounds and an oxygen saturation of 92% on room air. She was recovering from hip surgery and had some pain during therapy sessions, was weak with balance problems, and periodically was confused; her short-term memory was also impaired, making it difficult for her to remember instructions.

### Nursing Diagnosis #1
*Impaired Physical Mobility* related to auto accident.
**NOC:** Ambulation; Walking; Joint Movement: Active; Mobility Level; Self-Care; Activities Of Daily Living; Transfer Performance
**NIC:** Exercise Therapy; Ambulation; Joint Mobility; Positioning

### Expected Outcomes
The client will:
1. Walk at least 50 feet in hallway with walker or cane by the end of the month.
2. Safely ascend and descend steps using an assistive device correctly by the end of the month.

*(continues)*

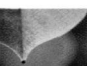

# CASE STUDY/NURSING CARE PLAN (continued)

## Planning/Interventions/Rationales
1. Give positive reinforcement during activity. *Promotes motivation and encouragement.*
2. Provide for periods of rest between therapy sessions. *Prevents fatigue and will enhance benefit of therapy.*
3. Medicate adequately for pain prior to therapy. *Makes it easier for client to bear weight and move.*
4. Walk client at least once on evening shift (physical therapy sessions are in the morning and afternoon). *Increases muscle strength and opportunity to reinforce skills learned in therapy.*

## Evaluation
Mrs. Abernathy walked two blocks safely. However, she was not safe going up and down stairs unless a person was there to "cue" her. There was no longer a fatigue problem if she took a nap each afternoon. Her pain was now controlled with two acetaminophen twice a day.

## Nursing Diagnosis #2
*Impaired Memory* related to auto accident.
**NOC:** Cognitive Orientation; Neurological Status: Consciousness; Memory
**NIC:** Memory Training

## Expected Outcomes
The client will:
1. Remember to take medications on the correct schedule by the end of the month.
2. Remember and follow instructions for hip precautions, and use the walker correctly on the stairs by the end of the month.

## Planning/Interventions/Rationales
1. Assess for depression or anxiety, which may contribute to memory loss. *Memory loss in older adults may be affected by depression, anxiety, and change of familiar surroundings.*
2. Provide alternative ways to help patient with memory loss, such as a time schedule written on a large piece of paper hung on the wall and a written medication schedule. *Written or pictorial language "cues" may help focus the client's memory more than verbal instructions.*
3. Frequently reorient client to surroundings, schedule and instructions. *Change of surroundings may cause confusion in older adults.*
4. Keep environment quiet with few distractions. *Distractions make it difficult to focus.*
5. Instruct and reinforce hip precautions. *Prevent hip dislocation during the healing process.*

## Evaluation
After weeks at home, Mr. Abernathy felt knowledgeable and confident in his role as caregiver. The community support services for home health aides and meals have been very satisfactory. Mrs. Abernathy is nearly independent now except for needing her walker on stairs. Since returning home, her short-term memory has returned to normal.

## Key Concepts

- Restorative nursing care is the process of teaching the client and caregiver the knowledge, rationale, and skills of self-care activities that will maximize the client's functional ability.
- Historically, restorative nursing care has developed as the process of teaching the client and caregiver the knowledge, rationale, and skills of self-care activities that will maximize the client's functional ability.
- Whether defined as disability, impairment, handicap, or functional impairment, the goal of rehabilitation is to prevent further deterioration or complications and to aid the client in recovering functional ability and resuming his life roles again.
- Restorative care settings have designed partnerships and alliances between types of facilities to return the client to the community in as cost-effective a way as possible.

- All age groups experience a wide variety of acute or chronic conditions which may require restorative care.
- The acuity level of restorative care classifies where the client is on the care continuum from being highly dependent on complex nursing care to being independent in self-care.
- Restorative nurses recognize the emphasis on self-care, overcoming deficits, independence, self-esteem, worth of the client, and the importance of client education as theorized in the Orem model.
- The client's right to become the expert in her own health care is a unique philosophy that focuses on self-care and independence in restorative nursing care.
- The nursing process in restorative nursing is integrated into the work of the interdisciplinary team, offering a more holistic view of the client.
- The nursing process is an organized, systematic process that is continual and ongoing throughout the rehabilitation process as the client adapts and his functional ability changes.
- Discharge planning must be initiated early in the nursing process by the entire interdisciplinary team, but the greatest share of the responsibility falls on the social worker and the nurse.
- Quality improvement in restorative care is evaluated by professional standards, current scientific knowledge, client outcomes, and cost-effectiveness.

## Review Questions and Activities

1. Describe the principles of restorative care and how they would impact the nursing care you are giving to your client.
2. What are some frequent comorbidities found in older adults that complicate their progress in restorative care?
3. Describe how Orem's self-care model applies to the restorative care client.
4. Describe the seven roles of the restorative care nurse.
5. Describe how assessment of the restorative care client differs from that of the acute care client.
6. Explain the Functional Instrument of Measurement and the Barthel Index.
7. You are doing discharge planning for a client who will leave the acute care hospital soon. The client had a stroke with left-sided weakness, poor balance, and inability to transfer to the commode without a two-person assist. The wife wants the client to come home, believing she can take care of him. What concerns would you discuss with the wife? What recommendations would you make?
8. Discuss how relocation to a different setting can be stressful to a client and her family.
9. What is the most important issue impacting restorative care today and in the future? Explain your answer.

## Web Resources

Association of Rehabilitation Nursing
http://www.rehabnurse.org
Cardiac Rehabilitation Program
http://www.holycrosshealth.org
Community Resources for Rehabilitation
http://www.contactdelaware.org
Medical Equipment for Rehabilitation Nursing
http://www.visionq.com
Rehabilitation Nursing
http://www.nursingspectrum.com

## References

Ackley, B. J., & Ladwig, G. B. (2002). *Nursing diagnosis handbook: A guide to planning care* (5th ed.). St. Louis: Mosby.

Alexander, T. T., Hiduke, R. J., & Stevens, K. A. (1999). *Rehabilitation nursing procedures manual.* (2nd ed.). New York: McGraw-Hill.

American Nurses Association & Association of Rehabilitation Nurses (1988). *Rehabilitation nursing: Scope of practice: process and outcome criteria for selected diagnoses.* Kansas City, MO: Author.

Bianchi, B. (2001). Understanding the proposed rules for acute rehabilitation prospective payment. *Rehabilitation Nursing, 26*(2), 44–50.

Black, T. (1999). Outcomes: What's all the fuss about? *Rehabilitation Nursing, 24*(5), 188–191.

Bonder, B. R., & Wagner, M. B. (2001). *Functional performance in older adults.* (2nd ed.). Philadelphia: F. A. Davis Co.

Buhrer, R. (2001). "E-health and rehabilitation nursing." *Rehabilitation Nursing, 26*(4), 128.

Cervizzi, K., & Edwards, P. A. (1999). Where is rehabilitation nursing documentation going? *Rehabilitation Nursing, 24*(3), 92.

Chin, P. S., Finocchiaro, D., & Rosebrough, A. (1998). *Rehabilitation nursing practice.* New York: McGraw-Hill.

Dean-Barr (1998). "Our vision for the future." *Rehabilitation Nursing, 23*(1), 6.

Derstine, J. B., & Hargrove, S. D. (2001). *Comprehensive rehabilitation nursing.* Philadelphia: Saunders.

Estes, M. (2002). *Health assessment & physical examination* (2nd ed.). Clifton Park, NY: Delmar Learning.

Grove, N. C., & Spier, B. E. (1999). Motivating the well elderly to exercise. *Journal of Community Health Nursing, 16*(3), 179–188.

Gunderson, A. (2000). Tertiary care: A changing environment. *Rehabilitation Nursing, 25*(5), 164–166.

Hoeman, S. (2002). *Rehabilitation nursing: Process, applications, & outcomes* (3rd. ed.). Philadelphia, Pennsylvania: W. B. Saunders Co.

Hogstel, M. (2001). Gerontology: Nursing care of the older adult. Clifton Park, NY: Delmar Learning.

Michael, K. (2001). A case for rehabilitation in palliative care. *Rehabilitation Nursing, 26*(3), 84.

Mullahy, C. M. (1995). *The case manager's handbook.* Rockville, MD: Aspen.

Neal, L. J. (1999). Research supporting the congruence between rehabilitation principles and home health nursing practice. *Rehabilitation Nursing, 24*(3), 115–121.

Neufeldt, V. (Ed.). (2001). *Webster's new world dictionary.* (5th college ed.). New York: Prentice-Hall.

Nightingale, F. (1859). *Notes on nursing: What it is, and what it is not.* London: Harrison & Sons.

Orem, D. (1995). *Nursing concepts of practice* (5th ed.). New York: McGraw-Hill.

Pearson, J. S. (2001). Extending a rehabilitation pathway to include multiple providers: Outcomes and pitfalls. *Rehabilitation Nursing, 26*(2), 54–57.

Resnick, B. (2000). Functional performance and exercise of older adults in long-term care settings. *Journal of Gerontological Nursing, 26*(3), 7–16.

Sine, R., Liss, S. E., Roush, R. E., Holcomb, J. D., & Wilson, G. (2000). *Basic rehabilitation techniques* (4th ed.). Gaithersburg, MD: Aspen.

Tappen, R. M. (2001). *Nursing leadership and management: Concepts and practice.* (4th ed.). Philadelphia: F. A. Davis.

Tellis-Nayak, M. (1998). The postacute continuum of care: Understanding your patient's options. *American Journal of Nursing, 98*(8), 44–48.

Thorne, S. (2000). Neurological rehabilitation nursing: A review of the research. *Journal of Advanced Nursing, 31*(5), 1029–1038.

Warner, P. M. & Hutchinson, C. (1999). Heart failure management. *Journal of Nursing Administration, 29*(7/8), 28–37.

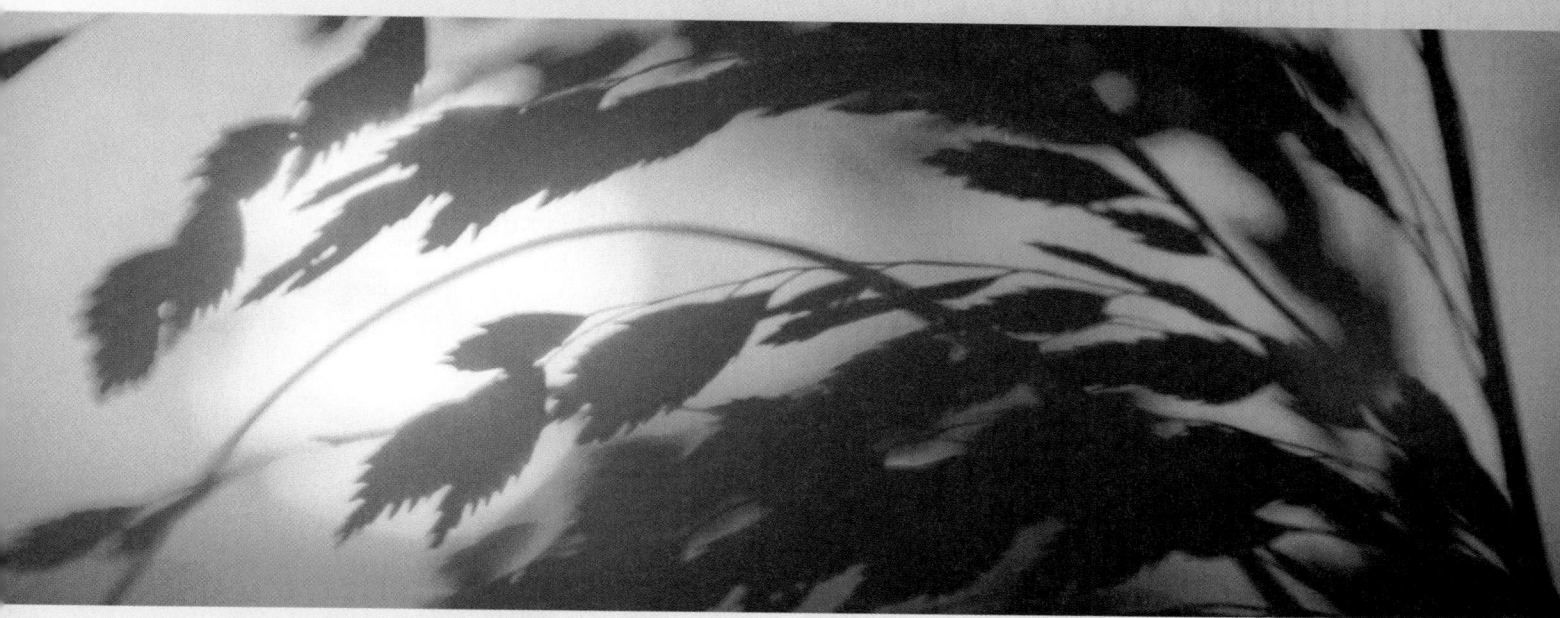

# CHAPTER 22

# Home Care

Valerie Lindquist Stalsbroten, RN, MN

*"Nursing is love in action, and there is no finer manifestation of it than the care of the poor and disabled in their own homes."*

(Lillian Wald)

# Chapter Competencies

*Upon completion of this chapter, the reader should be able to:*

1. Define home health care.
2. Identify the highlights in the history of home health nursing.
3. Describe the types of home health agencies, the services they offer, and the funding considerations for home health organizations.
4. Analyze the Medicare constraints on home care.
5. Apply the nursing process (i.e., assessment, nursing diagnoses, planning/intervention, evaluation) to care of the client in the home.
6. Evaluate the critical issues of home health care and the concepts of hospice care.
7. Discuss the safety and occupational hazards dimensions applicable to the home care setting.

# Key Terms

Conditions of Participation (COPs)
home health agencies
home health care
home health care nursing
hospice

Medicare certified
nonprofit agencies
Outcome and Assessment Information Set (OASIS)
Outcome Based Quality Improvement (OBQI)

palliative care
proprietary agencies
prospective payment system (PPS)
telehealth

Home health care began as a service addressing the needs of women and children in poverty, because morbidity and mortality were so high. Lack of knowledge, malnutrition, poor living conditions, and limited access to care contributed to these problems (Rosen, 1958). The value of home health care continued to be evident as visiting nursing expanded from crowded cities to rural areas serving young and old alike. In 1965, Medicare introduced home health care benefits for all recipients, not just for the elderly poor. Attending to people's health care needs in their homes has significantly affected the outcomes of clients' health throughout the age spectrum and for all income levels.

Emphasis has always been on improving the environment, teaching and training clients and caregivers, coordinating care, and collaborating with community services. A specific body of nursing knowledge is needed to have a positive impact on clients and families.

## Evolution of Home Health Care Nursing

**Home health care** is an organized, nonphysician health service provided by professionals to clients in their homes (Vladeck, 2000). Services can include nursing care, physical therapy, speech therapy, occupational therapy, nutri-

tional counseling, and medical social work. **Home health care nursing** has evolved over the years (Table 1-1 in Chapter 1) and is a subspecialty of community health nursing and can be offered to a variety of clients throughout the age spectrum. The main focus of home health care nursing is that of health restoration and promotion, whereas **hospice** nursing provides holistic care to terminal clients when cure is not a possibility. Rather, palliation of symptoms and quality of life issues are the primary goals of hospice care (Milone-Nuzzo, 2000).

## Medicare Legislation

With the implementation of Medicare benefits in 1965 as part of the Social Security Act, home health services became available to qualified elderly in their homes, not just the poor. In 1973, this benefit was extended to certain younger recipients with disabilities (National Association of Home Care [NAHC], 2001). Home health agencies were no longer dependent on donations to provide needed care. The evolution of home health in the United States has also been linked to the Medicare requirements, or **Conditions of Participation (COPs)**. This legislation impacted who could receive care and the payment system for that care. Since the first established rules and regulations, Medicare home health recipients must be homebound and require skilled services on an intermittent basis (Vladeck, 2000). The emphasis in home health nursing shifted from a predominance of mother-child recipients to the frail elderly.

### Prospective Payment System (PPS)

In 1983, further changes were made to the way Medicare reimbursed hospitals for inpatient stays. The introduction of the **prospective payment system (PPS)** paid hospitals according to the client's diagnosis, or diagnosis-related groups (DRGs), instead of the number of hospital days spent in the facility. Consequently, hospitals had more incentive to discharge clients early and refer them to home care for further follow-up. However, the states and the federal government tried to contain the costs for home care, denying reimbursement in many cases, and creating a growing number of frail elderly with limited financial circumstances in need of home care. The unmet needs were burgeoning, and Federal District Judge Stanley Sporkin ruled in a case entitled *Duggan v. Bowen* in 1988 (National Association for Home Care and Hospice, 2003) that the Health Care Financing Administration (HCFA) had abused its authority and violated the intent of the home care benefit. HCFA controls were loosened (Vladeck, 2000). As a result of this ruling, there was exponential growth in the home care industry. By 1997, the Medicare home care benefit again seemed to be spiraling out of control. Congress enacted the Balanced Budget Act (BBA), effectively resulting in a decrease in the number of Medicare beneficiaries served and a decrease in the overall number of visits per beneficiary. This paved the way for instituting a PPS reimbursement model to be applied to home health agencies (Vladeck, 2000). In addition, the HCFA transitioned to the Center for Medicare & Medicaid Services (CMS).

### Outcome and Assessment Information Set (OASIS)

A method to systematically collect data on client assessment, care planning, quality monitoring, and reimbursement was instituted in 2000. The **Outcome and Assessment Information Set (OASIS)** provides a consistent way to collect needed information on all Medicare home health beneficiaries. Data is collected electronically from all Medicare-certified agencies and is used to provide a foundation for **Outcome Based Quality Improvement (OBQI)**, a process to increase quality care and determine which services are contributing (or not contributing) to the outcomes of care (Vladeck, 2000).

### Other Reimbursement Sources

Medicare has become the largest single payer of home care services. Other public funding sources for home care include Medicaid, the Older Americans Act, Title XX Social Services Block Grants, the Veterans' Administration, and TRICARE (the military health system formerly known as the Civilian Health and Medical Program of the Uniformed Services, or CHAMPUS). Private insurance and individual out-of-pocket payments account for the large majority of other funding resources (National Association of Home Care [NAHC], 2001).

## Home Health Agencies and Organizations

Home health agencies, home care aide organizations, and hospices are known collectively as "home care organizations." **Home health agencies** (organizations that provide services utilizing health professionals in an individual's place of residence) and hospices provide skilled care through registered professionals. The home care aide organizations provide supportive care, such as attendant care, companionship, homemaking, shopping, and other types of assistance with activities of daily living (ADLs) that do not qualify as "skilled" care. Respiratory services, home medical equipment, and nutrition counseling are other areas of home health services (NAHC, 2001).

### Types of Agencies Described by Credentials

Three distinct credentials indicate an agency's compliance with specific standards set by the state, federal government, or an independent accrediting agency. First, a home care organization can seek licensure from the state, which differs from state to state. Issues such as staffing, policies, and procedures are addressed with licensure. The purpose is to ensure minimal standards are being observed by the agency. In states with these regulations, an agency cannot operate without a license. Not all states require licensure (Milone-Nuzzo, 2000).

Second, to receive funding from the Medicare program, an agency must be **Medicare certified**. This process requires that Medicare representatives visit the agency to survey charts, policies, procedures, billing practices, qualifications of care providers, and administrative structure. Since Medicare is a federally administered program, the same requirements are imposed on all Medicare-certified agencies in all states. In order to guarantee a specific standard, many insurance companies specify that they cooperate only with Medicare-certified agencies.

Third, the Joint Commission on Accreditation of Healthcare Organizations (JCAHO) and the Community Health Accreditation Program (CHAP) are the two accrediting agencies in the United States recognized by the federal government. Because the JCAHO and CHAP accreditation standards of excellence are more stringent than even the Medicare certification requirements, these two organizations have been given "deeming authority" by the federal government. Since the JCAHO and CHAP have deeming authority, the agency can consolidate the certification process and the accreditation procedures into a single inspection (accreditation from JCAHO and CHAP, 2002).

## Various Types of Home Care Organizations

Home health agencies can be described by type of administration and tax status. Historically, the first types of organizations that used trained nurses to administer home care (usually to the poor) were voluntary agencies financed by concerned citizens. These agencies became the **nonprofit agencies** and have a tax-exempt status. In order to be considered nonprofit, any income that appears to be in excess of operating costs must be reinvested in the agency—providing staff education, funding unreimbursed care, and making capital improvements. In addition, public, government, or official agencies provide home care that is supported by state and/or federal tax dollars. These agencies can include health departments. With the increase in home care, more private, **proprietary agencies** began to arise. These agencies were not tax-exempt, and profits did not have to be reinvested into the agency but could be used to reward investors. Finally, some hospitals and institutions began to provide care as an extension of the inpatient experience. These institution-based or hospital-based agencies may be serving a particular client population in a certain geographic area or those with a particular type of health insurance. They could be either nonprofit or proprietary in nature, depending on the parent institution. In addition, home care organizations offer a variety of services as shown in Table 22-1.

## Personnel Working in Home Care Environments

There are a variety of personnel types who work in home care environments. The categories of personnel are skilled services, nursing services, physical therapy services, speech therapy services, occupational therapy services, medical social worker services, and home health aide services.

### Skilled Services

Skilled services are delivered by a professional, licensed health care provider in the areas of nursing, physical therapy, occupational therapy, speech therapy, nutrition counseling, and medical social work. Under Medicare guidelines, certain skilled services can be the primary provider of services, able to "open" a case by initially assessing the client, establishing a plan of care, and subsequently supervising home care aides.

### Nursing Services

Nursing services (RN/LPN) include observation and assessment, teaching and training, performing direct

| TABLE 22-1    TYPES OF HOME CARE ORGANIZATIONS | |
| --- | --- |
| **Home Care Organization** | **Services Provided** |
| Home health | Health professionals under the direction of physician's orders. The professional services can include skilled nursing, physical therapy, occupational therapy, speech therapy, nutritional counseling, and social work. Home care aides and physical therapy assistants may be supervised by the health care professionals. |
| Hospice | Meets the needs of clients with terminal illnesses and limited life expectancies with an interdisciplinary team. The focus is on relieving pain, managing other physical symptoms, and meeting psycho-socio-spiritual needs. Bereavement care and grief support groups are often available to the caregivers following the client's death. |
| Home care aides | Provides the ADL care that does not require skilled nursing services, such as attendant care, homemaking, companionship, and shopping. |
| Private duty | Provides nursing and attendant care for significant periods of time, up to 24-hour continuous care. |
| Home medical equipment | Provides various types of equipment in the home. Equipment includes such things as electric beds, bathroom devices, oxygen delivery systems, respirators, phototherapy, and infusion therapy. |

Compiled from Milone-Nuzzo, P. (2000). Home health care. In C. Smith & F. Maurer (Eds.), *Community health nursing: Theory and practice* (2nd edition, pp. 842–869). Philadelphia: W. B. Saunders Company; NAHC (2001), http://www.nahc.org

skilled procedures, and management and supervision of the client's care. Skilled nursing includes both registered nurses (RNs) and licensed practical nurses (LPNs), but only the RN can "open" a case by being the nurse to assess the client and initiate a plan of care. The nurse may be the primary care provider in the home for Medicare purposes (NAHC, 2001).

## Physical Therapy (PT) Services

Physical therapy (PT) services concentrate on gait training and improving the mobility of large muscle groups. Joint and muscle pain can be addressed. The physical therapist may be the primary discipline in the home for Medicare purposes.

## Speech Therapy (ST) Services

Speech therapy (ST) services address the needs of clients who have difficulty with communication and swallowing. The speech therapist may be the primary discipline in the home.

## Occupational Therapy (OT) Services

Occupational therapy (OT) services concentrate on the fine motor movements and assist with managing ADL. Some occupational therapists are able to assist with swallowing difficulties. Adaptive equipment may be recommended by the occupational therapist. According to Medicare guidelines, the OT is not the primary care provider to "open" a case, but may continue as the only skilled care provider to supervise aides after other skilled services (RN, PT, ST) have established and completed their plan of care (NAHC, 2001).

## Medical Social Workers (MSW) Services

Medical social workers (MSW) services assist clients with accessing community services, financial services, and mental health services. The MSW can be a valuable resource in helping the client and caregivers to adjust to the physical, emotional, social, and financial challenges of an illness.

## Home Health Aide/Home Care Aide (HHA/HCA) Services

Home health aide/home care aide (HHA/HCA) services provide a variety of care interventions, depending on the level of training (Figure 22-1). Skilled services provide supervision for the HCA to be in the home. The three levels and responsibilities of home care aides are shown in Table 22-2.

## Hospice Care

The term *hospice* comes from the same root word as *hospitality* and was originally associated with a refreshing resting place for weary travelers. Today this term means a

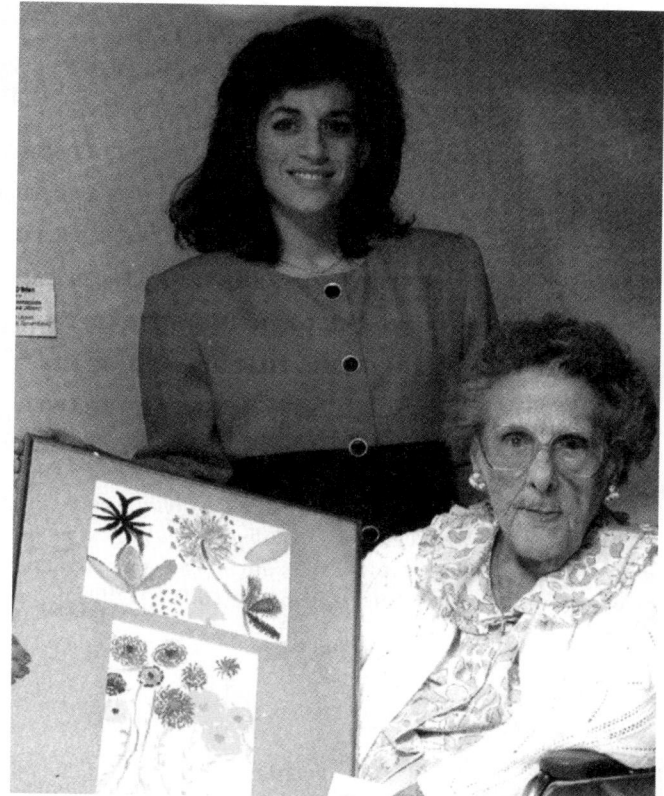

**Figure 22-1    Home health aide supporting client through caring activities**

| TABLE 22-2 | HOME CARE AIDES AND THEIR RESPONSIBILITIES |
|---|---|
| Level of Home Care Aide | Responsibilities |
| Home Care Aide | Assists with providing a safe home environment, but does not perform personal care for the client. |
| Home Care Aide II | Provides basic personal care such as bathing and ambulating. The HCA II cannot administer medications or provide wound care. |
| Home Care Aide III | Assists clients with medications, apply simple, nonsterile dressings, and continue with a rehabilitation plan that can include exercises. Certification is possible, and Medicare requires that all aide services are performed by an HCA III. |

NAHC, 2001. http://www.nahc.org

concept of care that provides comfort and quality of life to clients, and their significant others, who are facing life's final journey associated with terminal illness. The modern hospice movement was started by Dr. Cecily Saunders at St. Christopher's Hospice near London in 1967. The movement in the United States started as a home care program in New Haven, Connecticut, in 1974. Hospice is a concept of care for clients and their families who are facing end-of-life issues. Emphasis is on non-curative care, offering alternatives to aggressive therapeutic regimens. This type of care can be provided in any setting the client chooses, and offers a continuum of palliative and supportive services. Approximately 80% of hospice care is administered in homes or nursing homes. An interdisciplinary team addresses medical, psychosocial, and spiritual issues. There is a commitment to aftercare and bereavement services. Trained volunteers are an integral part of hospice care, helping to prevent caregiver burnout, providing respite care, and assisting with the grieving process (Hospice services, 2003; Williams & Wheeler, 2001).

## Palliative Care

**Palliative care** is slightly different from hospice care in that it emphasizes relief of physical symptoms when a cure for the underlying disease is not possible. These symptoms (Box 22-1) may or may not be part of an imminent terminal phase of the disease. In addition, the nursing care for clients during palliative care requires good problem-solving skills and sound judgment on the part of the nurse (see Box 22-2).

---

### BOX 22-1    PALLIATIVE CARE

The 10 most common symptoms during palliative care:

- Pain
- Easy fatigue
- Weakness
- Anorexia
- More than 10% of weight loss
- Lack of energy
- Dry mouth
- Constipation
- Dyspnea
- Early satiety

Hospice services, 2003, http://www.hospicefoundation.org

---

### BOX 22-2    PALLIATIVE CARE

*World Health Organization (WHO) Description of Palliative Care Focus:*

- Affirms life and regards dying as a normal process
- Neither hastens nor postpones death
- Provides relief from pain and other distressing symptoms
- Integrates the psychological and the spiritual aspects of care
- Offers a support system to help clients live as actively as possible until death
- Offers a support system to help the family cope during the client's illness and in their own bereavement

Williams, M. A., & Wheeler, M. S. (2001). Palliative care: What is it? *Home Healthcare Nurse, 19*(9).

---

# Home Care Based on Medicare Guidelines

Medicare requires skilled care that is reasonable and necessary, intermittent (as opposed to continuous) care, provided to clients who are homebound (justifying the need to receive the services in the home as opposed to the client obtaining the services at a clinic or other facility). The client must be under a physician's care, and the physician must certify the need for the home health care (Pfaadt, 2000).

## Skilled Care

Skilled care involves licensed professionals (RN, LPN, physical therapist, occupational therapist, and speech therapist) performing at least one of the following activities: 1) observation and assessment, 2) teaching and learning, 3) performance of skilled, direct hands-on care, and 4) management and evaluation of a client care plan (Pfaadt, 2000).

### Observation and Assessment

Observation and assessment depends upon the likelihood that the client's condition could change, requiring a skilled professional to anticipate new developments in health status (e.g., medication changes, the development of symptoms, signs of infection, and emergency room visits). During the assessment phase, the nurse formulates a nursing diagnosis and proposes a plan of care to improve health and minimize problems (Pfaadt, 2000).

## CLINICAL ALERT

### Identifying Multiple Medications in the Home

Be sure to ask the client to show you all the medications and vitamins he is currently taking and have him describe exactly how he takes them. Make special note of the names of physicians ordering the medicines. Sometimes clients may see several different doctors for a variety of concerns. Each individual doctor may be unaware that the client has received prescriptions from another source. It is often the home health nurse who gets a total picture of what the client is taking and whether he understands his treatment regimen.

Hitchcock, J., Schubert, P., & Thomas, S. (2003). *Community health nursing: Caring in action* (2nd ed.). Clifton Park, NY: Delmar Learning.

## LEGAL AND ETHICAL ISSUES

### Confidentiality in Home Health Nursing

Confidentiality is an important issue in home health nursing. Often the nurse calls clients from home or cellular phones. These lines should be secure and should be used in a location where client privacy and confidentiality are preserved. The nurse may do charting at home or keep records in the car. Any records should be secured and transported to the office as soon as possible. Fax phone numbers need to be checked for accuracy when communicating with the home health agency or physician offices. Client information should only be disclosed to family or insurance companies under defined written policies.

Kinsella, A. (2000). Take a reality check on telehealth: The nurse IS in the picture! *Home Healthcare Nurse, 18*(2), 89–92.

## Teaching and Learning

Teaching and learning have always been important aspects of home health nursing. The nurse must first assess the level of client and caregiver knowledge, their ability to learn, language barriers, available caregivers, limitations, the environment in which the care will be delivered, the health needs, and tasks to be addressed (Barry, 2000). The teaching plan must require the knowledge of a skilled nurse, be new information as well as reinforcement of previously learned information, and be related to the medical diagnosis. Documentation should indicate the need for learning, the receptiveness of the client and caregivers, and the progress made toward the learning goals (Pfaadt, 2000). In addition, confidentiality must also be maintained in all documentation. When teaching the client and caregivers to perform certain skilled tasks at home (e.g., maintaining respirators, performing wound care, administering injections), the learning goals should address the important concepts (e.g., safety issues, cleaning and maintenance of equipment, ordering supplies).

## LIFE SPAN CONSIDERATIONS

### Special Needs of the Elderly

The older client has special needs because the speed of processing information typically is slower, short-term memory can decline, and she may be more cautious in her responses (Barry, 2000). If the learning goals are not met within a certain time period, the extenuating circumstances should be noted in the chart. Alternate teaching methods and extended time frames may facilitate learning.

Hogstel, M. (2001). *Gerontology: Nursing care of the older adult.* Clifton Park, NY: Delmar Learning.

## Skilled Treatments and Procedures

Skilled treatments and procedures involve services that require the knowledge of a skilled or licensed nurse to prevent complications in high-risk clients. Therapies such as wound care, injections, intravenous therapy, peritoneal dialysis, and catheter management would be considered skilled treatment (Pfaadt, 2000).

## Management and Evaluation of a Client Care Plan

Management and evaluation (M&E) of a care plan requires the skilled nurse to coordinate care among several disciplines and supervise home health aides and other client caregivers. Usually the clients requiring M&E have complicated problems involving several medical diagnoses. The primary focus of M&E is to integrate care provided by a variety of professional and nonprofessional or unskilled caregivers to establish the medical safety of the client, and to prevent exacerbations and rehospitalizations (Pfaadt, 2000).

## LIFE SPAN CONSIDERATIONS

### High-Risk Pregnancies

Many women with high-risk pregnancies can be managed in their homes with the help of the home health nurse. Complications that require bed rest include such things as pregnancy-induced hypertension (PIH, also known as pre-eclampsia), preterm labor (labor that occurs between the 20th and 37th weeks of gestation), and ruptured membranes. The nurse monitors environmental, family, psychosocial, educational, and physiological needs. The ability to assess for deep tendon reflexes, fetal heart tones, fundal height, edema, and protein in the urine are essential nursing functions. The nurse should have tape measure, Doppler for fetal heart tones, scale, and urine dip sticks to assess the client adequately. The nurse can help the client and her family to adapt to the limitations imposed by a high-risk pregnancy by addressing the environmental constraints, social support systems, and coping mechanisms evident in the situation.

Kodadek, M. P., & Boland, M. L. (1998). Assessing the high-risk pregnant woman at home. *Home Healthcare Nurse, 16*(3), 157–163.

## Medicare Reimbursement for Care in the Home

Medicare will reimburse for intermittent home care, which is skilled nursing care provided on fewer than 7 days each week, or less than 8 hours each day (combined) for 21 days or less. Furthermore, intermittent care is home care delivered periodically and not continuously. The client should only require limited professional services in order to stay in the residence. Medicare will *not* pay for care longer than a regular visit to perform services. As an example, Medicare would not pay for a home care aide to stay for 8 hours or a 24-hour shift (Home-bound care, 2003).

In addition, Medicare classifies clients as being homebound and will pay for these services. A homebound client is defined as a person with a medical condition restricting the ability to leave the house except with assistance—or for whom it is medically inadvisable to leave the house. Recipients of home care may attend adult day care programs, therapeutic sessions, medical treatment, or religious services. The adult day care should be approved by CMS (Centers for Medicare & Medicaid Services, formerly HCFA). It is up to the home health agency to assure that the client is not disqualified by attending a nonaccredited service (Stoker, 2001).

## Home Health Visit and the Nursing Process: Phases of the Home Health Visit

Referrals for home health care are often made by physicians in outpatient clinics or by inpatient discharge planners directly to the home health agency; however, anyone can initiate a visit. Concerned neighbors, family members, even mail-carriers (who notice that the mail has not been collected for several days) may identify problems with the normal functioning of a client and seek help for that person. Contact is made with the client and family to set up a visit.

### Assessment

Components of assessment include taking a health history; examining medication regimens; performing the physical examination; interviewing the family, significant others, or caregivers; and identifying significant information from the client's record. It is essential to assess the client, the caregivers, the necessary legal and financial aspects, and the safety of the environment.

### Assessing the Client Using the SANE Model

In the first visits, it is important to perform a physical assessment, giving special attention to the medical conditions that qualify the client for care. One helpful tool to assess the functioning of the client uses the acronym *SANE* (senses, activity, neurological status, and emotional status). In addition to the physical assessment, the SANE model helps organize data collection regarding clinical and functional health status, especially in relation to the ability of the client and caregiver to learn new information (Barry, 2000).

### Assessing Functional Independence

The nurse may find the Katz Index of Independence in Activities in Daily Living useful. This tool assesses the functional status of the client and is helpful in measuring the progress of some home care goals. It takes into account the ability of the client to perform self-care tasks such as bathing, dressing, toileting, transferring, continence, and feeding. It can be used to determine the prior level of self-care and appropriate goals can be set accordingly (Shelkey and Wallace, 2001).

### Assessing a "Typical" Day

When the home health nurse initially assesses the client, she'll find it helpful to ask the client and caregiver to describe the unfolding of a typical day and how this has changed in light of current health issues (Roush & Cox, 2000). This helps the client and caregiver become aware of habitual patterns and activity. The client and caregiver start by narrating the morning activities and then progress through the day's activities, identifying what,

## CLIENT REFLECTIONS

### Difficulty Living with Family

Esther, a widowed 82-year-old, suffered compression fractures secondary to osteoporosis when she was doing light housework. No one responded to her calls for help, and she was unable to get to the phone. Her daughter-in-law, Anna, arrived 6 hours after the incident to bring her groceries and found her in extreme pain. After a visit to the emergency room, Esther was discharged to her daughter-in-law's care and a home health nurse to follow up for pain control. Anna's home had many stairs and a sunken living room, so it was difficult for Esther to move from room to room and nothing was wheelchair accessible. Anna has two active boys, ages 7 and 9. The nurse was able to speak with Esther about the difficulty they were having in controlling her pain. Esther's eyes began to tear up as she said, "I know they are trying their best to make me feel comfortable, but I am a prisoner in the guest bedroom. Will I ever be able to go back to my home? I love my grandchildren, but it is not easy to rest when they are home. I don't want them to know me as a cranky old lady! What can I do?"

What would you say to this client?

## BOX 22-3 THREE DIMENSIONS OF HOME

**Home as Familiar**
The place where one is comfortable and at ease because of the habitual nature of routines and physical arrangements

**Home as Center**
The place that is the center of the everyday experiences of space, time, and social life

**Home as Protector**
A place where privacy, identity, and safety can be preserved and protected; a refuge from the hazards of the outside world.

Roush, C. V., & Cox, J. E. (2000). The meaning of home: How it shapes the practice of home and hospice care. *Home Healthcare Nurse, 18*(6), 388–394.

### Assessing the Home Environment

The nurse must remember to assess the home environment for its impact on client care. For example, maintaining medical asepsis doing a dressing change may be difficult in many home environments. The nurse would need to assess the home for the best place that the client can do the procedure. There are several tools for assessing

where, how, and with whom activities take place. The nurse becomes aware of the caregiver's potential strain, as well as the client's level of functioning. It is important to gain perspective on how the client and caregivers view the concept of "home," as described in Box 22-3 (Roush & Cox, 2000).

### Assessing the Caregivers in Home Care

The family has an integral role in the care of the client at home. Unlike the hospital or other inpatient institutions where nurses and other members of the health care team are providing 24-hour care and monitoring, the home setting requires the family caregivers to shoulder these responsibilities. At home, the family members may need to be taught sophisticated technical skills (like administering total parenteral nutrition [TPN]), signs and symptoms of significant changes in the client's condition, and techniques for advocating for the client. It is important to assess the ability of the caregivers as a whole to cope with the stresses introduced when one or more members experience an alteration in health and independence (see Chapter 44, which expands on the concept of social support and identifies tools such as the Family Coping Index).

## CLIENT EDUCATION

### Caregiver Care

✓ If the caregiver is unable to provide care for the client, the feasibility of the client staying in the home is threatened.

✓ Analyze ways that the caregiver can receive help, either in direct care for the client or assistance with other roles such as carpooling, housecleaning, gardening, shopping, or car maintenance.

✓ Plan time for the caregiver. It is important for the caregiver to take the time to be renewed. In preserving health and well-being, it is possible for the loved one to remain in the home.

✓ Encourage health promotion in the caregiver. Exercise and socialization are important in maintaining an attitude that enhances the ability to care for the client.

Edwards, A. B., Zarit, S. H., Stephens, M., & Townsend, A. (2002). Employed family caregivers of cognitively impaired elderly: An examination of role strain and depressive symptoms. *Aging and Mental Health, 6*(1), 55–61.

## COMMUNITY/HOME CARE

### Home Safety Risk Appraisal

#### Infants

- Crib side rails stay in the up position while the infant is in the crib.
- Infants are not left unattended, especially on elevated surfaces or in the bath.
- Bath water temperature is 37.8° to 40.6°C (100° to 105°F). Check temperature for comfort with wrist.
- Environment is kept warm and draft free at bath time.
- Bottles are washed with soap and hot water, and formula is refrigerated.
- Toys are soft and have no detachable pieces.
- Car seat has a restraint strap and is used consistently.
- Stroller and carry seat are sturdy and have a restraint strap.
- Fire, police, and poison control numbers are posted by telephones.
- Caregivers know infant cardiopulmonary resuscitation (CPR).

#### Toddlers/Preschoolers

- Sharp objects are placed out of reach and out of sight.
- Poisons are labeled and placed in a locked cabinet.
- Medications and other toxins have childproof lids and are stored in a locked cabinet.
- Small, hard food objects (peanuts, candy) are kept in locked cabinets.
- Stairs and floor furnaces have gates or barriers.
- Doors and windows have safety locks.
- Electrical outlets are covered.
- Burners on the stove are not left on and unattended.
- Pots with hot liquids are placed on back burners, handles facing toward the back wall.
- Home and yard are free of poisonous plants.
- Play equipment is kept in proper functioning condition; toys have no small parts; crayons are nontoxic.
- Outdoor play is supervised in a fenced area with locks on gates.
- Car seat or seat belt is used consistently.
- Children are supervised when crossing the street.
- Caregivers know child CPR and Heimlich maneuver.

#### School-Age Children

- Play and sports are supervised.
- Play equipment is kept in proper functioning condition and free of hazards.
- Outdoor play is limited to soft surfaces.

- Bicycle helmet is worn consistently.
- Children are taught not to open the door or speak to strangers while at play.
- Firearms are kept unloaded and in locked cabinets.
- Seat belt is worn at all times.
- Caregivers know child CPR and the Heimlich maneuver.

#### Adolescents

- Firearm safety is taught.
- Seat belt is worn at all times.
- Teenagers take drivers' education and are cautioned about drinking and driving.
- Caregivers know adult CPR and the Heimlich maneuver.

#### Adults

- Firearms have safety latches.
- Smoke detectors and fire extinguishers are installed in the home.
- A nondrinking designated driver is chosen.
- Emergency phone numbers are readily available.
- Caregiver knows adult CPR and Heimlich maneuver.

#### Older Adults

- Stairs have adequate lighting and nonskid surfaces, and rails are in good condition.
- Throw rugs are not present.
- Hallways are uncluttered.
- Carpets are free from frayed ends/pieces.
- Phone cords and other cords are behind furniture.
- Bathtub has rails and a nonslip surface.
- Shower stall has a seat.
- Bathroom is free of drafts.
- Shoes fit properly and have nonskid soles.
- Home is adequately ventilated and heated.
- Home is free of space heaters.
- Pilot lights on gas appliances are functional.
- Electrical appliances are in good working condition.
- Food is properly refrigerated.
- Medications are kept in properly labeled containers with readable print.
- Emergency phone numbers are readily available.
- Fire and police departments are aware that older adult is home alone.
- Caregiver knows adult CPR and Heimlich maneuver.

## CLINICAL ALERT

### Appropriate Documentation

The adequacy of the nurse's documentation is often the determining factor in whether or not a reimbursement source will pay for the visit. Be aware of the requirements and limitations of the client's insurance plan. It is important to have all consents for service and other necessary documents signed by the client before initiating care. Clinical notes must be in compliance with the plan of care. Changes in client status must be clearly stated, and the subsequent need for revisions to the plan of care must be detailed.

Carelock, J., & Innerarity, S. (2001). Critical incidents: Effective communication and documentation. *Critical Care Nursing, 23*(4), 59–66.

the home. Overall, assessing the environment is essential to home care nursing.

## Assessing Legal and Financial Issues

When performing the initial assessment, the home care nurse must identify not only what the client and caregivers hope to receive from the experience, but also explain what services they can expect from the home care

## STOP AND THINK

### Family Roles and Caregiver Role Strain

● How does the compromised health of one individual in a family have an impact on the other members in that family?

● How do roles change?

● What accommodations need to be made in order to best care for the individual who is ill?

● What impact does the health and well-being of the caregiver have on the overall outcome of the situation?

● What kind of teaching and encouragement can the nurse provide in order to maximize the health and well-being of all concerned individuals?

agency and what limits may be placed on those services by their insurance, Medicare, Medicaid, and so on. The nurse must prepare the clients for discharge from home care, clearly stating goals that can be measured and achieved. Each subsequent visit must be purposeful and guided by the prescribed plan of care, documenting reasonable and necessary needs for service in the areas of observation and assessment, teaching and training, and skilled care and management. The nurse is in the position to ask if the client has a living will, who has durable power of attorney, and what resources the client and family might have for out-of-pocket payment. Since the home health nurse is the primary representative of the agency that the client has contact with, all legal, financial, and insurance-related topics must be addressed during the home visit.

## Nursing Diagnoses Related to Home Care

After the assessment has been made, the nursing diagnoses need to be identified. Problems can be actual situations that are currently treated, or the client can have potential complications that would put him "at risk" for developing further challenges to health. Risk for injury, risk for impaired skin integrity, and risk for infection are all pertinent nursing diagnoses. Of particular importance to home care are caregiver role strain or risk for caregiver role strain, ineffective management of therapeutic regimen, noncompliance, impaired home maintenance management, and deficient knowledge. In addition to individual nursing diagnoses, collaborative problems are identified by a health care team and require multiple discipline intervention (Carpenito, 2001).

## Planning and Outcome Identification

After the nursing diagnoses have been identified, the plan of care (POC) should be created. The Nursing Strategy box depicts specific concepts to incorporate into this plan of care.

## Implementation

The nurse puts the plan of care into action, collaborating with caregivers, community agencies, other members of the health care team, and the physician. Activities need to be coordinated, and documentation must reflect the care and coordination provided.

Skilled care should be identified for each client visit. The goals of the care plan need to be kept in mind, since the skilled care needs to directly relate to the medical reason for the nurse to be in the home. Each contact with the client must be recorded, including attempts to reach the client and family by telephone. Team meetings and family

## NURSING STRATEGY

### Concepts of a Home-Based Plan of Care

- Delineate why the care was justified.

- Identify the skilled nursing interventions that should be consistently performed on an intermittent basis.

- Specify other skilled disciplines to be involved in the care.

- Establish client-centered goals that are realistic, taking into consideration the level of functioning prior to the event that required home care.

- Develop outcomes that are measurable, keeping the criteria for discharge in mind.

- Involve the client, family, and other caregivers in all aspects of care planning.

Hitchcock, J., Schubert, P., & Thomas, S. (2003). *Community health nursing: Caring in action* (2nd ed.). Clifton Park, NY: Delmar Learning.

## NURSING STRATEGY

### Collaborating with Outside Resources

- It is critical for the home health nurse to be informed about the resources available to the client. It is important to assess the potential for family and friends, religious organizations, community centers, senior services, Red Cross, Salvation Army, food banks, and government services.

- Depending on the client's diagnosis, organizations such as the American Cancer Society, Muscular Dystrophy Association, ALS Society, Leukemia and Lymphoma Society, may be able to provide support groups, equipment, or other services.

- Response systems such as "Lifeline" may enable the client to stay at home. This type of system can activate the emergency medical system to check on the client in the event of an emergency.

Hitchcock, J., Schubert, P., & Thomas, S. (2003). *Community health nursing: Caring in action* (2nd ed.). Clifton Park, NY: Delmar Learning.

conferences that deal with a particular client's care need to become part of the client's permanent record.

### Telehealth

**Telehealth** is the use of telecommunications equipment and communications networks for transferring health care information between participants at different locations (Chaffe, 1999). Modern technology offers many opportunities to promote communication among the nurse, clinical specialists, clients, and caregivers. Many models exist for using technology to monitor the client's condition, teach information, and provide supportive care.

One method of home monitoring involves the interactive voice response (IVR). At a prearranged time, clients would receive an automated telephone message, asking specific questions about the client's condition. The client would respond by entering appropriate numbers on a Touch-Tone telephone. If the answers received were "outside the safety zone," the client would be immediately connected to a home health nurse or supervisor. Clients and caregivers can access the Visiting Nurses Association Health Education Library, which offers specific disease information and nutritional information at a time that is convenient for them. Clients using IVR exhibit more awareness of their disease process and the significant parameters that would indicate the need to consult professional help (Stricklin, Jones, & Niles, 2000).

Monitoring equipment can be directly connected to a computer. Videoconferencing can also enhance the telehealth experience. Stethoscopes, spirometers, glucometers, sphygmomanometers, scales, electrocardiograms, and pulse oximeters are potential ways to connect the client and the health care providers through special computer programs (Kinsella, 2000; Capone & Frantz, 2000). Telehealth can provide an intermediate step for the nurse who cannot be physically present for a performed procedure. The nurse can observe the client doing the activity by using video hookup (Figure 22-2). Insulin dosages can be double-checked. In addition to collecting data, it is possible to teleconference with clinical specialists who are

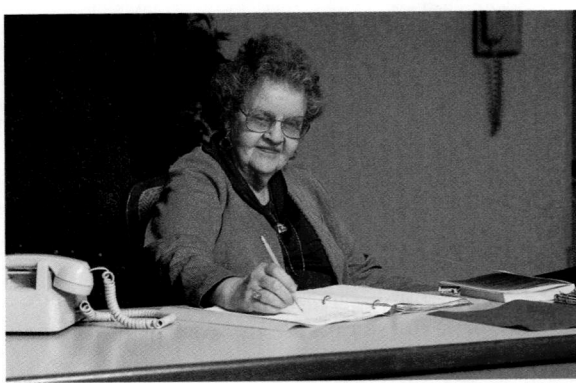

**Figure 22-2   Older client taking notes after connecting with her home health nurse via a telehealth connection.**

## RESEARCH FOCUS

**Title of Study:** Home Talk™/Healthy Talk: Improving patients' health status with telephone technology

**Study Purpose:** To study the client care outcomes, cost, and benefits of using telephone technology in the home care setting. The following areas were measured: (1) Client satisfaction, (2) knowledge of disease-specific information at the time of discharge from home health, (3) compliance with recommended lifestyle changes, (4) nurse-care contact time and productivity as reflected by home visits, telephone time, documentation, and travel time, and (5) acceptance of the technology by the nurse in his practice.

**Methods:** Home Talk™ is an interactive voice response system that uses disease-specific questions in a preprogrammed format. Clients receiving home health services for diabetes, congestive heart failure (CHF), hypertension, or chronic obstructive pulmonary disease (COPD) were included in the study. The system calls the client's home at a scheduled time and delivers the disease-specific questionnaire. The client responds to each question by using the Touch-Tone phone. Responses are scored by a computer. If a client's response to the questions falls outside of a predetermined "safety zone," a system is triggered so the client can be put in touch with a nursing supervisor for further investigation.

Specific information about nutrition and other health issues is also available by this method. First, a pilot study evaluated the validity of the questionnaire and the accuracy of the client responses. A home health nurse followed the initial telephone interactions with a visit within an hour. A 92% validity was established between client reports of the health condition and nurse observations. During the intervention phase, a prospective study examined the advantages and disadvantages of the Home Talk™ model as compared with the traditional home health visit. The final study compared hypertension and congestive heart failure (CHF) clients randomized into traditional (control) and Home Talk™ (experimental) groups for a 60-day monitoring period.

**Findings:** Client outcomes were similar in both groups. Compliance with the treatment regimen, exercise, and knowledge of the disease process were comparable. However, Home Talk™ clients were more aware of disease parameters and were able to express these thoughts in a more organized manner.

Productivity was significantly different for the two groups. The average Home Talk™ client received 11 visits, while the traditional (control) group received 15 visits in the same time frame. Total visit time was 496 minutes for the Home Talk™ group and 654 minutes for the control group. The Home Talk™ group used less time in nurse travel time, and the computer was able to document client responses at the time of the telephone voice interaction.

Client satisfaction was identical for both groups, with 72% being "very satisfied" and 28% reporting "satisfied." Nurse satisfaction was reported as "high" because of the feature that alerts the nursing supervisor to health changes. Intervention for potential problems could be more timely. Home Talk™ provided a means to reinforce teaching and offered the clients a sense of security about their own self-monitoring of their chronic disease.

**Implications:** Technology can be used to enhance nursing care. In an attempt to provide quality, cost-effective care, systems such as this may provide new options for selected clients. This could be a valuable opportunity to provide monitoring and feedback to clients in rural areas or those with limited resources. Computer documentation, client education, and nurse productivity are important avenues to explore as other applications are developed.

Stricklin, M., Jones, S., & Niles, S. (2000). Home Talk™/Healthy Talk: Improving patients' health status with telephone technology. *Home Healthcare Nurse, 18*(1), 53–62.

unable to make the actual home visit. For instance, a wound care specialist can directly visualize the wound while the home care nurse is at the client's bedside (Durtschi, 2001).

Telehealth nursing has many advantages, as shown in the Research Focus box. However, some clients would not be candidates for using telehealth technology. Those who do not want to learn the data collection methods would not experience a high degree of satisfaction with the service. Those with unreliable or inadequate phone or electric service can present time delays, lack of audio or visual clarity, and the need for repetition. The telehealth nursing visit can be perceived as unfriendly (Kinsella, 2000). Those home care nurses who rely on assessing the family and environment and having private conversations with the client or caregivers may need more in-person visit time.

## Evaluation

At each visit, the nurse should be assessing and reevaluating the plan of care. Progress toward the mutually established goals needs to be noted, and adjustments should be identified. The client and family should be prepared for discharge with each encounter by including them in the assessment of the treatment plan, and teaching them to look for signs of improvement or significant changes that should be reported to the physician.

## Issues Specific to Home Health and Hospice Nursing

Many people feel that home health nurses should have a minimum preparation of a BSN, because this type of education focuses more on community health (Townes & Cook, 2001). Because of a high likelihood that some clients will be discharged to the home with complicated medical equipment such as TPN, PCAs respirators, or peritoneal dialysis, it is necessary for the home health nurse to spend significant time in the inpatient setting working with this type of equipment. The nurse may be called upon to verbally walk the client through steps for troubleshooting machines over the telephone. This is only possible if the nurse is confident with such knowledge and skills (e.g., physical assessment, Medicare/Medicaid guidelines, disease processes, and case management).

## Certification

Certification is possible for home health nursing, hospice nursing, advanced practice nursing, and case management. If a nurse achieves certification, that nurse is recognized for proven competency and knowledge in his area. The American Nurses Credentialing Center (ANCC) offers a home health nursing certification process and exam to nurses with a BSN. Advanced certification is also available to clinical specialists who hold a master's degree or higher and meet other criteria (Narayan, 2002). In 1994, the National Board of Certification for Hospice and Palliative Nurses began certifying hospice nurses (Volker & Watson, 2001).

## Nurse Safety and Occupational Hazards

There are specific safety issues for the nurse in the home care environment. A list of guidelines for safety are as follows:

1. Appearance
   a. Wear uniform and name badge identifying you as a representative of the home health agency.
   b. Call clients in advance, confirming the time of the appointment and the directions to the residence.
   c. Request that pets be secured before your arrival.
   d. Do not carry a purse.

2. Traveling
   a. Keep car in good working order with over half a tank of fuel.
   b. Use a mobile phone to maximize communication and safety. Have a car charger attachment to run the phone off the car battery if necessary.
   c. Keep a blanket or sleeping bag in the car if you are traveling in winter.
   d. Keep a snack and drinking water in the car.
   e. Park in full view of the residence if possible.
   f. Always let the agency know your intended schedule. Notify the agency if there are changes to your schedule.
   g. If your car fails, call for help on the mobile phone. Notify the agency of car trouble. If no telephone is available, put a Call Police sign in the window. Do not accept rides from strangers.
   h. Walk in a professional, businesslike manner, and walk directly to the client's residence.
   i. Use common walkways and avoid isolated stairs and alleys.

3. Precautions during visits
   a. Standard precautions should always be in effect; handwashing is essential.
   b. Use good body mechanics.

Adapted from Hitchcock, J., Schubert, P., & Thomas, S. (2003). *Community health nursing: Caring in action* (2nd ed.). Clifton Park, NY: Delmar Learning; Hogstel, M. (2001). *Gerontology: Nursing care of the older adult*. Clifton Park, NY: Delmar Learning.

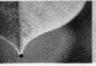 **CASE STUDY/NURSING CARE PLAN**

Mr. Wheeler is a 63-year-old executive who is counting the days to retirement. He lives at home with his wife, who is severely affected by arthritis. Mr. Wheeler has a fairly sedentary lifestyle and is about 30 pounds overweight. He fell at the airport while getting luggage to the curb and twisted his left knee. In falling, Mr. Wheeler hit his left leg on the suitcase, and this area continued to throb for a while after the incident. Two days after he returned home from his cross-country trip, Mr. Wheeler experienced sudden pain and significant swelling in the upper thigh and groin area of his left leg. He went to see his family physician, and was diagnosed with deep vein thrombosis. He was observed for 8 hours in the hospital, then discharged to home with a home health referral after receiving his first dose of low molecular weight heparin (LMWH).

*(continues)*

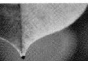

# CASE STUDY/NURSING CARE PLAN *(continued)*

The home health nurse is asked to follow Mr. Wheeler to continue his LMWH anticoagulation therapy and initiate warfarin. Mr. Wheeler is interested in trying to give himself his LMWH injections, so the home health nurse designs a teaching plan that includes monitoring for bleeding complications. The nurse draws blood for prothrombin (PT), partial thromboplastin time (PTT), and international normalized rate (INR) to monitor the anticoagulation therapy. Other labs may be added such as creatinine, as ordered. The client is assessed for pain, skin integrity, respiratory function, elimination function, and bleeding complications. Areas of teaching include environmental safety, diet, and activity. The need for home health aide assistance, durable medical equipment, and physical therapy is assessed and the appropriate requests and referrals made.

## Assessment

Client has deep vein thrombosis of left leg. The left leg is swollen, the pedal pulses are present bilaterally, and color is slightly more pale in left foot than the right foot. Client has pain at level of 4 on scale of 1 to 10. Client requires extensive teaching for follow-up care in the home setting.

## Nursing Diagnosis #1

*Deficient Knowledge* related to lack of information regarding disease process, diet, activity, and treatment regimen as evidenced by the deficiency of cognitive information related to anticoagulation therapy.
**NOC:** Knowledge of Anticoagulant Therapy
**NIC:** Teaching Concepts of Administering Anticoagulants

## Expected Outcomes

The client will:
1. Understand disease state, recognize need for medications, and understand treatments by end of first home visit.
2. Be able to recite schedule for anticoagulation therapy monitoring (blood draws), and demonstrate ability to perform self-injections by end of first home visit.
3. List signs and symptoms of excessive bleeding (e.g., blood in urine, change in stool color, nosebleeds, bruising) by end of first home visit.

## Planning/Interventions/Rationales

1. Assess client's previous knowledge of or skills related to present diagnosis and treatment regimen. *New skills are learned in the context of previously acquired knowledge and experiences.*
2. Evaluate client's learning through return demonstration in the skill of self-injection. *Efficacy of teaching is evident in the demonstration of critical thinking and psychomotor skills.*
3. Teach client about disease process and treatment regimen, presenting information that is most significant to the client first; introduce additional information after the initial learning needs have been met, such as giving self-injections. *The client has a priority for information he wants to learn. Addressing the areas of most significance to the client will aid learning. Information building begins with simple concepts, and moving on to explain more complex information.*
4. Discuss potential side effects of anticoagulation therapy. *It is imperative that the client is aware of safety information, early recognition of side effects, and appropriate actions to take in the event of complications.*

## Evaluation

Client verbalized information about disease process and treatment regimen. He understands the schedule for anticoagulation therapy. He performed self-injection of heparin with supervision and verbalized the side effects of anticoagulation therapy.

## Key Concepts

- Home health care nursing is a subspecialty of community health nursing and works in collaboration with the multidisciplined health care delivery system.
- Agencies providing home care may be licensed by the state, certified by the federal Medicare program, and certified by an independent accrediting body (e.g., JCAHO, CHAP).
- In order to receive Medicare funding for home care, the agency must follow Medicare guidelines and comply with all Medicare requirements.
- Nurses make nursing diagnoses after assessing the home health care client.
- The plan of care for home health clients is made after nursing diagnoses have been identified.
- Implementing nursing care to clients in their home environment presents challenges for the nurse, including readily accessible equipment and supplies

for providing care to the client, travel and personal safety, and communication with the home care agency.
- Evaluation of home health care is made from mutually agreed-upon goals between the nurse and the client.
- Home health nursing requires specific knowledge and skills because of the complexity of the clients' care.
- There are specific safety issues for the nurse in the home care environment.

## Review Questions and Activities

1. How has home health care nursing evolved?
2. What impact did Medicare legislation have on the development of home health in the United States?
3. What credentials are necessary for home health funding?
4. In what ways can home health be used throughout the life span?
5. What elements are important to include in a home health assessment?
6. Describe some innovations in telehealth that may be applied to the home health setting.
7. What is the difference between home health, hospice, and palliative care?
8. Describe the challenges the home health nurse faces that are not experienced in the controlled inpatient or clinic setting.

## Web Resources

Accreditation from JCAHO and CHAP
    http://www.jcaho.org
    http://www.chapinc.org
Assessment of Home Safety
    http://www.geri-ed.com
Homebound care
    http://www.ltcconnection.net
National Association of Home Care
    http://www.nahc.org
Medicare services
    http://www.ltcconnection.net
Public health nursing history
    http://www.redcross.org

## References

Accreditation from JCAHO and CHAP, 2002, http://www.jcaho.org/, http://www.chapinc.org/

Barry, C. B. (2000). Teaching the older patient in the home: Assessment and adaptation. *Home Healthcare Nurse, 18*(6), 374–387.

Capone, L., & Frantz, A. (2000). HHNA announces new telehealth special interest group. *Home Healthcare Nurse, 18*(8), 548.

Carelock, J., & Innerarity, S. (2001). Critical incidents: Effective communication and documentation. *Critical Care Nursing, 23*(4), 59–66.

Carpenito, L. J. (2001). *Nursing diagnoses: Application to clinical practice* (8th ed.). Philadelphia: Lippincott-Raven.

Chaffe, M. (1999) A telehealth odyssey. *American Journal of Nursing, 99*(7), 26–32.

Durtschi, A. (2001). Three patients' tele-home care experiences. *Home Healthcare Nurse, 19*(1), 9–11.

Edwards, A. B., Zarit, S. H., Stephens, M., & Townsend, A. (2002). Employed family caregivers of cognitively impaired elderly: An examination of role strain and depressive symptoms. *Aging and Mental Health, 6*(1), 55–61.

Hitchcock, J., Schubert, P., & Thomas, S. (2003). *Community health nursing: Caring in action* (2nd ed.). Clifton Park, NY: Delmar Learning.

Hogstel, M. (2001). Gerontology: Nursing care of the older adult. Clifton Park, NY: Delmar Learning.

Home-bound care, 2003, http://www.ltcconnection.net

Hospice services, 2003, www.hospicefoundation.org

Kinsella, A. (2000). Take a reality check on telehealth: The nurse IS in the picture! *Home Healthcare Nurse, 18*(2), 89–92.

Kodadek, M. P., & Boland, M.L. (1998). Assessing the high-risk pregnant woman at home. *Home Healthcare Nurse, 16*(3), 157–163.

Milone-Nuzzo, P. (2000). Home Health Care. In C. Smith & F. Maurer (Eds.), *Community health nursing: Theory and practice* (2nd edition, pp. 842–869). Philadelphia: W. B. Saunders Company.

National Association for Home Care & Hospice, 2003, http://www.nahc.org

Narayan, M. C. (2002). The benefits of certification as a clinical specialist in home health nursing. *Home Healthcare Nurse, 20*(1), 72.

National Association of Home Care, 2001, http://www.nahc.org

Pfaadt, M. (2000). A review of the basics—Understanding the categories of skilled nursing services. *Home Healthcare Nurse, 18*(5), 297–300.

Rosen, G. (1958). *A history of public health*. New York: MD Publications.

Roush, C. V., & Cox, J. E. (2000). The meaning of home: How it shapes the practice of home and hospice care. *Home Healthcare Nurse, 18*(6), 388–394.

Shelkey, M., & Wallace, M. (2001). Katz Index of Independence in Activities of Daily Living. *Home Healthcare Nurse, 19*(5), 323–324.

Stoker, J. (2001). Updated definition of homebound status. *Home Healthcare Nurse, 19*(5), 311.

Stricklin, M. L., Jones, S., & Niles, S. (2000). Home Talk/Health Talk: Improving patients' health status with telephone technology. *Home Healthcare Nurse, 18*(1), 53–62.

Townes, J., & Cook, P. (2001). Standards of practice: A measure of competence. *Home Healthcare Nurse, 19*(6), 383–386.

Vladeck, B. (2000). The storm before the calm before the storm. *Case Management Journals, 2*(4), 232–237.

Volker, B., & Watson, A. (2001). HPN develops end-of-life core curriculum. *Home Healthcare Nurse, 19*(6), 388.

Williams, M. A., & Wheeler, M. S. (2001). Palliative care: What is it? *Home Healthcare Nurse, 19*(9), 551–556.

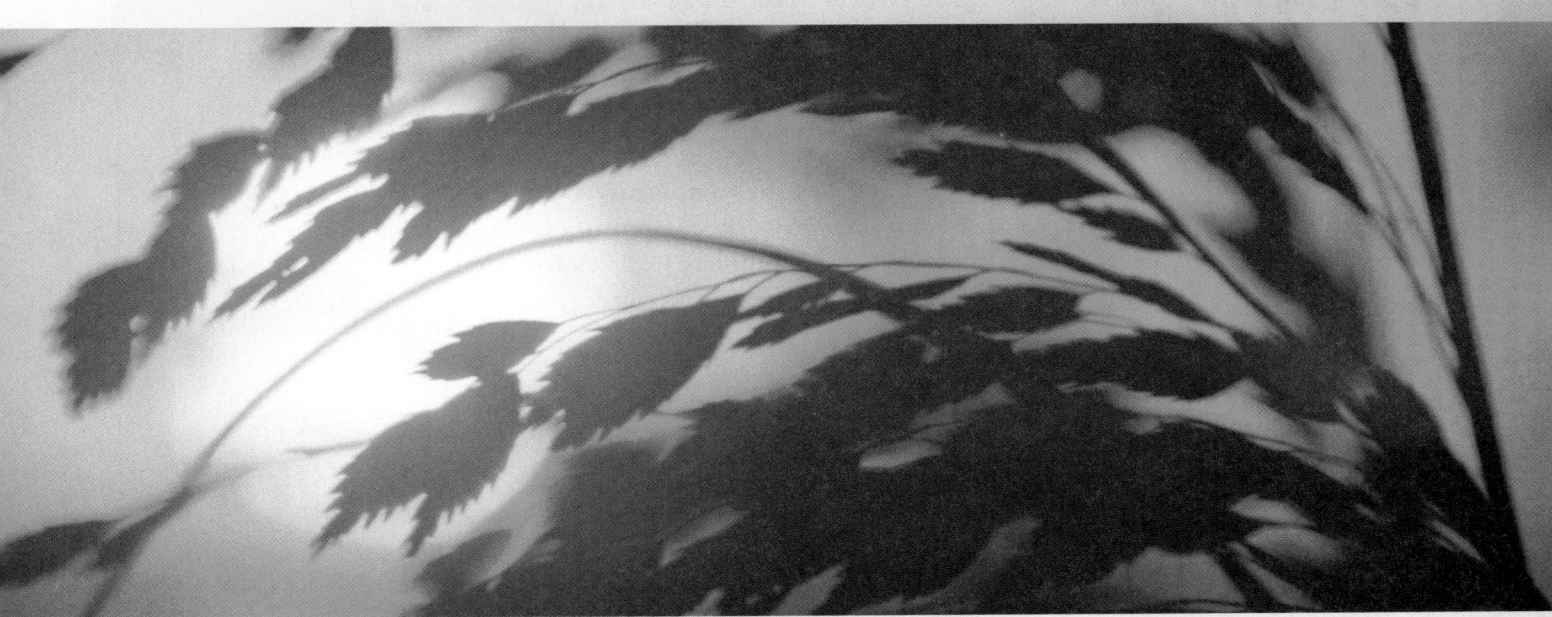

# CHAPTER 23

# Community Care

Wendy Neander, MSN, RN

*"We must be with those who have suffered and we must be with those who have tried to prevent suffering. This is the real community: it does not deny differences, but rather enhances and transcends them."*

(Elie Wiesel)

# Chapter Competencies

*Upon completion of this chapter, the reader should be able to:*

1. Describe the elements of a community.
2. Identify types of communities.
3. Identify and compare different frameworks for the delivery of community care to ensure community participation.
4. Identify and compare different nursing roles for community care.
5. Evaluate different settings in which nurses provide community care.
6. Discuss various partnerships that exist in community health care nursing.
7. Describe the nursing process with respect to community care.

# Key Terms

advocate
community
community development
    society (CDS)
community health nursing
community partnerships

consultation
critical social theory
epidemiology
facilitator
global migration
migrants

nurse epidemiologist
parish nursing
social marketer
telecare
telehealth

The concept of community has many meanings. A community can refer to a geographic location or a population of individuals who have common characteristics. Communities vary in size; they can be as intimate as a small group or as expansive as the global community that encompasses the world. **Community health nursing (CHN)** refers to the field of nursing that provides health care to a wide variety of populations (e.g., communities, groups). Community health nursing has a philosophy of delivering primary health care.

## Elements of Community

The elements of a community are contingent upon the definition used for community. For the purpose of this chapter, a **community** is defined as a group of people engaged in multifaceted relationships, sharing a common culture, with the capacity to act collectively over a period of time (Figure 23-1). In addition, a **community development society (CDS)** is an organization that identifies community as the building blocks for society. Therefore, when identifying the elements of a community, the nurse must first identify the community members. In addition, the nurse must identify whether or not the community members share a common locality in their cultural, economic, social, and political relationships.

In providing care, the nurse needs to discern what health issues, concerns, and needs are connected to which community. Traditionally, another element of communities was their geographic boundaries, which designated a community as a village, city, or urban or rural environment. The **global migration** occurring today is an ongoing trend: people crossing regions, countries, and international boundaries to reside and maintain themselves in new and unfamiliar places (McGuire, 1998).

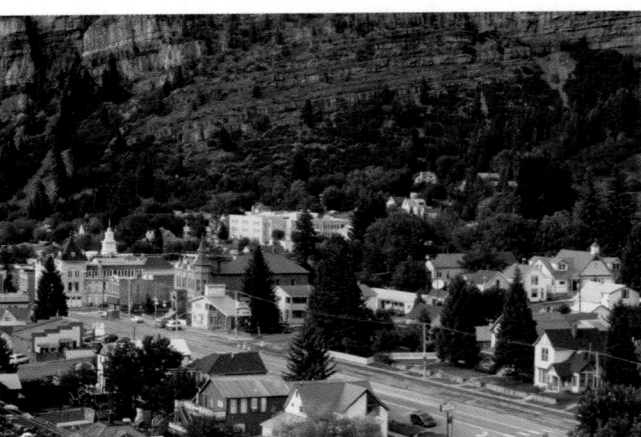

**Figure 23-1** A community shares common elements within its culture.

## NURSING STRATEGY

### Identifying the Members of a Community

The nurse answers the following basic questions to identify the members of a community:

1. Who are the people?
2. Do the people share a common locality (physical place)?
3. What is their shared culture?
4. What are their relationships?

Hitchcock, J., Schubert, P., & Thomas, S. (2003). *Community health nursing: Caring in action* (2nd ed.). Clifton Park, NY: Delmar Learning.

## CLIENT REFLECTIONS

### A Mid-Eastern Immigrant

Abdul, a 51-year-old man, fled from Iran 8 years ago. He comments, "I was very afraid in my country. There were many wars in my country, and I did not feel safe when living there. I came to the United States and worked for 2 years before I could send enough money to get my wife and two boys here. We love our freedom here (in the United States). Things are safer, and we will never leave this country. We don't know that many people here and much of our family is still in Iran, but this is our home now."

Migration creates a community of people who identify themselves by their displacement and not by a geographic boundary. These people are the immigrants and refugees of the world. They are a community distinct from communities that have lived more stable lives (DeSantis, 1999).

## Types of Communities

The rural villages of the world, women's shelters, group homes, schools, factories, urban neighborhoods, homeless shelters, community groups, religious groups, social clubs, and members of immigrant and refugee groups are all examples of communities (Figure 23-2). Within each of the preceding communities are smaller ones. For example, within a school a classroom can be considered a community. Communities are constantly changing and evolving. For example, the global events of today have created population shifts across borders, as people flee political strife

and war, look for economic opportunities to sustain themselves and their families, or search for a new life.

## Frameworks for Delivery of Community Care

Community care is extremely broad in its concepts. Therefore, it is helpful to have a framework to understand how community care is organized and delivered within the health care delivery system. Three frameworks (i.e., critical social theory, citizen ladder of participation theory, and ecological approach to health care theory) for community care are presented in the following section.

### Critical Social Theory Framework

**Critical social theory** (Stevens & Hall, 1992) has as its goal the liberation of people from health-damaging environmental conditions. In using critical social theory, the community care nurse recognizes the need for social change to alter health-damaging conditions. For example, addressing the HIV crisis requires the nurse to understand the societal norms as related to sexual activities.

When employing critical social theory in community practice, the nurse must ask critical questions to assess the situation and develop and implement a plan to respond to the health issue(s). Examples of critical questions the nurse can use in assessing the health issue are shown in the Nursing Strategy box.

### Citizen Ladder of Participation Framework

The citizen ladder of participation framework introduced by Sherry Arnstein (1969) is useful for community nursing. This framework identifies different levels of community involvement. The levels are named according to the degree

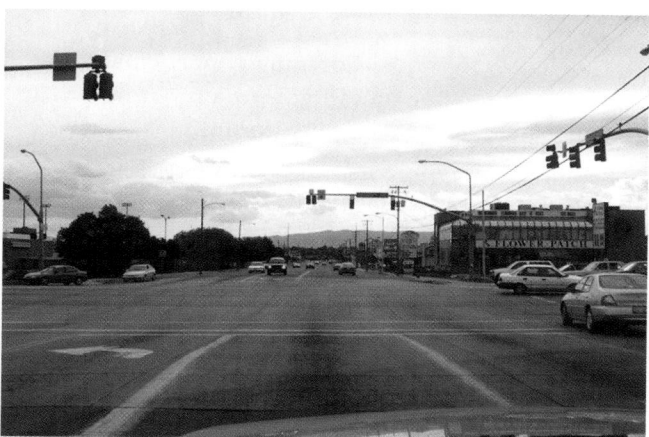

**Figure 23-2  An example of a small community as seen from a car.**

## NURSING STRATEGY

### Questions for the Nurse to Ask in Critical Social Theory

1. What is the issue, and who is defining the issue?
2. What is the history of the issue, and how did things get to be how they are?
3. Whose health is being damaged? Who benefits?
4. What are the inequities? Who has the political power?
5. How effective are certain programs, strategies, and policies?
6. What are the barriers to help and relief?
7. What strategies were tried? How successful were they?

Stevens, P. E., & Hall, J. M. (1992). Applying critical theories to nursing in the communities. *Public Health Nursing, 9*(1), 2–9.

### TABLE 23-1     FRAMEWORK FOR PARTICIPATION

| Levels of Community Participation | Description of Each Level |
| --- | --- |
| Informing | • Lowest degree of participation<br>• Emphasis is placed on a one-way flow of information from officials to citizens.<br>• Participants have little opportunity to influence the program designed for their benefit. |
| Consultation | • Ascertains citizens' views rather than simply giving them the organization's views.<br>• Offers no assurance that citizen concerns and ideas will be used. |
| Partnership | • Negotiation between citizens and powerholders<br>• Community care nurses have power by the nature of their positions. |
| Delegated Power | • Highest degree of community participation<br>• Citizens have the power and responsibility to assure accountability of a program or plan to the community. |
| Citizen Control | • Highest level of community involvement<br>• Community participants can govern a program or an institution. |

Arnstein, S. (July 1969). A ladder of citizen participation, *Journal of the American Institute of Planners, 13*(4) 216–223.

of community participation. The nurse can use the information about these levels of participation in working with communities. Table 23-1 describes the levels of community participation (from lowest to highest level of participation).

The citizen ladder of participation framework is useful for community care because a nurse can use the different levels in the framework to assess community participation in identified health issues. This framework can also be used to evaluate nursing actions and process in the community setting. For example, a nurse working on tobacco prevention can question whether the program has an impact while operating at the informing stage (i.e., strictly providing information) or if the program needs the higher level of citizen control. At this higher level, the community invites the nurse to participate in the institution or program as an expert or consultant to provide a tobacco prevention program.

## Ecological Framework

In 1976, Nancy Milio developed an ecological framework for health promotion and illness prevention that is applicable to present-day community care. This framework mainly assumes that all individual health care decisions are made within a social context. Therefore, health is both an individual and a societal responsibility. Using an ecological framework enables the nurse to perceive and understand structural barriers to health-promotion and illness-prevention behaviors of individuals and communities. An outline of Milio's framework is shown in Box 23-1.

The role of the nurse in Milio's framework includes:

1. Advocating for healthy public policy on a societal level
2. Increasing individuals' awareness of their options, and supporting them in the integration of healthy choices into their lifestyles (Milio, 1976).

## Nursing Roles in Community Health Care

In the delivery of community care, the nurse must be capable of varied nursing roles. One of the major differences between hospital and community care is the focus on groups or aggregates in the community setting. In this section, different community health nursing roles are presented.

## BOX 23-1 OUTLINE OF MILIO'S FRAMEWORK FOR AN ECOLOGICAL APPROACH TO HEALTH CARE

1. There is a strong relationship between individual health behavior and societal options.
2. The range of choices in community care is shaped by policy decisions, such as those made in a national health insurance plan.
3. Personal resources (e.g., money, time, knowledge) and societal resources (e.g., community programs and services) are important in community care.
4. Health-promoting choices must be readily available and less costly than health-damaging choices.

Milio, N. (1976). A framework for prevention: Changing health-damaging to health-generating life patterns. *American Journal of Public Health, 66*(5), 435.

## FOCUS ON WELLNESS

### Example of Citizen Control Level in a Smoking Cessation Program

Elements of a citizen control community smoking cessation program:

1. Identifying literature from organizations such as the American Cancer Society and distributing those to potential candidates
2. Encouraging a social support network for the person interested in quitting smoking; accountability partners are excellent extrinsic motivators
3. Informing friends and family that the person is ceasing smoking, as this enlarges the network for accountability issues

Arizona Smokers Helpline, 2001, http://www.ashline.org

## Educator

Community health nurses deliver varied types of educational programs to different community groups. For example, recent research has demonstrated that community nurses are effective dental health educators for families. Kowash, Pinfield, Smith, and Curzon (2000) found that nurses can substantially reduce tooth decay in underprivileged children. The study was carried out with the families of over 200 children born in a deprived area in England. Home visits were made every 3 to 6 months during a 3-year period. The families were given dental health advice by either a dental hygienist or a community nurse. The oral health of these children dramatically improved.

## Advocate

The advocacy role in community nursing fits with both Milio's (1976) framework for health promotion and prevention of illness, and critical social theory. As an **advocate**, the nurse takes action to achieve a goal on behalf of another. Nursing advocacy is directly related to care (Schroeter, 2000). Therefore, given the varied roles of the nurse in the community, advocacy may be individual or group focused. As an advocate, a nurse may request services or programs for individuals or groups to facilitate equal access of health services (Pan American Health Organization [PAHO], 2001). For example, in 1997, Nancy McPherson, a community health nursing manager in Edmonton, Canada, set up comprehensive services at the public clinic she ran based on an observed need. She observed that many single mothers did not know how to process their tax returns, resulting in loss of income

in the form of a child tax credit. McPherson incorporated income tax services into the clinic as mothers came for immunizations, parenting classes, and other standard community health services (Canadian Health Network, 2003).

## Researcher

In delivering community care, the nurse has a role as a researcher. Sometimes the role may involve conducting research in response to problems and questions that have arisen in practice. For example, Rew, Fouladi, and Yockey (2002) researched sexual health practices of homeless youth to generate knowledge that would enable them to provide culturally relevant interventions. In community care, the nurse also has the responsibility for dissemination of research findings both to colleagues and community members. This might entail reporting research findings that support nursing interventions for diabetic care or nutritional requirements to meet developmental needs of children.

## Consultant

As mentioned in Arnstein's model (1969), when full community participation occurs, the nurse becomes the consultant. **Consultation** is the act of two or more health care professionals deliberating together to make a decision. As a consultant, the nurse responds to requests from community-controlled health care programs to meet health needs and resolve health issues. Nurses also act as consultants to individuals. Telephone consultation is a way in which nurses share their expertise by providing information, support, or teaching in response to individual health

## LEGAL AND ETHICAL ISSUES

### Advocacy for Professional Reasons vs. Personal Reasons

The nurse must remember that the advocacy role denies personal beliefs and desires: ethically, the nurse must represent the client and the client's issues. For example, the nurse who personally does not believe in federally funded programs for nonworking single parents must still advise these persons of the available programs for funding possibilities.

concerns. For example, the new mother who calls the public health clinic asking for information about how to introduce solid foods to her infant receives nursing expertise that provides information to support parenting.

## Direct Care Provider

In the direct care provider role, the community nurse assesses an individual's health status and plans, implements, and evaluates care in a community setting. The care is provided in partnership with the individual. Home health and hospice care (see Chapter 22) are examples of direct care in the community. School and occupational health are other examples of environments where nurses provide direct care in the community (Hitchcock, Schubert, & Thomas, 2003). In addition, the **nurse epidemiologist** is a direct care provider role in which the nurse studies illnesses, their causes, and the illnesses distribution in groups of people. (Note: **epidemiology** is the study of the cause and distribution of diseases, disability, and death among populations.)

## Social Marketer

The nurse in the **social marketer** role uses marketing techniques and skills to promote healthy living as well as health promotion programs. Social marketing is the application of commercial marketing technologies to the analysis, planning, execution, and evaluation of programs designed to influence the voluntary behavior of target audiences in order to improve their personal welfare and that of society (Bryant, Lindenberger, Brown, Kent, Schreiber, Bustillo, & Canright, 2001).

The Texas supplemental nutrition program for women, infants, and children (WIC) used social marketing to increase participation in the program. Some of the marketing strategies used in Texas to increase participation included extended clinic hours, producing vouchers that looked more like bank checks and thus not as conspicuous when used to purchase food products, and a statewide media campaign about the program (Bryant et al., 2001).

## Facilitator

The **facilitator** role (the role of lessening the difficulty of a task) of the community health nurse includes working with groups or aggregates in addressing a community care need. To better serve the community, nursing interventions are group-focused instead of individual-focused. For example, a nurse working in the community may discover that several families express the same concern that their school crosswalks are dangerous. A community nurse's response to these concerns would be a group approach. The community nurse can discuss with the families their options of meeting together to design a coordinated community effort to make the crosswalk areas safer. Community nurses may facilitate the formation of a group or provide input into existing groups to address community needs (Hitchcock et al., 2003).

## Selected Settings for Community-Based Health Care

Community health nursing has had a history of providing community care to a variety of settings. Some examples of these community environments are schools, neighborhood/ community centers, 24-hour health lines, migrant clinics, rural community health services, correctional health, occupational/environmental health, and public/ community health clinics.

## Schools

The National Association of School Nurses (NASN) of the United States identifies the school nurse as a health expert who serves the school community (NASN, 2003). The school nurse provides comprehensive care that includes the prevention of illness, promotion of health, and interventions for injury and illness in the school setting (Figure 23-3). Additionally, the school nurse contributes to the development, implementation, and evaluation of health policies. The community served by a school nurse includes the students, staff, and families of the school community. In recognition of school nursing as a specialty area, the National Association of School Nurses defines the scope of practice in Box 23-2. Relatedly, school nursing is often affected by the economy and is a specialty area that needs community support. Brownson and Krueter (1997) identify the need for innovative partnerships among schools, university health science centers, community coalitions, and traditional public health agencies to develop collaborative strategies to ensure the continuance of school nursing.

## Neighborhood/ Community Centers

The community nursing role in a neighborhood can be one of outreach to determine health needs and communi-

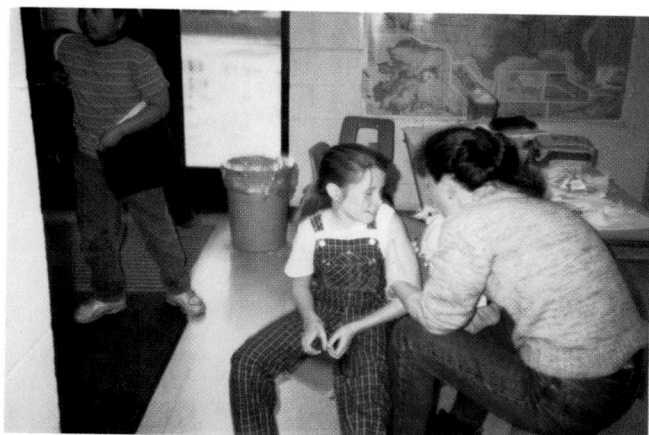

**Figure 23-3**    School nurses perform invaluable functions, as shown in this administration of an immunization program.

ty strengths. A wide variety of health promotion and prevention services is offered. Examples of neighborhood center health services are regularly scheduled blood pressure clinics or diabetic risk screening. Senior wellness clinics are also examples of community centers. In a senior wellness clinic, the nurses screen the elderly population for such things as hypertension, nutritional habits, and exercise and activity practices.

## Twenty-Four-Hour Health Lines (Telehealth)

Telehealth is an innovative approach that has enabled health care professionals to support chronic illness outside of the hospital. Telehealth has been identified as the way of the future for the delivery of multidisciplinary community care (Panahi & Shahtahmasebi, 1999). Chaffee (1999) defines **telehealth** as "the use of telecommunication equipment and communication networks for transferring health care information between participants at

---

**BOX 23-2    DEFINITION OF SCHOOL NURSING**

"School Nursing is a specialized practice of professional nursing that advances the well-being, academic success, and lifelong achievement of students. To that end, school nurses facilitate positive student responses to normal development, promote health and safety, intervene with actual and potential health problems, provide case management services, and actively collaborate with others to build student and family capacity for adaptation, self-management, self-advocacy, and learning."

National Association of School Nurses, 2003, http://www.nasn.org

---

different locations" (p. 38). In the telehealth model, nursing care and community support to clients at a distance is called **telecare**. Monitoring the daily living of individuals at risk by connecting telecommunication to other technologies, ranging from television cameras to alarm systems, is part of telecare (Roberts, Rigby, & Birch, 2000). For example, in the province of British Columbia, Canada, the Ministry of Health has established a 24-hour health line. This community service is managed by registered nurses (RNs). Residents of the province can call a toll-free number, available 24 hours a day, to speak with an RN. The RN answers questions related to illness symptoms, health concerns, a recommended course of action with respect to a health issue, when to see a health professional, and information about available health resources (Canadian Health Network, 2003).

## Migrant Clinic Health Services

**Migrants** (laborers who move from one location to another in pursuit of work) are often treated in migrant clinics, and their health care is an example of the community nursing role for mobile populations. The migrant clinician's network identifies health needs of the migrant population, develops programs, and disseminates information across the country. An example of a nurse-run program for migrant populations is TB NET. The TB NET program is a binational migrant tuberculosis referral and tracking project funded by the Pan American Health Organization and the governments of the United States of America and Mexico. It includes referrals and follow-up for individuals who potentially have tuberculosis upon return to their home country. The countries in which referrals have occurred include Mexico, Guatemala, Honduras, and Peru (DeSantis, 1999).

## Rural Community Health Services

Rural groups are aggregates for which community health nurses provide care. Rural populations can present a challenge to health care providers due to the access problems and poverty (Figure 23-4). Clients need to travel long distances for health care, and there is often a lack of available health care providers. Nurse midwives, nurse practitioners, and other advanced practice nurse specialists are examples of how community nurses meet rural health needs.

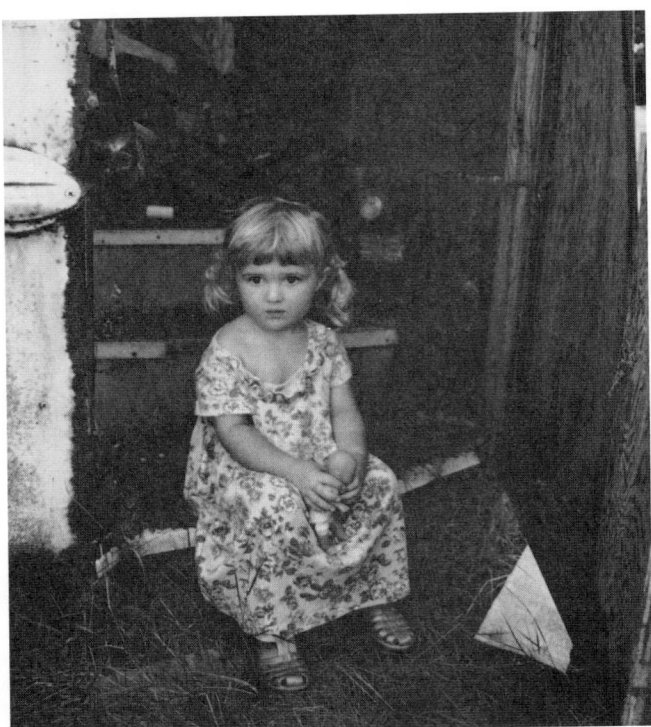

**Figure 23-4** Poor children are at tremendous risk for the physical, social, and emotional effects of living in communities of poverty. *Source: Photodisc*

## Correctional Health Nursing

Correctional health nursing provides nursing services to clients in correctional facilities (Figure 23-5). These settings include such agencies as prisons, youth detention centers, and parole divisions. These are challenging environments due to the scarce public resources available for personal health needs and the stigma associated with these populations. Nursing services range from brief ambulatory or emergent care to comprehensive health programs. The correctional health nurse provides care to all individuals regardless of the nature of their crimes or the duration of their incarceration (National Association of Correctional Nursing, 2003).

## Occupational/Environmental Health Nursing

Occupational health nurses execute the scope of occupational health practices. The role of the occupational health nurse is diversified and complex due to the changing nature of the work environment. Population-based nursing practice that focuses on outcome measurement, quality assurance, and advocacy is imperative to occupational nursing practice. The occupational health nurse is responsible for (1) primary health care delivery in the workplace, (2) health promoting nursing interventions, (3) health programs on employee productivity and morale, (4) strategies to reduce worker injury

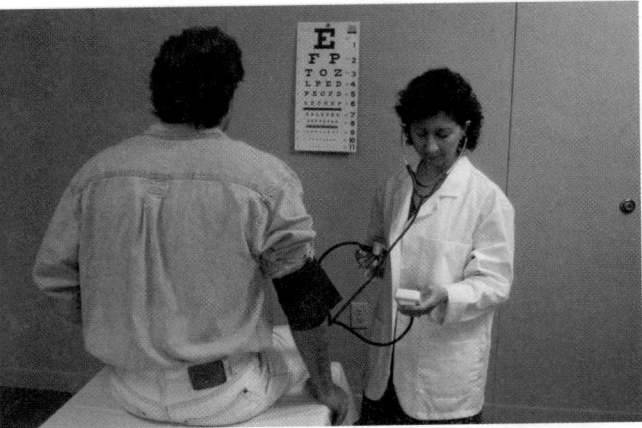

**Figure 23-5** Working in a correctional facility offers many challenges to the nurse; however, rewards can be found in opportunities to function as a group leader, innovator, teacher, planner, and caregiver.

and safety, (5) methods for addressing ethical issues related to workers' health, and (6) influencing rehabilitation in the work environment (Hitchcock et al., 2003).

## Public Health Care Services

Another common place for community nursing care is public health clinics. The public health nurse is an educator, case manager, and direct care provider who promotes health and prevents illness in different population groups. An example population served via public health clinics is pregnant adolescents. More than 1 million teenage girls become pregnant each year, and most of these pregnancies are not planned. This population has many health needs and many complications (e.g., low birth weight, premature births, sexually transmitted diseases) (Figure 23-6). Other subgroups of public health clients are the poor, substance abusers, those with mental health disorders, and migrant, rural, and minority groups.

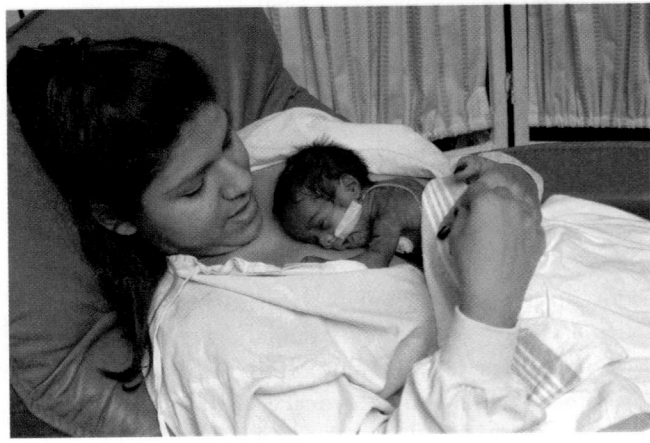

**Figure 23-6** A single, teenage mother who has delivered a preterm infant.

## RESEARCH FOCUS

**Title of Study:** Maternal employment and parent-child relationships in single-parent families of low-birth-weight preschoolers

**Study Purpose:** This study explores the differences in parent-child and family relationships of single mothers of low-birth-weight and full-term preschool children. Family environmental factors, such as the mother's employment, employment history, and employment attitude-behavior consistency, were studied in relation to family relationships.

**Methods:** Public health nurses collected data on single mothers with low-birth-weight and full-term preschool children. A total of 60 mothers with low-birth-weight children and 81 mothers of full-term preschool children were in the study. The data collected was demographics regarding employment, the Parenting Stress Index, Feetham Functioning Survey, and Home Observation for Measurement of the Environment.

**Findings:** Employed mothers provided more stimulating home environments and had more positive perceptions of their children. These results could be related to other effects such as education, income, and number of children. Mother-child relationships and family functioning were similar for families of preterm and full-term children.

**Implications:** Employment and gestational status had little effect on mother-child relationships. Public health nurses can examine studies such as this to develop intervention plans to address the specific needs of single mothers.

Youngblut, J., Singer, L., Madigan, E., Swegart, L., & Rogers, W. (1998). Maternal employment and parent-child relationships in single-parent families of low-birth-weight preschoolers. *Nursing Research, 47*(2), 114–121.

## Settings for Partnerships with Community Health Care Nursing

There are many settings where **community partnerships** (health care providers that bring together a large number of community-based agencies, health care clinicians, educational institutions, and public organizations to address the health needs of a specific community) are established among health care organizations and community health nursing. These connections provide the added benefit of resources, personnel, and administrative organizational structures.

## Homeless Care

One example of a community health partnership is Healthcare for the Homeless in Houston (HHH). HHH is a conglomerate of health care providers that brings together a large number of community-based agencies, health care clinicians, educational institutions, and public organizations to address the health needs of homeless people (Healthcare for the Homeless in Houston, 2001). The principles of HHH are shown in Box 23-3.

## Parish Nursing

Another example of an organization where partnerships exist in community-based nursing is **parish nursing**. Parish nursing is an organization whereby a religious or health care system coordinates RNs in providing nursing care to members of a church congregation. Parish nurses don't address just spiritual needs—they address the physical and emotional needs of their clients as well. The goal of parish nursing is not to provide home health care services, but to provide counseling, education, screening, and advocacy. In addition, parish nurses can coordinate volunteers, develop support groups, and make referrals to appropriate community resources (Hamlin, 2000).

## International Partnerships

International partnerships between well-developed countries and countries with underdeveloped health care systems are another kind of partnership in community health nursing. An example is L'Arche, an international organization that began in Canada. L'Arche has taken developmentally disabled persons out of institutions in impoverished countries and, with the support of their

### BOX 23-3 PRINCIPLES OF A HEALTH CARE PROGRAM FOR THE HOMELESS

1. Community-oriented primary care
2. Use of research to determine who are stakeholders, and needs and resources identification.
3. Health care is provided along with food, clothing, and shelter.
4. Hiring the homeless as researchers, to ensure they are part of the solution (i.e., what do the recipients of care identify as the needs).

Healthcare for the Homeless in Houston, 2001, www.homeless-healthcare.org

families, placed them in community homes where they can live normal lives. The L'Arche philosophy fits an important principle of community care nursing: to acknowledge and use individual and group strengths (International L'Arche Care, 2001).

# Nursing Process in Community Health Care

Community health nursing is built on the knowledge and professional practice of RNs. The goal of community health nurses is to preserve and improve the health of populations and communities worldwide. Community health nurses use the nursing process as they work with families and groups within a wide variety of communities. Community health nurses are in a position to contribute to the development of community-based systems that address the current and projected health needs of populations (Hitchcock et al., 2003).

## Assessment

The success of a community health care program hinges on a comprehensive assessment of group needs. A needs assessment enables the nurse to ascertain common concerns or appropriate interventions for the group (e.g., teaching strategies). Factors to consider when assessing a group for the purpose of a program or intervention are seen in the community assessment in Box 23-4 and in the Nursing Strategy box. In addition, many sources of data are available to use for a group needs assessment. First, the nurse can assess the client group with verbal questioning or short questionnaires. Second, the nurse can make observations of the group and others who work with the group (e.g., teachers at school, health care providers). Third, the nurse can review any client records that exist. Last, a literature review can also provide the nurse with valuable information on group interventions that have been used to respond to group concerns and health issues.

## Nursing Diagnosis

In community health nursing, the focus is on groups rather than on individuals; therefore, consideration is given to health promotion and wellness concepts for entire populations of individuals. When formulating nursing diagnoses, the nurse takes into consideration both health promotion and illness prevention for populations, as well as diagnoses aimed at illness management for the health of the community.

### Omaha System

The Visiting Nurses Association of Omaha, Nebraska, developed a system of nursing diagnoses in the 1970s (Martin & Scheet, 1992). This system was developed to identify physical factors and external health factors important to community health. The OMAHA system

allowed for flexibility in assigning diagnoses to groups as well as individuals. The OMAHA system has three components: (1) the problem classification scheme, (2) the intervention scheme, and (3) the problem rating scale for outcomes. The problem classification scheme is divided into four levels. The first level is called the *domain* and includes the four general areas of community health practice: environmental, psychosocial, physiological, and health-related behaviors. The second level, called the *problem*, consists of 40 nursing diagnoses that nurses are licensed to assign and treat and that are amenable to nursing intervention. The third level identifies *modifiers*, or terms used in conjunction with the problems. *Signs and symptoms* are the fourth level. They are used only with actual deficits.

The problem rating scale for outcomes "provides a framework for evaluating the client's problem-specific knowledge, behavior, and status at regular or predictable time intervals" (Martin & Scheet, 1992, p. 93). These components can be assessed on a continuum that provides five degrees of response, from the most negative to the most positive state of a problem.

## Planning

To develop a plan for working with clients in community health nursing, the first issue that a nurse must address is acceptance by the clients. Sometimes nurses may be perceived as threatening or as outsiders. Nurses may represent agencies, which are not respected or trusted. Therefore, time and care may be needed to establish rapport with the client group. Nurses can gain acceptance and establish rapport by participating in community activities and maintaining a nonthreatening presence over a period of time (Hitchcock et al., 2003). Given the information and data that have been collected through an assessment, the nurse needs to determine the main focus or priority for the client. The factors that the community health nurse must consider priority are listed in Box 23-5.

## Implementation

The interventions for community health nursing have been exemplified in the aforementioned nursing roles, settings of community-based nursing, and partnerships. In general, the goal of these methods of implementation is to improve the society's overall health status. The nurse must identify the need for change and implement interventions to accomplish this mission. Often, the nurse must identify policy changes and then recognize that social changes are needed.

## Evaluation

The evaluation of community health care has evolved greatly over the past 2 decades. Initially, evaluation was not well defined or controlled. Priorities were poorly established, and written standards for evaluation were unclear.

## BOX 23-4 COMMUNITY ASSESSMENT GUIDE: THE PLACE, THE PEOPLE, AND THE SOCIAL SYSTEM

The community health assessment guide is a tool that guides the community health nurse in the systematic collection of data about the characteristics of an identified community and the formulation of community health diagnoses about the community's assets and health problems and concerns. The guide provides a method for assessing relevant community parameters and identifies categories and subcategories that provide direction for the organization of data in a meaningful way.

Community _____ Date _____

### I. Overview
A. Description of the community
   1. History
   2. Type of community: urban, suburban, rural

### II. The Community as a Place
A. Description: general identifying data
   1. Location
   2. Topography
   3. Climate
B. Boundaries, area in square miles
C. Environment
   1. Sanitation: water supply, sewage, garbage, trash
   2. Pollutants, toxic substances, animal reservoirs or vectors, flora and fauna
   3. Air quality: color, odor, particulates
   4. Food supply: sources, preparation
D. Housing for special populations
   1. Types of housing (public and private)
   2. Condition of housing
   3. Percent owned, rented
   4. Housing for special populations
      a. Near homeless
      b. Homeless
      c. Frail elders
E. Leading industries and occupations

### III. The People of the Community
A. Population profile
   1. Total population for _____ (year of last census)
   2. Population density
   3. Population changes in past 10 years
   4. Population per square mile
   5. Mobility
   6. Types of families
B. Vital and demographic population characteristics
   1. Age distribution
   2. Sex distribution
   3. Race distribution
   4. Ethnic group composition and distribution

   5. Socioeconomic status
      a. Income of family
      b. Major occupations
      c. Estimated level of unemployment
      d. Percent below poverty level
      e. Percent retired
   6. Educational level
   7. Religious distribution
   8. Marriage and divorce rates
   9. Birth and death rates
C. Leading causes of morbidity
   1. Incidence rates (specific diseases)
   2. Prevalence rates (specific diseases)
D. Mortality characteristics
   1. Crude death rate
   2. Age-specific death rate
   3. Infant mortality rate
   4. Maternal mortality rate
   5. Leading causes of death

### IV. The Community as a Social System
A. Government and leadership
   1. Type of government (mayor, city manager, board of supervisors)
   2. City offices (location, hours, services, access)
B. Education
   1. Public educational facilities
   2. Private educational facilities
   3. Libraries
   4. Services for special populations
      a. Pregnant teens
      b. Adults with special problems
      c. Children and adults who are developmentally disabled
      d. Children and adults who are blind and/or deaf
C. Transportation
   1. Transport systems: bus, suburban train, private auto, air, streetcar, other
   2. Transportation provisions for special populations
      a. Elders
      b. Homeless/near homeless
      c. Adults with disabilities
D. Communication resources
   1. Newspapers
   2. Radio stations
   3. Television
   4. Key community leaders and/or decision makers
   5. Internet websites
   6. Other
E. Religious resources
   1. Churches and other religious facilities

*(continues)*

## BOX 23-4   COMMUNITY ASSESSMENT GUIDE: THE PLACE, THE PEOPLE, AND THE SOCIAL SYSTEM (*continued*)

2. Community programs and services (e.g., health ministries, parish nursing)
3. Major religious leaders

F. Recreation resources
1. Public and private facilities
2. Programs for special population groups
   a. People with disabilities
   b. Elders
   c. People with hearing or vision impairment
   d. Other

G. Community safety (protection)
1. Fire protection (describe)
2. Police protection, including county detention facilities (describe)
3. Disaster preparation

H. Stores and shops
1. Types and location
2. Access

I. Community health facilities and resources (see Section V)

### V. Community Health Facilities and Resources
(Resource access, availability, eligibility)

A. Health systems
1. Hospitals (type and services rendered): acute care facilities—emergency medical, surgical, intensive care, psychiatric
2. Rehabilitation health care facilities: physical conditions, alcoholism, and substance abuse
3. Home health services: hospice and home health agencies
4. Long-term care facilities (e.g., skilled nursing facilities)
5. Respite care services for special population groups
6. Ambulatory services
   a. Hospital ambulatory clinics
   b. Public health service clinics
   c. Nursing centers
   d. Community mental health centers
   e. Crisis clinics
   f. Community health centers
7. Special health services for targeted populations
   a. Preschool
   b. School age
   c. Adult or young adult
   d. Adults and children with handicaps (e.g., regional centers for developmentally disabled)
8. Other
   a. School health services
   b. Occupational health services

B. Public health and social services
1. Health departments (various programs)
2. Social services
   a. Department of social services
      (1) County level—location of suboffices
      (2) Official (public) social services, major programs (e.g., adult services, children's services, Welfare to Work)—eligibility, services rendered, location
   b. Social Security (USA)
      (1) Location and program availability
      (2) Eligibility

C. Voluntary health organizations
1. Cancer Society
2. Heart Association
3. Red Cross
4. Women's shelter
5. Suicide prevention
6. Rape crisis centers
7. Family service agency
8. Catholic Charities
9. Alzheimer's Association
10. Lung Association
11. Diabetes Association

D. Health-related planning groups
1. Area Agency on Aging
2. Senior coordinating councils
3. High-risk infant coordinating councils
4. Healthy Communities Coordinating Teams
5. Multipurpose agencies
6. Teen violence prevention planning teams

### VI. Summary

A. What are the major assets of the community and from whose perspective—health care provider's, community members', and so on?
1. The place
2. The people
3. The resources (availability, accessibility, acceptability; public and private)

B. What are the major health problems/needs?
1. The place
2. The people
3. The resources (availability, accessibility, acceptability; public and private)

C. Identify and propose the contributions of nurses, other health care providers, community leaders, community residents, and so on to the solutions

D. Which of the health problems/needs should be given priority—first, second, and third? Why?

From Hitchcock, J., Schubert, P., & Thomas, S. (2003). *Community health nursing: Caring in action* (2nd ed.). Clifton Park, NY: Delmar Learning.

## NURSING STRATEGY

### Factors the Nurse Considers When Assessing a Group

1. Gender, age, and ethnicity
2. Socioeconomic status (provides information on what resources may be available to group members)
3. Educational levels and literacy rates (helpful for determining handouts, posters, or other materials)
4. Support services and resources already available (determines what other programs are available and accessible to the group)

Hitchcock, J., Schubert, P., & Thomas, S. (2003). *Community health nursing: Caring in action* (2nd ed.). Clifton Park, NY: Delmar Learning.

## BOX 23-5　PRIORITIES FOR ASSESSMENT IN COMMUNITY HEALTH CARE

1. Number of people affected by the issue or problem
2. Severity of the issue or problem
3. Group's awareness of the issue or problem
4. Group's motivation to resolve or better manage the issue or problem
5. Nurse's ability to influence the issue or problem
6. Practical considerations, the nurse's individual skills, time, and resource constraints

Then in 1991, the American Public Health Association (APHA) published national standards and objectives in *Healthy People 2000* (American Public Health Association, 2003). These model standards allowed communities to set health objectives and to establish budgetary plans for addressing the health needs of their communities. Then the APHA updated the national standards with *Healthy People 2010*, which continues to address the health needs of communities with an outcome-driven system (Healthy People 2010, 2003).

# CASE STUDY/NURSING CARE PLAN

As a community health nurse, you have a referral from a school district to make a home visit to the Plotnik family, consisting of mother Stella, age 30, and her two children, Jane, age 3, and 6-month-old Susan. They live in a small two-bedroom apartment complex. Stella is a single parent who was recently divorced from her husband. Her major source of income is from social assistance. Because she finds it hard "to make ends meet," she is also caring for other children in her home to supplement her income. The community infant and pre-school nurse is concerned that Stella has not brought her children in for immunizations since Jane's initial series of DTaP (diptheria-tetanus-acellular pertussis) and IPV (inactivated polio) was completed at 6 months of age. Susan has had no immunizations. Stella tells you that Jane has generally been well with an occasional cold and flu, especially since Stella began caring for other children. Susan was a "colicky" baby but "seems to be growing out of it," although she is still "somewhat fussy." Stella tells you she hates injections, and she just doesn't have time to get the children immunized. The hours are limited at the community clinic, and "you have to wait forever." Stella tells you that her friends also don't have time to immunize their children. And, "besides, we are all healthy, and the children are growing well and developing similarly to their peers."

## Assessment

The community health nurse is caring for a family with a single-parent mother, a preschool 3-year-old child, and 6-month-old child. The family has financial limitations causing a lack of immunizations for the children and questionable health care services.

## Nursing Diagnosis #1

*Interrupted Family Processes* related to time constraint difficulty from single-parenting due to recent divorce

**NOC:** Family Coping; Family Functioning; Family Normalization

**NIC:** Family Integrity Promotion; Family Process Maintenance

*(continues)*

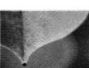 **CASE STUDY/NURSING CARE PLAN** (*continued*)

**Expected Outcomes**

The client will:

1. Describe the resources available for assistance and sources of support regarding single-parenting situation in first meeting with nurse.
2. Express feelings regarding the recent divorce and any effects these feelings might have on parenting style in first meeting with nurse.
3. Explore options for obtaining immunizations for children within 2 weeks.

**Planning/Interventions/Rationales**

1. Ask client the characteristics of extended family and friends. *Evaluates the resources of assistance that exist.*
2. Identify the support resources that exist for the client (e.g., church, school). *Evaluates the support resources, and makes mobilizing these resources possible.*
3. Explore client's feelings regarding recent divorce and how it has affected her parenting skills. *Identifying emotional effects of the divorce can be a first step in resolving problems of parenting associated with the divorce.*
4. Identify public health services to provide immunizations for the children. *Public health is often available for this type of treatment.*

**Evaluation**

Client verbalized that the grandparents of her children live close by, and she asked them to help her with the children. In addition, she was able to get friends from her church to assist her food stores by having a "food pounding" (donating groceries to her family). Client also was able to have children immunized at a free public health clinic within 2 weeks of seeing the community health nurse.

## Key Concepts

- It is important to identify the members of a community and to understand their common culture.
- Global migration has greatly affected the boundaries of community.
- Critical social theory, the citizen ladder of participation, and Milio's ecological approach to health care are three frameworks for the delivery of community care.
- Some of the nursing roles of community care are educator, advocate, direct care provider, and social marketer.
- Schools, neighborhood/community centers, and migrant clinics are examples of the settings in which community care takes place.
- Partnerships occur in community care, such as parish nursing, care of the homeless, and international partnerships.

## Review Questions and Activities

1. What are elements of a community?
2. What are several types of communities?
3. What are the primary differences among the three identified frameworks for community care?

4. What are several nursing roles commonly employed in community health nursing?
5. Where do nurses practice community health care? How do these settings compare to one another?
6. What are the advantages of developing partnerships internationally?
7. How do nurses assess community needs?
8. What are several nursing diagnoses specific to community-based care?

## Web Resources

American Public Health Association
http://www.apha.org
Arizona Smokers Helpline
http://www.ashline.org
Canadian Health Network
http://www.canadian-health-network.ca
Canadian Public Health Association
http://www.cpha.ca
Healthcare for the Homeless in Houston
http://www.homeless-healthcare.org
Healthy People 2010
http://phpartners.org

Immunization Initiatives
    http://www.aap.org
International L'Arche Care
    http://www.larche.org.uk
National Association of School Nurses
    http://www.nasn.org

# References

American Public Health Association (2003): http://www.apha.org

Arizona Smokers Helpline (2001): http://www.ashline.org

Arnstein, S. (July 1969). A ladder of citizen participation. *Journal of the American Institute of Planners, 13*(4), 216–223.

Brownson, R., & Krueter, M. (1997) Future trends affecting public health, *Journal of Public Health Management and Practice 3*(2), 47.

Bryant, C., Lindenberger, J., Brown, C. Kent, E., Schreiber, J., Bustillo, M., & Canright, M. (2001). A social marketing approach to increasing enrollment in a public health program: A case study of the Texas WIC program. *Human Organization, 60*(3), 234–246.

Canadian Health Network (2003): http://www.canadian-health-network.ca

Chaffee, M. (1999). A telehealth odyssey. *American Journal of Nursing, 99*(7), 27–32.

DeSantis, L. (1999). Building health communities with immigrants and refugees. *Journal of Transcultural Nursing, 9*(1), 20–31.

Hamlin, L. (2000). Faith and healing. *Vital Signs, 10*(27), 21–26.

Healthcare for the Homeless in Houston (2001): http://www.homeless-healthcare.org

Healthy People 2010 (2003): http://nnlm.gov/partners

Hitchcock, J., Schubert, P., & Thomas, S. (2003). *Community health nursing: Caring in action* (2nd ed.). Clifton Park, NY: Delmar Learning.

International L'Arche Care (2001): http://www.larche.org.uk

Kowash, M., Pinfield, A., Smith, J., & Curzon, M. (2000). Effectiveness in oral health of a long-term health education program for mothers with young children. *British Dental Journal, 188*(4), 201–205.

Martin, K., & Scheet, N. (1992). *The OMAHA system: Applications for community health nursing.* Philadelphia: W. B. Saunders Co.

McGuire, S. (1998). Global migration and health: Ecofeminist perspectives. *Advances in Nursing Science 21*(2), 1–16.

Milio, N. (1976). A framework for prevention: Changing health-damaging to health-generating life patterns. *American Journal of Public Health, 66*(5), 435.

National Association of Correctional Nursing (2003): www.correctionalnursing.org

National Association of School Nurses (2003): http://www.nasn.org

Pan American Health Organization (PAHO) (March 2001). Nursing services contributing to equity access, quality and sustainability in the health services. March 2001. *Organization and management of health systems and services, division of health systems and services development.*

Panahi G. R., & Shahtahmasebi, S. (1999) The implication of telemedicine for nursing. *Professional Nurse, 14*(2) 835–838.

Rew, L., Fouladi, R., & Yockey, R. (2002). Sexual practices of homeless youth. *Journal of Nursing Scholarship, 34*(2), 139–145.

Roberts, R., Rigby, M., & Birch, K. (2000). Telematics in healthcare: New paradigm, new issues. In R. Roberts, M. Rigby, & K. Birch (Eds.). *Taking health telematics into the 21st century.* Oxon, UK: Radcliffe Medical Press Ltd.

Schroeter, K. (2000). Advocacy in perioperative nursing practice. *AORN Journal, 71*(6), 1207-1210,1213,1215–1218.

Stevens, P. E., & Hall, J. M. (1992). Applying critical theories to nursing in the communities. *Public Health Nursing, 9*(1), 2–9.

Youngblut, J., Singer, L., Madigan, E., Swegart, L., & Rogers, W. (1998). Maternal employment and parent-child relationships in single-parent families of low-birth-weight preschoolers. *Nursing Research, 47*(2), 114–121.

Wiesel, E. (1994). *The Night Trilogy: Night Dawn the Accident.* New York: Noonday Press.

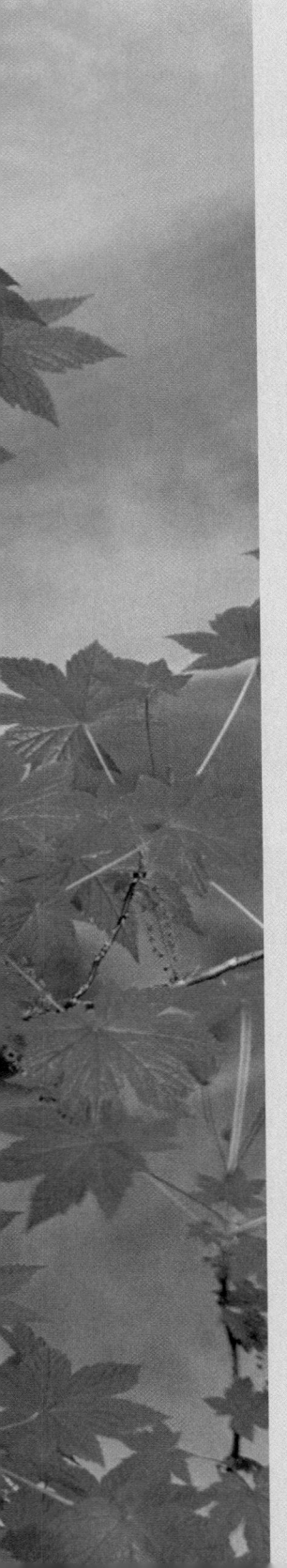

# V UNIT

# Leadership in Nursing

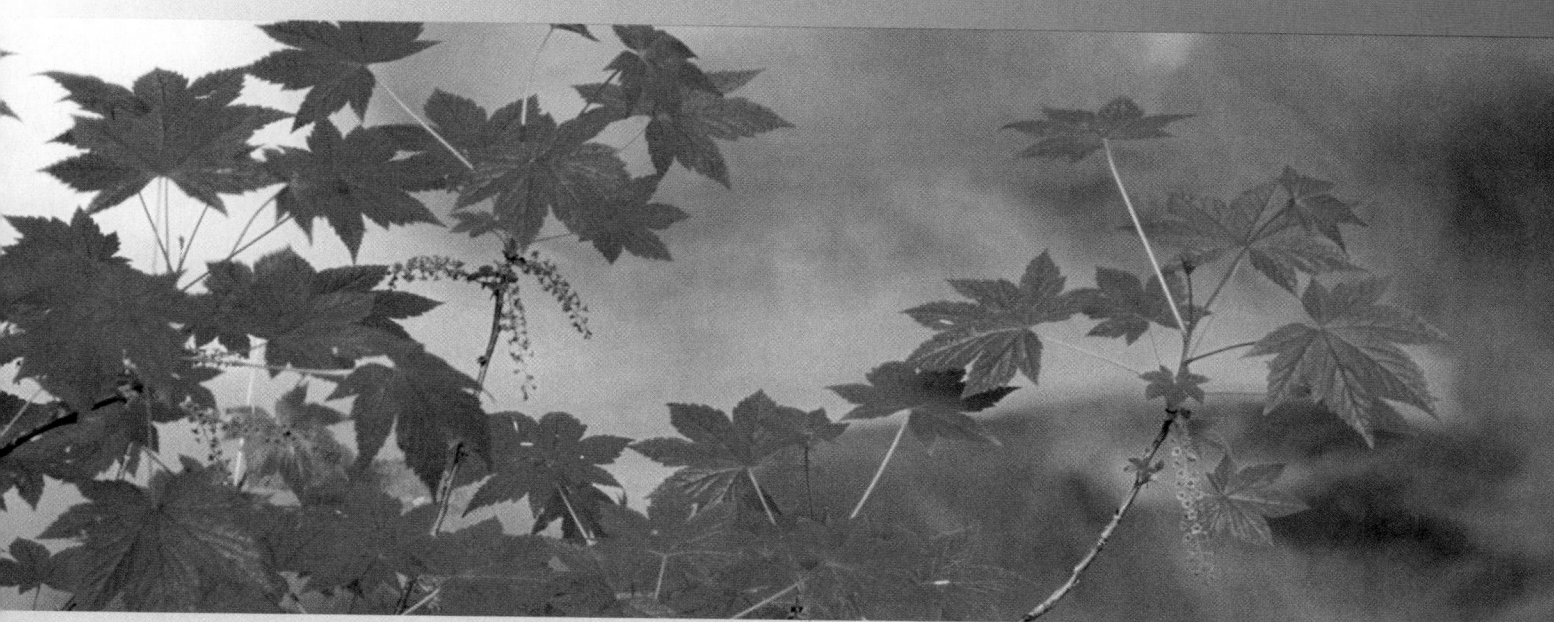

# CHAPTER 24

# Leadership, Delegation, and Collaboration

Leonard H. Friedman, PhD, MPH
Larry A. Mullins, FACHE, CFAAMA

*"Managers do things right—leaders do the right things."*

*(Warren Bennis and Burt Nannus, 1985)*

# Chapter Competencies

*Upon completion of this chapter, the reader should be able to:*

1. Analyze and define the role of leadership as it relates to nursing.
2. Identify the history of leadership theory.
3. Describe various frameworks that support leadership.
4. Compare and contrast nursing management versus nursing leadership.
5. Compare and contrast leadership styles.
6. Evaluate the use of different leadership styles in nursing.
7. Analyze a variety of leadership characteristics.
8. Identify the principles of conflict management and resolution.
9. Assess and describe resource management in nursing leadership.
10. Identify various leadership maxims for nursing.

# Key Terms

accommodation
autocratic leadership style
avoidance
budget
change
change agent
collaboration
consultative leadership style
credibility

delegation
democratic leadership style
direct expenses
emotional intelligence (EI)
indirect expenses
laissez-faire leadership style
leadership
leadership theory
management

negotiation
nursing leadership
participative leadership style
pressing
servant leadership
situational leadership
transformational leadership

The need for nursing leaders with an ability to delegate, collaborate, think creatively, and act boldly is more critical now than perhaps at any time in the past (Figure 24-1). There are two critical influences on the nursing profession and the need for nursing leaders. First, the predicted shortage of nurses has already started to occur, with some estimates of shortage running from 400,000 to 1,000,000 nurses. Second, the complexity of health care delivery suggests that there will be a growing need for nurse leaders to guide nursing through an increasingly complex health care environment (Lindholm, Sivberg, & Uden, 2000).

Nursing leaders are fundamentally no different from others who are asked to lead professional workers in highly complex and rapidly changing organizations. It is important to define what nursing leadership means and then examine how both classical and contemporary theories of leadership can be applied to nursing environments. Factors in the health care system that influence nursing leadership are continually shrinking reimburse- ment, growing sophistication in clinical technology, and an increasing militancy among physicians, payers, and clients.

# Definition of Nursing Leadership

Leadership is commonly defined as a process of influence in which the leader influences others toward goal achievement (Yukl, 1998). Influence is an instrumental part of leadership and means that leaders affect others, often by inspiring, enlivening, and engaging others to participate. The process of leadership involves the leader and the follower in interaction. What this means for nurses as professionals is that they function as leaders when they influence others toward goal achievement. Nurses are leaders. There are many more leaders in organizations than those who are in positions of authority. Each person has the potential to serve as a leader.

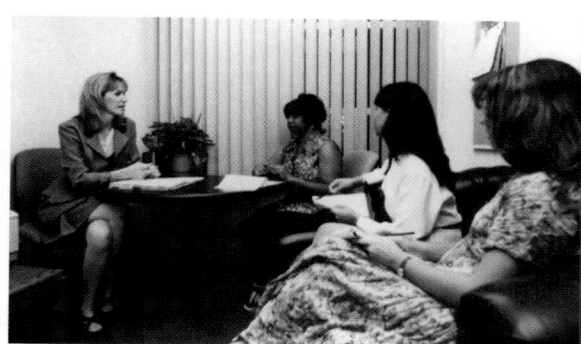

**Figure 24-1    Nurse leaders meeting together to make critical decisions**

New models of leadership for a constantly changing health care environment are continually explored. Empowering models of transformational leadership and the integration of new technology and new systems for the information age are also used. Students learn to design, manage, and evaluate health care systems with the potential for global application. Furthermore, student nurses are equipped with organizational skills that promote their ability to be partners in health care organizations to facilitate changes that improve practice and lead to changes in the health care system (Wheatley, 1999).

In an interesting definition of **nursing leadership**, the King Faisal Specialist Hospital and Research Center in Saudi Arabia characterizes nursing leadership as information about the individual patient, science of care, provision of care, outcome of care, cost of care, and organizational performance in order to design nursing systems. There is general agreement that more experience in nursing practice should translate both to enhanced professional expertise and, more important, to a willingness to mentor young nurses. A number of factors make nursing leadership challenging, including a wide variation of entry points into the field, increased scientific and clinical expertise required of nurses, nursing's role as the centerpiece of the hospital setting, and the need to recruit ever larger numbers of young nurses into the field.

# History of Leadership Theory

**Leadership theory** is a constantly evolving field that seeks to identify those traits or characteristics that distinguish leaders, and to clarify the relationship between the leaders and the followers. Current leadership theory also incorporates a study of the leaders' effectiveness within a culture specific to an organization or society. The study of modern leadership theory began in earnest during the early part of the 20th century when scientific management principles were first applied to the industrial workplace. Even though formal theories of leadership did not evolve until the 1900s, people have been studying leaders and their actions since the beginning of recorded time. Evidence of this is reflected in the writings of Aristotle where he comments that some are born to lead while others are born to follow. Throughout history, different classes of society were afforded leadership opportunities based more upon birthright than ability, and it was assumed that some people were "destined " to be leaders. Largely for this reason, their traits or characteristics were studied so that distinguished leaders could be identified and modeled. Most early studies of leadership focused on "Great Men" in history and what they did. This approach to leadership study highlighted great individuals with great accomplishments. Yet it missed studying those who may have had the potential to become leaders but, for whatever reason, did not.

Another theory that evolved was that leaders came about because "great events" were thrust upon them; because of these events, leaders were produced. The study was also limited to leaders of birth or circumstance, but did not include design. While the study of leadership is quite extensive with over 10,000 books and articles on the subject and over 850 definitions of leadership (Goleman, 2000), there is still not a clear definition of leadership. Much like medicine or nursing, leadership is as much an

## STOP AND THINK

### Becoming a Nursing Leader

- What characteristics of leadership do you believe nursing students need to develop for their future roles as nurse leaders?

- How does becoming a nurse leader relate to recruitment of persons into the nursing profession?

## STOP AND THINK

### Characteristics of a Leader

- In your opinion, are leaders born or made? Why?

- What "natural characteristics" do you have that will enhance your effectiveness as a leader?

- What "natural characteristics" do you have that need to be developed to increase your potential as an effective leader?

- Who has influenced you or developed you in your leadership traits?

art as a science and can best be defined by what it accomplishes or the value it creates for its followers and society. As Bennis and Nanus (1985) stated in their management classic, "True leaders have an uncanny way of enrolling people in their vision through their optimism—sometimes unwarranted optimism."

## Leadership Frameworks

Given the very dynamic nature of health care organizations, leaders might employ certain frameworks to increase their effectiveness and the performance of their followers. A number of recent authors suggest that this not only is possible, but has been demonstrated in a large number of different organizations. Among the more important new leadership frameworks pertinent for nursing are transformational leadership, servant leadership, emotional intelligence leadership, and Collin's leadership levels.

## Transformational Leadership

In 1978, James Burns defined **transformational leadership** as leadership that promotes the end values of justice, equality, and human rights, as well as endorses the modal values of honesty, loyalty, and fairness as its basis for influencing change. A number of papers written in recent years speak to the power of transformational leadership for nursing. Bowles and Bowles (2000) discovered that nurses who worked for managers trained in transformational leadership techniques were significantly more satisfied with their leaders than those who worked for managers not trained in these methods. Ohman (2000) writes about critical care nurse managers who are highly transformational, using inspiration, motivation, and vision to empower staff, rather than intervening only when problems arise. She finds significant positive relationships between transformational leadership and previous leadership experience. The transformational leader seeks to help staff achieve extraordinary performance rather than just achieve what is required (Dunham-Taylor, 2000).

## Servant Leadership

In 1970, Robert Greenleaf first used the phrase **servant leadership** to describe a belief that leadership should be based on the needs of others and on helping those served to become "healthier, wiser, more autonomous, and more likely themselves to become servants" (Greenleaf, 1998). Greenleaf in his study of multiple institutions and organizations concludes that great leaders are first great servants. Ten characteristics of servant-leaders are identified in Box 24-1. A number of authors believe the servant leadership approach is valuable in health care applications. For example, Wilson (1998) writes that servant leadership is being used successfully at Baptist Health System, and ser-

## BOX 24-1    CHARACTERISTICS OF SERVANT-LEADERS

- Listening receptively to what is being said by others
- Empathy (although not specifically sympathy)
- Healing one's self and relationship with others
- Awareness of both self and one's surroundings
- Persuasion as opposed to personal authority in an organization
- Conceptualization (sometimes called thinking outside the box)
- Foresight that allows the leader to understand the lessons from the past
- Stewardship that includes the use of openness and persuasion rather than control
- Commitment to the growth of people
- Building community among those who work within an institution

Greenleaf, R. K. (1998). *The power of servant leadership*. San Francisco, CA: Berrett-Koehler.

vant leadership is also viewed as central to the daily operations of Catholic Health Association hospitals in St. Louis (Clifton & McEnroe, 1994).

## Emotional Intelligence Framework for Leadership

In 1995, Goleman coined the term **emotional intelligence (EI)** in the popular business press as emotional considerations being a way of helping to explain leadership effectiveness (Goleman, 1998). With a nod toward the behavior model of leadership, Goleman posits that in his research, effective leaders have high degrees of EI. In recent years, the principles of EI have been described in various nursing journals. In one instance, EI is being used as the foundation for a BSN curriculum on leadership (Bellack, Morjikian, Barger, Strachota, Fitzmaurice, Lee, Kluzik, Lynch, & Tsao, 2001). Muller-Smith (1999) notes that EI is a tool that makes even the nurse with average technical skills a self-directed employee who is an asset to the organization. Strickland (2000) believes that EI is "twice as important as a person's intelligence quotient and technical skills combined." EI also adds directly to nursing's increased profitability, lower costs, and increased client satisfaction.

## Collin's Leadership Levels

Jim Collins (2001) led a research team studying leadership in Fortune 500 companies. Leadership attributes were identified as well as comparisons made in leadership behaviors and style. Collins describes a leadership hierarchy consisting of five levels, each one necessary to transform an organization from good to great. At the highest level, leadership focuses on the contributions of team members, which is a good fit for nurses, who typically work in a team or collaborative environment.

## Nursing Management Versus Nursing Leadership

*Leadership* and *management* are terms often used interchangeably; however, some significant differences exist. **Management** is the accomplishment of tasks either by oneself or by directing others (see Box 24-2). **Leadership** is the interpersonal process that involves motivating and guiding others to achieve goals. Management is about power, and leadership is about influence; the difference is control versus vision. Leaders inspire staff to contribute to the organization's mission. Every nurse, regardless of title or position, is a manager; each has the potential to be a leader. The future success of the nursing profession lies in the hands of capable leaders (Figure 24-2). These individuals must possess competencies that motivate, activate, and energize those with whom they interact. Active listen-

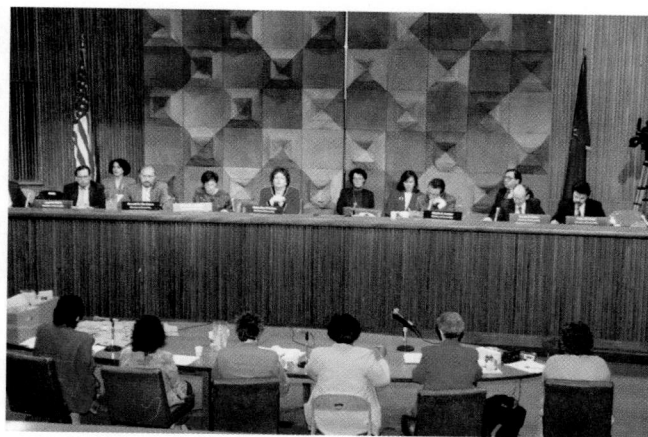

**Figure 24-2    Nurse leaders making a presentation before a state legislature; the future of the nursing profession depends on capable leaders representing nursing in a positive manner.** *Photo courtesy of the New York State Nurses Association*

ing, critical thinking, articulation of the relationship between costs and quality, goal setting, and quality care are characteristics the nursing profession needs (Anderson & McDaniel, 2000).

## Leadership Styles

Nurse leaders each have a particular style that tends to be consistent from one situation to the next. No single style is superior to another. Each leadership approach has its advantages and disadvantages. The effective leader will use **situational leadership**, which is a blending of styles based on current circumstances and events. The leader knows that behavior does not occur in a vacuum; thus, leadership styles are assumed according to the needs of the group and the tasks to be achieved. Rather than seek one ideal leadership style, Tannenbaum and Schmidt (1973) suggest that leadership styles exist along a continuum that ranges from autocratic to laissez-faire. Their model contrasts the use of authority by managers with the area of freedom for subordinates. The five leadership styles (autocratic, consultative, participative, democratic, and laissez-faire), in order of decreasing use of management authority and increasing subordinate freedom, are presented in the following section. (These styles of leadership are expanded on in Table 24-1.)

## Autocratic Leadership Style

The **autocratic leadership** style is leader-focused; that is, the leader maintains strong control, makes all decisions, and solves all problems. The leader dominates the group by issuing commands rather than making suggestions or seeking input (Lewin, 1939; Tannenbaum & Schmidt, 1973).

---

### BOX 24-2    ESSENTIAL FUNCTIONS OF EFFECTIVE MANAGERS

Essential functions that are performed by effective managers include

- Planning: Determining objectives and identifying methods that lead to achievement of those objectives

- Organizing: Using resources (human and material) to achieve predetermined outcomes

- Directing: Guiding and motivating others to meet the expected objectives

- Controlling: Using performance standards as criteria for measuring success, and taking corrective action, if necessary, to see that others comply with performance standards

- Decision making: Identifying a problem and deciding which alternatives can best meet the objectives

## TABLE 24-1    LEADERSHIP STYLES

| Style | Description | Leader Behaviors | Potential Impact on Group Members | Advantages | Disadvantages |
|---|---|---|---|---|---|
| Autocratic | Basic premise: leader knows best. Communication flows downward. | Controlling Directive Makes all decisions and solves all problems. Issues commands | Hostility Rebellion | Task oriented, high productivity. Facilitates a quick response. Often necessary in crisis situation. | Inhibits creativity and autonomy of members. Promotes mistrust and fear among followers. Members may become hostile or passive. |
| Consultative | Basic premise: leader informs members of best concepts. | Directive approach; teacher of information. | Increases knowledge levels | Promotes knowledge of members | May inhibit creativity; members can become dependent on leader. |
| Democratic ("Participative Leadership") | Basic premise: every member should have input. Communication is open and mutual. | Acts as a facilitator. Serves as a resource person. Encourages members' active participation. | Improved productivity. More opportunity for personal growth. Increased cooperation and teamwork. | Promotes empowerment of team members. Facilitates communication. Increased creativity and autonomy. | Time-consuming. May be less efficient (in quantifiable terms). Disagreements may happen as members express their viewpoints. |
| Laissez-Faire | Leadership responsibilities are assumed by group. Almost any behavior by the group is permissible due to the leader's lack of limit-setting and stated expectations. | Passive, non-directive approach. Provides little, if any, support, guidance, or feedback. Sets no limits. | Unmet tasks. Relationship needs of group members ignored. Apathy | Promotes autonomy and creativity in members. | May evoke passivity in team members. Aimless behavior often occurs. Chaos common. Inefficiency and low productivity. |

## Consultative Leadership Style

The **consultative leadership style** is based on the notion that leaders "sell" their decisions to subordinates. The concept of consultation is used, and the leader carefully explains the rationale for a decision and its effect on followers. The goal of the consultative style of leadership is to inform members and to allow questions by subordinates, thereby allowing greater understanding and acceptance of the decision (Tannenbaum & Schmidt, 1973).

## Democratic Leadership Style

The **democratic leadership style** is based on the belief that every group member should have input into development of goals and problem solving. The democratic leader acts primarily as a facilitator and resource person. Concern for each member of the group as a unique individual is demonstrated by the leader. Groups that adhere to this style of leadership often work well together as a team (Lewin, 1939; Tannenbaum & Schmidt, 1973).

The **participative style of leadership** is often considered as almost synonymous with the democratic style of leadership. Participative leaders present tentative decisions that may be changed if subordinates make a convincing case for an alternative. In the participative style, every person's viewpoints are considered valuable and everyone has equal voice in making decisions (Tannenbaum & Schmidt, 1973).

## NURSING STRATEGY

### Nursing Approaches and Leadership Styles

Descriptions of various leadership styles can also be used to explain differing nursing approaches to client care. For instance:

- The autocratic approach may not be successful with clients who have a high inner locus of control and are very independent in their personalities.

- Clients who may benefit more from the laissez-faire approach are those who are self-directive and make decisions well on their own.

- Sometimes, it may be beneficial for a client to have several members of the health care team together and use a participative approach, where the client's input is used in making health care decisions.

Heidenthal, P. (2003). *Nursing leadership & management.* Clifton Park, NY: Delmar Learning.

## CLIENT REFLECTIONS

### Leadership Style Used in a Coronary Care Unit

Mrs. Arnett had a coronary artery bypass graft (CABG) and was in your coronary care unit. She had to be ambulated frequently and required several staff members to assist her. She stated, "I was impressed with the way that the nurses kept each other informed of my different tubes and how they [the nurses] should move me together. They really worked well together, and I felt very safe when they came in together to work with me."

What approach (leadership style) do you think was used in this situation?

## Laissez-Faire Leadership Style

In the **laissez-faire leadership style**, the leader assumes a passive, nondirective, and inactive approach. Leadership responsibilities are either assumed by the members of the group or completely abdicated. All decision making is left to the group with the leader giving little, if any, guidance, support, or feedback. Almost any behavior by the group is permissible, due to the leader's lack of limit-setting and

stated expectations. The tasks are unmet, and the relationship needs of group members are ignored (Lewin, 1939; Tannenbaum & Schmidt, 1973).

## Leadership Characteristics

Leaders have many characteristics, and there is some debate about whether effective leaders are "born" versus effective leaders who learn behaviors of leadership. A compilation of important characteristics of effective leaders are discussed in the following sections.

### Effective Communication

Effective leadership relies heavily on the individual's ability to communicate well. An effective nurse leader will listen actively to others; articulate thoughts in an intelligent, persuasive manner; and differentiate aggressive, passive, and assertive behaviors in order to communicate appropriately in a given situation.

### Credibility

A leader motivates others by demonstrating enthusiasm and exerting influence. To be influential, the leader must be credible. **Credibility**, the quality or power of inspiring beliefs, is based on competence. From competence comes confidence. Individuals who know what they are doing and perform well are those who can influence others (Heidenthal, 2003).

## FOCUS ON WELLNESS

### Communicating the Concept of Wellness

Often the ability of the nurse to communicate clearly is a defining factor in creating a wellness orientation for the client. For example, in acute care settings the nurse must remember that wellness needs to be encouraged even though the client has acute care needs. Also, the nurse's assessment of the client's nonverbal cues as related to wellness orientation are important. For example, the client might look puzzled if the nurse uses phrases like "wellness" or "health promotion." In that event, the nurse would need to define what is meant in terms that are practical and relevant to the client.

Pender, J., Murdaugh, C., & Parsons, M. A. (2002). *Health promotion in nursing practice* (4th ed.). Upper Saddle River, NJ: Prentice-Hall.

## Collaboration

In health care, as in most industries today, effective team performance and **collaboration** (a partnership in which all parties are valued for their contribution) is the norm. Today, nurses work in multidisciplinary teams that form, dissolve, and reform in matrix structures, as the need requires. But simply bringing the best trained and most skillful people to the task at hand is often a futile and fruitless effort. In order for these teams to successfully collaborate and achieve the desired results, two things must occur. First, the team must agree on common goals. A conscious effort must be undertaken to structure goals that allow all group members to feel as though they are better off participating than not. In this "game," while "lose-lose," "win-lose," or "lose-win" scenarios are possible, the most desirable outcome is to structure "win-wins" for all the participants. Coupled with an intentional creation of mutually beneficial goals is the need to continually share information and resources. Decisions made by the group need to be transparent both to those within the group and those outside the group.

Experience teaches that trust is at the heart of any meaningful collaboration. In a recent study of the reasons for the failure or poor performance of otherwise well-designed integrated health systems, lack of trust between and among key stakeholders was found to be more important than misaligned economic incentives (Friedman & Goes, 2001). Trust is developed over a long period and is based on the alignment of words and actions. Kouzes and Posner (1995) found in their research that trust in effective teams was built on the vulnerability of team members and the willingness to carefully listen to what others were saying.

## Delegation

The nurse leader must be able to delegate effectively to coordinate the delivery of care. **Delegation** is the process of transferring a selected task in a situation to an individual who is competent to perform that specific task. Delegation is a multifaceted process involving communication, conflict resolution, feedback and evaluation, and knowledge of the person to whom a task is delegated. Delegation is a very helpful tool for nurse leaders in that it encourages team members to develop skills. Kouzes and Posner (1995) postulate that "we become the most powerful when we give our own power away" (p. 98). Leadership power is not a function of a title and a fancy office. Rather, it emanates from those who are led. There are many interventions with which to delegate power, responsibility, and authority.

As health care facilities restructure to address cost-containment issues, nurses delegate tasks to unlicensed assistive personnel (UAP) (e.g., nursing assistants, care partners, nurse extenders). RNs also delegate tasks to licensed practical or vocational nurses. The nurse practice

### NURSING STRATEGY

### Delegating Client Care

- Assess overall client assignments, and match with individual staff abilities.

- Discuss client assignments with staff, and ask for their input and suggestions at the beginning of the shift of care.

- Be willing to adjust client assignments as needs change in a nursing arena.

- Advise staff to ask others for assistance in client care situations and to keep the nurse manager informed of daily challenges.

- Show sensitivity to others, and offer visible support to peers and subordinates.

- Seek out ways to increase the number of decision choices and options.

Heidenthal, P. (2003). *Nursing leadership & management.* Clifton Park, NY: Delmar Learning.

acts define which aspects of care may be delegated and which must be performed by the RN. Because nurse practice acts vary among states, it is imperative that the nurse stay current with the rules and regulations regarding the delegation of nursing tasks.

## Critical Thinking

Another characteristic of an effective leader is the ability to think critically. This concept is covered thoroughly in Chapter 4 and can be reviewed. In general, the effective leader must apply critical-thinking skills on an ongoing basis.

### LEGAL AND ETHICAL ISSUES

### Critical Thinking and Delegation

Each nurse is responsible for knowing whether or not staffing is adequate to safely administer nursing care. A nurse needs to notify the nurse manager or supervisor if a client assignment is beyond her capabilities. The nurse should not continue to provide care when there is inadequate staffing, as this creates an unsafe client care environment.

Heidenthal, P. (2003). *Nursing leadership & management.* Clifton Park, NY: Delmar Learning.

## CLINICAL ALERT

### The Legalities of Delegation

Nurses must consult their state practice acts regarding the policies for safe practice and the roles of care providers in their settings. Delegation of specific tasks heavily depends on what a given professional is permitted to do. For example, in some states, personal care assistants may be allowed to perform skills that other states do not allow. The nurse is liable for knowing those differences that exist. Care givers must not be delegated tasks they are not legally allowed to perform. Ultimately, the safety and concern of the client is at stake.

Townes, J., & Cook, P. (2001). Standards of practice: A measure of competence. *Home Healthcare Nurse, 19*(6), 383–386.

# Conflict Management and Resolution

In their everyday duties, nurses are familiar with issues surrounding conflict and its resolution. The nature of health care is such that there is rarely one clear choice of a particular diagnosis or course of treatment. Nurses with similar training and experience can disagree on the best course of action. The expectation is that professionals will calmly, rationally, and openly discuss their options and come up with a mutually agreed-upon decision. However, while it is expected that group members will come into conflict with one another, conflict often is either treated as failure or may ultimately work to dissolve a previously well-functioning group. Many nurses actively try to avoid conflict, with the result that unresolved issues remain smoldering below the surface and negatively affect interactions between and among group members. Often, what passes for consensus is actually disengagement from the process (Eisenhardt, Kahwajy, & Bourgeois, 1997; Polzer & Neale, 2000).

## Levels of Conflict

Conflict can occur at one of three levels, including within the individual, between individuals within groups, and between groups. Individual conflict occurs when people are forced to choose between multiple alternatives. Accepting one alternative necessarily means rejecting all others. Conflict between individuals within groups is generally thought to be the most common form of conflict. Conflict between people and within groups is influenced by a number of variables including assumptions about one another, perceived (and often real) power gradients, past real or perceived injustices, and a host of other factors

both spoken and hidden below the surface. Finally, conflict between groups is becoming increasingly important as health care moves from the performance of individual professionals to the effective operation of teams of people. Sources of conflict between groups can result from differing beliefs, incompatible goals, or resource scarcity. The critical role of nursing leaders is to acknowledge that conflict exists and develop strategies to manage conflict (Heidenthal, 2003).

## Managing Conflict

Conflict is a natural part of every group and every organization. Nurse leaders must acknowledge that conflict exists regardless of their best efforts to stay clear of obvious problem areas. Also, some of the most effective organizations are those where teams are allowed to "have a good fight" as long as the process is carefully managed and the goal of high-quality client care remains the focus of all the members of the group. Conflict management is a highly individual activity with many strategies for resolution. The literature suggests that there are four principle strategies for handling conflict: accommodation, pressing, avoidance, and negotiation (Polzer & Neale, 2000).

### Accommodation

**Accommodation** is certainly a popular method of handling conflict. Just give the aggrieved party what they want and conflict is resolved. Unfortunately, this method more often than not creates more conflict, as other members of the group begin to question the motives and rationale for the decision (Polzer & Neale, 2000).

### Pressing

The next conflict management strategy is termed **pressing**, which is based on an assertive concern for self or group coupled with little or no concern for others. In the process of negotiation, this approach is frequently referred to as a "win-lose" strategy. The nurse manager might include threats and promises, irrevocable commitments, and (when appropriate) persuasive arguments as tools for managing conflict among individuals or groups. One common application of pressing is a quid pro quo approach where there is an exchange for support or acquiescence relative to the decision in question (Polzer & Neale, 2000).

### Avoidance

A third conflict management approach is **avoidance**. In order not to deal with an uncomfortable or difficult situation, some nurse managers may try to avoid it altogether with the assumption that given enough time, the issue will resolve itself and just go away. While conflict avoidance is sometimes a reasonable approach, using it as the only method is certain to create additional problems as systemic conflicts are allowed to grow in both size and complexity (Polzer & Neale, 2000).

## Negotiation

Finally, nurse managers may want to use **negotiation** as a way of navigating conflict. In this technique, the parties to a conflict decide what they must retain and what they are willing to give up in order to reach a compromise position. The goal of the nurse manager is to assist the parties in conflict to arrive at a point where they are satisfied that their needs are fulfilled and a "win-win" can be created (Polzer & Neale, 2000).

## Resource Management for Nurse Leaders

Resource management (of people, equipment, time) is an increasingly challenging task for nurse managers because of the tremendously increased expenses in today's health care delivery system. While managing human resources is an art unto itself and is probably the largest part of a nurse manager's job, some responsibilities for the allocation and control of resources go beyond just abiding by various labor laws and hiring practices. Financial management by nurse managers is vital for health care organizations, because expression of their strategic plans and objectives are operationalized in the various operating budgets developed for each and every department. Control of finances involves developing a strategy whereby nurse managers continually review financial performance and assess the reason for variation from stated budget objectives (Heidenthal, 2003).

## Financial Control Method of Budgeting

The primary financial control method for nurse managers is operationalizing a fiscally sound **budget** (a plan that provides formal quantitative expression for acquiring and distributing funds over the ensuing time period). Budgets are constructed of both revenues and expenses. At the department level, it may not be possible or desirable to estimate revenues for the provision of client services. However, the expense budget is a standard tool required of all nursing departments. All nurses must be aware of the expenses of their services and practice accordingly. The nurse manager will categorize expenses as being either direct or indirect. **Direct expenses** are those that are directly attributable to the department and will include both labor and nonlabor components. Examples of direct expenses are dressing supplies, nurse salaries, and medications. **Indirect expenses** are those costs allocated from the operation of the larger organization to the various service units. Examples of indirect expenses include information systems, administration, billing, housekeeping, and maintenance. According to JCAHO (2001), depart-

mental budgets need to be developed in collaboration with staff from respective services involved in care. The challenge to the nurse manager is creating a budget that is realistic and meets the fiscal demands of the total health care environment.

## Leadership Maxims for Nurses

Both the generalizability and specificity of nursing leadership lead to the development of three maxims that are useful to all nurses, from entry-level to the most experienced nurses. These simple rules have application at all levels of nursing organizations.

## Nursing Leadership Is Based on Values

Certain core values are essential to nursing leadership. One such core value is service to others. Other important

---

### BOX 24-3    CRITICAL ELEMENTS OF SELF-AWARENESS

- Communication—particularly the ability to carefully listen to what others are saying. While written and verbal communication is vital for any leader, listening intently to others may be even more important.

- Empathy—at its core, health care in general and nursing in particular are predicated on serving people at their moments of greatest need. Your job is to sense the moods and emotional needs of others and understand what they are experiencing. This ability to be empathetic with those you lead is at least as important.

- Balance—in your personal and professional lives. While work itself is important, relationships with family, friends, and loved ones may be equally important in your success as a leader.

- Attitude—the way others perceive you and the face you put on for the world to see. Your ability to keep a positive attitude sends a very powerful and persuasive message to those around you.

Adapted from Goleman, D. (1998). What makes a leader? *Harvard Business Review, 76*(6), 93–102.

values include self-sacrifice, social justice, and honesty. These core values ultimately define the nurse leader. Effective nurse leaders must not only understand their own values, but also be consistent in expressing them both in word and in action. Put another way, when nurse leaders fail to "walk their talk," they are seen as something less than credible. The combination of a clear and undiluted understanding of core values and the consistent application of those values increases the effectiveness of nursing leadership (Clifton & McEnroe, 1994).

## Nursing Leaders Are Change Agents

Leadership in nursing requires the nurse to be an agent for **change** (making something different from what it was). This goes beyond simply managing the change process and making sure that the various steps associated with the particular change activity occurs on time. The nurse leader must take the role of the **change agent** to not only respond to change processes but also instigate change. The reason for continuous change in health care is clear. From a systems perspective, the health care industry is an open system with inputs

from a vast number of sources (e.g., providers, payers, government agencies, regulators, manufacturers, clients). The role of the nurse leader is to anticipate change where possible and make sure the best systems are put into place to comply with the demands of the change driver. The nurse leader has the responsibility to decide what change is needed to propel the organization forward (Wheatley, 1999).

## Nursing Leaders Must Be Self-Aware

Bennis and Nanus in their classic work (1985) reported that successful leaders had a high degree of self-awareness. Numerous other leadership books also mention the tremendous value that self-awareness imparts to current and prospective leaders. Perhaps Socrates' recommendation of "Know thyself" was the primer for all leaders. More recently, Goleman (1998) suggests that self-awareness is one of the keys to emotional intelligence. The necessity for nurse leaders to achieve a high level of self-awareness is rooted in the need to be continually aware of the skills and attributes of the nurse. Self-awareness is particularly critical for nurse leaders in a number of aspects (see Box 24-3).

# CASE STUDY/NURSING CARE PLAN

Nurse manager, Nera, is making client assignments for her new graduate nurse, Judy, on her medical unit. Nera is assigning Mr. Agrwal to Judy. Mr. Agrwal is a very critical COPD (chronic obstructive pulmonary disease) client with respiratory complications accompanying acute bacterial pneumonia. Mr. Agrwal requires frequent nasotracheal suctioning, is somewhat tachypneic, has a decreased level of consciousness, has an oxygen saturation level of 88%, and has to have careful respiratory assessment and management. Judy expresses concern to her nurse manager about the care required, but agrees she needs the challenge of such a critical client. Nera reexamines the staffing for the day and decides to "shuffle" the client loads to enable Sherri, an experienced nurse, to have clients who are located close to Judy's clients. Then Nera asks Sherri to "work closely" with Judy. Furthermore, Nera communicates this decision to Judy and also asks Sherri and Judy to let her know "how it is going" at least twice during the shift of work.

## Assessment

Client is experiencing acute respiratory difficulties associated with bacterial pneumonia, and this is complicated with a history of a COPD. In addition, Mr. Agrwal has a decreased level of consciousness, which has likely resulted from a lowered oxygen saturation level of 88%. In addition, acid-base values are pH = 7.48, $CO_2$ = 49, $HCO_3$ = 24. And, from a leadership perspective, the nurse manager made an effective leadership decision in having an "expert" nurse (Sherri) mentor and help the "novice" nurse (Judy).

## Nursing Diagnosis #1
*Ineffective Airway Clearance* related to bacterial pneumonia and a history of COPD.
**NOC:** Respiratory Status: Ventilation; Respiratory Status: Airway Patency; Respiratory Status: Gas Exchange
**NIC:**  Airway Management; Airway Suctioning; Cough Enhancement

## Expected Outcomes
The client will:
1.  Demonstrate an increased air exchange by achieving an oxygen saturation level of at least 93% within 48 hours.
2.  Maintain a patent airway at all times.

*(continues)*

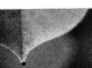

## CASE STUDY/NURSING CARE PLAN (continued)

### Planning/Interventions/Rationales

1. Auscultate breath sounds every 2 hours, and monitor constant pulse oximetry. *Assesses effectiveness of respiratory management and care.*
2. Provide nasotracheal suctioning every 2 hours and as needed. *Increases alveolar exchange by decreasing airway secretions.*
3. Maintain adequate hydration by monitoring intravenous fluids as ordered. *Prevents viscous secretions from accumulating.*

### Evaluation

Client maintained an oxygen saturation level of 94% within 48 hours and maintained a patent airway throughout hospitalization.

### Nursing Diagnosis #2

*Impaired Gas Exchange* as evidenced by lowered oxygen saturation levels and imbalances in acid-base values.

**NOC:** Respiratory Status: Gas Exchange; Respiratory Status: Ventilation; Tissue Perfusion: Pulmonary; Acid-Base Balance

**NIC:** Airway Management; Oxygen Therapy; Respiratory Monitoring; Acid-Base Management

### Expected Outcomes

The client will:

1. Demonstrate an increased air exchange by achieving an oxygen saturation level of at least 93% within 48 hours.
2. Demonstrate an improving acid-base balance by achieving pH and $CO_2$ within normal limits within 48 hours.

### Planning/Interventions/Rationales

1. Monitor constant pulse oximetry. *Assesses effectiveness of respiratory management and care.*
2. Assess respiratory rate, rhythm, and pattern, and encourage client to take deep breaths every 2 hours. *Deep breathing stimulates the airways, stimulates surfactant production, and expands the lung tissue surface, thus improving gas exchange.*
3. Monitor determinants of tissue oxygen delivery (e.g., pH, $CO_2$, $HCO_3$) daily. *Monitors acid-base balance, and detects abnormalities.*

### Evaluation

Client maintained an oxygen saturation level of 94% within 48 hours and achieved pH, $CO_2$, and $HCO_3$ within normal ranges within 48 hours.

## Key Concepts

- Nursing leadership is an essential component of the practice of nursing.
- Leadership theory has evolved from identifying the traits and behaviors of effective leaders to examining the particular organization and environment in which the leadership exists.
- Four current leadership frameworks are transformational leadership, servant leadership, emotional intelligence leadership, and Collin's leadership levels.
- Nursing leadership involves motivating others to achieve their goals, and it is different from nursing management, which is more narrow in focus and aimed at accomplishing specific tasks.
- Styles of leadership are autocratic, consultative, participative, democratic, and laissez-faire, which are often blended when used in nursing practice.

- Leadership characteristics include such concepts as communication, credibility, delegation, critical thinking, and conflict resolution.
- Identifying elements of resource management are fundamental concepts of quality nursing leadership.
- Three maxims for nursing leadership are based on values, change concepts, and self-awareness

## Review Questions and Activities

1. How is nursing leadership defined?
2. How has leadership theory been examined in the last century?
3. What are current leadership frameworks that potentially support the practice of nursing?

4. How are nursing management and nursing leadership different?

5. What are reasons for varying the styles of leadership used in nursing practice?

6. What characteristics of leadership are important to develop within nursing?

7. What principles of conflict management and resolution are used in nursing practice?

8. What is the nurse manager's role in resource management?

9. What leadership maxims are identified for use in nursing practice?

## Web Resources

American Association of Colleges of Nursing
http://www.aacn.nche.edu
American Nurses Association
http://www.ana.org
American Organization of Nurse Executives
http://www.aone.org
Health Resources and Services Administration of the Bureau of Health Professions, Division of Quality Assurance
http://www.npdb-hipdb.com
Joint Commission on Accreditation of Healthcare Organizations
http://www.jcaho.org
National Council of State Boards of Nursing
http://www.ncsbn.org
National League for Nursing
http://www.nln.org

## References

Anderson, R. A., & McDaniel, R. R. (2000). Managing health care organizations: Where professionalism meets complexity science. *Health Care Management Review, 25*(1), 83–92.

Bellack, J. P., Morjikian, R., Barger, S., Strachota, E., Fitzmaurice, J., Lee, A., Kluzik, T., Lynch, E., & Tsao. (2001). *Developing BSN leaders for the future: The Fuld leadership initiative for nursing.*

Bennis, W., & Nanus, B. (1985). *Leaders: The strategies for taking charge.* New York: HarperCollins.

Bowles, A., & Bowles, N. D. (2000). A comparative study of transformational leadership in nursing development units and conventional clinical settings. *Journal of Nursing Management, 8*(2), 69–76.

Burns, J. M. (1978). *Leadership.* New York: Harper Row.

Clifton, R. M., & McEnroe, J. J. (1994). A synergy of values. Catholic health care leaders must implement their organization's mission and model its values. *Health Progress 75*(5), 37–39.

Collins, J. (2002). Level 5 leadership: The triumph of humility and fierce resolve. *Harvard Business Review, 79*(1), 66–76.

Dunham-Taylor, J. (2000). Nurse executive transformational leadership found in participative organizations. *Journal of Nursing Administration, 30*(3), 241–250.

Eisenhardt, K., Kahwajy, J., & Bourgeois, L. (1997). How management teams can have a good fight, *Harvard Business Review, 75*(4), 77–85.

Friedman, L., & Goes, J. (2001) Have integrated health networks failed? *Frontiers of Health Services Management, 17*(4), 3–28.

Goleman, D. (1998). What makes a leader? *Harvard Business Review, 76*(6), 93–102.

Goleman, D. (2000). Leadership that gets results. *Harvard Business Review, 78*(2), 78–90.

Greenleaf, R. K. (1998). *The power of servant leadership.* San Francisco: Berrett-Koehler.

Heidenthal, P. (2003). *Nursing leadership & management.* Clifton Park, NY: Delmar Learning.

Joint Commission on Accreditation of Healthcare Organizations (2001). *Comprehensive accreditation manual for hospitals (CAMH): The official handbook.* Oakbrook Terrace, IL: Author.

Kouzes, J., & Posner, B. (1995). *The leadership challenge.* San Francisco: Jossey-Bass Publishers.

Lewin, K. (1939). Field theory and experiment in social psychology: Concepts and methods. *Journal of Sociology, 44*, 868–896.

Lindholm, M., Sivberg, B., & Uden, G. (2000). Leadership styles among nurse managers in changing organizations. *Journal of Nursing Management, 8*(6), 327–336.

Muller-Smith, P. (1999). Yet another workplace crisis. *Journal of Perianesthesia Nursing, 14*(4), 217–220.

Ohman, K. A. (2000). The transformational leadership of critical care nurse managers. *Dimensions of Critical Care Nursing, 19*(1), 46–54.

Pender, J., Murdaugh, C., & Parsons, M. A. (2002). *Health promotion in nursing practice* (4th ed.). Upper Saddle River, NJ: Prentice-Hall.

Polzer, J., & Neale, M. (2000). Conflict management and negotiation. In Stephen Shortell and Arnold Kaluzny (Eds.), *Health care management: Organization design and behavior* (4th ed.). Clifton Park, NY: Delmar Learning.

Strickland, D. (2000). Emotional intelligence: The most potent factor in the success equation. *Journal of Nursing Administration, 30*(3), 112–117.

Tannenbaum, R., & Schmidt, W. (1973). How to choose a leadership pattern. *Harvard Business Review, 51*(3), 162–180.

Townes, J., & Cook, P. (2001). Standards of practice: A measure of competence. *Home Healthcare Nurse, 19*(6), 383–386.

Wheatley, M. J. (1999). *Leadership and the new science: Discovering order in a chaotic world.* San Francisco: Berrett-Koehler.

Wilson, R. T. (1998). Servant leadership. *Physician Executive, 24*(5), 6–12.

Yukl, G. (1998). *Leadership in organizations* (4th ed.). Upper Saddle River, NJ: Prentice Hall.

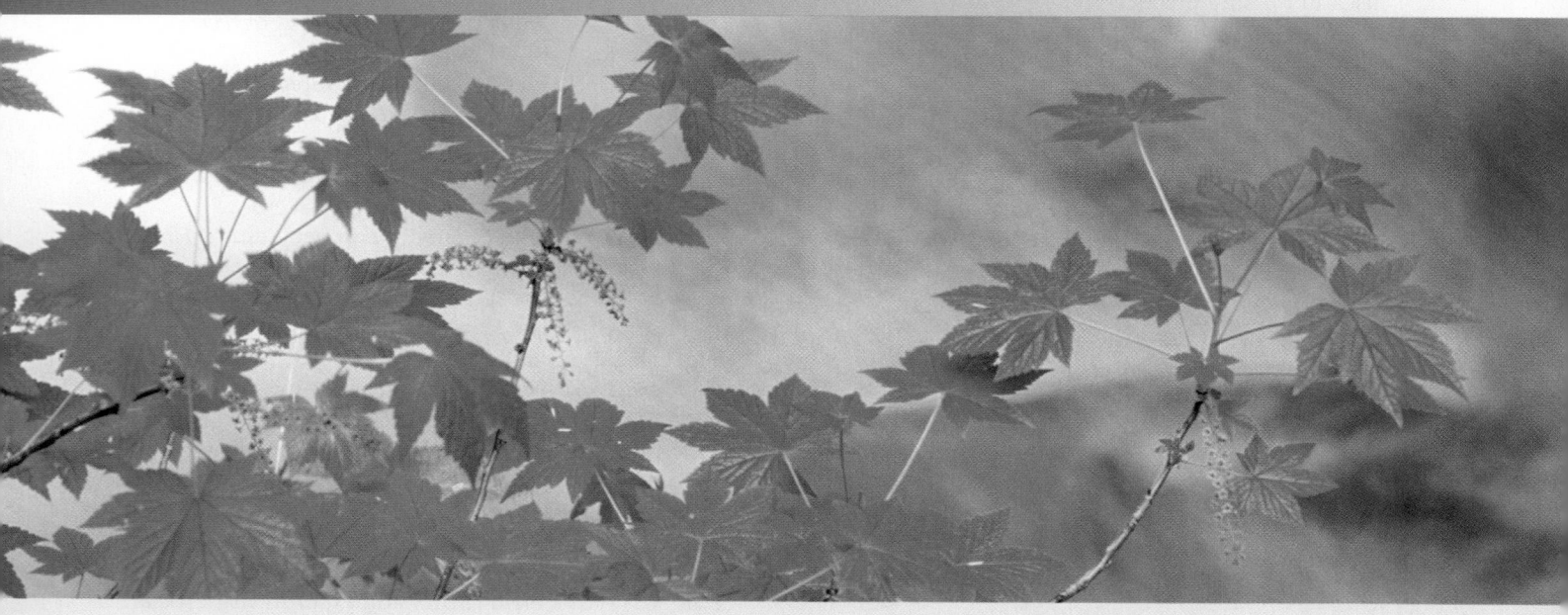

# 25 CHAPTER

# Management and Policy

## Deborah L. Fell-Carlson, BSN, RN, COHN-S, HEM

*"Addressing quality of care issues should be the most important concern of every practicing nurse. Nothing is more fundamental to our business than understanding what quality care is and how to deliver it cost-effectively."*

(Marilyn S. Fetter, 1998)

# Chapter Competencies

*Upon completion of this chapter, the reader should be able to:*

1. Describe the evolution of quality of care initiatives in health care.
2. Explain the impact of the Joint Commission on Accreditation of Hospitals and Healthcare Organizations.
3. Identify the traditional quality assurance framework.
4. Describe the process that occurs from quality assurance to quality improvement.
5. Evaluate the JCAHO accreditation survey process.
6. Strategize in regard to the future of health care as pertaining to issues of quality.
7. Describe the roles of government, citizens, and professional associations in the health care policy-making process.
8. Evaluate professional accountability in client safety and quality of health care.

# Key Terms

accreditation
algorithm
benchmark
clinical practice guidelines
Environment of Care
external customer
FOCUS PDCA
hazardous condition
health policies
internal customer

Joint Commission on
  Accreditation of Healthcare
  Organizations (JCAHO)
judicial decisions
near miss
operational decisions
outcome
peer review
political action teams
politics
procedures

process
professional organizations
quality assurance framework
quality improvement
rules and regulations
sentinel event
standard of care
structure
supplemental recommendation
Type I recommendation

Nursing is much different today than it was a decade ago, and is continuing to change at a surprisingly rapid rate. The entire health care field is changing. It is more turbulent, chaotic, high-tech, and highly regulated than ever before. Nurses at all levels and in all specialties have an essential role and important responsibility in the regulatory and policy-making process, serving as client advocates to safeguard quality of care during the change process.

Nurses today must deliver care within a framework of regulatory and policy guidelines originating from a variety of different governmental agencies and organizations. While this framework adds a dimension of administrative complexity to nursing care, it serves to guide caregivers to "do the right things right," for themselves, for coworkers, for the organization, for visitors, and most important, for the client.

This chapter will describe the quality assurance framework and trace the evolution of health care quality initiatives, leading the nurse to explore the impact of clinical practice guidelines and regulatory guidance on nursing

care and overall health care quality. The crucial role of the nurse as change agent, client advocate, and active participant in the policy-making process relevant to health care delivery, will be examined. The roles of government, professional organizations, and citizens in health policy development and analysis will be described, along with opportunity options for the practicing nurse to consider to effectively engage in policy-making activities.

## Quality in Health Care: A Glimpse of the Past

High-quality care is a reasonable client expectation. Nurses have long advocated for quality care on behalf of the client. Florence Nightingale (1820–1910) recognized the impact of the physical setting on client recovery, elaborating on the need for adequate ventilation, sunlight, cleanliness, and other healthful environmental considerations. She candidly proclaimed that nurses should be keenly observant and should develop sound clinical judgment (Figure 25-1). She

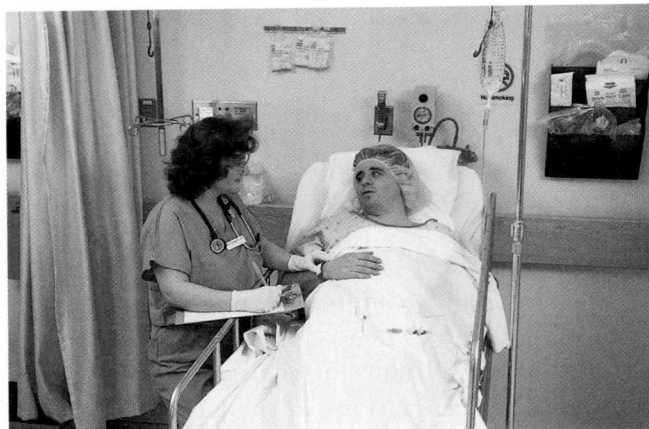

**Figure 25-1    A nurse practicing sound clinical judgment**

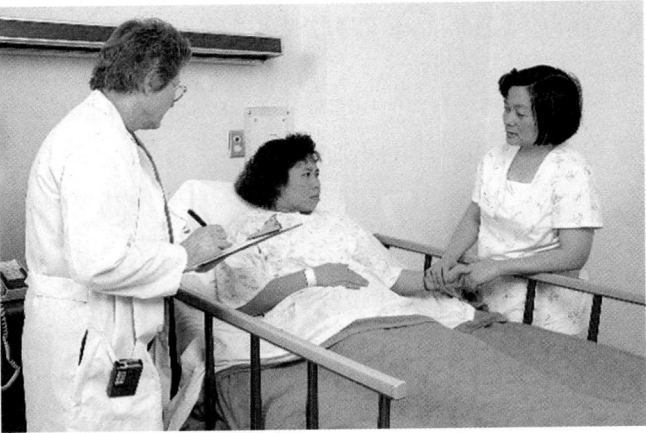

**Figure 25-2    A hospital JCAH accreditation**

held them accountable to develop and use assessment skills:

> Which of us has not heard fifty times, from one or another, a nurse, or a friend of the sick, aye, and a medical friend too, the following remark:—"So A is worse, or B is dead. I saw him the day before; I thought him so much better; there certainly was no appearance from which one could have expected so sudden a change." I have never heard anyone say, though one would think it the more natural thing, "There *must* have been *some* appearance, which I should have seen if I had but looked; let me try and remember what there was, that I may observe another time." No, this is not what people say. They boldly assert that there was nothing to observe, not that their observation was at fault. Let people who have to observe sickness and death look back and try to register in their observation the appearances which have preceded relapse, attack, or death, and not assert that there were none, or that there were not the *right* ones. (Nightingale, 1860)

## Quality Initiatives Through Accreditation—the History of the Joint Commission on Accreditation of Healthcare Organizations

Florence Nightingale's contributions to health care's quality environment paved the way for today's main health care accrediting and standard-setting organization, the **Joint Commission on Accreditation of Healthcare Organizations (JCAHO)**. **Accreditation** is recognition or approval bestowed by an authorized organization or agency (JCAHO, 2003, www.jcaho.com).

In the mid-1800s, Florence Nightingale demonstrated that quality could be measured by statistically measuring results of care, and thus revolutionized hospital care and provided the foundation for statistical measures in health care. In 1910, Ernest Codman, MD, expanded on this con-

cept, and developed a system to track clients, specifically to determine the effectiveness of treatments. If the treatment failed, the hospital pursued the reasons for the failure in an effort to avoid similar failures. This tracking system was incorporated into the American College of Surgeons (ACS) doctrine when the ACS was formally organized a few years later. The ACS published a directive entitled "The Minimum Standard" in 1917, outlining ACS hospital and physician standards of quality. The directive addressed such issues as complete, thorough documentation in the client record and a regular analysis of clinical experience based on client record review. The ACS began inspecting hospitals in 1918, according to this directive.

Standards of quality in health care continued to develop and improve, and in 1951, the ACS, the American Hospital Association, the American Medical Association, and the Canadian Medical Association formed the nonprofit organization called the Joint Commission on Accreditation of Hospitals (JCAH) (Figure 25-2). The JCAH began hospital accreditation in 1953, and began charging for accreditation survey services in 1964. The organization continued to evolve, developing a close alliance with the health-related agencies in the federal government. In 1965, Congress recognized JCAH accreditation as a **benchmark**, or standard of excellence, for hospital reimbursement for Medicare and Medicaid programs, effectively tying accreditation to funding eligibility.

## STOP AND THINK

### Issues of Accreditation

If accreditation is tied to federal and other third-party funding, what kind of an impact do you think loss of accreditation would have on the health care organization's ability to continue to operate?

# The Traditional Quality Assurance Framework

In the mid-1960s, around the time the JCAH started charging for hospital quality accreditation visits, Avedis Donabedian (1966) published what has become the traditionally held framework for quality assessment in health care. Donabedian's **quality assurance framework** is based on the premise that health care quality is most effectively measured by scrutinizing care in the domains of structure, process, and outcome. Predetermined criteria are developed to measure past performance. In 1970, the JCAH revised accreditation standards to shift the focus from minimum standards of quality to optimal standards of quality, providing an ideal opportunity to operationalize Donabedian's broad approach to assessing quality assurance. This changed the scope of the survey to include the entire organization, and registered nurses and administrators joined the JCAH survey team that same year to provide a nursing and management perspective.

## Structure

The **structure** in Donabedian's model (1996) encompasses the integrity of the infrastructure within the health care organization to determine if the resources needed to deliver high-quality care are sufficient and used efficiently. Examples include human resources, informational resources, facility resources, and technological resources. Evaluation of payment and billing systems and staffing models are also included. Donabedian more specifically defines *structure* as pertaining to "the settings in which [health care] takes place and the instrumentalities of which it is the product"(p. 73). This emphasis on structure as a component of care is consistent with Florence Nightingale's teachings on the healing environment.

## Process

Evaluating **process** is the most complex component of the Donabedian model. He defined *process* simply as whether what is now known as "good" medical care has been applied. Process evaluation is an examination of actual health care delivery activities. A variety of different procedures are benchmarked, or compared, against published practice guidelines developed by peer groups.

## Outcome

The last component, and the ultimate measure, of quality care, is client **outcome**. Donabedian defined *outcome* in terms of recovery, restoration of function, and of survival. The intent of outcome measures is to examine community health and disability relative to health care delivery.

Outcomes may be client-focused or provider-focused. Client-focused outcomes are either related to diagnosis, pertaining to the disease state outcome and changes in condition, or holistic, related to the client's response to or level of adaptation to a change in health (Jennings, Staggers, & Brosch, 1999). Provider-focused outcomes are related to provider proficiency and are normally measured by complication rates and appropriateness of interventions discovered through the **peer review** process. The peer review process involves pulling client charts based on certain criteria, and submitting those charts for review by a peer physician. This is a physician quality assessment process, but may reveal gaps in nursing practice as well.

In 1987, the organization expanded their scope of quality assurance activities and became the Joint Commission on Accreditation of Healthcare Organizations (JCAHO). Since that time, the scope of the JCAHO has continued to expand. Accreditation survey and support services are available to health care networks, hospitals, home care organizations, assisted living and long-term care facilities, ambulatory and behavioral health care organizations, and clinical laboratories. Approximately 19,000 surveys are conducted each year, and survey results remain tied to Medicare and Medicaid funding.

# From Quality Assurance to Quality Improvement

The quality assurance framework provides a tool for *measuring* quality of care, and while it does have a role in today's health care environment, it does not provide a mechanism for *correcting* the identified problems. **Quality improvement** is a multidisciplinary approach to process change—a powerful tool for change and measurable improvement. An adaptation of the well-known Deming/Shewhart model, often referred to as **FOCUS PDCA**, is used in many health care organizations to correct problems identified through application of the quality assurance framework. Problems are identified or **F**ound, and resolved by **O**rganizing a multidisciplinary team that **C**larifies the process and **U**ncovers the problem. A solution is **S**elected. The team is tasked with **P**lanning the improvement; **D**oing, or implementing, the improvement; **C**hecking, or monitoring, to ensure it corrected the problem; and **A**cting, to either return to the planning phase or to hold the gain. A clinical application of this model is illustrated in Table 25-1.

Quality improvement is customer-focused. Clients are not the only customers—staff, physicians, and nurses are also customers, and some customers are simultaneously suppliers and customers. All customers, internal and external, should be treated with respect and dignity. An **internal customer** is an individual employed by the organization who must depend on the efficiency and productivity of other employees to do his work. An example is a nurse who has requested an x-ray or laboratory test. An **external customer** is an individual who is not employed by the organization and who uses the services the organization provides (Geatti & Pegoraro, 1999).

## TABLE 25-1    FOCUS PDCA MODEL FOR CONTINUOUS QUALITY IMPROVEMENT
### EXAMPLE OF CLINICAL APPLICATION

| F | **Find**<br>*a problem or process to improve* | Traditional pain medication distribution method caused delay in medication administration, resulting in frustration, increased costs, client/physician dissatisfaction. |
|---|---|---|
| O | **Organize**<br>*an interdisciplinary team* | Key personnel or departments involved in the process are asked to participate and identify known "weak links" in structure or process domain: pharmacist, nurse educator, case manager, obstetrical department manager. |
| C | **Clarify**<br>*the current process* | Team members outline all steps of the process, with assistance from quality improvement nurse. |
| U | **Understand or uncover**<br>*causes for deviation from the process, or poor quality* | Team investigates the root cause through chart reviews, meetings with physicians and nurses. Problems identified: (1) Because of the variable nature of the unit activities, nurse often delayed in going to the cart to retrieve medication. (2) Physicians ordered wide variety of analgesia for each client, much of which did not get used. |
| S | **Select and start**<br>*with a methodology appropriate to the process and begin PDCA cycle* | Examine previously identified "weak links" and root causes. Decide on areas for improvement. Self-Administered Medication Packet selected as a strategy, thought to enhance independence and client satisfaction. |
| P | **Plan**<br>*the improvement* | Team develops specific action steps necessary to correct the problem. Packet preparation, physician orders, client education, documentation, policy development, and so on. |
| D | **Do**<br>*the improvement that has been planned and collect data.* | Implement the change. May include inservicing staff, purchasing of new equipment, and so on. Follow-up phone call within 72 hours. |
| C | **Check**<br>*the results* | Evaluate the data, and continue with data collection for ongoing monitoring. |
| A | **Act**<br>*to continue improvement efforts (i.e., returning to "Plan" step) or to hold the gain* | Change or maintain process as needed. |

Beger, D., Messenger, F., & Roth, S. (1999). Self-administered medication packets for patients experiencing vaginal birth. *Journal of Nursing Care Quality*, 13(4), 47–59.

## The JCAHO Accreditation Survey Process

JCAHO accreditation survey preparation requires an entire health care organization to function as a team. "Mock" surveys are often completed to help prepare staff for the survey experience. The triennial survey is comprehensive, evaluating every area of the organization over a period of days. This survey model allows for an additional, unannounced, random survey sometime between 9 and 30 months after the comprehensive survey. Currently under consideration is a proposal to divide the survey into two visits spaced 18 months apart, rather than one comprehensive visit every 3 years. The JCAHO mission in 2001 remains quality-based:

The mission of the Joint Commission on Accreditation of Healthcare Organizations is to continuously improve the safety and quality of care provided to the public through the provision of health care accreditation and related services that support performance improvement in health care organizations (JCAHO, 2001).

# The Role of the Nurse and Other Direct Care Caregivers

Nurses and other clinical staff members are key participants in the JCAHO survey. Surveyors conduct personal interviews to assess competency of staff in all departments, on all shifts. Staff members are assessed on *clinical* competencies, but are also evaluated on *organizational* competencies ranging from hazard recognition and emergency procedures necessary for client safety, to an understanding of the organizational mission, vision, and values. Clinical policies are scrutinized, staff are queried about the content of these policies, and staff are observed in an effort to determine if policies are followed (Fetter, 1998).

The competent nurse should not fear a JCAHO accreditation survey. Surveyors simply assess the nurse's ability to do the right things right in a safe environment while being prepared for contingencies. Professional accountability should motivate the nurse to remain knowledgeable about organizational and clinical policies, nursing practice guidelines, and additional information needed to deliver high-quality client care (Dozier, 1998).

## Management's Role

Management competency and leadership are assessed during the JCAHO survey process. JCAHO surveys evaluate administrative resources, policies, documentation, and internal consistency regarding whether or not organizational policies are followed. JCAHO emphasizes the management relationships to both client safety and client care. In addition, JCAHO processes of evaluation are used to credential medical staff and to scrutinize the educational programs.

## Organizational Safety and the JCAHO: Managing the "Environment of Care"

Nightingale and Donabedian emphasized the relationship of the care setting to client outcomes. The JCAHO also recognizes the importance of this and has recently created accreditation standards intended to improve safety in the care environment. These standards are called "**Environment of Care**" (**EOC**) standards, and provide a framework for a solid, comprehensive, organizational safety program. Nurses and other clinical personnel are responsible to assist in managing the EOC. Failure to do so may endanger the life of a client or the health of a coworker (Figure 25-3) (Maddox, Wakefield, & Bull, 2001).

OSHA and JCAHO have joined in recent years, which has resulted in an increased emphasis on employee safety and health in the EOC. This partnership has resulted in increased management attention to initiatives that create a safer, more healthful environment for staff, as well as clients and visitors. Nurses and other health care workers have been the primary beneficiaries of these initiatives.

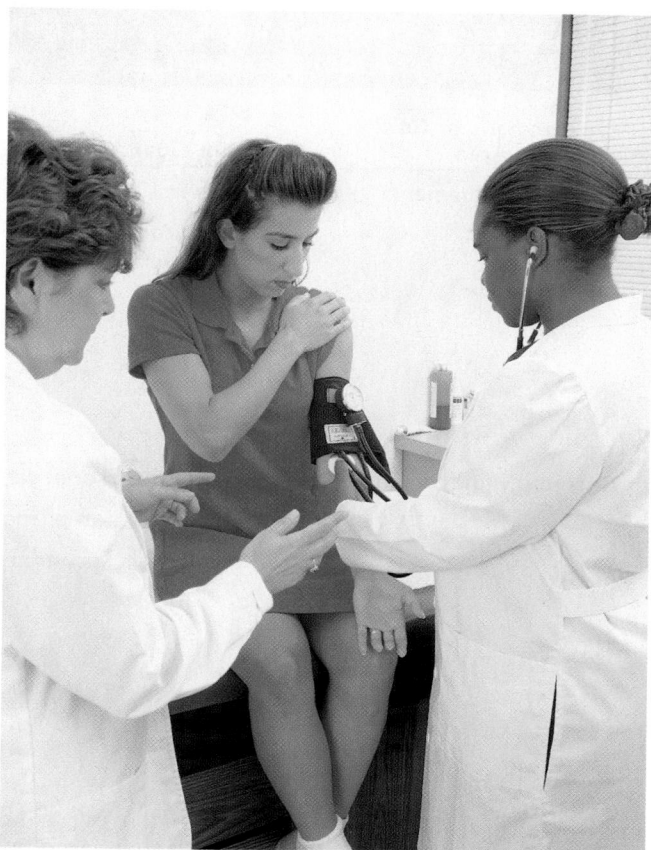

**Figure 25-3    A safe client environment**

A recent example of this partnership is the revision of the OSHA Bloodborne Pathogen Standard, requiring employers to actively seek safe needle or needleless technology, and to solicit employee input prior to purchase. Although this is likely to be a focus area if OSHA visits a facility for an inspection, the chances of an OSHA inspection are reasonably slim. The JCAHO, however, began evaluating compliance with this revised standard with each accreditation survey in early 2002. This type of JCAHO emphasis, with its tie to funding, will enhance employer compliance with OSHA standards.

The JCAHO separates the EOC into seven broad areas, with a program manager assigned to each area (JCAHO, 2001). These management areas include safety, security, utilities, emergency management, medical equipment, fire prevention, and hazardous materials and waste. Program managers are appointed by administration and are selected based on their knowledge of a particular area, as well as their availability to serve in this additional capacity. These appointments are normally an additional duty, over and above their primary position. The seven EOC areas are depicted in Table 25-2, along with examples of nursing responsibilities. As is evident, representatives from infection control, risk management, and professional development are often included on the EOC team as well.

## TABLE 25-2    THE SEVEN ENVIRONMENT OF CARE AREAS AND EXAMPLES OF NURSING ROLE

| Environment of Care Program Area | Program Goal | Examples of Nursing Role |
|---|---|---|
| Safety Management | Minimize risk of injury to clients, visitors, and staff. | • Observe work environment, and report hazards or safety concerns promptly.<br>• Participate on organization's safety committee.<br>• Attend safety training.<br>• Use safe work practices.<br>• Report all injuries promptly.<br>• Know policies and procedures. |
| Security Management | Physical and personal safety of staff; protection of material and property is secondary. | • Wear identification badge.<br>• Report hostile or suspicious activity.<br>• Participate in infant abduction drills.<br>• Exit with a coworker when leaving after dark.<br>• Secure personal valuables and sensitive equipment during the shift.<br>• Secure medications, needles, and syringes.<br>• Know bomb threat procedures.<br>• Know policies and procedures. |
| Utilities Management | Supply adequate air quality, lighting, water, and power to the client care environment. | • Know location of utility shutoffs, including oxygen shutoffs.<br>• Know which outlets and equipment systems have generator backup in the event of power failure.<br>• Know reporting procedures.<br>• Know policies and procedures. |
| Emergency Management | Management of situations that disrupt care. Includes contingencies for natural as well as man-made disasters. Phases: preparedness, mitigation (reduces loss), response and recovery (returning to normal operations) | • Be familiar with the Evacuation Plan and the overall Emergency Management Plan.<br>• Become familiar with characteristics of hazards most likely to occur in your region.<br>• Seek knowledge on actions necessary to protect your home and your family, and make appropriate plans, so you will be able to focus on your client.<br>• Participate in disaster drills.<br>• Know policies and procedures. |
| Medical Equipment Management | Training, use, storage, and care of medical equipment to ensure it does not endanger client. | • Maintain proficiency on clinical equipment.<br>• If a problem is found, take equipment out of service and tag it.<br>• Report equipment problems promptly.<br>• Know policies and procedures. |

*(continues)*

**TABLE 25-2    THE SEVEN ENVIRONMENT OF CARE AREAS AND EXAMPLES OF NURSING ROLE** (*continued*)

| Environment of Care Program Area | Program Goal | Examples of Nursing Role |
|---|---|---|
| Fire Prevention | Provide a fire-safe environment in which to deliver care. | • Keep hallways free of clutter and equipment.<br>• Do not block exit doorways.<br>• Know fire policies and procedures, including location of nearest fire pull and fire extinguisher.<br>• Know primary and alternate exit routes.<br>• Know where clients are to be taken in the event of fire. |
| Hazardous Materials and Waste Management | Safe storage, handling, and disposal of chemical, radiological, and biologic materials and wastes. | • Know the location and understand content of the Material Safety Data Sheets (MSDSs) for chemicals used in workplace, including chemotherapeutic drugs.<br>• Use proper protective equipment as prescribed on MSDS.<br>• Ensure labeling is present on all containers.<br>• Use proper disposal methods.<br>• Empty sharps containers when two-thirds full.<br>• Know policies and procedures. |

**Focus Areas Closely Related to Environment of Care**

| Focus Area | Goal | Examples of Nursing Role |
|---|---|---|
| Infection Control | Protect clients from suffering nosocomial infection. | • Follow proper isolation procedures, including appropriate use of negative pressure rooms.<br>• Use proper protective equipment appropriately.<br>• Wash hands frequently, and maintain own skin integrity.<br>• Know policies and procedures. |
| Education and Professional Development | Provide appropriate staff education. | • Attend training opportunities, including those related to safety and the Environment of Care.<br>• Advise manager of identified training needs.<br>• Seek opportunities to gain knowledge.<br>• Know policies and procedures. |
| Risk Management | Minimize client potential for injury related to hospital stay. | • Follow 5 rights of medication administration.<br>• Report all errors promptly.<br>• Be professionally accountable.<br>• Consider consequences, including legal, of everything you do.<br>• Know policies and procedures. |

JCAHO (1998). *Environment of care handbook*. Terrace, IL

## NURSING STRATEGY

### Creating a Healthier Environment for Health Care Providers

To conserve valuable human resources, the health care provider must:

- Stay physically fit to better meet the physical challenges of the position.

- Get adequate rest and take time to reenergize the mind, body, and soul.

- Report injuries promptly and seek care as needed.

- Stay home if affected by a communicable disease.

Murray, R., & Zentner, J. (2001). *Health promotion strategies through the life span* (5th ed.). Upper Saddle River, NJ: Prentice-Hall.

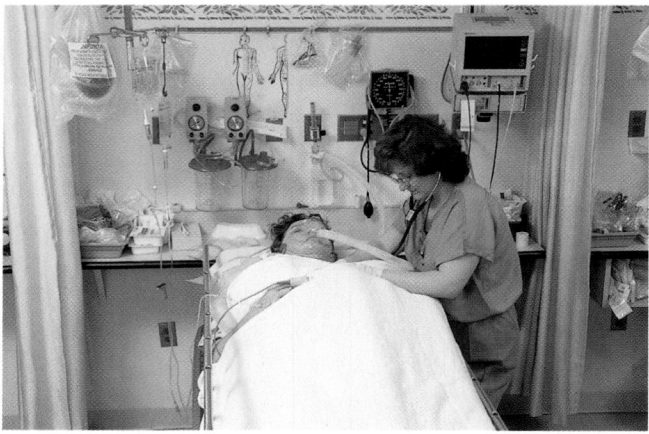

**Figure 25-4   A sentinel event**

## Survey Outcomes

Eligibility for Medicare and Medicaid, as well as other third-party reimbursements, are contingent upon JCAHO accreditation. In most organizations, these reimbursements comprise a large percentage of facility earnings. If such earnings are blocked through loss of accreditation, the future of the organization may be jeopardized. JCAHO accreditation is sought for reasons beyond funding. Accreditation is viewed as a quality benchmark by the public, and thus enhances the health care consumer confidence. It provides a structured, comprehensive assessment of organizational performance and motivates quality improvement activities.

There are several levels of JCAHO accreditation. "Accreditation with Full Standards Compliance" reflects compliance with JCAHO standards in all applicable program areas. "Accreditation with Requirements for Improvement" indicates that while most program areas were satisfactory, one or more areas have deficiencies that must be resolved within a given time frame in order to maintain accredited status. Organizations that are denied accreditation have failed to accomplish the process improvement initiatives necessary to meet accreditations standards.

The more serious deficiencies discovered during the survey process are identified as either Type I recommendations or supplemental recommendations.

A **Type I recommendation** is the most serious. This recommendation requires that the organization take action within a certain time frame to resolve the substandard finding in a particular performance area, document that action, and then demonstrate that the problem has been resolved.

**Supplemental recommendations** are issued when an area of noncompliance is identified, but it is not as serious

as a Type I. These, too, must be resolved in a timely fashion or accreditation status may be impacted. Process and documentation is similar to that required for a Type I.

A **sentinel event** is an unexpected event involving death or serious injury to a client (Figure 25-4). It also includes **near misses**, those situations where a deviation from a process does not actually harm the client, but could place the client at risk if it were to occur again. The term *sentinel* is used to communicate the urgency needed for investigation and response. Sentinel events trigger a thorough investigation of the root cause and require immediate process improvement initiatives to correct the underlying system defect. Performance monitoring continues until the organization is certain the deficiency is corrected. Health care organizations are encouraged to report sentinel events to the JCAHO to assist other organizations in preventing a similar event (Smith, 2001).

## The 21st Century— a Quality Revolution

A study by the Institute of Medicine, entitled *To Err Is Human: Building a Safer Health System*, was published in 2000. The report publicly—and candidly—revealed the magnitude of medical errors suffered by health care consumers in the United States. The scope of errors covered by the report was broad, and the severity of errors was hor-

## STOP AND THINK

### Legislation and Quality of Health Care

- Why do some issues generate legislative action while others do not?

- Do you think legislated health care policy is always of benefit to the client?

## RESEARCH FOCUS

**Title of Study:** To err is human: Building a safer health system

**Study Purpose:** To "break the cycle of inaction" by revealing the magnitude of the health care safety problem in the United States.

**Methods:** Methods included a literature review of pertinent, available articles on quality, medical errors, employee safety, and safety of pharmaceuticals. Two group meetings were held to solicit input from certain targeted groups, public testimony was solicited, and a survey was conducted by telephone to gather information on state reporting requirements. In addition, a paper on legal issues surrounding reporting was commissioned and is contained within the final report.

**Findings:** Medical errors are estimated to be the eighth leading cause of death in the United States. More people are fatally harmed by the health care system every year than die in motor vehicle crashes! Much can be learned by analyzing errors, but a mechanism must be developed to capture them. For this to be successful, the current atmosphere of blame must shift to an atmosphere toward improvement.

**Implications:** This research study indicates a need for a multifaceted, comprehensive approach to health care safety.

Kohn, L., Corrigan, J., & Donaldson, M. (2000). *To err is human: Building a safer health system*. Washington, DC: National Academy Press.

## CLINICAL ALERT

### Safe Medication Administration

The "5 Rights" of medication administration were developed to assist nurses in safe delivery of pharmaceuticals. Methodically checking to ensure that the nurse has the right medication, in the right dose, for the right route, to administer to the right client, at the right time, will improve accuracy of medication delivery (Figure 25-5). It is imperative that the nurse understand adverse effects and contraindications of all medication administered. This adds an extra measure of safety. Finally, if the nurse has any question regarding the interpretation of the physician order, the nurse should contact the physician to obtain clarification.

White, L., & Duncan, G. (2002). *Medical-surgical nursing: An integrated approach* (2nd ed.). Clifton Park, NY: Delmar Learning.

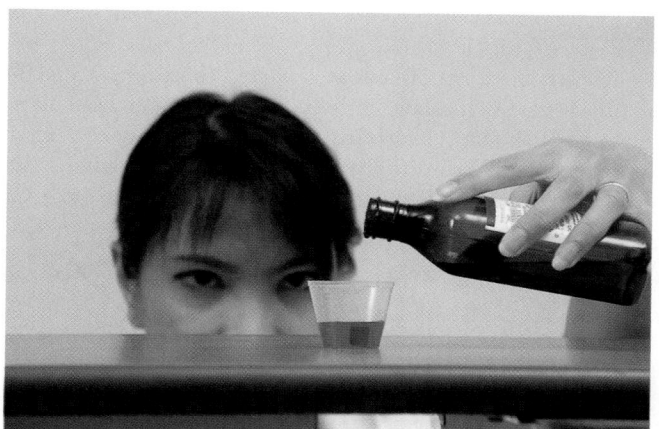

**Figure 25-5    A nurse giving medications**

rific. The report estimated that 44,000 or more Americans die each year from preventable adverse events related to health care.

A follow-up report, entitled *Crossing the Quality Chasm: A New Health System for the 21st Century*, was released by the Institute of Medicine later that same year. The scope of this report was not limited to a particular area of health care; instead, it addressed health care quality as a whole. While several areas for improvement were identified, the report was optimistic in its recommendations.

These reports rightly invoked passion in the American public, catapulting health care to the top of the legislative agenda. The outrage moved federal agencies and health care oversight organizations, including the JCAHO, to action, launching a revolutionary movement for health care quality improvement.

The report identified six goals for 21st-century health care delivery, outlined in Table 25-3. These goals, or dimen-

sions, are similar to the standards set forth by the JCAHO in the past, and are operationalized through a variety of policy-making agencies and organizations, including the JCAHO. The JCAHO has launched comprehensive client safety standards to emphasize these areas, and client advocacy legislation has been introduced in Congress.

## Health Policy

**Health policies** are written decisions directing or influencing the actions or decisions of others. They can take a variety of forms, including law, rules and regulation, operational decisions, or judicial rulings. Health policies impact health by altering health determinants such as lifestyle, socioeconomic status, and available services, ultimately changing the health of the affected population or individual (Garry, 2000).

## TABLE 25-3     INSTITUTE OF MEDICINE: DIMENSIONS FOR 21ST CENTURY HEALTH CARE

| | |
|---|---|
| Safe | Health care should be safe. Injuries to clients resulting from care intended to help them should be avoided. |
| Effective | Overuse and underuse of services should be avoided. Scientific knowledge should be used as a basis for service delivery; care should be provided to those who will benefit. |
| Client-centered | Care should be delivered in such a manner as to demonstrate respect and responsiveness to individual preferences, values, and needs. |
| Timely | Minimizing delays benefits those who give the care as well as those who receive it. |
| Efficient | Good stewardship of resources and minimizing waste, including waste of ideas and energy, should be pursued. |
| Equitable | Quality of care should be consistent regardless of gender, ethnic background, or socioeconomic status. |

Institute of Medicine (2000). *Crossing the quality chasm: A new health system for the 21st century.* Washington, DC: National Academy Press.

## Laws

Policies in the form of laws are enacted to achieve a specific objective. Such a law, Title XVIII of the Social Security Act, established a "Health Insurance Program for the Aged and Disabled," commonly referred to as "Medicare," to complement Social Security benefits.

## Rules, Regulations, Operational, and Judicial Decisions

**Rules and regulations** provide specific guidance for implementation of a law. In the above example, a law was passed to create a specific program. Rules and regulations are developed by the agency responsible to oversee the law-mandated program, which, in this case, is the federal Centers for Medicare and Medicaid Services (CMS). These rules and regulations may be quite lengthy, and contain detailed information to assist the health care organization through the implementation process.

**Operational decisions** have the same authority as rules and regulations, but tend to be less permanent. Finally, **judicial decisions** are authoritative decisions based on the interpretation of laws and are made by a judge.

## Health Policy Making, Implementation, and Analysis

In many ways, the health policy-making, implementation, and analysis process is similar to the continuous quality improvement model (FOCUS PDCA) previously discussed. There are some very special differences, however. In health care policy making, an issue with a proposed solution is presented to a legislator. *If the political climate is favorable*, the issue will be drafted as a bill and introduced in Congress. It enters the legislative process, and a regulation is developed to guide implementation. Once implemented, the policy impact is examined and reexamined, and modifications are made, as necessary, to achieve the desired result.

## The Nurse's Role in Health Policy Making

Nurses involved in the policy-making process serve as client advocates to entire populations of health care consumers. The nurse's role in this process is essential, whether through a professional organization, a political action team, or as an individual professional (Figure 25-6). **Professional organizations** are comprised of members engaged in the same professional pursuit, and often have the same goals and concerns. **Political action teams** are often developed within these organizations to collectively analyze or address a particular health policy issue of concern to the organization. Nurses who stay abreast of current legislative issues, whether individually or as a member of an organization, are in the position to mobilize in response to legislation impacting client care, before it becomes law (Pulcini, J., Mason, D., Solomon Cohen, S., Kovner C., & Leavitt, J., 2000).

One nurse can make a difference in the policy-making process. Attending and providing testimony at public hearings on new regulations, writing to congresspersons in support of or in opposition to a particular bill, and speaking at civic gatherings on health issues are effective ways to impact the policy-making process. A unified professional organization or other special interest group, however, speaks with a much more powerful voice. Nurses will gain professionally—collectively and as individuals—if they are active participants in their professional organiza-

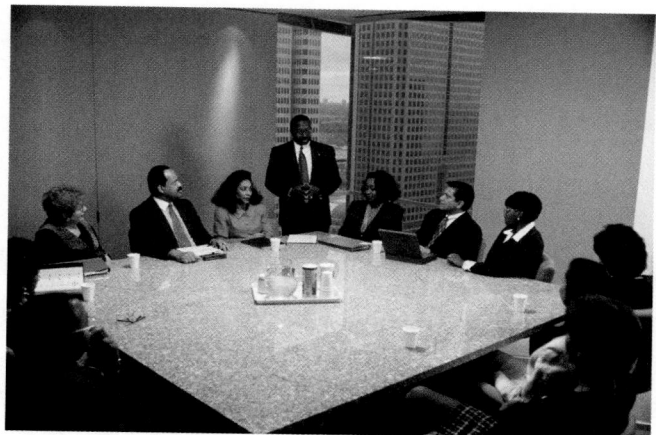

**Figure 25-6 A political action team.** *Courtesy of Photodisc*

tions. These organizations and groups provide powerful input to legislators.

The political and economic environments can change perceptions of a bill. In fact, the policy-making process can be impacted by politics at any point. **Politics**, the use of power to effect change, can either impede or propel the policy-making process.

## Organizational Policy Making and Excellence in Nursing Practice

Policies impacting client care implemented at the national and state levels, and those developed by the JCAHO, ultimately impact nursing practice at every level by imposing certain policy mandates to be integrated into client care in an effort to achieve an expected level of quality. Excellence in health care quality occurs, however, when an organization does not wait for mandates but moves toward excellence independently.

Health care policies at the organizational level *define* nursing practice. Tools to integrate the policy mandates and "best practices" into nursing care include standards of care, procedures, guidelines, and algorithms. If care is taken to ensure that each document is clear and concise, and reflects the care delivered within the organization, these documents can provide a framework for health care excellence and reduce liability. In the event of a lawsuit, these documents will define the organizational **standard of care**, against which the nurse will be measured. In the absence of organizational policies, the courts rely on expert medical witnesses, nursing literature, and standards of practice from professional organizations to assist in defining the standard of care for a particular situation. The "standard of care" has a broad scope, and reflects the expected physical, spiritual, emotional, and intellectual care of client population. It delineates the extent and character of the nurse's duty to the client. When health care organizations set policies in any form, especially clinical practice guidelines or procedures, they prescribe the specific standard of care expected at their organization.

**Clinical practice guidelines** are intended to standardize care by providing standards of nursing and medical care for clients with the same clinical problem. These guidelines are based on sound evidence derived from research, and can have an enormous impact on the length of stay, quality of care, and cost of treatment. Because they are evidence-based, only proven interventions are included and redundant services and interventions are eliminated. Current nationally published clinical practice guidelines by the Agency for Healthcare Research and Quality (AHRQ) typically have excellent client teaching components, and because they are considered to be a "consensus standard," they can be relied upon to reduce institutional and individual liability (Goes, Friedman, Seifert, & Buffa, 2000). The AHRQ is a federally funded agency, formerly known as the Agency for Health Care Policy and Research, with a mission to provide evidence-based outcome information and related information to assist health care professionals in making informed decisions. Clinical practice guidelines published by the AHRQ (2003) can be viewed and downloaded from their website.

## LIFE SPAN CONSIDERATIONS

### Assisting the Older Client to Obtain Health Care

Today's health care environment is very different than that of yesterday. Today's health care consumers, particularly the elderly, may need assistance navigating the health care regulatory maze they face. Frustration and hostility directed at you may actually reflect their fear of lost benefits, or embarrassment at their difficulty in understanding a particular process. By showing patience and respect as you explain things, you will effectively guide these clients through the health care system.

Hogstel, M. (2001). *Gerontology: Nursing care of the older adult.* Clifton Park, NY: Delmar Learning.

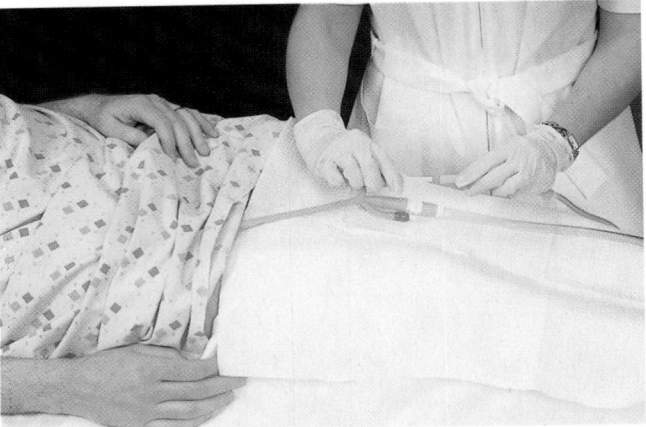

**Figure 25-7    Procedure: Connecting irrigation tubing to irrigation port of the catheter**

Professional organizations and private health care organizations have also published clinical practice guidelines. Clinical practice guidelines under consideration should be reviewed carefully to ensure they include documentation showing they are evidence-based, with current references from peer-reviewed journals.

Clinical practice guidelines may be comprised of one statement describing a standard for a certain population. This is most common in the public health arena, where a certain standard is set for a particular group. In the clinical setting, however, it is typical to see a group of statements relating to a specific clinical problem.

**Procedures** are specific step-by-step directions, which are based on sound science, on how to perform a specific clinical activity or technical skill, such as how to irrigate a urinary catheter (Figure 25-7). The procedure is quite narrow in scope when compared to the clinical practice guideline.

**Algorithms** are graphical representations, often in flowchart format, depicting a set of steps used in a particular clinical decision-making process. The steps are determined by an expert clinician, and then established as clinical rules. Algorithms may stand alone or may be incorporated into a clinical practice guideline. The initial sequence of the cardiopulmonary resuscitation process is an example of an algorithm.

Nurses who monitor the literature for "best practices" and become involved in the organizational policy-making process serve as advocates to clients by helping to shape a framework of excellence for client care delivery. Often, best practices are identified in the literature prior to being mandated through the formal policy-making process. The proactive nurse initiates action on these issues and seeks to be involved on the appropriate committees, working to implement best-practice policies at the lowest level (Johnson, 1999).

### Clinical Practices Committee

Organizational integration of best practices or health care policy mandates is challenging and can be frustrat-

## CLIENT REFLECTIONS

### Self-Administration of Insulin

Ms. Swiggert has been administering her own insulin at home. As she watches you draw up and carefully adjust the dose in the syringe, she comments, "I don't get that picky at home. I just draw it up about a third full and inject it somewhere handy. It seems to work all right, and it is ever so much faster!"

What resources might be available to you as you reassess Ms. Swiggert's educational needs?

## CLIENT EDUCATION

### Health Care and the Internet

Emphasize to your client that while the Internet is a convenient health care resource, not all health care information obtained from the Internet is accurate. Clients who delay treatment or self-treat with either ineffective or inappropriate modalities based on information obtained from the Internet may suffer unnecessarily as a result.

Tyson, T. (2000). The Internet: Tomorrow's portal to nontraditional health care services. *Journal of Ambulatory Care, 23*(2), 1.

## NURSING STRATEGY

### Reporting Errors

If you make an error, take the following action:

- Tend to the safety needs of your client.

- Report the incident promptly according to your organization's policy.

- Follow up with your manager to provide information necessary to discovering what actually occurred.

- Participate in the quality improvement process to correct the root cause (FOCUS PDCA).

King, K., & Teo, K. (2000). Integrating clinical quality improvement strategies with nursing research. *Western Journal of Nursing Research, 22*(5), 596–609.

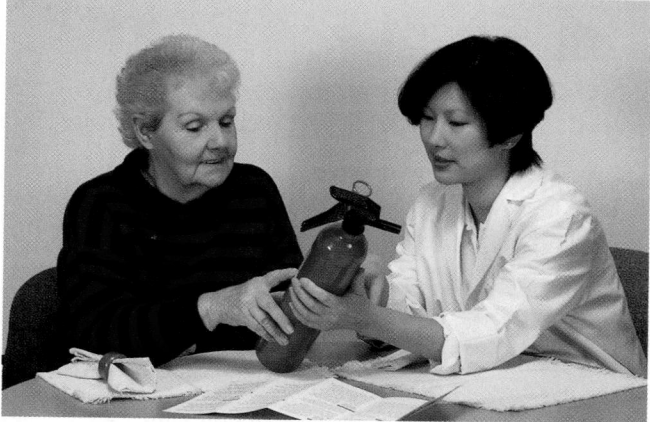

**Figure 25-8    Education of fire safety in the home is a vital emergency procedure.**

ing. It is also rewarding. When a nurse identifies a procedure or clinical practice guideline that needs to be changed, the change must be done with input from all affected parties. This is usually accomplished through the committee process, often through a clinical practices committee. It is necessary to obtain buy-in from stakeholders before beginning the policy-making process for a new and innovative concept. Nurses will do well to remember that in the private-sector health care organization, stockholders and board members are in powerful positions and can be instrumental in helping the nurse achieve the support needed to initiate an innovative policy change at the organizational level (Wakefield & Maddox, 2000).

## Professional Accountability

Professional accountability enhances quality and client safety. It is important to promptly report **hazardous conditions**—situations that increase the risk of a serious adverse client outcome unrelated to the disease condition. Nurses must know emergency procedures (Figure 25-8). All errors should be reported. The trending of minor errors may prevent a serious incident in the future. An error is any *unintended* act of omission (meaning something was not done that should have been), or commission (meaning something was done that should not have been done). The goal is not to place blame but to improve performance. Integrating best practices into all areas of nursing care fosters an environment whereby excellence in quality of care and innovation is expected, and adverse outcomes are the exception rather than the norm. Health care consumers deserve nothing less.

 ## CASE STUDY/NURSING CARE PLAN

Ms. Simons, a cheerful 79-year-old widow, is a retired schoolteacher. She is admitted for the removal of nasal polyps, a minor short-stay surgical procedure. As you are obtaining a surgical history upon her current admission, she states she was admitted about 10 years ago for a minor surgery, but that the procedure was not what she expected. In addition, she tells you that she developed an infection as a result of poor hygiene practices during the procedure. Now, Ms. Simons expresses considerable anxiety about the nasal polyps procedure and tells you she would like to know what will be happening to her. And she wants to have an assurance that "nothing bad will happen to her this time." The assurance of quality of care is a primary concern of Ms. Simons.

### Assessment

Client is currently admitted for a procedure and has fears and anxiety related to previous surgical procedures. She desires the health care providers to ensure her safety and allay her concerns during her current admission.

### Nursing Diagnosis #1

*Anxiety Related to Invasive Procedure* as evidenced by verbalization of apprehension.

*(continues)*

# CASE STUDY/NURSING CARE PLAN (continued)

**NOC:** Anxiety Control
**NIC:** Anxiety Reduction; Teaching: Procedure/Treatment

### Expected Outcome

The client will:

1. Verbalize a relief of anxiety during the first 24 hours of her admission.

### Planning/Interventions/Rationales

1. Provide reassurance and comfort to client at frequent intervals. *Decreases anxiety and fear levels.*
2. Provide clear, concise explanations regarding upcoming procedures. *Increases knowledge level and answers questions of client.*
3. Explain that clinical practice guidelines are developed by and will be practiced by her care providers. *Ensures procedure will be done appropriately and decreases anxiety.*

### Nursing Diagnosis #2

*Deficient Knowledge* related to invasive procedure as evidenced by request for information.
**NOC:** Knowledge: Treatment Procedure
**NIC:** Teaching: Preoperative; Teaching: Procedure/Treatment

### Expected Outcome

The client will:

1. Verbalize an understanding of upcoming invasive procedure by the end of the nurse's explanation of the procedure.

### Planning/Interventions/Rationales

1. Assess client's readiness to learn by assessing emotional response (anxiety). *Provides ongoing assessment of client in regard to anxiety level.*
2. Allow client to express intense emotions prior to teaching. *Encourages honest emotional outlet for client and development of therapeutic relationship with health care provider.*
3. Assess preferred learning mode. *Provides health care provider with the most appropriate method of teaching and educating client.*
4. Assess literacy level of client. *Ensures accurate use of communication and teaching aids by the health care provider.*
5. Use client teaching materials associated with clinical practice guideline. *Provides broad approach to client teaching and assists in providing optimum learning environment for the client.*

### Evaluation

Client expressed a relief from anxiety after discussing her concerns with the nurse. In addition, the client verbalized an understanding of the upcoming procedure immediately after discussing the procedure during the admission process.

## Key Concepts

- Quality of health care has evolved over several centuries to become a reasonable client expectation.
- The JCAHO has had a vital role in establishing the standards of care for hospitals and other agencies that the JCAHO accredits.
- Donabedian's quality assurance framework assisted health care quality to improve.
- Quality assurance has evolved into a multidisciplinary quality improvement model.
- JCAHO accreditation surveys assist the members of the health care organization to function as a team.

- Recommendations for improving the quality of health care for the 21st century are optimistic in the measures for improvement.
- Health policies may be in the form of laws, rules, regulations, and judicial or operational decisions. These policies, when they pertain to care, define nursing practice.
- Clinical practice guidelines, procedures, and algorithms are tools used to integrate health policy and best practices into nursing practice. These documents define the standard of care for an organization.
- Nurses are accountable and responsible to impact health policy by becoming involved individually or as a member of a professional organization.

# Review Questions and Activities

1. What impact has the JCAHO had on health care quality?
2. How has the relationship between the JCAHO and the CMS affected the emphasis on accreditation?
3. How can a nurse ensure that policies and procedures will not increase liability?
4. What is one advantage of clinical practice guidelines, and how do they impact care?
5. How does Donabedian's model for quality assurance differ from the quality improvement process used today?
6. What impact did the Institute of Medicine report on medical errors have on the general public?

# Web Resources

*A journey through the history of the joint commission*
   http://www.jcaho.org
*Crossing the quality chasm: a new health system for the 21st century.* Washington, DC: National Academy Press.
   http://www.nap.edu/books
*Notes on nursing: What it is, and what it is not.*
   http://digital.library.upenn.edu
*The minimum standard.*
   http://www.jcaho.org
The policy and politics of continued competence
*NursingWorld.*
   http://www.nursingworld.org

# References

Agency for Healthcare Research and Quality (AHRQ) (2003). Clinical practice guidelines. http://www.ahcpr.gov/clinic/cpgonline.htm

Beger, D., Messenger, F., & Roth, S. (1999). Self-administered medication packets for patients experiencing vaginal birth. *Journal of Nursing Care Quality, 13*(4), 47–59.

Donabedian, A. (1966). Evaluating the quality of medical care. *Milbank Memorial Fund Quarterly, 44,* 166–203.

Donabedian, A. (1996). The effectiveness of quality assurance. *International Journal for Quality in Health Care, 8*(4), 401–407.

Dozier, A. (1998). Professional standards: Linking care, competence, and quality. *Journal of Nursing Care Quality 12*(4), 22–29.

Fetter, M. (1998). Quality: The staff nurse's role. *MEDSURG Nursing, 7*(3), 130–131.

Garry, R. (2000). Benchmarking: A prescription for healthcare. *Journal of Nursing Administration, 30*(9), 397–398.

Geatti, S., & Pegoraro, M. (1999). Basic tools to integration in management and continuous quality improvement: Protocols and procedures. *EDTNA/ERCA Journal, 25*(2), 36–38.

Goes, J., Friedman, L., Seifert, N., & Buffa, J. (2000). A turbulent field: Theory, research, and practice on organizational change in health care. *The future of integrated delivery systems: Volume I* (pp. 131–169). Greenwich, CT: JAI/Elsevier, Inc.

Hogstel, M. (2001). *Gerontology: Nursing care of the older adult.* Clifton Park, NY: Delmar Learning.

Institute of Medicine (2000). Crossing the quality chasm: A new health system for the 21st century. Washington, DC: National Academy Press.

Jennings, B., Staggers, N., & Brosch, L. (1999). Health policy and systems: A classification scheme for outcome indicators. *Image: The Journal of Nursing Scholarship 31*(4), 381–385.

Johnson, C. (1999). Knock your socks off service. *Nursing Management, 30*(7), 16–20.

Joint Commission on Accreditation of Healthcare Organizations (JCAHO) (1998). *Environment of care handbook.* IL: Oakbrook Terrace.

Joint Commission on Accreditation of Healthcare Organizations (JCAHO) (2003). *Setting the standard for quality healthcare.* http://www.jcaho.org

King, K., & Teo, K., (2000). Integrating clinical quality improvement strategies with nursing research. *Western Journal of Nursing Research, 22*(5), 596–609.

Kohn, L., Corrigan, J., & Donaldson, M. (2000). *To err is human: Building a safer health system.* Washington, DC: National Academy Press.

Maddox, P., Wakefield, M., & Bull, J. (2001). Patient safety and the need for professional and educational change. *Nursing Outlook, 49,* 8–13.

Murray, R., & Zentner, J. (2001). *Health promotion strategies through the life span* (5th ed.). Upper Saddle River, NJ: Prentice-Hall.

Nightingale, F. (1860). *Notes on nursing: What it is, and what it is not.* http://digital.library.upenn.edu/women

*Norton v. Argonaut Insurance Co.* (2001). http://findlaw.com. 144S. 2d 249.

Pulcini, J., Mason, D., Solomon Cohen, S., Kovner C., & Leavitt, J. (2000) Health policy and the private sector, new vistas for nursing. *Nursing and Health Care Perspectives, 21*(1), 22–25.

Smith, A. (2001). Removing the fluff: The quality in quality improvement. *Nursing Economics, 19*(4), 185–188.

Tyson, T. (2000). The Internet: Tomorrow's portal to nontraditional health care services. *Journal of Ambulatory Care, 23*(2), 1.

Wakefield, M., & Maddox, P. (2000). Patient quality and safety problems in the U.S. health care system: Challenges for nursing. *Nursing Economics, 18*(2), 58–62.

White, L., & Duncan, G. (2002). *Medical-surgical nursing: An integrated approach* (2nd ed.) Clifton Park, NY: Delmar Learning.

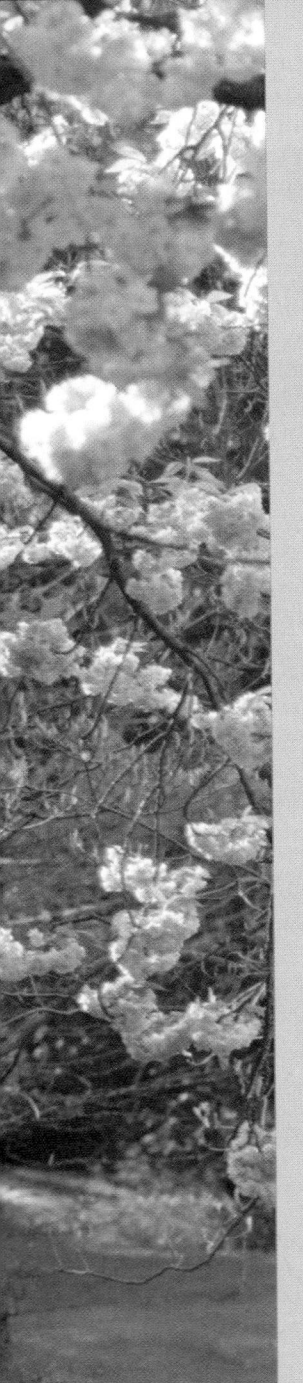

# UNIT VI

# Concepts of Therapeutic Nursing

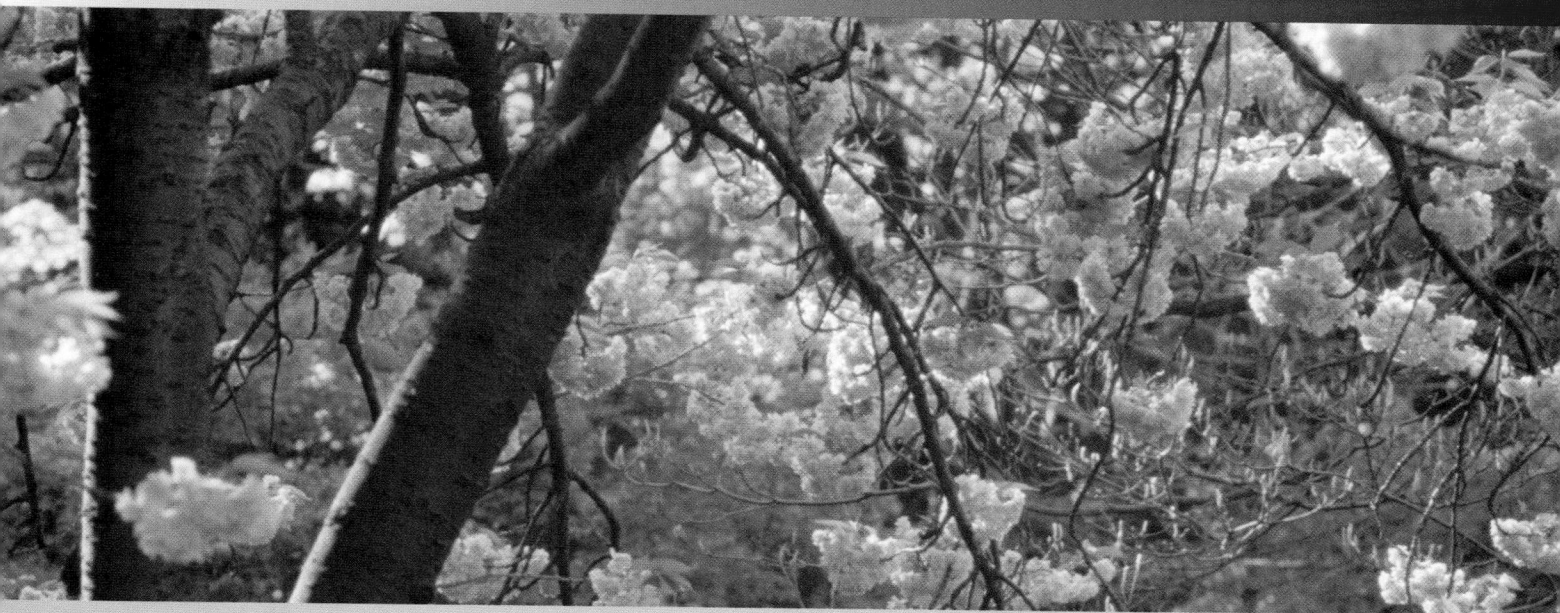

# CHAPTER 26

# Infection Control

## Fred Wilkins, RN, MN (C)

*". . . What nursing has to do is to put the patient in the best condition for nature to act upon him."*

(Florence Nightingale, 1859)

# Chapter Competencies

*Upon completion of this chapter, the reader should be able to:*

1. Identify the concepts of pathogens, infection, and colonization.
2. Understand the relationship among agent, host, and environment.
3. Describe the components of the chain of infection.
4. Discuss various factors that influence a microorganism's capability to produce an infectious disease.
5. Compare and contrast the nonspecific and specific immune defense mechanisms.
6. Describe localized and systemic infections.
7. Evaluate nosocomial infections as related to the health care delivery system.
8. Discuss the guidelines for standard precautions as related to infection control.
9. Evaluate the use of alternative therapies in infection control.

# Key Terms

| | | |
|---|---|---|
| acquired immunity | convalescent stage | nosocomial infections |
| active immunity | direct contact | passive immunity |
| agent | dirty objects | pathogens |
| airborne transmission | disinfectants | physical agent |
| anthropogenic | disinfection | portal of entry |
| antibodies | flora | portal of exit |
| antigen | fomite | prodromal stage |
| artificial immunity | germicide | reservoir |
| asepsis | handwashing | resident flora |
| aseptic technique | host | resident infectious agents |
| autoantigen | humoral immune response | sebum |
| barrier precautions | illness stage | spores |
| biological agent | immunity | Standard Precautions |
| cell-mediated immunity | immunoglobulins | sterilization |
| (cellular immunity) | incubation period | surgical asepsis |
| chemical agent | indirect contact | susceptible host |
| clean objects | infection | transient flora |
| cleansing | infection chain | transient infectious agents |
| colonization | infectious agent | vectorborne transmission |
| communicable agents | inflammation | vehicle transmission |
| communicable diseases | medical asepsis | virulence |
| compromised host | mode of transmission | |
| contact transmission | natural immunity | |

Client safety in the health care environment requires the reduction of microorganism transmission. Infection control practices are directed at controlling or eliminating sources of infection in the health care agency, home, or communities. Nurses are responsible for protecting clients and themselves by using infection control prac- tices (e.g., Standard Precautions). Nurses and clients must be educated on the types of infections, modes of transmis- sion, risks for susceptibility, and infection control prac- tices required to control or prevent further transmission. Infection control is vital to the health care delivery system and to the communities in which health care exists.

# Pathogens, Infection, and Colonization

Pathogenicity is the ability of a microorganism to produce disease. Microorganisms that cause diseases in humans are called **pathogens**. **Virulence** is the degree of pathogenicity of an infection's microorganism.

Infection and colonization are not synonymous. **Infection** is an invasion and multiplication of microorganisms in body tissue that results in cellular injury. These microorganisms are called **infectious agents**. In addition, **communicable agents** can be transmitted to a client by direct or indirect contact, through a vehicle (or vector), or by an airborne route, and result in **communicable diseases**. **Colonization** is the multiplication of microorganisms on or within a host that does not result in cellular injury. However, microorganisms that are colonized on a host may be a potential source of infection, especially if host susceptibility declines or the microorganism's virulence increases (White & Duncan, 2002).

Some microorganisms reside on the human body as normal flora. This is synonymous with colonization. **Flora** are the vegetation of microorganisms on the human body. There are two types of flora: resident and transient. **Resident flora** are microorganisms that are always present, usually without altering the client's health. Handwashing with soap and water alone is not sufficient to remove resident flora; there must be considerable friction, which is created by rubbing the hands and scrubbing the nails. **Transient flora** are episodic microorganisms. They attach to the skin for a brief period of time but do not continually live on the skin. Transient flora are usually acquired from direct contact with the microorganisms on environmental surfaces. Handwashing with soap and water is an effective means of removing transient flora.

# Agent, Host, and Environment

An **agent** is an entity that can cause disease. Agents that cause disease may be:

- **Biological agents:** Living organisms that invade the host, such as bacteria, viruses, fungi, protozoa, and rickettsia
- **Chemical agents:** Substances that can interact with the body, such as pesticides, food additives, medications, and industrial chemicals
- **Physical agents:** Factors in the environment that can cause disease, such as heat, light, noise, radiation, and machinery

In the chain of infection, the main concern is biological agents and their effects on the host.

A **host** is a simple or complex organism that can be affected by an agent. Generally, a human being is considered a host. A **susceptible host** is a person who lacks resistance to an agent and is thus vulnerable to disease. A **compromised host** is a person whose normal defense mechanisms are impaired and who is therefore susceptible to infection.

Interaction between agent and host occurs in the environment; the environment consists of everything other than the agent and host. Environmental factors that affect the chain of infection are water, food, plants, animals, housing conditions, noise, meteorological conditions, and environmental chemicals. Many of the conditions that promote the transmission of microorganisms are **anthropogenic**, reflecting changes in the relationship between humans and their environments (Todar, 2002).

The causes of most emerging infectious diseases are the same today as throughout recorded history: the transfer and dissemination of existing agents to new host populations (a process called "global microbial traffic"). For instance, cholera probably originated in Asia in ancient times; in the 19th century, it spread to Europe and the New World because of increased global travel. Cholera entered South America for the first time this century (1992) through the possible contaminated bilge water released from a Chinese freighter. The causes of emerging infectious diseases and outbreaks require careful consideration of environmental changes and especially of anthropogenic factors.

# Infection Chain

In order for a client to acquire an infection, a series of elements needs to be present. Each element or link is necessary to result in an infection. This process is known as the **infection chain** and contains six links: (1) microorganism (infectious agent), (2) source or reservoir, (3) portal of exit from reservoir, (4) mode of transmission, (5) portal of entry into host, and (6) susceptible host (Figure 26-1).

## Infectious Agents (Microorganisms)

Agents that produce infections can consist of bacteria, viruses, fungi, protozoa, and rickettsia. The ability of one of these microorganisms to infect a client is related to the virulence of the agent, the number of microorganisms present, the ability of the agent to enter and live in the client, and the susceptibility of the client.

### Resident Infectious Agents

There are two general types of infectious agents, resident and transient. **Resident infectious agents** are microorganisms that are always present on skin. These residents can be reduced through handwashing but not totally removed—although some antimicrobial agents are very effective at killing microbes on the skin.

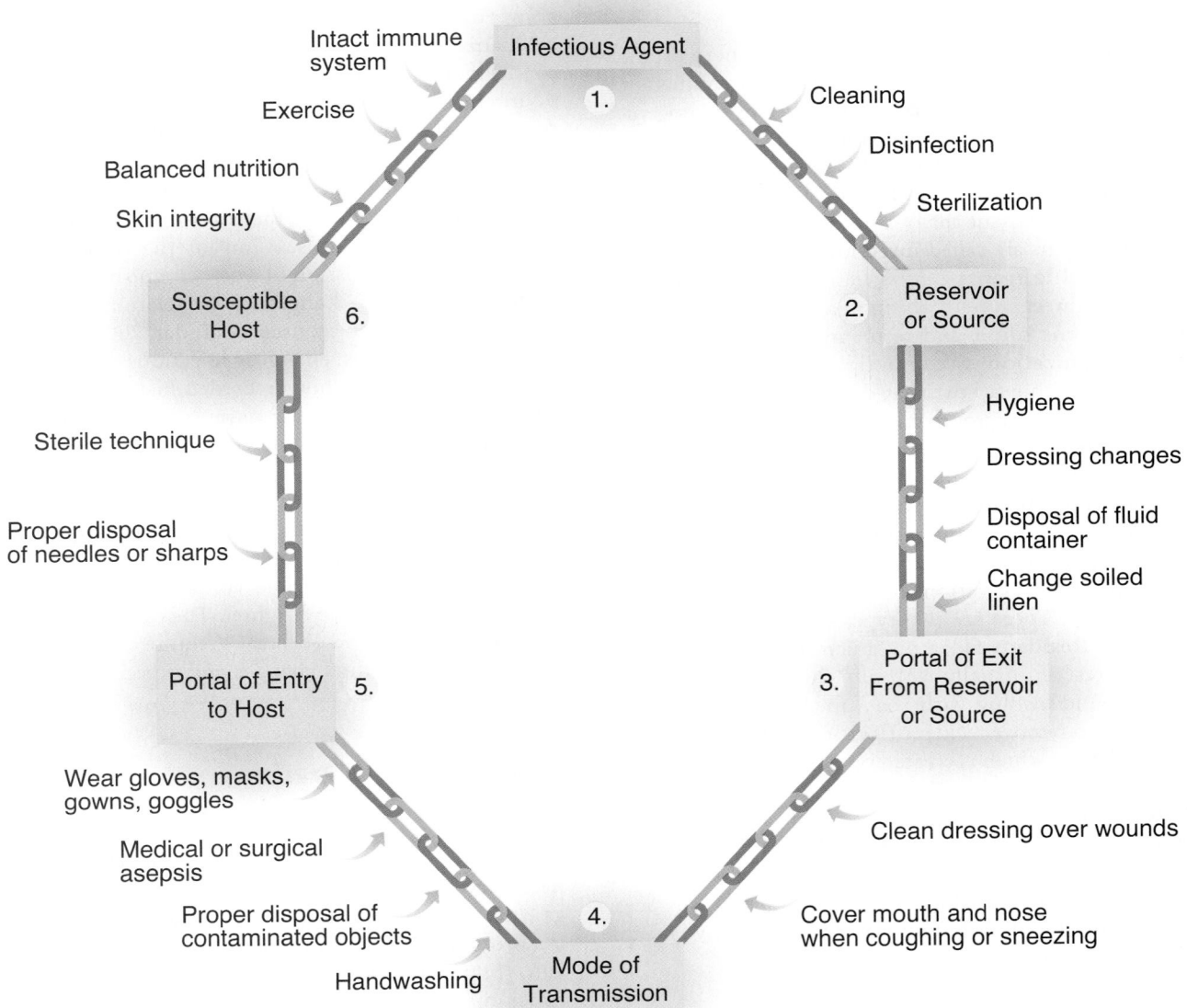

**Figure 26-1**   Breaking the chain of infection; preventive measures follow each critical link in the chain of infection.

## Transient Infectious Agents

**Transient infectious agents** are picked up via the skin from another person or object. This may occur when a nurse handles a dirty dressing and fails to adequately wash with an antimicrobial soap. These agents attach themselves to the skin and then may be transmitted to a susceptible host.

## Reservoir

A **reservoir** (or source) is required for the microorganism to survive. This is a place for the microorganism to live while awaiting a host. The reservoir may allow the organism to multiply, making it more dangerous. The human body is the most common reservoir. The intact skin of a hospital worker may function as the reservoir for many microorganisms. Besides the human body, other common reservoirs are food, plants, animals, and feces. In order to survive, the microbe needs food, oxygen (if aerobic), a viable temperature range (around 95°F), water, a pH of 5 to 8, and lack of sunlight. The human body makes an ideal reservoir for microbes. A nonsusceptible human may carry the microbe and not become infected. The chain of infection requires a **susceptible host** (an organism in which another organism is nourished and is vulnerable to a disorder or disease); therefore, a healthy person may be carrying harmful, deadly microbes, which would do great harm to a hospitalized client.

## Portal of Exit

The next link in the chain is the **portal of exit** (pathway by which pathogens leave the body of a host). The infectious agent leaves the reservoir by three methods: (1) direct contact, (2) indirect contact, and (3) airborne transmission.

### Direct Contact

**Direct contact** (transmission of a communicable disease from the host) is the most common portal of exit and occurs with touching, kissing, and sexual intercourse. Sources involved are skin, mucous membranes, urine, feces, reproductive tract, and blood. Droplets are also considered direct contact (Note: droplets are also considered airborne contaminants). During talking, saliva is emitted in the form of droplets. These droplets can easily contaminate another person during a conversation.

### Indirect Contact

**Indirect contact** (transmission of a communicable disease by any medium) occurs with the use of vehicles and vectors. A vehicle (**fomite**) is merely an object that has become contaminated with a microorganism. These may be objects such as toys, hospital supplies, instruments, dishes, cups, or surgical dressings. Other vehicles may include food, fluids, or even blood, when contaminated by the source. For example, the nurse hanging blood in the hospital may be the source of microbes that contaminate the blood product during transfusion. The microbes use the blood as a vehicle to enter the host. The food service worker may contaminate the drink of a customer. The drink then becomes the vehicle. While vehicles are usually objects or substances, vectors are usually insects. Vectors can carry microorganisms to a host, normally through a bite. The mosquito, for example, spreads West Nile virus (Ortolon, 2002).

### Airborne Transmission

**Airborne transmission** (transmission of infectious agents via airborne route) is usually considered when an infected person is coughing, thus producing airborne spread of infection. Unseen infectious agents can ride in the air on dust particles carried by the wind to a host in the form of droplet nuclei. These agents usually enter a person via the respiratory tract (e.g., common cold, flu virus).

## Mode of Transmission

The **mode of transmission** is the process that bridges the gap between the portal of exit of the biological agent from the reservoir, or source, and the portal of entry of the susceptible "new" host. Most biological agents have a primary mode of transmission; however, some microorganisms may be transmitted by more than one mode. Almost anything in the environment can become a potential means of transmitting infection, depending on the agent.

The most important and frequent mode of transmission is **contact transmission**, which involves the direct

## NURSING STRATEGY

### Decreasing Contaminants (Vehicles) to a Minimum in Client Care Settings

Nurses must take preventive actions to decrease the number of contaminants (vehicles) in their client care settings. The following are suggestions to achieve this goal:

1. Ask clients to have "gifts" such as flowers and cards placed in areas that are not close to the client's sleeping and sitting areas.
2. Create a place where friends can put their gifts, such as bookshelves, that might exist in the client's room or window ledge areas.
3. Encourage clients to keep personal items from their homes to a minimum.
4. Create a specific area for hospital supplies to be kept in the client's room (e.g., additional bedside table, supply cart).
5. Consistently remove hospital meal trays (e.g., dishes, cups, silverware) from the client's room immediately after use.

Adapted from Friedman, M., & Rhinhart, M. (2000). Improving infection control in home care: From ritual to science-based practice. *Home Healthcare Nurse, 18*(2), 34–39.

physical transfer of an agent from an infected person to a host through direct contact with a contaminated object or close contact with contaminated secretions. Sexually transmitted diseases are examples of diseases spread by direct contact.

**Airborne transmission** occurs when a susceptible host contacts droplet nuclei or dust particles that are suspended in the air. Vehicle and vectorborne transmission are indirect modes of transmission, because transmission occurs by an intermediate source. **Vehicle transmission** occurs when an agent is transferred to a susceptible host by contaminated inanimate objects such as water, food, milk, drugs, and blood. **Vectorborne transmission** occurs when an agent is transferred to a susceptible host by animate means such as mosquitoes, fleas, ticks, lice, and other animals.

## Portal of Entry

The **portal of entry** is the pathway by which infectious agents gain access to the body. The infectious agent often enters the body the same way it left the source. For example, a break in the natural skin barrier (a cut or wound) allows infectious agents to pass from the skin of the source directly to the skin of the host (Figure 26-2). A cough will

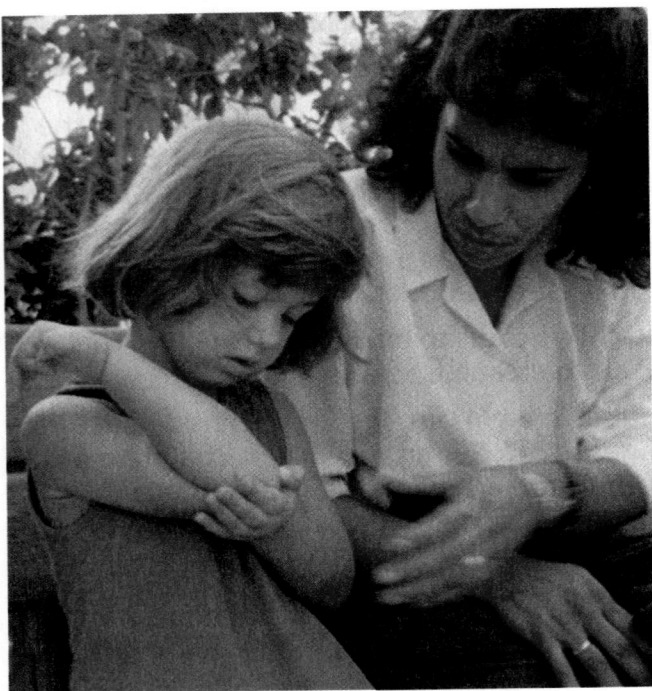

**Figure 26-2    School nurse examines a "portal of entry" (break in skin) for infection created from this child's minor accident.**

allow infectious agents to exit the source via the respiratory tract, and they can enter the host through inhalation.

## Susceptible Host

The last link in the chain of infection is that of the susceptible host. The hospitalized patient often has a reduced immune response, increasing susceptibility. The immune response describes a process, which involves the body's natural defense against infection, including specific and nonspecific mechanisms.

## Factors Influencing a Microorganism's Capability to Produce an Infectious Disease

The susceptibility of a person is related to age, heredity, level of stress, surgeries, nutritional status, and general health status, including medical diseases. One or more of these factors, coming together with microorganisms present in the health care facility, puts clients at risk.

## Age

Of all the factors that influence a microorganism to produce an infectious disease, age causes the greatest risk. The elderly acquire **nosocomial infections** (illness acquired while in a hospital) at two to five times the rate of other clients. As people age, their immune systems begin to

weaken. For example, it is recommended that the elderly get immunized annually for the flu because of their susceptibility to viral infections. On the other hand, the child before the age of 2 does not have a completely developed immune system and consequently is also more susceptible to disease (Potts & Mandleco, 2002).

## Heredity

Certain heredity traits increase susceptibility to infection. For example, agammaglobulinemia results in the absence of serum antibodies. A person with this disorder cannot form antibodies to fight infection. Other diseases may prevent the formation of immunoglobulins, reducing the body's defenses.

## Stress

Stress causes many responses in the body. The metabolic rate increases, using up stored energy. Blood cortisol is elevated, decreasing anti-inflammatory responses. If this stress is prolonged, elevated cortisone will decrease the body's ability to fight infection. Continued stress produces exhaustion, further depleting ability to ward off infection.

## Surgery

Surgery eliminates the primary barrier of intact skin to infection, predisposing clients to surgical site infections (formerly called surgical wound infections). The introduction of microorganisms into the wound produces a localized infection. The site becomes red, hot, and painful, and the infection can progress into a systemic infection. Once the microorganisms enter the bloodstream, symptoms such as fever, chills, low blood pressure, and even mental confusion may be apparent. Besides the wound itself, adjuncts to surgery can also carry additional risks of infection. For example, catheters placed into the urinary tract or blood vessels can introduce microorganisms. Tubes passed into the mouth and nose may introduce microorganisms into the body by allowing them to be inhaled into the lungs. The three most common types of hospital-acquired infections are urinary tract infections (UTIs) (34%), surgical site infections (17%), and pneumonia (lower respiratory infections) (13%). Since it is common for a surgical client to experience tubes in the bladder, mouth, and nose in addition to a surgical wound, it is easy to understand why the surgical client is at risk for infection (AORN, Inc., 2001).

## Nutrition

Adequate nutrition is essential for fighting off infections. For example, when protein consumption is insufficient, antibody production is reduced, greatly inhibiting the body's ability to ward off infection. Without necessary protein reserves, wound healing is also reduced.

## Health Status

General health status of the client greatly influences the client's susceptibility. For example, clients with disease of their immune system are at greater risk. Leukemia, AIDS, lymphoma, and aplastic anemia can weaken the body's response to infection. White blood cells normally able to trap microorganisms are not produced in the client with leukemia. Chronic diseases can predispose the client to infection related to generalized debilitation or inadequate nutrition.

# Normal Defense Mechanisms

A host's immune system serves as a normal defense mechanism to resist the transmission of infectious agents. A unique feature of the immune system is its ability to recognize "self" and "nonself"; that is, the immune system recognizes which agents are not consistent with the genetic composition of the host (self). These agents are usually referred to as antigens (nonself). **Antigens** are substances, usually proteins, that cause the formation of an antibody and react specifically with that antibody (e.g., allutinogen). An immune response is mounted against an antigen, which is recognized as nonself, to protect the body from infection. The immune defenses are categorized as nonspecific and specific immune defenses. Nonspecific and specific immune defenses work in harmony to defend the host from pathogens.

## Nonspecific Immune Defense

The nonspecific immune defense mounts a response to protect the host from all microorganisms; it is not dependent on prior exposure to the antigen. Nonspecific immune defenses are skin and normal flora; mucous membranes; sneeze, cough, and tearing reflexes; elimination and acidic environment; and inflammatory response.

### Skin and Normal Flora

Intact skin is the first line of defense against infection, serving as a physical barrier to infectious agents. Skin cells are shed along with potentially harmful microorganisms. Sebum is produced by the skin and contains fatty acids that kill some bacteria. The normal flora that reside on the skin compete with pathogenic flora for food and inhibit their multiplication. The balance of normal flora may become disrupted as a result of the inappropriate use of antibiotics, which allows pathogenic organisms to proliferate and cause infection or superinfection.

### Mucous Membranes and Sneeze, Cough, and Tearing Reflexes

Mucous membranes also function as a physical barrier to infectious agents. Mucus produced by these membranes entraps infectious agents and contains substances such as antibodies, lactoferrin, and lysozyme, which inhibit bacte-

rial growth. Cilia of the respiratory tract trap and propel mucus and microorganisms away from the lungs. The sneeze and cough reflexes physically expel mucus and microorganisms from the respiratory tract and oral cavity with force. Tears protect the eyes by continually flushing away microorganisms.

### Elimination and Acidic Environment

Elimination patterns and an acidic environment normally prevent microbial growth of pathogenic organisms. Resident flora of the large intestines prevent the growth of pathogens. The mechanical process of defecation evacuates the bowel of feces and microorganisms. Acidity of the urine prevents microbial growth. The flushing action of urination cleanses the bladder neck and urethra of microorganisms and prevents microorganisms from ascending into the urinary tract.

Normal vaginal flora prevent growth of several pathogens. At puberty, lactobacilli ferment and produce sugars in the vagina that lower the pH to an acidic range. The acidic environment of the vagina prevents pathogenic growth. Inappropriate use of antibiotics destroys the lactobacilli and its protective function.

### Inflammatory Response

**Inflammation** is a nonspecific cellular response to tissue injury or infection. Tissue injury caused by bacteria, trauma, chemicals, heat, or any other phenomenon releases multiple substances that produce dramatic secondary changes in the injured tissue. This entire complex of tissue changes and response to injury is referred to as the inflammatory process (Table 26-1). The inflammatory process has five stages that facilitate the localization, neutralization, and resolution of the offending agent within the damaged tissue. The result of the body's response to injury produces the characteristic local and systemic signs of inflammation.

The intensity of the inflammatory process is usually in proportion to the degree of tissue injury. For example, when staphylococci invade the tissues, they release lethal cellular toxins that cause the inflammatory process to develop quickly; the staphylococcal infection is characteristically walled off rapidly before the organism can multiply and spread. Streptococci, on the other hand, do not cause such intense local tissue destruction, and the walling-off process develops slowly, allowing the organism to reproduce and migrate. Therefore, the streptococci have a far greater tendency than do staphylococci to spread throughout the body and cause death, even though staphylococci are far more destructive to the tissue.

## Specific Immune Defense (The Immune Responses)

The specific immune defense mounts an immune response that is specific to the invading antigen and is labeled

## TABLE 26-1    STAGES OF THE INFLAMMATORY PROCESS

| Stage | Description | Result |
|---|---|---|
| 1 | Initial injury precipitates release of chemicals: histamine, bradykinin, serotonin, prostaglandins (reaction products of the complement and blood-clotting systems), and lymphokines (hormonal substances released by sensitized T cells). | Activates the inflammation process. |
| 2 | Increased blood flow to the inflamed area (erythema). | Produces characteristic signs of redness and increased warmth. |
| 3 | Increased capillary permeability with leakage of large quantities of plasma out of the capillaries into the damaged tissue; tissue spaces and lymphatics blocked by fibrinogen clots. | Initiates the inflammation process; infection is "walled off," and nonpitting edema occurs. |
| 4 | Damaged tissue infiltrated by leukocytes, which engulf the bacteria and necrotic tissue. After several days, these leukocytes eventually die and form a cavity of necrotic tissue and dead leukocytes (mainly neutrophils and some macrophages). | Produces purulent exudate (pus). |
| 5 | Destroyed tissue cells are replaced with identical or similar structural and functioning cells and/or fibrous tissue. | Promotes tissue healing or the formation of fibrous (scar) tissue, which may reduce the functional capacity of the tissue. |

**immunity** (defined as a specific defense mechanism used to combat infection). When foreign particles (antigens) enter the body, macrophages, monocytes, or neutrophils digest or phagocytize them. When an antigen originates from the body's own proteins, it is called an **autoantigen**. Some antigenic particles remain trapped inside the phagocytes and are sent to the lymph system or the spleen. The antigen is processed and released to the lymphocytes. This stimulates humoral immunity with the production of B lymphocytes or cell-mediated immunity with the production of T lymphocytes.

There are a number of types of immune responses. **Active immunity** results from antibodies that develop within the body to neutralize or destroy the infective agent. **Passive immunity** is acquired by the introduction of preformed antibodies, such as in utero when antibodies pass from the mother to the fetus. **Acquired immunity** results either from exposure to an antigen or from the passive injection of immunoglobulins. **Natural immunity** refers to the genetically determined response of protection (developing antibodies) within a specific species. For example, felines cannot contract the human disease of mumps. **Artificial immunity** is produced following a vaccine. The protection may not last a lifetime, so booster vaccinations may be required to maintain immunity (McCance & Huether, 2002).

## Humoral Immune Response

The **humoral immune response** is thought to attack bacteria and viruses at the extracellular level. This response is initiated when an antigen is recognized and attacked by a macrophage. The macrophage processes the antigen and gives it to a B lymphocyte. This allows the B lymphocyte to recognize the antigen as an enemy based on receptor sites located on the outer wall of the microbe invader. The B cell binds with the antigen, causing the formation of plasma and memory B cells. This process usually takes from 4 to 8 days. The plasma cells produce large amounts of antibodies. **Antibodies** are immunoglobulins produced by the body in response to bacteria, viruses, or other antigenetic substances; antibodies counteract and neutralize the effects of antigens, and destroy bacteria and other cells (agglutinin is one type of antibody). **Immunoglobulins** are plasma protein cells that produce large amounts of antibodies in five different classes (IgM, IgG, IgA, IgD, and IgE). These immunoglobulins (antibodies) circulate throughout the bloodstream for the purpose of destroying antigens in the immune responses (Todar, 2002).

## Cell-Mediated Immune Response

**Cell-mediated immunity (cellular immunity)** is initiated when the antigen stimulates the release of activated T cells. Cellular immunity is especially important to fight pathogens that survive inside cells (some bacteria and viruses), fungal infections, and tumors. There are three types of T cells: cytotoxic T cells, helper T cells, and suppressor T cells. The cytotoxic T cells seek out the infection site, attacking the cell membrane of the pathogen. They release a cytotoxic substance that kills the pathogen. These cells also release a substance called lymphokine, which attracts phagocytes to the area. Lymphokines also keep the phagocytes in the area, continuing to fight the infection. Once the antigens have been destroyed, the lymphokines are no longer released and disappear. Memory T cells remain in the area. Like memory B cells, these cells contain information that helps to identify and attack the invader if it reappears.

Helper T and Suppressor T cells assist with both humoral antibody response and cell-mediated immunity. These cells provide the start and stop of the immune response, virtually regulating the system. When the ratio is altered in one way or another, certain disease processes are allowed to occur. For example, the number of suppressor cells decreases with many autoimmune conditions, causing an overactive immune response. The opposite occurs when human immunodeficiency virus (HIV) attacks helper T cells. They prevent the body from mounting a defense against infections and tumors (McCance & Huether, 2002).

Other cells that are neither T nor B cells are called natural killer cells (NK). These cells do not require activation by exposure to an antigen. They are involved with the destruction of virally transformed cells, resistance to infection, tumor resistance, and resistance to various infections. These cells are primarily important in warding off the development of tumors by attacking malignant cells. Both humoral and cellular immunity are required to destroy potential infections and tumors in order to maintain good health.

## Localized Versus Systemic Infections

Activation of the immune response indicates the occurrence of infection. Infection results from tissue invasion and damage by an infectious agent. The two types of infectious responses are (1) localized infections, which are limited to a defined area or single organ with symptoms that resemble inflammation (redness, tenderness, and swelling); and (2) systemic infections, which affect the entire body and involve multiple organs. These types of infections progress through stages of infection as shown in Box 26-1.

The **incubation period** is the time interval between an infectious agent's entry in the host and the onset of symptoms. During this time period, the infectious agent invades the tissue and begins to multiply to produce an infection.

The **prodromal stage** is the time interval from the onset of nonspecific symptoms until specific symptoms of

---

### BOX 26-1    FOUR STAGES OF INFECTION (LOCALIZED OR SYSTEMIC)

- Incubation
- Prodromal
- Illness
- Convalescence

---

the infectious process begin to manifest. During this period, the infectious agent continues to invade and multiply in the host. A client may also be infectious to other persons in this time period.

The **illness stage** is when the client is manifesting specific symptoms of an infectious process. The period of time from when acute symptoms begin to disappear until the client returns to the previous state of health is referred to as the **convalescent stage** (Kerstein, 1997).

## Nosocomial Infections

Nosocomial infections usually appear 3 days after a client is admitted to a health care setting. Between 5% and 15% of the clients admitted to hospitals in the United States will acquire a nosocomial infection. Regardless of the work setting—hospital, ambulatory clinic, nursing home, dialysis center, freestanding surgery center, or rehabilitation facility—nosocomial infections will occur. About one-quarter to one-third of these infections can be prevented if health care workers use appropriate precautions (Eggimann, 2001). The combination of microorganisms with clients who have increased susceptibility to infection leads to the transmission of infectious diseases.

Since 1% of nosocomial infections end in death, rapid diagnosis and treatment is essential. More important than diagnosis is prevention. High-risk procedures

---

### CLINICAL ALERT

#### Incubation Period

Always check the incubation period of an infection by asking the client when exposure occurred and how long it was before symptoms developed. Depending on the infectious agent, a client may be able to transmit the infection to another person.

Todar, K. (2002). Immune defense against microbial pathogens. *Todar's Online Textbook of Bacteriology.* http://www.textbookof-bacteriology.net.

## FOCUS ON WELLNESS

### Prodromal Stage

When a client is experiencing prodromal clinical manifestations, she should be encouraged to participate in the following health promotive behaviors with the explanation that the illness stage may be prevented or subdued:

1. stress management activities
2. intake of a well-balanced nutritional diet and perhaps a multivitamin in the event that appetite is decreased during this stage
3. maintenance of well-hydrated state, including fruit juices that contain vitamin C
4. good sleep habits and rest periods
5. ingestion of such products as echinacea, eucalyptus, herbal teas, and other wellness-oriented or comfort-promoting substances

National Center for Complementary and Alternative Medicine (NCCAM), 2003. http://nccam.nih.gov

## RESEARCH FOCUS

**Title of Study:** Infection control: New hand hygiene practices reduce drug-resistant germs in Washington, DC, hospital

**Study Purpose:** There is extremely poor compliance in health care workers using consistent hand-washing techniques. This study's primary goal was to determine if staff could use alcohol-based hand-rubs (e.g., foam, gel, lotion), which are much less time-consuming than soap and water handwashing, and reduce nosocomial infection rates.

**Methods:** A 2-year study began at a VA medical center (an inner-city, tertiary-care teaching hospital with 167 acute and 120 long-term care beds). Five hundred alcohol-based dispensers were installed in all inpatient rooms and outpatient clinic rooms, and the infection control team gave educational presentations to all clinical staff. No other changes in infection control practice were made during the time of the study. No change was made in hand soap availability at this inner-city facility.

**Findings:** The rates of new nosocomial cases of vancomycin-resistant enterococcus (VRE), methicillin-resistant *Staphylococcus aureus* (MRSA), and *Clostridium difficile* colitis (CD) decreased with the distribution of an alcohol-based hand rub. Over the 2-year period of the study, the number of new cases of MRSA decreased by 21%, and the number of vancomycin-resistant enterococcus (VRE) decreased by 43%. The number of CD cases decreased about 22%. In addition to significantly reducing the number of cases of new, hospital-acquired, drug-resistant germs, the alcohol-based hand-rub was very popular with the busy staff.

**Implications:** In the future, there is the possibility that alcohol-based hand-rubs could take the place of handwashing techniques. The new aseptic technique could take less time for staff, and ultimately lead to more client contact time for nurses and reduced rates of nosocomial infections.

Shultz, M. (2002). Infection control: New hand hygiene practices reduce drug-resistant germs in Washington, DC, hospital. *TB & Outbreaks Weekly.* Atlanta Publishing Co.

identified as possible sources of infection, such as urinary catheterization, should be done only when necessary and then removed as soon as possible (Table 26-2). Equipment and instruments should be cleaned or sterilized using strict standards of care. Health care workers should use frequent handwashing, since this one factor is the single, most important event related to prevention of nosocomial infections (Rizzo, 1999). However, recent research is also showing the benefits to using alcohol-based hand-rubs.

Most recently, there is a surgical asepsis risk of Creutzfeldt-Jakob disease ("mad cow disease") originating in the perioperative setting (Joint Commission on the Accreditation of Healthcare Organizations, 2002).

## Ensure Asepsis

Nurses are responsible for providing the client with a safe environment, which includes preventing the transmission of nosocomial infections. **Asepsis** is the absence of microorganisms. Providing nursing care using aseptic technique decreases the risk and spread of nosocomial infections. **Aseptic technique** is the infection control practice used to prevent the transmission of pathogens. Two types of asepsis are medical and surgical.

### Medical Asepsis

**Medical asepsis** uses practices to reduce the number, growth, and spread of microorganisms. Medical asepsis is also referred to as "clean technique." Objects are generally referred to as "clean" or "dirty" in medical asepsis. **Clean objects** are considered to have the presence of some microorganisms that are usually not pathogenic. **Dirty** (soiled) **objects** are considered to have a high number of

## TABLE 26-2    NOSOCOMIAL INFECTIONS

| Site of Infection | Causes |
|---|---|
| **Urinary Tract** | |
| *Escherichia coli* | Catheterization technique |
| Enterococcus species | Contamination of closed drain system |
| *Pseudomonas aeruginosa* | Inadequate handwashing |
| **Surgical Sites** | |
| *Staphylococcus aureus* | Inadequate handwashing |
| Enterococcus species | Improper dressing change technique |
| *Pseudomonas aeruginosa* | |
| **Pneumonia** | |
| *Staphylococcus aureus* | Inadequate handwashing |
| *Pseudomonas aeruginosa* | Improper suctioning tech |
| Enterobacter species | |

## CLINICAL ALERT

### Mad Cow Disease

In the summer of 2001, the Joint Commission on Accreditation of Healthcare Organizations (JCAHO) issued a Sentinel Alert related to exposure to variant Creutzfeldt-Jakob disease (CJD). This degenerative disease caused by prions (malformed proteins) is linked to "mad cow" disease. The Sentinel Alert warned hospitals to review their policies on cleaning and sterilization of instruments used on clients known to have CJD. Recommendations have been made from the extreme of "throwing the instruments away" to a combination of soaking in sodium hydroxide solutions and steam sterilization at high temperatures and for long periods. This topic will likely remain a great concern with the fear of the spread of this disease.

Bren, L. (2002). FDA continues work to help prevent mad cow disease. *FDA Consumer, 36*(3), 31–32; Gray, G., Kreindel, S., Ropeik, D. (2002). Mad cow disease risk in the United States. Does perceived threat overshadow true likelihood of occurrence? *Postgraduate Medicine, 111*(2), 13–16.

microorganisms, with some that are potentially pathogenic. Common medical aseptic measures used for clean or dirty objects are handwashing, gloving, changing linens daily, and cleaning floors and hospital furniture daily.

### Handwashing

**Handwashing** is the rubbing together of all surfaces and crevices of the hands using a soap or chemical and water. Handwashing is a component of all types of isolation precautions and is the most basic and effective infection control measure that prevents and controls the transmission of infectious agents. The Centers for Disease Control and Prevention (CDC) (2003) recommends vigorous scrubbing with warm, soapy water for at least 15 seconds to prevent the transfer of germs; high-risk areas, such as nurseries, usually require about a 2-minute handwash. Soiled hands usually require more time (CDC, 2000).

The three essential elements of handwashing are soap or chemical, water, and friction (see Procedure 26-1 for the proper steps of handwashing). Soaps that contain antimicrobial agents are frequently used in high-risk areas such as emergency departments and nurseries. Friction is the most important element of the three because it physically removes soil and transient flora.

Handwashing should be performed after arriving at work, before leaving work, between client contacts, after removing gloves, when hands are visibly soiled, before eating, after excretion of body waste (urination and defecation),

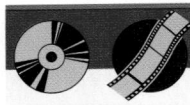

**PROCEDURE 26-1**    **Handwashing**

## EQUIPMENT NEEDED

- Soap
- Sink
- Paper or cloth towels
- Running water

## IMPLEMENTATION—ACTION/RATIONALE

| ACTION | RATIONALE |
|---|---|
| 1. Remove jewelry. Wristwatch may be pushed up above the wrist (midforearm). Push sleeves of uniform or shirt up above the wrist at midforearm level. | 1. Provides access to skin surfaces for cleaning. Facilitates cleaning of fingers, hands, and forearms. |
| 2. Assess hands for hangnails, cuts, or breaks in the skin, and areas that are heavily soiled. | 2. Intact skin acts as a barrier to microorganisms. Breaks in skin integrity facilitate development of infection and should receive extra attention during cleaning. |
| 3. Turn on the water. Adjust the flow and temperature. Temperature of the water should be warm. | 3. Running water removes microorganisms. Warm water removes less of the natural skin oils than does hot water. |
| 4. Wet hands and lower forearms thoroughly by holding under running water. Keep hands and forearms in the down position with elbows straight. Avoid splashing water and touching the sides of the sink. | 4. Water should flow from the least contaminated to the most contaminated areas of the skin. Hands are considered more contaminated than arms. Splashing of water facilitates transfer of microorganisms. Touching of any surface during cleaning contaminates the skin. |
| 5. Apply about 5 ml (1 teaspoon) of liquid soap. Lather thoroughly. | 5. Lather facilitates removal of microorganisms. Liquid soap harbors less bacteria than bar soap. |
| 6. Thoroughly rub hands together for about 10 to 15 seconds. Interlace fingers and thumbs and move back and forth to wash between digits. Rub palms and back of hands with circular motion (see Figure 26-3). Special attention should be provided to areas such as the knuckles and fingernails, which are known to harbor organisms (Figure 26-4). | 6. Friction mechanically removes microorganisms from the skin surface. Friction loosens dirt from soiled areas. |

**Figure 26-3    Lather thoroughly, and rub hands together.**

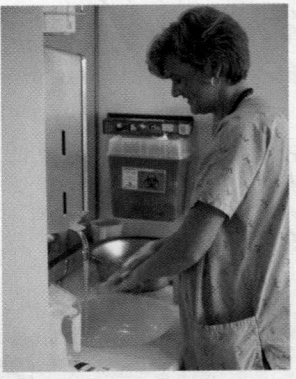

**Figure 26-4    Give special attention to fingernails and knuckles.**

*(continues)*

## PROCEDURE 26-1 (continued)

| ACTION | RATIONALE |
|---|---|
| 7. Rinse with hands in the down position, elbows straight. Rinse in the direction of forearm to wrist to fingers. | 7. Flow of water rinses away dirt and microorganisms. |
| 8. Blot hands and forearms to dry thoroughly. Dry in the direction of fingers to wrist and forearms. Discard the paper towels in the proper receptacle. | 8. Blotting reduces chapping of skin. Drying from cleanest (hand) to least clean area (forearms) prevents transfer of microorganisms to cleanest area. |
| 9. Turn off the water faucet with a clean, dry paper towel. | 9. Prevents contamination of clean hands by a less clean faucet. |

after contact with body fluids, before and after performing invasive procedures, and after handling contaminated equipment.

### Surgical Asepsis

**Surgical asepsis**, or sterile technique, consists of those practices that eliminate all microorganisms and spores from an object or area. Spores are single-celled microorganisms or microorganisms in the resting or inactive stage. Surgical asepsis refers to handwashing, the donning of surgical attire (caps, masks, and eyewear), handling of sterile instruments and equipment, and establishing and maintaining sterile fields.

Surgical asepsis is practiced by the nurse in the operating room, during labor and delivery, and for many diagnostic and therapeutic interventions at the client's bedside. Common nursing procedures that require sterile technique are:

- All invasive procedures, either intentional perforation of the skin (injections, insertion of intravenous needles or catheters) or entry into a bodily orifice (tracheobronchial suctioning, insertion of a urinary catheter)
- Nursing measures for clients with disruption of skin surfaces (changing a surgical wound or intravenous site dressing) or destruction of skin layers (trauma and burns)

### Sterile Field

The nurse needs to establish and maintain a sterile field when performing those procedures that require sterile technique, such as changing burn dressings or large wound dressings. Agency policy and supplies vary in different health care settings. Review the agency's policy and gather all the necessary supplies before preparing the sterile field.

Sterile dressing packages can be either commercially prepared or agency wrapped. When opening the package, allow the edges of the wrapper to drop down and away from the package (see Procedure 26-2) (Altman, 2004) The sterile field must be kept free of microorganisms by placing only sterile items inside the field. When adding additional supplies to the field, avoid reaching across a sterile field. Gently drop additional supplies onto the sterile field, making sure that the supply wrapper does not touch the field; always open packages away from the field to prevent crossover and contamination.

When the sterile field is prepared, always face the field and keep sterile objects above waist level to avoid the risk of field contamination. Behaviors such as talking, sneezing,

## CLINICAL ALERT

### Handwashing

Wash hands before and after every client contact. The most common cause of nosocomial infections is contaminated hands of health care providers.

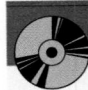

**PROCEDURE 26-2**

## Surgical Asepsis:
## Preparing and Maintaining a Sterile Field

### EQUIPMENT NEEDED

- Antimicrobial soap for handwashing
- Sterile materials (antiseptic solution, bowl, dressing, instruments)
- Additional sterile supplies (culture swab, gauze, or dressings to complement the type of procedure to be performed)

- Sterile drape (may be contained in dressing tray)
- Sterile solution
- Package of proper-sized sterile gloves
- Container for disposal of waste materials (follow agency policy, colored bag that designates infectious waste products)

### IMPLEMENTATION—ACTION/RATIONALE

| ACTION | RATIONALE |
|---|---|
| 1. Gather equipment for the type of procedure:<br><br>  **a.** Select only clean, dry packages marked sterile, and read listing of contents.<br><br>  **b.** Check the package for integrity and expiration date. | 1. Prevents break in technique during procedure. If the package is moist or outdated, it is considered contaminated and must be discarded. |
| 2. Select a clean, easily accessible area in the client's environment to establish the sterile field. | 2. Promotes access to the sterile field during the procedure. |
| 3. Explain procedure to the client; provide specific instructions if client assistance is required during the procedure. | 3. Gains client's understanding and cooperation during the procedure. |
| 4. Inquire about and attend to the client's toileting needs. | 4. Prevents break in technique during the procedure. |
| 5. Hospital environment: If the procedure is to be performed at the client's bedside, the client should be in a private room or moved to a clean treatment room. | 5. Minimizes microorganisms in the environment. |
| 6. Home environment: Secure privacy and remove pets from the room. | 6. Puts the client at ease and promotes a clean environment. |
| 7. Position client and attend to comfort measures; the client's position should provide you easy access to the area and facilitate good body mechanics during the procedure. | 7. Helps the client relax and prevents movement during the procedure; prevents reaching, decreasing the risk of contamination and back strain. |
| 8. Wash hands; refer to Procedure 26-1. | 8. Prevents transmission of infection. |
| 9. Place sterile package (drape or tray) at waist height in the center of the clean, dry work area. | 9. Prevents reaching over exposed sterile items when wrapper is removed. |
| 10. Remove the wrapper, pulling away from the body (Figure 26-5). | 10. Prevents contamination. |

*(continues)*

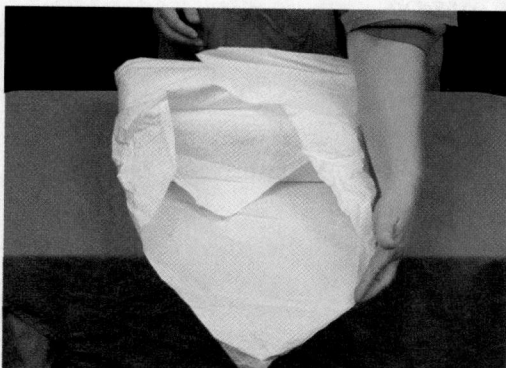

**Figure 26-5   Open the first flap of a sterile wrapped package.**

11. Grasp the folded top edge with fingertips of one hand.

12. Remove the drape by lifting up and away from all objects while it unfolds; discard the outer wrapper with other hand.

13. With free hand, grasp the other drape corner, keeping it away from all objects.

14. Lay the drape on the surface, with the drape bottom first touching the surface farthest from you; step back and allow the drape to cover the surface (see Figure 26-6).

11. Edges are considered unsterile.

12. If the drape touches an unsterile object, it is contaminated and must be discarded.

13. Avoids contamination.

14. Prevents you from reaching over the sterile field; stepping back decreases risk that drape will touch your uniform.

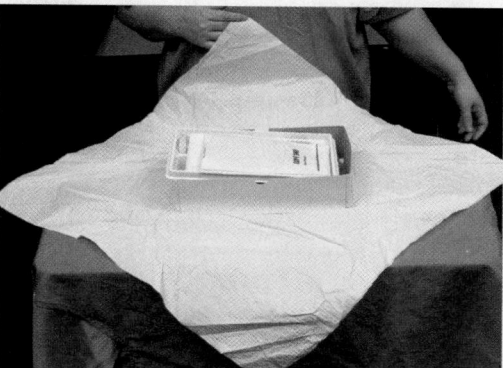

**Figure 26-6   Place drape on the surface by first placing the bottom portion of drape farthest from oneself and then placing the top portion of drape over the work surface.**

15. Open and place the tray on the work surface so that the top flap of the sterile wrapper opens away from you.

15. Prevents reaching over the sterile items.

*(continues)*

## PROCEDURE 26-2 (continued)

16. Reach around the tray; with thumb and index fingertips grasping the wrapper's top flap, gently pull up, then down to open over the surface.

17. Repeat the same steps to open the side flaps.

18. Grasp the corner of the bottom flap with fingertips, step back, and pull flap down.

19. While facing the sterile field, step back, remove the outer wrapper, and grasp the item in your nondominant hand so that the top flap will open away from you.

20. With your dominant hand, open the flaps as previously described (see Figure 26-7).

21. With your dominant hand, pull the wrapper back and away from the sterile field and place the item onto the field (see Figure 26-8).

16. Only the edges of the field can be contaminated; pulling up frees the top folded flap.

17. Keeps the arm from reaching over the sterile field.

18. Creates a sterile work surface.

19. Keeps your dominant hand free; item remains sterile.

20. Prevents reaching over the sterile item.

21. Prevents the wrapper from touching the sterile field.

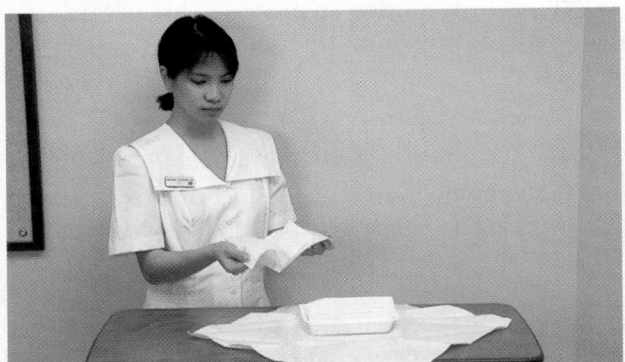

**Figure 26-7   Grasp the flaps of the wrapped supply and pull downward.**

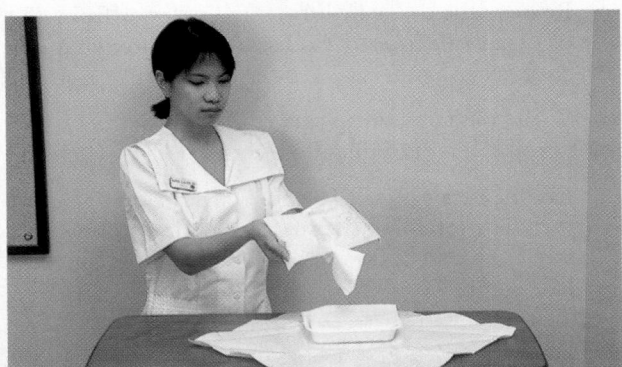

**Figure 26-8   Add contents to the sterile field by holding the package 6 inches (15 cm) above the field and allowing the contents to drop onto the field.**

22. When adding additional gauze or dressings to the sterile field, open the package as directed; grasp the top flaps of the wrapper and pull downward; then drop the contents onto the center of the field.

23. Read the labels and strengths of all solutions three times prior to pouring.

24. Remove the lid from the bottle of solution and place the sterile side up onto a clean surface.

25. Hold the bottle, label in palm of hand, 4 to 6 inches (10–15 cm) over the container on the sterile field; slowly pour the solution into the container to avoid splashing.

22. Prevents contamination of item and sterile field.

23. Ensures proper solution and strength.

24. Inverting the lid prevents contamination of the inner surface.

25. Prevents the label from getting wet; if the solution splashes onto the label, the field is contaminated because moisture conducts microorganisms from the nonsterile surface.

*(continues)*

## PROCEDURE 26-2 (*continued*)

26. Replace the lid on the container, label the container with the date and time, and initial the container if retained for reuse.

27. Wash hands and don nonsterile gloves.

28. With dominant hand, grasp forceps from the sterile field, making sure only the handles of the forceps are touched.

29. Hold forceps above waist level throughout the procedure.

30. Keep forceps tips pointing downward when adding, arranging, or removing items to the sterile field during the sterile procedure.

31. Dispose of contaminated items in colored plastic bag.

32. Wash hands and perform open gloving (see Procedure 26-3).

33. Continue with procedure, keeping gloved hands above waist level at all times, touching only items on the sterile field.

34. If using a solution to cleanse a site, use the sterile forceps to prevent contamination of gloves; dispose of forceps after use.

35. Postprocedure, dispose of all contaminated items in colored plastic bag.

36. Remove gloves by grasping the outside of one cuff with the other gloved hand; pull glove off, turning it inside out. Dispose in plastic bag with other contaminated items.

37. Using the fingers of your ungloved hand, slip fingers, palm up, inside the cuff and peel the glove off, inside out. Dispose of glove in colored plastic bag.

38. Reposition the client.

39. Clean the environment; wash hands.

40. In the client's medical record, document the procedure, findings (description of infected area), and the response of the client.

---

26. Sterility of the solution will be lost if exposed to air for an extended period of time.

27. Prevents transmission of infection to client.

28. Prevents contamination of sterile items.

29. Keeps forceps in your view, and decreases the risk of contamination.

30. Gravity will prevent any liquids from flowing back and forth between forceps tips and handle held in ungloved hand.

31. Alerts other health care workers of contaminated waste, decreasing their risk of infection.

32. Prevents transmission of infection.

33. Decreases chance of contamination. Any item below waist level and out-of-sight is considered contaminated.

34. Prevents field contamination.

35. Decreases risk of transmission of infection to all health care workers.

36. Minimizes your risk of contact with infectious wastes on the gloves.

37. Outside of the glove does not touch your skin and contaminate it.

38. Promotes client comfort.

39. Prevents transmission of infection.

40. Demonstrates compliance with sterile procedure and the effectiveness of therapy.

---

and coughing should be avoided to maintain the field's sterility; if the client is unable to cooperate, explain why a face mask is needed and apply.

Care of a wound requires a sterile dressing change to promote wound healing and to prevent infection. Assess the wound during the dressing change for infection (redness, edema, pain at the incision line, and purulent drainage from the wound) and progression of healing. See Chapter 36 for a complete discussion of wound care.

Wound care often requires the use of a sterile solution to cleanse the wound during a dressing change. Maintain the sterility of the solution by handling the container to keep the inside of the container sterile. When the lid to the container is removed, place the sterile side up and pour some of the solution into a nonsterile container before adding to the sterile container on the field. Gently pour the sterile solution into the sterile container to avoid wetting the field. The sterile technique is maintained throughout wound care; if the sterile field becomes wet or damp, discard all supplies and prepare a new sterile field (Atiyeh, Ioannovich, Al-Amm, & El-Musa, 2002).

### Donning Sterile Gloves

There are two methods for applying sterile gloves: open and closed. The open method is used most frequently when performing procedures that require the sterile technique such as dressing changes (see Procedure 26-3 for applying sterile gloves by the open method). The closed method is used when the nurse wears a sterile gown.

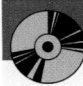

**PROCEDURE 26-3**    **Applying Sterile Gloves via the Open Method**

## EQUIPMENT NEEDED

▪ Package of proper-sized sterile gloves (Figure 26-9)

## IMPLEMENTATION—ACTION/RATIONALE

| ACTION | RATIONALE |
|---|---|
| 1. Wash hands. | 1. Prevents transmission of infection. |
| 2. Read the manufacturer's instructions on the package of sterile gloves; proceed as directed in removing the outer wrapper from the package (Figure 26-10) and in placing the inner wrapper onto a clean, dry surface (Figure 26-11). Open inner wrapper to expose gloves (Figure 26-12). | 2. Different manufacturers package gloves differently; the instructions will tell you how to properly open to avoid contamination of the inner wrapper; any moisture on the surface will contaminate the gloves. |

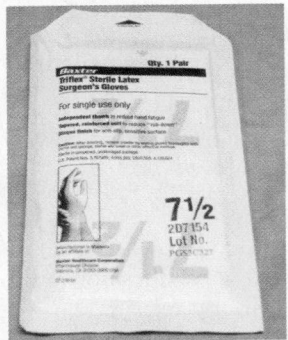

**Figure 26-9    Sterile gloves**

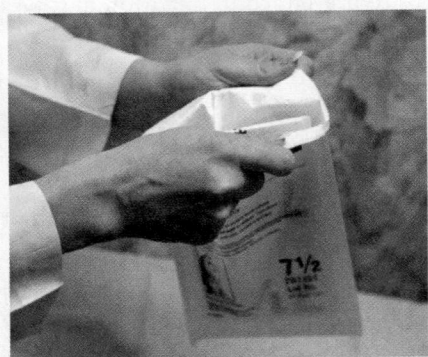

**Figure 26-10    Remove the outer wrapper of the sterile glove package.**

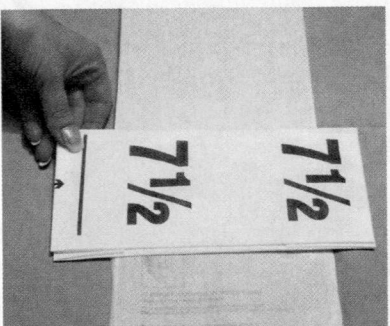

**Figure 26-11    Place the gloves in the inner wrapper on clean, dry surface.**

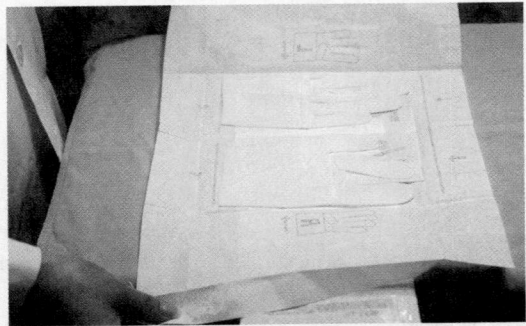

**Figure 26-12    Open the inner wrapper to expose gloves.**

*(continues)*

## PROCEDURE 26-3 (*continued*)

3. Identify right and left hand; glove dominant hand first.

4. Grasp the 2-inch- (5-cm-) wide cuff with the thumb and first two fingers of the nondominant hand, touching only the cuff (Figure 26-13).

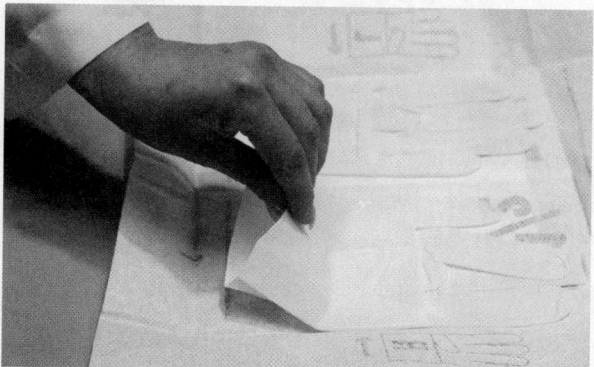

**Figure 26-13    Grasp first cuff with the nondominant hand.**

5. Gently pull the glove over the dominant hand, making sure the thumb and fingers fit into the proper spaces of the glove (Figure 26-14). Hold hands above the waist while applying glove. Once dominant hand is gloved, keep hands visible and above waist to prevent accidental contamination.

6. With the gloved dominant hand, slip your fingers under the cuff of the other glove, gloved thumb abducted, making sure it does not touch any part on your nondominant hand (Figure 26-15). Be careful not to drag glove or touch gloved dominant hand with ungloved nondominant hand.

7. Gently slip the glove onto your nondominant hand, making sure the fingers slip into the proper spaces (Figures 26-16 and 26-17).

3. Dominant hand should facilitate motor dexterity during gloving.

4. Maintains sterility of the outer surfaces of the sterile glove.

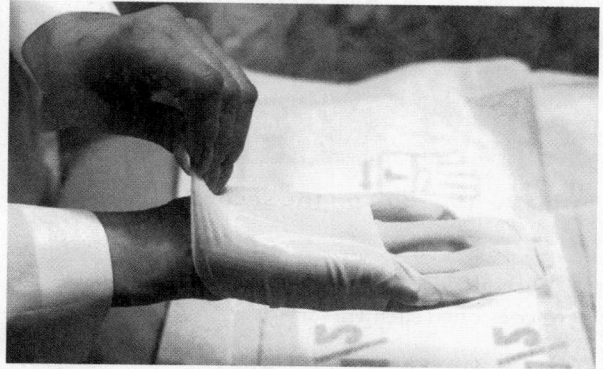

**Figure 26-14    Pull the glove over the dominant hand.**

5. Prevents tearing the glove material; guiding the fingers into proper places facilitates gloving.

6. Cuff protects gloved fingers, maintaining sterility.

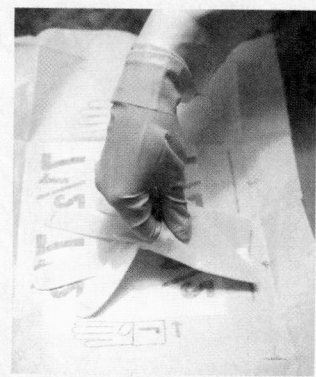

**Figure 26-15    Slip fingers under the cuff of the second glove.**

7. Contact is made with two sterile gloves.

*(continues)*

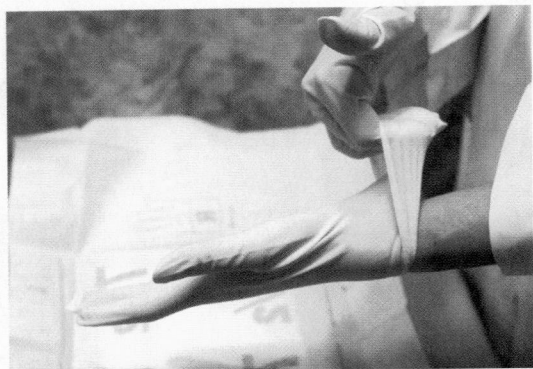

**Figure 26-16    Pull on the second glove.**

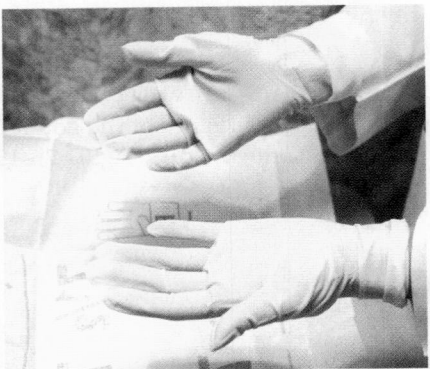

**Figure 26-17    Make sure all fingers are in the proper spaces.**

8. With gloved hands, interlock fingers to fit the gloves onto each finger.

   If the gloves are soiled, remove by turning inside out as follows:

9. Slip gloved fingers of the dominant hand under the cuff of the opposite hand, or grasp the outer part of the glove at the wrist if there is no cuff.

10. Pull the glove down to the fingers, exposing the thumb (Figure 26-18).

8. Promotes proper fit over the fingers.

9. Contact is made with two sterile gloves.

10. Frees the thumb for the next step.

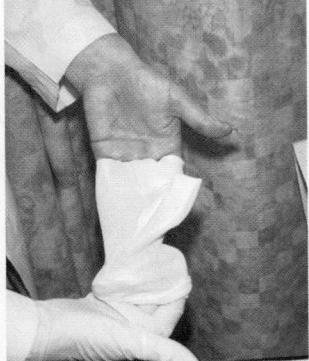

**Figure 26-18    Peel glove down to fingers, exposing one thumb.**

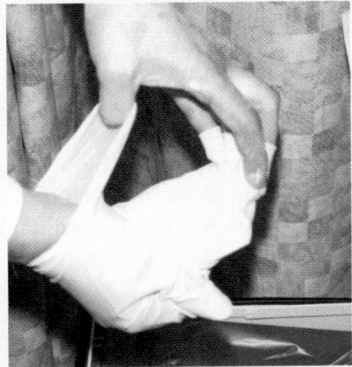

**Figure 26-19    Slip uncovered thumb into the opposite glove.**

11. Slip the uncovered thumb into the opposite glove at the wrist, allowing only the glove-covered fingers of the hand to touch the soiled glove (Figure 26-19).

12. Pull the glove down over the dominant hand almost to the fingertips, and slip the glove on to the other hand (Figure 26-20).

11. Contact is made with two sterile gloves.

12. Removes glove without contact with soiled surfaces.

*(continues)*

**PROCEDURE 26-3** (*continued*)

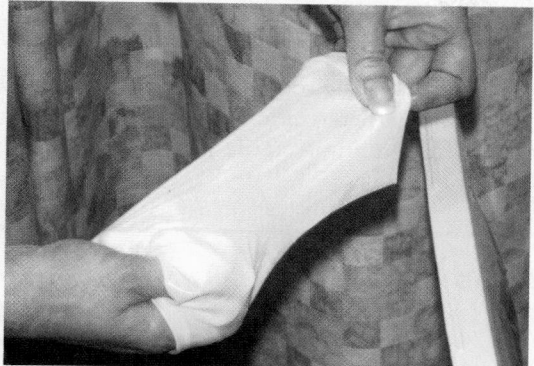

**Figure 26-20   When soiled gloves are removed correctly, only the inside clean surface of one glove is exposed.**

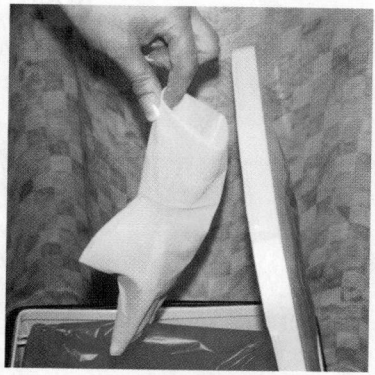

**Figure 26-21   Dispose of gloves in appropriate receptacle.**

13. With the dominant hand touching only the inside of the other glove, pull the glove over the dominant hand so that only the inside (clean surface) is exposed.

14. Dispose of soiled gloves according to institutional policy and wash hands (Figure 26-21).

13. Exposes only the clean surface of the gloves.

14. Prevents the transfer of microorganisms.

### Donning Surgical Attire

Surgical nurses are required to wear a surgical mask and a clean cloth or paper cap that covers all of the hair. After the cap is applied, the nurse positions the mask to cover the nose and mouth (see Procedure 26-4). Protective eyewear (glasses or goggles) is worn during all procedures that pose a threat of splashing body fluids into the eyes.

### Surgical Handwashing

Surgical handwashing or scrub is used to remove soil and most transient microorganisms from the skin. Nurses working in the operating room perform surgical handwashing to decrease the client's risk for an infection. The

## LIFE SPAN CONSIDERATIONS

### Gloving

- When gloving to care for a confused or restless client, make sure you open the gloves away from the client, so accidental contamination does not occur.

- Seek assistance restraining or holding a client in position prior to applying sterile gloves.

## COMMUNITY/HOME CARE

### Gloving in the Home

- Caregivers may shy away from the cost of sterile gloves and be tempted to perform procedures at home with clean gloves or find other ways to "cut corners." Be supportive as you listen to their concerns. Even with insurance, the costs associated with illness are often overwhelming to a caregiver on a limited budget. Make sure an adequate supply of gloves is available, and educate the caregiver on the need for proper technique to prevent infection.

- Uncluttered tabletop space is often at a premium in the home care setting. If you need space to lay out supplies or open your glove package, bring along a TV tray or stand. You can quickly set it up and take it down in the client care area.

## CLINICAL ALERT

### Disposable Equipment

Disposable equipment should be discarded after use. The materials used for disposable equipment cannot be thoroughly cleaned and are not intended for reuse.

skin on the nurse's hands and arms should be intact (free of lesions). Agency policy determines how to perform the scrub with regard to method and timing (see Procedure 26-5 for the basic principles in performing surgical hand-washing [surgical scrub]).

### Gowning and Closed Gloving

Nurses in the operating room and special procedure areas such as cardiac catheterization labs use the closed gloved method when donning a sterile gown. After the surgical

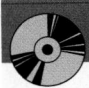

**PROCEDURE 26-4**   **Donning a Cap and Mask**

### EQUIPMENT NEEDED

■ Cap
■ Mask

■ Mask with a face shield, if necessary

### IMPLEMENTATION—ACTION/RATIONALE

| ACTION | RATIONALE |
|---|---|
| 1. Wash hands. | 1. Reduces transmission of microorganisms. |
| 2. Apply cap to head, being sure to tuck hair under cap. Males with facial hair should use a hood to cover all hair on head and face. | 2. Protective garments prevent the transmission of organisms from the nurse to the client. The cap also protects the nurse from infectious pathogens. |
| 3. Secure mask around mouth and nose (Figure 26-22). For masks with strings: | 3. Barrier garments prevent the transmission of organisms between nurse and client. Mask will prevent organisms from entering or escaping around nose. |
| a. Hold mask by top and pinch metal strip over bridge of nose. | |
| b. Pull two top strings over ears and tie at upper back of head. | |
| c. Tie two lower ties around back of neck so that bottom of mask fits snugly under chin (Figure 26-23). | |

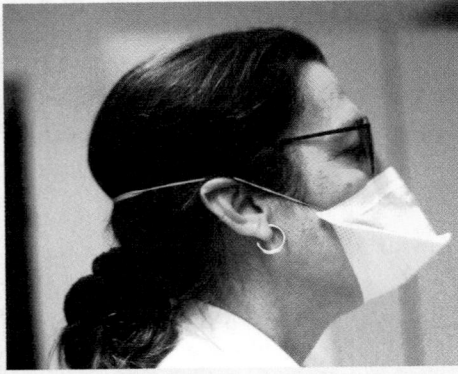

**Figure 26-22**   **Secure mask around mouth and nose.**

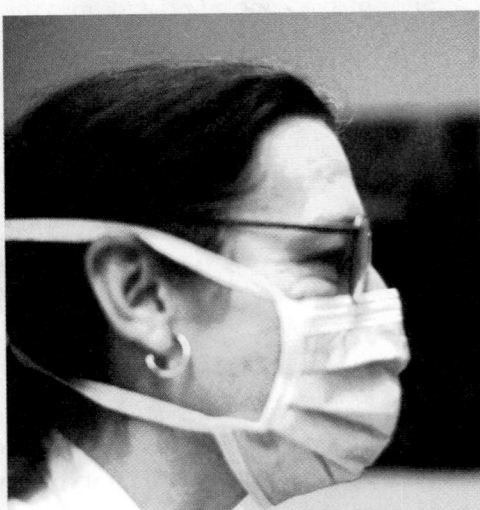

**Figure 26-23**   **Bottom of the mask should fit snugly under chin.**

*(continues)*

## PROCEDURE 26-4 (*continued*)

4. Enter the client's room, and explain the rationale for wearing a cap and mask.

5. After performing necessary tasks, remove cap and mask before leaving room.

   a. Untie bottom strings of mask first, then top strings, and lift off of face. Hold mask by strings and discard.

   b. Grasp top surface of cap and lift from head.

6. Wash hands after removing mask.

4. Minimizes anxiety and feelings of isolation.

5. Reduces transmission of organisms.

   a. Prevents contaminated surface of mask from contacting uniform.

   b. Minimizes contact of hands to hair.

6. Reduces transmission of microorganisms.

---

scrub, the nurse proceeds to don the sterile gown and gloves using the closed method (see Procedure 26-6). The sterile gown serves as a barrier to decrease the risk of wound contamination. The sterile gown also allows the nurse to move freely in the environment with sterile drapes and objects.

## LIFE SPAN CONSIDERATIONS

### Applying a Mask

#### Pediatric Clients

- A child may feel more confused and isolated if those caring for him are wearing a mask and cap. Allowing the child to play with a mask and cap will help the child become more comfortable with them.
- The nurse should show the child her face from the doorway before putting on the mask and cap.
- Younger children may feel they are being punished for being sick. Discuss the child's feelings at regular intervals to be sure the reason for the cap and mask is understood.
- Provide a cap and mask for the child's favorite stuffed toy to wear as well.

#### Geriatric Clients

- Older clients who are confused may become more confused if they are unable to identify the person behind the mask.
- Elderly clients who lip-read may have difficulty understanding a person wearing a mask. Make sure alternative communication devices are available, such as a pad and pencil or a computer. Make sure hearing aid is in place.

### Reduce or Eliminate Infectious Agents

Transmission of microorganisms to clients may also occur through contact with inanimate objects. Cleansing, disinfecting, and sterilizing can break this link in the chain of infection by reducing or destroying microorganisms on objects. Cleansing, disinfection, and sterilization are usually the responsibility of nursing, housekeeping, and central supply departments. These infection control practices can and should also be practiced in the home care setting.

### Cleansing

**Cleansing** is the removal of soil or organic material from instruments and equipment used in providing client care. Nurses are involved in cleansing instruments after assisting with or performing an invasive procedure. Reusable objects are cleansed prior to sterilization and disinfection to reduce the amount of contamination and loosen the material on the object. Cleansing involves the use of water, mechanical action, and sometimes a detergent. Contaminated objects are cleaned using a soft-bristled brush to scrub the surface. The steps for proper cleansing are:

1. Rinse object under cold water since warm water causes proteins in organic material to coagulate and stick.
2. Apply detergent and scrub object under running water with soft-bristled brush.
3. Rinse the object under warm water.
4. Dry the object prior to sterilization or disinfection.

Cleansing presents a potential hazard to the nurse through splashing of contaminated material onto the body or into eyes. Nurses should wear gloves, masks, and goggles during cleansing.

### Disinfection

**Disinfection** is the elimination of pathogens, except spores, from inanimate objects. **Disinfectants** are chemical solutions used to clean inanimate objects. Bedpans,

| PROCEDURE 26-5 | **Surgical Scrub** |
|---|---|

## EQUIPMENT NEEDED

▰ Surgical scrub items (antimicrobial soap, two brushes, and nail file) (Figure 26-24)

▰ Sterile towel

▰ Surgical shoe covers (booties) and cap, face mask, sterile gown, and proper-size gloves

## IMPLEMENTATION—ACTION/RATIONALE

| ACTION | RATIONALE |
|---|---|

### Preparing for Surgical Handwashing

1. Remove rings, chipped nail polish, watch, and earrings that do not fit under a surgical cap.

2. Use a deep sink with side or foot pedal to dispense antimicrobial soap and control water temperature and flow.

3. Have two surgical scrub brushes and nail file.

4. Apply surgical shoe covers and cap to cover hair and ears completely.

5. Apply mask (Figure 26-25).

1. Decreases resident and transient microorganisms.

2. Prevents hands and forearms from touching a soiled surface.

3. Enhances mechanical friction during the scrub.

4. Prevents introduction of contaminants into environment.

5. Provides a respiratory barrier.

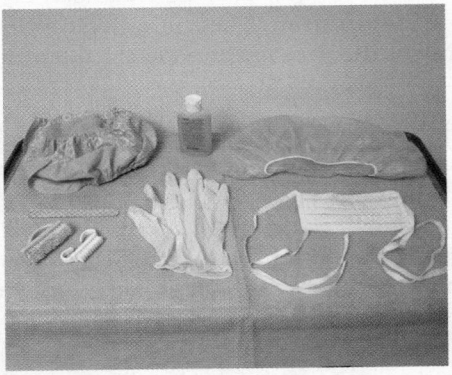

**Figure 26-24    Surgical scrub items**

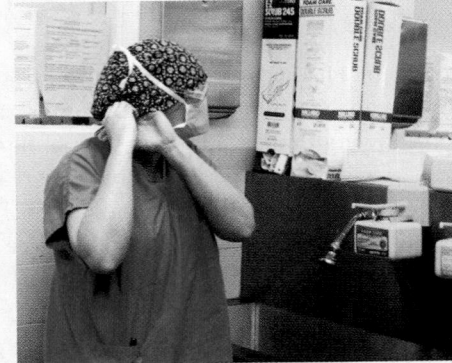

**Figure 26-25    Apply cap and mask.**

6. Before beginning the surgical scrub:
   a. Open the sterile package containing the gown; using aseptic technique, make a sterile field with the inside of the gown's wrapper.
   b. Open the sterile towel and drop it onto the center of field.
   c. Open the outer wrapper from the sterile gloves and drop the inner package of gloves onto the sterile field beside the folded gown and towel.

7. At a deep sink with foot or knee controls (Figure 26-26), turn on warm water; under flowing water, wet forearms and hands (from elbows to finger-

6. Preparing the sterile items prior to the scrub decreases the risk of contaminating scrubbed hands.

7. Water should flow from the least contaminated (forearms) to the most contaminated (hands).

*(continues)*

**PROCEDURE 26-5 (*continued*)**

tips), keeping arms and hands above elbow level during entire procedure (do not allow uniform to get wet).

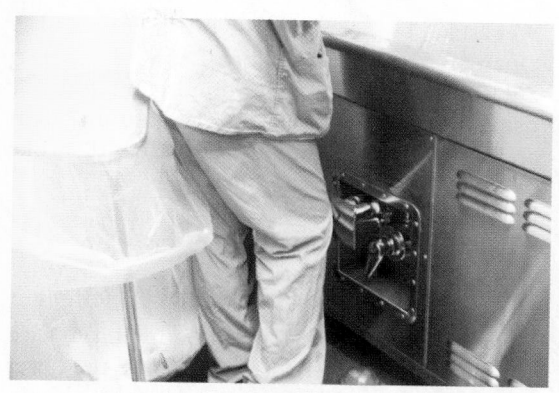

**Figure 26-26**    Handwashing sink with knee controls

8. Apply a liberal amount of soap onto hands and rub hands and arms to 2 inches above elbows (Figures 26-27 and 26-28).

8. Reduces number of microorganisms on hands.

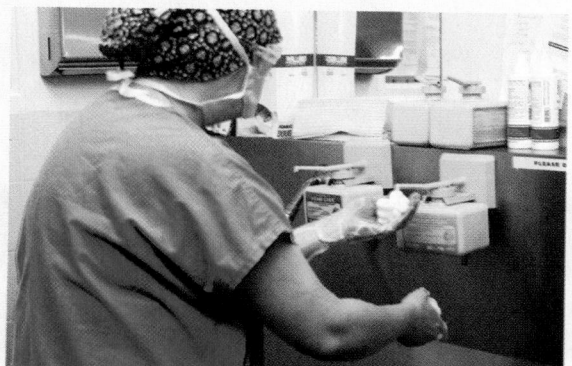

**Figure 26-27**    Apply a liberal amount of soap.

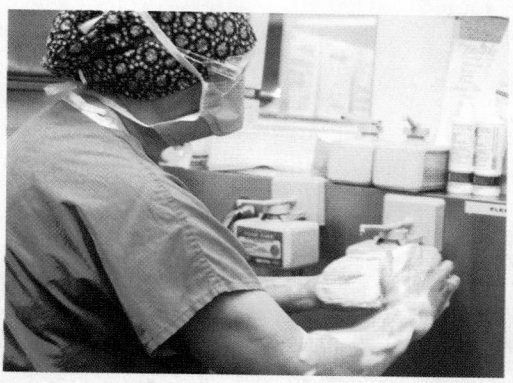

**Figure 26-28**    Scrub hands and arms.

9. Use nail file under running water, clean under each nail of both hands, and drop file into sink when finished (Figure 26-29).

9. Removes dirt that harbors microorganisms.

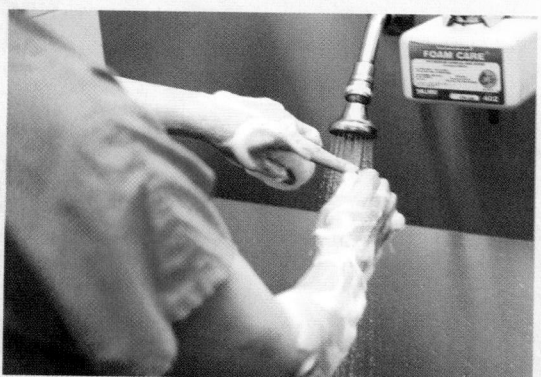

**Figure 26-29**    Use a nail file under running water to clean fingernails.

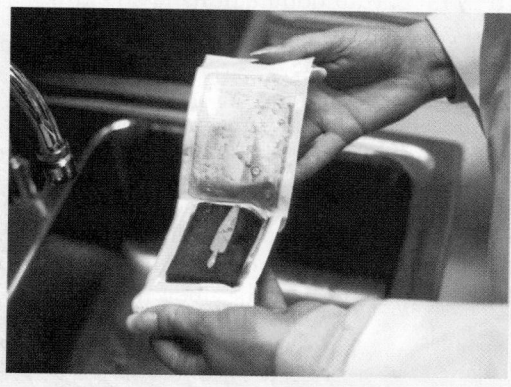

**Figure 26-30**    Prepackaged scrub brush

*(continues)*

**PROCEDURE 26-5 (continued)**

10. Wet and apply soap to scrub brush, if needed. Open prepackaged scrub brush if available (Figure 26-30). With brush in your dominant hand and using a circular motion, scrub nails and all skin areas of nondominant hand and arm (10 strokes to each of the following areas):
    a. Nails
    b. Palm of hand and anterior side of fingers

11. Rinse brush thoroughly, reapply soap.

12. Continue with scrub of nondominant arm with a circular motion for 10 strokes each to the lower, middle, and upper arm; drop brush into the sink.

13. Maintaining the hands and arms above elbow level, place the fingertips under running water and thoroughly rinse the fingers, hands, and arms (allow the water to run off your elbow into the sink); take care not to get your uniform wet (Figure 26-31).

10. Removes resident bacteria from the skin's surfaces; the circular motion mechanically removes microorganisms. Scrubbing the nondominant hand first sets a routine you can remember if you should get interrupted during the scrub.

11. Decreases transfer of microorganisms.

12. Decreases transfer of microorganisms from the arm; dropping the brush avoids contamination.

13. Allows flow of water to cleanse from the area of least contamination to the area of most contamination. Water conducts microorganisms, and keeping uniform dry aids in maintaining sterility of gown.

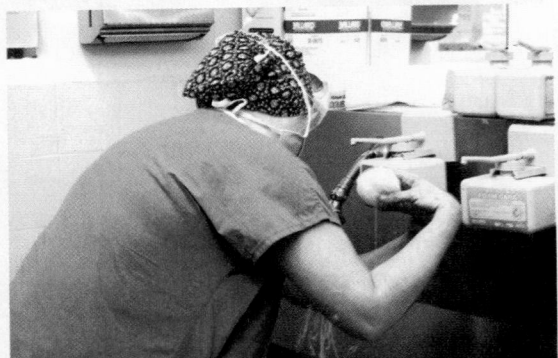

**Figure 26-31  Thoroughly rinse fingers, hands, and arms.**

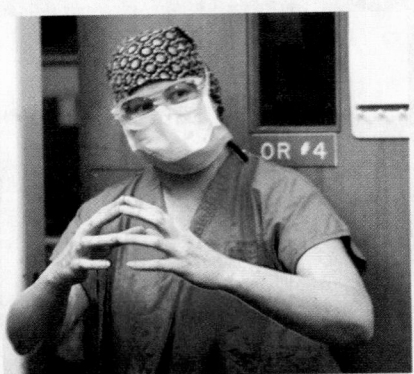

**Figure 26-32  Keep arms flexed and proceed to area.**

14. Take the second scrub brush and repeat Actions 10 to 13 on your dominant hand and arm.

15. Keep arms flexed and proceed to area (operating or procedure room) with sterile items (Figure 26-32).

16. Secure sterile towel by grasping it on one edge, opening the towel, full length, making sure it does not touch your uniform.

17. Dry each hand and arm separately; extend one side of the towel around fingers and hand and dry in a rotating motion up to the elbow (Figure 26-33).

14. See Rationales 10 to 13.

15. Prevents water from flowing from least (elbows) to most (hands) clean area.

16. Maintains the sterility of the towel.

17. Prevents contamination by drying from cleanest to least clean area.

*(continues)*

## PROCEDURE 26-5 (*continued*)

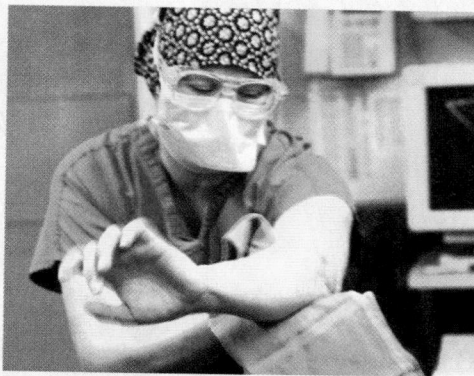

**Figure 26-33    Dry arms up to the elbows.**

| ACTION | RATIONALE |
|---|---|
| 18. Reverse the towel and repeat the same action on the other hand and arm, thoroughly drying the skin. | 18. Prevents contamination of the gown. |
| 19. Discard the towel into a linen hamper. | 19. Keeps the environment clean. |

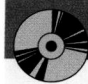

## PROCEDURE 26-6    Applying Sterile Gloves via the Closed Method

### EQUIPMENT NEEDED

- Sterile gown
- Sterile and proper-sized gloves

### IMPLEMENTATION—ACTION/RATIONALE

| ACTION | RATIONALE |
|---|---|
| **Gowning** | |
| 1. The sterile gown is folded inside out. | 1. Allows ungloved hands to touch only the inside. |
| 2. Grasp the gown inside the neckline, step back, and allow the gown to open in front of you; keep the inside of the gown toward you; do not allow it to touch anything (Figure 26-34). | 2. Keeps the outside of the gown sterile. |
| 3. With hands at shoulder level, slip both arms into the gown; keep your hands inside the sleeves of the gown (Figure 26-35). | 3. Prevents the gown from touching nonsterile objects; allows sterile items to come in contact only with other sterile items. |
| 4. The circulating nurse will step up behind you and grasp the inside of the gown, bring it over your shoulders, and secure the ties at the neck and waist. | 4. Prevents any part of the gown from touching a nonsterile object; provides complete coverage of undergarments. |

*(continues)*

**PROCEDURE 26-6 (*continued*)**

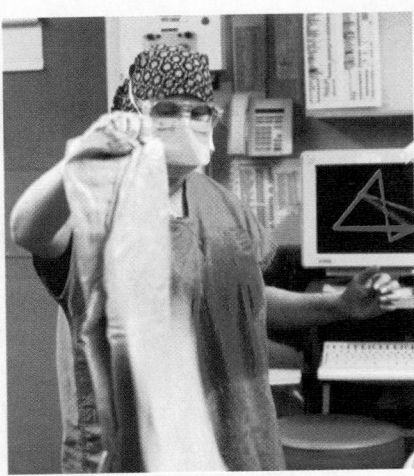

**Figure 26-34    Allow the gown to fall open.**

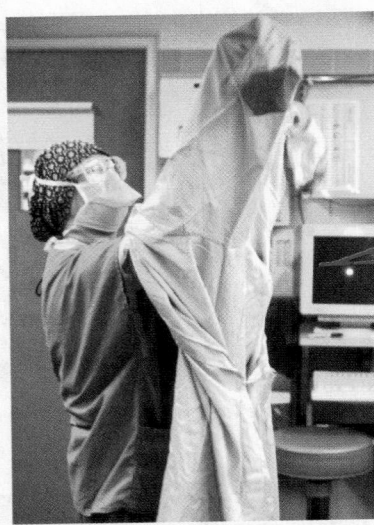

**Figure 26-35    Slip both arms into the gown.**

## Closed Gloving

5. With hands still inside the gown sleeves, open the inner wrapper of the gloves on the sterile gown field (Figure 26-36).

5. Maintains sterility of the gloves.

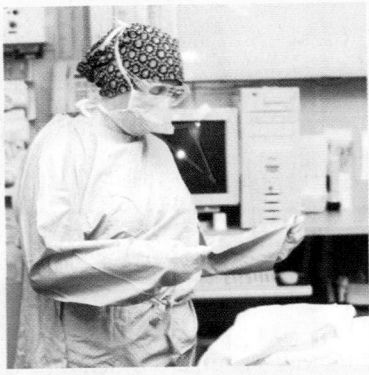

**Figure 26-36    Keep hands inside the gown sleeves when opening gloves. Handle the gloves through the fabric of the gown.**

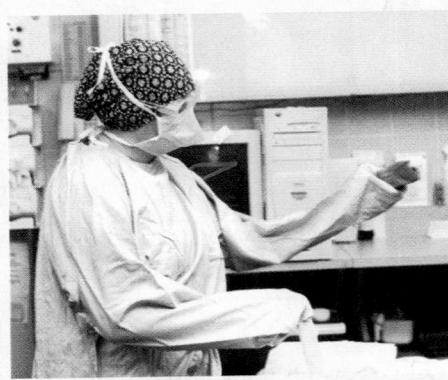

**Figure 26-37    Grasp the cuff of the glove.**

6. With your nondominant sleeved hand, grasp the cuff of the glove for the dominant hand and lay it on the extended dominant forearm (Figure 26-37); with palm up, place the palm of the glove against the sleeved palm, with fingers of the glove pointing toward elbow (see Figure 26-38).

6. Only sterile items come in contact with each other.

7. Manipulate the glove so that the sleeved thumb of your dominant hand is grasping the cuff; with your nondominant hand, turn the cuff over the end of dominant hand and gown's cuff.

7. Prevents the hands from contaminating the sterile glove.

*(continues)*

**PROCEDURE 26-6** (*continued*)

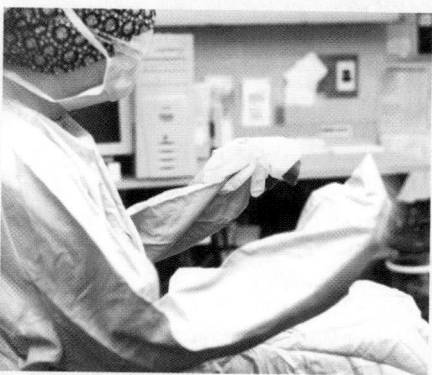

**Figure 26-38    Keep the fingers of the glove facing the elbow.**

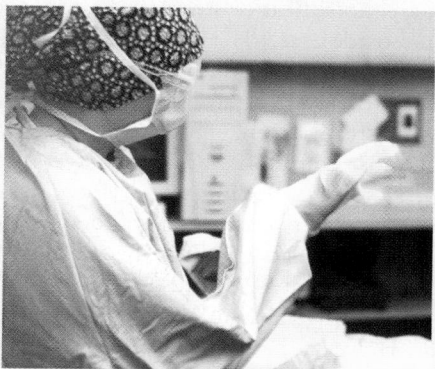

**Figure 26-39    Extend fingers into the glove.**

8. With sleeved nondominant hand, grasp the cuff of the glove and the gown's sleeve of the dominant hand; slowly extend the fingers into the glove, making sure the cuff of the glove remains above the cuff of the gown's sleeve (Figure 26-39).

9. With the gloved dominant hand, repeat Actions 7 and 8 (Figures 26-40 and 26-41).

8. Provides a closed sterile method for gloving; the glove cuff over the gown prevents contamination of the operative field with microorganisms.

9. Only sterile items can touch each other.

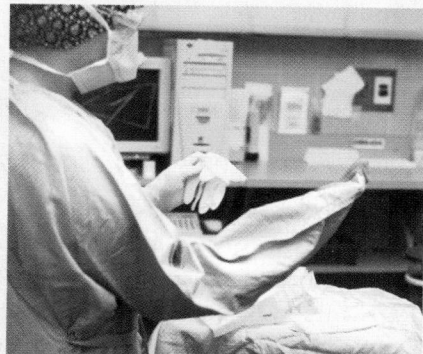

**Figure 26-40    Place the second glove on the gown.**

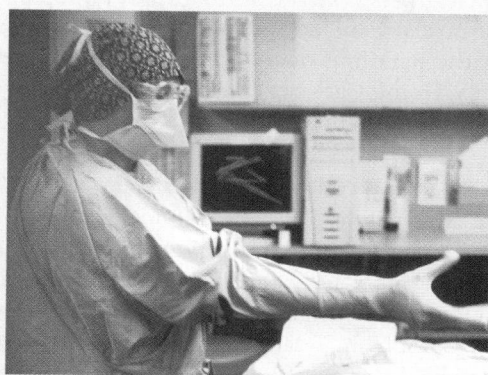

**Figure 26-41    Extend the fingers into the second glove.**

10. Interlock gloved fingers; secure fit.

10. Promotes dexterity of gloved hands.

blood pressure cuffs, linens, stethoscopes, thermometers, and some types of endoscopes are disinfected in the hospital setting. The U.S. Environmental Protection Agency (EPA) licenses (registers) disinfection products and monitors the products to ensure they work as claimed on the label (Environmental Protection Agency, 2003). Common disinfectants are alcohol, sodium hypochlorite, quaternary ammonium, phenolic solutions, and glutaraldehyde. In the home, Lysol and bleach are common disinfectants that are capable of eliminating several pathogens. A **germicide** is a chemical that can be applied to both animate and inanimate objects for the purpose of eliminating pathogens. Antiseptic preparations such as alcohol and silver sulfadiazine are germicides and may be used on skin.

## Sterilization

**Sterilization** is the total elimination of all microorganisms including spores. Instruments that are used for invasive procedures must be sterilized. Methods of achieving sterilization are moist heat or steam, radiation, chemicals, and ethylene oxide gas. The method of sterilization depends on the type of contamination, amount of contamination, and object to be sterilized.

Autoclaving sterilization, which uses moist heat or steam, is the most common sterilization technique used in the hospital setting. Boiling water is not an effective sterilization measure as some viruses and spores can survive boiling water. Objects that have been boiled in water for 15 to 20 minutes at 121°C (249.8°F) are considered clean but not sterilized (United States Department of Labor, 2003). However, boiling water is still the best and most common sterilization measure used in the home. For example, boiling baby bottles and nipples makes them safe for use.

## Home Health Care Considerations

"While many home care policies and procedures are developed with the best of intentions, they frequently lack a scientific basis and have been perpetuated over the years" (Friedman & Rhinehart, 2000, p. 99). Home care and hospice nurses are faced with significant challenges when adapting acute care infection control practice to the home care setting such as cleaning and disinfecting equipment and using clean versus sterile technique. Common practice of home care organizations requires special practice regarding the handling of the *nursing supply bag*; see the Community/Home Care box for basic nursing bag technique procedure that may be followed.

## Disposal of Infectious Waste

All health care facilities must have guidelines for the disposal of infectious waste materials. Always observe the biological hazard symbol and handle all infectious materials as a hazard.Occupational Safety and Health Administration (OSHA) regulations mandate that "immediately after use, sharps shall be disposed of in closable, puncture-resistant, disposable containers that are leakproof on the sides and bottom and are labeled or color coded." Dispose of soiled and infectious items in the home; do not place in car to dispose elsewhere.

Not all waste generated in a health care setting is infectious. Infectious waste, by definition, may contain pathogenic organisms and is regulated by the EPA. This waste is referred to as regulated medical waste, and constitutes about 10% to 15% of waste generated in a typical hospital. The definition of regulated medical waste varies from state to state, but consistently includes discarded absorbent material saturated with blood, discarded body parts, cultures and related materials, and sharps. Consult local environmental protection authorities for additional information.

---

## COMMUNITY/HOME CARE

### Supply Bagging in the Home

- Place the bag on a clean, dry surface.

- Wash hands with soap and running water prior to direct client contact. For MRSA or VRE clients, wash hands with antibacterial soap and running water. Cleanse hands with a waterless product if running water is not available.

- Remove the necessary supplies from the nursing bag, and place them on a clean, dry surface.

- Perform client care.

- Clean and disinfect semicritical equipment such as an oral thermometer with a 70% isopropyl alcohol prep pad, and return the equipment to the supply bag.

- Clean noncritical equipment such as a blood pressure cuff, stethoscope, or scale if soiled and return to the bag. If the client is infected or colonized with MDR bacteria, and equipment has not been designated for the client's individual use, clean and disinfect the equipment with a disinfectant of the home care or hospice organization's choice prior to replacing the noncritical items in the bag.

- Remove personal protective items such as a gown and gloves if worn.

- Wash hands with soap and running water prior to direct client contact. For MRSA or VRE clients, wash hands with antibacterial soap and running water. Cleanse hands with a waterless product if running water is not available, and wash hands with soap and running water as soon as possible.

Adapted from Friedman, M., & Rhinehart, E. (2000). Improving infection control home care: From ritual to science-based practice. *Home Healthcare Nurse, 18*(2), 99–106.

---

When disposing of infectious waste:

- Wear gloves.
- Use the proper containers (red or one labeled with the biological hazard symbol as required by the facility), leakproof plastic bags for waste from client areas (soiled

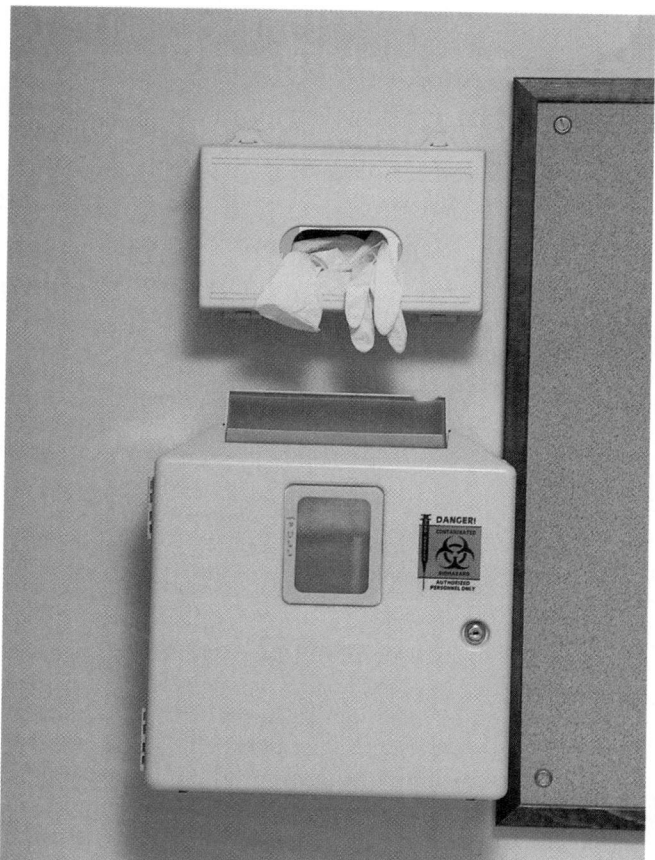

**Figure 26-42   Sharps disposal and infectious waste container**

dressings, gloves, linen), and sharps containers for needles, scalpels, and other sharp instruments or devices (Figure 26-42).

- Ensure that all infectious waste is properly labeled.
- Use care when handling plastic bags to avoid punctures and tearing.
- Disinfect carts used to carry infectious waste.
- Dispose of waste in designated areas only.
- Wash hands after disposing of hazardous materials.

Containers for contaminated sharps should be readily accessible to personnel and maintained in an upright position.

Many of the caregiver's exposures to hepatitis B virus (HBV) and human immunodeficiency virus (HIV) have been related to contamination by sharp objects. Thus the rationale for appropriate use of sharps containers (National Institute for Occupational Safety and Health, 1999).

# Guidelines for Standards Precautions

A tremendous number of diseases can be transmitted from one person to another. Also, health care personnel can practice careful techniques to not contaminate them-

## CLINICAL ALERT

### Needle Disposal

Used needles should not be recapped, bent, or broken. Needles should be placed in a puncture-resistant marked or color-coded container close to the work site. Correct disposal decreases the risk of needle punctures to caregivers. Replace container when two-thirds full.

selves or others. These techniques are labeled **Standard Precautions** (guidelines recommended by the CDC to reduce the risk of infection). Standard precautions are applied to many body substances in all settings (see Box 26-2). **Barrier precautions** are used to minimize the risk of exposure to blood and body fluids. Barrier precautions consist of personal protective equipment, such as masks, gowns, and gloves used to create a barrier between the person and the microorganism that prevents transmission of the microorganism.

## CLINICAL ALERT

### Standard Precautions

Standard Precautions must be practiced with all clients, since this is the most effective method to decrease the risk of infection for clients and caregivers.

Centers for Disease Control and Prevention, 2003. http://www.cdc.gov

## BOX 26-2   BODY SUBSTANCES TO WHICH STANDARD PRECAUTIONS APPLY

- Blood
- All body fluids, secretions, excretions, and contaminated items regardless of whether or not they contain visible blood
- Nonintact skin
- Mucous membranes

Daniels, R. (2003). *Delmar's manual of laboratory and diagnostic tests.* Clifton Park, NY: Delmar Learning.

## TABLE 26-3    TRANSMISSION-BASED PRECAUTIONS

| Category | Private Room | Gloves | Gowns | Masks |
|---|---|---|---|---|
| Contact precautions | If possible; cohort if not available | Required | If anticipate contact with soiled items; client is incontinent; diarrhea, ileostomy, colostomy, wound drainage | Not required |
| Droplet precautions | If possible; cohort or maintain separation of 3 feet | Not required | Not required | Required when within 3 feet |
| Airborne precautions | Required. Negative air pressure, 6 to 12 air changes per hour, keep door closed, discharge air outdoors or HEPA filter | Not required | Not required | N95 respirator required for known or suspected tuberculosis and measles varicella if not immune |

The CDC (2003) has established transmission-based precautions to be used in addition to Standard Precautions. These guidelines are based on routes of entry (i.e., contact, droplet, and airborne transmission). Transmission-based precautions are to be used for specific syndromes that are highly suspicious for infections until a diagnosis is confirmed (Table 26-3).

## Role of Health Care Personnel and Health Agencies in Infection Control

Nurses focus on breaking the chain of infection by applying proper infection control practices to interrupt the mode of transmission. Interrupting or blocking the

### COMMUNITY/HOME CARE

#### Maintaining Standard Precautions in the Home Setting

The nurse must remember to take adequate supplies for maintaining Standard Precautions when in the home setting. Examples are "waterless" soap foams, gloves, and plastic bags that can be used as "dirty supply containers." The nurse may have to create a "waste basket" from the plastic bags as opposed to using the client's trash containers. In addition, the client and family members must be taught to practice Standard Precautions when handling contaminated materials.

agent, portal of exit, or portal of entry; destroying the agent; or decreasing the host's susceptibility can also break the chain of infection. Refer to Figure 26-1, which shows preventive measures that break the chain of infection. Host susceptibility depends on the immune system to function as a defense mechanism. Nurses should get vaccinated to prevent the potential of HBV. Although 10,000 new cases of HBV, formerly called serum hepatitis, are reported each year in the United States, HBV is considered one of the most underreported diseases in the country. Risk factors associated with HBV infection among health care workers include the frequency of blood and needle exposures. This is no small figure: the CDC estimates that hospital workers receive 384,325 percutaneous injuries involving contaminated sharps yearly (Farley, 2001). In order to protect health care workers against HBV infections, OSHA has established standards relative to vaccination programs.

Nurses use isolation precautions to protect the host's normal defense mechanisms by preventing the transmission of pathogens (nosocomial infections). Isolation precautions include barrier protections that break the chain of infection. When the nurse cares for a client in isolation, additional precautions are used along with handwashing and gloves. A mask and eye protection (or face shield) are worn to protect the mucous membranes of the eyes, nose, and mouth during interventions that are likely to produce splashes or sprays of blood, body fluids, secretions, and excretions. A nonsterile gown is also worn to protect the skin and clothing against splashes or sprays.

Nurses caring for clients with tuberculosis (caused by the tubercle bacillus *Mycobacterium tuberculosis*) are required to wear special masks, since transmission occurs between individuals through respiratory contact (Manangan, Simonds, Pugliese, Kroc, Banerjee, Rudnick, Steingraber, & Jarvis, 1998). There are two types of tuberculosis masks: high-efficiency particulate air (HEPA) mask used for suspected or confirmed multidrug-resistant (MDR) tuberculosis; and the disposable submicrometer mask used for confirmed tuberculosis. These masks form a tight-fitting seal against particulates 1–5 um in size.

Isolation precautions are usually ordered by the physician; however, nurses may initiate these precautions whenever there is a nursing diagnosis related to the infections process—for example, *Risk for Infection* related to decreased resistance of immune system. Most agencies require nurses to obtain a culture from a draining body area and to initiate isolation precautions when positive cultures are reported. Once isolation precautions have been instituted, visitors and all personnel should comply with the agency's policy regarding isolation precautions. The nurse is responsible to reinforce adherence to isolation. Signs should be posted in a prominent location outside the client's room indicating the type of isolation precautions, preparation prior to entering the room, and the necessary supplies that should be readily available (Lutwick, 1999).

Clients in isolation should be placed in a private room with adequate ventilation and have their own supplies. Personal belongings should be kept to a minimum, and health care providers should use disposable supplies and equipment. All articles leaving the room, such as soiled linen and collected specimens, should be labeled and either placed in impermeable bags or double-bagged. Home health nurses should provide the client and family with appropriate written isolation instructions relative to the specific precautions.

Isolation precautions are for the client's protection; however, clients who are placed on isolation precautions may experience psychological discomfort (Figure 26-43). Nurses should be alert for symptoms of anxiety, depression, rejection, guilt, or loneliness. Clients should be educated on which isolation precautions will be practiced and their purposes. Nurses should encourage clients to verbal-

## LEGAL AND ETHICAL ISSUES

### Isolation Precautions

Where were the nurses? Cox, Diamond, Hatlie, Pugliese, & Wilson (2002) cited a nursing home that was fined $75,000 for isolating a 36-year-old stroke client with human immunodeficiency virus (HIV) for 9 months. The client filed a complaint with the division of human rights. Who should have been the advocate for this client? What would you have done if you had been working in this nursing home? Other issues related to client confidentiality have been raised related to isolation signs indicating a particular illness. Signs should not indicate the actual disease of the client.

Cox, J. L., Diamond, L. H., Hatlie, M. J., Pugliese, G., Wilson, N. J. (2002). Overview of the partnership symposium 2001: Patient safety—stories of success. *Joint Commission Journal on Quality Improvement. 28*(6), 283–286.

ize their feelings regarding the isolation precautions and provide the client with intellectual stimulation. Family members and close friends should be encouraged in preventing the client's feelings of isolation and loneliness. The following Client Education box lists several psychological interventions.

### Blood-borne Pathogen Exposure

The risk for blood-borne pathogens in the health care setting is an increasing concern for health care providers. In the fall of 1999, OSHA issued an update that supersedes

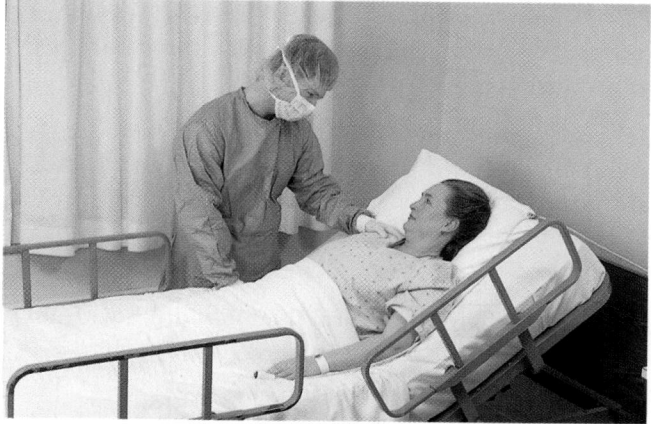

**Figure 26-43    This nurse is interacting with a client who requires isolation precautions. Although both the client and nurse are observing isolation precautions, they are still able to communicate with one another. In planning the care of this client, what would the expected outcomes of these interventions be?**

## CLIENT EDUCATION

### Psychological Interventions for Clients Requiring Isolation Precautions

✓ Explain isolation procedure and rationale.
✓ Discuss client's feelings about isolation procedures.
✓ Convey a sense of empathetic understanding.
✓ Permit visitors in accordance with isolation precautions, and teach visitors about isolation precautions.
✓ Support existing coping mechanisms.
✓ Visit with the client.

Davies, H., & Rees, J. (2000). Psychological effects of isolation nursing: Mood disturbance. *Nursing Standard, 14*(28), 35–38.

the one issued in 1992 regarding the risk for blood-borne pathogens to health care providers. OSHA's new directive recognizes the advances made in medical technology, such as improved safety equipment and devices (see Box 26-4); better methods of treatment following exposure; and more concise policy interpretations. These advances decrease the risks of health care worker exposure to blood-borne pathogens, specifically the human immunodeficiency virus (HIV) and hepatitis B and C (Bending, 2000). OSHA requires that all health care agencies make available the hepatitis B vaccine and vaccination series to all employees.

## Exposure Control Plan

Each health care facility is required by law (OSHA) to have an exposure control plan. This plan begins with Standard Precautions and moves to postexposure prophylaxis. With all exposure to pathogens, the area is to be cleaned thoroughly with soap and water and the incident reported to the occupational health nurse. Specific follow-up for blood-borne pathogens may include HIV antibody, HBV antigen, and HCV antigen testing of the client and the nurse; administration of prophylactic medication(s); and postexposure follow-up and counseling. The CDC recommends postexposure prophylaxis only in the cases of highest risk. This involves deep injury with bleeding from a hollow-bore contaminated needle or any exposure to blood or bodily fluids with a high HIV viral load. Postexposure prophylaxis is not recommended for percutaneous sticks or membrane contract with solid suture needles or splashes to eye or mouth in persons with low HIV viral loads.

---

### BOX 26-4    SPECIFIC PRECAUTIONS WHEN HANDLING VARIOUS EQUIPMENT

1. Capillary puncture: Blood is obtained in a microtube. The ends are sealed and the tube placed in a plastic biohazard bag for transport to the laboratory.

2. Venipuncture: Blood is obtained directly from the vein into vacuum tubes or by syringe and transferred to a vacuum tube. The vial is to be placed in a biohazard bag for transport to the laboratory. If a pneumonic tube system is used to transport tubes, they must be doubled-bagged. Most institutions do not allow blood to be transported via pneumonic tube systems.

3. Biopsies:
   a. Laboratory transport: The tissue biopsy is placed in a sterile container with fixative. The container is closed. This container is placed in a plastic biohazard bag for transport to the laboratory. An example of this would be stereotactic breast biopsy tissue.
   b. Bedside slide preparation: Sometimes the biopsied material is placed on a slide, a slide smear is made, and fixative is added to the slide. The slide is then placed into a container for holding. The container is placed in a plastic biohazard bag for transport to the laboratory. An example of this would be bone marrow biopsies.

4. Urine specimens: Urine should be collected in a clean container. The container should be placed in a plastic biohazard bag for transport to the laboratory. For 24-hour specimens, a large container is kept on ice for collection of the urine. There is usually a preservative in this container, so if it spills, the laboratory should be notified immediately for proper instructions on cleanup.

5. Stool specimens: Feces should be collected in a dry, clean container such as a bedpan or commode. (A plastic "hat" that fits in the toilet to measure urine could also be used but it needs to be clean.) Unless otherwise specified, the entire specimen should be transferred to a container (clean denture holder works well) with a clean tongue blade. The specimen is covered and placed into a plastic biohazard bag. The bag is transported immediately to the laboratory.

6. Bodily fluids: For example, spinal fluid, pericardial fluid, synovial fluid, or pleural fluid is withdrawn from the corresponding body areas via needle and syringe. The sterile fluid is placed in sterile vial(s), which are sealed. The vials are placed in plastic biohazard bags and transported to the laboratory.

7. Cultures: The area to be cultured (e.g., throat, conjunctiva, wound) is swabbed with a sterile swab. Moistening the swab with sterile normal saline can sometimes increase the likelihood of obtaining microbes with the swabbing. The swab is placed in a vial and sealed. The sealed vial is placed in a plastic biohazard bag and transported to the laboratory.

Daniels, R. (2003). *Delmar's manual of laboratory and diagnostic tests.* Clifton Park, NY: Delmar Learning.

# Alternative Therapies Used to Treat Infections

The American Nurses Association recognizes holistic, complementary, and alternative practices for the client in regard to treating infections. More and more clients are seeking alternative therapy for common medical conditions, mainly chronic conditions (Spratto & Woods, 2004). Hospitals are becoming more responsive to client demands by incorporating new practice models to allow the client choices and requests for alternative options as part of a holistic approach to both curing and healing. The Massachusetts and Louisiana state boards of nursing have issued statements regarding the role and scope of registered nurse practice and holistic care. Documentation of the client's alternative or complementary practices should be included in the health history to ensure an integration of alternative and conventional care. Nurses need to have knowledge of herbal products and their effects to avoid possible adverse reactions when prescribed drugs are used in combination with the client's herbal regimen (Ernst, 2002). A brief discussion regarding herbal baths and the use of herbs for infections is presented.

## Herbs for Infections

Herbs are used in two ways for infections. Through their antimicrobial action, they work directly against microbes. They also augment and vitalize the body's own defenses. Although research may not always be available to explain how herbs work, many plants have a direct toxic effect upon microbes. The best antimicrobials that can be used safely to combat infections include echinacea, eucalyptus, garlic, myrrh, nasturtium, thyme, wild indigo, and wormwood (Hoffman, 1998, p. 115).

---

## NURSING STRATEGY

### Herbal Baths

Herbal baths are a safe home method of treatment for all clients, especially infants and the elderly, and can be made just for the specific part of the body, such as the hands, hips, or feet, or can be a full body bath. A bath made from freshly grated gingerroot tea stimulates circulation, alleviates aches and pains, breaks a cold, helps arthritis, and warms the body. To calm the mind and relax the body, combine equal parts of lavender, rose, chamomile, and skullcap in the bathwater. To stimulate circulation and relieve fever and chill, combine equal parts bayberry bark, ginger, and prickly ash, and one-fourth part cayenne pepper in the bathwater. Clients using herbs in bathwater for the first time should do a simple patch test to rule out a possible allergic response.

Tierra, L. (1997). *The herbs of life: Health and healing using Western and Chinese techniques.* Freedom, CA: The Crossing Press.

---

# CASE STUDY/NURSING CARE PLAN

## Case Study Nursing Care Plan

Mr. Cartier, a 48-year-old mill worker, comes into an urgent care center with a puncture wound to his left hand. He states a rusty file broke off into his hand while he was sharpening a saw. The left hand has an old towel wrapped around it, and the palm is red with serosanguineous drainage; the hand is swollen, tender to the touch, and generally dirty. As Mr. Cartier is assessed, he states he has had no immunizations since childhood and does not remember when he had his last tetanus injection. The nurse gives careful attention to adhering to Standard Precautions while taking off the towel and cleaning the wound. In addition, the nurse disposes of the old towel in the blood-borne pathogen containers designed for use with contaminated fluids.

## Assessment

A 48-year-old mill worker has a puncture wound of the left hand that requires medical asepsis. The wound is about 3/4-inch deep, 1/4-inch long, and 1/4-inch wide. It is obviously contaminated with wood shavings, grease, and dirt. The client's vital signs are stable (B/P = 138/76, P = 74, R = 16, T = 98.6°F), and he has no other problems.

## Nursing Diagnosis #1

*Risk for Infection* related to lack of immunization (tetanus) and site trauma with penetration of microorganisms

**NOC:** Immune Status; Knowledge: Infection Control; Risk Control; Risk Detection

**NIC:** Immunization/Vaccination Administration; Infection Control; Infection Protection

*(continues)*

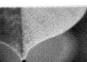

# CASE STUDY/NURSING CARE PLAN (continued)

## Expected Outcomes

The client will:

1. Maintain noninfected left hand wound area.
2. Receive immunization for tetanus before discharge.

## Planning/Interventions/Rationales

1. Assess wound, cleanse wound area, apply pressure dressing to the area, and dress the wound appropriately after suturing. *Prepares the area for suturing and keeps the area from continued bleeding.*
2. Administer tetanus immunization as per prescriber's order. *Prophylaxis for tetanus and further complications of wound infection.*

## Evaluation

Client was given tetanus immunization. Wound remained infection-free. Client's wound area was sutured with three sutures. The area was dressed with gauze, and the client was given dressing supplies to take home.

## Nursing Diagnosis #2

*Deficient Knowledge* related to understanding of the rationale to have tetanus immunization.
**NOC:** Knowledge of: Disease Process; Health Behaviors; Infection Control; Immunization Treatments
**NIC:**   Teaching: Disease Process; Teaching: Individual

## Expected Outcomes

The client will:

1. Explain the disease process of tetanus and the need for immunization by the time of discharge.
2. Discuss the implications of his work environment with the potential risk of future contamination requiring health care assistance.

## Planning/Interventions/Rationales

1. Observe client's ability and readiness to learn information about tetanus immunizations. *Education in self-care takes into account physical, sensory, and psychosocial factors.*
2. Determine client's previous knowledge of tetanus immunizations. *New information is assimilated into prior knowledge level.*
3. Determine client's understanding of the information provided on tetanus immunizations. *Evaluates the effectiveness of the teaching/learning instruction time.*

## Evaluation

Client received information regarding tetanus immunizations and was able to restate pertinent aspects of the teaching/learning presentation. He was also able to evaluate his work setting and discussed methods of preventing similar accidents in the future.

# Key Concepts

- Microorganisms that cause disease are labeled pathogens.
- The infection chain has six links: infectious agent, reservoir, portal of exit, mode of transmission, portal of entry, and susceptible host.
- Infectious agents are carried by direct transmission, indirect transmission, and airborne transmission.
- Many factors (e.g., age, heredity, stress) influence a microorganism's capability to produce infections in an individual.
- The immune response is a specific defense mechanism used in fighting infection.

- The inflammatory response is a nonspecific cellular response to infection.
- There are four stages of localized and systemic infections (i.e., incubation, prodromal, illness, and convalescence).
- Nosocomial infections are hospital-acquired infections.
- Medical and surgical asepsis are common techniques used to prevent contaminates from spreading.
- There are specific guidelines for standard precautions to prevent health care personnel from contracting diseases.
- There are specific care procedures to prevent the spread of disease through three routes (contact, droplet, and airborne).

- An exposure control plan must be followed anytime that a health care worker potentially comes in contact with a blood-borne pathogen.
- Alternative methods of treating infection are available for clients (e.g., herbal products, herbal baths).

## Review Questions and Activities

1. List the six "links" of the chain of infection.
2. What factors increase persons' susceptibility for acquiring an infection?
3. Of these, which factor causes the greatest risk for acquiring an infection?
4. List two nonspecific defenses the body uses to fight infection, and describe how they work.
5. What are specific defenses with which the body fights infection?
6. What is the single most important preventive measure against nosocomial infections?
7. Which type of aseptic technique is used in setting up a sterile procedure—medical or surgical?
8. What is an incubation period?
9. A client with HBV is added to a home health nurse's caseload. What considerations should the nurse take as related to Standard Precautions in the home environment?
10. A client admitted to the intensive care unit has been diagnosed with methicillin-resistant *Staphylococcus aureus* (MRSA). The MRSA is transmitted by direct contact. What isolation precautions are necessary to break the chain of infection?

## Multimedia Links

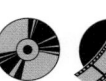 

Altman *Basic Care DVD: Handwashing*
Altman *Basic Care video: Handwashing*
Altman *Basic Care DVD: Preparing a Surgical Site*
Altman *Basic Care DVD: Applying Sterile Gloves via the Open Method*
Altman *Basic Care DVD: Donning and Removing Clean and Contaminated Gloves, Cap, and Mask*
Altman *Basic Care DVD: Surgical Scrub*
Altman *Basic Care DVD: Applying Sterile Gloves via the Closed Method*

## Web Resources

Centers for Disease Control and Prevention
    http://www.cdc.gov
Environmental Protection Agency
    http://www.epa.gov
National Center for Complementary and Alternative Medicine (NCCAM)
    http://nccam.nih.gov.

Safety and infection control site
    http://www.woundcare.org
United States Department of Labor
    http://www.dol.gov

## References

Altman, G. (2004). *Delmar's fundamental & advanced nursing skills* (2nd ed.). Clifton Park, NY: Delmar Learning.

AORN, Inc. (2001). Recommended practices for maintaining a sterile field. In *Standards, recommended practices, and guidelines* (pp. 221–225). Denver: AORN, Inc.

Atiyeh, B. S., Ioannovich J., Al-Amm, C. A., & El-Musa, K. A. (2002). Management of acute and chronic open wounds: The importance of moist environment in optimal wound healing. *Current Pharmaceutical Biotechnology, 3*(3).

Bending, K. (2000). Workplace safety: A personal responsibility. *Advances for Nurses, Special Edition,* 23–24.

Bren, L. (2002). FDA continues work to help prevent mad cow disease. *FDA Consumer, 36*(3), 31–32.

Centers for Disease Control and Prevention (2000). CDC: *Media Relations Why is Handwashing Important?* http://www.cdc.gov/ncidod/nicd.htm.

Centers for Disease Control and Prevention (CDC), 2003 http://www.cdc.gov

Cox, J. L., Diamond, L. H., Hatlie, M. J., Pugliese, G., & Wilson, N. J. (2002). Overview of the partnership symposium 2001: Patient safety—stories of success. *Joint Commission Journal on Quality Improvement, 28*(6), 283–286.

Daniels, R. (2003). *Delmar's manual of laboratory and diagnostic tests.* Clifton Park, NY: Delmar Learning.

Davies, H., & Rees, J. (2000). Psychological effects of isolation nursing: Mood disturbance. *Nursing Standard, 14*(28), 35–38.

Eggimann, P. (2001). Infection control in the ICU. *Critical Care Reviews.*

Environmental Protection Agency, 2003 http://www.epa.gov

Ernst, E. (2002). The risk-benefit profile of commonly used herbal therapies: Ginkgo, St. John's wort, ginseng, echinacea, saw palmetto, and kaya. *Annals of Internal Medicine, 136*(1): 42–53.

Farley, K. (2001). Evaluating the risks of bloodborne pathogens. *Point of View, 40*(3), 16–21.

Friedman, M., & Rhinhart, M. (2000). Improving infection control in home care: From ritual to science-based practice. *Home Healthcare Nurse, 18*(2), 34–39.

Gray, G., Kreindel, S., & Ropeik, D. (2002). Mad cow disease risk in the United States. Does perceived threat overshadow true likelihood of occurrence? *Postgraduate Medicine, 111*(2), 13–16.

Hoffman, D., (1998). *The new holistic model.* Boston: Element.

Joint Commission on the Accreditation of Healthcare Organizations (JCAHO) (2002). *Accreditation manual.* Chicago: Author

Kerstein, M. D. (1997). The scientific basis for wound healing. *Advances in Wound Care: The Journal for Prevention and Healing, 10*(3), 30–37.

Lutwick, S. L. (1999). Isolation. In D. Olendorf, C. Jeryan, & K. Boyden (Eds.), *The Gale Encyclopedia of Medicine* (5 vols.). Michigan: Farmington Hills.

Manangan, L., Simonds, D., Pugliese, G., Kroc, K., Banerjee, S., Rudnick, J., Steingraber, K., Jarvis, W. (1998). Are U.S. hospitals making progress in implementing guidelines for prevention of *Mycobacterium tuberculosis* transmission? *Archives of Internal Medicine, 158*(13), 1440–1445.

McCance, K. L., & Huether, S. E. (2002). *Pathophysiology: The biologic basis for disease in adults & children* (4th ed.). St. Louis: Mosby.

National Center for Complementary and Alternative Medicine (NCCAM), 2003: http://nccam.nih.gov.

National Institute for Occupational Safety and Health (1999). Curbing needlestick injuries. *Journal of Healthcare Protection Management, 15*(1), 78–82.

Nightingale, F. (1859). *Notes on nursing: What it is and what it is not.* Printed by Harrison and Sons, London, 1946.

Ortolon K. (2002). West Nile arrives. *Texas Medicine, 98*(11), 48–51.

Potts, N., & Mandleco, B. (2002). *Pediatric nursing: Caring for children and their families.* Clifton Park, NY: Delmar Learning.

Rizzo, T. (1999). *Gale encyclopedia of medicine: Hospital-acquired infections.* Michigan: Gale Group.

Spratto, G. & Woods, A. (2004). *PDR Nurse's Drug Handbook.* Clifton Park, NY: Delmar Learning.

Shultz, M. (2002). Infection control: New hand hygiene practices reduce drug-resistant germs in Washington, DC, hospital. *TB & Outbreaks Weekly,* Atlanta Publishing Co.

Tierra, L. (1997). *The herbs of life: Health and healing using Western and Chinese techniques.* Freedom, CA: The Crossing Press.

Todar, K. (2002). Immune defense against microbial pathogens. *Todar's Online Textbook of Bacteriology,* Atlanta Publishing Co.

United States Department of Labor, 2003 http://www.dol.gov

White, L., & Duncan, G. (2002). *Medical-surgical nursing: An integrated approach* (2nd ed.). Clifton Park, NY: Delmar Learning.

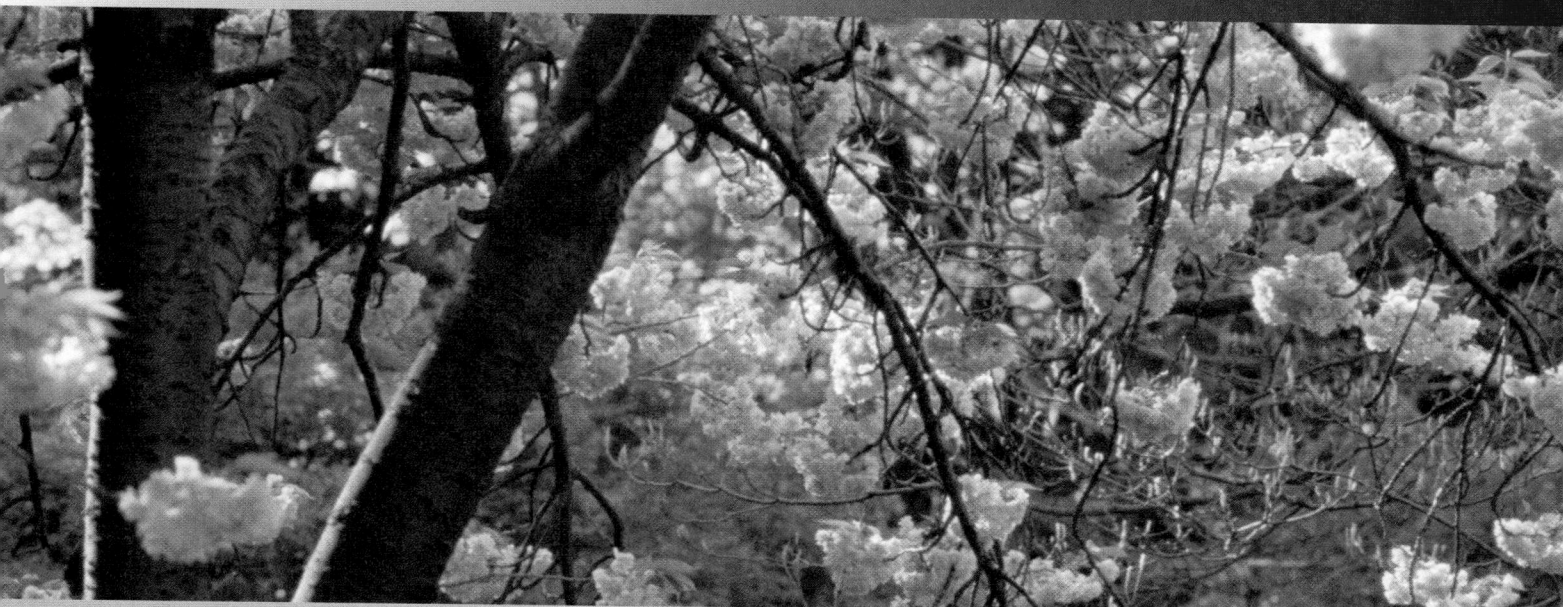

# CHAPTER 27

# Health Assessment

## Sharon M. Rayman, RN, MS, CPTC, CCTC

*"In dwelling upon the vital importance of sound observation, it must never be lost sight of what observation is for. It is not for the sake of piling up miscellaneous information or curious facts, but for the sake of saving life and increasing health and comfort."*

(Florence Nightingale, 1859)

# Chapter Competencies

**Upon completion of this chapter, the reader should be able to:**

1. Describe the physiological mechanisms governing temperature, pulse, respiration, and blood pressure.
2. Select the appropriate equipment used to take the vital signs and perform a physical examination.
3. Identify the normal age-related variations for vital sign measurements.
4. Use the four basic psychomotor techniques of physical examination.
5. Demonstrate a basic systematic, head-to-toe, and body systems approach for conducting a physical examination.
6. Identify what elements of the physical examination are important to document and to report.
7. Develop a nursing care plan based upon systematic collection of health assessment data from a specified case study.

# Key Terms

adventitious breath sounds
aneurysm
angina
aphasia
apnea
apnea monitor
arthritis
ascites
atherosclerosis
atrophy
auscultatory gap
basal metabolic rate (BMR)
baseline values
blood pressure
bradycardia
bradypnea
bronchial sounds
bronchovesicular sounds
bruits
cachexia
cardiac output
conduction
convection
costal (thoracic) breathing
crackles
crepitus
cyanosis
cystocele
degree
dermatome map

diaphoresis
diaphragmatic (abdominal) breathing
diastole
dullness
dyspnea
dysrhythmia
edema
eupnea
evaporation
expiration (exhalation)
external respiration
extinction
Glasgow Coma Scale (GCS)
goniometer
graphesthesia
heaves
hemodynamic regulation
hypertension
hypertonicity
hypertrophy
hyperventilation
hypotension
hypotonicity
hypoventilation
insensible heat loss
inspiration (inhalation)
integumentary system
internal respiration
ischemia

murmur
myocardial infarction
nystagmus
orthostatic hypotension (postural hypotension)
osteoarthritis
osteoporosis
oximeter
piloerection
pleura
pleural friction rub
pulse
pulse deficit
pulse oximetry
pulse pressure
pulse quality
pulse rate
pulse rhythm
pulse volume
pyrexia
pyrogens
radiation
regurgitation
respiration
rhonchi
Snellen chart
stenosis
stereognosis
stridor
stroke volume

*(continues)*

# Key Terms (continued)

systole
tachycardia
tachypnea
tactile fremitus
thermoregulation

thrills
tympany
vasoconstriction
vasodilation
vesicular sounds

vital capacity
vital signs
wheezes

Assessment to establish a database about a client's physical and emotional well-being, intellectual functioning, social relationships, and spiritual condition is a major component of nursing care. The client database consists of the nursing health history as presented in Chapter 11 and the physical assessment as presented in this chapter.

Health and physical assessment, an essential nursing function, is performed on every client. A health assessment can be any of three types: (1) a comprehensive assessment, such as when a client is admitted to a health care facility; (2) an assessment of a body system, such as the gastrointestinal system; or (3) assessment of a body part, such as the heart. Health assessment is aimed at establishing a database against which subsequent data can be compared to evaluate physiological functioning of the body, to detect problems related to altered function, and to identify factors that may place the client at risk for developing health problems. This chapter presents the preparations that are important to conducting a health assessment; the key data elements that are fundamental to establishing baseline values of the client's normal physiological functioning and common deviations, measurements, and evaluation of these functions; and the techniques used to perform a systematic head-to-toe physical examination.

## Preparing for the Health Assessment

The client and the environment require special consideration. Because the client will experience some anxieties regarding the examination, it is important for the nurse to keep the client informed while performing the examination. The nurse needs to be organized and demonstrate respect for the client's apprehension about physical exposure during the examination.

Although some uneasiness may be experienced when learning how to perform a physical examination, it is important that the nurse appear calm, organized, and competent at the bedside. The nurse should review the agency's physical examination/assessment form before meeting with the client. This process ensures that the nurse can fully explain the actions that will be performed and prevents omission of any area required to be assessed. The nurse usually takes the assessment form to the bedside to record the data to ensure accuracy of documentation.

## Environment

The nurse should review the health and psychosocial assessment data before visiting the client so that the environment will accommodate any special needs of the client. Adjust the environment to allow for placement of the equipment on a surface that is clean and free from movement at the bedside. Check to make sure that nothing is on the floor that would place the client at risk for falling.

The room needs to be quiet, warm, without drafts, and adequately lit. Depending on the setting, make the necessary adjustments to ensure privacy. Inform other personnel about the time of the examination to avoid interruptions, which are frustrating to both the client and the nurse.

## Equipment

Wash hands and gather the necessary equipment. Equipment should be gathered before entering the client's room. However, certain pieces of equipment, such as sphygmomanometer or ophthalmoscope/otoscope, may be permanently installed in the examination and inpatient rooms. The nurse should observe what equipment is in the client's room during the first visit with the client. The necessary equipment for clients who are maintained on isolation precautions should be kept inside the room, because items should not be taken in or out of isolation rooms.

All pieces of equipment should be maintained to function accurately. Table 27-1 describes the common types of equipment used to assess the vital signs. Table 27-2 presents the common equipment needed to conduct a physical examination. Secure enough clean gloves to change as needed throughout the examination to avoid cross-contamination.

## Positioning and Draping

The nurse should position the client to ensure accessibility to the body part being assessed. Table 27-3 presents the positions used in conducting a physical examination and discusses what areas are assessed with the client in each position. Although all the positions for a complete physical examination are included, it is not the expectation of this chapter for the beginning nursing student to

## TABLE 27-1    EQUIPMENT USED FOR VITAL SIGN MEASUREMENT

| Instrument | Description |
| --- | --- |
| **Thermometer** | |
| Glass | Mercury in glass, calibrated with Centigrade or Fahrenheit measurements |
| Oral 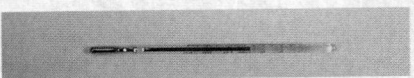 | Slim tip |
| Rectal 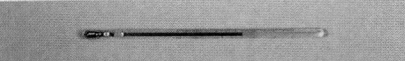 | Stubby, pear-shaped tip |
| Electronic 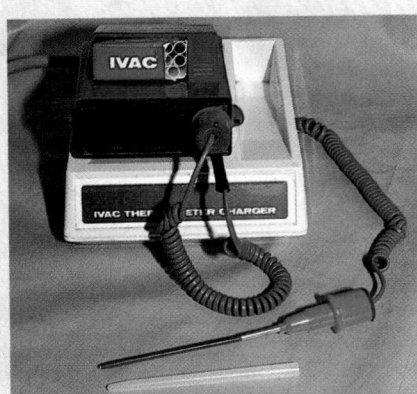 | Battery-powered display unit with a sensitive probe (blue for oral and red for rectal) covered with a disposable plastic sheath for individual use |
| Disposable (chemical), single-use 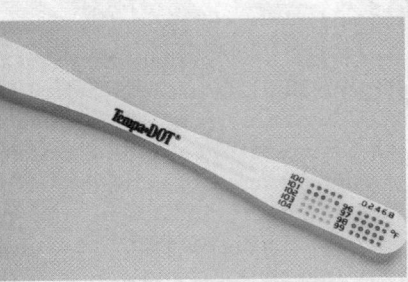 | Thin strips of plastic with chemically impregnated dots that change color to reflect temperature |
| Tympanic 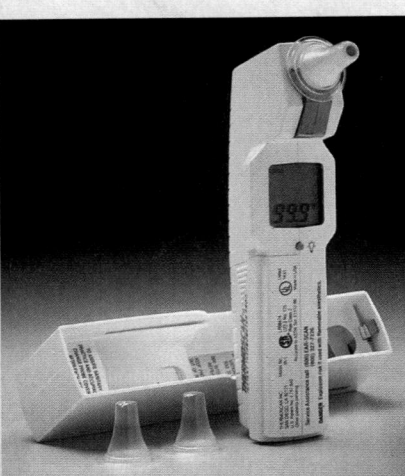 | Battery-powered display unit with disposable speculums and infrared-sensing electronics *Courtesy of The Gillette Company* |

*(continues)*

## TABLE 27-1    EQUIPMENT USED FOR VITAL SIGN MEASUREMENT *(continued)*

| Instrument | Description |
| --- | --- |
| **Stethoscope** | |
| Acoustic 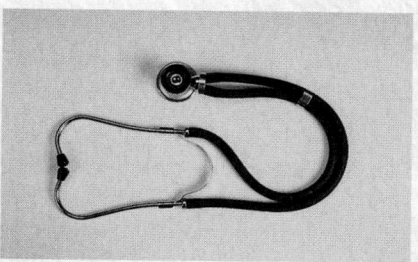 | Closed cylinder that prevents dissipation of sound waves and amplifies the sound through a diaphragm. Flat-disc diaphragm transmits high-pitched sounds, and the bell-shaped diaphragm transmits low-pitched sounds. |
| Ultrasound (Doppler) 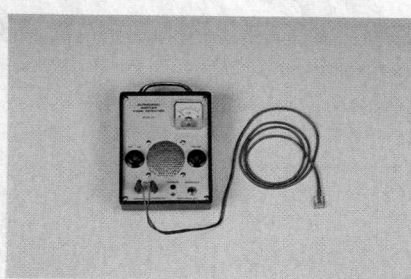 | Battery-operated headset with earpieces attached to a volume-controlled audio unit and ultrasound transducer that detects movement of red blood cells through a vessel |
| **Sphygmomanometer** | |
| Mercury manometer 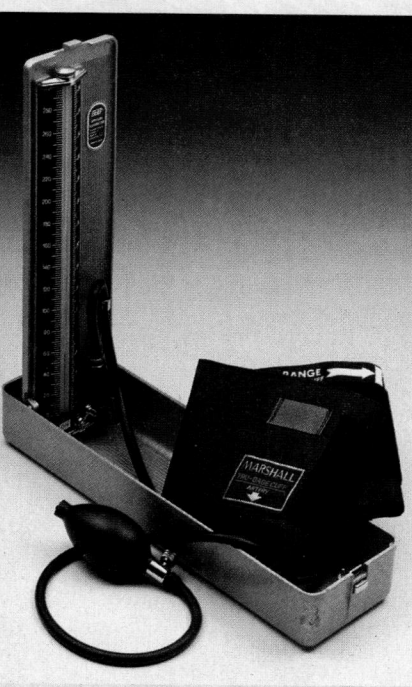 | Wall or portable unit that contains a mercury-filled glass column, calibrated in millimeters; the mercury rises and falls in response to pressure created when the cuff is inflated. *Courtesy of Omron Healthcare* |

*(continues)*

## TABLE 27-1    EQUIPMENT USED FOR VITAL SIGN MEASUREMENT (*continued*)

| Instrument | Description |
| --- | --- |
| Aneroid manometer  | Portable unit with a glass-enclosed gauge containing a needle to register millimeter calibration and a metal bellows within the gauge that expands and collapses in response to pressure variations from the inflated cuff |

perform a complete physical examination. For example, the lithotomy position is included for performing a vaginal examination; however, the discussion of the assessment of the female genitalia does not explain how to insert a vaginal speculum because that is usually within the scope of advanced practice nursing.

The primary purpose of draping the client is to prevent unnecessary exposure during the examination. Feelings of embarrassment elicit tension and restlessness and will decrease the client's ability to cooperate. The drapes also prevent the client from being chilled.

The drape may be cloth or paper—for example, a bath blanket, sheet, or towel. The client's gown can be rearranged to expose and cover different body parts. When the client is in a sitting, supine, dorsal recumbent, Sims', or prone position, use a gown or towel to cover the upper chest and a bath blanket or sheet to cover the rest of the body.

Although you will not be expected to place the client in the lithotomy position to conduct an internal vaginal examination, you may be expected to assist another practitioner with this examination. Draping a client in the lithotomy position requires a sheet and boots. The nurse should apply the boots, if available, to cover each of the client's feet and legs. Fold and place the sheet in a diamond-shaped arrangement over the body: top diamond under chin with opposite corner pointing toward the toes and lateral corners pointing toward the sides of the table. Ask the client to flex her knees, and with the lateral corners of the sheet, wrap it in a spiral fashion around the legs and feet. The bottom corner covers the perineum and is folded back over the abdomen to expose the perineum when the examination begins.

## Conducting the Health and Physical Assessment

A complete health assessment is initiated by performing a health history (as reviewed in Chapter 11) and a physical assessment. The physical assessment is initiated by performing a general survey, and height, weight, and vital signs measurements. These initial observations can provide data about the client's general state of health as well as provide important information that will guide the nurse on how to proceed with the physical examination. The physical examination may involve a complete head-to-toe physical examination, a focused examination of a body system, or a focused examination of a body part. The procedure can vary according to the age of the client, the severity of the illness, the preferences of the nurse, the location of the examination, and the agency's procedures. The physical examination is conducted in an aseptic, systematic, and efficient manner that requires the fewest position changes for the client.

### General Survey

Assessment begins at the initial contact with the client. The initial data from the general survey begins with a review of the client's primary health concerns. The nurse makes initial observations regarding the client's physical

---

### NURSING STRATEGY

#### Assessment with Clients Requiring Special Considerations

Certain clients such as infants and children, the elderly, clients who are disabled, and clients who have been abused will require special consideration during the health assessment process. Determine the client's ability to participate before conducting the examination. To allay client fears and anxiety, allow family members or significant others, with the client's approval, to remain with the client during the examination.

Estes, M. (2002). *Health assessment & physical examination* (2nd ed.). Clifton Park, NY: Delmar Learning.

## TABLE 27-2    EQUIPMENT AND SUPPLIES USED FOR A PHYSICAL EXAMINATION

| Instrument | Description/Usage |
|---|---|
| Aromatic substances (vanilla, coffee) | Test first cranial nerve (olfactory) |
| Cotton balls | Assess sensory system for light touch |
| Gloves | Reduce risk for transmission of microorganisms |
| Laryngeal mirror | Metal instrument with mirror to inspect pharynx and oral cavity |
| Ophthalmoscope | Lighted instrument attached to a battery tube to visualize the eye's interior |
| Otoscope | Special ear speculum that attaches to an ophthalmoscope to visualize external and middle ear (eardrum) |

*(continues)*

## TABLE 27-2 EQUIPMENT AND SUPPLIES USED FOR A PHYSICAL EXAMINATION (continued)

| Instrument | | Description/Usage |
|---|---|---|
| Penlight | | Flashlight to test pupillary reaction to light and third, fourth, and sixth cranial nerves (oculomotor, trochlear, and abducens) |
| Percussion hammer | | Instrument with rubber head to test reflexes |
| Safety pin | | Disposable sharp object to assess pain, sensory system |
| Tape measure | | Calibrated in cm to measure circumference |
| Tongue depressor | | Wooden tongue blade to inspect oral cavity and stimulate gag reflex to assess ninth and tenth (glossopharyngeal and vagus) cranial nerves |
| Tuning fork | | Metal fork that vibrates when tapped and is used to perform Rinne test to assess eighth (acoustic) cranial nerve |
| Lubricant | | Facilitates insertion of instruments into body cavities |
| Drape | | Covers exposed body parts |

## TABLE 27-3    POSITIONING FOR A PHYSICAL EXAMINATION

| Position | Body Part Assessed | Key Points/Contraindications |
|---|---|---|
| Sitting | Head, neck, back, posterior thorax and lungs, anterior thorax and lungs, breast, axillae, heart, extremities | Client can expand lungs; nurse can inspect symmetry. *Institute risk precautions for elderly and debilitated clients.* |
| Supine | Head, neck, anterior thorax and lungs, breast, axillae, heart, abdomen, extremities | Client relaxed; decreases abdominal muscle tension; nurse can palpate all peripheral pulses. *Contraindicated in clients with cardiopulmonary alterations.* |
| Dorsal recumbent | Head, neck, anterior thorax and lungs, breast, axillae, heart | Client comfortable; increases abdominal muscle tension. *Contraindicated in abdominal assessment.* |
| Sims' | Rectum and vagina | Relaxes rectal muscles. *Painful for clients with joint deformities.* |
| Prone | Posterior thorax and lungs, hip | Assessment of hip extension. *Contraindicated in clients with cardiopulmonary alterations.* |
| Knee-chest | Rectum | Maximal rectal exposure. *Contraindicated in clients with respiratory alterations.* |
| Lithotomy | Female genitalia, rectum, genital tract | Maximal genitalia exposure; embarrassing and uncomfortable for client. *Contraindicated in clients with joint disorders.* |

## LIFE SPAN CONSIDERATIONS

- When assessing infants, children, and older clients, it is important to know the normal changes that are associated with life span development.

- Refer to Chapters 17 and 19 for information about caring for the pediatric and geriatric client, respectively.

### Clients Who Are Disabled

When assessing a client who is disabled, the nurse should adapt interactions to the client's ability. For instance:

- hearing impairment—offer a written questionnaire

- intellectual impairment—use pictures or simple, direct sentences

- physical disability—ascertain the client's level of independence and feelings about the disability

### Clients Who Have Been Abused

When assessing clients, be observant for signs of abuse, especially in children and the elderly. The nurse should be familiar with state laws and agency policies for reporting suspected abuse. Observe for:

- psychological symptoms: not wanting to be touched, lack of eye contact, unwillingness to talk about bruises, burns, or other injuries

- physical symptoms: inspect for healed scarring or burns

Estes, M. (2002). *Health assessment & physical examination* (2nd ed.). Clifton Park, NY: Delmar Learning.

## STOP AND THINK

### What Is Cleanliness?

Cleanliness is highly valued by mainstream American society. However, in some cultures, a daily bath is not perceived as necessary or desirable. In fact, some cultures do not define natural body odors as offensive. It is important to consider the client in the context of cultural beliefs before labeling a client.

- Define the terms *dirty*, *unkempt*, and *foul-smelling*.

- Discuss how these value-laden terms can cloud the assessment process.

- Discuss how care can be affected by labeling a client as "dirty," "unkempt," or "foul-smelling."

- Observe for problems: assess the area or body system in detail during the physical examination.

Document the general survey data in an organized format to portray a clinical picture of the client. Proper terminology and agency-approved abbreviations should be used when recording assessment data.

## Measurement of Height and Weight

Measuring height and weight is as important as assessing the client's vital signs. Routine measurement provides data related to growth and development in infants and children and signals the possible onset of alterations that may indicate illness in all age groups. The client's height and weight are routinely taken on admission to acute care facilities and on visits to physicians' offices, clinics, and in other health care settings.

### Height

Measurement of height is expressed in inches (in.), feet (ft), centimeters (cm), or meters (m). See Box 27-1 for conversion equivalents from one system to another.

A scale for measuring height, calibrated in either inches or centimeters, is usually attached to a standing weight scale. This type of scale is used for measuring the height of children and adults. The nurse should ask the client to stand erect on the scale's platform. The metal rod attached to the back of the scale should be extended to gently rest on the top of the client's head, and the measurement should be read at eye level.

When measuring an infant's length, the nurse should place the child on a firm surface. Extend the knees, with

appearance, mood and behavior, signs and symptoms of distress, vital signs, and height and weight. During the general survey, it is important to make the following observations:

- Observe for signs of distress: labored breathing, pallor or cyanosis, guarding of painful site, flushing, sweating, facial grimacing, signs of anxiety such as inattention, nail biting, no eye contact.
- Observe physical presence: chronological age versus observed age, body symmetry, development and posture, body fat, stature, motor activity, body and breath odors.
- Observe psychological presence: dress, grooming, and personal hygiene; mood and behavior; speech patterns and voice intonation; facial expressions; reaction to persons and environment.

| BOX 27-1 | CONVERSION EQUIVALENTS FOR HEIGHT MEASUREMENT |
| --- | --- |

| | |
| --- | --- |
| 1 in. = 2.5 cm | 1 cm = 0.4 in. |
| 1 ft = 30.5 cm or 0.3 m | 1 m = 39.4 in. or 3.28 ft |

| BOX 27-2 | CONVERSION EQUIVALENTS FOR WEIGHT MEASUREMENT |
| --- | --- |

| | |
| --- | --- |
| 1 lb = 0.45 kg | 1 kg = 2.2 lb |
| 1 oz = 28.4 g | 1 g = 0.35 oz |

the feet at right angles to the table. Measure the distance from the vertex (top) of the head to the soles of the feet with a measuring tape. The procedure usually requires two nurses: one to hold the infant still and the other to measure the length. If the nurse needs to perform the measurement without assistance, an object should be placed at the infant's head, the infant's knees should be extended, and a second object should be placed at the infant's feet. Lift the infant and measure the distance between the two objects.

Height increases gradually from birth to the prepubertal growth spurt. Girls usually reach their adult height between the ages of 16 and 17 years, whereas boys usually continue to grow until the ages of 18 to 20 years. The older adult usually decreases in height as a result of a gradual loss of muscle mass and changes in the vertebrae that occur in conditions such as **osteoporosis** (a process in which reabsorption exceeds accretion of bone).

### Weight

Measurement of weight is expressed in ounces (oz), pounds (lb), grams (g), or kilograms (kg); see Box 27-2 for conversion equivalents. Weight increases gradually from birth until the prepubertal growth spurt. Height and weight changes occur in the adolescent's torso. The resulting redistribution of body fat gives the body an adult appearance (see Box 27-3 for the normal ranges of body height and weight according to age). The loss of muscle mass and changes in dietary habits usually cause weight loss in the elderly.

When a client has an order for "daily weight," the weight should be obtained at the same time of the day on the same scale, with the client wearing the same type of clothing. Standing scales are used for clients who can bear their own weight. The Nursing Strategy box describes the procedure for scale calibration and weight measurement.

Several types of scales, such as stretcher, chair, and bed scales, are available for clients who are unable to bear weight or are confined to a bed. For a scale that is equipped with a mechanical lift, a sheet should be placed between the client's skin and the surfaces of the belts.

Infants can be weighed on platform or cradle scales. Before weighing the infant, the nurse should make sure the room is warm. The infant's clothing and diaper should then be removed, and the nurse should place a light blanket on the scale's surface. The nurse should face the infant, keeping one hand over the top of the infant to prevent accidental injury while adjusting the scale with the other

| BOX 27-3 | NORMAL AGE-RELATED VARIATIONS IN HEIGHT AND WEIGHT |
| --- | --- |

| Age | Height | Weight |
| --- | --- | --- |
| Newborn | 50 cm (20 in.) | 3.38 kg (7.5 lb) |
| 1-6 mo | 63 cm (25 in.) | 2 × birth weight |
| 6-12 mo | 71 cm (28 in.) | 3 × birth weight |
| Toddler | 75-83 cm (30-33 in.) | 15 kg (33 lb) |
| Preschooler | 100 cm (40 in.) | 18.2-20.5 kg (40-45 lb) |
| School-age | 115-140 cm (46-56 in.) | 35.5-38.6 kg (75-85 lb) |
| *Growth Spurt* | | |
| Girls 8-14 yr | 120-160 cm (48-64 in.) | 40.9-63.6 kg (90-140 lb) |
| Boys 10-16 yr | 125-170 cm (50-68 in.) | 40.9-68.2 kg (90-150 lb) |

hand. The reading should be noted as quickly as possible, and the nurse should return the infant to the crib and dress the child.

### Nursing Considerations

Accurate recordings of weight are imperative because they are used in drug dosage calculations and to evaluate the effectiveness of drug, fluid, and nutritional therapy. Weights above the normal range may indicate obesity or fluid retention. Weights below the normal range may indicate malnutrition, delayed growth and development, or **cachexia** (weight loss marked by weakness and emaciation that usually occurs with a chronic illness such as tuberculosis or cancer). Height is compared with weight to evaluate growth of infants and children.

### Documentation

The height and weight measurements are recorded on the appropriate form, such as the admit assessment form. Daily weights are usually recorded on the vital signs record. If the weight is taken at a different time or on a different scale, the variation should be recorded. (See Procedure 38-8 for the specifics of using a hydraulic lift.)

## NURSING STRATEGY

The following are nursing interventions for scale calibration and weight measurement:

### The Standing Scale (Figure 27-1)

- Set both weight indicators to zero (Figure 27-2A).

- When calibrated, the balance beam will be at the midway point.

- With the client standing on the scale, move the weight indicators on the balance beam until the tip of the beam registers in the middle of the mark (Figure 27-2B).

### Digital Display Scale (stretcher, chair, mechanical lift, bed scales)

- The display should read zero. Follow manufacturer's instructions for calibration.

- Digital scales will automatically display the weight

Estes, M. (2002). *Health assessment & physical examination* (2nd ed.). Clifton Park, NY: Delmar Learning.

## COMMUNITY/HOME CARE

### Weighing in the Home

The client who needs to monitor daily weights should be instructed to weigh at the same time each day, usually in the morning prior to oral intake; wear similar weight clothing for each measurement; maintain a written log of serial measurements; and seek assistance from family members if visual or physical problems interfere with accurate measurement and reading.

Altman, G. (2004). *Delmar's fundamental & advanced nursing skills* (2nd ed.). Clifton Park, NY: Delmar Learning.

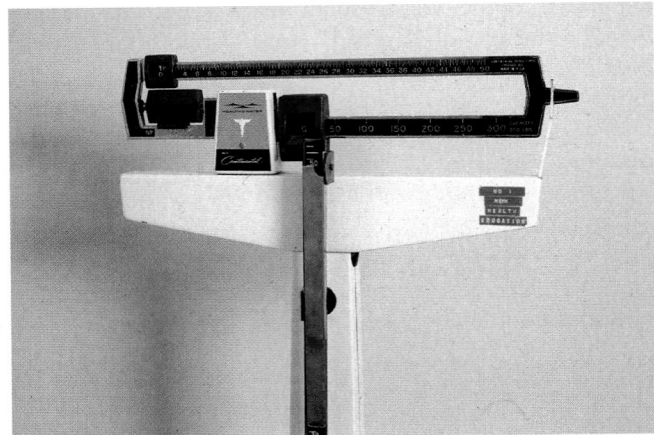

**A.**

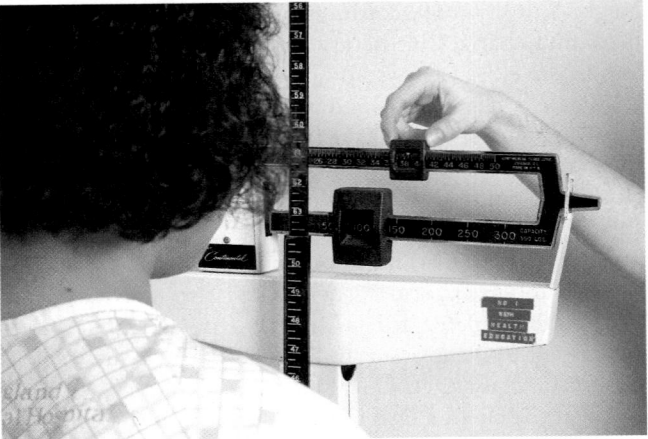

**B.**

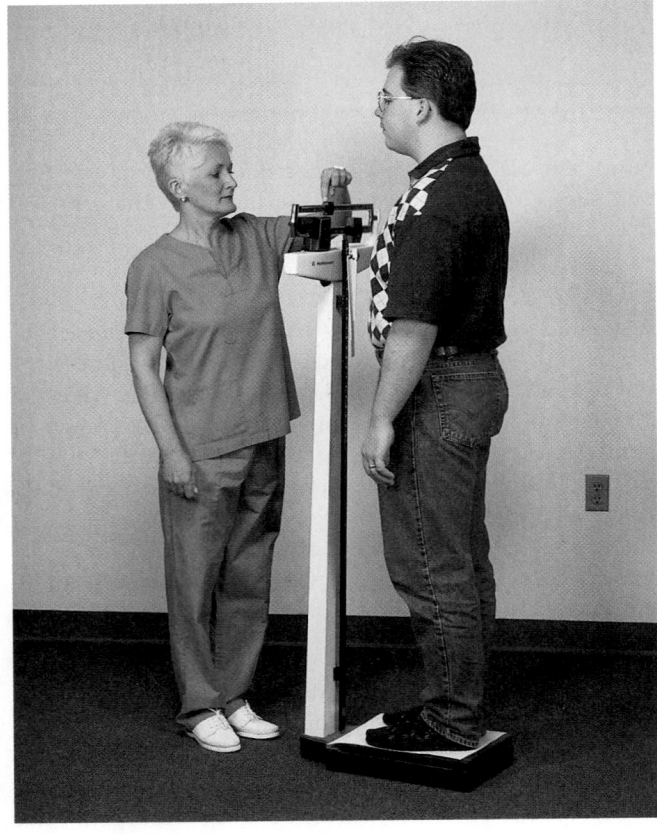

**Figure 27-1**   Weighing a client on a standing scale

**Figure 27-2**   Calibrating the scale and weighing the client. A. Set both weight indicators to zero. B. With the client standing on the scale, move the weight indicators on the balance beam until the tip of the beam registers in the middle of the mark.

# Vital Signs

The "taking of **vital signs**" refers to measurement of the client's body temperature (T), pulse (P) and respiratory (R) rates, and blood pressure (BP). Vital signs are fundamental to physical assessment (the first step in the physical examination) to establish baseline values of the client's cardiorespiratory integrity. **Baseline values** establish the norm against which subsequent measurements can be compared. Variations from normal findings may indicate potential problems with the client's health status. Nurses should confirm "normal" measurements with clients because the perception of what is normal may vary among clients.

Vital signs are taken whenever the client is admitted to a health care facility or service, for example, home health care, clinic, or other ambulatory setting, and on a routine basis in the hospital. The frequency of vital sign measurements for the hospitalized client is determined by the client's health status, physician orders, and the established standards of care for the particular clinical setting or service. Whenever a change is suspected in the client's status, the nurse should measure the vital signs, regardless of the setting.

The sequence for recording vital signs measurement in the nurses' notes is T-P-R and BP. Agencies usually have special graphic forms used to record vital signs findings. These forms facilitate data comparison at a glance because the data are plotted on a graph.

## Physiological Function

Healthy people have the ability to meet their own needs; however, during illness, people need assistance (in proportion to the degree of dysfunction) in meeting their basic needs. The assessment of physiological functioning provides specific data regarding the client's current condition. Data analysis allows the nurse to plan nursing care that is responsive to the preventive and restorative needs of the client. See Chapters 11 through 15 for a complete discussion of the steps of the nursing process.

### Thermoregulation

**Thermoregulation** is the body's physiological function of heat regulation to maintain a constant internal body temperature. The heat of the body is measured in units called **degrees**. The "core" internal temperature of 98.6° Fahrenheit (F) (37° centigrade [C]) does not vary more than 1.4°F (0.77°C) and is higher than the skin and external temperature. In contrast, the skin temperature rises and falls in accordance with changes in environmental temperature.

### Heat Production

Heat is produced in the body's cells through food metabolism that results in the release of energy. The body converts energy supplied by metabolized nutrients to energy forms that can be used directly by the body. One form of this energy is thermal energy for regulation of body temperature. Energy is measured in terms of heat. A kilocalorie is an energy value (heat measure) of a given food; 1 kilocalorie equals 1,000 calories (the amount of heat required to raise the temperature of 1 kilogram of water 1°C). This type of heat liberation is usually expressed as the metabolic rate and measured as the **basal metabolic rate**, or **BMR** (the rate of energy use in the body needed to maintain essential activities). See Chapter 35 for a complete discussion of calories, kilocalories, and metabolic rate.

Factors that affect the metabolic rate of heat liberation, such as age and exercise, are discussed later in this chapter. The thyroid hormones thyroxine and triiodothyronine increase basal metabolism by breaking down glucose and fat. Muscular activity also produces heat from the breakdown of carbohydrates and fats and through shivering.

Body temperature is controlled by balancing metabolic heat production with heat loss. Most heat production comes from the deep tissue organs (brain, liver, and heart) and the skeletal muscles. The skin, subcutaneous tissues, and fat of the subcutaneous tissues serve as heat insulators for the body. Sweat glands in the dermis are innervated by sympathetic nerves of the autonomic nervous system and are controlled by the anterior hypothalamus to regulate sweating.

When body heat rises, the hypothalamus transmits impulses to reduce body heat by triggering perspiring, **vasodilation** (the widening of blood vessels), and the inhibition of heat production. The opposite physiological functioning occurs in response to a decrease in body heat. In this situation the hypothalamus transmits impulses to stimulate heat production through **vasoconstriction** (the narrowing of blood vessels), muscle shivering, and **piloerection** (hairs standing on end).

### Heat Loss

Most body heat is lost from the skin's surface to the environment by the processes of radiation, conduction, convection, and evaporation as presented in Table 27–4. **Insensible heat loss** is the heat that is lost through the continuous, unnoticed water loss that occurs with vaporization, accounting for 10% of basal heat production. Evaporation accounts for the greatest heat loss when body heat increases.

### Behavioral Control of Body Temperature

In addition to the heat production and heat loss mechanisms described above, the body has another potent mechanism for temperature control, known as behavioral control. In response to the body's signaling conditions of either being overheated or too cold, the person makes appropriate environmental adjustments to reestablish comfort. Guyton & Hall (2001) recognize this mechanism as the most effective mechanism for body heat control in severely cold environments.

## TABLE 27-4    METHODS OF HEAT LOSS

| Method | Characteristics | Example |
|---|---|---|
| **Radiation:** Loss of heat in the form of infrared rays | All objects that are not at absolute zero radiate heat rays from the surface of one object to the surface of another object that is not in physical contact with the first object. | If the temperature of the body is greater than the surroundings, heat is lost from the body to the environment. A nude person in a room with normal temperature will lose about 60% of total heat loss by radiation. |
| **Conduction:** Loss of heat to an object in contact with the body | Heat is lost to other objects that are cooler than the skin. As much as 15% of the body's total heat loss is transferred to the air. Once the temperature of the air adjacent to the skin equals the skin temperature, there is no further loss of body heat. | Bathing a client in cool or tepid water will lower the client's temperature. |
| **Convection:** Movement of heat away from the body's surface | Convection accompanies conduction when the warmed air or water is replaced with cooler elements. | The use of fans enhances convected heat loss by air. Water adjacent to the skin can absorb far greater quantities of heat than can air. Clothing entraps air next to the skin, decreasing heat loss from the body by conduction and convection. |
| **Evaporation:** Continuous insensible water loss from the skin and lungs when water is converted from a liquid to a gas | It takes approximately 0.58 calories of heat for a gram of water to evaporate. | Insensible water loss is continuous. Insensible loss occurs regardless of body temperature; thus, it is not a major regulator of temperature. |

## Respiration

**Respiration** is the act of breathing. Respiration is defined by physiological functioning as:

- **External respiration**—the exchange of oxygen and carbon dioxide between the alveoli of the lungs and the pulmonary blood system
- **Internal respiration**—the interchange of oxygen and carbon dioxide between the circulating blood and cells throughout the body
- **Inspiration** (inhalation)—the intake of air into the lungs
- **Expiration** (exhalation)—the movement of gases from the lungs to the atmosphere
- **Vital capacity**—the amount of air exhaled from the lungs after a minimal full inspiration

The following five major physiological pulmonary functions provide oxygen to the tissues and remove carbon dioxide:

1. Ventilation—the inflow and outflow of air between the atmosphere and the lung alveoli.
2. Circulation—the quantity of blood flowing through the lungs is approximately 4-6 L/min.
3. Diffusion—the exchange of oxygen and carbon dioxide between the alveoli and the blood.
4. Transport—the carrying of oxygen and carbon dioxide in the blood and body fluids to and from the cells.
5. Regulation—the neurogenic system that adjusts the rate of alveolar ventilation to meet the demands of the body. The arterial blood oxygen pressure ($Po_2$) and arterial blood carbon dioxide pressure ($Pco_2$) may be altered during times of strenuous exercise and other types of respiratory stress. See Chapter 39 for a complete discussion about oxygenation.

The mechanics of pulmonary ventilation depend on abdominal recti and internal intercostal muscles that cause lung expansion and contraction. Normal breathing is accomplished by:

1. The downward and upward movement of the diaphragm to lengthen or shorten the chest cavity
2. The elevation and depression of the ribs to increase and decrease the anteroposterior diameter of the chest cavity

Children and men normally breathe with their diaphragm muscles; adult women generally breathe with their upper chest muscles (Barkauskas, Bauman, & Darling-Fisher, 2002).

## Hemodynamic Regulation

**Hemodynamic regulation** is the physiological function of blood circulating to maintain an appropriate environment in tissue fluids. Circulation transports nutrients to the tissues, removes waste products, and carries hormones from one part of the body to another. When the body's circulatory needs change, the heart rate either accelerates or decelerates. This is a compensatory mechanism under the control of the cardiac centers that are located in the medulla of the brain stem. The sensory receptors in the tissues transmit impulses to the cardiac centers, which in turn trigger a change in the heart rate through the sympathetic and parasympathetic nervous systems that innervate the heart. When the physiological needs of the tissues are met, the heart rate returns to normal.

Systemic circulation supplies blood to all the tissues of the body except the lungs (which is accomplished through pulmonary circulation). Approximately 84% of the entire blood volume is in the systemic circulation, with the heart containing 7% and the pulmonary vessels containing 9%. The circulatory system is composed of:

- Arteries—large vessels that transport systemic blood under high pressure to the tissues
- Arterioles—the smallest branches of the arterial system that act as control valves to release blood into the capillaries
- Capillaries—thin-walled vessels permeable to small molecular substances that exchange fluids, nutrients, electrolytes, hormones, and other substances between the blood and interstitial fluid
- Venules—vessels that collect blood from the capillaries and gradually coalesce into progressively larger veins
- Veins—vessels that transport systemic blood from the tissues back to the heart and serve as a reservoir for extra blood

The normal physiological function of the cells requires continuous blood flow and appropriate volume and distribution of blood to the cells that need nutrients. This is accomplished through the heart's contraction and ejection of blood into the aorta and the distensibility of the arterial system. The combination of the arterial distensibility and resistance reduces the pressure pulsations, allowing continuous blood flow to the tissues. The dynamics of distensibility and resistance maintain a constant blood flow; otherwise, blood would flow to the tissues only during **systole** (phase in which the ventricles contract to eject blood) with an absence of blood flow during **diastole** (phase in which ventricles are relaxed and no blood is being ejected).

The cardiac cycle has two phases: systole and diastole. At the onset of systole, an increase in ventricular pressure causes the mitral and tricuspid valves to close. The closing of these valves produces the first heart sound ($S_1$).

Ventricular pressure continues to increase until it exceeds the pressure in the pulmonary artery and the aorta, causing the aortic and pulmonic valves to open and allowing the ventricles to eject blood into these arteries. Ventricular emptying and relaxation cause a decrease in the ventricular pressure and closure of the aortic and pulmonic valves. Closure of these valves produces the second heart sound ($S_2$). During diastole, the pressure in the ventricles is less than that in the atria, causing the mitral and tricuspid valves to open and allowing blood to flow from the atria into the ventricles until the end of diastole, when the atria contract to send the rest of the blood into the ventricles. Ventricular filling causes an increase in pressure that closes the mitral and tricuspid valves (the beginning of systole) and starts another cardiac cycle.

**Stroke volume** is the measurement of blood that enters the aorta with each ventricular contraction. With each ventricular contraction, the heart ejects 60–70 ml of blood into the aorta. **Cardiac output** is the volume of blood pumped by the heart in 1 minute and is measured by multiplying the heart rate by the ventricle's stroke volume. For example, a client with a heart rate of 80 beats per minute times a stroke volume of 60 ml of blood would have a cardiac output of 4,800 ml. **Pulse pressure** is a measurement of the ratio of stroke volume to compliance (total distensibility) of the arterial system.

### Pulse

The **pulse** is the bounding of blood flow in an artery that is palpable at various points on the body. The pulse is caused by the stroke volume ejection and distension of the walls of the aorta, which creates a pulse wave as it travels rapidly toward the distal ends of the arteries. As the pulse wave reaches a superficial peripheral artery and travels over an underlying bone or muscle, the pulse can be palpated by applying gentle pressure over a pulse point (a specific area where the peripheral pulses can be palpated). Figure 27–3 shows the location of pulse points throughout the body.

### Blood Pressure

Both the blood pressure and pulse are measurements that determine the volume of ejected blood into the arterial system with each ventricular contraction. **Blood pressure** is the measurement of pressure pulsations exerted against the blood vessel walls during systole and diastole. It is measured in terms of millimeters of mercury (mm Hg). In a healthy young adult, the pressure at the height of each pulse (the systolic pressure) is approximately 120 mm Hg, and the pressure at the lowest point of each pulse (diastolic pressure) is approximately 80 mm Hg. The pulse pressure is the difference between these pressures, which is 40 mm Hg. If 1 mm Hg caused a vessel originally containing 10 ml of blood to increase its volume by 1 ml, the distensibility would be 0.1/mm Hg, or 10%/mm Hg (Guyton & Hall, 2001).

The body has four hemodynamic regulators for blood pressure control:

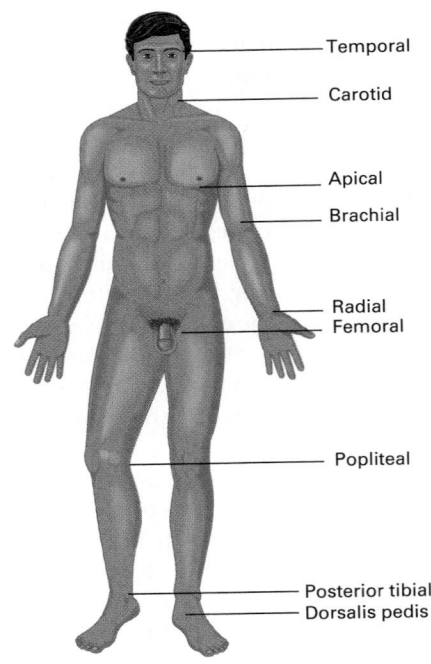

**Figure 27-3**    **Pulse points**

1. Blood volume—the volume of blood in the circulatory system. Blood pressure is proportional to the blood volume. Hemorrhage causes a loss in blood volume that in turn lowers the blood pressure. Rapid infusion of intravenous fluids causes an increase in volume and subsequent rise in pressure.
2. Cardiac output—the major factor that influences systolic pressure.
3. Peripheral vascular resistance—the size and distensibility of the arteries, which is the most important determinant of diastolic pressure. Arterial resistance (decreased distensibility) is encountered when the left ventricle pumps blood from the heart under pressure during the systolic phase. The arteries contain smooth muscles that allow them to contract, which decreases their compliance (tone) and causes resistance. The varying degrees of tone allow some of the arterioles to remain constricted while others dilate to protect the body's circulatory system from accommodating a greater blood capacity than the actual blood volume. If all of the arterioles were to dilate at one time, there would not be enough blood to fill them.
4. Viscosity—the thickness of the blood based on the ratio of proteins and cells to the liquid portion of blood. The greater the viscosity, the harder the heart must work to pump blood, with a resultant increase in blood pressure.

These regulators work in unison to create a constant blood pressure. For instance, when the blood volume decreases, the body compensates with an increased heart rate and vasoconstriction that increases peripheral resistance to maintain normal pressure and functions of the vital organs.

Blood pressure is a result of the cardiac output and peripheral vascular resistance. Normal arteries expand during systole and contract during diastole, creating two distinct pressure phases:

- Systolic blood pressure is a measurement of the maximal pressure exerted against arterial walls during systole (when myocardial fibers contract and tighten to eject blood from the ventricles), primarily a reflection of cardiac output.
- Diastolic blood pressure is a measurement of pressure remaining in the arterial system during diastole (period of relaxation that reflects the pressure remaining in the blood vessels after the heart has pumped), primarily a reflection of peripheral vascular resistance.

Serial blood pressure readings provide significant clinical data relative to the client's cardiovascular and fluid volume status. See Chapter 34 for a complete discussion of maintenance of fluid volume.

## Factors Influencing Vital Signs

Several factors can cause changes in one or more of the vital signs: age, gender, heredity, race, lifestyle, environment, medications, pain, and other factors such as exercise and metabolism, anxiety and stress, postural changes, diurnal variations, and hormones.

### Age

The normal values and variations in vital sign measurement are usually based on age (see Boxes 27-4 to 27-6 that present age-related changes in temperature, pulse, and respiration). In newborns, thermoregulation and the respiratory center are immature. The newborn's temperature fluctuates with the environment. Clothing must be ade-

| **BOX 27-4** | **NORMAL AGE-RELATED VARIATIONS IN BODY TEMPERATURE** | | |
|---|---|---|---|
| **Age** | **Measurement Route** | **Normal Range** | |
| | | **Celsius** | **Fahrenheit** |
| Newborn | Axillary | 35.5–39.5°C | 96.0–99.5°F |
| 1 yr | Oral | 37.7°C | 99.7°F |
| 3 yr | Oral | 37.2°C | 99.0°F |
| 5 yr | Oral | 37.0°C | 98.6°F |
| Adult | Oral | 37.0°C | 98.6°F |
| | Axillary | 36.4°C | 97.6°F |
| | Rectal | 37.6°C | 99.6°F |
| 70+ yr | Oral | 36.0°C | 96.8°F |

## BOX 27-5    NORMAL AGE-RELATED VARIATIONS IN RESTING PULSE

| Age | Normal Range | Average Rate/Minute |
|-----|-------------|---------------------|
| Newborn | 100–170 | 140 |
| 1 yr | 80–170 | 120 |
| 3 yr | 80–130 | 110 |
| 6 yr | 75–120 | 100 |
| 10 yr | 70–110 | 90 |
| 14 yr | 60–110 | 90 |
| Adult | 60–100 | 80 |

## BOX 27-6    NORMAL AGE-RELATED VARIATIONS IN RESTING RESPIRATION

| Age | Normal Range | Average Rate/Minute |
|-----|-------------|---------------------|
| Newborn | 30–50 | 40 |
| 1 yr | 20–40 | 30 |
| 3 yr | 20–30 | 25 |
| 6 yr | 16–22 | 19 |
| 14 yr | 14–20 | 17 |
| Adult | 12–20 | 18 |

## BOX 27-7    NORMAL AGE-RELATED VARIATIONS IN BLOOD PRESSURE

| Age | Systolic (mm Hg) | Diastolic (mm Hg) | Average |
|-----|------------------|-------------------|---------|
| Newborn | 65–95 | 30–60 | 80/60 |
| Infant | 65–115 | 42–80 | 90/61 |
| 3 yr | 76–122 | 46–84 | 99/65 |
| 6 yr | 85–115 | 48–64 | 100/56 |
| 10 yr | 93–125 | 46–68 | 109/58 |
| 14 yr | 99–137 | 51–71 | 118/61 |
| Adult | 100–140 | 60–90 | 120/80 |
| Elderly | 100–160 | 60–90 | 130/80 |

quate to maintain body heat. For example, the newborn's head should be covered because up to 30% of body heat can be lost through the head. The newborn's respiratory rate is from 30 to 50 breaths per minute with a slightly irregular rhythm.

In the elderly, the efficiency of thermoregulation is reduced by the physiological changes of aging, including loss of subcutaneous fat, decreased sweat gland activity, reduced metabolism, and poor vasomotor control. Financial status and environmental conditions experienced by the elderly may also affect diet, activity, and ability to control the external temperature.

The normal aging process causes changes in the elderly person's respiratory functions. Major physiological alterations include:

- Ventilation—Bony changes in the thorax and vertebrae and the decline in respiratory and abdominal musculature reduce the ability of the lungs to distend.
- Circulation and diffusion—The increase in dead air space in the respiratory tree decreases the quantity of blood flowing through the lungs and gaseous exchange.
- Transport—**Atherosclerosis** (plaques in the inner walls of arteries) and **dysrhythmia** (irregular heartbeat) reduce the amount of blood flow available to tissues.

- Regulation—The inability of lung function to perform maximal breathing for extended periods of time reduces the rate of alveolar ventilation to meet the demands of the body.

See Chapter 19 for a complete discussion of the physiological changes that occur in the elderly.

Blood pressure varies throughout life (see Box 27-7). From early childhood throughout adolescence, the blood pressure varies according to body size. An adult's blood pressure continues to increase with age.

## Gender

Women usually experience greater temperature fluctuations than men because of hormonal changes. Temperature variations occur during the menstrual cycle mainly in response to the progesterone level. As the progesterone level increases during ovulation, temperature gradually rises. During menopause, the instability of the vasomotor controls may cause periods (30 seconds to 5 minutes) of intense body heat and sweating. Males in general have higher blood pressure than do females of the same age.

## Heredity

Although many studies have been conducted to relate hereditary factors to specific cardiovascular disease occurrence, the results are often inconclusive regarding the influence of heredity versus environmental factors. For example, studies have been conducted to relate elevated blood cholesterol levels to a single gene. Giger and Davidhizar (1999) describe studies of Jews and non-Jews and compare Ashkenazi Jews with Asian Jews based on the theory that elevated blood cholesterol levels may be caused by a single gene. These studies indicate a higher occurrence of elevated blood cholesterol levels among Jews than among non-Jews and that Ashkenazi Jews may have a higher frequency of the gene than Asian Jews. The conclusions of these studies indicate a need for further studies to be done to determine the frequency of heart disease among Jews, as well as the interplay between heredity and environment (Giger & Davidhizar, 1999).

## Race

Some ethnic groups are more susceptible than others to hemodynamic alterations. The incidence of hypertension is higher in African Americans than in European Americans. For example, African American men over the age of 35 have higher blood pressure than do European American men of the same age.

## Lifestyle

Lifestyle factors, such as cigarette smoking, cause chronic changes in the lungs as manifested by impaired ventilation. Stimulants such as caffeinated beverages and tobacco elevate heart rate. The effects of exercise and stress are discussed below.

## Environment

Environmental factors such as temperature and noise level can alter heart rate. Acid rain and industrialized areas are often associated with a high occurrence of respiratory conditions, such as infections and chronic lung diseases.

Primary prevention is a major role of occupational (industrial) health nurses. A health screening examination relies heavily on vital sign measurements and physical examination findings. The occupational health nurse should perform health screening examinations that focus on the short-term results of certain environmental conditions (diseases) and monitor for the development of chronic trends; see Box 27-8 for screening criteria.

## Medications

Some medications can directly or indirectly alter the pulse, respirations, or blood pressure. Digitalis preparations (cardiac glycosides) decrease the pulse rate. Narcotic analgesics (pain medications) can depress the rate and depth of respirations and lower the blood pressure.

## CLINICAL ALERT

### Vital Signs and Medications

Always ask clients what medications they are currently taking and be aware of the side effects of any medications you administer. Certain drugs may either increase or decrease pulse rate and blood pressure. If the drug alters the client's pulse, respiration, or blood pressure, provide appropriate client teaching so that the client is able to compensate for the variations in these functions.

---

### BOX 27-8    HEALTH SCREENING CRITERIA

The performance of a health screening examination is justified when the disease being screened for has:

- A significant effect on the longevity or the quality of life

- A sufficiently high prevalence rate to justify the cost of the screening program

- Been shown to have better therapeutic results if detected in the early stage and worse results with delayed detection and treatment

- A significant asymptomatic period allowing an opportunity for detection and treatment that will reduce the rate of morbidity and mortality

- An acceptable method of treatment

Data from Edelman, C. L., & Mandle, C. L. (2001). *Health promotion throughout the life span* (5th ed., p. 231). St. Louis: Mosby-Yearbook.

## Pain

Each person reacts to pain in varying degrees. With acute pain, sympathetic stimulation increases the heart rate, which increases the cardiac output and vasoconstriction, causing an increased peripheral vascular resistance. These changes result in increased pulse and respiratory rates, depth of respirations, and blood pressure. Chronic pain causes parasympathetic stimulation and decreases the pulse rate. See Chapter 42 for a complete discussion about pain and measures to promote comfort.

## Other Factors

Table 27-5 presents the effects of exercise and metabolism, anxiety and stress, postural changes, and diurnal (daily) variations (also called circadian) on the vital sign measurements. Routine exercise increases metabolism and heat production and strengthens the cardiac muscles. The normal untrained person can increase cardiac output fourfold with exercise, and the trained athlete can increase cardiac output about sixfold (Guyton & Hall, 2001).

Anxiety and stress stimulate the sympathetic nervous system to:

- Increase the production of epinephrine and norepinephrine, with a resultant increase in metabolic activity and heat production
- Increase the heart rate, which, in turn, increases the cardiac output and causes vasoconstriction with a subsequent increase in peripheral vascular resistance

## TABLE 27-5   FACTORS INFLUENCING VITAL SIGNS

| Factor | Temperature | Pulse | Respiration | Blood Pressure |
|---|---|---|---|---|
| Exercise and metabolism | Increases | Short-term: increases Long-term: lowers the resting rate and return time to the resting rate postexercise | Rate and depth increase | Increases |
| Anxiety and stress | Increases | Increases | Increases | Increases |
| Postural changes | No change | Increases with sitting or standing; decreases when lying down | Decreases with stooped or slumped positions due to decreased chest expansion | Decreases with sitting or standing |
| Diurnal variations (Circadian rhythm) | Lowest level: 0400–0600 h Highest level: 2000–2400 h | Decreases during sleep | None | Lowest level: early morning Highest level: late afternoon or early evening |

Sympathetic stimulation causes an increase in the pulse rate and blood pressure. See Chapter 47 for a complete discussion about stress, anxiety, and adaptation.

Postural changes occur in response to stimulation of the baroreceptors (spray-type nerve endings of the autonomic nervous system) that are located in the walls of the arteries. The baroreceptor reflex is the primary mechanism for maintaining a relatively constant arterial pressure. When a person stands up after lying down, the arterial pressure in the head and upper part of the body immediately tends to fall. This falling pressure elicits an immediate baroreceptor reflex, resulting in strong sympathetic discharges throughout the body. This response minimizes the decrease in pressure in the head and upper body (Guyton & Hall, 2001). The person's blood pressure decreases when a person goes from a lying to a sitting or standing position. However, the pulse is lower in a lying position and increases in a sitting or standing position.

Each person has a different temperature pattern, with a normal variance ranging from 0.5°–1°C (0.9°–1.8°F) for a 24-hour period. Table 27-6 identifies the extremes of temperature variation.

The skin temperature rises and falls with a change in environmental temperature. Infants and older adults are most susceptible to environmental changes because their temperature-regulating mechanisms are less effective. Warm environments decrease conduction and increase body temperature, which, in turn, increases the metabolic rate, resulting in an increased pulse rate. Improper clothing in cold climates may lead to a decrease in body temperature through radiation and conductive heat loss that results in shivering to raise the body temperature.

Other factors can contribute to the vital signs' being above or below the established normal limits. Review of the client's health history data will reveal pertinent information regarding the factors that influence the vital signs.

## Body Temperature

Body temperature is measured during the routine physical examination by using one of the instruments described in Table 27-1. Frequent monitoring is required for clients who have or are at risk for infection; for example, postoperative clients or those with suppressed white blood cell count. Accuracy of temperature measurement is essential because it guides nursing and medical decision making and interventions.

### Temperature Scales

The nurse should consistently measure and record the temperature using either the centigrade or Fahrenheit scale as defined in specific health care agency policies. A centigrade-calibrated scale ranges from 34°–42°C, and a Fahrenheit-calibrated scale ranges from 94°–108°F. Conversions from one scale to another are based on the formula that 0°C is equal to 32°F (see Box 27-9).

### Sites

Although the physician may order a specific site to measure the temperature, nursing judgment usually determines the best site based on the client's age and physical and mental condition. Traditional sites for measuring the body's internal (core) temperature are oral (OT), rectal (RT), and axillary (AT), using either glass or electronic thermometers.

## TABLE 27-6    ALTERATIONS IN THERMOREGULATION

| Alteration | Definition | Characteristics |
|---|---|---|
| Heat exhaustion | An increase in body temperature (38°–40°C; 100.4°–104.0°F) in response to environmental conditions that, in turn, causes **diaphoresis** (profuse perspiration) | Loss of excessive amounts of water and sodium from perspiring leads to thirst, nausea, vomiting, weakness, and disorientation. |
| Heat stroke | A critical increase in body temperature (41°–44°C) resulting from exposure to high environmental temperatures | Dry, hot skin is the most important sign. The person becomes confused or delirious, and experiences thirst, abdominal distress, muscle cramps, and visual disturbances. Loss of consciousness occurs if untreated. |
| Hypothermia | A body temperature of 35°C or lower resulting from cold weather exposure or artificial induction | Decrease in metabolism leads to impaired mental functioning and depressed pulse, respirations, and blood pressure; can result in cardiac arrest if untreated. |
| Frostbite | Freezing of the body's surface areas (earlobes, fingers, and toes) in extremely low temperatures | Circulatory impairment may be followed by gangrene. |

Advances in clinical thermometry provide other devices and sites, such as thermistors for pulmonary artery temperature (PAT) and infrared thermometers for ear canal temperature (ET). ET is the most common site used for temperature measurements in adults because it is a safe and efficient method; however, it is less sensitive in detecting fever in infants and young children. ET should not be used in infected or draining ears or if adjacent lesions or incisions exist. The most reliable measure of core temperature is PAT. Since PAT requires placement of a thermodilution pulmonary artery catheter, it is impractical for routine care.

Oral and rectal temperature measurements are higher than axillary because the measuring device is in contact with the mucous membrane. Rectal measurements are higher than oral because of the seal created by the anal sphincter, which decreases contact with environmental air. With the availability of electronic measuring devices, a glass thermometer should never be used for oral readings if there is danger that the client will bite and break the thermometer.

The axilla is commonly used as a site for infants and children with disabilities because it is the safest, even though least accurate, method. Axillary or rectal sites are used for clients who are uncooperative, comatose, or who have a nasogastric or feeding tube in place.

### Assessing Body Temperature

Assess the client for the most appropriate site, and gather the necessary equipment. When checking the client's oral temperature, the nurse should confirm that the client has neither consumed hot or cold food or beverage nor smoked for 15 to 30 minutes before the measurement. Mouth breathing and tachypnea may also cause an inaccurate oral reading. The nurse should wear nonsterile gloves to protect the nurse's hands from contamination by body secretions and to reduce transmission of microorganisms.

When using a glass thermometer stored in a disinfectant solution, the nurse should rinse it under cold water to remove the solution. Hot water should not be used on the thermometer, because it will cause the mercury to expand and could break the thermometer. Procedure 27–1 describes the actions involved in measuring body temperature according to site.

### Alterations in Thermoregulation

When heat production exceeds heat loss and body temperature rises above the normal range, **pyrexia** occurs. This condition is caused by an elevation of the body's set-point in the hypothalamus. When the body's temperature rises above 37.4°C (101°F) orally or 38°C (100.4°F) rectally, the client is said to be febrile.

## BOX 27-9    CENTIGRADE AND FAHRENHEIT CONVERSION FORMULAS

- Centigrade to Fahrenheit conversion: multiply the centigrade reading by 9/5 and add 32: °F = (°C × 9/5) + 32

- Fahrenheit to centigrade conversion: deduct 32 from the Fahrenheit reading and multiply by 5/9: °C = (°F − 32) × 5/9

## CLINICAL ALERT

### Temperature Measurement Sites

Rectal temperature measurement is contraindicated in clients with cardiovascular alterations because the thermometer may stimulate the vagus nerve and cause an irregular cardiac rhythm. It is also contraindicated in leukemia and rectal surgery clients because the insertion of the thermometer may traumatize the mucosa or incision line, causing bleeding.

**Pyrogens** (bacteria, viruses, fungi, and some antigens) are endogenous or exogenous substances that cause fever. When a pyrogen enters the body, it causes an increased production of white blood cells and raises the set-point of the hypothalamus. It takes the body several hours to generate and conserve sufficient heat to achieve the new set-point. It is during this time that the person experiences the clinical symptoms of chills and shivering. When the temperature and set-point are equal, chills subside and fever is manifested clinically. The fever cycle continues until the body overcomes the pyrogen either naturally or through clinical intervention (e.g., administration of antibiotics).

Age, gender, and hormonal levels can influence "normal" physiological function. These factors account for the differences in individual temperature measurements relative to fever. When a person is exposed to extreme environmental conditions, several alterations in thermoregulation can occur. Table 27–6 discusses the alterations that can occur in thermoregulation.

### Nursing Considerations

The nurse should place the client experiencing heat exhaustion in a cool environment. The goal of nursing care is to stop diaphoresis by administering fluid and electrolytes as prescribed by a physician. See Chapter 34 for a complete discussion of fluid and electrolyte therapy.

Victims of heat stroke do not perspire because of severe electrolyte loss and impaired hypothalamic function. Heat stroke victims are usually discovered outdoors. Emergency measures must be instituted to lower the temperature during transport to an emergency center. Nursing's primary role relative to heat stroke is prevention. The nurse is usually involved in teaching preventive measures, such as drinking liquids before, during, and after exercise; avoiding strenuous exercise in humid, hot weather; and wearing light-colored, loose-fitting clothing and covering the head when working outdoors in hot climates.

Hypothermia and frostbite victims found injured in cold weather or who were immersed in cold water are treated while in transit to an emergency center with heating blankets and instillation of warm fluids into the stomach. Nursing's role is to teach preventive measures to groups at risk, such as the homeless, and to parents or guardians of mentally ill or handicapped clients who live in cold environments.

### Documentation

Record the temperature measurement and the site on the designated medical record form. Schmitz and colleagues (1995) identify the importance of both consistency in the measurement process for the purpose of establishing a client's temperature trend and awareness of the method used when interpreting clinical data. Temperature measurements are usually plotted on a graph to identify alteration patterns, such as sharp elevations and declines in temperature (a condition known as spiking).

## LIFE SPAN CONSIDERATIONS

### Obtaining Temperatures

#### Pediatric Variations

- Infants and children may lie supine with knees flexed toward the abdomen as the nurse inserts the rectal thermometer.

- It may be more accurate to measure pulse and respirations before temperature if the child becomes agitated during temperature taking.

- Glass thermometers are not the best choice for young children. Tympanic or chemical strip thermometers are much less invasive, and less anxiety producing.

- When using the chemical strip thermometer, allow the child to place the strip, and help you time the strip by holding your watch. Clean your watch before and after.

#### Geriatric Variations

- Geriatric clients may be confused and unable to follow directions; be attentive and give clear, concise instructions when taking an oral temperature.

- Elderly clients may be more comfortable lying on their side with legs slightly flexed when taking a rectal temperature. Keep one hand on the thermometer and one hand on the client's hip so that you can detect if he starts to roll over. Place a pillow at the client's back for extra support if needed.

- Baseline temperatures of elderly clients may be below the normal range; therefore increases should be compared to baseline.

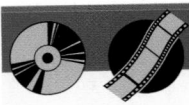

## PROCEDURE 27-1    Taking a Temperature

### EQUIPMENT NEEDED

- Thermometer (Figure 27-4)
  — Glass, oral, or rectal, at client's bedside
  — Electronic thermometer with disposable protective sheath
  — Tympanic membrane thermometer with probe cover
  — Disposable, single-use chemical strip thermometer
- Lubricant for rectal and glass thermometer
- Two pairs of nonsterile gloves
- Tissues

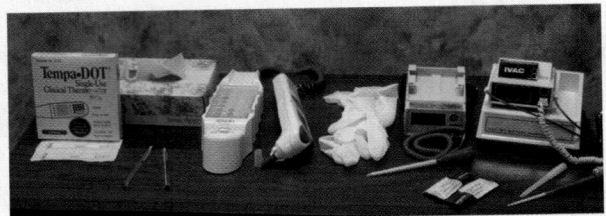

**Figure 27-4    Many types and brands of thermometers are available to assess temperature.**

### IMPLEMENTATION—ACTION/RATIONALE

| ACTION | RATIONALE |
|---|---|
| 1. Review medical record for baseline data and factors that influence vital signs. | 1. Establishes parameters for client's normal measurements, provides direction in device selection, and helps determine site to use for measurement. Vital signs are measured in the order of temperature, pulse, and respiration (TPR) and blood pressure (BP), usually without interruptions, so as to provide the nurse with an objective clinical database to direct decision making. |
| 2. Explain to the client that vital signs will be assessed. Encourage client to remain still and refrain from drinking, eating, and smoking. | 2. Encourages participation, allays anxiety, and ensures accurate measurements. Cold or hot liquids and smoking alter circulation and body temperature. |
| 3. Assess client's toileting needs and proceed as appropriate. | 3. Prevents interruptions during measurements, communicates caring, and promotes client comfort. |
| 4. Gather equipment. | 4. Facilitates organized assessment and measurement. |
| 5. Provide for privacy. | 5. Decreases embarrassment. |
| 6. Wash hands and apply gloves. | 6. Hands are washed before and after every contact with a client to reduce the transmission of microorganisms. Gloves are worn to avoid contact with bodily secretions and to reduce transmission of microorganisms. |
| 7. Position the client in a sitting or lying position with the head of the bed elevated 45°–60° for measurement of all vital signs except those designated otherwise. | 7. Promotes comfort and improves site access for all measurements. Activity and movement can elevate heart and respiratory rates. |
| 8. Remove gloves and wash hands. | 8. Reduces transmission of microorganisms. |

*(continues)*

### Oral Temperature: Glass Thermometer

9. Select correct color tip of thermometer from client's bedside container (Figure 27-5).

9. Identifies correct device.

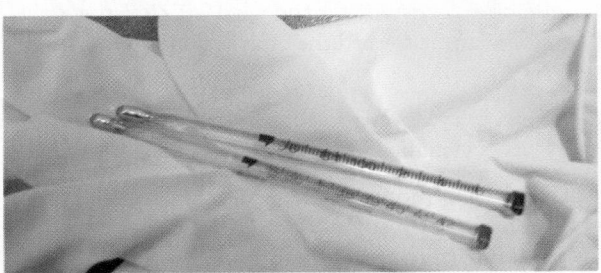

**Figure 27-5    Oral (blue tip) and rectal (red tip) glass thermometers.**

10. Remove thermometer from storage container and cleanse under cool water.

10. Cleansing removes disinfectant, which can irritate oral mucosa. Cool water prevents expansion of the mercury.

11. Use a tissue to dry thermometer from bulb's end toward fingertips.

11. Wipe from area of least contamination to most contaminated area.

12. Read thermometer by locating mercury level. It should read 35.5°C (96°F).

12. Thermometer must be below normal body temperature to ensure an accurate reading.

13. If thermometer is not below normal body temperature reading, grasp thermometer with thumb and forefinger and shake vigorously by snapping the wrist in a downward motion to move mercury to a level below normal.

13. Shaking briskly lowers level of mercury in column. Because glass thermometers break easily, make sure that nothing in the environment comes in contact with the thermometer when shaking it.

14. Place thermometer in client's mouth under the tongue and along the gumline to the posterior sublingual pocket. Instruct client to hold lips closed (Figure 27-6).

14. Ensures contact with large blood vessels under the tongue. Prevents environmental air from coming in contact with the bulb.

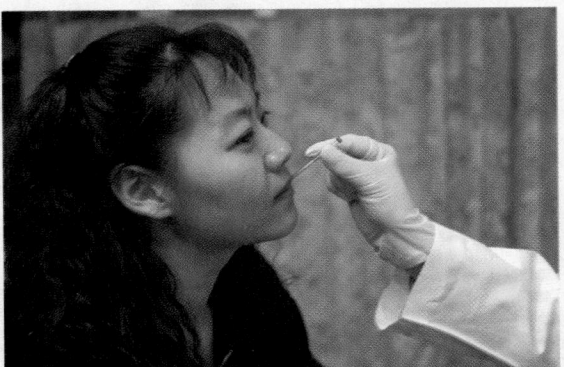

**Figure 27-6    Place bulb of thermometer in the posterior sublingual pocket. Have client close mouth around thermometer.**

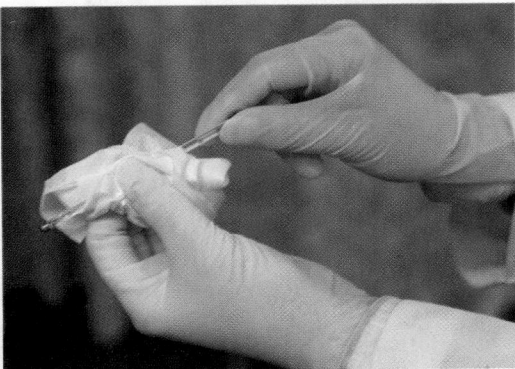

**Figure 27-7    Wipe the thermometer with a tissue from the fingers toward the bulb.**

*(continues)*

15. Leave in place as specified by agency policy, usually 3–5 minutes.

16. Remove thermometer and wipe with a tissue away from fingers toward the bulb's end (Figure 27-7).

17. Read at eye level and rotate slowly until mercury level is visualized.

18. Shake thermometer down, and cleanse glass thermometer with soapy water, rinse under cold water, and return to storage container.

19. Remove and dispose of gloves in receptacle. Wash hands.

20. Record reading and indicate site as "OT."

21. Wash hands.

### Oral Temperature: Electronic Thermometer

22. Repeat Actions 1 to 8.

23. Place disposable protective sheath over probe (Figure 27-8).

24. Grasp top of the probe's stem. Avoid placing pressure on the ejection button.

25. Place tip of thermometer under the client's tongue and along the gumline to the posterior sublingual pocket lateral to center of lower jaw (Figure 27-9).

15. Thermometer must stay in place long enough to ensure an accurate reading.

16. Mucus on thermometer may interfere with disinfectant solution's effectiveness. Wipe from area of least contamination to most contaminated area.

17. Ensures an accurate reading.

18. Mechanical cleansing removes secretions that promote growth of microorganisms. Hot water may cause coagulation of secretions and cause expansion of mercury in thermometer.

19. Reduces transmission of microorganisms.

20. Accurate documentation by site allows for comparison of data.

21. Reduces transmission of microorganisms.

22. See Rationales 1 to 8.

23. Reduces transmission of microorganisms.

24. Pressure on the ejection button releases the sheath from the probe.

25. Sublingual pocket contains superficial blood vessels.

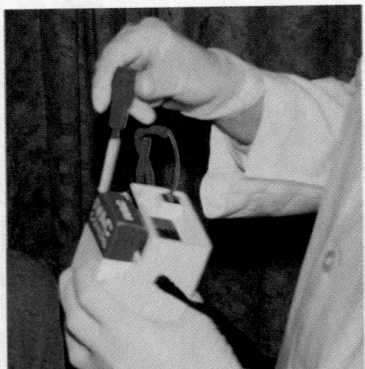

**Figure 27-8** **Place disposable sheath over probe.**

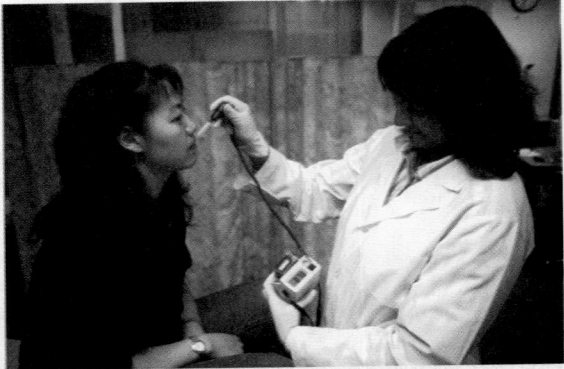

**Figure 27-9** **Place probe tip in the posterior sublingual pocket.**

26. Instruct client to keep mouth closed around thermometer.

26. Maintains thermometer in proper place and decreases amount of time required for an accurate reading.

*(continues)*

**PROCEDURE 27-1 (*continued*)**

27. Thermometer will signal (beep) when a constant temperature registers (Figure 27-10).

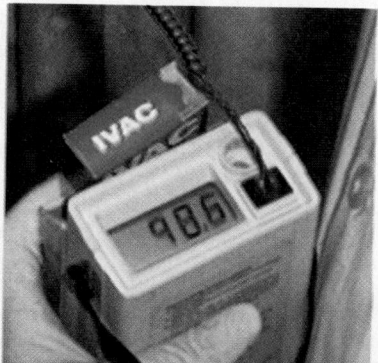

**Figure 27-10   Listen for audible beep signal when temperature registers.**

28. Read measurement on digital display of electronic thermometer. Push ejection button to discard disposable sheath into receptacle and return probe to storage well.

29. Inform client of temperature reading.

30. Remove gloves and wash hands.

31. Record reading and indicate site "OT."

32. Return electronic thermometer unit to charging base.

33. Wash hands.

### Rectal Temperature

34. Repeat Actions 1 to 8.

35. Place client in the Sims' position with upper knee flexed. Adjust sheet to expose only anal area.

36. Place tissues in easy reach. Apply gloves.

37. Prepare the thermometer.

38. Lubricate tip of rectal thermometer or probe (a rectal thermometer usually has a red cap).

39. With dominant hand, grasp thermometer. With other hand, separate buttocks to expose anus (Figure 27-11).

40. Instruct client to take a deep breath. Insert thermometer or probe gently into anus: infant, 1.2 cm (0.5 inches); adult, 3.5 cm (1.5 inches). If resistance is felt, do not force insertion.

27. Signal indicates final temperature reading.

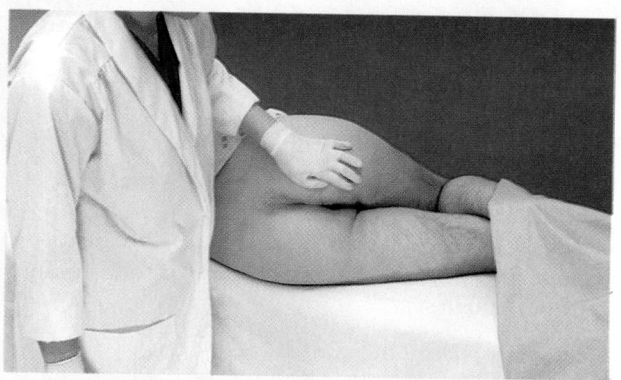

**Figure 27-11   Preparation for the insertion of a rectal thermometer**

28. Reduces transmission of microorganisms. Ensures that the electronic system is ready for next use.

29. Promotes client's participation in care.

30. Reduces transmission of microorganisms.

31. Accurate documentation by site allows for comparison of data.

32. Ensures charging base is plugged into electrical outlet and ready for next use.

33. Reduces transmission of microorganisms.

34. See Rationales 1 to 8.

35. Proper positioning ensures visualization of anus. Flexing knee relaxes muscles for ease of insertion.

36. Tissue is needed to wipe anus after device is removed.

37. Ensures a smooth procedure and an accurate reading.

38. Promotes ease of insertion of thermometer or probe.

39. Aids in visualization of anus.

40. Relaxes anal sphincter. Gentle insertion decreases discomfort to client and prevents trauma to mucous membranes.

(*continues*)

## PROCEDURE 27-1 (continued)

**41.** Hold in place for 2 minutes.

**41.** Prevents trauma to mucosa and breakage of glass thermometer.

**42.** Wipe secretions off glass thermometer with a tissue. Dispose of tissue in a receptacle.

**42.** Removes secretions and fecal material for visualization of mercury level. Prevents transmission of microorganisms.

**43.** Read measurement and inform client of temperature reading.

**43.** Promotes client's participation in care.

**44.** While holding glass thermometer in one hand, use other hand to wipe anal area with tissue to remove lubricant or feces. Dispose of soiled tissue. Cover client.

**44.** Prevents contamination of clean objects with soiled thermometer, decreases skin irritation, and promotes client comfort. Prevents embarrassment.

**45.** Cleanse thermometer.

**45.** Reduces transmission of microorganisms.

**46.** Remove and dispose of gloves in receptacle. Wash hands.

**46.** Reduces transmission of microorganisms.

**47.** Record reading and indicate site as "RT."

**47.** Accurate documentation by site allows for comparison of data.

### Axillary Temperature

**48.** Repeat Actions 1 to 8.

**48.** See Rationales 1 to 8.

**49.** Remove client's arm and shoulder from one sleeve of gown. Avoid exposing chest.

**49.** Exposes axillary area.

**50.** Make sure axillary skin is dry; if necessary, pat dry.

**50.** Removes moisture and prevents a false low reading.

**51.** Prepare thermometer.

**51.** Ensures accurate use of thermometer.

**52.** Place thermometer or probe into center of axilla. Fold client's upper arm straight down and place arm across client's chest.

**52.** Puts device in contact with axillary blood supply. Maintains the device in proper position.

**53.** Leave glass thermometer in place as specified by agency policy (usually 6 to 8 minutes). Leave an electronic thermometer in place until signal is heard.

**53.** Device must stay in place long enough to ensure an accurate reading. Signal indicates final temperature reading.

**54.** Remove and read thermometer.

**54.** Allows accurate reading of temperature.

**55.** Inform client of temperature reading.

**55.** Promotes client's participation in care.

**56.** Cleanse glass thermometer. Shake thermometer down, and cleanse glass thermometer with soapy water, rinse under cold water, and return to storage container.

**56.** Prevents transmission of microorganisms and breakage of glass thermometer.

**57.** Assist client with replacing gown.

**57.** Promotes comfort.

**58.** Record reading and indicate site as "AT."

**58.** Promotes accurate documentation for data comparison.

**59.** Wash hands.

**59.** Reduces transmission of microorganisms.

*(continues)*

## PROCEDURE 27-1 (*continued*)

### Disposable (Chemical Strip) Thermometer

**60.** Repeat Actions 1 to 8.

**61.** Apply tape to appropriate skin area, usually forehead.

**62.** Observe tape for color changes.

**63.** Record reading and indicate method. Remove and discard tape.

**64.** Wash hands.

### Tympanic Temperature: Infrared Thermometer

**65.** Repeat Actions 1 to 8.

**66.** Position client in seated or Sims' position.

**67.** Remove probe from container and attach probe cover to tympanic thermometer unit (Figure 27-12).

**68.** Turn client's head to one side. For an adult, pull pinna upward and back; for a child, pull down and back. Gently insert probe with firm pressure into ear canal (Figure 27-13).

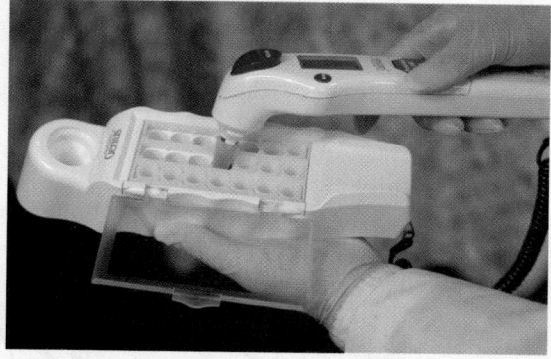

**Figure 27-12** Attach disposable probe cover to unit.

**69.** Remove probe after the reading is displayed on digital unit (usually 2 seconds).

**70.** Remove probe cover and replace in storage container.

**71.** Return tympanic thermometer to storage unit.

**72.** Record reading and indicate site as "ET."

**73.** Wash hands.

**60.** See Rationales 1 to 8.

**61.** Tape must be in direct contact with the client's skin.

**62.** Color indicates temperature reading (refer to the manufacturer's instructions).

**63.** Promotes accurate documentation for data comparison.

**64.** Reduces transmission of microorganisms.

**65.** See Rationales 1 to 8.

**66.** Promotes access to ear.

**67.** Prevents contamination.

**68.** Provides access to ear canal. Gentle insertion prevents trauma to external canal. Firm pressure is needed to ensure probe will record an accurate temperature.

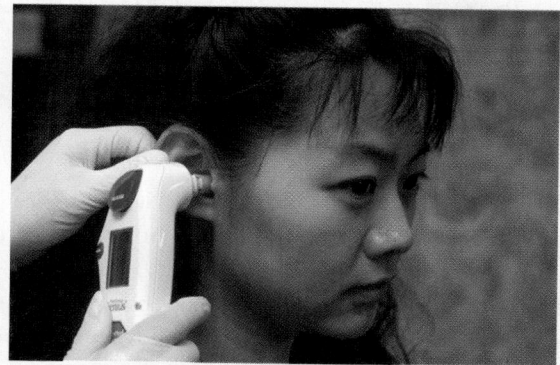

**Figure 27-13** Insert temperature probe into ear canal.

**69.** Reading is displayed within seconds.

**70.** Protects damage to the reusable probe.

**71.** Recharges batteries of unit for future use.

**72.** Promotes accurate documentation for data comparison.

**73.** Reduces transmission of microorganisms.

## COMMUNITY/HOME CARE

### Temperature Measurements in the Home Environment

#### Home Care Variations

- Working equipment may not be available in the home care setting. The nurse should come prepared with working equipment, including a thermometer appropriate to the client.

- The temperature and ventilation of the room may affect the client's temperature.

#### Long-Term Care Variations

- Long-term care clients more often have physical limitations that must be considered when choosing the route to use in measuring the internal temperature. When considering route in a long-term care client, consider the possibility of a stoma where the rectum has been surgically closed or perhaps severe contractures that would make client positioning and cooperation difficult and painful.

##  LIFE SPAN CONSIDERATIONS

### Temperature Regulation

Infants and older clients have ineffective or altered thermal regulation. Infants produce body heat but are unable to conserve heat produced. Thus, environmental temperatures affect their body temperature. Older clients respond poorly to environmental temperature extremes due to altered circulation, decreased heat-producing activities, altered sensations, and structural and functional changes in the skin.

McCance, K. L., & Heuther, S. E. (2002). *Pathophysiology: The biologic basis for disease in adults and children* (4th ed.). St. Louis: Mosby.

## Pulse

Pulse assessment is the measurement of a pressure pulsation created when the heart contracts and ejects blood into the aorta. Assessment of pulse characteristics pro-

vides clinical data regarding the heart's pumping action and the adequacy of peripheral artery blood flow.

### Sites

There are multiple pulse points (Figure 27-3). The most accessible peripheral pulses are the radial and carotid sites. Because the body shunts blood to the brain whenever a cardiac emergency such as hemorrhage occurs, the carotid site should always be used to assess the pulse in these situations.

Variances exist among health care agencies regarding which pulse sites to assess. The common sites for each type of assessment are:

- Complete physical assessment—apical and all bilateral peripheral pulses
- Initial assessment—apical and bilateral peripheral radial and dorsalis pedis pulses
- Routine vital sign assessment—apical and radial pulses in adults and apical and temporal pulses in infants and children

Disorders that alter the client's cardiovascular status require different pulse point assessments (Table 27-7). Whenever circulation is compromised, the corresponding pulse point should be assessed.

### Assessing Pulse Rate

The nurse should begin the assessment by speaking with the client about the normal pulse rate. The client's medical record should be reviewed for baseline data, if available, and any medications that could affect the heart rate should be noted. Because physical activity increases the heart rate, ensure that the client rests 5 to 10 minutes before the pulse is assessed.

Clinical data regarding the efficacy of blood circulation to an extremity are obtained by assessing the characteristics (quality, rate, rhythm, and volume) of the peripheral pulses. These attributes are described in the section entitled Pulse Characteristics. Palpate a peripheral pulse by placing the first two fingers on the pulse point with moderate pressure. A firm pressure will obliterate the pulse; if the pressure is too light, the pulse cannot be felt.

A Doppler ultrasound stethoscope (DUS) is used on superficial pulse points to detect and magnify heart sounds and pulse waves when the peripheral pulse cannot be palpated. The DUS, which has an earpiece similar to that of a stethoscope, is connected by a cord to a volume-control audio unit with an ultrasound transducer.

Normal radial and apical pulses are identical in rate. The stethoscope is used to auscultate the heart's rate and rhythm. The stethoscope should be placed on the fifth intercostal space at the midclavicular line. Count the rate for a full minute, noting the regularity (rhythm).

## TABLE 27-7    PULSE POINT ASSESSMENT

| Pulse Point | Assessment Criteria |
| --- | --- |
| Temporal: over temporal bone, superior and lateral to eye | Accessible; used routinely for infants and when radial is inaccessible |
| Carotid: bilateral, under lower jaw in neck along medial edge of sterno-cleidomastoid muscle | Accessible; used routinely for infants and during shock or cardiac arrest when other peripheral pulses are too weak to palpate; also used to assess cranial circulation |
| Apical: left midclavicular line at fourth to fifth intercostal space | Used to auscultate heart sounds and assess apical-radial deficit |
| Brachial: inner aspect between groove of biceps and triceps muscles at antecubital fossa | Used in cardiac arrest for infants, to assess lower arm circulation, and to auscultate blood pressure |
| Radial: inner aspect of forearm on thumb side of wrist | Accessible; used routinely in adults to assess character of peripheral pulse |
| Ulnar: outer aspect of forearm on finger side of wrist | Used to assess circulation to ulnar side of hand and to perform the Allen's test |
| Femoral: in groin, below inguinal ligament (midpoint between symphysis pubis and anterosuperior iliac spine) | Used to assess circulation to legs and during cardiac arrest |
| Popliteal: behind knee, at center in popliteal fossa | Used to assess circulation to legs and to auscultate leg blood pressure |
| Posterior tibial: inner aspect of ankle between Achilles tendon and tibia (below medial malleolus) | Used to assess circulation to feet |
| Dorsalis pedis: over instep, midpoint between extension tendons of great and second toe | Used to assess circulation to feet |

## CLINICAL ALERT

### Carotid Pulse Assessment

When assessing a carotid pulse, apply light pressure to only one carotid artery to avoid disruption of cerebral blood flow.

apical and radial pulses for a minute. This procedure is usually performed by two nurses; however, it can be performed by one nurse if necessary.

### Pulse Characteristics

A normal pulse has defined characteristics: quality, rate, rhythm, and volume (strength or amplitude). **Pulse quality** refers to the "feel" of the pulse, its rhythm and forcefulness.

**Pulse rate** is an indirect measurement of cardiac output obtained by counting the number of apical or peripheral pulse waves over a pulse point. A normal pulse rate for adults is between 60 and 100 beats per minute. **Bradycardia** is a heart rate less than 60 beats per minute in an adult. **Tachycardia** is a heart rate in excess of 100 beats per minute in an adult.

**Pulse rhythm** is the regularity of the heartbeat. It describes how evenly the heart is beating: regular (the beats are evenly spaced) or irregular (the beats are not evenly spaced). Dysrhythmia (arrhythmia) is an irregular rhythm caused by an early, late, or missed heartbeat.

**Pulse volume** is a measurement of the strength or amplitude of force exerted by the ejected blood against the arterial wall with each contraction. The pulse volume is normally the same with each beat. It is described as normal (full, easily palpable), weak (thready and usually rapid), or strong (bounding). There are various scales for measuring pulse volume. To facilitate data comparison of this measurement, a standard pulse volume scale should be used. Box 27-10 on page 577 contains the two most commonly used scales. Procedure 27-2 describes the actions and rationale involved with assessing pulse rate and characteristics.

### Nursing Considerations

An irregular pulse rate, if not previously documented in the medical record, should be reported immediately. The following equipment is used to identify the type of dysrhythmia causing the irregular heartbeat:

- Electrocardiogram (ECG or EKG) provides an electrical representation of the heart's activity. The primary pacemaker of the heart is the sinoatrial (SA) node. If another site within the heart initiates the electrical activity, the ECG tracing will identify the area serving as the pacemaker.
- A Holter monitor is a portable device worn for a 24-hour interval to identify the dysrhythmia pattern.
- Cardiac telemetry transmits the heart's electrical activity to a site for continuous monitoring.

When an irregular peripheral pulse is present, the nurse needs to assess for a **pulse deficit** (condition in which the apical pulse rate is greater than the radial pulse rate). A pulse deficit results from the ejection of a volume of blood that is too small to initiate a peripheral pulse wave. When a discrepancy exists between the apical and radial pulses, the deficit is assessed by simultaneously measuring the

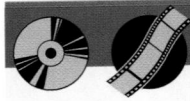

## PROCEDURE 27-2    Taking a Pulse

### EQUIPMENT NEEDED

- Watch with a second hand (Figure 27-14)
- Stethoscope
- Alcohol swab
- Gloves

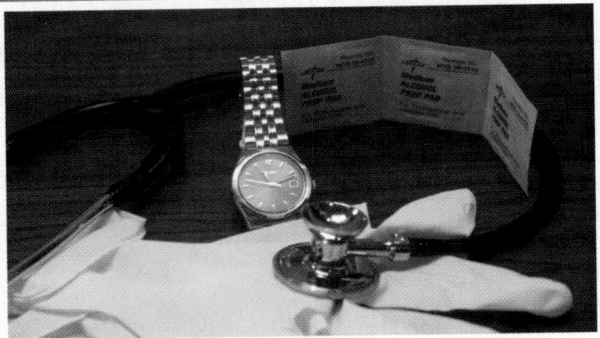

**Figure 27-14    A watch with a second hand is used to count pulse. Use a stethoscope to assess apical pulse. Gloves and alcohol swabs reduce the transmission of microorganisms.**

## IMPLEMENTATION—ACTION/RATIONALE

| ACTION | RATIONALE |
|---|---|
| **Taking a Radial (Wrist) Pulse** | |
| 1. Wash hands. | 1. Reduces transmission of microorganisms. |
| 2. Inform client of the site(s) at which you will measure pulse. | 2. Encourages participation and allays anxiety. |
| 3. Flex client's elbow and place lower part of arm across chest. | 3. Maintains wrist in full extension and exposes artery for palpation. Placing client's hand over chest will facilitate later respiratory assessment without undue attention to your action. (It is difficult for any person to maintain a normal breathing pattern when someone is observing and measuring.) |
| 4. Support client's wrist by grasping outer aspect with thumb. | 4. Stabilizes wrist and allows for pressure to be exerted. |
| 5. Place your index and middle finger on inner aspect of client's wrist over the radial artery and apply light but firm pressure until pulse is palpated (Figure 27-15). | 5. Fingertips are sensitive, facilitating palpation of pulsating pulse. Feel your own pulse if palpating with thumb. Applying light pressure prevents occlusion of blood flow and pulsation. |
| 6. Identify pulse rhythm. | 6. Palpate pulse until rhythm is determined. Describe as regular or irregular. |
| 7. Determine pulse volume. | 7. Quality of pulse strength is an indication of stroke volume. Describe as normal, weak, strong, or bounding. |
| 8. Count pulse rate by using second hand on watch (Figure 27-16). | 8. An irregular rhythm requires a full minute of assessment to identify the number of inefficient cardiac contractions that fail to transmit a pulsation, referred to as a "skipped" or irregular beat. |

*(continues)*

## PROCEDURE 27-2 (continued)

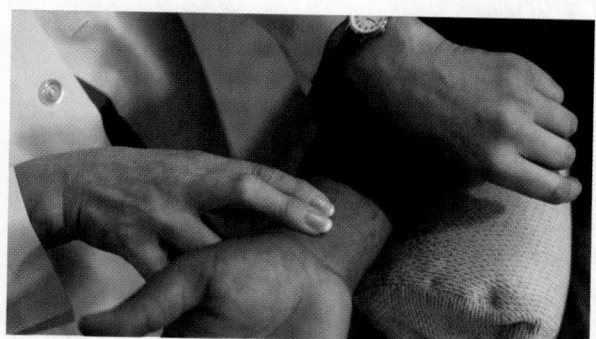

**Figure 27-15** Place index and middle fingers over radial artery.

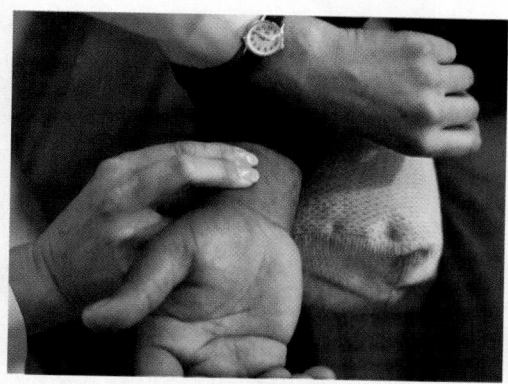

**Figure 27-16** Count pulse rate for 30 seconds. Multiply by 2.

For a regular rhythm, count number of beats for 30 seconds and multiply by 2.

For an irregular rhythm, count number of beats for a full minute, noting number of irregular beats.

### Taking an Apical Pulse

9. Wash hands.

10. Cleanse earpiece and diaphragm of stethoscope with an alcohol swab.

11. Put stethoscope around your neck.

12. Raise client's gown to expose sternum and left side of chest.

13. Locate apex of heart:
    - With client lying on left side, locate suprasternal notch.
    - Palpate second intercostal space to left of sternum.
    - Place index finger in intercostal space, counting downward until fifth intercostal space is located.
    - Move index finger along fourth intercostal space left of the sternal border and to the fifth intercostal space, left of the midclavicular line to palpate the point of maximal impulse (PMI) (Figure 27-17).
    - Keep index finger of nondominant hand on the PMI.

14. Inform client that you are going to listen to his heart. Instruct client to remain silent.

15. With dominant hand, put earpiece of the stethoscope in your ears and grasp diaphragm of the stethoscope in palm of your hand for 5 to 10 seconds.

9. Reduces transmission of microorganisms.

10. Decreases transmission of microorganisms from one practitioner to another (earpiece) and from one client to another (diaphragm).

11. Ensures stethoscope is nearby for frequent use.

12. Allows access to client's chest for proper placement of stethoscope.

13. Identification of landmarks facilitates correct placement of the stethoscope at the fifth intercostal space in order to hear point of maximal impulse.
    - Ensures correct placement of stethoscope.

14. Elicits client support. Stethoscope amplifies noise.

15. Dominant hand facilitates psychomotor dexterity for placement of earpiece with one hand. Heat warms metal or plastic diaphragm and prevents startling client.

*(continues)*

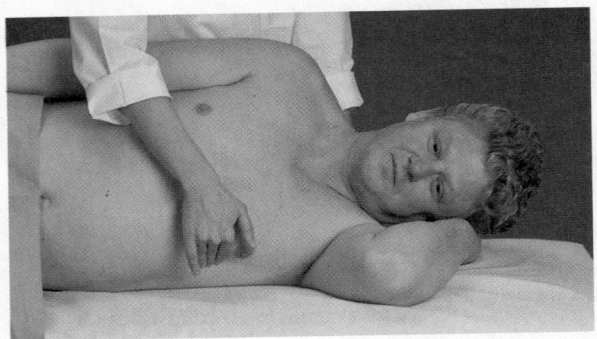

**Figure 27-17**   **Palpating the apical pulse**

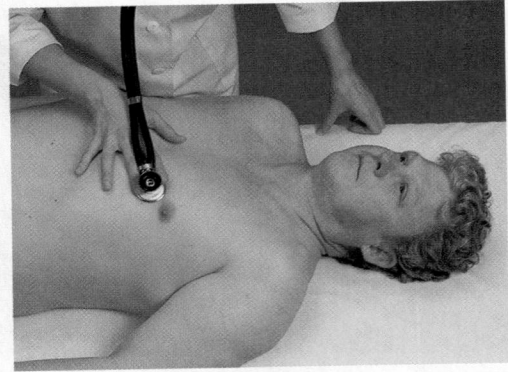

**Figure 27-18**   **Place diaphragm of stethoscope over the PMI to hear the heart rate.**

16. Place diaphragm of stethoscope over the PMI and auscultate for sounds $S_1$ and $S_2$ to hear lub-dub sound (Figure 27-18).

16. Movement of blood through the heart valves creates $S_1$ and $S_2$ sounds. Listen for a regular rhythm (heartbeats are evenly spaced) before counting.

17. Note regularity of rhythm.

17. Establishment of a rhythmic pattern determines length of time to count the heartbeats to ensure accurate measurement.

18. Start to count while looking at second hand of watch. Count lub-dub sound as one beat:
    • For a regular rhythm, count rate for 30 seconds and multiply by 2.
    • For an irregular rhythm, count rate for a full minute, noting number of irregular beats.

18. Ensures sufficient time to count irregular beats.

19. Share your findings with client.

19. Promotes client participation in care.

20. Record by site the rate, rhythm, and, if applicable, number of irregular beats.

20. Record rate and characteristics at bedside to ensure accurate documentation.

21. Wash hands.

21. Reduces transmission of microorganisms.

Clients on certain cardiac medications, such as cardiovascular agents and cardiac glycosides, need to monitor their pulse rate. Clients receiving cardiovascular agents (verapamil hydrochloride) and cardiac glycosides (digoxin) may experience an irregular pulse or pulse rate change that should be reported to their physician. In addition, clients who follow an exercise regimen should assess their pulse rate to measure their heart's response to the exercise. Routine or regular exercise lowers the resting and activity pulses. When teaching clients how to monitor their own heart rate, nurses should show them the procedure in assessing the radial or carotid pulse points.

### Documentation

All pulse measurements are documented by recording in the client's medical record on the appropriate forms (e.g., the vital sign flow sheet). Documentation of pulses should include site, rate, rhythm, pulse volume, and instrumentation if other than a stethoscope. If the pulse rhythm is irregular, describe the dysrhythmia (irregularity). Dysrhythmias may consist of irregular beats that

## BOX 27-10    PULSE VOLUME SCALE

### 3-Point Scale

| Scale | Description of Pulse |
|-------|----------------------|
| 0 | absent |
| 1+ | weak and thready |
| 2+ | normal |
| 3+ | bounding |

### 4-Point Scale

| Scale | Description of Pulse |
|-------|----------------------|
| 0 | absent |
| 1+ | weak and thready |
| 2+ | normal |
| 3+ | increased |
| 4+ | bounding |

Guyton, A., & Hall, J. E. (2001). *Textbook of medical physiology* (10th ed.). Philadelphia: W. B. Saunders Company.

## LIFE SPAN CONSIDERATIONS

### Taking Pulses Across the Life Span

**Pediatric Variations**

- Radial pulses on infants are not reliable because of the small size of the client and the rapid heart rate normal in infants. A temporal or apical pulse is preferable.

- The PMI in an infant is usually located at the third to fourth intercostal space near the sternum.

- A child may be more comfortable sitting on her parent's lap while having her pulse assessed.

- A curious child may be more cooperative if she can listen to her own heart with a stethoscope.

**Geriatric Variations**

- Tremors in geriatric clients can interfere with evaluating the radial pulse accurately.

- An apical or carotid pulse might be the better option in older clients.

## COMMUNITY/HOME CARE

### Obtaining Pulses in Different Settings

**Home Care Variations**

- The home care environment can be distracting for the nurse and the client. The television and loud music can make it difficult to hear an apical pulse and can artificially elevate the client's pulse rate.

- Be sure that the client is sitting or lying quietly before taking her pulse.

- Clients can be taught to assess their own pulse especially when taking cardiac medications.

**Long-Term Care Variations**

- The relative immobility of most long-term care clients puts them at risk of decreased peripheral circulation. Pedal pulses are an important part of the nursing examination in long-term care clients.

either are random or are present in a regular pattern. Immediately report any newly identified dysrhythmia and its characteristics to the client's physician (Estes, 2002).

## Respirations

Respiratory assessment is the measurement of the breathing pattern. Respirations should be assessed in every vital sign evaluation. A baseline should be established so comparisons can be made. A respiratory assessment can provide valuable information about a client's physical or emotional health.

### Sites

Normal breathing is slightly observable, effortless, quiet, automatic, and regular. It can be assessed by observing chest wall expansion and bilateral symmetrical movement of the thorax. Another method the nurse can use to assess breathing is to place the back of the hand next to the client's nose and mouth to feel the expired air.

### Assessing Respirations

When assessing respirations, ascertain the rate, depth, and rhythm of ventilatory movement. The nurse should assess the rate by counting the number of breaths taken per minute. Note the depth and rhythm of ventilatory movements by observing for the normal thoracic and abdominal movements and symmetry in chest wall movement. Normal respirations are characterized by a rate ranging from 12 to 20 breaths per minute. Procedure 27-3 describes the actions involved in assessing respirations.

One inspiration and expiration cycle is counted as one breath. The nurse should observe the rise and fall of the chest wall and count the rate by placing the hand lightly on the chest to feel its rise and fall.

### Movement of the Diaphragm

When the chest wall moves, so do the lungs, because the lungs are attached to the inner wall of the thoracic cavity by the outer layer of the **pleura** (lining of the chest cavity). The movement of the chest wall should be even and regular, without noise and effort. On inspiration the chest changes shape and expands as the rib cage is raised and the diaphragm is lowered. Before inspiration, the pressure inside the chest cavity is negative (–4.5 to –9.0 mm Hg below atmospheric pressure). Air flows along the concentration gradient from a higher atmospheric pressure to the lower intrathoracic pressure.

The opposite action occurs with expiration. The muscles relax, causing the rib cage to lower, and the diaphragm to rise, compressing the chest. Intrathoracic pressure decreases to –3 to –6 mm Hg to allow the air to escape into the atmosphere.

### Characteristics of Normal and Abnormal Breath Sounds

Different respiratory wave patterns are characterized by their rate, rhythm, and depth.

**Rate**    Respiratory rate is measured in breaths per minute. One respiratory cycle consists of one inhalation and one expiration. Respiratory rates vary for different age groups, with newborns averaging 40 breaths per minute to adults averaging 18 breaths per minute. Anxiety, exercise, medications, fever, and altitude may affect respiratory rate. **Eupnea** refers to respirations that are easy with a normal rate of breaths per minute that are age-specific. **Bradypnea** is a respiratory rate of 10 or fewer breaths per minute. **Tachypnea** is a respiratory rate greater than 24

breaths per minute. **Apnea** is the absence of breathing (White & Duncan, 2002).

**Rhythm**    The rhythm (or pattern) of respirations is evaluated for regularity or irregularity. Normal respirations are regular and even in rhythm. However, there are a wide variety of rhythms that exist in relation to different pathologies. For example, head injuries may cause an irregular respiratory rhythm (Cheyne-Stoke respirations) or a diabetic complication can cause a client to breath deep and rapid (Kussmaul breathing).

**Depth**    The depth of each respiration is normally about the same during rest. The depth of respirations normally varies from shallow to deep. **Hypoventilation** is characterized by shallow, slow respirations. **Hyperventilation** is characterized by deep, rapid respirations.

**Chest Wall Movements**    The nurse can also observe alterations in the movement of the chest wall: **costal (thoracic) breathing** occurs when the external intercostal muscles and the other accessory muscles are used to move the chest upward and outward; **diaphragmatic (abdominal) breathing** occurs when the diaphragm contracts and relaxes as observed by movement of the abdomen. **Dyspnea** refers to difficulty in breathing as observed by labored or forced respirations through the use of accessory muscles in the chest and neck to breathe. Dyspneic clients are acutely aware of their respirations and complain of shortness of breath.

### Nursing Considerations

Respiratory alterations may cause changes in skin color as observed by a bluish appearance in the nailbeds, lips, and skin. The bluish color (**cyanosis**) results from reduced oxygen levels in the arterial blood. Changes in the level of consciousness may also occur with decreased oxygen levels. Dyspneic clients will assume a forward-leaning position to increase the expansion capacity of the lungs.

Clients with respiratory alterations require additional nursing assessment. Noninvasive oxygen assessment can be performed with an **oximeter** (a machine that measures the oxygen saturation of the blood through a probe clipped to the fingernail or earlobe) or an **apnea monitor** (a machine with chest leads that monitors the movement of the chest). Both noninvasive machines have alarm features that are set to specific parameters. For example, if the client's respirations fall below 6 breaths per minute, the apnea monitor alarm will sound. The apnea monitor is used in the home environment for apneic clients; when the alarm sounds, it wakes the person and causes him to breathe.

**Pulse oximetry** offers a noninvasive means for approximating oxygenation saturation. Because of its safety and noninvasiveness, it is routinely used in various health care settings and in the home-care setting to spot and trend arterial oxygen saturation. Experience and clinical judgment help the skilled practitioner relate oximetry readings

**PROCEDURE 27-3**    **Counting Respirations**

## EQUIPMENT NEEDED

■ Watch with a second hand (Figure 27-19)          ■ Stethoscope if needed

## IMPLEMENTATION—ACTION/RATIONALE

| ACTION | RATIONALE |
|---|---|
| 1. Wash hands. | 1. Reduces transmission of microorganisms. |
| 2. Be sure chest movement is visible. Client may need to remove heavy clothing. | 2. Facilitates observation of chest wall and abdominal movements. |
| 3. Observe one complete respiratory cycle. If it is easier, place the client's hand across her abdomen and your hand over the client's wrist. | 3. Helps determine what constitutes a breath. Helps to determine what to count. Hand rises and falls with inspiration and expiration. |
| 4. Start counting with first inspiration while looking at the second hand of a watch (Figure 27-20). <br> • Infants and children: count a full minute. <br> • Adults: count for 30 seconds and multiply by 2. If an irregular rate or rhythm is present, count for 1 full minute. | 4. Respiratory rate is one complete cycle (inspiration and expiration). <br><br> • Infants and children usually have an irregular rate. |

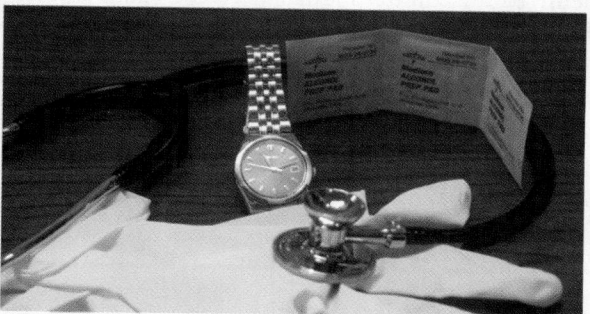

**Figure 27-19**   A watch with a second hand is used to assess respirations.

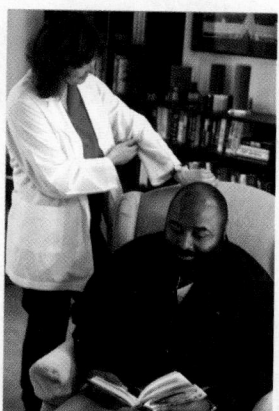

**Figure 27-20**   Count inspirations for a full 30 seconds.

| | |
|---|---|
| 5. Observe character of respirations: <br> • Depth of respirations by degree of chest wall movement (shallow, normal, or deep) <br> • Rhythm of cycle (regular or interrupted) | 5. Reveals volume of air movement into and out of the lungs. |
| 6. Replace client's gown if needed. | 6. Prevents embarrassment and chilling. |
| 7. Record rate and character of respirations. | 7. Record rate and characteristics at bedside to ensure accurate documentation. |
| 8. Wash hands. | 8. Reduces transmission of microorganisms. |

## LIFE SPAN CONSIDERATIONS

### Evaluating Respirations

**Pediatric Variations**

- Counting respirations in small children should be done by observation.

- Give a small child a toy or something to distract her while you count her respirations.

- Infants or newborns at risk for respiratory arrest may need an apnea monitor at home.

**Geriatric Variations**

- Geriatric clients may be confused, restless, or eager to talk, so it may be difficult to get an opportunity to count quiet, at-rest respirations.

- Ask the client to sit quietly while you take her pulse or perhaps distract her with television or other activities.

to client condition. A range of 95% to 100% is considered normal oxygen saturation. Procedure 27-4 describes the actions involved in measuring oxygen saturation of the blood by using a pulse oximeter (Altman, 2004).

### Documentation

Document the assessment findings for the respiratory rate, depth, rhythm, and character on the appropriate form (e.g., the vital sign flow sheet). Report a respiratory rate outside the normal age range, an irregular rhythm,

inadequate depth, or any abnormal characteristics such as dyspnea.

## Blood Pressure

Blood pressure measurement is performed during a physical examination, at initial assessment, and as part of routine vital signs assessment. Depending on the client's condition, the blood pressure is measured by either a direct or an indirect technique. The direct method requires an invasive procedure in which an intravenous catheter with an electronic sensor is inserted into an artery and the artery-transmitted pressure on an electronic display unit is read. The indirect method requires use of the sphygmomanometer and stethoscope for auscultation and palpation as needed.

### Sites

The most common site for indirect blood pressure measurement is the client's arm over the brachial artery. When the client's condition prevents auscultation of the brachial artery, the nurse should assess the blood pressure in the forearm or leg sites (see Box 27-11).

When pressure measurements in the upper extremities are not accessible, the popliteal artery, located behind the knee, becomes the site of choice. The nurse can also assess the blood pressure in other sites, such as the radial artery in the forearm and the posterior tibial or dorsalis pedis artery in the lower leg. Because it is difficult to auscultate sounds over the radial, tibial, and dorsalis pedis arteries, these sites are usually palpated to obtain a systolic reading.

### Assessing Blood Pressure

Selecting the proper equipment and following procedural technique are basic to ensuring an accurate reading.

---

**PROCEDURE 27-4**     **Administering Pulse Oximetry**

### EQUIPMENT NEEDED

- Pulse oximeter (Figure 27-21)
- Alcohol wipe or soap and water
- Proper sensor
- Nail polish remover if necessary

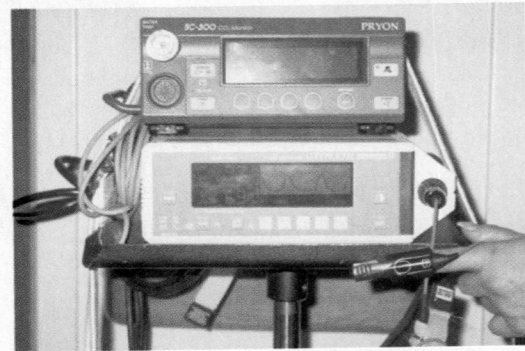

**Figure 27-21     Pulse oximeter**

*(continues)*

PROCEDURE 27-4 (continued)

## IMPLEMENTATION—ACTION/RATIONALE

| ACTION | RATIONALE |
|---|---|
| 1. Wash hands. | 1. Reduces the transmission of microorganisms. |
| 2. Select an appropriate sensor. Sensors are commonly used for the fingertips. | 2. The sensor should be selected based on the size of the person and the site to be used. |
| 3. Select an appropriate site for the sensor. Fingers are most commonly used; however, toes (Figure 27-22), ear lobes, nose, forehead (Figure 27-23), hands, and feet can be used. Assess for capillary refill and proximal pulse. If the client has poor circulation, use an earlobe, forehead, or nasal sensor instead. In children, sensors may be used on the hand, foot, or trunk. If elderly clients have thickened nails, pick another site. | 3. Decreased circulation alters the $O_2$ saturation measurement. |

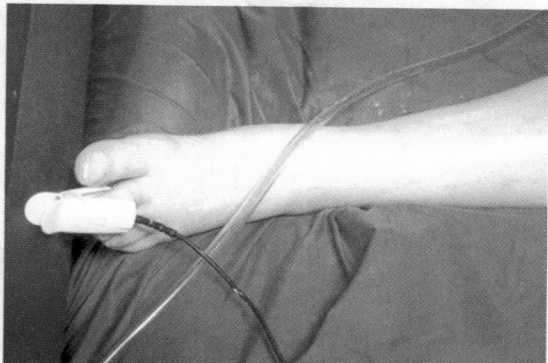

**Figure 27-22    Pulse oximeter sensor placed on a toe**

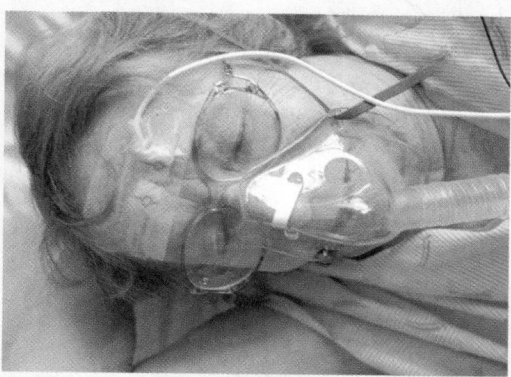

**Figure 27-23    Pulse oximeter sensor placed on the forehead**

| | |
|---|---|
| 4. Clean the site with an alcohol wipe. Remove artificial nails or nail polish if present or select another site. Clean any tape adhesive. Use soap and water if necessary to clean site. | 4. Polish and artificial fingernails alter the results. |
| 5. Apply the sensor. Make sure the photo detectors are aligned on opposite sides of the selected site (Figure 27-24). | 5. Proper application is necessary for accurate results. |
| 6. Connect the sensor to the oximeter with a sensor cable. Turn on the machine. Initially a tone can be heard, followed by an arterial wave-form fluctuation with each arterial pulse. In most oximeters if the battery is low, a low-battery light illuminates when 15 minutes of battery life is remaining. Oximeters should remain plugged in even when not in use (Figure 27-25). | 6. The tone and waveform fluctuation indicate that the machine is detecting blood flow with each arterial pulsation. |

*(continues)*

## PROCEDURE 27-4 (continued)

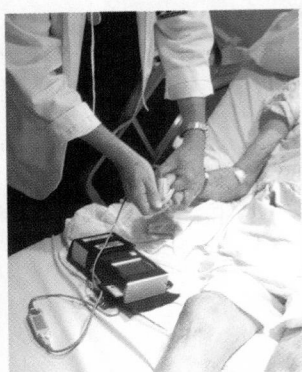

**Figure 27-24    Apply the sensor to the selected site.**

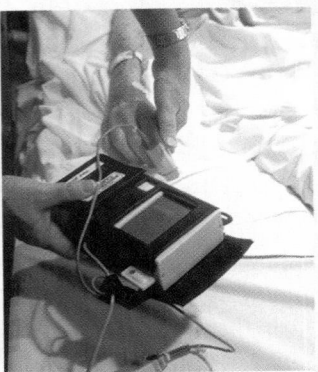

**Figure 27-25    Follow the manufacturer's instructions when taking an oximetry reading.**

7. Adjust the alarm limits for high and low $O_2$ saturation levels according to the manufacturer's directions. Pulse rate limits most often can also be set. Adjust volume.

7. The alarms indicate that the saturation levels or pulse rates are out of the designated levels and alert the nurse of abnormal $O_2$ saturation levels and pulse rates.

8. If taking a single reading, note the results (Figure 27-26). If the oximeter is being used for constant monitoring, move the site of spring sensors every 2 hours and adhesive sensors every 4 hours.

8. Prevents skin breakdown from pressure and skin irritation from the adhesive.

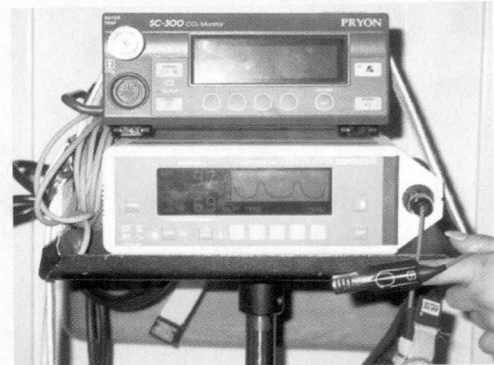

**Figure 27-26    Note the results on the oximeter.**

9. Cover the sensor with a sheet or towel to protect it from exposure to bright light.

9. Ambient light sources such as sunlight or warming lights may interfere with the sensor and alter the $SaO_2$ results.

10. Notify the physician or qualified practitioner of abnormal results.

10. Low $SaO_2$ levels require medical attention because permanent tissue damage may result from low oxygen saturation.

11. Record the results of $O_2$ saturation measurements according to physician's or qualified practitioner's order or protocol. Include in the documentation the type of sensor used, the site of application, the hemoglobin levels, and your assessment of the client's skin at the sensor site.

11. Communicates the findings to the other members of the health care team and contributes to the legal record by documenting the care given to the client.

## BOX 27-11    CONTRAINDICATIONS FOR BRACHIAL ARTERY BLOOD PRESSURE MEASUREMENT

When the client has any of the following, *do not* measure blood pressure on the involved side:

- Venous access devices, such as an intravenous infusion or arteriovenous fistula or graft for renal dialysis

- Surgery involving the breast, axilla, shoulder, arm, or hand

- Injury or disease to the shoulder, arm, or hand, such as trauma, burns, or application of a cast or bandage

---

## COMMUNITY/HOME CARE

### Pulse Oximeters in the Home

Because they are portable, pulse oximeters may be used in home care to monitor oxygen needs. When home care clients are to be monitored for oxygen saturation levels with exercise, it is imperative that the pulse oximetry reading is taken during or right after ambulation. Otherwise, the reading will not give a true picture of the client's oxygen requirements.

Hogstel, M. (2001). *Gerontology: Nursing care of the older adult.* Clifton Park, NY: Delmar Learning.

---

Psychomotor skills, acquired with practice, are needed to manipulate the blood pressure equipment. Procedure 27-5 describes the actions involved in assessing blood pressure.

A sphygmomanometer is a device used to measure indirect blood pressure. A sphygmomanometer consists of a mercury or aneroid manometer and a cuff that contains an inflatable rubber bladder connected to two pieces of rubber tubing. One piece of tubing connects the bladder to the manometer or gauge, and the second tubing is attached to a pressure bulb with a release valve to inflate

## LIFE SPAN CONSIDERATIONS

### Pulse Oximetry Variations

#### Pediatric Variations

- Finger sensors are generally not sized appropriately for children and hence not intended for neonatal or pediatric use. Adhesive sensors can be used on the hand or feet of children or on the hand of the neonate.

- Children may pull off sensors and activate alarms.

#### Geriatric Variations

- Elderly clients may have poor peripheral circulation and require other than finger sensors.

- Elderly clients may have thickened nails, which can lead to inaccurate readings if finger sensors are used.

---

and deflate the cuff. When pressure is applied to the bulb, air enters the bladder and inflates the cuff.

The sphygmomanometer wears with usage. If there is a defect in any part of the system, the blood pressure reading will be inaccurate. The aneroid gauge needle or mercury in the manometer column should be at a zero reading when the cuff is deflated and should rise evenly when pressure is applied to the bulb. The valve should turn freely and all tubing should be intact, with secured connections to prevent air from leaking out of the system.

An accurate reading also requires the correct width of the blood pressure cuff as determined by the circumference of the client's extremity. The bladder cuff must encircle the width and length of the site. According to the American Heart Association (1997), the bladder width should be approximately 40% of the circumference or 20% wider than the diameter of the midpoint of the extremity. To measure the width of the bladder, the nurse should place the cuff lengthwise on the client's extremity and extend the width to cover 40% of the extremity's circumference. The length of the sphygmomanometer bladder should be twice the width. Table 27-8 recommends bladder sizes based on different arm circumferences. A falsely elevated reading will result if the bladder is too narrow, and a falsely low reading will result if it is too wide.

Electronic sphygmomanometers are used by clients for self-measurements. A stethoscope is not required because the device electronically inflates and deflates the cuff while simultaneously reading and displaying the systolic and diastolic pressures. The electronic device is useful for clients who must monitor their own pressure at home. However, it must be recalibrated routinely to ensure an accurate reading.

### Auscultation

A stethoscope is used to auscultate the blood pressure (hear the sounds created by blood flowing through the artery). As presented in Procedure 27-5, the blood pressure cuff is inflated 30 mm Hg higher than the palpated

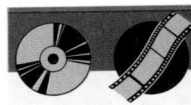

| PROCEDURE 27-5 | **Taking Blood Pressure** |

## EQUIPMENT NEEDED

- Stethoscope (Figure 27-27)
- Mercury sphygmomanometer with bladder and cuff
- Gloves if required
- Alcohol swabs

## IMPLEMENTATION—ACTION/RATIONALE

| ACTION | RATIONALE |
|---|---|

### Auscultation Method Using Brachial Artery

1. Wash hands.

2. Determine which extremity is most appropriate for reading. Do not take a pressure reading on an injured or painful extremity or one in which an intravenous line is running.

3. Select a cuff size that completely encircles upper arm without overlapping (Figure 27-28).

1. Reduces transmission of microorganisms.

2. Cuff inflation can temporarily interrupt blood flow and compromise circulation in an extremity already impaired or a vein receiving intravenous fluids.

3. Provides equalization of pressure on the artery to ensure accurate measurement.

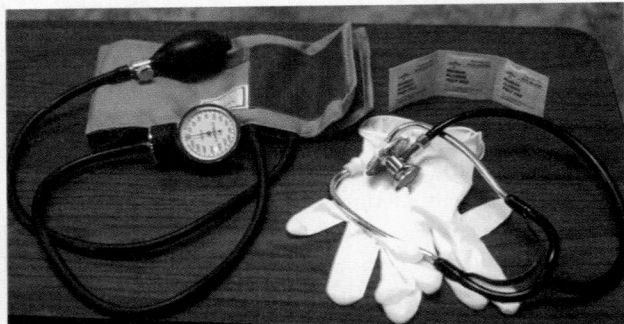

**Figure 27-27 Sphygmomanometer, stethoscope, and gloves**

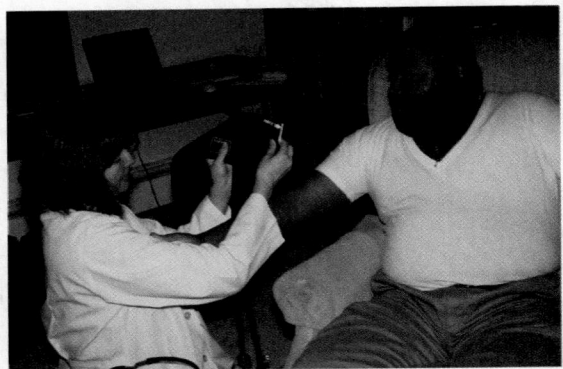

**Figure 27-28 Select proper cuff size. An obese client may need a larger size to obtain an accurate reading.**

4. Move clothing away from upper aspect of arm.

5. Position arm at heart level; extend elbow with palm turned upward.

6. Make sure bladder cuff is fully deflated and pump valve moves freely.

7. Locate brachial artery in the antecubital space (Figure 27-29).

8. Apply cuff snugly and smoothly over upper arm, 2.5 cm (1 inch) above antecubital space with center of cuff over brachial artery (Figure 27-30).

4. Ensures accurate measurement.

5. Blood pressure increases when arm is below level of heart and decreases when arm is above level of heart.

6. Equipment must function properly to obtain an accurate reading.

7. Designates placement of stethoscope.

8. Ensures even pressure distribution over brachial artery. Prevents tubing from being constricted and allows visualization of aneroid manometer dial.

*(continues)*

## PROCEDURE 27-5 (*continued*)

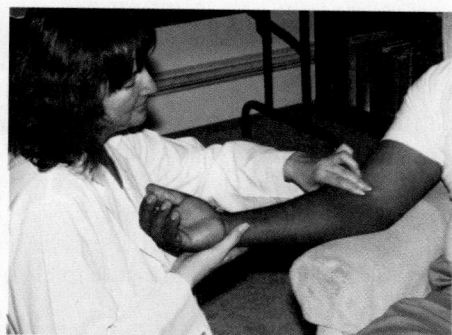

**Figure 27-29** Palpate the brachial artery to determine placement of the stethoscope.

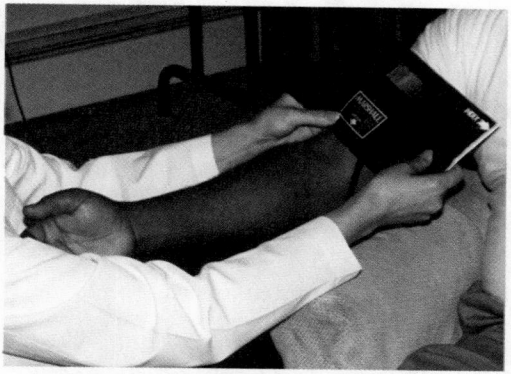

**Figure 27-30** Center the blood pressure cuff over the brachial artery.

9. Connect bladder tubing to manometer tubing. If using a portable mercury-filled manometer, position vertically at eye level.

10. Palpate brachial artery, turn valve clockwise to close and compress bulb to inflate cuff to 30 mm Hg above point where palpated pulse disappears, then slowly release valve (deflating cuff), noting reading when pulse is felt again.

11. Insert earpieces of stethoscope into ears with a forward tilt, ensuring diaphragm hangs freely.

12. Relocate brachial pulse with your nondominant hand and place bell or diaphragm chestpiece directly over pulse. Chestpiece should be in direct contact with skin and not touch cuff (Figure 27-31).

13. With dominant hand, turn valve clockwise to close. Compress pump to inflate cuff until manometer registers 30 mm Hg above diminished pulse point identified in Action 10 (Figure 27-32).

9. Maintains closed system; supports accurate reading of mercury level in manometer.

10. Inflates the cuff's bladder with pressure and temporarily impairs flow of blood through artery. Provides an estimate of maximum pressure required to measure systolic pressure.

11. Enhances sound transmission from chestpiece to ears.

12. Sound is heard best directly over artery; decreases muffled sounds that cause inaccurate reading. Bell chestpiece is more sensitive to low-frequency sound that occurs with pressure release.

13. Prevents air leak during inflation. Ensures the cuff is inflated to a pressure greater than the client's systolic pressure.

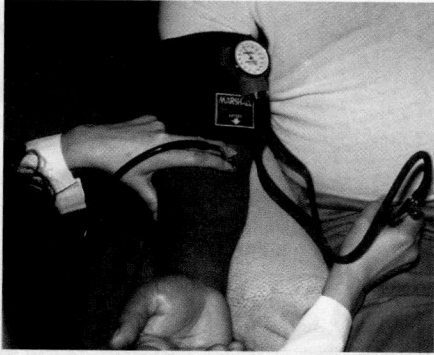

**Figure 27-31** The stethoscope chestpiece should not touch the blood pressure cuff.

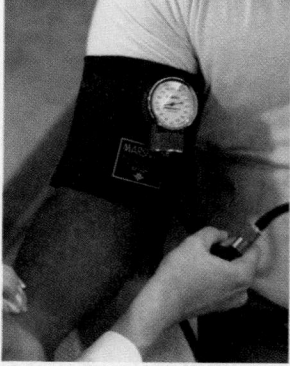

**Figure 27-32** Compress the pump to inflate the blood pressure cuff.

*(continues)*

## PROCEDURE 27-5 (*continued*)

14. Slowly turn valve counterclockwise so that mercury falls at a rate of 2–3 mm Hg per second. Listen for five phases of Korotkoff's sounds while noting manometer reading (for more information about Korotkoff's sounds, see Box 27-12).
    I    A faint, clear tapping sound appears and increases in intensity.
    II   Swishing sound
    III  Intense sound
    IV   Abrupt, distinctive muffled sounds
    V    Sound disappears

14. Maintains constant release of pressure to ensure hearing first systolic sound. Identify manometer readings for each of the five phases.
    - Identify two consecutive tapping sounds to confirm systolic reading.
    - Phase IV is regarded by the American Heart Association (AHA) as the best indicator of diastolic pressure in children (AHA, 1997).
    - Phase V is regarded by the AHA as the best index of diastolic blood pressure in clients over age 13 (AHA, 1994).

15. Deflate cuff rapidly and completely.

15. Prevents arterial occlusion and client discomfort of numbness or tingling.

16. Remove cuff or wait 2 minutes before taking a second reading (Figure 27-33).

16. Releases trapped blood in the vessels.

17. Inform client of reading.

17. Promotes client's participation in care.

18. Record reading.

18. Ensures accuracy.

19. If appropriate, lower bed, raise side rails, place call light in easy reach.

19. Promotes client safety.

20. Put all equipment in proper place.

20. Fosters maintenance of equipment.

21. Wash hands.

21. Reduces transmission of microorganisms.

### Palpation Method Using Brachial or Radial Artery

22. Palpate brachial or radial artery with fingertips of one hand (Figure 27-34). Inflate cuff to 30 mm Hg above point at which pulse disappears.

22. Ensures accurate detection of true systolic pressure when cuff is deflated.

23. Deflate cuff slowly as you note on the manometer when the pulse is again palpable.

23. Ensures accurate reading.

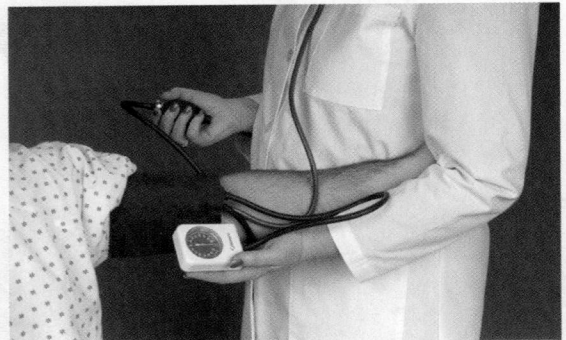

**Figure 27-33  Deflate the cuff completely and wait at least 2 minutes before taking a second reading.**

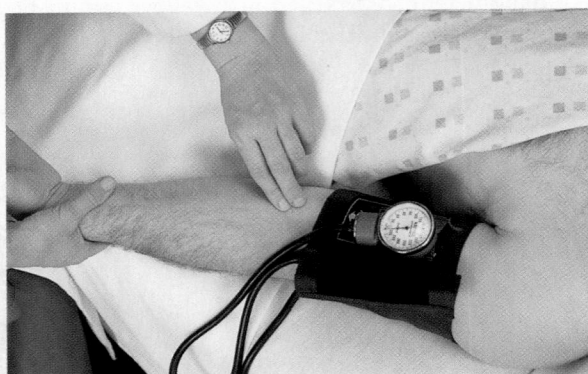

**Figure 27-34  Palpate the brachial artery with index and middle fingers below the blood pressure cuff.**

(*continues*)

## PROCEDURE 27-5 *(continued)*

24. Deflate cuff rapidly and completely.

25. Remove cuff or wait 2 minutes before taking a second reading.

26. Inform client of reading.

27. Record reading.

28. Wash hands.

24. Prevents arterial occlusion and client discomfort of numbness or tingling.

25. Releases trapped blood in the vessels.

26. Promotes client's participation in care.

27. Ensures accuracy.

28. Reduces transmission of microorganisms.

---

pressure so that the inflated pressure causes the artery to collapse; blood flow ceases, and sound is absent on auscultation. As the pressure is released from the bladder, blood begins to flow through the artery and creates the first sound, which is the systolic pressure.

The Korotkoff sounds are named after the Russian surgeon who first identified the five distinct phases of sound heard with a stethoscope during auscultation. Korotkoff's sounds are correlated to the pressure dynamics of measurement.

## LIFE SPAN CONSIDERATIONS

### Blood Pressure Measurement

#### *Pediatric Variations*

- Small children may be uncooperative with the procedure and need the assistance of a parent to hold still.

- A cuff that fits adequately may not be available.

- It may be preferable to use the popliteal artery when taking a child's blood pressure.

- BP varies with size when a child reaches adolescence.

- Take BP first, before other anxiety or pain-producing procedures.

#### *Geriatric Variations*

- Elderly clients may have lost muscle mass and their upper arms may be quite thin. Be sure to adjust the cuff size to accommodate the client's arm.

- Many elderly clients have a history of hypertension and are taking antihypertensive medications.

Bilateral readings should be done with the initial blood pressure assessment. A pressure variance of 5–10 mm Hg normally exists between arms. The arm with the higher reading should be used for routine measurements.

When measuring a popliteal blood pressure, the nurse should select a cuff wide and long enough to fit the girth of the thigh. Although the American Heart Association does not specify cuff sizes for thigh BP readings, the association emphasizes that the cuff should be wider and longer than an arm cuff to allow for the greater girth. Place the client in a supine position with the legs in a nondependent position for at least 10 minutes. (A prone position is also acceptable.) Apply the bladder cuff to the client's thigh with the center of the bladder over the

### COMMUNITY/HOME CARE

#### Taking Blood Pressures in the Home

#### *Home Care Variations*

- Use the same cuff the client normally uses for his home readings.

- Compare home readings to readings from a cuff you know is properly calibrated.

- Assess the client's financial ability to buy his own sphygmomanometer.

- Consider use of an electronic BP cuff if the client has a hearing deficit.

#### *Long-Term Care Variations*

- Be aware of any injuries, disease process, or appliances that may contraindicate a blood pressure reading at the chosen site.

## TABLE 27-8 GUIDELINES FOR SPHYGMOMANOMETER SELECTION

| Midpoint* Arm Circumference** | Bladder Cuff Width** | Bladder Length** |
|---|---|---|
| 5–7.5 (newborn) | 3 | 5 |
| 7.5–13 (infant) | 5 | 8 |
| 13–20 (child) | 8 | 13 |
| 24–32 (average adult) | 13 | 24 |
| 32–42 (large adult) | 17 | 32 |

\* Distance between the acromion and olecranon processes
\*\* Measurement in centimeters (cm)

## BOX 27-12 KOROTKOFF SOUNDS CORRELATED TO PRESSURE DYNAMICS

| Phase | Pressure Dynamics |
|---|---|
| I. Clear, soft tapping that increases to a thud or loud tap (systolic sound) | 1. Ventilation |
| II. Tapping changes to a soft, swishing sound | 2. Circulation |
| III. Clear tapping sound returns | 3. Diffusion |
| IV. Muffled, blowing sound (diastolic sound in children or physically active adults) | 4. Transport |
| V. Disappearance of muffled, blowing sound (second diastolic sound) | 5. Regulation |

popliteal artery. Wrap the cuff snugly, and place it far enough above the popliteal fossa to allow for auscultation of arterial sounds. Help the client slightly flex the knee and abduct the hip; this position will facilitate palpation of the pulse and placement of the stethoscope. Place the diaphragm of the stethoscope over the area where the pulse was palpated and follow the same procedure as presented for brachial artery auscultation. When the BP cuff is removed, inspect the area, and note abnormalities such as bruising, hematoma, or skin tear. Document in the medical record the systolic and diastolic BP, the site, and the size of the BP cuff. "Systolic readings in the thigh may be 10–40 mm Hg higher than in the arm, but diastolic readings are generally the same" (Rice, 1999, p. 58).

### Palpation

When the client's hemodynamic regulation is compromised to the degree that Korotkoff sounds cannot be heard, such as occurs with myocardial infarction or shock, the blood pressure has to be monitored by palpation or direct measurement. To palpate the systolic blood pressure, apply the cuff over the brachial artery, inflate the cuff, place the fingers over the radial artery, slowly release the pressure, and note the reading on the manometer when the first pulse (systole) is felt. With palpation, it is difficult to assess the diastolic pressure. Direct measurement is obtained with insertion of an intravenous catheter.

### Hypotension

**Hypotension** refers to a systolic blood pressure less than 90 mm Hg or 20–30 mm Hg below the client's normal systolic pressure. Hypotension is caused by a disruption in hemodynamic regulation, such as:

- Decreased blood volume (e.g., hemorrhage)
- Decreased cardiac output (e.g., myocardial infarction [heart attack])
- Decreased peripheral vascular resistance (vascular dilation) (e.g., shock)

A hypotensive client manifests symptoms relative to the degree of hypotension regardless of the cause.

One of the initial compensatory responses to a falling blood pressure is an increased pulse rate. For example, if a blood vessel cauterized during surgery begins to bleed internally at the point at which the circulating blood volume is compromised, the heart will automatically beat faster to compensate for the decreased circulating volume. If the falling pressure is untreated, the body's compensatory mechanisms will fail and the client will exhibit the symptoms of shock: cool, clammy skin; fast, thready pulse; a gradual decrease in urinary output; and disruption to cerebral blood flow that causes confusion, progressing to coma.

**Orthostatic hypotension (postural hypotension)** refers to a sudden drop of 25 mm Hg in systolic pressure and 10 mm Hg in diastolic pressure when the client moves from a lying to a sitting or a sitting to a standing position. Orthostatic hypotension usually occurs with aging and is a common antiadrenergic side effect of several medications, such as chlorpromazine hydrochloride.

Clients with orthostatic hypotension should be advised to rise slowly from a supine position and to sit down immediately if they feel faint.

### Hypertension

**Hypertension** refers to a persistent systolic pressure greater than 135–140 mm Hg and a diastolic pressure greater than 90 mm Hg. Diagnosis of hypertension is based

## NURSING STRATEGY

### Orthostatic Hypotension

When measuring the blood pressure of a client who experiences orthostatic hypotension:

1. Place the client in a supine position for 2 to 3 minutes. This allows the blood pressure to stabilize.
2. Assess and record the blood pressure and pulse.
3. Assist the client to a sitting or standing position and wait 1 minute. Reassess the blood pressure and pulse.
4. Record results. A drop in blood pressure of 30 mm Hg systolic or a rise in pulse of 40 beats per minute indicates abnormal orthostatic vital signs that should be reported.

Roper, M. (1996). Back to basics: Assessing orthostatic vital signs. *American Journal of Nursing, (96)*8, 43–46.

on the average of two or more readings taken at each of two or more visits after an initial screening. Classifications of hypertension for adults have been developed with recommended medical follow-up (see Box 27-13).

A number of physiological changes occur as a result of hypertension. The arterial walls thicken and lose their elasticity, which, in turn, increases resistance to blood flow. Hypertrophy of the left ventricle develops. These changes place the client at risk for a myocardial infarction or stroke. Malignant hypertension is a diastolic pressure higher than 120 mm Hg. With this condition, the client complains of severe headaches, blurred vision, and confusion (Keele-Smith & Price-Daniel, 2001).

### Nursing Considerations

Before checking a blood pressure, review the client's chart for brachial artery contraindications and make sure that the client has not exercised or eaten for the past 30 minutes. Clients who have recently eaten, ambulated, or experienced an emotional upset will have a falsely high blood pressure reading. When the vital signs are taken correctly in sequence (T-P-R and BP), the client should be calm from sitting or lying quietly.

Faulty techniques that constrict blood flow will produce a false high pressure reading:

- A cuff too narrow for the extremity
- A cuff that does not fit snugly around the extremity
- A cuff that is deflated too slowly

Other false high readings occur when the mercury column in the manometer is not positioned flat on a firm surface or is read above eye level or the extremity is below the heart's apex level.

False low readings occur when the extremity is above the heart's apex level, the cuff is too wide for the extremity, or the mercury column in the manometer is read below eye level. If the nurse fails to recognize the **auscultatory gap**, the temporary disappearance of sounds at the end of Korotkoff phase I and beginning of phase II, the systolic pressure is read at a false low pressure.

### Documentation

The nurse should record the blood pressure measurement on the appropriate form. If the brachial artery is not used for the measurement, indicate the site when recording the

## BOX 27-13    CLASSIFICATION OF BLOOD PRESSURE FOR ADULTS AGES 18 AND OLDER, WITH RECOMMENDED FOLLOW-UP (FOR PERSONS NOT TAKING ANTIHYPERTENSIVE DRUGS AND NOT ACUTELY ILL)

| Category | Systolic (mm Hg) | | Diastolic (mm Hg) | Follow-up recommended |
|---|---|---|---|---|
| Optimal | < 120 | and | < 80 | Recheck 2 years |
| Normal | < 130 | and | < 85 | Recheck 2 years |
| High normal | 130–139 | or | 85–89 | Recheck 1 year |
| **Hypertension** | | | | |
| Stage 1 | 140–159 | or | 90–99 | Confirm within 2 months |
| Stage 2 | 160–179 | or | 100–109 | Evaluate within 1 month |
| Stage 3 | 180 or higher | or | 110 or higher | Evaluate immediately or within 1 week depending on clinical situation |

Data from the National High Blood Pressure Education Program; National Heart, Lung, and Blood Institute; National Institutes of Health (1997). The sixth report of the Joint National Committee on Detection, Evaluation, and Treatment of High Blood Pressure. *Archive of Internal Medicine, 157*(2413), 2.

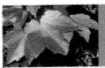

## RESEARCH FOCUS

**Title of Study:** Effects of crossing legs on blood pressure measurement

**Study Purpose:** The purpose of this study was to determine if blood pressure measurement in a well senior population is affected by the leg crossed at the knee as compared with feet flat on the floor.

**Methods:** A repeated-measures, crossover design was used. One hundred and three senior citizens (50 to 92 years of age) from two local senior citizen centers participated in the study. A written protocol for taking blood pressure was adapted from the American Heart Association and the National Heart Foundation. Subjects were randomly assigned to one of two protocols. One protocol had clients sitting with feet flat on the floor for 3 minutes. Blood pressure was then measured. Clients were then asked to cross one leg over the knee for 3 minutes. Blood pressure measurement was then repeated. The other protocol was just the reverse of the one previously described.

**Findings:** Blood pressure readings were significantly higher when legs were crossed versus uncrossed.

**Implications:** Instructing clients to keep legs uncrossed and feet flat on the floor is important when measuring blood pressure and should be incorporated into nursing practice.

Keele-Smith, R., & Price-Daniel, C. (November 2001). *Effects of crossing legs on blood pressure measurement.* Oral presentation at the Sigma Theta Tau International 36th Biennial Convention, Indianapolis, IN.

results. If the pressure was obtained by palpation, record "80 systolic by palpation."

Monitoring blood pressure changes in relation to T-P-R measurements is one of the major responsibilities of the registered nurse. One element of critical thinking is having concrete, objective clinical data, as provided by vital sign measurements, to direct decision making.

## The Physical Examination

The physical examination is a systematic means of collecting objective assessment data. Objective data may be used to verify findings from the subjective assessment data obtained from the health history or to determine the meaning of the findings. Although the health history assessment, general survey, vital signs assessment, and physical examination are often conducted as separate procedures, the information is synthesized to identify and explain the client's health status and problems. The complete assessment data are used to:

- Ascertain the client's perceived and actual level of health and physiological function
- Identify factors placing the client at risk and to determine areas of preventive nursing and health promotion
- Confirm health deviations, disease, or inability to perform the activities of daily living
- Identify the need for additional testing, evaluation, or follow-up care
- Evaluate the outcomes of treatment and therapy

The examination should be performed according to the agency's policy. Policy may vary from one agency to another.

The physical examination is done in a sequential, head-to-toe manner to ensure a thorough assessment of each system. This method enables the nurse to assess all areas and decreases the number of times the nurse and the client have to change positions.

With experience, the nurse will become proficient with performing the physical examination. The experienced nurse examiner will be able to integrate assessment into all aspects of providing client care. For example, while weighing the client, observe posture, motor activity, gait, stature, grooming, breath and body odors, mood, and behavior (Estes, 2002).

## Techniques

Chapter 11 introduced the assessment techniques of inspection, palpation, percussion, and auscultation; this section demonstrates how these techniques are used in performing a physical examination. The specific techniques used to assess each body system are identified and explained within the context of the assessment. While practicing how to conduct a physical examination, refer to the following assessment tables to reinforce appropriate techniques for each system.

The nurse should use the senses of sight, hearing, smell, and touch when gathering information during the physical examination pertinent to the client's clinical status. The nurse uses the sense of sight by visually inspecting the client's body parts and assessing the client's normal behaviors and adaptive coping behaviors to alterations in functions. For example, the skin is inspected for color, tone, and texture, as well as scars, lesions, abrasions, and rashes. Throughout the examination, the nurse should visually observe the client's general body appearances, such as movement, motor dexterity, contour and symmetry of the body, and deformities.

The nurse uses the sense of touch when performing palpation. The skin is thinner on the backs of the hands and more sensitive to temperature changes. The back of the hand can be used to assess skin temperature over an inflamed joint or a leg with impaired circulation. The fingerpads are also sensitive and are used to palpate the size, position, and consistency of various body parts, such as lymph nodes and breast tissue. Figure 27-35 demonstrates how to perform light palpation.

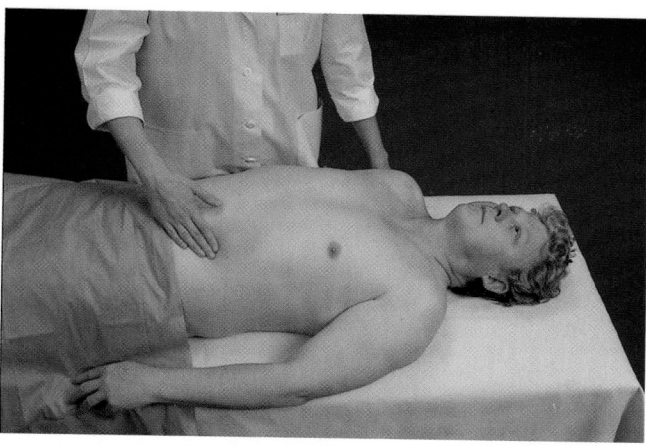

**Figure 27-35    Light palpation**

Learning the technique of percussion is challenging; it can be practiced on any surface. Refer to Figure 27-36, and practice percussion as follows:

1. Hyperextend the middle (pleximeter) finger of the nondominant hand and press its distal phalanx and joint firmly on the surface to be percussed (Figure 27-36A). Only the distal phalanx and joint should be touching the surface. Having other parts of the hand in contact with the surface will damp the vibrations.
2. Position the forearm of the dominant hand close to the surface, with the hand cocked upward, as shown in Figure 27-36B, with the middle finger partially flexed, relaxed, and poised to strike.
3. With a quick, sharp, but relaxed *wrist* motion, strike the pleximeter finger with the tip of the right plexor finger of the dominant hand, as shown in Figure 27-36C. Only the wrist joint is flexed, not the finger or elbow.
4. Quickly withdraw the plexor finger to avoid damping the vibration.

5. Strike one or two blows in one location, then move on, using the lightest percussion that will produce a clean note.

If the client becomes fatigued, encourage frequent rest periods. Adjust the client's position for comfort without compromising the ability to visualize the area of assessment.

The nurse uses the sense of hearing during the physical examination when performing auscultation. A stethoscope allows the nurse to listen to sounds produced in the heart, lungs, abdomen, and blood vessels.

Throughout the entire examination, the nurse uses the senses of hearing and smell. Besides auscultation, the nurse should listen to what clients say relative to their health status during the examination. Smell is used to investigate any environmental, body, or fluid odors, such as drainage from a wound.

## Integumentary System

The **integumentary system** (skin, hair, scalp, and nails) provides the body with external protection, regulates temperature, and is a sensory organ for pain, temperature, and touch. The sebaceous and sweat glands are considered appendages of the skin. Nurses should routinely assess the skin of elderly and debilitated clients for primary lesions that can lead to the development of secondary lesions such as pressure ulcers.

To facilitate learning and psychomotor proficiency, the integumentary system is assessed separately. However, once skills are established, the integumentary system assessment can be integrated into the examination of other systems. Table 27-9 presents the specific areas of the integumentary system to be examined and the normal and key findings of this assessment.

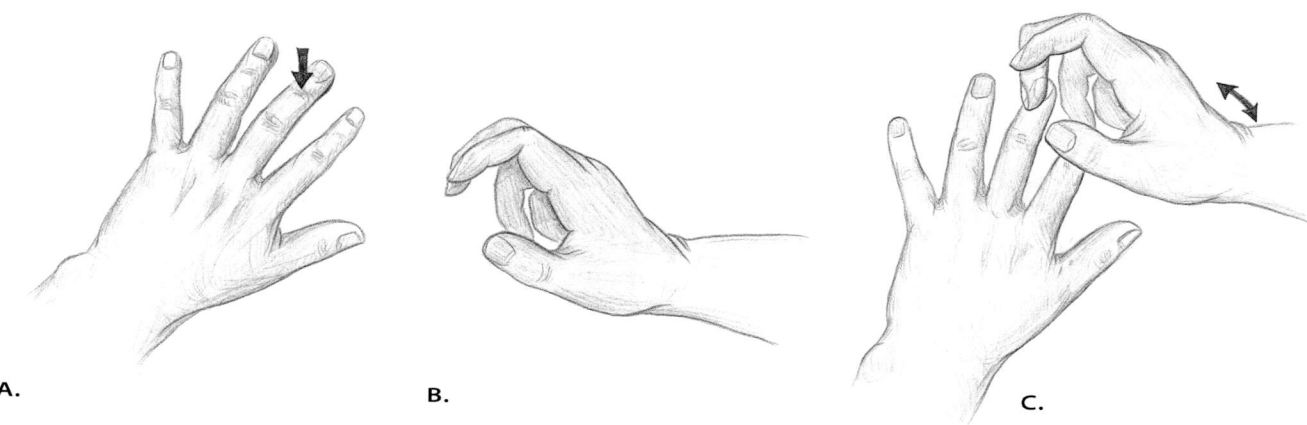

**A.**                              **B.**                              **C.**

**Figure 27-36    Percussion. A. Hyperextend the pleximeter finger and press the distal phalanx and joint firmly on the surface to be percussed. B. Cock the hand upward with the middle finger partially flexed and poised to strike. C. Strike the pleximeter finger with the tip of the right plexor finger.**

## TABLE 27-9 ASSESSMENT OF INTEGUMENTARY SYSTEM: NORMAL AND KEY FINDINGS

| Area of Assessment/*Normal Findings* | Key Findings |
|---|---|
| **Skin: Inspect and Palpate** | |
| 1. Color: inspect variations in skin color under natural sunlight to ensure accuracy in findings. *Color varies from light to ruddy pink or dark brown, or is yellow with olive overtones, with uniform skin color except in sun-exposed areas or normally lighted pigmented areas (nailbeds, palms, lips) in dark-skinned people.* | 1. The presence or absence of certain substances in the circulatory system or the deposition of substances in the skin are indications of disease processes. See Box 27-14 for common alterations in skin color. |
| 2. Lesions: note color, size, and anatomic location and distribution; palpate the lesions with fingerpads for mobility, contour (flat, raised, or depressed), and consistency (soft or durable). *Freckles, skin tags in elderly, and some types of birthmarks and moles are normal.* | 2. Vascular and purpuric lesions are discussed in Table 27-10. Primary skin lesions, such as a vesicle, can give rise to secondary lesions, for example, erosion and crusting, as in chickenpox. See Table 27-11 for the different types of primary and secondary skin lesions. Refer to Nursing Strategy box. |
| 3. Moisture (wetness and oiliness): note amount and distribution. *Moisture varies with activity, body and environmental temperature, and humidity in skinfolds and the axillae.* | 3. Excessive moisture or perspiration (hyperhidrosis) is usually caused by hyperthermia, infection, hyperthyroidism, strong emotions, menopause; excessive dryness often occurs in dehydration. Bromidrosis (body odor) is usually caused by bacterial decomposition of perspiration on the skin. |
| 4. Temperature: palpate with back (dorsum) of hand, noting uniformity of warmth. *Temperature should be uniform and within normal range.* | 4. Generalized hyperthermia is seen in fever; generalized hypothermia is seen in shock; localized hyperthermia is seen with an infection; localized hypothermia is characteristic of arteriosclerosis. |
| 5. Texture (quality, thickness, suppleness): palpate with fingerpads in different areas. *Texture is not uniform; for example, palms and soles are usually thicker than other areas, which are smooth, soft, and flexible. Wrinkled, leathery skin in the elderly results from the normal aging process, with decreased collagen, subcutaneous fat, and sweat glands.* | 5. Generalized roughness is seen in hypothyroidism. |
| 6. Mobility and turgor (elasticity): assessing mobility and turgor measures the elasticity of skin to determine the degree of hydration:<br>a. Palpate dependent areas (sacrum, feet, ankles) for mobility by applying pressure with fingers, noting degree of indentation (Figure 27-37). If indentation occurs, firmly apply pressure with your thumb for 5 seconds: Rate the degree of **edema** (accumulation of fluid in intercellular spaces) by assessing the depth of indentation. Edema may be described on a scale as follows: 0 = no pitting, 1+ = trace/mild (2 mm) pitting, 2+ = moderate (4 mm) pitting, 3+ = deep/severe (6 mm) pitting, 4+ = very deep/severe (greater than 8 mm) pitting. Become familiar with the agency's edema rating scale.<br>b. Pinch a fold of skin on the sternal area using your thumb and forefinger (Figure 27-38). Note the speed with which it returns into place (turgor).<br>*Absence of indentation in dependent areas and the resilience of the skin to spring back to its previous state after being pinched.* | 6. Dependent edema gives the skin a stretched, shiny appearance. The degree of pitting edema reflects the depth of indentation. Edema is usually caused by direct trauma or impairment of venous return. Failure of the skin to reassume its normal contour or shape after being pinched indicates dehydration, which places the client at risk for skin breakdown. *Tenting* is the term used to describe skin that remains in a pinched position. |

*(continues)*

## TABLE 27-9    ASSESSMENT OF INTEGUMENTARY SYSTEM: NORMAL AND KEY FINDINGS (continued)

**Area of Assessment/*Normal Findings***

**Key Findings**

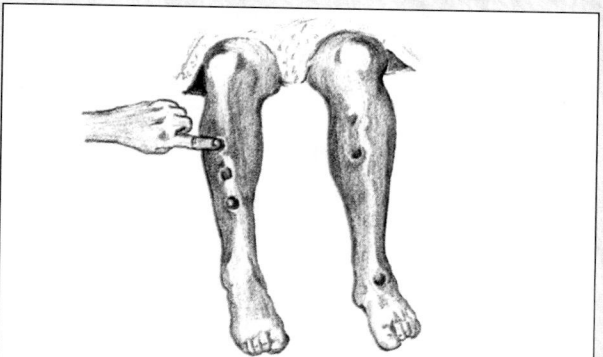

**Figure 27-37    Assessing for edema**

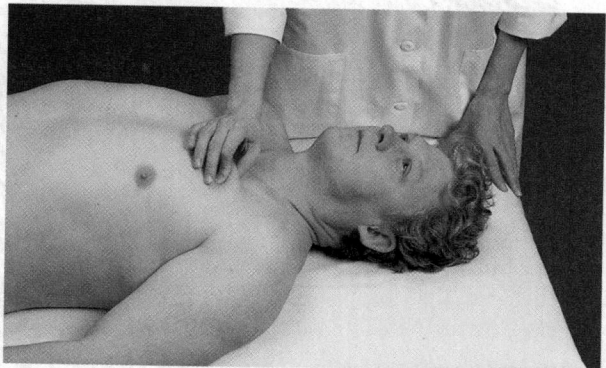

**Figure 27-38    Assessing skin turgor**

### Hair: Inspect and Palpate

1. Color and distribution of scalp hair, eyebrows, eyelashes, and on body surface. *Color varies from dark black to pale blonde based on the amount of melanin present.*

2. Texture and oiliness. *Thin, straight, coarse, thick, or curly. Shiny and resilient.*

3. Note infestation. *Free of infestation.*

### Scalp: Inspect and Palpate

1. Part the hair repeatedly all over the scalp and inspect for scaliness and scars. *The scalp should be shiny and smooth without lesions, lumps, or masses.*

2. Place the fingerpads on the scalp at the front and palpate down the midline and each side for tenderness, lesions, lumps, or masses. *Absence of redness or scaliness.*

### Nails: Inspect and Palpate

1. Note the nail color, shape, and texture. *Nailbed is highly vascular with a pink color in light-skinned clients and longitudinal streaks of brown or black pigmentation in dark-skinned clients. Angle between the fingernail and base is about 160°. When palpated, the nail base is firm.*

2. Test for capillary refill by pressing two or more nails between your thumb and index finger. Note the degree of blanching and return to normal color. *When pressure is released from the nail, it promptly returns to its normal color.*

3. Inspect the tissue surrounding nails for lesions. Tissue surrounding the nail is intact.

1. As melanin production decreases, hair turns gray. Color may be chemically changed. Alopecia (hair loss) and hirsutism (excessive body hair) are considered abnormal. Hair loss may be the result of chemotherapy, radiation therapy, infection, hormone disorders, or inadequate nutrition. Vellus hair loss may be due to decreased oxygenation of peripheral tissues. Excessive hair growth may be due to hormone disorders.

2. Thin, brittle, dull hair may be indicative of malnutrition, hyper/hypothyroidism, chemicals, or infections.

3. *Pediculus capitis, P. corporis,* and *P. pubis* are lice that adhere to head, body, and pubic hair. The eggs are white ovoid nits.

1. Sebaceous cysts or trauma deformities.

2. Dry flaking, scaling occurs in seborrhea (dandruff) and psoriasis (red patches covered by thick, dry, silvery, adherent scales that result from excessive development of epithelial cells).

1. Refer to Table 27-12 for abnormalities and variations of the nailbed.

2. Delayed return of nailbed color may indicate circulatory impairment.

3. Paronychia (inflammation of the skin around the nail) is described in Table 27-12.

From Estes, M. (2002). *Health assessment & physical examination* (2nd ed.). Clifton Park, NY: Delmar Learning.

## Skin

The skin is the largest organ system of the body, its surface area covering approximately 20 square feet in the average adult. The skin's thickness, influenced by age, varies from 0.2–1.5 mm. Skin assessment provides a noninvasive window to observe the body's physiological functions.

Lesions of the skin vary from superficial, involving only the epidermis, to penetrating the dermis or subcutaneous layers of the skin. Table 27-10 presents common vascular lesions, and Table 27-11 describes the common skin lesions.

## Hair and Scalp

Hair is distributed over the body except for the palmar and plantar surfaces, lips, nipples, and the glans penis. The amount and texture of hair vary with age, sex, race, and body part.

- Vellus: Fine, unpigmented hair that covers most of the body.
- Terminal hair: Coarser, darker hair of scalp, eyebrows, and eyelashes; axillary and pubic hair becomes terminal with the onset of puberty.

---

## CLINICAL ALERT

### Skin Palpation

When palpating the skin, wear gloves to prevent the transmission of microorganisms, *because lesions are not always visible on general inspection.*

---

Men have coarser, thicker chest and facial hair growth than women.

The scalp should be smooth, clean, and intact. It should be free of lumps or tender areas.

## Nails

The nail plate (translucent tissue that covers the distal portion of the digits and provides protection) changes with many disease processes, as presented in Table 27-12.

## Head and Neck

Areas to be included in the head and neck examination are the skull, face, eyes, ears, nose, mouth, pharynx, and neck. The carotid artery assessment is conducted either as part of the neck examination or with peripheral artery assessment. Inspection and palpation are used throughout this assessment. Auscultation is used if the carotid arteries are assessed as part of this examination. Table 27-13 presents the specific areas of the head and neck to be examined and the normal and key findings of this assessment.

## Skull and Face

Assessment of the skull and face involves inspection and palpation. The client's face has its own unique characteristics

---

### BOX 27-14    COMMON ALTERATIONS IN SKIN COLOR

- Melanin (naturally occurring brown pigment) is *increased* in exposed areas or points of pressure—for example, nipples, palmar creases, recent scars—and with Addison's disease and some pituitary tumors. It is *decreased* in albinism (congenital inability to form melanin) and vitiligo (acquired loss of melanin).

- Cyanosis (bluish discoloration in the lips, mucous membranes, and nails) results from an increased amount of reduced hemoglobin in the blood caused by a cold environment or heart or lung disease.

- Jaundice (yellowish discoloration) results from increased bilirubin levels caused by red blood cell hemolysis in liver disease as observed first in the sclera and mucous membranes and then generalized.

- Carotenemia (yellowish discoloration) is described as normal as a result of increased levels of carotenoid pigments in the palms, soles, and face from a diet high in carotene. Also occurs in diseases such as myxedema, hypopituitarism, and diabetes.

---

## NURSING STRATEGY

### Evaluate Skin Lesions by Using the ABCDE Mnemonic

A = Asymmetry (Is the lesion symmetrical or asymmetrical?)

B = Border (Are the edges of the lesion regular or irregular?)

C = Color (Is the color of the lesion even, varied, or multicolored?)

D = Diameter (Has the diameter of the lesion increased in size? Over what period of time?)

E = Elevation (Is the lesion even with the skin or raised?)

## TABLE 27-10    VASCULAR AND PURPURIC LESIONS OF THE SKIN

| Findings | Body Area Assessed | Key Points |
|---|---|---|

**Vascular**

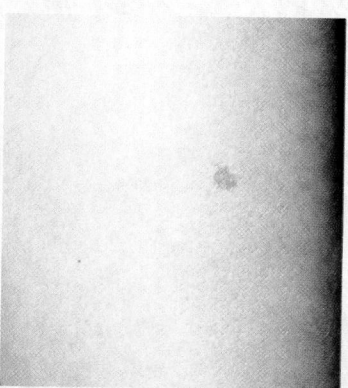

Cherry angioma: Ruby red, 1–3 mm, round lesion.

Trunk and extremities

Pressure with a pinpoint edge causes partial blanching. Increase in size and number and may become brownish with age.

Spider angioma: Fiery red lesion up to 2 cm with a central body surrounded by erythema and radiating legs.

Face, neck, arms, and upper trunk

Occurs normally in some people. May occur with pregnancy, vitamin B deficiency, or liver disease.

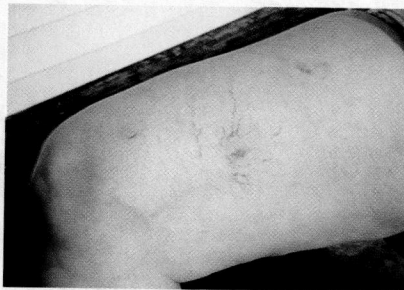

Venous star: Bluish, varying in size from small to 1–2 inches. May resemble a spider or be linear, irregular, and cascading.

Areas with superficial veins: legs and anterior chest

Indicates an increased pressure in superficial veins—for example, varicose veins.

**Purpuric**

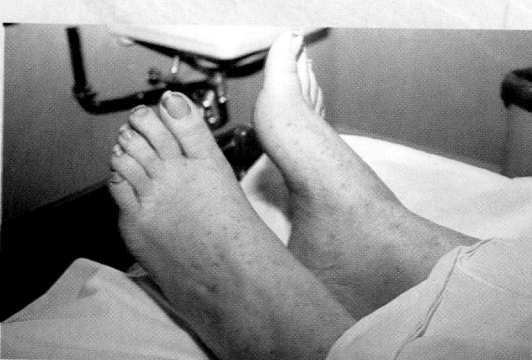

*Courtesy of Dr. Mark Dougherty, Lexington, KY*

*(continues)*

## TABLE 27-10     VASCULAR AND PURPURIC LESIONS OF THE SKIN (*continued*)

| Findings | Body Area Assessed | Key Points |
|---|---|---|
| Petechia: Reddish purple, flat round lesion, 1–3 mm in size. | Variable distribution in areas with superficial blood supply | May indicate vitamin C deficiency, blood clotting disorders, liver disease, or drug reactions. |
| Ecchymosis (bruise): Purplish blue, fading to green, yellow, and brown in time. | Area of blood vessel trauma | Results from injury or with bleeding disorders. |

Estes, M. (2002). *Health assessment & physical examination* (2nd ed.). Clifton Park, NY: Delmar Learning.

influenced by factors such as race, state of health, emotions, and environment.

### Eyes

Active client participation is needed for the various eye tests. To prevent client weakness or discomfort, the eye tests are separated by assessment of the eye's external anatomic structures. The nurse should practice holding and using the index finger to rotate the dial for the five lens settings of the ophthalmoscope before conducting the examination.

The assessment of visual acuity is a simple, noninvasive procedure that is performed with the use of a **Snellen chart** (a chart that contains various-sized letters with standardized numbers at the end of each line of letters) (Figure 27-39). The standardized numbers (called the denominator) indicate the degree of visual acuity when the client is able to read that line of letters at a distance of 20 feet.

### Ears

Physical assessment of the ears consists of auditory screening, inspection and palpation of the external ear, and otoscopic assessment. The nurse should observe the client for signs of hearing difficulty during the physical examination, such as turning the head, lipreading, and speaking in a loud voice. If the client is wearing a hearing aid, ask if it is turned on, when the batteries were last changed, and if the device causes any irritation to the ear canal.

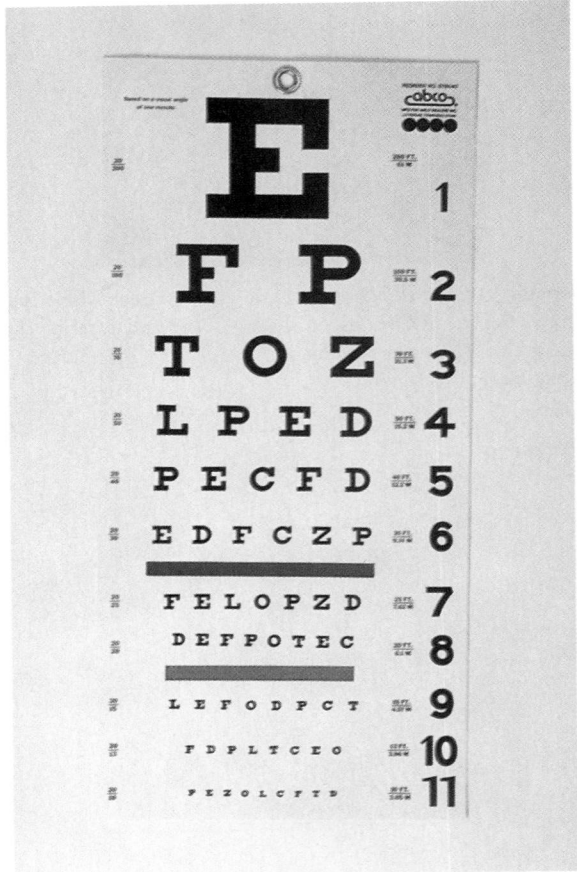

**Figure 27-39     Snellen chart**

## TABLE 27-11    COMMON SKIN LESIONS

**Primary Lesions**

| Nonpalpable | Palpable | Fluid-Filled Cavities within the Skin |
|---|---|---|

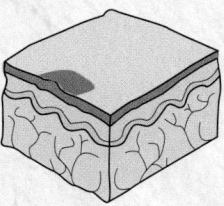

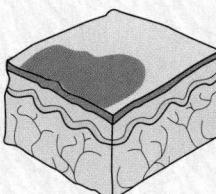

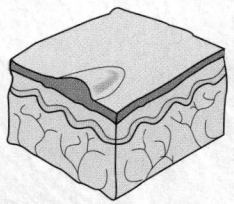

Macule: localized changes in skin color < 1 cm in diameter (e.g., freckle)

Papule: solid, elevated lesion < 0.5 cm in diameter (e.g., elevated nevi)

Vesicle: elevated mass containing serous fluid accumulation between the upper layers of the skin (e.g., herpes simplex and zoster, chickenpox, second-degree burns)

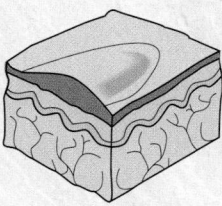

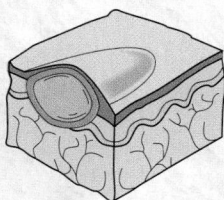

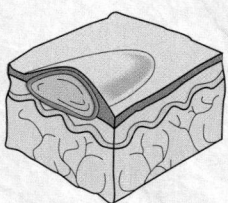

Patch: localized changes in skin of < 1 cm (e.g., vitiligo, stage 1 of pressure ulcer)

Plaque: solid, elevated lesion > 0.5 cm in diameter (e.g., psoriasis)

Bullae: same as vesicle only > 0.5 cm (e.g., contact dermatitis, large second-degree burns, bulbous impetigo, pemphigus)

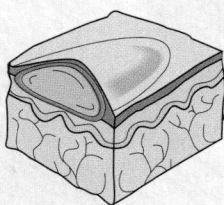

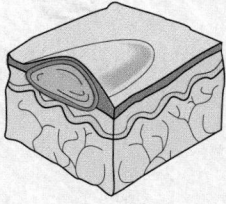

Nodule: solid and elevated; extends deeper than papule into the dermis or subcutaneous tissues, 0.5–2.0 cm (e.g., lipoma, erythema, cyst)

Pustule: pus-filled vesicle or bullae, < 0.5 cm in diameter (e.g., acne, impetigo, carbuncles)

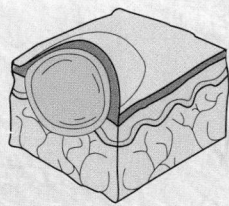

Cyst: subcutaneous or dermis mass (e.g., sebaceous or epidermoid cyst)

*(continues)*

## TABLE 27-11     COMMON SKIN LESIONS (continued)

### Secondary Lesions

| Above the Skin Surface | Below the Skin Surface | Below the Skin Surface |
|---|---|---|
| 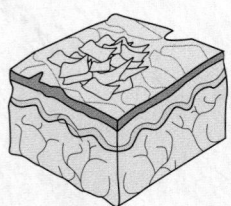 Scales: flaking of the skin's surface (e.g., dandruff, psoriasis) | 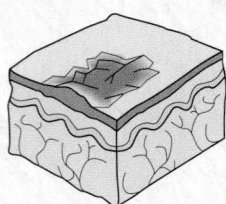 Erosion: loss of epidermis (e.g., ruptured chickenpox vesicle) | 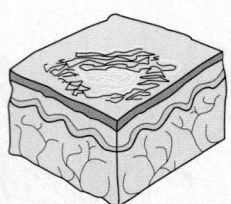 Scar: fibrous tissue that replaces dermal tissue after injury (e.g., surgical incision) |
| 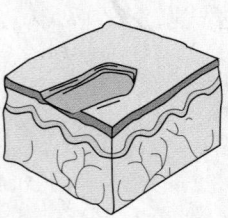 Crust: dried serum, blood, or pus on skin's surface (e.g., impetigo) | 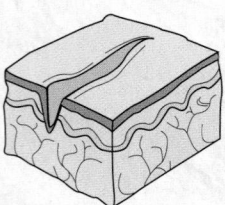 Fissure: linear crack in the epidermis that can extend into the dermis (e.g., chapped hands or lips, athlete's foot) | 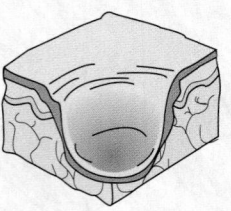 Keloid: enlarging of a scar past wound edges due to excess collagen formation (more prevalent in dark-skinned persons) (e.g., scar) |
| 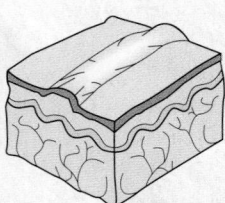 Atrophy: thinning of skin surface and loss of markings (e.g., striae, aged skin) | 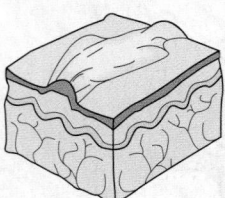 Ulcer: depressed lesion of the epidermis and upper papillary layer of the dermis (e.g., stage 2 pressure ulcer) | 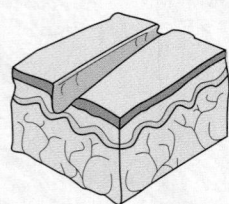 Excoriation: loss of epidermal layers exposing the dermis (e.g., abrasion) |

## TABLE 27-12     VARIATIONS OF THE NAILBED

| 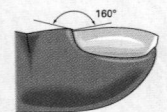 | 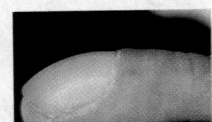 | 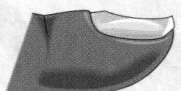 | 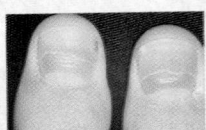 | 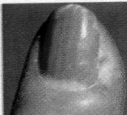 |
|---|---|---|---|---|
| Normal nail: Has an angle of approximately 160° between the fingernail and nail base; nail feels firm when palpated. | Clubbing: Hypoxia causes an angle greater than 180° between the fingernail and nail base; nail feels springy when palpated. *Courtesy of Robert A. Silverman, MD, Pediatric Dermatology, Georgetown University* | Koilonychia (Spoon nail): Characterized by concave curves; associated with iron deficiency anemia. | Beau's line: Characterized by transverse depression in the nails; associated with injury and severe systemic infections. *Courtesy of Robert A. Silverman, MD, Pediatric Dermatology, Georgetown University* | Paronychia: Characterized by an inflammation at the nail base (may be swollen, red, or tender); associated with trauma and local infection. |

## TABLE 27-13 ASSESSMENT OF HEAD AND NECK: NORMAL AND KEY FINDINGS

| Area of Assessment/*Normal Findings* | Key Findings |
|---|---|
| **Skull: Inspect and Palpate** | |
| 1. Inspect skull for shape, symmetry, size in proportion to body and position. *Rounded, symmetrical, normocephalic, upright.* | 1. Asymmetry, or enlarged skull size may be indicative of hydrocephalus and Paget's disease. |
| 2. Palpate with fingerpads, beginning in frontal area and continuing over parietal, temporal, and occipital areas for contour, masses, depressions, and tenderness. *Smooth, nontender, free of masses or depressions.* | 2. Hard or soft masses are abnormal and may be indicative of carcinomas or lymphomas. Softening of outer bone layer may be caused by hydrocephalus or demineralization of bone secondary to rickets, hypervitaminosis A, or syphilis. |
| **Face: Inspect** | |
| 1. Inspect facial features for expression, shape, and symmetry of eyebrows, nasolabial fold, placement of nose, eyes, and ears. *May be oval, round, or square. Symmetrical facial features and movement.* | 1. a. Asymmetry may be indicative of cranial nerve VII damage, a stroke, or Bell's palsy.<br>b. Sunken temples, eyes, and cheeks are indicative of dehydration and malnutrition. (Refer to Box 27-15 on page 614 for a description of common abnormal faces.) |
| 2. Inspect for edema and masses | 2. Puffy, swollen appearance anterior to ear lobes and above angles of jaw may indicate parotid gland enlargement. |
| **Eyes: Inspect and Palpate** | |
| 1. Assess visual acuity (Figure 27-40).<br>    a. Position Snellen chart 20 feet in front of client.<br>    b. Remove corrective lenses, if appropriate.<br>    c. Instruct client to cover one eye and read lines, starting with top of chart from left to right (Figure 27-39); note the line where the client correctly reads more than half the letters.<br>    d. Record results as a fraction sc (without correction), 20/distance number, and the number of letters missed for the eye test.<br>    e. Repeat Steps a–d for other eye.<br>    f. If appropriate, repeat Steps a–e with client wearing corrective lenses, record result cc (with correction). *Normal vision, based on the Snellen chart, is 20/20 (at a distance of 20 feet the normal eye can read the chart).* | 1. A value of 20/40 means that a client can read at a distance of 20 feet what a person with normal vision can read at a distance of 40 feet (see Box 27-16 for common refractive errors). |
| 2. Test extraocular muscle movements:<br>    a. Place client in sitting position facing you (Figure 27-41 A & B).<br>    b. Instruct client to hold head still.<br>    c. Ask client to follow an object (finger, pen, penlight) with eyes.<br>    d. Move object through six fields of gaze (Figure 27-41 C–H).<br>    e. Observe for parallel eye movement.<br>    f. Pause during upward and lateral gaze fields to detect involuntary rhythmic oscillation of eyes. | 2. Asymmetrical movement or the presence of nystagmus results from local injury to eye muscles and supporting structures or may indicate neurologic impairment. |

*(continues)*

**TABLE 27-13 ASSESSMENT OF HEAD AND NECK: NORMAL AND KEY FINDINGS (continued)**

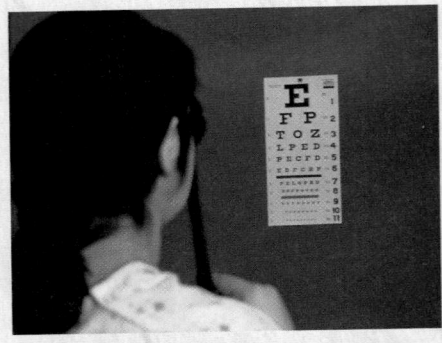

Figure 27-40 Assessing visual acuity

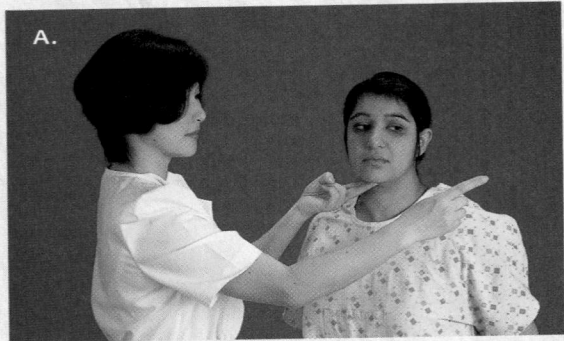
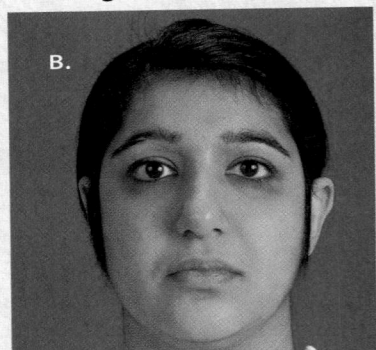

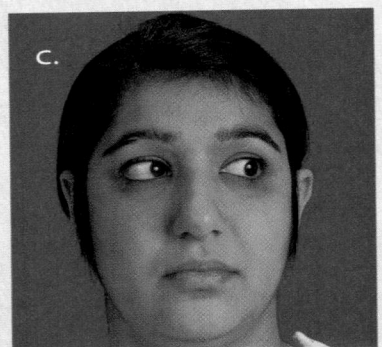
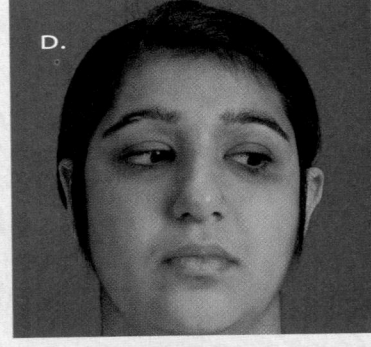
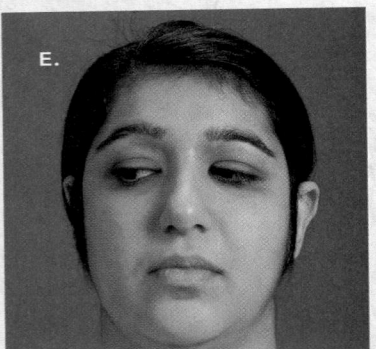

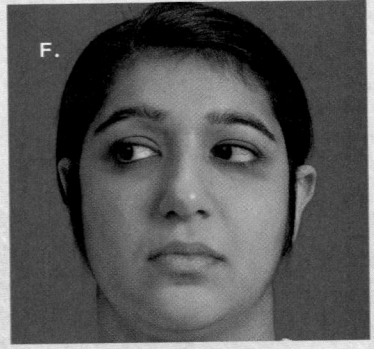
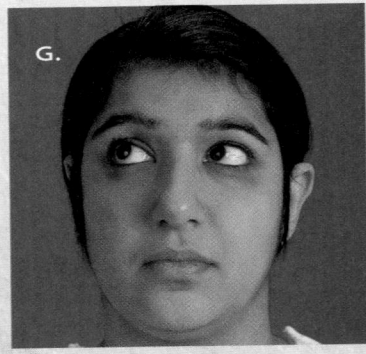
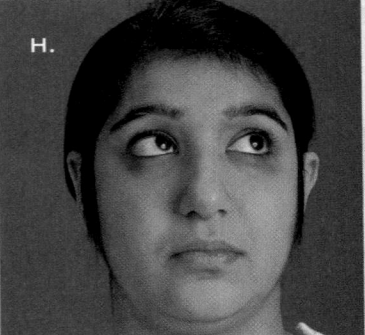

Figure 27-41 Testing extraocular muscle function. A. Basic position. B. Normal resting position. C. Conjugate left lateral gaze. D. Left down and lateral gaze. E. Right down and lateral gaze. F. Conjugate right lateral gaze. G. Right up and lateral gaze. H. Left up and lateral gaze.

*(continues)*

## TABLE 27-13   ASSESSMENT OF HEAD AND NECK: NORMAL AND KEY FINDINGS (*continued*)

| Area of Assessment/*Normal Findings* | Key Findings |
|---|---|
| g.  Note position of upper eyelid in relation to the iris and eyelid lag as the client's eyes move from up to down.<br><br>h.  Move the object forward to about 5 inches in front of the client's nose at the midline and observe for convergence.<br><br>i.  Record results. *Eye movements should be symmetrical as both eyes follow the direction of the gaze and converge on the held object as it moves toward the nose. The upper eyelids cover only the uppermost part of the iris and are free from* **nystagmus** *(involuntary, rhythmical oscillation of the eyes.) A few beats of nystagmus with extreme lateral gaze can be normal* (Estes, 2002). | |

3. External anatomic structures (Figure 27-42).

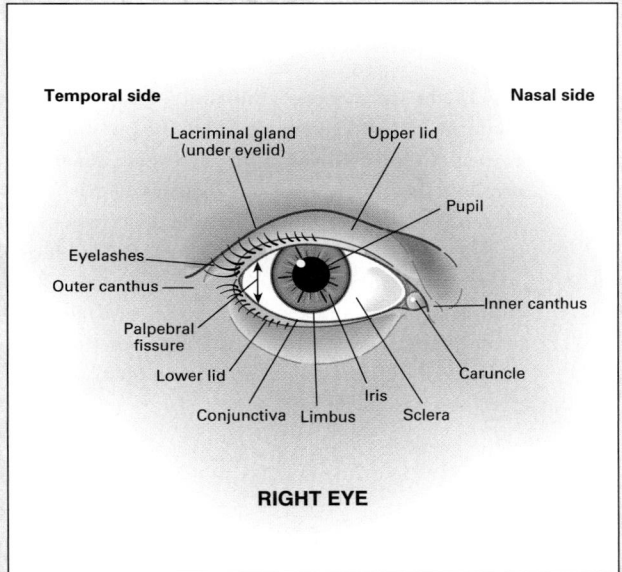

Temporal side                                      Nasal side

Lacriminal gland (under eyelid)     Upper lid

Pupil

Eyelashes

Outer canthus

Inner canthus

Palpebral fissure

Lower lid                                          Caruncle

Conjunctiva  Limbus   Iris   Sclera

**RIGHT EYE**

**Figure 27-42    External structures of the eye**

| Area of Assessment/*Normal Findings* | Key Findings |
|---|---|
| a.  Observe upper eyelid. *Upper eyelid should overlap iris.*<br><br>b.  Check eyes and eyelids for inflammation, crusting, edema, or masses. *Eyes and eyelids should be free from inflammation, crusting, edema, or masses.*<br><br><br><br><br><br><br><br>c.  Inspect and palpate lacrimal glands and sacs for swelling. If lacrimation is excessive:<br>(1) Check for blockage of the nasolacrimal duct by pressing against inner orbital rim of lacrimal sac. | a.  Upper eyelid should not overlap pupil.<br><br>b.  Red lid margins with yellowish scales result from an inflammation of the eyelids (blepharitis). Presence of inflammation, crusting, edema, or masses may indicate acute hordeolum (sty), a painful, red infection of a hair follicle of the eyelashes; chalazion (chronic inflammatory lesion of the meibomian gland); or basal cell carcinoma (papule with a pearly border and a depressed or ulcerated center) of the lower lid.<br><br>c.  Swelling of lacrimal sac indicates dacryocystitis (inflammation) or tumor. Regurgitation of tears through the puncta indicates blockage of lacrimal duct. |

(*continues*)

## TABLE 27-13    ASSESSMENT OF HEAD AND NECK: NORMAL AND KEY FINDINGS (*continued*)

| Area of Assessment/*Normal Findings* | Key Findings |
|---|---|
| (2) Inspect duct blockage by palpating on the lacrimal sac and observing for regurgitation of fluid. *Lacrimal gland should not be palpable. Tears flow freely from the lacrimal gland over the cornea and conjunctiva to the lacrimal duct.*<br><br>d. Inspect bulbar and palpebral conjunctiva and sclera.<br>　(1) Instruct client to look upward while you depress lower lid with your thumb.<br>　(2) Inspect for color, redness, swelling, exudate, or foreign bodies. *Bulbar [". . . conjunctiva, covering the sclera,"] is transparent with small blood vessels visible. Palpebral conjunctiva, covering the inside of the upper and lower eyelids, is pink and moist. Sclera should be white with some superficial blood vessels in light-skinned clients and grayish blue to yellow with tiny brown patches in dark-skinned clients.*<br><br>e. Inspect cornea, lens, pupil, iris, and anterior chamber.<br>　(1) Stand in front of client.<br>　(2) Shine penlight directly on cornea.<br>　(3) Move light laterally and view cornea from that angle; note color, discharge, and lesions.<br>　(4) Look at pupil and note size and shape (see Box 27-17 on page 614).<br>　(5) Shine penlight directly on pupil to assess the lens and its color.<br>　(6) Look at iris for size, and ability of the pupils to react to light.<br>　(7) Anterior chamber is the compartment between the cornea and iris. This space between must be adequate enough to let aqueous fluid out of the eye. Shine a light obliquely through anterior chamber from lateral side toward nasal side. Observe the distribution of light in the anterior chamber.<br>*Cornea are moist, shiny, and clear; lens are transparent; pupils are black, round, and equal diameter, ranging from 2–6 mm. Entire iris should illuminate when shining light laterally to nasally.*<br><br>f. Test pupillary responses to light and reaction to accommodation in a dimly lit room.<br>　(1) Instruct client to look straight ahead.<br>　(2) Bring the penlight from the side of the client's face to directly in front of the pupil (Figure 27-43A).<br>　(3) Note the quickness of response to light.<br>　(4) Shine light into same eye, observing response of opposite pupil for equality of size (Figure 27-43B). | d. Bright red conjunctiva with crusty drainage occurs with conjunctivitis (contagious infection of the conjunctiva). It may be bacterial, viral, or allergic. A pale conjunctiva usually indicates anemia. Bright red patch on the exposed bulbar conjunctiva is a subconjunctival hemorrhage that may result from trauma or sudden increase in venous pressure possibly due to coughing, sneezing, anticoagulant therapy, or uncontrolled hypertension.<br><br>e. A grayish, ulcerated area on cornea is abnormal; it may be due to a bacterial infection. Arcus senilis, a bilateral, benign degeneration of the peripheral cornea and normal variation with aging clients, presents as a hazy gray ring, 2 mm in width around the limbus. Opacity of the lens (loss of transparency) occurs with cataracts, caused most commonly by aging. Cloudy pupils occur with cataracts. If the angle is too narrow, or drainage is inadequate, the pressure of the aqueous fluid in the anterior chamber increases, and glaucoma develops.<br><br>f. Altered pupillary reaction time and equality occur with increased intracranial pressure, lesions involving the third cranial nerve, trauma, or some medications. Pupillary constriction occurs with inflammation of the iris or in response to medication (e.g., pilocarpine or morphine). Pupillary dilation may occur with trauma, neurologic disorders, glaucoma, or in response to medication (e.g., atropine). |

*(continues)*

| TABLE 27-13 | ASSESSMENT OF HEAD AND NECK: NORMAL AND KEY FINDINGS (continued) |
|---|---|

| Area of Assessment/*Normal Findings* | Key Findings |
|---|---|

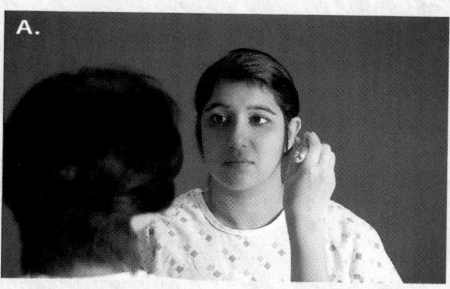

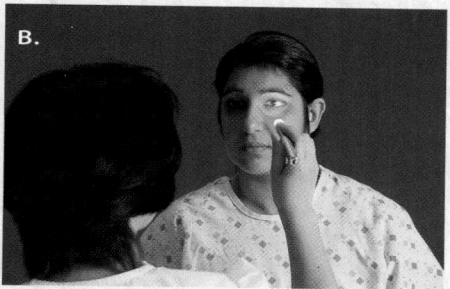

**Figure 27-43**   A. Move penlight from side of client's face to eye. B. Shine penlight into the eye and observe response of the opposite pupil.

(5) Repeat Steps 2 to 4, opposite eye.

(6) Instruct client to gaze at your finger held 4 to 6 inches from her nose, then to glance at a distant object while you note pupillary reflex.

(7) Move the finger toward the bridge of the client's nose, noting response of both pupils.

(8) Record results PERRLA (pupils equal, round, reactive to light and accommodation).
*Pupil should constrict quickly in direct response to light and the opposite pupil should also constrict. Pupils should be equal in size. Pupillary accommodation causes constriction in response to objects that are near, and dilation occurs to accommodate distant vision, with symmetrical convergence of eyes.*

4. Test visual fields (Confrontation Test)
   a. Sit or stand 2 feet in front of client with your eyes at the same level as the client's.
   b. Instruct client to cover the right eye while you cover your left eye, and ask client to look into your eye directly opposite to create one vision field.
   c. Hold your free hand at arm's length, equidistant from you and the client. Move your hand or an object into your and the client's field of vision from nasal, temporal, superior, inferior, and oblique angles.

4. Defects in the visual field can be associated with tumors, strokes, or neurologic diseases such as glaucoma or retinal detachment.

*(continues)*

## TABLE 27-13    ASSESSMENT OF HEAD AND NECK: NORMAL AND KEY FINDINGS (continued)

| Area of Assessment/*Normal Findings* | Key Findings |
|---|---|
| d. Instruct client to tell you when your finger becomes visible.<br>e. Note if you see the finger before the client does.<br>f. Repeat Steps c and d for each field of vision.<br>g. Record results, indicating eye tested.<br>h. Repeat Steps b–g with other eye. *Consensual peripheral vision should occur when the nurse's finger comes into the client's visual field.* | |
| 5. Inspect fundus with ophthalmoscope. (Fundus examination requires advanced assessment skills of a nurse practitioner.)<br>  a. Set ophthalmoscope at 0 diopters.<br>  b. Instruct client to gaze at a designated point on the far wall, keeping both eyes open during the examination.<br>  c. With your right hand, hold the ophthalmoscope 10 inches from the client and use your right eye to examine the client's right eye. Rest your left hand on client's forehead.<br>  d. Shine the light on the pupil and locate the red reflex (bright, orange glow).<br>  e. Slowly move the ophthalmoscope closer until the retina is seen. While rotating the lens, dial to focus on the internal structures (Figure 27-44).<br>  f. Assess the size, color, and clarity of the optic disc.<br>  g. Carefully follow the blood vessel central to the optic disc into each of the four quadrants, observing for lesions (hemorrhages or exudates).<br>  h. Inspect the appearance of the macula, lateral to optic disc.<br>  i. Repeat Steps a–h using your left eye and left hand to examine the client's left eye. | 5. Changes in color, size, or clarity of the margins of the optic disc or the identification of lesions should be recorded and reported; a follow-up examination by an ophthalmologist should be scheduled. |

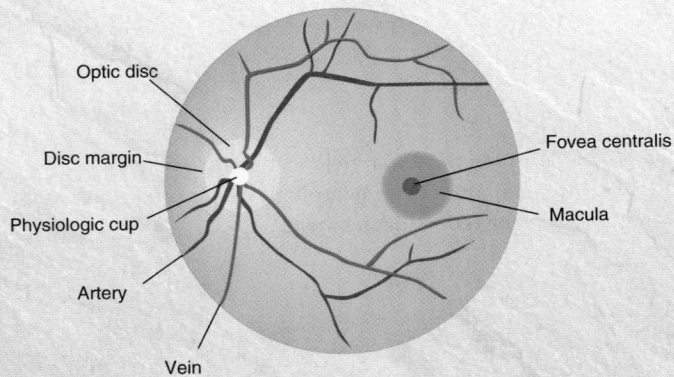

**LEFT EYE**

**Figure 27-44    Landmarks of the retina**

(continues)

## TABLE 27-13    ASSESSMENT OF HEAD AND NECK: NORMAL AND KEY FINDINGS (continued)

| Area of Assessment/*Normal Findings* | Key Findings |
|---|---|
| j.  Record findings. *Red reflex is present. Optic disc is pinkish orange, with a yellow-white excavated center known as the physiologic cup. The ratio of the cup diameter to that of the entire disc is 1:3. Disc border may be sharp, or rounded to a more blended border. Four main vascular branches come from the disc; each branch consists of an arteriole and venule. Venules are darker in color and four times the size of the arterioles. Arterial-to-venous width is a ratio of 2:3 or 4:5.* | |

**Ears: Inspect and Palpate**

| | |
|---|---|
| 1.  Examine external ears, called auricle or pinna, for placement, symmetry, color, discharge, and swelling (Figure 27-45). *Symmetrical, with upper attachment at eye-corner level (lateral canthus), flesh color.* | 1.  Ears set below lateral canthus occur with congenital anomalies (e.g., Down syndrome). Redness indicates inflammation or fever. Yellow or green discharge, itching, or pain occurs with middle ear infections (otitis media). |

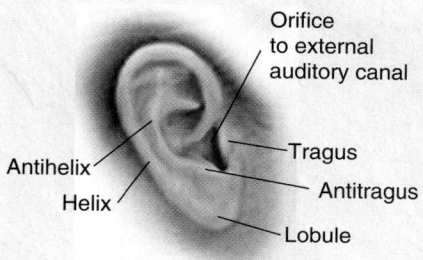

Orifice to external auditory canal

Tragus

Antitragus

Antihelix

Helix

Lobule

**Figure 27-45    External structures of the ear**

| | |
|---|---|
| 2.  Palpate the auricle between thumb and index finger, noting lesions or tenderness by moving auricle up and down. With index and middle fingers, palpate mastoid tip, noting any tenderness. Press inward on tragus, noting any tenderness. *Firm, smooth, free from lesions and pain.* | 2.  Auricular pain is common with acute otitis externa (external air infection). Mastoid tenderness is associated with middle ear inflammation (mastoiditis). Tragus swelling or tenderness may indicate inflammation of the external or middle ear. Keloids (scar tissue) on the ear lobe may result from ear piercing. Yellow or green discharge may indicate infection. |
| 3.  Otoscopic assessment.<br>  a.  Select largest speculum to comfortably fit the client's ear canal.<br>  b.  Tip client's head away from the ear being assessed and straighten ear canal by grasping and pulling the auricle upward, back, and slightly outward, if client is older than 3 years old. For infants and children under the age of 3, pull auricle down and back.<br>  c.  Hold otoscope securely in dominant hand, rest back of dominant hand against side of client's face, and slowly insert speculum. | 3.  Buildup of cerumen, a normal moist, waxy yellow substance that turns hard, dry, and dark yellow-brown when impacted, may cause temporary hearing loss. Swollen or reddened canal with discharge occurs with infection. Nontender, nodular swelling deep in the ear canal suggests osteoma (usually a benign tumor composed of bone tissue). Red, bulging tympanic membrane indicates acute purulent otitis media; whitish appearance on tympanic membrane results from pus in the middle ear. Perforations of the tympanic membrane result from infection or trauma. Scarring may be a result from chronic ear infections. Tympanostomy |

*(continues)*

## TABLE 27-13    ASSESSMENT OF HEAD AND NECK: NORMAL AND KEY FINDINGS (continued)

| Area of Assessment/Normal Findings | Key Findings |
| --- | --- |
| d. Examine the canal for earwax, foreign bodies, discharge, scaliness, redness, or swelling. If wax or a foreign body is present, stop the examination and make referral to qualified specialist.<br><br>e. Inspect the tympanic membrane by sliding speculum slightly down and forward. If membrane is not visible, gently pull the auricle slight farther to straighten the canal.<br><br>f. Identify the color, light reflex, umbo, the short process, and long handle of the malleus. Note perforations, lesions, bulging or retraction of the membrane, dilation of blood vessels, bubbles, or fluid level (Figure 27-46). | tubes may be surgically placed for prolonged otitis media with effusion. |

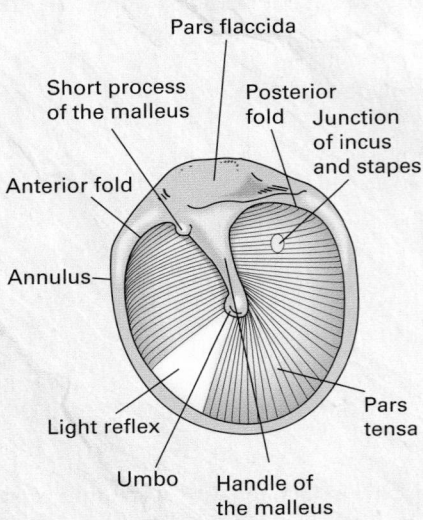

**Figure 27-46    Tympanic landmarks**

Pars flaccida

Short process of the malleus

Posterior fold    Junction of incus and stapes

Anterior fold

Annulus

Light reflex

Umbo    Handle of the malleus

Pars tensa

| Area of Assessment/Normal Findings | Key Findings |
| --- | --- |
| g. Gently withdraw the speculum and repeat procedure in opposite ear. *Cerumen, a waxy yellow or brown substance, is normal. Ear canal is pinkish and dry. Intact tympanic membrane, translucent or pearly gray. Light reflex is seen at 5 o'clock in right ear and 7 o'clock in left ear.*<br><br>4. Test auditory acuity.<br>  a. Whispered voice test:<br>    (1) Instruct client to occlude one ear with finger and repeat the words when heard.<br>    (2) Nurse stands 1 to 2 feet away from client, out of view to avoid client lip-reading, and softly whispers numbers on side of open ear. Increase voice volume until client identifies words correctly. | a. Inability to hear words may indicate a high-frequency hearing loss (e.g., resulting from excessive exposure to loud noises). |

(continues)

**TABLE 27-13    ASSESSMENT OF HEAD AND NECK:
NORMAL AND KEY FINDINGS** (*continued*)

| Area of Assessment/*Normal Findings* | Key Findings |
|---|---|
| (3) Repeat procedure on other ear.<br>(4) Record results. *Client should be able to repeat whispered words.* | |
| b. Weber test:<br>  (1) Strike tuning fork (512 Hz) against your fist or pinch the prongs together.<br>  (2) Hold the base (handle) of the vibrating fork with your thumb and index finger and place the base of the fork on the top of the head at the midline (Figure 27-47).<br>  (3) Ask client if the sound was heard centrally or toward one side.<br>  (4) Record results. *Sound perceived equally in both ears; results indicate a "negative" Weber test.* | b. Results "positive" from Weber test when sound lateralizes to affected ear with a unilateral conductive hearing loss. Occurs with impacted cerumen, perforated tympanic membrane, serum or pus in the middle ear, or fusion of the ossicles. Sound can also lateralize to unaffected ear with sensorineural hearing loss. Occurs with inner ear disorders, auditory nerve damage, or results from repeated, prolonged loud noise or effects of ototoxic drugs. |

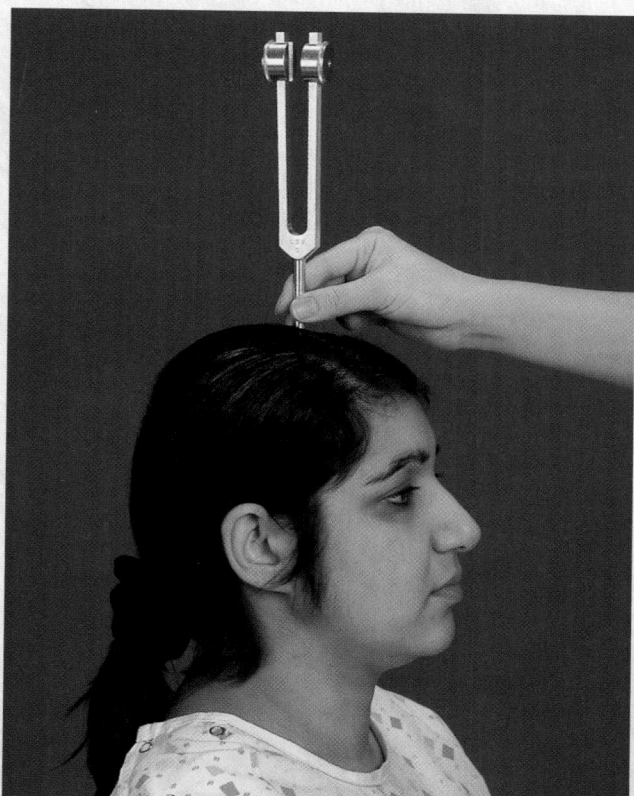

**Figure 27-47    Weber test: place the base of the tuning fork on the top of the client's head.**

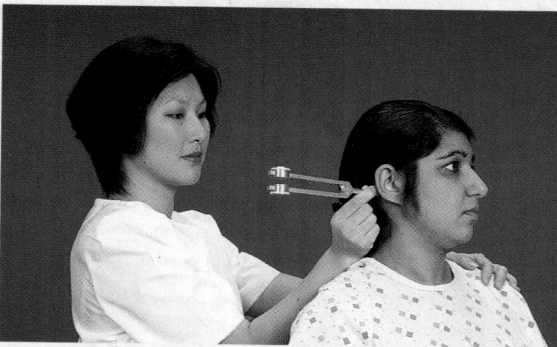

A.

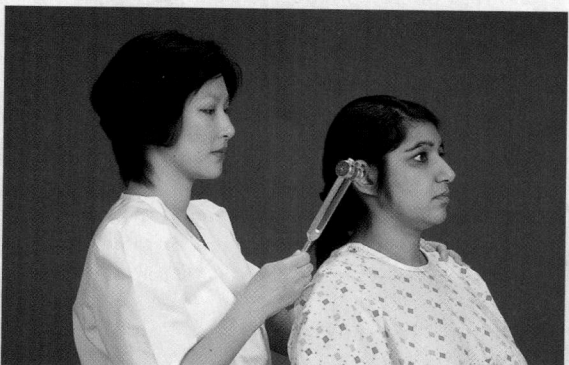

B.

**Figure 27-48    Rinne test: A. Place the base of the fork on the mastoid process. B. Place tuning fork in front of ear canal.**

(*continues*)

## TABLE 27-13   ASSESSMENT OF HEAD AND NECK: NORMAL AND KEY FINDINGS (*continued*)

| Area of Assessment/*Normal Findings* | Key Findings |
|---|---|
| c. Rinne test:<br>  (1) Vibrate prongs of tuning fork and place base of fork on mastoid process of ear being tested and note the time on your watch. Instruct the client to indicate if the sound is heard, and ask the client to tell you when the sound stops (Figure 27-48A)<br>  (2) When the client says that the sound has stopped, move the vibrating fork in front of the ear canal, noting the length of time sound is heard (Figure 27-48B).<br>  (3) Record results.<br>  (4) Repeat test, opposite ear.<br>  *Sound heard longer in front of the right auditory meatus than on the mastoid process because air conduction is twice as long as bone.* | c. Bone conduction is equal to or greater than air conduction. Occurs with conductive hearing loss resulting from diseases, obstruction, or damage to outer or middle ear. |
| **Nose and Sinuses: Inspect, Palpate, and Percuss**<br>1. Inspect the nose for symmetry, deformity, flaring, or inflammation and discharge from the nares. *Located symmetrically, midline of the face, and is without swelling, bleeding, lesions, or masses.* | 1. Swollen or broken as a result of trauma or surgery. |
| 2. Test patency of each nostril.<br>  a. Instruct the client to close the mouth and apply pressure on one naris and breathe.<br>  b. Repeat test on opposite naris. *Each nostril is patent.* | 2. Air cannot move through the nostril. May occur with a deviated septum, foreign body, upper respiratory infection, allergies, or nasal polyps. |
| 3. Inspect the nasal cavities with a penlight.<br>  a. Tilt the client's head in an extended position.<br>  b. Place nondominant hand on client's head. Using your thumb, lift the tip of the nose.<br>  c. With the lit penlight, assess each nostril: note color of anterior nares, nasal septum for deviation, perforation, lesions, or bleeding, and inspect for swelling, discharge. *Mucosa is pink or dull red without swelling or polyps. Septum is midline and intact. A small amount of clear watery discharge is normal.* | 3. Rhinitis, red, swollen mucosa with copious clear, watery discharge occurs with a cold. Discharge becomes purulent if a secondary bacterial infection develops. Pale, edematous mucosa with clear, watery discharge occurs with allergies or hay fever. A normal mucosa with clear, watery nasal discharge that tests positive for glucose following head injury or nasal, sinus, or dental surgery usually indicates the leakage of cerebrospinal fluid. If present, stop the exam and make a referral to a qualified specialist immediately. |
| 4. Palpate the nasal sinuses (Figures 27-49 and 27-50) by applying gentle, upward pressure on frontal and maxillary areas, avoiding pressure on the eyes. Percuss area with middle or index finger and note the sound. *Nontender, air-filled cavities, resonant to percussion.* | 4. Pain or tenderness may be caused by viral, bacterial, or allergic processes that cause inflammation and obstruction, eliciting a dull sound. |
| **Mouth and Pharynx: Inspect and Palpate**<br>1. Stand 12 to 18 inches in front of client and smell the breath. *Breath should smell fresh.* | 1. Halitosis (foul-smelling breath) occurs with tooth decay or disease of gums, tonsils, or sinuses or with poor oral hygiene (see Box 27-18 on page 614 for common abnormal breath odors). |
| 2. Observe the lips for color, moisture, swelling, or lesions. Instruct client to open mouth. With a tongue depressor, retract the buccal mucosa and note color, hydration, | 2. Pale or cyanotic lips may indicate systemic hypoxemia. Dry, cracked lips occur with dehydration or exposure to weather. Swollen lips (angioneurotic |

*(continues)*

## TABLE 27-13    ASSESSMENT OF HEAD AND NECK: NORMAL AND KEY FINDINGS (*continued*)

| Area of Assessment/*Normal Findings* | Key Findings |
|---|---|

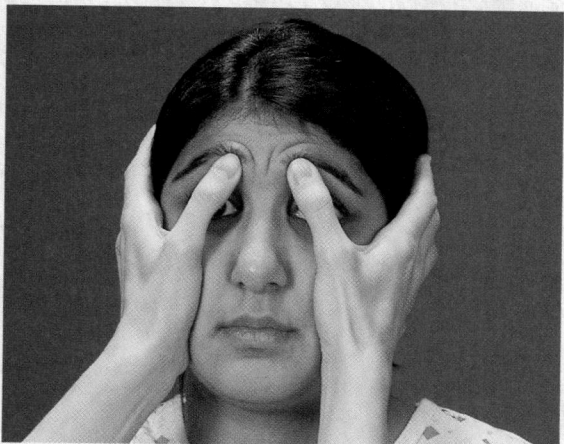

**Figure 27-49    Palpating frontal sinuses**

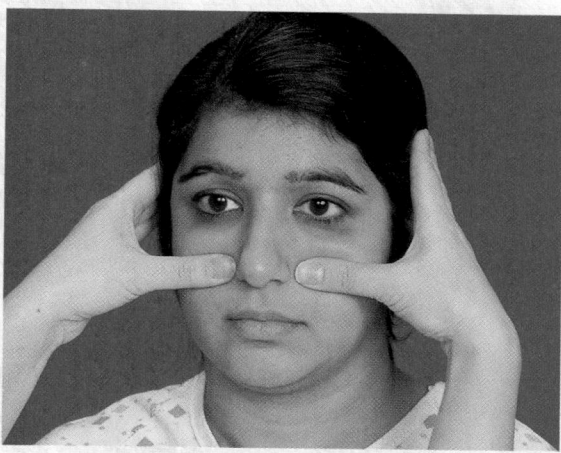

**Figure 27-50    Palpating maxillary sinuses**

inflammation, or lesions (Figure 27-51). Invert lower lip with your thumbs on inner oral mucosa, note muscle tone; repeat with upper lips using thumbs and index fingers. *Lips and mucosa should be pink, firm, and moist without inflammation or lesions.*

3. If present, remove dentures. Retract the cheeks with a tongue depressor and inspect gums (gingivae). Note color, edema, retraction, bleeding, and lesions. Palpate the gums with the tongue blade for texture. *Gums are pink, smooth, moist, and firm.*

4. Instruct client to clench teeth. Note position and alignment. Inspect teeth: use tongue depressor to expose the molars. Note tartar, cavities, extraction, and color. *Properly aligned, smooth, white, and shiny.*

5. Instruct client to protrude the tongue.

   a. Inspect dorsum of tongue. Note color, hydration, texture, symmetry, presence or absence of fasciculations (Figure 27-52).

edema) result from allergic reactions (e.g., medication or food; see Box 27-19 on page 614 for common lip lesions).

3. Pale gums that bleed easily may indicate periodontal disease or vitamin C deficiency.

4. Chalky white discoloration of teeth's enamel indicates early formation of dental caries (cavities). Brown or black discoloration indicates formation of caries.

5. Enlarged tongue may indicate glossitis or stomatitis or may occur with myxedema, acromegaly, or amyloidosis. Deep red, smooth surface occurs with glossitis caused by vitamin $B_{12}$, iron, or niacin deficiency or as a side effect from chemotherapy. Thick white coating with red, raw surface is candidiasis (thrush) indicating immunosuppression. Lesions on ventral surface or hardened areas or ulcerations on the lateral surface may indicate cancer.

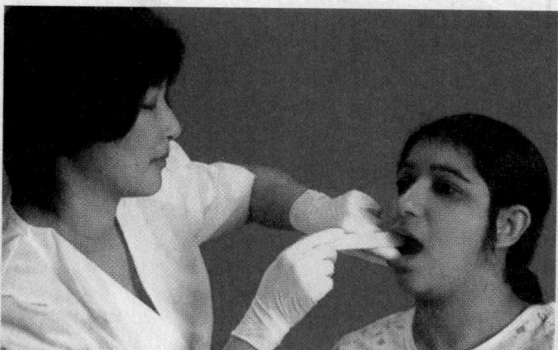

**Figure 27-51    Inspecting buccal mucosa**

*(continues)*

## TABLE 27-13     ASSESSMENT OF HEAD AND NECK: NORMAL AND KEY FINDINGS (continued)

| Area of Assessment/*Normal Findings* | Key Findings |
| --- | --- |

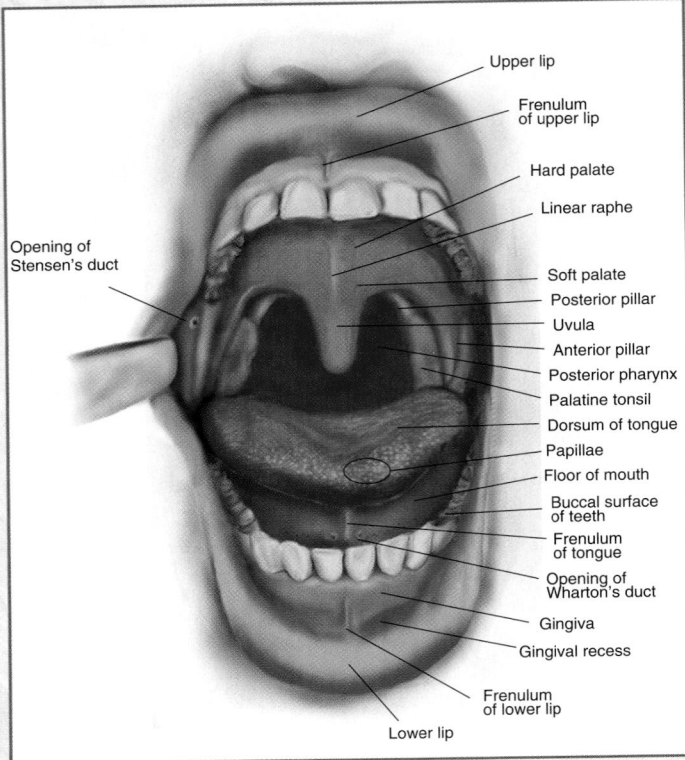

**Figure 27-52    Structures of the tongue**

b.  With penlight, inspect sides and ventral surface. Note size, texture, nodules, or ulcerations.

c.  Grasp tongue with gauze. Gently pull it to one side and palpate the full length of tongue.

d.  With penlight, inspect floor of mouth, salivary glands, and duct openings. *When protruded, tongue lies midline, medium red or pink in color, moist and smooth along lateral margins, with free mobility. The dorsal surface is slightly rough (taste buds) and free of lesions. The ventral surface is highly vascular, smooth, moist, and free of lesions.*

6.  Inspect the hard and soft palate with penlight.
    a.  Instruct client to extend head backward and hold mouth open.
    b.  Inspect the hard palate (roof of mouth), located anteriorly, and the soft palate, which extends posteriorly to pharynx. Note color, shape, lesions. *Palates are concave and pink. Hard palate has ridges; soft palate is smooth.*

7.  Inspect the pharynx using a tongue depressor and penlight.
    a.  Explain procedure to the client.
    b.  Instruct client to tilt head back and open mouth.

6.  Cleft palate (maxillary processes fail to fuse prenatally) is a congenital defect. Red, swollen, tender palates indicate infection. Eroded lesion on hard palate may indicate cancer.

7.  Reddened, edematous uvula and tonsillar pillars with yellow exudate indicate pharyngitis. Swollen, gray membranes and tonsillar enlargement may result from acute tonsillitis, infectious mononucleosis, or diphtheria.

*(continues)*

## TABLE 27-13    ASSESSMENT OF HEAD AND NECK: NORMAL AND KEY FINDINGS (continued)

| Area of Assessment/*Normal Findings* | Key Findings |
|---|---|
| c. With your nondominant hand, place tongue depressor on middle third of tongue. With dominant hand, shine light into back of throat.<br><br>d. Instruct client to say "ah." Note the position, size, and appearance of tonsils and uvula.<br><br>e. If palate and uvula fail to rise symmetrically with phonation, inform client about eliciting gag reflex (touch the posterior one-third of tongue with blade to stimulate the gag reflex) and inspect as stated in Step 7d. *With phonation, the soft palate and uvula rise symmetrically. The pharynx is pink, vascular, lesion-free. Tonsil size is evaluated using grading scale (Figure 27-53).* | 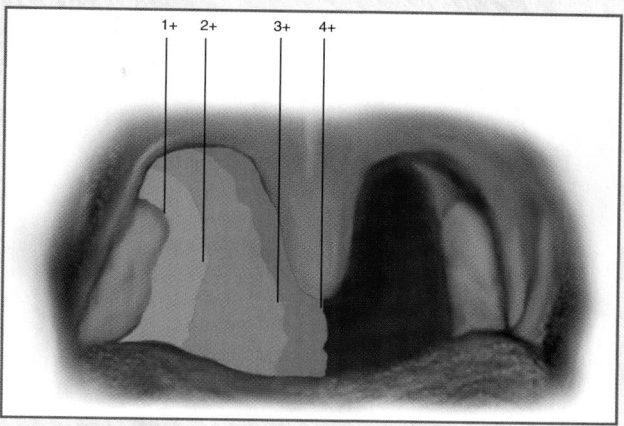<br><br>**Figure 27-53    Grading of tonsils**<br>**1+ tonsils are visible.**<br>**2+ tonsils are between pillars and uvula.**<br>**3+ tonsils are touching uvula.**<br>**4+ one or both tonsils extend to midline of the oropharynx.** |

### Neck: Inspect, Palpate, and Auscultate

1. Inspect for symmetry and musculature. Instruct client to:
   a. Flex chin to chest and to each side and shoulder to test anterior sternocleidomastoid muscle.
   b. Hyperextend the neck backward to test posterior trapezia. *Muscles are symmetrical with head in central position. Movement through full range of motion without complaint of discomfort or limitation.*

2. Palpate lymph nodes. Instruct the client to relax and flex neck slightly forward.
   a. Stand in front of seated client.
   b. Methodically palpate both sides of face and neck simultaneously. With gentle pressure, move pads and tips of middle three fingers in small circular motion. Follow a systematic sequence (Figure 27-54) beginning with the the preauricular, postauricular, occipital, submental, submandibular, and tonsillar nodes. Move down to the neck, palpate anterior cervical chain, the posterior cervical chain, and the supraclavicular nodes.
   c. Note size, shape, mobility, consistency, and tenderness. *Lymph nodes should not be palpable. Small, movable nodes are insignificant.*

3. Inspect and palpate trachea.
   a. Note position.
   b. Place thumbs and index fingers on sides of trachea. Apply gentle pressure and palpate. *Midline position above the suprasternal notch.*

**Key Findings:**

1. Pain with flexion or rotation of head is associated with muscle spasm that may be caused by inflammation of muscles, meninges, or diseases of the vertebrae. Prominent lateral deviation of sternocleidomastoid muscles (torticollis) is commonly associated with inflammation of viral myositis or trauma (e.g., sleeping with head in unusual position). Decreased range of motion is commonly associated with degenerative osteoarthritis.

2. Palpable nodes may result from a variety of diseases, most commonly an infectious process or malignancy.

3. Lateral displacement may be caused by a neck or mediastinum mass or pulmonary disorders.

*(continues)*

## TABLE 27-13    ASSESSMENT OF HEAD AND NECK: NORMAL AND KEY FINDINGS (continued)

| Area of Assessment/*Normal Findings* | Key Findings |
|---|---|

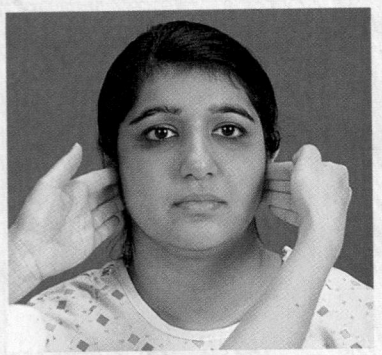

**A. Preauricular**

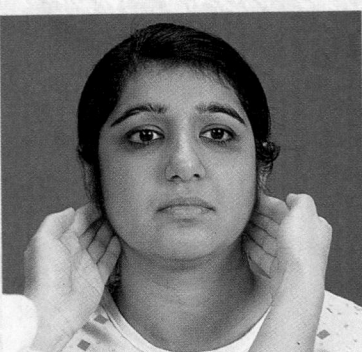

**B. Postauricular**

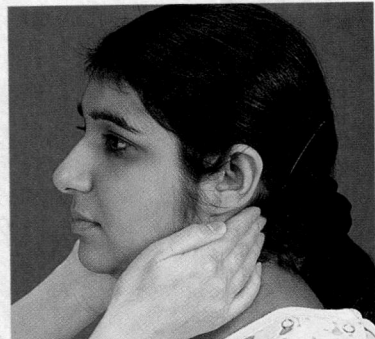

**C. Occipital**

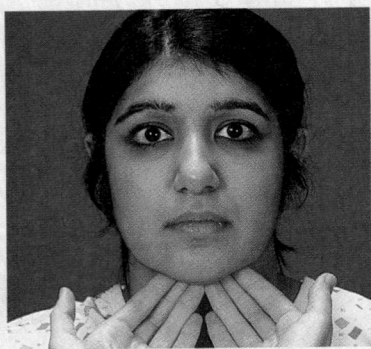

**D. Submental**

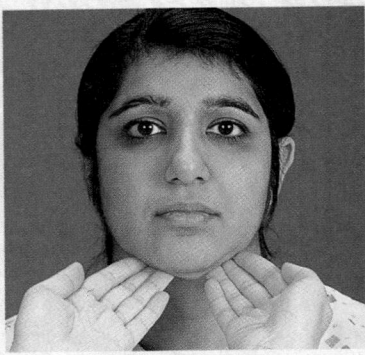

**E. Submandibular**

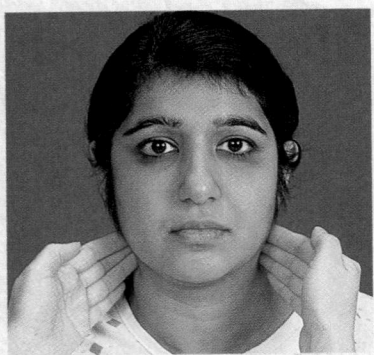

**F. Tonsilar**

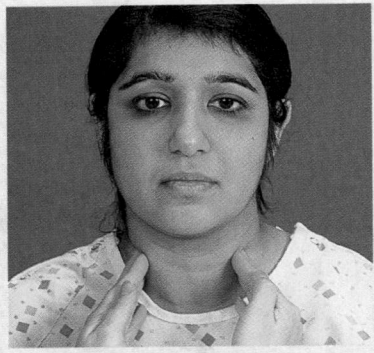

**G. Anterior cervical chain**

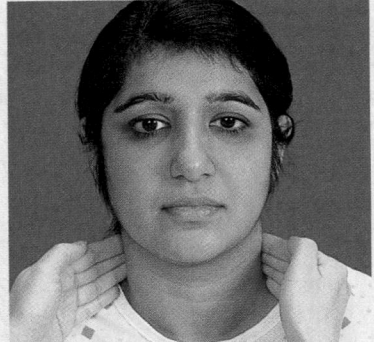

**H. Posterior cervical chain**

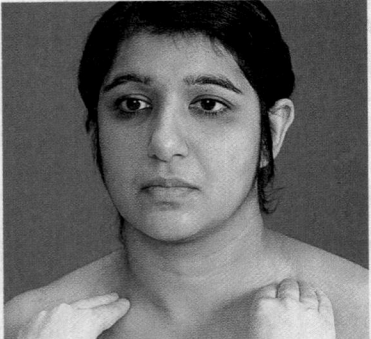

**I. Supraclavicular**

**Figure 27-54    Palpation of lymph nodes**

4. Palpation of the thyroid may be approached anterior or posterior to the seated client (Figure 27-55).
   a. Posterior approach (Figure 27-55A)
      (1) Stand behind client, place thumbs on nape of neck and bring fingers anteriorly around neck with their tips resting over the tracheal rings.
      (2) Ask client to tilt chin forward to relax neck muscles and swallow.

4. Masses or enlargement during swallowing may indicate a goiter (enlarged thyroid gland) or thyroid nodules indicating thyroid disease. Vibrations or bruits heard on auscultation occur with increased turbulence in a vessel and are caused by increased vascularization of the gland (enlarged toxic goiter).

*(continues)*

## TABLE 27-13    ASSESSMENT OF HEAD AND NECK: NORMAL AND KEY FINDINGS (*continued*)

Area of Assessment/*Normal Findings*                    Key Findings

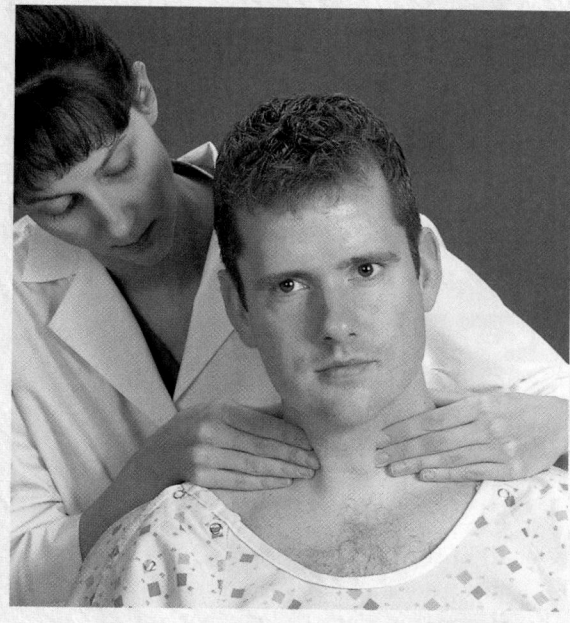

A.

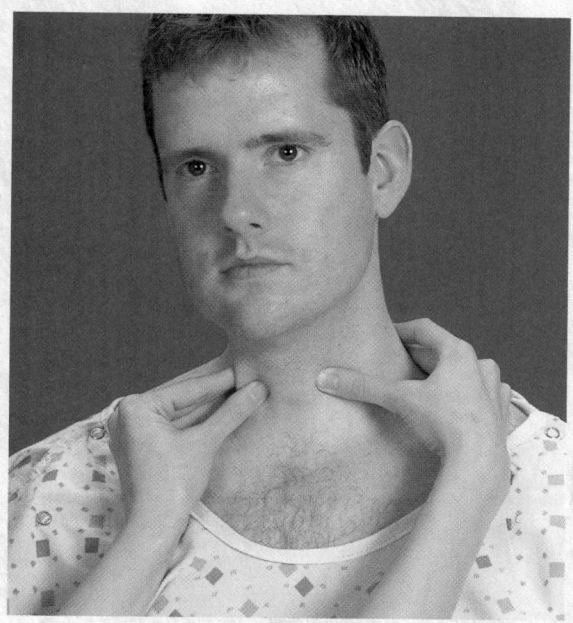

B.

**Figure 27-55    Palpating the thyroid: A. Posterior approach. B. Anterior approach**

(3) Palpate the isthmus rise under your fingers and feel each lateral lobe before and while client swallows.

(4) Ask client to flex neck forward and to left, and displace thyroid cartilage to right with tips of your left fingers. Note any bulging of gland.

(5) Press fingers of left hand against left side of thyroid cartilage to stabilize it while palpating with the fingers of your right hand while the client swallows.

(6) Note consistency, nodularity, or tenderness as gland moves upward.

(7) Repeat Steps 4 through 6 on the opposite side.

b. Anterior approach (Figure 27-55B)

(1) Stand in front of client.

(2) Instruct client to tilt chin forward, and place your right thumb on thyroid cartilage and displace the cartilage to the right.

(3) Grasp the elevated, displaced right lobe with thumb and fingers of left hand and palpate for consistency, nodularity, or tenderness as client swallows.

(4) Repeat Steps 2 to 3 on the opposite side.

(5) If gland appears enlarged, place the bell of the stethoscope over gland and listen for vascular sounds such as a soft, rushing sound, or bruit.
*Thyroid cannot be visualized. It may or may not be felt. If felt, it should be smooth, soft, nontender, and not enlarged.*

From Estes, M. (2002). *Health assessment & physical examination* (2nd ed.). Clifton Park, NY: Delmar Learning.

## BOX 27-15     COMMON ABNORMAL FACES

- Exophthalmos is the protrusion or bulging of the eye that results from an increased pressure in the eye's orbit (e.g., from tumor or inflammation).

- Acromegaly is characterized by an elongated head with prominent forehead, nose, and lower jaw and enlarged nose, lips, and ears resulting from excessive growth hormone.

- Cushing's syndrome is a round or "moon" face with excessive hair growth (mustache and sideburns); it occurs in clients with excessive production of adrenal hormones or in clients taking adrenal hormone medications.

- Clients with chronic renal failure have pale, swollen tissue around their eyes.

- Parkinson's disease causes decreased facial mobility and expressions, producing a masklike face; results from progressive, degenerative, neurologic disorders.

## BOX 27-16     COMMON REFRACTIVE ERRORS

- Myopia (nearsightedness): elongation of the eyeball or an error of refraction that causes the parallel rays to focus in front of the retina.

- Hyperopia (farsightedness): an error of refraction in which rays of light entering the eye are brought into focus behind the retina.

- Presbyopia (farsightedness): an error of refraction resulting from a loss of elasticity of the lens of the eye.

- Astigmatism: an unequal spherical curve of the cornea that prevents the light rays from being focused directly in a point on the retina.

## BOX 27-17     PUPIL SIZE IN MILLIMETERS

## BOX 27-18     COMMON ABNORMAL BREATH ODORS

- Acetone breath ("fruity" smell) is common in malnourished or diabetic clients with ketoacidosis.

- Musty smell is caused by the breakdown of nitrogen and presence of liver disease.

- Ammonia smell occurs during the end stage of renal failure from a buildup of urea.

## BOX 27-19     COMMON LIP LESIONS

- Herpes simplex (cold sores or fever blisters) are painful vesicular lesions that rupture and crust over.

- Chancre (primary lesion of syphilis) is a reddish round, painless lesion with a depressed center and raised edges that appears on the lower lip.

- Squamous cell carcinoma (most common form of oral cancer) usually involves the lower lip and may appear as a thickened plaque, ulcer, or warty growth.

## Nose and Sinuses

Assessment is limited to inspection and palpation of the external nose and nasal passages using a penlight. An examination with a nasal speculum to inspect the nasal chambers is usually performed only by an advanced nurse practitioner because the nasal chambers are lined with respiratory mucosa. Clients with nasal impairments are at risk of developing respiratory infections. Sinus assessment is limited to palpation of the frontal and maxillary sinuses. Transillumination of the sinuses is usually limited to advanced practitioners.

## Mouth and Pharynx

Physical assessment of the oral cavity includes the breath, lips, tongue, buccal mucosa, gums and teeth, hard and soft palates, and pharynx. If the client is wearing dentures or removable orthodontia, remove these devices before examination to visualize and palpate the gums. The oral cavity can yield significant information regarding the client's health, because systemic diseases may manifest initially in the oral cavity.

## Neck

Physical examination of the neck includes the neck muscles, lymph nodes of the head and neck, thyroid gland, and trachea. The lymph nodes are normally not easily palpable. If the client has an enlarged thyroid gland, the blood supply will be increased, causing a fine vibration that can be auscultated with the diaphragm of the stethoscope.

## Thorax and Lungs

Chest assessment begins with inspection, proceeds to palpation and percussion, and then moves to auscultation. Assessment of the thorax and lungs enables the nurse to evaluate the client's ability to breathe and to exchange air. Changes in the respiratory system can occur gradually or quickly. In clients with chronic lung or pulmonary disease, such as emphysema, asthma, and bronchitis, changes are often gradual in an effort to increase lung expansion.

It is important to observe the client's posture. A client with breathing difficulties will often assume a bending forward position with arms thrust forward. This position is an attempt to reduce the effort to breathe and to expand the chest fully.

### Thorax (Chest Landmarks)

Figure 27-56 depicts the landmarks of the thorax.

Landmarks are imaginary lines that are based on anatomic structures such as the spine and sternum. These landmarks assist with visualizing the underlying organs for percussion and auscultation and for accurate documentation of findings. The angle of Louis is a landmark for identifying the ribs in the midclavicular line. Each

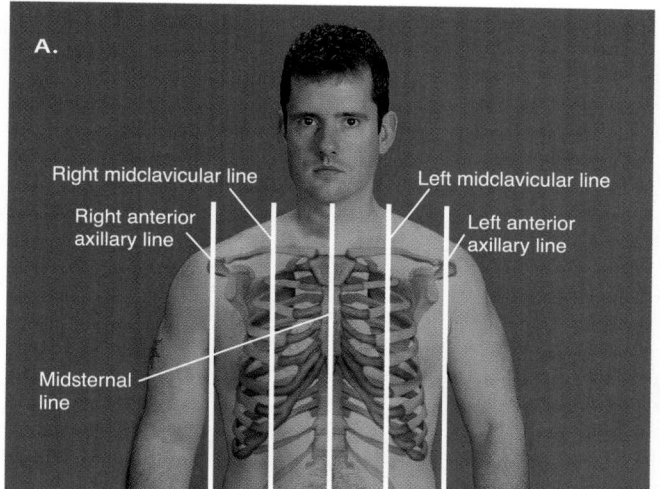

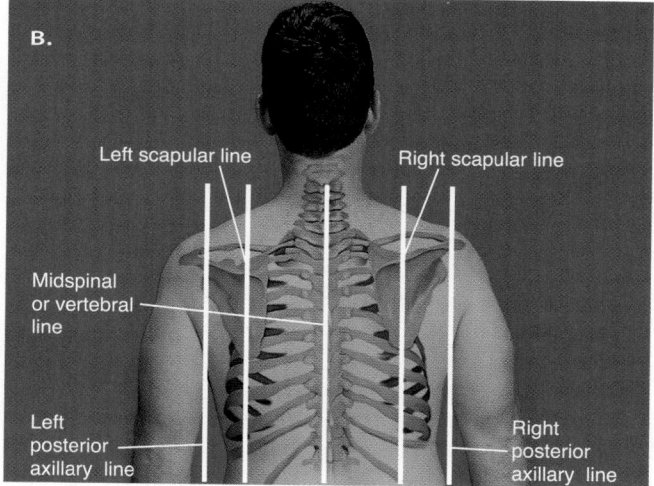

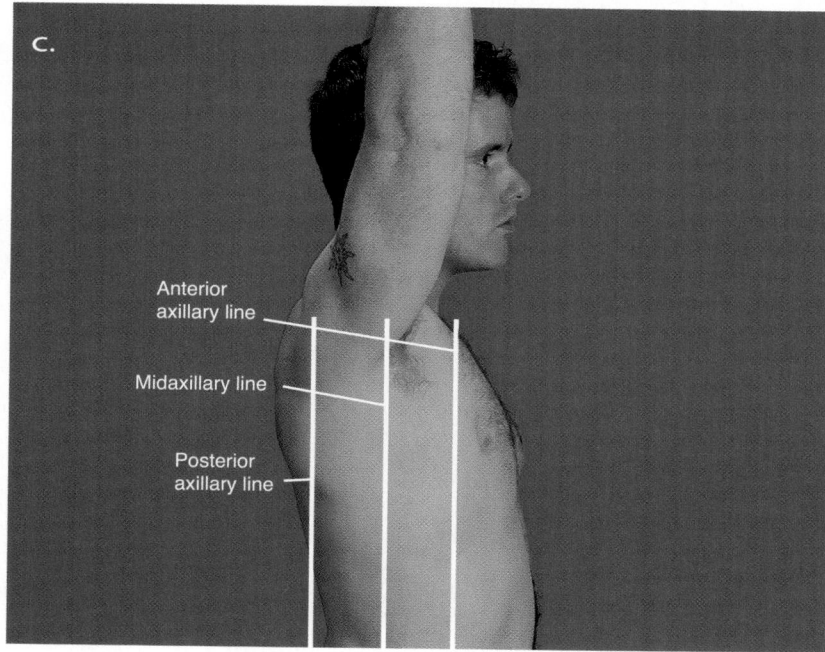

**Figure 27-56** **Landmarks of the thorax: A. Anterior thorax. B. Posterior thorax. C. Right lateral thorax**

intercostal space is named for the number of the rib directly above it; that is, the space between the third and fourth ribs is the third intercostal space. When used together, landmarks and intercostal spaces identify the specific lobes of the lungs for percussion and auscultation.

## Breath Sounds

Respiratory auscultation reveals the presence of normal and abnormal breath sounds. During auscultation, the client should be instructed to breathe only through the mouth, because mouth breathing decreases air turbulence that could interfere with an accurate assessment. Figure 27-57 shows the anterior, posterior, and right lateral positions of the lung lobes. Table 27-14 presents the specific areas of the thorax and lungs to be examined and the normal and key findings of this assessment. See Box 27-20 on page 621 for common terms associated with respiratory assessment.

There are three distinct types of normal breath sounds with their own unique pitch, intensity, quality, location, and relative duration in the inspiratory and expiratory phases of respiration:

- **Vesicular sounds:** soft, breezy, and low-pitched sounds heard longer on inspiration than expiration that result from air moving through the smaller airways over the lung's periphery, with the exception of the scapular area
- **Bronchovesicular sounds:** medium-pitched and blowing sounds heard equally on inspiration and expiration from air moving through the large airways, posteriorly between the scapula and anteriorly over bronchioles lateral to the sternum at the first and second intercostal spaces
- **Bronchial sounds:** loud and high-pitched sounds with a hollow quality heard longer on expiration than inspiration from air moving through the trachea

These normal breath sounds must be auscultated over the correct location—for example, bronchial sounds over the trachea. Otherwise, bronchial sounds in clients with emphysema are heard in the peripheral lung areas where normal vesicular sounds should be heard.

Breath sounds that are not normal are described as either abnormal or **adventitious breath sounds** (superimposed sounds on the normal vesicular, bronchovesicular, and bronchial breath sounds). Abnormal breath sounds are characterized by decreased or absent sounds. See Box 27-21 on page 621 for a description of the five types of adventitious breath sounds.

During the assessment of the thorax and lungs, the nurse should monitor the client for symptoms of hyperventilation (light-headedness or dizziness). If this occurs, assist the client in restoring a normal breathing pattern. Continue with the assessment when the client's dizziness is gone and breathing is normal.

## Heart and Vascular System

The heart and vascular system assessment is conducted through physical assessment of the heart and the extremities. The assessment techniques used are inspection, palpation, and auscultation. The nurse should review the client's profile relative to the health history for cardiac risk factors. Risk factors that clients have no control over are age, gender, race, and family history. However, many risk factors associated with cardiovascular disease are lifestyle practices that clients can control or modify. These include avoiding tobacco use, blood pressure control management, dietary practices to reduce cholesterol and sugar intake, estrogen replacement in postmenopausal women, regular physical exercise habits, and weight management (American Heart Association, 1997; Woods, 2002).

### Heart

The heart is located directly behind the sternum, with the left ventricle projecting into the left chest. Inspection, palpation, and auscultation are performed in a systematic

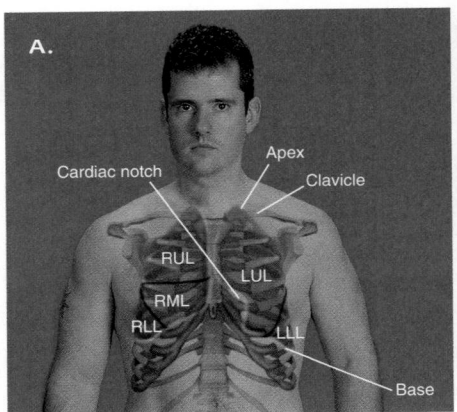
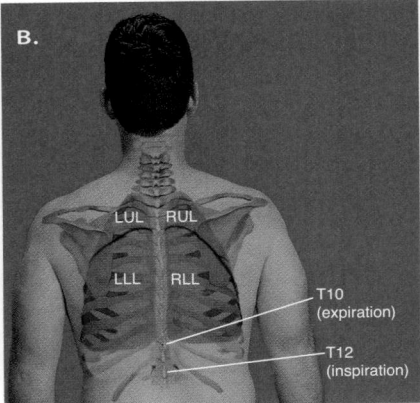
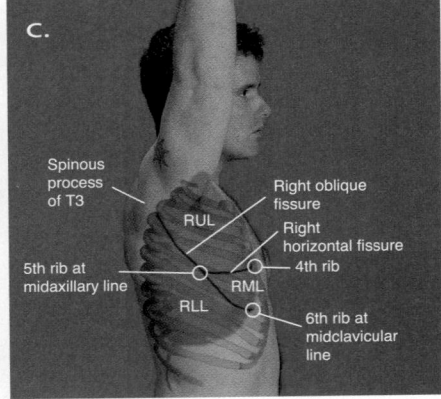

**Figure 27-57**     **Positions of the lung lobes: A. Anterior view with ribs. B. Posterior view with ribs. C. Right lateral view with ribs**

## TABLE 27-14    ASSESSMENT OF THORAX AND LUNGS: NORMAL AND KEY FINDINGS

| Area of Assessment/*Normal Findings* | Key Findings |
|---|---|
| **Posterior Chest: Inspect, Palpate, Percuss, and Auscultate**<br>Place client in a sitting position, arms folded across chest (separates scapulae), back exposed. Refer to Figure 27-56 to review landmarks.<br>1. Inspect posterior thorax.<br>  a. Assess shape and symmetry. Note rate and rhythm of respirations, movement of chest wall with deep inspiration and full expiration, and signs of distress.<br>  b. Estimate the anteroposterior diameter in proportion to lateral diameter. *Respirations are quiet, effortless, and regular, 12 to 20 breaths per minute. Thorax rises and falls in unison with respiratory cycle. Ribs slope across and down, without movement or bulging in the intercostal spaces. The adult ratio of anteroposterior to lateral diameter ranges from 1:2 to 5:7.*<br>2. Palpate.<br>  a. Lesions or areas of pain; palpate and note tenderness.<br>  b. Thoracic expansion at 10th rib: place thumbs close to client's spine and spread hands over thorax (Figure 27-58). Note divergence of thumbs, feel for range and symmetry of movement during deep inhalation and full exhalation.<br>  c. Place ulnar aspect of your open hand at right apex of lung and place the hand at each location as shown in Figure 27-59. Instruct client to say "99" and palpate for **tactile fremitus** (vibrations created by sound waves). Note areas of increased or decreased fremitus. | 1. Structural changes that occur in the thorax are discussed in Chapter 39. Defined horizontal slope of ribs occurs with emphysema. Bulging in the intercostal spaces indicates increased effort of breathing (e.g., emphysema). Retraction of intercostal spaces during inspiration indicates airway obstruction (e.g., asthma). Impairment in respiratory movement occurs with lung or pleural disease.<br><br>2. Tenderness may result from a fractured rib. Unilateral decreased thoracic expansion occurs on the affected side (e.g., pneumonia or pneumothorax). Bilateral decreased expansion occurs when alveoli do not fully expand (e.g., emphysema or pleurisy). Absent or decreased fremitus occurs when voice is decreased, in presence of bronchus obstruction, or by fluid, air, or solid tissue in the pleural space. Fremitus is increased over areas of consolidated lung. |

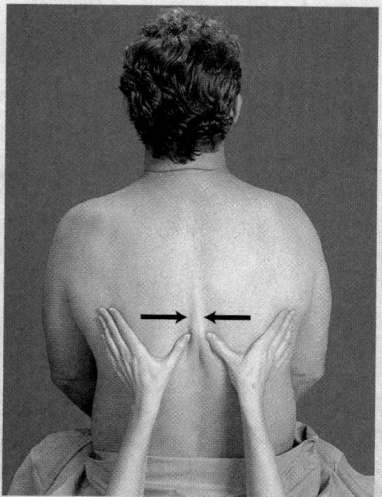

**Figure 27-58    Palpating posterior thoracic expansion**

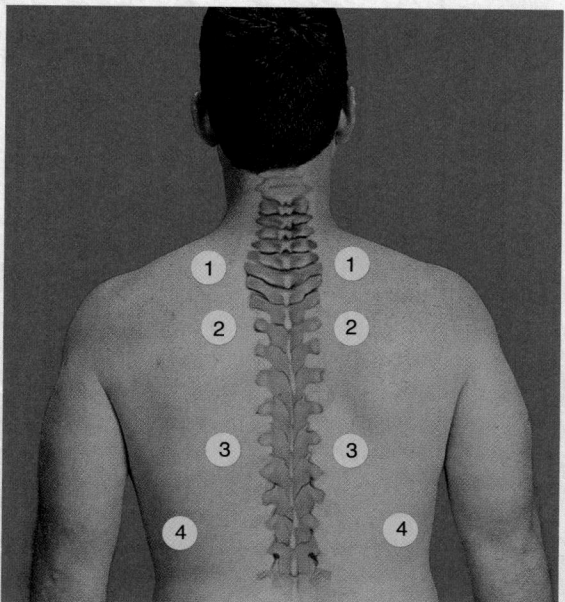

**Figure 27-59    Palpation pattern for tactile fremitus: Posterior thorax**

*(continues)*

## TABLE 27-14  ASSESSMENT OF THORAX AND LUNGS: NORMAL AND KEY FINDINGS (*continued*)

| Area of Assessment/*Normal Findings* | Key Findings |
|---|---|
| d. Move hands from side to side, from right to left, with client repeating the words with the same intensity every time you place your hands on the back. *Thumbs should separate an equal distance (3 to 5 cm) and in the same direction during thoracic expansion and meet in the midline on expiration. Posterior thorax is free from tenderness, lesions, and pulsations. Fremitus is equal on both sides of thorax, strongest at the level of tracheal bifurcation.* | |
| 3. Percuss chest systematically (Figure 27-60). <br> a. Start at lung apices. Move hands from side to side across the top of each shoulder. Note sound produced from each percussion strike and compare with contralateral sound. <br> b. Continue downward and posterolateral every other intercostal space. Note intensity, pitch, duration, and quality of percussion. *Air-filled lungs create a resonant sound. Identify contralateral sound; bones (e.g., ribs or spine) create a flat sound. Thorax is more resonant in children and thin adults.* | 3. Hyperresonance in adults occurs in pneumothorax, emphysema, or asthma. Dull sound is created in solid or fluid-filled structures (e.g., pneumonia, pleural effusion, or tumors). Pleural fluid sinks to lowest part of pleural space (posteriorly in a supine client). <br><br> 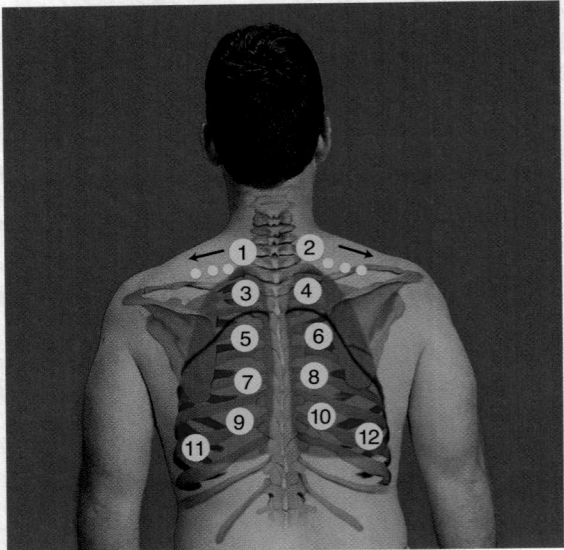 <br> **Figure 27-60  Percussion pattern of posterior thorax** |
| 4. Auscultate posterior and lateral surfaces. <br> a. Place diaphragm of stethoscope on right lung apex. Instruct client to inhale and exhale deeply and slowly when the stethoscope is felt on the back. Repeat on left lung apex. <br> b. Move downward every other intercostal space and auscultate, placing stethoscope in the same position on both sides. <br> c. Auscultate the lateral aspect by placing the stethoscope directly below the right axilla, instructing the client to breathe only through the mouth and to inhale and exhale deeply and slowly. Proceed downward, every other intercostal space on the same side. | 4. Decreased breath sounds caused by an inability to inhale and exhale deeply (e.g., emphysema or by an obstruction; atelectasis or foreign object). Absent breath sounds (e.g., empyema, hemothorax, pneumothorax, or pneumonectomy). See Box 27-21 for a description of adventitious breath sounds. |

(*continues*)

## TABLE 27-14 ASSESSMENT OF THORAX AND LUNGS: NORMAL AND KEY FINDINGS (continued)

| Area of Assessment/*Normal Findings* | Key Findings |
|---|---|

d. Repeat Step c on left side. *Posterior sounds: bronchovesicular and vesicular sounds; lateral: vesicular sounds. A large chest will produce decreased breath sounds.*

**Anterior Chest: Inspect, Palpate, Percuss, and Auscultate**
Place client in a sitting or supine position.
1. Instruct client to inhale deeply and exhale fully. Inspect anterior thorax for:
  a. Symmetry and depth of movement
  b. Rhythm of respirations
  c. Slope of ribs and musculoskeletal deformities *Scapula at same height. Thorax rises and falls in unison with respiratory cycle, ribs at a 45° angle with sternum. Inspiratory breath sounds are not audible at a distance of more than 2 to 3 cm from the mouth.*

2. Palpate.
  a. Place fingerpads on right apex, above the clavicle. Proceed downward to each rib and intercostal space and note tenderness, pulsation, masses, and crepitance. Repeat on left side.
  b. Assess respiratory excursion by placing your thumbs along each costal margin with hands on lateral rib cage (Figure 27-61). Instruct client to inhale deeply; note divergence of thumbs on expansion; feel range and symmetry of respiratory movement.
  c. Palpate for tactile fremitus as shown in Figure 27-62. Repeat steps discussed above for posterior palpation for tactile fremitus, gently displacing female breasts as necessary. Note that fremitus is usually decreased or absent over the precordium. *Same as normal findings for posterior palpation.*

3. Symmetrically percuss anterior surface as shown in Figure 27-63.
  a. Percuss 2 to 3 strikes along right lung apex: repeat on left lung apex. Proceed downward, percussing in every other intercostal space going from right to left in same position on both sides. Displace breast tissue as necessary.
  b. Assess in each thoracic area.
    (1) Resonant-lung field
    (2) Cardiac dullness: third to fifth intercostal spaces left of sternum
    (3) Liver dullness: place your pleximeter finger parallel to upper border of expected liver dullness in right midclavicular line; percuss downward.
    (4) Gastric air bubble: repeat procedure performed for liver dullness on left side. *Resonant sound over lung tissue (hyperresonance in children and thin adults). Cardiac, liver, and gastric silhouettes emit dull sound. Ribs sound flat.*

**Key Findings**

1. One scapula higher than the other occurs with scoliosis. Rib angle less than 45° occurs with emphysema, bronchiectasis, and cystic fibrosis. Bulging of intercostal spaces on expiration occurs with an expiratory obstruction (e.g., emphysema, tension pneumothorax, and tumors). Retraction on inspiration obstructs free inflow of air (e.g., asthma, tracheal/laryngeal obstruction, or tumor).

2. Pulsations may indicate a thoracic aortic aneurysm. Tenderness may result from a fractured rib. Unilateral decreased thoracic expansion occurs on the affected side (e.g., pneumonia or pneumothorax). Bilateral decreased expansion occurs when alveoli do not fully expand (e.g., emphysema or pleurisy). **Crepitus** (a grating or crackling sensation caused by two rough surfaces rubbing together, as in subcutaneous emphysema) occurs when air escapes the lung and is trapped in subcutaneous tissue. It is palpated as a crackling sound from any condition that interrupts the pleurae (e.g., pneumothorax or thoracic surgery).

3. Dullness over lung tissue indicates fluid-filled or solid areas (e.g., pneumonia or tumors). Because pneumonia typically occurs in right middle lobe, unless you displace the breast, you may miss the abnormal percussion note.

*(continues)*

**TABLE 27-14    ASSESSMENT OF THORAX AND LUNGS: NORMAL AND KEY FINDINGS** (*continued*)

| Area of Assessment/*Normal Findings* | Key Findings |
|---|---|

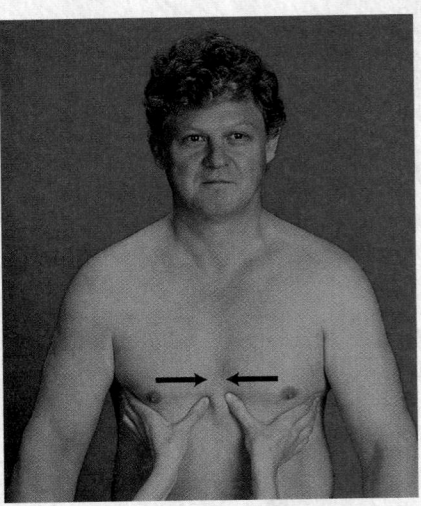

**Figure 27-61    Palpating anterior thoracic expansion**

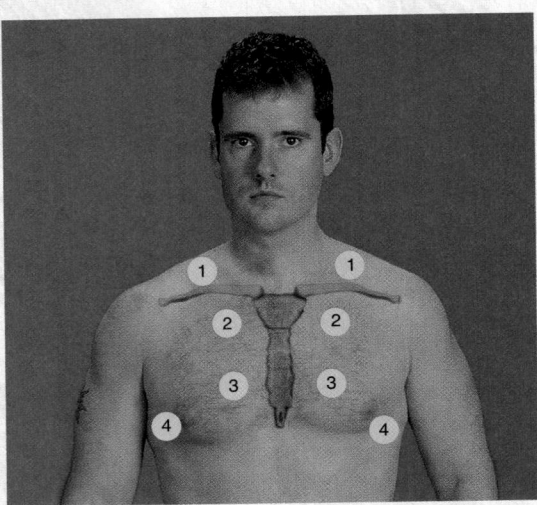

**Figure 27-62    Palpation pattern for tactile fremitus: Anterior thorax**

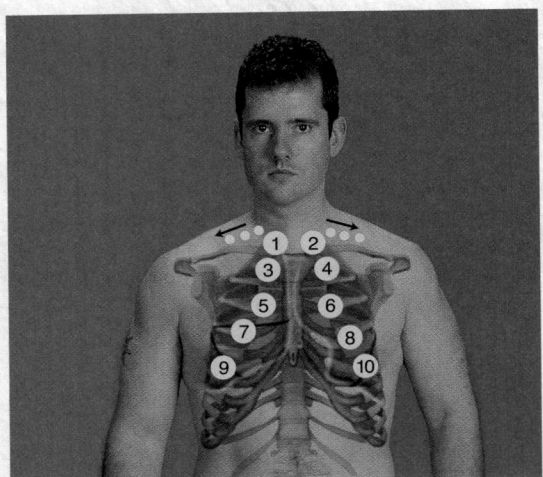

**Figure 27-63    Percussion pattern for anterior thorax**

4. Auscultate anterior surface: instruct client to breathe through mouth and compare symmetrical areas of the lungs, from above downward.
   a. Listen to breath sounds. Note intensity and identify variations from normal.
   b. Identify any added sounds by location on chest wall and time in the respiratory cycle.
   c. If breath sounds are diminished, ask client to breathe hard and fast with mouth open. *Anterior sounds: bronchial, bronchovesicular, and vesicular sounds. A large chest will produce decreased breath sounds.*

4. Decreased breath sounds caused by an inability to inhale and exhale deeply (e.g., emphysema or by an obstruction; atelectasis or foreign object). Absent breath sounds (e.g., empyema, hemothorax, pneumothorax, or pneumonectomy). See Box 27-21 for a description of adventitious breath sounds.

From Estes, M. (2002). *Health assessment & physical examination* (2nd ed.). Clifton Park, NY: Delmar Learning.

## BOX 27-20    COMMON TERMS ASSOCIATED WITH RESPIRATORY ASSESSMENT

- **Asthma:** recurring episodes of labored breathing, wheezing on expiration, and a productive cough of viscous mucoid bronchial secretions
- **Atelectasis:** collapse of lung tissue and decreased gas exchange
- **Bronchiectasis:** dilatation and destruction of the bronchial walls
- **Emphysema:** loss of alveolar elasticity and decreased gas exchange
- **Empyema:** accumulation of pus in a body cavity such as a pleural cavity
- **Hemothorax:** accumulation of blood and fluid in the pleural cavity
- **Pleural effusion:** accumulation of fluid in interstitial and air spaces of lungs
- **Pleurisy:** inflammation of the pleura
- **Pneumonia:** inflammation of the lungs
- **Pneumothorax:** collection of air in the pleural space that causes lungs to collapse

## BOX 27-21    ADVENTITIOUS BREATH SOUNDS

- **Crackles:** heard predominantly on inspiration over the base of the lungs as an interrupted fine crackle (dry, high-pitched crackling, popping sound of short duration) that sounds like a piece of hair being rolled between the fingers in front of the ear or a coarse crackle (moist, low-pitched crackling, gurgling sound of long duration) that sounds like water going down the drain after the plug has been pulled on a full tub of water
- **Rhonchi:** heard predominantly on expiration over the trachea and bronchi as a continuous, low-pitched musical sound
- **Wheezes:** heard predominantly on expiration all over the lungs as a continuous sonorous wheeze (low-pitched snoring) or sibilant wheeze (high-pitched musical sound)
- **Pleural friction rub:** heard on either inspiration or expiration over the anterior lateral lungs as a continuous creaking, grating sound
- **Stridor:** heard predominantly on inspiration as a continuous crowing sound

manner using certain cardiac landmarks. The cardiac landmarks, as seen in Figure 27-64, are defined as follows:

1. Aortic area is the second intercostal space (ICS) to the right of the sternum.
2. Pulmonic area is the second ICS to the left of the sternum.
3. Erb's point is located in the third ICS to the left of the sternum.
4. Tricuspid area (right ventricular area or septal area) is the fifth ICS to the left of the sternum.
5. Mitral area (left ventricular or apical area) is the fifth ICS at the left midcavicular line.

Whereas the mitral area is correlated anatomically with the apex of the heart, the aortic and pulmonic areas are correlated anatomically with the base of the heart. Assessment proceeds either from the base of the heart to the apex or from the apex to the base. When auscultating for cardiac sounds ($S_1$ and $S_2$) listen for:

- $S_1$, which is usually a quieter sound than $S_2$ in the aortic and pulmonic areas
- A split $S_2$ sound that may be heard in the pulmonic area during inspiration

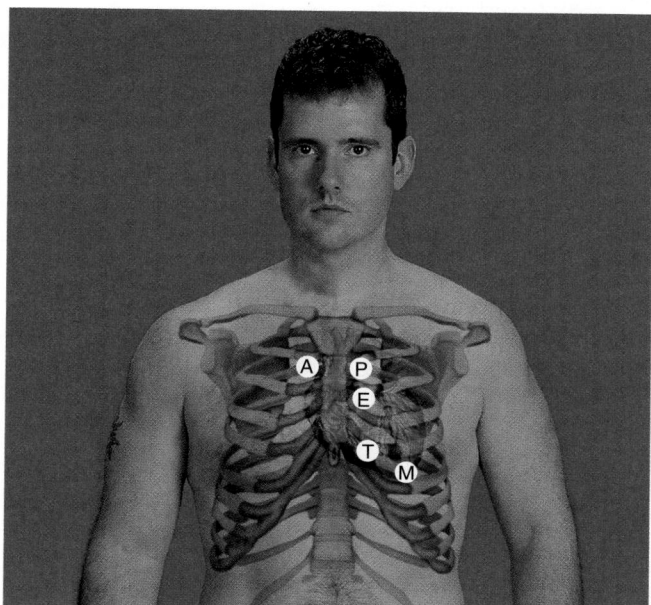

**Figure 27-64    Cardiac landmarks:** A, aortic area; P, pulmonic area; E, Erb's point; T, tricuspid area; M, mitral area

## CLINICAL ALERT

### Cerebrospinal Fluid Drainage

Clear or bloody drainage from the ear may indicate leakage of cerebrospinal fluid. If present, stop the examination and make a referral to a qualified specialist.

- $S_1$, which is usually louder than $S_2$ in the tricuspid and mitral areas
- A split $S_2$ sound that may be heard in the tricuspid area

Additional heart sounds ($S_3$ and $S_4$) may be heard during auscultation. $S_3$ (also called a ventricular gallop) may be heard in the tricuspid and mitral areas during the early to mid-diastole following the $S_2$ sound. $S_3$ is heard best when the client is in the left lateral recumbent position, and the sound resembles the pronunciation of the word *Kentucky* (lub-dub-by). $S_4$ (also called atrial diastolic gallop) may be heard in the tricuspid and mitral areas during the late phase of diastole, before $S_1$ of the next cardiac cycle. $S_4$ is heard best when the client is in the supine position, and the sound resembles the pronunciation of the word *Tennessee* (le-lub-dub).

An $S_3$ can be a normal physiological sound in children and young adults; in adults it may be indicative of cardiac dysfunction (Estes, 2002). An $S_4$ may occur with or without any evidence of cardiac decompensation or it can be indicative of decompensation that is seen in conditions that increase the resistance to filling because of poorly compliant ventricles such as coronary artery disease and heart failure (Estes, 2002).

There are distinct abnormal findings found on palpation and auscultation. During palpation the nurse should assess for **thrills** (vibrations that feel similar to what one feels when a hand is placed on a purring cat) and **heaves** (lifting of the cardiac area secondary to an increased workload and force of left ventricular contraction). Abnormal heart sounds relative to **stenosis** (a narrowing or constriction of a blood vessel or valve) or **regurgitation** (the backward flow of blood through a diseased heart valve, also known as insufficiency) can be heard during auscultation as a click (a high-pitched systolic sound created by the opening of the valve) or a **murmur** (swishing or blowing sounds of long duration heard during the systolic and diastolic phases created by turbulent blood flow through a valve). Other abnormal sounds heard on auscultation are a pericardial friction rub (high-pitched, multiphasic, scratchy or grating sound that does not change with respirations) and **bruits** (blowing sounds that are heard when the blood flow becomes turbulent as it rushes past an obstruction) (Guyton & Hall, 2000).

Murmurs are characterized by their:

- Location: area where the murmur is heard loudest (e.g., mitral, pulmonic).
- Radiation: transmission of sound from a specific valve to other adjacent structures (mitral murmurs can radiate to the axilla).
- Timing: phase in the cardiac cycle. If the murmur occurs simultaneously with the pulse, it is a systolic murmur. If the murmur is not related to the pulse, it is a diastolic murmur.
- Intensity: the loudness or intensity (see Box 27-22 for a grading of murmurs).
- Quality: sound produced (harsh, rumbling, blowing, or musical).
- Pitch: high, medium, or low (auscultated with the bell of stethoscope for low-pitched murmurs and the diaphragm for high-pitched murmurs).
- Configuration: pattern that the murmur makes over time; described as crescendo (soft to loud), decrescendo (loud to soft), crescendo-decrescendo (soft to loud to soft), and plateau (sustained sound) (Estes, 2002).

Table 27-15 presents the specific areas to be examined and the normal and key findings of assessment of the heart and vascular system. See Box 27-23 on page 626 for common terms associated with cardiac assessment.

### Vascular System

To assess blood perfusion of peripheral vessels and skin, the nurse should note changes in skin temperature, color, and sensation and in the pulses. Feeling the toes for warmth and color provides important information relative to peripheral circulation and tissue perfusion. Because the position of the extremities can affect the skin temperature and appearance, always assess extremities at heart level and at normal room and body temperature. Peripheral pulses should be compared bilaterally, and changes in strength and quality should be noted (Estes, 2002).

## BOX 27-22 GRADES AND CHARACTERISTICS OF MURMURS

Grade I: Barely audible

Grade II: Audible immediately

Grade III: Moderate intensity

Grade IV: Loud, may be associated with a thrill

Grade V: Loud, with palpable thrill, audible with stethoscope in contact with chest wall

Grade VI: Louder, heard without stethoscope, palpable thrill

From Estes, M. (2002). *Health assessment & physical examination* (2nd ed.). Clifton Park, NY: Delmar Learning.

## TABLE 27-15    ASSESSMENT OF HEART AND VASCULAR SYSTEM: NORMAL AND KEY FINDINGS

| Area of Assessment/*Normal Findings* | Key Findings |
|---|---|
| **Heart: Inspect, Palpate, and Auscultate**<br>Place client in supine or slightly elevated position. Expose anterior thorax using a drape. Stand at client's right side with light shining from opposite side to eliminate shadows.<br>1. Inspect anterior thorax, precordium area: note pulsations, heaves, or retractions. *Absence of visible pulsations, heaves, or retractions.*<br>2. Inspect and palpate each of the cardiac landmarks for apical impulses. Use fingerpads to palpate pulsations and ball of the hand to palpate thrills or heaves (see Figure 27-64 for landmarks). | 1. Visible pulsations, heaves, or retractions require additional inspection with palpation to identify exact location and timing in relation to cardiac cycle (systole or diastole). |
|   a. Aortic area (second intercostal space to right of sternum): note pulsation, thrill, or vibration of aortic valve closure. |   a. Thrill may indicate aortic stenosis or regurgitation. |
|   b. Pulmonic area (second left intercostal space): note pulsation, thrill, or vibration of pulmonic valve closure. |   b. Thrill may indicate pulmonic stenosis or regurgitation. |
|   c. Third left intercostal space: note pulsation, thrill, or vibration of pulmonic valve closure. |   c. Erb's point pulsations may indicate a left ventricular aneurysm or enlarged right ventricle. |
|   d. Right ventricular area (left, lower half of sternum and parasternal area): assess for a diffuse lift, heave, or thrill. |   d. Thrill may indicate a tricuspid stenosis or regurgitation; a heave may also be present. |
|   e. Apex of heart (fifth intercostal space just medial to midclavicular line): note pulsation, thrill, or heave. *No pulsations, thrills, or heaves should be palpated in aortic, pulmonic, Erb's point, or tricuspid areas. An apical impulse (heard after first heart sound, lasting for half of systole) occurs in 50% of adult population. Mitral thrill or heave is absent.* |   e. Thrill may indicate mitral stenosis or regurgitation. A heave (sustained apex beat) may result from left ventricular hypertrophy. |
| 3. Palpate high in epigastric region for pulsations. *Strong pulsations thrusting upward against the fingerpads are caused by the aorta.* | 3. Large pulsations and a mass may indicate an abdominal aortic aneurysm. Notify the nursing supervisor immediately if you detect signs of an aneurysm. |
| 4. Begin auscultation using the diaphragm of stethoscope for transmission of high-frequency sounds. Listen to several "lub dub" cycles in all five cardiac landmarks twice: first identify $S_1$ and $S_2$, then listen for $S_3$ and $S_4$ and murmurs and friction rubs. | 4. Diminished $S_2$ may indicate aortic stenosis and an intensified $S_2$ may indicate arterial hypertension. Ejection click following $S_1$ can be heard with aortic stenosis caused by calcified valve. |
|   a. Locate aortic valve landmark (second intercostal space, right sternal border) and listen for $S_2$. | |
|   b. Auscultate pulmonic valve (second intercostal space, left sternal border), listening for $S_2$. *Regular intervals of time occur with a regular rhythm: time between $S_1$ and $S_2$ (systole) and then the time between $S_2$ and the next $S_1$ (diastole) with a distinct silent pause between $S_1$ and $S_2$. Aortic $S_2$ heralds onset of diastole, corresponds with "dub" sound, and is louder than $S_1$. In the pulmonic area a split of the $S_2$ sound is usually heard every fourth or fifth beat (aortic and pulmonic components). Splitting of $S_2$ occurs on inspirations because of a* |   b. A split $S_2$ that is abnormally wide on inspiration indicates delayed closure of the pulmonic valve resulting from a delay in the electrical stimulation of the right ventricle (e.g., right bundle branch block). A pulmonic ejection click (heard loudest on expiration) is caused by the opening of a diseased pulmonic valve. A loud pulmonic $S_2$ is caused by an elevated pressure in the pulmonary artery. A diminished pulmonic $S_2$ occurs with a calcified or thickened valve (e.g., pulmonic stenosis). A split |

*(continues)*

## TABLE 27-15    ASSESSMENT OF HEART AND VASCULAR SYSTEM: NORMAL AND KEY FINDINGS (continued)

| Area of Assessment/Normal Findings | Key Findings |
|---|---|
| *greater negative intrathoracic pressure when the venous return to the right side of the heart increases; thus, pulmonic closure is delayed because of the extra time needed for increased blood volume to pass through the valve. Aortic $S_2$ is louder than pulmonic $S_2$ because of the greater pressures in the left side of the heart.* | pulmonic $S_2$ that is abnormally wide or occurs with every $S_2$ is usually indicative of an abnormality. |
| c.  Erb's point (third left intercostal space): auscultate for murmurs. | c.  Murmurs may indicate stenosis or regurgitation of a valve. |
| d.  Tricuspid area (fifth intercostal space, left sternal border): assess for $S_1$. Instruct client to hold her breath. *$S_1$ is split because the mitral valve closes slightly before the tricuspid valve. When the client holds her breath, the splitting disappears.* | d.  A wide split $S_1$ during inspiration that is still heard on expirations is due to an electrical malfunction (e.g., right bundle branch block or a structural alteration, mitral stenosis). |
| e.  Mitral area (fifth intercostal space, left midclavicular line): assess for $S_1$. If you are unable to distinguish between $S_1$ and $S_2$, palpate carotid artery while assessing mitral landmark; you will hear $S_1$ with each carotid pulse beat. *$S_1$ heralds the onset of systole ("lub" sound) and is louder than $S_2$ at this landmark.* | e.  A variable $S_1$ sound (soft or loud) occurs when diastolic filling time varies (e.g., tachycardia or atrial fibrillation). |
| 5.  Place client on left side. Use the bell of stethoscope (low-pitched sounds) and assess all five anatomic areas for extra heart sounds ($S_3$ and $S_4$ gallops, clicks, and rubs). *$S_3$ is heard in children and young adults under the age of 30 or in the third trimester of pregnancy. $S_4$ may occur without any evidence of cardiac decompensation. Gallops, clicks, and rubs are absent.* | 5.  $S_3$ (ventricular gallop) occurs after $S_2$ at the end of ventricular diastole and may be one of the earliest clinical findings of cardiac dysfunction (e.g., congestive heart failure). $S_4$ may indicate cardiac decompensation (e.g., coronary artery disease or myocardial infarction). |
| 6.  Epigastric area: place client in supine position. Place bell of stethoscope over visible aortic pulsations and auscultate for 10 to 15 seconds. *Bruits are absent.* | 6.  A bruit in the epigastric area indicates turbulent blood flow as seen in the presence of an aneurysm. |
| **Vascular System: Inspect, Palpate, and Auscultate**<br>Place client in supine position with head of bed elevated 30° to 45°. Use a drape and uncover only those areas that are being assessed. If skin is not assessed as a separate system, inspect the skin for color, texture, temperature, and edema during this part of the examination.<br>1.  Assess carotid pulse: | |
| a.  Inspect right carotid artery along margin of the sternocleidomastoid muscle. *Absence of kinks or bulging.* | a.  Kinking or bulging may indicate hypertension or arteriosclerotic artery. |
| b.  Palpate carotid artery at lower half of neck (to avoid carotid sinus) by instructing client to turn head toward right side (relaxes sternomastoid muscle) and placing fingerpads of index and middle fingers around medial edge of sternocleidomastoid muscle. | b.  Decreased pulsations may indicate arterial narrowing or occlusion. |
| c.  Auscultate carotid artery with bell of stethoscope. Instruct client to hold breath and listen for bruits. | c.  Bruits may indicate distribution of blood flow from arterial narrowing or occlusion. |
| d.  Repeat Steps 1a–c on left side. *Pulses are equal in rate and rhythm with a strong, thrusting quality. No blowing or swishing sound is heard on auscultation.* | |

*(continues)*

## TABLE 27-15    ASSESSMENT OF HEART AND VASCULAR SYSTEM: NORMAL AND KEY FINDINGS (continued)

| Area of Assessment/*Normal Findings* | Key Findings |
|---|---|
| 2. Identify bilateral external and internal (deep, along carotid artery) jugular veins with head of bed elevated 45° (avoid hyperextension or flexion of neck).<br>  a. Inspect right internal jugular vein.<br>  b. Measure the vertical distance in centimeters from the sternal angle (angle of Louis) to top of distended neck vein to obtain an indirect jugular venous pressure.<br>  c. Repeat Steps 2a and b on left side. *Measurement of 1–2 cm above the angle of Louis with head of bed elevated 45°.* | 2. Distended jugular veins (> 2 cm) with client in a sitting position may be related to fluid volume overload (rapid infusion of an intravenous solution). Elevated jugular venous pressure, when accompanied with a third heart sound are the most specific signs of heart failure (Agency for Health Care Policy and Research, 1994). |
| 3. Assess blood pressure; refer to Procedure 27-5. | |
| 4. Inspect and palpate bilateral peripheral pulses (locate pulse points as discussed in Figure 27-3 and Table 27-7. Starting with the temporal artery, proceed in a sequential pattern with the upper extremities (brachial, radial, and ulnar pulses), then the lower extremities (femoral, posterior tibial, and dorsalis pedis pulses). Note rate, quality, rhythm, and volume of pulses. If you are unable to palpate a pulse, use a Doppler or ultrasound stethoscope to amplify the sound. *Bilateral equality and symmetry of peripheral pulses.* | 4. Markedly diminished or absent pulses may indicate arterial occlusion; e.g., Buerger's disease (thromboangiitis obliterans). |

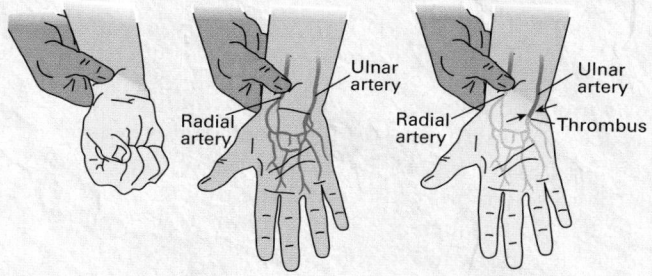

<table>
<tr><td>

5. Assess tissue perfusion:
  a. Perform the Allen test to determine patency of radial and ulnar arteries. Instruct client to rest hands in lap (Figure 27-65).
    (1) Compress both the radial and ulnar arteries.
    (2) Firmly compress arteries and instruct client to open the hand.
    (3) Note color of palms.
    (4) Release one artery and note the color of the palm.
    (5) Then Steps 1–4 are repeated for the other artery on the same hand. The procedure is then performed on the other hand. *Palms should turn pink promptly.*
  b. Inspect both legs from the groin and buttocks to feet. Note venous enlargement, redness or discoloration, and ulcers over saphenous veins. *Skin intact, free from venous engorgement and pain.*
  c. Check for Homan's sign by slightly bending client's knee and sharply dorsiflexing the client's foot. If client feels pain in calf area of leg, the test is positive. Repeat on opposite leg. *Absence of calf pain.*

</td><td>

**Figure 27-65    Allen test: A. Pallor is initiated by compressing the radial artery with the client's fist clenched. B. A patent ulnar artery reveals the return of palm perfusion despite radial artery compression. C. An occluded ulnar artery results in continued pallor of the hand while the radial artery is still compressed.**

  a. Persistence of pallor when one artery (e.g., radial) is manually compressed indicates occlusion of the other artery—for example, ulnar.
  b. Edema or ulceration are indicative of venous stasis. Tenderness or pain, warmth, redness, or discoloration indicates superficial thrombophlebitis. Dilated and tortuous veins are varicosities.
  c. A positive Homan's sign may indicate thrombophlebitis or deep vein thrombosis (DVT).

</td></tr>
</table>

**Lymphatic System: Inspect and Palpate**

| | |
|---|---|
| 1. Assess epitrochlear nodes.<br>  a. Client may be seated or supine.<br>  b. Support client's hand; with other hand, reach behind the elbow and place your fingerpads in the | 1. If a palpable node is present, note its size, shape, consistency, tenderness, and mobility. Enlarged, hardened, tender nodes may be indicative of infection or metastatic disease. |

*(continues)*

| TABLE 27-15 | ASSESSMENT OF HEART AND VASCULAR SYSTEM: NORMAL AND KEY FINDINGS (continued) |
| --- | --- |

| Area of Assessment/*Normal Findings* | Key Findings |
| --- | --- |
| groove between the biceps and the triceps muscles superior to medial condyle of humerus. | |
| c. Palpate for presence of nodes on both upper extremities. *Normally not palpable.* | |
| 2. Assess superficial inguinal nodes. | 2. If a palpable node is present, note its size, shape, consistency, tenderness, and mobility. Enlarged, hardened, tender nodes may be indicative of infection or metastatic disease. |
| a. Client is supine. If client is obese, place in frog-leg position to gain access to inguinal nodes. | |
| b. Palpate in the groin area, moving down toward the inner thigh. The vertical group of nodes lies close to the upper portion of the great sapheneous vein. The horizontal group lies below the inguinal ligament. *Normally not palpable.* | |

From Estes, M. (2002). *Health assessment & physical examination* (2nd ed.). Clifton Park, NY: Delmar Learning.

## Lymphatic System

The lymphatic system retrieves excess fluid from the tissue spaces and returns it to the blood stream. Lymphatic drainage enters the venous system at the subclavian veins via the right lymphatic duct and the thoracic duct. The right lymphatic duct drains the right side of the head and neck, thorax, heart, right arm, lung, and the right upper lobe of the liver. The thoracic duct drains the rest of the body.

Lymph nodes are small oval clumps of lymphatic tissue located at intervals along the vessels. Most nodes are arranged in groups. They are located deep and superficial in the body. The superficial nodes are accessible to inspection and palpation. The facial and cervical nodes drain the head and neck. The axillary nodes drain the breast and upper arm. The epitrochlear node is located in the antecubital fossa and drains the hand and lower arm. The inguinal nodes in the groin drain most of the lymph of the lower extremity, the external genitalia, and anterior abdominal wall. Assessment of the lymphatic drainage of the upper and lower extremities is performed during examination of the vascular system.

| BOX 27-23 | COMMON TERMS ASSOCIATED WITH CARDIAC ASSESSMENT |
| --- | --- |

- **Aneurysm:** localized (aortic) abnormal dilation of a blood vessel wall

- **Angina:** pain in the chest, neck, and/or arm resulting from myocardial ischemia

- Arteriosclerosis: buildup of plaques in the inner layers of the walls of large-to-medium-sized arteries

- Atrial fibrillation: rapid, random contractions of the atria with irregular ventricular beats

- Buerger's disease (thromboangiitis obliterans): an occlusion of a medium to small artery in the leg or foot that becomes inflamed and thrombotic

- Bundle branch block: conduction abnormality of the cardiac impulse through the bundle of His fibers

- Congestive heart failure: circulatory congestion caused by a cardiac disorder

- Coronary artery disease: any abnormal condition that may affect the arteries of the heart

- **Ischemia:** local and temporary lack of blood supply to the heart

- **Myocardial infarction:** necrosis of the heart muscle

- Thrombophlebitis: inflammation of a vein with a formed blood clot

## CLINICAL ALERT

### Homan's Sign

The Homan's sign has a low sensitivity for thrombophlebitis (less than 20% of all DVTs). This assessment technique is not routinely used by all health care providers.

## Breasts and Axillae

The breasts of men and women need to be inspected and palpated. Men have some glandular tissue beneath each nipple, a potential site for malignancy, whereas mature women have glandular tissue throughout the breast. In females, the largest portion of glandular breast tissue is located in the upper outer quadrant of each breast and extending into the axilla, called the tail of Spence. The majority of breast tumors are located in this upper outer breast quadrant and axillary area (American Cancer Society, 2002). A thorough explanation of breast self-examinations is provided in Chapter 46.

Inspection and palpation are used to assess the female and male breasts and axillae, and palpation is used for the axilla and lymph nodes.

The breasts are divided into four quadrants, inclusive of the tail of Spence, by lines crossing at the nipples as shown in Figure 27-66. These quadrants are used in a sequential fashion during assessment. Figure 27-67 shows a cross section of breast tissue.

Palpation of the supraclavicular, infraclavicular, and axillary nodes is included in the assessment of the breasts. The pattern of lymph drainage is illustrated in Figure 27-68. Note that not all the lymphatics drain into the axil-

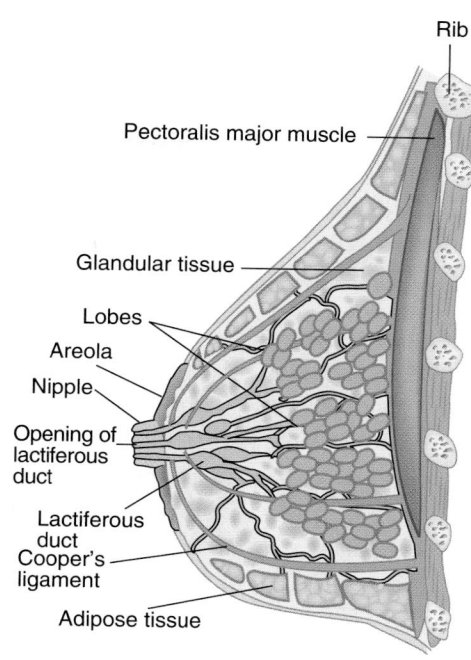

**Figure 27-67    Cross section of the left breast**

la; therefore, depending on the location of a malignant lesion, the spread of cancer cells may occur directly to the infraclavicular nodes, deep into the chest or abdomen, or even to the opposite breast.

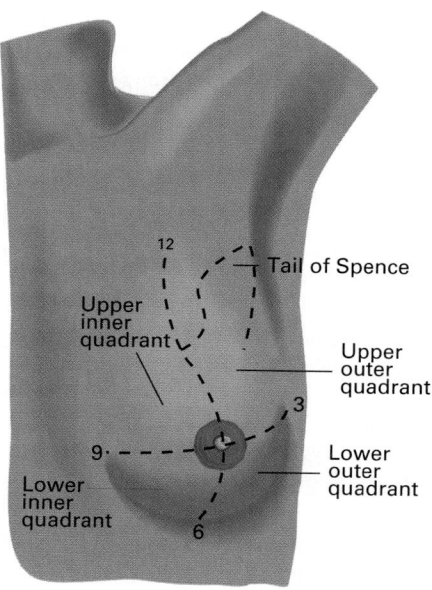

**Figure 27-66    Quadrants of the left breast**

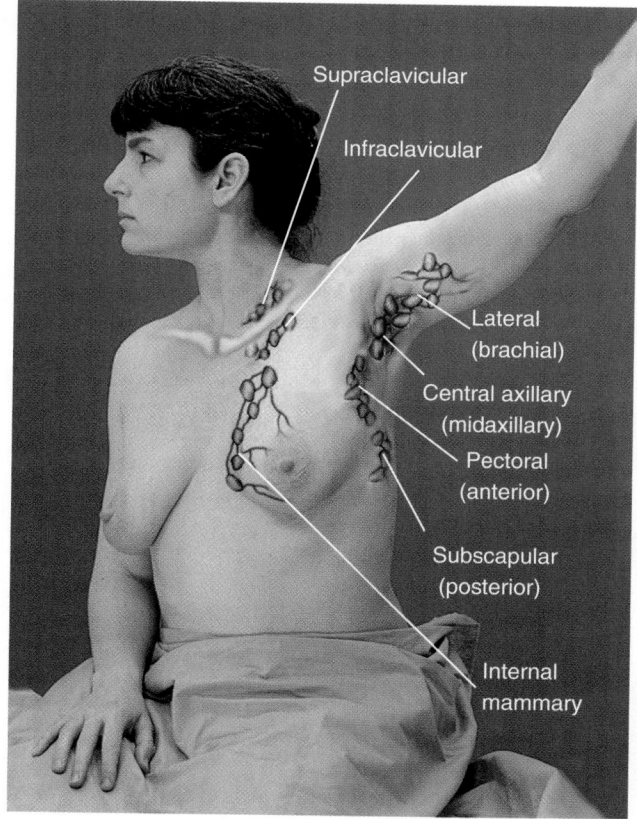

**Figure 27-68    Drainage patterns of the left breast**

### Breast Self-Examination (BSE)

The nurse should use the time during the assessment to educate the client about BSE and encourage the client to ask questions. BSE is discussed in detail in Chapter 46.

## Abdomen

Physical examination of the abdomen requires knowledge about the abdominal wall, viscera, vasculature, and anatomical mapping. Examination of the abdomen provides significant data relative to the various functions of the gastrointestinal, cardiovascular, and genitourinary systems (Table 27-16).

The examiner locates and describes abdominal findings in a client by using two common methods of subdividing the abdomen: regions and quadrants as shown in Figures 27-69 and 27-70.

To facilitate validity of observations and enhance client comfort, ask the client to empty the bladder prior to the examination. Then assist the client to a supine

### TABLE 27-16 ASSESSMENT OF ABDOMEN: NORMAL AND KEY FINDINGS

| Area of Assessment/*Normal Findings* | Key Findings |
|---|---|
| **Abdomen: Inspect, Auscultate, Percuss, and Palpate**<br>Place client in a supine position with knees flexed over a pillow, hands at sides or across chest. Undrape client from xiphoid process to symphysis pubis to expose the abdomen.<br>1. Stand at right side of client.<br>  a. Inspect abdomen from rib margin to pubic bone. Note contour and symmetry (observing for peristalsis, pulsations, scars, striae, or masses).<br>  b. Inspect umbilicus for contour, location, signs of inflammation, or hernia.<br>  c. Observe for smooth, even respiratory movement.<br>  d. Observe for surface motion (visible peristalsis).<br>  e. Inspect epigastric area for pulsations. *Contour is flat or rounded and bilaterally symmetrical. Umbilicus is depressed and beneath the abdominal surface. Abdomen rises with inspirations and falls with expirations, free from respiratory retractions. Visible peristalsis slowly traverses the abdomen in a slanting downward movement as observed in thin clients. Pulsations of the abdominal aorta are visible in the epigastric area in thin clients.*<br>2. Auscultate the abdominal quadrants for bowel sounds (high-pitched) using the diaphragm of the stethoscope.<br>  a. Begin by placing the diaphragm on the RLQ. Listen for a full minute to the frequency and character of the bowel sounds.<br>  b. Repeat Step a, proceeding in sequence to RUQ, LUQ, and LLQ.<br>  c. Listen at least 5 minutes before concluding the absence of bowel sounds. *High-pitched sounds, heard every 5 to 15 seconds as intermittent gurgling sounds in all four quadrants as a result of air and fluid movement in the gastrointestinal tract. Bowel sounds should always be heard at the ileocecal valve area.* | Promotes relaxation of the abdominal muscles.<br><br>1. A convex symmetrical profile reveals either a protuberant abdomen (results of poor muscle tone from inadequate exercise or obesity) or distension (taut stretching of skin across abdominal wall). Asymmetry may indicate a mass, bowel obstruction, enlargement of abdominal organs, or scoliosis. Umbilicus bulging may indicate a hernia. Old scars are flat with a shiny appearance, blending with client's pigmentation; new scars are raised and reddened. Atrophic lines or streaks reveal linea albicantes (striae) that occur with tumors, obesity, ascites, and pregnancy. Engorged or dilated veins around the umbilicus are associated with circulatory obstruction of superior or inferior vena cava. Uneven respiratory movement with retractions may indicate appendicitis. Strong peristaltic movement may indicate intestinal obstruction. Marked pulsations in epigastric area may indicate an aortic aneurysm.<br>2. Hypoactive or diminished bowel sounds are soft and low and widely separated so that only one or two are heard in a 2-minute interval. Hypoactive is normal the first few hours after general anesthesia. Hypoactive sounds may indicate decreased motility of the bowel, such as occurs with peritoneal irritation or paralytic ileus. Absent bowels sounds (none heard for 3 to 5 minutes) may signal paralytic ileus, peritonitis, or an obstruction. Hyperactive (loud, audible, gurgling sounds similar to stomach growling; sounds also called borborygmi) may occur with diarrhea or hunger. Rushed, high-pitched, or tingling sounds suggest air or fluid under pressure; this may occur in the early stages of an intestinal blockage when heard in the portion of the bowel that precedes the obstruction (Estes, 2002). |

*(continues)*

## TABLE 27-16  ASSESSMENT OF ABDOMEN: NORMAL AND KEY FINDINGS (continued)

| Area of Assessment/*Normal Findings* | Key Findings |
|---|---|
| 3. Auscultate with bell of stethoscope over the aorta, epigastric area, renal arteries, and femoral arteries. Note bruits over each area. *Free from audible bruits.* | 3. A bruit over an abdominal vessel reveals turbulent blood flow suggestive of an aortic aneurysm or partial obstruction (e.g., renal or femoral stenosis). |
| 4. Percuss all quadrants in a systematic fashion (Figure 27-71). Begin percussion in RLQ, move upward to RUQ, cross over to LUQ, and down to LLQ. Note when tympany changes to dullness. *Tympany is heard because of air in the stomach and intestines. Dullness is heard over organs (e.g., the liver).* | 4. Dullness over the stomach or intestines may indicate a mass or tumor, **ascites** (excessive fluid accumulation in the abdominal cavity), or full intestines. |
| 5. Perform light palpation. Never palpate over areas where bruits are auscultated. | 5. Tenderness and increased skin temperature may indicate inflammation. Large masses may be due to tumors, feces, or enlarged organs. |
|   a. Instruct client to cough. If client experiences a sharp twinge of pain in a quadrant, palpate that area last. | |
|   b. With client's hands and forearms on a horizontal plane, use fingerpads to depress the abdominal wall 1 cm in all four quadrants. Begin palpation in RLQ, move upward to RUQ, cross over to LUQ, and down to LLQ. Note texture and consistency of underlying tissue. *Should feel smooth with consistent softness.* | |

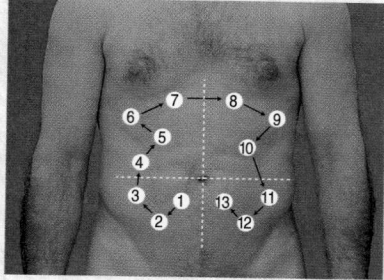

**Figure 27-71  Directional pattern of abdominal percussion**

Estes, M. (2002). *Health assessment & physical examination* (2nd ed.). Clifton Park, NY: Delmar Learning.

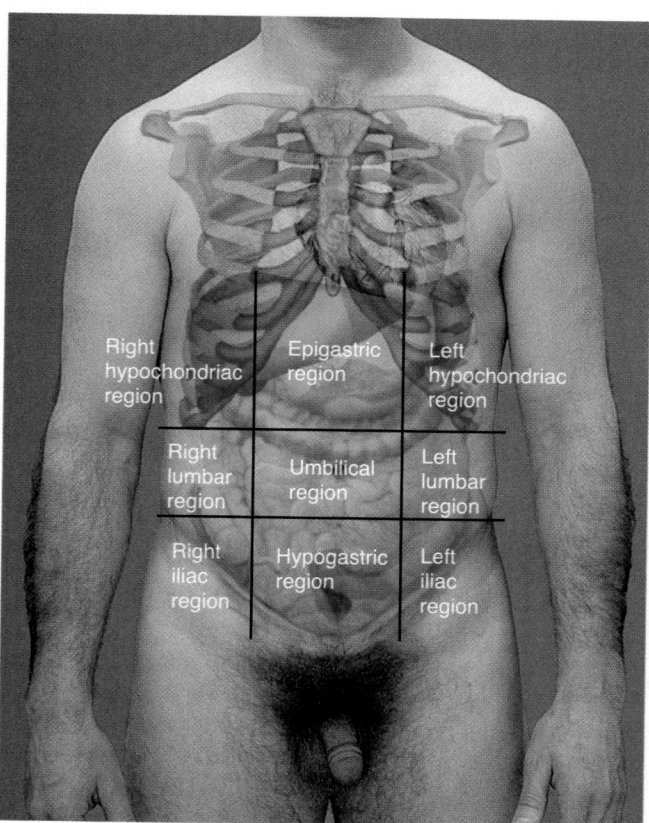

Figure 27-69  Abdominal regions

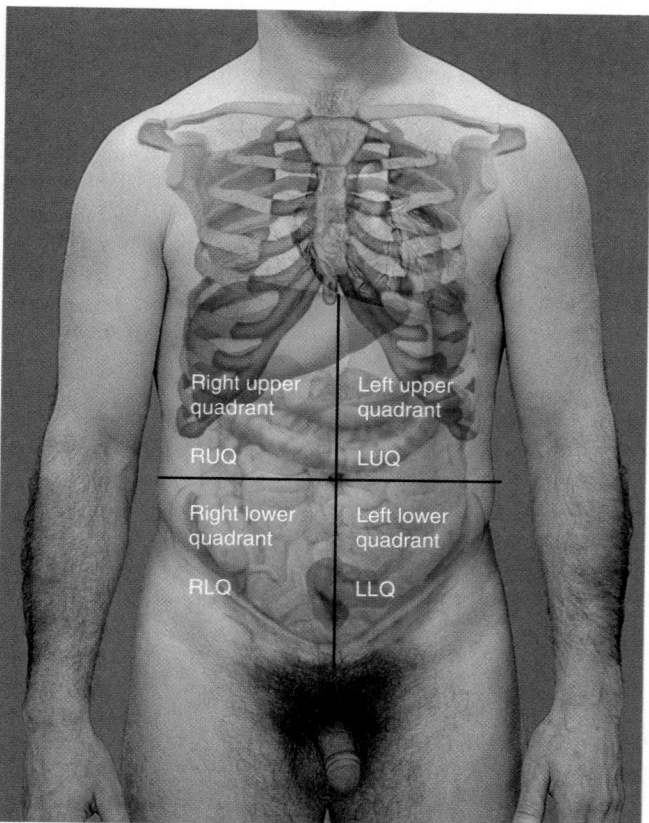

Figure 27-70  Abdominal quadrants

## CLINICAL ALERT

### Sequence to Assess the Abdomen

The assessment sequence for abdominal assessment is inspection, auscultation, percussion, and palpation. Auscultation is performed second because palpation and percussion can alter the bowel sounds.

position with arms at the sides and a small pillow beneath the head and knees. The room and equipment used for the abdominal assessment should be warm. All of these measures are implemented to facilitate relaxation of the client's abdominal muscles (Carpenito, 2002).

## NURSING STRATEGY

### Preparing Client for Speculum Examination of Vagina

1. Assemble equipment.

   - Drapes, gloves, vaginal speculum of correct size, warm water or lubricant, and supplies for cytology studies

2. Prepare client.

   - Instruct no intercourse or douching 24 hrs prior to procedure.

   - Procedure takes approximately 5 minutes.

3. Support client during procedure.

   - Drape and assist into lithotomy position.

   - Explain procedure as needed.

   - Encourage client to take deep breaths to relax pelvic muscles.

4. Monitor and assist client after procedure.

   - Assist client from lithotomy position.

   - Assist with perineal care as needed.

   - Monitor and observe discharge from vagina.

5. Document procedure.

   - Date, time, name of examiner

   - Assessment findings

Estes, M. (2002). *Health assessment & physical examination* (2nd ed.). Clifton Park, NY: Delmar Learning.

Auscultate the four quadrants when assessing bowel sounds and listening for vascular bruits. Assessment should always begin in the right lower quadrant (RLQ). Table 27-16 presents the specific areas of the abdomen to be examined and the normal and key findings of this assessment.

The nurse should percuss all four quadrants in the same systematic fashion. Visualize each organ in the corresponding quadrant; note when **tympany** (a low-pitched sound of long duration) changes to **dullness** (a high-pitched sound of short duration).

Light palpation of the abdomen is done in all four quadrants, beginning in the RLQ for resistance, tenderness, and rebound tenderness. Deep palpation is not addressed because this assessment technique usually requires supervision during the learning process. If any of the abdominal organs (gallbladder, liver, spleen, fecal-filled colon, or flatus-filled cecum) can be palpated, it is abnormal and should be reported to the nursing supervisor.

## Female Genitalia and Anus

Assessment of the female genitalia uses the techniques of inspection and palpation for the external genitalia and anus. Table 27-17 presents the specific areas of the female external genitalia and anus to be examined and the normal and key findings of this assessment. Speculum assessment of the internal genitalia is not presented in Table 27-17 because this function is usually within the scope of advanced practice registered nurses or registered nurses prepared in expanded roles. However, the generalist nurse often assists with this

### BOX 27-24     COMMON ABNORMAL LESIONS OF THE EXTERNAL FEMALE GENITALIA

- Chancre: a reddish, round ulcer with a depressed center and raised edges that appears during the primary phase of syphilis at the site where the treponema enters the body. It lasts for 4 weeks, then disappears.

- Condyloma acuminatum: white, dry, painless growth (wart) that has a narrow base that is caused by the human papillomavirus.

- Condylomata lata: raised, round, wartlike plaque with a moist surface covered by a gray exudate that appears during the secondary stage of syphilis.

- Herpes simplex: small, red vesicles that fuse together to form a large ulcer that may be painful and itchy.

## TABLE 27-17    ASSESSMENT OF FEMALE EXTERNAL GENITALIA AND ANUS: NORMAL AND KEY FINDINGS

| Area of Assessment/*Normal Findings* | Key Findings |
|---|---|
| **Female External Genitalia and Anus: Inspect and Palpate**<br><br>Place client in lithotomy position with knees flexed perpendicular to bed. Instruct client to relax thighs to allow each leg to abduct to side. The client's head may be elevated for comfort. Place drape over client's torso and thighs to expose external genitalia. Don gloves. | If client has difficulty assuming the lithotomy position, place in a left lateral or Sims' position with buttocks near the edge of bed with right knee flexed. |
| 1. Inspect the mons pubis and vulva. Touch the thigh before advancing to the perineum (extremely sensitive and tender).<br>    a. Observe skin coloration and condition of mons pubis and vulva.<br>    b. Separate the labia majora with thumb and index finger of dominant hand. Note color, lesions, or trauma.<br>    c. Palpate the labium between thumb and index finger of dominant hand for swelling, induration, pain, or discharge from a Bartholin gland. *Skin over the mons pubis is clear except for nevi and hair distribution. The labia majora and minora are symmetrical, with a smooth to wrinkled, unbroken, slightly pigmented skin surface, free from ecchymosis, excoriation, nodules, swelling, rash, and lesions. Sebaceous cysts (nontender, yellow-colored nodules less than 1 cm) may be present.* | 1. Ecchymosis over mons pubis or labia may be due to blunt accidental trauma or intentional abuse. Rashes over the mons pubis or labia have multiple origins (e.g., contact dermatitis or infestations). Labial swelling may be due to a hematoma, Bartholin's cyst, or obstruction of lymphatic system. Broken areas of the skin may be due to ulcerations or abrasions secondary to infections or trauma (see Box 27-24). A painless mass with pruritus or a cauliflower-like growth is suspicious of malignancy. Venous prominence (varicose veins) of the labia may be due to a congenital predisposition, prolonged standing, or pregnancy. |
| 2. Inspect the clitoris using the dominant thumb and index finger: separate the labia minora laterally to expose the prepuce of the clitoris. Note the size and condition. *Approximately 2 cm long and 0.5 cm in diameter; free from lesions.* | 2. Enlarged (hypertrophy) clitoris may indicate female pseudohermaphroditism caused by androgen excess. The clitoris is the common site for a chancre lesion. |
| 3. Using dominant thumb and index finger, separate the labia minora laterally to expose the urethral meatus to inspect the shape, color, and size. Avoid touching the meatus, because touching it may cause pain and urethral spasm. *Midline, slit-like opening, free of discharge, swelling, or redness; about the size of a pea.* | 3. Discharge of any color indicates a urinary tract infection. Swelling or redness around the urethral meatus indicates a possible infection of the Skene's glands, urethral caruncle or carcinoma, or prolapse of the urethral mucosa. |
| 4. Keeping the labia minora retracted laterally, inspect the vaginal introitus: instruct the client to bear down while you note patency and bulging. *Introitus mucosa is pink and moist with a clear to white discharge that contains white clumps of epithelial cells. Free of foul odor and bulging.* | 4. Pale color and dryness reveal atrophy from topical steroids or aging. Foul-smelling discharge of any color may indicate vaginitis or cervicitis. External tear of the vaginal introitus may indicate trauma from sexual activity or abuse. Bulging of the anterior wall may indicate a **cystocele** (protrusion of the urinary bladder through the wall of the vagina) due to weakness of supporting tissues and ligaments. |
| 5. Inspect the perineum and anus. Note texture and color of perineum and color and shape of anus. *Perineum is smooth, intact, and slightly darkened. The anus is dark pink to brown and puckered, usually with skin tags.* | 5. Fissure or tear results from area trauma, abscess, or unhealed episiotomy. Venous prominence of anal area indicates external hemorrhoids (varicose dilatation of a vein of the inferior hemorrhoidal plexus covered with modified anal skin). |

From Estes, M. (2002). *Health assessment & physical examination* (2nd ed.). Clifton Park, NY: Delmar Learning.

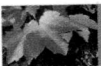

## RESEARCH FOCUS

**Title of Study:** Something to talk about: Sexual risk communication between young women and their partners

**Study Purpose:** To describe sexual risk communication between young women and their male sexual partners, and examine its impact on women's perceptions of sexual risks.

**Methods:** The study and results reported were part of a larger descriptive, retrospective study in which data were collected from young women and their male partners via telephone interviews. Participants of this study included 93 unmarried, sexually active heterosexual women between the ages of 17 and 26 years, and 82 of their male sexual partners. The sample was predominantly white; all other ethnic groups were underrepresented.

**Findings:** Nearly all of the women described their partners as "no risk" or "low risk," despite the fact that nearly half never discussed their partner's sexual risk histories. Women gave three primary reasons why sexual risk was not discussed: did not know the partner well enough/too embarrassed to ask; "knew" the partner was low risk/no need to discuss it, and did not think of it.

**Implications:** Nurses should adopt and promote the premise that all sexually active women are at some risk for sexually transmitted diseases (STDs), including human immunodeficiency virus (HIV). Furthermore, sexually active women should be advised to distinguish between what they think they know about their partners and what they actually know. As client advocates, nurses should help women recognize the need to protect themselves from STD/HIV.

Hutchinson, M. K. (1998). Something to talk about: Sexual risk communication between young women and their partners. *Journal of Obstetric, Gynecologic, and Neonatal Nursing, 27*(2), 127–133.

comfort and by empowering the client through education and participation in the assessment process, the nurse offers a path for the client in the management of her own health care. Most states require that a male nurse be accompanied by a female nurse or assistant during a gynecologic examination.

## Male Genitalia, Anus, and Rectum

Assessment of the male genitalia includes the essential organs (testes and male gonads), the accessory organs (seminal vesicles and bulbourethral glands), several ducts (epididymis, ductus [vas] deferens, ejaculatory), and the urethra. The supporting structures include the scrotum, penis, and spermatic cord. The anorectal examination allows for assessment of both the rectum and prostate gland. Table 27-18 presents the specific areas of the male genitalia, anus, and rectum to be examined and the normal and key findings of this assessment.

Female nurses may feel anxious about examining the male genitalia. If a nurse feels uncomfortable about this assessment, she needs to work through her feelings about sexuality and reproduction before she can talk comfortably with the client (Collins & Diego, 2000).

Some health care agencies do not allow nurses to perform a digital examination of the anus and rectum. Nurses must check the agency's policies relative to this

## BOX 27-25    COMMON ABNORMAL LESIONS OF THE EXTERNAL MALE GENITALIA

- **Candidiasis:** multiple, discrete, flat pustules with scaling and surrounding edema that are superficial mycotic infections of moist cutaneous sites associated with diabetes mellitus, deficiencies in systemic immunity, and antibiotic therapy

- **Chancroid:** tender, ulcerated, exudative, papular lesion with an erythematous halo surrounding edema and a friable base that results from small breaks in epidermal tissue and inoculation of *Hemophilus ducreyi*

- **Tinea cruris:** erythematous plaques with scaling, papular lesions with sharp margins caused by fungal infections of the groin

*Note:* Chancre, condyloma acuminatum, and herpes simplex are common abnormal lesions of the external male genitalia. These lesions are described in Box 27-24 for common abnormal lesions of the external female genitalia.

examination and needs to be familiar with the responsibilities that are involved in assisting with this procedure.

Assessment of the genitalia may produce feelings of fear, anxiety, indignity, and loss of control in many women. These feelings may be reduced by the sensitivity of the nurse before, during, and after the assessment. The nurse must respect the client's wishes regarding privacy and take into consideration cultural issues concerning this aspect of health assessment. For example, many Middle Eastern women will remain veiled during an assessment. By using techniques to diminish client dis-

## TABLE 27-18  ASSESSMENT OF MALE GENITALIA, ANUS, AND RECTUM: NORMAL AND KEY FINDINGS

| Area of Assessment/*Normal Findings* | Key Findings |
|---|---|
| **Male External Genitalia and Anus: Inspect and Palpate**<br><br>Place client supine, with legs spread slightly, or in standing position. Don gloves.<br>1. Assess the glans penis, urethral meatus, and scrotum.<br>  a. Instruct uncircumcised clients to retract the foreskin. Inspect the anterior and posterior surfaces by lifting the penis. Note lesions, swelling, or inflammation (client can replace the foreskin).<br><br>  b. Palpate the shaft of the penis using thumb and first two fingers to assess the entire length of penis. Note pulsations, tenderness, swelling, masses, or plaques.<br>  c. Inspect the urethral meatus. Note location and color, and observe for discharge (culture any discharge).<br><br><br><br>  d. Inspect the scrotum by displacing the penis to one side to assess the scrotal skin. Lift up the posterior side. Note lesions, inflammation, and swelling.<br>  e. Begin scrotal palpation by gently palpating the right testicle between your thumb and first two fingers. Proceed to the epididymis, then to the spermatic cord from the epididymis, and to the external ring, noting consistency, presence of tenderness or masses. Repeat on left side.<br><br><br><br><br><br><br><br>  f. Teach testiclar self-examination. *Foreskin retracts easily. Glans penis varies in size and shape. A small amount of smegma (white "cottage cheese" substance) may be present. Pulsations are present on the dorsal sides of the penis. The meatus is centrally located and pink. Scrotal skin appears rugated and thin and hugs the testicles firmly in the young male and becomes elongated and flaccid in the elderly. The left scrotal sac is lower than the right. Testicles are sensitive to pressure, firm, ovoid,* | If the client has difficulty in the supine position, elevate the head of the bed.<br>1. a. Uncircumcised men can develop phimosis (foreskin cannot be retracted over the glans penis). Paraphimosis occurs when retracted foreskin causes proximal constriction to glans and the penis distal to the foreskin becomes swollen and gangrenous. Priapism is a continuous and pathologic erection of the penis.<br>  b. Absent pulsations indicate vascular insufficiency associated with systemic disease, localized trauma, or disease that interrupts blood flow. See Box 27-25.<br><br>  c. Meatus that opens dorsally on penis (epispadias) occurs mainly with chordee (a congenital defect that results in ventral curvature of penis). Congenital defects, epispadias, and hypospadias (congenital defect in which the meatus opens on the underside of the penis) cause displacement of the meatus.<br>  d. and e. Painless swelling that is unilateral with a hard, fixed nodule may indicate a cancerous mass. An extremely sensitive, enlarged testicle may indicate a testicular torsion (twisting). Swollen, indurated, tender epididymis indicates epididymitis (inflammation). Warm scrotal skin, tenderness, and an acute onset of swelling indicates orchitis (inflammation of the testes) that is associated with mumps. Enlarged, reddened scrotum with taut skin and nonpalpable contents is scrotal edema. A large pear-sized mass in the scrotum (hydrocele) causes the skin to stretch with a shiny, erythematous appearance from the accumulation of fluid between the two layers of the tunica vaginalis. A bluish discoloration of the scrotal mass that disappears with supine positioning is a varicocele. Undescended testicle (cryptorchidism) is usually unilateral. The testicle remains in the inguinal canal.<br>  f. Provides for early detection and treatment of testicular cancer. |

*(continues)*

## TABLE 27-18 ASSESSMENT OF MALE GENITALIA, ANUS, AND RECTUM: NORMAL AND KEY FINDINGS (continued)

| Area of Assessment/*Normal Findings* | Key Findings |
|---|---|

*smooth, and equal in size bilaterally. The epididymis should be distinguishable from the testicle, and the spermatic cord feels smooth and round.*

2. Inspect and palpate the inguinal and femoral areas with client standing.
   a. Instruct the client to strain down. Observe for bulges.
   b. Begin palpation on the client's right side.
      (1) Using your right hand, invaginate (telescope) loose scrotal skin with index finger. Follow spermatic cord upward to opening of external inguinal ring.
      (2) Ask client to cough or strain down. If mass is present, it will touch your finger.
   c. Repeat palpation on client's left side with your left hand. *Inguinal area is smooth, free from swelling or bulges.*

3. Examine the anal and rectal area with the client in a side-lying position. Spread the buttocks with your nondominant hand.
   a. Inspect sacrococcygeal and perineal areas. Observe for excoriation, rashes, inflammation, and nodes.
   b. Palpate any nodules for tenderness.
   c. Lubricate gloved index finger of dominant hand. Instruct client to strain down while inspecting anus for hemorrhoids, fissures, excoriation, and growths. As client strains down, place pad of index finger over anus.
   d. As sphincter relaxes, insert finger pad into the anal canal, pointing toward umbilicus. Note sphincter tone, tenderness, or nodules.
   e. Insert finger further and palpate as much of rectal wall as possible in sequence (right lateral, posterior, left lateral surfaces), noting nodules, irregularities, or undue tenderness.
   f. Palpate surface of prostate gland (lateral lobes and median sulcus). Extend fingerpad above prostate gland and instruct client to strain down. Note size, shape, consistency, and mobility of prostate. Withdraw finger and wipe anal area. *Perineum and sacrococcygeal area is smooth, intact, and free of feces and mucus. Anal mucosa is deeply pigmented, coarse, moist, and hairless. Anal opening should be closed. Rectal sphincter has good tone, and rectal wall is smooth. Prostate gland is small (about the size of a chestnut), smooth, mobile, and median sulcus is palpable.*

2. Oval swelling at the pubic tubercle just above the inguinal ligament indicates an inguinal hernia (portions of the bowel or omentum protrude through the external inguinal ring). A mass medial to the femoral vessels and inferior to the inguinal ligament is indicative of a femoral hernia (portions of the bowel or omentum protrude through the femoral wall).

3. Fissure or tear results from trauma or abscess. Venous prominence of anal area indicates external hemorrhoids. A soft, nontender, enlarged prostate may reveal benign prostatic hypertrophy that occurs with the loss of androgens (e.g., as with aging). Firm, hard, or indurated nodules on prostate may indicate acinar adenocarcinoma. A firm, tender, or fluctuant mass may reveal a prostatic abscess that has a high occurrence with diabetes mellitus clients and is caused mainly by *Escherichia coli*. A tender, warm prostate may indicate acute bacterial prostatitis associated with a bladder infection (e.g., *E. coli*).

From Estes, M. (2002). *Health assessment & physical examination* (2nd ed.). Clifton Park, NY: Delmar Learning.

part of the physical examination. Nursing students should have a qualified registered nurse with them the first time they perform a digital examination. After this procedure has been done, the color of feces on your gloved finger should be noted. Bright red or tarry, black stools are indicative of bleeding and should be reported. Usually a sample of the feces is tested for occult blood.

Middle-aged white men are at highest risk for testicular cancer; early detection and treatment decrease mortality rates. Monthly testicular self-examination (TSE) allows for early detection of testicular cancer. The nurse should teach the client during the scrotal examination about TSE. The Client Education box highlights the content for teaching testicular self-examination.

## Musculoskeletal System

The musculoskeletal system provides the client with the ability to maintain and change position in response to both internal and external stimuli. Muscle tone and bone strength allow the client to maintain an upright and erect position. The musculoskeletal system consists of bones, joints, skeletal muscles, and supportive connective tissue (Figure 27-72).

Inspection, palpation, range of motion (ROM), and muscle testing are performed on the major skeletal muscles and joints by comparing paired muscles and joints. Table 27-19 and Figure 27-73 present the specific areas of the musculoskeletal system to be examined and the normal and key findings of this assessment. This table is not

meant to be a complete examination to assess complaints or musculoskeletal disease.

A complete musculoskeletal examination requires the full assessment of range of motion. A **goniometer** is a protractor with two movable arms (Figure 27-74) used to measure the angle of a skeletal joint during range of motion.

Skeletal muscles provide contour for the body and promote joint mobility. Muscle contour is affected by the exercise and activity patterns of the client. **Hypertrophy** refers to an increase in muscle size and shape due to an increase in muscle fiber. **Atrophy** refers to thin, flabby muscles due to a reduction in muscle size and shape. Increased muscle tone (**hypertonicity**) causes resistance with joint movement. **Hypotonicity** refers to a flabby muscle with poor tone.

Joints are normally nontender and move freely. **Arthritis** is an inflammation of the joints that causes pain and swelling. Degenerative joint disease or **osteoarthritis** (the most common type of degenerative arthritis, in which the joints become stiff and tender to touch) causes the joints to undergo degenerative changes. ROM and activities of daily living are compromised by the loss of joint mobility. Crepitus is often palpated in joints affected by degenerative joint disease (White & Duncan, 2002).

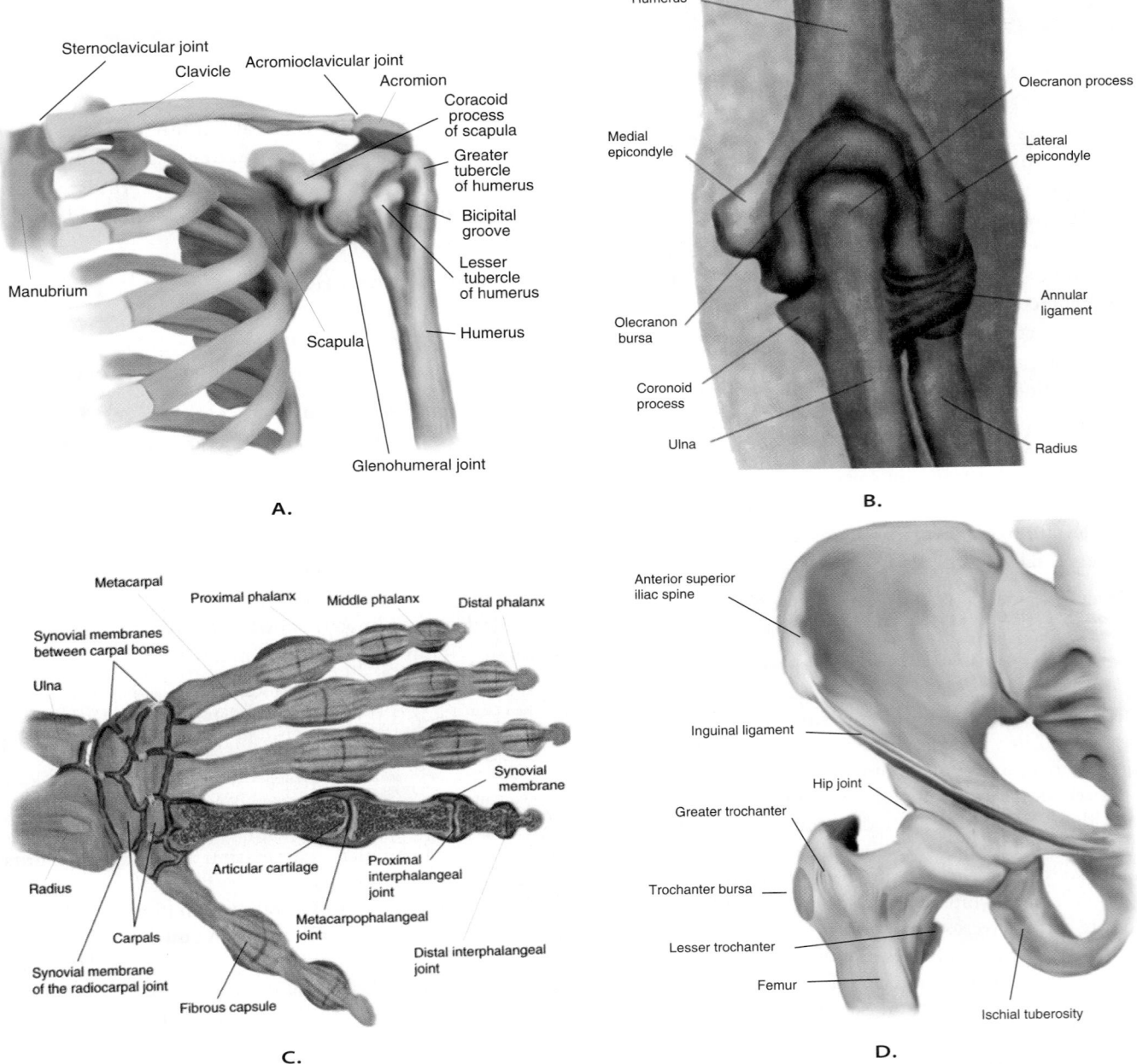

**Figure 27-72    The musculoskeletal system: A. Shoulder. B. Elbow. C. Wrist and hand. D. Hip, E. Leg. (*continues*)**

## Neurologic System

A complete neurologic examination includes an assessment of mental status, sensation, cranial nerves, motor functioning, cerebellar function, and reflexes. See Chapter 42 for a complete discussion of cranial nerve function. Clients with minor or intermittent neurologic symptoms may require only a screening assessment, as outlined in Table 27-20.

### Mental Status

The mental status assessment should be done during the interview and health history. A complete assessment should be performed if the client exhibits any signs of neurologic deficit (see Box 27-26).

### Physical Appearance and Behavior

Pertinent information relative to mental status is assessed by observing the client's posture and movements, dress and grooming, facial expressions, and affect. The nurse should observe the client's ability to wait patiently. Note the gait and posture (relaxed, slumped, or stiff).

The client should appear relaxed but with the appropriate amount of concern regarding the assessment. The client should exhibit an erect posture, smooth gait, and symmetrical body movements.

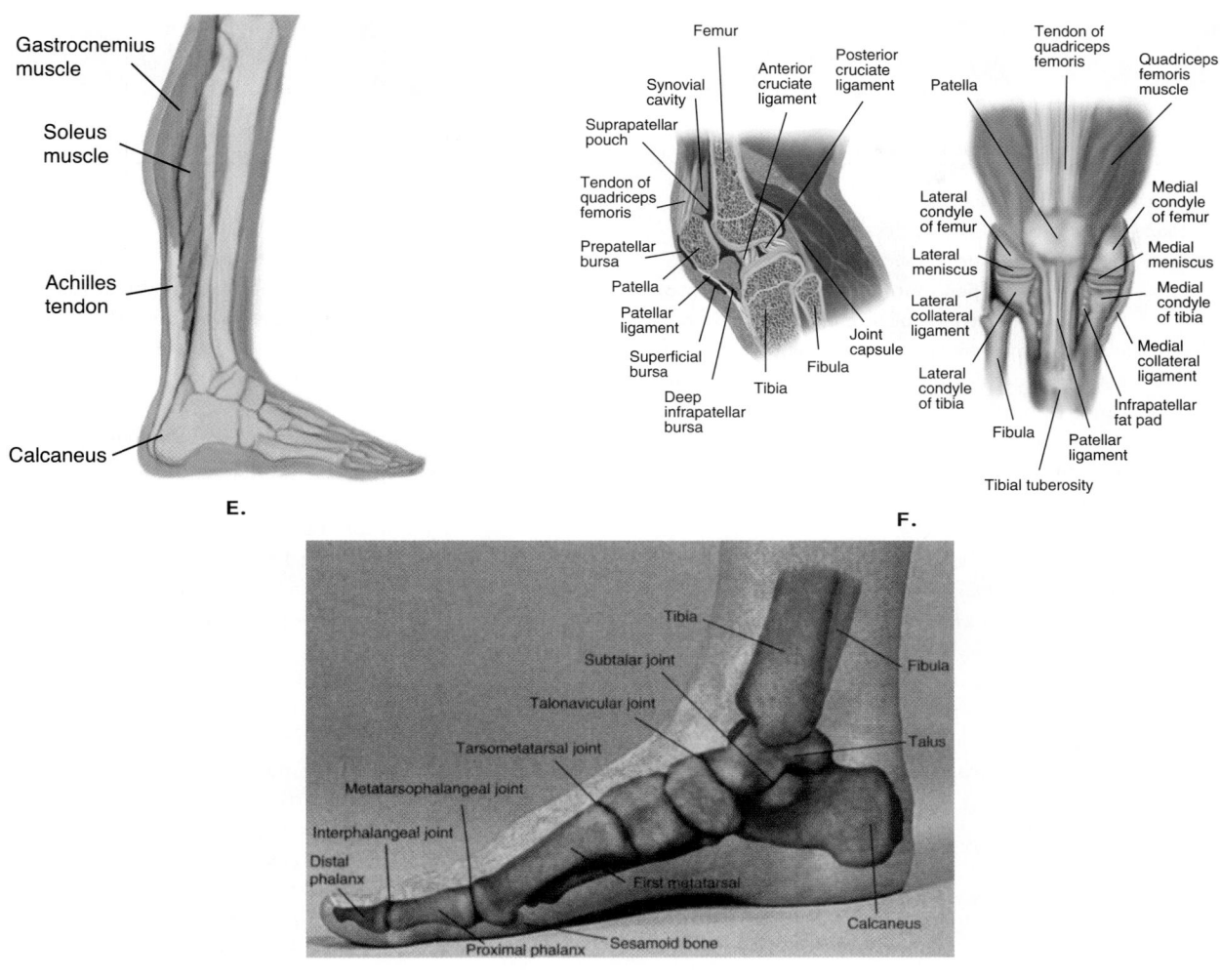

**Figure 27-72    The musculoskeletal system: E. Leg. F. Knee. G. Ankle and foot**

Dress and grooming are influenced by the client's economic status, age, home situation, and cultural background. Information obtained from the health history assists the nurse in determining appropriate dress and grooming for each client. It is also helpful to ask clients directly about their grooming routines and clothing choices.

Facial expressions should be symmetric and appropriate to the content of the conversation. Facial expressions may demonstrate anxiety or depression. The nurse should observe the client's verbal and nonverbal behaviors and note if the client's affect appears labile, blunted, or flat.

### Communication

Communication skills should be assessed throughout the entire interview, health history, and physical examination. The client should be able to produce spontaneous, coherent speech with an effortless flow and normal inflections, volume, pitch, articulation, rate, and rhythm. The message should make sense. Comprehen-

sion of language should be intact, and the client's ability to read and write should be commensurate with educational level.

**Aphasia** is an impairment of language functioning that results from injury to the cortex. Aphasia is classified as sensory (receptive), motor (expressive), or global (mixed sensory and motor). In receptive aphasia, auditory comprehension is impaired as well as is the content of speech. The client is unaware of the deficits, and his ability to name people and objects is severely impaired. With expressive aphasia, speech is slow and hesitant, the client has difficulty selecting and organizing words, and writing is impaired. Phrases are repeated. Oral and written comprehension are severely impaired with global aphasia.

### Level of Consciousness

Consciousness is the level of awareness of the self and the environment. Conscious behavior requires arousal, or wakefulness and awareness, or cognition and affect. Awareness is

## TABLE 27-19     ASSESSMENT OF MUSCULOSKELETAL SYSTEM: NORMAL AND KEY FINDINGS

| Area of Assessment/*Normal Findings* | Key Findings |
| --- | --- |
| **Inspect and Palpate**<br>Place client in a sitting position to provide comfort.<br>1. Assess the head and neck.<br>  a. Ask client to open mouth as you apply light pressure with fingerpads of dominant hand 2 to 3 inches away from the temporomandibular joint. Listen for crepitation and note any limitation of range of motion of jaw.<br>  b. Inspect neck, noting symmetry, deformities, and abnormal posture.<br>  c. Palpate cervical spine, paravertebral muscles, and trapezii for tenderness.<br>  d. Assess ROM of neck. *A click occurs when mouth opens. Lower jaw protrudes without deviating to the side and moves 1 to 2 cm with lateral movement. Head and neck are erect and straight. Alignment is straight in the cervical spine. Movements done with ease.* | 1. a. Tenderness, limited range of motion (ROM), and crepitus reveal temporomandibular joint dysfunction that occurs secondary to arthritis, malocclusion, dislocation, poorly fitting dentures, and myofacial dysfunction.<br><br>  b. Lateral tilting of the head and neck indicates degenerative joint disease.<br>  c. Aching pain and tightness of muscles may be associated with chronic postural strain, tension, or depression.<br>  d. Pain and limited movement may be caused by herniation of a cervical intervertebral disc, arthritis, or degenerative joint disease. |
| 2. Assess hands and wrists.<br>  a. Inspect for swelling, redness, nodules, deformity, or muscular atrophy.<br><br>  b. Test ROM.<br><br><br><br><br><br>  c. Assess strength of hand grasp.<br>    (1) Place your dominant index and middle fingers in the client's dominant hand and your nondominant index and middle fingers in the client's nondominant hand.<br>    (2) Instruct the client to squeeze your fingers as hard as possible.<br>    (3) Release grasp on client's hands.<br>  d. Palpate medial and lateral aspects of each interphalangeal joint between your thumb and index finger. Note tenderness, bony enlargement, swelling, or bogginess.<br>  e. Use your thumb to palpate the metacarpophalangeal joints, just distal to and on each side of knuckles.<br><br><br>  f. Palpate each wrist joint with your fingers underneath the client's hands and your thumbs on the dorsum of client's hand. *Move your thumbs from side to side. Fingers, hands, and wrists are straight. Joints are smooth, movement is easy, and strength is felt on grasp.* | 2. a. Hard, painless nodules on the dorsolateral aspects of the distal interphalangeal joints (Heberden's nodes) are the main sign of degenerative joint disease or osteoarthritis.<br>  b. Flexion contracture that affects the little, ring, and middle fingers (Dupuytren's contracture) may limit full extension of the fingers. Limited movement of all fingers is associated with arthritis.<br>  c. Weakness of opposition of thumb and ipsilateral finger against resistance indicates median nerve disorders.<br><br><br><br><br><br><br><br><br>  d. Enlargement of interphalangeal distal joints is associated with degenerative joint disease. Bony enlargement with tender, swollen interphalangeal proximal joints is associated with acute rheumatoid arthritis.<br>  e. Painful, swollen, and boggy metacarpophalangeal joints, with ulnar deviation of deformed fingers, are associated with chronic rheumatoid arthritis.<br>  f. Bilateral swelling of wrist suggests rheumatoid arthritis. Round, nontender swelling near the tendon sheaths or joint capsules that is more prominent on the dorsum of the hand and wrist when flexed is a ganglia (cystic growth). |
| 3. Assess elbows.<br>  a. Support the client's forearm, elbow partially flexed: | 3. Painful, asymmetrical elbow with forearm out of alignment is associated with a dislocation or subluxation of the elbow. Red, warm, swollen, and tender |

*(continues)*

## TABLE 27-19    ASSESSMENT OF MUSCULOSKELETAL SYSTEM: NORMAL AND KEY FINDINGS (*continued*)

| Area of Assessment/*Normal Findings* | Key Findings |
|---|---|
| (1) Inspect and palpate each elbow, extensor surface of ulna, and olecranon process. Note tenderness, swelling, or nodules.<br>(2) Palpate both sides of olecranon groove for tenderness or swelling.<br>(3) Palpate the lateral epicondyle for tenderness.<br>b. Assess ROM. *Elbows are at the same height and symmetrical in appearance. Movements should be done with ease.*<br><br>4. Assess shoulders.<br>  a. Inspect anterior shoulder and girdle for symmetry. Note swelling, atrophy, or deformity.<br>  b. Inspect and palpate scapulae and related muscles posteriorly.<br>  c. Palpate the following areas on each side and note tenderness:<br>    (1) Sternoclavicular joint<br>    (2) Acromioclavicular joint<br>    (3) Shoulder<br>    (4) Biceps groove<br>    (5) Greater tubercle of humerus<br>  d. Assess ROM. *Shoulders are equal in height, and movements should be done with ease.* | olecranon process indicates arthritis. A boggy, soft, or fluctuant swelling with tenderness in the grooves between the olecranon process and the epicondyles on either side indicates a synovial inflammation. Localized tenderness and pain during ROM indicate epicondylitis (inflammation of muscle tissue surrounding elbow) that results from repetitive motion (e.g., swinging a racquet, tennis elbow).<br><br>4. Increased outward prominence of scapula is indicative of a serratus anterior muscle injury or weakness. Painful, decreased movement with swelling and asymmetry are associated with degenerative joint disease, arthritis, or injury, which may trigger bursitis (an inflammation of the bursa). Pain with swelling at the distal end of clavicle is associated with an acromioclavicular joint separation (separated shoulder). Shoulder subluxation and dislocation are common athletic injuries that result when the glenohumeral joint pops out of the socket. |
| 5. Assess feet and ankles with client in a supine position.<br>  a. Inspect for swelling, calluses, corns, nodules, or deformity.<br>  b. Palpate anterior surface of ankle joint. Note tenderness, bogginess, or swelling. Palpate the Achilles tendon for nodules.<br>  c. Palpate metatarsophalangeal joints and metatarsal head in the sole of each foot, compressing joint between thumb and finger for tenderness.<br>  d. Assess ROM. *Foot is in alignment with lower leg.* | 5. Nontender thickening of skin on sole of foot is a callus, which is caused by pressure. Painful, conical thickening of skin over bony prominences is a corn (also caused by pressure). Painful, swollen, red, and warm first metatarsophalangeal joint usually indicates acute gouty arthritis. Ankle pain, decreased ROM, and crepitation occur with a sprain or fracture secondary to injury. |
| 6. Assess knees.<br>  a. Inspect for contour, alignment, and deformity; atrophy of quadriceps muscles; and loss of normal hollows around patella.<br>  b. Palpate suprapatellar pouch on each side of quadriceps. Note tenderness, thickening, or bogginess. Compress suprapatellar pouch.<br>  c. Palpate each side of patella over joint space and near femoral epicondyles for structural abnormalities, tenderness, thickening, or edema. *Knees are in alignment with each other and do not protrude medially or laterally.* | 6. Bilateral inward deviation toward midline of the knees is genu valgum (knock knees). Bilateral outward deviation away from the midline is genu varum (bow legs). Thickening, bogginess, or swelling indicates synovial effusion (excessive synovial joint fluid). |
| 7. Assess hips and spine with the client in a standing position.<br>  a. Inspect for symmetry of the iliac crests and buttocks.<br>  b. Observe the client's posture and gait. Note position of trunk in relation to legs; foot drop; shuffling or limp; cervical, thoracic, and lumbar curves.<br>  c. Place client in supine position and palpate the hips (Figure 27-73). | 7. Unequal iliac crests and lateral curvature of the thoracic or lumbar vertebrae is scoliosis. The chin tilted downward onto the chest, with abdominal protrusion, indicates kyphosis (excessive convexity of the thoracic spine). Excessive concavity of the lumbar spine is lordosis. |

*(continues)*

## TABLE 27-19    ASSESSMENT OF MUSCULOSKELETAL SYSTEM: NORMAL AND KEY FINDINGS (continued)

| Area of Assessment/*Normal Findings* | Key Findings |
|---|---|
| d. Test ROM. *Iliac crests and buttocks are symmetrical with each other. Stance is upright, with parallel alignment of hips and shoulders. Gait is natural, with arms swinging freely at sides and head leading the body. Spine has a cervical concavity, thoracic convexity, and lumbar concavity.* | 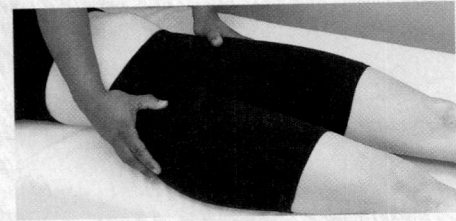 |

**Figure 27-73    Palpation of the hips**

From Estes, M. (2002). *Health assessment & physical examination* (2nd ed.). Clifton Park, NY: Delmar Learning.

## TABLE 27-20    NEUROLOGIC SCREENING ASSESSMENT

| Area of Assessment | Assessment Parameter | Outcome Findings |
|---|---|---|
| Mental status/level of consciousness | Note general appearance, affect, speech content, memory, logic, judgment, and speech patterns during the health history. Perform the Glasgow Coma Scale (GCS) (see Chapter 41) with motor assessment component and pupil assessment. | If any abnormalities are evident, perform a full mental status assessment. If the GCS < 15, perform a full assessment of mental status. If motor assessment is abnormal or asymmetrical, perform a complete motor and sensory assessment. |
| Sensation | Assess pain and vibration in the hands and feet with light touch on the limbs. | If deficits are identified, perform a complete sensory assessment. |
| Cranial nerves (CNs) | Assess CN II, III, IV, VI: visual acuity, gross fields, funduscopic, pupillary reactions, and extraocular movements. Assess CN VII, IX, X, XII: facial expression, gross hearing, voice, and tongue. | If any abnormalities exist, perform complete assessment of all 12 CNs. |
| Motor system | Assess muscle tone and strength, abnormal movements, and grasps. | If deficits are noted, perform a complete motor assessment. |
| Cerebellar function | Observe the client's gait and ability to walk heel-to-toe and to perform shallow knee bends. Perform Romberg's test: ask the client to stand erect, feet together and arms at side, first with eyes open, then closed. The nurse should stand close to the client to catch the client in the event of a fall. Note the client's ability to maintain balance with eyes open and closed for 20 seconds with minimum swaying. | If any deficits exist, perform a complete cerebellar assessment. |
| Reflexes | Assess the muscle stretch reflexes and the plantar response. | If an abnormal response is elicited, perform a complete reflex examination. |

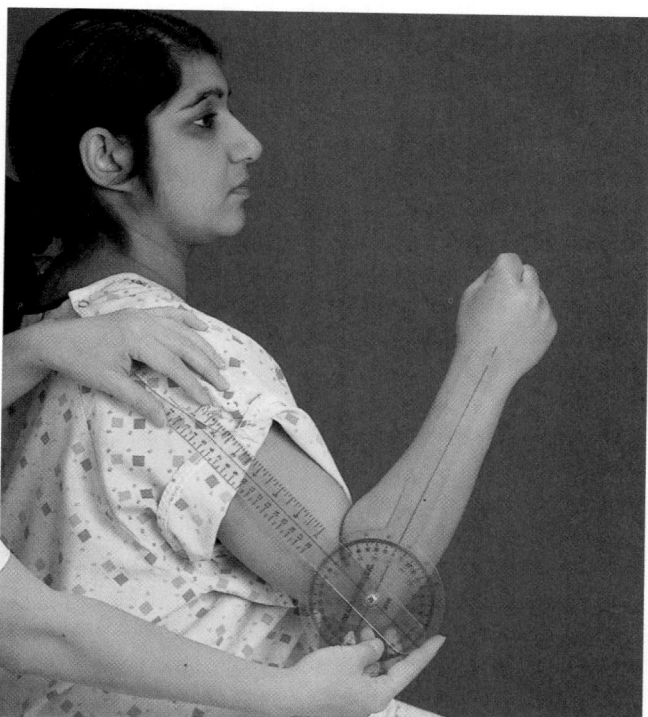

**Figure 27-74    Use of goniometer to measure joint ROM**

a higher-level function of the cerebral cortex that includes judgment and thinking, which are usually assessed as part of the cognitive assessment.

The **Glasgow Coma Scale** (GCS) is an international scale used in grading neurologic responses to determine

---

**BOX 27-26    NEUROLOGIC DEFICITS REQUIRING A COMPLETE ASSESSMENT**

- Known brain lesion (stroke, tumors, trauma)

- Suspected brain lesion (new seizures, headaches, behavioral changes)

- Memory deficits

- Confusion

- Vague behavioral complaints (by significant others if client is unaware or denies behavioral changes)

- Aphasia

- Irritability

- Emotional lability

- Change in level of consciousness

---

the client's level of consciousness. Figure 27-75 is an example of a neurologic flow sheet, which includes the Glasgow Coma Scale.

## Cognitive Abilities and Mentation

Assessment of cognitive function includes testing for attention, memory, judgment, insight, spatial perception, calculation, abstraction, thought process, and thought content. See Chapter 41 for a complete discussion about assessment of these abilities.

## Sensory Assessment

Sensation should be tested early in the neurologic assessment because of the detail involved and the need for client cooperation. If the client becomes fatigued, the findings may be unreliable. The assessment is divided into three sections:

- Exteroceptive sensations: superficial sensations that originate in the sensory receptors in the skin and mucous membranes (light touch, pain, heat, and cold)
- Proprioceptive sensations: deep sensations that originate in the sensory receptors in the muscles, joints, tendons, and ligaments (motion, position, and vibration sense)
- Cortical sensations: sensations that compose cerebral integration and discrimination abilities—**stereognosis** (ability to identify objects by manipulation and touch), **graphesthesia** (ability to identify numbers, letters, or shapes drawn on the skin), two-point discrimination (a test to determine at a given site how close two points can be brought together before being felt as one), and **extinction** (ability to discriminate the points of distance when two body parts are simultaneously touched)

The sensory **dermatome map** (cutaneous area whose sensory receptors and axons feed into a single dorsal root of the spinal cord) is used to assess the major sensory nerves (Figure 27-76). The map of dermatomes is helpful in identifying the areas of pain and altered sensation. Although several dorsal roots may receive inputs from a single dermatome, the map is helpful in identifying where a neurologic lesion may exist. For example, pain localized in the posterior area of the neck would suggest a possible lesion in the third cervical spinal cord segment.

The assessment is carried out with the client's eyes closed to note the client's ability to perceive the sensation. The nurse should observe the client's reactions by watching for facial grimacing or withdrawal of the stimulated extremity. Compare the client's sensation on the corresponding areas bilaterally. The nurse should note the proximal to distal sensory differences on all four extremities, evaluate whether any sensory deficits follow a dermatome distribution, and map the borders of any area exhibiting changes in sensation.

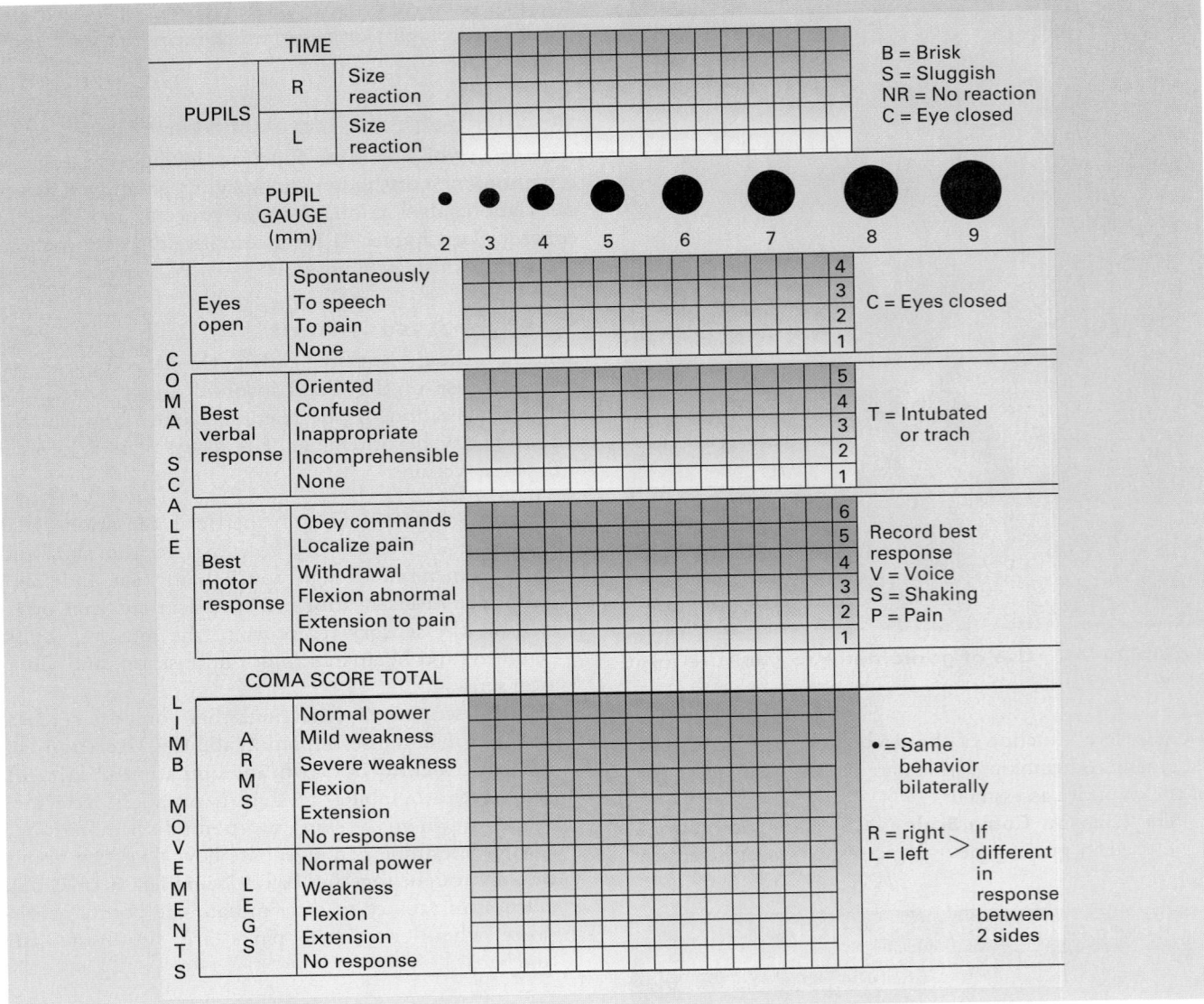

**Figure 27-75    Neurologic flow sheet, including Glascow Coma Scale**

## Cranial Nerves Assessment

A complete assessment of the 12 cranial nerves is necessary for a baseline assessment, if a tumor of a specific cranial nerve is suspected, or when periodic assessment is required after surgery or radiation treatments. An abbreviated cranial nerve assessment is an integral part of a neurologic screening.

Pupil assessment (cranial nerve III, oculomotor) is included in the screening assessment and is tested with the trochlear and abducens (cranial nerves IV and VI) because all three cranial nerves supply the muscles of the eye, as previously discussed in Table 27-13.

## Motor Assessment

The assessment of the motor system involves testing for muscle size, tone, and strength under voluntary movements. Cerebellar assessment can be done either with motor testing or separately as follows.

## Cerebellar Assessment

Cerebellar assessment includes observation of coordination, station or balance, and gait. Cerebellar muscular activity requires the motor coordination of various muscle groups to execute smooth, precise, and harmonious movements. Coordination is an integrated process that involves complicated neural integration of the motor and premotor cortex, basal ganglia, cerebellum, vestibular system, posterior columns, and peripheral nerves.

## Coordination

Equilibratory coordination is concerned with maintenance of an upright stance and depends on the vestibular, cerebellar, and proprioceptive systems. Nonequilibratory coordination is concerned with smaller movements of the extremities and involves the cerebellar and proprioceptive mechanisms.

To test coordination the nurse should position the client comfortably with eyes open. Clients who wear glass-

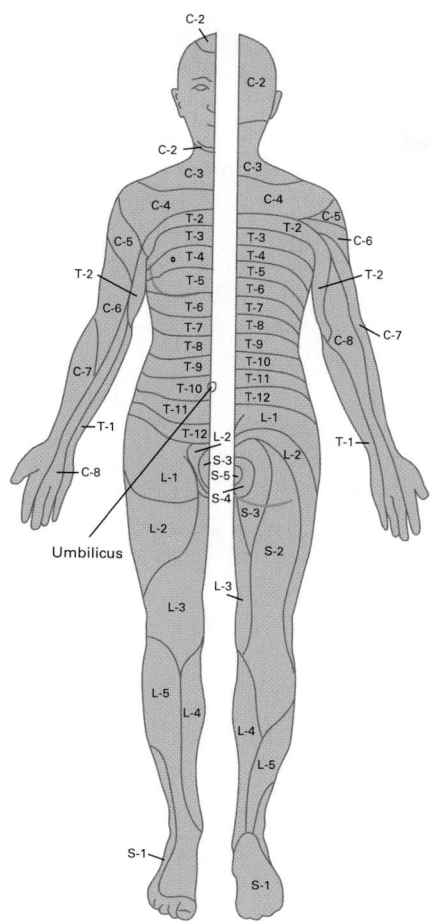

**Figure 27-76**   **Dermatome map**

es should be wearing their glasses before coordination is assessed. Instruct the client to first touch the index finger to the nose, then to alternate rapidly with the index finger of the opposite hand. Ask the client to close her eyes and continue to rapidly touch her nose with alternate index fingers. Tell the client to open her eyes and ask her to touch her finger to her nose and to touch the nurse's index finger, which is held about 18 inches away from the client. The test is repeated with the client using the opposite hand. Throughout testing, the nurse should observe for intention tremor or over- or undershooting of the client's finger.

To assess rapid alternate movements of the upper extremities, ask the client to alternately pat her knees with rapid supinating and pronating of the hands. Test the lower extremities for rapid alternating movement by asking the client to rapidly extend the ankle ("tap your foot") and to place the heel just below the knee on the shin of the opposite leg and slide it down to the foot.

The client should be able to rapidly alternate touching finger to nose and moving finger from nose to the nurse's finger in a coordinated fashion. Also, the client should be able to perform alternating movements in a purposeful,

rapid, coordinated manner. The client should demonstrate the ability to purposefully and smoothly run her heel down the shin.

## Gait and Posture

The performance of Romberg's test is described in Table 27-20. A positive Romberg sign exists if the client becomes unsteady and tends to fall with the eyes closed.

The assessment of gait begins when the client enters the room and continues throughout the examination. The nurse must consider the client's age, activity level, and degree of alertness. The tandem walk is tested by having the client walk in a straight line touching the ground heel-to-toe. The arms should be held at the side and the eyes should be open. Note the client's posture and ability to maintain balance. Posture should be upright with a narrow base and the gait smooth with arms swinging opposite the movement of the legs. Heel-to-toe walk should be in a straight line without losing balance.

## Reflex Assessment

A reflex action is a specific response to an adequate stimulus that occurs without conscious control. The stimulus can occur in a joint, muscle, or skin and is transmitted through the sensory and motor pathways of the reflex arc and specific spinal cord segments. Each muscle contains a muscle spindle (small sensory unit) that controls muscle tone and detects changes in the length of the muscle fibers.

To elicit a muscle stretch reflex, the nurse should briskly tap the client's tendon with a reflex hammer, thereby stretching the muscle and tendon and lengthening the spindle. The spindle transmits the signal along the afferent neurons to the dorsal roots where it synapses. Following synapse in the cord, the anterior motor neurons trigger an impulse on efferent neurons to the endplates of the skeletal muscle, causing the reflex response.

Normal reflexes are classified into two main categories: muscle stretch (deep tendon) reflexes (DTR) and superficial (cutaneous) reflexes. When testing reflexes, clients should be relaxed and positioned so that their extremities are symmetrical. The nurse should hold the reflex hammer loosely between the thumb and index finger and strike the tendon with a brisk motion from the wrist. The reflex hammer should make contact with the correct point on the tendon in a quick, direct manner.

Table 27-21 discusses the assessment of common DTRs: biceps, triceps, brachioradialis, patellar, Achilles, and plantar (Babinski). When testing the reflexes, the nurse should observe the degree and speed of response of the muscle after the reflex hammer makes contact. Grading of reflexes is presented in Box 27-27. The reflex responses between the right and left sides should be compared. The normal response to taps in the correct area should elicit a brisk (++ or +++) contraction of the muscles involved.

## TABLE 27-21 ASSESSMENT OF COMMON DEEP TENDON REFLEXES

| Type | Assessment | Normal Reflex |
|------|-----------|---------------|
| Biceps 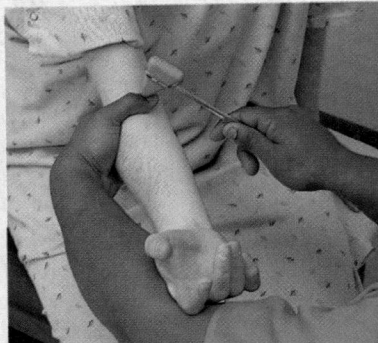 | Flex client's arm between 45° and 90°. Place your thumb firmly on the biceps tendon just above the crease of antecubital fossa and tap thumb with reflex hammer. | Flexion of arm at elbow |
| Triceps 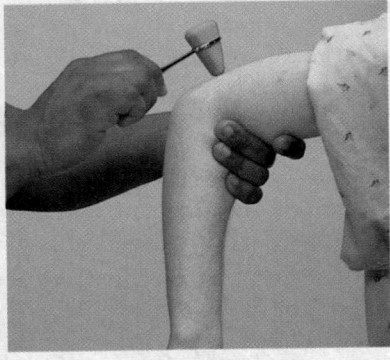 | Flex client's arm between 45° and 90°. Tap triceps tendon just above elbow. | Extension of elbow |
| Brachioradialis 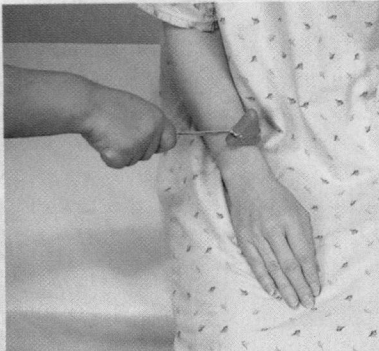 | Flex client's arm 45° and place in lap with the arm in semipronation. Tap brachioradialis tendon on thumb side of wrist. | Flexion of forearm |

(continues)

| TABLE 27-21 | ASSESSMENT OF COMMON DEEP TENDON REFLEXES (*continued*) | |
|---|---|---|

| Type | Assessment | Normal Reflex |
|---|---|---|
| Patellar 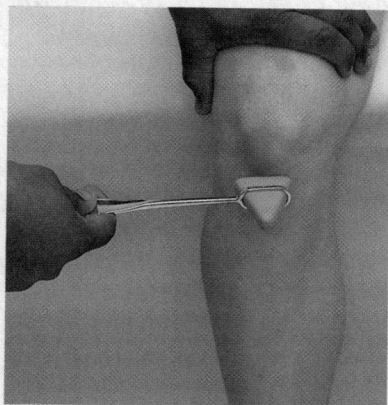 | Ask client to sit in a chair or on edge of bed with legs hanging freely or in a supine position with knee flexed. Tap patellar tendon just below the patella. | Extension of leg below the knee |
| Achilles 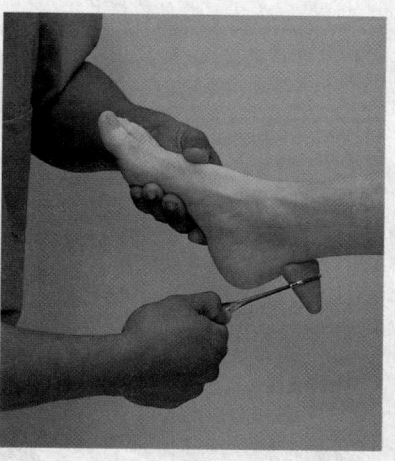 | Ask client to sit with feet dangling and partially dorsiflexed or in a supine position with leg flexed at knee and thigh externally rotated. Tap the Achilles tendon just above heel. | Plantar flexion of foot |
| Plantar (Babinski) 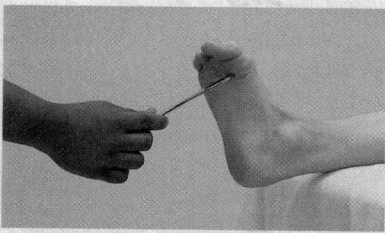 | Position the client's ankle firmly against the bed and slowly stroke client's sole with the handle of the reflex hammer. | Bending of the toes downward |

## BOX 27-27    REFLEX GRADING SCALE

| Scale | Response |
|-------|----------|
| 0 | Absent |
| + | Present but diminished |
| ++ | Normal |
| +++ | Mildly increased but not pathologic |
| ++++ | Markedly hyperactive; clonus may be present |

# Care of the Client After the Examination

A physical examination is taxing on the client, especially if the complete assessment is performed in one session. The nurse should assess the client's needs after this process and respond appropriately. The nurse should also dispose of soiled articles in the proper container, clean and store equipment appropriate for the setting, and put all furniture back in its original place. Thanking the client for cooperating during the physical examination demonstrates concern and caring.

## Home or Outpatient Setting

If the physical examination is conducted in the home environment, the nurse should acknowledge the client's need to rest before dressing. The client should be offered assistance with either toileting or dressing. If a family member is in the home, the nurse should notify that person that the assessment is completed. If the client is home alone, the nurse should verify before leaving that the client is capable of caring for his own needs. The nurse should telephone the client within 2 hours after leaving to answer any questions about the examination (Hitchcock, Schubert, & Thomas, 2003).

In an outpatient setting, assess whether the client needs assistance in dressing. After the client is dressed, discuss the experience by inviting questions and comments. Listen carefully to the client's remarks, and provide information regarding the assessment. The nurse should make certain that the client is capable of driving home or should secure safe transportation if needed.

## Acute or Extended Care Setting

Nursing students should check with their instructors or supervisors before conducting the assessment to ascertain the amount of information that they can share with the client during and after the examination. This varies in different agencies and according to the admitting physician. It is best to secure this information before beginning the examination.

## STOP AND THINK

### Physical Examination: Benefit and Implications

- With the emphasis on cost containment in health care and the expanding roles of nurses as case managers for managed care companies, what do you think are the implications for accurate assessment data?

- Can you relate the health care implications of preventive nursing to assessment and cost controls?

- How does performance of thorough physical examination ensure the holistic care of the client?

After concluding the assessment, the nurse should dispose of soiled articles and clean and store the equipment. The bed should be returned to a low position, side rails up, and call light in place. Quietly check on the client several times within the 2 to 3 hours after assessment to monitor the client's condition.

## Data Documentation

Health care agencies have specific forms for recording the assessment findings. Review these forms before initiating the assessment, and record the findings on the appropriate form as the data are gathered. This practice ensures accuracy in documentation of findings. Some data (e.g., vital signs) may need to be recorded on two or more forms.

Reporting information is a critical part of documentation. If findings that require immediate attention—for example, bright red blood or a change in the nature and character of a previous symptom—are detected, report the findings to the nursing supervisor and document in the medical record the actions taken.

Documentation should reflect the objective data obtained from the examination regarding the client's current condition. Avoid phrases such as the *client appears lethargic*; rather, record the GCS score. If the data identify areas in which the client is at risk, such as a 35-year-old woman with a family history of breast cancer, use the appropriate resources for prevention—for example, BSE and the American Cancer Society's guidelines for early detection of breast cancer. Likewise, abnormal findings should be addressed in planning the nursing care and client outcomes.

# CASE STUDY/NURSING CARE PLAN

Ms. Hernandez is a 76-year-old Hispanic female widow, a retired hairdresser, previously in good health, and lives alone in a one-bedroom apartment. She is brought into the emergency room by her next-door neighbor, who found her lying on the floor, confused, sweaty, and who reports that it was "very hot in the apartment." It is a hot (100°F, humid 95%) summer afternoon. Ms. Hernandez states, "I am very tired, weak, and sick to my stomach."

## Assessment

Evaluation reveals a 76-year-old Hispanic female who was found lying on the floor by her neighbor. The client is confused, febrile, dehydrated, nauseated, diaphoretic, tachypneic, and tachycardiac. She is very weak and unable to sit or stand.

## Nursing Diagnosis #1

*Deficient Fluid Volume* related to diarrhea, hyperthermia, and anorexia as evidenced by T = 102.4°F, BP 100/50, flushed clammy skin, and no urine output.
**NOC:** Fluid Balance; Hydration; Nutritional Status; Food and Fluid Intake
**NIC:**  Fluid Management; Hypovolemia Management; Shock Management: Volume

## Expected Outcomes

The client will:
1. Maintain fluid balance as evidenced by no tenting, and by moist mucous membranes.
2. Demonstrate a continuous balance of intake and output.
3. Maintain a temperature to 98.6°F or lower within 24 hours.

## Planning/Interventions/Rationales

1. Evaluate fluid status in relation to dietary intake by measuring hourly intake and output. *Most fluid enters the body through drinking; water in foods.*
2. Encourage client to drink amount of prescribed fluids by (a) identifying client preferences, (b) placing fluids within each reach, and (c) allowing creativity in selecting fluid sources. *Oral fluid replacement is indicated for mild fluid deficit. Older clients have a decreased sense of thirst and may need ongoing reminders to drink.*
3. Assess skin turgor at clavicle and oral mucous membranes for signs of rehydration. *Older clients tend to have flaccid skin; therefore the best place to assess for tenting is along the clavicle. The tongue will be less furrowed when rehydrated.*
4. Monitor hemoglobin, serum electrolytes, and urine osmolality, and report abnormal values. *Elevated hemoglobin and blood urea nitrogen, and increased urine-specific gravity suggest fluid deficit.*

## Evaluation

Client experiences no tenting, oral mucous membranes are moist, vital signs are within normal range for client's age, and urine output is greater than 30 cc/hr.

## Nursing Diagnosis #2

*Activity Intolerance* related to generalized weakness as evidenced by reports of weakness, fatigue, weak grips and pushes, inability to sit or stand, shallow respirations, and respiratory rate of 32.
**NOC:** Endurance; Energy Conservation; Activity Tolerance; Self-Care: Activities of Daily Living
**NIC:**  Energy Management; Activity Therapy

## Expected Outcomes

The client will:
1. Demonstrate increased endurance as evidenced by ability to sit, stand, and ambulate without assistance within 48 to 72 hours.
2. Perform activities of daily living within 24 to 48 hours.
3. Maintain a respiratory rate between 12 and 20.
4. Identify community resources to contact for assistance with cooling her apartment within 36 hours.

*(continues)*

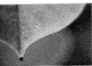

# CASE STUDY/NURSING CARE PLAN (continued)

## Planning/Interventions/Rationales

1. Assess the cause of the activity intolerance. Determine if fatigue and weakness occurred in conjunction with the fluid volume deficit. *Determining the cause can direct appropriate interventions.*

2. Monitor and record client's ability to tolerate activity: note pulse rate, blood pressure, use of accessory muscles, and skin color before and after activity. *Heart rate and blood pressure responses to changes in positions from supine to standing can vary widely.*

3. If appropriate within 4 hours, gradually increase activity at 2-hour intervals, allowing client to assist with sitting and standing and then to ambulation. *Gradually increasing activity helps maintain muscle strength, tone, and endurance.*

## Evaluation

Client is able to sit, stand, and ambulate without assistance; perform activities of daily living. Her respirations are diaphragmatic at a rate of 14 to 20. The home health social worker will make a home visit within 24 hours to assess environmental conditions of her apartment.

## Key Concepts

- Health and physical assessment, an essential nursing function, is performed on every client and can be performed in all health care settings, and for all age groups to gather pertinent, comprehensive data.
- All equipment used for assessment should be in working order and gathered prior to the initiation of the examination.
- Baseline values establish the norm; variations from normal may indicate possible problems with the client's health status.
- The assessment of physiological functioning provides specific data regarding the client's current condition.
- Thermoregulation is the body's physiological function of heat regulation to maintain a constant internal body temperature.
- Hemodynamic regulation is the body's physiological function of blood circulation to maintain an appropriate environment in all the tissue fluids.
- The pulse is caused by the stroke volume ejection and distension of the walls of the aorta, which creates a pulse wave as it travels rapidly toward the distal ends of the arteries.
- Blood pressure is the measurement of pressure pulsations exerted against the blood vessel walls during cardiac systole and diastole. It is measured in terms of millimeters of mercury (mm Hg).
- Several factors cause changes in one or more of the vital signs: age, sex, exercise and metabolism, anxiety and stress, postural and diurnal variations, hormones, pain, medications, and alterations in physiological functions.
- The normal values and variations in vital signs measurement are usually based on age.

- All pieces of equipment used to measure the vital signs and perform a physical assessment should be maintained to function accurately.
- Clinical data regarding the efficacy of blood circulation to an extremity are obtained by assessing all the characteristics (rate, quality, rhythm, and volume) of the peripheral pulses.
- When assessing ventilation, ascertain the rate, depth, and rhythm of ventilatory movement.
- Before checking a blood pressure, review the client's chart for brachial artery contraindications and make sure that the client has not exercised or eaten for the past 30 minutes.
- The physical examination provides a complete picture of the client's physiological functioning; when combined with a health and psychosocial assessment it forms a database to direct decision making.
- Because the client will experience some anxieties regarding the examination, it is important for the nurse to keep the client informed while performing the examination.
- The primary purpose of draping the client is to prevent unnecessary exposure during the examination; feelings of embarrassment will elicit tension and restlessness and will decrease the client's ability to cooperate.
- The physical examination is done in a sequential, head-to-toe fashion to ensure a thorough assessment of each system; when you gain proficiency in performing the physical examination, you will be able to integrate assessment into routine care.
- Assessment begins from the moment you come in contact with the client; data obtained from the health history will assist in identifying areas of alteration.

- Know the agency's policies relative to performing and documenting a physical assessment.
- Use the landmarks and visualize the internal organs when assessing the thorax, heart, and abdomen.
- The order of abdominal assessment is inspection, auscultation, percussion, and palpation, because palpation and percussion can alter the bowel sounds.
- Nurses play a major role by teaching breast self-examination (BSE), testicular self-examination (TSE), and by supporting clients in achieving healthier lifestyles believed to decrease the risk factors of cancer.
- If you feel uncomfortable about assessing the genitalia, you need to work through your own feelings about sexuality and reproduction before you can talk comfortably with the client; work through any reluctance you may have about discussing sexual situations.
- Reporting information is a critical part of documentation; if you assess findings that require immediate attention, report the findings to your supervisor and document your action in the medical record.
- Documentation should reflect the objective data obtained from the examination regarding the client's current condition.

## Review Questions and Activities

1. Ms. Reynolds is 33 years old; her vital signs measurements are OT—37.0°C (98.6°F), P—96/min., R—22/min., and BP—144/90. Which of these measurements are outside the normal ranges?
2. You are assigned to care for Mr. Warren, a 77-year-old client in a long-term care facility. When you enter his room to take his vital signs, you note that the fan is on high speed and blowing directly over him. He is sweating, and the bed linens are damp. What type of reading would you expect to find when you take his temperature? Why is the fan on? What type of heat loss from the skin surface is being increased: radiation, conduction, convection, or evaporation?
3. Mrs. Gray is 55 years old and had a right mastectomy 9 months ago. What implications would the mastectomy have on your assessment (vital signs and examination)?
4. What hemodynamic function is compromised when the lips and nailbeds have a bluish discoloration?
5. What normal sounds should you hear when you percuss the posterior aspect of the apex of the right lung?
6. Are bronchial breath sounds upon auscultation of the lung periphery normal?
7. What type of palpating technique should you use to assess an obese client or a client with large breasts?

8. Match the adventitious breath sound in Column A with the description that best describes it in Column B.

COLUMN A

_____ 1. Fine crackle

_____ 2. Coarse crackle

_____ 3. Sonorous wheeze
_____ 4. Sibilant wheeze

_____ 5. Pleural friction rub
_____ 6. Stridor

COLUMN B

a. Moist, low-pitched crackling, gurgling sound of long duration
b. Creaking, grating sound
c. Crowing sound
d. Dry, high-pitched crackling, popping sound of short duration
e. Low-pitched snoring sound
f. High-pitched musical sound

9. Describe how the examination technique sequencing is different when examining the abdomen, and give the rationale.
10. What risk factors can be modified to help reduce the risk for getting cancer?

## Multimedia Links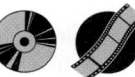

Altman *Basic Care DVD: Taking a Temperature*
Altman *Basic Care Video: Vital Signs*
Altman *Basic Care DVD: Taking a Pulse*
Altman *Basic Care DVD: Counting Respirations*
Altman *Advanced Care DVD: Administering Pulse Oximetry*
Altman *Basic Care DVD: Taking Blood Pressure*

## Web Resources

American Cancer Society
    http://www.cancer.org
American Heart Association
    http://www.americanheart.org
North American Nursing Diagnosis Association
    http://www.nanda.org

## References

Agency for Health Care Policy and Research (AHRQ) (1994). USDHHS Publication No. 94-0612. Rockville, MD: U.S. Department of Health and Human Services.

Altman, G. (2004). *Delmar's fundamental & advanced nursing skills* (2nd ed.). Clifton Park, NY: Delmar Learning.

American Cancer Society (2001). *Breast cancer facts & figures 2001–2002*. Atlanta: Author.

American Cancer Society (2002). *Cancer prevention & early detection facts & figures 2002*. Atlanta: Author.

American Heart Association (1997). Guide to primary prevention of cardiovascular diseases. http://www.americanheart.org

Barkauskas, V. H., Baumann, L. C., & Darling-Fisher, C. S. (2002). *Health & physical assessment* (3rd ed.). St. Louis: Mosby.

Carpenito, L. J. (2002). *Nursing diagnosis: Application to clinical practice* (9th ed.). Philadelphia: Lippincott.

Collins, A. M., & Diego, L. (2000). Mental health promotion and protection. *Journal of Psychosocial Nursing, 38*(1), 27–32.

Edelman, C. L., & Mandle, C. L. (2001). *Health promotion throughout the life span* (5th ed.). St. Louis: Mosby-Yearbook.

Estes, M. (2002). *Health assessment & physical examination* (2nd ed.). Clifton Park, NY: Delmar Learning.

Giger, J. N., & Davidhizar, R. E. (1999). *Transcultural nursing assessment and intervention* (3rd ed.). St. Louis: Mosby-Yearbook.

Guyton, A., & Hall, J. E. (2001). *Textbook of medical physiology* (10th ed.). Philadelphia: W. B. Saunders Company.

Hitchcock, J., Schubert, P., & Thomas, S. (2003). *Community health nursing: Caring in action*. Clifton Park, NY: Delmar Learning.

Hogstel, M. (2001). *Gerontology: Nursing care of the older adult*. Clifton Park, NY: Delmar Learning.

Hutchinson, M. K. (1998). Something to talk about: Sexual risk communication between young women and their partners. *Journal of Obstetric, Gynecologic, and Neonatal Nursing, 27*(2), 127–133.

Keele-Smith, R., & Price-Daniel, C. (November 2001). *Effects of crossing legs on blood pressure measurement*. Oral presentation at the Sigma Theta Tau International 36th Biennial Convention, Indianapolis, IN.

McCance, K. L., & Heuther, S.E. (2002). *Pathophysiology: The biologic basis for disease in adults and children* (4th ed.). St. Louis: Mosby.

National High Blood Pressure Education Program; National Heart Lung, and Blood Institute; National Institutes of Health (1997). The sixth report of the Joint National Committee on Detection, Evaluation, and Treatment of High Blood Pressure. *Archive of Internal Medicine, 157*: 2413–2422.

Nightingale, F. (1859). *Notes on nursing: What it is and what it is not*. Printed by Harrison and Sons, London, 1946.

Rice, K. L. (1999). Measuring thigh BP. *Nursing99, 29*(8), 58–59.

Roper, M. (1996). Back to basics: Assessing orthostatic vital signs. *American Journal of Nursing, 96*(8), 43–46.

Schmitz, T., Bair, N., Falk, M., & Levine, C. (1995). A comparison of five methods of temperature measurement in febrile intensive care patients. *American Journal of Critical Care, 4*(4), 286–292.

White, L., & Duncan, G. (2002). *Medical-surgical nursing: An integrated approach* (2nd ed.). Clifton Park, NY: Delmar Learning.

Woods, A. (2002). High cholesterol. *Nursing 2002, 32*(6), 56–57.

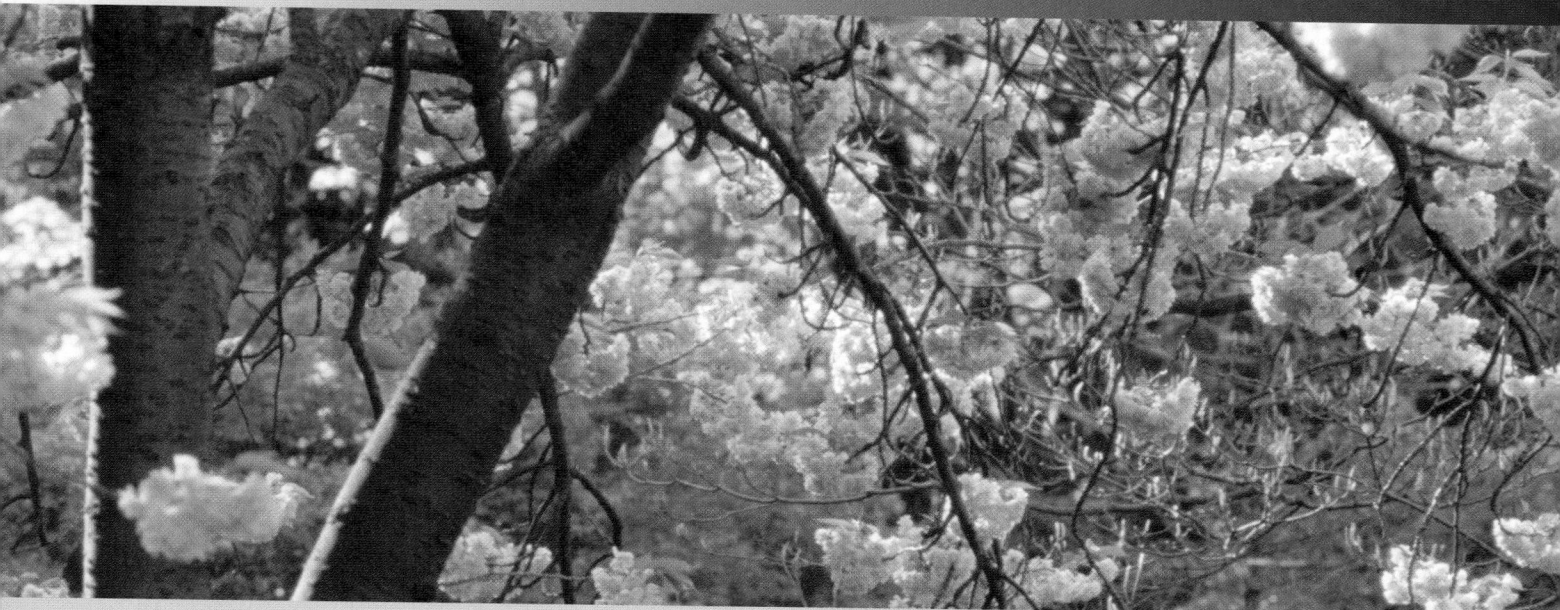

# CHAPTER 28

# Client Education

## Sandra B. Holmes, RN, BSN, MA (C)

*"The great aim of education is not knowledge, but action."*

(Herbert Spencer)

# Chapter Competencies

*Upon completion of this chapter, the reader should be able to:*

1. Describe the elements of the teaching-learning process as related to client education.
2. Discuss the nurse's responsibilities related to client teaching.
3. Explain how learning principles vary throughout the life span.
4. Relate the teaching-learning process to the nursing process.
5. Evaluate teaching strategies in applying the teaching-learning process with clients.

# Key Terms

affective domain
auditory learner
cognitive domain
kinesthetic learner
learning

learning plateau
learning style
philosophy
psychomotor domain
readiness for learning

self-efficacy
teaching
teaching-learning process
teaching strategies
visual learner

Client education is an integral part of nursing care. It is the nurse's responsibility to assist the client to identify the learning needs and resources that will restore and maintain an optimal level of functioning. This chapter offers an overview of the teaching-learning process, including learning barriers and teaching responsibilities of nurses. Client education is extremely important today in a health care environment that demands cost-effective measures. With shorter hospital stays, clients are being discharged to the home or other health care settings in more critical conditions than ever before. Client education, a hallmark of quality nursing care, is a fiscally responsible intervention that encourages health care consumers to engage in self-care and to develop healthy lifestyle practices.

## The Teaching-Learning Process

The **teaching-learning process** is a planned interaction promoting behavioral change that is not a result of maturation or coincidence. **Teaching** is an active process in which one individual shares information with others to provide them with the information to make behavioral changes. Teaching refers to all the activities used by a teacher to assist the learner to absorb new information; it consists of activities that promote change. Teaching is a goal-directed process that provides the opportunity for learning (Figure 28-1).

**Learning** is the process of assimilating information with a resultant change in behavior. Nurses and clients have shared responsibilities in the teaching-learning process. Knowledge is power. By sharing knowledge with clients, the nurse empowers clients to achieve their maximum level of wellness. The teaching-learning process will be familiar to nurses in that it mirrors the steps of the nursing process: assessment, identification of learning needs (nursing diagnosis), planning, implementation of teaching strategies, and evaluation of learner progress and teaching efficacy.

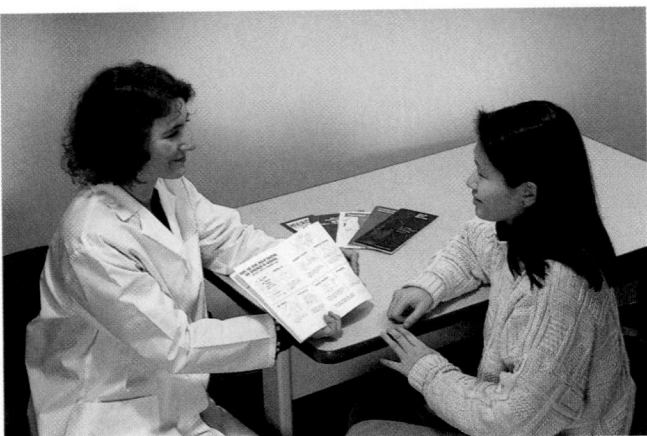

**Figure 28-1** A nurse involves a client in the teaching-learning process. The nurse is using a manual that explains potential dietary plans for the client's nutritional needs.

## Purposes of Client Teaching

According to Edelman and Mandle (2002), the goal of health education is to help individuals achieve optimum states of health through their own actions. Teaching, one of the most important nursing functions, addresses clients' need for information. Often, a knowledge deficit about the course of illness and/or self-care practices hinders a client's recovering from illness or engaging in health promotion behaviors. The nurse's charge is to help bridge the gap between what a client knows and what a client needs to know in order to achieve optimum health.

Client teaching is done for a variety of reasons (Table 28-1). Client education focuses on the client's ability to practice healthy behaviors. The client's ability to care for self is enhanced by effective education.

To be more effective teachers, nurses need a basic understanding of learning theories. There are many schools of thought (theories) about how people learn. Table 28-2 provides an overview of major learning theories.

Each nurse needs to develop an individual **philosophy** (statement of beliefs that is the foundation for behavior) of learning. When formulating a philosophy about teaching-learning, nurses need to consider the common beliefs about learning listed in Box 28-1.

## Facilitators of Learning

Certain fundamental principles of education can be used by nurses to facilitate client learning. Knowles (1984) stated four basic assumptions about adult learners, which are applicable to client education:

- *Assumption:* An individual's personality develops in an orderly fashion from dependence to independence. *Nursing Application:* Plan teaching-learning activities that promote client participation, thus encouraging independence; this increases client control and self-care through empowerment.
- *Assumption:* Learning readiness is affected by developmental stage and sociocultural factors. *Nursing Application:* Conduct a thorough psychosocial assessment before planning the teaching-learning activities.
- *Assumption:* An individual's previous learning experiences can be used as a foundation for further learning. *Nursing Application:* Perform a complete assessment to determine what the client already knows and build on that knowledge base.
- *Assumption:* Immediacy reinforces learning. *Nursing Application:* Provide opportunities for immediate application of knowledge and skills. Incorporate feedback as a continuous part of each nurse-client interaction.

Table 28-3 describes key learning principles.

It is a good idea to keep in mind that **learning plateaus**, or peaks in effectiveness of teaching and depth of learning, will occur in relation to the client's motivation, interest, and perception of relevance of the material. Frequent reinforcement of learning through immediate feedback and continual reassessment of effectiveness will enhance the value of the learning process for both the teacher and the learner. Making the information acquisition process as user-friendly as possible will also increase satisfaction and success. This can be done by organizing content from the simple to the complex and from the familiar to the new, making learning as creative and interesting as possible, and adopting a flexible approach to allow the learning process to be dynamic.

---

### TABLE 28-1    CLIENT EDUCATION TOPICS

| Health Promotion | Health Restoration |
|---|---|
| • Parenting skills | • Medication information |
| • Nutrition | • Community resources |
| • Exercise | • Information about treatment modalities |
| • Family planning | |
| **Disease/Injury Prevention** | **Facilitating Coping** |
| • Immunizations | • Safe use of medical equipment |
| • Health screenings | • Dietary modifications |
| • Smoking cessation | • Information about the disease process |
| • Breast self-examination | • Counseling related to anger, grief, self-esteem |
| • Safety measures (e.g., car seat/restraining devices) | • Stress management |

## TABLE 28-2  OVERVIEW OF LEARNING THEORIES

| Theorist | Description |
| --- | --- |
| John Watson | Learning is: A result of conditioning and experiences. Encouraged by changing the environment. |
| Ivan Pavlov | The learner is passive, controlled by the environment. |
| B. F. Skinner | Teaching is the deliberate manipulation of the environment. |
| Edward L. Thorndike | Learning can be transferred from one situation to another. Assessment of learner's behavior is necessary. |
| John Dewey | The learner must have an understanding of the goals. Education should promote learner independence. |
| Jerome Bruner | Learning is affected by culture and value system. The learner is an active participant in the learning process. |
| Robert Gagne | Learning occurs in an orderly fashion, from the simple to the complex, from the concrete to the abstract. |
| Albert Bandura | Behavior is regulated by internal mechanisms, such as self-efficacy. |

## STOP AND THINK

### Your Beliefs About Learning

Consider the information presented in Table 28-2 and Box 28-1.

- Which statements mirror your own philosophy about learning?

- Which statements are most congruent with a nursing philosophy that views clients not as recipients of care but as partners in the caring and healing process?

## BOX 28-1  BELIEFS ABOUT LEARNING

- Each individual has the capacity to learn; learning ability varies from person to person and is situational.
- The pace of learning varies with each person.
- Learning is a continuous process, occurring throughout the life cycle.
- Learning can occur in formal and informal settings and interactions.
- Learning is an individualized process.
- Learning new information is based on previous knowledge and experiences.
- Motivation and readiness are necessary for learning to occur.
- Prompt feedback facilitates learning.

## Barriers to Learning

Receiving information does not, in and of itself, guarantee that learning will occur. Several barriers can impede the learning process. In a nursing situation, learning barriers can be classified as either internal (psychological or physiological) or external (environmental or sociocultural). Examples of these barriers are shown in Box 28-2.

The nurse must assess for the presence of barriers to facilitate the learning process. Specific assessment information is presented later in this chapter.

## Domains of Learning

Bloom, in his classic work (1977), identified three areas or domains in which learning occurs: the **cognitive domain** (intellectual understanding), the **affective domain** (emotions and attitudes), and the **psychomotor domain** (motor skills). Each domain responds to and processes information in very different ways. Table 28-4 briefly describes the three domains of learning through clinical examples.

## Teaching Strategies

Nurses need to be sensitive to all three domains of learning when developing effective teaching plans and to use **teaching strategies**, or techniques to promote learning, that will tap into each of the domains. For instance, teaching a diabetic client how and why to measure the proper daily balance of insulin against glucose levels is within the cognitive domain. Helping this client learn how to self-administer insulin falls within the psychomotor domain, and seeing that the client learns to view diabetes as only

## TABLE 28-3    PRINCIPLES OF LEARNING

| Principle | Explanation |
|---|---|
| Relevance | The material should be:<br>• Meaningful to client<br>• Easily understood by client<br>• Related to previously learned information |
| Motivation | Client should:<br>• Want to learn<br>• Perceive value of information |
| Readiness | Client should be able and willing to learn. |
| Maturation | Client should be developmentally able to learn and have requisite cognitive and psychomotor abilities. |
| Reinforcement | Feedback to learner should be:<br>• Positive<br>• Immediate |
| Participation | Active involvement promotes learning. |
| Organization | The material should:<br>• Incorporate previously learned information<br>• Be presented in sequence of simple to complex |
| Repetition | Retention of material is reinforced by practice, repetition, and presentation of same material in a variety of ways. |

## BOX 28-2    BARRIERS TO LEARNING

**External Barriers**

**Environmental**
- Interruptions
- Lack of privacy
- Multiple stimuli

**Sociocultural**
- Language
- Value system
- Educational background

**Internal Barriers**

**Psychological**
- Anxiety
- Fear
- Anger
- Depression
- Inability to comprehend

**Physiological**
- Pain
- Fatigue
- Sensory deprivation
- Oxygen deprivation

## TABLE 28-4    DOMAINS OF LEARNING

| Domain | Definition | Clinical Example |
|---|---|---|
| Cognitive | Learning that involves the acquisition of facts and data. Used in problem solving and decision making. | Client states the name and purpose of prescribed medications. |
| Affective | Learning that involves changing attitudes, emotions, beliefs. Used in making judgments. | Client accepts that he has a chronic illness. |
| Psychomotor | Learning that involves gaining motor skills. Uses physical application of knowledge. | Client gives self an injection. |

Learning Domains, 2003. http://tip.psychology.org

one part of an entire individual stimulates the affective domain.

Although teaching opportunities arise with any interaction with a client, the nurse must do advanced planning for a formal teaching session. Most educators agree that a combination of teaching strategies is most beneficial for learning to take place. Proper assessment of the client's learning needs and the way clients learn best are imperative for a teaching session to be successful. A variety of teaching strategies is presented in this section (i.e., discussion, demonstration, role-playing, visual aids, programmed instruction, computer-assisted instruction).

### Discussion

Discussion is the exchange of information both verbally and nonverbally. It involves audience participation. It requires the nurse to focus on building some sort of conversation before focusing on expanding that conversation. Discussion is effective for large groups, as it pools ideas and experiences from diverse backgrounds, allowing everyone to participate in an active process of exchanging information. It is the nurse's responsibility to act as facilitator to keep the discussion on track. Discussion also is effective for one-to-one interactions. Some clients prefer this method, especially if the topic is sensitive.

### Demonstration

Demonstration and return demonstration provide a realistic learning experience. Demonstrations should be as realistic as possible. Adequate time should be allowed for this type of teaching strategy. Demonstration combined with lecture or discussion is a practical strategy when teaching a new skill—for example, insulin injection, use of equipment, wound care, or exercise. Return demonstration allows for evaluation of the client's learning.

### Role-Playing

Role-playing allows the client to apply knowledge in a simulated environment. The nurse sets the stage, then the client plays out the scenario with the nurse or another learner. This can be very effective with adolescents. For example, a teenage boy can rehearse with a partner what he will say to his parents when telling them his girlfriend is pregnant.

Role-playing is also beneficial for small children (Figure 28-2). It allows them the opportunity to deal with their fear and negative emotions about illness or hospitalization. Game playing is also very useful when dealing with small children or clients with developmental delay (Antai-Otong, 2003).

### Visual Aids

Visual aids come in many forms, allowing the nurse to select the one(s) most appropriate for the client. These include flip charts, slides, television programs, pamphlets, and books, to name a few. It is important that the nurse does not rely solely on the use of visual aids. They should be used in conjunction with other teaching strategies.

### Programmed Instruction

Programmed instruction, often referred to as "canned" (audio) presentations, is intended for use without the nurse. This can be effective for some clients, but the nurse needs to do a thorough assessment of the client and the instruction to make sure the two are compatible.

### Computer-Assisted Instruction

Computer-assisted instruction is a relatively new aid available to nurses. The programs can be personalized to the client. The options for this form of instruction are growing daily. They, however, come with a price. Depending on the type of computer equipment, the cost can run into the thousands. Clients also need to have some basic computer skills, and some may feel intimidated by the "modern technology."

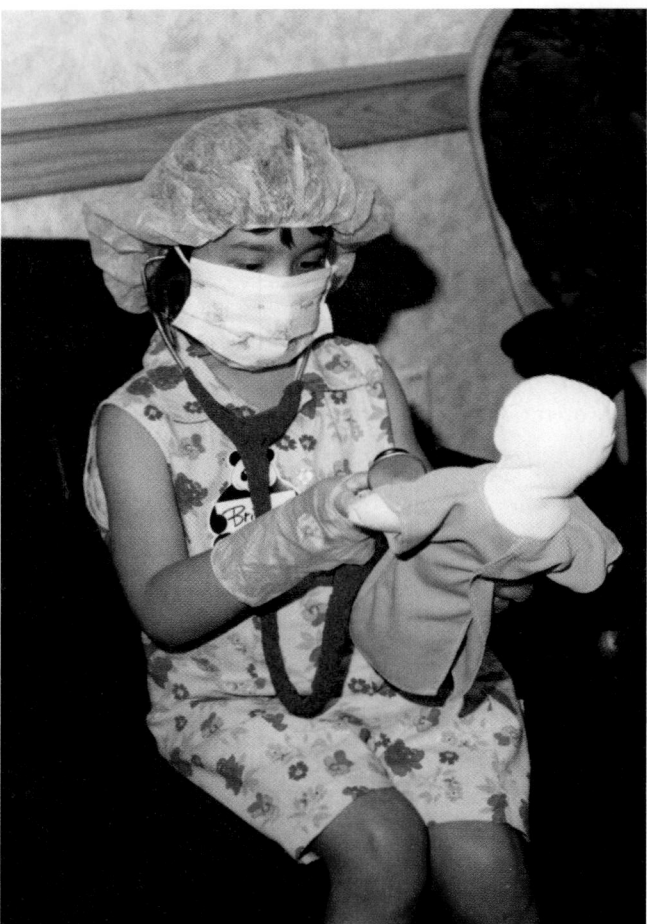

**Figure 28-2   Hospitalized child using doll in her role-playing activity**

## Professional Responsibilities Related to Teaching

Through teaching, the nurse empowers clients in their self-care abilities. Teaching is the tool for providing information to clients about specific disease processes, treatment methods, and health-promoting behaviors.

### Legal Aspects

The American Nurses Association, in its *Social Policy Statement* (1995), identifies health teaching as an essential function of nursing. Each state has its own definition of nursing practice; in most states, teaching is a required function of nurses.

Client teaching is also mandated by several accrediting bodies, such as the Joint Commission for Accreditation of Healthcare Organizations (JCAHO, 2002). The American Hospital Association's *Patient's Bill of Rights* (1980) calls for the client's understanding of health status and treatment approaches. Informed consent for treatment procedures can be given only by clients who are well informed. The nurse assesses the client's level of understanding about

## LEGAL AND ETHICAL ISSUES

### Client Education and the Law

The nurse must remember the legal ramifications of client education. Specific considerations are the informed consent, characteristics of the client (e.g., age, mental condition, anxiety), appropriate language of the information, and the timing of presenting the information. The nurse must present the information in wording that is understandable to the client and ask the client for clarifications regarding the information.

Dempski, K. M., & Killion, S. W. (2001). *Legal & Ethical Issues in Nursing.* Thorofare, New Jersey: SLACK, Inc.

### TABLE 28-5   LEARNING NEEDS IN VARIOUS PHASES OF CARE

| Primary: Health Maintenance | Secondary: Diagnosis and Treatment | Tertiary: Follow-up |
|---|---|---|
| Disease prevention | Disease process | Care at home |
| Health care services availability | Methods of care and treatment | Medications |
| | | Dietary modifications |
| Growth and development | Health care setting | Activity |
| | | Rehabilitation plans |
| Safety | | Prevention/ recurrence of complications |
| First Aid | | |
| Nutrition | | |
| Hygiene | | |

treatment methods and corrects any knowledge deficits. The nurse is often a physician interpreter to the client—explaining in easily understood terms, clarifying, and referring.

Teaching supports behavior change that leads to positive adaptation. Thus, teaching involves decreasing the fear of change. Reducing anxiety and anticipatory stress is an important component of teaching.

Client teaching is an essential function of every professional nurse regardless of the practice setting. Table 28-5 outlines learning needs as they relate to the three phases of nursing care: primary, secondary, and tertiary. Clients who are hospitalized need information regarding their condition, the hospital environment, and expectations regarding treatment (Boyd, Graham, Gleit, & Whitman, 1998).

## Documentation

The nurse is legally responsible to document client education in the medical record. From a legal perspective, if the nurse teaches the client but fails to document it, then the educational activities never occurred. Documentation of the teaching-learning event should include a summary of the learning need, the plan of action, implementation of the plan, and evaluation of the results. The evaluation phase is crucial. It must include whom the nurse instructed. The nurse must document concrete evidence that the desired outcome was achieved, and what steps were taken if the outcome was not achieved. The medical record must contain evidence that the client, caregiver, or significant other has actually learned the material taught. Documentation of teaching promotes continuity of care and facilitates accurate communication to other health care colleagues (Carelock & Innerarity, 2001).

Many different approaches can be used to document client teaching. Figure 28-3 provides one example of documentation for client teaching in an inpatient setting. For a sample form documenting teaching in the home setting, see Figure 28-4.

## Learning Throughout the Life Span

One basic assumption underlies teaching effectiveness—*all people are capable of learning.* This ability to learn varies from person to person and from situation to situation. Most clients—because of anxiety, pain, or other stressors related to illness—have only limited adaptive resources. They may not have much energy or interest to invest in learning.

Learning needs and learning abilities change throughout life. The client's chronological age and developmental stage greatly influence the ability to learn. The principles of learning discussed earlier in this chapter have relevance to learners of all ages. However, teaching approaches must be modified according to the client's developmental stage and level of understanding. Specific information about teaching children, adolescents, and older adults is described in the following sections. Table 28-6 lists teaching strategies for different age groups.

### Children

**Readiness for learning** (evidence of willingness to learn) varies during childhood according to maturational level. Responding to knowledge deficits of young children requires that the nurse work closely with the

# Tulane
## UNIVERSITY
### Medical Center

## PATIENT TEACHING PROTOCOL

LEVEL: Interdependent

TITLE: Teaching the Patient with Diagnosis of Gastrointestinal (GI) Bleed

COMMENT KEY    S = Successfully meets outcome
N = Needs further instruction
U = Unable to comprehend
* = See Nursing Progress Note for Patient/Family Education

| OUTCOME STANDARDS TO BE MET PRIOR TO DISCHARGE: | DATE / INITIALS | | |
|---|---|---|---|
| | INITIATED | MET | NOT MET |
| PHYSIOLOGIC:    Patient will be free of evidence of GI bleed. | | | |
| PSYCHOLOGIC:    Patient will express fears and concerns with diagnosis of GI bleed and procedures to be performed. | | | |
| COGNITIVE:    Patient will verbalize understanding of information presented. | | | |

| PATIENT LEARNING OUTCOMES (PLO) | Information to be Presented/ Patient Learning Activities | Date Time | PLO # | Initials | | Comment (See Key) |
|---|---|---|---|---|---|---|
| | | | | Nurse | Pt. | |
| 1. Patient will verbalize understanding and compliance with diagnostic procedures and treatment measures. | 1. Discuss with patient and offer literature for various tests/procedures ordered:<br>– Colonoscopy<br>  Barium Enema<br>  EGD<br>  Gastrointestinal Series (upper GI)<br>  Sigmoidoscopy<br>– Nasogastric Tube if applicable<br>– NPO, clear liquids<br>– Collection of Stool specimens for blood<br>– Intake and output recorded<br>– IV fluids if ordered<br>– Medications | | | | | |
| 2. Patient will verbalize those signs/symptoms to report to nurse/M.D. | 2. Discuss with patient those signs and symptoms to be reported:<br>– Severe abdominal pain<br>– Abdominal swelling<br>– Cramping<br>– Increased nausea/vomiting, diarrhea or bleeding<br>– Increased weakness | | | | | |
| 3. Patient will verbalize fears, concerns, and anxieties regarding diagnosis, procedures, and prognosis. | 3. Encourage patient to ventilate fears, feelings, and concerns during hospital stay and provide emotional support prn. | | | | | |

**Figure 28-3    Documentation form for client teaching: Inpatient setting.** *Courtesy of Tulane Medical Center*

# RIVER REGION HOME HEALTH SERVICES, INC.
## PSYCHIATRIC NURSE PROGRESS NOTE

PATIENT NAME _____ MR# _____ _____ IN _____ OUT _____

NURSE NAME _____ _____ DAY _____ DATE _____

VSBP _____ T _____ P _____ R _____ WT _____ DIET _____

Nutritional Status _____ Heart/Lung Status _____

Neuro Oriented X _____ PEERL _____ Homebound Status _____

Physical Status _____

_____

Assess Degree of Existing Problem: (1) Mild, (2) Moderate, (3) Severe

| | | | | | |
|---|---|---|---|---|---|
| Somatic Concern | ____ | Emotional Withdrawal | ____ | Anxiety | ____ |
| Depressive Mood | ____ | Hostility | | Uncooperativeness | ____ |
| Blunted Affect | ____ | Lack of Insight | ____ | Delusions | ____ |
| Suicidal Ideation | ____ | Motivational Disability | | Hallucinations | ____ |
| Impaired Memory | ____ | Rx Non–Compliance | ____ | Socialization | ____ |
| Communication | ____ | Mannerisms & Posturing | | | |
| ADL's | ____ | Unusual Thought Concern | ____ | | |
| Conceptual Disorganization | ____ | | | | |

SN Assessment/Intervention/Teaching: _____

_____

_____

Teaching: _____

_____

_____

Feedback to Teaching: _____

_____

_____

Changes: Meds/Plan of Care: _____

Aide Supervision AS/PAS: _____
Reason HHA Needed: _____
Comments Regarding Care: _____

_____

HOME HEALTH ASSISTANT _____

Current Requisition in Home _____
Completes Assignment _____
Rapport with Patient _____

Planning:   Continue Same Plan _____
            Increase Visits _____
            Decrease Visits _____
            Discharge Planning _____

PATIENT _____

Appearance _____
Bathed Completely _____
Body Alignment _____
PT/FMY Satisfied _____
Room Tidy _____
Personal Hygiene _____

**Figure 28-4**   Documentation form for client teaching: Home health. *Courtesy of River Region Home Health Services, Inc., Louisiana*

## TABLE 28-6    TEACHING ACROSS THE LIFE SPAN

| Teaching Strategy | Nursing Implications |
| --- | --- |
| **Infants**<br><br>• Be consistent in actions.<br><br>• Use brightly colored toys and objects.<br><br>• Role-play nurturing behavior for parent to model. | • Teach the primary caregivers.<br><br>• Emphasize the need for consistency in approach.<br><br>Learning needs: safety, growth and development concepts, infant care, nutrition, sleep patterns, skin integrity (diaper rash) |
| **Toddlers**<br><br>• Play with appropriate medical equipment and supplies (e.g., Band-Aids, surgical caps).<br><br>• Use child's comfort toy.<br><br>• Positive simple commands<br><br>• Picture books<br><br>• Coloring books<br><br>• Puppets, dolls<br><br>• Audio tapes | • Involve parents to decrease child's anxiety level.<br><br>• Use words easily understood by the child without being condescending.<br><br>• Assess for signs of sensory overload (toddlers tire quickly); avoid trying to teach when the child is overwhelmed or irritable.<br><br>Learning needs: safety, immunizations, nutrition, dental hygiene |
| **Preschoolers**<br><br>• Provide immediate reinforcers (rewards) for positive behavior (e.g., smiley-face stickers).<br><br>• Encourage play.<br><br>• Books and coloring books<br><br>• Music, singing, audiotapes | • Preschoolers often use words without fully understanding their meanings.<br><br>• Feelings are expressed through actions instead of words.<br><br>Learning needs: immunizations, safety, nutrition, dental hygiene, parenting skills |
| **School-Aged Children**<br><br>• Toys<br><br>• Computer games<br><br>• Books<br><br>• Demonstration<br><br>• Role-play | • Able to follow simple directions<br><br>• Understand the use of symbols<br><br>• Often seek approval by doing the "right" thing<br><br>• Assess child's reading ability.<br><br>Learning needs: safety, hygiene, nutrition, socialization with peers |
| **Adolescents**<br><br>• Printed material (at appropriate literacy level) | • Peer approval is important; group sessions may be useful unless the material to be taught is too threatening. |

*(continues)*

## TABLE 28-6    TEACHING ACROSS THE LIFE SPAN (continued)

| Teaching Strategy | Nursing Implications |
|---|---|
| **Adolescents (continued)**<br><br>• Role-play<br><br>• Demonstration | • Maintain privacy.<br><br>• Assess for and correct any misinformation.<br><br>• A sense of invulnerability leads to an "it can't happen to me" attitude.<br><br>• Emphasize immediate benefit of learning information.<br><br>Learning needs: physiological changes, sexuality (including contraception), substance abuse prevention, self-esteem, automobile safety, prevention of sports injuries |
| **Young Adults**<br><br>• Printed materials appropriate to literacy level<br><br>• Discussion<br><br>• Demonstration<br><br>• Role-play | • Content must be perceived as relevant to young adults.<br><br>• Strong need for independence; provide choices.<br><br>• Encourage input into decision making.<br><br>Learning needs: nutrition, exercise, stress management, time management, sexuality issues (i.e., contraception), some may need parenting skill classes |
| **Middle-Aged Adults**<br><br>• Printed materials geared to level of comprehension<br><br>• Discussion<br><br>• Demonstration<br><br>• Role-play | • Increased awareness of personal vulnerability<br><br>• Generally, a recognition of the need for lifestyle changes<br><br>• Assess reading skills.<br><br>Learning needs: nutrition, exercise, stress management, warning signs of illness |
| **Older Adults**<br><br>• Assess for reading skills.<br><br>• Frequent repetition<br><br>• Demonstration<br><br>• Discussion<br><br>• Assess learning style and match with corresponding materials. | • May need large-print materials<br><br>• Often a strong desire for independence; offer choices<br><br>• Chronic illness (i.e., arthritis) may impair mobility and dexterity.<br><br>• Aging does not lead to an overall decreased intelligence.<br><br>Learning needs: loss and grief, disease-specific information, stress management, socialization skills, elimination patterns, dental hygiene |

Adapted from Hunt, R., & Zurek, E. L. (1997). *Introduction to community-based nursing*. Philadelphia: Lippincott.

## NURSING STRATEGY

### Guidelines for Teaching Children

- Make sure the client is comfortable.

- Encourage caregiver participation.

- Assess developmental level. Do not equate age with developmental level.

- Assess client's learning readiness and motivation.

- Assess client's psychological status.

- Determine self-care abilities of client and caregiver.

- Use play, imitation, and role-playing to make learning fun and meaningful.

- Use different visual stimuli such as books, chalkboards, and videos to convey information and check understanding.

- Use terms that are easily understood by the client and caregiver.

- Provide frequent repetition and reinforcement.

- Develop realistic goals that are consistent with developmental abilities.

- Verify client's understanding of information presented.

## STOP AND THINK

### Adolescents

Adolescents are especially sensitive to discrepancies between an adult's actions and words.

- How does this apply to you as a beginning practitioner of nursing?

- What messages do you send to others by your health behaviors?

- Are your health behaviors consistent with what you teach your clients?

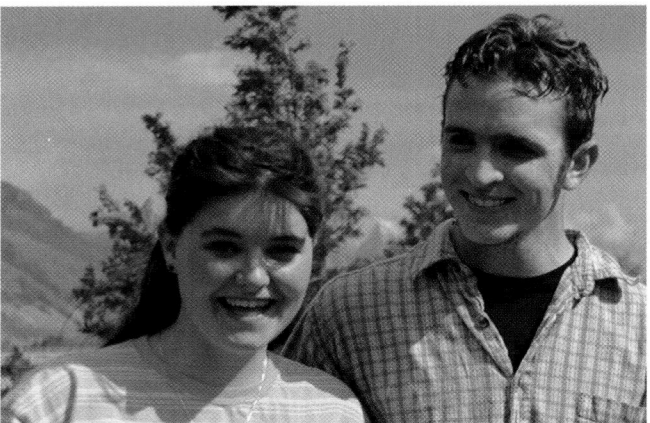

**Figure 28-5** The relationships that adolescents develop are very important. Learning about concepts such as intimacy becomes a significant aspect in the adolescent stage of development.

child's caretaker; including the family or significant others in teaching is essential when caring for young children (Potts & Mandleco, 2002).

Young children learn primarily through play, which can be incorporated into teaching activities. For example, puppets, toys, and coloring books can be effective teaching tools for the young child.

Older children can also benefit from the use of art materials and medical supplies (e.g., medicine cups, putting bandages on dolls). While the child is involved in play, the nurse is alleviating anxiety by teaching the child what to expect regarding treatment procedures.

## Adolescents

As children approach adolescence, they are better able to conceptualize relationships between things. Usually, reading skills and comprehension ability have advanced, and the adolescent can understand more complex information. One of the strongest influences on an adolescent is peer support (Figure 28-5); therefore, group meetings are

often useful in teaching. Nurses also teach by acting as role models. Nurses relate to adolescents on their level by trying to understand how they think. Listening allows the nurse to hear the adolescent's feedback relative to learning needs. It is also important to focus on the present when teaching adolescents and to be aware of their need to maintain control. "Independence is crucial to adolescents. By enlisting teens as active participants in their health care and encouraging them to participate in other activities, you can increase independence and decrease noncompliance" (Muscari, 1998, p. 29). The Nursing Strategy box provides additional guidelines for teaching adolescents.

## Older Adults

Aging is accompanied by many physiological changes. As a result of these changes, some older adults have perceptual impairments such as impaired vision and hearing. The nurse must assess for perceptual changes and adjust teaching materials accordingly. For example, provide large-print

## NURSING STRATEGY

### Guidelines for Teaching Adolescents

- Show respect for adolescents by recognizing that they still have to gain the knowledge and experience of adulthood while struggling to break away from the grasp of childhood.

- Boost adolescents' confidence by asking their input and opinions on health care matters.

- Encourage adolescents to explore their own feelings about self-concept and independence.

- Be sensitive to the peer pressure many adolescents face.

- Help adolescents identify their positive qualities and build on those.

- Use language that is clear yet appropriate to the health care setting.

- Gear teaching to the adolescent's developmental level.

- Engage adolescents in problem-solving activities to encourage independent and informed decision making.

## LIFE SPAN CONSIDERATIONS

### Guidelines for Teaching Older Adults

- Make sure the client is comfortable. Pain, fatigue, and hunger can impair learning.

- Assess client's learning readiness and motivation; also assess developmental level. Do not equate age with developmental level.

- Assess client's psychological status. Depression, severe anxiety, and denial interfere with learning.

- Determine client's self-care abilities.

- Use terms that are easily understood by the client. Avoid talking down to the client; a condescending, paternalistic manner impedes learning.

- Determine the time of day in which the client is better able to concentrate.

- Assess for perceptual impairments and individualize teaching strategies accordingly.

Adapted from Beare, P. G., & Myers, J. L. (1999). *Principles and practices of adult health nursing* (3rd ed., p. 111.). St. Louis: Mosby.

written material and make sure the client can hear all your instructions and directions. The Life Span Considerations box provides guidelines for teaching older adults.

## Teaching-Learning and the Nursing Process

The teaching-learning process and the nursing process are interdependent. Both are dynamic and consist of the same phases: assessment, diagnosis, planning, implementation, and evaluation. Figure 28-6 compares the nursing process and the teaching-learning process. See Chapter 12 for more information about the nursing process.

## Assessment

The nurse should assess each learning situation for every client. Primary and secondary data sources are used by nurses for assessment of learning needs. See Chapter 11 for a discussion of these sources. Communicating with the client and family or significant others is the foundation of assessment related to learning. Several factors need to be considered during assessment, including:

- Learning styles
- Learning needs
- Potential learning needs
- Ability to learn
- Readiness to learn
- Client strengths
- Previous experience and knowledge base

### Learning Styles

Each individual has a unique way of processing information. The manner in which an individual incorporates new data is called **learning style**. Some people learn by processing information visually (**visual learners**), others by listening to words (**auditory learners**), and others by doing (**kinesthetic learners**). The nurse should use a variety of techniques, such as lecture, discussion, small group work, role-playing, modeling, return demonstration, imitation, problem solving, games, and question-and-answer sessions, to match different learning styles of clients. A good way to discover a client's learning style is to ask the client, "What helps you to learn?" or "What kinds of things do you enjoy doing?"

**TEACHING-LEARNING PROCESS**

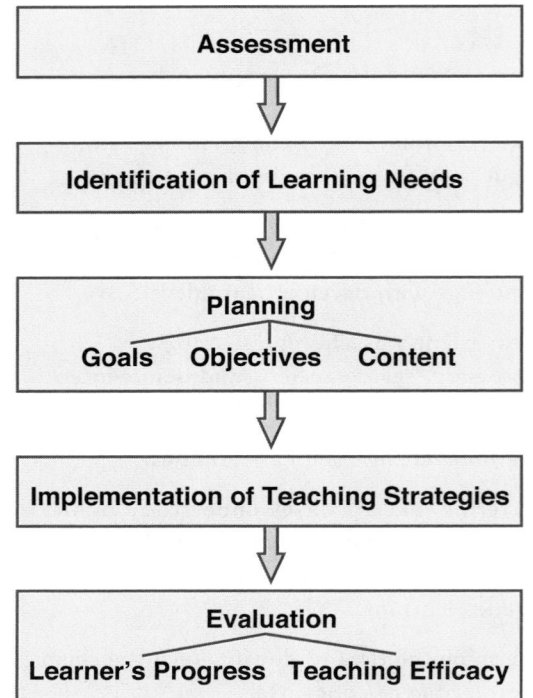

**NURSING PROCESS**

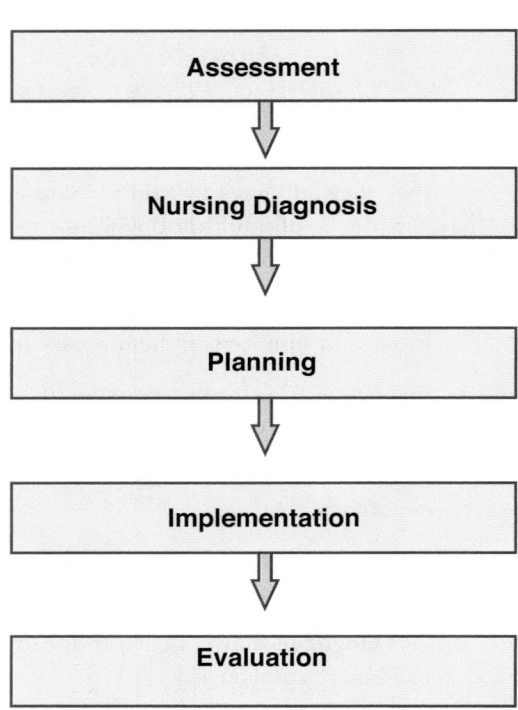

**Figure 28-6    Teaching-learning process and nursing process: A comparison**

## Learning Needs

Everyone who receives health care services has some need for learning. Client teaching may be indicated when a client:

- Expresses a need for information to make decisions
- Has a need for new skills
- Desires to make modifications in lifestyle
- Is in an unfamiliar environment

Comprehensive assessment is a mutual process between client and nurse. A crucial step in teaching is to determine the client's learning needs—what the client needs to know and what the client already knows. The nurse must evaluate the client's knowledge about the content that is to be taught. This previous knowledge can then be used as a foundation for new concepts. If the client is misinformed, the nurse develops a remediation plan for learning. Determination of the client's learning needs is accomplished in a variety of ways, including:

- Questioning the client directly
- Observing client behaviors
- Interacting with the client's family or significant others

It is imperative that the nurse address the client's immediate need for knowledge first. This is facilitated by assessing the client's perception of learning needs and prioritizing those needs on the basis of client input and status.

## Potential Learning Needs

The nurse also assesses for potential learning needs so that anticipatory planning can be done to avert a relapse in the recovery process and to maintain wellness. Some examples of anticipatory learning needs include:

- Mrs. Stone is pregnant for the first time. *Potential Learning Need:* Infant care
- Mr. Carpenter has just been diagnosed with diabetes that is currently controlled by dietary modifications. He has been told that he may have to take insulin daily in the future. *Potential Learning Need:* Self-administration of insulin

## Ability to Learn

The nurse assesses the client for characteristics that will hinder or facilitate learning. One such characteristic is the client's developmental stage. For example, do not automatically assume that a client who is 34 years old has mastered the developmental tasks of earlier stages. Age is not synonymous with developmental level; observation of behavior provides the clearest clue to developmental level.

The client's maturity level greatly influences the ability to learn information. Every developmental stage is characterized by unique skills and abilities that affect the response to various teaching tools. Developmental stage

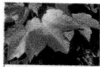

## RESEARCH FOCUS

**Title of Study:** Meeting patients' information needs before and after discharge from hospital

**Study Purpose:** To build a client-centered account of information needs, focusing on discharge from the hospital

**Methods:** Clients participated in a semi-structured interview process—the first shortly before discharge and then at 1, 4, and 8 weeks after their return home—to investigate their perceptions and experiences.

**Findings:** After discharge, clients adopted a variety of strategies for resolving uncertainties, including reliance on common sense and lay advice. Clients were generally not clear about the role and responsibility of hospital and community staff for the provision of information once the client had been discharged.

**Implications:** The authors suggest that this study questions the idealistic assumption that the individual information needs of all clients can be comprehensively identified and met. Many of these needs may not become evident until after the client returns home and identifies an "information gap." Informal opportunities for client education arise at many levels, beginning in the preadmission phase through hospitalization and discharge. Further research regarding client education is indicated.

Tierney, A. J., Worth, A., & Watson, N. (2000). Meeting patients' information needs before and after discharge from hospital, *Journal of Clinical Nursing, 9*(6), 14–19.

## NURSING STRATEGY

### Learning Needs Assessment

Questions for the nurse to ask in determining the learning needs of the client:

- Does the client express uncertainty and/or anxiety over an upcoming procedure?

- Is the client able to tell you about medications, purposes, and side effects?

- Can the client describe necessary lifestyle modifications?

- Does the client perform self-care activities correctly?

- Is the client able to demonstrate necessary treatment procedures (e.g., colostomy irrigations, injections, blood glucose monitoring)?

participating in return demonstration of a dressing change. Some behaviors that indicate lack of client readiness are anxiety, avoidance, denial, lack of participation in discussion or demonstration, and lack of participation in self-care activities.

Closely related to readiness is client motivation. Individuals must believe that they need to learn the information before learning occurs. Does the client perceive

| TABLE 28-7 | FACTORS INFLUENCING LEARNING READINESS | |
| --- | --- | --- |
| **Capability** | **Comfort** | **Motivation** |
| Maturity level | Basic physiological needs met | Care for self |
| Physical ability | | Get well |
| Cognitive ability | Feelings of safety and security | Achieve a higher level of wellness |
| Attitude | Low degree (or absence of) pain | Know and understand |
| | Pleasant surroundings with few distractions | Return to work |
| | | Please others |
| | Rapport with caregiver | Be a "good patient" |
| | | Avoid complications and relapse |

greatly determines the type of data to be taught, the method(s) to be used, the language that is used, and the location for teaching. In addition to developmental stage, assessment should include evaluation of the client's cognitive skills, problem-solving abilities, and attention span.

### Readiness to Learn

Another characteristic to be assessed is the client's learning readiness. Table 28-7 shows some factors that influence readiness.

Readiness is closely related to growth and development; for example, does the client have the requisite cognitive and psychomotor skills for learning a particular task? Can the client comprehend the information? Learning readiness is present when the client asks questions. Another indicator that the client is ready to learn is client participation in learning activities, such as actively

## CLINICAL ALERT

### Checking Literacy

"Lscean uyro sdhna. Seu yver dloc rweat."

The preceding statement is what many of your clients will see when you give them printed educational materials. Be sure to assess the client's ability to comprehend written materials, and avoid making assumptions about your clients' literacy level. Check for comprehension through return explanation of the written material.

## STOP AND THINK

### How Do You Learn?

● What motivates you to study?

● How do you prepare yourself to learn new material?

● What helps you to perceive material as relevant?

● Identify some ways you can assist your client to perceive the material as relevant.

relevance (meaningfulness) in the current information to be taught? If an individual sees the information as being personally valuable, the information is more likely to be learned. However, if the client does not think that the content is relevant, learning is not likely to occur. Relevance is determined individually; the nurse must assess the personal meaning of learning content for each client.

Albert Bandura, a psychologist, described the concept of **self-efficacy** (a belief that one will succeed in attempts to change behavior) as having a profound influence on motivation (1977). If clients feel they will not achieve the goals, they will lack motivation to try. To maximize motivation, keep the teaching-learning goals realistic. Break the content down into small steps that are achievable and provide feedback on the progress.

### Client Strengths

Identifying the client's strengths and limitations provides a foundation for realistic expectations. An understanding of the client's strengths and weaknesses allows the nurse to plan successful teaching-learning experiences. Determination of client strengths assists the nurse in selecting appropriate teaching methods.

### Previous Experience and Knowledge Base

The client has a knowledge base acquired through life experiences. Previous knowledge affects the client's attitudes about learning and perception of the importance of information to be learned and is related to the client's type of educational experiences.

Certainly when considering a client's previous knowledge, the nurse recognizes that culture plays an important role in knowledge acquisition. Attitudes (which are derived from a cultural context) toward what is appropriate to learn and who should teach may require alterations in the nurse's approach. The nurse's sensitivity to cultural values affects every aspect of the teaching-learning process.

## Nursing Diagnosis

Several nursing diagnoses can apply to the client when barriers to the learning process exist. When lack of knowledge is the primary barrier to learning, the diagnosis of *Deficient Knowledge* is applicable. For example:

- A client who does not understand how to use crutches for assisted ambulation may have the diagnosis of *Deficient Knowledge: Crutchwalking*, related to inexperience as evidenced by multiple questions and hesitancy to walk.
- A client who has had a colostomy and will be discharged soon may have a diagnosis of *Deficient Knowledge: Follow-Up Care* related to colostomy care and maintenance as evidenced by requests for information.

Deficient knowledge may also be a component of many other nursing diagnoses in which risk or impaired behavior exists. For instance, *Risk for Infection* may relate to a client's compromised health status; this risk can be modified or reduced through certain physical and environmental changes and also through proper client education. A client presenting with a diagnosis of a *Self-Care Deficit: Bathing* may need assistance acquiring the physical supplies to remedy the deficit, as well as instruction in techniques related to present physical and mental abilities (Ackley & Ladwig, 2002).

## Planning and Outcome Identification

Informal teaching can occur in any setting at any time; formal teaching is planned and goal directed. Teaching is a goal-directed, purposeful process, which means that teaching-learning activities must be planned. Learning is the process by which a person acquires or increases knowledge in a way that is measurable. It is the nurse's responsibility to adequately plan a formal teaching session. The teaching plan closely resembles a nursing care plan; both use the nursing process as a guide. Planning, an ongoing phase of the teaching process, involves consideration of the following:

- What to teach
- How to teach
- Who will teach and who will be taught
- When teaching will occur
- Where teaching will be done

"Meeting the patient educational needs of the consumer is one well-recognized aspect of quality care. Delivering quality care does not happen by chance, rather, it requires intense planning" (Patyk, Gaynor, & Verdin, 2000, p. 14).

Determination of *what* to teach is done through comprehensive assessment. The content to be taught depends greatly on the client's knowledge base, readiness to learn, and current health status.

Deciding *how* to teach involves matching teaching strategies with client's learning needs, readiness, and ability. The nurse who is an effective teacher uses methods that capture the client's interest. A variety of teaching methods can be used to match the client's learning styles.

Planning also means deciding *who* will teach the client. Effective client education is the result of a multidisciplinary effort. However, the nurse is the coordinator of the health care team's teaching activities. Responsibility for planning a comprehensive teaching approach, from admission to postdischarge, remains with the nurse. Continuity of care is greatly affected by the teaching plan. The "who" part of planning also means determining who should be taught. In addition to the individual client, the nurse must determine who else in the family needs to be taught about the illness and recovery process.

Timing of *when* to teach should be carefully considered. The nurse recognizes that *every* interaction with the client is an opportunity for informal teaching. Whenever a client asks a question, there is an opportunity for teaching. These windows of teaching opportunities must be used.

## CLIENT REFLECTIONS

### Demonstration as a Teaching Technique

Mr. Van Eck, age 54, has colon cancer. He comments about the client education related to his new ostomy, "I really appreciate my [enterostomal] nurse showing me how to put on my [ostomy] bag. She [the nurse] really told me how to apply the bag. She also told me it was common to have the feelings I had about the bag. I wouldn't have made it without her teaching. She really understood how I felt."

Why was this method of instruction received so well?

Nothing destroys a client's motivation for learning more quickly than hearing such comments as "Ask your doctor that" or "We'll talk about that later; right now take your medicine." The best time for teaching is when the client is comfortable—physically and psychologically.

In addition to capitalizing on informal teaching time, the nurse must plan time during which formal teaching can be done. Teaching must match the pace of the client's progress. Some clients learn more quickly than others; some need more repetition. Timing of the teaching session is crucial. The more information presented, the more a client is likely to forget. Therefore, teaching sessions must be kept brief to avoid overwhelming the client. Throughout the teaching session, use repetition and frequently ask the client questions to allow you to pace the delivery of information.

The location for teaching activities must also be well-planned. *Where* teaching occurs affects the quality of learning. Some factors to be considered in determining the location of teaching include provision for privacy and availability of equipment. Selection of teaching methods is often determined by the location. For example, videos can often be used effectively in inpatient settings; however, the same information may need to be presented with flip charts or brochures in the home setting.

An important part of planning in the teaching-learning process is goal setting. The client and family or significant others must be involved in setting goals. Mutually determined learning goals promote learning. Specific learning goals should include these elements:

- Measurable behavioral change
- Time frame
- Methods and intervals for evaluation

Teaching-learning goals must be realistic, that is, based on the abilities of the learner and the teacher (Pesut, 1999).

Establishing teaching-learning goals involves setting priorities. See Chapter 13 for a description of the process of establishing goals. One way to prioritize goals is to teach the "need-to-know" information (that which is necessary for survival) before moving on to the "nice-to-know" content. For example, Mrs. Stone, who is in her first trimester of pregnancy, *must* know guidelines for diet and exercise ("need-to-know" goal); learning about infant care can occur later in the pregnancy ("nice-to-know" goal).

## Teaching Vulnerable Populations

When planning to teach individuals with special needs, it is important that the usual teaching strategies be modified according to the client's individual needs. This section describes education of individuals who experience developmental delays, chronic illness, low literacy skills, and sensory impairments.

### Developmental Delays

Individuals with limited cognitive abilities have a medical diagnosis of mental retardation if the IQ level is 70 or less

(American Psychiatric Association, 2000). The client's learning depends upon the degree of cognitive impairment, so teaching strategies must be selected accordingly. For example, a client who has mild mental retardation (IQ level of 50–70) may be able to learn by discussion of simple concepts that are stated in easily understood terms. Note that it is important to use concrete language and frequent repetition with clients in this category; the use of simple games is often effective. On the other hand, a client who is profoundly mentally retarded (IQ level below 25) may be unable to learn in the traditional sense. Frequent communication and repetition are required when working with a client with this degree of mental impairment.

### Chronic Illness

Clients who experience chronic illness (such as arthritis, hypertension, diabetes, asthma) have many learning needs, both actual and potential. Some chronic disorders, such as arthritis, may impair mobility and thus interfere with learning psychomotor skills as a result of decreased flexibility and dexterity of the fingers. Other chronic illnesses, such as diabetes, require ongoing assessment of the client's level of understanding about self-care (e.g., diet, exercise, and lifestyle changes). Essential hypertension, another chronic disease process, often leads to client's noncompliance with the prescribed treatment regimen. Ongoing education related to antihypertensive medication helps improve compliance.

### Low Literacy Skills

It is imperative that nurses assess the reading and comprehension abilities of clients before using printed educational materials. The majority of health care teaching involves the use of printed materials. However, approximately one in five Americans is functionally illiterate, which translates to more than 20 million American adults who cannot read (Hunt & Zurek, 1997). It is a common mistake to equate the highest educational level achieved with reading level. Typically, individuals read at three to five grade levels lower than their achieved educational level.

### Sensory Impairments

Many clients have sensory impairments as a result of illness, injury, or the aging process. Effective nurses modify their teaching approaches in order to accommodate such impairments. A common mistake many people make when talking with someone who has a sensory impairment is to talk loudly. Screaming and yelling do not help the person who has auditory or visual impairments. See the accompanying Nursing Strategy box for guidelines in working with clients who have visual, auditory, or memory impairments.

## Implementation

Implementation of the teaching plan may not go as envisioned. The nurse must constantly assess the client's

---

## NURSING STRATEGY

### Guidelines for Teaching Clients with Sensory Impairments

***For memory-impaired clients:***

- Use repetition.
- Use a variety of cues (verbal, written, pictures, and symbols).

***For visually impaired clients:***

- Provide large-print materials.
- Provide prescription eyeglasses and magnifying glasses.
- Provide adequate lighting while reducing glare.

***For hearing-impaired clients:***

- Face the client directly when you speak.
- Use short sentences and words that are easily understood.
- Use signals to reinforce verbal information— point, gesture, demonstrate.
- Eliminate distracting noises or activities from the environment as much as possible.

***For all clients:***

- Encourage client involvement and participation.
- Ask for feedback and listen actively.
- Provide frequent feedback.

Adapted from Beare, P. G., & Myers, J. L. (1999). *Principles and practice of adult health nursing* (3rd ed.). St Louis: Mosby.

---

response during this phase. Fatigue, pain, fear, and ambivalence can alter the client's ability to learn. The nurse needs to speak in terms the client understands, be specific on what is to be covered, and keep the message short and concise. The client may become bored or confused if too much information is given in one setting. Questions and interactive dialogue can help keep the client engaged.

There are several characteristics of nurses that influence the outcome of the teaching-learning process. Nursing self-awareness, an all-important first step in teaching, focuses on the concepts discussed in the following sections. The Nursing Strategy box provides some implementation guidelines for making teaching more meaningful to clients.

## CLINICAL ALERT

### Client Education and the Elderly

The nurse must constantly evaluate older clients for potential memory impairment or other clinical manifestations of common disorders like Alzheimer's disease.

## Knowledge Base

It is impossible for nurses to teach if they lack the knowledge or skills that are to be taught. Staying current in knowledge and proficient in skills is the first step to maintaining efficacy and credibility as a teacher. It is impossible for one individual to be an expert in every area of nursing. Therefore, knowing when to refer the client to others for teaching can augment learning.

## NURSING STRATEGY

### Guidelines for Effective Client Teaching

- Assess client's knowledge and needs.

- Focus on client's perceived needs.

- Relate material to prior knowledge.

- Encourage client's active participation.

- Provide opportunity for immediate application of knowledge or skill.

- Expect learning plateaus to occur.

- Reinforce learning frequently.

- Provide immediate feedback to facilitate learning.

- Ensure a comfortable environment.

- Organize content from the simple to the complex, building on what the client already knows.

- Use a variety of teaching methods.

- Emphasize verbal instructions with writing and pictures.

- Stay flexible in your approach.

- Be creative!

## Interpersonal Skills

Effective teaching is based on the nurse's ability to establish rapport with the client. "Information in itself does not ensure health-promoting behavior. There is no substitute for a relationship between you and your patients" (Gallagher & Zeind, 1998, p. 16AAA). The nurse who is empathic to the client shows sensitivity to the client's needs and preferences. An atmosphere in which the client feels free to ask questions promotes learning. Activities that help establish an environment conducive to learning include:

- Showing genuine interest in the client.
- Including the client in *every* step of the teaching-learning process.
- Using a nonjudgmental approach.
- Communicating at the client's level of understanding.

"Learning should take place in an environment that fosters mutual trust, respect, and helpfulness. Creating such an environment takes a conscious effort on your part" (Hansen & Fisher, 1998, p. 58). In other words, deliberately plan to communicate a sense of empathy and caring; see Chapter 4 for more information on these therapeutic factors.

## Teaching Clients at Home

Clients, and their families, who are recovering at home also have significant learning needs. A primary role of the home health nurse is to teach the client how to care for himself at home; this often involves teaching family members how to provide care (Figure 28-7). Home-based clients need information regarding their chronic illness, accident, or injury. They also need to learn how to achieve and maintain a maximum state of wellness. Accurate teaching plans for the home-based client and family are established by assessing multiple factors, some of which are listed in Table 28-8 (Clark, 2003).

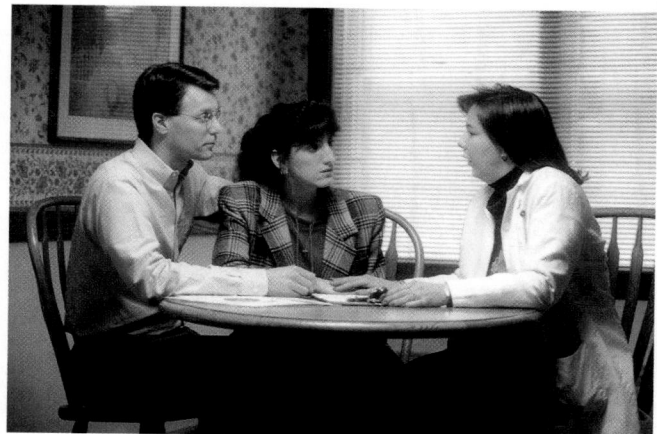

**Figure 28-7**    A nurse is teaching these two family members about the home care for their elderly relative who is recovering from a recent surgery. *Courtesy of Bellevue, The Woman's Hospital, Niskayuna, New York*

## TABLE 28-8  FACTORS AFFECTING LEARNING NEEDS OF HOME HEALTH CLIENTS

| Type | Example |
| --- | --- |
| Environmental | • Accessibility of home to client with physical disability |
| | • Need and availability of equipment and supplies |
| | • Space to accommodate special needs of client |
| | • Need for information about environmental cleanliness as it relates to health |
| | • Need for assistance with self-care activities |
| Economic | • Ability to purchase medications, equipment, and supplies |
| | • Available financial assistance |
| Support system | • Persons available to assist with caregiving |
| | • Caregiver's deficient knowledge regarding necessary care |
| Community resources | • Resources in the immediate area |
| | • Awareness of and access to support services |
| | • Available respite to the family |

## Evaluation

Evaluation of teaching-learning is a twofold process:

1. Determining what the client has learned
2. Assessing the nurse's teaching effectiveness

### Evaluation of Learning

Evaluation is the last step of the teaching process. It is a continuous and crucial step in the teaching process. Evaluation includes determining if the teaching session was successful and if the client learned the intended information. Evaluation also provides the needed evidence that the client received and understood the educational material. The nurse can ascertain this information by asking these questions:

• Is there a change in behavior?

## COMMUNITY/HOME CARE

### Discharge Planning

Preparing the client and family for home care begins not at the time of hospital discharge but rather with hospital admission. The nurse's effective teaching is the link to thorough follow-up care in the home. Discharge planning considers the current learning needs for clients and caregivers as well as potential needs after discharge. Thus, teaching includes consideration of community resources and possible referral.

• Is the behavior change related to learning activities?
• Is further change necessary?
• Will continued behavior change promote improved health?

The accompanying Nursing Strategy box provides guidelines for evaluating the client's achieved learning.

### Evaluation of Teaching

A major purpose of evaluation is to assess the effectiveness of the teaching activities and decide which modifi-

 **STOP AND THINK**

### Communicating Effectively with the Client

Imagine meeting Mrs. Clancy on your morning rounds. You say to her, "Good morning, Mrs. Clancy, I'm here to take your *vital signs*. Remember you are *npo*, so the water you requested is *contraindicated*. We will *dangle* you before we *ambulate* you to go *void* and *defecate*. All of your meds for pain are *prn*, but you can have the Tylenol *q4* and the OxyContin *bid*."

This would be reasonable if talking to another nurse, but imagine what Mrs. Clancy is thinking. Remember to communicate with clients in a language they understand.

● How would you translate the above interaction so Mrs. Clancy understands?

● How would you determine she has received and understands what you are saying?

## NURSING STRATEGY

### Evaluation of Learning

- Did the client meet mutually established goals and objectives?

- Can the client demonstrate skills?

- Have the client's attitudes changed?

- Can the client cope better with illness-imposed limitations?

- Does the family understand health problems and know how to help?

## NURSING STRATEGY

### Evaluation of Teacher Effectiveness

- Was content presented clearly and at the client's level of comprehension?

- Was the presentation (session) interesting?

- Did the nurse use a variety of teaching aids?

- Were the teaching aids appropriate for the client and the content?

- Was client participation encouraged?

- Was the nurse supportive?

- Did the nurse communicate an interest in the client and in the material?

- Did the nurse give frequent feedback and allow for immediate return demonstration?

- Were learning objectives stated in behavioral terms (i.e., easy to evaluate)?

cations, if any, are necessary. When learning objectives are not met, reassessment is the basis for planning modification of teaching-learning activities. Several activities can evaluate teaching effectiveness, including the following:

- Feedback from the learner
- Feedback from colleagues
- Situational feedback
- Self-evaluation

Evaluation is facilitated through the use of goals that are measurable and specific. Use of the accompanying Nursing Strategy box facilitates evaluation of teacher effectiveness.

Client education has been proven to decrease the length of hospital days, improve the general quality of care, decrease visits needed from home care, and improve client adherence to the plan of care (Gallagher & Zeind, 1998; Hitchcock, Schubert, & Thomas, 2003).

## CASE STUDY/NURSING CARE PLAN

Miranda is a 23-year-old who has been an insulin-dependent diabetic since she was 15. Compliance with her diet, exercise, and insulin regime has always been difficult for Miranda. As a teenager, Miranda didn't want to be seen as different, which was a barrier to her compliance. More recently, Miranda learned she is three months pregnant. She is very concerned about the health of her baby and the potential complications related to the fact that she has diabetes. Miranda comes to your outpatient diabetic education class for instruction on how to take care of herself and her developing baby. During your assessment of Miranda, you discover she could improve the technique for giving insulin injections. She also does not have a good understanding of her diabetic diet.

### Assessment

Client lacks both knowledge of proper insulin injection technique and understanding of her diabetic diet. She is expressing a desire to become proficient and educated in diabetic care for herself and the well-being of her unborn baby. Client's blood glucose level was 192 at the clinic, and she could not verbalize the normal range of her blood glucose levels.

*(continues)*

# CASE STUDY/NURSING CARE PLAN (continued)

## Nursing Diagnosis #1

*Deficient Knowledge* related to insulin injection technique and American Diabetic Association (ADA) diet as evidenced by uncontrolled blood sugars and client's demonstration of improper injection technique.

**NOC:** Knowledge of Diabetes and Medication Therapy; Health Behaviors; Treatment Regimen

**NIC:** Teaching: Individual; Teaching: Diabetes Management

### Expected Outcomes

The client will:

1. Explain and return-demonstrate correct insulin injection technique (cognitive and psychomotor domains) during visit to clinic. *Learning mode of demonstration is valid for learning physical skills.*
2. Verbalize confidence in self-administration of correct insulin dosages. *Self-confidence increases level of performance.*
3. Learn self-care of diabetes as shown through her attendance at diabetic education classes. *Reflects internal motivation and adherence to treatment regimen.*
4. Explain and identify proper foods for ADA diet. *Verifies knowledge and retention of disease process information.*

### Planning/Interventions/Rationales

1. Ask client, through the interview process, what teaching strategies (discussion, visual aids, etc.) are the most effective ways for her to learn. *Matching teaching strategies to learning styles and needs increases likelihood of a successful and productive educational experience.*
2. Explain briefly mechanics of proper insulin injection techniques and rationale for such. *Knowledge of the correct technique for insulin injection will help the client understand the mechanics of administering insulin.*
3. Demonstrate proper insulin injection techniques. *Proper injection technique is vital for insulin to work properly. Observing proper technique will help Miranda be able to perform it properly.*
4. Encourage client to have her husband learn proper insulin technique and ADA diet. *He will be able to give injection confidently if necessary and can help reinforce with her the proper technique. He will also be able to help with meal planning.*

### Evaluation

Client verbalizes proper sequence and technique for insulin injection. Client performs return demonstration of drawing up and administering insulin using sterile and proper technique, requiring minimal verbal cueing. Correctly identifies proper food for her prescribed ADA diet.

## Key Concepts

- Client education is done to help individuals achieve optimum states of health.
- The teaching-learning process is a planned interaction promoting behavioral change that is not a result of maturation or coincidence.
- Teaching supports behavior change that leads to positive adaptation.
- Learning is the process of assimilating information with a resultant change in behavior.
- Learning occurs in three domains: the cognitive (intellectual), the affective (emotional), and the psychomotor (motor skills).
- Learning readiness is affected by developmental and sociocultural factors, and is a lifelong process occurring in every developmental stage.
- Elements for documenting client education include the content taught, teaching methods used, who was taught, and response of the learners.
- The teaching-learning process and the nursing process are interdependent dynamic processes.
- Evaluation of the teaching-learning process involves two aspects: (1) determination of what the client has learned and (2) efficacy of the teacher.
- Identify teaching strategies for client education.

## Review Questions and Activities

1. Give an example of each of the three domains of learning.

2. List four barriers to learning. What nursing interventions would you implement to overcome each barrier?

3. Why is it important for the nurse to use more than one teaching method?

4. Write your own philosophy of learning.

5. What are some of your own learning needs right now? How are they being addressed?

6. Compare the teaching roles of the nurse in different practice settings, such as hospitals, extended care facilities, clinics, schools, industries, home environments, and health maintenance organizations.

7. Develop a flow sheet for client teaching to use in one of your clinical agencies.

8. Identify two learning needs of a selected client. What will you do to help the client overcome the knowledge deficits?

9. Is it ethical for a nurse to attempt to get a client to change beliefs under the guise of teaching? Think of the many areas in which your value system may conflict with the beliefs of your clients. Whose belief system is "right"? Which belief system should prevail? Should you "teach" a client the "right" attitude or belief?

10. Have you or has anyone in your family ever had a health-related learning need that was dealt with inadequately? If so, (1) Why do you think that happened? (2) How did you feel as a result?

## Multimedia Links

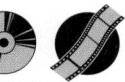

Christensen *Core Concept Videos: Client Education*

## Web Resources

American Association of Diabetes Education
  http://www.aadenet.org
American Geriatrics Patient Education Forum
  http://www.americangeriatrics.org
American Nurses Association
  http://www.nursingworld.org
Learning Domains
  http://tip.psychology.org
National Institutes of Health
  http://www.nih.gov
Stanford University Patient Education Research Center
  http://www.stanford.edu
U-Write Patient Education Handouts
  http://www.u-write.com

## References

Ackley, B. J. & Ladwig, G. B. (2002). *Nursing diagnosis handbook: A guide to planning care* (5th ed.). St. Louis: Mosby.

American Hospital Association (1980). *A patient's bill of rights.* Chicago: Author.

American Nurses Association (1995). *Nursing: A social policy statement.* Washington, DC: Author.

American Psychiatric Association (2000). *Diagnostic and statistical manual of mental disorders* (4th ed.). Washington, DC: Author.

Antai-Otong, D. (2003). *Psychiatric nursing: Biological and behavioral concepts.* Clifton Park, NY: Delmar Learning.

Bandura, A. (1977). *Social learning theory.* Englewood Cliffs, NJ: Prentice Hall.

Beare, P. G., & Myers, J. L. (1999). *Principles and practice of adult health nursing* (3rd ed.). St. Louis: Mosby.

Bloom, B. S. (1977). *Taxonomy of educational objectives: The classification of educational goals, Handbook I: Cognitive domain.* New York: Longman.

Boyd, M. D., Graham, B. A., Gleit, C. J., Whitman, N. I. (1998). *Health teaching in nursing practice: A professional model* (3rd ed.). Stamford, CT: Appleton and Lange.

Carelock, J., & Innerarity, S. (2001). Critical incidents: Effective communication and documentation. *Critical Care Nursing, 23*(4), 59–66.

Clark, M. J. (2003). *Community health nursing, caring for populations* (4th ed.). Cranbury, New Jersey: Pearson Education, Inc.

Dempski, K. M., & Killion, S. W. (2001). *Legal & Ethical Issues in Nursing.* Thorofare, New Jersey: SLACK, Inc.

Edelman, C. L., & Mandle, C. L. (2002). *Health promotion throughout the life span* (5th ed.). St. Louis: Mosby.

Gallagher, S., & Zeind, S. M. (1998). Bridging patient education and care. *American Journal of Nursing, 98*(9), 16AAA–16DDD.

Hansen, M., & Fisher, J. C. (1998). Patient-centered teaching from theory to practice. *American Journal of Nursing, 98*(1), 56–60.

Hitchcock, J., Schubert, P., & Thomas, S. (2003). *Community health nursing: Caring in action.* Clifton Park, NY: Delmar Learning.

Hunt, R., & Zurek, E. L. (1997). *Introduction to community-based nursing.* Philadelphia: Lippincott.

Joint Commission for Accreditation of Healthcare Organizations (2002). *Accreditation manual.* Chicago: Author.

Knowles, M. S. (1984). *The adult learner: A neglected species* (3rd ed.). Houston: Gulf Publishing.

Muscari, M. E. (1998). Rebels with a cause: When adolescents won't follow medical advice. *American Journal of Nursing, 98*(12), 20–30.

Patyk, M., Gaynor, S., & Verdin, J. (2000). Patient education resource assessment: Project management. *Journal of Nursing Care Quality, 14*(2), 14–20.

Pesut, D. (1999). *Clinical reasoning: The art and science of critical and creative thinking.* Clifton Park, NY: Delmar Learning.

Potts, N., & Mandleco, B. (2002). *Pediatric nursing: Caring for children and their families.* Clifton Park, NY: Delmar Learning.

Spencer, H. (1884). The Man Versus the State, with Six Essays on Government, Society, and Freedom. London: Williams and Norgate.

Tierney, A. J., Worth, A., & Watson, N. (2000). Meeting patients' information needs before and after discharge from hospital. *Journal of Clinical Nursing, 9*(6), 14–19.

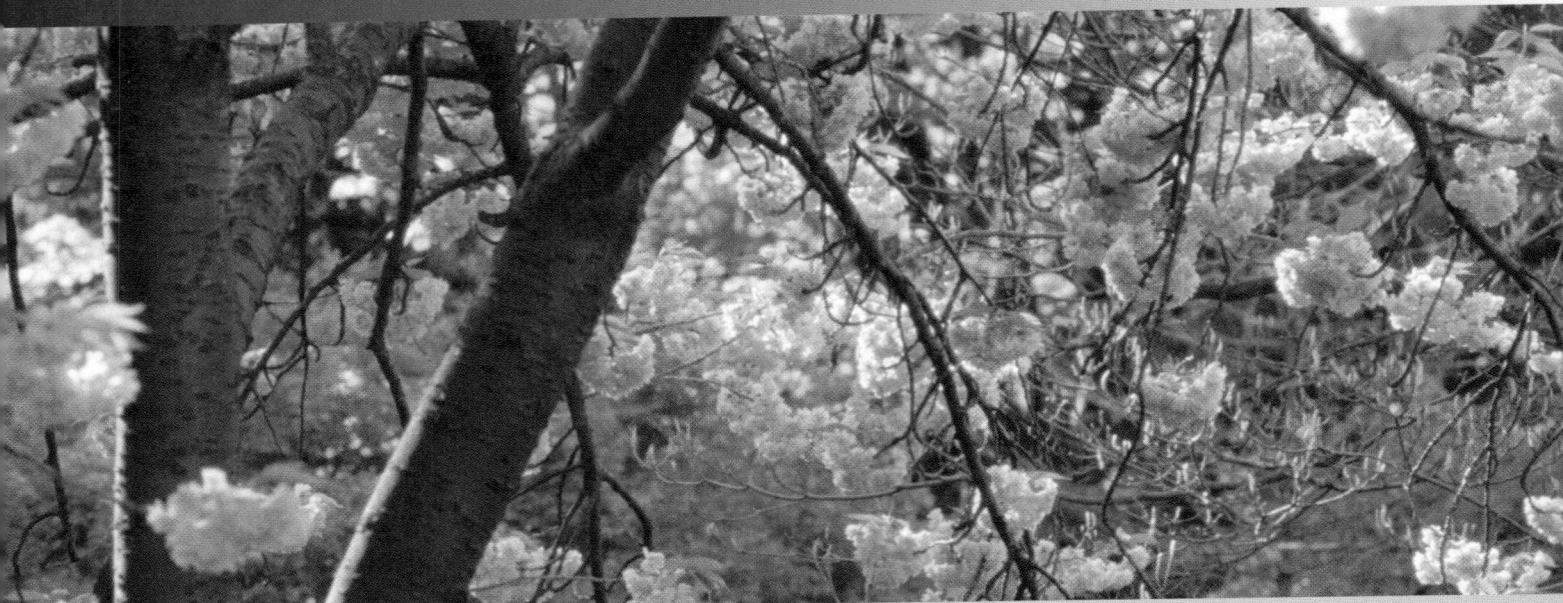

# Diagnostic Testing

## Crisamar J. Anunciado, MS, FNP, RN, C

*"Look with all your eyes, look."*

*(Jules Verne, 1873)*

# Chapter Competencies

*Upon completion of this chapter, the reader should be able to:*

1. Identify the role of diagnostic testing.
2. Describe nursing care for the care of the client before, during, and after noninvasive and invasive diagnostic procedures.
3. Discuss the common specimen collection methods.
4. Describe the radiologic studies commonly used in diagnostic testing.
5. Describe the following diagnostic procedures: ultrasonography, magnetic resonance imaging, electrodiagnostic studies, endoscopy methods, and aspiration/biopsy.
6. Evaluate the nursing process for the common diagnostic procedures.

# Key Terms

agglutination
agglutinin
agglutinogen
Allen test
amniocentesis
analyte
aneurysm
angiography
anions
antibody
antigens
arteriography
ascites
aspiration
atherosclerotic plaque
bacteremia
barium
barium enema
barium swallow
biopsy
bronchography
cardiac catheterization
cations
central line
cholangiography
cholinesterase
computed tomography (CT)
conscious sedation
contrast medium
culture
cystography

cytology
digital subtraction angiography
disseminated intravascular coagulation (DIC)
Doppler
echocardiogram
electrocardiography (ECG or EKG)
electroencephalogram (EEG)
electrolyte
endoscopy
enzyme
erythrocyte
erythrocyte sedimentation rate (ESR)
fluoroscopy
general anesthesia
glucose-6-phosphate dehydrogenase (G6PD)
glycosylated hemoglobin $A_1$
hematuria
hemoconcentration
hemoglobin electrophoresis
hemolysis
incidence
intravenous pyelogram
invasive
ketone
late potentials
leukocytes
lipoproteins
local anesthesia

lumbar puncture
lymphangiography
magnetic resonance imaging (MRI)
mammography
myelography
necrosis
noninvasive
occult
oliguria
oral cholecystography
paracentesis
Papanicolaou test
peripherally inserted central catheter (PICC)
phagocytosis
phlebotomist
pneumothorax
polyp
port-a-cath
predictive value
radiography
red cell indices
regional anesthesia
sensitivity
signal-averaged electrocardiography (SAECG)
specificity
spherocytes
stress test
thallium
thoracentesis

*(continues)*

# Key Terms (continued)

| | | |
|---|---|---|
| thrombus | T-tube | venipuncture |
| transducer | type and crossmatch | venography |
| trocar | ultrasound | venous access device (VAD) |
| troponin | urobilinogen | void |

With the arrival of health care reform, reimbursement practices such as managed care, and medicolegal concerns, health care is redefining the importance of history taking and physical examinations with a decreasing reliance on diagnostic tests. In the last two decades, before reform acts, health care relied heavily on the use of diagnostic testing to determine the nature of the client's condition.

Health care providers rely primarily on a thorough history and physical examination to make a diagnosis. Findings from the history and physical will help determine any further action needed to confirm or rule out a diagnosis. Laboratory and diagnostic testing will aid the clinician or practitioner in several ways. Tests are helpful in screening or identifying the risk factors for occult disease. Early detection of risk factors can lead to early intervention and treatment, possibly reducing morbidity and mortality. In addition, diagnostic tests are helpful in establishing or confirming a diagnosis. Early diagnoses are confirmed by some tests after onset of signs and symptoms, others aid in making differential diagnoses of various possible diseases, and others help determine the activity or stage of the disease. Diagnostic tests are also helpful in managing the client's illness. Tests can help (1) evaluate the severity of disease, (2) estimate prognosis, (3) monitor the course of the disease (progression, stability, resolution), (4) detect disease recurrence, and (5) select drugs and adjust therapy (Tierney, McPhee, & Papadakis, 2000).

The role of the nurse is to teach the client, family, and significant others about the diagnostic procedure, the steps to be taken in preparation for the specific test, and the care following the procedure. The nurse is also sometimes called to assist or perform the required invasive or noninvasive procedure, depending on the type and complexity of the test. Nonetheless, the nurse must be knowledgeable in the implication of the tests to deliver appropriate nursing care.

This chapter discusses the most common diagnostic tests. The terms *test* and *procedure* are used interchangeably throughout the chapter. The term *practitioner* is used in this chapter to refer to either the physician or other authorized prescribers. Most state boards of nursing allow advanced practice registered nurses to order and perform certain diagnostic tests.

## Noninvasive and Invasive Diagnostic Testing

Diagnostic tests are either noninvasive or invasive. **Noninvasive** means the body is not entered with any type of instrument. The skin and other body tissues, organs, and cavities remain intact. **Invasive** means accessing the body's tissue, organ, or cavity through some type of instrumentation procedure.

## Nursing Care of the Client

Diagnostic testing can be an important element of the assessment piece in the nursing process. Assessment data are used to formulate the nursing diagnosis, create a plan of care, and establish outcome measures in collaboration with the client and other members of the interdisciplinary health care team.

### Preparing a Client for Diagnostic Testing

The nurse plays a key role in scheduling and preparing the client for diagnostic testing. The emphasis of preparation is on appropriate test selection, proper client preparation, and client education (Daniels, 2003). When tests are not scheduled correctly, the client is inconvenienced. It may also delay interventions, which places the client's health at risk. The institution is also at risk to lose money. Table 29-1 presents a sample protocol of the nursing care to prepare a client for diagnostic testing.

The nursing care contained in the protocol provides a systemic format, based on the nursing process, to prepare the client for most diagnostic studies. During the

## CLINICAL ALERT

### Diagnostic Testing: Safety Measures

Use Standard Precautions whenever performing invasive and noninvasive testing to protect your health and safety, as well as that of other health care providers and the client.

## TABLE 29-1   PROTOCOL: PREPARING THE CLIENT FOR DIAGNOSTIC TESTING

| | |
|---|---|
| *Purpose* | To increase the reliability of the test by providing client teaching on why the test is being performed, what the client can expect during the test, and the outcomes and side effects of the test |
| | To decrease the client's anxiety about the test and the associated risk |
| *Level* | Independent |
| *Supportive Data* | Increasing the client's knowledge promotes cooperation, enhances the quality of the testing, and decreases the time required to perform the study in a safe, efficient, and cost-effective manner. |
| | Proper physical preparation prevents delays. |
| *Assessment* | Check to be sure the client is wearing an identification band. |
| | Review the medical record for allergies and previous adverse reactions to dyes and other contrast media, a signed consent form, and the recorded findings of diagnostic tests relative to the procedure. |
| | Assess for presence, location, and characteristics of physical and communicative limitations or preexisting conditions. |
| | Monitor the client's knowledge of why the test is being performed and what to expect during and after testing. |
| | Monitor vital signs for clients scheduled for invasive testing to establish baseline data. |
| | Assess client outcome measures relative to the practitioner's preferences for preprocedure preparations. |
| | Monitor level of hydration and weakness for clients who are NPO (nothing by mouth), especially geriatric and pediatric populations. |
| *Report to Practitioner* | Notify the practitioner of any allergy, previous adverse reactions, or suspected reaction following administration of dye, contrast media, or medications. |
| | Notify practitioner of any client or family concerns you were not able to alleviate. |
| | Notify the practitioner immediately for any usual signs and symptoms noted during the physical examination that may place the client at risk for any complications during the test. |
| *Interventions* | Clarify with practitioner if regularly scheduled medications are to be administered. |
| | The NPO status is determined by the type of test. |
| | Administer cathartics or laxatives as denoted by the test's protocol; however, there must be a specific practitioner order to give children and infants a laxative. Instruct clients who are weak, especially geriatric clients, to call for assistance to bathroom. |
| | Teach relaxation techniques, such as deep breathing and imagery. |
| | Establish intravenous (IV) access if necessary for procedure. |
| *Evaluation* | Evaluate client's knowledge of what to expect. |
| | Evaluate client's anxiety level. |
| | Evaluate client's level of safety and comfort. |
| | Monitor that someone will accompany a child to the department where the test is to be performed and remain with the child during the tests if not at risk of harmful exposure. |

*(continues)*

**TABLE 29-1    PROTOCOL: PREPARING THE CLIENT FOR DIAGNOSTIC TESTING** *(continued)*

| | |
|---|---|
| *Client Teaching* | Discuss the following with the client and family as appropriate to the specific test: |
| | • Explain reason for test and what to expect |
| | • An estimation of how long the test will take |
| | • NPO (If oral medication to be taken, how much water to drink) |
| | • Cathartics or laxative: how much, how often |
| | • Sputum: cough deeply, do not clear throat |
| | • Urine: voided, clean-catch specimen, time to collect |
| | • No objects (jewelry or hair clips) to obscure x-ray film |
| | • Barium: taste, consistency, aftereffects (stools lightly colored for 24 to 72 hours, can cause obstruction/impaction) |
| | • Iodine: metallic taste, delayed allergic reaction (itching, rashes, hives, wheezing, and breathing difficulties) |
| | • Positioning during the test |
| | • Positioning posttest (e.g., angiography)—immobilize limb |
| | • Posttest, encourage fluids if not contraindicated |
| *Documentation* | Record the following in the client's medical record: |
| | • Practitioner notification of allergies or suspected adverse reaction to contrast media |
| | • Presence, location, and characteristics of symptoms |
| | • Teaching and the client's response to teaching |
| | • Response to interventions (client's outcomes) |

assessment of the client, make sure the client is wearing an identification band (Figure 29-1). The identification band is a key factor to ensure client safety in all health care settings.

Other key nursing measures to ensure client safety are to establish baseline vital signs, identify known allergies, and assess the effectiveness of teaching. In the ambulatory and outpatient centers, the nurse might have only one opportunity to assess and record the vital signs; it is important for the nurse to confirm that these findings are *normal values* for the client. To accurately assess the client's response to anesthetic agents and the procedure, the nurse has to compare the vital signs taken during and after the procedure with the baseline data.

The client needs to know what to expect during the procedure. Teaching can increase the client's level of cooperation and should decrease the degree of anxiety. The client's family should also know what will happen during the procedure and approximately how long the procedure normally lasts. In addition, there may be special considerations for pediatric clients.

Reference is made to Table 29-1 throughout this chapter. This protocol provides you with the direction and guidance needed to plan nursing care. Nurses must also know the institution's protocols and procedures because these are not standardized in all practice settings.

## Care of the Client During Diagnostic Testing

Although the care of the client needs to be individualized for a specific procedure, general guidelines for client care

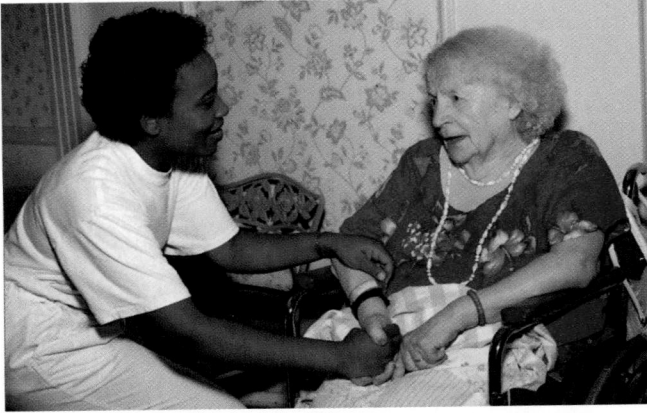

**Figure 29-1**    The nurse is asking the resident her name after checking the identification band in preparation for a diagnostic procedure.

during a procedure are given in Table 29-2. Protocols are used to assist the nurse with client care.

Standard Precautions are initiated when exposure to body fluids presents a threat to the safety of the caregiver. Protective barriers, such as gloves and a gown, should be used during invasive procedures. The nurse is responsible for labeling any specimen with the client's name, room number (hospitalized clients), date, time, and source of the specimen. Some specimens may need to be taken immediately to the laboratory or placed on ice (e.g., arterial blood gases) (Daniels, 2003).

In order to promote the client's comfort and cooperation during diagnostic tests, nurses must consider the management of procedural pain. Although not all procedures are painful, advances in diagnostic and therapeutic

studies have placed clients at risk for painful procedures. Clients who are repeatedly subjected to painful procedures without adequate analgesia become anxious and anticipate pain; if pain is experienced during one procedure, the client is reluctant to return for the same procedure or other tests. Consideration must be given to the adverse physiological effects of unrelieved pain, even if the pain is temporary (McCaffery & Pasero, 1999).

Careful attention should be given to client populations who may be at high risk for undertreated pain, such preterm or full-term infants, children, and the elderly. Vulnerable clients who are critically ill, victims of traumatic injury, paraplegic or quadriplegic, chronically ill, cognitively impaired, comatose, or unconscious are also at a special risk (McCaffery & Pasero, 1999).

| TABLE 29-2 | PROTOCOL: CARE OF THE CLIENT DURING DIAGNOSTIC TESTING |
|---|---|
| Purpose | To increase cooperation and participation by allaying the client's anxiety and to provide the maximum level of safety and comfort during a procedure |
| Level | Interdependent |
| Supportive Data | Increasing the client's participation and comfort encourages relaxation of muscles to facilitate instrumentation. |
| | Proper preparation of the client ensures efficient use of time during the test and reliable results. |
| Assessment | Check the client's identification band to ensure the correct client. |
| | Review the medical record for allergies. |
| | Assess the preprocedure sedatives administered to the client before the administration of anesthesia during the procedure. |
| | Assess airway maintenance and gag reflex if a local anesthetic is sprayed into the client's throat. |
| | Assess vital signs throughout the procedure and compare with baseline data. |
| | Assess the client's ability to maintain and tolerate the prescribed position. |
| | Assess the client's comfort level to ensure the effectiveness of the anesthetic agent. |
| | Assess for related symptoms indicating complications specific to the procedure (e.g., accidental perforation of an organ). |
| Report to Practitioner | Notify the practitioner if the client has any concerns or questions that you were not able to resolve. |
| | Notify the practitioner if the client has family members present and where they are waiting during the procedure. |
| | Notify the practitioner when the client is positioned properly and the anesthetic agent has been administered to the client. |
| Interventions | Institute Standard Precautions or appropriate aseptic technique for the specific test. |
| | Report to all personnel involved with the test any known client allergies. |
| | Place client in the correct position, drape, and monitor to ensure that breathing is not compromised. |
| | Remain with the client during the administration of anesthesia. |

*(continues)*

## TABLE 29-2    PROTOCOL: CARE OF THE CLIENT DURING DIAGNOSTIC TESTING (*continued*)

| | |
|---|---|
| *Interventions (continued)* | Assist the client to relax during insertion of the instrument by telling the client to breathe through the mouth and to concentrate on relaxing the involved muscles. |
| | Explain what the practitioner is doing so that the client will know what to expect. |
| | Label and handle the specimen according to the type of materials obtained and the testing to be done. |
| | Report to the practitioner any symptoms of complications. |
| | Secure client transport from the diagnostic area. |
| | Posttest in the diagnostic area: |
| | 1. Assist client to a comfortable, safe position. |
| | 2. Provide oral hygiene and water to clients who were NPO for the test, if they are alert and able to swallow. |
| | 3. Remain with the client awaiting transport to another area. |
| *Evaluation* | Evaluate client's ventilatory status and tolerance to the procedure. |
| | Evaluate client's need for assistance. |
| | Evaluate client's understanding of what was performed during the procedure. |
| | Evaluate client's understanding of findings identified during the procedure. |
| | Evaluate client's knowledge of what to expect after the procedure. |
| *Client Teaching* | Discuss the following with the client and family as appropriate to the specific test: |
| | • Explain what occurred during the procedure. |
| | • Answer questions and concerns of the client or family member. |
| | • Explain what to expect during the immediate recovery phase. |
| | • Explain what to report to the nurse during the immediate recovery phase. |
| *Documentation* | Record in the client's medical record: |
| | • Who performed the procedure |
| | • Reason for the procedure |
| | • Type of anesthesia, dye, or other medications administered |
| | • Type of specimen obtained and where it was delivered |
| | • Vital signs and other assessment data, such as client's tolerance of the procedure or pain/discomfort level |
| | • Any symptoms of complications |
| | • Who transported the client to another area (designate the names of persons who provided transport and place of destination) |
| | If the procedure requires the administration of a dye, ensure the client is not allergic to the dye; if the client has not received the dye before, perform the skin allergy test according to the drug manufacturer's instructions that accompany the medication. |
| | Maintain the client's airway and keep resuscitative equipment available. |

## LIFE SPAN CONSIDERATIONS

### Implications for Pediatric Clients Prior to Diagnostic Procedures

Prior to some diagnostic procedures, pediatric clients may require sedation to enhance the ability of the procedure to be performed. The child should be placed on a blanket for comfort and simple instructions should be given to the parents or caregivers. Emphasis should be on the safety afforded the child during the procedure. In addition, the family members are instructed as to the length of time the procedure will take and where the family members can wait during the procedure.

Potts, N., & Mandleco, B. (2002). *Pediatric nursing: Caring for children and their families.* Clifton Park, NY: Delmar Learning.

Recognizing that diagnostic procedures are performed in various settings, intravenous conscious sedation (conscious sedation) is often used to manage pain during diagnostic testing.

**Conscious sedation** is a minimally depressed level of consciousness during which the client retains the ability to maintain a continuously patent airway and respond appropriately to physical stimulation or verbal commands. The nurse managing conscious sedation is usually functioning in an expanded role that requires additional education and demonstrated ability beyond basic education.

Ongoing assessment of the client's status is required during the procedure. Always assess the patency of the client's airway, which may be compromised by the client's position, anesthesia, or the procedure itself. During an invasive procedure, the nurse needs to monitor for signs and symptoms of accidental perforation of an organ (e.g., sudden changes in vital signs).

The nurse has additional responsibilities:

- Preparing the room (e.g., adequate lighting)
- Gathering and charging for supplies used during the procedure
- Testing the equipment to ensure it is functional and safe
- Securing proper containers for specimen collection

Practitioners usually have *preference cards* within the diagnostic testing area that specify the type of equipment to be used, the position to place the client, and the type of sedation or anesthesia.

### Care of the Client After Diagnostic Testing

Nursing care postprocedure is directed toward restoring the client's prediagnostic level of functioning (Table 29-3). Nursing assessment and interventions are based mainly on the nature of the test and whether or not the client received anesthesia. Anesthesia can be administered in one of three ways:

- **Local anesthesia**—client loses sensation to a localized body part—spraying the back of the throat with lidocaine to decrease the gag reflex
- **Regional anesthesia**—client loses sensation in an area of the body—laparoscope for a tubal sterilization
- **General anesthesia**—client loses all sensation and consciousness—major surgical procedures

The client is monitored closely for signs of respiratory distress and bleeding. Some diagnostic procedures require that the vital signs be measured every 15 minutes for the first hour, then gradually decreased in frequency until the client is stable (alert and vital signs within the client's normal range).

Some diagnostic tests require the use of medications that are excreted through the kidneys; the nurse monitors the client's intake and output for 24 hours. The client is taught how to monitor intake and output. Instruct the client to report **hematuria** (presence of blood in the urine). Clients receiving radioactive iodine must have their urine collected and properly discarded in a special container, according to agency policy for handling radioactive medical wastes.

When clients are discharged after diagnostic tests, they should receive written instructions. Most agencies have discharge forms for the nurse to document teaching regarding medications, dietary and activity restrictions, and signs and symptoms to be reported immediately to the practitioner. Clients may also need to have follow-up appointments made for them.

## Laboratory Tests

Common laboratory studies are usually simple measurements to determine how much or how many **analytes** (a substance dissolved in a solution, also called a solute) are present in a specimen. Laboratory tests are ordered by practitioners to:

- Detect and quantify the risk of future disease
- Establish and exclude diagnoses
- Assess the severity of the disease process and determine the prognosis
- Guide the selection of interventions
- Monitor the progress of the disorder
- Monitor the effectiveness of the treatment

Nurses are often the first to view results of laboratory studies, and they need to know the terminology regarding laboratory tests: purpose, process, procedure, and normal test values. The clinical value of a test is related to:

1. **Sensitivity**—the likelihood that a diseased client has a positive result. 100% sensitivity means that all clients with a given disease will have positive results and clients without the disease will have negative results.
2. **Specificity**—the likelihood that a healthy individual will have negative results. 100% specificity means that

## TABLE 29-3 PROTOCOL: CARE OF THE CLIENT AFTER DIAGNOSTIC TESTING

| | |
|---|---|
| *Purpose* | To restore the client's prediagnostic level of functioning by providing care and teaching relative to what the client can expect after a test and the outcomes or side effects of the test |
| *Level* | Independent |
| *Supportive Data* | Increasing the client's participation and knowledge of expected outcome measures after a diagnostic test |
| | Proper postprocedure care and client teaching alerts the client to what signs and symptoms need to be reported to the practitioner. |
| *Assessment* | Check the identification band and call the client by name. |
| | Assess the client closely for signs of airway distress, adverse reactions to anesthesia or other medications, and other signs that may indicate accidental perforation of an organ. |
| | Assess body area(s) where a biopsy was performed for bleeding. |
| | Assess the client's color and skin temperature. |
| | Assess vascular access lines or other invasive monitoring devices. |
| | Assess the client's ability to expel air if air was instilled during a gastrointestinal test. |
| | Assess the client's knowledge of what to expect during the recovery phase. |
| *Report to Practitioner* | Notify the practitioner of any signs of respiratory distress bleeding or changes in vital signs; adverse reactions to anesthetic, sedative, or dye; and other signs of complications. |
| | Notify the practitioner regarding client or family concerns or questions that you are not able to answer. |
| | Notify the practitioner when any results are obtained from the diagnostic test. |
| | Notify the practitioner when the client is fully alert and recovered for an order to discharge. |
| *Interventions* | Implement the practitioner's orders regarding the postprocedure care of the client. |
| | Institute Standard Precautions or surgical asepsis as appropriate to the client's care needs. |
| | Position the client for comfort and accessibility to perform nursing measures. |
| | Monitor vital signs according the frequency required for the specific test. |
| | Observe the insertion site for a hematoma or blood loss; replace pressure dressing, as needed. |
| | Monitor the client's urinary output and drainage from other devices. |
| | Enforce activity restrictions appropriate to the test. |
| | Schedule client appointments as directed by the practitioner. |
| *Evaluation* | Evaluate the client's respiratory status to any anesthetic agents. |
| | Evaluate the client's tolerance of oral liquids. |
| | Evaluate the client's understanding of procedural findings or the time frame that written results should be reported to the practitioner. |
| | Evaluate the client's knowledge of what to expect after discharge. |

*(continues)*

## TABLE 29-3   PROTOCOL: CARE OF THE CLIENT AFTER DIAGNOSTIC TESTING (*continued*)

| | |
|---|---|
| *Client Teaching* | Based on client assessment and evaluation of knowledge, teach the client or family about the following: |
| | • Dietary or activity restrictions |
| | • Signs and symptoms that should be reported immediately to the practitioner |
| | • Medications |
| *Documentation* | Record in the client's medical record on the appropriate forms: |
| | • Assessment data, nursing interventions, and achievement of client expected outcomes |
| | • Client or family teaching and demonstrated level of understanding |
| | • Written instructions given to the client or family members |

all clients without a given disease will have negative results (Tierney et al., 2000).

3. **Incidence**—the prevalence of a disease in a population or community. The predictive value of the same test can be different when applied to people of differing ages, genders, and geographic locations.

4. **Predictive value**—the ability of screening test results to correctly identify the disease state. A true-positive correctly identifies persons who actually have the disease, whereas a true-negative correctly identifies persons who do not actually have the disease.

Laboratory test results are based on *normal range values*. Le Système International d'Unités (SI), the International System of Units, is an international normal range reference established for reporting laboratory results (Daniels, 2003). For example, the SI reference range for reporting red blood cell count for a woman is 4.0 to $5.2 \times 10^{12}/L$; the conventional range would appear as 4,000,000 to 5,200,000/mm³ of blood.

It is also important to consider factors that may affect laboratory test results, such as age, sex, weight, diet, medication use, activity level, smoking, alcohol intake, and time of day. Test sensitivity and specificity may also be affected by these factors. Therefore, it is also important to look at the client's entire clinical status in determining the client's disease state (Daniels, 2003).

## Specimen Collection

The scheduling and sequencing of laboratory tests is an important function of the nurse. All tests requiring **venipuncture** (the puncturing of a vein with a needle to aspirate blood) are grouped together so that the client is subjected to only one venipuncture. Fasting laboratory and radiologic studies are scheduled on the same day so that the client has to fast for only one day. Appropriate scheduling increases the client's comfort level and satisfaction.

"Communication errors account for more incorrect results than do technical errors" (Fischbach, 2004, p. 13). Accuracy in laboratory testing requires that:

• The practitioner's order is transcribed onto the correct requisition form.
• All information requested should be written onto the form (e.g., the client's full name and medical number).
• Pertinent data that could influence the test's results, such as medication taken, must be included.
• Collection of the specimen from the correct client is confirmed by the identification band.
• Laboratory results are placed on the correct client's medical record.

The risk for errors increases when clients have the same last name. Always check the full name of the client and the medical record number before placing the laboratory results report onto a chart.

Point of care testing (POCT) is a common practice in critical care settings and is proving to be a cost-effective, quality intervention for both clients and agencies. With advances in POCT technology over the past two decades, critical care nurses can perform a blood analysis and within seconds to minutes have a measurement upon which to

## CLINICAL ALERT

### Documentation

Document on the laboratory requisition slip and in your nurses' notes any difficulty you experience while collecting the specimen. Such problems may be indicative of adverse effects that clients may experience due to the nature of the test and are conditions that must be reported and treated immediately.

change or implement an intervention. Schallom (1999) suggests that nurses be involved in the implementation and evaluation process of POCT, since accuracy of the test is contingent on correct calibration and correct usage by the test performer. The following advantages are inherent in POCT (McConnell, 1999; Schallom, 1999):

- Prompt client diagnosis, treatment, and monitoring by decreasing turnaround time (TAT)
- Decreasing the risk for error by eliminating many of the steps in conventional laboratory testing
- Decreasing prolonged hospital stays and avoiding unnecessary hospitalizations by facilitating appropriate triage from emergency departments and prehospital settings
- Decreasing delays or cancellations of surgical procedures due to unavailable laboratory results, and the actual time the client spends in surgery
- Minimizing blood loss due to phlebotomy since POCT devices usually require only a few microliters or drops of blood versus 25 to 125 microliters per day for the critically ill client due to laboratory testing

Studies regarding POCT's clinical and financial value have revealed positive results: improved overall day-stay unit operations and client services, and earlier therapeutic decision-making time that required blood test results for emergency room clients (McConnell, 1999). Although studies have proven positive results in settings where the client's condition is acute and unstable, critical care applications may be quite different from that on a general medical/surgical unit. Studies will need to document the usefulness of POCT as a quality intervention in nonacute care settings.

## Venipuncture

Venipuncture can be performed by various members of the health care team. Laboratories employ a **phlebotomist** (an individual who performs venipuncture) to collect blood specimens; however, it is the responsibility of a nurse to know *how* to perform a venipuncture. Nurses routinely perform venipuncture in the home, long-term care settings, and hospital critical care units (Procedure 29-1).

Venipuncture can be performed by using either a sterile needle and syringe or a vacuum tube holder with a sterile two-sided needle. Test tubes are used to collect blood specimens. Test tubes have different-colored stoppers to indicate the type of additive in the test tube. Collecting tubes are universally color-coded as follows:

- Red—no additive
- Lavender—EDTA (ethylenediaminetetra-acetic acid)
- Light blue—coagulation tubes
- Green—sodium heparin
- Gray—fluoride oxalate
- Black—sodium oxalate

There are three sources of venipuncture variability that can cause inaccurate results. **Hemoconcentration** is the reduced volume of plasma water and the increased concentration of blood cells, plasma proteins, and protein-

## CLINICAL ALERT

### Preventing Hemoconcentration

Keep to a minimum both the length of time a client stands before venipuncture and the length of time of tourniquet application during venipuncture. These actions lower the risk of hemoconcentration and increase the rate of accuracy in laboratory tests.

bound constituents. It occurs with increased capillary hydrostatic pressure that causes water to shift from the intravascular into the interstitial space.

Hemoconcentration can be caused from prolonged standing or a prolonged time of application of a tourniquet during venipuncture. Alterations in the circulating blood volume can also cause hemoconcentration, such as occurs with dehydrated and burned clients.

**Hemolysis** is the breakdown of red blood cells and the release of hemoglobin. Hemolysis occurs with the rapid flow of blood through small-bore needles and exposure to large negative pressures. A negative pressure exists inside the collecting test tubes and syringe. To minimize the possibility of hemolysis, use a large-bore needle, moderate flow rates, and moderate negative pressures.

The third source of variability occurs when a blood specimen is drawn from a site above an intravenous infusion. The specimen is contaminated with intravenous solutions. Blood should be drawn from the client's other arm or below the infusion site.

Venipuncture is an invasive procedure. Health care providers performing venipuncture are at risk for the transmission of blood-borne organisms, such as human immunodeficiency virus (HIV) and hepatitis. HIV is the

## LEGAL AND ETHICAL ISSUES

### Diagnostic Testing and Confidentiality

Mr. Takahashi comes to the Ambulatory Surgery Clinic for his preoperative diagnostic testing. You overheard the staff saying that Mr. Takahashi has had a history of hepatitis. Your instructor gathers all the student nurses and says, "Who needs the experience of performing a venipuncture?" Two of your classmates indicate to the instructor that they have not had the opportunity to perform this procedure. Should you say anything to the instructor? Would you share with your classmates Mr. Takahashi's history? If you said something, would this be a breach of client confidentiality?

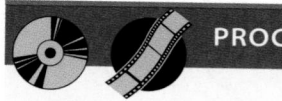

## PROCEDURE 29-1

# Performing Venipuncture (Blood Drawing)

## EQUIPMENT NEEDED

- Disposable gloves (Figure 29-2)
- Alcohol swabs
- Rubber tourniquet
- Sterile 2 × 2 gauze pads
- Band-Aid or adhesive tape (precut)
- Appropriate blood collection tubes
- Labels for each collection tube with the appropriate client information included
- Completed laboratory requisition forms

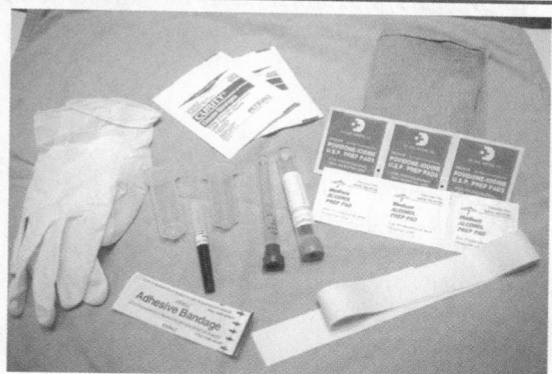

**Figure 29-2    Nonsterile gloves, sponges, povidone-iodine, alcohol swabs, blood collection tubes, vacutainer tube, vacutainer needle, and rubber tourniquet.**

## IMPLEMENTATION—ACTION/RATIONALE

| ACTION | RATIONALE |
|---|---|
| 1. Greet client by name and validate client's identification. | 1. Proper client identification ensures safety for the client and the nurse. |
| 2. Explain the procedure to the client. | 2. Client rights dictate that any action be explained to the client. The client always has the right to refuse a procedure. Information decreases anxiety. |
| 3. Bring equipment to bedside or client exam room (Figure 29-2). Transfer client to the procedure room, especially for small children, since it is important to keep their hospital room a "safe haven." | 3. Provides an organized approach to the procedure. |
| 4. Close curtain or door. | 4. Provides privacy. |
| 5. Raise or lower bed/table to comfortable working height. | 5. Maintains good body mechanics for the nurse during the procedure. |
| 6. Wash hands. | 6. Reduce transmission of microorganisms. |
| 7. Position client's arm; extend arm to form a straight line from shoulder to wrist. Place pillow or towel under upper arm to enhance extension. Client should be in a supine or semi-Fowler's position. | 7. Helps stabilize the arm. The bed should support the client's body (when possible) in case client should feel faint during the procedure. |
| 8. Apply disposable gloves. | 8. Reduces the risk of infection to both the client and the nurse (Standard Precautions). |

*(continues)*

## PROCEDURE 29-1 (continued)

9. Apply the tourniquet 3 to 4 inches above the venipuncture site. Most often the antecubital fossa site is used. The tourniquet should be able to be removed by pulling the end with a single motion.

9. Tourniquet provides improved visibility of the veins as they dilate in response to decreased venous return of blood flow from the extremity to the heart.

10. Check for the distal pulse. If there is no pulse felt, then the tourniquet is applied too tightly and must be reapplied more loosely.

10. If the pressure is too tight, it may impede arterial flow to the extremity.

11. Have client open and close fist several times, leaving fist clenched prior to venipuncture.

11. Increases the venous distension and enhances visibility of the vein. Vigorous motion, however, may result in hemoconcentration of the specimen.

12. Maintain tourniquet for only 1 to 2 minutes.

12. Prolonged time may increase client discomfort and alter some laboratory results (e.g., falsely elevated serum potassium).

13. Identify the best venipuncture site through palpation; the ideal site is a straight prominent vein that feels firm and slightly rebounds when palpated. Palpate potential site.

13. Straight, intact veins are easier to puncture. A thrombosed vein is rigid, or rolls easily, and is difficult to stick.

14. Select the vein for venipuncture. (If the tourniquet has been on too long, release it and let the client rest for 1 to 2 minutes before reapplying the tourniquet.)

14. Allowing the client to rest increases client comfort and ensures accurate laboratory results.

15. Prepare to obtain the blood sample. Technique varies depending on equipment used:
    • Syringe method: Have syringe with appropriate needle attached.

    • Vacutainer method: Attach double-ended needle to vacutainer tube and have the proper blood specimen tube resting inside the vacutainer. Do not puncture the rubber stopper yet.

15.

    • A needle with a very small bore can damage the red cells as the blood is drawn, leading to inaccurate test results.
    • The long end of the needle is used to puncture the vein, and the short end enters the blood tube.

16. Cleanse the venipuncture site with alcohol swab, using a circular method at the site and extending the motion 2 inches beyond the site (Figure 29-3). Allow the alcohol to dry.

16. The alcohol and mechanical cleaning motion cleans the skin surface of bacteria that may cause infection at the site. Allowing the alcohol to dry reduces the stinging sensation that the client may experience.

17. Remove the needle cover and warn that client will feel the needle stick for a few seconds.

17. Clients will be better able to control their reaction if they know what to expect.

18. Place the thumb or forefinger of the nondominant hand 1 inch below the site and pull the skin taut.

18. Helps stabilize the vein during insertion.

(continues)

## PROCEDURE 29-1 (continued)

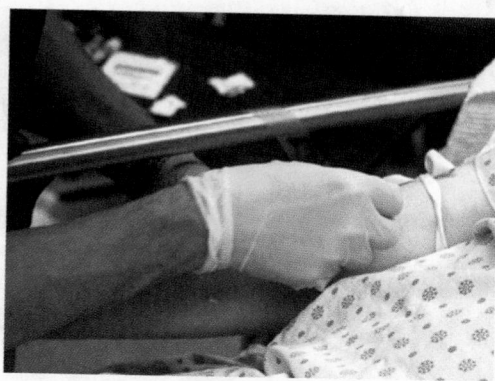

**Figure 29-3** After applying the tourniquet, cleanse the skin at the venipuncture site. Do not let the tourniquet stay on longer than 2 minutes. If you need more time, remove the tourniquet for a couple of minutes to allow the client to rest, and begin again.

19. Hold syringe needle or vacutainer at 15°–30° angle from the skin with the bevel up.

19. This angle reduces the chance of penetrating though the vein during insertion. The needle causes less trauma to the skin and vein when the bevel is up during insertion.

20. Slowly insert needle/vacutainer (Figure 29-4).

20. Prevents puncture through the other side of the vein.

21. Technique varies depending on equipment used:
    • Syringe method: Gently pull back on syringe plunger and look for blood return. Obtain desired amount of blood into the syringe.
    • Vacutainer method: Hold vacutainer securely and advance specimen tube into needle of holder. Be careful not to advance the needle into the vein. The blood should flow into the collection tube. After the collection tube is full, grasp the vacutainer firmly, remove the tube, and insert additional specimen collection tubes as indicated (Figures 29-4 and 29-5).

21.
    • If blood does not appear, the needle is not in the vein.

    • Pushing the needle through the stopper breaks the vacuum and causes the flow of blood into the collection tube. Failure of blood to appear in the collection tube indicates the vacuum in the tube has been lost or the needle is not in the vein.

22. After the specimen collection is completed, release the tourniquet.

22. Reduces bleeding from pressure when the needle is removed.

23. Apply 2 × 2 gauze over the puncture site without applying pressure and quickly withdraw the needle from the vein.

23. Positions the gauze for removal and helps to gently prevent the skin from pulling with the needle removal.

24. Immediately apply pressure over the venipuncture site with the gauze for 2 to 3 minutes or until the bleeding has stopped. Tape the gauze dressing over the site (or apply the Band-Aid).

24. Direct pressure stops the bleeding and minimizes formation of a hematoma.

*(continues)*

**PROCEDURE 29-1** (*continued*)

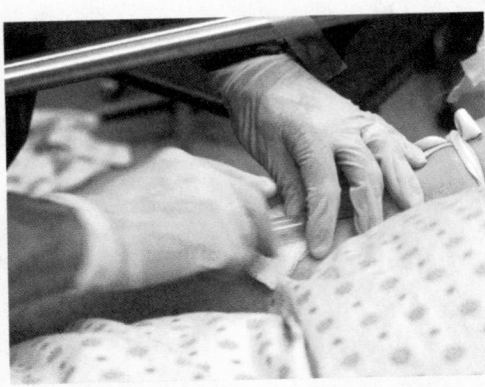

**Figure 29-4    Hold the vacutainer and needle assembly securely and press the specimen tube into the holder. The needle inside the holder will pierce the specimen tube and blood should begin to flow into the tube.**

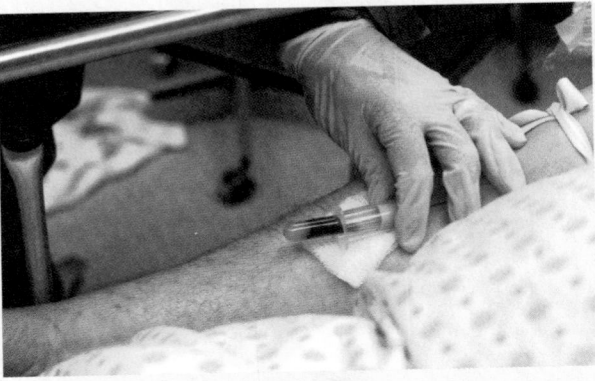

**Figure 29-5    Allow the tube to fill with blood. When it is full, remove the tube and insert additional tubes if needed.**

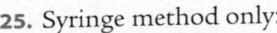

25. Syringe method only:

    • Using one hand, insert the syringe needle into the appropriate collection tube and allow vacuum to fill. You may also remove the stopper from each vacutainer collection tube, remove the needle from the syringe, fill the tube, and replace the stopper.

26. If any of the blood tubes contain additives, gently rotate back and forth 8 to 10 times.

27. Inspect the client's puncture site for bleeding. Reapply clean gauze and tape if necessary.

28. Assist client into a comfortable position. Return bed into low position with guard rails up if appropriate.

29. Check tubes for any external blood and decontaminate with alcohol as appropriate.

30. Check tubes for proper labeling. Place tubes into appropriate bags/containers for transport to the laboratory.

31. Dispose of needles, syringe, and soiled equipment into proper container.

32. Remove and dispose of gloves.

25. Using a one-handed method to fill the syringe helps reduce the chance of needle-stick injury.
    • The alternative method allows you to control the speed and amount of fill in the collection tubes.

26. Ensures that the additive is properly mixed throughout the specimen.

27. Keeps site clean and dry.

28. Provides comfort and safety for the client.

29. Prevents contamination to other equipment and personnel.

30. Ensures the specimens are properly identified.

31. Prevents spread of disease and needle-stick injury.

32. Reduces transmission of microorganisms.

*(continues)*

**PROCEDURE 29-1** (*continued*)

33. Wash hands after the procedure.

34. Send specimens to the laboratory.

33. Reduces transmission of microorganisms.

34. Facilitates timely handling of specimens and accurate results.

causative agent for acquired immunodeficiency syndrome (AIDS). Extreme care should be taken whenever there is a possibility for exposure to blood and body substances. State laws and the Occupational Health and Safety Agency (OSHA) mandate hospitals and other health care institutions to follow stringent regulations for needle-stick injury prevention. It is important to follow these guidelines when performing venipuncture.

Correct selection and preparation of equipment and vein provides for a safe and efficient venipuncture. Review of the client's health history and physical assessment data will assist in identifying special client considerations. If the client has a bleeding disorder or is taking anticoagulant therapy, apply pressure to the puncture site for 3 to 5 minutes after the removal of the needle.

### Arterial Puncture

Assessment of arterial blood gases (ABG) reveals the ability of the lungs to exchange gases by measuring the partial pressures of oxygen ($PO_2$) carbon dioxide ($PCO_2$) and evaluates the pH of arterial blood. Blood gases are ordered to evaluate:

- Oxygenation
- Ventilation and the effectiveness of respiratory therapy
- Acid-base level of the blood

Arterial blood samples are drawn from a peripheral artery (e.g., radial or femoral) or from an arterial line. The arterial blood sample is collected in a 5 ml heparinized syringe. The syringe is then rotated to mix the blood with the heparin to prevent clotting. The blood sample is placed on ice to reduce the rate of oxygen metabolism.

In some agencies it is within the scope of nursing practice to perform radial artery puncture; however, femoral artery puncture is usually performed only by an advanced practitioner. An increased risk of hemorrhage exists with a femoral puncture. Although it is not common practice for

student nurses to draw ABG samples, students often have to assist with the procedure and care for the client after the procedure.

Arterial punctures should not be performed:

- If the client is hyperthermic
- Immediately after breathing and suctioning treatments
- If there have been changes on ventilator settings

Arterial samples are also contraindicated in the following conditions:

- Anticoagulant therapy
- Clotting disorders
- Symptomatic peripheral vascular disease
- Negative Allen test

An **Allen test** is performed to measure the collateral circulation to the radial artery.

Regardless of who performs the arterial puncture, the nurse is responsible for assessing the client for symptoms of bleeding or occlusion postpuncture. Direct pressure must be applied to the puncture site until all bleeding has stopped, a minimum of 5 minutes. Ensure that all bleeding has stopped before releasing the pressure. Symptoms of impaired circulation include:

- Numbness and tingling
- Bluish color
- Absence of a peripheral pulse

### Capillary Puncture

Skin punctures are performed when small quantities of capillary blood are needed for analysis or when the client has poor veins. Capillary puncture is also commonly performed for blood glucose analysis, discussed later in this chapter.

## CLINICAL ALERT

### Arterial Blood Gases

Arterial blood gases should not be drawn within 20 minutes after any respiratory treatment to *ensure accurate determination of the client's actual blood gases.*

## CLINICAL ALERT

### Postarterial Puncture

Instruct the client to notify you immediately if any pain or numbness occurs in the arm or leg after arterial puncture, as these symptoms indicate impaired circulation.

The common sites for capillary punctures are the:

- Heel—most common site for neonates and infants
- Fingertip—the inner aspect of palmar fingertip used most commonly in children and adults
- Earlobe—when the client is in shock or the extremities are edematous

To perform a skin puncture, assemble the equipment, prepare the client, and select the appropriate site (Procedure 29-2). Figure 29-6 shows a capillary puncture of a fingertip.

### Central Lines

Some clients have a central venous access device or central line. A **central line** is an intravenous (IV) device, which is inserted into the superior vena cava through several kinds of veins. The most common veins used are (1) subclavian, (2) internal jugular, (3) external jugular,

---

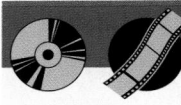

### PROCEDURE 29-2    Skin Puncture

## EQUIPMENT NEEDED

- Antiseptic—70% isopropanol or povidone-iodine
- Sterile 2 × 2 gauze
- Sterile lancet
- Hand towel or absorbent pad

- Microhematocrit tubes or micropipette (collection tubes)
- Nonsterile gloves

## IMPLEMENTATION—ACTION/RATIONALE

| ACTION | RATIONALE |
|---|---|
| 1. Wash hands. | 1. Decreases transmission of microorganisms. |
| 2. Check client's identification band. | 2. Ensures correct client. |
| 3. Explain procedure to client. | 3. Allays anxiety and encourages cooperation. |
| 4. Prepare supplies:<br>  • Open sterile packages.<br>  • Label specimen collection tubes.<br>  • Place in easy reach. | 4. Ensures efficiency. |
| 5. Don gloves. | 5. Decreases the health care provider's exposure to blood-borne organisms. |
| 6. Select site:<br>  • Lateral aspect of the fingertips in adults/children | 6. Avoids damage to nerve endings and calloused areas of the skin. |
| 7. Place the hand or heel in a dependent position; apply warm compresses if fingers or heel are cool to touch. | 7. Increases the blood supply to the puncture site. |
| 8. Place hand towel or absorbent pad under the extremity. | 8. Prevents soiling the bed linen. |
| 9. Cleanse puncture site with an antiseptic and allow to dry; use 70% isopropanol if client is allergic to iodine. | 9. Reduces skin surface bacteria; povidone-iodine must dry to be effective. |
| 10. With nondominant hand, apply light pressure by gently squeezing the area above/around the puncture site. Do not touch puncture site. | 10. Increases blood supply to puncture site; maintains asepsis. |
| 11. With the sterile lancet at a 90° angle to the skin, use a quick stab to puncture the skin (about 2 mm deep) (Figure 29-6). | 11. Provides a blood sample with minimal discomfort to the client. |

*(continues)*

**PROCEDURE 29-2** (*continued*)

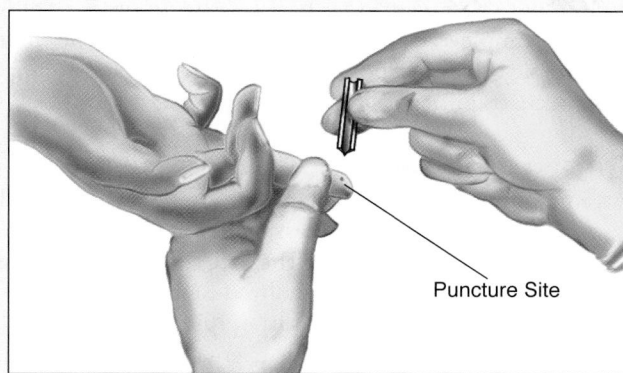

**Figure 29-6   Capillary puncture of fingertip**

12. Wipe off the first drop of blood with a sterile 2 × 2 gauze; allow the blood to flow freely. If blood does not flow freely, gently "milk" the finger or heel from proximal to distal to move blood to the puncture site. (Do not squeeze the finger or heel to obtain a specimen.)

12. Pressure at the puncture site can cause hemolysis.

13. Collect the blood into the tube(s). If a platelet count is to be collected, obtain this specimen first.

13. Allows blood collection; avoids aggregation of platelets at the puncture site.

14. Apply pressure to the puncture site with a sterile 2 × 2 gauze.

14. Controls bleeding.

15. Place contaminated articles into a sharps container.

15. Reduces risk for needle stick.

16. Remove gloves; wash hands.

16. Reduces transmission of microorganisms.

17. Position client for comfort with call light in reach.

17. Provides for comfort and communication.

(4) cephalic, (5) basilic, (6) cephalic antecubital, (7) basilic antecubital, or (8) median antecubital. Central lines (Figure 29-7) are inserted when peripheral access cannot be obtained, when peripheral access cannot sustain the type of intravenous drug therapy prescribed, or to withdraw blood for analysis.

Nurses need to know the type and location of the central line catheter. Various types of **venous access devices**

**(VAD)** are available in the market. Percutaneous catheters are commonly used in the hospital as well outpatient settings. **Peripherally inserted central catheters (PICC)** are also used for specific types of IV therapy. VADs are made of different types of materials and are available in single, double, triple, or even quadruple lumens. The diameter and length of the lumens vary due to the need for infusion of hypertonic and viscous solutions. The proximal port is usually the best line to use for blood withdrawal since this provides the least contaminated specimen from the IV solutions infusing through the other lumens (Daniels, 2003). Lumens without continuous infusion of fluids are capped with an infusion plug and flushed with a heparinized solution (10 to 100 units of heparin in 1 mL saline) every 8 hours or per agency's protocol (Phillips, 2001). Heparin prevents obstruction of the catheter lumen with a blood clot. The first sample of blood drawn from the central line cannot be used for diagnostic testing; it must be discarded. The amount of discard volume

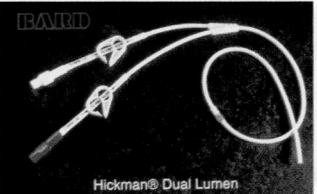

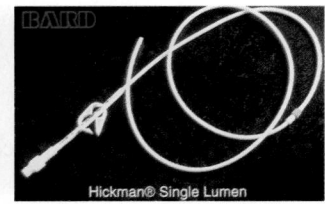

**Figure 29-7   Hickman catheter** *Photo provided by Bard Access Systems. Hickman is a registered trademark of Bard Access Systems.*

## NURSING STRATEGY

### Obtaining a Blood Sample from a Central Line

- Gather equipment (the sizes of the needle and syringe to obtain the blood sample are determined by the amount of blood needed for the test and the type and size of central line catheter).

- Check the client's identification band.

- Wash hands and don gloves to prevent exposure to blood-borne organisms.

- Select a port that is not used routinely for an infusion.

- Cleanse the port of the lumen with an antiseptic.

- Insert the needle into the port and aspirate the discard volume according to agency protocol; dispose of the syringe containing the discard blood into a sharps container.

- Access the port and withdraw the blood sample.

- Apply the same principles used in venipuncture to prevent the hemoconcentration and hemolysis of blood when withdrawing the sample.

- Transfer the sample into the correct collection tubes and discard the contaminated needle and syringe into the sharps container.

- Instill the required heparin solution to prevent the lumen from clotting.

- Transport specimen to the laboratory.

- Remove gloves, wash hands.

## COMMUNITY/HOME CARE

### Central Line

Clients in the home environment usually have a central line in place for prolonged therapy. Because one of the primary complications of central venous catheter insertion is infection, the nurse must be alert for signs of infection (e.g., fever) exhibited by the client.

---

is directly related to the dead space (catheter size). The agency's protocol should indicate the volume to discard relative to the type and size of catheter.

The nursing care of central lines requires strict sterile technique. The practitioner has to write an order to allow a blood sample to be obtained from a central line. Refer to the Nursing Strategy box for how to draw a blood sample from a central line.

### Implanted Port

An implanted port (often labeled a **port-a-cath**) is another type of central venous access, which has been available since 1983. It was named for the fact that it is implanted under the skin. It was originally designed for oncology clients on long-term chemotherapy (Phillips, 2001). Implantable ports are used for clients who require long-term drug or fluid therapy. The port, which is available as a single or dual port system, is usually made of stainless steel, titanium, or plastic. The catheter attached to the port is either made of silicone or polyurethane (Bard Access Systems, 2002). Implantable ports are placed typically below the right or left clavicle on the first or second intercostal space. Intraperitoneal or intra-arterial placements have also been used (Phillips, 2001). The implanted port is used for the same purpose as the central lines.

Blood can be withdrawn for sampling by accessing the port using strict sterile technique. The best port for blood draws is the proximal port. If the proximal port is used for infusion, select the port not used for infusion. To obtain an uncontaminated sample, the infusion of drugs or fluids should be held while obtaining a blood specimen. Then the catheter is flushed with saline to clear the catheter of blood. Afterward, a heparinized solution is infused to prevent clot development in the lumen. Accessing a port should only be performed by a nurse with proper education. Students are not usually taught how to access an implanted port.

### Urine Collection

The kidneys are responsible for maintaining homeostasis of the body's buffering systems and the volume, and ionic and osmotic composition of its fluid compartments; refer to Chapter 34 for a complete discussion of the composition of fluid compartments. "Although the results of kidney functions are reflected in analyses of blood, the mechanisms by which normalcy of body fluids is preserved can be

## CLINICAL ALERT

### Urine Collection

As with blood, all urine collection requires the use of Standard Precautions to prevent the transmission of microorganisms among nurses, clients, and other health care providers.

understood only through studies of urine" (Kirschbaum, Sica, & Anderson, 1999, p. 597).

Urine can be collected for various studies. The type of testing determines the method of collection. The different methods of urine collection are:

- Random collection (routine analysis)
- Timed collection
- Collection from a closed urinary drainage system
- Clean-voided specimen

The urine from a closed urinary drainage system is a sterile specimen. Client teaching depends on the client's age, the method of collection, and, in some instances, the location of the client. Initiate the protocol for preparing the client for testing (see Table 29-1). The method of collection should be written on the laboratory requisition.

### Random Collection

The practitioner usually writes the order for a UA (routine urine analysis), which is also called a random collection. It can be collected at any time using a clean cup. The urine does not have to be collected in a sterile container. Instruct the client to urinate into the specimen cup or into a clean bedpan or urinal. Wearing gloves, transfer the urine into a clean container. Seal the lid tightly, label, and place in a biohazard bag for transport to the laboratory. Submit the specimen immediately to the laboratory to prevent the growth of bacteria or changes in the urine's analytes (substances).

### Timed Collection

Timed collection is done over a 24-hour period. The urine is collected in a plastic gallon container that contains preservative(s), some of which are caustic. The laboratory usually adds the preservatives to the container. If the analyte to be studied is light sensitive, a dark plastic container is necessary.

Provide the client with specific instructions. The client is told to **void** (the process of urine evacuation) and discard the specimen at the beginning of the collection. The 24-hour collection begins with the first discarded voiding. For example, if the client voided at 0930 hours (24-hour clock time frame), discard the urine and mark the time as the start time. Save all the urine from that time on until 0930 hours of the following day. The client may void into a clean container, then transfer the urine into the collection bottle. Instruct the client to void prior to passing stool since feces may contaminate the specimen. Advise the client not to drop toilet paper into the container used to catch the urine.

The collection container should be refrigerated or kept on ice throughout the 24 hours. This retards bacterial growth and stabilizes the analytes. The last urine collection, 0930 hours, should be a complete, forced voiding at the exact timed period. Seal the labeled container tightly and take immediately to the lab.

### Collection from a Closed Drainage System

A sterile specimen can be collected from a client with an indwelling Foley catheter with a closed drainage system. A sterile specimen is used to culture the urine. *The urine specimen should not be obtained from the drainage bag.* The analytes in the urine drainage bag change; this will cause inaccurate results. Bacteria grow quickly in the drainage bag.

The catheter's closed drainage tubing has an aspiration port that is used for a sterile specimen collection (Procedure 29-3).

### Clean-Voided Specimen

Clean-voided (clean-catch or midstream) specimen collection is done to secure a specimen uncontaminated by skin flora. A clean-voided specimen should be obtained on first voiding in the morning. Most adult clients are capable of following instructions to perform this test.

## NURSING STRATEGY

### Clean-Voided Specimen, Female

1. Check the client's identification band.
2. Instruct the client on the procedure.
3. Wash hands and don gloves if the client needs assistance with the procedure.
4. Instruct to:
   - Sit with legs separated on the toilet.
   - Open sterile container, placing lid up on a firm surface within easy reach.
   - Using thumb and forefinger, separate the labia.
   - With labia separated, using a downward stroke, cleanse one side of the labia with the towelette, discard the towelette, repeat procedure on the other side with the second towelette, and make sure the labia stays separated throughout the procedure.
5. Begin to urinate in the toilet and place the collection cup under the stream of urine after a good flow of urine has been started. Fill the container halfway with urine.
6. Place sterile lid back onto container, label, and transport to laboratory.

Altman, G. (2nd ed.). (2004). *Delmar's fundamental & advanced nursing skills.* Clifton Park, NY: Delmar Learning.

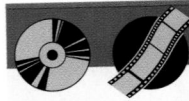

**PROCEDURE 29-3**

# Obtaining a Residual Urine Specimen from an Indwelling Catheter

## EQUIPMENT NEEDED

- Nonserrated clamp or rubber band (Figure 29-8)
- Nonsterile gloves
- Syringe with needle (1 inch), 10 cc
- Specimen container, plastic bag, and labels
- Povidone-iodine swabs

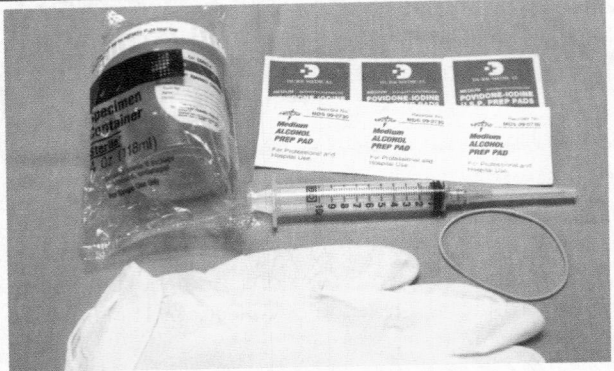

**Figure 29-8** Specimen container, syringe, nonsterile gloves, and a rubber band are used to obtain a urine specimen from an indwelling container.

## IMPLEMENTATION—ACTION/RATIONALE

| ACTION | RATIONALE |
|---|---|
| 1. Wash hands. | 1. Reduces transmission of microorganisms. |
| 2. Check physician's or qualified practitioner's order. | 2. Determines test and container needed for the specimen. |
| 3. Explain procedure to the client and provide privacy. | 3. Informs client and maintains client dignity. |
| 4. Check for urine in the tubing. | 4. Determines if there is sufficient urine in the collecting tubing for a specimen. Urine from the collection bag should not be used for sterile specimens. |
| 5. If more urine is needed, clamp the tubing using a nonserrated clamp or a rubber band for 10 to 15 minutes (Figure 29-9). | 5. Collects 10 cc of urine, which is needed for most urinalysis. |
| 6. Put on clean gloves. | 6. Practices Standard Precautions. |
| 7. Clean sample port with a povidone-iodine swab. | 7. Prevents entrance of microorganisms into the system. |
| 8. Insert sterile needle and syringe into the sample port or catheter at a 45° angle and withdraw 10 ml of urine (Figure 29-10). | 8. Obtains specimen with sufficient volume for most urine tests. |
| 9. Put urine into sterile container and close tightly, taking care not to contaminate the lid of the container. | 9. Prevents contamination of specimen and spill of urine. |
| 10. Remove clamp and rearrange tubing, avoiding dependent loops. | 10. Reestablishes urine flow and drainage into the system. |

*(continues)*

**PROCEDURE 29-3** (*continued*)

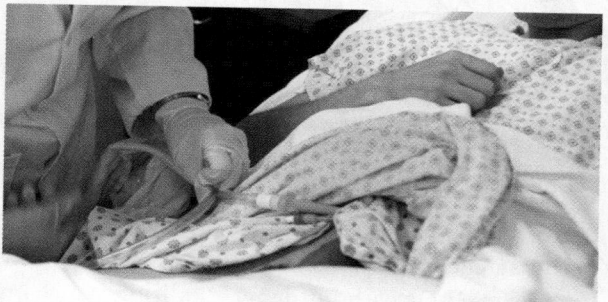

**Figure 29-9    Clamp the tubing by folding it over and securing it with a rubber band to collect an adequate sample.**

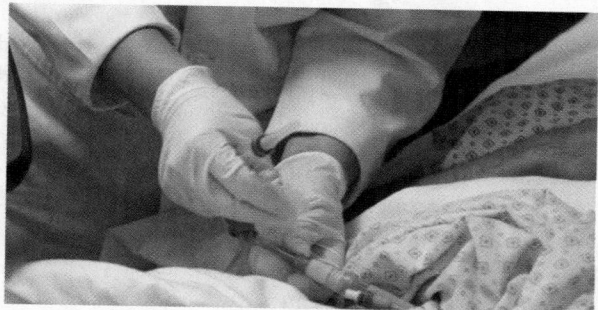

**Figure 29-10    Cleanse the sample port and insert a sterile needle and syringe into the sample port.**

11. Label specimen container, put it in a plastic bag, and send to the laboratory.

12. Wash hands.

13. Record procedure on flowsheet or approved agency form.

11. Ensures right test and controls transfer of pathogens.

12. Reduces transmission of microorganisms.

13. Maintains continuity of care.

Different aseptic techniques are used for women and men. Poor technique in cleaning the perineum can contaminate the specimen. Instruct the female client to cleanse from the front to the back.

Instruct the male client to perform the same procedure except for the cleansing of the perineal area; men should cleanse from the tip of the penis downward. The Nursing Checklist describes the procedure for obtaining a clean-voided specimen from a man.

When obtaining a clean-voided specimen from infants and small children, secure assistance.

 **NURSING STRATEGY**

### Clean-Voided Specimen, Infant and Child

1. Check the identification band.
2. Explain the procedure to family member present with infant or child. If the child can cooperate, tell child what to do before having someone hold her in position.
3. Wash hands and don gloves.
4. Place in a supine position with hips externally rotated.
5. Have parent or assistant flex and abduct the knees; hold the knees throughout the procedure.
6. Cleanse the perineal area as you would for an adult.
7. Place a sterile collection bag over the perineum or penis and scrotum; apply a diaper.
8. Remove the collection bag immediately after voiding.
9. Transfer the urine into the labeled collection container, close lid tightly, and place in biohazard bag for immediate transport to the laboratory.

 **NURSING STRATEGY**

### Clean-Voided Specimen, Male

1. Check the client's identification band.
2. Instruct the client on the procedure.
3. Wash hands and don gloves if the client needs assistance with the procedure.
4. If uncircumcised, retract the foreskin and hold retracted.
5. Cleanse the head of the penis with a towelette using a circular motion. Cleanse the meatus and glans, beginning with the urethral opening, and make one complete circle around the penis, moving down the glans shaft.
6. Discard the towelette.
7. Repeat the procedure until all three towelettes have been used.

## Stool Collection

Explain to the client why the stool specimen is being collected. Instruct the client to defecate into a clean bedpan or container, discarding tissue into the toilet. Stools can be collected for either a one-time defecation or over 24, 48, or 72 hours. If a specimen is needed over a prolonged period of time, all stools must be placed into a container and refrigerated. Once collected, label the container with the client's name, date, time, and the test to be performed on the specimen. All stool specimens are placed in a biohazard bag before transport to the laboratory.

## Hematologic System

Understanding the hematologic system requires a knowledge of the blood's composition and its functions. Table 29-4 discusses the origin, normal range values, and the major function for each of the three types of cells found in blood:

- Red blood cells (**erythrocytes**)
- White blood cells (**leukocytes**)
- Platelets

Forty to 45% of the blood's volume is composed of blood cells; the remaining blood volume is plasma as shown in Figure 29-11. Plasma is part of the body's extracellular fluid system, consisting of water and analytes. Blood proteins form the largest portion of the plasma analytes. The average plasma volume for a normal adult is 3 L.

## Red Blood Cells

Red blood cells (RBCs), in embryonic life, are produced first in the yolk sac until the middle trimester; then the liver becomes the main organ of RBC production. RBC production becomes the exclusive function of the bone marrow by the end of gestation, after birth, and throughout life. RBC bone marrow site production changes with age:

- From birth to age 5—all bone marrow
- Five to 20 years—the shaft of the long bones (tibia and femur)
- After 20 years—the membranous bones (ilia, ribs, sternum, and vertebrae). As part of the normal aging process, the production of RBCs decreases with age.

Functions of the RBCs include:

- Transporting oxygen carrying hemoglobin

### CLINICAL ALERT

#### Stool from a Client with Hepatitis

When collecting a stool specimen from a client with hepatitis, write on the lab requisition form that the client has hepatitis. This increases the laboratory personnel's awareness to be extra careful when handling the specimen.

### STOP AND THINK

#### Overcoming Embarrassment

You are cleansing the genitals of a client to obtain a clean-catch urine sample. How would you feel about performing this type of procedure if the client were a man? A woman? What methods would you use to maintain your professional role while still respecting and caring for the client? How would you maintain your nurse-client relationship without becoming too personal? Or without depersonalizing the client so that he or she becomes uncomfortable?

- Transporting carbon dioxide in the form of sodium bicarbonate
- Being an acid-base buffer for whole blood

## White Blood Cells

Six types of white blood cells (WBCs, leukocytes) are found in the blood.

- Neutrophils
- Basophils
- Lymphocytes
- Eosinophils
- Monocytes
- Plasma cells

The polymorphonuclear cells, neutrophils, eosinophils, and basophils have a granular appearance, hence the name granulocytes or polys. The granulocytes and monocytes

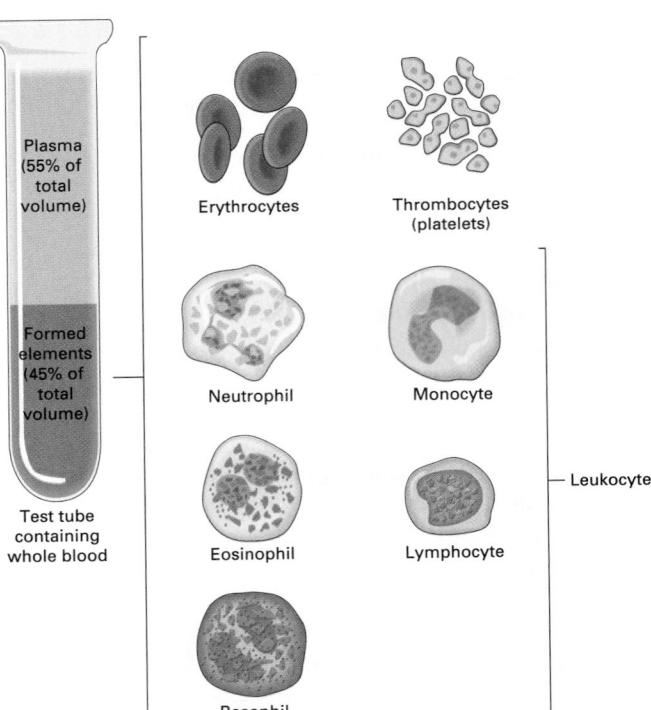

**Figure 29-11    Blood cells**

## TABLE 29-4   TYPES OF BLOOD CELLS

| Cell | Origin | Range SI Units* | Major Function |
|---|---|---|---|
| Erythrocytes | Bone marrow | F: $4.0–5.2 \times 10^{12}$/L<br>M: $4.5–5.9 \times 10^{12}$/L | Transport hemoglobin |
| Leukocytes | Granulocytes<br>Monocytes<br>Bone Marrow<br><br>Lymphocytes<br>Plasma cells<br>Lymph tissue | $4.5–11.0 \times 10^{9}$/L | The body's protective system |
| Platelets | Bone Marrow from megakaryocytes | $150–300 \times 10^{9}$/L | Vascular repair |

*Data for normal range SI units from Daniels, R. (2003). *Delmar's manual of laboratory and diagnostic tests.* Clifton Park, NY: Delmar Learning.

are responsible for **phagocytosis** (process by which certain cells engulf and dispose of foreign bodies). The lymphocytes and plasma cells function mainly as the body's immune system.

The WBCs are formed and stored in the bone marrow until needed by the body. Table 29-5 presents laboratory studies for a complete blood count with SI values and when each analyte is either increased or decreased in clinical situations.

### Red Cell Indices

**Red cell indices** measure the size and hemoglobin content of the RBCs. The RBC indices are:

- Mean corpuscular volume (MCV)—size of erythrocytes
- Mean corpuscular hemoglobin (MCH)—amount of each hemoglobin in each erythrocyte (by weight)
- Mean corpuscular hemoglobin concentration (MCHC)—percentage of erythrocyte occupied by hemoglobin

The indices are diagnostic in determining the type of anemia. For example, an elevated MCHC means that **spherocytes** (smaller, thicker red cells) are present; this occurs in acquired hemolytic anemia.

### Platelets

Platelets are fragments of a seventh type of WBC found in the bone marrow, the megakaryocytes. Platelets maintain hemostasis and blood coagulation by being the active mechanism of the blood in vascular repair. The active factors necessary for blood to coagulate are found in the cytoplasm of platelets. Blood coagulation is a comprehensive, sequential process of the body's response to injury.

The blood coagulation flowchart (Figure 29-12) reviews the key elements of vascular constriction and coagulation. Prothrombin (factor II) is a plasma protein, formed in the liver, and requires vitamin K for synthesis. It is activated when blood vessels are damaged. Prothrombin activator causes the conversion of prothrombin into thrombin, which then causes fibrinogen to form threads. This whole process takes 10 to 15 seconds.

Prothrombin activator is the governing element in blood coagulation. Prothrombin time (PT) measures the defects in this extrinsic clotting mechanism, specifically fibrinogen (factor I), prothrombin (factor II), and factors V, VII, and X (Daniels, 2003).

Many factors affect PT, as shown in Table 29-6.

Partial thromboplastin (PTT) or activated partial thromboplastin time (aPTT) measures the intrinsic clotting mechanism factors (I, II, V, X, XI, XII). There are five primary screening tests to diagnose suspected coagulation disorders (Daniels, 2003):

1. Platelet count, size, and shape
2. Bleeding time—the ability of platelets to function normally and the ability of capillaries to constrict their walls, prolonged with deficiencies in platelets and other clotting factors
3. PTT—measures the ability of the blood to clot, prolonged with any intrinsic factor deficiencies such as hemophilia A (factor VIII) and hemophilia B (factor X)
4. PT—measures the total quantity of prothrombin in the blood, monitors the effectiveness of coumarin therapy, prolonged with deficiencies in the extrinsic factors and vitamin K
5. Fibrinogen level—investigates abnormal PT and APTT and to screen for **disseminated intravascular coagulation (DIC)** (an acquired hemorrhagic syndrome characterized by uncontrolled formation and deposition of thrombi) and fibrin-fibrinogenolysis; levels increase with acute inflammatory reactions, trauma, coronary heart disease and cigarette smoking and decrease in liver disease, DIC, cancer, primary fibrinolysis, and congenital hypofibrinogenemia.

## TABLE 29-5   COMPLETE BLOOD COUNT WITH CLINICAL SIGNIFICANCE

| Analyte | SI Range | Increased | Decreased |
|---|---|---|---|
| Red blood cell count | F: 4.0–5.2 × $10^{12}$/L<br>M: 4.5–5.9 × $10^{12}$/L | Dehydration, induced hypoxia, polycythemia | Anemias, hypothyroidism, leukemias |
| Hemoglobin (Hb):<br>Whole blood<br>Fetal Plasma | F: 120–150 g/L,<br>M: 139–163 g/L<br>0–75 mg/L < 0.01 | Chronic obstructive lung disease, polycythemia, high altitudes burns, shock | Anemia, severe hemorrhage |
| Hematocrit (Hct) | F: 0.36–0.46<br>M: 0.41–0.53 | Dehydration, polycythemia | Leukemia, hemorrhage |
| Mean red cell Hb | 26–34 pg/RBC | Macrocytosis | Microcytic hypochromic anemia |
| Mean red cell Hb concentration | 310–370 g/L | Spherocytosis | Chronic iron deficiency anemia |
| Mean red cell volume | 80–100 fl | Aplastic anemia, cirrhosis, folic acid & vitamin $B_{12}$ | Chronic iron deficiency, thalassemias, chronic anemia |
| White blood cell (WBC):<br>Total count | 4.5–11.0 × $10^9$/L | Acute leukemia, infections, surgery, trauma | Acute chronic leukemias, aplastic anemia, agranulosytosis |
| WBC Differential | % of total WBC | | |
| Band neutrophils | 0–0.06% | Severe bacterial disease | |
| Segmented neutrophils | 0.31–0.76% | Diabetic acidosis, infarctions, inflammatory diseases, malignancies | |
| Lymphocytes | 0.14–0.44% | Chronic lymphocytic leukemia | Lupus erythematosus, Hodgkin's disease |
| Monocytes | 0.02–0.11% | Chronic inflammatory diseases | |
| Eosinophils | 0–0.04% | Allergies, parasites | |
| Basophils | 0–0.02% | Myelofibrosis | |
| Platelets | 150,000–450,000 mm³ | High altitude, cirrhosis, iron deficiency | Bone marrow malignancies, DIC, anemias |

Data for normal range SI units from Daniels, R. (2003). *Delmar's manual of laboratory and diagnostic tests.* Clifton Park, NY: Delmar Learning.

Thrombin time (TT) measures the fibrinogen portion of the hemostatic mechanism; it is infrequently used today to evaluate the fibrinogen-to-fibrin reaction. Direct measurements of fibrinogen level and the increasing use of other tests have decreased the usefulness of TT (Daniels, 2003).

### Sickle Cell Test

Sickle cell test (hemoglobin S) is used to identify the sickle cell trait and sickle cell disease. A negative result, which is normal, indicates the absence of hemoglobin S. The presence of sickle cells causes a positive result, thus requiring hemoglobin

electrophoresis to determine the presence of the genetically transmitted deficit. Figure 29-13 shows the difference in the shape between a normal RBC and a sickle-shaped RBC.

**Hemoglobin electrophoresis** refers to a laboratory test that uses an electromagnetic field (an anode [+] and a cathode [–], which are separated by cellulose acetate or starch gel) to identify various types of hemolytic anemia. Electrophoresis distinguishes between genetically transmitted homozygous and heterozygous hemoglobin S, which is responsible for sickle cell anemia. For example, if both genes carry hemoglobin S, it is called homozygous

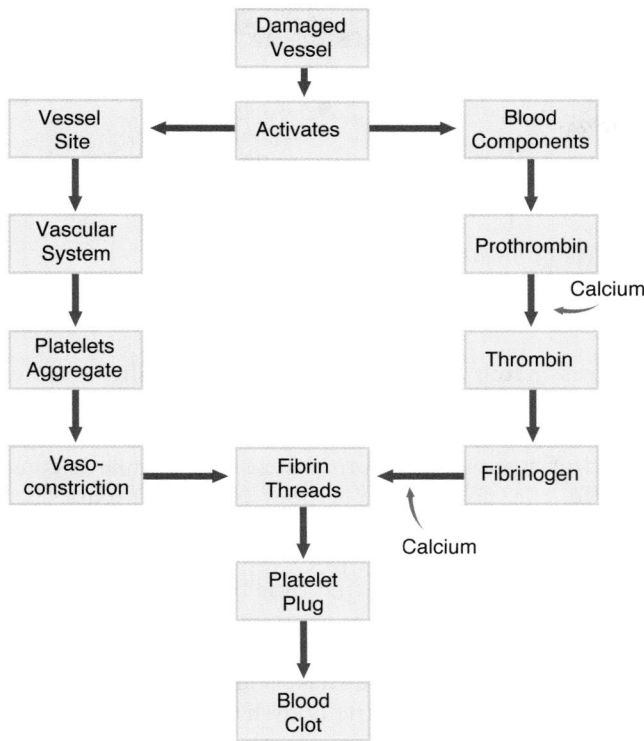

**Figure 29-12   Blood coagulation flowchart**

| TABLE 29-6 | FACTORS THAT AFFECT PT |
| --- | --- |
| Increase PT | Decrease PT |
| • Alcohol intake | • High-fat diet |
| • Drugs: | • Drugs: |
| • Allopurinol | • Anabolic steroids |
| • Aminosalicylic acid | • Barbiturates |
| • Barbiturates | • Chloral hydrate |
| • Beta-lactam antibiotic | • Digitalis |
| • Cephalothins | • Diphenhydramine |
| • Chloral hydrate | • Estrogen |
| • Chloramphenicol | • Griseofulvin |
| • Chlorpromazine | • Metaproterenol |
| • Cholestyramine | • Oral contraceptives |
| • Cimetidine | • Rifampin |
| • Clofibrate | • Vitamin K |
| • Colestipol | |
| • Glucagon | |
| • Heparin | |
| • Methyldopa | |
| • Neomycin | |
| • Oral anticoagulants | |
| • Propylthiouracil | |
| • Quinidine | |
| • Quinine | |
| • Salicylates | |
| • Sulfonamides | |

Daniels, R. (2003). *Delmar's manual of laboratory and diagnostic tests.* Clifton Park, NY: Delmar Learning.

and the client has sickle cell disease; however, if only one gene has the abnormal hemoglobin S and the other gene has the normal hemoglobin A, the client is heterozygous, having the sickle cell trait. Electrophoresis is also used to identify fetal hemoglobin and distinguish between thalassemia minor and major.

Sickle cell anemia is a blood disorder with multiple, recurring symptoms that not only causes the client pain from the clumping of RBCs in the joints but has widespread effects on other systems.

Other common laboratory tests that measure hematologic functions are presented in Table 29-7.

## Type and Crossmatch

A **type and crossmatch** is a laboratory test that identifies the client's blood type and determines the compatibility of blood between a potential donor and recipient (client). There are four basic blood types—A, B, AB, and O—that are determined by the presence or absence of A or B antigens as seen in Figure 29-14. **Antigens** are substances, usually proteins, that cause the formation of and react specifically with antibodies. **Antibodies** are immunoglobulins produced by the body in response to bacteria, viruses, or other antigenic substances. Type A and type B are antigens that are classified as **agglutinogens**, which are substances that cause **agglutination** (clumping of RBCs). **Agglutinins** are specific kinds of antibodies whose interaction with antigens is manifested as agglutination.

## CLINICAL ALERT

### Drug Effect on Prothrombin Time

Be sure to list the drugs the client is taking on the laboratory requisition for the PT test, as some drugs affect the PT.

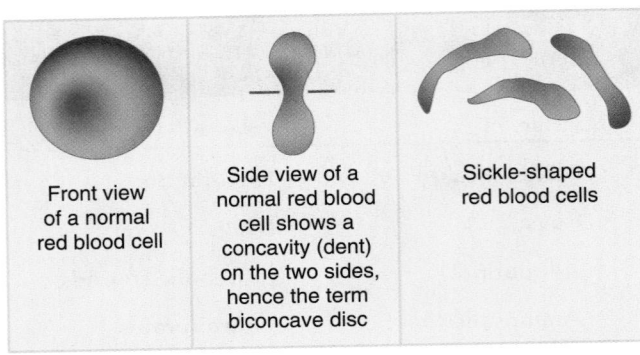

**Figure 29-13** Differences in shape are apparent in a normal red blood cell (biconcave disc) and a sickle-shaped red blood cell (crescent-shaped).

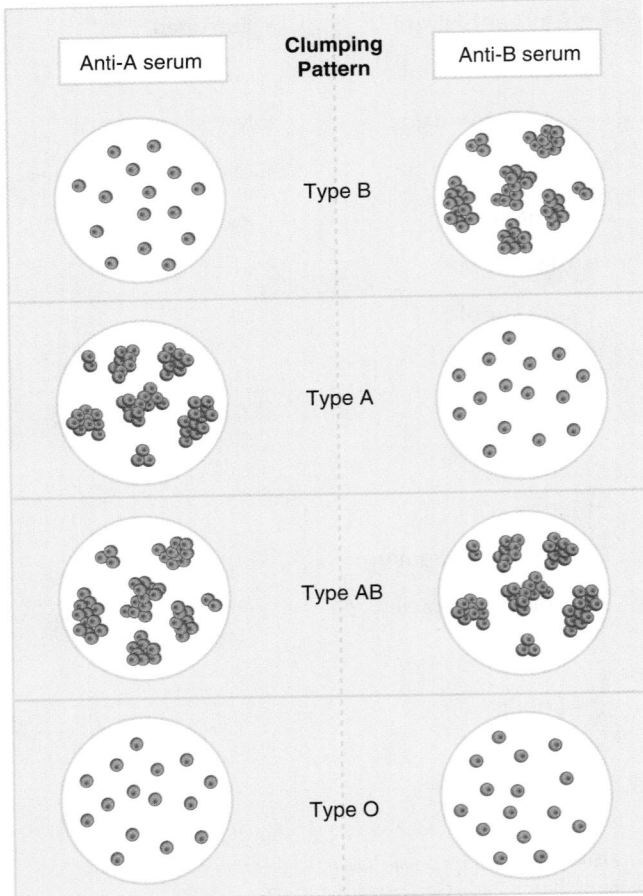

**Figure 29-14    Blood types**

Blood types are also designated as either positive or negative, depending on the presence or absence of the Rh factor. Rh factor refers to an antigen found on the RBC. Rh positive means the antigen is present; Rh negative means the antigen is absent.

When factoring the four basic blood types with either Rh positive or Rh negative factor, there are eight possible combinations (see Box 29-1). An individual's blood type is determined by heredity.

## BOX 29-1    BASIC BLOOD TYPES

- A positive
- B positive
- AB positive
- O positive
- A negative
- B negative
- AB negative
- O negative

Crossmatch determines the compatibility of the donor's blood with that of the recipient. In the laboratory, a sample of the recipient's blood is mixed with the blood of a possible donor. If the blood sample is compatible, the mixed sample does not agglutinate. For example, blood type A negative means that the person's blood contains the A antigen but does not contain the anti-Rh agglutinins. The first time the person is exposed to A-positive blood, either through a transfusion or by giving birth to an Rh-positive child, agglutination does not occur because the body has no antibodies against the antigen. However, once the body has had time to build up antibodies (agglutinins), agglutination will occur (Figure 29-14).

### Blood Chemistry

Blood chemistry analytes can be ordered separately or as profile groups (panels) that consist of 4 to 20 biochemical tests performed on a few milliliters of serum with an instrument called a sequential multiple analyzer (SMA). The studies are referred to as SMA panels based on the number of analytes being tested; refer to Box 29-2.

### Blood Glucose

Glucose is a simple sugar formed from the digestion of carbohydrates and used by the cells for energy. Insulin is needed to transport glucose into the cells.

Glucose measurement is performed by either skin puncture or venipuncture, and fasting blood sugar (FBS) or nonfasting (usually 2 hours postprandial). The normal fasting value is 70–115 mg/dl and less than 120 mg/dl postprandial. The 2-hour postprandial blood sugar is drawn 2 hours after the client eats a meal. This test is used to screen for diabetes mellitus; if the results are abnormal, the practitioner may order a glucose tolerance test.

A glucose tolerance test is the most accurate test for diagnosing hypoglycemia and hyperglycemia (diabetes mellitus). The client is asked to fast until the test begins. The test is conducted as follows:

- Initial blood and urine specimens are obtained.
- An oral loading dose of glucose is administered.
- Blood and urine specimens are obtained at 30 minutes, 1 hour, 2 hours, 3 hours, and sometimes 4 hours after loading dose.

## TABLE 29-7    HEMATOLOGIC FUNCTION STUDIES

| Test/Normal Range | Diagnostic Value |
|---|---|
| Erythrocyte sedimentation rate (ESR or sed rate) Westergren: F: < 50 yr 0–25 mm/h > 50 yr 0–30 mm/h M: < 50 yr 0–15 mm/h > 50 yr 0–20 mm/h | **Erythrocyte sedimentation rate** (ESR) is the rate with which the RBCs settle in saline/plasma over a specified time period. ESR is diagnostic for temporal arteritis, polymyalgia rheumatica, and possibly for rheumatoid arthritis. ESR is increased in chronic renal failure, malignant disease, bacterial infection, inflammatory disease, necrotic tissue diseases, hyperfibrinogenemia, macroglobulinemia, and severe anemias. ESR is decreased in sickle cell anemia, spherocytosis, hypofibrinogenemia, and polycythemia vera. |
| Haptoglobin 0.10–0.30 g/L 12–35 µmol/L | Haptoglobins bind with free hemoglobin released from the destruction of RBCs, conserving iron. *Decreased in* any condition causing hemolysis of RBCs: hemolytic anemias (sickle cell anemia, hereditary spherocytosis, erythroblastosis fetalis), thalassemia, liver disease, transfusion reactions, systemic lupus erythematosus, prosthetic heart valve implants. *Increased with* acute and chronic infections, inflammation, malignancies, steroid therapy, rheumatoid arthritis, ulcerative colitis, peptic ulcer, oral contraception, pregnancy. |
| Glucose-6-phosphate dehydrogenase (G6PD) (red blood cell) F: 7.4–9.4 IU/g hemoglobin Whites 6.5–9.3 IU/g hemoglobin African-Americans M: 7.4–9.4 IU/g hemoglobin Whites 6.6–10.8IU/g hemoglobin African-Americans | **G6PD** is an enzyme in RBCs that metabolizes glucose. The test measures enzyme deficiencies that are hereditary, sex-linked conditions carried on the female X chromosome, which causes hemolytic anemia. Clinical disease traits are found in males. *Increased in* pernicious anemia, megaloblastic anemia, chronic blood loss, myocardial infarction, hepatic coma, and hyperthyroidism. *Decreased in* G6PD deficiency, hemolytic anemia, and unusual nonspherocytic anemias. |
| Osmotic fragility 0.30%–0.45% saline < 0.30% saline > 0.50% saline | Test measures the fragility of RBCs to aid in the diagnosis of hereditary spherocytosis. *Increased in* hereditary spherocytosis, spherocytosis resulting from autoimmune hemolytic anemia, severe burns, chemical poisoning, erythroblastosis fetalis, transfusion reactions, prosthetic heart valve transplantation. *Decreased in* sickle cell and iron deficiency anemia, polycythemia vera, hemoglobin C disease, thalassemia major, liver disease, obstructive jaundice, or splenectomy. |
| Reticulocyte count (results reported in % of total erythrocytes) Adults 0.5–2.0% Children 0.5–2.0% Infants 0.5–3.5% Newborns 2.5–6.0% | Used to differentiate between hypoproliferative and hyperproliferative anemias; to assess blood loss and bone marrow response to therapy. *Increased in* hemolytic and sickle cell anemia; hereditary spherocytosis; treatment of anemias from iron, vitamin $B_{12}$, and folic acid deficiencies. *Decreased in* aplastic, iron deficiency and untreated pernicious anemias; chronic infection; radiation therapy. |

Daniels, R. (2003). *Delmar's manual of laboratory and diagnostic tests.* Clifton Park, NY: Delmar Learning.

## BOX 29-2    SMA PANELS

| SMA-4 | Red blood cells | Hemoglobin |
| | White blood cells | Hematocrit |
| SMA-6 | Sodium | Bicarbonate |
| | Potassium | Glucose |
| | Chloride | Blood urea nitrogen |
| SMA-12 | Total protein | Glucose |
| | Albumin | Uric acid |
| | Calcium | Creatinine |
| | Blood urea nitrogen | Total bilirubin |
| | Inorganic phosphate | Alkaline phosphatase |
| | Cholesterol | Aspartate amino transferase (AST) |
| SMA-20 | Glucose | Bilirubin, direct |
| | Blood urea nitrogen | Bilirubin, indirect |
| | Creatinine | Lactic dehydrogenase |
| | Uric acid | AST |
| | Sodium | Alanine aminotrans- ferase (ALT) |
| | Potassium | Alkaline phosphate |
| | Chloride | Albumin |
| | Bicarbonate | Total protein |
| | Calcium | Cholesterol |
| | Phosphorus | Triglycerides |

Data from Daniels, R. (2003). *Delmar's manual of laboratory and diagnostic tests.* Clifton Park, NY: Delmar Learning.

Figure 29-15 is a graphic presentation of the results of a glucose tolerance test, showing results that indicate hyperglycemia, normal glucose, and hypoglycemia.

Glucose results reveal deficits in either the digestion of carbohydrates or glucose metabolism (e.g., diabetes mellitus). Drugs, especially diuretics and steroids, can cause physiological changes resulting in elevated blood glucose values. Clients receiving intravenous fluids with a high glucose content need to have their glucose levels monitored for hyperglycemia.

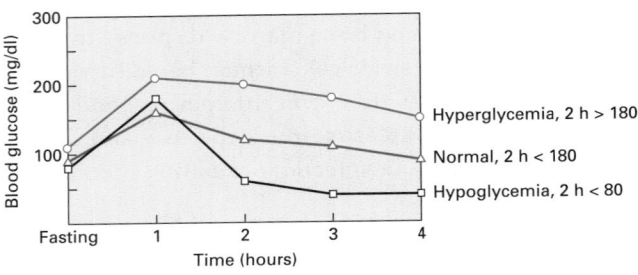

Glucose Tolerance Test (GTT) Graph

**Figure 29-15    Glucose tolerance test (GTT) graph**

## RESEARCH FOCUS

**Title of Study:** Diurnal variation in fasting plasma glucose: Implications for diagnosis of diabetes in patients examined in the afternoon

**Study Purpose:** To document diurnal variation in fasting plasma glucose levels in adults not known to have diabetes, and to examine the applicability to afternoon-examined clients based on the diagnostic criteria for diabetes.

**Methods:** Participants were selected from the U.S. population-based Third National Health and Nutrition Examination Survey (1988–1994). All participants were 20 years of age or older who had no previously diagnosed diabetes. The participants were randomly assigned to morning or afternoon examinations, and fasted prior to blood sampling.

**Findings:** The two groups did not differ in age, body mass index, waist-to-hip ratio, physical activity index, and other factors. The mean fasting plasma glucose levels were higher in the morning group than in the afternoon group.

**Implications:** The results of this study indicate that if current diabetes diagnostic criteria are applied to clients seen in the afternoon, approximately half of all cases of undiagnosed diabetes in these clients will be missed.

Troisi, R. J., Cowie, C. C., & Harris, M. I. (2000). Diurnal variation in fasting plasma glucose: Implications for diagnosis of diabetes in patients examined in the afternoon. *Journal of the American Medical Association, 284*(24), 3157–3159.

**Glycosylated hemoglobin $A_1$** measurement (Hb $A_1$) is abnormally high in clients with diabetes mellitus. About 98% of the hemoglobin in the red blood cells (RBCs) are Hb $A_1$. Seven percent of hemoglobin A is Hb $A_1$, which combines strongly with glucose in the process called glycosylation. The major form of glycohemoglobin is Hb $A_{1c}$ (see Box 29-3). Since glycohemoglobins circulate within the RBCs that have a life span of 120 days, they reflect the

## BOX 29-3    VALUES FOR Hb $A_{1C}$

| Adult/elderly: | 4% to 8% |
| Child: | < 7% |
| Good diabetes control: | 7% |
| Poor diabetes control: | 13%–20% |

Daniels, R. (2003). *Delmar's manual of laboratory and diagnostic tests.* Clifton Park, NY: Delmar Learning.

state of glycemia over 8 to 12 weeks. The Hb A$_{1c}$ is used to assess glycemic control.

## Serum Electrolytes

An **electrolyte** is an element or compound that, when dissolved in water or another solvent, separates into ions and provides for cellular reactions. Some electrolytes act on the cell membrane, allowing for the transmission of electrochemical impulses in nerve and muscle fibers. Other electrolytes determine the activity of different enzymatically catalyzed reactions that are necessary for cellular metabolism.

**Cations** are ions that have a positive charge: sodium (Na$^+$), potassium (K$^+$), calcium (Ca$^{++}$), and magnesium (Mg$^{++}$). **Anions** are ions that have a negative charge: chloride (Cl$^-$) and phosphate (HPO$_4^{--}$).

The routine electrolyte laboratory tests are presented in Table 29-8. These tests measure the serum concentration of sodium, potassium, calcium, chloride, magnesium, and phosphate. See Chapter 34 for a detailed discussion of the intracellular and extracellular functions of electrolytes.

## Blood Enzymes

**Enzymes** are globular proteins produced in the body that catalyze chemical reactions within the cells by promoting the oxidative reactions and synthesis of various chemicals, such as lipids, glycogen, and adenosine triphosphate (ATP). Enzyme tests play a key role in diagnosing the degree of tissue damage mainly to the myocardium and, to a lesser degree, to the brain.

Elevations in plasma levels of intracellular enzymes occur during myocardial **necrosis** (tissue death as the result of disease or injury). Enzymes are released into the bloodstream in proportion to the degree of cellular damage. Table 29-8 discusses the common alterations of electrolytes and their clinical significance.

Enzymes are not used as single diagnostic values in determining a diagnosis but are viewed in relation to other diagnostic studies. The results from several diagnostic procedures will assist the practitioner in determining the cause of clinical symptoms.

Creatine phosphokinase (CPK) is an enzyme used to convert creatine to phosphocreatine and adenosine diphosphate (ADP) to ATP. ATP provides energy to the cells to carry on metabolism. CPK levels indicate the degree of normal tissue catabolism. Elevated values of CPK reflect the damage that has occurred in tissue with a high CPK content. For example, the myocardium has a high CPK content; when the client has a myocardial infarction, CPK is elevated because the heart's tissue has been damaged, requiring ATP to repair the damaged myocardium.

Creatine phosphokinase has three isoenzymes of differing molecular structure that are present in different tissue (Table 29-9). The isoenzymes provides clinical data to the practitioner in diagnosing the site and extent of tissue injury.

Aspartate aminotransferase (AST) is one of two enzymes that catalyze the transfer of the nitrogenous portion of an amino acid to an acid residue. It is an intracellular enzyme found mainly in the liver, heart, skeletal muscles, kidney, pancreas, and RBCs. The normal range is:

- Adults/children      4–36 IU/L
- Newborns             4 times as high as those of adults.

Blood for AST is drawn to determine:

- A recent myocardial infarction (together with the CPK and lactic dehydrogenase levels)
- Acute hepatic disease
- The client's progress and prognosis in cardiac and hepatic diseases

Certain drugs may increase the AST (Box 29-4). Remember to note drugs on the laboratory requisition when a client is taking a drug that can influence the results of testing.

Lactic dehydrogenase (LDH), a cellular enzyme that contributes to carbohydrate metabolism, catalyzes the reversible conversion of muscle pyruvic acid into lactic acid. The diagnostic value of serum LDH is limited because it is present in almost all body tissue; however, through electrophoresis, five isoenzymes can be related to specific tissue (Table 29-10).

The percent of isoenzymes changes with tissue damage. For example, in an acute myocardial infarction, the LHD$_1$ becomes greater than LDH$_2$ 12 to 48 hours postinfarction.

α-Hydroxybutyrate dehydrogenase (HBD) is the total LDH forced to act on α-ketobutyric acid rather than lactic or pyruvic acid. It is a serum measurement used when the assay of isoenzymes of LDH is not available in the laboratory. Once a myocardial infarction has been diagnosed, the HBD has clinical significance by indicating the duration of tissue injury. HBD will remain elevated up to 2 weeks after infarction.

**Troponin** complex are cardiac-specific proteins involved in muscle contraction. It has three components: troponin T aids in the binding to actin and tropomysin; troponin I inhibits the ATPase of actimyosin; and troponin C contains binding sites for calcium ions involved in contraction. Troponin levels, specifically troponin I (cTnI) and troponin T (cTnT) become elevated within 6 hours of myocardial damage, peaks at 10 to 24 hours, and remains elevated for 5 to 7 days or longer. The American Heart Association (AHA) and the American College of Cardiology (ACC) are incorporating troponin testing, along with other cardiac enzyme testing, in the diagnosis of acute myocardial infarction (AMI). The enzymatic criteria for the diagnosis of AMI per AHA/ACC guidelines are shown in Box 29-5.

Alkaline phosphatase (a zinc-dependent enzyme) influences bone calcification and lipid and metabolite transport. The normal plasma range is 30 to 120 IU/L. Alkaline phosphatase is used to detect:

## TABLE 29-8    ROUTINE SERUM ELECTROLYTES

| Electrolyte/Normal Range | | Clinical Significance |
|---|---|---|
| **Sodium Normal Values** | | *Increased:* excessive intake of sodium without water; salt water drowning; high solute concentration (tube feeding, IV, hyperali-mentation) without fluid correction; diarrhea; diabetes insipidus; primary aldosteronism; renal failure; Cushing's syndrome. *Decreased:* excessive intake of water without sodium (oral, IV therapy, tap water enemas); heart failure, cirrhosis; nephrosis and massive diuretic therapy, SIADH, and Addison's disease. |
| Adult/elderly: | 136–145 meq/L | |
| Child: | 136–145 meq/L | |
| Infant: | 134–150 meq/L | |
| Newborn: | 134–144 meq/L | |
| **Potassium Normal Values** | | *Increased:* high potassium intake (oral, IV therapy, rapid infusion of aged blood); renal disease; drugs (adrenal steroids, potassium-conserving diuretics, potassium penicillin, chemotherapeutic agents); Addison's disease; burns and other massive tissue trau-ma; metabolic and respiratory acidosis; crush injury to tissues; hemolysis; transfusion of hemolyzed blood; infection; and dehy-dration. *Decreased:* drugs (diuretics, digitalis); metabolic alkalosis; primary aldosteronism; Cushing's disease; vomiting and gastric suction; burns; diuretics; renal tubular disease; licorice ingestion; ascites; renal artery stenosis; cystic fibrosis; trauma; and surgery. |
| Adult/elderly: | 3.5–5.0 meq/L | |
| Child: | 3.4–4.7 meq/L | |
| Infant: | 4.1–5.3 meq/L | |
| Newborn: | 3.9–5.9 meq/L | |
| Possible critical values: | | |
| Adult: | < 2.5 or 6.5 meq/L | |
| Newborn: | < 2.5 or > 8 meq/L | |
| **Calcium Normal Values** | | *Increased:* hyperparathyroidism; bone catabolism (multiple myelo-ma, leukemia, bone tumors); immobility; vitamin D intoxication; Addison's disease; and acromegaly. *Decreased:* renal failure; sprue; pancreatitis; Crohn's disease; hyperphosphatemia; drugs (aminoglycosides, antacids containing aluminum, caffeine, cis-platin, corticosteriods, loop diuretics, mithracin, phosphate, vita-min D deficiency, osteomalacia, pancreatitis, and fat embolism). |
| Total calcium | | |
| Child: | 8.8–10.10.8 mg/dl | |
| Adult: | 9.0–10.5 mg/dl | |
| Ionized calcium: | | |
| Newborn: | 4.20–5.58 mg/dl | |
| 2 months–18 years | 4.80–5.52 mg/dl | |
| Adult | 4.5–5.6 mg/dl | |
| **Chloride Normal Values** | | *Increased:* hyperparathyroidism; drugs (ammonium chloride, ion exchange resin, phenylbutazone); metabolic acidosis; respiratory acidosis; dehydration; eclampsia; anemia; and multiple myelo-ma. *Decreased:* prolonged vomiting and gastric suction; diarrhea; diuretics (ethacrynic acid and furosemide); overhydration; Addison's disease; diuretic therapy; burns; and hypokalemia. |
| Adult/elderly: | 90–110 meq/L | |
| Child: | 90–110 meq/L | |
| Newborn: | 96–106 meq/L | |
| Premature infant: | 95–110 meq/L | |
| Possible critical values: | < 80 or > 115 meq/L | |
| **Magnesium Normal Values** | | *Increased:* chronic renal failure; drugs (magnesium sulfate, antacids, enemas containing magnesium, sedatives); acute adrenalcortical insufficiency; uncontrolled diabetes; and Addison's disease. *Decreased:* chronic diarrhea and alcoholism; nontropical sprue; steatorrhea; hereditary malabsorption; star-vation; bowel resection; diuretics (mannitol, urea, glucose); hypoparathyroidism; alcoholism; and diabetic ketoacidosis. |
| Adult: | 1.2–2 meq/L | |
| Child: | 1.4–1.7 meq/L | |
| Newborn: | 1.4–2 meq/L | |
| Possible critical values: | < 0.5 or > 3 meq/L | |
| **Phosphate Normal Values** | | *Increased:* renal insufficiency; intake, IV solutions and enemas; blood transfusion; muscle necrosis; hypoparathyroidism; liver disease; rhabdomyolysis; sarcoidosis; and hemolytic anemia. *Decreased:* alcohol withdrawal; hyperventilation; diabetic ketoaci-dosis; phosphate-binding antacids; rickets; osteosarcoma; mal-nutrition; sepsis; and chronic alcoholism. |
| Adult: | 3.5–4.5 mg/dl | |
| Child: | 4.5–6.5 mg/dl | |
| Newborn: | 4.3–9.3 mg/dl | |
| Possible critical values: | < 1 mg/dl | |

Daniels, R. (2003). *Delmar's manual of laboratory and diagnostic tests.* Clifton Park, NY: Delmar Learning.

## TABLE 29-9 CPK ISOENZYMES

| Isoenzyme | Normal Range* | | Tissue Source |
|---|---|---|---|
| CPK₁ (BB) | 0% | 0 IU/l | Primarily in brain/indicative of cerebrovascular accident |
| CPK₂ (MB) | 0% | 0–7 IU/l | Exclusively in myocardium/indicative of myocardial infarction |
| CPK₃ (MM) | 100% | 5–70 IU/l | Found in skeleton and myocardium/skeletal muscle disorders |

*Data for normal range values from Daniels, R. (2003). *Delmar's manual of laboratory and diagnostic tests*. Clifton Park, NY: Delmar Learning.

## TABLE 29-10 LDH ISOENZYMES

| Isoenzyme | Range of % of Total LDH | Tissue Source |
|---|---|---|
| LDH₁ | 17–33 | Primarily in heart, kidneys, RBCs |
| LDH₂ | 27–37 | Primarily in heart, kidneys, RBCs |
| LDH₃ | 18–25 | Primarily in lungs, to a lesser extent in pancreas, thyroid, adrenal glands, lymph nodes |
| LDH₄ | 3–8 | Liver and skeletal tissue |
| LDH₅ | 0–5 | Liver and skeletal tissue |

Data for normal range values from Daniels, R. (2003). *Delmar's manual of laboratory and diagnostic tests*. Clifton Park, NY: Delmar Learning.

- Osteoblastic activity
- Hepatic tumors or abscess
- Impaired zinc status
- The response of vitamin D in the treatment of deficiency-induced rickets

Certain drugs can cause a mild to moderate elevation in the alkaline phosphatase (Box 29-6).

Acid phosphatase is an enzyme found primarily in the adult male prostate gland. It is used clinically to distinguish between encapsulated and metastatic carcinoma of the prostate gland. If the cancer cells are contained within a capsule, the acid phosphatase levels remain normal (0.2–0.8 IU/L).

Glucose-6-phosphate dehydrogenase is an RBC enzyme. The normal range and the clinical significance were shown in Table 29-7.

The main proteolytic enzymes for digestion are contained in the pancreatic juices (trypsin, chymotrypsin, and carboxypeptidase). The common laboratory tests for measuring the digestive enzymes are presented in Table 29-11.

**Cholinesterase** is an enzyme, manufactured in liver, that is responsible for the breakdown of acetylcholine and other choline esters. The normal range for cholinesterase in adults and children is 8–18 IU/L. It is elevated in diabetes, hyperthyroidism, and nephrotic syndrome. Decreases in cholinesterase can result from severe

## BOX 29-4 DRUGS THAT CAN ELEVATE ASPARTATE AMINOTRANSFERASE (AST)

- Antibiotics
- Contraceptives
- Cortisone
- Digitalis
- Flurazepam
- Guanthidine
- Indomethacin
- Isoniazid
- Mithramycin
- Narcotics
- Pyridoxine
- Rifampin
- Salicylate
- Theophylline
- Vitamin A

## BOX 29-5 ENZYMATIC CRITERIA FOR THE DIAGNOSIS OF ACUTE MYOCARDIAL INFARCTION (AMI)

- Serial increase, then decrease of plasma CK-MB, with changes greater than 25% between 2 values
- CK-MB is greater than 10–13 U/L or greater than 5% total CK activity
- Increase in CK-MB activity is greater than 50% between any two samples, separated by at least 4 hours.
- If only a single sample is available, CK-MB is more than twofold.
- Beyond 72 hours, an elevation of troponin T or I or LDH-1 is greater than LDH-2.

Daniels, R. (2003). *Delmar's manual of laboratory and diagnostic tests*. Clifton Park, NY: Delmar Learning.

## BOX 29-6    DRUGS THAT CAN ELEVATE ALKALINE PHOSPHATASE

- Allopurinol
- Antibiotics
- Ergosterol
- Estrogen
- Isoniazid
- Methyldopa
- Methyltestosterone
- Oral contraceptives
- Phenothiazine tranquilizers
- Procainamide
- Propranolol
- Sulfonamides
- Tolbutamide

## TABLE 29-11    DIGESTIVE ENZYMES

| Enzymes | Reference Range | Clinical Significance |
|---|---|---|
| Alanine amino-transferase | 0–30 IU/L | Hepatocellular damage |
| Aldolase | 0–8 IU/L | Anemia (hemo-lytic and mega-loblastic); granulocytic leukemia; metastatic carci-noma; skeletal muscle tissue damage |
| Amylase | Total: 40–220 IU/L | Pancreatitis |
| Aspartate amino-transferase | 0–35 IU/L | Hepatitis; infec-tious mononucle-osis; cirrhosis |
| Lipase | 0–1 Cherry-Crandell U/L | Acute pancreatitis |
| 5-Nucleotidase | 0–17 U/L | Biliary cirrhosis; extrahepatic obstruction; hepatic carcinoma |

Data for normal range values from Daniels, R. (2003). *Delmar's manual of laboratory and diagnostic tests*. Clifton Park, NY: Delmar Learning.

anemias and infections, exposure to some insecticides, liver disease, malnutrition, shock, and uremia.

## Blood Lipids

Coronary heart disease (CHD) is the number one killer of both men and women in the United States. According to the National Center for Health Statistics (NCHS), some 7 million Americans suffer from CHD and more than 500,000 Americans die of heart attacks each year caused by CHD (NCHS, 1999). The National Cholesterol Education Program (NCEP) and the American Heart Association have published guidelines and recommendations regarding the need to improve laboratory detection of hypercholesterolemia and treatment. Total blood cholesterol is the most common measurement of blood cholesterol. Cholesterol is measured in milligrams per deciliter of blood (mg/dl). Blood cholesterol for adults is classified by levels.

Exogenous cholesterol is present in the diet and absorbed into the gastrointestinal tract. Endogenous cholesterol is formed in the liver and other cells in the body. As much as 80% of cholesterol is converted into cholic acid to form bile salts. Cholesterol is also needed:

- Throughout the body for the formation of membranes
- By the adrenal glands to form adrenocortical hormones
- By the ovaries to form progesterone and estrogen
- By the testes to form testosterone
- By the skin to provide a water-soluble barrier

Cholesterol and other fats cannot dissolve in the blood; they have to be transported to and from the cells by special carriers called **lipoproteins** (blood lipids bound to protein). The types of lipoproteins are described below, but the ones to be most concerned about are low-density lipoprotein (LDL) and high-density lipoprotein (HDL).

- Chylomicrons—mainly ingested triglycerides
- Very low-density lipoproteins (VLDLs)—mainly endogenous triglycerides
- Low-density lipoproteins (LDLs)—moderate amounts of phospholipids with 50% cholesterol
- High-density lipoproteins (HDLs)—50% protein

LDL is the major cholesterol carrier in the blood. When too much LDL circulates in the blood, it can slowly build up in the walls of the arteries feeding the heart and brain. The buildup of LDL and other substances causes the formation of **atherosclerotic plaque**, a thick,

## CLINICAL ALERT

### Blood Enzyme Tests

Client must be fasting 1 to 2 hours before having a serum amylase drawn. If the client has eaten and received a narcotic at the same time, the serum results could be invalidated.

hard deposit that can clog the arteries in the heart and brain. A **thrombus** (a blood clot) can develop around the plaque that blocks the flow of blood to part of the heart muscle and causes a myocardial infarction (MI). If the thrombus blocks the flow of blood to part of the brain, it results in a cerebrovascular accident (CVA). High levels of LDL cholesterol (more than 130 mg/dl) increase the risk for CHD; this type of cholesterol is often called bad cholesterol.

HDL accounts for one-third to one-fourth of blood cholesterol and carries the cholesterol away from the arteries and back to the liver, where it is removed from the blood. HDL removes excess cholesterol from atherosclerotic plaques, slowing their growth. HDL is known as good cholesterol because a high level of HDL seems to decrease the risk of CHD.

Triglycerides are the chemical form in which most fat exists in food as well as in the body; they account for more than 90% of dietary intake and comprise 95% of fat stored in tissues (Fischbach, 2004). Triglycerides are insoluble in water and are the main plasma glycerol ester. An increase in triglyceride levels can be detected by plasma measurements; this test evaluates suspected atherosclerosis and measures the body's ability to metabolize fat.

Table 29-12 shows the relationship of lipids to a client being at risk for CHD. The practitioner must examine all of the lipid levels together. For instance, a client whose total cholesterol, LDL cholesterol, and triglycerides are all slightly elevated and whose HDL is slightly decreased is at a greater risk for CHD than someone whose cholesterol is elevated but whose HDL is also high.

The nurse must prepare clients for the lipid level testing. Education guidelines can be found in the Client Education box. Diurnal variation causes triglycerides to be lowest in the morning and highest around noon (Fischbach, 2004).

Several factors can affect the test results. The client's position, such as lying down, causes a redistribution between vascular and extravascular compartments. For instance, after 5 minutes in a recumbent position, total

## CLIENT EDUCATION

### Lipid Level Testing

✓ Eat a regular diet 3 to 7 days before the test.

✓ Fast 12 to 14 hours before the test.

✓ Refrain from vigorous exercise 24 hours before the test.

✓ Refrain from caffeine and nicotine 24 hours before the test.

✓ Per practitioner order, withhold drugs 24 hours before the test (many drugs affect the serum triglycerides level).

✓ Be aware that repeat tests may be necessary to confirm elevated levels, because results can vary 15% or more from day to day.

plasma cholesterol may be significantly reduced (10 to 15% decrease after 20 minutes). Recent trauma and severe infections may decrease the cholesterol level by 10% to 30%. Because pregnancy increases the HDL, LDL, and VLDL levels 20% to 30%, postpone testing 3 to 4 months postdelivery.

### Therapeutic Drug Monitoring

Therapeutic drug monitoring is performed when a quantitative relationship exists between the drug concentration and drug response or toxicity is known. For a drug concentration to be significant:

- It must be determined in a blood sample drawn after the drug has been completely absorbed from the oral or intramuscular route.
- It has had an opportunity to be distributed to its site of action.
- Its steady state has been reached (e.g., four to five half-lives must have passed).

| TABLE 29-12 | RELATIONSHIP OF LIPIDS TO CORONARY HEART DISEASE (CHD) RISK | | |
|---|---|---|---|
| Lipid | Desirable Level | Borderline CHD Risk | High CHD Risk |
| Cholesterol | < 200 mg/dl | 200–239 mg/dl | > 240 mg/dl |
| LDL Cholesterol | < 130 mg/dl | 130–159 mg/dl | > 160 mg/dl |
| HDL Cholesterol | > 40 mg/dl | 35–40 mg/dl | < 35 mg/dl |
| Triglyceride | < 250 mg/dl | 250–500 mg/dl | > 500 mg/dl |

Data from Daniels, R. (2003). *Delmar's manual of laboratory and diagnostic tests.* Clifton Park, NY: Delmar Learning.

For instance, with digoxin (a cardiac medication, administered on a daily schedule) the absorption and distribution phases may take 6 to 12 hours to complete. For a meaningful interpretation, the blood specimen should be drawn at least midway through the elimination phase (6 hours before the next dose). If the specimen is drawn just before the next dose, one obtains a trough concentration, whereas a specimen drawn 6 to 12 hours after dosing yields a peak concentration. For digoxin, the swing between peak and trough would be expected to be minimal because the drug is given at intervals that are less than the drug's terminal half-life (42 ± 19 hours). Generally, such sampling is most significant after steady state has been reached (about 8 days for digoxin). Trough and peak sampling help the practitioner to determine the dose rate, keeping the drug level below toxic value.

## Arterial Blood Gases

Blood gas results are reported in millimeters of mercury (Hg). Normal ABG ranges are:

- $PO_2$  75–100 mm Hg
- $PCO_2$  35–45 mm Hg
- pH  7.35–7.45

The clinical interpretation of gases studies the relationship between the gases. For example, a low $PO_2$ combined with a high $PCO_2$ may indicate bronchiole obstruction or that the alveoli are filled with fluid. In both situations, there is an impairment of gaseous exchange. See Chapter 39 for a complete discussion.

## Urine Tests

The primary function of the kidneys is to rid the body of waste products and to maintain homeostasis through regulation of the acid-base balance, fluid and electrolyte balance, and arterial blood pressure. Urine leaves the kidneys through the ureters. Peristaltic waves move the waste products through the ureters to the bladder. Normally, the bladder stores 200–400 ml of urine; however, its capacity is greater.

Urinalysis (UA) is an essential part of an examination for both diagnostic and preventive purposes. A UA is easy to collect and can be a valuable screening procedure. The kidneys have the ability to regulate sodium and urine concentration and dilution in accordance with the needs of the individual. The main urine constituents are water, urea, uric acid, creatinine, ammonia, sulfates, sodium, potassium, chloride, calcium, magnesium, and phosphate. Other kidney filtrates found in the urine include hormones, vitamins, and medications. The urine may also contain other constituents indicative of disease such as RBCs and WBCs, casts, crystals, mucus, bacteria, protein, glucose, and ketones. See Table 29-13 for normal values.

Although laboratories provide a wide range of urine tests, some types of tablet, tapes, and dipstick tests for UA can be performed outside the laboratory setting (Table 29-13). Kerr, Marshall, and Sinclair (1999) conducted a study

to determine if there was a difference in the urine results obtained by the emergency department physician as compared with the results obtained by a trained laboratory technician. On comparison, the results were similar for both dipstick and microscopic components of urinalysis: red blood cell urinalysis and microscopy, leukocyte esterase, and nitrite testing; however, emergency physicians were not able to consistently perform UA for microscopic white cells and bacteria, and testing for proteinuria.

## Urine pH

The pH is governed by the hydrogen ion concentration of the urine. Disorders such as diabetes mellitus, dehydration, diarrhea, emphysema, and starvation make the urine acidic. Chronic renal failure, renal tubular acidosis, urinary tract infections, and salicylate poisoning cause the urine to be alkaline.

## Specific Gravity

Specific gravity measures the number of solutes in a solution. Urea and uric acid (the by-products of nitrogen metabolism) have the greatest influence on the specific gravity of urine. A urinometer and cylinder are used to measure the specific gravity. The urinometer has a specific gravity scale and a weighted mercury bulb. A fresh urine specimen is poured into the cylinder. The nurse inserts and twirls the urinometer into the cylinder. The depth of the urinometer is determined by the concentration of dissolved analytes. When the urinometer stops spinning, the nurse reads the urinometer at eye level.

The specific gravity increases with conditions that increase the loss of fluids from the body, such as diabetes mellitus, gastrointestinal fluid losses, third-space fluid accumulation, and fear or anxiety. Decreases in the specific gravity result from renal disease. When the amount of urine increases and the specific gravity decreases, there is an absence of the antidiuretic hormone (ADH), usually triggered by diabetes insipidus (a disorder of the posterior pituitary gland).

## Urine Glucose

When the blood levels of glucose exceed the renal threshold (180 mg/dl), glucose spills into the urine. Multiple agents are available for measuring the glucose content of urine. These agents are not as accurate a test method as blood glucose levels.

Some of the reducing agents can measure other products, such as protein and blood, along with the glucose (Clinitest and Clinistix). Each product has specific step-by-step instructions for performing the test and reading the results. Teach the client how to perform these urine tests.

## Urine Ketones

**Ketones** are products of fatty acid metabolism and are completely metabolized by the liver under normal conditions. The most common cause of ketonuria is diabetes.

## TABLE 29-13   NORMAL URINE FINDINGS

| | |
|---|---|
| Appearance | Clear |
| Color | Amber yellow |
| Odor | Aromatic |
| pH | 4.6–8.0 (average 6.0) |
| Protein | None or up to 8 mg/dl<br>50–80 mg/dl (at rest)<br>< 250 mg/dl (exercise) |
| Specific gravity | Adult: 1.005–1.030 or usually 1.010–1.025<br><br>Elderly: values decrease with age<br><br>Newborn: 1.001–1.020 |
| Leukocyte esterase | Negative |
| Nitrites | Negative |
| Ketones | Negative |
| Crystals | Negative |
| Casts | None present |
| Glucose | Negative |
| White blood cells (WBC) | 0–4 per low-power field |
| WBC casts | Negative |
| Red blood cells (RBC) | Up to 2 |
| RBC casts | None |

Daniels, R. (2003). *Delmar's manual of laboratory and diagnostic tests.* Clifton Park, NY: Delmar Learning.

However, with strenuous exercise, starvation, and sustained febrile and hypoxic conditions, an increase in fatty acid metabolism causes ketoacidosis, resulting in ketone bodies in the urine.

## Urine Cells and Casts

Normally the urine is free from blood cells and casts. When the renal system is impaired as in renal damage or failure, nephritis, and stones and infections in the urinary tract, the following can occur:

- Bleeding with resulting RBCs in the urine
- Accumulation of epithelial cells with cast formation
- WBCs, which indicate infections

## Stool Tests

Stool analysis is used to determine the various constituents of the stool for diagnostic purposes such as diseases of the gastrointestinal tract, the liver, and the pancreas. Normal constituents of the stool are urobilinogen, porphyrins, sodium, chloride, potassium, and small amounts of nitrogen and lipids. The most frequent tests ordered on feces include leukocytes, blood, fat, ova and parasites, and pathogens.

### Urobilinogen

**Urobilinogen** is derived from the normal bacterial action of intestinal flora on bilirubin. It is increased with severe hemolysis of RBCs and decreased with most biliary obstructions.

### Occult Blood

When blood is invisible on inspection, it is said to be **occult**; it is blood that can only be detected through a microscope or by chemical means. In the gastrointestinal tract, the digestive process acts on blood, making it occult. Random sampling for occult blood is done to diagnose gastrointestinal bleeding, ulcers, and malignant tumors. Colorectal cancer is a leading cause of cancer deaths in the United States. Most colorectal cancers begin as a **polyp**, a small abnormal growth of tissue, in the wall of the colon. As the polyp grows, it may cause bleeding from the rectum, blood in the stool, or a change in the shape of the stool. Screening for colorectal cancer begins with fecal occult blood testing. The 2003 U.S. Preventive Services Task Force (USPSTF, 2003b) strongly recommends colon cancer screening by fecal occult blood testing for both men and women at 50 years of age or older. Any person age 50 years or older but asymptomatic is considered average risk for colorectal cancer. The risk factors increase when one or more of the following exist:

- Close relative(s) who have had colorectal cancer or an adenomatous polyp
- Family history of adenomatous polyposis
- Family history of hereditary nonpolyposis colorectal cancer
- History of adenomatous polyps
- History of colorectal cancer
- Inflammatory bowel disease

See Box 29-7 for the complete set of guidelines for colorectal screening as developed by the American Cancer Society, the American College of Gastroenterology, and the American Society of Gastrointestinal Endoscopists.

When the practitioner is using occult blood to confirm suspicions of a gastrointestinal disorder, the client is placed on a 3-day diet free of meat, poultry, and fish to decrease the possibility of a false-positive result. Fresh fruits and vegetables such as melons, turnips, horseradish, and others can also cause a false positive. Common drugs that can cause a positive test for occult blood are salicylate, steroids, and indomethacin.

## BOX 29-7    GUIDELINES FOR COLORECTAL SCREENING

| Risk Category | Recommendations |
|---|---|
| Average | Fecal occult blood screening yearly, starting at 50 years of age |
| | Flexible sigmoidoscopy every 5 years or colonoscopy every 10 years or double-contrast barium enema every 5 to 10 years |
| Increased Risk | Same as above, but screening is initiated when the client is 40 years of age |
| | Genetic counseling/testing |
| | In a gene carrier, flexible sigmoidoscopy every 12 months, beginning at puberty |
| | Genetic counseling/testing |
| | Examination of the entire colon every 1 to 2 years, starting when the client is 20 to 30 years old |
| | Examination of the entire colon yearly after the client is 40 years old |
| | Colonoscopy 3 years after initial examination, with subsequent examinations, depending on the types of polyps detected |
| | Complete examination 1 year after colon surgery; if normal, reexamination of colon in 3 years; if still normal, reexamination in 5 years |
| | Surveillance colonoscopy every 1 to 2 years, beginning after 8 years of disease in the client with pancolitis and after 15 years in the client with left colon involvement only |

From Johnson, B. A. (1999). Flexible sigmoidoscopy for colorectal cancer. *American Family Physician*, Jan. 15, 1999.

## Parasites

The gastrointestinal tract can harbor parasites and their eggs (ova). Some of these parasites are harmless, whereas others cause clinical symptoms. With the exception of pinworms (which can enter the body through both the oral and anal routes), all other common parasites gain portal entry through the mouth by ingestion of contaminated water or food. Roundworm, hookworm, whipworm, tapeworm, *Trichinella spiralis,* and *Entamoeba histolytica* are common parasites found in the United States.

## Culture and Sensitivity Tests

**Culture** refers to the growing of microorganisms to identify the pathogen. Culture and sensitivity (C&S) tests are performed to identify both the nature of the invading organisms and their susceptibility to commonly used antibiotics. Sensitivity allows the practitioner to select the appropriate antibiotic therapy. All C&S specimens should be taken immediately to the laboratory.

## Blood Culture

**Bacteremia** is the condition of bacteria in the blood. The blood culture should be obtained while the client is experiencing chills and fever. A series of three venipuncture collections is performed using strict sterile technique; change the needle after the specimen is collected before injecting the blood sample into the test tube.

## Swab (Throat) Culture

The throat normally colonizes many organisms. Throat cultures serve to isolate and identify such pathogens as ß-hemolytic streptococci, *Staphylococcus aureus,* meningococci, gonococci, *Bordetella pertussis,* and *Corynebacterium diphtheria.* A throat swab is commonly done to identify streptococcal infections, which, if untreated, can cause rheumatic fever or glomerulonephritis.

To obtain a throat swab, use a wooden blade to depress the tongue and swab the white patches, exudate, or ulcerations of the throat with a sterile applicator. Avoid touching other parts of the mouth with the swab. Once obtained, place the applicator in a sterile container.

## Sputum Culture

Sputum tests are done for culture, smear, and cytology. Sputum is created by the mucous glands and goblet cells of the tracheobronchial tree and is raised by coughing. Sputum is sterile until it reaches the throat and mouth where it comes in contact with normal flora. Sputum can be obtained by tracheobronchial suctioning and transtracheal aspiration, producing a more accurate identification of pulmonary organisms.

A sputum smear will identify the same organism found in a culture plus eosinophils, epithelial cells, and other substances. Smears are helpful in diagnosing asthma (eosinophils) and fungal infection. The specimen needs to be refrigerated if it cannot be taken immediately to the laboratory.

Sputum can also be examined for **cytology** (the study of cells). It is performed to diagnose cancer of the lungs. The specimen should be collected early in the morning after a deep cough.

## Urine Culture

Urinary C&S tests are performed whenever a urinary tract infection is suspected. Organisms enter the urinary system by one of two ways:

1. Ascending urinary tract infections are associated with *Escherichia coli* and *Candida albicans* from the rectum, vagina, and catheterization.
2. Descending sources are caused from staphylococcus and streptococcus entering the urinary system from the blood.

## Stool Culture

Stool C&S is performed to identify bacterial infections. If the client has diarrhea, a rectal swab can be taken as a specimen; fecal material must be visible on the swab for the laboratory to perform the test.

## Wound Culture

Clinical specimens taken from abscesses or infected wounds reveal a variety of aerobic and anaerobic microorganisms. Because anaerobic microorganisms are the preponderant microflora in humans and are consistently present in the upper respiratory, gastrointestinal, and genitourinary tracts, they are also likely to invade other parts of the body to cause severe, and sometimes fatal, infections (Fischbach, 2004). Pathogens are likely to be present in the following wound specimens: pus, necrotic tissue, debrided material, postoperative wound drainage, lower-extremity ulcers, and pressure ulcers. Use Standard Precautions when obtaining a wound culture. Most wounds require some form of preparation prior to culturing a wound.

## Bone Marrow

Bone marrow specimens are examined by either culture or smear for identification of microorganisms. Smear slides are prepared at the client's bedside by the nurse.

## Papanicolaou Test

**Papanicolaou test** (smear method of examining stained exfoliative cells), commonly called a Pap smear, is done to evaluate the cell maturity, metabolic activity, and morphologic variations of the cervical tissue. Papanicolaou testing can also be used for tissue specimens from other organs, such as bronchial aspirations and gastric secretions.

Cervical Pap smear testing is recommended every 2 to 3 years after the onset of sexual activity. Annual testing is indicated for women:

- Over 40 years of age
- With a family history of cervical cancer
- With a previous positive test

To increase the accuracy of a cervical specimen, the client should be told to avoid intercourse, douches, and vaginal creams for 24 hours before the test. The vaginal speculum should not be lubricated. This test should not be performed if the client is menstruating because the specimen will be unsuitable for cytologic study.

# Radiologic Studies

**Radiography** (the study of x-rays or gamma ray-exposed film through the action of ionizing radiation) is used by the practitioner to study internal organ structure. **Fluoroscopy** (the immediate, serial images of the body's structure and function) is used to demonstrate the motion of organs when used with **contrast medium** (a radiopaque substance that facilitates roentgen imaging of the body's internal structures). X-rays are valuable to the practitioner in either formulating a diagnosis (e.g., pneumonia) or as a tool to determine if other studies are necessary (e.g., lung lesion requiring biopsy to differentiate between a benign or malignant tumor).

Certain radiologic tests will require a contrast medium that could interfere with other diagnostic studies. Barium and iodine are commonly used contrast media. Laboratory blood samples measuring the thyroid function should be drawn before an intravenous pyelogram (IVP) where radioactive iodine dye is administered. If the client needs both an IVP and barium enema, the IVP is done first because the barium is likely to decrease the visualization of the kidneys.

Precautions need to be taken to ensure client safety, particularly in the elderly. It is essential during history taking that the client be questioned about the possibility of pregnancy, asthma, and allergic reactions to contrast media (iodine) as well as to other foods and drugs. If the client has never received iodine, this should be noted on the requisition.

## Chest X-Ray

The most common radiologic study is the noninvasive, non-contrasted chest x-ray. The best results are obtained when the films are taken in the radiology department; however, a portable chest x-ray can be performed at the bedside.

Radiographic projection positions of chest x-ray films are taken from various views (Figure 29-16). Multiple views of the chest are necessary for the practitioner to assess the entire lung field. To prepare the client for a chest x-ray,

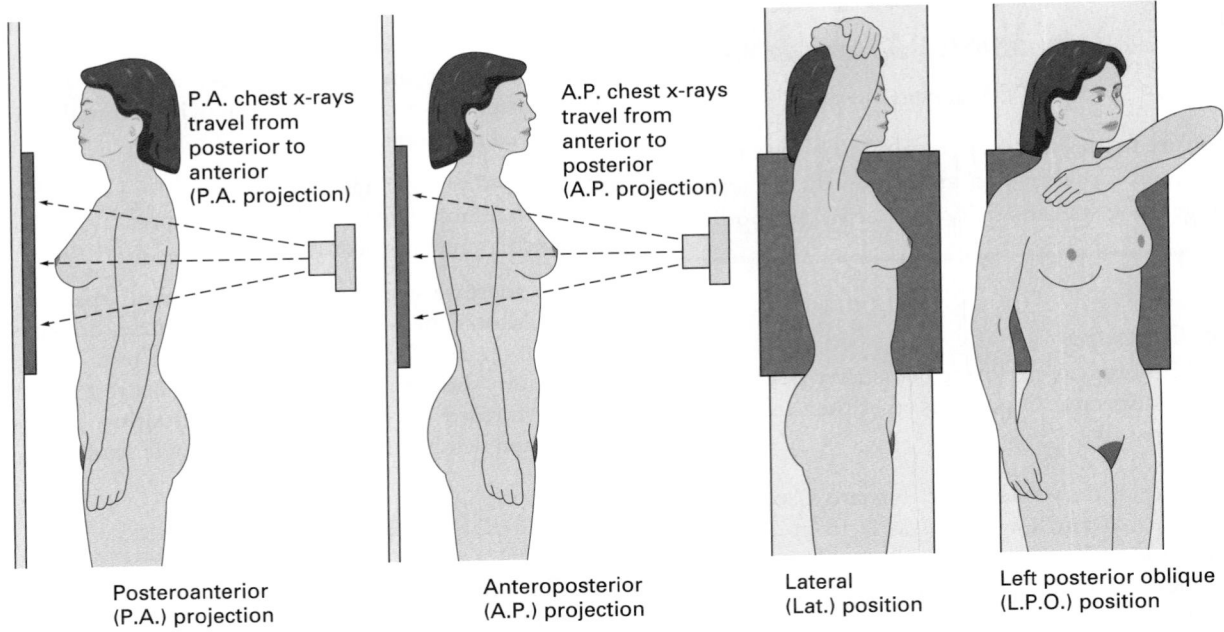

**Figure 29-16    Radiographic projection positions**

remove metal objects (jewelry) and all clothing from the waist up and replace with a gown. Metal will appear on the x-ray film, thereby obscuring visualization of parts of the chest. Pregnant women are draped with a metal apron to protect the fetus.

Chest films can indicate the following alterations and diseases:

- Lesions (tumors, cysts, masses) in the lung tissue, chest wall, bony thorax, or heart
- Inflammation of lung tissue (pneumonia, atelectasis, abscesses, tuberculosis), pleura (pleuritis), and pericardium (pericarditis)
- Fluid accumulation in the lung tissue (pulmonary edema, hemothorax), pleura (pleural effusion), and pericardium (pericardial effusion)
- Bone deformities and fractures of the rib and sternum
- Air accumulation in the lungs (chronic obstructive pulmonary disease, emphysema), and pleura (pneumothorax)
- Diaphragmatic hernia

## Kidney-Ureter-Bladder

A kidney-ureter-bladder, also known as a KUB (x-ray of the abdomen), is used to visualize the kidney, ureter, and bladder and sometimes the gallbladder, liver, and spleen. The results can reveal congenital abnormalities, enlarged organs, lesions, and obstructions.

## Mammography

**Mammography** (a low-dose radiographic study of breast tissue) is used to reveal congenital abnormalities and

lesions. The American Cancer Society (2002) recommends a baseline mammogram by age 40, followed by a mammogram every 2 years until age 50, and every year after age 50.

## Skeletal X-Rays

Skeletal x-rays are taken of any bony processes to reveal congenital abnormalities, fractures, joint and spine abnormalities, and degeneration (arthritis).

## Computed Tomography

**Computed tomography (CT)** is the radiologic scanning of the body with x-ray beams and radiation detectors that transmit data to a computer that transcribes the data into quantitative measurement and multidimensional images of the internal structures. Figure 29-17 demonstrates the directions of sagittal, transverse, and coronal planes taken during CT scanning.

CT scan may be performed with or without intravenous (IV) contrast media. A written consent from the client is required with the used of IV contrast media. An abdominal or pelvic CT scan will also usually require the client to take barium sulfate, an oral contrast, between 1 and 4 hours prior to the procedure, and immediately before the procedure to allow the contrast to pass through the intestines (Daniels, 2003). Because the client will be positioned on the scanning table and told to remain motionless, the client's cooperation is essential during the scanning. Prepare the client with an explanation and pictures of what to expect. Assess the client's ability to relax and review imagery relaxation. Sedation can be administered with an order from the practitioner.

## CLINICAL ALERT

### Computed Tomography

Because of the use of contrast media during CT to improve the images yielded by the equipment, the nurse must observe the client after the procedure for indicators of allergic dye reactions such as respiratory distress, urticaria, hives, nausea, vomiting, decreased production of urine (**oliguria**) and decreased blood pressure.

Clients who will receive a contrast medium need to be kept NPO 2 to 4 hours before the test. The client should void before the test, unless the pelvic area is to be studied. A full bladder enhances visualization of the pelvic area.

## Barium Studies

**Barium** (a chalky white contrast medium) is an oral preparation that allows for roentgenographic visualization of the internal structures of the digestive tract. The results of barium studies can reveal congenital abnormalities; lesions; spasm, reflux, stricture, and obstruction; inflammation and ulceration; varices; and fistula. General client preparation for barium studies should include:

- Placing the client on NPO status after midnight
- Administering a laxative the evening before and enemas the morning of the test
- Forcing fluid postprocedure
- Follow-up 2 to 3 days postprocedure to ensure the client has had a normal brown stool

Postprocedure barium will be expelled in the stool, making it milky white. Fluids are forced to help with the excretion of barium. If the barium is not completely excreted, it can cause an intestinal obstruction.

### Barium Swallow

**Barium swallow** (also called esophography) is a fluoroscopic visualization of the esophagus following the ingestion of barium sulfate. Implement the nursing care discussed above for a client having a barium study.

### Upper Gastrointestinal Study

Upper gastrointestinal (UGI) study is a fluoroscopic visualization of the stomach and small bowel following the ingestion of barium sulfate. In addition to the general preparation of the client for a barium study, also instruct the client:

- Not to smoke 24 hours before the procedure (smoking causes an increased production of gastric juices)
- That during the procedure (which will last approximately 2 hours), pictures will be taken at 30-minute intervals with the client in different positions

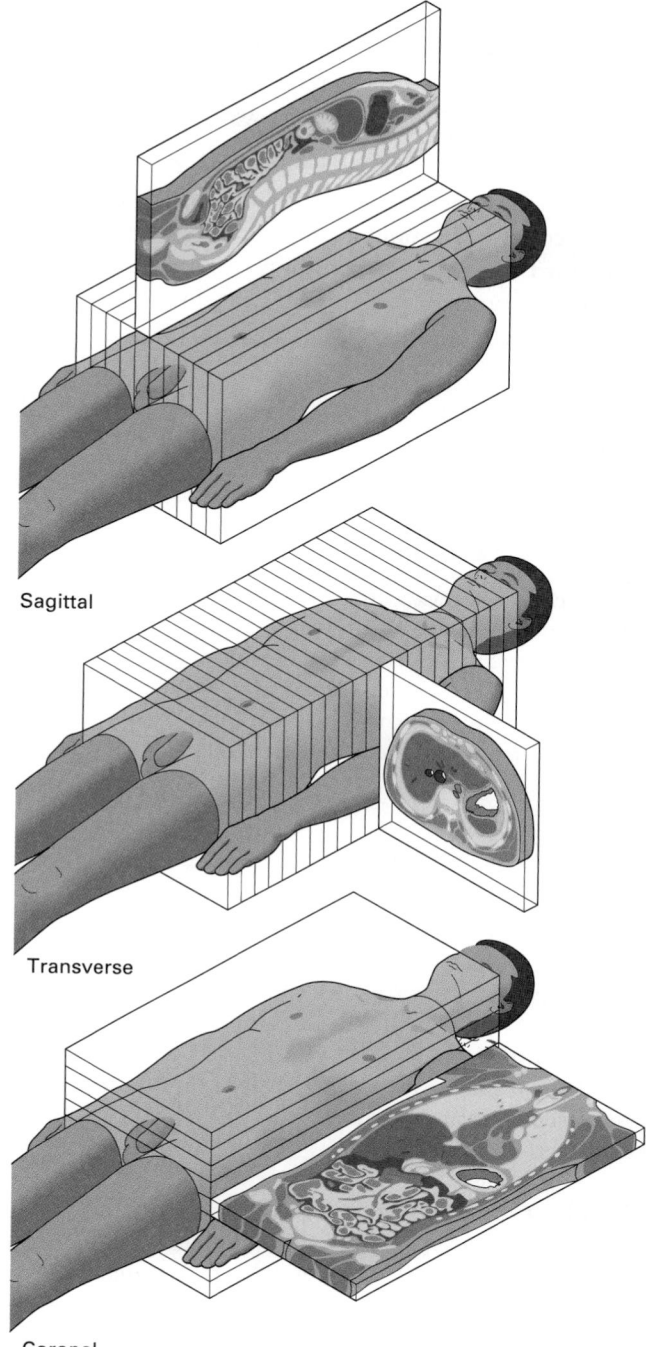

Sagittal

Transverse

Coronal

**Figure 29-17    Computed tomography (CT)**

### Barium Enema

**Barium enema** (a rectal infusion of barium sulfate) is the roentgenographic study of the lower intestinal tract. The colon should be free of all fecal material to allow for maximum visualization. Instruct the client:

- To eat a low residue diet 2 days prior to the test
- That during the procedure various positions will need to be assumed on the table to facilitate movement of the barium in the intestines

## CLINICAL ALERT

### Enema

Clients with severe abdominal pain, ulcerative colitis, or a history of a megacolon should have a written order before enemas can be administered, because these conditions would normally prohibit the use of standard bowel preparation procedures such as administration of laxatives and cleansing enemas.

- That the test will take about 1 hour
- That the postprocedure cleansing enemas will be given to help remove the barium

## Angiography

**Angiography** allows visualization of the vascular structures through the use of fluoroscopy with a contrast medium. It is performed in radiology or diagnostic studies departments. The test reveals the blood flow to the heart, lungs, brain, kidneys, and lower extremities. It is also useful in diagnosing an **aneurysm** (weakness in the wall of a blood vessel).

## Arteriography

**Arteriography** is the radiographic study of the vascular system following the injection of a radiopaque dye through a catheter. The practitioner uses fluoroscopy to thread the catheter through a peripheral artery into the area to be studied, such as the aorta or the cerebral, coronary, pulmonary, renal, iliac, femoral, or popliteal arteries. The client is placed on a cardiac monitor. Dye is injected in a vascular catheter with a rapid sequence of films to visualize the vasculature.

### Cardiac Catheterization

**Cardiac catheterization** is a radiographic study with the use of a contrast medium injected into a vascular catheter that is threaded into the heart and coronary or pulmonary vessels. The client is placed in a supine position and connected to a cardiac monitor.

The peripheral site, either the groin or brachial area, is prepped and injected with xylocaine. A catheter is inserted and threaded:

- Right-sided catheterization—into the right atrium, ventricle and pulmonary artery
- Left-sided catheterization—into the aorta to the coronary arteries or the left ventricle

The study includes pressure measurements, blood gas sampling, and viewing the integrity of the heart's valves. For postcatheterization procedures, see the Nursing Strategy box.

## RESEARCH FOCUS

**Title of Study:** Financial impact of elimination of routine chest radiographs in a pediatric intensive care unit

**Study Purpose:** To determine the change in chest radiograph use if each chest radiograph requires a separate order and clinical indications

**Methods:** A prospective, nonrandomized, controlled design with an intervention study was conducted in a pediatric intensive care unit (PICU) at a children's hospital. The study comprised 3,727 PICU clients treated between 1992 and 1996. The study's interventions were a change in ordering practice: no standing orders for routine daily morning chest radiographs; each radiograph required a written order and clinical indication for ordering the chest radiograph. During a 29-month control phase when routine daily chest radiographs were obtained for all intubated clients, 1.026 chest radiographs per client day were performed. After the intervention, the ratio dropped to 0.653 chest radiographs per client day, a decrease of 36.4% and a cost savings of $45,476.

**Findings:** The study results demonstrated the outcome of an evaluation and subsequent change in radiology ordering practice; the change resulted in decreased variability in ordering practice, fewer chest radiographs per client, and a cost savings to the clients and payers.

**Implications:** This study is the beginning effort to validate the need for diagnostic testing versus standing orders for routine testing. Other routine tests need to be studied regarding outcome measures that include client safety and health promotion.

Price, M. B., Grant, M. J., & Welkie, K. (1999). Financial impact of elimination of routine chest radiographs in a pediatric intensive care unit. *Critical Care Medicine, 27*(8), 1588–1593.

## Digital Subtraction Angiography

**Digital subtraction angiography** is a computerized imaging of the vasculature with visualization on a monitor screen after the intravenous injection of iodine through a catheter. The results reveal the presence of vascular malformations (stenosis, occlusion, obstruction, ulceration, plaques, and aneurysms), lesions, and emboli.

## Lymphangiography

**Lymphangiography** is a radiographic study of the lymphatic system after a catheter injection of an oil-based dye.

## CLIENT REFLECTIONS

### Worried About a CT Scan

Mr. Tillotson is about to have a CT scan as one of several diagnostic procedures associated with his non-Hodgkins lymphoma. He states, "I've heard friends of mine say that I will be locked in a big tube (CT machine) for a long time. I have problems with claustrophobia and tight places, so I am pretty worried. My hip hurts and I am concerned that the pain will make me move and that will make the test bad—and I don't want to have to repeat the CT scan."

What would you say to this client?

A lymphatic vessel is first identified with an intradermal injection of a blue dye into either the foot or hand, depending on the area to be studied. The results reveal the presence of a lymphoma, metastatic disease, and the degree of edema in lymphatic tissue.

## Venography

**Venography** is a radiographic study of the venous system of the lower extremities after the injection of an iodine contrast agent. A venogram reveals both the presence and degree of trauma or disease (e.g., incompetent valves) to a vein, soft tissue compression, and the presence of thrombi.

## LIFE SPAN CONSIDERATIONS

### Performing Radiologic Studies in the Elderly

Older persons may find it somewhat difficult to remain motionless during lengthy radiologic studies or to assume certain positions on their own. For example, some x-rays require the client to stand upright during the procedure. The care providers must take precautions to support the client during the procedure, especially if the older client is fatigued or ill. In addition, the older client may easily get cold while lying down on a flat x-ray table. Care should be implemented to cover the client with blankets whenever possible during this type of situation.

Daniels, R. (2003). *Delmar's manual of laboratory and diagnostic tests.* Clifton Park, NY: Delmar Learning.

## NURSING STRATEGY

### Postcatheterization Care

Postcatheterization care should include:

1. Assessment of the client's laboratory results to include complete blood count (CBC), platelet count, prothrombin time (PT), international normalized ratio (INR), and partial thromboplastin time (PTT).
2. Assessment of the client's electrocardiogram (ECG) rhythm and vital signs.
3. Administration of medications to maintain systolic blood pressure 150 mm Hg.
4. Assessment of the client's extremity distal to the arterial sheath for quality and strength of pulses, color, temperature, sensation, and movement.
5. Administration of pain medication to ensure client's comfort.
6. Monitoring of client's hemodynamic status before, during, and after sheath removal.
7. Assessment for complications such as hematoma, bleeding, pseudoaneurysm, vagal response, hemodynamic instability, and impaired perfusion to the extremity distal to the site of sheath removal, and angina.

Daniels, R. (2003). *Delmar's manual of laboratory and diagnostic tests.* Clifton Park, NY: Delmar Learning.

## Dye Injection Studies

Iodine is a common dye used in radiographic studies. Iodine injection might cause the client to experience temporary symptoms of shortness of breath, nausea, and a warm, hot-flushed sensation. Most dye injection studies are invasive, requiring written consent. General guidelines for a client receiving a dye injection study should include:

- Preprocedure—NPO 6 to 12 hours before testing.
- Postprocedure—drink 2,500 ml of water daily to encourage dye excretion. Notify the practitioner of decreased urinary output, bleeding, and signs of infection.

Test findings can reveal congenital abnormalities, lesions, inflammation, stones, obstruction, and organ-specific disorders.

## Cholangiography

**Cholangiography** is the roentgenographic procedure visualizing the integrity of the biliary system by a radiopaque contrast medium. There are three methods of performing a cholangiogram: intravenous, percutaneous, and direct injection into a **T-tube** (an artificial drain placed in common bile duct during surgery). The client is placed NPO 8 to 12 hours before the test with a cleansing enema the evening before.

## Intravenous Cholangiography

Intravenous Chologaffin (contrast agent) is administered with photographs taken every 15 to 30 minutes until the common bile ducts are visualized. If the gallbladder has not been removed, a fatty meal is given the evening before. The x-ray films are taken to show the contraction of the dye in the gallbladder.

## Percutaneous Cholangiography

The percutaneous method for performing a cholangiogram requires the contrast agent to be injected directly into the liver tissue. A venous catheter or long needle is inserted into the liver tissue during fluoroscopy. For this method, the client must have a normal prothrombin time and platelet count before the procedure.

Postprocedure the client is placed on bed rest. Assess the insertion site for bleeding. Clients are at risk for bile peritonitis. Instruct the client to report immediately to the practitioner if any of the following symptoms occur: abdominal pain, distension and rigidity; chills and fever; and nausea or vomiting.

## T-Tube Cholangiography

T-tube cholangiography requires the instillation of iodine to visualize the patency of the hepatic and common bile ducts. The client is at risk for bile peritonitis.

## Oral Cholecystography

**Oral cholecystography** is the visualization of the gallbladder and presence of stones through the administration of radiopaque iodine tablets. The evening before the test, the client eats a fatty meal and takes the iodine tablets 5 minutes apart with 8 ounces of water. The number of tablets administered is based on weight.

## Cystography

**Cystography** is a radiographic study that uses an aqueous iodine contrast agent instilled into the bladder through a urinary catheter. It is used to visualize the bladder, urethra,

and ureteral openings. Postprocedure, instruct the client on how to monitor urinary output and to notify the practitioner of bleeding, decreased output, and signs of infection.

## Intravenous Pyelogram

An **intravenous pyelogram** (IVP) is a series of x-ray films of the kidneys, ureters, and bladder following the administration of an intravenous iodine preparation. The test may reveal organ specific disorders such as hydronephrosis, polycystic disease, chronic pyelonephritis, and acute renal failure.

## Bronchography

**Bronchography** is a radiographic study of the trachea and bronchi following the injection of a contrast agent through a catheter. Before the insertion of the catheter, the client is given a local anesthetic agent to sedate the gag and swallow reflex. The test may reveal bronchiectasis.

## Myelography

**Myelography** is the study of the spinal cord and its surrounding subarachnoid spaces through the use of radiography and Pantopaque (contrast agent). *Strict aseptic technique is used throughout the procedure.* This test is performed in the radiology department with the client on a tilt table.

To inject the Pantopaque dye, the practitioner has to access the subarachnoid space by performing a posterior lumbar puncture.

The practitioner inserts a needle with a stylet between the vertebrae to access the subarachnoid space. The stylet is removed, and a pressure reading is taken of the cerebrospinal fluid (CSF). If the CSF pressure is elevated, the test is stopped. Otherwise, the dye is injected. The table is tilted into various up and down positions. Changing position allows the dye to flow within the subarachnoid space. X-ray films are taken to reveal compression or herniated intervertebral discs and tumors.

# Ultrasonography

**Ultrasound** (echogram) is a noninvasive study that uses high-frequency sound waves to visualize deep body structures. This test should be scheduled before any studies using a contrast medium or air to ensure accuracy, because an ultrasound *does not* require any contrast medium. The client is instructed to lie still during the procedure.

Ultrasound is used to evaluate the brain, thyroid gland, heart, vascular structure, abdominal aorta, spleen, liver, gallbladder, pancreas, and pelvis. An ultrasound is commonly done during pregnancy to evaluate the size of the fetus and placenta; a full bladder is needed to ensure visualization. Instruct the mother to drink 3 to 4 glasses (200–350 ml) of water 1 hour before the exam and to hold voiding until after the pelvic ultrasound.

A coupling agent (lubricant) is placed on the surface of the body area to be studied to increase the contact between the skin and the **transducer** (instrument that converts electrical energy to sound waves). The transducer emits waves that travel through the body tissue and are reflected back to the transducer and recorded. The varying density of body tissues deflects the waves into a differentiated pattern on an oscilloscope. Photographs can be taken of the sound wave pattern on the oscilloscope.

## Echocardiograms

**Echocardiography** is a noninvasive procedure used to evaluate the function and structures of the heart. This procedure is used to diagnose pericardial effusion, valvular heart disease, subaortic stenosis, myocardial wall abnormalities, cardiac tumors, infarction, and aneurysms. Echocardiography is also a method of choice in cardiac stress testing. During the exercise or chemical stress test, the ischemic muscles are evident. A newer form of echocardiography is by insertion of an endoscopic probe through the esophagus, referred to as transesophageal echocardiography (TEE).

## Doppler Ultrasonography

**Doppler** (a handheld transducer) transmits high-frequency sound waves to the artery or vein being studied. The sound waves strike the moving RBCs and are reflected back to the transducer, which amplifies the sound and produces a graphic recording. Doppler ultrasonography reveals blood clots and peripheral vascular disease.

## Magnetic Resonance Imaging

**Magnetic resonance imaging** (MRI) is a noninvasive diagnostic scanning procedure that places the client in a magnetic field instead of ionizing radiation. MRI is based on the behavior of hydrogen atoms in the body that are placed in a magnetic field and disturbed by radiofrequency signals. MRI provides better contrast between normal tissue and pathologic tissue than CT scan. MRI is useful in evaluating lesions, and changes in the body's organs, tissues, and vascular and skeletal structures. MRI is contraindicated for clients with implantable metal objects (pacemakers, infusion pumps, aneurysm clips, etc.) and for clients who weigh 300 lbs., or are confused/agitated, claustrophobic, or unstable requiring continuous life support.

## Radioactive Studies

Radionuclide imaging (nuclear scanning) uses radionuclides (or radiopharmaceuticals) to image the morphologic and functional changes in the body's structure. A scintigraphic scanner is placed over the area of study to detect the radiation emission and to produce a visual image of the structure on film. Radiopharmaceutical agents are administered by various routes with consideration given to time delays of absorption. The results reveal congenital abnormalities, lesions, skeletal changes, infections, and gland and organ enlargement.

## Electrodiagnostic Studies

These diagnostic tests use devices to measure the electrical activity of the heart, brain, and skeletal muscles. Electrical sensors (electrodes) are placed at certain anatomic points to measure the tone, velocity, and direction of the impulses. The impulses are then transmitted to an oscilloscope or printed on graphic paper.

## Electrocardiography

An **electrocardiogram** (**ECG** or **EKG**) is a graphic recording of the heart's electrical activity. The client may be asked not to smoke or drink caffeinated beverages 24 hours before the test. Nicotine and caffeine can affect the heart rate.

Electrodes are applied to the chest wall and extremities. A lubricating gel applied to the electrodes increases the conduction of electrical activity between the skin and electrode. The client is instructed to lie still during the painfree test. The test can reveal abnormal transmission of impulses and electrical position of the heart's axis.

A portable cardiac monitor (Holter monitor) is a device that records the heart's electrical activity. It produces a continuous recording over a specified period of time (e.g., 24 hours). The portable unit allows the client to ambulate and perform regular activities. Clients are instructed to maintain a log of activities that occur when they feel their heart beating faster or irregularly. The practitioner reviews the ECG tracing in relation to the client's log to determine if certain activities, such as walking, are associated with abnormal transmission of impulses.

### Signal-Averaged Electrocardiography
**Signal-averaged electrocardiography (SAECG)** is a surface ECG that amplifies **late potentials** (the electrical activity that occurs after normal depolarization of the ventricles). The test requires a specialized ECG machine and small computer to detect the late potentials. It is performed on clients who have had a myocardial infarction. The test reveals the client's risk for ventricular tachycardia.

## Stress Test

A **stress test** measures the client's cardiovascular response to exercise tolerance. It demonstrates the ability of the myocardium to respond to increased oxygen requirements (the result of exercise) by increasing the blood flow to the coronary arteries.

The client is connected to an ECG machine and asked to walk on a treadmill. Continuous ECG recordings are made of the client's heart response (rate, electrical activity, and cardiac recovery time) to frequent changes in the treadmill's speed and slope. The test is stopped immediately if the client experiences any symptoms of decreased cardiac output (chest pain, dyspnea, fatigue, or ischemic changes on the ECG monitor). Chemical stress test may be performed if the client is unable to walk. Dipyridamole (Persantine), adenosine, and dobutamine are coronary vasodilators that are used for this test. Pacing stress test is another form of stress testing used for clients with permanent pacemakers.

## Thallium Test

**Thallium** (a radionuclide that is the physiological analogue of potassium) is normally absorbed into normal myocardial tissue from the circulating blood. During the test, thallium is administered intravenously to detect damaged myocardial tissue (necrotic or ischemic). Because thallium is not absorbed by the damaged tissue, the degree of heart damage can be estimated.

There are two types of thallium tests: resting imaging or stress imaging. Resting imaging is performed a few hours after myocardial infarction. The thallium is injected and an ECG tracing is performed. Stress imaging (thallium stress test) is performed while the client is on the treadmill with ECG monitoring. At peak stress the intravenous thallium is injected; scanning is done 3 to 5 minutes postinjection. The test is stopped immediately if the client becomes symptomatic for ischemia.

## Electroencephalography

An **electroencephalogram** (EEG) is the graphic recording of the brain's electrical activity. The procedure is painless and takes about an hour. The test is performed in a quiet, nonstimulating environment. It can reveal the presence and type of seizure disorder and intracranial lesion. The absence of brain's electrical activity is used to confirm death.

During the procedure, electrodes are placed on the client's scalp. The electrodes transmit the impulses from the brain to an EEG machine. The machine amplifies the brain's impulses and makes a recording of the waves on strips of paper.

## Endoscopy

**Endoscopy** is the visualization of a body organ or cavity through a scope. The procedure is performed with an endoscope (a metal or fiber-optic tube) being inserted directly into the body structure to be studied. A light at the end of the scope allows the practitioner to assess for lesions and structural problems. The endoscope has an opening at the distant tip that allows the practitioner to administer an anesthetic agent, lavage, suction, and biopsy tissue. Common endoscopic procedures are presented in Table 29-14.

General client preparation and positioning depend on the structure being studied as discussed in Table 29-14. As with all invasive procedures, the client needs to sign a consent form and the nurse needs to establish baseline vital signs before administering sedative agents.

Postprocedure the nurse monitors the vital signs, observes for bleeding, and assesses for procedural risks (e.g., return of the gag and swallowing reflexes following an esophagogastroduodenoscopy with local anesthesia).

## Aspiration/Biopsy

**Aspiration** is performed to withdraw fluid that has abnormally collected or to obtain a specimen. Aseptic technique and Standard Precautions are used during aspiration. Aspiration diagnostic studies are invasive; implement the protocols for diagnostic tests. A local anesthetic is administered in the area being studied to decrease the client's discomfort when the skin is pierced by the needle.

A stylet needle with an outer, hollow-bore needle is used to pierce the skin. Once the needle is in place, the stylet is withdrawn, leaving only the outer needle to aspirate the fluid. A tissue **biopsy** (excision of a small amount of tissue) can be obtained during aspiration or with other diagnostic tests (e.g., bronchoscopy). A biopsy can be taken from most of the body's tissue.

## Amniocentesis

**Amniocentesis** is the withdrawal of amniotic fluid to obtain a sample for specimen examination. The amniotic

### STOP AND THINK

#### Participating in Diagnostic Testing

A client comes to an outpatient clinic for a laparoscopy to retrieve an egg for in vitro fertilization. You are to assist the practitioner with this procedure. How would you handle this situation if your own religious beliefs were in conflict with the procedure being performed? Would it make any difference to you if the client had had an abortion as a teenager?

## TABLE 29-14    ENDOSCOPIC PROCEDURES

| Procedure/Area Studied | Preparation/Position | Clinical Significance |
| --- | --- | --- |
| Arthroscopy—examine joint structures, primarily the knee | Instruct client to fast after midnight; test is usually performed under local anesthesia, may be done under spinal or general anesthesia if surgery is necessary. Position the joint for accessibility. | Diagnose a torn meniscus, patellar, condylar, and synovial disorders; perform surgery. Also used to monitor the progression of a disease or effectiveness of therapy. |
| Bronchoscopy—examine the bronchus and bronchial tree | Instruct client to fast 6 to 12 hours before the test; test is usually done under local anesthesia. Position client supine or sitting upright. | Identify the origin of bleeding, lesions, or obstruction; collect a specimen for bacteriologic and cytologic examination (diagnosis abnormal cells); remove foreign bodies, lesions, mucus plugs, or excessive secretions. |
| Colonoscopy—examine the large intestine | Instruct client to maintain a clear liquid diet for 48 hours before the test, take the prescribed laxative the evening before the examination; place client on left side with knees flexed and drape. | Identify origin of bleeding or lesions; evaluate inflammatory and ulcerative bowel disease and recurrence of polyps or malignant lesions. |
| Colposcopy—examine the cervix and vagina following a positive Pap smear | No restriction on food or liquids. Place client in lithotomy position. | Evaluate abnormal cytology or grossly suspicious lesions and to perform a biopsy or take photographs of suspicious lesions. |
| Cystoscope (see cystourethroscopy) | | |
| Cystourethroscopy—uses two instruments: a cystoscope to examine the bladder and ureter openings, urethroscope to examine the bladder neck and the urethra | Food and fluids are restricted only if the client is to receive general anesthesia; regional anesthesia is usually given. Place client in a lithotomy position. | Identify bladder lesions and urethral strictures, ulcers, inflammation, and an enlarged prostate gland. |
| Esophagogastroduodenoscopy (EGD)—examine the esophagus, stomach, and upper duodenum | Instruct client to fast 6 to 12 hours before the test. An intravenous tranquilizer may be given, then a local anesthetic is sprayed into the back of the throat to decrease the gag reflex (swallowing will seem difficult). Place client in a sitting position. | Identify diverticula, varies, Mallory-Weiss syndrome, esophageal rings and hiatal hernia, and esophageal and gastric stenoses. When combined with histologic and cytologic tests may indicate acute or chronic ulcers, benign or malignant tumors, and inflammatory disease. |

*(continues)*

## TABLE 29-14    ENDOSCOPIC PROCEDURES (continued)

| Procedure/Area Studied | Preparation/Position | Clinical Significance |
| --- | --- | --- |
| Laparoscopy—examine the peritoneal cavity: pelvis and abdomen | Instruct client to fast 8 hours before the surgery; the test is performed either with a local or general anesthetic agent. Place the client in a lithotomy position; catheterize the client to ensure the bladder is empty (avoids puncture of the bladder during the test with the laparoscope). | Used to detect cysts; adhesions; fibroids; and infections of the uterus, fallopian tubes and ovaries; ectopic pregnancies; and liver lacerations and cirrhosis. May also be used for lysis of adhesions, ovarian biopsy, tubal sterilization, foreign body removal, and fulguration of endometriotic implants. |
| Proctosigmoidoscopy—three steps: 1. Digital examination to dilate the anal sphincters to detect obstruction that might hinder passage of the endoscope 2. A sigmoidoscope to examine the distal sigmoid colon and rectum 3. A proctoscope to examine the lower rectum and anal canal | Instruct client according to physician orders relative to dietary restrictions and bowel preparation (these are usually based on physician preference). If the client has rectal inflammation, a local anesthetic agent is applied to decrease discomfort. Secure the client to a tilting table that rotates into horizontal and vertical positions. | Identify internal hemorrhoids, hypertrophic anal papillae, polyps, fissures, fistulae, and rectal and anal abscesses. |

fluid increases during pregnancy from 50 ml at the end of the first trimester to an average of 1,000 ml near term. This test is indicated when:

- Maternal age exceeds 35
- A spontaneous abortion occurred with a previous pregnancy
- There is a family history of genetic, chromosomal, or neural tube defects

The amniocentesis is performed when the amniotic fluid volume reaches 150 ml, usually after the 16th week of pregnancy.

There are no restrictions on fluids or food. The procedure usually lasts 10 to 15 minutes. Instruct the mother to void to prevent the risk of puncturing a full bladder. Position the client supine and assesses the fetal heart tones.

The abdomen is prepped and injected with lidocaine hydrochloride (a local anesthetic agent). The practitioner withdraws 10–20 ml amniotic fluid by transabdominal needle aspiration. Postprocedure the nurse monitors the client's vital signs, fetal heart tones, and assesses for signs of labor. Instruct the client to notify the practitioner of any signs of labor or infection.

## Bone Marrow Aspiration/Biopsy

The sternum and iliac crest are the common sites for bone marrow puncture. During a bone marrow puncture, a fluid specimen (aspiration) or a core of marrow cells (biopsy) can be obtained. Both tests are commonly done concurrently to obtain the best marrow specimen. The

test can reveal anemias or cancer, such as leukemia, multiple myeloma, or Hodgkin's disease, or the client's response to chemotherapy.

There are no restrictions on fluids or food before the puncture. The nurse should explain the procedure to elicit the client's support during the procedure. The client must lay perfectly still throughout the procedure. The client is usually fearful; allay the client's fear with relaxation methods or sedation. Infants and small children are restrained by holding them throughout the procedure.

Client positioning is determined by the site to be used, supine (sternum) or side-lying (iliac crest). The site is prepped for puncture to decrease the skin's normal flora. Explain to the client that pressure may be experienced as the specimen is withdrawn. The client should not move when the specimen is being withdrawn; a sudden movement may dislodge the needle.

Postprocedure the client should be on bed rest for an hour. The nurse monitors vital signs to assess for bleeding (rapid pulse rate, low blood pressure). Instruct the client to report to the practitioner any bleeding or signs of inflammation.

## Paracentesis

**Paracentesis** is the aspiration of fluid from the abdominal cavity. This test can either be diagnostic, therapeutic, or both. For instance, with end-stage liver or renal disease there is **ascites** (an accumulation of fluid in the abdomen). Pressure caused from the ascites can interfere with breathing and gastrointestinal functioning.

## CLINICAL ALERT

### Taking the Pressure Reading

The client should be relaxed and quiet during the initial pressure reading; *straining increases the CSF.*

Aspiration in this instance is therapeutic. If a culture specimen is taken, it is also diagnostic.

Have the client void and obtain a body weight before the procedure. Place the client in a high Fowler's position in a chair or sitting on the side of the bed. The skin is prepped, anesthetized, and punctured with a **trocar** (a large-bored abdominal paracentesis needle). The trocar is held perpendicular to the abdominal wall and advanced into the peritoneal cavity. When fluid appears, the trocar is removed, leaving the inner catheter in place to drain the fluid. Observe the client for pressure changes that can result from the rapid removal of fluid.

Postprocedure apply a sterile dressing to the puncture site. Monitor the client for changes in vital signs and electrolytes. Instruct the client to record the color, amount, and consistency of drainage on the dressing after discharge.

## Thoracentesis

**Thoracentesis** is the aspiration of fluids from the pleural cavity. The pleural cavity normally contains a small amount of fluid to lubricate the lining between the lungs and pleura. Infection, inflammation, and trauma may cause an increased production of fluid, which can impair ventilation.

Position the client with arms crossed and resting on a bedside table to allow access to the rib cage. Instruct the client not to cough during insertion of the needle. The practitioner selects, preps, and anesthetizes the puncture site. The needle is usually inserted into the intercostal space at the location of maximum dullness to percussion. Posteriorly, the site should be above the ninth rib, and laterally, above the seventh rib.

During the procedure, monitor the client for symptoms of a **pneumothorax** (collection of air or gas in the pleural space causing the lungs to collapse), such as dyspnea, pallor, tachycardia, vertigo, and chest pain. Postprocedure observe for cardiopulmonary changes and a mediastinum shift as assessed by vital signs and bloody sputum.

## Cerebrospinal Fluid Aspiration

**Lumbar puncture** ("spinal tap") is the aspiration of cerebrospinal fluid (CSF) from the subarachnoid space. The specimen is examined for organisms, blood, and tumor cells. A spinal tap is also performed:

- To obtain a pressure measurement when blockage is suspected

- During a myelogram, as discussed earlier
- To instill medications (anesthesia, antibiotics, or chemotherapy)

A spinal tap is contraindicated in clients with increased intracranial pressure, hemorrhagic diathesis, and an infection at the proposed puncture site.

Place the client in a lateral recumbent position with the craniospinal axis parallel to the floor and flat of the back perpendicular to the procedure table. Have the client assume a flexed knee-chest position to bow the back. This position separates the vertebrae. Most clients will require assistance in maintaining this position throughout the procedure. To assist, the nurse stands facing the client with one hand across the client's posterior shoulder blades and the other hand over the buttocks.

The practitioner selects, preps, and anesthetizes the puncture site (usually interspace L3-L4, L4-L5, or L5-S1). The needle and stylet are inserted into the midsagittal space and advanced through the longitudinal subarachnoid space (Figure 29-18).

Once in the subarachnoid space, the stylet is removed, leaving the needle in place. An initial CSF pressure reading is taken:

- A three-way stopcock with a manometer (calibrated column) is securely connected to the spinal needle.
- The stopcock is opened toward the manometer to allow the CSF to rise in the column. Under normal conditions, the CSF will fluctuate in the column with respirations.
- When the CSF stabilizes, a pressure reading is taken.

If the pressure reading is greater than 200 mm $H_2O$ or falls quickly, only 1 or 2 ml CSF is obtained for analysis. If the pressure is less than 200 mm $H_2O$, an adequate specimen sampling is withdrawn slowly.

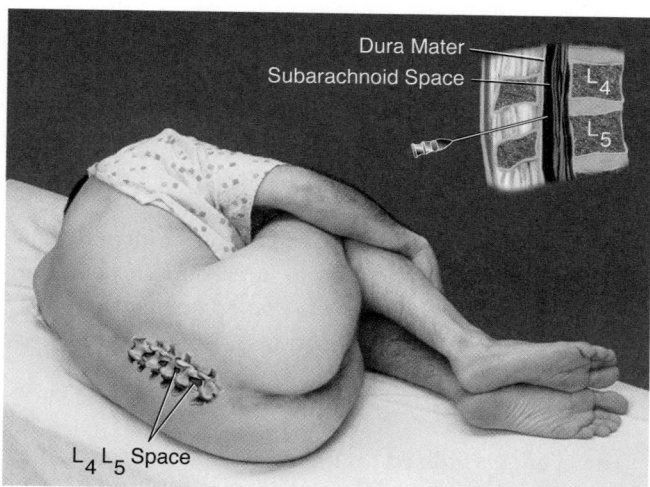

**Figure 29-18    Lumbar puncture: position of client and insertion of the needle into the subarachnoid space as shown**

After the pressure reading is taken, the stopcock is turned to allow the CSF to slowly flow into a sterile test tube. A sterile cap is placed on the test tube, and the sample is transported to the laboratory for analysis. Rapid withdrawal of CSF can cause a transient postural headache. Throughout the procedure, monitor the client's cardiorespiratory status.

Postprocedure, pressure is applied and then a sterile bandage. Assess the bandage for leakage of CSF and the client's neurologic and cardiorespiratory status. A postural headache is the most common complication of a lumbar puncture; using a small-bore spinal needle minimizes the chances of a headache.

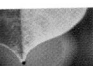

# CASE STUDY/NURSING CARE PLAN

Mrs. Cynthia Reyes is a 56-year-old female who is admitted to the medical floor due to blood in the stool and abdominal pain for 3 days. She primarily will be assessed with a variety of laboratory and diagnostic tests. A review of systems reveals bowel habit changes, loss of appetite, weight loss of more than 10 pounds, and fatigue for 2 months. Mrs. Reyes' past medical history includes primary hypertension, obesity, gastroesophageal reflux disease, and constipation. The client's medications include HCTZ 25 mg po qd, Omeprazole 20 mg po qd prn, and Metamucil prn. The client's nutritional intake is usually high in fat, low in fiber, and less than two servings of fruits and vegetables per day. Her fluid intake consists primarily of sodas, tea or coffee, and possibly 2 cups of water per day. Mrs. Reyes' activity is sedentary, and her social history includes working as a clerical assistant for 25 years. She has been smoking cigarettes for 20 years, has an occasional alcohol intake of 2 to 3 drinks per week, and denies the use of illicit drugs.

## Assessment
Client has gastrointestinal bleeding and recent history of abdominal pain. Her vital signs are temperature 98.2, pulse 69, respiration 18, and blood pressure 112/56. Bowel sounds normal on four quadrants, tympanic to percussion, no CVA tenderness, pain elicited on palpation of left lower quadrant, palpable mass noted on left lower quadrant area. Client's skin color is pink and has good turgor. Rectal exam reveals 3 cm by 4 cm palpable lesion with stool positive for occult blood. Neurologic system shows client to be awake, alert, and oriented × 3. A psychosocial assessment reveals her to appear nervous, crying, and fearful; client states she has not been in the hospital since her husband died 10 years ago.

## Nursing Diagnosis
*Acute Pain* related to colorectal mass.
**NOC:** Comfort Level; Medication Response; Pain Control
**NIC:** Analgesic Administration; Conscious Sedation; Pain Management; Patient-Controlled Analgesia Assistance

## Expected Outcomes
The client will:
1. Decrease pain level from 7 to 3 (on scale of 1 to 10) within 24 hours.
2. Relate an improvement of pain as evidenced by an increase in daily activities within 48 hours.

## Planning/Interventions/Rationales
1. Evaluate pain frequently by asking client to rate pain on scale of 1 to 10. *Provides ongoing assessment of pain that is measurable.*
2. Reduce or eliminate the factors that increase the pain experience. *Decreases overall pain response.*
3. Collaborate with client to initiate noninvasive pain relief measures. *Broadens measures to decrease pain and incorporates nonmedication approaches to pain relief.*
4. Administer pain medications, and assess response to the medications. *Provide optimal pain relief and reduces side effects.*

## Evaluation
The client verbalized that her pain was a 2 (scale of 1 to 10) within 24 hours. She took analgesics every 4 hours as ordered and had no side effects.

## Key Concepts

- Most invasive procedures require the client's written consent and a thorough understanding of the reasons the test is being performed. Nurses explain the purpose of the diagnostic test and the reasons it has been ordered.
- Nurses prepare clients for diagnostic testing by ensuring client understanding and compliance to preprocedural requirements.
- Clients, families, and significant others need to be involved in the testing process; advise them of the estimated time the procedure requires.
- Nurses teach the client how to perform relaxation and imagery techniques to cope with the discomfort and anxiety experienced during procedures.
- After a procedure, the nurse provides care and teaches the client what to expect following a diagnostic test and the outcomes or side effects of the test.
- Specimen collection methods include punctures such as venipuncture, arterial puncture, capillary puncture, catheter insertion, and bone marrow aspiration. Specimens collected by noninvasive methods include urine, stool, sputum, throat tissue, and cervical tissue.
- Invasive procedures include endoscopy, angiography, aspiration, biopsy, and other procedures in which body cavities are punctured.
- Noninvasive procedures include radiography, fluoroscopy, mammography, computed tomography, radioisotope scanning, ultrasonography, magnetic resonance imaging, and electrodiagnostic studies.
- The role of the nurse in diagnostic procedures is to facilitate the scheduling of diagnostic tests, perform client teaching, perform or assist with procedures, and assess the client for adverse responses to the procedures.
- Nurses should schedule diagnostic procedures to promote client comfort and cost containment.
- Standard Precautions are used when obtaining a specimen for diagnostic examination or assisting with an invasive procedure
- Before the procedure the nurse is responsible for assessing the client's preparation for testing.
- After the procedure, the nurse assesses the client for secondary procedural complications and provides any necessary nursing interventions.

## Review Questions and Activities

1. Why would a nurse practitioner order a white blood cell differential as opposed to a white blood cell count?
2. With invasive procedures, the body is entered with some type of instrumentation; there is a puncture site. If you fall down and a nail pierces your leg, you have a puncture site. What are you at risk for immediately after the incidence and 48 to 72 hours postinjury? Can you relate the body's physiological response to an invasive procedure to a puncture injury?
3. Explain how the three sources of venipuncture variability can cause inaccurate laboratory results.
4. What is a normal prothrombin time (PT)? PT is a comparative test that measures the client's PT to the control time. Both the PT and control time results are reported. One example of the use of a PT is to measure the effectiveness of prescribed anticoagulant therapy. In this case, the therapeutic range is 2 to 2.5 times the control time, which is 12 to 14 seconds. If the control time is 12 seconds, what would you expect the client's PT to be?
5. If your blood type is AB positive, what are the possible blood types of your parents? Can you receive Rh-negative blood? Explain your answer.
6. What are the physiological effects of acetylcholine on the nervous system? Why should the practitioner be notified about a decreased level of cholinesterase for a client scheduled to receive succinylcholine for either major surgery or electroconvulsive therapy?
7. Which client is more at risk for coronary heart disease? Mrs. Silipo, a 59-year-old who is postmenopausal with a cholesterol of 185 mg/dl, LDL of 131 mg/dl, HDL of 25 mg/dl, and triglycerides of 250 mg/dl. Mr. Joseph, a 55-year-old who smokes occasionally with a cholesterol of 220 mg/dl, LDL of 157 mg/dl, HDL of 37 mg/dl, and triglycerides of 249 mg/dl.
8. You are counseling Maria Rodriguez regarding the symptoms and risk factors of large radiation exposures. She is receiving radiation therapy for breast cancer. Where in her medical record should the potential risk factors be addressed?
9. What specific teaching should be done for a client undergoing arteriography? Evaluate the need for teaching based on the procedure. Refer to the protocol on preparing the client for diagnostic testing for appropriate teaching interventions.
10. Plan the postprocedural care for a cardiac catheterization client using the protocol for care of the client after diagnostic testing.

## Multimedia Links

Altman *Basic Care DVD: Collecting a Clean-Catch, Midstream Urine Specimen*

Altman *Basic Care Video: Specimen Collection*

Altman *Basic Care DVD: Testing Urine for Specific Gravity, Ketones, and Occult Blood*

Altman *Basic Care DVD: Performing a Skin Puncture*

Altman *Basic Care DVD: Measuring Blood Glucose Levels*

Altman *Basic Care DVD: Collecting Nose, Throat, and Sputum Specimens*

Altman *Basic Care DVD: Testing for Occult Blood with a Hemoccult Slide*

Altman *Intermediate Care DVD: Obtaining a Residual Urine Specimen from an Indwelling Catheter*

Altman *Intermediate Skills Video: Nutrition & Elimination II: Catheter Care*

Altman *Intermediate Care DVD: Obtaining an Arterial Blood Gas Specimen*

Altman *Intermediate Care DVD: Obtaining a Wound Drainage Specimen for Culturing*

Altman *Advanced Care DVD: Performing Venipuncture (Blood Drawing)*

Altman *Advanced Skills Video: Circulatory I: Venipuncture and Starting IV Therapy*

Altman *Advanced Care DVD: Administering an Electrocardiogram*

Altman *Advanced Care DVD: Magnetic Resonance Imaging (MRI)*

Altman *Advanced Care DVD: Assisting with Computed Tomography (CT) Scanning*

Altman *Advanced Care DVD: Assisting with a Liver Biopsy*

Altman *Advanced Care DVD: Assisting with a Thoracentesis*

Altman *Advanced Care DVD: Assisting with an Abdominal Paracentesis*

Altman *Advanced Care DVD: Assisting with a Bone Marrow Biopsy/Aspiration*

Altman *Advanced Care DVD: Assisting with a Lumbar Puncture*

Altman *Advanced Care DVD: Assisting with Amniocentesis*

Altman *Advanced Care DVD: Assisting with Bronchoscopy*

Altman *Advanced Care DVD: Assisting with a Gastrointestinal Endoscopy*

Altman *Advanced Care DVD: Assisting with a Proctosigmoidoscopy*

Altman *Advanced Care DVD: Assisting with Arteriography*

Altman *Advanced Care DVD: Positron-Emission Tomography Scanning*

## Web Resources

American Cancer Society
  http://www.cancer.org
American Radiological Nurses Association
  http://www.rsna.org
BreastCancer.Net
  http://www.breastcancer.net
FDA Center for Devices and Radiological Health
  http://www.fda.gov

## References

Altman, G. (2004). *Delmar's fundamental & advanced nursing skills* (2nd ed.). Clifton Park, NY: Delmar Learning.

American Cancer Society (2002). *Breast cancer stats and figures.* Atlanta, GA: Author.

Bard Access Systems (2002). http://www.crbard.com

Daniels, R. (2003). *Delmar's manual of laboratory and diagnostic tests.* Clifton Park, NY: Delmar Learning.

Fischbach, F. (2004). *A manual of laboratory and diagnostic tests* (7th ed.). Philadelphia: Lippincott.

Johnson, B. A. (1999). Flexible sigmoidoscopy for colorectal cancer. *American Family Physician*, Jan. 15, 1999.

Kerr, S., Marshall, C., & Sinclair, D. (1999). Emergency physicians versus laboratory technicians: Are the urinalysis and microscopy results comparable? A pilot study. *Journal of Emergency Medicine, 17*(3), 399–404.

Kirschbaum, B., Sica, D., & Anderson, P. (1999). Urine electrolytes and the urine anion and osmolar gaps. *Journal of Laboratory and Clinical Medicine, 133*(6), 597–604.

McCaffrey, M., & Pasero, C. (1999). *Pain: Clinical manual* (2nd ed.). St. Louis: Mosby.

McConnell, E. A. (1999). Hold the lab in the palm of your hand. *Nursing Management, 30*(5), 57–59.

National Center for Health Statistics (NCHS) (1999). *Final data for 1997*, PHS 99–1120, 47(19), 108.

Phillips, L. D. (2001). *Manual of I.V. therapeutics* (3rd ed.). Philadelphia: F. A. Davis Company.

Potts, N., & Mandleco, B. (2002). *Pediatric nursing: Caring for children and their families.* Clifton Park, NY: Delmar Learning.

Price, M. B., Grant, M. J., & Welkie, K. (1999). Financial impact of elimination of routine chest radiographs in a pediatric intensive care unit. *Critical Care Medicine, 27*(8), 1588–1593.

Schallom, L. (1999). Point of care testing in critical care. *Critical Care Nursing Clinics of North America, 11*(1), 99–106.

Tierney, L. M., McPhee, S. J., & Papadakis, M. A. (Eds.) (2000). *Current medical diagnosis & treatment* (39th ed.). Boston: McGraw-Hill Company.

Troisi, R. J., Cowie, C. C., & Harris, M. I. (2000). Diurnal variation in fasting plasma glucose: Implications for diagnosis of diabetes in patients examined in the afternoon. *Journal of the American Medical Association, 284*(24), 3157–3159.

U.S. Preventive Services Task Force (USPSTF) (2003). http://www.ahcpr.gov

USPSTF. (2003a). Screening breast cancer. http://www.ahcpr.gov/clinic/uspstf/uspsbrca.htm

USPSTF (2003b). Screening colorectal cancer. http://www.ahcpr.gov/clinic/uspstf/uspscolo.htm

USPSTF (2003c). Screening cervical cancer. http://www.ahcpr.gov/clinic/uspstf/uspscerv.htm

Verne, Jules (1984). *Around the World in Eighty Days.* New York: Bantam Books.

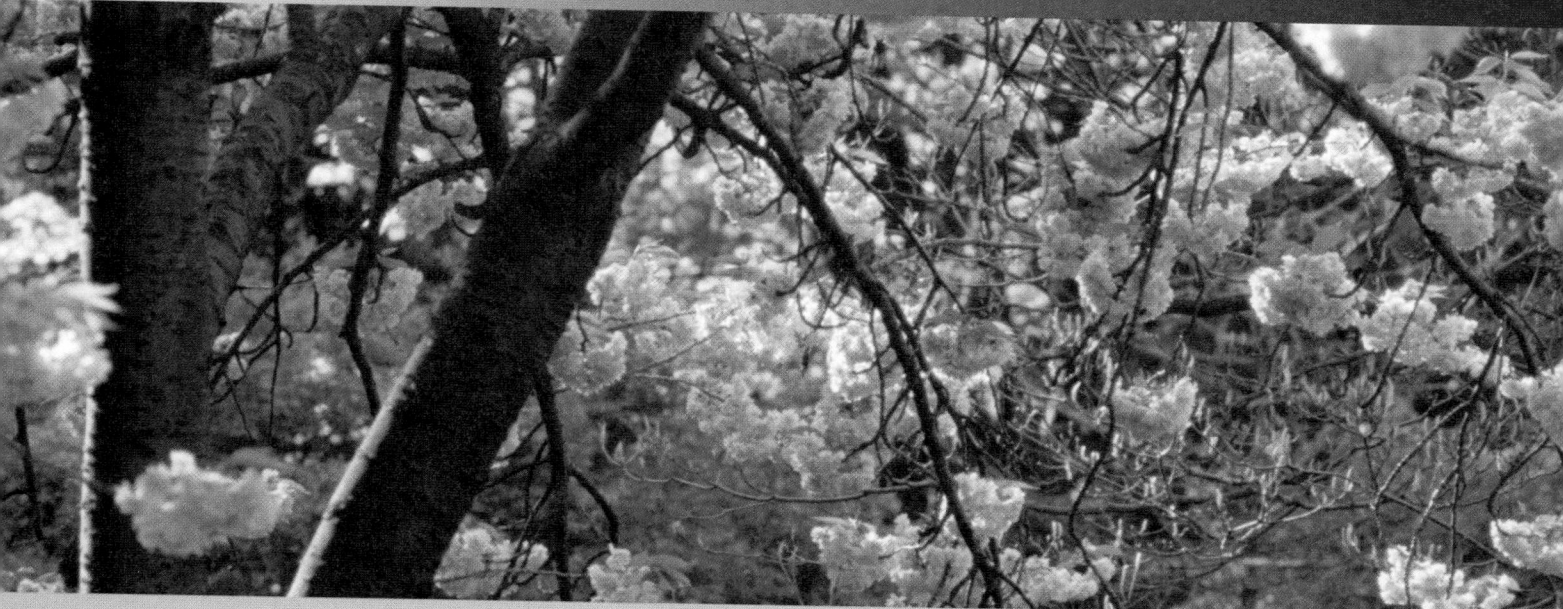

# CHAPTER 30

# Medication Administration

## Marilyn Housel Poysky, RN, MSN, CS

*"Increased collaboration among health care providers demands in-depth understanding of drug actions, interactions, therapeutic and adverse effects, and the exercise of judgment in drug administration."*

*(Gutierrez, 1999)*

# Chapter Competencies

*Upon completion of this chapter, the reader should be able to:*

1. Define the key terms and abbreviations frequently used in medication administration.
2. Describe the influence of drug standards and legislation on medication administration.
3. Discuss the nurse's legal responsibilities in preparation and administration of medications.
4. Explain the principles of pharmacokinetics, including absorption, distribution, metabolism, and excretion of drugs.
5. Describe the factors that can affect a medication's actions.
6. Differentiate among allergic reaction, side effect, toxic effect, and idiosyncratic reaction to medications.
7. Describe the differences between the types of medication orders.
8. Correctly calculate appropriate dosage for medications as prescribed.
9. Discuss principles of safe medication administration including the five rights of medication administration.
10. Correctly explain procedures for the different methods of medication administration, including the choice of route and site.
11. Analyze the use of the nursing process in medication administration, including the assessment of the client's medication history.
12. Develop teaching guidelines for clients regarding medication in the home.

# Key Terms

| | | |
|---|---|---|
| absorption | idiosyncratic reaction | plateau |
| addiction | infiltration | prn (as necessary) orders |
| adverse reaction | intradermal (ID) | residual |
| aspiration | intramuscular (IM) | side effects |
| biotransformation | intravenous (IV) | stat order |
| buccal | medication | stock supplied |
| compliance | medication interaction | subcutaneous (SC or SQ) |
| controlled substance | medicine | sublingual |
| chemical dependence | metabolism | sustained release |
| dissolution | Nurse Practice Act | therapeutic range |
| distribution | onset of action | toxic effect |
| drug | parenteral | transdermal |
| drug incompatibility | patency | trough |
| drug tolerance | peak plasma level | unit dose form |
| duration | pharmacodynamics | vesicant |
| excretion | pharmacokinetics | Z-track technique |
| half-life | phlebitis | |

Alteration in health related to acute or chronic conditions lead clients to seek relief of their symptoms through various treatment options. One modality frequently used to help alleviate symptoms and restore health is a medication regime. Medications are substances prescribed by the client's health care practitioner to help in the treatment, relief, or cure of the cause of the client's health alteration or in the prevention of an alteration.

Nurses play an essential role in the administration of, education about, and evaluation of the effectiveness of prescribed medications. The nurse's role changes with the setting of the client. In the home or community setting, clients take their own medication as prescribed by the health care practitioner. Nurses are responsible for educating the client about her medications and their possible side effects as well as for evaluating the outcome of the prescribed therapy in restoring and maintaining the client's health. In the acute care setting, nurses spend a great deal of time administering medications and evaluating their effectiveness. Nurses are responsible for teaching clients how to take their medications safely when they are discharged.

Medication administration requires specialized knowledge, judgment, and nursing skill based on the principles of pharmacology. The focus of this chapter is to assist the student in applying knowledge of pharmacology and in acquiring skills in the safe administration of medications. The nursing process is used to direct nursing decisions relative to safe drug administration and to ensure compliance with standards of practice.

# Drug Standards and Legislation

A drug is a chemical substance intended for use in the diagnosis, treatment, cure, mitigation, or prevention of a disease. When a drug is given to a client, there is an intended specific effect. The terms *drug*, *medication*, and *medicine* are often used interchangeably by health care providers and lay persons. However, the term **drug** is basically defined as any substance that can modify one or more of the body's functions (Taber's, 2002, p. 570). The term can be used for legal and illegal substances that are used recreationally by the public for a desired effect, such as amphetamines or cocaine. On the other hand, a **medication** (or **medicine**) is a drug that is used for a therapeutic effect.

## Federal Standards and Legislation

Standards have been developed to ensure drug uniformity so that the effects of the medication are predictable. The Pure Food and Drug Act of 1906 designated the *United States Pharmacopeia* (USP) and the *National Formulary* (NF) as the official references to establish drug standards. The act also gave the federal government the authority to enforce these standards. The *British Pharmacopeia* is the Canadian complement to the USP and the *Canadian Formulary* provides a listing of drugs commonly used in Canada.

The federal Food, Drug, and Cosmetic Act of 1938 empowered the Food and Drug Administration (FDA) to test all new drugs for toxicity before granting a pharmaceutical company approval to market a drug. The federal Food, Drug, and Cosmetic Act of 1938 was amended in 1952 to distinguish prescription (legend) drugs from nonprescription (over-the-counter) drugs and to regulate the dispensing of prescriptions.

The FDA is empowered to regulate the manufacture, sale, and effectiveness of medicines. It approves which new medicines are allowed to be available to the public after analyzing the results of three-phase clinical trials for the safety and efficacy of the medication. The agency is also responsible for recalling medications when further data shows they are unsafe. In 1993, the MedWatch program was initiated by the FDA to encourage doctors, nurses, and other health care providers to report when a medication causes untoward side effects. Through the MedWatch program, data from across the nation can be compiled, and warnings or even recalls can be done more quickly by the FDA.

The Harrison Narcotic Act of 1914 classified habit-forming drugs as narcotics and began regulating these substances. This law and other drug abuse laws have been replaced with the Comprehensive Drug Abuse Prevention and Control Act (Controlled Substance Act) of 1970. This act defines a *drug-dependent person* in terms of physical and psychological dependence and provides for strict regulation of narcotics and other controlled drugs such as barbiturates through the establishment of five categories of scheduled drugs (see Box 30-1). Any controlled substance must be recorded by the dispensing pharmacist and by the nurse giving the medication. The Drug Enforcement Administration (DEA) employs pharmacists to inspect all types of records, including prescriptions, to detect the illicit distribution of these substances.

## State and Local Legislation

The nurse's functions and responsibilities are legally defined by each state's **Nurse Practice Act**. In general, most Nurse Practice Acts give the nurse a broad range of

---

## BOX 30-1    CONTROLLED SUBSTANCES

- Schedule C-I: High abuse potential, no current accepted medical use (e.g., heroin, marijuana, and LSD)

- Schedule C-II: High abuse potential for severe dependence (e.g., narcotics, amphetamines, dronabinol, and some barbiturates)

- Schedule C-III: Less abuse potential than schedule II drugs for moderate dependence (e.g., nonbarbiturate sedatives, nonamphetamine stimulants, and limited amounts of certain narcotics)

- Schedule C-IV: Lower abuse potential than schedule III drugs for limited dependence (e.g., sedatives, antianxiety agents, and nonnarcotic analgesics)

- Schedule C-V: Limited abuse potential (e.g., codeine used as antitussive and antidiarrheals)

responsibilities under the prescriptive authority of a licensed physician or physician's assistant. In some states, advanced practice nurses also may be licensed for prescriptive authority. The nurse is responsible for knowing the boundaries set by the state Nurse Practice Act in the particular state of practice. A health care institution may develop policies that are more restrictive than the Nurse Practice Act but cannot expand the scope of practice outlined by the state legislation. The primary intent of all state Nurse Practice Acts is to protect the public by defining required education and skill levels of all state-licensed nurses.

State and local regulations of medications must conform with federal legislation. States, however, have the power to enforce additional regulations that impose stricter control of substances. For example, the Controlled Substance Act has codeine in antitussives as a schedule V drug, but an individual state that identifies abuse of antitussives with codeine may place this drug in the schedule II category, which is more restrictive (Reiss, Evans, & Broyles, 2002).

## Health Care Institution Regulations

All health care institutions are required to meet minimum standards set by federal, state, and local agencies. In addition to these standards, most institutions have established specific policies that regulate administration of medication within the institution. Institutional policies are typically more restrictive and more specific than federal and state regulations. Furthermore, health care institutions are trying to prevent problems stemming from medication administration. For example, institutional policies may set the times for medication administration (medications ordered for every 8 hours are given at 0600 [6 A.M.], 1400 [2 P.M.], and 2200 [10 P.M.]) to prevent omission of irregularly timed doses. To prevent overuse of antibiotics, institutional policies may automatically discontinue all antibiotics after 5 days unless reordered by the health care provider.

## Medication Names

Medications can be identified by their chemical, generic, or trade names. The *chemical name* is a precise description of the drug's composition (chemical formula) but is rarely used in clinical practice. The *generic name* is the drug name assigned by the United States Adopted Names Council to the manufacturer who first develops the drug. Drugs with a proven therapeutic value are listed in the USP and NF by their generic names. When a pharmaceutical company markets the medication, the company assigns a *trade name*, also called a *brand* or *proprietary* name; therefore, one generic drug may have several trade names based on the number of companies marketing the drug. For example,

| TABLE 30-1 | EXAMPLES OF TRADE AND GENERIC DRUG NAMES |
|---|---|
| **Trade Name** | **Generic Name** |
| Bayer | Aspirin |
| Benadryl | Diphehydramine hydrochloride |
| Zovirax | Acyclovir |
| Ancef, Kefzol, Zolicef | Cefazolin |

ibuprofen is a generic name; common trade names for this drug are Advil, Excedrin IB, Motrin, and Nuprin. See Table 30-1 for additional examples of trade and generic names. Having multiple names has created confusion for both the public and health care providers and creates a greater risk for errors. Many medication names have only slight differences in pronunciation and spelling. Medications may be ordered by either their generic or trade name, and nurses must carefully check the name and spelling, using a drug reference guide or formulary if necessary (Reiss, Evans, & Broyles, 2002).

## Classification of Medications

Medications are commonly classified by the body system that they interact with (e.g., cardiovascular) or in accordance with therapeutic usage (e.g., antihypertensive or antianginal medications) (Deglin & Vallerand, 2002). For example, in the antianginal classification the medications are in three major categories depending on their general action: beta-adrenergic blocking agents, calcium channel blockers, and nitrates and nitrites. Medications with multiple therapeutic uses are usually classified in accordance with their most common usage.

## Forms of Medication Preparations

Drugs are available in many forms for administration by a specific route (see Box 30-2). The route refers to how the drug is absorbed: oral, buccal, sublingual, rectal, parenteral (hypodermic routes), topical, and inhalation.

Drugs prepared for administration by one route should not be substituted by other drug forms. For example, when a client has difficulty swallowing a large tablet or capsule, *the nurse should not administer an oral solution or elixir of the same drug without first consulting the physician, because a liquid may be more easily and completely absorbed, producing a higher blood level than a tablet.*

The nurse should be aware of the various drug forms and how they are administered. Certain drug preparations

## BOX 30-2    FORMS OF MEDICATION PREPARATIONS

### Oral Solids

- Tablets: compressed or molded substances, to be swallowed whole, chewed before swallowing, or placed in the buccal pocket or under the tongue (sublingual)
- Capsules: substances encased in either a hard or a soft soluble container or gelatin shell that dissolves in the stomach
- Caplets: gelatin-coated tablets that dissolve in the stomach
- Powder and granules: finely ground substances, usually mixed with water or juice
- Troches, lozenges, and pastilles: designed to dissolve in the mouth
- Enteric-coated: coated tablets that dissolve in the intestines, rather than stomach, to decrease gastric irritability; never crushed
- Time-release capsules: encased substances that are further enclosed in smaller casings that deliver a drug dose over an extended period of time; never chewed or pulverized
- Sustained-release: compounded substances designed to release a drug slowly to maintain a steady blood medication level; never chewed or pulverized

### Topical

- Powder: lightly dusted on skin
- Liniments: substances mixed with an alcohol, oil, or soapy emollient that is applied to the skin
- Ointments: semisolid substances for topical use
- Pastes: semisolid substances, thicker than an ointment, absorbed slowly through the skin
- Transdermal patches: contain medication that is absorbed through the skin over an extended period of time
- Suppositories: gelatin substances designed to dissolve when inserted in the rectum or vagina

### Inhalants

- Inhalations: drugs administered by the nasal or oral respiratory route for a local or systemic effect

### Solutions

- Solutions: contain one or more soluble chemical substances dissolved in water; can be used orally, topically, or if sterile, can be injected parenterally
- Enemas: aqueous solutions for rectal instillation
- Douches: aqueous solutions that function as a cleansing or antiseptic agent that may be dispensed in the form of a powder with directions for dissolving in a specific quantity of warm water
- Suspensions: particle or powder substances that must be dissolved in a liquid (shaken vigorously) before administration
- Emulsion: a two-phase system in which one liquid is dispersed in the form of small droplets throughout another liquid
- Syrups: substances dissolved in a sugar liquid
- Gargles: aqueous solutions
- Mouthwashes: aqueous solutions that may contain alcohol, glycerin, and synthetic sweeteners and surface-active flavoring and coloring agents
- Nasal solutions: aqueous solutions in the form of drops or sprays
- Optic (eye) and otic (ear) solutions: aqueous solutions that are instilled as drops
- Elixirs: nonaqueous solutions that contain water, varying alcohol content, and glycerin or other sweeteners

require special consideration regarding administration. For example:

- Chewable tablets are designed to be chewed before swallowing because chewing enhances gastric absorption.
- Buccal and sublingual medications must be allowed to dissolve completely before the client can drink or eat.
- Suspensions and emulsions should be administered immediately after shaking and pouring from the bottle.

## Pharmacokinetics

For a medication to achieve a therapeutic effect, it must proceed from the point of entry into the body to the tissue with which it will react. The effectiveness is further affected by the dosage of the medication and the amount of time the medication spends in the body before it is excreted.

**Pharmacokinetics** refers to the study of the absorption, distribution, metabolism, and excretion of drugs to determine the relationship between the dose of a drug and the drug's concentration in biologic fluids. The knowledge of pharmacokinetics is used by health care providers in medication management to maintain a therapeutic drug level in the blood and to prevent alterations in the absorption or excretion of the medication.

The physician, when ordering a medication, is concerned mainly with dose and route to produce the most therapeutic effects; physicians, pharmacists, and nurses are all involved in identifying appropriate times for drug administration and for avoiding interactions with other substances that could alter the drug's actions. Physicians and nurses monitor the client's response to the drug's action. Drug actions are dependent on four properties: absorption, distribution, metabolism, and excretion.

## Absorption

The degree and rate of **absorption**, or passage of a drug from the site of administration into the bloodstream, depend on several factors: the drug's physicochemical effects, its dosage form, its route of administration, its interactions with other substances in the digestive system, and various client characteristics such as age. Oral preparations, such as tablets and capsules, must first disintegrate into smaller particles for gastric juices to dissolve and prepare the drug for absorption in the small intestines. **Dissolution** is the rate at which a drug becomes a solution. After ingestion, a pill, capsule, or caplet must disintegrate before it can be dissolved and then absorbed by the body for therapeutic use. The more rapid the rate of dissolution, the more quickly the medication can be absorbed. Oral drugs in liquid form are more readily absorbed by the gastrointestinal tract than are tablets. **Sustained release** medications are specifically coated so that the medication is released more slowly over a longer period of time. Figure 30-1 shows the process of absorption of solid drugs.

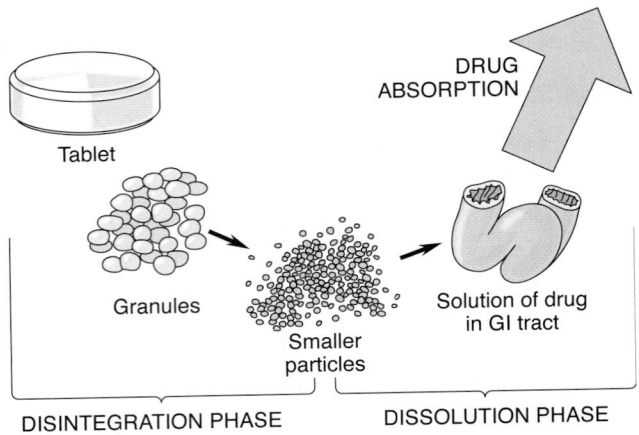

**Figure 30-1    Phases of solid drug absorption**

Drugs administered intramuscularly are absorbed through the muscle into the bloodstream. Suppositories are absorbed through the mucous membranes into the blood. Intravenous drugs are immediately active because of their direct injection into the blood.

Blood flow to the absorption site is a major factor in drug absorption. A rich blood supply facilitates absorption, whereas a poor blood supply will slow absorption. **Sublingual** (under the tongue) medications, such as Nitrostat (for angina), are absorbed more quickly than are medications such as insulin that are injected into subcutaneous tissue. A person in shock, which results in poor peripheral circulation, may not absorb intramuscular medications as well as a person with normal circulation. Circulation is enhanced by exercise, so a diabetic who has exercised hard may experience low blood sugar (hypoglycemia) because of more rapid absorption of the insulin from increased peripheral circulation (Deglin & Vallerand, 2002).

The solubility of the drug is also a factor in absorption. To be absorbed, the drug must be in a liquid form. The more soluble the drug, the faster it will be absorbed. Because cells have a fatty acid layer, drugs that are more lipid in content are absorbed more rapidly. Chemicals and minerals that are insoluble in the gastrointestinal tract, such as barium salts, are not absorbed. When injected into the muscle, drugs with an oily base such as streptomycin (anti-infective) are absorbed more slowly than are drugs dissolved in a water base. Another factor is drug concentration; drugs that are highly concentrated such as epinephrine tend to be absorbed more quickly.

The pH of the drug is another factor in absorption. A drug that is acidic (such as aspirin) can be more easily absorbed in an acidic environment such as gastric content. A drug that is more basic in composition is not absorbed in the stomach but passes on to the small intestine, where it is absorbed.

Another factor affecting absorption is the ingestion of food before taking oral medications. Interactions of some medications with food change the chemical structure of the drug, thereby affecting absorption. For example, tetracycline (an anti-infective) should not be taken with dairy products. Clients taking warfarin (an anticoagulant) should avoid or limit their intake of food high in vitamin K, which is an antidote for warfarin. Some medications, when given together, interact with each other to impair absorption.

The administration time of dosages needs to be regulated to ensure adequate absorption of drugs. For example, it may be best to take certain medications a half-hour before meals. The nurse needs to use this knowledge to be sure prescribed medications are administered properly (Reiss, Evans, & Broyles, 2002).

## Distribution

**Distribution** refers to the movement of medications from the blood into various body fluids and tissues. The rate at which the drug reaches the specific site of action is affected by blood flow, cell membrane permeability, and the protein-binding capacity of the medication.

How fast the drug reaches the organs and tissues depends on the cardiac output (blood flow) of the person. When conditions exist that decrease blood flow (as in cardiogenic shock) or when circulation to the tissue is poor (as in peripheral vascular disease from atherosclerosis), the distribution of the drug will be slowed. When conditions exist that increase blood flow (such as strenuous exercise), distribution will be facilitated.

To be distributed to the tissue, the drug must cross the cell membrane. Some membranes act as a barrier for distribution of medications. The blood brain barrier, for example, allows only fat-soluble medications to pass through (e.g., alcohol, general anesthetics, penicillin G).

Once the medication enters the circulation, much of it binds to proteins, especially albumin. This protein binding decreases the amount of free drug available to reach the site of action. The protein-drug molecule is trapped in the blood flow because it is too large to diffuse through the cell membrane. While medications vary in the extent to which they bind with proteins, most drugs have some protein binding properties. Some diseases (such as malnutrition or liver disease) cause a decrease in circulating albumin, which results in more available drug. This can result in increased distribution of the drug (enhanced pharmacological effect) and toxicity if not carefully monitored.

The body composition also affects the distribution of medications. Many drugs are prescribed based on body weight. An increase in body fat (e.g., in an obese person) causes longer drug duration because of slower distribution. The less a person weighs, the higher the concentration of medication in the circulation, which results in a more powerful drug effect. This needs to be monitored very closely in the elderly who have changes in body composition naturally related to aging and often lose weight due to a decreased appetite.

## Metabolism

After the medication is absorbed and distributed, the process of **metabolism** (also known as **biotransformation**) inactivates the medication and changes it into a form that can be excreted more easily. The liver is the primary source of biotransformation, although the lungs, kidney, blood, and intestines also biotransform some medications (Gutierrez, 1999). The rate of metabolism is determined by the presence of enzymes in the liver cells that detoxify the drugs. Diseases that affect the liver (such as cirrhosis) affect the body's ability to biotransform medications. Other conditions that affect metabolism are blood flow to the liver, the presence of other substances that affect liver function, and age. If drug metabolism is inhibited, there will be a buildup of the medication, causing a cumulative effect. This will be exhibited as prolonged response to a normal dose of medication. If metabolism is enhanced (as in high fevers), the medications will be inactivated faster than expected, resulting in a shorter response to medications.

There is a growing understanding of genetic factors that influence enyzmes involved in medication metabolism. For example, nearly half of the population in the United States have an autosomal recessive trait that slows the acetylation phase of biotransformation (Gutierrez, 1999, p. 65). These people metabolize medications more slowly and are more likely to show toxicity unless given lower doses of medication. Most drug research trials and studies have focused on Caucasian male subjects. Studies are beginning to discover differences in required drug levels among races such as in African Americans taking antihypertensive drugs. There is also recognition that many medications metabolize differently in women than in men.

### LIFE SPAN CONSIDERATIONS

#### Differences in Pediatric Pharmacokinetics

- Absorption of oral medications is often delayed in young infants because they have less gastric acidity until about 3 years of age. However, acid-labile medications such as penicillin may absorb more rapidly.

- Infants have a lower capacity of protein-binding; therefore, a greater amount of "free" drug can circulate, which can cause side effects or drug toxicity.

- Infants' urine is less acid, which affects the elimination rate of some medications that are more readily excreted in acid urine.

Gutierrez, K. (1999). *Pharmacotherapeutics: Clinical decision-making in nursing.* Philadelphia: W. B. Saunders Company.

## LIFE SPAN CONSIDERATIONS

### Differences in Geriatric Pharmacokinetics

- Body composition changes can impact drug distribution. Many older clients have less lean muscle mass and body water and have more fat. Fat-soluble medications, which dissolve in fat, will have a longer half-life and longer duration of action. Water-soluble medications are more concentrated because there is less body water.

- Decreased liver or kidney function in older clients can slow elimination of medication and increase the concentration of metabolites. Thus older clients are more apt to experience side effects and drug toxicities.

- H-antagonist or proton-pump inhibitor medications for gastric acid reflux (GERD) will affect the absorption of many other medications. Iron and calcium are absorbed less readily, whereas enteric-coated medications will be absorbed faster.

Gutierrez, K. (1999). *Pharmacotherapeutics: Clinical decision-making in nursing.* Philadelphia: W. B. Saunders Company.

## Excretion

**Excretion** is the process in which drugs are eliminated from the body. Excretion occurs primarily through the liver/biliary system and the kidneys. Some gaseous compounds exit through the lungs. Sweat glands, the skin, breast glands, and tear ducts excrete minute amounts of some medications. For breast-feeding women, however, even small amounts of excreted medication are of concern for the infant.

Factors that affect the kidneys' ability to excrete drugs include maturity of the kidneys, circulation, and disease. As kidney function decreases, there can be an accumulation of drugs, which can result in toxicity. If the kidneys are not functioning normally, a decreased dosage of medications may be needed. Adequate fluid intake aids in the elimination of drugs in a healthy individual.

## Types of Medication Action

Medication action refers to the **pharmacodynamic** changes in cellular biochemistry that the drug causes at the site of action. The medication may cause changes to occur in the cellular environment, such as osmolarity or pH changes in the surrounding fluids. It is thought that the majority of drugs attach to cell receptors on the cell surface and alter specific cellular functions such as depression of membrane functions, blockage of a type of cell receptor, or inhibition or acceleration of cellular enyzme functions (Reiss, Evans, & Broyles, 2002). However, with a number of medications even the site of action is not known. The medication action may be local at the cellular or organ level, systemic—affecting changes throughout the body—or both local and systemic. For example, when diphenhydramine hydrochloride (Benadryl) cream is applied to the skin, it elicits only a local effect; however, when this drug is administered in a tablet or injectable form, it causes both systemic and local effects.

## Medication Management of Drug Levels

The purpose of medication management is to produce the desired drug action by maintaining a constant drug level within the therapeutic range. **Therapeutic range** is defined as the range of drug concentration in the blood that gives the desired effect without causing serious side effects or toxicity. Drug action is based on the half-life of a drug.

A drug's **half-life** refers to the time it takes the body to eliminate half of the blood concentration level of the original drug dose and correlates roughly with duration of action (Deglin & Vallerand, 2002). For example, if a drug has a half-life of 6 hours, 50% of the drug's original dose is present in the blood 6 hours after administration; in 12 hours after administration, 25% of the original drug is present. Because of a drug's half-life, repeated doses are often required to maintain the drug level at the therapeutic level over a 24-hour interval.

The nurse should understand other terms used to describe drug action: onset, peak plasma level, trough, duration, and plateau. **Onset of action** is the time it takes the body to respond to a drug after administration. Onset is affected by route of administration and pharmokinetic factors already discussed. A **peak plasma level** is the highest blood concentration of a single drug dose before the elimination rate equals the rate of absorption. Once the peak plasma level is achieved, the blood concentration level will decrease steadily unless another drug dose is given. The peak drug level is measured by doing a blood draw a half hour to an hour after a dose of the medication is given. **Trough** is the lowest blood serum concentration of a drug in a person's system. This is measured immediately before the next scheduled dose. Peak and trough drug levels are very important for medications that have high toxicity risks for permanent kidney damage or ear damage causing deafness. By knowing a client's peak and trough levels, the medication dose can be adjusted to maintain a therapeutic drug level while avoiding a toxic level. **Duration** is the time a drug remains in the system in a concentration great enough to have a therapeutic effect.

Table 30-2 defines the common terms associated with the medical management of medication administration. If a series of scheduled drug doses are administered, the blood concentration level is maintained; maintenance of a certain level is called a **plateau**.

# Factors That Alter Medication Action

The goal of prescribing a medication is to have a therapeutic response with alleviation of symptoms or a decrease in the disease process, with as few unpredictable responses or untoward effects as possible. However, there is great variation in responses to a medication among individuals. Some of the factors that can alter medication action include interaction with the client's other medications, diet, renal and liver function, genetic factors, and amount of body fat.

## Medication Interaction

**Medication interaction** refers to the effect one drug can have on another. Medication interactions may occur when one drug is administered in combination with a second drug or when a short time interval exists between the administration of two different drugs. Drugs can be combined deliberately to produce a positive effect, as when hydrochlorothiazide (a potassium-depleting diuretic) is combined with spironolactone (a potassium-sparing diuretic) to maintain a normal blood level of potassium. A positive drug combination can also occur when one drug, such as a preoperative medication, is deliberately given to potentiate the action of another drug.

Not all drug combinations are therapeutic. Some drug combinations can interfere with the absorption, effect, or excretion of other drugs. For example, calcium products and magnesium-containing antacids can cause inadequate absorption of tetracycline (antibiotic) in the digestive tract.

## Food and Drug Interactions

Medication management requires avoidance of possible food and drug interactions. There are three primary types of food and drug interaction:

1. Certain drugs may interfere with the absorption, excretion, or use in the body of one or more nutrients.
2. Certain foods may increase or decrease the absorption of a drug into the body.
3. Certain foods may alter the chemical actions of drugs, preventing their therapeutic effect on the body.

Most interaction problems occur with the use of diuretics, oral antibiotics, and anticoagulant and antihypertensive drugs (see Box 30-3). Clients on sodium-restricted diets should be advised to consult with a pharmacist regarding the sodium content in prescription and over-the-counter drugs. Some drugs can contain almost one-half the total daily allowance of sodium. Alcohol is also considered a drug. Small amounts of alcohol interact with many drugs, such as antibiotics, antihistamines, anticoagulants, and sleeping pills. Food and drug interactions can vary depending on the dose and the form in which the drug is taken and the client's age, sex, body weight, nutritional status, and specific medical condition.

## Client Factors Influencing Drug Action

Individual client characteristics such as genetic factors, gender, age, height and weight, and physical and mental conditions can influence the action of drugs on the body. Sometimes mistaken for drug allergies, genetic factors can interfere with drug metabolism and produce an abnormal sensitivity to certain drugs.

The nurse should consider age-related factors that can influence drug action and dosing. For example, neonates and infants have underdeveloped gastrointestinal systems, muscle mass, and metabolic enzyme systems and inadequate renal function; older clients often experience decreased hepatic or renal function and diminished muscle mass.

The physician often correlates the client's age, height, and weight when determining the dosage for many drugs. The nurse should make sure that this information is accurately recorded in the client's medical record. The amount

| TABLE 30-2 | COMMON TERMS ASSOCIATED WITH MEDICAL MANAGEMENT |
|---|---|
| Half-life | The time it takes the body to eliminate half the blood concentration level of the original drug dose |
| Onset | The time it takes the body to respond after medication administration |
| Peak plasma level | The time it takes for a drug to reach the highest blood concentration after a plasma level single dose before elimination rate equals the rate of absorption |
| Trough | The lowest blood serum concentration immediately before the next scheduled dosage |
| Duration | The time a drug remains in the system in a therapeutic concentration |
| Plateau | Blood concentration level maintained after a series of scheduled drug doses is administered |
| Therapeutic range | The drug level range at which the medication can effectively and safely accomplish the desired effect |

## BOX 30-3    COMMON FOOD AND DRUG INTERACTIONS

### Drug Effects on Nutritional Status

- Abuse of antacids can lead to phosphate depletion, which can cause a vitamin D deficiency, resulting in osteomalacia, or softening of the bones due to loss of calcium.

- Excessive use of diuretics may result in the loss of electrolytes, especially potassium, that places clients with cardiac conditions at a higher risk for serious rhythm problems. Potassium loss is greatest in clients taking digitalis as well as diuretics, making the heart more sensitive to the drug.

- Prolonged use of oral contraceptives by women may cause folacin and vitamin C deficiencies if their diets are inadequate in these nutrients.

- Hydralazine (antihypertensive drug) can deplete the body's supply of vitamin $B_6$.

### Food Effects on Drug Absorption

- Calcium in milk and milk products may decrease the absorption of certain antibiotics such as tetracycline.

- Certain liquids such as soda pop or high-acid fruit or vegetable juices can cause an increase in the stomach acidity that can dissolve some drugs before they reach the intestine. Because most drugs are absorbed in the intestines, this interaction will decrease the amount of drug that can be absorbed into the body.

- Certain foods such as fatty foods can increase the rate of absorption of some drugs (e.g., griseofulvin, an antifungal).

### Food Effects on Drug Utilization

- The effects of anticoagulants can be decreased by certain foods in the liver such as green leafy vegetables that contain vitamin K, which is used by the body to promote blood clotting.

- Aged or fermented foods such as aged cheese, chicken livers, and other foods can decrease the metabolism in the body of monoamine oxidase inhibitors that are used to treat depression and high blood pressure.

- Long-term use of licorice and licorice-flavored candy or drugs can counteract the effect of high blood pressure medication.

of body fat may also alter drug distribution because some drugs such as digoxin (inotropic) are poorly distributed to fatty tissues.

The client's physical condition can also alter the effects of drugs. For example, in an edematous client the drug must be distributed to a larger volume of body fluids than for a nonedematous client; therefore, the edematous client may require a larger drug dose to produce the drug action, whereas a dehydrated client would require a smaller dosage. Diseases that affect liver and renal functions can alter the metabolism and elimination of most drugs.

## Nontherapeutic Drug Actions

Drug effects other than those that are therapeutically intended and expected may occur with almost all medications. Some are mild and transitory, others severe and potentially dangerous. The nurse must monitor for the following types of drug actions in clients and report them to the health care provider who ordered the medication.

### Side Effects

**Side effects** are nontherapeutic, though often predictable, actions that a low percentage of clients may experience with a specific medication. Examples of side effects are nausea, dizziness, sleepiness, or constipation. Most side effects are mild, although some may progress to a serious problem, such as continuing nausea causing the client to be dehydrated. Some side effects can be treated such as using an antiemetic medication for nausea. However, clients may find the side effects intolerable and refuse to take the medication (Reiss, Evans, & Broyles, 2002).

### Adverse Reactions

**Adverse reactions** are serious reactions of the client to the medication and are generally sufficient reason for the health care provider to discontinue the medication. Examples of adverse effects are bone marrow depression, coma, or hepatic or kidney damage evidenced by elevated laboratory values. Red-man syndrome (RMS) is an extremely serious adverse reaction, most commonly seen in clients receiving vancomycin, but it can occur with other antibiotics (Reiss, Evans, & Broyles, 2002). Clinical trials of new drugs are meant to detect and eliminate medications that cause adverse reactions, but not all reactions are apparent during the trials. It is imperative that all adverse reactions be reported to the FDA through the MedWatch program.

### Toxic Effects

A **toxic effect** occurs when the body cannot readily metabolize a drug, causing the drug to accumulate in the blood. Toxic effects can result after prolonged intake of high doses of medication or after only one dose. They can occur if the client has poor hepatic or kidney function, lacks the genetic code of an enzyme necessary for metabolism to occur, or if the dose is too large for the body-fat ratio or body surface of the individual. A few medications have another medication that is an antidote to the toxic effect. For example, vitamin K may be given to counteract a high drug level of coumadin. Narcan can be given to counteract the effects of narcotic opioids.

### Drug Allergy

A drug allergy is an antigen-antibody immune reaction that occurs when an individual who has been previously exposed to a drug has developed antibodies against the drug. The type of reaction may be mild such as skin rash, urticaria, and a headache. However, any reaction must be quickly assessed as it can progress quickly to anaphylaxis. The most common medications causing anaphylaxis are penicillin and all the cephalosporins (Carroll, 2001). Anaphylaxis is an immediate, life-threatening reaction to a drug, such as to penicillin, characterized by respiratory distress, sudden severe bronchospasm, and cardiovascular collapse. If emergency measures such as administration of epinephrine, bronchodilators, and antihistamines are not instituted immediately, anaphylaxis can be fatal.

A medication should never be given to a client who has a known allergy to the medication. The nurse should also be aware that there can be cross-hypersensitivity between some classes of medications, such as between penicillin and cephalosporins. Clients should be taught to keep a record of their medication allergies with them at all times in order to avoid being inadvertently reexposed. Those with known severe allergies should wear an identification arm band or neck tag with the name of the known medication on it, which alerts health care providers in case the client is unconscious.

Identification bracelets or neck chains are available from the nonprofit MedicAlert organization at 1-888-633-4298 or http://www.medicalert.org (2002).

### Idiosyncratic Reaction

An idiosyncratic reaction is a highly unpredictable response that may be manifested by overresponse, underresponse, or an atypical response. Because of its rare occurrence, it is impossible to predict beforehand the chances of this type of reaction.

## STOP AND THINK

### Allergic Reactions

- What are the signs and symptoms of a mild allergic reaction?

- What are the early symptoms of an anaphylactic reaction?

- What nursing interventions do you need to take immediately?

### Drug Tolerance

Drug tolerance occurs when the body becomes so accustomed to a specific drug that larger doses are needed to produce the desired therapeutic effect. For example, cancer clients with severe pain may require larger and larger doses of morphine to control the pain as the body builds up a tolerance to the morphine.

## Routes of Medication Administration

Medications may be administered via the following routes: oral, parenteral, topical, inhalants, and intraocular. Each of these routes of medication administration is presented in the following section.

## Oral Route

Most drugs are administered by the oral route because it is the safest, most convenient, and least expensive method. The medicine is swallowed with fluid or given by gastrointestinal tube. The disadvantage of the oral route is that it is slower acting than the other routes, such as injectables. Drugs may not be given orally to clients with gastrointestinal intolerance or those on NPO (nothing by mouth) status. Oral drugs should be given with caution to clients who have difficulty swallowing, such as a client who has had a cerebrovascular accident (stroke). Oral administration is also precluded by unconsciousness unless a gastrointestinal tube is used.

When small amounts of drugs are required, the **buccal** (cheek) or sublingual (under the tongue) route is used. Drugs administered through these routes act quickly because of the oral mucosa's thin epithelium and large vascular system, which allows the drug to quickly be absorbed by the blood.

Certain oral drugs are prepared for sublingual or buccal administration to prevent their destruction or transformation in the stomach or small intestines. Buccal drugs are designed to be placed in the buccal pocket (superior-posterior aspect of the internal cheek next to the molars) for absorption by the mucous membrane of the mouth. Sublingual medications are designed to dissolve quickly when placed under the tongue. Nitroglycerin, an antianginal medication, is given sublingually during an episode of chest pain for its quick absorption and action to relieve the angina. The client should not swallow the buccal or sublingual medication but allow it to dissolve.

## Parenteral Route

By definition, **parenteral** means introduction of a medication by injection into a body tissue. Sterile technique is always used for any medication injection. The four routes that nurses commonly use to administer parenteral medications are:

- **Intradermal (ID)** is an injection into the dermis.
- **Subcutaneous (SC or SQ)** is an injection into the subcutaneous tissue.
- **Intramuscular (IM)** is an injection into the muscle.
- **Intravenous (IV)** is an injection into a vein.

Other parenteral routes, such as intrathecal or intraspinal, intracardiac, intrapleural, intra-arterial, and intra-articular, are used by physicians and in some cases by advanced practice registered nurses for medication administration.

## Topical Route

Topical medications are given to deliver a drug either for a local effect on the skin or mucous membrane or for absorption into the blood stream for a systemic effect. Although a large number of topical drugs are applied to the skin, other topical drugs include eye, nose and throat, ear, and rectal and vaginal preparations.

Topical medications that are meant for a local effect are usually creams, lotions, or ointments for the skin. There are also solutions for mucous membranes and suppositories for rectal and vaginal cavities. Some solutions meant for local treatment can still be absorbed in small amounts, resulting in some systemic effects.

Medications meant for systemic absorption include pastes such as nitropaste (antihypertensive, antianginal) and transdermal patches for fentanyl (pain medication), estrogen, nitroglycerin, and other medications. The patches are impregnated with the medication and have tiny membranes that slowly allow the medication to pass through to the skin and be absorbed. Patches can last from 24 to 72, hours according to the manufacturer's instructions.

The client may complain of a burning sensation when the nurse instills eye or nasal drops because the cornea of the eye and nasal mucous membranes are often sensitive to medications. Eyedrops should never be applied onto the sensitive cornea.

## Inhalant Route

Inhalants such as oxygen and most general anesthetics deliver gaseous or volatile substances that are almost immediately absorbed into the systemic circulation. The inhalants are delivered into the alveoli of the lungs, which promote fast absorption owing to:

- The permeability of the alveolar and vascular epithelia
- An abundant blood flow
- A very large surface area for absorption

Oropharyngeal handheld inhalers deliver topical drugs to the respiratory tract to create local and systemic effects. There are three types of inhaler: metered-dose inhaler or nebulizer, turbo-inhaler, and nasal inhaler. They are explained later in this chapter (Togger & Brenner, 2001).

## Intraocular Route

Intraocular medications are administered by applying a clear, flexible, elliptical-shaped disk similar to a contact lens to the conjunctival sac. This provides continuous treatment of diseases such as open-angle glaucoma. Pilocarpine, a medication to treat glaucoma, can be administered in this manner. The disk can remain in the patient's eye for up to a week. This route increases compliance and decreases the number of times a client must administer medication.

# Professional Roles in Medication Administration

The health care practitioner determines the therapeutic drug plan and conveys the plan to others by initiating orders or a prescription. Each state has laws regarding who has prescriptive authority, which may include not only physicians but physician's assistants (PA) and advanced practice nurses such as nurse practitioners and clinical nurse specialists. In long-term care facilities and hospitals, medication orders are written on the client's order sheet in the medical record. In the community, medication orders are written on legal prescription pads. Increasingly, orders can be written at computer terminals in many settings. When allowed by organizational policy, the prescriber may also give medication orders via telephone or as a verbal order (Haack & Yocum, 2002).

If the prescriber gives a medication order orally, either directly or over the telephone, the nurse enters the information on the client's medical record. This information includes the name of the health care practitioner who ordered the medication, the name of the medication, the dosage, the frequency, the route of administration, and the nurse's name. Most institutions require the prescriber to confirm oral orders within 24 hours; the nurse is responsible for ensuring that the verbal order is clear. It often helps for the nurse to repeat the order to the prescriber to make sure it was interpreted as intended. See Chapter 16 for a complete discussion of written and verbal orders and the role of the nurse in transcribing orders.

The pharmacist processes the prescriber's orders, clarifies any entries that are unclear, and prepares the medications for administration. The pharmacist is responsible for filling prescriptions and for making sure they are valid entries. Pharmacists also assess medication plans, monitoring for incompatibilities and, at times, recommending the best time to administer a medication to obtain therapeutic benefit such as Lovastatin (cholesterol-lowering drug), which is most effective if taken in the evening. The pharmacist participates in calculating the appropriate dosage of certain medications such as anti-infective drugs (e.g., gentamicin). These dosages are based on the patient's body weight and kidney function and may be adjusted during the course of therapy by the pharmacist with the health care practitioner's consent. Nurses frequently consult with pharmacists in determining compatibility if intravenous medications are to be administered simultaneously. Pharmacists also answer medication-related questions for both nurses and clients.

The nurse's role is to use the nursing process to assess the client's health history, administer the medication safely, and to evaluate the effect of the medication on the client, including monitoring for side effects and adverse reactions.

Nurses spend a great deal of time with their clients and have specific knowledge and skills that qualify them to administer medication and to evaluate a medication's effectiveness. Nurses understand why particular medications are ordered for clients and what physiological changes may result from the medication that cause a therapeutic effect. Because of their knowledge, skills, and frequent client contact, nurses can readily assess changes in a client's condition and can determine whether it is appropriate to administer a medication on the basis of the client's condition.

In addition, nurses are responsible for teaching clients to self-administer medications such as insulin and for assessing the client's ability to self-administer correctly. Before discharge, nurses teach clients about the medications they will be taking at home and how to assess for side effects and adverse reactions.

## Types of Medication Orders

Depending on their purpose, medications can be prescribed as stat, single-dose, standing, and prn orders.

### Stat Orders

When the prescriber writes orders, the nurse should read all of the orders to determine if any stat orders have been prescribed. A **stat order** is an order for a single dose of medication to be given immediately. Stat drugs are often prescribed in emergency situations to modify a serious physiological response; a stat dose of nitroglycerin may be ordered for a client experiencing chest pain. The nurse should assess and document the client's response to all stat medications.

### Single-Dose Orders

Single-dose orders are onetime medications or may require the administration of drops or tablets over a short period of time. The nurse should administer single-dose orders only once, either at a time specified by the health care practitioner or at the earliest convenient time. These drugs are often prescribed in preparation for a diagnostic or therapeutic procedure; for example, radiopaque tablets may be administered in preparation for a gallbladder test, or a onetime order may be given for a preoperative medication.

### Standing Orders

Standing orders are also referred to as *scheduled orders* because they are administered routinely as specified until the order is canceled by another order. The standing orders stay in effect until the prescriber discontinues or modifies the dosage or frequency with another order or until a prescribed number of days has elapsed as determined by agency policy.

A standing medication is ordered at specific times to maintain the therapeutic blood level of the medication. For example, antibiotics must be given around the clock at regular intervals to maintain a therapeutic blood level, whereas Coumadin (an anticoagulant) needs to be given only once daily (qd). Most agencies have specific times for once daily, three times a day (t.i.d.), and other scheduled medication times to help coordinate pharmacy preparation times and to prevent an accidental omission of a medication dose. For example, t.i.d. drugs may be administered at 0800, 1400, and 2000 or at 0900, 1500, and 2100. Medications ordered qd may have a specified time identified in the order, such as Isophane (NPH) Insulin 10 U SC qd at 0600, or they may be given at the agency's designated time, for example, Lanoxin 0.25 mg PO qd 0900. However, the nurse may need to adjust the specific hours of a client's medication if a dose is missed while the client is at a test or a new medication arrives.

When the order specifies the number of days or the number of dosages of the drug the client is to receive, the order has an automatic stop date to discontinue the drug. For example, the order may read tetracycline 250 mg PO q6h for 5 days. The nurse should execute this order by administering 250 mg tetracycline orally every 6 hours for 5 days for a total of 20 doses. Day one begins with the administration of the drug and the time the first dose is given. If the first dose of tetracycline is given on a Tuesday at 1200, then every 6 hours, the last dose will be given on Sunday at 0600. Although the medication is given over 6 consecutive days, it totals 20 doses as ordered. Most agencies have an automatic stop date to discontinue certain medications, such as 5 or 7 days for antibiotics and 48 or 72 hours for narcotics.

## prn Orders

A drug may be ordered on a **prn** (as needed) basis as circumstances indicate. The drug is administered when, in the nurse's judgment, the client's condition requires it. Before administering a prn medication, the nurse must thoroughly assess the client, using both objective and subjective data in determining the appropriateness of administering the medication. This type of order is commonly written for analgesics, antiemetics, and laxatives.

The order written by the prescriber indicates how frequently a prn medication can be given. A nurse cannot administer a prn medication more frequently than the order indicates without consulting with the prescriber for a change in that order. Examples of prn orders are meperidine (a narcotic analgesic) 75 mg IM q3–4 hours prn incisional pain and Tylenol 650 mg q4 hours prn headache. When the prn medication has been administered, the nurse documents the assessment and the time of administration. In addition, the nurse is responsible for monitoring the effectiveness of the medication and documenting the effect in the client's medical record. The nurse administers the pain medication on the basis of the assessment of the client's pain and as specified in the order.

## Parts of the Medication Order

All orders should be written clearly and legibly, and the order should contain seven parts:

1. The name of the client
2. The date and time when the order is written
3. The name of the drug to be administered
4. The dosage
5. The route by which it is to be administered and special directives about its administration
6. The time of administration and frequency
7. The signature of the person writing the order, such as the physician or advanced practice registered nurse

Medication prescriptions written in settings other than acute care facilities may also specify whether the generic or trade name of the drug is to be dispensed, the quantity to be dispensed, and how many times the prescription can be refilled.

Most agencies have a listing of abbreviations officially accepted for use in the agency. The agency's medical records department maintains the official listing of abbreviations adopted by the medical staff; only abbreviations from the official list can be used in any part of the client's medical record. See Table 30-3 for a list of common abbreviations used in medication orders.

## Medication Administration Record

After the prescriber has written the medication order in the client's medical record, the nurse transcribes (hand-writes) the exact order onto another part of the medical record called the medication administration record (MAR). After the day of admission, the MAR is usually computer-generated in the pharmacy and the nurse transcribes new orders daily as they are written. (A computer-generated MAR form is shown in Figure 30-2.) The MAR contains the client's medication orders for each day the client is in the health care institution. The nurse records on the MAR the date and time when each dose is given and initials the entry.

| TABLE 30-3 | COMMON ABBREVIATIONS USED IN MEDICATION ORDERS |
|---|---|
| **Abbreviation** | **Meaning** |
| a.c. | before meals |
| ad lib | freely, as desired |
| b.i.d. | two times a day |
| c̄ | with |
| cap | capsule |
| DC | discontinue |
| elix | elixir |
| h | hour |
| hrly | hourly |
| h.s. | at bedtime |
| ID | intradermal |
| IM | intramuscular |
| IV | intravenous |
| IVPB | intravenous piggyback |
| OD | right eye |
| od | every day |
| OS | left eye |
| OU | each eye |
| p.c. | after meals |
| PO | by mouth |
| per | by |
| prn | as needed |
| q | every |
| qd | every day |
| q2h | every 2 hours |
| q.i.d. | four times a day |
| qod | every other day |
| qs | sufficient quantity |
| SC or SQ | subcutaneous |
| stat | immediately |
| supp | suppository |
| susp | suspension |
| tab | tablet |
| t.i.d. | three times a day |
| Tr or tinct | tincture |

# Systems of Medication Measurement

Medication administration requires the nurse to have a knowledge of weight and volume measurement systems. In North America, there are three systems of measurement used in medication management: metric, apothecary, and household. The apothecary system is rarely used.

## Metric System

The metric, or decimal, system is a simple system of measurement based on units of 10. The basic units can be multiplied or divided by 10 to form secondary units. The decimal point is moved to the right for calculating multiples, and the decimal point is moved to the left for division.

The basic units of measurement in the metric system are the meter (linear), the liter (volume), and the gram (mass). When the metric system is used, a zero is always placed in front of the decimal for values less than 1 (e.g., 0.5) to prevent error.

## Measurement Conversions within the Metric System

Because the metric system is based on units of 10, dose equivalents within the system are computed by simple arithmetic, either dividing or multiplying. For example, to change milligrams to grams (1,000 mg equals 1 g) or milliliters to liters (1,000 ml equals 1 L), divide the number by 1,000:

$$250 \text{ mg} = x \text{ g}$$
(move the decimal point three places to the left)
$$x = 0.25 \text{ g}$$
or
$$500 \text{ ml} = x \text{ L}$$
(move the decimal point three places to the left)
$$x = 0.5 \text{ L}$$

**PHARMACY MAR**

| START | STOP | MEDICATION | SCHEDULED TIMES | OK'D BY | 0001 HRS. to 1200 HRS. | 1201 HRS. to 2400 HRS. |
|---|---|---|---|---|---|---|
| 08/31/xx 1800 SCH | | PROCAN SR 500 MG TAB-SR 500 MG Q6H PO | 0600 1200 1800 2400 | JD | 0600 GP 1200 GP | 1800 MS 2400 JD |
| 09/03/xx 0900 SCH | | DIGOXIN (LANOXIN) 0.125 MG TAB 1 TAB QOD PO ODD DAYS-SEPT. | 0900 | JD | 0900 GP | |
| 09/03/xx 0900 SCH | | FUROSEMIDE (LASIX) 40 MG TAB 1 TAB QD PO | 0900 | JD | 0900 GP | |
| 09/03/xx 0845 SCH | | REGLAN 10 MG TAB 10 MG AC&HS PO GIVE ONE NOW! | 0730 1130 1630 2100 | JD | 0730 GP 1130 GP | 1630 MS 2100 MS |
| 09/04/xx 0900 SCH | | K-LYTE 25 MEQ EFFERVESCENT TAB 1 EFF. TAB BID PO DISSOLVE AS DIR. START 9-4 | 0900 1700 | JD | 0900 GP | 1700 GP |
| 09/03/xx 1507 PRN | | NITROGLYCERIN 1/50 GR 0.4 MG TAB-SL 1 TABLET PRN* SL PRN CHEST PAIN | | JD | | |
| 09/03/xx 1700 PRN | | DARVOCET-N 100* 1 TAB Q4-6H PO PRN MILD-MODERATE PAIN | | JD | | |
| 09/03/xx 2100 PRN | | MEPERIDINE*(DEMEROL) INJ 50 MG Q4H IM PRN SEVERE PAIN W PHENERGAN | | JD | | 2200 (H) MS |
| 09/03/xx 2100 PRN | | PROMETHAZINE (PHENERGAN) INJ 50 MG Q4H IM PRN SEVERE PAIN W DEMEROL | | JD | | 2200 (H) MS |

| Gluteus | Thigh |
|---|---|
| A. Right | H. Right |
| B. Left | I. Left |
| Ventro Gluteal | |
| C. Right | J. Right |
| D. Left | K. Left |
| E. Abdomen | 1|2 / 3|4 |

| Nurse's Signature | Initial |
|---|---|
| 7-3  G. Pickar, R.N. | GP |
| 3-11  M. Smith, R.N. | MS |
| 11-7  J. Doe, R.N. | JD |

Allergies: NKA

Diagnosis: CHF

| | |
|---|---|
| Patient: | Patient, John D. |
| Patient #: | 3-81512-3 |
| Admitted: | 08/31/xx |
| Physician: | J. Physician, MD |
| Room: | PCU-14 PCU |

**Figure 30-2    Computerized pharmacy medication administration record**

To convert grams to milligrams or liters to milliliters, the nurse multiplies the number by 1,000:

$$0.005 \text{ g} = x \text{ mg}$$

(move the decimal point three places to the right)

$$x = 5 \text{ mg}$$

or

$$0.725 \text{ L} = x \text{ ml}$$

(move the decimal point three places to the right)

$$x = 725 \text{ ml}$$

The nurse may need to convert the volumes of liters and milliliters for enemas and irrigating solutions such as for bladder and wound irrigations. Intravenous solutions are sterile, prepackaged solutions dispensed in volumes as ordered by the health care practitioner, such as 50 ml, 100 ml, 250 ml, 500 ml, and 1,000 ml (1 liter).

## Apothecary System

The apothecary system, which originated in England, is based on the weight of one grain of wheat. Therefore, the basic unit of weight is the grain (gr), and the basic unit of volume is the minim (the approximate volume of water that weighs a grain). The grain is expressed in fractions such as morphine gr 1/4. The minim (*m*) is the smallest unit of volume, followed in ascending order by the fluid dram (*D*), fluid ounce (*Z*), pint (pt), quart (qt), and gallon (gal).

## Household System

The household system of measurement is similar to the apothecary system of liquid measures and is the least accurate of the three systems. The units of liquid measure are drop (gtt), teaspoon (tsp), tablespoon (Tbsp), cup, and glass. Household units are often used to inform clients of the size of a liquid dose. Home health nurses often have to convert a liquid dose to an approximate household unit.

As shown in Table 30-4, the USP recognizes the use of the teaspoon as the ordinary practice for household med-

ication administration and states that the teaspoon may be regarded as representing 5 ml (American Hospital Formulary Service, 1996). Household spoons are not appropriate when accurate measurement of a liquid dose is required; therefore, the USP recommends that a calibrated oral syringe or dropper, which can be purchased at the neighborhood pharmacy, be used for accurate measurement of liquid drug doses.

## Drug Dose Calculations

Several formulas may be used by the nurse when calculating drug doses. One formula uses ratios based on the *dose on hand* and the *dose desired*. For example, cephalexin (antiinfective cephalosporin) 500 mg PO q.i.d. (dose desired) is ordered by the health care practitioner; the dose on hand is 250 mg/5 ml. The formula is as follows (Springhouse Corporation, 2002):

$$\frac{250 \text{ mg (dose on hand)}}{5 \text{ ml (dose on hand)}} \qquad \frac{500 \text{ mg (dose desired)}}{x \text{ (dose desired)}}$$

(cross-multiply)

$$250 \, x = 5 \times 500$$

$$\frac{5 \times 500}{250}$$

$$x = 10 \text{ ml}$$

The ratio formula can be used in calculating dosages. For example, the health care practitioner orders heparin (anticoagulant) 10,000 units SC; the dose on hand is 40,000 units/ml:

$$\frac{40,000 \text{ units}}{1 \text{ ml}} \qquad \frac{10,000 \text{ units}}{x}$$

(units cancel out)

$$40,000 \, x = 10,000$$

$$x = \frac{10,000 \text{ units}}{40,000 \text{ units}}$$

$$x = \frac{1}{4}$$

$$x = 0.25 \text{ ml}$$

### Pediatric Dosages

Metabolism of medications is different in infants and children than in adults. Body surface is more important in infants and children than weight or height, because body surface influences the metabolic rate, fluid balance, and renal and cardiovascular functions. For example, the cardiovascular changes from infancy through childhood influence the uptake and distribution of medications (Gutierrez, 1999, p. 9). In addition, many organ systems have immature physiological functions in the very young. Several rules have been devised to calculate infants' and children's dosages such as *Young's Rule, Clark's Rule*, and *Fried's Rule*, but these rules give only approximate dosages. Even when pediatric drug dosages are calculated on body surface area, weight, and age of the child, they are based on

| TABLE 30-4 | APPROXIMATE METRIC SYSTEM AND HOUSEHOLD EQUIVALENTS |
|---|---|

| Metric | | Household |
|---|---|---|
| 5 ml | = | 1 teaspoon |
| 15 ml | = | 1 tablespoon |
| 30 ml | = | 1 ounce |
| 500 ml | = | 1 pint |
| 1,000 ml | = | 1 quart |

a proportion of the usual adult dose (approximate). Regardless of the method used in calculating pediatric drug dosages, the nurse should realize that dosages are approximate and often need adjustment based on the child's response. The nurse should recheck all doses using a pediatric drug reference. If the nurse has any questions or concern about the medication or dose, the prescriber or pharmacist should be consulted before the nurse gives the medication.

The body surface area method of determining pediatric doses is based on the body surface area of an adult weighing 150 lb. The body surface area of an adult weighing 150 lb is 1.73 square meters. The approximate child dose is calculated as follows:

$$\frac{\text{Body surface area of child}}{\text{Body surface area of adult}} \times \text{adult dose}$$

$$= \text{approximate child dose}$$

$$\frac{\text{Body surface area of child (m}^2) \times \text{adult dose}}{1.73 \text{ m}^2}$$

$$= \text{approximate child dose}$$

Nomograms based on height and weight are used to compute the body surface area. Nomograms are used primarily in calculating pediatric drug dosages; however, they are also used when calculating some adult drug dosages, such as aminoglycosides and antineoplastic agents.

## Medication Storage and Distribution

Medications are dispensed by the pharmacy to nursing units through various methods to accommodate the agency's medication system. Once the pharmacy delivers the medications to a nursing unit, the nurse is responsible for their safe storage. All medications must *always* be stored in a locked, secure place and never left out unattended. Hospitals and long-term care facilities have locked cabinets, medicine carts, and medicine rooms for secure storage until it is time to dispense the medication.

Many hospitals are using computer-controlled dispensing units for secure storage of medications on each unit (Figure 30-3). These are controlled through a computer in the pharmacy that has the client's medication orders. Using a secure password and the touch screen, the nurse selects the medication needed, the drawer with the medication opens, and the computer keeps a record of who took out the medication.

In hospitals, regularly scheduled drugs for each client are usually dispensed in a **unit dose form**. Unit dose is a system of packaging and labeling each dose of medication by the pharmacy or manufacturer. It provides a method to check the name and dose of the medication both as it is withdrawn from the storage unit and again at the bedside

before it is given to the client. A variation is the blister or bingo pack of medication used in long-term care facilities. These packs have 25 to 50 doses of the medication individually packaged on a large card. A dose is separated from the card after the name of the medication is checked with the MAR. This form is cost-effective for agencies where there is no in-house pharmacy.

In some institutions, certain drugs are **stock supplied** (dispensed in large quantities in a labeled bottle or jar) and stored in a locked medication room. However, preparing medications from a stock supply is time-consuming and has a high potential for medication errors. Therefore, it is seldom used in today's health care facilities (Smeltzer, 2001).

Certain intravenous fluids and medications must be stored in the medication refrigerator to preserve the integrity of the drug. The Public Health Department and accrediting agencies mandate that only drugs can be stored in the medication refrigerator.

## Narcotics and Controlled Substances

Health care agencies have forms to record the supply on hand and the administration of narcotics and controlled substances in accord with federal regulations. These forms usually require the recording of the following information for each drug administered:

- Name of the client receiving the drug
- Amount of the drug used
- Time the drug was administered
- Name of the prescribing health care practitioner
- Name of the nurse administering the drug

Nursing practice usually requires that nurses count the narcotics and controlled substances at specified intervals. For example, at the change of shifts, one nurse who is going off duty counts the drugs with a nurse coming on duty. Each drug used must be accounted for on the narcotic record. When the narcotic count does not check, the nurse must report the discrepancy immediately. Narcotics and controlled substances are kept in a double-locked

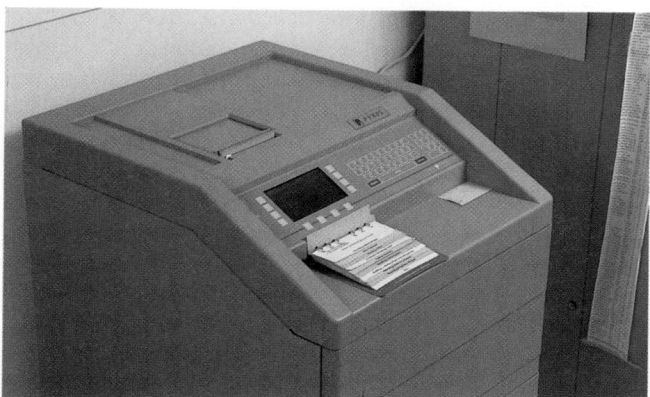

**Figure 30-3   Computer-controlled dispensing unit**

drawer, box, room, or medication-dispensing cart. The law requires these safety precautions in the use of narcotics and controlled substances to aid in the control of drug misuse. If for any reason a narcotic has to be discarded, a second person should act as a witness and that person should also sign the narcotic sheet (Smeltzer, 2001).

## Drug Abuse in Health Care Professionals

In the United States, more than 15% of those over the age of 18 have serious substance abuse issues, with two-thirds primarily abusing alcohol and one-third abusing nonalcoholic substances (Griffith, 1999). Substance abuse often leads to chemical dependence and addiction. **Chemical dependence** is a physiological neuroadaptation to the substance, requiring continued doses to prevent physiological withdrawal symptoms. **Addiction** is a state of psychological and physiological dependence that creates a craving for and preoccupation with the substance, to the detriment of the person's health, family, and work. Chemical dependence and addiction require professional treatment (Box 30-4).

Nurses and other health care providers (physicians, dentists, and pharmacists) can be at risk for substance abuse because of their access to drugs such as benzodiazepines (Valium, Librium), sedative hypnotics (Nembutal), amphetamines (Dexedrine, Benzedrine), and narcotics (meperidine, morphine, oxycodone). The incidence of substance abuse in nurses is difficult to document; however, it appears to reflect the same incidence as in the general population with 8% to 15% who are chemically dependent on alcohol, drugs, or both (Griffith, 1999).

The difficulty of obtaining factual data for the number of chemically addicted nurses is often related to the reluctance of professionals to report one another. Nurses often exhibit "enabling" behaviors that "protect" the impaired nurse by covering mistakes, excuses for absences, and other suspicious behaviors. The nurse who is abusing substances often takes elaborate steps to hide it in the workplace, especially if they are dependent on their work site for access to drugs. Those who are addicted to prescription drugs may display suspicious behaviors, such as insisting on carrying the narcotic keys and volunteering to administer all of the narcotics during the shift. Although it may be uncomfortable to report an addicted colleague, nurses have a moral responsibility to report the situation to the appropriate authority.

In 1983, Florida was the first state to enact a "diversion" law as an alternative to disciplinary proceedings against substance abusers. Florida's diversion program is called the Intervention Project for Nurses and has served as a model for other states to create similar programs such as impaired nurse programs. These programs provide support, confidentiality, and stringent on-the-job monitoring and allow the nurse to maintain licensure as long as the nurse complies with the program. An impaired nurse pro-

| BOX 30-4 | CHARACTERISTICS OF DRUG-ADDICTED NURSES IN THE WORKPLACE |
| --- | --- |

- Exhibit extreme and rapid mood swings
- Always wear long sleeves
- Sign out more controlled drugs than anyone else
- Report frequent spills and breakage of controlled drugs
- Commit multiple medication errors
- Practice illogical or sloppy charting
- Are frequently absent from work
- Come to work early and stay late
- Frequently use sick leave

gram is a welcomed alternative for nurses with addictive behaviors and has increased the reporting of nurses with addiction problems. (Contact your state board of nursing office to inquire about alternative programs to disciplinary measures.)

## Safe Medication Administration

In order to administer a medication safely, the nurse must be alert and think critically about several important factors.

### Interpretation of Medication Order

The nurse is responsible and held accountable for questioning any medication order if in the nurse's judgment the order is unclear or in error. Medication orders may be incorrectly written by the prescriber. A single letter changed in the spelling of a medication can change it to a different, but incorrect, medication for the client. Examples are the names of *amrinone* and *amiodarone* (both cardiac medications). Handwritten orders have a much higher potential for error because of the legibility of the order. Verbal orders can be easily misheard. An incorrect dose may have been written. The nurse must be certain that the drug ordered is spelled correctly, the dose is appropriate, and the medication is relevant to the client's health problems. Drug references should be consulted for clarification of the medication's purposes and normal doses (Osborne, Blais, & Hayes, 1999).

## RESEARCH FOCUS

**Title of Study:** State policies and nurses with substance use disorders

**Study Purpose:** The study investigated the outcomes of two types of policies used by state boards of nursing for nurses with substance use disorders (SUD). One type of policy was the traditional, disciplinary method. The other type was use of board-sanctioned alternative programs designed to treat and rehabilitate the nurses.

**Method:** 219 participants were recruited, approximately half in each type of policy approach. The participants were from all levels of nursing practice, including LPN, vocational, registered, and advanced practice nurses. Questionnaires were used for demographic, licensure, and work description data. A Maintenance of Abstinence questionnaire was completed each month by the participants of the 6-month study.

**Findings:** There was no difference in the relapse rates between the two programs. Less than 15% of nurses in either group had one or more relapses. Alcohol and crack cocaine were most commonly used during relapse. Relapse is considered part of the recovery process by experts in substance abuse recovery. A statistically significant higher number of nurses (76%) in the alternative rehabilitation program were allowed to work, compared to the disciplinary program (49%). Those prohibited from working most likely lacked health insurance and financial means for treatment.

**Implications:** The alternative rehabilitation programs worked as well as the traditional, disciplinary approach. The alternative programs were more humane and based on the recovery model for substance abuse recommended by Healthy People 2010.

Haack, M. R., & Yocum, C. J. (2002). State policies and nurses with substance use disorders. *Journal of Nursing Scholarship, 34*(1), 89–94.

## CLINICAL ALERT

### Refusal of Medications

The nurse has the right and responsibility to refuse to give a medication that would appear to endanger the client.

## The Five Rights of Medication Administration

To protect the client from medication errors, nurses have traditionally used as a guideline the "five rights" of drug administration (see Box 30-5).

### Right Medication

Before administering any medication, the nurse compares the medications listed on the MAR with the prescriber's order. When administering a medication, the nurse should check the label written on the container or unit dose package against the MAR at least three times before giving the drug. The nurse should:

1. Check the medication label when removing the medication from the storage unit.
2. Check the medication label with the MAR again.
3. Check the medication label and MAR with the client's name band at the bedside.

The nurse should give only medications that the pharmacist or nurse has prepared and checked. The nurse should not give medications that have been removed from their unit dose package or drawn up in a syringe by anyone else. The nurse who administers the medication is the responsible party should an error occur. If a client questions a medication to be administered, the nurse should never ignore the question. Clients are active participants in their care and usually know when a medication is different from that usually taken. The nurse should withhold this medication until the order can be rechecked. Frequently,

| BOX 30-5 | FIVE RIGHTS OF MEDICATION ADMINISTRATION |
|---|---|

1. Right medication
2. Right dose
3. Right client
4. Right route
5. Right time

When the nurse is not able to read or understand the order or has concern about the safety of the medication, the prescriber should be contacted for clarification. The nurse should not *guess* what the person who wrote the order is trying to communicate. A drug error has serious legal implications if the nurse involved could have been expected to have noted the error on the basis of knowledge and experience.

the medication order has changed, but the client question can stop an error before it occurs.

The client has the right to refuse the medication. However, if clients understand the actions of the medication, they may be willing to take the medication. If it is refused, the medication should be discarded rather than returned to the original container. Unit-dose medications that have not been opened can be returned to the locked storage unit.

## Right Dose

The unit-dose system was implemented to help decrease medication errors. However, there are times when medications on hand are in a larger volume or strength than needed. Careful calculation is especially important when the health care practitioner orders a unit of measurement different from what is supplied by the pharmacy.

The nurse must know how to reduce the risk of error by correctly calculating doses and having them double-checked before administration. Policy in some agencies, for instance, mandates that two nurses check insulin dosages to ensure accuracy. After calculations have been completed, the nurse should prepare the medication using appropriate measurement devices such as graduated measuring cups, syringes, and droppers.

To cut a pill in half, the pill should be scored (manufactured with an indented line) and the nurse should use a pill cutter to make a clean break. This practice will prevent overdosage or underdosage of a medication. If the medication has to be crushed with a mortar and pestle, the nurse should thoroughly cleanse the pestle after each use. Cleansing the pestle will avoid the mixing of different medications and will prevent the client from receiving minute amounts of a medication that may cause serious adverse effects.

## Right Client

The nurse should correctly identify the client by asking the client to state her full name and checking the MAR with the client's identification armband (Figure 30-4). Never identify a client solely by calling the person's name, because some clients may be confused and will answer to any name. Identification bracelets that become blurred or are missing for any reason should be replaced. The nurse needs to obtain a new identification band for the client. Verify the identification by asking the client to state his full name before placing the new band on the client's arm. Be alert to same last names or similar sounding names. Some institutions mark charts or client rooms with an "alert" symbol to help staff avoid name errors.

## Right Route

The route of the medication is specified in the written order. The nurse should consult the prescriber whenever a route is not identified in the prescription, when the route indicated differs from the recommended one, or when the

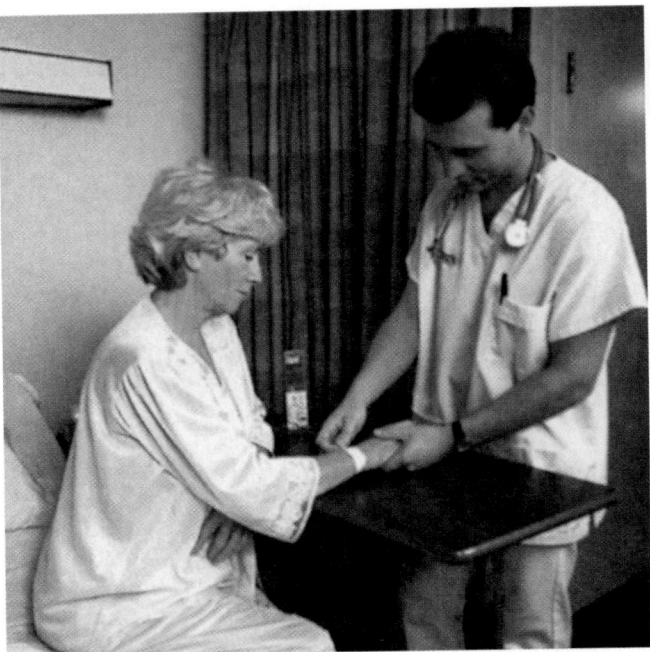

**Figure 30-4   Check a client's identification band before administering medication.**

nurse questions the choice of route prescribed. For example, the nurse should not substitute an oral medication for an intramuscular medication simply because the oral medication is available and the intramuscular one is not.

Injecting a medication designed to be administered orally can cause adverse reactions such as a sterile abscess at the injection site. Medications for parenteral injections should be prepared from medications designed for this purpose. Manufacturers of medications label medications that can be used for parenteral injections as "for parenteral use only."

## Right Time

The fifth right is giving the medication at the correct time and frequency that it is ordered. Nurses should be aware of the general principles of drug timing, such as which medications need to be given before meals or around the clock. The pharmacist or prescriber should be consulted for discrepancies between the order and the manufacturer's recommendation for timing (Figure 30-5).

> ## CLINICAL ALERT
> ### Administering Medication Safely
>
> Never give medications that another nurse has prepared unless it is in a sealed unit dose package. Always double-check the order before giving it yourself.

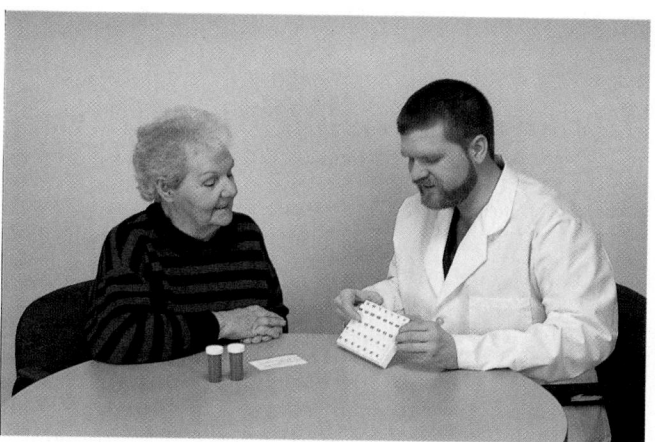

**Figure 30-5    A pill box correlated to the days of the month can help the client follow her medication regimen.**

Hospitals usually have routine times for typical daily, b.i.d., and other scheduled medications. Generally, the medication should be given within half an hour before or after the scheduled time. Keeping medications on the normal institutional schedule helps prevent omissions, especially if a dose coincides with shift change, when it can be easily forgotten. When a client is NPO for a test or unable to take the medication for other reasons, the nurse should call the prescriber to get verification that the medication can be held or orders for it to be given by a different route.

## Documentation of Medication Administration

A critical element of medication administration is documentation. The standard is "if it was not documented, it was not done." Many medication errors can be avoided with appropriate documentation. The nurse responsible for administering the medication must document on the MAR the time the medication was given and initial it (Figure 30-2). Usually, space is available for a full signature on the record.

If the client refuses to take a medication or was unable to take it, the nurse must indicate that a dose was missed. In some hospitals, a circle is placed around the time the medication was scheduled to be given. The nurse should write in the record why the dose was missed and notify the prescriber.

## Medication Errors

Concern about medical errors has increased across the United States. Frequent articles in both professional journals and the lay press have been published in recent years (Karch & Karch, 2001). Medication errors have involved manufacturers, prescribers, systems of naming and labeling medications, institutional systems of orders and med-

ication distribution, as well as the professional practice of individual health care professionals.

To help prevent medication errors, the nurse can practice a number of important double- and triple-checks, which have been discussed. These include correct interpretation of the medication order, correct dosage calculation, following the five rights of medication administration, documenting, and knowing the client's health and medication history. Additional safety tips for medication administration are noted in the Nursing Strategy box (Smeltzer, 2001).

There are many examples of medication errors. For example, if a wrong medication is administered or a correct medication given to the wrong client or at the wrong time, it would be a medication error. If a medication is given at too fast a rate or by the wrong route, it is an error. If a medication is not charted when it is given, it is an error. Medication errors include incorrect dose calculations, incorrect orders or mistakes in transcribing orders, and mistakes from sound-a-like or look-a-like names. All medication errors need to be documented in a variance or incident report and the health care practitioner notified promptly. The nurse must monitor the response of the client to the medication (or to its omission). If an antidote is needed, the prescriber needs accurate information to make appropriate care decisions.

Incident or variance report forms are sent to the institution's committee (Risk Management or Continuous Quality Control) that studies client safety issues. In July 2001, the Joint Commission on Accreditation of Healthcare Organizations (JCAHO) set new standards for client safety and medication errors. Hospitals are required to implement an organization-wide system for promoting safety and identifying potential errors. Hospitals are now required to tell clients and families about outcomes of care, including adverse events (Cavanaugh, 2001). Health care agencies must study ways that the institution's system can be improved to prevent further errors. This approach should remove the practice of blaming one person, which causes fear and cover-up of errors.

It is important for the institution not only to track medication errors and improve its system, but also to have a national tracking system for medication errors. The United States Pharmacopia (USP) gathers and shares data about potential and actual medication errors. It issues warnings to the FDA, the Institute for Safe Medication

## NURSING STRATEGY

### Safety Tips in Medication Administration

- Have a second nurse or pharmacist check your medication calculation.

- Check the placement of the decimal point of the dose ordered or calculated. There is a big difference between 2 mg and 0.2 mg.

- Know your client's health and medication histories. Question any order that does not seem to be relevant.

- If the handwriting in the order is not clear, ask the prescriber for clarification.

- Never rush or hurry when preparing medications. If interrupted, start the double-check over for the five rights: medication, dose, time, route, and client. Concentrate when preparing and administering the medication.

- Be alert to sound-a-like and look-a-like medication names.

- Take the MAR to the bedside to double-check the client's name.

- Do not leave any medications at the client's bedside.

- Immediately initial the medication record for the medications you have given.

- Enlist the client as part of the "safety net" by teaching him about the medication purposes and side effects. Always double-check the order if the client says he hasn't had that medication before.

- Keep up-to-date drug references on the unit, use them, and consult with the pharmacist.

- Educate yourself. Continue to increase your pharmacology knowledge. Read updates on new medications as well as reports published about potential and actual medication errors.

Adapted from Reiss, B., Evans, M., & Broyles, B. (2002). *Pharmacological aspects of nursing care.* Clifton Park, NY: Delmar Learning.

## LEGAL AND ETHICAL ISSUES

### Would You Report a Colleague's Medication Error?

Medication errors happen even to very competent nurses. It is not uncommon to find an error made by a colleague. Asking for response from readers of *RN* journal, Haddad received a variety of comments (Haddad, 2001). When the client's immediate safety was an issue, readers believed that the error must be reported so that monitoring and orders for antidotes could correct the problem. However, if client safety did not seem to be compromised, nurses stated they often did not report the error, because they were concerned that the colleague would face reprisals. Others disagreed, stating that if they were the one who had made the error, they would want to be told so they could correct their practice and prevent future errors. Haddad concluded that reprisals should not be part of the agency's reporting system; then there would be forthright reporting and the agency's medication systems could be evaluated to prevent future errors.

Haddad, A. (2001). Ethics in action. *RN, 64*(9), 25–28.

an actual or potential error by calling the number in the Nursing Strategy box. The health care professional and the institution can remain anonymous (Karch & Karch, 2001, p. 25). In addition the federal Patient Safety and Errors Reduction Act of 2001 included appropriations for the establishment of a National Patient Safety Database to be used for research on improvement of client safety (Cavanaugh, 2001).

## The Nursing Process in Medication Administration

Medication administration is more than technical procedures. It involves critical thinking that is guided by the nursing process, which provides a central focus on the client.

### Assessment

Medication administration is based on assessment data obtained by reviewing the client's health history, eliciting a drug history, performing a physical examination, and obtaining and interpreting relevant laboratory results. Assessment is an ongoing process and requires the knowledge, skills, and abilities of a licensed professional.

Practices, and all health care professionals about types of medication errors that are occurring and recommends how to prevent them. Any health care provider can report

## NURSING STRATEGY

### Medication Error Reporting

To report medication errors, the nurse can:

Report an actual or potential medication error by calling 1-800-23-ERROR or online at http://www.usp.org.

## Health History

The client's health history is obtained by the nurse when conducting the interview assessment and by reviewing the client's medical record. The nurse should identify all chronic diseases and disorders and correlate these data with the drugs prescribed by the health care practitioner. Because the client may have more than one health care practitioner, the admitting health care practitioner might not be aware of all the drugs the client is taking, including over-the-counter medications. It is the nurse's responsibility to gather this information and document it on the client's chart.

Preexisting conditions such as liver and kidney dysfunction may require drug alteration because they prolong drug action, thereby increasing the potential for toxicity. The nurse needs to elicit this type of information during the health history so that these clients can be closely monitored for signs of adverse reactions to drugs (Estes, 2002).

## Medication History

A medication history is obtained on admission to a health care facility. The medication history should contain specific questions about the client's background: allergies, prescription and over-the-counter drugs, use of herbal and supplement therapies, health history, pregnancy and lactation status, biographical data, lifestyle and beliefs, and sensory and cognitive status. See Chapter 27 for a complete discussion of taking a health history. If the client is unable to answer the questions, the nurse should contact a family member to obtain the data. Data from the health history and the medication history are used by nurses in determining the client's plan of care and learning needs.

## Allergies

The nurse should inquire about all food and drug allergies. If the client has had an allergic reaction to a drug, the nurse should have the client describe the details of the reaction: name of the drug; dosage, route, and number of times the drug was taken before the reaction; onset of the reaction; and manifestations of the reaction. The nurse should question the client about possible contributing factors to the allergic reaction, such as concurrent use of stimulants (tobacco, alcohol, or illegal drugs), or significant changes in diet.

The nurse should also ask about allergies to foods because drugs may contain the same elements or nutrients that cause allergic reactions to some foods. For example, clients who are allergic to shellfish may also experience a reaction to drugs containing iodine. Vaccines are commonly derived from chick embryos and would be contraindicated in clients with allergies to eggs.

Allergies to food and drugs, including over-the-counter drugs, should be noted in the client's record, in the admission note, on the medication administration record (MAR), and on the history and physical examination forms. The pharmacy should be notified of any drug or food allergies. In hospitals, clients wear allergy alert bands that list all medications to which the person is allergic. Nurses in all settings should discuss the use of medical alert bracelets by clients with allergies. These bracelets would inform health care providers of allergies should the person not be able to speak for himself.

## Prescription Medications

The nurse should have the client identify all current prescription medications and describe:

- Why the medication was prescribed and by whom
- The medication's dosage, route, and frequency
- The client's knowledge of the medication's action: side and adverse effects, when to notify the health care practitioner, and special administration considerations such as with or without foods

If the client is receiving any medication that requires monitoring before administration such as insulin (antidiabetic hormone), the nurse needs to make sure the client is checking blood sugar and that the results are within normal limits.

## Over-the-Counter Medications

Clients usually have to be questioned separately about nonprescription drugs because they often fail to identify these drugs when asked to list all the medications they take routinely. For example, the nurse must determine if the client takes aspirin, antacids, or laxatives routinely. The client should describe the dosage, route, and frequency of these drugs. Because many drugs are available in topical form, the nurse should also inquire about the use of creams, ointments, patches, or sprays. Clients admitted to inpatient facilities should be asked if they have any prescription or over-the-counter medications with them. The nurse needs to explain that all medications will be given by the nurse in order to prevent confusion about doses or medication interactions. The client's personal supply should be sent home with a family member or locked in the medication cart until the client's discharge.

The nurse should explain to the client in a sensitive manner why these questions are necessary in order to allay any anxieties that might arise from this nature of questioning. Depending on the dosage and frequency, nonprescription drugs may have a profound effect on the client's treatment.

## Herbals and Alternative Therapies

It is estimated that 1 out of every 3 Americans uses one or more herbal products (White & Foster, 2000). Problems can arise if herbal products are used improperly or in combination with drugs. Nurses need to know which herbs can alter the activity of certain drugs. For example, garlic and ginkgo may increase the effects of blood thinners, whereas goldenseal, Oregon graperoot, and barberry may counteract short-acting blood thinners. Refer to Chapter 31 for additional information on the safe, effective use of herbal medicines.

## Biographical Data

The client's biographical data, including age, education, occupation, and insurance coverage, may influence the nursing care plan and teaching plan. These data are also used by the nurse when helping a client develop a drug regimen that complements the client's daily routine.

## Pregnancy and Lactation Status

Because of the teratogenic danger of many medications causing abnormal embryonic development and the passage of drug metabolites through breast milk, the nurse should always ascertain whether a premenopausal woman is using a birth control method, is pregnant, or is breast-feeding.

---

### FOCUS ON WELLNESS

## Herbal Therapies

Many people are taking herbals to treat or prevent diseases or their symptoms. Others seek to counteract the effects of aging. However, there is little research on the efficacy or safety of herbs (O'Neil, 1999). Some herbs, such as ephedra, are unsafe for clients with hypertension, cardiac disease, or cerebrovascular disease, putting them at higher risk for heart attacks, strokes, and seizures. In addition, little is known about medication-herbal interactions. St. John's wort, a popular herb used for depression, alters the metabolism of numerous medications, including immune suppressants and anticoagulants (Mayo Clinic, 2000). Nurses should warn all clients to tell their health care practitioner what herbals they are taking. Clients need to be aware that there is great variation in quality and strength between different brands and even in different batches made by the same company (Mayo Clinic, 2000).

---

## Culture and Lifestyle

Health care providers need to be aware of and sensitive to cultural variations that may affect clients in their care (Kudzma, 1999). The client's culture affects her attitudes and beliefs about her health, use of the health care system, use of medications, and her daily activity patterns. For example, knowing a client's cultural beliefs about the yin and yang (hot and cold) of illness can help the nurse avoid conflicts about the treatment plan and nursing interventions. Some clients may use folk remedies that can alter a medication's metabolism. For example, the herb ginseng can act as an accelerant or inhibitor of certain medications. Knowing the client's cultural and personal food preferences can help the nurse plan the medication's schedule and teach the client about food and medication interactions.

A client's lifestyle can also determine dietary habits and nontherapeutic use of tobacco, alcohol, and illegal drugs. For example, a client who is homeless may have very irregular eating patterns and poor nutrition, which can alter the absorption and metabolism of medications.

## Sensory and Cognitive Status

The nurse should assess for and inquire about sensory deficits such as vision or hearing impairments, weakness or paralysis, or loss of sensation in one or more extremities. These deficits may impair a client's ability to comply with a prescribed drug plan, administer a subcutaneous injection, break a scored tablet, or open a medication container.

The nurse should assess the client's cognitive abilities throughout the drug history interview by noting whether the client is alert and oriented and interacts appropriately. Clients who are not able to express their thoughts coherently or who exhibit impaired memory function will require special consideration by the nurse when planning the client's care and teaching plan. See Chapter 41 for a complete discussion of sensory and cognitive impairments.

## Physical Examination

The nurse conducts a physical assessment to identify those body systems that may be affected by a particular drug the client is currently taking or will be taking. The nurse assesses the client's condition before administering any drug to establish the client's baseline, or normal, health status. For example, the nurse assesses the client's apical pulse before administering Lanoxin (inotropic) so that the heart rate after receiving the drug can be compared with the baseline measurement.

## Diagnostic and Laboratory Data

Common laboratory values, such as electrolytes, blood urea nitrogen, creatinine, glucose, complete blood count, and a white blood cell count, are usually monitored over a period of time to identify trends and to measure the body's response to medications. Blood drug levels are monitored to ensure the medication is within therapeutic range. Laboratory results are evaluated on the basis of the client's clinical condition, physical assessment, and drug therapies. See Chapter 29 for a complete discussion of laboratory testing.

## Nursing Diagnosis

The nurse analyzes the assessment data to determine the client's ability to self-administer medications and to identify any potential or actual drug-related problems. Once the nurse identifies the actual or potential problems, relevant nursing diagnoses can be formulated. The common nursing diagnoses specifically related to medication administration are (Ackley & Ladwig, 2002):

- *Deficient Knowledge*
- *Ineffective Therapeutic Regimen Management*
- *Ineffective Health Maintenance*
- *Impaired Physical Mobility*
- *Disturbed Sensory Perception*
- *Impaired Swallowing*
- *Impaired Memory*
- *Noncompliance*

The related factor(s) for each nursing diagnosis should be identified because the nursing interventions may be different. For example, if the nursing diagnosis is "*Impaired Memory* related to over-sedation from medications," the nursing intervention will be different than if the diagnosis is related to short-term memory loss. In the first example, the nurse will attempt to get a change in medication orders to decrease the sedation symptoms. In the second, the nurse will determine with the client, and possibly a family member, how to set up a medication schedule with reminders, such as the use of a Mediset and a timer, so that the client can remember to take the medications.

Selecting the most appropriate nursing diagnosis will identify the client's teaching needs.

## Planning

Nurses need to carefully plan nursing care activities to ensure safe administration of medications. Reviewing scheduled diagnostic tests, laboratory results, and the overall plan of care helps to ensure that clients receive medications at the appropriate times and that medications that should not be given are withheld until their administration can be clarified with the health care practitioner. For example, digoxin might be withheld if the lab test indicates an above-normal level. Medication administration is a good time for nurses to incorporate client teaching. Adequate planning provides for questions and discussion by the client and demonstration of skills learned. Planning ahead ensures that enough time is allocated for the client to accomplish all the desired tasks in a timely manner.

## Outcome Identification

The nurse develops client goals based on the nursing diagnosis. In the inpatient setting, some goals may be short-term-focused on achieving immediate treatment goals, monitoring labs, and treating mild side effects. However, because most clients go back to their community setting and must be able to safely self-administer their medications, a major focus is on client education.

### Client Education

The client needs to understand the purpose of the medications, adhere to the medication schedule and self-monitor for side effects. In addition, the client must understand the potential for medication interactions from over-the-counter medications and relevant food-medication interactions. The client may need assistance in developing a drug schedule that promotes compliance and complements his lifestyle. Client teaching needs to begin, even when the client is acutely ill, because he is in the hospital for such a short time. Each time the nurse gives a medication, the name and purpose of the medication should be discussed with the client.

For some medications, the techniques of self-administration or monitoring must be taught. For example, a newly diagnosed client who is insulin-dependent must be taught blood glucose monitoring and subcutaneous injection for insulin. Clients must learn how to take and record their blood pressure and pulse when taking blood pressure and cardiac medications.

Client teaching should include a family member if possible. A family member can help clarify and reinforce the importance of taking a medication. If the client becomes unable to administer it or monitor himself, the family member will have sufficient knowledge to do it.

Examples of outcomes for a client needing to learn insulin administration are (Strowig, 2001):

- Client will correctly state the actions of insulin in the body.
- Client will prepare the correct dose of insulin in a syringe three times before discharge.
- Client will state the reasons for rotating the injection sites and demonstrate the correct technique of self-injecting insulin three times before discharge.
- Client will correctly identify the onset of action and peak plasma level for the type of insulin prescribed.
- Client will correctly perform glucometer testing.
- Client will describe the signs of hypoglycemia and the appropriate actions to take.

The nurse plans what nursing interventions are needed to accomplish the client education goals. A teaching plan with specific steps and a time frame for accomplishing it should be started as soon as possible. Teaching an inpatient client should always begin before the day of discharge, or the client will feel overwhelmed. Most institutions have pamphlets or client teaching manuals to help illustrate the content to be covered. Written materials that are correct for the client's reading level should be selected. Demonstrations should be broken into segments so the client and family member can practice, ask questions, and return-demonstrate the skill.

Documentation of client teaching should clearly include what content was covered and the client's ability to understand or return-demonstrate. Client education goals may not be fully accomplished in the acute setting, and the community home or clinical nurse will need to follow up and complete the teaching.

## Implementation

The administration of medication requires diligence and concentration by the nurse with all of the safety guidelines discussed earlier in the chapter. Medications are administered in accordance to set procedures for each route. In addition, drug manufacturers may have additional specific guidelines for certain medications, such as droperidol (requires ECG monitoring) and bactrim (mix only with sterile water). A drug reference should always be consulted when giving medications. Refer to the procedures in the last part of this chapter for the specific steps in administering medications for each route.

## CLIENT EDUCATION

### Implementation: Client Teaching

The American Nurses Association and various governing bodies support written medication information for clients that is "scientifically accurate, unbiased in content and tone, sufficiently specific and comprehensive, presented in an understandable and legible format, timely, up to date, and useful." Written medication information should:

✓ Be appropriate to client literacy levels
✓ Reflect print size appropriate to client's visual abilities
✓ Give straightforward instructions
✓ Include brand and trade names
✓ Prominently display drug warnings
✓ Outline indications for use, contraindications, and precautions
✓ List possible adverse reactions and risks, storage, and use

From American Nurses Association (March/April, 1997). *The American Nurse*, 29(2), 11.

## Evaluation

The nurse is responsible for ongoing evaluation of the client's response to medication. This evaluation requires knowledge of the therapeutic action, side effects, and adverse reactions that can occur. Changes in a client's health status can also change the way a client responds to medications. For example, clients who develop renal failure do not excrete medications well, causing toxic effects. Many medications have sedative side effects that can cause the client to be at risk for falls or for poor gas exchange due to a depressed respiratory rate. These side effects need immediate nursing interventions.

Client learning must be evaluated to be sure that the teaching was effective and that the client understands how to adapt the information to his home setting. Nurses in the community setting need to evaluate their clients' ongoing ability to manage their own medication regimen. They need to discuss the regimen with the client and family and observe client technique in self-administering medications and self-monitoring procedures.

The client's compliance with the therapeutic medication regimen can be associated with the client's understanding of why a medication was ordered and how it can decrease the likelihood of getting a disease or lessen the effects of an existing disease. However, clients may stop taking the medication for other reasons as well. If a hypertensive client is asymptomatic, it may be difficult for the client to understand the need to take prescribed medications. If the medication is taken, the dose may be altered at the discretion of the client. Medications are costly, and the client may be on a fixed income or unemployed. If the medication does not provide prompt relief, the client may consider the medication useless and discontinue it. The medication may be discontinued if the client experiences undesirable side effects such as dizziness, impotence, or weight gain. After consulting with the client and the caregiver, the nurse can make suggestions that may improve compliance.

## CLIENT REFLECTIONS

### A Diabetic Sent Home With Medications

Mr. Scott was newly diagnosed with adult diabetes after being hospitalized for a hyperglycemic crisis. After being stabilized, he was discharged. Upon returning to his home, he stated to his wife, "I was sent home with so many medicines that I am having trouble organizing them. They gave me written instructions, but I don't really understand them. I feel overwhelmed."

What would you say to this client?

## Medications in the Home Environment

- Help the client remove outdated prescriptions and over-the-counter drugs from medication cabinets. The chemical composition may change over time, causing a different drug action.

- "Translate" instructions for taking medications into clear layman terms. For example, b.i.d. should not be "twice a day," which the client may interpret as two pills whenever she wants. Instead it should be "one tablet in the morning when you get up and one tablet in the evening, about 12 hours later." Be sure it fits a realistic schedule for her sleep and eating patterns, as some clients have very different schedules.

- Assess for visual or cognitive problems that may cause noncompliance with the therapeutic plan. Use a mechanism such as a paper clock, reminder calendar, or a pill box with compartments for days of the week.

- Encourage the client or caregiver to maintain drug refills to decrease the risk of missing scheduled medications.

- Be sure the client has a list of potential side effects and the phone number of the prescriber to report them.

Karch, A. M., & Karch, F. E. (2001). Take part in the solution. *American Journal of Nursing, 101*(10), 25.

policies for specific medications must also be followed by the nurse. For example, a few intravenous medications such as dilantin require administration with an inline filter (Gahart & Nazareno, 2001).

## Oral Administration

Oral administration of drugs is the most common route; however, there are potential risk factors that the nurse must consider. Before administering oral drugs, the nurse should assess the client's ability to take the medication as prescribed. This assessment includes the client's gag reflex, state of consciousness, and presence of nausea and vomiting.

The nurse should protect the client against aspiration when administering any form of oral drug. **Aspiration** refers to the inhalation of regurgitated gastric contents into the pulmonary system. If a client has a weak gag reflex or difficulty swallowing water, medication can be inhaled during medication administration. To prevent aspiration, the nurse confirms the client's gag reflex and ability to swallow. In addition, the client's head must be raised to 90 degrees (high Fowler's position) when swallowing the medication. When administering an oral drug, the nurse prepares the medication, correctly identifies the client, and provides some form of liquid. See Procedure 30-1 for administering an oral medication. The nurse should remain with the client until *all* of the medications have been swallowed. If there is doubt that the client has swallowed the pill, the nurse should don a nonsterile glove and visually inspect the client's mouth with a tongue depressor.

## Sublingual and Buccal Administration

Sublingual and buccal drugs are types of oral medications. Certain drugs are given by these routes to prevent their destruction or transformation in the stomach or small intestines. The nurse should assess the integrity of the mucous membranes by inspecting underneath the client's tongue and in the buccal cavity. If the membranes are excoriated or

Documentation of the nurse's evaluation in the medical record is very important. In addition, the nurse needs to be clear what nursing interventions helped alleviate side effects and compliance problems. Learning outcomes must also be clearly documented.

## Medication Administration Procedures

The following pages outline the steps and rationale for the administration of medications by the oral, parenteral, topical, and inhalation routes (see Procedure 30-1). Additional guidelines by manufacturers or institutional

## Points to Remember in Administering Oral Medications

Prevent aspiration when giving medications orally by mouth or tube by ensuring that the client (1) is alert, (2) has a gag reflex, (3) is able to swallow, and (4) is in a high Fowler's position (90 degrees) unless contraindicated clinically.

Reiss, B., Evans, M., & Broyles, B. (2002). *Pharmacological aspects of nursing care* (6th ed.). Clifton Park, NY: Delmar Learning.

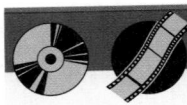

**PROCEDURE 30-1**

# Administering Oral, Sublingual, and Buccal Medications

## EQUIPMENT NEEDED

- Physician's or qualified practitioner's order for the medication
- Medication administration record (MAR)
- Medication cart or dispensing computer
- Medication tray

- Disposable medication cups
- Glass of water, juice, or other liquid
- Drinking straw
- Mortar and pestle, if needed
- Paper towels

## IMPLEMENTATION—ACTION/RATIONALE

| ACTION | RATIONALE |
|---|---|
| 1. Wash hands and put on clean gloves. | 1. Reduces the number of microorganisms. |
| 2. Arrange the medication tray and cups in the medication room or on the medication cart outside the client's room. | 2. Organizing medications and equipment saves time and reduces the possibility of error. |
| 3. Unlock the medication cart or log on to the computer. | 3. Medications need to be safeguarded. |
| 4. Prepare the medication for one client at a time following the five rights. Select the correct drug from the medication drawer according to the MAR (Figure 30-6). Calculate the drug dosage if needed. | 4. The five rights are right client, right time, right medication, right dose, and right route. Comparing the MAR with the label reduces error. Double-checking reduces error in calculation. |

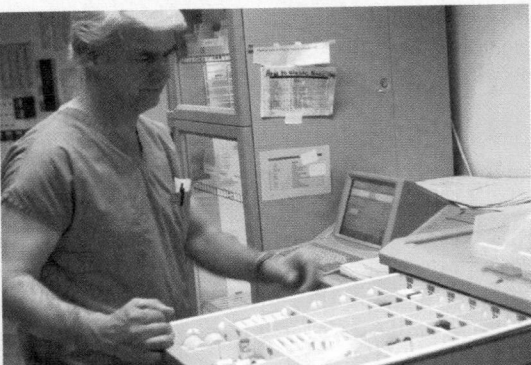

**Figure 30-6   Prepare oral medications following the five rights—right client, time, medication, dose, and route.**

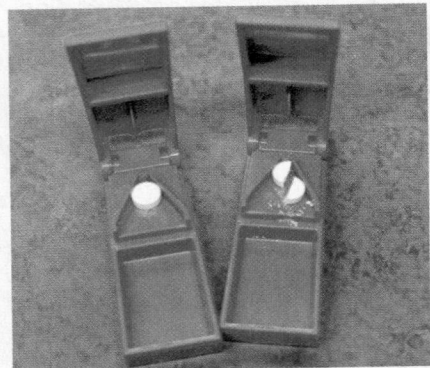

**Figure 30-7   Scored tablets may be broken, if necessary.**

| | |
|---|---|
| 5. To prepare a tablet or capsule: Pour the required number of tablets or capsules into the bottle cap and transfer the medication to a medication cup without touching them. | 5. Avoids wasting expensive medications and avoids contamination of medication. |
| • Scored tablets may be broken, if necessary, using gloved hands or a piliating device (Figure 30-7). | • Tablets that are not scored are not meant to be broken. The medication's effectiveness would be diminished if the tablet were broken or crushed. |
| • A unit-dose tablet should be placed directly into the medicine cup without opening it. | • The wrapper maintains cleanliness and identification until it is administered. |

*(continues)*

## PROCEDURE 30-1 (continued)

- For clients with difficulty swallowing, some tablets may be crushed into a powder using a mortar and pestle or by being placed between two paper medication cups and ground with a blunt object, then mixed in a small amount of applesauce or custard. Be aware that time-released or specially coated medications must not be crushed. Check with the pharmacy if you are uncertain (Figure 30-8).

- A large tablet is usually easier to swallow if it is ground and mixed with soft food.

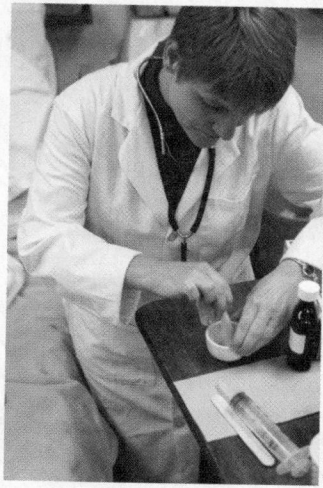

**Figure 30-8**   Some medications may be crushed and mixed with a soft food such as applesauce, for clients with difficulty swallowing.

6. To prepare a liquid medication: Remove the bottle cap from the container and place cap upside down on the cart. Hold the bottle with the label up and the medication cup at eye level while pouring (Figure 30-9). Fill the cup to the desired level using the surface or base of the meniscus as the scale, not the edge of the liquid on the cup. Wipe lip of bottle with paper towel.

6. Placing the bottle cap upside down on the cart prevents contamination of the inside of the container. Holding the bottle with the label up keeps spilled liquid from obliterating the label. Holding the medication cup at eye level ensures an accurate dose. Wiping the lip of the bottle prevents the bottle cap from sticking.

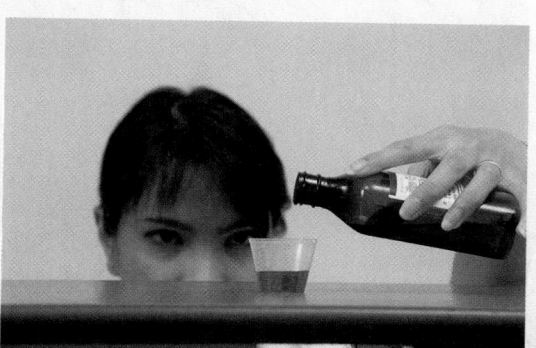

**Figure 30-9**   Measure oral medications at eye level.

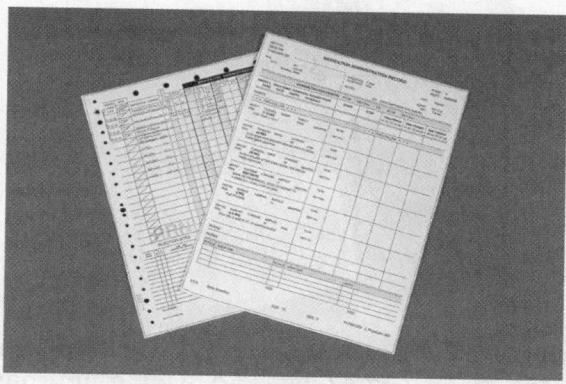

**Figure 30-10**   Controlled-substance laws require records of each narcotic dose dispensed.

7. To prepare a narcotic, obtain the key to the narcotic drawer and check the narcotic record for the drug count when signing out the dose (Figure 30-10).

7. Controlled-substance laws require records of each dose dispensed.

(continues)

## PROCEDURE 30-1 (*continued*)

8. Check expiration date on all medications.
   - Double-check the MAR with the prepared drugs.
   - Return stock medications to their shelf or drawer.
   - Place MARs with the client's medications.
   - Do not leave drugs unattended.

8. Expired medications may lose their effectiveness.
   - Reduces risk of error.

   - Ensures safety of stock medications.
   - Ensures identification of medications.
   - Drugs are safeguarded by nurse.

9. Administer medications to client: Observe the correct time to give the medication.

   - Identify the client by reading the client's name bracelet, repeating his name, and/or asking him to state his name (Figure 30-11).

   - Check the drug packaging if it is present to ensure the medication type and dosage.
   - Assess the client's condition and the form of the medication.
   - Perform any assessment required for specific medications such as a pulse or blood pressure.
   - Explain the purpose of the drug and ask if the client has any questions.
   - Assist the client to a sitting or lateral position.
   - Allow client to hold the tablet or medication cup.
   - Give a glass of water or other liquid, and straw if needed, to help the client swallow the medication (Figure 30-12).

9. Ensures the therapeutic effect of the drug when given within 30 minutes of the prescribed time. (*Right time.*)
   - Identification bracelets made at the time of admission are the most reliable source of identification even if the client is unable to state his name. (*Right client.*)
   - Prevents giving the wrong medication or wrong dose. (*Right medication, right dose.*)
   - Allows you to assess the route of the medication and if this route is appropriate. (*Right route.*)
   - Determines whether the medication should be given at that time or not.
   - Improves compliance with drug therapy.

   - Prevents aspiration during swallowing.
   - Client becomes familiar with medications.

   - Promotes client comfort in swallowing and can improve fluid intake.

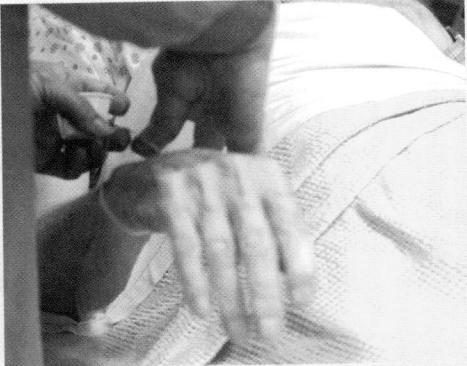

**Figure 30-11    Identify the client by reading the client's name bracelet and asking his name before administering medication.**

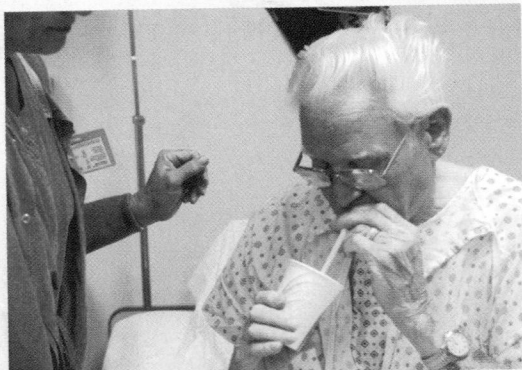

**Figure 30-12    Allow the client to hold the tablet, and give water or juice to help him swallow the medication.**

   - For *sublingual* medications, instruct client to place medication under the tongue and allow it to dissolve completely.

   - Drug is absorbed through the mucous membranes into the blood vessels. If swallowed, the drug may be destroyed by gastric juices or detoxified in the liver too quickly so that its intended effects will not occur.

*(continues)*

## PROCEDURE 30-1 (*continued*)

- For *buccal* administration of drugs, instruct the client to place the medication in the mouth against the cheek until it dissolves completely.
- For oral medications given through a *nasogastric tube,* crush tablets or open capsules and dissolve powder with 20–30 ml of warm water in a cup. Be sure medication will still be properly absorbed if crushed and dissolved. Check placement of the feeding tube or nasogastric tube before instilling anything but air into the tube.
- Remain with the client until each medication has been swallowed or dissolved.

- Assist the client into a comfortable position.

10. Dispose of soiled supplies and wash hands.

11. Record the time and route of administration on the MAR and return it to the client's file.

12. Return the cart to the medicine room; restock the supplies as needed. Clean the work area.

- Promotes local activity on mucous membranes.

- Allows medication administration via NG or feeding tube. Ensures that the medication is absorbed and used correctly.

- Nurse is responsible for ensuring that the client receives the dose and does not save it or discard it.
- Maintains client's comfort.

10. Reduces transmission of organisms.

11. Prevents administration error.

12. Assists other staff in completing duties efficiently.

---

## COMMUNITY/HOME CARE

### Medication Administration

#### Home Care Variations

- Clients need to be compliant in order to successfully self-administer their medications.

- Clients may benefit from a special medication container with compartments for times of the day and days of the week to assist them in remembering and complying with the medication schedule.

#### Long-Term Care Variations

- Maintain medication cart with a mortar and pestle, spoons, and a supply of applesauce.

- Keep a record on each client's MAR of how the client needs medications given.

---

painful, the nurse should withhold the medication and notify the health care practitioner. Some buccal drugs may irritate the mucosa, requiring the nurse to use alternate sides of the mouth to prevent irritation of the mucosa.

Sublingual and buccal administration of drugs (Figure 30-13) requires the nurse to use Standard Precautions because the nurse's hand may come into contact with oral secretions. See the Nursing Strategy box for administering sublingual and buccal drugs. Drugs given by these routes are quickly absorbed by the mucosa's thin epithelium and the abundant blood supply.

## Administration Through Tubes

When the client is unconscious or unable to swallow, many oral medications may be given through gastric or intestinal tubes. The tube is nasogastric when it is inserted through a nostril and into the stomach. These tubes include very small-bore feeding tubes. When a tube is surgically inserted through the abdominal wall into the stomach, it is called a percutaneous endoscopic gastrostomy (PEG) tube. Either small-bore feeding tubes or PEG tubes may be advanced into the jejunum by the health care practitioner. Having the tip of the tube in the jejunum helps

## LIFE SPAN CONSIDERATIONS

### Medication Administration

#### Pediatric Variations

- Liquid oral medications are the preferred route of administration for children.

- Solid preparations such as tablets and capsules are not recommended for children less than 5 years old.

- An oral syringe (without needle), plastic cup, and teaspoon for dispensing liquid medication are helpful in administering medications to pediatric clients.

- Offering carbonated beverages poured over finely crushed ice after giving medications to a client may reduce nausea in both children and adults.

- Use small amounts of flavorings when mixing with medications.

#### Geriatric Variations

- Older clients may be more at risk for fluid overload; if so, any fluid intake restrictions should be considered when giving oral medications.

- Older clients may have increased difficulty swallowing and therefore be at greater risk of aspiration.

- Older clients should be encouraged to take one tablet at a time and not rush.

- Older clients may have dry mouth due to loss of elasticity in oral mucosa or reduction in parotid gland secretion.

- Difficulty swallowing may be due to delayed esophageal clearance.

- Physiological changes with aging may include reduction in gastric acidity and stomach peristalsis and reduced colon motility, which may slow drug absorption and excretion.

prevent aspiration. See Chapter 35 for a complete discussion on these tubes. Regardless of the type of tube, the client should be in a Fowler's or high Fowler's position, unless contraindicated by the clinical condition, while medications are administered. The client should remain in the Fowler's position for 30 minutes thereafter to help prevent aspiration.

The nurse should assess the client for the presence of bowel sounds and check the tube for **patency** (openness), placement, and residual before administrating a medica-tion (see Nursing Strategy box on administering medications through a gastric or intestinal tube). The administration of drugs is contraindicated when the tube is obstructed, the tube is improperly placed, there is a **residual** (gastric contents) of more than 100 ml, the client is vomiting, or if bowel tones are absent.

It is preferable to instill liquid medications into tubes, especially PEG tubes that have a small lumen. Tablets can clog the tube unless they are very finely crushed and dissolved in 30 ml of water. Capsules are prepared for administration by opening the capsule and emptying the contents into 30 ml water.

The nurse should question the prescriber if oily medications and enteric-coated or sustained-release tablets are ordered, because these drug forms should not be given through a tube. Oily preparations may cling to the sides of the tube and resist mixing with the irrigating solution. Crushing enteric-coated or sustained-release tablets destroys their intended effect.

## Parenteral Administration

Parenteral medications are given through a route other than the alimentary canal; these routes are intradermal (ID), subcutaneous (SC or SQ), intramuscular (IM), and

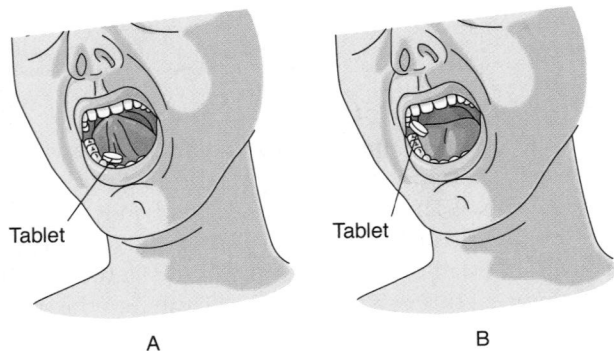

Tablet

A

Tablet

B

**Figure 30-13    A. Sublingual administration of a tablet; B. Buccal administration of a tablet**

## NURSING STRATEGY

### Administering Sublingual and Buccal Drugs

- Follow the five rights of safe drug administration.

- Wash your hands and don nonsterile gloves.

- Assess the client's knowledge of the drug and its action.

- Explain the procedure to the client, and allow the client time to ask questions.

- Offer the client a sip of water and explain to the client that liquids cannot be taken until the tablet is completely dissolved.

- Never crush a buccal or sublingual medication.

- To give a drug sublingually, ask the client to open the mouth and lift the tongue; place the drug under the client's tongue. Give the client the following instructions:

  —Keep the medication under the tongue until it dissolves completely to ensure absorption.

  —Avoid chewing the tablet or touching the tablet with the tongue to prevent accidental swallowing.

  —Do not smoke before the drug has completely dissolved, because nicotine has a vasoconstriction effect that slows absorption.

- To give a drug buccally, instruct the client to open the mouth wide, and place the tablet between the client's cheek and teeth. Give the client the following instructions:

  —Keep the medication in place until it dissolves completely to ensure absorption.

  —Do not drink liquids for an hour, because some tablets take up to an hour to dissolve.

  —Do not smoke before the drug has completely dissolved, because nicotine has a vasoconstriction effect that slows absorption.

- Remove gloves and dispose in a proper receptacle; wash hands.

- Document the medication administration on the MAR. When the client is receiving repeated doses of a buccal medication, the nurse should indicate the site, such as right buccal cavity, to prevent irritation of the same site.

## NURSING STRATEGY

### Administering Medications Through a Gastric or Intestinal Tube

1. Assess client for bowel tones and vomiting.
2. Assess tube for patency and placement: Put on gloves and inject 20 ml air into tube with a syringe, while auscultating with the stethoscope over the epigastrium. Listen for a "whish" or "rumble"noise. (Sometimes, this noise is not heard with small-bore feeding tubes. Draw back on the syringe plunger to aspirate for gastric fluids as a second evidence for gastric placement.
3. Assess residual by aspirating stomach or intestinal contents. Return fluid to the stomach. If there are 100 ml, more than one-half the previous feeding or one-half the hourly rate, consult the health care practitioner. Remove gloves and document amount of residual.
4. Prepare the medications. If medication is a tablet, crush finely and mix with 10 ml water. Do not crush enteric-coated or sustained-release medications, but consult the prescriber for a different medication order (Miller, 2000).
5. Move client into Fowler's or high Fowler's position unless clinical condition contraindicates. (Client must be at 30 degrees or higher to prevent aspiration.)
6. Put on gloves. If client is receiving a continuous tube feeding, stop the infusion and flush with 10–20 ml water. Do not mix medications with tube feeding, or solution may congeal in the tube.
7. Administer medications. It is preferable to let them flow in by gravity by pouring them into a 60 ml syringe without the plunger; small-bore tubes require gentle administration using the plunger. Flush afterward with 20–30 ml water. Restart tube feeding if it is continuous.
8. Leave client in Fowler's or high Fowler's for 30 minutes.
9. Document medications and amount of water used for flushes.
10. For clients who have a nasal gastric tube to suction to decompress gastric contents, medications can be administered through the tube. Disconnect tube from suction, administer medications, flush with water, and clamp for 20 to 30 minutes while medication is absorbed. Reconnect to suction. Never use the pigtail air vent for flushing or administration of medications.

Altman, G. (2004). *Delmar's fundamental & advanced nursing skills* (2nd ed.). Clifton Park, NY: Delmar Learning.

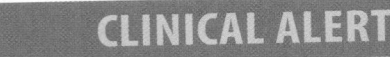

---

## CLINICAL ALERT

### Medication Abbreviations

Sustained-release medications may be identified by these abbreviations in their name: SR, ER (extended release), contin (continuous acting), EL (extended length), CR (controlled release), and TR (time release).

Miller, D., & Miller, H. (2000). To crush or not to crush. *Nursing 2000, 30*(2), 51.

---

## CLINICAL ALERT

### Prefilled Syringe

Always check the dose in a prefilled syringe with the order, and discard any extra medication.

---

intravenous (IV). Other routes such as intra-arterial or spinal are only accessed by specially trained professionals. Many clients have broadly classified the parenteral route into one category: "injections" or "shots." The nurse should provide the client with an explanation of the various routes used when administering parenteral drugs. To prepare and administer parenteral medications, the nurse must have knowledge of the special equipment, use manual dexterity and sterile technique, and follow Standard Precautions. An injection is an invasive procedure because it breaks the skin barrier. As such, it must be performed using proper aseptic technique to prevent risk of infection.

### Equipment

Nurses use special equipment such as syringes, needles, ampules, and vials when administering parenteral medications.

### Syringes

A syringe has three basic parts: the tip, which connects with the needle; the barrel, or outside part, which contains measurement calibrations; and the plunger, which fits inside the barrel and has a rubber tip (Figure 30-14). The nurse must ensure that the syringe tip, inside of the barrel, shaft and rubber plunger tip, and shaft of the needle are kept sterile. When handling the syringe, the nurse should touch only the outside of the barrel and the plunger's handle.

Most syringes are disposable, made of plastic, and individually packaged for sterility. There are several types of syringes, such as the standard, insulin, and tuberculin syringes (Figure 30-15). When a medication is incompati-

ble with plastic, it is usually prefilled in a single-dose glass syringe. Syringes are often prepackaged with the commonly used needle size and gauge.

The *standard syringe* comes in 3-, 5-, and 10-ml sizes. The measurement calibrations (scales) are usually printed in milliliters or cubic centimeters (cc). The equivalent measurement is 1 cc = 1 ml. Syringes come packaged with and without needles.

The *insulin syringe* is designed specially for use with the ordered dose of insulin. Most insulin is usually made in a concentration of U 100 in 1 cc (U 100/cc) by the manufacturer. However, some rare exceptions are manufactured in concentrations of U 500/cc. Some insulins for infants are U 10/cc. Outside the United States, insulin may be U 40 (American Diabetes Association, 1999). The insulin syringe should always match the concentration of insulin. For example, a U 100 syringe should be used for U 100 insulin. Check the labeling on both the insulin bottle and the syringe to see that the units per cc are the same. Insulin syringes come in sizes that hold 0.5 ml (50 units) to 1.0 ml (100 units). Insulin syringes that hold 0.5 ml are the easiest to read and are therefore used for low dosages. Insulin syringes usually have a permanently attached needle that is very thin (26–30 gauge) and short (¼ inch).

The *tuberculin syringe* is a narrow syringe, calibrated in tenths and hundredths of a milliter (up to 1 ml) on one scale and in sixteenths of a minim (up to 1 minim) on the other scale. Originally this syringe was designed to administer the tuberculin drug, but it is commonly used today to administer small or precise doses, such as pediatric dosages. The tuberculin syringe should be used for doses 0.5 ml or less.

*Prefilled single-dose syringes* (Figure 30-16) should not be confused with a unit dose. For example, if the health care practitioner orders diazepam (Valium) 5 mg IM as a preoperative sedative and the prefilled single-dose contains

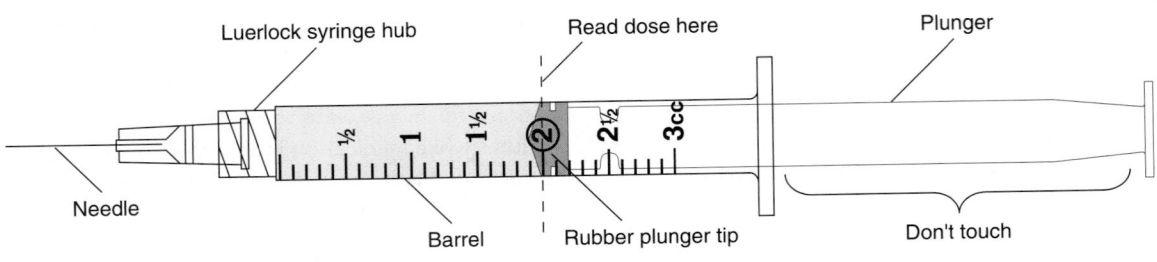

**Figure 30-14   The parts of a syringe**

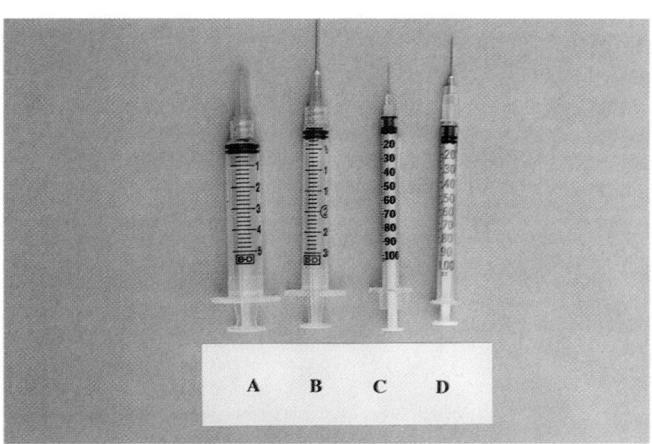

**Figure 30-15    Types of syringes: A. Standard 5 cc syringe with Luer cap; B. Standard 3 cc syringe with needle; C. U 100 insulin syringe; D. Tuberculin syringe**

10 mg/2 ml, the nurse must calculate dosage (5 mg/1 ml) and discard 1 ml from the syringe before administration.

## Needles

Most needles are disposable, made of stainless steel, and individually packaged for sterility. Reusable needles are seldom used, except in certain areas such as surgery and special procedure rooms.

The needle has three basic parts: the hub, which fits onto the syringe; the shaft, which is attached to the hub; and the bevel, which is the slanted part at the tip of the shaft. Needles come in various lengths, from ¼ inch to 3 inches, and with gauges that range from 28 to 14 (Figure 30-17).

The *gauge* of the needle refers to the diameter of the shaft; the larger the gauge number, the smaller the diameter of the shaft. Large-gauge needles produce less trauma to the body's tissue; however, the nurse has to consider the viscosity of a solution when selecting the gauge.

The *shaft of the needle* determines its length. The nurse selects the length of the needle on the basis of the client's

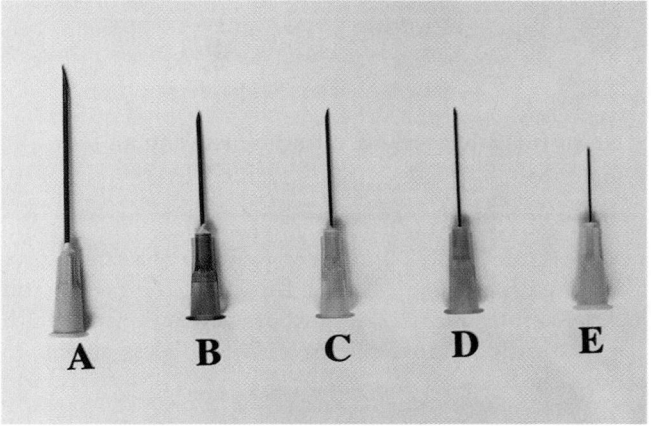

**Figure 30-17    Needles of various lengths from ¼ inch to 3 inches**

muscle development and weight and the type of injection, such as intradermal versus intramuscular.

The needle may have a short or long *bevel*. The length of bevel selected is based on the type of injection. Long bevels are sharp and produce less pain when injected into the subcutaneous or muscle tissues; however, a short-bevel needle must be used for intradermal and intravenous injections to prevent occlusion of the bevel either by the tissue or by a blood vessel wall (Figure 30-18). A filter needle has a filter inside to prevent drawing up small particles of glass or rubber in ampoules or vials. After drawing up the medication, the filter needle should be removed and discarded in the sharps box and a new unfiltered needle put on.

When the nurse removes a needle from its sterile wrapper, the hub of the needle should be immediately attached to the hub of the syringe to prevent contamination. Likewise, the protective cover should remain on the needle's shaft until the nurse is ready to use the needle.

After administering an injection, the nurse should not recap the needle; used needles should be disposed of in the proper receptacles, such as a sharps container, to prevent needle sticks. Agencies have sharps containers in all client

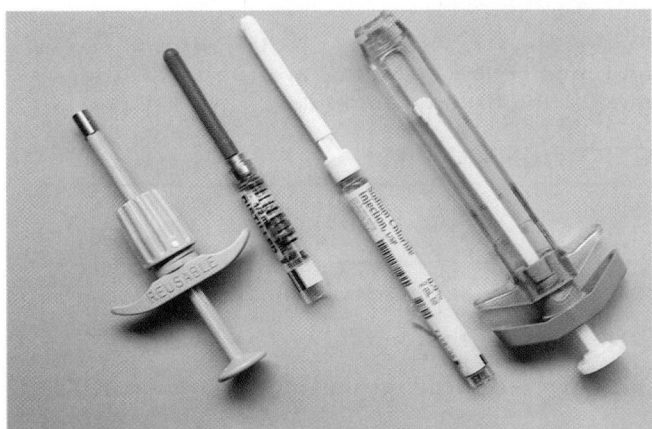

**Figure 30-16    Prefilled single-dose syringes and their holders**

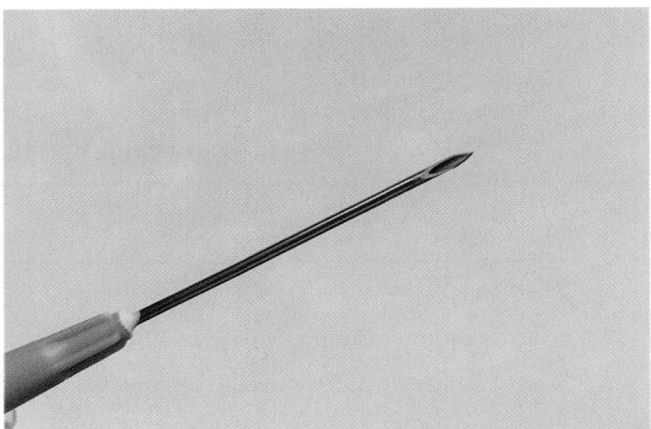

**Figure 30-18    The bevel is the slanted tip of the needle, facing upward.**

## CLINICAL ALERT

### Needle Recapping

Never recap a needle after administering an injection.

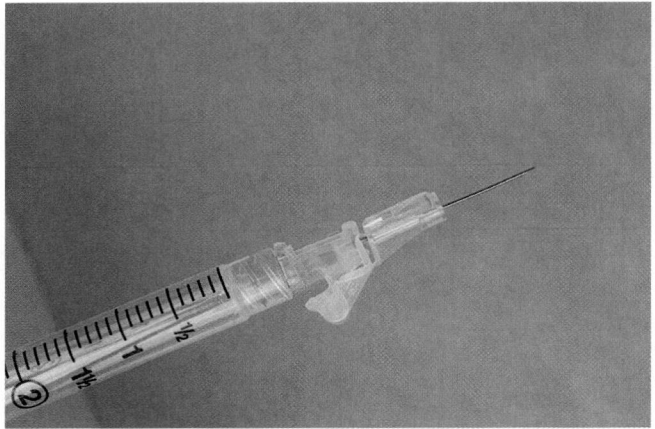

**Figure 30-19** **A safety needle: The plastic hinge is pushed with the finger after the injection, and a cover locks over the needle tip.**

care areas. See Figure 30-19 for an example of a safety cover for a needle; when pushed, it flips over the needle and locks. Recently many states are passing laws that health care institutions must change to a needleless system to protect the workers.

### Ampoules and Vials

Drugs for parenteral injections are sterile preparations. Drugs that deteriorate in solution are dispensed as tablets or powders and dissolved in a solution immediately before injection. Drugs that remain stable in a solution are dispensed in ampoules and vials in an aqueous or oily solution or suspension.

Ampoules are glass containers of single-dose drugs (Figure 30-21). The glass container has a constriction in the stem to facilitate opening the ampoule. See Procedure 30-2 for removing a drug from an ampoule. Because many drugs are irritating to the subcutaneous tissue, the nurse should change the needle on the syringe after withdrawing a drug from an ampoule.

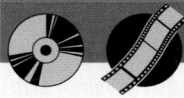

### PROCEDURE 30-2
# Withdrawing Medication from an Ampoule

## EQUIPMENT NEEDED

- Medication ampoule (Figure 30-20)
- Sterile gauze pad or alcohol pad
- Syringe with filter needle
- Replacement needle
- Clean work space
- Medication administration record (MAR)

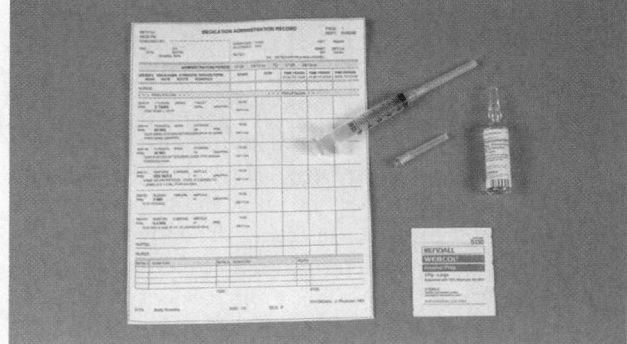

**Figure 30-20** **Syringes, needles, alcohol wipes, and medication ampoules are used to withdraw medication from an ampoule.**

## IMPLEMENTATION—ACTION/RATIONALE

### ACTION

1. Wash hands.

2. Select appropriate ampoule (Figure 30-21).

3. Select syringe with filter needle (Figure 30-22).

### RATIONALE

1. Decreases the transmission of microorganisms.

2. Ensures client receives correct medication.

3. Filter needle entraps any glass fragments.

*(continues)*

## PROCEDURE 30-2 (continued)

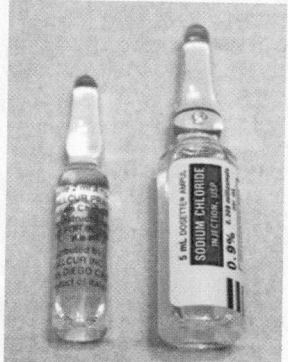

**Figure 30-21    Medication ampoules**

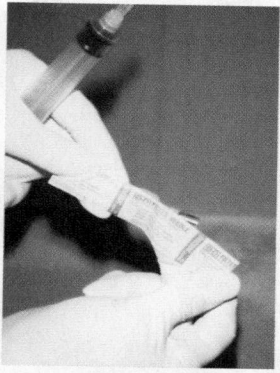

**Figure 30-22    Select a syringe and a filter needle.**

4. Obtain a sterile gauze pad.

5. Select and set aside the appropriate length of needle for planned injection.

6. Clear a work space.

7. Observe ampoule for location of the medication.

8. If the medication is trapped in the top, flick the neck of the ampoule repeatedly with your fingernail while holding the ampoule upright (Figure 30-23).

9. Wrap the sterile gauze pad around the neck and snap off the top in an outward motion (Figure 30-24).

4. Using a gauze pad prevents the nurse from being cut on the jagged edge of the broken ampoule.

5. Accurate needle length ensures the medication is administered where it is intended.

6. Prevents contamination of microdroplets that may spill when the ampoule is broken.

7. The medication frequently becomes trapped in the top of the ampoule.

8. Flicking the neck and top of the ampoule moves the medication into the body of the ampoule.

9. The gauze prevents the nurse from being cut by the jagged edge of the broken ampoule. The outward motion provides added safety for the nurse.

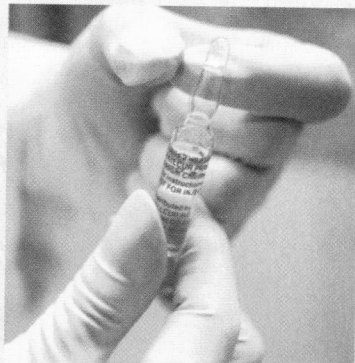

**Figure 30-23    Flick the neck of the upright ampoule to dislodge medication from the top of the vial.**

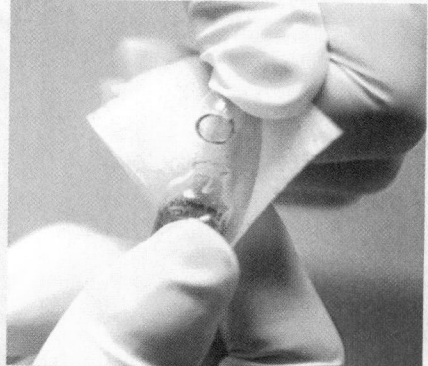

**Figure 30-24    Wrap gauze or alcohol pad around the neck to protect fingers. Snap off the top in a quick outward motion.**

*(continues)*

## PROCEDURE 30-2 (*continued*)

10. Invert ampoule and place the needle into the liquid. Gently withdraw medication into the syringe (Figure 30-25).

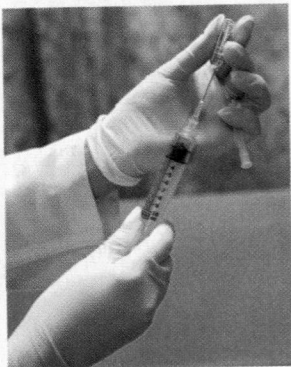

**Figure 30-25    Invert ampoule and gently draw the liquid into the syringe.**

11. Alternately, place the ampoule on the counter, hold and tilt slightly with the nondominant hand. Insert the needle below the level of liquid and gently draw liquid into the syringe, tilting the ampoule as needed to access all the liquid.

12. Remove the filter needle and replace with the injection needle (Figure 30-26).

13. Dispose of filter needle and glass ampoule (including lid) in appropriate container (Figure 30-27).

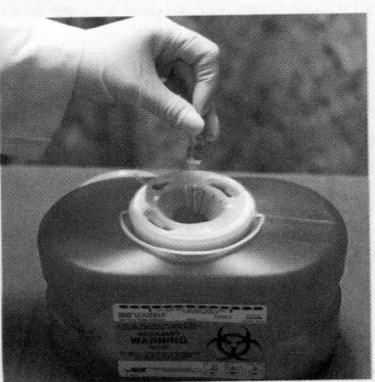

**Figure 30-27   Dispose of the filter needle, ampoule, and ampoule top in an appropriate container.**

14. Label the syringe with drug, dose, date, and time.

15. Wash hands.

10. Inverting the ampoule allows all of the medication to be withdrawn into the syringe. Surface tension will hold the medication in the ampoule until the negative pressure of the syringe barrel draws it into the syringe.

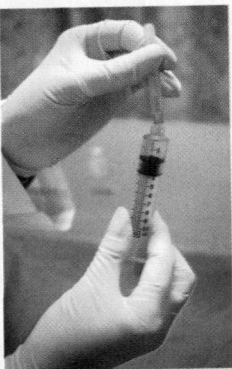

**Figure 30-26    Remove the filter needle and replace with the injection needle.**

11. While it is more difficult to read the syringe calibrations, it is easier to hold the ampoule steady. Choose the method most comfortable for you.

12. The filter needle is designed to trap glass particles and must not be used for client injections.

13. Needles or sharp glass objects must always be disposed of in puncture- and leak-proof containers in order to provide safety for clients and health care workers.

14. Prevents medication errors from taking place.

15. Decreases the transmission of microorganisms.

## LIFE SPAN CONSIDERATIONS

### Ampoules

**Pediatric Variations**

- Keep this and all medications out of the reach of children.

- If the setting requires drawing up the medication at the bedside, do not leave the empty ampoule within the reach of a child.

- Make sure all sharps go completely into the sharps container and that a small hand cannot reach into the opening.

**Geriatric Variations**

- If an older adult is drawing up medication from an ampoule, assess that his vision is adequate to see the contents of the ampoule and to check for glass. Check that he can clearly read the syringe calibrations and the medication label.

## COMMUNITY/HOME CARE

### Ampoules

**Home Care Variations**

- Correct disposal of a used ampoule in the home health setting is extremely important as it has sharp and jagged edges and may cut someone. A glass jar or metal container with a small mouth may be used. Make sure there is a lid that fits. Label the container clearly, and place where it is accessible to the caregiver. Empty the container regularly.

- Change the needle prior to injection if you suspect any contamination has occurred or if there is irritating medication on the outside of the needle.

**Long-Term Care Variations**

- Change the needle prior to injection if you suspect any contamination has occurred or if there is irritating medication on the outside of the needle.

- Empty sharps containers regularly.

The nurse should consider the use of a needle filter when withdrawing medication from an ampoule or vial. Reiss, Evans, & Broyles (2002) suggest that the last few drops of the drug be left in an ampoule or vial; some studies have found foreign substances, such as glass and rubber, in the containers that could be drawn into the syringe.

Single- or multiple-dose rubber-capped drug containers are called vials. The vial is usually covered with a soft metal cap that can be easily removed. See Procedure 30-3 for removing a drug from a vial. If giving an IM or SC injection, the nurse should change the needle on the syringe after withdrawing a drug from a vial. Inserting the needle through the rubber cap of the vial can dull the needle or remove the needle coating that helps it glide through the skin.

Compatible medications can be mixed in the same syringe. Refer to compatibility charts or check with the pharmacist to determine if the medications can be mixed. If medications are going to be mixed, care must be exercised not to contaminate one medication with the other in their respective vials. See Procedure 30-4 for mixing insulins in one syringe. The nurse must calculate and measure carefully to be sure the final dose is accurate.

### Intradermal Injection

**Intradermal (ID)** or intracutaneous injections are typically used to diagnose tuberculosis, identify allergens, and administer local anesthetics. The site below the epidermis is the location for administering ID injections; drugs are absorbed slowly from this site. The sites commonly used for ID injection are the inner aspect of the forearm (if it is not highly pigmented or covered with hair), upper chest, and upper back beneath the scapula. Only small amounts of water-soluble medication should be used for subcutaneous injections.

The drug's dosage for an ID injection is usually contained in a small quantity of solution (0.01–0.1 ml). A 1-ml tuberculin syringe with a short bevel, 25–27-gauge, ³⁄₈- to ¹⁄₂-inch-needle is used to provide accurate

## CLINICAL ALERT

### Expiration Dates

Manufacturers are required by law to put the expiration date on all drugs. The nurse should check the expiration date to ensure that the drug is current. Outdated drugs should be returned to the pharmacy for proper disposal.

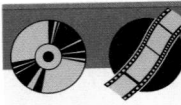

## PROCEDURE 30-3    Withdrawing Medication from a Vial

## EQUIPMENT NEEDED

- Medication vial (Figure 30-28)
- Syringe with needle
- Alcohol sponge pad
- Gloves (optional)
- Clean work space
- Medication administration record (MAR)

## IMPLEMENTATION—ACTION/RATIONALE

| ACTION | RATIONALE |
|---|---|
| 1. Wash hands. Apply gloves (optional). | 1. Decreases the transmission of microorganisms. |
| 2. Select the appropriate vial (Figure 30-29). | 2. Prevents medication errors. |

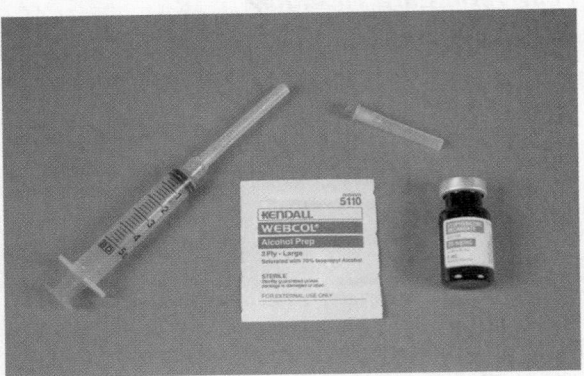

**Figure 30-28    Syringe, needle, vial of medication, and alcohol wipe are used to withdraw medication from a vial.**

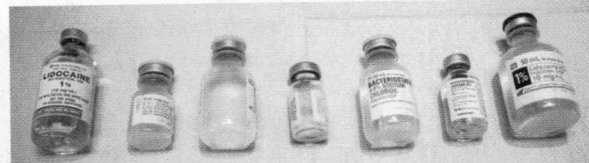

**Figure 30-29    Carefully select the medication ordered.**

| | |
|---|---|
| 3. Verify physician's or qualified practitioner's orders. | 3. Prevents medication errors. |
| 4. Check expiration date. | 4. Avoids giving expired medication, which may have altered potency. |
| 5. Determine the route of medication delivery and select the appropriate size syringe and needle. | 5. The route of medication delivery is essential to knowing what size syringe and needle will be needed. |
| 6. While holding the syringe at eye level, withdraw the plunger to the desired volume of medication. | 6. Holding the syringe at eye level makes it easier to read the syringe calibrations and increases accuracy. |
| 7. Clean the rubber top of the vial with a 70% alcohol pad. Use a circular motion starting at the center and working out. | 7. Ensures that the center of the rubber top is the cleanest area for needle entry. Reduces potential contamination with microorganisms. |
| 8. Using sterile technique, uncap the needle (Figure 30-30). | 8. Prevents spread of microorganisms. |

*(continues)*

PROCEDURE 30-3 (continued)

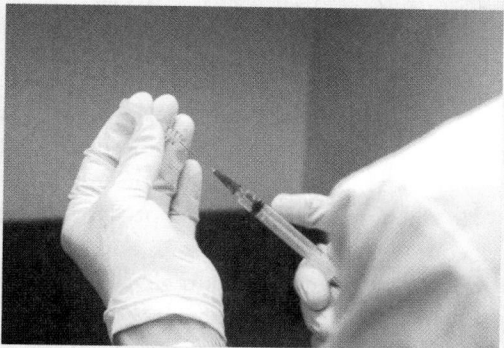

**Figure 30-30    Using sterile technique, uncap the needle.**

9.  Lay the needle cap on a clean surface.

10. Placing the needle in the center of the vial, inject the air slowly. Do not cause turbulence.

11. Invert the vial and slowly, using gentle negative pressure, withdraw the medication. Keep the needle tip in the liquid.

12. With the syringe at eye level, determine that the appropriate dose has been reached by volume (Figure 30-31).

13. Slowly withdraw the needle from the vial. Follow the institution's policy regarding recapping needles (Figure 30-32).

9.  Prevents spread of microorganisms.

10. Adding air prevents the buildup of negative pressure in the vial. Injecting quickly may cause turbulence, which can result in air bubbles forming within the vial, which could affect the accuracy of the volume of liquid being withdrawn.

11. Decreases the number of air bubbles that tend to form with unsteady, fast, jerky motions. Keeping the needle tip in the liquid prevents drawing in air.

12. Ensures client receives the ordered dose of medication.

13. Avoids splatter of medication and potential contamination of nearby supplies. Keeps the needle sterile.

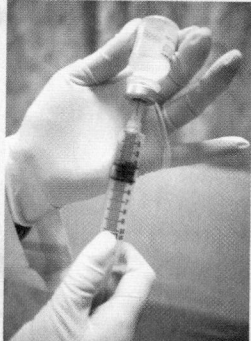

**Figure 30-31    Invert the vial and slowly withdraw the medication until the appropriate dosage has been reached.**

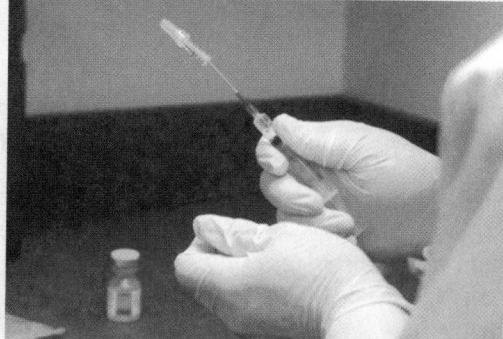

**Figure 30-32    Follow the institutional policy regarding recapping needles.**

14. Using ink, mark the current date and time and initials on the vial.

15. Label the syringe with drug, dose, date, and time.

16. Wash hands.

14. Prevents using a medication that has been opened too long per hospital protocol.

15. Prevents medication errors.

16. Decreases the transmission of microorganisms.

## LIFE SPAN CONSIDERATIONS

### Vials

**Pediatric Variations**

- Keep this and all medications out of the reach of children, especially on an unattended medication cart.

- If the setting requires drawing up the medication at the bedside, do not leave capped needles within reach of a child.

- Make sure all sharps go completely in the sharp container and that a small hand cannot reach into the opening.

**Geriatric Variations**

- If an older adult is drawing up medication from a vial, assess that her vision is adequate to read the syringe calibrations and the vial label.

- Assess that the client has the flexibility in her hands to manipulate the syringe and hold the vial.

measurement. If repeated doses are ordered, the site should be rotated. ID injections are administered into the epidermis layer by angling the needle 10 to 15 degrees to the skin. See Procedure 30-5 for administering intradermal injections.

## COMMUNITY/HOME CARE

### Vials

**Home Care Variations**

- Correct disposal of used vials and needles in the home health setting is extremely important to avoid needle-stick injury or cuts from broken glass. Sharps boxes are often not available in the home setting. An empty labeled bleach container can make a useful and safe sharp object container. Encourage clients to return their filled bleach containers to a medical facility instead of dispensing in the trash.

- Periodically reassess the client's or caregiver's technique when withdrawing medication from a vial to evaluate for any lapses in technique.

- Teach the client or caregiver to question any vial of medication that looks different (color, amount, consistency, label) than normal.

**Long-Term Care Variations**

- Multiuse vials should be checked regularly for expiration, labeling with date they were opened, and any changes in appearance of the medication.

- Multiuse vials are more prone to contamination than single-use vials. Take care not to contaminate the contents of a vial. If there is any doubt, throw it out.

---

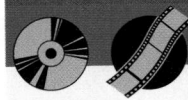  **PROCEDURE 30-4**    # Mixing Medications from Two Vials into One Syringe

### EQUIPMENT NEEDED

- Medication administration record (MAR)
- Medication vials (Figure 30-33)
- Syringe
- Alcohol wipes

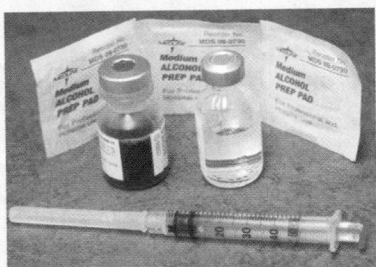

**Figure 30-33** Syringe with needle, vials, and alcohol wipes used to draw two medications into one syringe

*(continues)*

**PROCEDURE 30-4** (*continued*)

## IMPLEMENTATION—ACTION/RATIONALE

| ACTION | RATIONALE |
|---|---|
| 1. Check MAR against the physician's or qualified practitioner's written orders. | 1. Ensures accuracy in the administration of the medication. |
| 2. Check for drug allergies. | 2. Decreases risk of allergic reaction such as hives, urticaria, or anaphylactic shock. |
| 3. Wash your hands. | 3. Decreases transmission of microorganisms. |
| 4. Gather the equipment needed. Prepare the medication for one client at a time. | 4. Promotes organization. Ensures that the right client receives the right medications. |
| 5. Check need for one medication to be drawn up before the other. | 5. Determines the order in which medications will be drawn up. |
| 6. Determine the total medication volume (in milliliters) you will have in the syringe when you have finished drawing both medications into the syringe. | 6. Determines how much of the second medication will need to be drawn into the syringe. |
| 7. Swab the top of each vial with alcohol (Figure 30-34). | 7. Decreases the transmission of microorganisms. |

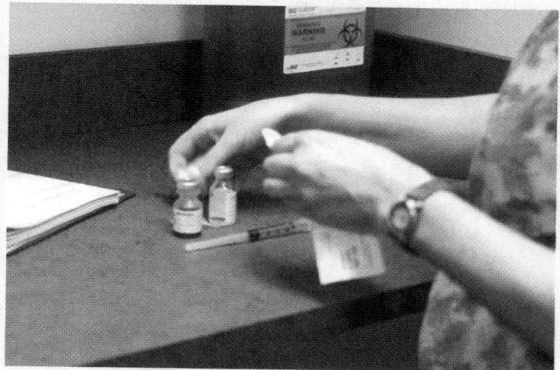

**Figure 30-34    Swab the top of each vial with alcohol.**

| | |
|---|---|
| 8. Draw air into the syringe equal to the amount of medication to be drawn up from the second vial (Figure 30-35). Inject air into the second vial and remove the syringe and needle from the vial (Figure 30-36). | 8. Avoids creating a vacuum in the second vial. When you draw medication from the second vial, you will not be able to inject air at that time, because your syringe will already contain medication from the first vial. If you inject air, you will also risk injecting medication and contaminating the second vial. |
| 9. Draw air into the syringe equal to the amount of medication to be drawn up from the first vial. Inject air into the first vial. Keep the needle and syringe in the vial (Figure 30-37). | 9. Avoids creating a vacuum in the first vial. |

*(continues)*

### PROCEDURE 30-4 (*continued*)

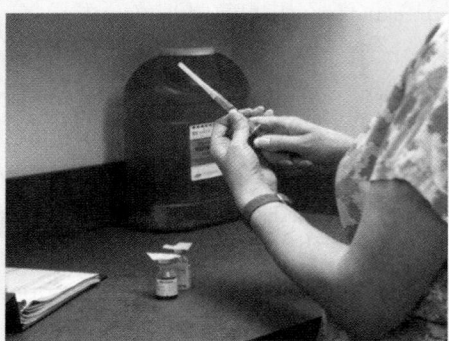

**Figure 30-35**   Draw air into the syringe equal to the amount of medication to be drawn up from the second vial.

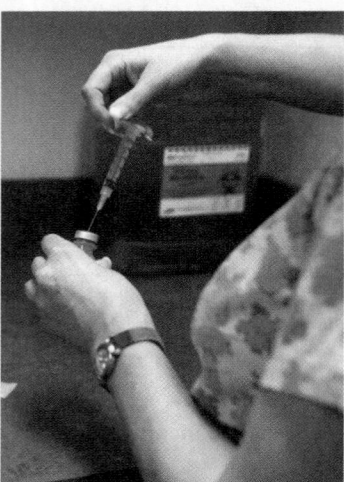

**Figure 30-36**   Inject the air into the second vial.

10. Pulling back on the plunger, withdraw the correct amount (in milliliters) of medication from the first vial (Figure 30-38).

10. Draws up the first medication.

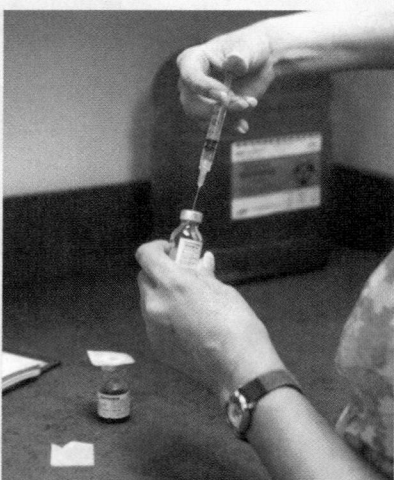

**Figure 30-37**   Inject air into the first vial.

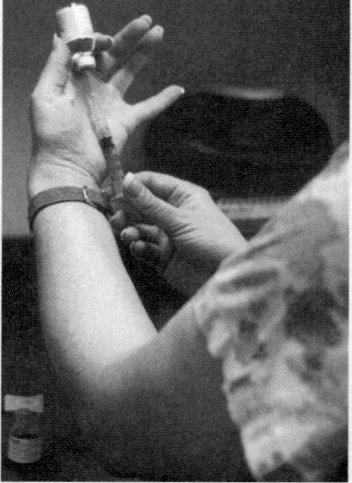

**Figure 30-38**   Withdraw the correct amount of medication from the first vial.

11. Remove the syringe from the first vial and insert it into the second vial. Withdraw medication from the second vial to the volume (in milliliters) total of both medications summed together (Figures 30-39 and 30-40).

12. Either leave the needle in the second vial until just prior to injecting the medication or follow the institution's policy regarding recapping needles.

11. Draws up the second medication. Drawing up medication equal to the total of both medications ensures the correct amount of second medication is withdrawn.

12. Prevents needle-stick injuries.

*(continues)*

**PROCEDURE 30-4 (continued)**

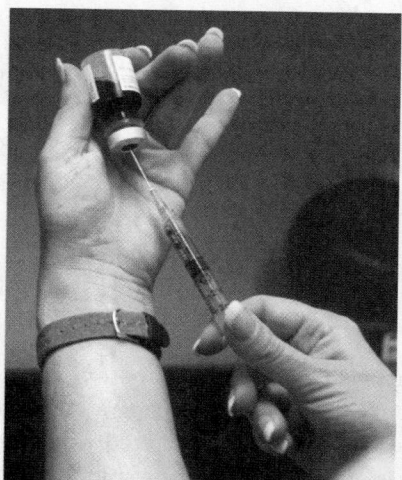

Figure 30-39    Withdraw medication from the second vial to the volume of both medications summed together.

13.  Wash hands.

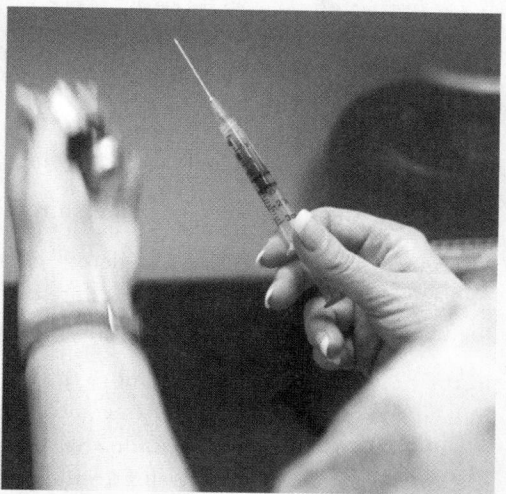

Figure 30-40    Double-check the syringe to make sure it contains medication equal to the total volume of both medications summed together.

13.  Reduces the transmission of microorganisms.

---

## LIFE SPAN CONSIDERATIONS

### Mixing Medications

*Pediatric Variations*

- Determine with the doctor, parent, and hospital policy at what age a child or adolescent may begin to participate in the preparation and administration of their own medications.

- Check manual dexterity and motor skills.

- Determine areas where the child can participate, such as observation, play-therapy, and hands-on activities, with supervision.

- Allow the child to participate in the process as much as possible.

*Geriatric Variations*

- Vision must be clear enough to assure that the correct dose of medication is drawn up.

- Manual dexterity must also be checked because of the difficulty drawing up medications.

- Write down instructions in a step-by-step format in large print to help clients with vision or short-term memory difficulties self-administer the medication.

- Follow up teaching immediately to verify the client can perform the skill. Follow up in 1 to 2 weeks to verify client has retained the skill correctly.

## COMMUNITY/HOME CARE

### Mixing Medications

*Home Care Variations*

- Care must be taken in this setting to assure the client is comfortable with the skill and that all needed supplies are available.

- Make sure medication vials are clearly labeled and the client or caregiver can read the labels.

- Check that the medication is being stored in a safe place at the proper temperature.

- Assess the client or caregiver to determine that they understand the basics of medication safety. For example, can they locate the expiration date on the vials? Remind them to question, and not to administer, medications that have been improperly stored, look discolored, or do not look like their usual medication.

- In the home care setting, it is more difficult to replace medications if an error has contaminated a vial. The client, nurse, or caregiver needs to know the exact procedure for quickly replacing a medication during the day or after-hours should the need arise. This will reduce the anxiety associated with mixing medications from two vials as well as reduce the temptation to overlook a possible contamination or mixing medication error.

- Make sure lighting is adequate to see the calibration numbers on the syringe.

*Long-Term Care Variations*

- A client who self-administers the same medication over time may need a "refresher" course on how to correctly maintain her technique. This will reduce the temptation to adopt "short-cuts," such as not adequately cleaning the vial stopper. It may reduce the risk of damage to skin integrity, infection, or medication errors due to poor technique.

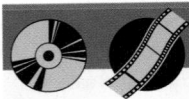

**PROCEDURE 30-5**    ## Administering an Intradermal Injection

### EQUIPMENT NEEDED

- Tuberculin syringe, 1 ml (Figure 30-41)
- Needle (25–27 gauge, 1/4–5/8 inch)
- Antiseptic or alcohol swabs
- Medication ampoule or vial
- Medication card or medication administration record
- Disposable gloves

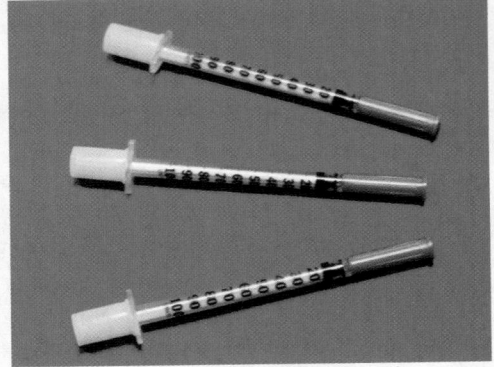

**Figure 30-41    Syringes come in many sizes. Select the 1 ml tuberculin syringe for intradermal injections.**

*(continues)*

**PROCEDURE 30-5** (*continued*)

## IMPLEMENTATION—ACTION/RATIONALE

| ACTION | RATIONALE |
|---|---|
| 1. Wash hands and put on clean gloves. | 1. Reduces the transmission of microorganisms. |
| 2. In the inpatient setting, close door or curtains around bed and keep gown or sheet draped over body. In the outpatient setting, close door to exam or treatment room. Identify client. | 2. Provides privacy. Assures medication is given to right client. |
| 3. Select injection site.<br>• Inspect skin for bruises, inflammation, edema, masses, tenderness, and sites of previous injections.<br>• Forearm site should be 3 to 4 fingerwidths below antecubital space and one handwidth above wrists on inner aspect of forearm. | 3. Injection site should be free of lesions. Repeated daily injections should be rotated. Assures a clear site for interpreting results. |
| 4. Select ¼- to ⅝-inch, 25–27-gauge needle (Figure 30-42). | 4. Ensures that needle will be injected into the intradermis. |
| 5. Assist client into a comfortable position. Forearm site: Relax the arm with elbow and forearm extended on a flat surface. Distract client by talking about an interesting subject. | 5. Relaxation minimizes discomfort. Distraction reduces anxiety. |
| 6. Use antiseptic swab in a circular motion to clean skin at site. | 6. Circular motion and mechanical action of swab remove secretions containing microorganisms. |
| 7. While holding the swab between fingers of nondominant hand, pull cap from needle. | 7. Swab remains accessible during procedure. Prevents contamination of needle. |
| 8. Administer injection:<br>• With nondominant hand, stretch skin over site with forefinger and thumb.<br>• Insert needle slowly at a 5- to 15-degree angle, bevel up, until resistance is felt; then | 8.<br>• Needle penetrates tight skin easier than loose skin.<br>• Ensures needle tip is in the dermis. |

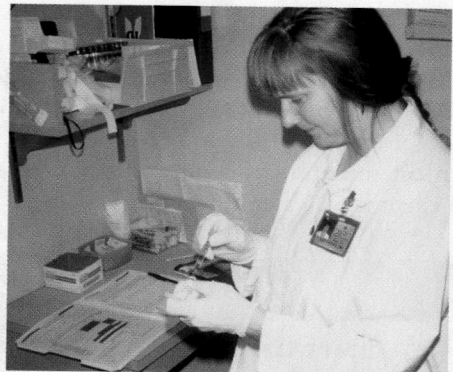

**Figure 30-42    Select a ¼-inch to ⅝-inch, 25–27-gauge needle for the injection.**

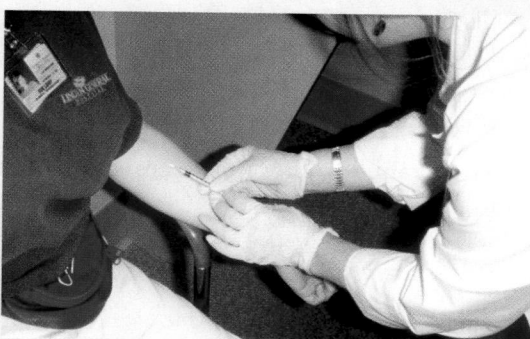

**Figure 30-43    Note a small bleb, like a mosquito bite, forming under the skin surface as the medication is injected.**

(*continues*)

## PROCEDURE 30-5 (*continued*)

advance to no more than ⅛ inch below the skin. The needle tip should be seen through the skin.

- Do not aspirate. Slowly inject the medication. Resistance will be felt.
- Note a small bleb, like a mosquito bite, forming under the skin surface (Figure 30-43).

9. Withdraw the needle while applying gentle pressure with the antiseptic swab.

10. Do not massage the site.

11. Assist the client to a comfortable position.

12. Discard the uncapped needle and syringe in a safe receptacle.

13. Remove gloves and wash hands.

14. Document procedure, if indicated.

- Dermal layer is tight and does not expand easily when fluid is injected.
- Indicates the medication was deposited in the dermis.

9. Supporting tissue around injection site minimizes discomfort.

10. Prevents medication from being dispersed into the tissue and altering test results.

11. Promotes comfort.

12. Decreases risk of needle stick.

13. Reduces transmission of organisms.

14. Maintains continuity of care.

## LIFE SPAN CONSIDERATIONS

### Intradermal Injections

#### *Pediatric Variations*

- Distracting a child so he does not see the syringe and needle may help relieve anxiety.

- Lightly tap the skin before inserting the needle. This may decrease pain by focusing the child's attention on the touch rather than the needle. Be sure not to contaminate the clean site.

- Elicit the child's cooperation to sit still and enlist the parent's or caregiver's help to assist the child to remain still. Discuss a reward, such as a play opportunity after the injection, to elicit cooperation.

- Draw a rabbit, cat, or flower around the site instead of just a circle.

#### *Geriatric Variations*

- Aging skin may be fragile. Use extra caution and guide the needle into position slowly. Apply gentle pressure when withdrawing the needle.

### Subcutaneous Injection

**Subcutaneous (SC or SQ)** injections are commonly used in the administration of medications such as insulin and heparin, because these drugs are absorbed slowly, to produce a sustained effect. SC injections place the medication into the subcutaneous tissue, between the dermis and the muscle. The amount given varies but should not exceed 1.0 ml. If using the abdominal site, injections should not be closer than 2 inches to the umbilicus. It should be noted that the speed of absorption of the medication varies with the site, the abdomen having the fastest absorption.

If repeated drug doses are given, the client or nurse should rotate within an anatomical site before moving to the next site (American Diabetes Association, 1999). This gives less variation in day-to-day absorption. Because medication is irritating to the subcutaneous tissue, hard painful lumps (lipohypertrophy) can develop beneath the skin if sites are not rotated. Absorption of medication from areas of lipohypertrophy is poor. Teaching the client to document injection sites on a diagram at home can help the client keep a rotation pattern.

## CLINICAL ALERT

### Aspirating the Syringe

Do not aspirate on the plunger when giving heparin; *doing so may cause excessive bleeding because heparin is an anticoagulant.*

## NURSING STRATEGY

### Variations for Insulin Injection

- Aspiration before injection is optional (ADA, 1999).

- Monitor for clinical manifestations of hypoglycemia.

- For self-administration at home, clients are not taught to wipe with alcohol, which many diabetic educators state causes toughening and drying of the skin (Fleming, 1999).

- Studies have shown that clients doing self-injection through clothing have had no symptoms of infection (Fleming, 1999).

- Insulin can be stored at room temperature for 1 month.

- A growing number of clients are using insulin pens at home. Ninety-five percent of European diabetics use them (Fleming, 2000). There are two types of insulin pens: prefilled pens that are discarded when empty, and reusable pens in which a new cartridge of insulin can be inserted. Many types of insulin come in pens. A dial is turned to the desired dose, and the client injects the dose by pushing the top of the pen. Clients are advised not to reuse needles. Convenience and easy dosage calculation using the dial are two of the benefits of insulin pens. A drawback is the greater cost, but they are sometimes covered by insurance.

## CLINICAL ALERT

### Prevention of Hypoglycemic Reactions

Always check the blood glucose level and ascertain when the client will be eating before giving insulin. Rapid-acting insulin should be injected within 15 minutes before a meal.

needle is used. A child will require a short needle, and an obese person may require a longer needle to ensure placing the medication in the subcutaneous tissue. The length of the needle should be approximately half the width of the pinched skinfold. See Procedure 30-6 for the technique used in administering an SC injection.

### Intramuscular Injection

**Intramuscular (IM)** injections are used to promote rapid drug absorption and to provide an alternate route when the drug is irritating to subcutaneous tissue. The IM route enhances the absorption rate because there are more blood vessels in the muscles than in subcutaneous tissue; however, the absorption rate may be affected by the client's circulatory status (Box 30-6).

The nurse should determine the maximum volume to inject on the basis of the site and the client's muscle development:

- 2.5–3 ml for a large muscle (gluteus medius) in a well-developed adult
- 1–2 ml for less developed muscles in children, elderly, and thin clients
- 0.5–1.0 ml for the deltoid muscle

If the volume ordered is more than the maximum amount for one site, it must be divided between two different sites.

Only insulin syringes should be used for insulin. Other subcutaneous injections should be given with a 0.5–3-ml syringe using a 25–29-gauge needle. The length of the needle should be $3/8$ to $5/8$ inch, depending on the client's body weight and amount of subcutaneous tissue (Fleming, 1999).

The medication is administered by angling the needle 45 or 90 degrees to the skin. The client's body weight will influence the angle used for injection. As a general rule, to reach subcutaneous tissue, if you can grasp 2 inches of tissue between two fingers, insert the needle at a 90-degree angle. If only 1 inch of tissue can be grasped between the fingers, use a 45 degree angle to administer the medication.

The length of the needle may also vary with body weight. Normally for SC injections, a 25-gauge, $5/8$-inch

| BOX 30-6 | COMMON INTRAMUSCULAR INJECTION SITES AND MUSCLES |
|---|---|
| *Site* | *Muscle* |
| Dorsogluteal | Gluteus maximus |
| Ventrogluteal | Gluteus medius |
| Anterolateral aspect of thigh | Vastus lateralis |
| Upper arm | Deltoid |

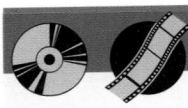

**PROCEDURE 30-6**    ## Administering a Subcutaneous Injection

## EQUIPMENT NEEDED

- Syringe appropriate for the medication being given (Figure 30-44)
- Needle (25–27 gauge, ³/₈–⁵/₈ inch)
- Antiseptic or alcohol swabs

- Medication ampoule or vial
- Medication record
- Disposable gloves

## IMPLEMENTATION—ACTION/RATIONALE

| ACTION | RATIONALE |
|---|---|
| 1. Wash hands and put on clean gloves. | 1. Reduces the number of microorganisms. |
| 2. Close door or curtains around bed and keep gown or sheet draped over body. Identify client. | 2. Provides privacy. Assures medication is given to right client. |
| 3. Select injection site.<br>• Inspect skin for bruises, inflammation, edema, masses, tenderness, and sites of previous injections.<br>• Use anatomic landmarks (Figure 30-45). | 3. Injection site should be free of lesions.<br>• Repeated daily injections should be rotated.<br><br>• Avoids injury to underlying nerves, bone, or blood vessels. |

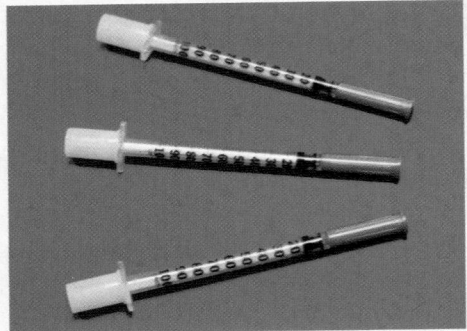

**Figure 30-44    100-unit insulin syringes are used to administer insulin subcutaneously.**

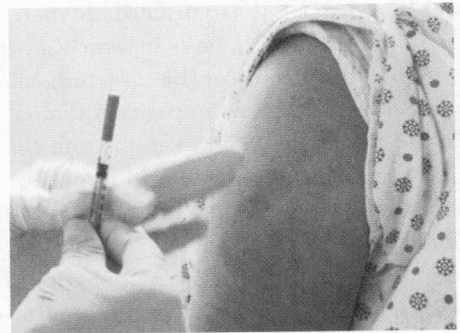

**Figure 30-45    Select injection site. Inspect for bruises, tenderness, swelling, or other skin conditions prior to administering the injection.**

| | |
|---|---|
| 4. Select needle size:<br>• Measure skinfold by grasping skin between thumb and forefinger.<br>• Be sure needle is one-half the length of the skinfold from top to bottom. | 4. Ensures that needle will be injected into subcutaneous tissue. |
| 5. Assist client into a comfortable position:<br>• Relax the arm, leg, or abdomen.<br>• Distract client by talking about an interesting subject or explaining what you are doing step by step. | 5. Relaxation minimizes discomfort. Distraction reduces anxiety. |
| 6. Use antiseptic swab to clean skin at site. | 6. Circular motion and mechanical action of swab remove microorganisms. |

*(continues)*

**PROCEDURE 30-6** (*continued*)

7. While holding swab between fingers of nondominant hand, pull cap from needle.

8. Administer injection:
   - Hold syringe between thumb and forefinger of dominant hand like a dart.
   - Pinch skin with nondominant hand (Figure 30-46).

   - Inject needle quickly and firmly (like a dart) at a 45- to 90-degree angle (Figure 30-47).

7. Swab remains accessible during procedure. Prevents contamination of needle.

8.
   - Quick, smooth injection is easier with proper position of syringe.
   - Needle penetrates tight skin easier than loose skin. Pinching skin elevates subcutaneous tissue.
   - Quick, firm injection minimizes discomfort.

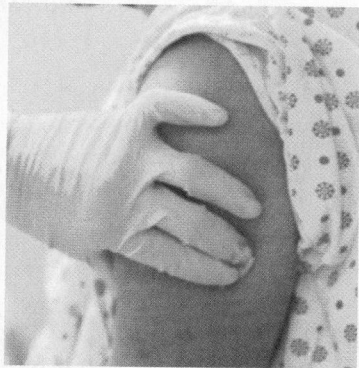

**Figure 30-46    Pinch the skin with the nondominant hand.**

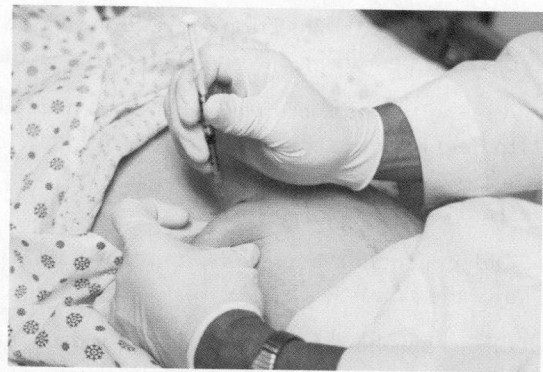

**Figure 30-47    When injecting at a 90-degree angle, hold the syringe like a dart and pierce the skin quickly and firmly.**

   - Release the skin.
   - Grasp the lower end of the syringe with nondominant hand and position dominant hand to the end of the plunger. Do not move the syringe.
   - Pull back on the plunger to ascertain that the needle is not in a vein. If no blood appears, slowly inject the medication. (Aspiration is contraindicated with some medications; check with the pharmacy if you are unclear.)

9. Quickly withdraw the needle while applying pressure with the antiseptic swab. Do not push down on the needle with the swab while withdrawing it, as this will cause more pain.

10. Gently massage the site. Some medications should not be massaged. Ask the pharmacy if you are unclear.

11. Assist the client to a comfortable position.

12. Discard the uncapped needle and syringe in a disposable needle receptacle.

13. Remove gloves and wash hands.

   - Injection requires smooth manipulation of syringe parts. Movement of syringe may cause discomfort.

   - Aspiration of blood indicates intravenous placement of needle so procedure may have to be abandoned.

9. Supporting tissue around injection site minimizes discomfort.

10. Stimulates circulation and improves drug distribution and absorption.

11. Promotes comfort.

12. Decreases risk of needle stick.

13. Reduces transmission of microorganisms.

## LIFE SPAN CONSIDERATIONS

### Subcutaneous Injections

#### Pediatric Variations

- Distracting a child so he does not see the syringe and needle may help relieve anxiety.

- Lightly tapping the skin before inserting the needle may decrease pain by focusing the child's attention on the touch rather than the needle. Make sure not to tap the clean area, so it does not become contaminated.

- Demonstrate the injection procedure on a doll or teddy bear using a syringe without a needle.

- A parent or another caregiver may be needed to help hold the child for a safe procedure.

#### Geriatric Variations

- Older clients have less subcutaneous tissue and the skin is less elastic.

- Clients may have an increased need for daily subcutaneous injections such as insulin or heparin.

## COMMUNITY/HOME CARE

### Subcutaneous Injections

#### Home Care Variations

- A safe method of disposing needles and syringes should be maintained, especially if children or animals are present.

#### Long-Term Care Variations

- Clients who receive subcutaneous injections over long-term periods should be taught to rotate injection sites to prevent the buildup of scar tissue and poor absorption at any one site.

- Periodically reassess the client's injection technique. Over the long term, clients can become careless with technique. Be sure the client continues to use the proper technique.

There are four common sites for administrating IM injections. Injection sites are identified by using appropriate anatomic landmarks (Figure 30-48).

The primary site for administering an IM injection in clients over 7 months old is the ventrogluteal (VG) site. The gluteus medius is a well-developed muscle, free of major nerves and large blood vessels. Research shows that injuries—including fibrosis, nerve damage, abscess, tissue necrosis, muscle contraction, gangrene, and pain—have been associated with all the common sites (e.g., dorsogluteal, deltoid, and vastus lateralis) *except* the VG site (Beyea & Nicoll, 1996, p. 35).

The nurse should avoid using the deltoid and dorsogluteal sites in infants and children. There is a risk of striking the sciatic nerve when using the dorsogluteal site. The deltoid muscle is not well developed in infants and children.

The nurse will need to decide on the gauge and length of the needle on the basis of the consistency of the solution, the site, and how far the needle must be injected to reach the muscle. A 21–23-gauge needle will accommodate the consistency of most drugs and will minimize tissue injury and subcutaneous leakage. The needle's length is determined by the site and the amount of subcutaneous tissue.

- 1½-inch needle, VG site for average-sized adults
- 1-inch needle, VG site for children
- 1-inch needle, deltoid or vastus lateralis

An obese client usually requires a 2–3-inch needle to ensure that the needle will reach a large muscle such as the gluteal muscle. For example, for a client weighing 100 pounds, use a needle 1 to 1½ inches long; usually for a child use only a 1-inch needle. It is important to consider the size of the client when determining the needle length; some children are large, and some adults are small. The nurse should administer an IM injection at a 90-degree angle. See Procedure 30-7 for administering an intramuscular injection.

### Air Lock Technique

Injecting a small amount of air immediately after the medication is injected into the muscle is thought to help prevent the medication from leaking back into the subcutaneous tissue through the needle tract. It can be used with both the Z-track (discussed in next section) and non-Z-track techniques. It is important to first eliminate all air from the syringe and accurately measure the medication. Then a 0.1- or 0.2-ml bubble of air is drawn into the syringe. It is also important to inject the medication at a 90-degree angle (best done with the client lying down)

## CLINICAL ALERT

### Air Lock Technique

The optional air lock technique is used only in intramuscular injections.

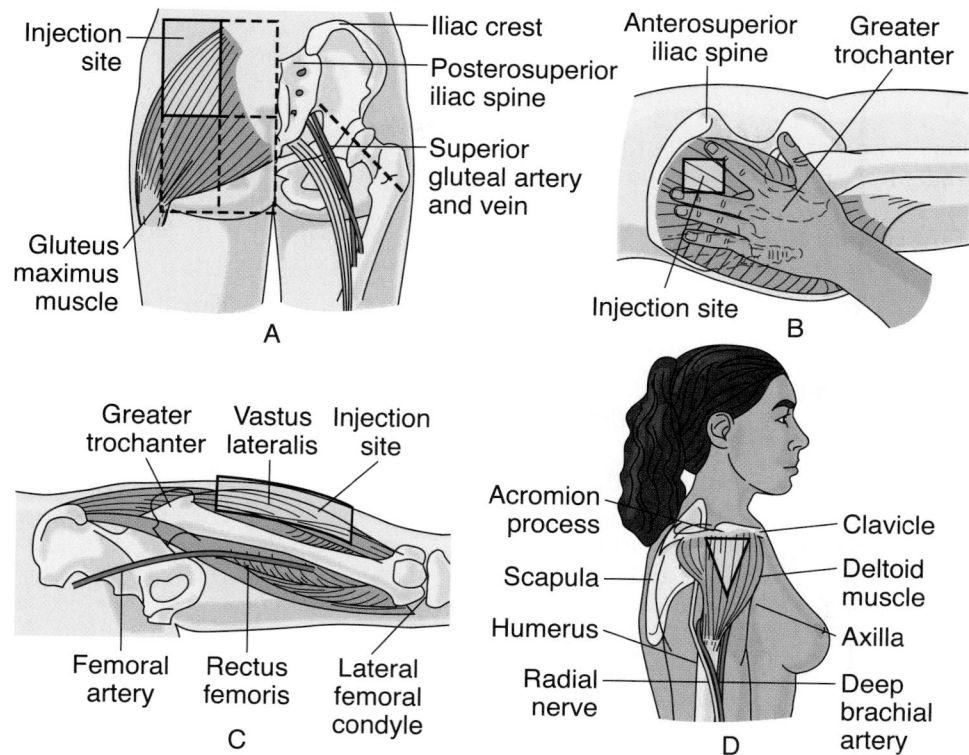

**Figure 30-48**    **Intramuscular injection sites: A. Dorsogluteal: Place hand on ilia crest and locate the pos-terosuperior iliac spine. Draw an imaginary line between the trochanter and the iliac spine; the injection site is the outer quadrant. B. Ventrogluteal: Place palm of left hand on right greater trochanter so that index finger points toward anterosuperior iliac spine; spread first and middle fingers to form a V; injection site is the middle of the V. C. Vastus lateralis: Identify greater trochanter; place hand at lateral femoral condyle; injection site is middle third of anterior lateral aspect. D. Deltoid: Locate the lateral side of the humerus from two to three fingerwidths below the acromion process in adults or one fingerwidth below the acromion process in children.**

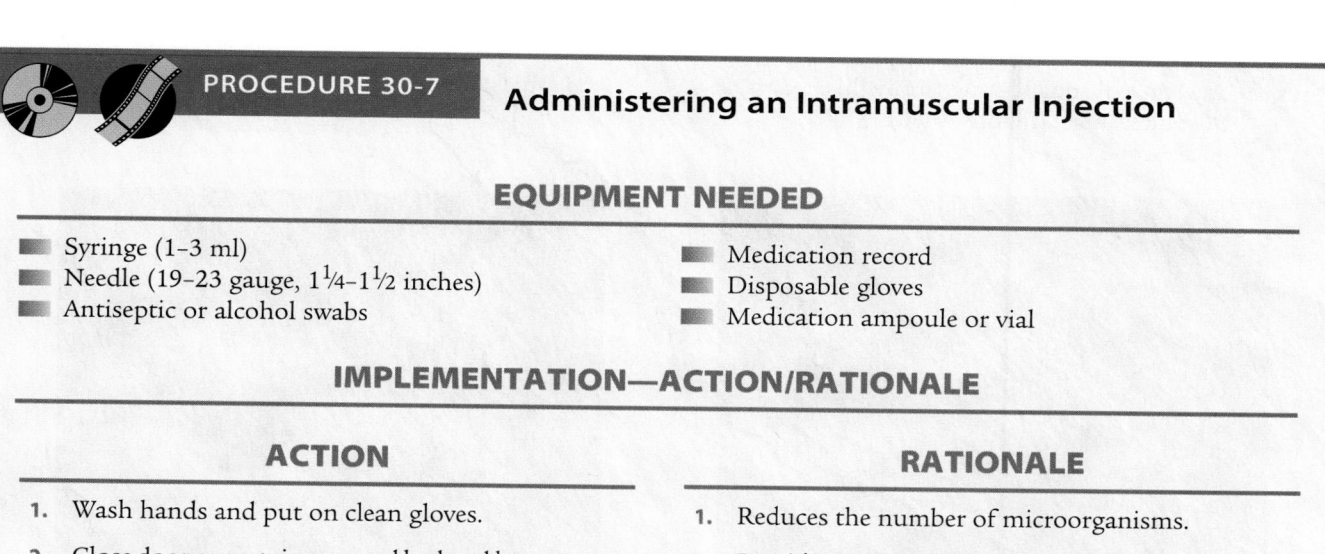

PROCEDURE 30-7    **Administering an Intramuscular Injection**

## EQUIPMENT NEEDED

- Syringe (1–3 ml)
- Needle (19–23 gauge, $1\frac{1}{4}$–$1\frac{1}{2}$ inches)
- Antiseptic or alcohol swabs

- Medication record
- Disposable gloves
- Medication ampoule or vial

## IMPLEMENTATION—ACTION/RATIONALE

| ACTION | RATIONALE |
|---|---|
| 1. Wash hands and put on clean gloves. | 1. Reduces the number of microorganisms. |
| 2. Close door or curtains around bed and keep gown or sheet draped over body. Identify client. | 2. Provides privacy. Assures medication is given to the right client. |
| 3. Select injection site. | 3. Injection site should be free of lesions. |

*(continues)*

## PROCEDURE 30-7 (*continued*)

- Inspect skin for bruises, inflammation, edema, masses, tenderness, and sites of previous injections.
- Use anatomic landmarks.

4. Select needle size: Assess size and weight of client and site to be used.

5. Assist client into a comfortable position:
   - For vastus lateralis, lie flat or supine with knee slightly flexed.
   - For ventrogluteal, lie on side or back with knee and hip slightly flexed.
   - For dorsogluteal, lie prone with feet turned inward or on side with upper knee and hip flexed and placed in front of lower leg.
   - For deltoid, stand with arm relaxed at side or sit with lower arm relaxed on lap or lie flat with lower arm relaxed across abdomen (Figure 30-49).
   - Distract client by talking about an interesting subject.

6. Use antiseptic swab to clean skin at site.

7. While holding swab between fingers of nondominant hand, pull cap from needle.

8. Administer injection:
   - Hold syringe between thumb and forefinger of dominant hand like a dart.
   - Spread skin tightly, or pinch a generous section of tissue firmly—for cachectic patients.
   - Inject needle quickly and firmly (like a dart) at a 90-degree angle (Figure 30-50).
   - Release the skin.

- Repeated daily injections should be rotated.

- Avoids injury to underlying nerves, bone, or blood vessels.

4. Ensures that needle will be injected into the muscle.

5. Relaxation minimizes discomfort. Distraction reduces anxiety.

6. Circular motion and mechanical action of swab remove secretions containing microorganisms.

7. Swab remains accessible during procedure. Prevents contamination of needle.

8.
   - Quick, smooth injection is easier with proper position of syringe.
   - Needle penetrates tight skin easier than loose skin.
   - Quick, firm injection minimizes discomfort.

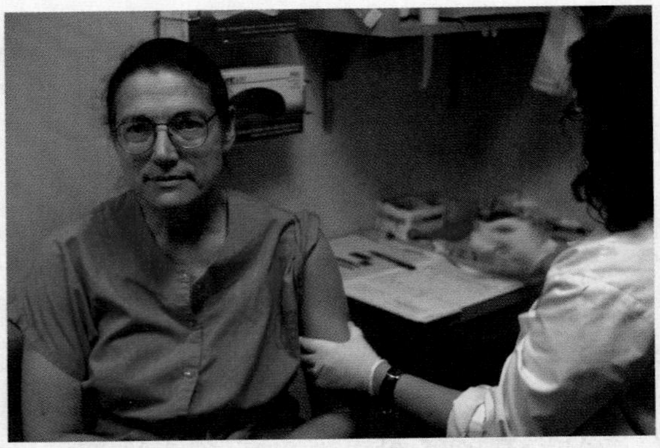

**Figure 30-49** **Have the client stand or sit with arm relaxed at side.**

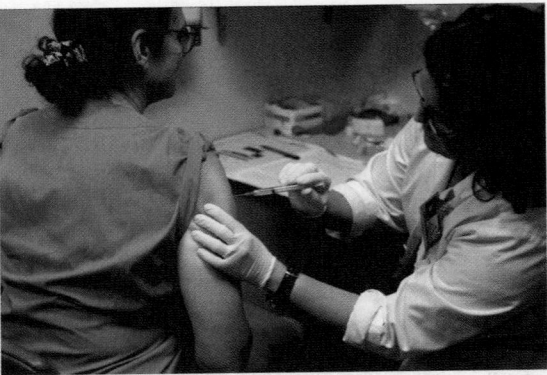

**Figure 30-50**    **Inject needle quickly and firmly at a 90-degree angle.**

*(continues)*

## PROCEDURE 30-7 (continued)

- Grasp the lower end of the syringe with non-dominant hand and position dominant hand to the end of the plunger. Do not move the syringe.

- Pull back on the plunger to ascertain if needle is in a vein. If no blood appears, slowly inject the medication.

9. Quickly withdraw the needle while applying pressure with the antiseptic swab.

10. Gently massage the site.

11. Assist the client to a comfortable position.

12. Discard the uncapped needle and syringe in a safe receptacle.

13. Remove gloves and wash hands.

- Injection requires smooth manipulation of syringe parts. Movement of syringe may cause discomfort.

- Aspiration of blood indicates intravenous placement of needle so procedure may have to be abandoned.

9. Supporting tissue around injection site minimizes discomfort.

10. Stimulates circulation and improves drug distribution and absorption.

11. Promotes comfort.

12. Decreases risk of needle stick.

13. Reduces transmission of microorganisms.

# LIFE SPAN CONSIDERATIONS

## IM Injections

### Pediatric Variations

- No more than 1 ml of medication should be injected into the muscle of a small child. Small infants should not be given more than 0.5 ml IM.

- A tuberculin syringe and a ½- to 1-inch, 25–27-gauge needle are more appropriate for infants who require small doses of medications.

- Distracting a child so she does not see the syringe and needle may help relieve anxiety.

- Lightly tapping the skin before inserting the needle may decrease pain by focusing the child's attention on the touch rather than the needle.

- Parents can comfort their child after an injection.

- Band-Aids with cartoon pictures help soothe a child after an injection.

- Assistance may be required to help the child hold still.

### Geriatric Variations

- Older clients who have had a cerebrovascular accident may have muscle atrophy.

- Older clients may require shorter and smaller-gauged needles due to muscle atrophy.

- Older clients should receive no more than 2 ml of medication.

## COMMUNITY/HOME CARE

### IM Injections

#### Home Care Variations

- Clients need an approved method of discarding needles and syringes when giving injections at home.

#### Long-Term Care Variations

- If the client requires routine doses of IM medication, be sure to rotate the sites to prevent tissue damage and poor absorption of the medication.

- Reassess the client's need for ongoing IM medications regularly. It may be more appropriate to deliver the medication via a different route.

with the syringe in a vertical position to the floor and the air bubble at the plunger tip. Otherwise, the air bubble is not injected last.

### Z-Track Technique

The **Z-track (zigzag) technique** refers to a method used in administering IM injections (see Procedure 30-7). This technique was traditionally used when administering Imferon, an iron preparation, which can cause permanent discoloration in the subcutaneous tissue. Today, the technique is used commonly when administering ventrogluteal and dorsogluteal injections.

When administering a Z-track injection, the nurse should place the client in the prone position; then pull the skin to one side, insert the needle at a 90-degree angle, and administer the medication. Spreading the skin, a common method formerly used for IM injections, increases the risk that medication will leak into the needle track and the subcutaneous tissue; this risk is virtually eliminated using the Z-track technique, making it the technique of choice (Altman, 2004). The nurse waits 10 seconds and withdraws the needle at the same angle of insertion; the site should not be massaged because massaging could cause tissue irritation.

Table 30-5 summarizes the basics of intradermal, subcutaneous, and intramuscular injections.

### Intravenous Injections

The intravenous (IV) route is used when a rapid drug effect is desired or when the medication is irritating to tissue. This route is also useful when the gastrointestinal system is not functioning or the peripheral circulation is decreased, making absorption unpredictable with other routes. IV administration provides immediate release of

medication into the bloodstream; consequently, it can be dangerous. IV medications are administered by one of the following methods:

- Intravenous fluid container
- Volume-control administration set
- Intermittent infusion by piggyback or partial fill
- Intravenous push (IVP or bolus)

See Chapter 34 for a discussion of other IV delivery systems.

### Assessment

When administering IV medications, the nurse should assess the patency of the infusion system and the condition of the injection site for signs of complications such as **infiltration** (leakage of solution into surrounding tissues, causing swelling and discomfort at the IV site) and **phlebitis** (inflammation of a vein). See Chapter 35 for a complete discussion of these IV complications. Some IV medications or solutions with high or low pH or high osmolarity are irritating to veins and can cause phlebitis. **Vesicants** are medications which, if they infiltrate through the vein into surrounding tissues, can cause serious tissue destruction, necessitating months of treatment and even surgical intervention (Skokal, 2001). Vesicants include not only chemotherapy medications but also more common medications such as vancomycin and the electrolytes potassium chloride and calcium gluconate.

Before administering any IV medication, the nurse should note the client's allergies, drug or solution incompatibilities, the amount and type of diluent needed to mix the medication, and the client's general condition to establish a baseline for administering medication.

### Checking for Medication Incompatibility

**Drug incompatibilities** cause an undesired chemical or physical reaction between a drug and solution, between two medications, or between a drug and the container or tubing. It is essential for the nurse to check if the medication to be injected is compatible with all other solutions cur-

## TABLE 30-5   SUMMARY OF INTRADERMAL, SUBCUTANEOUS, AND INTRAMUSCULAR INJECTIONS

| Type of Injection | Purpose | Site | Needle Size | Maximum Dose | Angle of Insertion |
|---|---|---|---|---|---|
| Intradermal | Injects medication below the epidermis; drugs are absorbed slowly; typically used for diagnosis of tuberculosis and allergens | Inner aspect of forearm; upper chest; upper back | Syringe with short bevel; 25–27-gauge; 3/8 to 1/2-inch | 0.01 to 0.1 ml | 45° |
| Subcutaneous | Injects medication between dermis and muscle; absorbed slowly; typically used for insulin and anticoagulants | Abdomen; lateral and anterior aspects of upper arm and thigh; scapular area on back; ventrogluteal area | 25-gauge, 5/8-inch needle (varies by size of person) | 0.5–1.0 ml | 45° or 90° |
| Intramuscular | Used to promote rapid drug absorption and to provide an alternate route when drug is irritating to SC tissue | Ventrogluteal; dorsogluteal; anterolateral aspect of thigh (vastus lateralis); upper arm (deltoid) | The gauge and length of needle are selected on the basis of medication volume and viscosity and client's body size | Well-developed adult: 3 ml in a large muscle; infant and small child: 0.5–1.0 ml; children and elderly: 1–2 ml; deltoid muscle: 0.5–1 ml | 90° |

rently infusing. For example, hydration solutions and additives such as potassium or sodium bicarbonate should be checked for compatibility, as well as other medications being currently infused, such as the patient-controlled analgesia (PCA) medication. Compatibility of flushes must be considered, because some medications, such as amphotericin B, are not compatible with normal saline. Amphotericin B can only be infused with dextrose water or flushed with sterile water. A drug incompatibility can cause either a visually apparent change such as a milky fluid or microscopic (unseen) crystallization. The nurse must check online pharmacology resources or textbook references for compatibility. Unless it is clearly stated as compatible, the medication should be treated as incompatible and infused separately from other fluids or medications.

Some drugs are incompatible with plastic bags or tubing. For example, insulin is absorbed by IV bags and tubing. Some medications also need to be infused with a filter. Consult drug references or agency policy.

### Adding Medication to an Intravenous Solution

Nurses rarely add medications directly into IV bags because most hospital pharmacies manage IV mixtures. Generally, the only medications that nurses may add to an intravenous solution are potassium chloride or Solu-B, a vitamin. These medications should always be added to full IV bags, not partially full bags, or the increased concentration of medication could be dangerous for the client (Figure 30-51).

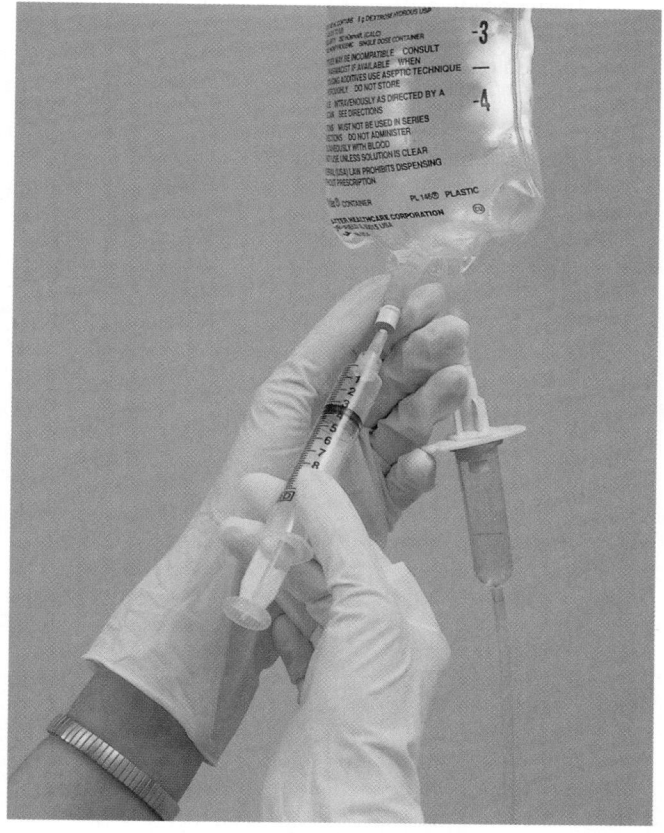

**Figure 30-51   Adding a medication to an intravenous fluid container**

## Adding Medication to a Volume-Control Administration Set

A volume-control set is used to administer small volumes of IV solution. These devices have various names as determined by the manufacturer, such as Soluset, Metriset, Volutrol, or Buretrol. To administer a drug by this method, the nurse should:

- Withdraw the prescribed amount of medication into a syringe that is to be injected into the volume-control set.
- Cleanse the injection port of a partially filled volume-control set with an alcohol swab.
- Inject the prepared medication into the port of the volume-control set.
- Add 50–100 ml solution from the primary hydration solution bag into the Volutrol set and reclamp primary bag.

- Gently mix the solution in the volume-control chamber.
- Calculate and set the rate the medication should be infused.
- After the medication is infused, refill the Volutrol with solution from the primary hydration bag and reset the infusion rate to the prescribed rate.

## Administering Medications by Intermittent Infusion

A common method of administering IV medications is by using a secondary, or partial-fill additive bag, often referred to as an IV piggyback (IVPB). A secondary line is a complete IV set (fluid container and tubing with either a microdrip or a macrodrip system) connected to a Y-port of a primary line (see Procedure 30-8). The primary line maintains venous access. The IVPB is used for medication administration. See

---

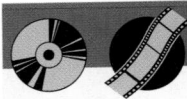

**PROCEDURE 30-8**

## Administering Medications via Secondary Administration Sets (Piggybacks)

### EQUIPMENT NEEDED

- Disposable gloves
- Medication prepared in a labeled infusion bag
- Short microdrip or macrodrip tubing set for piggyback (needleless system preferred) (Figure 30-52)
- Sterile needles, 21 or 23 gauge, if needleless system not available
- Antiseptic swab
- Adhesive tape
- IV pole
- Medication administration record

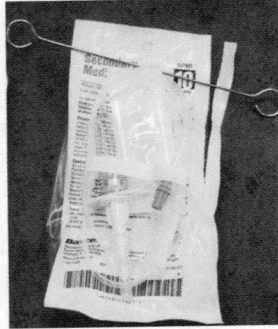

**Figure 30-52** IV tubing set for piggyback administration

### IMPLEMENTATION—ACTION/RATIONALE

| ACTION | RATIONALE |
|---|---|
| 1. Check physician's or qualified practitioner's order. | 1. Ensures accurate administration of medication. |
| 2. Wash hands. *Gloves are not necessary if you are adding fluids to an existing infusion line.* | 2. Reduces the transmission of microorganisms. |
| 3. Check client's identification bracelet. | 3. Ensures medication is given to the correct client. |
| 4. Explain procedure and reason drug is being given. | 4. Information decreases anxiety. |
| 5. Prepare medication bag:<br>• Close clamp on tubing of infusion set.<br>• Spike medication bag with infusion tubing (Figure 30-53).<br>• Open clamp (Figure 30-54).<br>• Allow tubing to be filled with solution to evacuate air from tubing (Figure 30-55). | 5.<br><br>• Prevents leakage of solution.<br>• Provides a method of infusing the medication into the system.<br>• Allows the solution to fill the tubing.<br>• Prevents air embolus. |

*(continues)*

**PROCEDURE 30-8 (*continued*)**

6. Hang piggyback medication bag above level of primary IV bag. One way to do this is to lower the primary bag using an extender (found in the piggyback tubing package (Figure 30-56).

6. Relationship between height of the bags affects the flow rate to the client.

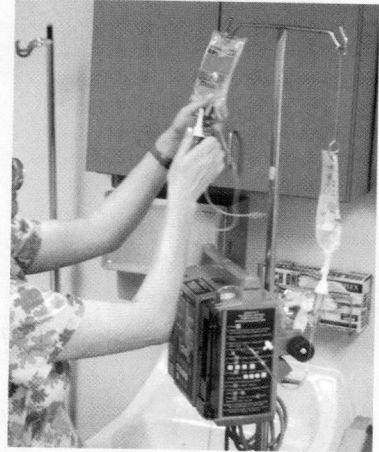

**Figure 30-53    Spike the medication bag with the infusion tubing.**

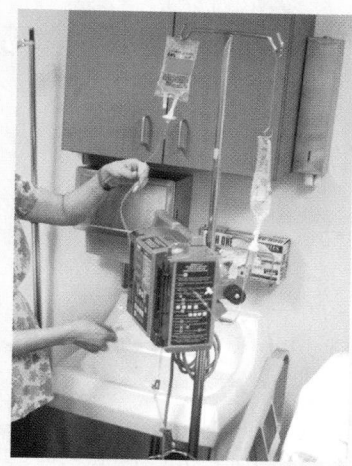

**Figure 30-54    Open the clamp on the IV tubing.**

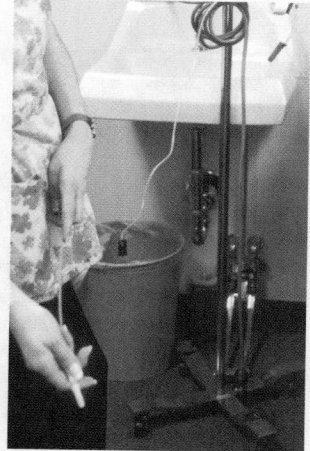

**Figure 30-55    Allow the tubing to fill with solution.**

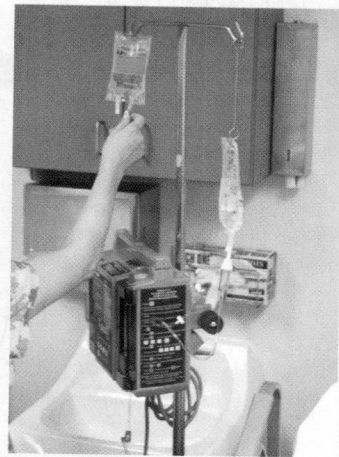

**Figure 30-56    Hang the piggyback bag higher than the primary IV bag.**

7. Connect piggyback tubing to primary tubing at Y-port:
   - For needleless system, remove cap on port and connect tubing (Figure 30-57 and 30-58)
   - If a needle is used, clean port with antiseptic swab and insert small-gauge needle into center of port.
   - Secure tubing with adhesive tape.

8. Administer the medication:
   - Check the prescribed length of time for the infusion.

7. Ensures medication in piggyback bag is infused.
   - A needleless system is preferred to prevent accidental needle sticks.
   - A small-gauge needle does less damage to the rubber stopper on the port.

   - Prevents accidental removal of tubing.

8.
   - Each medication has a recommended rate for IV piggyback administration.

*(continues)*

**PROCEDURE 30-8** (*continued*)

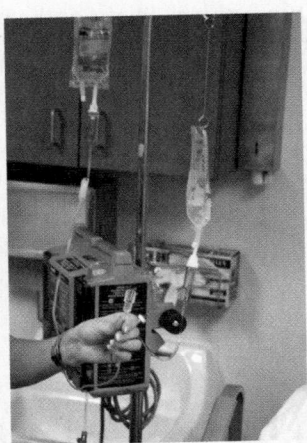

**Figure 30-57     Remove the cap on the needleless system port.**

- Regulate the flow rate of the piggyback by adjusting the regulator clamp (Figure 30-59).
- Observe whether backflow valve on piggyback has stopped flow of primary infusion during drug administration (Figure 30-60).

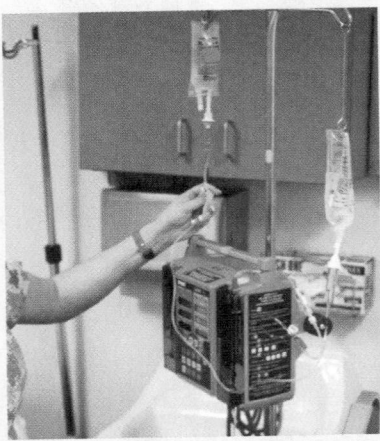

**Figure 30-59     Regulate the flow rate of the piggyback by adjusting the regulator clamp.**

9. Check primary infusion line when medication is finished:
   - Regulate primary infusion rate.
   - Leave secondary bag and tubing in place for next drug administration.

10. Dispose of all used materials and place needles in needle disposal container.

11. Wash hands.

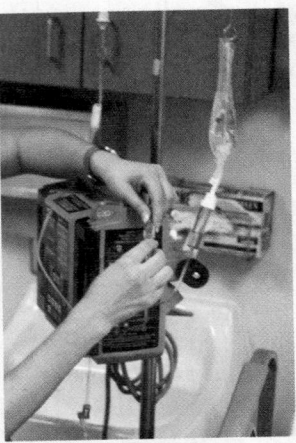

**Figure 30-58     Connect the needleless system tubing.**

- Medication infuses through primary line.
- Prevents backup of medication into primary infusion line.

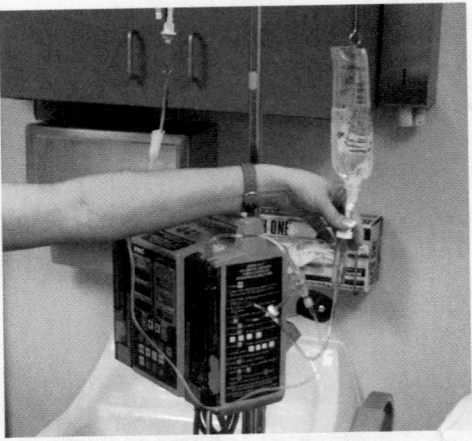

**Figure 30-60     Double-check that the primary infusion has stopped flowing.**

9.

- Reestablishes primary infusion.
- Reduces risk for entry of microorganisms by repeated changes of tubing.

10. Reduces transmission of microorganisms.

11. Reduces transmission of microorganisms.

## LIFE SPAN CONSIDERATIONS

### IV Injections

#### Pediatric Variations

- Giving a medication to a child through an established IV may be less traumatic than an IM or subcutaneous injection.

- Special precautions need to be taken to maintain an intact IV in very young clients.

- Adaptation to promote optimum mobility for a child while piggyback medication is infusing will increase the child's compliance with the procedure.

#### Geriatric Variations

- The veins of older clients may be more fragile and sensitive to irritating solutions.

## COMMUNITY/HOME CARE

### IV Injections

#### Home Care Variations

- Medications can be given by IV piggyback at home after teaching caregiver and client how to perform the procedure.

#### Long-Term Care Variations

- Clients who are receiving IV medication over the long term generally have central lines in place to prevent repeated trauma to their peripheral veins. The procedure for administering a piggyback medication through a central line is the same.

Chapter 34 for a complete discussion of primary and secondary lines. When the IVPB medication is incompatible with the primary IV solution, the nurse must flush the primary IV tubing with normal saline before and after administering the medication. (Some medications, such as Valium, are incompatible with normal saline, and sterile water should be used for a flush.)

**Intermittent Infusion Devices or Locks**   When the client requires only the administration of IV medications without the infusion of solutions, an intermittent infusion device is inserted into a peripheral needle or catheter in the client's vein. This device is commonly referred to as a heparin or saline lock (Figure 30-61). A lock provides continuous access to venous circulation, eliminating the need for a continuous IV, and it increases the client's mobility.

The device can be used to infuse intermittent IVPB or IV push medications, or it can be converted to a primary IV. A major consideration for inserting a lock device is that it provides venous access in case of an emergency. Lock devices are routinely used with cardiac clients.

When a lock is used intermittently, it is generally flushed every 8 hours to maintain its patency (patency refers to being freely opened). Most agencies use saline to flush a peripheral lock. However, some agencies require a diluted dose of heparin (10 units/ml). Lock devices are also used on central lines; usually a heparinized saline (10 units/ml to 100 units/ml) flush is used. Agency policy should always be followed for concentration and amount. Because a medication may be incompatible with heparin, a flush of normal saline (or sterile water depending on

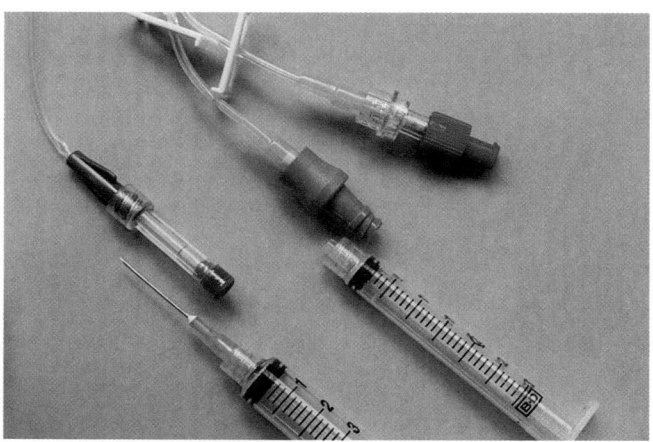

**Figure 30-61   Heparin and saline lock equipment**

## STOP AND THINK

### IV Titrating of Medications

- Your client has an IV titration (push) dose of 80 mg methylprednisolone ordered. The vial states there is 125 mg of medication in 2 ml.

- How much medication should you draw up?

- How fast should it be injected?

- Is it compatible with the D5 1/2 normal saline hydration fluid and the Dilaudid PCA (patient-controlled analgesia) that are currently infusing?

## CLINICAL ALERT

### IV Infusion Rate

Know the correct rate that an IV medication should be infused or injected. Double-check any medication infusing by gravity to be certain that the rate has not changed by the client changing position or accidentally kinking the tubing.

medication compatibility) should be given before and after the medication is administered (Barbone, 1999).

### Administering IV Push Medications

The method of medication administration by IV bolus or IV push injection is determined by the type of IV system. For example, an IV push medication can be injected into a peripheral or central line through a lock device (Figure 30-61) or a continuous infusion line (Figure 30-62). When giving an IV push medication into a continuous infusion line that is running by gravity and has no back check valve, the nurse should pinch the IV tubing above the injection port while slowly giving the medication. This will prevent the medication from going up into the bag instead of into the client. The hydration rate should be checked after the tubing is unpinched, but it will usually not have to be reset if the roller clamp has not been used. Most pump tubing has a back check valve feature (check with the manufacturer if in doubt) and stopping the primary is not necessary, unless the solution is incompatible with the medication.

It is imperative that the nurse knows the specific time (rate) that the medication should be injected and whether the medication should be diluted. Intravenous medications quickly circulate to the heart and other central organs, and too fast an injection can cause serious effects. Consult IV drug references or the pharmacist if uncertain. The nurse should know the specific effects of the medication and monitor the client closely during and after the injection for drug reactions.

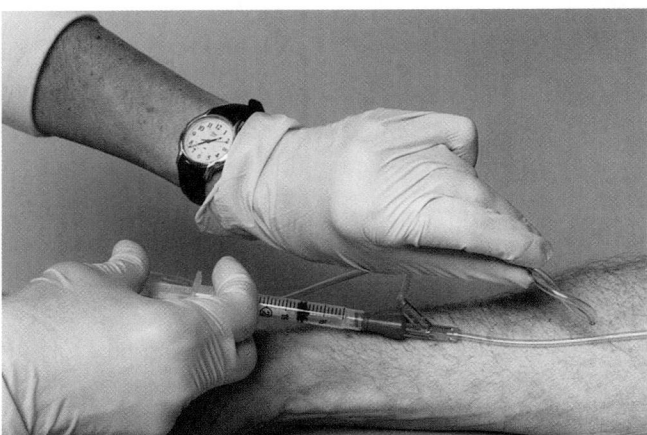

**Figure 30-62   An IV push medication given in a continuous infusion line**

## Topical Administration

Topical medications may be administered to the skin, eyes, ears, nose, throat, rectum, and vagina. The medication generally provides a local effect but can also cause systemic effects. Topical medications are usually ordered two or three times a day to achieve their therapeutic effect. The nurse should check with the client and the medical record for any known allergies.

Because secretions are produced by the skin and mucous membranes, the nurse should *always* implement Standard Precautions by wearing gloves when applying a topical drug. In addition, if the nurse is not wearing gloves, some medications can be absorbed through the nurse's skin and affect the nurse systematically. For example, nitropaste can cause a headache and a drop in blood pressure.

### Skin Medications

Skin medications are usually given to relieve pruritus (itching), to protect the skin, to prevent or treat an infection, to provide local anesthesia, or to create a systemic effect. They come in forms of lotions, pastes, ointments, creams, powders, aerosol sprays, and patches.

A **transdermal** medication is made to be absorbed through the skin for the purpose of causing a systemic effect. A common transdermal medication is nitropaste, which is prescribed in "inches" and measured out by the nurse onto a paper marked in half-inch increments. The paper is then turned over and applied to the skin with tape. However, most transdermal medications are manufactured in patches, which have small pores allowing timed-release of the medication through the skin over a 24–72-hour period.

Before applying a topical preparation, the nurse should assess the condition of the skin for any open lesions, rashes, or areas of erythema and skin breakdown. If the medication is applied by patch or is nitropaste, the former dose should be removed and the skin wiped.

Body oils may interfere with the adhesive properties of patches or tape. The skin should be cleansed and dried well, unless contraindicated by a specific order. It should be thoroughly dry before applying a new medication dose. When applying a new dose, rotate to a new site without body hair. Sign the patch with the date, time, and initials.

When a cream is applied, the nurse should use a sterile tongue blade *each time* to dip into the medication. This prevents cross-contamination of the medication. The medication can then be transferred to the nurse's gloved fingers, unless it is an open surgical wound or burn that must be treated with sterile technique.

## CLINICAL ALERT

### Application of Topical Medications

Always wear gloves when applying a topical medication in any form to prevent absorption of the medication through your skin.

## Eye Medications

Eye medications, often referred to as ophthalmic medications, refer to drops, ointments, and disks. These drugs are used for diagnostic and therapeutic purposes—to lubricate the eye or socket for a prosthetic eye and to prevent or treat eye conditions such as glaucoma (elevated pressure within the eye) and infection. Diagnostically, eyedrops can be used to anesthetize the eye, dilate the pupil, and stain the cornea to identify abrasions and scars.

The nurse should review the abbreviations used in medication orders to ensure that the medication is instilled in the correct eye. Cross-contamination is a potential problem with eyedrops. The nurse should adhere to the following safety measures to prevent cross-contamination:

• Each client should have his own bottle of eyedrops. Clients should never share eye medications.
• Discard any solution remaining in the dropper after instillation.

• Discard the dropper if the tip is accidentally contaminated, as by touching the bottle or any part of the client's eye. The risk of transferring infection from one eye to the other is increased if the tip touches any part of the client's eye.

See Procedure 30-9 for administering eye medications. The nurse should insert medication disks at bedtime because they usually cause blurring of the eyes on insertion. Standard Precautions are used when eye care and medications are being administered, because of the potential contact with bodily secretions.

### Ear Medications

Solutions ordered to treat the ear are often referred to as *otic* (pertaining to the ear) drops or irrigations. Eardrops may be instilled to soften earwax, to produce anesthesia, to treat infection or inflammation, or to facilitate removal of a foreign body, such as an insect. External auditory canal irriga-

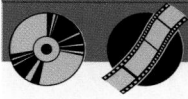

PROCEDURE 30-9 | **Administering Eye and Ear Medications**

## EQUIPMENT NEEDED

### Eye Medication

■ Medication administration record (MAR)
■ Eye medication
■ Tissue or cotton ball
■ Nonsterile gloves (if needed)

### Ear Medication

■ Medication administration record (MAR)
■ Medication
■ Cotton-tipped applicator
■ Tissue

## IMPLEMENTATION—ACTION/RATIONALE

| ACTION | RATIONALE |
|---|---|
| **Eye Medication** | |
| 1. Check with the client and the chart for any known allergies or medical conditions that would contraindicate use of the drug. | 1. Prevents occurrence of adverse reactions. |
| 2. Gather the necessary equipment. | 2. Promotes efficiency. |
| 3. Follow the five rights of drug administration. | 3. Promotes safety. |
| 4. Take the medication to the client's room and place on a clean surface. | 4. Decreases risk of contamination of bottle cap. |
| 5. Check client's identification armband. | 5. Accurately identifies client. |
| 6. Explain the procedure to the client; inquire if the client wants to instill medication. If so, assess the client's ability to do so. | 6. Reduces client's anxiety and enhances collaboration; some clients are used to instilling their own medication. |
| 7. Wash hands, don nonsterile gloves if needed. | 7. Decreases contact with bodily fluids. |
| 8. Place client in a supine position with the head slightly hyperextended. | 8. Minimizes drainage of medication through the tear duct. |

*(continues)*

## PROCEDURE 30-9 (continued)

### Instilling Eyedrops

9. Remove cap from eye bottle and place cap on its side.

10. Squeeze the prescribed amount of medication into the eyedropper.

11. Place a tissue below the lower lid.

12. With dominant hand, hold eyedropper $1/2$ to $3/4$ inch above the eyeball; rest hand on client's forehead to stabilize.

13. Place hand on cheekbone and expose lower conjunctival sac by pulling down on cheek.

14. Instruct the client to look up and drop prescribed number of drops into center of conjunctival sac (Figure 30-63).

15. Instruct client to gently close eyes and move eyes. Briefly place fingers on either side of the client's nose to close the tear ducts and prevent the medication from draining out of the eye (Figure 30-64).

9. Prevents contamination of the bottle cap.

10. Ensures correct dose.

11. Absorbs the medication that flows from the eye.

12. Reduces risk of dropper touching eye structure, and prevents injury to the eye.

13. Stabilizes hand and prevents systemic absorption of eye medication.

14. Reduces stimulation of the blink reflex; prevents injury to the cornea.

15. Distributes solution over conjunctival surface and anterior eyeball.

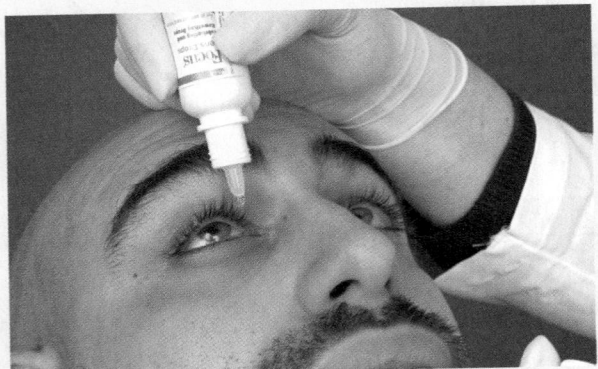

Figure 30-63   Instruct the client to look up. Administer prescribed number of drops into the center of the conjunctival sac.

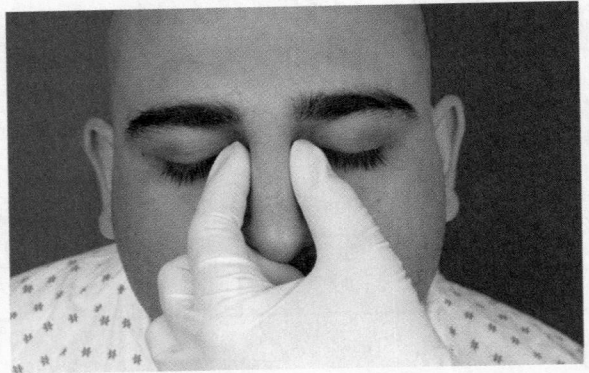

Figure 30-64   Placing the fingers on the sides of the client's nose closes the tear ducts and prevents the medication from draining out of the eye.

16. Remove gloves; wash hands.

17. Record on the MAR the route, site (which eye), and time administered.

### Eye Ointment Application

18. Repeat Actions 1 to 8.

19. Lower lid:
    • With nondominant hand, gently separate client's eyelids with thumb and finger and grasp lower lid near margin immediately below the lashes; exert pressure downward over the bony prominence of the cheek.

16. Reduces the transmission of microorganisms.

17. Provides documentation that the medication was given.

18. See Rationales 1 to 8.

19.
    • Provides access to the lower lid.

*(continues)*

**PROCEDURE 30-9** (*continued*)

- Instruct the client to look up.

- Apply eye ointment along inside edge of the entire lower eyelid, from inner to outer canthus.

20. Upper lid:
    - Instruct client to look down.
    - With nondominant hand, gently grasp client's lashes near center of upper lid with thumb and index finger, and draw lid up and away from eyeball.
    - Squeeze ointment along upper lid starting at inner canthus.

21. Repeat Actions 16 and 17.

**Medication Disk**

22. Repeat Actions 1 to 8.

23. Open sterile package and press dominant, sterile gloved finger against the oval disk so that it lies lengthwise across fingertip.

24. Instruct the client to look up.

25. With nondominant hand, gently pull the client's lower eyelid down and place the disk horizontally in the conjunctival sac.
    - Then pull the lower eyelid out, up, and over the disk.
    - Instruct the client to blink several times.
    - If disk is still visible, repeat steps.
    - Once the disk is in place, instruct the client to gently press the fingers against the closed lids; do not rub eyes or move the disk across the cornea.
    - If the disk falls out, rinse it under cool water and reinsert.

26. If the disk is prescribed for both eyes (OU), repeat Actions 23 to 25.

27. Repeat Actions 15 to 17.

**Removing an Eye Medication Disk**

28. Repeat Actions 3 and 5 to 8.

29. Remove the disk:
    - With nondominant hand, invert the lower eyelid and identify the disk.
    - If the disk is located in the upper eye, instruct the client to close the eye, and place your finger on the closed eyelid. Apply gentle, long, circular strokes;

---

- Reduces stimulation of the blink reflex and keeps cornea out of way of medication.
- Ensures drug is applied to entire lid.

20.
- Keeps cornea out of way of medication.

- Ensures medication applied to entire length of lid.

21. See Rationales 16 and 17.

22. See Rationales 1 to 8.

23. Promotes sticking of disk to fingertip.

24. Reduces stimulation of the blink reflex and keeps cornea out of way of medication.

25. Allows the disk to automatically adhere to the eye.

- To secure the disk in the conjunctival sac.

- To allow the disk to settle into place.
- To ensure correct placement of the disk.
- To secure disk placement. To prevent corneal scratches.

- Preserves medication. This is not a sterile procedure.

26. Ensures both eyes are treated at the same time.

27. See Rationales 15 to 17.

28. See Rationales 3 and 5 to 8.

29.
- Exposes the disk for removal.

- Safely moves the disk to the lower conjunctival sac.

(*continues*)

instruct client to open the eye. Disk should be located in corner of eye. With your fingertip, slide the disk to the lower lid, then proceed.
- With dominant hand, use the forefinger to slide the disk onto the lid and out of the client's eye.

30. Remove gloves; wash hands.

31. Record on the MAR the removal of the disk.

- Safely removes the disk without scratching the cornea.

30. Reduces transmission of microorganisms.

31. Provides documentation that the disk was removed.

## ACTION

### Ear Medication

1. Check with client and chart for any known allergies.

2. Check the MAR against the physician's or qualified provider's written orders.

3. Wash your hands.

4. Calculate the dose (Figure 30-65).

5. Use the identification armband to properly identify the client (Figure 30-66).

6. Explain the procedure to the client.

## RATIONALE

1. Prevents the occurrence of hypersensitivity reactions.

2. Ensures accuracy in identification of the medication.

3. Reduces the transfer of microorganisms.

4. Ensures the administration of the correct dose.

5. Ensures correct client.

6. Enhances cooperation.

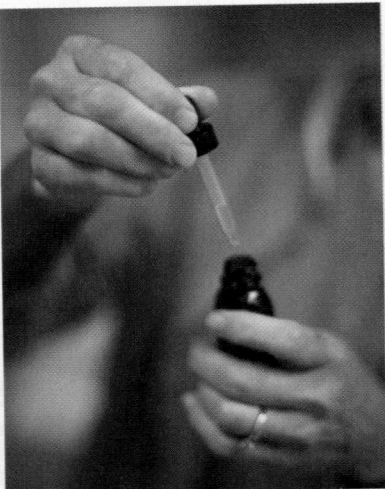

**Figure 30-65** Calculate the correct dose and draw medication into the ear dropper.

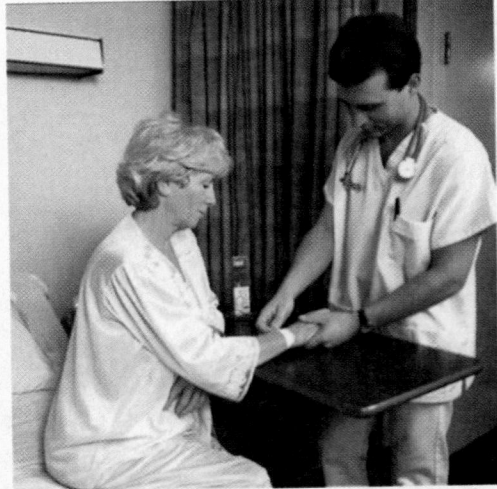

**Figure 30-66** Check the client's identification band before administering medication.

7. Place the client in a side-lying position with the affected ear facing up.

8. Straighten the ear canal by pulling the pinna down and back for children less than 3 years of age or upward and outward in adults and older children.

7. Facilitates the administration of the medication.

8. Opens the canal and facilitates introduction of the medication.

*(continues)*

## PROCEDURE 30-9 (*continued*)

9. Instill the drops into the ear canal by holding the dropper at least ½ inch above the ear canal (Figure 30-67).

9. Prevents injury to the ear canal.

10. Ask the client to maintain the position for 2 to 3 minutes.

10. Allows for distribution of the medication.

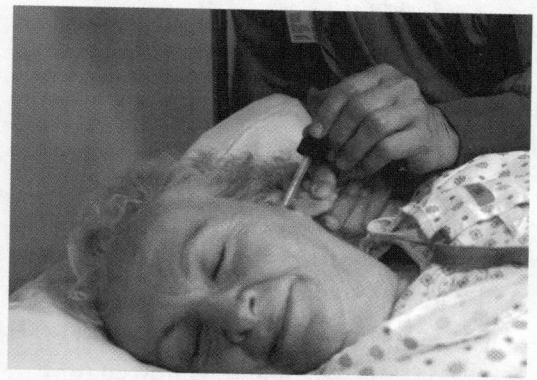

**Figure 30-67   Slowly instill the drops, holding the dropper at least ½ inch above the ear canal.**

11. Place a cotton ball on the outermost part of the canal.

11. Prevents the medication from escaping when the client changes to a sitting or standing position.

12. Wash hands.

12. Reduces the transmission of microorganisms.

13. Document the drug, number of drops, time administered, and ear medicated.

13. Documenting the actions of the nurse will reduce the number of medication errors.

# LIFE SPAN CONSIDERATIONS

## Eye and Ear Medications

### Pediatric Variations

- Children tend to rub their eyes and noses when tired. A child with an eye infection, such as pinkeye, can easily cross-contaminate from one eye to another. Parents need to be taught the importance of keeping the child's hands away from the eyes as well as keeping the child's hands and eyes clean.

### Geriatric Variations

- Older clients may be treated with eyedrops for glaucoma or cataracts. These conditions make it difficult to read the small print on eyedrop bottles. Be sure to mark the bottles in an easily identifiable manner so the client will be sure to get the right medication at the right time in the correct eye.

- Small bottles may be hard to hold if the older client has reduced fine motor skills, trembling, or reduced sensation in his hands. The nurse can help the client devise ways of stabilizing the bottle by bracing the other fingers of the hand on the face (for eyedrops) or the side of the head (for eardrops). The nurse can demonstrate how to make an eyedrop or eardrop bottle easier to hold by wrapping it with a cloth to increase its diameter.

## COMMUNITY/HOME CARE

### Eye and Ear Medications

**Home Care Variations**

- Clients who use eyedrops routinely at home can become careless about identifying the right medication for the right time and the right use. Help the client mark the eyedrop bottles so they are clearly identifiable.

- Contact lens wearers have been known to confuse eyedrop bottles with liquid glue or nail adhesive bottles. Be sure the client is aware of the similarity and teach the client to carefully identify anything before putting it in the eyes.

- Make sure there is adequate lighting in the home care setting. A client who is having trouble with vision may have difficulty seeing medication in the dropper or reading the medication labels. Good lighting makes it easier to read and see without eyestrain.

**Long-Term Care Variations**

- Long-term care clients who are self-medicating may be reluctant to dispose of outdated or contaminated eyedrops/eardrops. Explain the importance of not using contaminated or outdated medications.

- The risk of contamination of an eyedrop or eardrop bottle rises if that bottle is used repeatedly, especially if proper technique is not followed. Make sure that proper technique is taught and reinforced for caregivers and clients in the long-term care setting.

tions are usually performed for cleaning purposes and less frequently for applying heat and antiseptic solutions. The internal ear is very sensitive to changes in temperature. Sudden changes can cause nausea and dizziness. Eardrops and irrigation fluids should be at room temperature.

Before instilling a solution into the ear, the nurse should inspect the ear for signs of drainage, an indication of a perforated tympanic membrane. Eardrops are usually contraindicated when the tympanic membrane is perforated. If the tympanic membrane is damaged, all procedures must be performed using sterile aseptic technique; otherwise, medical asepsis is used when instilling medications into the ear (see Procedure 30-9). Medication should never be forced into the ear canal, especially if it is occluded (as by wax). Forcing medication into an occluded eardrum can injure the eardrum.

Certain conditions have contraindications for specific drugs; for example, hydrocortisone eardrops are con-

traindicated in clients with a fungal infection or a viral infection such as herpes.

### Nasal Medications

Nasal instillations can be performed with different preparations: drops or nebulizers (atomizer or aerosol). Nasal drugs are administered to produce one or more of the following effects: to shrink swollen mucous membranes, to loosen secretions and facilitate drainage, and to treat infections of the nasal cavity or sinuses. Because many of these products are nonprescription drugs, clients should be taught their correct usage. For example, nasal decongestants are common over-the-counter drugs used to shrink swollen mucous membranes; however, when these drugs are used in excess, they may have a reverse or rebound effect by increasing nasal congestion.

The nasal sinuses (frontal, ethmoid, maxillary, and sphenoid sinuses) communicate with the nasal fossae and are lined with mucous membranes similar to those that line the nose. Nose drops can be instilled to remain in the nasal passage, to reach the ethmoid and sphenoid sinuses, or to reach the frontal or maxillary sinuses. Location is determined by the degree of hyperextension and position of the head during instillation. Although the nose is considered a clean (not sterile) cavity, because of its connection with the sinuses, the nurse uses medical asepsis when performing nasal instillations.

Nebulizers (inhalers) are used to deliver a fine mist containing medication droplets. The nurse should administer or assist clients with the usage of atomizers and aerosols:

## CLINICAL ALERT

### Systemic Effects of Eyedrops

The nurse should apply pressure to the inner canthus when instilling eyedrops that have potential systemic effects such as atropine and timolol maleate (Timoptic). Gentle pressure over the inner canthus prevents the medication from flowing into the tear duct, thereby decreasing the absorption rate of the drug.

## COMMUNITY/HOME CARE

## Nasal Medications

### Home Care Variations

- If nasal congestion persists, clients may have chronic sinus infections that require the adjunct of humidifiers or different medications.

- Saline nose sprays or drops may be effective for simple nasal congestion or as adjunct therapy and can be made by dissolving 1 teaspoon of salt in 1 pint of warm water.

- Saline solutions should not be kept over 24 hours because bacterial growth will occur. Clients should assess temperature and report long-lasting sinus headaches.

### Long-Term Care Variations

- Tolerance can develop with some nasal decongestants and therefore cannot be used on a routine basis.

- Other categories of drugs may be needed.

- Clients with persistent nasal congestion should seek medical attention and be evaluated for allergies, chronic sinus problems, or other health problems.

- Instruct the client to clear the nostrils by blowing the nose.
- Client should be in an upright position with head tilted back slightly.

*Atomizer*
- Occlude one nostril to prevent air from entering the nasal cavity and to allow the medication to flow freely in the open nostril.
- Insert the atomizer tip into the open nostril and instruct the client to inhale, then squeeze the atomizer once, and instruct the client to exhale.

*Aerosol*
- Shake the aerosol well before each use.
- Grasp between thumb and index finger and insert the adapter tip into one nostril while occluding the other nostril with a finger, then press the adapter cartridge firmly to release one measured dose of medication.
- Repeat the preceding steps as ordered for the other nostril.

- Instruct the client to keep head tilted backward for 2 to 3 minutes and to breathe through the nose while the medication is being absorbed.

When the client is discharged with a nasal inhaler, the nurse should teach the client how to store and use the device. Refer to Procedure 30-10 for information on administering nasal medication.

### Respiratory Inhalant Medications

Respiratory inhalants are delivered by devices that produce fine droplets, which are inhaled deep into the respiratory tract. These droplets are absorbed almost immediately through the alveolar epithelium into the bloodstream. Respiratory inhalants are used to produce anesthesia during surgery and to treat respiratory diseases and symptoms such as bronchospasm, allergic reactions, and asthma.

Respiratory inhalant medications produce both local and systemic effects. The desired local effects are decreased mucus congestion and inflammation (corticosteroids), liquification of bronchial secretions (mucolytics), and dilation of the bronchials (bronchodilators) to increase airway patency. The main systemic effect of concern is the potential stimulation of the heart by the beta-agonist bronchodilators, causing tachycardia and possible arrhythmias. Bronchodilators are contraindicated in clients with a history of tachycardia. Bronchodilators also have drug interactions with anticoagulants.

Respiratory inhalants are usually delivered by handheld devices including nebulizers, metered-dose inhalers (MDI) (Figure 30-68), dry powder turbo-spinners, or nasal inhalers (already discussed under nasal medications). Except for the nebulizer, these devices are small and can fit into a purse or pocket.

The nebulizer produces very fine droplets by forced air (or oxygen, if needed by the client) under high pressure (available in wall outlets in hospitals) or by an electrical machine, which is portable and used both in hospitals and at home. Inhalants by this method go deep into the bronchial system and require little client effort other than keeping the lips around the mouthpiece and breathing through the mouth. It can be converted to a mask to deliver nebulized inhalants for clients who are unconscious or otherwise unable to use the mouthpiece (Figure 30-69). Either the nurse—or if at home, the client or caregiver—

## CLINICAL ALERT

### Respiratory Medications

Be sure the client knows which respiratory medication is short-acting and used for "rescue" when symptoms develop or worsen. Long-acting medications have no effect in an emergency flare-up or exacerbation of symptoms.

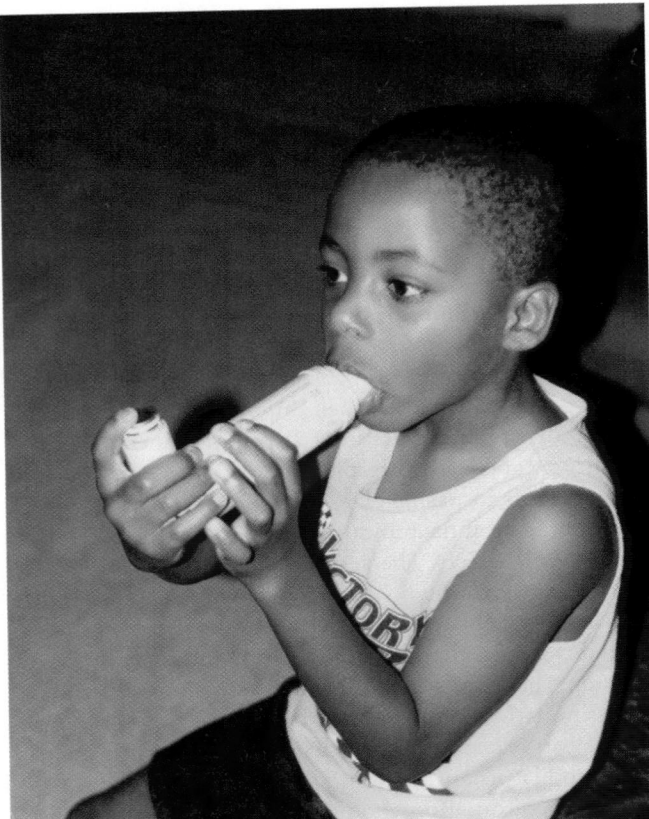

**Figure 30-68**   **Child using an MDI with a spacer and mouthpiece**

must assemble the mouthpiece, insert the medication dose, and rinse the mouthpiece afterward.

The turbo-spinner is used with certain medications that are very fine powders encased in a capsule. The capsule is inserted into the device and punctured when the device is closed. The fine powder is distributed into the bronchial tree when the client inhales deeply through the device. The client must be able to insert the capsule into the device.

Most inhalants for respiratory disorders are delivered by the MDI. The medication is in a small metal canister that is inserted into a plastic mouthpiece. When the canis-

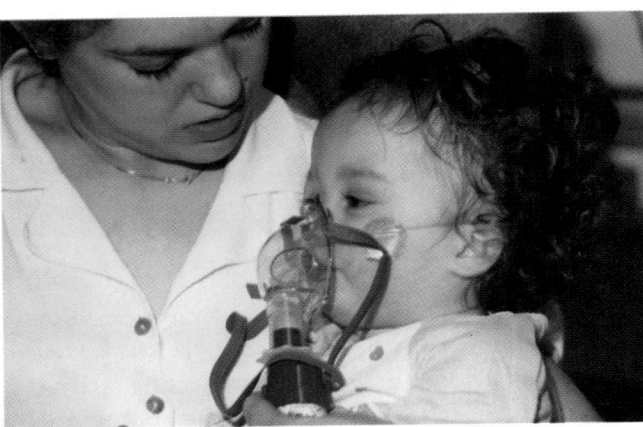

**Figure 30-69**   **Nebulizer medications—using a mask to deliver the inhalants to this child**

## COMMUNITY/HOME CARE

### Home Care Applications for Respiratory Inhalants

- Keep dry-powder inhalers dry; humidity clumps the powder.

- Keep extra capsules or canisters on hand to prevent running out of medication.

- Wait 1 to 5 minutes between inhalations.

- If there are multiple inhalant medications, doing them in the correct order will make each dose more effective. The short-acting bronchodilator medication should be used first.

- Calculate number of doses in an MDI canister, and mark on calendar when it needs to be changed.

- When inserting a new MDI canister, prime with two or three puffs or client will not receive the full dose when first using it.

- If client is inhaling corticosteroid medications, have the client rinse the mouth afterward to decrease the chance of developing thrush.

Togger, D. A., & Brenner, P. S. (2001). Metered dose inhalers. *American Journal of Nursing, 101*(10), 26–32.

ter is pressed, a propellant causes a "puff" of medication to come out. The dose is a measured amount for each puff (hence the name "metered"); the number of puffs to be taken is prescribed. The client must be able to perform several important steps in rapid sequence or the medication will not be delivered effectively. These steps include exhaling, then placing lips around the mouthpiece, and inhaling deeply while pressing down on the canister (Figure 30-73 A, B). The ability to compress the canister for dose delivery can be affected by hand strength (which diminishes with age), flexibility (difficult with arthritis), and disease related to weakness (such as neurologic disease).

The use of a "spacer" or "aerochamber" can help overcome the difficulty in using the MDI for many clients (Figure 30-73 C). The spacer is attached to the mouthpiece of the MDI. The patient then can exhale, place lips on the spacer mouthpiece, compress the canister once (the medication is held by the spacer), and then inhale deeply.

The nurse should ensure that the client knows how to use the inhaler correctly so that the prescribed medication dose is delivered. See Procedure 30-11 for teaching a client how to use an MDI. It has been documented in research

## COMMUNITY/HOME CARE

### Considerations for Use of Nasal Inhalers

- Provide the client with the manufacturer's directions for the specific type of inhaler, such as how to replace a medication cartridge for a nasal aerosol.

- Inhalers should be stored at room temperature.

- Aerosols are prepared under pressure and should not be punctured or placed in an incinerator.

- Instruct the client not to allow other people to use the inhaler.

- Caution the client about overuse that could cause a rebound effect, making the condition worse.

- Ensure that the client is knowledgeable about the expected and adverse effects of the drug. Some of these drugs do not produce therapeutic effects for several days, and some require 2 weeks of continuous use before the drug effects appear.

- Provide the client with a telephone number to call if assistance is needed.

---

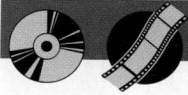 **PROCEDURE 30-10**  ## Administering Nasal Medications

### EQUIPMENT NEEDED

- Medication in spray, drops, or aerosolized form (Figure 30-70)
- Gloves
- Tissue as needed
- Dropper as needed

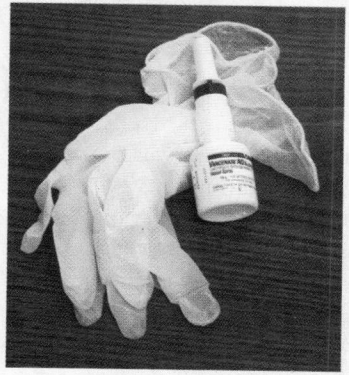

**Figure 30-70   Nasal medication spray; wear gloves when administering nasal medications to a client.**

### IMPLEMENTATION—ACTION/RATIONALE

| ACTION | RATIONALE |
|---|---|
| 1. Wash hands. Wear a mask if the client is coughing or sneezing. | 1. Reduces transmission of microorganisms. Respiratory-related microorganisms are easily transferred by the hands and air droplets. |
| 2. Explain the purpose of the medication and the desired position (Figure 30-71). | 2. The client will be more compliant with medication if she understands the purpose and proper use of medication. Proper positioning is necessary with nose drops so the drops will reach the area of treatment by gravity with the client assuming a dependent position. |

*(continues)*

## PROCEDURE 30-10 (continued)

3. Explain to the client the sensation of the local effects of the medication, such as burning, tingling, and effect on taste buds. If drops are used, explain to the client that a sensation of medication may be felt in the posterior oral pharynx.

4. If a nasal inhaler is prescribed, explain the manufacturer's directions and how inhalers work. Follow the five rights of drug administration (check identification and orders at five different stages of administration).

5. Have the client assume a comfortable position. If inhalers are to be used, this will generally be an upright position. If drops are to be instilled, the client should assume the appropriate position to medicate specific sinuses that need treatment. Before the instillation of drops or the use of an inhaler, ask the client to blow his nose and clear the nostrils of discharge as much as possible. Squeeze nose drops into dropper.

6. Have the client exhale and close one nostril.

7. Ask the client to inhale while the spray is pumped or sprayed into the first nostril (Figure 30-72). If nose drops are used, insert nasal dropper only about $3/8$ inch into the nostril, keeping the tip of the dropper away from the sides of the nostril. Insert the prescribed dosage of medication into the nostril. Discard any unused medication in dropper.

3. Some nasal medications cause undesirable tastes. If this occurs, the physician or qualified practitioner may order other medications or encourage mouthwashes after treatment. Warning of post-nasal sensations of the medication will prepare the client. Some clients may feel a quick sensation of choking. This can be frightening if the client has not been alerted to this consequence.

4. Clients will be more compliant if they understand the use of the inhalers and that a fine cold mist will be released into the nasal passage via a pressurized container. Nasal medications that are prescribed must be considered to have the same safety precautions of administration as any medication.

5. Nose drops are effective only if they reach the areas to be medicated. The client should be as comfortable as possible; otherwise he may not stay in the desired position an adequate time. If the client is in a position with the neck hyperextended, a pillow or support by the nurse's hand under the neck may be necessary. Medications can only be effective if they are in contact with the mucous membranes. If large amounts of discharge are present, medications cannot be effective.

6. Since the client will be asked to inhale with the use of nasal medication, exhalation will first be necessary.

7. Nasal medications are more effective if instilled during inhalation, since they will be carried and distributed farther into the nasal passages. Droppers should be kept away from the nostril to avoid inserting bacteria into the medication bottle. Discard excess medication for the same reason.

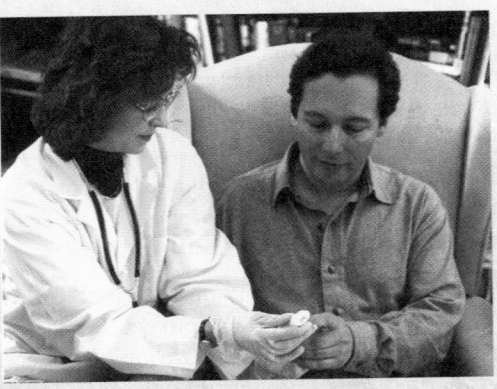

**Figure 30-71**    Explain the purpose of the medication to the client.

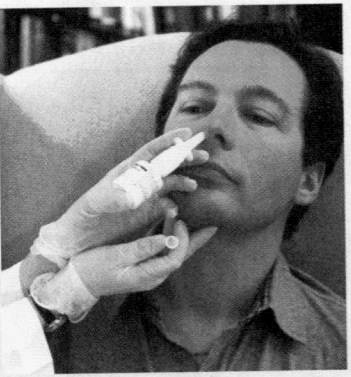

**Figure 30-72**    Ask the client to inhale while the spray is administered into the nostril.

*(continues)*

## PROCEDURE 30-10 (*continued*)

8. Ask the client to blot excess drainage from the nostril; however, do not have the client blow his nose.

8. Blowing the nose will remove medication and therefore should not be done. However, excess medication should be removed from dripping out of the nostrils onto the facial areas in order to avoid discomfort.

9. Repeat the procedure on the other nostril.

9. Most often both nostrils contain congestion and therefore need to be treated.

10. Help the client resume a comfortable position. If nose drops are used, the client should stay in the appropriate position as indicated by manufacturer's suggestions, generally 5 minutes. Ask the client to breathe through the nose after the decongestion administration. It may be necessary to occlude one nostril at a time and breathe deeply.

10. Nose drops need positions that by gravity will allow medications to reach areas of desired treatment.

11. Remove all soiled supplies and dispose according to universal precautions. Wash hands carefully.

11. Proper disposal decreases the chance of transmission of microorganisms. Respiratory diseases are especially easily transmitted.

12. Evaluate the effect of the medication in 15 to 20 minutes.

12. It is necessary to note if the medication is effective without adverse side effects; otherwise, other medications may be considered. If the client experiences bothersome or unpleasant symptoms, such as a bad taste, other medications may be considered. Clients generally will not comply with medications that have too many unpleasant side effects.

13. Wash hands.

13. Reduces transmission of microorganisms.

# LIFE SPAN CONSIDERATIONS

## Nasal Medications

### Pediatric Variations

- Small children may not be cooperative and may need to be restrained. Sometimes the use of a reward system may be beneficial.

- Position infants using a football hold and slightly hyperextend the neck.

### Geriatric Variations

- Older clients may not be able to tolerate positions with the head dependent for long periods of time; therefore, pump sprays may be more useful.

- Aerosolized containers may be too difficult for older clients to apply the appropriate pressure needed to be effective.

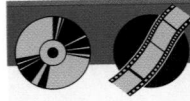

**PROCEDURE 30-11**

## Teaching Self-Administration with a Metered-Dose Inhaler

### EQUIPMENT NEEDED

- Medication administration record (MAR)
- Inhaler
- Nonsterile gloves
- Wash basin or sink to rinse mouth
- Tissue (optional)

### IMPLEMENTATION—ACTION/RATIONALE

| ACTION | RATIONALE |
|---|---|
| 1. Check with the client and the chart for known allergies or medical conditions that would contraindicate the use of the drug. | 1. Prevents occurrence of adverse reactions. |
| 2. Check the MAR against written health care practitioner orders. | 2. Ensures accuracy in identification of medication. |
| 3. Gather necessary equipment. | 3. Promotes efficiency. |
| 4. Wash your hands. | 4. Reduces the transmission of microorganisms. |
| 5. Follow the five rights of medication administration. Check the client's identification band. | 5. Ensures correct client. |
| 6. Review with the client the purpose of each prescribed medication. | 6. Some clients have several inhalants ordered and need to be taught the correct sequence. For example, fast-acting bronchodilators (albuteral sulfate) are taken before slower-acting bronchodilators (iprotropium bromide). |
| 7. Allow the client to hold and manipulate the canister. Explain how the canister fits into the inhaler. Have the client demonstrate insertion of the canister. | 7. Nurse can assess client's ability to manipulate inhaler, and client can become more comfortable with task. |
| 8. Explain metered-dose concept to client, and discuss frequency of prescribed medications. | 8. Client needs to understand dangers of overuse related to adverse reactions. |
| 9. Explain that the inhaler must be shaken before each use. | 9. Medication must be mixed with aerosol propellant to ensure correct dosage of medication. |
| 10. Remove the mouthpiece and cap from the bottle and insert the stem into the small hole on the flattened portion of the mouthpiece. | 10. Facilitates medication administration. |
| • Client should grasp the inhaler with thumb and first two fingers. | • Proper hand position facilitates use of the inhaler. |
| 11. Instruct the client to exhale, place the mouthpiece into the mouth, and ensure that the lips form a tight seal around the mouthpiece (Figure 30-73A). | 11. Tight seal prevents escape of medication. |
| 12. Instruct the client to firmly push the cylinder down against the mouthpiece only once (Figure 30-73B), while slowly inhaling until the lungs feel full. | 12. Releases the medication; as client inhales, medication is distributed into the airway. |

*(continues)*

**PROCEDURE 30-11 (continued)**

13. Ask the client to remove the mouthpiece while holding breath for about 10 seconds and then to exhale slowly through pursed lips.

    - If the client had difficulty coordinating the inhalation and medication dispensing, an aerochamber may be added (Figure 30-73C).

13. Allows the medication to reach the alveoli.

    - An aerochamber provides dead space for the medicated mist while the client inhales slowly and deeply.

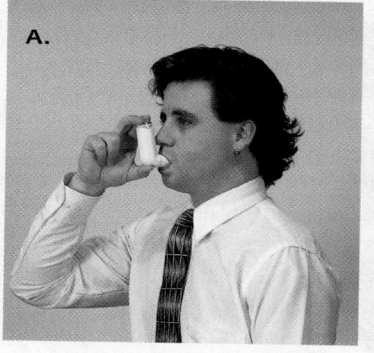
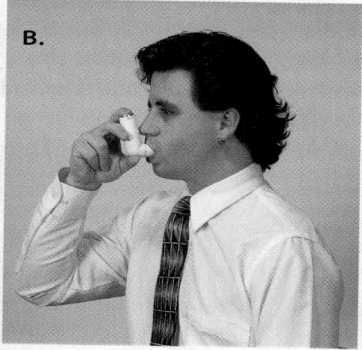
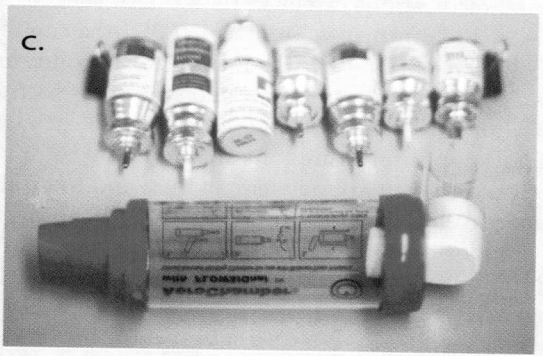

**Figure 30-73   Self-administration with a metered-dose inhaler: A. Insert mouthpiece into mouth, forming a tight seal with the lips. B. Push the cylinder down and inhale. C. Aerochamber and nebulizer medications**

14. Repeat doses as ordered, waiting 1 minute between puffs.

14. Allows for maximal absorption and effect of first dose before another is taken.

15. Inform client that a mouthwash can be used to remove the taste of the medication.

15. Promotes client comfort.

16. Show client how to wash the mouthpiece under tepid running water to remove secretions.

16. Accumulation of medication around mouthpiece can interfere with delivery of next metered dose.

17. If two or more metered-dose medications are ordered, wait 5 to 10 minutes between inhalations or as specifically ordered by the health care practitioner.

17. Drugs must be inhaled sequentially to maximize therapeutic effect.

18. Record on the MAR the drug's name, dose, date, and time of medication.

18. Provides documentation that medication was given.

19. Observe for effectiveness of the medication and relief of client symptoms.

19. Evaluates effectiveness of medication.

studies that only 21% of clients who use inhalers do all the steps correctly (Togger, 2001). In addition, clients' ability seems to decline over time, perhaps becoming negligent in following all the steps. In addition, Benner's research shows that while nurses are the main health professionals (58%) teaching the use of the MDI, nurses need additional training in the steps, which were updated by the National Institutes of Health (NIH) in 1997 (Togger, 2001). The most frequent mistakes were proper inhalation and breath-holding techniques.

It is very important to teach the client how to correctly calculate the number of doses used and when to change to a new canister. Even though propellant is still remaining in the canister, there may be less or no medication in the dose delivered. Some clients have been taught to float the canister in water to see if it is empty. The correct method taught by the National Heart, Lung and Blood Institute (NHLBI), however, is based on the number of doses prescribed per day multiplied by the number of doses in the canister when full, which is stated on the label (Togger,

2001). For example, if the client is ordered to have two puffs 3 times a day, that would equal six doses (puffs) a day. If the canister states there are 200 doses in a full canister, dividing 200 by 6 will be 33 days of use.

Careful discharge instructions and observation of the client performing the task are important for continued therapeutic effect at home. The website for the NHLBI has some excellent teaching materials for health professionals and clients on the handheld devices.

## Rectal Medications

Rectal medications can be in the form of enemas, suppositories, and ointments. See Chapter 37 for a complete discussion of enema administration. Rectal ointments are used to treat local conditions and symptoms such as pain, inflammation, and itching caused from hemorrhoids. Rectal suppositories are cone-shaped masses of substances designed to melt at body temperature and to produce the intended effect at a slow and steady rate of absorption.

Suppositories provide a safe and convenient route for administering drugs that interact poorly with digestive enzymes or have a bad taste or odor. They are also used to provide temporary relief for clients who cannot tolerate oral preparations: for example, to relieve nausea and vomiting. Suppositories are also used to induce relaxation, relieve pain and local irritation, reduce fever, and stimulate peristalsis and defecation in clients who are constipated.

Rectal suppositories are contraindicated in cardiac clients because insertion may stimulate the vagus nerve, causing cardiac dysrhythmias (abnormal heart patterns). These drugs are also avoided in clients recovering from rectal or prostate surgery because they may cause pain on insertion and trauma to the tissues.

The nurse should assess the rectum for irritation or bleeding and check sphincter control. Some clients may experience problems in retaining the suppository. The nurse should instruct such a client to remain in the Sims' position for at least 15 minutes or should place the client on the abdomen, if the condition allows, and hold the buttocks closed. The health care practitioner should be notified when the client is unable to retain a suppository so that another route can be ordered.

Suppositories are often stored in the refrigerator to preserve the integrity of the drug form. A softened suppository is difficult to insert; to harden a suppository, place it under cold running water while it is still in its original wrapper. The nurse should follow the five rights of medication administration and Standard Precautions when administering rectal instillations. See Procedure 30-12 for the procedure on inserting a rectal suppository.

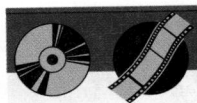

**PROCEDURE 30-12** **Administering Rectal Medications**

## EQUIPMENT NEEDED

- Medication (suppository or medicated enema)
- Water-soluble lubricant (Figure 30-74)
- Gloves
- Tissue or washcloth
- Bedpan if client is physically immobile
- Medication administration record

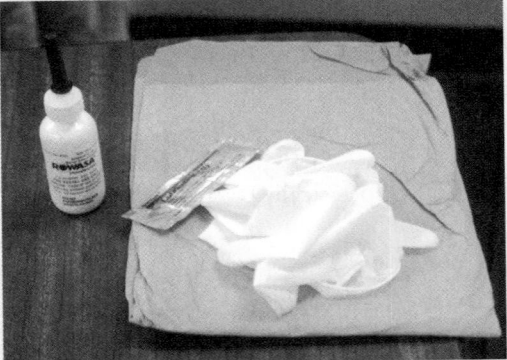

**Figure 30-74** **Protective pad, gloves, lubricant, and rectal medication**

## IMPLEMENTATION—ACTION/RATIONALE

| ACTION | RATIONALE |
|--------|-----------|
| 1. Assess the client's need for the medication. | 1. Allows nurse to determine effectiveness of the medication. |
| 2. Check physician's or qualified practitioner's written order. | 2. Ensures safe and accurate administration of medication. |

*(continues)*

## PROCEDURE 30-12 (*continued*)

3. Check the medication administration record against the medication order, verifying correct client, medication, dose, route, and time.

4. Check for any drug allergies.

5. Review the client's history for any previous surgeries or bleeding.

6. Gather the equipment needed for the procedure before entering the client's room.

7. Assess the client's readiness to receive the medication. Encourage visitors to leave until the procedure is completed and close door or curtain.

8. Wash hands.

9. Apply disposable gloves (Figure 30-75).

10. Ask the client his name and check identification band.

11. Assist client into correct position; side-lying Sims' position, preferably the left side with upper leg drawn up toward chest.

12. Visually assess the client's external anus.

13. Remove suppository from wrapper and lubricate rounded end along with insertion finger. If a medicated enema is used, lubricate the enema tip if it is not prelubricated (Figure 30-76).

3. Ensures accuracy and decreases chance of medication error.

4. Decreases risk of allergic reaction.

5. Contraindications for rectal administration may be discovered.

6. Prevents numerous trips to gather supplies and helps the procedure flow smoothly.

7. Promotes privacy and maintains self-image.

8. Reduces transmission of microorganisms.

9. Prevents contact with fecal material.

10. Ensures correct client.

11. The descending colon is on the left side; this is a more anatomically correct position. This position exposes the anus to identify placement.

12. Determines presence of any active bleeding.

13. Lubrication decreases friction and decreases discomfort.

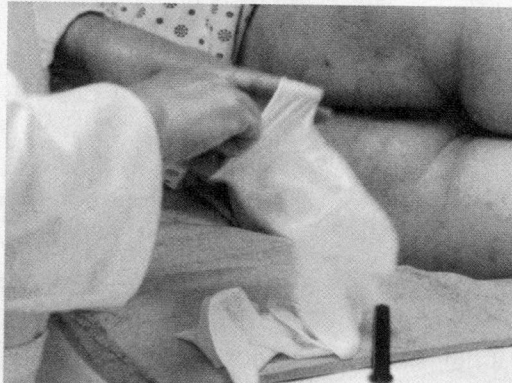

**Figure 30-75    Apply gloves prior to administering rectal medications.**

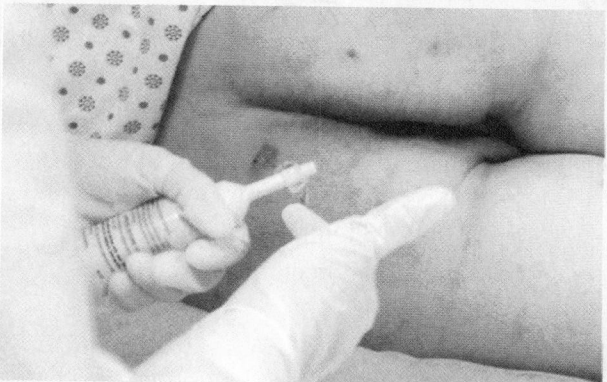

**Figure 30-76    Lubricate the enema tip if it is not prelubricated.**

14. Tell client he will experience a cool sensation and pressure during administration. Encourage slow deep breaths.

15. Retract buttocks with nondominant hand, visualizing the anus (Figure 30-77). Using the dominant index finger, slowly and gently insert the suppository through the anus, past the

14. Prepares the client for administration. Relaxes the rectal sphincter.

15. Slow insertion minimizes pain. Correct placement ensures adequate absorption and less chance for expulsion of medication.

*(continues)*

## PROCEDURE 30-12 (*continued*)

internal sphincter, and against the rectal wall. Depth of insertion will differ if client is a child or infant. If instilling a medicated enema, gently insert the enema tip past the internal sphincter and instill the contents by slowly squeezing (Figure 30-78).

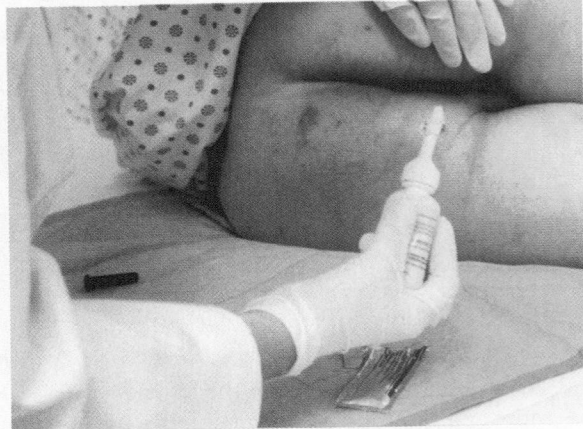

**Figure 30-77**   **Retract the buttock and visualize the anus.**

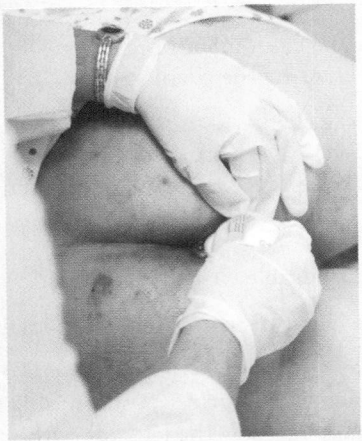

**Figure 30-78**   **Gently insert the enema tip and instill the contents by slowly squeezing the bottle.**

16. Remove finger or enema tip and wipe client's anal area with a washcloth or tissue.

17. Discard gloves.

18. Wash hands.

19. Discuss with client a 10-minute time frame to remain in bed or on side.

20. Place call light in client's reach if administering suppository containing laxative to assist once client has sensation to defecate.

21. Record administration of medication.

22. Document effectiveness or any side effects of treatment on nursing flow sheet or progress note if applicable.

16. Removes lubricant externally. Promotes cleanliness and comfort.

17. Reduces transfer of microorganisms.

18. Reduces transfer of microorganisms.

19. Keeps suppository or medicated fluid in place for better absorption.

20. Gives client control over situation and nurse response once sensation to defecate occurs.

21. Provides documentation of administration of medication.

22. Communicates with other caregivers the effectiveness of treatment.

## Vaginal Medications

Medications inserted into the vagina are in the form of suppositories, creams, gels, ointments, foams, or douches. These medications may be used to treat inflammation, infections, and discomfort, or as a contraceptive measure.

Vaginal creams, gels, or ointments usually come with a disposable tubular applicator with a plunger to insert the drug. Standard Precautions are always used by the nurse when inserting suppositories. Body temperature causes the suppository to melt and be absorbed. Suppositories are usually inserted with the index finger of a gloved hand; however, small suppositories may come with an applicator and the suppository is placed in the applicator's tip. Many clients prefer to insert their own vaginal suppository. In this case, provide privacy for the client. See Procedure 30-13 for administering a vaginal suppository. After insertion of these preparations, the client may notice drainage and should be informed that this is expected. If a suppository is

# LIFE SPAN CONSIDERATIONS

## Rectal Medications

### Pediatric Variations

- Consider the age of the client when explaining the procedure. Provide simple and brief explanations and answer questions honestly, facilitating open communication.

- Never leave the medication unsupervised near the client.

- After the medication has been inserted into the rectum, press the buttocks together for several minutes to prevent expulsion.

- Provide extra assurance of privacy for adolescent clients during the procedure.

### Geriatric Variations

- Absorption may vary in older adults.

- Elderly are more prone to constipation due to such factors as insufficient fluid intake, insufficient dietary fiber and bulk, decreased activity or sedentary lifestyle, or side effects of medications.

- Older clients may be physically unable to self-administer the medications and require assistance.

- Fecal impaction may occur more often, interfering with suppository placement.

- If suppository is a laxative, provide bedpan or bedside commode if client is immobile or at risk to not make it to the bathroom on time.

# COMMUNITY/HOME CARE

## Rectal Medications

### Home Care Variations

- Teach client or family members the procedure of administration. If the rectal suppository is ordered on an as-needed basis, teach the caregivers how to determine whether the medication is needed.

- Make sure rectal suppositories are stored correctly in the home setting, refrigerated if needed, and discarded when they have expired.

### Long-Term Care Variations

- Review medications given over extended periods of time to determine any long-term side effects that might occur.

- Review with primary caregivers how to assess and document these side effects.

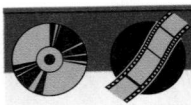

**PROCEDURE 30-13** | **Administering Vaginal Medications**

## EQUIPMENT NEEDED

- Vaginal medication: cream, foam, jelly, or suppository (Figure 30-79)
- Applicator (if needed)
- Water-soluble lubricating jelly (for suppository)
- Nonsterile gloves
- Perineal pad
- Paper towel, toilet tissue, or tissue paper
- Washcloth and warm water (optional)

## IMPLEMENTATION—ACTION/RATIONALE

| ACTION | RATIONALE |
|---|---|
| 1. Verify orders. | 1. Prevents medication errors. |
| 2. Ascertain if the client has ever had vaginal medications before and understands the procedure. | 2. Enables understanding and compliance. |
| 3. Ask the client to void. | 3. Provides for client comfort during the procedure. |

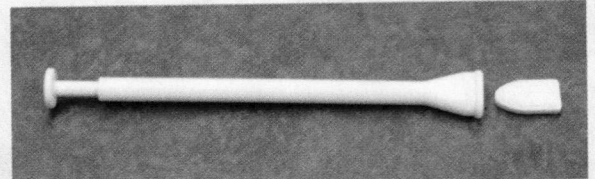

**Figure 30-79   Vaginal medication and applicator.**

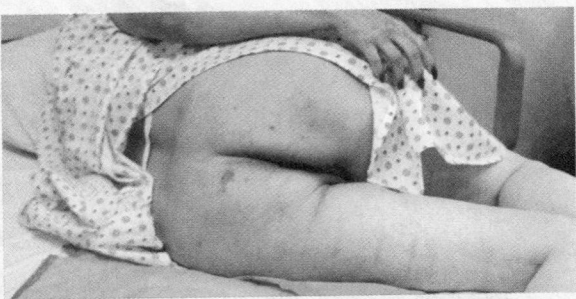

**Figure 30-80   This client is placed in a Sims' position for administering vaginal medications.**

| | |
|---|---|
| 4. Wash hands. | 4. Reduces transmission of microorganisms. |
| 5. Arrange equipment at client's bedside. | 5. Promotes organization. |
| 6. Provide complete privacy by closing door and curtains. | 6. This procedure can be embarrassing, and this protects the client's privacy. |
| 7. Assist the client into a dorsal-recumbent or Sims' position (Figure 30-80). | 7. Allows positioning for administration and for medication to remain in vagina. |
| 8. Drape the client as appropriate, such as over the client's abdomen and lower extremities. | 8. Provides privacy. |
| 9. Position lighting to illuminate vaginal orifice. | 9. Assists in visualization of vagina and proper administration of medication. |
| 10. Assess the perineal area for redness, inflammation, discharge, or foul odor. | 10. Provides baseline data. |
| 11. If using an applicator, fill with medication. If using a suppository, remove the suppository from the foil and position in the applicator (applicator is optional) (Figure 30-81). An applicator may be used for suppositories or a gloved finger may be used. The foil is discarded. Apply water-soluble lubricant to suppository or applicator (optional for applicator). | 11. The medication is prepared for insertion. Lubricant provides comfort and ease of insertion. |

*(continues)*

## PROCEDURE 30-13 (*continued*)

12. For suppository, with nondominant hand, retract the labia (Figure 30-82).

12. Allows visualization of the vaginal orifice and eases insertion of medication.

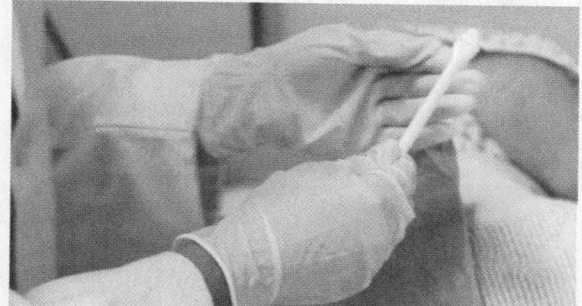

**Figure 30-81    Place the suppository in the applicator.**

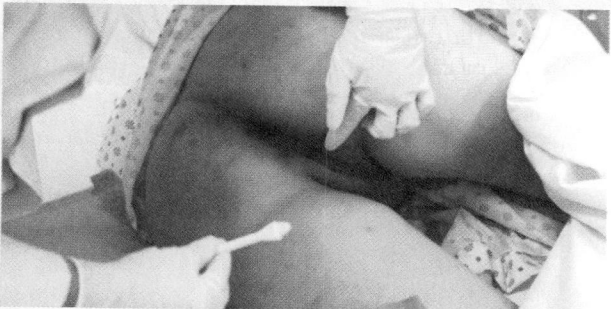

**Figure 30-82    Retract the labia with the nondominant hand.**

13. With dominant hand, insert the applicator 2 to 3 inches into the vagina, sliding the applicator posteriorly (Figure 30-83). Push the plunger to administer the medication (Figure 30-84). With a suppository, insert the tapered end first with the index finger or applicator along the posterior wall of the vagina (approximately 3 inches).

13. Medication must be inserted completely to provide coverage of the entire vagina. When medication is deposited at the posterior end of the vagina, gravity will allow medication to move toward the orifice.

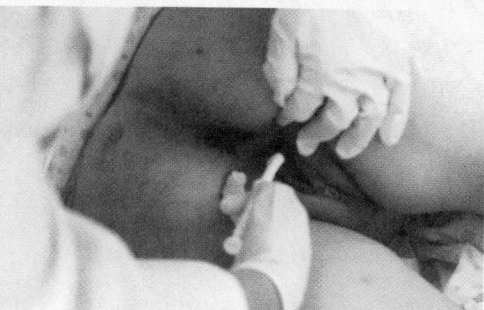

**Figure 30-83    Slide the applicator 2 to 3 inches into the vagina.**

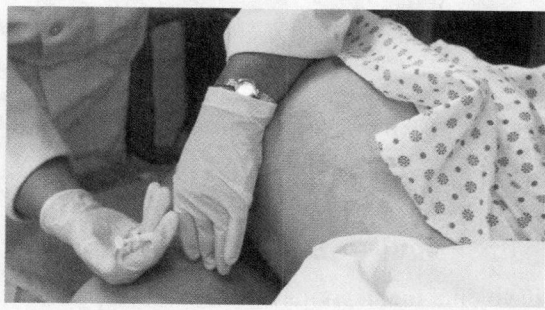

**Figure 30-84    Push the plunger to administer the medication.**

14. Withdraw the applicator and place on a towel.

14. Reduces the transmission of microorganisms.

15. If administering a douche or irrigation:
    - Warm solution to slightly above body temperature (105°–110°F). Check using the back of the hand or the wrist.
    - Position the client in a semirecumbent position on a bedpan, on a toilet seat, or in a tub.
    - Apply lubricant to the irrigation nozzle and insert approximately 3 inches into the vagina.
    - Hang the irrigant container approximately 2 feet above the client's vaginal area.

    - Open the clamp and allow a small amount of solution to flow into the vagina.

15.
    - Avoids burning the client. The mucous membranes of the vagina are sensitive.

    - Provides comfort during procedure and allows for appropriate drainage of irrigation solution.
    - Provides comfort.

    - Height is necessary for drainage by gravity. If the container is too high, the flow will be too forceful and uncomfortable.
    - Allows the client to evaluate the temperature.

*(continues)*

## PROCEDURE 30-13 (continued)

- Move the nozzle and rotate around the entire vaginal area. If the labia are inflamed, allow the solution to flow over the labia as well. If the client is on the toilet seat, alternate between closing off the labia and allowing solution to be expelled.

- Rotation allows for irrigation throughout vagina. Closing off labia allows medication to stay in and flush total vagina.

16. Wipe and clean the client's perineal area, including the labia, from the front to the back with toilet tissue. Some clients may prefer that the perineal area is also cleaned with a washcloth and warm water.

16. Provides comfort for client and avoids spread of infective agents to perineal area.

17. Apply a perineal pad.

17. Protects client from discomfort of drainage and spread of infection or irritation to perineal area.

18. Wash the applicator (if reusable) with soap and warm water and store in appropriate container in client's room.

18. Applicator can only be used for individual clients; however, some applicators and inducers are reusable and must be appropriately cleaned and stored to prevent reinsertion of infective agents.

19. Remove gloves and wash hands.

19. Reduces the transmission of microorganisms.

20. Instruct the client to remain flat for at least 30 minutes.

20. Allows maximum contact between the medication and the vaginal mucous membranes.

21. Raise side rails and place the call light in reach.

21. Provides for client comfort and safety.

---

##  LIFE SPAN CONSIDERATIONS

### Vaginal Medications

#### Pediatric Variations

- Vaginal medications can be very embarrassing for children. The staff need to be extremely sensitive to the child's privacy.

- Inappropriate touching can be an issue with children. Have a trusted female family member or a second staff member present when giving vaginal medications to children.

#### Geriatric Variations

- The labia may be more difficult to hold apart in older clients.

- Older clients may be more sensitive to temperature variations of irrigation fluids.

- Assess the client's previous use of vaginal irrigations since some older clients may use douches frequently.

## COMMUNITY/HOME CARE

### Vaginal Medications

#### Home Care Variations

- Assess the home environment to see if there is a place where equipment can be properly cleaned and stored.

- Instruct the client or the client's caregiver on how to administer the medication, if necessary.

#### Long-Term Care Variations

- The client's ability to assume a Sims' or recumbent position may be limited. Alternative positioning or medication administration may be necessary.

- Most vaginal medications were not designed to be used over long periods. Regular reevaluation of the need for a vaginal medication should be performed.

## CLINICAL ALERT

### Tampon Use

Clients should be instructed not to use tampons after the insertion of vaginal medications, because the tampon can absorb the medication and decrease the drug's effect.

given to treat infection, tell the client that the drainage may be foul smelling. The nurse should advise the client to wear a perineal pad to prevent soiling of the underpants.

Sterile technique is usually required if there is an open wound when administering a vaginal douche (irrigation). Douches are ordered to apply antimicrobial solutions, to remove offensive or irritating discharge, to reduce inflammation, and to prevent hemorrhage with warm or cold irrigations. The nurse should ensure that the client does not have an allergy to iodine, because many vaginal preparations contain povidone-iodine.

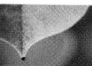

# CASE STUDY/NURSING CARE PLAN

Mrs. Landry, a 45-year-old, was admitted to your floor with a diagnosis of deep vein thrombosis. The client noticed swelling of her left leg about a week ago but decided to treat it at home. Four days later, the lower leg was very edematous, warm, and painful to move. After an office visit, the client was admitted to the hospital. This is Mrs. Landry's first hospitalization. On examination you find that the left leg is warmer than the right. The left thigh circumference is 3 inches larger than the right. The physician ordered a heparin IV drip after a loading dose bolus was given. The drip contained 10,000 units heparin in 500 ml of D5W at 10 ml/h (200 units/h). 10 mg Coumadin (oral) was also ordered for the evening of admission, with orders for daily prothrombin (PT) blood draws and subsequent evening doses to be given until the PT is at a therapeutic blood level with an international normalized ratio (INR) of 2–2.5. It is anticipated the drug level will be at this level by the third or fourth day, the IV heparin will be discontinued, and the patient discharged home on daily Coumadin doses for 3 months with weekly monitoring of the PT and INR.

### Assessment

The client is a 45-year-old with a diagnosis of deep vein thrombosis. She has a very edematous left leg, which is inflamed and 3 inches larger than the right leg. The client has been admitted to an acute care facility for anticoagulant therapy.

### Nursing Diagnosis #1

*Ineffective Tissue Perfusion* related to the development of venous thrombi in the deep femoral vein.
**NOC:** Circulation Status; Tissue Perfusion: Peripheral
**NIC:** Circulatory Care: Arterial Insufficiency

### Expected Outcomes

The client will:

1. Report an absence of pain within 48 hours.
2. Demonstrate an absence of edema within 48 hours.
3. Experience the same degree of skin temperature in both legs.

### Planning/Interventions/Rationales

1. Maintain on bed rest. *Reduces the possibility of embolus; may decrease the pain and swelling.*
2. Elevate the legs above the heart. *Elevation facilitates venous return and decreases the edema.*
3. Measure the circumference of the left thigh and compare with that of the right thigh. *Measuring the circumference provides a quantitative reference point that can be used to evaluate the swelling.*
4. Apply moist heat to the affected extremity. *Heat provides an analgesic effect; it decreases venospasms and pain.*
5. Administer the heparin drip at 200 units/h. *Heparin prevents the conversion of fibrinogen to fibrin and prothrombin to thrombin, thereby limiting the extension of the thrombus.*
6. Monitor the partial thromboplastin time (PTT). *The partial thromboplastin time is used to monitor heparin therapy, because heparin, a short-acting anticoagulant, increases the PTT.*

*(continues)*

# CASE STUDY/NURSING CARE PLAN (continued)

7. Administer the evening dose of Coumadin. *Coumadin is an oral medication that interferes with the synthesis of vitamin-K-dependent clotting factors (II, VII, IX, X).*

8. Monitor prothrombin (PT) and INR. *Prothrombin is increased by Coumadin and must be in the therapeutic range of × 1.3–1.5 the normal for the medication to be effective. INR is a standardized system for reporting the PT throughout the United States and Europe.*

## Evaluation

The client still has pain after 48 hours at a 3 on a scale of 1 to 10. However, there is a complete decrease in swelling and no warmth of the left leg within 48 hours of the anticoagulant therapy.

## Nursing Diagnosis #2

*Ineffective Protection* related to abnormal blood profiles (i.e., anticoagulant).

**NOC:** Immune Status; Coagulation Status

**NIC:** Bleeding Precautions; Infection Control

## Expected Outcomes

The client will:

1. Not demonstrate evidence of bleeding from gums or nose, in urine or stool, or under the skin.
2. Maintain the prothrombin time (PT) or international normalized ratio (INR) within therapeutic range.

## Planning/Interventions/Rationales

1. Advise the client to withhold the medication in the event that bleeding occurs and to notify the physician immediately. *The dose may need to be adjusted.*
2. Encourage the client to discontinue smoking. *Smoking has a tendency to increase the metabolism of the medication, necessitating an increase in the dose.*
3. Advise the client to watch food intake. *Foods high in fat and foods rich in vitamin K can interfere with the PT.*
4. Warn against taking oral contraceptive medication. *There may be a decrease in anticoagulant effect due to the increased production of clotting factors with oral contraceptives.*
5. Warn against taking aspirin and other over-the-counter medications. *Aspirin may increase the risk of bleeding; it inhibits platelet formation.*

## Evaluation

The client has no bleeding from the gums, nose, stool, or skin. In addition, the PT and INR are within the therapeutic range.

## Key Concepts

- The *United States Pharmacopeia and National Formulary* outline drug standards for usage in the United States.
- The Food and Drug Administration tests all drugs for toxicity before granting a company the right to market a drug.
- The pharmacokinetics of drugs includes absorption, distribution, metabolism, and excretion.
- Safe drug administration is facilitated by following the five rights: right drug, right dose, right client, right route, and right time.
- The oral administration route is the safest and least expensive administration route.
- Parenteral drugs are injected through intradermal (ID), subcutaneous (SC or SQ), intramuscular (IM), or intravenous (IV) routes.

- Oral solutions should be poured and measured at eye level to ensure accuracy.
- Although the prescriber will determine the dose and route of a parenteral drug, the nurse is responsible for choosing the correct gauge and length of the needle to be used.
- Federal legislation, the state's Nurse Practice Act, and the health care institution's policies define the role of the nurse in administering medications.
- Medications are identified by their chemical, generic, and trade names.
- Medications are commonly classified by the body system with which they interact.
- Medications are available in many forms (e.g., oral, buccal, topical).
- Pharmacodynamics refers to the changes in cellular biology that medications cause at the site of action.

- Several different systems of measurement are used in the administration of medications (e.g., metric, household).
- Medications are stored and distributed in established systems that enhance safe administration (e.g., computer-controlled dispensing).
- The nurse is responsible for correctly interpreting the order or clarifying any questions about it with the prescriber.
- The nursing process guides the nurse in the client assessment, plan of client education outcomes, and evaluation of the effects of the medication regimen.
- Before administering medications, the nurse must be aware of the client's health history, medication history such as allergies, and the current labs and physical assessment data.
- Client education about the medication's purpose, therapeutic action, potential side effects, and contraindications is a very important part of the nursing process.
- Medication errors need to be reported to avoid compromising client safety and studied to identify what can be changed to prevent future errors.

## Review Questions and Activities

1. Mrs. Adams is a 76-year-old client being discharged from the hospital with cancer of the lungs. Mrs. Adams elected not to have surgery and was given her first chemotherapy before discharge. She is not accustomed to taking medications. Before the onset of symptoms that necessitated her admission to the hospital, Mrs. Adams considered herself in good health, only bothered with the discomfort of arthritis in her hands. She is being discharged on the following medications:
   - Sulfamethoxazole (sulfonamide anti-infective) 500 mg/5 ml susp PO b.i.d.
   - Granisetron (antiemetic) 1 mg PO q12h
   - Morphine 30 mg PO q4h, prn for pain

   Describe the nursing interventions that should be included in Mrs. Adams's discharge teaching relative to medication self-administration and other appropriate nursing actions.

2. A client receiving doxycycline, a tetracycline, 100 mg PO daily should avoid which of the following food groups?

| Group A | Group B | Group C |
| --- | --- | --- |
| Beef liver | Buttermilk | Aged meat |
| Brussels sprouts | All cheese | Avocados |
| Cabbage | Pizza | Caffeine |
| Oils | Yogurt | Chicken liver |
| Kale | Ice cream | Cola drinks |
| Arugula | Milk | Raisins |
| Spinach | | Soy sauce |

3. You are preparing to give an IV dose of vancomycin to a client who has an IV of $D_5$ 1/2 NS infusing and a Dilaudid PCA.
   a. Name at least 2 things you would assess about the client's IV site.
   b. Discuss what drug incompatibilities you would check.
   c. Where would you find the correct rate for infusion of this medication?
   d. What would you assess about the client's medication history?

4. Demonstrate (or discuss) the steps you would go through to calculate, draw up, and give a subcutaneous heparin injection of 6,000 units. The heparin is in a vial labeled "8,000 Units in 1 cc."

## Multimedia Links

Altman *Intermediate Care Video: Medication Administration I*
Altman *Intermediate Care Video: Medication Administration II: Routes of Administration*
Altman *Intermediate Care Video: Medication Administration III: Parenteral Medication*
Altman *Intermediate Care Video: Medication Administration III: Parenteral Medication*
Altman *Intermediate Care Video: Medication Administration IV: Intravenous Medication*
Altman *Intermediate Care DVD: Administering Oral, Sublingual, and Buccal Medications*
Altman *Intermediate Care DVD: Withdrawing Medication from an Ampoule*
Altman *Intermediate Care DVD: Withdrawing Medication from a Vial*
Altman *Intermediate Care DVD: Mixing Medications from Two Vials into One Syringe*
Altman *Intermediate Care DVD: Administering an Intradermal Injection*
Altman *Intermediate Care DVD: Administering a Subcutaneous Injection*
Altman *Intermediate Care DVD: Administering an Intramuscular Injection*
Altman *Intermediate Care DVD: Adding Medications to an IV Solution*
Altman *Intermediate Care DVD: Administering Medications via Secondary Administration Sets (Piggyback)*
Altman, *Intermediate Care: Administering Medications via IV Bolus or IV Push*
Altman *Intermediate Care DVD: Administering Medications via Volume Control Sets*
Altman *Intermediate Care DVD: Administering Ear and Eye Medications*
Altman *Intermediate Care DVD: Administering Skin/Topical Medications*
Altman *Intermediate Care DVD: Administering Nasal Medications*
Altman *Intermediate Care DVD: Administering Nebulized Medications*

Altman *Intermediate Care DVD: Administering Rectal Medications*

Altman *Intermediate Care DVD: Administering Vaginal Medications*

Altman *Intermediate Care DVD Administering Medication via Z-Track Injection*

Altman *Intermediate Care DVD: Managing Controlled Substances*

## Web Resources

American Diabetes Association
  http://www.diabetes.org
Federal Drug Administration's MedWatch Program
  http://www.fda.gov
Mayo Clinic Health Information
  http://www.mayoclinic.com
Medic Alert Organization
  http://www.medicalert.org
National Institute on Drug Abuse
  http://www.nida.nih.gov
Office of Dietary Supplements, National Institutes of Health
  http://dietary-supplements.info.nih.gov
U.S. Food & Drug Administration
  http://www.fda.gov

## References

Ackley, B. J., & Ladwig, G. B. (2002). *Nursing diagnosis handbook: A guide to planning care* (5th ed.). St. Louis: Mosby.

Altman, G. (2004). *Delmar's fundamental & advanced nursing skills* (2nd ed.). Clifton Park, NY: Delmar Learning.

American Diabetes Association (ADA) (1999). Insulin administration. *Diabetes Care, 22* (Supplement 1), 583–586.

American Hospital Formulary Service (1996). *AHFS drug information 96.* Bethesda, MD: American Society of Hospital Pharmacists.

American Nurses Association (March/April, 1997). *The American Nurse, 29*(2), 11.

Barbone, M. (1999). A tip of the cap to intermittent infusions. *Nursing 99, 29*(2), 53–54.

Beyea, S. C., & Nicoll, L. H. (1995). Administration of medication via intramuscular route: An integrative review of the literature and research-based protocol for the procedure. *Applied Nursing Research, 8*(1), 23–33.

Carroll, P. (2001). Anaphylaxis. *RN, 64*(12), 45–49.

Cavanaugh, M. L. (2001). New regulations focus on medical errors. *RN, 64*(4), 71–74.

Deglin, J. H., & Vallerand, A. H. (2002). *Davis's drug guide for nurses* (7th ed.). Philadelphia: F. A. Davis Company.

Estes, M. (2002). *Health assessment & physical examination* (2nd ed.). Clifton Park, NY: Delmar Learning.

Fleming, D. R. (1999). Challenging traditional insulin injection practices. *American Journal of Nursing, 99*(2), 72–74.

Fleming, D. R. (2000). Mightier than the syringe. *American Journal of Nursing, 100*(11), 44–48.

Gahart, B. L., & Nazareno, A. R. (2001). *Intravenous medications.* St. Louis: Mosby.

Griffith, J. (1999). Substance abuse disorders in nurses. *Nursing Forum, 34*(4), 19–28.

Gutierrez, K. (1999). *Pharmacotherapeutics: Clinical decision-making in nursing.* Philadelphia: W. B. Saunders Company.

Haack, M. R., & Yocum, C. J. (2002). State policies and nurses with substance use disorders. *Journal of Nursing Scholarship, 34*(1), 89–94.

Haddad, A. (2001). Ethics in action. *RN, 64*(9), 25–28.

Karch, A. M., & Karch, F. E. (2001). Take part in the solution. *American Journal of Nursing, 101*(10), 25.

Kudzma, E. C. (1999). Culturally competent. *American Journal of Nursing, 99*(8), 46–51.

Mayo Clinic. (2000). *Your guide to herbal supplements.* Rochester, MN: Mayo Clinic.

Miller, D., & Miller, H. (2000). To crush or not to crush. *Nursing 2000, 30*(2), 50–52.

O'Neil, C. K., Avila, J. R., & Fetrow, C. W. (1999). Herbal medicines: Getting beyond the hype. *Nursing 99, 29*(4), 58–61.

Osborne, J., Blais, K., & Hayes, J. S. (1999). Nurses' perceptions: When is it a medication error? *Journal of Nursing Administration, 29*(4), 33–38.

Reiss, B., Evans, M., & Broyles, B. (2002). *Pharmacological aspects of nursing care* (6th ed.). Clifton Park, NY: Delmar Learning.

Skokal, W. A. (2001). Extravasation. *RN, 64*(9), 57–61.

Smeltzer, J. (2001). Take 10 giant steps to medication safety. *Nursing 2001, 31*(11), 49–53.

Springhouse Corporation (2002). *Dosage calculations made incredibly easy!* Springhouse, Pennsylvania: Springhouse, Co.

Strowig, S. (2001). Diabetes update: Insulin therapy. *RN, 64*(9), 38–44.

Thomas, C. (Ed.) (2002). *Tabler's cyclopedic medical dictionary* (19th ed.). Philadelphia: F. A. Davis.

Togger, D. A., & Brenner, P. S. (2001). Metered dose inhalers. *American Journal of Nursing, 101*(10), 26–32.

White, L. B., & Foster, S. (2000). *The herbal drugstore.* Emmaus, PA: Rodale.

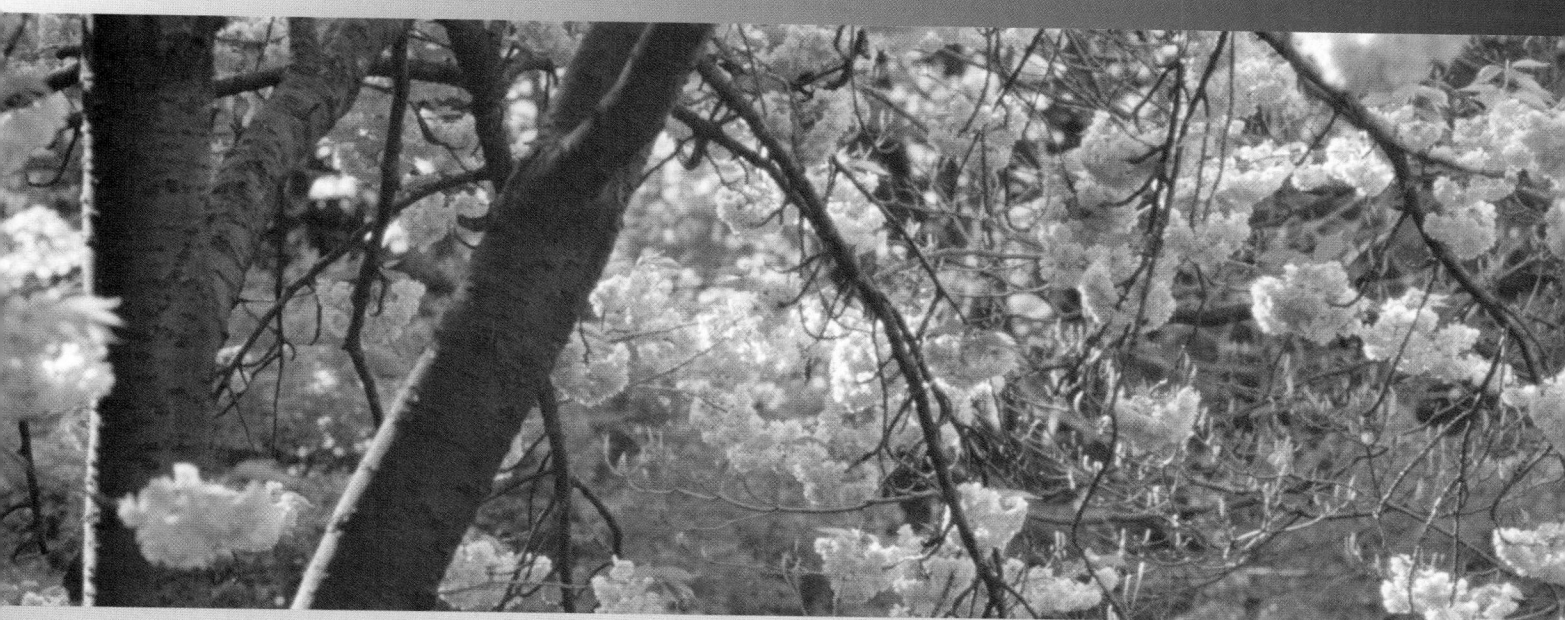

# CHAPTER 31

# Alternative and Complementary Therapies

## Debra L. Topham, PhD, RN, CNS, ACRN

*"My road to healing had two parts. The first part was simply learning to calm down the body/mind . . . . The second level of healing involved changing my negative perceptions about certain events in my life so that I could learn to experience things differently."*

*(Borysenko & Borysenko, 1994)*

# Chapter Competencies

*Upon completion of this chapter, the reader should be able to:*

1. Identify the principles of allopathic medicine.
2. Describe the historical roots of current complementary and alternative medicine.
3. Discuss the contemporary trends of the mind/body connection and the effect of this connection.
4. Identify the concept of holism and its relationship to nursing practice.
5. Describe various complementary and alternative medicine modalities used in client care.
6. Describe the therapeutic benefits of various complementary and alternative medicine modalities.
7. Discuss the use of complementary and alternative medicine modalities throughout the life cycle.

# Key Terms

acupressure
acupuncture
allopathic
alternative therapies
aromatherapy
Ayurveda
biofeedback
bodymind
centering
chakra
chiropractic
complementary therapies
effleurage
endorphins
friction

healing touch
holism
homeopathy
imagery
integrative therapy
meditation
moxibustion
music-thanatology
neuropeptides
neurotransmitters
nutraceuticals
petrissage
phytonutrients
prana
psychoneuroimmunology

reflexology
reiki
relaxation response
rolfing
shaman
shamanism
shiatsu
Tao
tapotement
therapeutic massage
therapeutic touch
touch
vibration

Western society tends to think of health care in terms of medical, surgical, and other technological interventions. However, in many other cultures—both past and present—healing has been promoted by nonallopathic approaches.

The use of **alternative therapies** (treatment approaches that are not accepted by mainstream medical practice) and **complementary therapies** (treatment approaches that can be used in conjunction with conventional medical therapies) is becoming more prevalent among the general public. Americans annually spend billions of dollars out-of-pocket to pay for alternative and complementary therapies. Many insurance companies have increased coverage of these therapies, including chiropractic therapy, massage, and acupuncture. This chapter discusses complementary/alter-native medicine (CAM) modalities that are currently being used in holistic nursing practice. Nurses are encouraged to critically evaluate CAM modalities before recommending or implementing these approaches.

## Allopathic Medicine

Western medicine, referred to as **allopathic** medicine, is relatively new in that it was begun about 200 years ago. Its fundamental principle is that body and mind are separate entities. Allopathic medicine views the human as a collection of separate body parts. This medical approach views health as the absence of disease and sees the goal of treatment as curing the disease or "fixing" the problem (such as trauma). The Western medical model focuses on ridding the body of symptoms induced by disease or injury.

The allopathic system is effective when aggressive treatment is needed for an emergency situation. State-of-the-art technology and advanced surgical techniques have become true lifesavers for many in our society. However, with its emphasis on curing disease, allopathic medicine overlooks the crucial role of energy, emotions, and thoughts. Allopathic medicine has been less effective in treating chronic conditions such as hypertension and arthritis. "Alternative medicine is especially effective for people with chronic, debilitating illnesses for which conventional medicine has few, if any, answers" (Fontaine, 2000, p. 6).

# Historical Roots of CAM Modalities

For as long as history has been recorded, people have tried to cure ills and relieve pain. Early cave drawings depict healers practicing their art. Primitive healers attributed the cause of mysterious diseases to magic and superstition; as a result, religious beliefs and health practices became intertwined. Remedies and practices that are based in ancient traditions are being rediscovered and used by contemporary holistic healers. This section discusses the impact of ancient healing practices on current use of CAM modalities.

## Influences from Ancient Greece

The ancient Greek culture perceived health as the maintenance of balance in all dimensions of life. In Greek mythology, Asclepius was the god of healing. Temples, called Asclepions, were beautiful places for people to rest, restore themselves, and worship. The elaborate healing system consisted of myths, symbols, and rites administered by rigorously trained priest-healers.

## Influences from the Far East

Healing systems from the Far East integrated mind, body, and spirit into a system of balanced energy between the individual and the universe. The concept of a life force or life energy permeates Eastern philosophies. In Chinese culture, the life force was known as *chi*; in Indian culture, it was known as *prana*; and in Japanese culture, it is known as *qi*. Chinese (traditional Chinese medicine) and Indian (Ayurveda) medical systems have most heavily influenced CAM modalities in allopathic medicine. The concept of the human body is looked at much differently among Western cultures, Eastern cultures, and Indian cultures (Figure 31-1).

### China

The traditional Chinese healing system is based on the **Tao**. The Tao is a spiritual belief system based upon the teachings of Lao Tzu. In essence, it is believed that everything is the Tao and the Tao is found in everything. This leads to the belief in the oneness of all things in nature. Life energy (*chi*) flows through both the universe and the person, thus creating a wholeness among all things and people. *Chi* provides warmth, protection from illness, and vitality. *Chi* flows along an invisible system of meridians (pathways) that link Chinese medicine's five organ systems together. Illness and injury can alter the flow of this energy. The *chi* flow can be enhanced by stimulating points along the meridians.

Acupuncture, acupressure, Chinese herbs, Qi Gong (breath work), and tai chi (moving meditation) are all modalities within the field of traditional Chinese medicine (TCM) that act by enhancing the flow of chi. This enhanced chi flow leads not only to healing, but also to prevention of imbalances that can lead to disease. Specific TCM modalities will be discussed later in this chapter.

### India

**Ayurveda**, a healing system based on Hindu and Indian philosophy, embraces the concept of an energy force in the body that seeks to maintain balance or harmony. From the Ayurvedic perspective, the body and mind are filled with a vital energy (*prana*) that is the life force. "Like all enlightened healing methods, Ayurveda emphasizes prevention above curing disease" (Goldberg, 1999, p. 68). The life energy (*prana*) is transported through the body by a "wind" or *vata*. Vata regulates every type of movement. Table 31-1 shows the types of vata in the human body.

The Hindu concept of chakras refers to seven primary energy centers in the physical body. A **chakra** is a concentrated area of energy. The chakras are vertically aligned through the center of the body from the crown of the head to the pelvis. Chakras influence the physical body, emotions, mental patterns, and spiritual awareness. Each chakra has specific functions and a corresponding relationship to body structures and organs.

Prevention of illness and restoration of health through inner search and spiritual growth are the primary goals in the Ayurvedic system. Union of the Divine and the Truth occurs through the physical and meditative practice of yoga. In contemporary practice, Ayurvedic interventions may consist of yoga, herbs, diet, exercise, steam baths, acupuncture, cathartics, and detoxifying massage.

## Shamanistic Tradition

**Shamanism** refers to the practice of entering altered states of consciousness with the intent of helping others. The **shaman** (a folk healer-priest who uses natural and supernatural forces to help others) has an extensive knowledge of herbs, is skilled in many forms of healing, and serves as guardian of the spirits. Illness is considered to be the result of spirit loss. Shamans have the power to

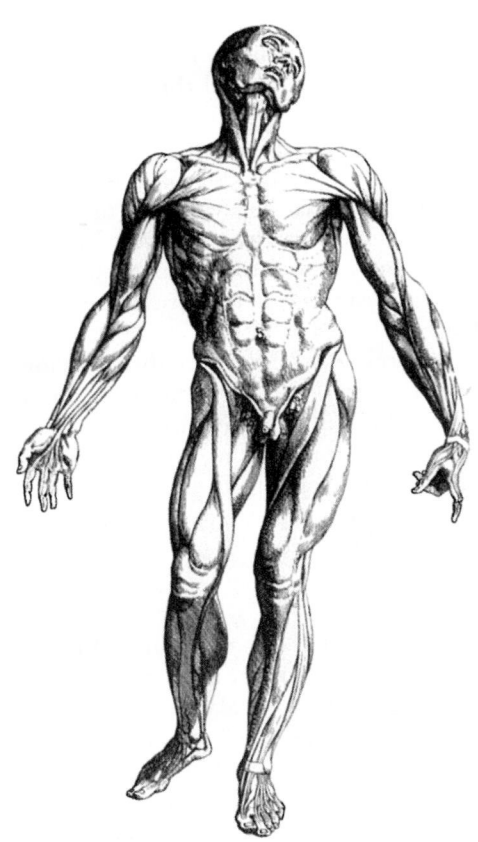

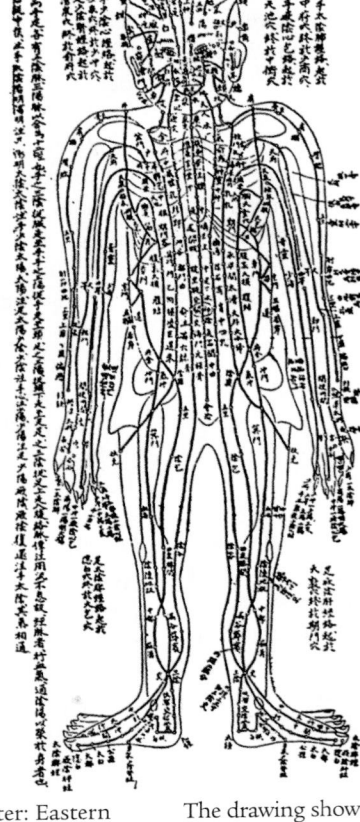

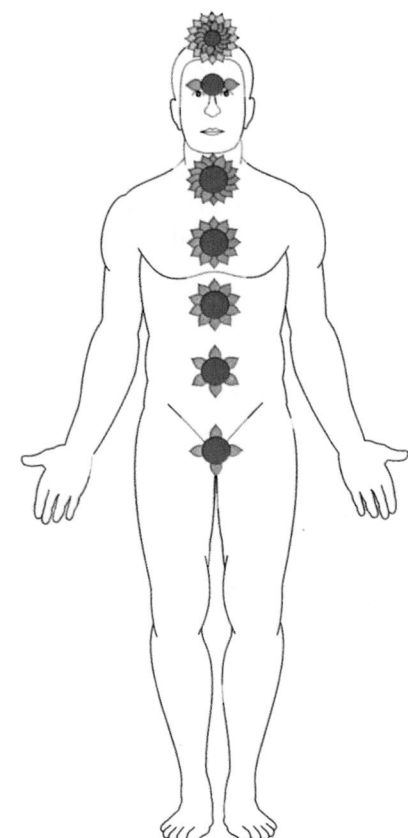

Left: Western sci-
entific concept of
the human body as
made up of interre-
lated systems of
muscles, tissues,
bones, nerves,
blood vessels, cells,
and organs

The drawing
shown was done by
Vesalius in the
16th century, and
is based on
anatomical obser-
vations obtained
by dissection of
the human body.

Center: Eastern
philosophical con-
cept of the human
body as a complex
network of meridi-
ans, which are
pathways for dis-
tributing vital
energy called *qi*

The drawing shown
is a meridian map
dating from 200 B.C.
Ancient Eastern
healers did not con-
cern themselves
with the actual
physical makeup of
the body.

Right: Indian spiri-
tual concept of the
human body as a
complex of energy
centers and chan-
nels that distribute
vital energy, called
*prana*, throughout
the body

The drawing shown
is a modern depic-
tion. While India
possesses many
ancient medical
texts, it has virtual-
ly no ancient tradi-
tion of illustrative
medical drawings.

**Figure 31-1    Concepts of the human body.** *From* **Essential anatomy: For healing and martial arts (p. 9)** *by*
*M. Tedeschi, 2000, Trumbull, CT: Weatherhill. Reprinted with permission of Weatherhill.*

| TABLE 31-1 | VATA IN THE HUMAN BODY |
|---|---|
| **Types of *Vata*** | **Regulatory Effect** |
| *Prana vata* | Nervous system |
| *Udana vata* | Cognitive skills, speech, and memory |
| *Samana vata* | Digestion |
| *Vyana vata* | Circulation |
| *Apana vata* | Excretion |

Adapted from Goldberg, B. (1999). *Alternative medicine: The
definitive guide.* Tiburon, CA: Future Medicine Publishing.

heal by working with the spirits to encourage their full
return to the individual. The shaman functions as both
healer and priest.

Seeking wisdom about the universe, a relationship
with the creator, and avoidance of death are all accomplished through ritualized processes that are performed
by the shaman. The shaman's practice may incorporate
special objects such as power animals, totems, and fetish-
es as well as ritual songs, dances, food, and clothing. Sleep
deprivation, ritual chants, isolation, imagery, drumming,
and hallucinogenic drugs may be used to create a trance-
like state that is the vehicle through which the shaman
contacts the spirit world. It is on behalf of the client that
the shaman requests spiritual healing. It is believed the
spiritual healing will lead to physical and emotional healing. (See Table 31-2 for a comparison of allopathic and
CAM modalities.)

| TABLE 31-2 | COMPARISON OF ALLOPATHIC AND CAM MODALITIES | |
|---|---|
| **Allopathic Perspective** | **CAM Perspective** |
| Health is absence of disease. | Health is a state of well-being characterized by mind-body balance. |
| Focus is on cure of disease. | Emphasis is on health maintenance and disease prevention through lifestyle choices. |
| Mind and body are treated as separate entities. | Mind and body are one; what affects one affects the other. |
| Disease results from causative agents, usually external. | Disease originates from within and is the result of imbalances that occur in response to unhealthy lifestyle and/or inner disharmonies. |
| Healing depends on outside agents to cure the disease. | The body has a natural ability to heal itself. |
| Treatment consists of drugs, surgery, and radiation. | Treatment consists of a variety of noninvasive therapies. |
| Healing is aggressive, quick, and seeks to destroy the invading agents. | Healing is a slow, natural process. |
| The physician has a a paternalistic relationship with the client. | The practitioner and client have a collaborative, equal-power relationship. |

Adapted from Fontaine, K. L. (2000). *Healing practices: Alternative therapies for nursing.* Upper Saddle River, NJ: Prentice Hall; Froemming, P. (1998). *The best guide to alternative medicine.* Los Angeles: Renaissance Books; Goldberg, B. (1999). *Alternative medicine: The definitive guide.* Tiburon, CA: Future Medicine Publishing.

# Contemporary Trends

The contemporary public perception of CAM modalities has been changing over the past few decades. In the late 1960s and early 1970s, the "natural," "new age," and "self-help" movements began to attract adherents, first among consumers and later among health care practitioners. During that time, there was a growing trend toward rejection of allopathic medicine because of its perceived invasiveness, painfulness, cost, and ineffectiveness. A rekindled interest in Eastern religions, lifestyle, and medicine has fueled the use of contemporary holistic, CAM modalities in allopathic medicine.

Ever increasing numbers of consumers who are seeking natural and safe approaches to health care are using CAM modalities. The goals of CAM are numerous, including the following (Rimmer, 1998):

- Health promotion
- Pain relief
- Treatment of chronic illness
- Spiritual growth
- Disease prevention

There is an increasing prevalence of the use of CAM modalities in the United States. Forty percent of those surveyed in one study (Astin, 1998) reported use of some form of alternative therapies. The growing interest in complementary therapies is evidenced by the increased sale of natural substances, such as herbs and vitamins, which has become a multimillion-dollar industry over the last few years (Rimmer, 1998).

According to Eisenberg (1998), up to 54% of adults (83 million people) in the United States used one or more types of alternative medicine in the previous year. Sixty percent of these health care consumers did not tell their primary care provider about their use of alternative therapies. In total, 629 million visits were made to alternative healers in 1997. Approximately $27 billion were paid by consumers as out-of-pocket expenditures on alternative therapies.

Several factors have contributed to the increased use of CAM modalities in the United States. Many health care consumers want to be more involved in their own healing and see CAM modalities as a way to promote this autonomy and control (Collins, 2000). Astin (1998) found that predictors of CAM use include persons with higher education, poorer health status, certain health problems (anxiety, chronic pain, back problems, urinary tract infections, chronic fatigue syndrome, addictions, arthritis, headaches), and a holistic view of health.

Nurses are encouraged to teach clients to use the best of all systems in order to promote positive health outcomes. The term **integrative therapy** (a clinical approach that combines allopathic medicine with techniques from Eastern medicine) is becoming more prevalent in the United States. The integrative approach "neither rejects conventional medicine nor embraces alternative medicine uncritically" (Froemming, 1998, p. xi).

As a result of the public's increased use of CAM, the unethical behavior of some CAM practitioners, and a lack of scientific evidence to either support or refute the efficacy of CAM modalities, the federal government established an Office of Alternative Medicine (OAM) in 1992. The OAM is now the National Center for Complementary and Alternative Medicine (NCCAM) in the National Institutes of Health (NIH). Its mission is to conduct and support research and training, and to disseminate information on

CAM modalities to the public and health care practitioners. Since its inception, the NCCAM has greatly increased the amount of federally funded research that explores the efficacy and therapeutic benefits of CAM. Clinical trials are underway in nearly every CAM modality. For a listing of clinical trials, go to the NCCAM (2003) website at http://nccam.nih.gov.

## Mind-Body Research

The allopathic medical model was founded on the dualistic belief that the mind and body are separate entities. However, **psychoneuroimmunology** (PNI), an emerging field of science, is studying the complex relationship between the mind and body, specifically the cognitive/affective system in the brain, neurologic system, and immune system. Psychoneuroimmunologists are investigating how the brain transmits signals along the nerves to enhance the body's normal immune functioning. PNI research supports the idea that the human mind and psychosocial support can alter physiology.

All body cells have receptor sites for **neuropeptides** (amino acids produced in the brain and other sites in the body that act as chemical communicators) that are released when **neurotransmitters** (chemical substances produced by the body that facilitate nerve transmission) signal emotions in the brain. Thus, it is possible for cells to be directly affected by emotions. In other words, people can affect their health by what they think and feel. The intermeshed complex system of psyche and body chemistry is now referred to as the **bodymind** (inseparable connection and operation of thoughts, feelings, and physiological functions).

## Holism and Nursing Practice

The concept of holism builds on the mind-body connection and adds a spiritual dimension. **Holism** refers to the concept that the whole is greater than the sum of its parts. Since Florence Nightingale's time, nursing has been holistic in its approach to client care. Holism encompasses consideration of the physiological, psychological, sociocultural, intellectual, and spiritual aspects of each individual. Holistic nursing can be described as the art and science of caring for the whole person, knowing that each person is unique in all expressions of self. As holistic healers, nurses often employ CAM modalities to promote clients' well-being. Box 31-1 lists concepts basic to a holistic philosophy of caring.

## The Nature of Healing

The word *healing* is derived from the Anglo-Saxon word *hael*, which means to make whole, to move toward, or to become whole. It is important to establish that healing is not the same as curing (ridding one of disease) but is a process that activates the individual's healing forces from within (Box 31-2). As a healing facilitator, the nurse enters into a relationship with

---

### BOX 31-1 HOLISTIC CONCEPTS

- Mind and body are one, not separate.
- People are responsible for their own choices.
- People have the power to solve their own problems.
- Well-being is multifaceted—physical, emotional, mental, and spiritual.

---

### BOX 31-2 AN EXPERIENCE OF HOLISTIC HEALING

**Finding Peace and Inner Strength**

I am much more at peace and much healthier when I listen chiefly to my own body signals and hardly at all to the messages from the media, medical experts, or even social activists and alternative healing groups. . . . One of my first acts when in danger is to reach out for help to mother or father, to doctors, to friends, to pills and potions, to books, anything to hold onto or lean upon, like the drowning man to straws. The real source of my strength and healing is from within and it is important for me to go there, stay there, live there, see from there, meet and make peace with whatever comes from there and do my reaching from there from my body. I think when some of my friends got sick, the fear and desperation took them a long way out from their bodies in search of a cure. So much of their hope was invested in external possibilities that they almost abandoned their bodies— as if they could flee what is happening inside. I think it is necessary to go back down and deep within yourself to face and feel and own your own experience. I realize I can't send something else down to do battle in my place. No miracle, no surgeon's knife, no megavitamin, no medicine or macrobiotic diet, no crystal energy, no faith healer's touch, or shaman's prayer—nothing is of any value at all unless I am there fully present . . . Without one foot in the past, the other in the future. I think of healing a little differently than I used to—it's not about living forever or curing disease. It is about living and feeling fully the whole spectrum from joy to sadness, however long that is, dying with a sense of peace, whenever that comes.

*Anonymous*

the client and can assist the client by offering to be a guide, change agent, or instrument of healing (a means by which healing can be achieved, performed, or enhanced). Gilkeson (2000) describes healing by saying, "healing potential exists in each of us . . . it is important to recognize that it is not so much that the 'healer' heals another person, but rather that he triggers the other person's own self-healing potential" (p. 6). From a nursing perspective, the nurse facilitates the client's healing by assisting and supporting the client. Nightingale said it best when she wrote, "and what nursing has to do . . . is to put the patient in the best condition for nature to act upon him" (1860, p. 133).

## CAM Modalities

Many CAM modalities are used in holistic nursing practice. These modalities are categorized as mind-body, body-movement, spiritual, nutritional, and other methodologies (see Table 31-3). Although different in technique, many of the CAM therapies have common ideological threads, as shown in Box 31-3.

## Mind-Body Techniques

Mind-body techniques are methods by which an individual can consciously control some functions of the sympathetic nervous system (for example, heart rate, respiratory rate, and blood pressure). Mind-body techniques include relaxation, meditation, imagery, biofeedback, and hypnosis.

---

**BOX 31-3 CONCEPTUAL THREADS SHARED AMONG CAM INTERVENTION METHODS**

- The whole system must be considered if the *parts* of the individual are to be helped to function.

- The person is integrated and related to her surroundings.

- There exists some life force or energy that can be used in the healing process.

- Ritual, prescribed practice, and skilled practitioners are integral parts of holistic healing interventions.

---

### Relaxation

When confronted with a stressor, the body's flight-or-fight response is stimulated. As a result, the body releases epinephrine, speeds up metabolism, and increases heart and respiratory rate. It has been found that relaxation techniques offer a way for a person to reduce the flight-or-fight response, returning the body to a normal physiological state.

Cardiologist Herbert Benson (1975) studied the effects of meditation on individuals. He then incorporated the

---

## TABLE 31-3 CATEGORIES OF CAM MODALITIES

| Mind-Body | Body Movement | Energy and Body Work | Spiritual | Nutritional and Diet | Other |
|-----------|---------------|----------------------|-----------|----------------------|-------|
| • Relaxation | • Exercise | • Therapeutic Touch | • Faith Healing | • Nutraceuticals | • Aromatherapy |
| • Meditation | • Yoga | • Healing Touch | • Prayer | • Vitamins and Supplements | • Humor |
| • Imagery | • Tai chi | • Reiki | • Shamanism | • Herbs | • Pet Therapy |
| • Biofeedback | • Chiropractic Therapy | • Acupuncture | | | • Music |
| • Hypnosis | | • Acupressure | | | • Homeopathy |
| | | • Therapeutic Massage | | | |
| | | • Shiatsu | | | |
| | | • Rolfing | | | |
| | | • Reflexology | | | |
| | | • Touch | | | |

National Center for Complementary and Alternative Medicine. (NCCAM). (2003). http://nccam.nih.gov.

basic elements of meditation into the therapeutic process he called the **relaxation response**, a state of increased arousal of the parasympathetic nervous system, which leads to a relaxed physiological state. Benson employed the relaxation response with individuals experiencing high blood pressure and heart disease. While initially trying to avoid a mystical flavor in his work, Benson later discovered that the techniques were more effective if individuals focused on an inspirational prayer or phrase. The basic elements of the relaxation response are shown in Box 31-4.

"Relaxation techniques are skills anyone can use. These skills can be taught to clients when educating them about nutrition and exercise" (Grotbo, 1999, p. 24KK). One method for achieving relaxation is progressive muscle relaxation (PMR), which is the alternate tensing and relaxing of muscles. Aids to relaxation training include music or nature sounds, hypertonic saline relaxation tanks, isolation chambers, yoga, and imagery.

Nurses can use relaxation techniques in their work with clients to reduce pain and stress. Relaxation techniques are also an essential aspect of cognitive behavioral therapy when treating people with phobias, fear, and depression.

## Meditation

The practice of **meditation** (quieting the mind by focusing one's attention) can bring about remarkable physiological changes. People who meditate strive for a sense of oneness within themselves and a sense of relatedness to a greater power and the universe (Figure 31-2).

A person can be guided into a meditative or relaxed state by using breath coaching (assisting client to become aware of or focus on breathing and thus slow it). Nurses can teach this modality to clients by using verbal cues, counting the client's inhalations and exhalations, and showing the client how to take slow, deep breaths. Some therapeutic benefits of meditation are:

- Stress relief
- Relaxation
- Reduced levels of lactic acid
- Decreased oxygen consumption

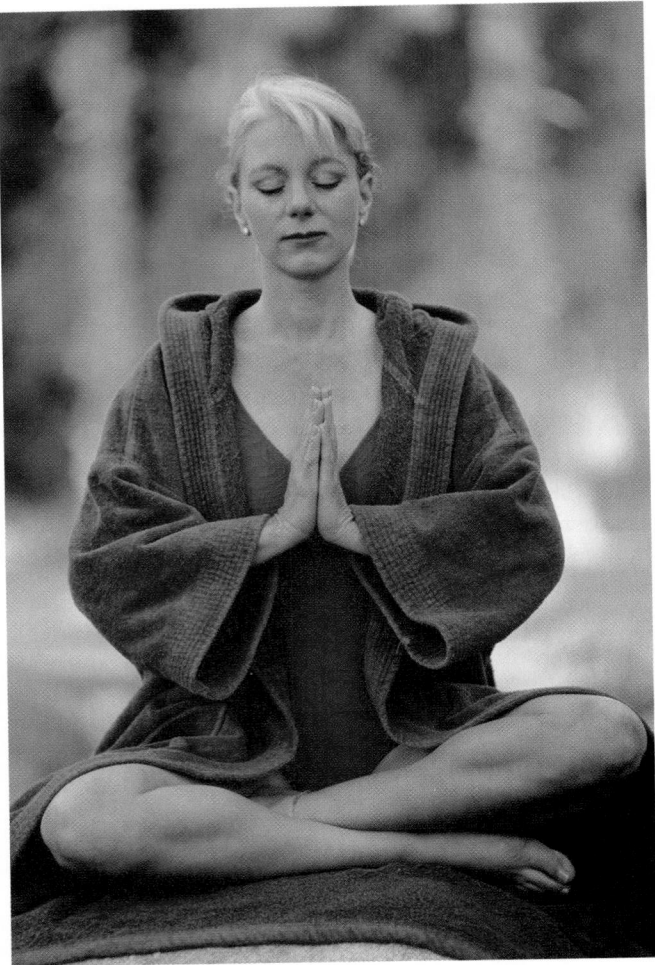

**Figure 31-2   Clients may find relief from anxiety through meditation. *Courtesy of PhotoDisc***

- Slowed heart rate
- Decreased blood pressure
- Improved functioning of immune system

## Imagery

**Imagery** is the use of one's senses to create an image in one's mind. The practitioner encourages the client to use as many of the senses as possible in order to enhance the formation of vivid images. Table 31-4 presents examples of images that can be evoked by the five senses.

Imagery is not a new concept in nursing. In the mid-1800s, Nightingale wrote in *Notes on Nursing* about nurses helping the ill to alter their thoughts through images of nature, such as a bouquet of flowers (Nightingale, 1860). Imagery has been used effectively by nurses with clients of all ages in settings as varied as schools, homes, hospitals, and nursing homes (Hoffart & Keene, 1998).

Nurses can create guided imagery for many clients who are capable of hearing and understanding the nurse's suggestions of meaningful and physiologically correct images. For example, a nurse can show a chart of the stages of bone

---

**BOX 31-4   ELEMENTS OF THE RELAXATION RESPONSE**

- A quiet environment
- Comfortable position
- Focused attention
- Passive attitude
- Practice

| TABLE 31-4 | INCORPORATING ALL FIVE SENSES INTO IMAGERY | | | |
| --- | --- | --- | --- | --- |
| Visual | Auditory | Kinesthetic | Gustatory | Olfactory |
| See the dark blue sky. | Hear the babbling brook. | Feel yourself floating on a cloud. | Taste the tartness of the freshly cut lemon. | Smell the salt air at the ocean. |

healing to a client who has suffered a fracture and ask the client to imagine this sequential activity in her body.

Imagery has been found to reduce pain and anxiety during procedures, decrease the need for medication and/or restraints, and promote relaxation (Hoffart & Keene, 1998).

### Biofeedback

**Biofeedback** is a mechanism of providing feedback of physiological process to help clients learn how to manipulate those responses through mental activity. It was developed by experimental psychologists and rehabilitation clinicians in the 1960s. Biofeedback allows a person to see the effect of the mind over the body. Froemming (1998) describes biofeedback as "[a] method of gaining conscious control over many bodily reactions involved in creating wellness by monitoring your own emotional state with specially designed equipment" (p. 224). While attached to sensory devices that measure such bodily responses as skin temperature, blood pressure, galvanic skin resistance, and electrical activity in the muscles, the individual imagines stressful experiences. The person's physiological responses are then measured and recorded. Subsequent physiological responses to the relaxation response are also recorded. The individual receives an interpretation of these responses and is taught methods for practicing relaxation, while using feedback from the physiological measures to alter his stress response.

Biofeedback has been found to enhance relaxation in tense muscles, relieve tension headaches, reduce bruxism (grinding of the teeth), reduce the pain of temporomandibular joint syndrome, and relieve backache. Temperature biofeedback is useful in training people to purposefully warm their hands to treat Raynaud's disease (a circulatory disorder), to lower blood pressure, and to prevent or relieve migraine headaches.

### Hypnosis

Therapeutic hypnosis induces altered states of consciousness or awareness (a trance) during which the person is more receptive to suggestion. A hypnotic state also enhances the client's ability to form images.

In 1955, the British Medical Association approved hypnotherapy as a valid medical intervention. The American Medical Association did likewise in 1958. Approximately 15,000 American physicians currently use hypnosis in conjunction with conventional medical interventions (Goldberg, 1999).

Once the client is in a hypnotic state, the practitioner offers the client therapeutic suggestions. Therapeutic use of suggestion is the heart of hypnosis. Suggestions can be phrased directly ("You will feel more comfortable") or indirectly ("You may feel different"). Once aroused from the hypnotic state, the client's behavior may be affected according to the therapeutic suggestion introduced during the hypnotic state. For example, if the suggestion was to not smoke, a client may decrease the amount of cigarettes smoked or stop smoking entirely.

Hypnosis is a potentially effective and powerful tool for altering pain, anxiety, and some physiological processes. Although hypnosis is useful as an adjunct to treatment, it does not magically cure such problems as nicotine addiction, alcoholism, and eating disorders, and should be used in conjunction with other modalities.

---

## CLIENT EDUCATION

### Teaching Meditation to Clients

✓ Have the client assume a relaxed position; usually sitting upright in a chair with feet flat on the floor or sitting upright on the floor with legs crossed. The client can be lying in bed.

✓ Have the client use a soft gaze at an object in the distance (the object will not be in focus).

✓ Have the client repeat a word or short phrase, such as "relax" or "breathe."

✓ Have the client inhale and exhale slowly through the nose while repeating the phrase.

✓ Instruct the client that if the mind starts to wander or intrusive thoughts enter, he just needs to go back and focus on the word or phrase.

Transcendental Meditation Resource. (2002). http://www.tm.org

---

## CLINICAL ALERT

### Precaution for Imagery

Imagery is not recommended for clients who are emotionally unstable.

Nurses wishing to use hypnosis in their practice must be aware of the guidelines concerning this modality in the scope of practice as defined by the respective state boards of nursing. Advanced training in hypnosis is also necessary. In most states, licensure or certification is required to practice as a hypnotist.

## Body and Movement Manipulation Strategies

As the name implies, body-movement therapies employ techniques for moving or manipulating various body parts to achieve therapeutic outcomes. There are many body-movement strategies. The more common strategies of movement and exercise, yoga, tai chi, and chiropractic treatment are discussed in the following sections.

### Movement and Exercise

Movement, as a therapeutic intervention and health-promoting activity, is associated with athletic exercise and dance. Although the primary goal of exercise is fitness (muscle strength, flexibility, endurance, and cardiovascular and respiratory health), there are many other positive outcomes of exercise.

Nurses can help clients use movement as therapy in a variety of ways, such as range-of-motion exercises, water exercises, physical therapy, and stretching exercises. It is an effective method through which people of all ages can improve their level of functioning. Some of the therapeutic benefits of exercise are as follows (Rechtschaffen & Cohen, 1999):

- Improves circulation
- Enhances respiratory function
- Promotes elimination

## LEGAL AND ETHICAL ISSUES

### Referring Clients to Participate in Exercise Programs

Nurses must remember to carefully assess clients prior to directing them to be involved in exercise programs. For example, a client who has a slight history of cardiovascular risk factors could develop arrhythmias without a cardiac workup. Or, the client who has a history of noninsulin diabetes needs to be educated as to the changes in calorie consumption if exercise patterns are suddenly changed. The nurse would be legally responsible for suggesting an exercise program that results in negative consequences for a client with a preexisting condition.

Adapted from Burkhardt, M., & Nathaniel, A. (2002). *Ethics & issues in contemporary nursing* (2nd ed.). Clifton Park, NY: Delmar Learning.

## STOP AND THINK

### Movement Programs Across the Life Span

- What movement program would you recommend for an 8-year-old?

- What movement program would you recommend for a 20-year-old?

- What movement program would you recommend for a 45-year-old?

- What movement program would you recommend for a 70-year-old?

- Besides age, what other factors would influence your recommendations?

- Stimulates the release of **endorphins** (brain chemicals that boost mood and help fight depression)
- Helps regulate metabolism
- Enhances immune function

Numerous self-help books, videotapes, magazines, and so on are available to assist clients with learning about exercise and movement strategies. For a sedentary client, a complete physical exam is recommended before beginning any new exercise regimen, especially if the client is over 40 years old. Clients should be referred to appropriate professionals to assist in learning proper movement and exercise techniques. These would include, but are not limited to, exercise physiologists, personal trainers, physical therapists, and dance instructors.

### Yoga

Many cultures believe that particular forms of movement keep the body's life forces in correct balance and flow. Yoga and tai chi are examples of ancient ritual movements that enhance overall health, including spiritual enlightenment and well-being. Both of these approaches require concentration, strength, flexibility, and use of symbolic movements. Yoga has its historical roots in Hindu culture around 3000 B.C. It was introduced into Western cultures in the 1800s. The three main elements of yoga are breathing, movement, and posture. Yoga involves completing a series of postures carried out in sequential order; Figure 31-3 illustrates some basic yoga postures. "By promoting disciplined focus on mind and body, yoga is said to enable a greater consciousness of daily life and of its divine origins" (Cassileth, 1998, p. 249).

Yoga postures are designed to benefit the physical body. Spiritual benefits are realized when breathing techniques and meditation are incorporated into yoga practice. This enhances the flow of **prana** or life energy. While self-help tapes are useful, clients should be directed to an experi-

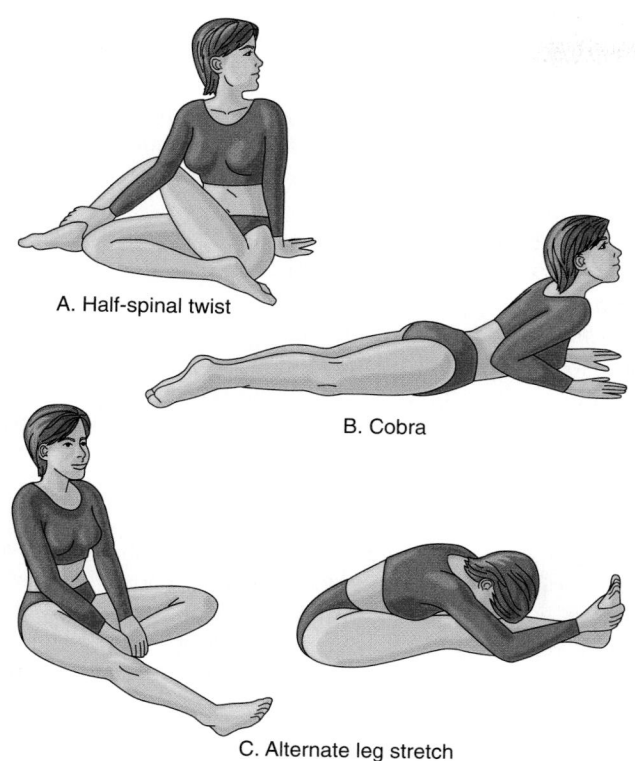

A. Half-spinal twist

B. Cobra

C. Alternate leg stretch

**Figure 31-3 Yoga postures**

enced yoga teacher to learn correct postures and techniques. This will enhance the benefits of yoga practice.

### Tai Chi

Tai chi originated in 13th-century China as a form of movement therapy practiced by Taoist monks. It is often described as a moving meditation, with the goal of gaining balance in the mind, body, and spirit. Tai chi is based on the philosophy of the quest for harmony with nature and the universe through the laws of complementary (yin and yang) balance. When balance exists, everything functions effortlessly, spontaneously, perfectly, and in accordance with the laws of nature. Tai chi consists of a series of sequential dancelike moves connected in a smooth flowing process.

As with other forms of chi manipulation, tai chi improves chi flow through meridians of the body. In this manner, tai chi enhances health and promotes healing. People who regularly perform tai chi believe it enhances stamina, agility, and balance and that it boosts energy and confers a sense of well-being. Tai chi has been shown to lower blood pressure and heart rate in people in cardiac rehabilitation programs, and it is also a method for improving balance and thus reducing falls, especially helpful in older adults (Fontaine, 2000).

### Chiropractic Therapy

Chiropractic therapy was begun in 1895 by Daniel Palmer. Palmer found that deliberate and specific manipulation of the spine could improve a client's health. The major principle underlying **chiropractic** therapy (the promotion of healing through manipulation of the spinal column) is that the brain sends vital energy to every organ in the body via the nerves originating in the spinal column. Disease results from interferences along these pathways; therefore, manipulation of the spinal column is useful in alleviating a variety of ills. Removing the blocks with quick thrusts and adjustments of the spine allows the body to restore its innate recuperative power.

The American Medical Association (AMA) has a long history of skepticism about chiropractic therapy, condemning it as unscientific in the 1960s. In 1987, the AMA lost a court battle to limit chiropractic therapy. Since then, chiropractic therapy has gradually been accepted by the medical community. Chiropractors are staff members of some medical centers/hospitals and are commissioned to military branches as health care providers (Goldberg, 1999). As with any CAM modality, nurses should encourage clients considering the use of chiropractic services to seek the services of board-certified chiropractic physicians. Overwhelming research evidence supports the use of chiropractic therapy for the treatment of acute lower back pain as well as other back injuries.

## Energy and Body Work

A category of CAM modalities that has been incorporated into nursing within the past 30 years is energy and body work therapies. Energy work is a group of techniques that work with the body's energy field by the use of the hands to direct or redirect the energy to enhance balance within the field. These modalities have been found to be effective for many client problems and can be used to restore balance in all aspects of a person's health. Energy therapies can be used with persons of all ages.

Energy therapies have their roots in traditional Chinese, ancient Eastern, and Native American philosophies. The fundamental concept is that individuals are composed of a life force, a source of energy that is not confined to physical skin boundaries. "Energywork, by its nature, brings us face to face with the spiritual" (Gilkeson, 2000, p. 3). Figure 31-4 illustrates the energy field that extends beyond a person's physical body. Collinge (1998) lists the following as commonly accepted beliefs about energy and healing:

- All things are manifestations of energy.
- Energy comes from one universal source.
- Life depends on the movement of energy.
- People consist of several energy fields that interact with the environment.
- Interpersonal relationships are influenced by energy exchanges.

An individual's energy field consists of layers of energy that are in constant flux. The energy layers can be diminished or otherwise adversely affected by any type of illness,

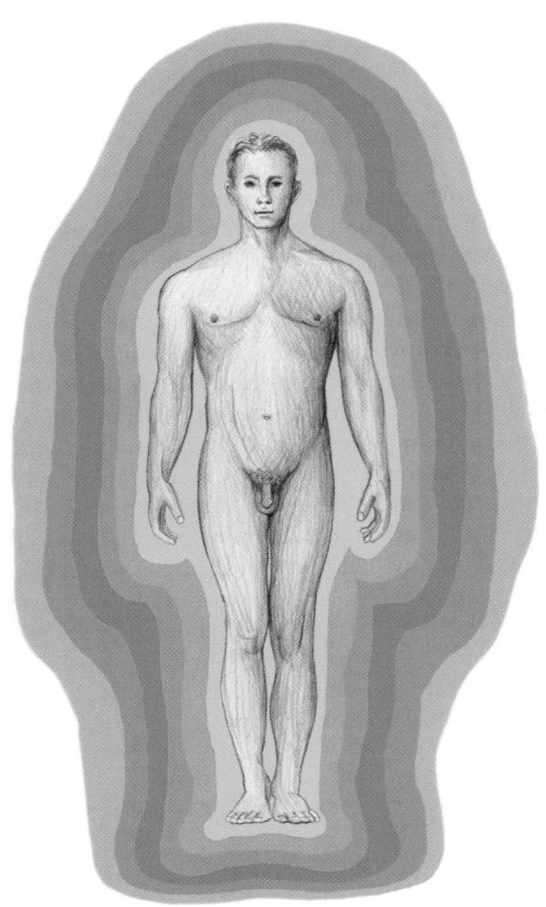

**Figure 31-4   Layers of the human energy field extending beyond the physical boundaries**

trauma, or distress. The energy system can also be positively affected by the intentionally directed use of the hands of a practitioner.

Holistic nurses were integral in helping the North American Nursing Diagnosis Association (2003) to establish the diagnosis *Disturbed Energy Field*. See Box 31-5 for an explanation of this diagnosis.

Many energy therapies are being used by nurses today. These therapies are being effectively integrated into holistic practice. "Western bodywork looks on your body as a machine in need of repair and manipulations. Eastern bodywork looks on your body as an energy field in need of constant balancing to function well" (Rush, 2000, p. 133). Therapeutic touch, healing touch, reiki, acupuncture, and acupressure are some examples discussed in this section.

## Energy Therapies

A variety of energy therapies are ascribed to in alternative healing practices. They provide complementary interventions for the nurse to consider in caring for clients. The following energy therapies are discussed in this section: therapeutic touch, healing touch, reiki, acupuncture, and acupressure.

### Therapeutic Touch

**Therapeutic touch** (TT), which is similar to the ancient healing practices (such as the laying on of hands), consists of assessing alterations in a person's energy field and

---

## NURSING STRATEGY

### Experiencing an Energy Field

To experience your energy field, do the following:

1. Rub your hands together until the heat from the friction is very warm.
2. Hold your hands 1 to 2 inches apart and move slightly in and out.
3. Once you can feel the energy, play by moving your hands more than 2 inches apart or manipulating the energy you feel.
4. Experiment with another person by having both rub the hands together until they are very warm and then hold your hands approximately 2 inches from the other person's hands.

Gaudiano, B. G., & Herbert, J. D. (2000). Can we really tap our problems away? A critical analysis of thought field therapy. *Skeptical Inquirer, 32*(3), 32–38.

---

## BOX 31-5   ENERGY-RELATED NURSING DIAGNOSES

*Nursing Diagnosis*
Disturbed Energy Field

*Definition*
A disruption of the flow of energy surrounding a person's being that results in disharmony of the body, mind, and/or spirit

*Defining Characteristics*
- Movement in the energy field (wave/spike/tingling/dense/flowing)
- Sounds (tone/words)
- Temperature change (warmth/coolness)
- Visual changes (image/color)
- Disruption of the field (vacant/hold/spike/bulge)

*Related factors*
- To be developed

From North American Nursing Diagnosis Association. (2003). *Nursing diagnoses: Definitions and classification: 2003–2004.* Philadelphia: Author.

using the hands to direct energy to achieve a balanced state. The practice of TT was developed in the early 1970s by Dolores Krieger, PhD, RN (1993), then professor of nursing at New York University, and Dora Kunz, a noted healer. TT is based on four assumptions that are shown in Box 31-6.

The TT process is readily learned in workshops, can be done with hands either on or off the body in the energy field, complements medical treatments, and has reasonably consistent and reliable results (Figure 31-5). Table 31-5 presents the five-phase process of TT.

Research has been documenting the effectiveness of therapeutic touch in wound healing, relaxation, and immunological functioning. Gordon and Merenstein (1998) found that therapeutic touch can decrease knee pain caused by arthritis. Research participants who received TT reported significantly less pain and improved function than those in the control group.

### Healing Touch

**Healing touch** (HT) is an energy-based therapeutic modality that alters the energy field through the use of touch. HT was developed by Janet Mentgen, a nurse, in the 1980s. In 1993, HT was established as a certification program of the American Holistic Nurses Association (AHNA). The AHNA curriculum includes varied techniques for use of HT in general balancing of the body's energy field, relaxation, and for specific problems such as headaches, spinal problems, and pain.

Table 31-6 lists the five steps of HT. HT recognizes the need for follow-up or sequential treatments as well as discharge planning and referral to assist the client in adequately meeting goals.

In both TT and HT, the practitioner uses **centering** (a process of bringing oneself to an inward focus of serenity) before initiating treatment. Centering is a useful tool to employ before performing any treatment or before any situation that may be stressful or difficult (such as a major school examination).

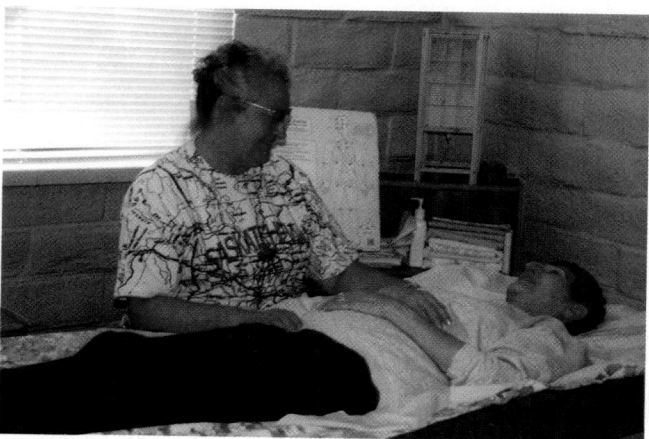

**Figure 31-5    Nurse administering therapeutic touch**

---

### BOX 31-6    FOUNDATIONAL CONCEPTS OF THERAPEUTIC TOUCH

- A human being is an open energy system.

- Anatomically, a human being is bilaterally symmetrical.

- Illness is an imbalance in an individual's energy field.

- Human beings have natural abilities to transform and transcend their conditions of living.

From Krieger, D. (1993). *Accepting your power to heal: The Personal practice of therapeutic touch.* Santa Fe, NM: Bear & Company Publishing.

---

### Reiki

**Reiki** is one of many forms of energy work that also resembles the "laying on of hands." Traditional reiki was founded in the 1800s when Mikao Usui, a Christian minister in Japan, sought to explain how Jesus could heal through the laying on of hands. Usui studied a healing tradition of using hands by Buddhist monks. Through his study and meditation, the system of traditional reiki was founded. Reiki has three levels of practitioners, with the reiki master or master teacher being the highest level. Level I reiki practitioners are prepared to provide healing work at the physiological level and work with the client physically present. Level II reiki practitioners are prepared to provide healing on the emotional and spiritual levels and in absentia. The Level III reiki practitioner is more skilled and can advance to becoming a reiki teacher. While anyone can learn the hand positions of reiki, reiki attunements from a master teacher are necessary to prepare the practitioner for work with clients. Reiki attunements open the crown chakra, enhancing universal energy flow through the practitioner.

Reiki is used for physical, emotional, and spiritual healing. The practitioner does not use her energy to heal the client, but rather acts as a conduit for the universal energy to flow into the person. A typical reiki session involves the practitioner laying hands over the seven chakras of the body, both anterior and posterior, and the feet. The universal energy then flows through the chakras, opening the energy flow in the individual so that he might heal.

There is some research, mostly anecdotal, that supports the benefits of reiki treatment. Reiki has been found to calm physiological function, increase red and white blood cell production, enhance pain relief, and reduce anxiety. Because reiki works on physical, emotional, and spiritual levels, opening emotional blockages could result in the client reexperiencing emotional traumas. The reiki practitioner should be aware of this and

## TABLE 31-5    PHASES OF THERAPEUTIC TOUCH

| Phase | Definition | Techniques |
|---|---|---|
| Centering | • Bringing body, mind, and emotions to a quiet, focused state of consciousness<br><br>• Being still<br><br>• Being nonjudgmental | Become centered by use of:<br><br>• Controlled breathing<br><br>• Imagery<br><br>• Meditation |
| Assessment ("Scanning") | • Using the hands to determine the nature of the client's energy field<br><br>• Being attuned to sensory cues (e.g., warmth, coolness, static, pressure, tingling) to detect changes in client's energy | • Hold hands 2 to 6 inches away from person's energy field while moving the hands from the head to the feet in a rhythmic, symmetrical manner. |
| Unruffling ("Clearing") | • Facilitating the symmetrical and rhythmic flow of energy through the field | • Use slightly more vigorous hand movements from midline while continuing to move in a rhythmic and symmetrical manner from the head to the feet. |
| Treatment ("Balancing," "Rebalancing," or "Intervention") | • Projecting, directing, and modulating energy on the basis of the nature of the living energy field<br><br>• Assisting to reestablish order in the system | • Because each practitioner experiences the living energy field uniquely, the law of opposites serves as a guideline for intervening (e.g., if a pulling or drawing sensation is detected, then direct energy to the depleted area until it feels replenished).<br><br>• Continue to assess, clear, and balance the field while remaining centered.<br><br>• Reassess the field. |
| Evaluation | • Using professional, informed, and intuitive judgment to determine when to end the session | • Elicit feedback from the client.<br><br>• Give the client an opportunity to rest and integrate the process. |

Note: The phases, although learned sequentially by beginners, are dynamic and often are performed concurrently and repetitively by experienced practitioners. Adapted from Nurse Healers-Professional Associates, Inc. (1992). *Therapeutic touch: Teaching guidelines: Beginner's level Krieger/Kunz method.* New York: Author.

ensure that the client has support to process emotional trauma after a reiki session. Based upon early research, the NCCAM has been conducting clinical trials in the use of reiki since 2000.

Reiki practitioners are not licensed. Reiki practitioners do receive certificates from their reiki master verifying that they have completed reiki training. Nurses should educate clients to request to see the certificate. As with any CAM modality, nurses should seek proper education, training, and certification prior to performing reiki energy work. An excellent source to find out more about reiki is the book *Essential Reiki* by Diane Stein (1995).

### Acupuncture

**Acupuncture** is the use of needles inserted at specific points on the body (meridians) to promote healing (Figure 31-6). Acupuncture is done to enhance the energy flow throughout the body. Treatment focuses on correcting the flow of *chi* (energy) when imbalances or blockages occur. TCM practitioners believe that meridians conduct *chi* between the body's surface and internal organs. In the case of pain, acupuncture points are believed to stimulate the central nervous system to release chemicals into the muscles, spinal cord, and brain. These chemicals either alter the experience of

## TABLE 31-6    STEPS OF HEALING TOUCH

| Step | Description | Nursing Guidelines |
|---|---|---|
| Initial Interview | • Provides the working base for energetic interventions and functions as an intake assessment. | • Introduce yourself.<br><br>• Explain enough about your work so that a feeling of confidence can begin to develop.<br><br>• Determine the main problem or reason for treatment.<br><br>• Identify relevant health history: hospitalizations, diseases, injuries, diagnoses, medications (past and present) including use of recreational drugs, nicotine, alcohol, caffeine, vitamins, and herbs. All of these factors can influence the energy field. |
| Assessment | • In wellness, the energy flows evenly from head to toe without blocks, breaks, unevenness, or temperature variations. Any disruption of the flow reflects disharmony in that area. | • Approach the client from a centered state.<br><br>• Begin by determining the shape of the energy field by slowly scanning its outer edges.<br><br>• Start 3 to 4 feet away from the body and move toward it using the palms until you can determine the actual outline of the energy field.<br><br>• Continue the assessment by feeling the vital layer 1 to 6 inches off the skin.<br><br>• Identify areas in relation to the physical body where the field is different, perhaps not as vibrant or as smooth as in other areas. |
| Documentation | • Begins with the initial client contact. | • Mentally take note of all sensations, even the ones that may seem very subtle.<br><br>• A picture of the energy pattern is usually easy to execute by drawing the perceived pattern on a simple outline of the body.<br><br>• Areas of energetic differences can be drawn in, as can injuries, swelling, scars, or the track of a pain ridge. |
| Intervention | • The healer can choose many healing interventions in this sequence: therapeutic touch, full body techniques, and localized and specific techniques. | • During the intervention, which may last 20 to 30 minutes, all of the healer's skill and experience are used. |
| Completion and Grounding | • After completion of the interventions, carefully ground the client to help restore balance and promote integration.<br><br>• Carefully determine that the client is fully alert if the client will leave after the session. | Grounding can be done in a variety of ways, including:<br><br>• Hold the feet until you sense a flow and a connection with the client and sense that the client's energy is back in the feet.<br><br>• Brush down the body from head to toe and down the arms toward the ground. Repeat briskly several times.<br><br>• Give a suggestion: "Feel your fingers, and your toes; now gently move them until you return to full awareness in this room."<br><br>• Reassess the energy field at this time and document the changes.<br><br>• Spend some time with the client to obtain feedback. Focus on what the client experienced. Talking helps the client to feel grounded. |

## The Positive Effects of Reiki Therapy

Jane was a 58-year-old woman admitted for uncontrolled nausea and vomiting secondary to chemotherapy. She was dying of metastatic breast cancer, but her primary focus was on reducing her nausea, pain, and anxiety. When admitted to the hospital's oncology unit, she requested to have therapeutic touch, as it had been used with her at another medical center. The nurses didn't know of anyone who did therapeutic touch, but did know a reiki practitioner. The reiki practitioner saw Jane that night, explained reiki, and administered a reiki treatment. The next morning, Jane proclaimed, "That was wonderful. I slept through the night for the first time in ages." She still had some slight nausea, but did not require any medications through the night for pain, anxiety, or nausea.

What would you suggest as some next steps for Jane?

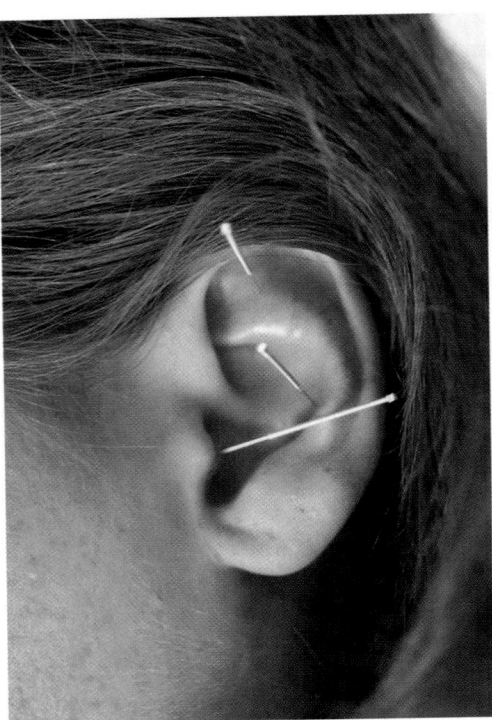

**Figure 31-6    Acupuncture needles inserted for treatment of depression** *Courtesy of PhotoDisc*

pain or produce other chemicals that lessen pain (National Institutes of Health, 1997).

Acupuncture is one of the oldest, most commonly used medical procedures in the world. It originated in China over 5,000 years ago and is effective in treating a variety of health problems. Acupuncture is rapidly gaining acceptance in mainstream allopathic medicine. As of 1997, an estimated one-third of certified acupuncturists in the United States are medical doctors (Culliton, 1997). The use of acupuncture needles is officially approved for use by licensed practitioners.

One of the major reasons Americans use acupuncture is for relief of chronic pain, especially pain caused by arthritis or low back disorders (Bullock, Pheley, Kiresuk, Lenz, & Culliton, 1997). Several studies on acupuncture have been sponsored by the NCCAM, including:

- A small randomized controlled clinical trial that showed more than half the women with a major depressive episode who received acupuncture therapy improved significantly (Allen, 1998) (Figure 31-6).
- Another study found that **moxibustion** (application of heat from certain burning substances, such as herbs, at acupuncture points on the body) applied to pregnant women with breech presentations significantly increased the number of normal head-first births (Cardini & Weixin, 1998).

### Acupressure

Acupressure is similar to acupuncture in its application and its effect. The difference is that rather than using fine, solid needles to stimulate acupuncture points, the

practitioner uses consistent and firm pressure from fingers or other devices. Antiemetic armbands can be applied to the wrists, and beads on the bands place pressure on the acupuncture point that is specific to relief of nausea.

### Body Work Therapies

One of the most universal CAM modalities is various forms of touch. **Touch,** simply defined, is the means of perceiving or experiencing through tactile sensation. According to anthropologist Montague (1986), touch is the earliest sense to develop in humans, and thus it provides a basic means of interacting with others and the environment. Tactile stimulation is necessary for survival and the healthy behavioral development of an individual (Bowlby, 1984). Touch carries with it taboos and prescriptions. It was used in all ancient cultures and shamanistic traditions for healing. The advent of scientific medicine and Puritanism led many healers away from the purposeful use of touch. Some cultures are very comfortable with physical touch; others specify that touch may be used only in certain situations within specified parameters. In addition, the use of gloves by health care providers adds to the difficulty of contact and the use of therapeutic touch.

Because touch involves personal contact, the nurse must be sure to convey positive intentions. When in doubt, the nurse should withhold touch until effective communication with the client has been established. Touch has several important uses in nursing practice in that it:

## RESEARCH FOCUS

**Title of Study:** Preoperative intradermal acupuncture reduces postoperative pain, nausea and vomiting, analgesic requirement, and sympathoadrenal responses

**Study Purpose:** The purpose of the study was to determine if the stimulation of acupuncture points in the preoperative period would reduce postoperative pain.

**Methods:** Preoperative abdominal surgery clients were randomly assigned to an acupuncture group or a control group. Acupuncture needles were placed in the experimental group members prior to induction of anesthesia. They were removed postoperatively. Both groups received postoperative analgesia through epidural morphine. Morphine use, incision pain at rest, incision pain with coughing, visceral pain, nausea, and plasma cortisol and epinephrine levels were measured in recovery and 4 days thereafter in both groups.

**Findings:** Researchers found that from the recovery room on, clients in the acupuncture group reported good pain relief. Acupuncture clients used 50% less morphine, had 30% less nausea, and plasma cortisol and epinephrine concentrations were less in clients who received acupuncture in recovery and on the first postoperative day.

**Implications:** When used preoperatively, acupuncture is effective in enhancing pain relief, while reducing nausea and stress (as indicated by cortisol and adrenaline levels), in abdominal surgery clients. Therefore, acupuncture may be a technique that nurses can support as a preoperative intervention option for clients. In addition, this research study adds to the need for nurses to think positively toward alternative therapies.

Kotani, N., Hashimoto, H., Sato, Y., Sessler, D. I., Yoshioka, H., Kitayma, M., Yasuda, T., & Matsuki, A. (2001). Preoperative intradermal acupuncture reduces postoperative pain, nausea and vomiting, analgesic requirement, and sympathoadrenal responses. *Anesthesiology, 95*(2), 349–356.

- Is an integral part of assessment
- Promotes bonding between nurse and client
- Is an important means of communication, especially when other senses are impaired
- Assists in soothing, calming, and comforting
- Helps keep the client oriented

## STOP AND THINK

### Using Gloves When Applying Therapeutic Touch

1. How has the use of latex gloves, decreasing the amount of skin-to-skin contact, affected client care?
2. What are the implications for judicious use of gloves?
3. How might decreased skin-to-skin contact affect the nurse-client relationship?

### Therapeutic Massage

**Therapeutic massage** is the application of pressure and motion by the hands with the intent of improving the recipient's well-being. Massage increases muscle circulation, promotes removal of toxins, and leads to muscular relaxation. It involves kneading, rubbing, and using friction. The primary techniques used to perform a massage are described in Box 31-7.

For the past 30 years, many touch therapies have been assimilated into mainstream nursing practice. Massage therapy is now recognized as a highly beneficial modality and is prescribed by a number of physicians. In addition, most states now have licensing requirements for massage practitioners. While only licensed massage therapists can perform therapeutic massage, nurses and physical therapists commonly use massage techniques to promote client relaxation and healing.

Traditionally, back rubs have been administered by nurses to provide comfort to hospitalized clients. Today, they are considered standard practice. Massage techniques can be used with all age groups and are especially beneficial to those who are immobilized. A back rub or massage can promote relaxation, increased circulation of the blood and lymph, and relief from musculoskeletal stiffness, pain, and spasm. Research (Beeken, Parks, Cory, & Montopoli, 1998) suggests that individuals with chronic obstructive

## CLINICAL ALERT

### Contraindications for Touch

It is important to know when *not* to touch. It may be difficult for persons who have been neglected, abused, or injured to accept touch therapy. Touching those who are distrustful or angry may escalate negative behaviors. Persons with burns or overly sensitive skin may not benefit from touch.

### BOX 31-7   BASIC MASSAGE TECHNIQUES

**Effleurage:**
- The whole hand is used.
- Gliding and long rhythmic strokes are used.
- Firm, even-pressured strokes are directed toward the heart to assist blood return.
- Lighter pressure is used when moving away from the heart.

**Petrissage:**
- Pressing, squeezing, kneading, and rolling movements by both hands (use entire hand) are used.
- Deep circulation is enhanced.
- C-shaped motions stimulate the muscle body.
- Promotes muscle relaxation.

**Friction:**
- Thumb pads, heel of hand, or fingertips are used.
- Focused, deep, circular motions are used.
- Penetrates deeper muscle layers.
- Is done after effleurage and petrissage.

**Tapotement:**
- Palms, fingertips, and knuckles are used.
- Brisk, vigorous, rhythmic, percussive movements are used.
- Hands alternately tap, cup, slap, and pummel muscles.
- Invigorates and stimulates tired muscles.

**Vibration:**
- Very fine, rapid, shaking movements are administered by the entire hand.
- Stimulates or relaxes muscles.

### CLINICAL ALERT

#### Precautions with Massage

- Massage should be used with caution for people with heart disease, diabetes, hypertension, or kidney disease because increased circulation in these conditions may be harmful.

- Massage should never be attempted in areas of circulatory abnormalities such as aneurysm, varicose veins, necrosis, phlebitis, or thrombus or in areas of soft-tissue injury, open wounds, inflammation, joint or bone injury, dermatitis, recent surgery, or sciatica.

### Shiatsu

**Shiatsu** is a combination of acupressure, massage, and joint manipulation. It is based on a Japanese methodology but is heavily influenced by TCM. *Shiatsu* literally means "finger pressure." As with acupuncture, the focus of the shiatsu practitioner is to unblock *chi* flow by application of pressure, massage, and manipulation along meridians in the body. As with all CAM modalities, the shiatsu practitioner must be grounded and focused to promote the client's healing. Being grounded and focused also aids the practitioner in not taking on the client's energy.

### Rolfing

**Rolfing** is a form of deep tissue massage and manipulation to correct body posture. The rolfing practitioner focuses on one specific body part and applies pressure to loosen connective tissue or fascia. This results in lengthening and relaxation of the fascia. This results in the body's correct alignment being restored. Usually 10 sessions are required to completely restore body alignment. It is believed that the corrected body alignment allows the body to restore natural healing.

### Reflexology

**Reflexology** is rooted in ancient healing arts. Egyptian wall paintings from approximately 2300 BC show the use of reflexology. Contemporary use of reflexology is credited to the work of William H. Fitzgerald, an American physician, who, in the early 1900s, discovered that applying pressure to certain parts of the fingers could relieve pain in other body parts (Cassileth, 1998). In the 1930s, Eunice Ingham discovered that certain points on the feet were more responsive to pressure and provided better pain relief than points on the hand.

The fundamental concept of reflexology is that the body is divided into 10 equal, longitudinal zones that run the length of the body from the top of the head to the tip of the toes. These 10 zones are correlated with the 10 fingers and toes. The foot is viewed as a microcosm of the entire body. Reflexology theory posits that illness

lung disease benefit from massage therapy. The subjects in this study experienced positive changes in heart rate, oxygen saturation, and blood pressure as a result of massage. Procedure 31-1 describes the techniques involved in performing a massage. Boards of Nursing in some states (e.g., Louisiana, Massachusetts) state that it is within the scope of nursing practice for nurses to employ complementary therapies, including massage (Louisiana State Board of Nursing, 1999; Massachusetts Board of Registration in Nursing, 1997). The National Association of Nurse Massage Therapists (NANMT) was established in 1990 to promote professional ethical standards for nurse massage therapists. The NANMT-established standards reflect those of the American Nurses Association.

**PROCEDURE 31-1**          **Therapeutic Massage**

## EQUIPMENT NEEDED

- Flat sheet (Figure 31-7)
- 1 or 2 pillows
- Lotion or oil
- Bath blanket or light coverlet
- Towel
- Tape or CD player

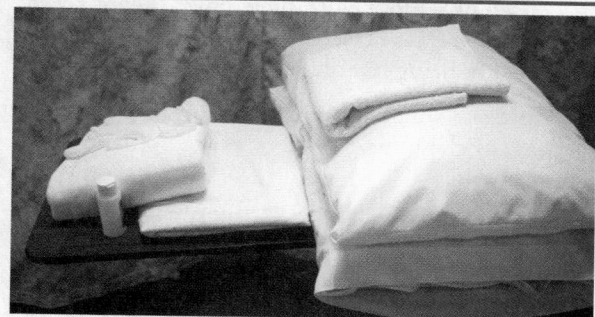

**Figure 31-7    Lotion or oil is used to reduce friction. Towels and light blankets are used to keep the client warm and comfortable.**

## IMPLEMENTATION—ACTION/RATIONALE

| ACTION | RATIONALE |
|---|---|
| 1. Set room temperature at approximately 75°F. Provide low or indirect lighting, privacy, and background music. | 1. Maintains client's body heat, protects privacy, and promotes relaxation. |
| 2. Prepare the massage table or hospital bed by placing a clean sheet on the surface. Adjust the surface height. | 2. Both the massage table and hospital bed can be adjusted so that the height of the work surface can be raised or lowered as necessary. |
| 3. Remove your rings and watches. Wash hands. | 3. Avoids scratching the client and reduces the transmission of microorganisms. |
| 4. Explain the procedure to the client. | 4. Prepares the client for the treatment. |
| 5. Assist the client to either a prone, supine, or sitting position, depending on client's condition (Figure 31-8). | 5. Appropriate position enables the nurse to apply the necessary amount of pressure to the back without causing discomfort to the client. |

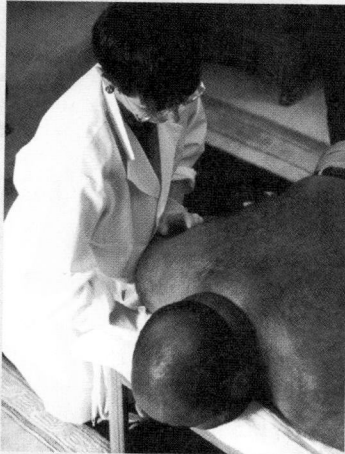

**Figure 31-8    Position the client sitting or prone. Assess for comfort prior to beginning the procedure.**

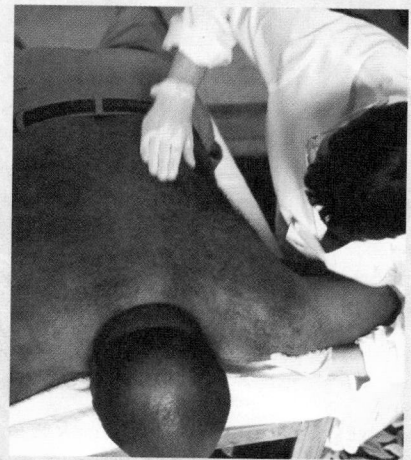

**Figure 31-9    Massage gently but firmly, keeping your hands in contact with the client's skin.**

*(continues)*

## PROCEDURE 31-1 (*continued*)

6. Loosen or remove clothing from the client's back and arms. Drape the client with a sheet to cover areas not being treated directly.

6. Exposes parts of the back on which the massage will be performed. Draping untreated parts of the back helps keep the client warm.

7. Squeeze a small amount of lotion or oil into the palm of the hand to warm before applying to the client.

7. Cold lotion or oil can cause discomfort to the client.

8. Begin with light to medium effleurage at lower back and continue upward following muscle groups, being careful to avoid the spine and spinal processes. Move hands up toward the base of the neck and continue outward over the trapezius muscles with circular motions, over and around shoulders and upper arms, and return with lighter downward strokes laterally over the latissimus dorsi to the upper gluteals. Use slow, rhythmic movements, keeping in contact with the skin at all times. Check pressure. Continue the effleurage for approximately 3 minutes (Figure 31-9).

8. Prevents damage to internal structures, stimulates circulation, and promotes relaxation.

9. Continue treatment, if appropriate, with gentle petrissage (see explanation in text; Figure 31-10) to major muscle groups in the back, shoulders, and upper arms (Figure 31-11).

9. Enhances circulation, stimulates muscles, and promotes relaxation.

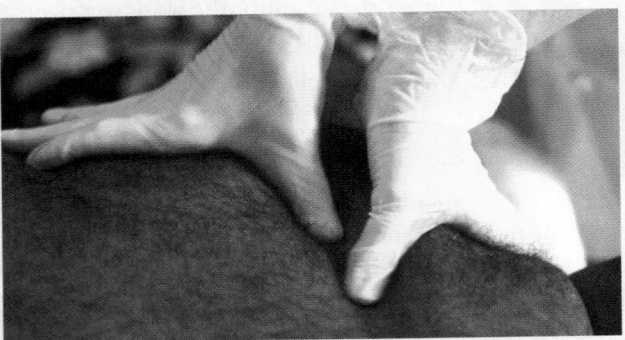

**Figure 31-10** Petrissage involves pressing, squeezing, kneading, and rolling hand movements.

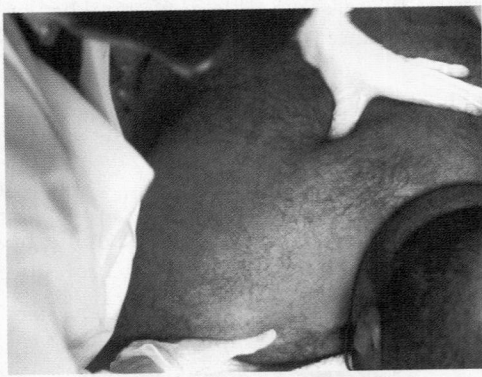

**Figure 31-11** As the massage continues, move outward from the neck to the upper back and shoulders.

10. Use friction on particular muscle groups where tension is being held.

10. Penetrates deeper muscle layers, thus promoting further relaxation.

11. Use tapotement to stimulate any muscle groups that may be fatigued (Figure 31-12).

11. Invigorates and stimulates tired muscles.

12. Finish treatment with effleurage (Figure 31-13).

12. Assists with relaxation and provides a sense of completion.

13. Wipe any excess lotion or oil from skin with a towel, or use a small amount of warm soap and water to clean the client's skin, taking care to dry it completely.

13. Promotes and maintains skin integrity.

*(continues)*

## PROCEDURE 31-1 (continued)

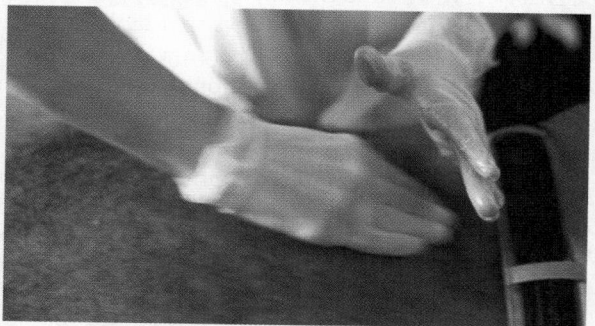

**Figure 31-12** Use hands to tap, cup, slap, and pummel muscles to stimulate fatigued muscle groups.

14. Assist client into a comfortable position for a period of rest or sleep.

15. Document treatment, client's response, and skin assessment data.

16. Wash hands.

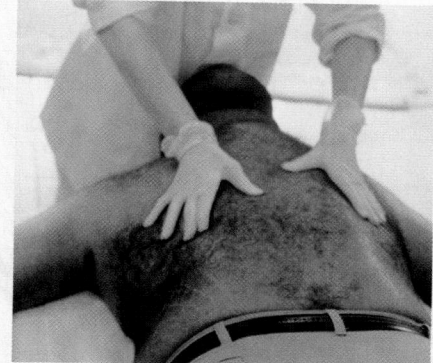

**Figure 31-13** Finish the massage with effleurage—long, gliding, rhythmic strokes.

14. Allows client to fully experience the therapeutic benefit of massage.

15. Communicates pertinent data to other members of treatment team; promotes continuity of care.

16. Reduces the transmission of microorganisms.

---

## LIFE SPAN CONSIDERATIONS

### Therapeutic Massage

#### Pediatric Variations

- Pediatric clients are often fearful of strange situations and strange people. Therapeutic massage is contraindicated in these clients.

- Pediatric clients who have been neglected or abused may respond negatively to therapeutic massage.

#### Geriatric Variations

- Geriatric clients are more likely to be confused and may misinterpret the intent of the therapeutic massage. They may become combative or react in other inappropriate ways.

- Geriatric clients are more likely to be immobilized. Therapeutic massage is especially beneficial for these clients.

- Massage over bony prominences in an older person with thin skin may increase the potential of developing a pressure sore. Very carefully and gently massage the skin around these areas.

manifests itself in calcium deposits and acids in the corresponding part of the person's foot. Pressing specific points on the foot stimulates energy movement and produces relaxation, reduces stress, and promotes health by relieving pressures and accumulation of toxins in the corresponding body part (Figure 31-14).

Massage of specific points on the feet and hands promotes energy flow to corresponding organs and body parts. Reflexology has been shown to be effective in stress relief. It is believed to facilitate healing in the body organs and to restore balance to the body.

### COMMUNITY/HOME CARE

### Therapeutic Massage

- The home care setting is often more relaxing for the client and can increase the effectiveness of therapeutic massage. Provide for privacy.

- Clients in long-term care are sometimes in the position of receiving decreased contact and human touch. Therapeutic massage is one method of increasing clients' level of awareness and involvement in the surrounding world.

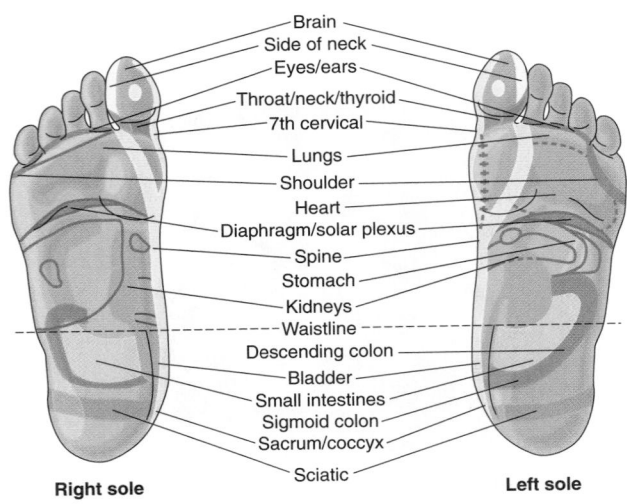

Brain
Side of neck
Eyes/ears
Throat/neck/thyroid
7th cervical
Lungs
Shoulder
Heart
Diaphragm/solar plexus
Spine
Stomach
Kidneys
Waistline
Descending colon
Bladder
Small intestines
Sigmoid colon
Sacrum/coccyx
Sciatic

**Right sole**          **Left sole**

**Figure 31-14** **Foot reflexology charts.** *Reproduced with permission from* **Better health with foot reflexology.** *Copyright 1983 by Dwight C. Byers. Ingham Publishing, Inc., POB 12642, St. Petersburg, FL 33733-2642.*

## Spiritual Modalities

A basic premise of spiritual modalities is that one's health is dependent upon the spiritual aspects of oneself. When the body or mind is disrupted or unhealthy, it reflects a spiritual imbalance. Thus spiritual interventions will facilitate whole-body healing. See Chapter 48 for a discussion of the relationship between spirituality and health. The idea that there is a relationship between spirituality and health is not new. "At the core of many holistic modalities are spirituality and healing, which encompass a person's values, meaning, and purpose in life . . . The concept of spirit implies a quality of transcendence, a guiding force,

---

### LIFE SPAN CONSIDERATIONS

#### Spirituality in Older Clients

Older adults may have a well-developed sense of their spirituality, or they may have never confronted their spiritual concerns until diagnosed with a serious or terminal illness. Furthermore, older adults tend to be more involved in religious activities and to state that religion is very important in their daily lives. Consequently, spiritual modalities in older clients may be easier to implement than in other age groups.

Davidhizar, R., Bechtel, G. A. & Cosey, E. J. (2000). The spiritual needs of hospitalized patients. *American Journal of Nursing,* 100(7), 24C–D.

---

or something outside the self and beyond the individual nurse or patient" (Dossey, 1998).

The role of the spirit in healing is witnessed in all cultures. The inseparable link between the state of one's soul (life energy or spirit) and the state of one's health is accepted by many cultures. Healers believe that biologic changes are a result of therapeutic changes in a person's soul or spirit. Scientists, specifically psychoneuroimmunologists, are beginning to validate that there are inner mechanisms of healing within individuals.

Health maintenance implies having a balanced spiritual life. Dossey and Dossey (1998) quote a study that examined factors contributing to successful coronary artery bypass surgery. The best single predictor of survival was the degree of religious faith and spiritual meaning in the client's life. "Over 250 studies now show that religious practice—the specific religion doesn't seem to matter—is correlated with greater health and increase longevity" (Dossey & Dossey, 1998, p. 37).

### Faith Healing

At the heart of spiritual or faith healing is the practitioner's belief that one has to purify one's self and reach a state of unity with God or a Higher Power. This process, based on religious belief, is usually done through prayer. During preparation for healing, the practitioner adapts a passive and receptive mood in order to be a channel for divine power. To benefit from the healer's intervention, the ill person is best healed if she has faith in the healer and/or the deity that the healer represents.

### Healing Prayer

When individuals pray, they believe they are communicating directly with God or a Higher Power. Prayer is an integral part of a person's spiritual life and, as such, can affect well-being. Florence Nightingale (1860) recognized that prayer helps connect individuals to nature and the environment. Many religions adhere to established rituals for organized prayer. For example, Tibetan Buddhists use prayer wheels—wooden and metal cylinders with prayers written on them. Islam has five periods of prayer scheduled daily. Some religious groups, such as Christian Scientists, rely on prayer in lieu of conventional medical therapy due to the belief that prayer alone can heal disease (Cassileth, 1998). "Research has shown that religious practices such as worship attendance and prayer have significant health and survival implications" (Fontaine, 2000, p. 346). Medical research is currently investigating the effects of prayer on physical health. The exact mechanism for the effect of prayer on healing is not known. However, "people are nourished by life-affirming beliefs and philosophies. They meditate and say prayers that elicit physiological calm and a sense of peacefulness, both of which contribute to longer survival" (Fontaine, 2000, p. 346). Cassileth (1998) states:

There is no doubt about the numerous benefits of prayer and spirituality: solace in times of suffering, uncertainty, and loss; a community of people who share one's values and beliefs; principles to help guide us through difficult situations. These benefits are helpful and healing in the deepest sense of the term. (p. 312)

Larry Dossey (1998), a physician, is so strongly convinced of prayer's effect on health that he postulates that treatment plans should include prayer.

## Shamanism

As previously described in this chapter, shamanism is a form of spiritual healing. With the increased interest in CAM modalities, many clients are turning to shamans to assist in healing and well-being. Shamans, both priest and healer, work with a variety of modalities to enhance healing, but spiritual guidance underlies all shamanic practice. The shaman connects with spiritual guides and seeks healing on behalf of the client.

## Nutritional and Diet Therapies

In the last 30 years, nutritional interventions for prevention and treatment of disease have received increased interest from consumers and health care providers. Allopathic researchers have been able to clearly demonstrate a link between diet and cardiac disease, diabetes, and some forms of cancer, specifically gastrointestinal cancers. Based upon this research, allopathic practitioners recommend a diet high in fiber, low in fat, and high in fruits and vegetables. Nutritional therapies discussed here will be focused on CAM therapies, which have less, but increasing, scientific support.

### Nutraceuticals

Currently, many foods are being studied for their medicinal value. **Nutraceuticals** refer to any natural substances found in plant or animal foods that act as protective or healing agents. **Phytonutrients** refer to those chemicals found in plants; see Table 31-7 for a listing of the major phytonutrients and their actions.

Foods that are being investigated by the National Cancer Institute for possible cancer preventive qualities include carrots, celery, citrus fruits, flaxseed, garlic, licorice root, parsley, and soybeans.

The best source of nutrients is fresh whole foods, preferably eaten in their natural form. The standard Western diet lacks many essential nutrients due to processing and contains many harmful additives. In contrast, the TCM diet contains fresh, semiraw, and slightly cooked ingredients. "Ultimately, one might say there is much wisdom in the ancient Chinese view of food. The Chinese diet emphasizes natural food alchemy taking place inside the body by virtue of food enzyme activity, instead of the synthetic food alchemy that we now accept in the package processed goods the Western consumer has been conditioned to buy" (Froemming, 1998, p. 45).

## Vitamins and Supplements: Antioxidants and Free Radicals

Vitamins and other supplements have long been believed to be effective in promoting health. While a healthy, balanced diet should provide all the vitamins and minerals the body needs, many Americans eat unbalanced diets and thus need vitamin supplementation. Vitamins and minerals for supplementation are different than vitamins used for CAM. Vitamins and minerals in CAM traditionally are used in doses higher than recommended daily doses of vitamins and minerals. Research has just begun on the health benefits of vitamins and minerals used in CAM.

Vitamins C and E, and beta-carotene which converts to vitamin A, may prevent heart disease and some forms of cancer. Antioxidants exert several beneficial effects, including prevention of cancer, reduction of heart disease, and possible retardation of the aging process (Ferguson & Ferguson, 2000, p. 28). Antioxidants neutralize free radicals, preventing them from damaging cells or altering DNA. Sources of dietary antioxidants include vitamin C (in fruits and vegetables), vitamin $B_6$ (whole grains), vitamin A (metabolized from beta-carotene), beta-carotene (yellow-orange pigment in fruits and vegetables), and vitamin E (in polyunsaturated oils, butter, and eggs). The antioxidants devour free radicals (unstable molecules that alter genetic codes and trigger the development of cancer growth in cells).

Other vitamins, minerals, trace elements, and enzymes are being investigated for possible therapeutic value. See Chapter 35 for a thorough discussion of the essential vitamins, their functions, and major sources.

Other supplemental vitamins, minerals, and trace elements have been studied or are being studied for their health benefits. For instance, calcium supplements are believed to be beneficial in prevention of osteoarthritis, while it is also believed to have a sedative effect if taken before bedtime. Chromium is believed to play a role in blood sugar regulation via enhancement of fat metabolism. Folic acid is commonly prescribed in early pregnancy as it enhances neurodevelopment of the fetus. Iron supplements aid in treating some forms of chronic anemia. A final example of beneficial supplements is the omega-3 fatty acids. Omega-3 fatty acids, most commonly found in fish oils, have been found to support immune system function and help mediate allergic response, especially in persons with allergy-induced asthma (Roth & Townsend, 2002).

## CLINICAL ALERT

### Fat-Soluble Vitamins

Fat-soluble vitamins (e.g., vitamins A and E) are stored in the body. Ingestion of large amounts of these vitamins in supplement form can lead to serious adverse health effects.

## TABLE 31-7   ACTIONS AND SOURCES OF MAJOR PHYTONUTRIENTS

| Phytonutrient | Sources | Actions |
|---|---|---|
| Ascorbic acid | Citrus fruits, broccoli, most fruits and vegetables | Binds iron, preventing it from becoming a cancer-causing preoxidant |
| Capsaicin | Red chili peppers | Helps prevent carcinogens from binding with DNA at the cellular level |
| Catechins | Green tea, black tea | Reduces the risk of gastrointestinal cancers |
| Fiber lignans | Soybeans, flaxseed, nuts | Inhibits growth of tumors |
| Fiber pectins | Apples, pears, plums, prunes | Improves colon health; encourages growth of beneficial intestinal flora |
| Lycopene | Tomatoes, tomato sauce | Protects against prostate cancer; helps block UVA and UVB rays |
| Phytoestrogens | Soy products, alfalfa sprouts | Helps reduce menopausal symptoms; may block some cancers (i.e., breast, prostate) |
| Phytosterols | Plant oils, corn, sesame, soy, safflower, pumpkin, wheat | Inhibits uptake of cholesterol from foods; blocks hormonal role in cancer production |
| Protease inhibitors | Soybeans and soy products, eggs, cereals, potatoes | Protects against negative effects of radiation and free radical damage; prevents activation of certain genes that cause cancer |
| Sulfur compounds | Onions, garlic | Lowers blood pressure; improves immune system response; fights infections; antimicrobial effect; lowers cholesterol; reduces triglycerides |

Data from Froemming, P. (1998). *The best guide to alternative medicine.* Los Angeles: Renaissance Books; Mayo Clinic. (2000). *Women's Healthsource, 4*(2), 1–2; Weil, A. (2000). *Eating well for optimum health: The essential guide to food, diet, and nutrition.* New York: Alfred A. Knopf.

### Herbal Therapy

Herbal medicine has been a powerful tool in folk healing for centuries. Medicinal herbs have been catalogued for thousands of years. The earliest record of herbal remedies was found in ancient Egypt. More than 500 herbal remedies were recorded on papyrus during that time.

Herbal remedies are prevalent throughout the world. Most herbs that are used are indigenous to various cultures. Only recently have herbs been transported for use by persons of other cultures. Outside of industrialized countries, herbs may be the primary form of medication.

Herbal medicine, also known as botanical medicine or phytotherapy, uses plant extracts for therapeutic outcomes. Many holistic practitioners incorporate the use of herbs into their practice.

Learning about herbal treatment is similar to learning pharmacology. Herbs work because of their chemical composition. Different herbs contain different compounds that can strengthen the immune system, alter the blood chemistry, or protect specific organs against

### NURSING STRATEGY

#### Tips for the Use of Herbs

- During client assessment, assess use of herbs, herbal teas, vitamins, minerals, and other over-the-counter supplements.

- Discuss the risks and benefits of herbs and supplements.

- Refer the client to a qualified herbalist if client is using herbs and has not already seen an herbalist.

Robbers, J., & Tyler, V. (1999). *Tyler's herbs of choice.* New York: Haworth Herbal Press.

### Using Herbs to Promote Health and Healing

Share these tips with your clients:

✓ Do not self-prescribe herbs. Consult with a qualified herbalist prior to using herbs. Many states are moving to certification or licensure of herbalists.

✓ Report herb use to your primary care provider and pharmacists. Some herbs and allopathic medications can cause serious drug interactions (Table 31-10).

✓ Take the herbs as recommended by the herbalist. Do not take any herb for extended periods of time. Herbs are used with the idea of returning the body to a healthy state. Overuse of herbs can lead to a new imbalance in the body.

Herbal Remedies. (2003).  http://www.nhlmedical.org

disease. Peppermint oil may help relieve the symptoms of irritable bowel syndrome by exerting a relaxant effect on the muscles of the gastrointestinal tract (Pittler & Ernst, 1998). "Herbal immune system enhancers help the body fight common viral illnesses and assist in preventing the overuse of antibiotics" (Collins, 2000, p. 3). Echinacea is frequently used for its immune-enhancing properties. However, it should not be taken longer than 8 to 10 consecutive weeks due to the potential for liver toxicity. Table 31-8 lists medicinal uses of commonly used herbs.

In the past decade, more than 53,000 natural products were tested by the National Cancer Institute. Approximately one-third of all new cancer therapies are derived from natural sources (Cassileth, 1998). Many drugs commonly used today were folk remedies derived from plants. For example, salicin, the active chemical ingredient found in white willow bark, has been used by TCM practitioners and Native Americans for pain relief. This same salicin is a precursor to salicylic acid, an ingredient in aspirin.

Herbs are not to be used indiscriminately, as their use may result in some negative outcomes. Some individuals may experience allergic reactions to certain herbs (Table 31-9).

Consumers need to be taught the following regarding herbs and allergies: to recognize the potential for developing allergic reactions to herbs, to identify the indicators of such reactions, and to immediately stop using the herb if allergic symptoms occur.

Individuals using herbs need to understand that problems can occur when taking herbal products and medications concurrently. The chemical constituents of herbs may alter the effects of some medications (Table 31-10).

## Other CAM Modalities

The mind-body, body-movement manipulation, energy and body work, spiritual, and nutritional treatment modalities are not the only available CAM modalities. Others, such as aromatherapy, homeopathy, humor, pet therapy, and music therapy, are being used as methods to improve health status.

### Aromatherapy

**Aromatherapy** is defined as the therapeutic use of concentrated essences or essential oils that have been extracted from plants and flowers. When diluted in a carrier oil for massage or in warm water for inhalation, essences may be stimulating, uplifting, relaxing, or soothing. Essential oils help relax the mind and the body by promoting balance between the sympathetic and parasympathetic nervous systems. They stimulate the production of endorphins and rejuvenate the immune system (Froemming, 1998). "Essential oils enter the body in several ways. They can be absorbed through

## NURSING STRATEGY

### Guidelines for Using Aromatherapy

● Always dilute essential oils in a carrier oil.

● Do a skin patch test for sensitivity before applying essential oils to the skin.

● Avoid contact with the eyes.

● Inhale essential oils only for short periods of time.

● Store in dark glass bottles, tightly capped and away from heat and sunlight.

● Store only in glass containers, not plastic.

● Use only pure essential oils, not synthetics.

## CLINICAL ALERT

### Precautions with Essential Oils

Some essential oils can trigger asthma attacks or epileptic seizures, cause harm to people with cancer, or elevate or depress blood pressure. Instruct clients with asthma, cancer, epilepsy, or hypertension, or those who are pregnant to avoid the use of essential oils.

## TABLE 31-8    MEDICINAL VALUE OF HERBS

| Herb | Medicinal Use(s) | Herb | Medicinal Use(s) |
|---|---|---|---|
| Aloe vera (Aloe vera) | • Promotes wound healing<br>• Minor cuts and abrasions<br>• Burns | Ginger (continued) | • Stimulates circulation in feet and hands<br>• Expectorant<br>• Helps relieve indigestion and flatulence<br>• Diarrhea |
| Calendula (Calendula officinalis) | • Promotes wound healing<br>• Cuts, abrasions<br>• Minor burns<br>• Sunburn<br>• Acne<br>• Athlete's foot<br>• Oral thrush (as a mouthwash)<br>• Vaginal thrush (as a douche) | Ginkgo (Ginkgo biloba) | • Enhances cerebral blood flow<br>• Mild depression<br>• Dementia<br>• Impotence<br>• Peripheral vascular insufficiency<br>• PMS<br>• Memory impairment |
| Celery seed (Apium graveolens) | • Cholesterol-lowering effect<br>• Dizziness, headache<br>• Diuretic effect | Lavender (Lavandula angustifolia) | • Headache<br>• Reduces muscle spasms<br>• Increases relaxation |
| Chamomile (Matricaria chamomilla; Anthemis nobilis) | • Produces a calming effect<br>• Nausea<br>• Tension headache | Milk thistle (Silybum marianum) | • Liver disorders<br>• Hepatitis<br>• Cirrhosis<br>• Gallstones |
| Dandelion (Taraxacum officinale) | • Produces a diuretic effect<br>• Helps decrease edema (especially that of premenstrual water retention)<br>• Indigestion | Peppermint (Mentha × peperita) | • Headache<br>• Sinus congestion<br>• Digestive aid |
| Eucalyptus (Eucalyptus globulus) | • Antibacterial<br>• Produces a decongestant effect | Saint John's wort (Hypericum pereforatum) | • Mild to moderate depression<br>• Sleep disorders<br>• Viral infections |
| Evening primrose (Oenothera biennis) | • Atopic eczema<br>• Asthma<br>• Migraine<br>• PMS symptoms (e.g., mood swings, breast pain, and tenderness)<br>• Arthritis | Sage (Salvia officinalis) | • Antibacterial properties |
| Feverfew (Tanacetum parthenium) | • Migraine headache | Thyme (Thymus vulgaris, T. serphyllum) | • Antibacterial properties<br>• Helps relieve symptoms of common cold<br>• Antispasmodic effect on bronchioles<br>• Relieves cystitis<br>• Antifungal effect (especially when applied as a lotion for athlete's foot<br>• As a mouthwash for oral thrush |
| Garlic (Allium sativum) | • Decreases cholesterol<br>• Helps protect against and treat respiratory infections<br>• Expectorant in cases of bronchitis or a cold | Valerian (Valeriana officinalis) | • Sedative effect<br>• Counters insomnia |
| Ginger (Zingiber officinale) | • Nausea (especially effective with motion sickness and morning sickness associated with pregnancy) | White willow (Salix alba) | • Headache<br>• Fever<br>• Muscular aches and pains |

Note: This information is not intended to be a guide for self-medication or the treatment of others. Consult a health care practitioner trained in the use of herbs before consuming any herb for medicinal purposes.

Adapted from Goldberg, B. (1999). *Alternative medicine: The definitive guide.* Tiburon, CA: Future Medicine Publishing; Ody, P. (1999). *100 great natural remedies: Using healing plants at home.* New York: Barnes & Noble; Tierra, M. (1998). *The way of herbs.* New York: Pocket Books.

## TABLE 31-9  POSSIBLE REACTIONS TO CERTAIN HERBS

| Botanical | Reaction |
| --- | --- |
| Apricot | Contact allergy |
| Arnica | Contact allergy |
| Celery | Photosensitivity |
| Garlic | Systemic reaction |
| Motherwort | Photosensitivity |
| Tansy | Systemic reaction |

Data from Mustalish, S. H. (2000). Avoiding allergic reactions in children from botanical medicines. *Integrative Medicine Consult, 1,* 6.

## BOX 31-8  CONDITIONS RESPONSIVE TO AROMATHERAPY

- Stress and anxiety-related problems
- Muscular and rheumatic pains
- Digestive disorders (e.g., nausea)
- Female sexual health conditions (e.g., PMS, postpartal problems, and menopausal symptoms)
- Skin conditions

the skin and passed into the circulatory system. Oils can also be inhaled, passing into the bloodstream through the lungs, or by causing signals to be transmitted through the nervous system directly into the limbic system of the brain" (Walters, 1999, p. 16).

Aromatherapists use concentrated oils derived from roots, bark, or flowers of herbs and other plants to treat specific ailments. The aromas cause physiological, psychological, and pharmacological reactions within a person (Schnaubelt, 1999). Aromatherapy is used to treat a variety of conditions and promote a sense of well-being (see Box 31-8).

Some essential oils have antibacterial properties and are found in a wide variety of pharmaceutical preparations. Essential oils should be used intelligently and with caution.

## TABLE 31-10  INTERACTIONS BETWEEN HERBS AND MEDICATIONS

| Herbal Product | Drug | Effect When Combined |
| --- | --- | --- |
| Aloe | • Thiazide diuretics and corticosteroids<br>• Cardiac glycosides and antiarrhythmic agents | • Enhanced potassium loss<br>• Potentiated by potassium loss |
| Belladonna | Tricyclic antidepressants, amantadine, quinidine | Increased anticholinergic effect |
| Brewer's yeast | MAO inhibitor antidepressants | Increased blood pressure |
| Danshen | Warfarin | • Increased warfarin bioavailability<br>• Increased prothrombin time |
| Ginkgo | Warfarin, heparin | Increased risk of bleeding |
| Licorice root | • Acetaminophen<br>• Antihypertensives<br>• Estrogens<br>• Fludrocortisone<br>• Thiazide diuretics and corticosteroids | • Accelerated acetaminophen excretion<br>• Decreased antihypertensive effect<br>• Increased estrogenic effect<br>• Increased blood pressure<br>• Enhanced potassium loss |

Adapted from Blumenthal, M., Goldberg, A., & Brinkman, J. (Eds.) (2000). *Herbal medicine: Expanded commission E monographs.* Newton, MA: Integrative Medicine Communications; Lilley, L. L., & Gunk, R. (1998). Grapefruit and medication: Help your patient understand potential dangers of food–drug interactions. *American Journal of Nursing, 98*(12), 10.

## Humor

Of all the complementary interventions presented in this chapter, humor is the one that can be used most often to promote wellness (Figure 31-15). Humor is a frequently used CAM modality. Fritz (1998) questioned clients with chronic cancer pain about self-initiated, nondrug measures that they used to cope with pain. The clients rated laughing as the most effective type of therapy.

Humor has many therapeutic outcomes, including:

- Increased ability to cope with pain
- Enhanced immune functioning
- Reduced preprocedural anxiety

Former chairman of the Task Force in Psychoneuroimmunology at the School of Medicine at UCLA, Norman Cousins, related how he enhanced his recovery from an incurable connective tissue disorder, ankylosing spondylitis, by the daily watching of films and movies that made him laugh (Cousins, 1979). Humor can be used effectively to relieve anxiety and promote relaxation, improve respiratory function, enhance immunological function, and decrease pain by stimulating the production of endorphins.

It is important to determine the client's perception of what is humorous in order to avoid offending. Differentiation between humorous and offensive situations varies greatly from culture to culture and person to person. Nurses can use humor with clients in a variety of ways. A humor cart (portable cart or carrier filled with joke books, magic tricks, and funny videos) is easy to use and allows clients to select their own humor tools for health. The type of humor should be age-appropriate and culturally sensitive.

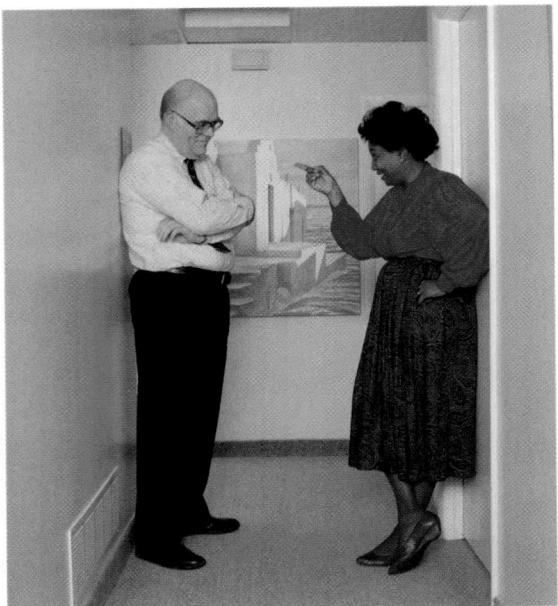

**Figure 31-15** Humor and laughter are effective means of promoting wellness.

---

### NURSING STRATEGY

## Using Humor as a Therapeutic Intervention

- Establish a trusting nurse-client relationship.

- Conduct a humor assessment to determine the type of humor appreciated by the client and the client's usual response to humor.

- Follow the client's lead in the type of humorous strategies used (i.e., jokes, satire, puns).

- Involve the family and significant others in the humor.

- Use humor as an adjunct, not a substitute, for pain medication.

- Continually evaluate the humor strategy for its effectiveness.

Data modified from Smith, N., & Oliver, N. (1998). Using humor while caring for patients. *American Journal of Nursing*, *98*(12), 14.

---

### Pet Therapy

The use of animals to enhance health status has a long history. In Britain in the 18th and 19th centuries, pets were used in institutions to give a sense of meaning and purpose to people institutionalized because of developmental delays. Florence Nightingale (1860) stated that "a small pet is often an excellent companion for the sick, for long chronic cases especially" (p. 36). The therapeutic use of pets may be particularly helpful with older people. "Many health care professionals are finding that loneliness may be as serious as cancer and heart disease for older adults" (Fontaine, 2000, p. 391). Playing with and/or petting animals can help people feel less isolated. Jennings (1998) found that blood pressure tends to decrease when people talk to their pets (Figure 31-16). Pet therapy is currently used as adjunctive treatment for people in both acute and long-term care settings.

There are many uses for pet therapy. It can be implemented to help overcome physical limitations, improve mood, decrease blood pressure, improve socialization skills, and improve self-esteem.

### Music

Music enters the bodymind through the auditory sense. Therapeutic use of music consists of playing music to elicit positive changes in behavior, emotions, or physiological responses. Music complements other treatment modali-

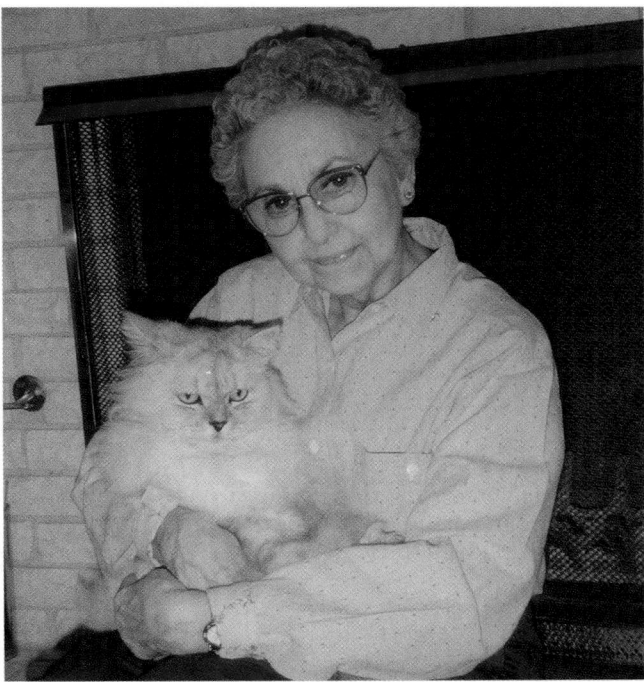

**Figure 31-16   Interacting with pets can lead to therapeutic benefits.**

ties and encourages clients to become active participants in their health care and recovery.

Music is a good adjunct to use with imagery as it can add to the relaxation response and, therefore, heighten images. Music can be used to relax or stimulate. "Music has been used for everything from lulling infants to sleep to stirring warriors to battle" (Grotbo, 1999, p. 24JJ). Music is used for celebrations, spiritual ceremonies, entertainment, and recreation. In hospitals in India, traditional Indian music is used to help restore balance in body rhythms (Fontaine, 2000). The healing power of music has been extensively studied. Campbell (1998) states that Mozart's music alters the energetic fields in the human brain and thus alters an individual's inner rhythms. The therapeutic benefit derived from music will be flavored by the client's perceptions and cultural backgrounds. The basic elements of music—rhythm, pitch, and intensity—are transmitted by sensory impulses from the cochlea to the thalamus, where they are mediated, then to the cerebral cortex, affecting the autonomic nervous system (Grotbo, 1999).

Listed here are some ways in which music has been used as a therapeutic intervention (Campbell, 1998):

- Music is used by hospice nurses to reduce clients' pain and ease the transition to death.
- Neonatal nurses often use lullabies to calm infants who are on ventilators or are irritable.
- Many labor and delivery nurses provide tape players and cassettes of relaxing music to clients.
- Relaxing music is often played in rehabilitation units.

- People with rheumatoid arthritis used guided imagery and music for 18 weeks and reported a reduction in pain as well as an improved ability to ambulate.
- Children with attention deficit disorder (ADD) who listened to Mozart had better attention spans, improved mood control, decreased impulsivity, and improved social skills.

Music on audiocassette used with a tape player and headphones can be a very useful tool for clients who may be immobilized, who must wait for diagnostic tests, or who undergo the perioperative experience. Some clients request that their music and tape player accompany them during surgery. Pleasurable sounds and music can reduce stress, perception of pain, anxiety, and feelings of isolation. To promote relaxation, select music that is repetitive and low-pitched, keeping in mind client preferences and cultural influences. Rhythm is most soothing when it has a 3/4 beat. Relaxation is induced by repetition of music, such as lullabies and chants. Music can also be especially useful in helping adolescent clients relax (Covington & Crosby, 1997).

Although music is therapeutic for people at all stages of the life cycle, **music-thanatology** is a holistic and palliative method for use of music with dying clients. Music-thanatology is used to help dissipate obstacles to the client's peaceful transition to death.

### Homeopathy

**Homeopathy**, the treatment of disease with minute drug dosages, was created by a German physician, Samuel Hahnemann, in the early 1800s. The term *homeopathy* is derived from the Greek terms *homoios*, which means "like," and *pathos*, which means "pathology." The basis of homeopathy is the belief that "like causes like." Thus a substance is given to activate an illness, which then stimulates the body's normal defense system to eliminate the illness. Hahnemann believed that symptoms of illness are a part of the curative process and that allopathic medicines stifled the innate curative process in the client. A homeopathic remedy is an extremely diluted form of a medication that serves to stimulate the client's defenses to fight disease and thus to heal.

## Nursing and CAM Modalities

Nurses play an important role in educating consumers about CAM modalities by providing information about the safety and efficacy of such methods. "In this new millennium, a major challenge facing nursing will be the promotion of integrative care in which clients use the best of CAM and conventional medicine. An integrative approach to practice will demand that nurses promote integration rather than replacement of conventional care" (Eliopoulous, 2000, p. 2). Education is a major function of nursing and is greatly needed as consumers try to determine which CAM methods to use. Consumers should be taught to recognize the signals of fraudulent practice and to avoid healers who:

- Promise immediate relief or success
- State that their way is the only sure therapy
- Refuse to work with other health care providers
- Claim to have all the answers
- Place more priority on money than the client's well-being (Tiedge, 1998)
- Use testimonials that claim amazing results
- Make statements using phrases such as "miraculous cure," "scientific breakthrough," or "secret ingredient" (Federal Trade Commission, 1998)

Many clients do not discuss their use of CAM techniques with their primary care providers because they fear ridicule or censure (Fontaine, 2000). It is imperative that nurses establish a setting in which clients feel free to express all issues related to their health. "When we nurses demonstrate an openness to clients' questions and self-care ideas without judgment, we can learn a lot more about our clients and help them find the treatments that work best for them" (Collins, 2000, p. 3).

Holistic nurses individualize every intervention on the basis of the client's unique needs. From the time before birth until the moment of death, people of all ages experience trauma, stress, and life challenges, and may benefit from CAM modalities (Collins, 2000). Table 31-11 provides suggestions for the use of complementary modalities throughout the life span.

Nurses using CAM modalities must maintain technical expertise, interpersonal skills, and critical thinking abilities related to CAM modalities. In addition to these requisite competencies, Fontaine (2000) states, "We need scientific principles, methods, and skills, but we also need to teach people ways to become more self-reliant as we shift in the role from caregiver to healer" (p. 17).

## Nurse as Instrument of Healing

When the nurse serves as an instrument of healing, the objective is to help clients call forth their inner resources for healing. In order to accomplish this goal, nurses must develop the following attributes:

- Knowledge base: Initially established in nursing school and then continuously expanded through lifelong learning
- Intentionality: A conscious direction of goals that is essential in helping the healer to focus
- Respect for differences: Demonstrated by honoring clients' culturally based health beliefs
- Ability to model wellness: Tending to own needs and attempting to stay as healthy and balanced as possible

Nurses can use many CAM modalities without advanced preparation. Imagery, relaxation, meditation, massage, touch, prayer, humor, music, and pet therapy are all CAM modalities that are available to all nurses. Nurses who are interested in performing reiki, therapeutic touch, healing touch, hypnosis, biofeedback, and other such modalities need additional education and training. In some cases, certification and/or licensure through individual states may be required.

| TABLE 31-11 | CAM MODALITIES FOR USE THROUGHOUT THE LIFE SPAN |
|---|---|
| **Population** | **Recommended Complementary Therapies** |
| Premature infants | • Massage (with modifications)<br>• Energy therapies<br>• Sound (e.g., recorded human heartbeat)<br>• Gentle movement<br>• Touch (stroking, skin-to-skin contact) |
| Infants | • Massage (with modifications)<br>• Energy therapies<br>• Music (e.g., lullabies)<br>• Movement (e.g., rocking) |
| Toddlers and preschoolers | • Massage<br>• Energy therapies<br>• Music (e.g., playing and listening to songs, singing)<br>• Movement |

*(continues)*

## TABLE 31-11  CAM MODALITIES FOR USE THROUGHOUT THE LIFE SPAN (*continued*)

| Population | Recommended Complementary Therapies |
| --- | --- |
| Toddlers and preschoolers (*continued*) | • Play (all activities should be age-appropriate)<br>• Humor<br>• Imagery<br>• Storytelling<br>• Art/drawing<br>• Aromatherapy (with precautions) |
| School-Aged children | • Massage<br>• Energy therapies<br>• Music (playing and listening)<br>• Movement (e.g., dance)<br>• Play (all activities should be age-appropriate)<br>• Humor (e.g., riddles, jokes)<br>• Imagery<br>• Storytelling<br>• Art/drawing<br>• Aromatherapy (with precautions)<br>• Hypnosis<br>• Yoga<br>• Tai chi<br>• Pet therapy |
| Adolescents | All modalities discussed in this chapter, as appropriate to condition |
| Adults | All modalities discussed in this chapter, as appropriate to condition |
| Women during childbirth | • Massage (emphasis on lower back and legs)<br>• Energy therapies<br>• Breath coaching<br>• Imagery<br>• Hypnosis |
| Older people | • Massage (lighter pressure and modifications for body's status)<br>• Aromatherapy (with precautions)<br>• Heat and cold applications (with precautions)<br>• Any other modalities discussed in this chapter, as appropriate to condition and with precautions |
| Terminally ill | • Massage<br>• Reflexology<br>• Energy therapies<br>• Music-thanatology<br>• Prayer<br>• Any other modalities discussed in this chapter, as appropriate to condition and with precautions |

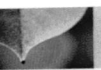

# CASE STUDY/NURSING CARE PLAN

Mr. Clark is a 48-year-old male with a history of stress and chronic, low back pain who comes to a nurse practitioner (NP) for advice. Mr. Clark rates the pain ranging from 4 to 6 on a scale of 1 to 10, is unable to complete a full range of motion with his back movements, and has a variety of "job-related stressors." The NP discusses Mr. Clark's previous management therapies, and finds that he has only seen his "family doctor," has had traction applied several times, sleeps on a firm mattress, and occasionally has taken muscle relaxants. These treatments do not get rid of the back pain, and Mr. Clark states the pain seems to slowly be "getting worse." In addition, Mr. Clark states that he "lifts things at work, which doesn't help my back." The NP suggests that Mr. Clark see a physical therapist and a chiropractor for evaluation, and a naturopath for potential herbal remedies for both the pain and the stress.

## Assessment
Client is a 48-year-old male with unresolved back pain. His blood pressure is 144/88, and pulse is 86. He cannot bend over with a complete range of motion and grimaces when asked to make these motions. The client continues to work in a labor-intensive position, which aggravates his back pain.

## Nursing Diagnosis
*Chronic Pain* related to unresolved back pain.
**NOC:** Pain Level; Pain Control; Comfort Level; Pain: Disruptive Effects
**NIC:** Pain Management; Analgesic Administration

## Expected Outcomes:
The client will:
1. Report a pain level of no greater than 3 each day.
2. Participate in stress-reduction activities daily.
3. Make appointments with a physical therapist, chiropractor, and naturopath within the week.

## Planning/Interventions/Rationales
1. Have client record his pain level daily using a scale of 1 to 10. *Allows for objective measurement and quantification of pain level.*
2. Educate the use of noninvasive methods of reducing pain and stress levels (e.g., relaxation techniques, heating applications, and therapeutic massage) to be used daily. *Decreases pain response.*
3. Follow up contact in 3 days to see if client has scheduled appointments with complementary/alternative care providers. *Assesses motivation of client to explore CAM providers.*

## Evaluation:
Client recorded a pain level each day below 3. He applied heat to his lower back twice a day and stated it "made his back feel better." In addition, the client was able to see a chiropractor within 2 days, and made an appointment with a physical therapist for the following week.

# Key Concepts

- Ever increasing numbers of health care consumers are using CAM modalities.
- Psychoneuroimmunology is the study of how the body and mind are connected and how beliefs, thoughts, and emotions affect health.
- Holistic nursing practice encompasses consideration of each client as a unique and whole being with physiological, psychological, sociocultural, intellectual, and spiritual components.

- Healing is not curing but rather is regaining balance and finding harmony and wholeness as changes take place from within the individual.
- No one can heal another, but a nurse can support healing for a client.
- CAM modalities can be categorized as mind-body, body-movement, energy and body work, nutritional therapies, spiritual therapies, and other modalities.
- Nurses should only practice CAM modalities for which they are prepared.

- Assessment of CAM modalities, especially herb use, should be a part of every health assessment.

## Review Questions and Activities

1. What CAM modalities would be appropriate for each of the following holistic dimensions: physical, emotional, social, and spiritual?
2. What two ancient healing traditions have influenced the development of CAM modalities?
3. What emerging field of science offers theoretical support for the efficacy of CAM modalities?
4. What conditions have been found to be improved through the use of acupuncture?
5. Which nursing organization supports the use of CAM modalities?

## Multimedia Links

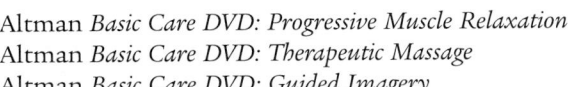

Altman *Basic Care DVD: Progressive Muscle Relaxation*
Altman *Basic Care DVD: Therapeutic Massage*
Altman *Basic Care DVD: Guided Imagery*

## Web Resources

American Holistic Nurses Association
   http://ahna.org
Association for the Advancement of Applied
   Psychoneuroimmunology
   http://www.hometown.aol.com
Herb Research Foundation
   http://www.herbs.org
National Center for Complementary and Alternative
   Medicine (NCCAM)
   http://nccam.nih.gov
Transcendental Meditation Resource
   http://www.tm.org

## References

Allen, J. B. (1998). An acupuncture treatment study for unipolar depression. *Psychological Science, 9,* 397–401.

Altman, G. (2004). *Delmar's fundamental & advanced nursing skills* (2nd ed.). Clifton Park, NY: Delmar Learning.

Astin, J. A. (1998). Why patients use alternative medicine: Results of a national study. *Journal of American Medical Association, 279*(19), 1548–1553.

Beeken, J. E., Parks, D., Cory, J., & Montopoli, G. (1998). The effectiveness of neuromuscular release massage therapy in five individuals with chronic obstructive lung disease. *Clinical Nursing Research, 7*(3), 309–325.

Benson, H. (1975). *The relaxation response.* New York: William Morrow.

Blumenthal, M., Goldberg, A., & Brinckman, J. (Eds.) (2000). *Herbal medicine: Expanded commission E monographs.* Newton, MA: Integrative Medicine Communications.

Borysenko, J., & Borysenko, M. (1994). *The power of the mind to heal.* Carson, CA: Hay House, Inc.

Bowlby, J. (1984). *Attachment and loss: Volume 1: Attachment* (2nd ed.). London: Penguin Books.

Bullock, M. L., Pheley, A. M., Kiresuk, T. J., Lenz, S. K., & Culliton, P. D. (1997). Characteristics and complaints of patients seeking therapy at a hospital-based alternative medicine clinic. *Journal of Alternative and Complementary Medicine, 3*(1), 31–37.

Burkhardt, M., & Nathaniel, A. (2002). *Ethics & issues in contemporary nursing* (2nd ed.). Clifton Park, NY: Delmar Learning.

Byers, D. C. (1983). *Better health with foot reflexology.* St. Petersburg, FL: Ingham Publishing Co.

Campbell, J. (1998, January/February). The riddle of the Mozart effect. *Natural Health,* 114–119.

Cardini, F., & Weixin, H. (1998). Moxibustion for correction of breech presentation: A randomized controlled trial. *Journal of the American Medical Association, 280,* 1580–1584.

Cassileth, B. R. (1998). *The alternative medicine handbook: The complete reference guide to alternative and complementary therapies.* New York: W. W. Norton.

Collinge, W. (1998). *Subtle energy.* New York: Warner Books.

Collins, S. B. (2000). Integrating CAM into a community healthcare setting: *Jin Shin Jyutsu. Integrative Medicine Consult, 1*(1), 3.

Cousins, N. (1979). *Anatomy of an illness.* New York: Norton.

Covington, H., & Crosby, C. (1997). Music therapy as a nursing intervention. *Journal of Psychosocial Nursing and Mental Health Services, 35*(3), 34–37.

Culliton, P. D. (1997, November 3–5). *Current utilization of acupuncture by United States patients.* Paper presented at the National Institutes of Health Consensus Development Conference on Acupuncture, Bethseda, MD.

Davidhizar, R., Bechtel, G. A. & Cosey, E. J. (2000). The spiritual needs of hospitalized patients. *American Journal of Nursing, 100*(7), 24C–D.

Dossey, B. M. (1998). Holistic modalities and healing moments. *American Journal of Nursing, 98*(6), 44–47.

Dossey, B. M., & Dossey, L. (1998). Attending to holistic care. *American Journal of Nursing, 98*(8), 35–38.

Eisenberg, D. M. (1998). Trends in alternative medicine use in the United States, 1990–1997. *Journal of the American Medical Association, 280*(18), 1569–1576.

Eliopoulos, C. (2000). A unique healing and leadership role: The nurse and integrative medicine. *Integrative Medicine Consult, 1*(1), 2.

Federal Trade Commission (1998). *Fraudulent health claims: Don't be fooled.* http://www.ftc.gov

Ferguson, L., & Ferguson, J. (2000). Pass the antioxidants, please. *Advances for nurses; job watch 2000, special edition,* 28.

Fontaine, K. L. (2000). *Healing practices: Alternative therapies for nursing.* Upper Saddle River, NJ: Prentice Hall.

Fritz, D. (1998). Noninvasive pain control methods used by cancer outpatients. *Oncology Nursing Forum (Suppl.),* 108.

Froemming, P. (1998). *The best guide to alternative medicine.* Los Angeles: Renaissance Books.

Gaudiano, B. G., & Herbert, J. D. (2000). Can We Really Tap Our Problems Away? A Critical Analysis of Thought Field Therapy. *Skeptical Inquirer, 32*(3), 32–38.

Gilkeson, J. (2000). *Energy healing: A pathway to inner growth.* New York: Marlowe & Company.

Goldberg, B. (1999). *Alternative medicine: The definitive guide.* Tiburon, CA: Future Medicine Publishing.

Gordon, A., & Merenstein, J. H. (1988). The effects of therapeutic touch on patients with osteoarthritis of the knee. *Journal of Family Practice, 47*(4), 271.

Grotbo, A. C. (1999). Giving your patients some time out. *American Journal of Nursing, 99*(7), 24HH–24KK.

Herbal Remedies. (2003). http://www.nhlmedical.org

Hoffart, M. B., & Keene, E. P. (1998). The benefits of visualization. *American Journal of Nursing, 98*(12), 44–47.

Jennings, R. L. (1998). Animals and cardiovascular health. In C. C. Wilson & D. C. Turner (Eds.), *Companion animals in human health* (pp. 161–171). Thousand Oaks, CA: Sage.

Kotani, N., Hashimoto, H., Sato, Y., Sessler, D.I., Yoshioka, H., Kitayama, M., Yasuda, T., & Matsuki, A. (2001). Preoperative intradermal acupuncture reduces postoperative pain, nausea and vomiting, analgesic requirement, and sympathoadrenal responses. *Anesthesiology, 95*(2), 349–356.

Krieger, D. (1993). *Accepting your power to heal: The personal practice of therapeutic touch.* Santa Fe, NM: Bear & Co. Publishing.

Lilley, L. L., & Gunk, R. (1998). Grapefruit and medication: Help your patient understand potential dangers of food-drug interactions. *American Journal of Nursing, 98*(12), 10.

Louisiana State Board of Nursing (1999). *Declaratory statement regarding the role and scope of practice of registered nurses performing holistic nursing practice and complementary therapies.* Metairie, LA: Author.

Massachusetts Board of Registration in Nursing (1997). *Advisory ruling: Holistic nursing practice and complementary therapies.* Boston: Author.

Mayo Clinic (2000). Phytoestrogens: Getting your hormones from plants. *Women's Healthsource, 4*(2), 1–2.

Montague, A. (1986). *Touching: The human significance of the skin* (3rd ed.). New York: Perennial Library.

Mustalish, S. H. (2000). Avoiding allergic reactions in children from botanical medicines. *Integrative Medicine Consult, 1*(1), 16.

National Center for Complementary and Alternative Medicine (NCCAM) (2003). http://nccam.nih.gov

National Institute of Health (1997). *Frequently asked questions about acupuncture.* Bethesda, MD: National Institutes of Health.

Nightingale, F. (1860). *Notes on nursing: What it is and what it is not.* London: Harrison & Sons.

North American Nursing Diagnosis Association (2003). *Nursing diagnoses: Definitions and classification 2003–2004.* Philadelphia: Author.

Nurse Healers–Professional Associates, Inc. (1992). *Therapeutic touch: Teaching guidelines: Beginner's level Krieger/Kunz method.* New York: Author.

Ody, P. (1999). *100 great natural remedies: Using healing plants at home.* New York: Barnes & Noble.

Pittler, M. H., & Ernst, E. (1998). Peppermint oil for irritable bowel syndrome: A critical review and meta-analysis. *American Journal of Gastroenterology, 93*(7), 1121.

Rechtschaffen, S., & Cohen, M. (1999). *Vitality and wellness.* New York: Random House.

Rimmer, L. M. (1998). What every home healthcare nurse should know about complementary therapy. *Home Healthcare Nurse, 16*(11), 760–765.

Robbers, J., & Tyler, V. (1999). *Tyler's herbs of choice.* New York: Haworth Herbal Press.

Roth, R., & Townsend, C. (2002). *Nutrition & diet therapy* (8th ed.). Clifton Park, NY: Delmar Learning.

Rush, A. K. (2000). *Bodywork basics.* New York: Random House.

Schnaubelt, K. (1999). *Advanced aromatherapy: The science of essential oil therapy.* Rochester, VT: Inner Traditions.

Smith, N., & Oliver, N. (1998). Using humor while caring for patients. *American Journal of Nursing, 98*(12), 14.

Stein, D. (1995). *Essential reiki: A complete guide to an ancient healing art.* Freedom, CA: The Crossing Press, Inc.

Tedeschi, M. (2000). *Essential anatomy: For healing and martial arts.* Trumbull, CT: Weatherhill.

Tiedge, L. B. (1998). Alternative health care: An overview. *Journal of Obstetric, Gynecologic and Neonatal Nursing, 27*(5), 557–562.

Tierra, M. (1998). *The way of herbs.* New York: Pocket Books.

Transcendental Meditation Resource (2002). http://www.tm.org

Walters, C. (1999). *Aromatherapy: A basic guide.* New York: Barnes & Noble.

Weil, A. (2000). *Eating well for optimum health: The essential guide to food, diet, and nutrition.* New York: Alfred A. Knopf.

# Nursing of Human Function

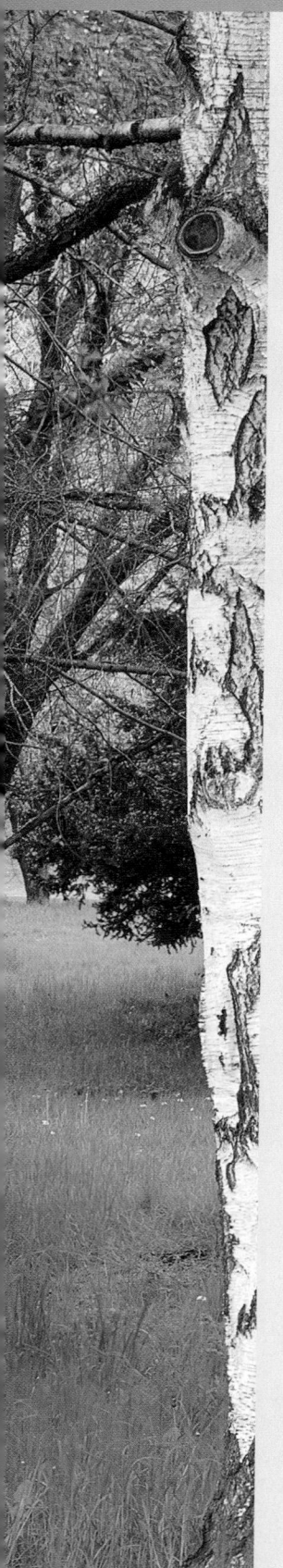

# VII UNIT

# Health Perception and Health Maintenance

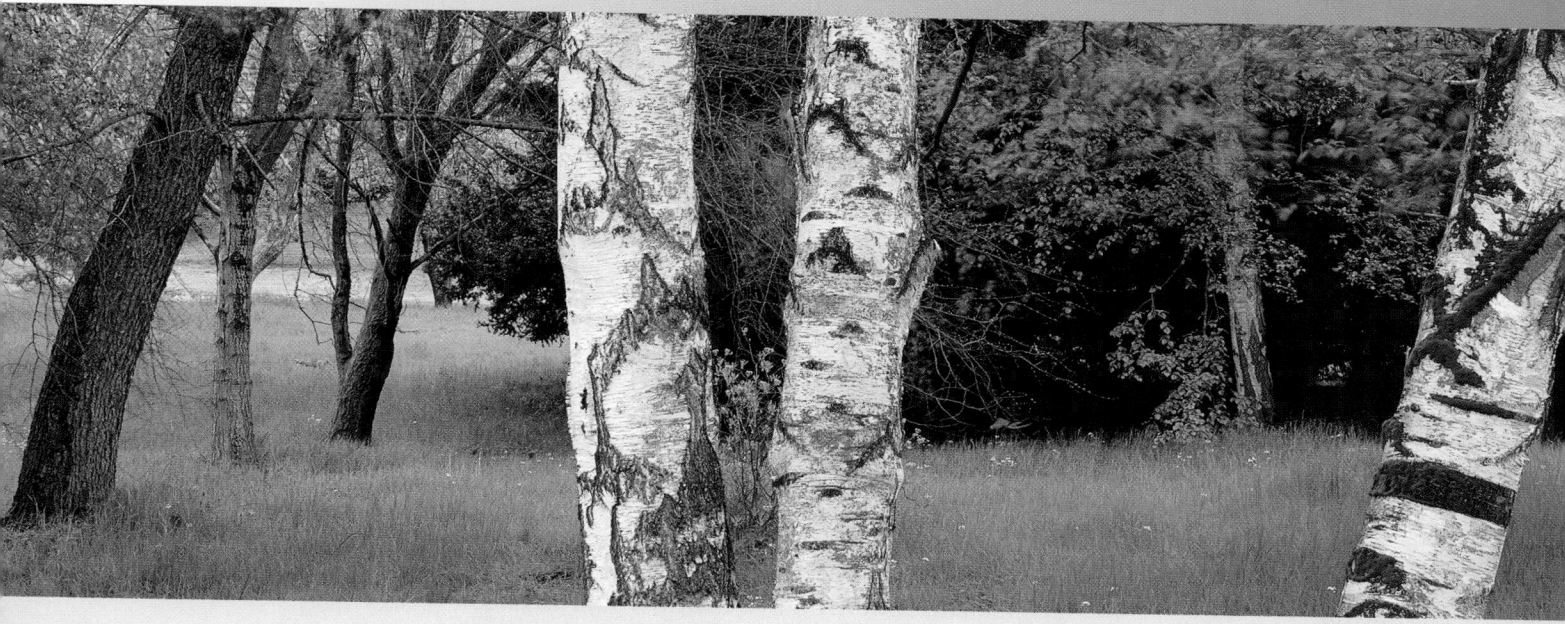

# CHAPTER 32

# Health Maintenance, Health Promotion, and Wellness

Wendy Neander, RN, MSN
Sandra B. Holmes, RN, BSN, MA(c)

*"Illness is the night-side of life, a more onerous citizenship.*
*Everyone who is born holds dual citizenship, in the kingdom of the*
*well and the kingdom of the sick. Although we all prefer to use only*
*the good passport, sooner or later each of us is obliged, at least for*
*a spell, to identify ourselves as citizens of that other place."*

(Susan Sontag, 1988)

# Chapter Competencies

*Upon completion of this chapter, the reader should be able to:*

1. Differentiate health, illness, and wellness.
2. Explain the relationship of variables such as lifestyle, locus of control, self-efficacy, health care attitudes, environment, and economic resources to health behaviors.
3. Describe the concept of normal health maintenance.
4. Compare and contrast the concepts of health promotion and disease prevention.
5. Explain global and international initiatives on health promotion and wellness.
6. Identify the assessment phase of the nursing process in health maintenance.
7. Discuss nursing diagnoses and implementation strategies appropriate for the health maintenance pattern.
8. Explain the importance of evaluation in health maintenance.

# Key Terms

acute illness
adaptation
basic human need
behavior
body image
chronic illness
disease prevention
empowerment
health
health maintenance

health maintenance activities
health-promoting behaviors
health promotion
health-seeking behaviors
high-level wellness
holism
homeostasis
homosexuality
illness
locus of control

modeling
motivation
perception
psychoneuroimmunology
self-concept
self-efficacy
sex roles
sexuality
spirituality
wellness

Health and illness can be defined in many ways. Health is a concept that includes physical and mental status, emotional well-being, and spiritual well-being. Historically, Western cultures defined health as the absence of illness. It is easier to measure illness than it is to measure health because definite parameters can be used to determine whether an individual has symptoms indicative of disease processes. In 1946, the World Health Organization (WHO) defined health as a state of complete physical, mental, and social well-being and not merely the absence of disease or infirmity. The WHO definition has not been revised, changed, or amended since 1948 (World Health Organization, 2002). What criteria are used for determining one's health? Is health merely the absence of disease, or is health more comprehensive?

In addition to examining these questions, this chapter describes health maintenance, health promotion, and disease prevention activities with an emphasis on nursing's role. There is a discussion of models of health, holism, basic human needs, and the physiological, psychological, sociocultural, intellectual, spiritual, and sexual dimensions of the individual.

# Health, Illness, and Wellness

**Health**, the process through which a person seeks to maintain an equilibrium that promotes stability and comfort, is a dynamic process that varies according to a person's perception of well-being. The traditional definition of health as the absence of illness is a narrow concept. **Illness** is the inability of an individual's adaptive responses to maintain physical and emotional balance that subsequently results in an impairment of functional abilities. **Wellness** is the condition in which an individual functions at optimal levels. An in-depth discussion of wellness appears later in this chapter.

Health is a global term because it refers to every aspect of a person's life, including:

- Physical status
- Emotional well-being
- Social relationships
- Intellectual functioning
- Spiritual condition

## Models of Health

There are several theoretical models of health, as shown in Table 32-1. These models help clarify the link between the states of well-being and illness and clients' responses to these processes.

The American Holistic Nurses Association (2003) describes health as a maintenance of harmony and balance among body, mind, and spirit. Balance refers to **homeostasis**, which is an equilibrium among psychological, physiological, sociocultural, intellectual, and spiritual needs. The process by which a person adjusts to achieve homeostasis is called **adaptation**. When people describe their health status, basically three areas are considered:

- Presence or absence of symptoms (physical and emotional)
- How they feel (emotionally and physically)
- What they are able to do (ability to function)

Health can be studied both in individuals and in groups (e.g., families and communities). Health status is influenced by the factors seen in Box 32-1.

An individual, within the context of the family unit, gives meaning to health and makes adjustments necessitated by the illness. A family's adaptation to changes in health status is strongly influenced by each member's personal resources and social support systems.

### Cultural Influence on Health

Health-related concepts evolve within the context of one's culture; that is, culture affects how an individual views health and illness. One's cultural background influences health-related behaviors and expectations of treatment when illness occurs. For example, how an individual cares for self is directly related to cultural norms. "It is essential for the nurse to provide cultural care by acquiring knowledge about the cultural practices and beliefs of the family and community and their effects on health" (Collins & Diego, 2000, p. 29). See Chapter 5 for a complete discussion of cultural beliefs and behaviors affecting health.

### Family Influences on Health Care

The changing composition of the family in today's world creates a challenge in defining and identifying the role of family in influencing health care (see Chapter 44 for further expansion on the topic of family relationships). Traditionally, the family unit was defined by marriage, blood, or adoption. The family is not an isolated unit; it exists and functions in the context of a society that in

recent generations, with industrialization and urbanization, has been undergoing radical changes. For example, in the United States the percentage of single mothers has increased 25% from 1990 to 2000. This group of single mothers is not the traditional stereotype of the unwed teenager of past generations (Kantrowitz & Wingert, 2001). It is important for nurses to recognize the variation in family structure when assessing family and individual health.

Because health is defined uniquely by each client's culture, the nurse must assess the family's health definitions and beliefs. Generally, families are the first to identify

---

### BOX 32-1 INFLUENCES ON HEALTH STATUS

- Beliefs and attitudes
- Cultural factors
- Environmental factors
- Lifestyle behaviors
- Political systems
- Socioeconomic status
- Religious factors

Adapted from Murray, R., & Zentner, J. (2001). *Health promotion strategies through the life span* (5th ed.). Upper Saddle River, NJ: Prentice-Hall.

---

### COMMUNITY/HOME CARE

#### Single-Parent Family

When counseling new parents concerning their status of becoming a single-parent family, the home health nurse must first recognize the difficulty of this situation. The nurse must then remember to support the parent in this new "busy position." Encouraging the single parent to form a network with others in similar positions can be valuable. In addition, the nurse can brainstorm with the new parent about interventions such as shared babysitting, and activities with other single parents that the parent can take the new child to (e.g., church, social groups).

Potts, N., & Mandleco, B. (2002). *Pediatric nursing: Caring for children and their families.* Clifton Park, NY: Delmar Learning.

## TABLE 32-1    THEORETICAL PERSPECTIVES OF HEALTH

| Model | Theorist | Assumptions |
|---|---|---|
| Clinical model | Traditional perspective | • Health is absence of illness.<br><br>• Individuals who are not "sick" (i.e., experiencing a disease) are healthy. |
| Health-belief model | Rosenstock | • Expectations direct behaviors that lead to fulfillment of the expectations.<br><br>• Group values exert influence on beliefs about health.<br><br>• Beliefs may change as a person grows and develops. |
| High-level wellness model | Dunn | • Health is influenced by the interaction among the individual, family, and community.<br><br>• Health is viewed as an attempt toward achieving one's fullest potential. |
| Social learning theory | Bandura<br><br>Rosenstock | • Beliefs strongly influence actions.<br><br>• Behavior is influenced by expectations and reinforcements (or incentives). |
| Host-agent-environment model ("Ecologic" model) | Leavell and Clark | • Health depends on the interaction of host, agent, and environment.<br><br>• Balance among these elements results in health.<br><br>• Illness occurs when there is an imbalance in one of the three elements.<br><br>• Model is used most often in predicting risk of illness. |
| Health promotion model | Pender | • People engage in health-promoting behavior when they:<br> 1. Value health<br> 2. Perceive health as being within their control<br> 3. Can identify benefits in self-care behaviors<br> 4. Have a positive perception of their health status<br><br>• Health-promoting behavior is influenced by:<br> 1. An individual's inherited and acquired characteristics<br> 2. Significant others, who model the behavior, expect the behavior to occur, and facilitate the behavior<br> 3. Families, peers, and health care providers |

Data from Bandura, A. (1977). *A social learning theory*. Englewood Cliffs, NJ: Prentice Hall; Becker, M. H. (1974). The health belief model and sick role behavior. *Health Education Monogram, 2*, 409–419; Dunn, H. (1961). *High-level wellness*. Arlington, VA: R. W. Beatty; Leavell, H., & Clark, A. E. (1965). *Preventive medicine for doctors in the community*. New York: McGraw-Hill; Rosenstock, I. (1974). Historical origin of the health belief model. In M. H. Becker (Ed.), *The health belief model and personal health behavior*. Thorofare, NJ: Charles B. Slack.; Edelman, C. & Mandle, C. (2002). *Health promotion throughout the life span* (5th ed.). St. Louis: Mosby; Pender, N., Murdaugh, C., & Parsons, M. (2002). *Health promotion in nursing practice* (4th ed.). New Jersey: Prentice Hall.

signals of impending illness. Also, families help determine the following:

• Whether to seek treatment
• What type of treatment is appropriate
• Who should provide the treatment or care
• Where the treatment or care should be provided

Families are often the major caregivers for their relatives. Extended families and communities have traditionally acted as a buffer against excessive stress and illness. Lack of social support from family or significant others results in psychological and spiritual isolation, which negatively impacts a person's physiological state. Thus, it is important to help clients identify, strengthen, and use their social support systems. Sometimes, families need guidance to optimize health behaviors. Nursing assessment *must* include the client's (including the family's) perspective of the *most* pressing problem.

## Illness Perspectives

Illness means different things to different people. It is more than just the existence of physical signs and symptoms. Illness is the result of a disease (either physiological or psychological) or injury that affects functioning, and occurs when there is an inability to meet one's needs.

There are two major classifications of illness: acute and chronic. An **acute illness** is a disruption in functional ability usually characterized by a rapid onset, intense manifestations, and a relatively short duration. Acute illnesses are usually reversible. A **chronic illness** is a disruption in functional ability usually characterized by a gradual, insidious onset with lifelong changes that are usually irreversible. Chronic illnesses last a long time, frequently throughout the individual's life. An example of an acute illness is influenza. Arthritis is an example of a chronic illness. It is possible for a person to have both a chronic illness and an acute illness at the same time—for example, the person with diabetes (chronic) who also develops pneumonia (acute).

Chronic illness affects individuals across the life span. Up to 10% of children in the United States have a chronic illness. "The impact of these disorders become most dramatic

## LIFE SPAN CONSIDERATIONS

### Cardiovascular Disease

The World Health Organization estimates that 25% more healthy life years will be lost to cardiovascular (CV) disease globally by 2020. High blood pressure alone causes about 50% of CV disease worldwide. High cholesterol causes about 33%. Inactive lifestyles, tobacco use, and low fruit and vegetable intake account for 20% each. The CV disease risks overlap, and thus the total percentages are greater than 100%. One individual may be at risk from both high cholesterol and high blood pressure.

World Health Organization (2002). *World health report 2002: Reducing risks, promoting health lifestyles.* Geneva, Switzerland.

during adolescence, and you can play a critical role in addressing their concerns and fostering more normal development in children" (Muscari, 1998b, p. 20). Adolescents experiencing chronic illnesses need two major nursing interventions: support and education.

Even though many older individuals have multiple chronic conditions, it is important to remember that chronicity is *not* an experience unique to the older client. However, as life expectancy continues to increase, a growing number of people are living with chronic illness. The implications for nursing are far-reaching. "As care in the home for acute and chronically ill clients continues to expand, advanced practice nurses will continue to integrate psychosocial care with physical care" (Collins & Diego, 2000, p. 28). Some of the goals of caring for people with chronic illnesses include:

* Coping with lifestyle changes and the subsequent modification of self-care activities
* Coping with long-term discomfort or pain
* Establishing or maintaining a sense of personal control
* Maintaining a positive self-esteem (Edelman & Mandle, 2002)

## Wellness Perspectives

Wellness further describes health status. It allows health to be placed on a continuum from one's optimal level ("wellness") to a maladaptive state ("illness"), as shown in Figure 32-1.

Wellness is a dynamic process that is ever changing. The well person usually has some degree of illness and the ill person usually has some degree of wellness. This concept of a health continuum negates the idea that wellness and illness are opposite because they may occur simultaneously in the same person in varying degrees. The classic

## CLIENT EDUCATION

### Wellness Practices in Recovering Cardiac Clients

Nurses should remember to inform chronically ill clients about participation in wellness activities. For example, clients recovering from cardiac surgeries benefit greatly from the following wellness practices:

✓ Engaging in a regimen of physical conditioning with a gradual increase in activity levels

✓ Walking daily, increasing distance and time as prescribed

✓ Developing regular eating patterns, modifying calories, fat, and sodium as recommended

✓ Using personal strengths to compensate for limitations

✓ Alternating activity with rest periods—some fatigue is normal and expected during convalescence

Goodman, H. (1997). Patients' perception of their education needs in the first six weeks following discharge after cardiac surgery. *Journal of Advanced Nursing, 25*(6), 1241–1251.

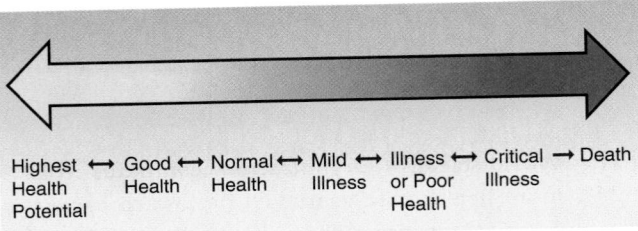

**Figure 32-1    Health continuum**

description of wellness was developed by Dunn in the early 1960s. According to Dunn (1961), **high-level wellness** means functioning to one's maximum health potential while remaining in balance with the environment.

# Health Behaviors and Variables Influencing Health

To understand how people influence their health status, it is important to know about health behaviors. **Behavior** is defined as the observable response of an individual to external stimuli. An important concept to remember when caring for clients is that *all behavior has meaning*. In other words, behavior is the individual's attempt to achieve satisfaction of needs. Nurses must sometimes act as detectives to determine the need(s) underlying client behavior. Thorough assessment is the key for nurses in determining the meaning of client behavior. **Health-seeking behaviors** are those activities directed toward attaining and maintaining a state of well-being. Many variables also influence health behaviors (see Box 32-2).

## Lifestyle

Individuals determine their health status through their actions (Figure 32-2). Lifestyle consists of a person's usual daily activities and routines that are acceptable practices in the person's life. Such routines and habits influence health status (Figure 32-3). For example, consumption of large amounts of caffeine, cigarette smoking, consistent intake of high-fat foods, and a sedentary routine can adversely affect health status. Lifestyles are developed within one's family and one's cultural environment. The family is the primary influence on a child's development of health-promoting (or health-defeating) behaviors.

When lifestyle modifications are necessary to improve health, many individuals have difficulty implementing the suggested changes. Individuals are less likely to comply with recommended lifestyle changes if there is a perception of increased inconvenience and cost. Also, the required degree of change in lifestyle may affect compliance. "A person is more likely to comply when he perceives the severity of an illness and his susceptibility to complications; when he believes in the reliability of his health care providers; and when he trusts the benefits of the prescribed therapy" (Muscari, 1998a, p. 27).

---

**BOX 32-2    VARIABLES INFLUENCING HEALTH BEHAVIORS**

Several variables influence health, including:

- Lifestyle
- Perceived locus of control
- Perceived ease or difficulty in accomplishing a task (self-efficacy)
- Health care attitudes
- Self-concept
- Cognition
- Age and developmental levels
- Gender
- Previous experiences with the health care system
- Environment
- Economic resources

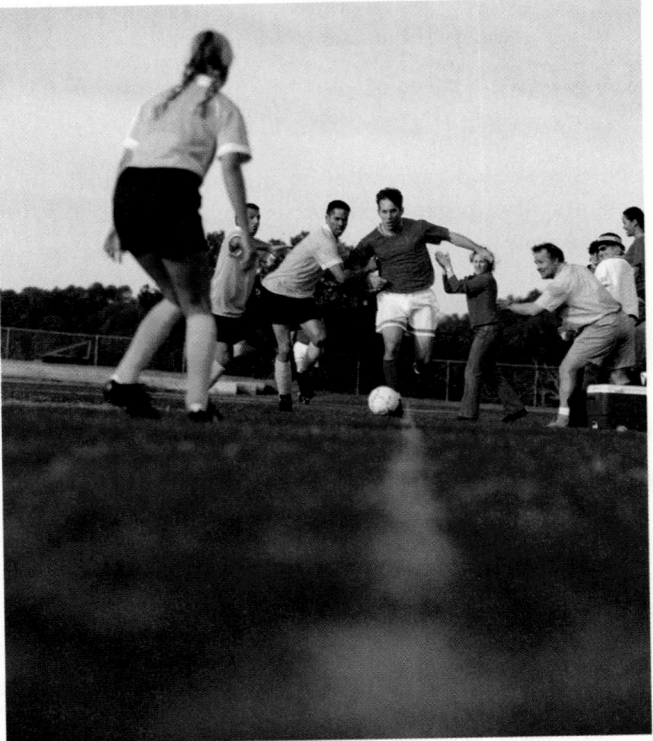

**Figure 32-2    A lifestyle that incorporates physical activity adds to the wellness of the participating individuals.**

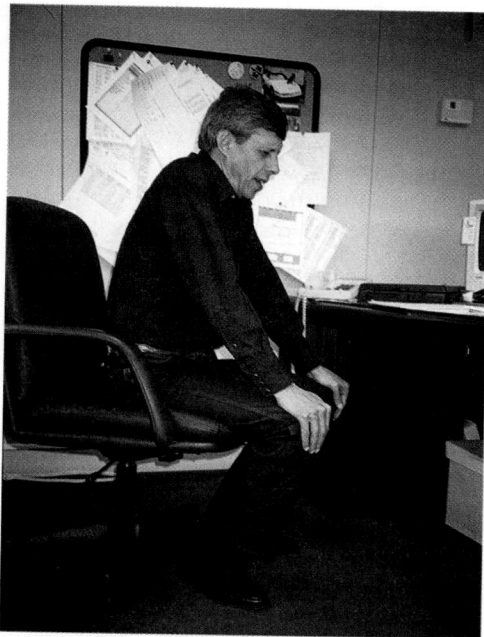

**Figure 32-3    A client in an orthopneic position to cope with negative effects of smoking**

## Locus of Control

**Locus of control** refers to individuals' sense of control over events and situations affecting their lives. A person with an external locus of control feels like a victim with little, if any, control over life events. However, a person with an internal locus of control feels able to influence significant events and occurrences affecting self; that is, they see themselves as responsible for their own lives. Thus, those with an internal locus of control are more willing to make lifestyle changes that will lead to wellness.

### CLINICAL ALERT

#### Obesity in Children

Obesity has become one of the most prevalent concerns affecting the health of Canadian and American children. The percentage of overweight American children has doubled since 1980 (National Center for Health Statistics, 2000). A similar trend in children is evident in Canada with a doubling of the percentage of obese children between 1981 and 1996. The U.S. government Healthy People 2010 initiative aims for a reduction in childhood obesity rates from 11% to 5% by 2010.

Covington, C., Cybulski, M., Davis, T., Duca, G., Farrel, E., Kasgorgis, M., Kator, C., & Sell, T. (2001). Kids on the move: Preventing obesity among urban children. *American Journal of Nursing, 101*(3), 73–75, 77, 79, 81–82.

### CLIENT REFLECTIONS

#### Self-Esteem and Locus of Control

Barbara, age 23, was raised with her mother and a stepfather. She states, "My mother treated me with love, but I don't like myself because my stepfather scolded me all the time and said I would never amount to anything." Barbara also states, "I can't get past my feelings of low self-esteem because of all the mean things he said to me."

What would you say to this client? (Hint: remember the variable of locus of control.)

## Self-Efficacy

Psychologist Albert Bandura (1977) coined the term **self-efficacy** to describe an individual's perception of one's own ability to perform a certain task. Self-efficacy has a powerful impact on initiating behavior change.

When clients are able to make informed decisions about their health behaviors and feel that they are successful in these areas, they are more likely to attempt behavior change. Thus, an essential component of nursing care is to provide opportunities for clients to achieve this level of self-motivation. For example, when teaching a client how to self-administer injections, the nurse breaks the task down into small manageable objectives and has the client do a return demonstration. The client receives immediate feedback, which encourages further success.

Self-efficacy is a form of self-confidence that leads to successful behavior performance; it is a strong influencing factor on behavior (Borsody, Courtney, Taylor, & Jairath, 1999). As described by Bandura (1986), self-efficacy encompasses two types of expectations:

1. *Outcome expectations:* Beliefs about whether behavior will produce desirable results
2. *Efficacy expectations:* Beliefs the person has about her own ability to perform the behavior

Health implies moving toward self-care, in other words, becoming and remaining independent. Self-responsibility, as it relates to health-promoting activities, is a fairly new concept to the majority of Americans. For years, individuals have

### STOP AND THINK

#### Barriers to Wellness

Identify specific behaviors that promote a person's ability to stay healthy. What are some behaviors that create barriers to wellness?

looked to physicians to "fix things" and "make it better." Only when individuals enter into active partnerships with their primary health care provider (nurse, physician, or other healer) will self-responsibility for health become a reality.

## Health Care Attitudes

Beliefs are powerful shapers of behavior. Health behaviors are based on beliefs. Attitudes about health and personal vulnerability (which are initially learned in the family unit) greatly influence behavior. Socialization (which occurs within the family) influences the development of beliefs about health care. These beliefs determine the person's willingness to participate in health care. For example, if the person believes in the use of herbs or folk healers, such nontraditional health care practices could either enhance or interfere with traditional treatment approaches.

There may also be some gender differences in beliefs regarding health care.

Nurses must be sensitive to the fact that all clients do not share the same beliefs about health care issues. Using a nonjudgmental attitude helps the nurse to be more accepting of clients with diverse beliefs and behaviors.

## Self-Concept

**Self-concept** is an individual's perception of self. It includes **self-esteem** (an individual's perception of self-worth) and **body image** (perception of physical self). The relationship between self-concept and health is strong.

Self-concept influences individuals' health behaviors in that people who think highly of themselves will tend to take care of themselves. On the other hand, a person with a negative self-concept will engage in reckless or self-destructive behaviors that endanger health. Persons with a

low self-concept frequently ignore their own needs because they are perceived to be less important than the needs of other people.

Self-concept is dynamic and may change according to health status. Not only does self-concept influence health, but changes in health status may influence self-concept. For example, consider the person who has lost a limb due to amputation. This person's self-concept would be altered as a result of the physical change.

## Cognition

A person's cognitive abilities can facilitate or obstruct healthy behavior. A person is more likely to perform a behavior if he understands the implications of consistent healthy lifestyles. However, deficiencies in cognition can be a barrier to compliance of health behavior. For example, poor vision interferes with written instructions about health behavior. In addition, deafness interferes with understanding oral instruction (Estes, 2002). Also, educational and knowledge level will also affect the way a client receives and interprets instructional information. When planning health maintenance activities, the nurse must first assess clients' cognitive capabilities to understand their level of health, perceived barriers, perceived susceptibility, their definition of health, and perceived control over their health status.

## Age and Developmental Levels

Each age has specific developmental considerations related to health maintenance. For example, physiological changes with aging predispose the client to altered health status. Older age groups tend to practice health maintenance behaviors more often than their younger counterparts (Figure 32-4). Clients realize they are not invincible, and by changing their health behaviors, can enjoy healthier lives. In addition, all age groups can benefit from adopting positive health behaviors. For example, although infants and children are dependent on others for health maintenance, they are beginning to learn health behaviors from their caregivers. Earlier ages provide an ideal opportunity to teach and encourage behaviors that will lead to a lifetime of effective health maintenance and potentially decrease the risk for health-behavior-related diseases (Mosher, Youngman, & Day, 1999).

## Gender

Gender is a determinant of health. Gender differences start at birth. Male infant death rates are higher than females. Men tend to participate in more risk-taking behaviors. Men still use alcohol and smoke more than women; however, this gender gap is rapidly getting smaller. Women have a longer life expectancy than men, perhaps as much as 6 years. Women have historically provided and sought the health care for their families. Women experience more acute and chronic health issues requiring med-

---

## STOP AND THINK

### The Media and Health Beliefs

The media are extremely powerful in shaping attitudes and beliefs. Here are some examples of how various media discourage health-promoting behaviors:

- Advertising foods with high sugar, salt, and fat content

- Promoting alcohol use

- Encouraging use of tobacco products

What other examples can you identify? Recently, there seems to be an emerging trend to advertise healthier lifestyles. What examples come to mind?

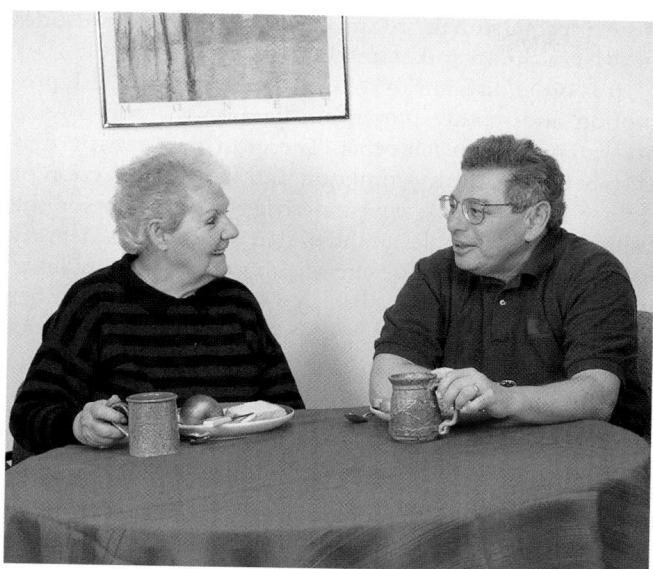

**Figure 32-4    Sharing meals is a wonderful means for older adults to meet their physical and interdependence needs, as one aspect of their positive health maintenance.**

ical attention (e.g., pregnancy). Home pregnancy kits are available commercially, allowing women to find out early on if they are pregnant, allowing for health-promotion activities to be practiced or established early in the pregnancy. Early pregnancy detection allows the developing fetus a greater opportunity to be born healthy. Women have access to over-the-counter medications for certain conditions such as yeast infections. Women are also more likely to seek alternative forms of health care (Littleton & Engebretson, 2002).

## Previous Experiences with the Health Care System

A negative experience with the health care system may cause the individual to refuse to seek treatment at the same facility. Since some insurance companies dictate which providers can be used, this may prevent that person from seeking needed health care. Conversely, if the client or family member had a positive response to previous contacts with the health care system, they are more likely to seek assistance and treatment (Hitchcock, Schubert, & Thomas, 2003).

## Environment

Air, water, and soil quality are all necessary to sustain life. Poor air quality can lead to increases in asthma and other respiratory problems. The quality of the water impacts the quality of soil used to grow food. Contamination of the water supply has negative effects on human consumption. Safe, accessible, and affordable housing, and safe, accessible schools, roads, and workplaces are necessary for health maintenance (Pender et al., 2002).

## Economic Resources

Financial resources increase the ability to provide the necessary commodities for health and well-being. These commodities for good health include adequate housing, food, clothing, utilities, and access to health care. The poor are at greater risk for health problems. They may not be able to afford basic, safe housing, let alone health care (Hitchcock et al., 2003).

# Health Maintenance

**Health maintenance** is defined as behavior directed toward maintaining a current level of health. **Health maintenance activities** are the activities and behaviors an individual performs to maintain or improve a current level of health.

## Characteristics of Health Maintenance

The client can do more to maintain health than anyone else. There are no "quick fixes" or "shortcuts" to be successful in achieving health maintenance. To be successful in changing health behavior, the client must take time to prepare and plan. Often the outcomes of health-related behaviors are the primary focus. However, it is important to also examine the role of motivation and attitudes about health status and the ability to change health status. Normal health maintenance can be conceptualized by three characteristics: (1) perception, (2) motivation, and (3) maintenance, which are examined as follows (Edelman & Mandle, 2002).

### Perception

The ability of a client to adopt and maintain healthy behaviors depends on the client's **perception** (i.e., a person's sense and understanding of the world) of his current health status, and his level of knowledge regarding the effect of the behaviors and how to maintain these behaviors. First, the client must identify the behavior(s) to be maintained or changed. If the client does not perceive a problem with his current health maintenance activities, it would be futile for the nurse to try to intervene at this point. The nurse first must work with the client to show how the lack of health-promotive activities is not beneficial (Murray & Zentner, 2001).

### Motivation

**Motivation** (i.e., the internal drive or externally arising stimulus to action or thought) to maintain a current level of health or achieve an optimal level of health must come from the client. Other factors can help or hinder the client's success for behavior management. Environment, support or nonsupport from friends and family, and genetic makeup all affect the person's ability to manage healthy behaviors. A friend suffering a heart attack or developing a chronic illness may energize a person to reevaluate her current health practices. At this point, the motivation for change may be high, but the person may lack the knowledge of how to undertake this change in behavior. A motivated person will seek health information, activities, and groups or organizations that support achieving wellness. The challenge to the nurse is to identify the client's level of motivation. Then the nurse must provide interventions that increase the client's motivation (Edelman & Mandle, 2002).

### Maintenance

The maintenance of new health behaviors is very challenging for clients. Learning a new behavior is not difficult; the difficulty comes in maintaining the behavior. In order for the new behaviors to be beneficial, they must be practiced for the long term. Once new health behaviors have been adopted, it is crucial to have the tools needed to maintain them. Time and preparation are required to maintain healthy behaviors.

## Health Promotion and Disease Prevention

Two basic components of health maintenance are health promotion and disease prevention or health protection. **Health promotion** is behavior motivated by the desire to increase the levels of health and well-being and actualize or maximize the health potential of individuals, families, groups, communities, and society. **Disease prevention or health protection** is behavior motivated by a desire to actively avoid illness, detect it early, or maintain functioning within the constraints of an illness (Figure 32-5). Health promotion includes activities undertaken by

health professionals to promote health and includes health education and counseling.

It is often difficult to differentiate between health promotion and disease prevention because the two overlap and complement each other. The most important difference between health promotion and health protection or disease prevention is the underlying motivation for the behavior. For example, an individual who lives a sedentary lifestyle may begin an exercise program (health maintenance) and continue this behavior after attainment of her goals, because she feels better practicing these behaviors (health promotion).

## Health Promotion

Health promotion begins with the mindset to shape a healthy lifestyle. Health promotion is the process of enabling people to increase control over their health and to improve their health through development of human resources and behaviors that maintain or enhance well-being. From an individual standpoint, health promotion means the practice of positive health behaviors (see Box 32-3). Health promo-

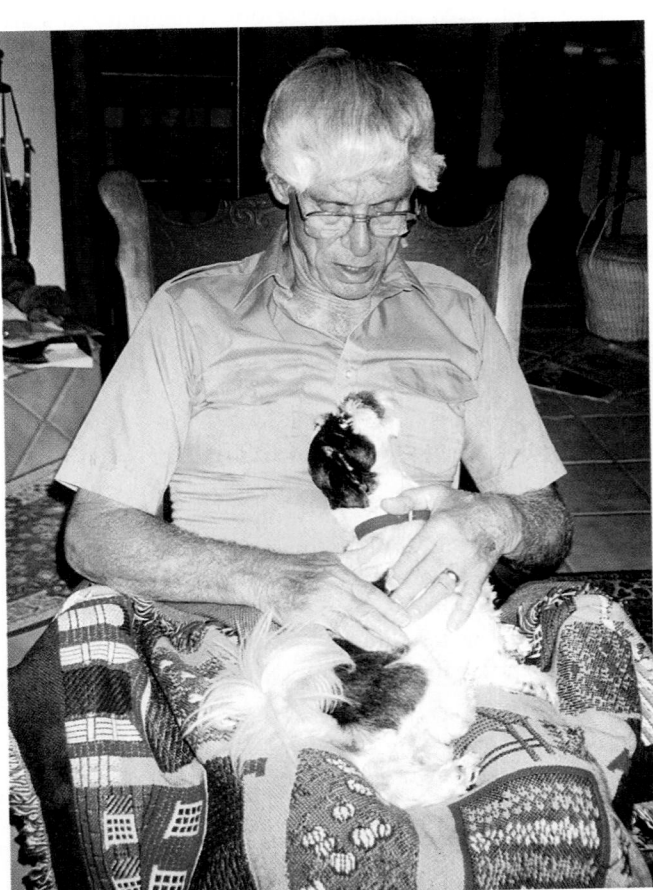

**Figure 32-5** Pet therapy is one method of a health-promotive behavior to provide positive health benefits for the prevention of disease. *Photo courtesy of John White, Corpus Christi, TX*

tion also includes avoidance of unhealthy behaviors (e.g., smoking, drug use, and excessive consumption of alcohol). Health-promotion efforts intervene with healthy rather than ill populations to help maximize their health status. Individuals who participate in health-promotive behaviors strive toward a high level of wellness rather than just being disease free (Pender et al., 2002).

## Disease Prevention or Health Protection

Disease-prevention or health-protection behaviors and activities are for the protection of people from the ill effects of actual or potential health threats. The three levels of prevention activities are addressed more specifically in Chapter 2 (i.e., primary prevention, secondary prevention, and tertiary prevention).

## Health Promotion on a Global Level

On global, national, and local levels, health promotion is still being developed, with the World Health Organization leading the way with international conferences and meetings and dissemination of successful health-promotion strategies, programs, and policies (Flynn, 1997). In 2000, the World Health Organization (WHO), the Pan American Health Organization (PAHO), and the Ministry of Health of Mexico hosted the Fifth Global Conference on Health Promotion (5GCHP). The 5GCHP took forward the priorities for health promotion in the 21st century, which were identified at the Fourth Global Conference on Health Promotion in Jakarta in 1997 and confirmed by the Health Promotion Resolution adopted by the World Health Assembly in May 1998. The priorities are shown in Box 32-3.

---

**BOX 32-3**    **PRIORITIES FOR HEALTH PROMOTION IN THE 21ST CENTURY**

1. Promoting social responsibility for health.
2. Increasing community capacity and empowering the individual.
3. Increasing investments for health development.
4. Securing an infrastructure for health promotion.
5. Strengthening the evidence base for health promotion.
6. Reorienting health systems and health services.

World Health Organization (2002). *World health report 2002: Reducing risks, promoting health lifestyles.* Geneva, Switzerland.

---

## International Community Health Promotion Developed by "Healthy Cities" Movement

The World Health Organization developed a "Healthy City" plan for identifying health-promotion strategies for communities. In this social ecological plan (model), the responsibility for health is shared by the community, including decision making with respect to health issues (Flynn, 1997). The international Healthy Cities movement was officially launched by the WHO European office in 1986 as a vehicle to stimulate local-level, health-promotion activities to reach the goal of "Health for All in the Year 2000." A healthy city is defined as:

> one that is continually creating and improving those physical and social environments and expanding those community resources which enable people to mutually support each other in performing all the functions of life and in developing to their maximum potential (Hancock & Duhl, 1988, p. 24).

The Healthy Cities movement supports the concept that many factors that make healthy people do not lie within the jurisdiction of the health care system. A Healthy City is a collaborative effort of the entire community, not just the health professionals. Community decisions about health must involve local people whose lives will be affected by these decisions. Involving local people includes focusing on those who are hard to reach such as poor, homeless, young, and older populations. A Healthy City acknowledges public, private, and nonprofit responsibility for health.

Being the closest level of government to the people, the city is an ideal level for shared decision making with respect to health issues. Local decision makers in a Healthy City emphasize health, broadly defined in terms of quality of life. The definition emphasizes prevention of community problems and the development of people. Health includes all aspects of people's lives. Housing, education, religion, employment, nutrition, leisure and recreation, health and medical care, good transportation, a clean and green environment, and safety are all factors that contribute to a healthy community. To date, approximately 3,000 municipalities are participating in the Healthy Cities movement (Québec World Health Organization [WHO], 1998).

## Health Promotion in the United States

The United States Public Health Service (1990), in its Healthy People 2000 initiative, focused on the individual's responsibility in promoting health. The individual is viewed as having the ability to influence her own health and also that of the country.

In 1979, the U.S. Department of Health and Human Services mobilized public health agencies to work toward developing healthier Americans. This initiative, Healthy People, is now in its third decade and is called Healthy People 2010 (Chrvala & Bulger, 1999). The program, coordinated by the U.S. Public Health Service, will focus efforts on allowing equal access of all Americans to preventive health care services. Most states use the Healthy People framework to guide the development and implementation of local health policies and programs. Healthy People 2010 recognizes the need to focus on improving the quality of life, as well as reducing disparities in the type of health care services received by Americans (Wilson, 1999).

Healthy People 2010 has established the four objectives that are to be emphasized through the efforts of health care agencies, both public and private, for the next 20 years; see Table 32-2.

## Assessment

The first functional health pattern (Gordon, 1997) is health perception–health management. The focus of this health pattern is the client's own perception of health and well-being, and how the client manages his health (health maintenance). Applying the nursing process is instrumental in addressing the strategies for alterations in health maintenance. The nurse must begin with the assessment phase of the nursing process.

The focus of assessing health maintenance is determining the client's health status. Examples of objective data for assessing health maintenance include such things as the potential or actual risk factors for ineffective health maintenance, and laboratory and diagnostic tests. Subjective data obtained from asking questions (and listening) assists the nurse to identify functional and dysfunctional patterns of health maintenance (see Box 32-4 and refer to Chapter 11 for further information on assessment strategies).

## Risk Factor Identification in Health Maintenance

Identifying risks that could decrease health is essential in the assessment of health maintenance. Risks to health behavior can be physical, environmental, or psychological behaviors that increase an individual's vulnerability to disease or injury. Risk factors also include the following inter-related categories: genes, physiology, age, physical environment, and lifestyle. These factors vary in intensity,

### TABLE 32-2    HEALTHY PEOPLE 2010 OBJECTIVES

| Objective | Description | Examples |
|---|---|---|
| Promote healthy behaviors | Focuses on behaviors resulting from personal choice | • Physical activity<br>• Nutrition<br>• Tobacco use |
| Promote healthy and safe communities | Addresses programs that have an impact on individual health through education and community-based programs | • Environmental health<br>• Food safety<br>• Occupational health<br>• Injury prevention<br>• Violence prevention |
| Improve systems for personal health and public health | Emphasizes the need for all citizens to have access to health care services (goal: to reduce racial and ethnic disparities) | • Maternal, infant, and child<br>• Family planning<br>• Medical product safety<br>• Health education<br>• Public health infrastructure |
| Prevent and reduce diseases and disorders | Outlines specific interventions related to chronic, prevalent health problems | • Cancer<br>• Cardiovascular disease<br>• Stroke<br>• Arthritis<br>• Mental illness |

Data from Chrvala, C. A., & Bulger, R. J. (1999). Leading health indicators for Healthy People 2010: Final report, Division of Health Promotion and Disease Prevention, Institute of Medicine; Wilson, L. M. (1999). Healthy people—a new millennium: Progress and comparison on the Healthy People 2000 and Healthy People 2010 objectives. *JONAs Healthcare Law, Ethics, and Regulation, 1*(2), 29–32.

## BOX 32-4    QUESTIONS FOR THE NURSE TO ASK IN ASSESSING HEALTH MAINTENANCE

- How do you feel about your current status of health?

- What do you do to maintain or improve your health?

- What factors keep you from being healthy?

Pender, J., Murdaugh, C., & Parsons, M. A. (2002). *Health promotion in nursing practice* (4th ed.). Upper Saddle River, NJ: Prentice-Hall.

## STOP AND THINK

### Laboratory and Diagnostic Tests

- Why is it important for the client to know both the normal and abnormal values of the diagnostic test?

- What are potential resources for a client to "learn more" about a specific diagnostic test?

## CLINICAL ALERT

### Health Maintenance Involving Diagnostic Tests for Diabetes

Clients with diabetes may not take appropriate measures when their blood glucose readings are high. These clients must be taught parameters for which they should contact their health care providers. For example, readings above 300 mg/dl and clinical manifestations such as nausea and vomiting, abdominal pain, severe fatigue, and muscle cramps should be reported to the health care provider. Out-of-control diabetic crises require immediate attention and management to prevent severe complications.

Daniels, R. (2003). *Delmar's manual of laboratory and diagnostic tests*. Clifton Park, NY: Delmar Learning.

and multiple risk factors may interact to develop additional risk factors. Assessing the client's knowledge of his risk factors can lead to the identification of health-promotion and disease-prevention activities. The nurse should assess for cues during the nursing history process that warn of the presence of a risk factor. Many tools are available for risk identification, and the nurse must carefully assess for potential or actual risk factors (Edelman & Mandle, 2002).

## Laboratory and Diagnostic Tests and Health Maintenance

Laboratory data (e.g., cholesterol levels, blood glucose, urine studies) are important pieces of information in assessing health maintenance. Health-maintenance behaviors may be measured with varieties of diagnostic tests and equipment, such as pregnancy tests, blood glucose monitors, thermometers, body fat calculators, and sphygmomanometers (Figure 32-6). It is important for nurses to make sure clients know the proper use and maintenance of the equipment. It is also necessary to educate clients on what to do with the results obtained from these tests. Clients may monitor blood pressure at home, but never contact the health care provider with elevated readings. Clients may think they are practicing health-maintenance activities appropriately, while in reality, they may be putting their health in jeopardy.

## Nursing Diagnosis

Alterations in health maintenance are caused by a client's inability to perform the daily functions needed to maintain health. The nurse's role is to first assess the client and then to select the appropriate nursing diagnosis pertinent to the client's condition. The selected nursing diagnosis will be identified by the defining characteristics of the client's condition (see Box 32-5). Several nursing diagnoses are typical for the functional health pattern of health maintenance. These nursing diagnoses are *Ineffective Health*

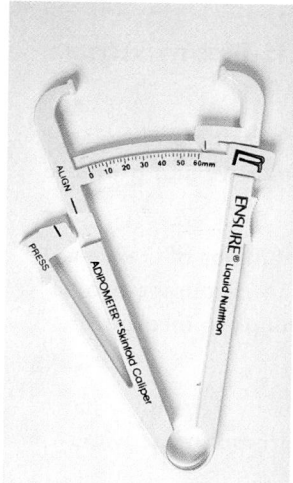
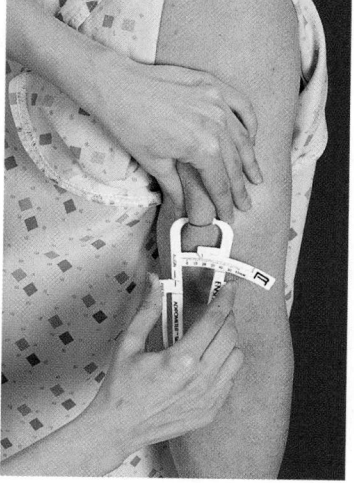

**Figure 32-6**    **Body fat measurement device**

## BOX 32-5    DEFINING CHARACTERISTICS FOR INEFFECTIVE HEALTH MAINTENANCE

The following are typical defining characteristics for the nursing diagnoses in alterations in health maintenance:

- Impairment of personal support systems

- Observed inability to take responsibility for meeting basic health practices

- Demonstrated lack of knowledge

- Failure to recognize important symptoms reflective of altered health state

- Lack of health-seeking behaviors

- Inadequate resources (e.g., equipment, finances, care providers)

## BOX 32-6    CLIENT OUTCOMES FOR INEFFECTIVE HEALTH MAINTENANCE

Examples of client outcomes for ineffective health maintenance are:

- Follows mutually acceptable health care maintenance plan

- Meets goals for health care maintenance

- Describes positive health-maintenance behaviors

- Identifies available resources for meeting health-maintenance alterations

*Maintenance, Health-Seeking Behavior, Noncompliance, Deficient Knowledge,* and *Ineffective Therapeutic Regimen Management.* After selecting the nursing diagnoses, the nurse identifies the risk factors that contribute to the client's dysfunctional health maintenance. Expected outcomes are developed to direct the client in pursuit of health, and the nurse devises interventions with the client to improve health status. An example of correct use of health-maintenance nursing diagnoses is seen in this chapter's case study.

## Planning and Outcome Identification

In identifying goals and planning nursing care for clients with alterations in health maintenance, the nurse considers client outcomes for each nursing diagnosis and each client. The goals that are developed will be individualized to reflect the client's capabilities and limitations. In many ineffective health-maintenance situations, the desired outcomes of care are best accomplished in small increments.

The client outcomes for an individual client are developed from the assessment data that led to the most appropriate nursing diagnosis (see Box 32-6). For example, if a diabetic client is dependent on insulin and becomes unemployed, the desired outcome for interventions could be obtaining the necessary resources to enable purchasing the insulin in order to not miss any doses of the medication. Achievement of the outcome resolves the problem for the client.

## Implementation

Nurses play a key role in promoting health and wellness. Through health promotion and risk reduction, the individual develops behavior patterns that promote a healthy lifestyle and reduce the risk of disease.

The challenge for nurses is to ensure policies and programs are conducive to health promotion. For example, it is not just a class on proper nutrition to enable people to change unhealthy eating patterns, but also the economic and structural resources that are required for good nutrition.

Another challenge for nurses is to find a way to motivate individuals and families to develop health-promoting behaviors. When behaviors that once worked for the individual are no longer effective, the individual must

 **STOP AND THINK**

### Inexpensive Health-Promoting Behaviors

Several behaviors, such as walking and breastfeeding, are relatively inexpensive and promote health.

- What are some other examples of inexpensive behaviors that nurses can encourage people of all socioeconomic groups to incorporate into their lifestyles?

- What reasons should the nurse give for participating in these health-promoting activities?

## NURSING STRATEGY

### Strategies for Health Promotion

| Health Promotion Strategies | Health Promotion IS NOT | Health Promotion IS |
| --- | --- | --- |
| Creating supportive environments | Recommending stress management courses for men | Creating an environment that includes men in a team approach to decision making regarding stress management |
| Strengthening community action and participation | Creating a women's group around an outside agenda | Responding to issues identified by women in partnership with other groups and community members |
| Developing healthy public policy | Imposing a policy that has been developed without consultation of the affected individuals and communities | Developing effective smoking restrictions in consultation with the affected individuals and communities |
| Developing personal skills | Giving an adolescent a pamphlet or fact sheet about risky health behaviors | Offering a program that develops adolescent skills for decision making related to risky health behaviors |
| Reorienting health care services | A health care organization setting program priorities for families | Families defining their own health issues and creating the solutions |

Adapted from Pender, J., Murdaugh, C., & Parsons, M. A. (2002). *Health promotion in nursing practice* (4th ed.). Upper Saddle River, NJ: Prentice-Hall.

give up the old behaviors to be able to adopt new, healthier ones. Teaching is an intervention for promoting health along with the supportive economic and structural conditions necessary for changing a behavior (Figure 32-7). An essential component of teaching is encouraging clients to make necessary lifestyle changes to promote health.

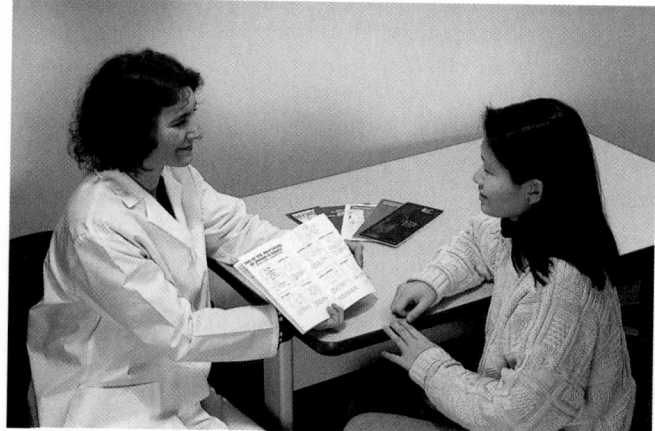

**Figure 32-7    To promote the health of this new juvenile diabetic client, the nurse is providing her with information necessary to change her behavior.**

## CLIENT EDUCATION

### Resources Required for Good Nutrition

The home health nurse can make the following statements to direct clients with limited resources to improve their nutrition intake:

✓ You plan to go to your local food store with $30.
✓ Can you walk to the store or do you have a car?
✓ Is there a bus or other form of public transportation you can take to get there?
✓ How much do you have to pay for transportation costs?
✓ How many fruits and vegetables can you purchase with the money remaining after transportation costs?
✓ How many packages of instant macaroni and cheese can you purchase with the money remaining after transportation costs?
✓ Compare your potential purchases with daily caloric and nutritional requirements for children and adults as recommended in daily food guides.

Motivation is a key component of achieving and maintaining health. Nurses can better help clients engage in healthy behaviors by considering the client's beliefs and experiences when planning care. Many factors help clients feel motivated to change health behaviors:

- Perception of self as able to succeed (self-efficacy)
- Belief that health status will improve
- Response to their attempts to change in the form of feeling healthier and receiving confirmation of these changes from others

## Health Promotion and Vulnerable Populations

Risk factors that threaten the health of individuals include teen parenting, poverty, and chronic disease (Olds, Henderson, Kitzman, & Cole, 1999). The health of certain population groups is threatened (Table 32-3). Especially vulnerable groups include:

- Children
- Older people
- Those who are economically disadvantaged
- Those who are immunocompromised
- The homeless
- Immigrants and refugees

One primary variable affecting health promotion is socioeconomic status. Middle- and upper-income families are more likely to demonstrate healthy behaviors as they have the financial means to purchase nutritional foods, buy exercise equipment, and pay for recreation. The monies of lower socioeconomic families are typically used in meeting basic needs such as food, shelter, and acute medical care. Health-promoting options must be affordable and readily available to people of all economic levels. Political involvement is one avenue for nursing to advance the health status of all. Nurses must be actively involved in shaping delivery of health care to influence the establishment of resources for underserved, disenfranchised groups.

Another variable affecting health is age. Older individuals tend to describe themselves as well when they are physically active, relatively free from pain, and able to maintain meaningful social ties. Maintaining independence and quality of life are of great importance for most elders. Nurses can promote self-care activities with elders to facilitate their wellness.

## The Individual as a Holistic Being

When implementing nursing interventions in clients with health-maintenance considerations, the nurse must remember that the individual is a holistic (**holism** is the belief that individuals function as complete units that cannot be reduced to the sum of their parts) being.

Due to the interwoven nature of the body and mind, it is impossible to separate physiological needs from psychosocial ones. **Psychoneuroimmunology** (the study of the complex relationship between the cognitive, affective,

| TABLE 32-3 | EXAMPLES OF LIFE SPAN CONSIDERATIONS FOR NURSING CONSIDERATIONS IN INEFFECTIVE HEALTH MAINTENANCE | |
|---|---|---|
| Developmental Stage | Common Problem Areas | Interventions |
| Fetus/Newborn/Infant | Hostile environment (e.g., alcohol use) | Identify poor health practices of mother. |
| | Inadequate nutrition | Teach mother the value of breast-feeding and feeding formulas with good nutrients. |
| Toddler/Preschooler/ School-Aged Child | Accidents/injuries | Educate regarding safety practices (e.g., wearing helmets, seat belts) (Figure 32-8) |
| Adolescence | Peer pressure and unhealthy choices (Figure 32-9) | Encourage open, honest communication with parents and guardians. Educate as to the consequences of poor choices. Identify healthy behaviors and activities. |
| Adulthood | Stress/chronic illness/financial pressure | Teach stress-management techniques. Education in physical self-examination practices. Encourage health care provider input and routine physical examinations. |

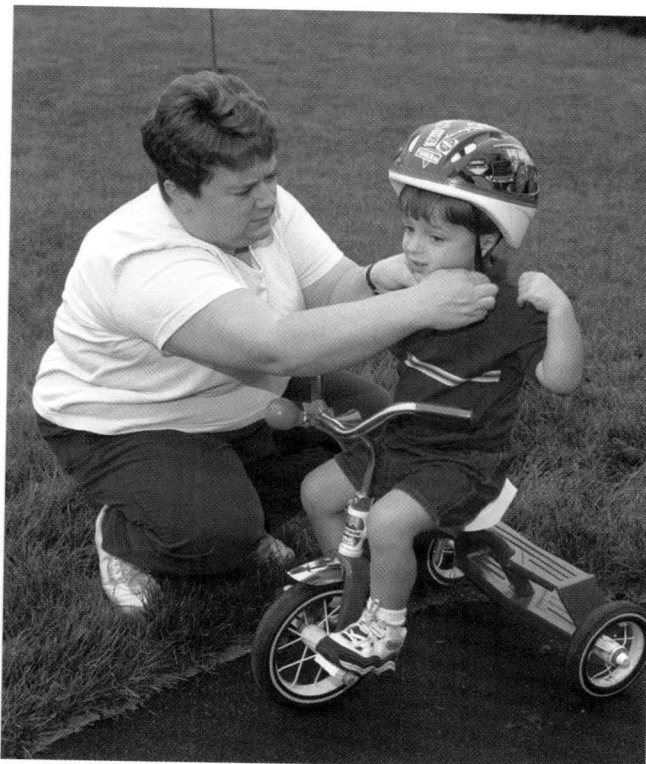

**Figure 32-8** The use of safety equipment such as safety helmets helps to protect children from injury.

and physical aspects of individuals) is based on recognition of the concept that mind, body, and spirit are one. "Our biology and our minds are in constant communication" (Leighton, 1998, p. 36). For example, a person who is physically ill also experiences psychosocial disruptions. On the other hand, when a person is anxious or depressed, physical manifestations occur. "In the natural world, there is no mind-body split. Rather, mind, body, and spirit are intricately connected" (Edmands, Hoff, Kaylor, Mower, & Sorrel, 1999, p. 35).

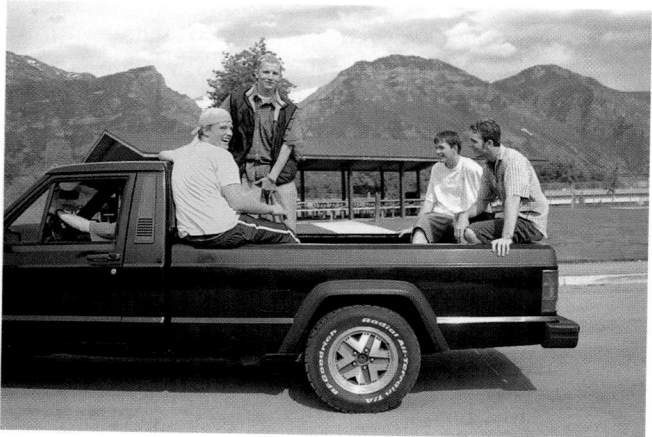

**Figure 32-9** Peer pressure often causes adolescents to engage in risky behavior.

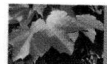

## RESEARCH FOCUS

**Title of Study:** Health promotion and participatory action research with South Asian women

**Study Purpose:** To examine South Asian immigrant women's health-promotion issues. The study objectives included the generation of knowledge to understand the effects of psychological, cultural, and personal factors upon participants' health as perceived by them and strategies for change to enable participants to take control of their health and reduce health risks.

**Methods:** The study was conducted over a 3-year period. It was a qualitative study guided by critical social theory. Participatory action research (PAR) was the research model used. In this model, researchers and study participants share power and decision making. Two groups of South Asian women (women from India and women of Indian origin) who had immigrated to Canada participated in the project. The qualitative data were generated through focus groups. Reflexive and dialectical critiques were used as methods of analyzing qualitative data. The data were interpreted through a reiterative process, and dominant themes were identified.

**Findings:** The researchers discovered the following three themes that influence participants' health: (1) the importance of maintaining culture and tradition, (2) placing family needs before self, and (3) surviving by being strong. An issue for the participants was intergenerational conflict leading to alienation of family members. The participants identified workshops as a strategy to promote health and resolve conflict. Over the 3-year period, workshops developed by the participants included the following topics: respect, religion, culture, marriage, dating, and parenting in Canada.

**Implications:** The research process empowered participants to develop and share knowledge, which was paramount in developing strategies to promote health. The findings indicated that family health affects women's health. They also showed that threats to cultural values can be destabilizing to the family and the community. Appropriate cultural interventions to maintain traditional values can decrease health risks and promote well-being in immigrant communities.

Choudhry, U. K., Jandu, S., Mahl, J., Singh, R., Sohi-Pabla, H., & Mutta, B. (2002). Health promotion and participatory action research with South Asian women. *Journal of Nursing Scholarship, 34*(1), 75–81.

The practice of body-mind medicine is not new and is rooted in the origins of healing, as shown in the following examples:

- Hippocrates taught doctors to establish trust with their patients.
- Hippocrates taught doctors to observe the emotional states of patients.
- Socrates suggested that curing the soul leads to healing.
- The fundamental principle of traditional Chinese medicine is to honor the spirit (Leighton, 1998).
- Florence Nightingale recognized "the need to honor the physiological and spiritual aspects of our patients" (Dossey & Dossey, 1998, p. 35).

This holistic viewpoint guides the total care of the individual as a *complete being* rather than fragmented care focused on parts of the person. Only when nurses treat clients as individuals and not as "cases" to be "cured" do nurses respond in a holistic, caring way. A major role for nurses is to put the *caring* back into the process of healing. In the holistic model, "health is seen as the achievement of a full and happy life characterized by social and spiritual connection, mental and emotional balance, and a healthy body" (Leighton, 1998, p. 36).

## Needs and Health

To implement holistic nursing interventions in health maintenance situations, the nurse takes into account the existing human needs. Since human beings are not merely physiological creatures, basic human needs occur in the emotional, sociocultural, intellectual, and spiritual realms as well as the physiological realm. The entire person (body, mind, and spirit) is influenced by satisfaction of needs. Figure 32-10 illustrates the various human dimensions in which needs occur. A variety of needs emerge, are met, and reemerge in each area of a person's life.

A need is anything that is absolutely *essential* for one's existence. **Basic human needs** (also known as universal needs) are those that are necessary for every person's survival. Table 32-4 provides an overview of basic needs.

Maslow (1970) classified human needs as they occur on a tier with the most basic needs at the foundation of the hierarchy (Figure 32-11). These basic needs must be met before the individual can satisfy higher-level needs. For example, an individual who is starving must be fed before achieving the need for acceptance. An individual with a deficient self-esteem and who is hemorrhaging must have the biologic needs met first. The satisfaction of basic needs enhances wellness. Conversely, an impairment in the satisfaction of basic needs can result in a client's altered health status.

## STOP AND THINK

### Holistic Nurturing

How do you nourish each dimension of your being? In other words, how do you feed your body? Your mind? Your spirit?

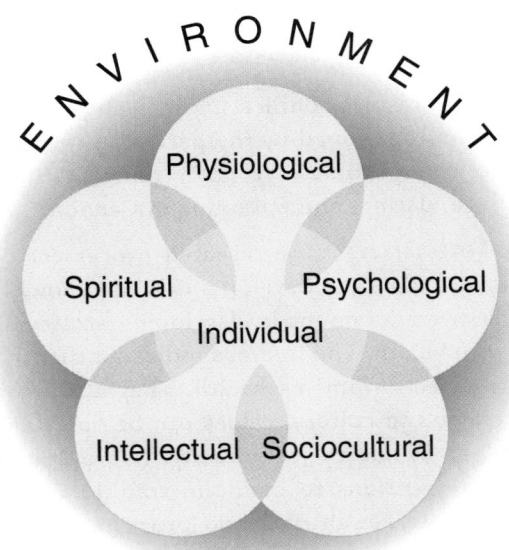

**Figure 32-10** **Holistic perspective of the individual**

| TABLE 32-4 | BASIC HUMAN NEEDS |
|---|---|
| **Need** | **Example** |
| Physiological | Oxygen, water, food, temperature (shelter and clothing), elimination, sleep, activity, and sex |
| Psychological | Self-esteem, feelings of security, happiness, sadness |
| Sociocultural | Feelings of belonging, relationships |
| Intellectual | Thinking, learning |
| Spiritual | Being connected to others, having a sense of purpose |

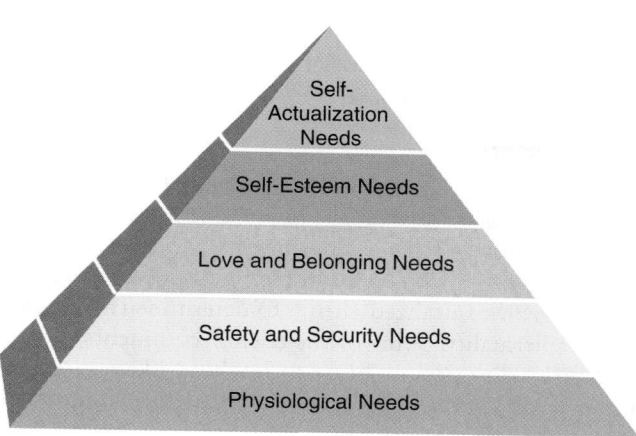

**Figure 32-11    Maslow's hierarchy of needs**

The following section describes implementing nursing care in addressing the basic needs related to the physiological, psychological, sociocultural, intellectual, spiritual, and sexual dimensions.

## Physiological Dimension

Providing physiological care focuses on the achievement of the basic needs of a client. The nurse must assess the client for the alterations that are occurring and then provide interventions to meet the client's needs. There are many physiological needs in health maintenance, and several examples of physiological interventions are provided in this section.

## Physical Self-Examination Techniques

Physical self-examination is a health maintenance behavior that doesn't require any special equipment, but requires proper instruction on the correct procedure. Breast self-exams, testicular exams, and skin exams should begin at age 18 for women and age 15 for

## STOP AND THINK

### Prioritizing Needs

Jane Thompson visits the public health clinic because of severe headaches. During the interview, the nurse practitioner learns that Jane and her three children frequently have no place to sleep because she has no income. Identify Ms. Thompson's problems. Using Maslow's hierarchy, which problem would be of the first priority? How do you determine which problem to address first?

men. The exams should be performed monthly. The nurse encourages the client to select a day that is easy to remember (e.g., the first day of the month). Then the nurse instructs the client on the correct technique of the self-exam. In addition, a return demonstration by the client is essential to ensure the client performs the exam properly (Estes, 2002). It is important that the nurse instructs the client in what to look for and what action to take if an abnormal finding is identified (see Chapter 46 for specific information of breast and testicular self-examinations).

## Health Maintenance in Nutrition Management Behaviors

Inadequate nutritional intake affects the activities of daily living. The exact number of health problems that can be directly attributed to the diet are unknown. Throughout the life cycle, nutritional needs change in relation to growth, development, and activity levels. In children, hunger compromises the ability to learn. Hungry children have a higher absentee rate, and when they do attend school, they have a difficult time concentrating. Inadequate nutrition can have a lasting effect on a child's cognitive development. Inadequate nutrition in adults impairs their ability to concentrate, which in turn can lead to poor work performance. Energy levels are also compromised. Inadequate nutrition also weakens a person's immune system, increasing susceptibility to illness and disease. Nursing interventions include such things as educating the client with information regarding food groups and recommended nutrients, selecting a diet plan that meets the client's nutrition needs, advising the client to keep a food journal to monitor the dietary intake, assisting the client and family to access resources for obtaining nutritious food, and teaching the client the clinical manifestations associated with nutrient deficiencies or excess (Roth & Townsend, 2002).

## Health Maintenance and Alterations in Sleep Patterns

Another health maintenance problem that affects activities of daily living is the lack of sleep. Sleep accomplishes restoration of physical well-being, relieves anxiety and stress, and restores the ability to cope and concentrate on activities of daily living. Poor sleep patterns can affect a person's ability to concentrate at work and school, resulting in a negative effect on their performance. Exercise, smoking, alcohol consumption, illness, and stress can all affect a person's sleep patterns. The nurse can suggest that the client monitor sleep patterns and keep a journal of hours of sleep for each 24-hour period (Idzikowski, 2000). In addition, the client can be encouraged to establish a routine bedtime to facilitate the transition from wakefulness to sleep (for further specific nursing interventions refer to Chapter 40).

## Psychological Dimension

Individuals have psychological needs for security, a sense of belonging, and self-esteem. Nursing actions that promote a sense of emotional comfort include the following:

- Treating the client as a unique individual
- Protecting confidentiality and privacy
- Using touch and personal space in a therapeutic manner
- Recognizing and respecting cultural differences
- Decreasing anxiety through stress management techniques

Goals for clients experiencing unmet psychological needs usually revolve around the following issues:

- Improve self-esteem
- Establish trusting relationships
- Develop social skills
- Cope with losses

## Sociocultural Dimension

As social creatures, all people rely on others to some extent. "The need for others seems as vital to our health as food and shelter" (Leighton, 1998, p. 35). Research (Dossey & Dossey, 1998) has shown that social connection is correlated with positive health outcomes. It is difficult for some people to ask for help or to accept assistance when it is offered. It is important for nurses to assess the client's degree of dependence. Often, the nurse becomes involved in a balancing act in an effort to maintain equilibrium between the client's needs for dependence and independence.

**Empowerment** is a process of enabling others to do for themselves. It consists of encouraging the client to be an active participant in treatment rather than a passive recipient of care. Nurses empower clients by teaching them and their families how to develop skills for self-care and for healthier living (see Chapter 23 for more discussion of the concept of empowerment).

## Intellectual Dimension

The intellectual dimension consists of cognitive functions such as judgment, orientation, memory, and the ability to take in and process information. Refer to Chapter 41 for information on cognition and perception.

Piaget conducted landmark studies on children to determine how children think at various developmental stages; refer to Chapter 17 for a complete discussion of cognitive development.

Intellectual functioning can be impaired by multiple factors, including infection, exposure to toxins, substance abuse, trauma, and psychological problems. It is important for nurses to determine the client's intellectual abilities in order to communicate effectively. Using words that are easily comprehended by the client and implementing teaching strategies appropriate to developmental level promotes client learning.

## Spiritual Dimension

**Spirituality** is multidimensional in that it refers to one's relationship with one's self, a sense of connection with others, and a relationship with a higher power or divine source. Spirituality assists a person in determining the sense of meaning or purpose in one's life. It is an integral component, or core, of one's being. Spirituality is somewhat difficult to define, as it is determined at an individual level. A survey conducted by Moeller (1999) interviewed hospitalized clients to determine their meaning of spirituality. Some of the clients' comments included "spirituality ties my heart to my head like a ligament and is strong and flexible," and "spirituality is hope there is something better" (p. 6).

Spirituality is *not* the same as religion, which refers to a set of beliefs and practices associated with a particular church, synagogue, mosque, or other formal organized group. Spirituality is a personal, individualized set of beliefs and practices that are not church related (see Chapter 48 for an in-depth discussion of the spiritual dimension of health).

## Sexual Dimension

**Sexuality** is a complex human characteristic that refers not just to genital sex but to all the aspects of being male or female, including feelings, attitudes, beliefs, and behavior. It is an essential part of one's personality. Sexuality is a pervasive aspect of the total self from birth to death and is an important aspect of health for people of all ages. Sexuality includes a person's attitudes toward relationships with people of the same sex, relationships with those of the opposite sex, and about touching and being touched. The ways people dress, talk, and relate to others are indicators of their sexuality.

**Sex roles** are culturally determined patterns associated with being male and female. These patterns are developed as a result of cultural expectations, customs, norms, habits, and traditions. For example, the differences between the sexes are evident in the ways infants are treated during their first days of life. Infant boys and infant girls are talked to, handled, and, many times, dressed differently. In many cultures, the role of the man is to be strong and protective, whereas the woman is expected to be passive and nurturing. Sex roles change as societal norms change and may be accepted or rejected by individuals (see Chapter 46 for an in-depth discussion of the sexual dimension of health).

# Evaluation

Evaluation is essential in the health-maintenance health pattern of an individual. The client and nurse together must measure how well the client has achieved the goals specified in the plan of care. Factors that contribute to the client's ability to achieve the goal are identified. This is also when goals may need to be reevaluated and adjusted accordingly.

# CASE STUDY/NURSING CARE PLAN

Sheila is a 44-year-old female who works as a receptionist in a large accounting firm. She has three children; ages 16, 18, and 21. Since her divorce 12 years ago, she has been a single mother. Sheila is concerned about her weight and her family history of high blood pressure and diabetes. She knows that exercising would be good for her, but she "just can't see how to fit it into her busy schedule." Working full time and being a single parent leaves her feeling exhausted. She lives in a small house in a neighborhood with a high crime rate, causing her to feel unsafe. She has come to your clinic to have a long overdue physical examination. At the end of her visit, she is scheduled to return for another appointment in 2 weeks.

## Assessment

Client is 5 feet 3 inches, weighs 172 pounds., blood pressure is 160/94, and her fasting blood glucose is 183 mg/dl. She has many external stressors in her life: single mother, unsafe neighborhood, no regular exercise program. She acknowledges she needs to make changes in her life and is prepared to do so. Her father suffered a stroke at 66 years of age, from which he subsequently died. Her mother has diabetes and high blood pressure.

## Nursing Diagnosis #1

*Ineffective Health Maintenance* related to lack of knowledge in basic health practices.
**NOC:** Health Beliefs: Perceived Resources; Health-Promoting Behavior; Health-Seeking Behavior
**NIC:**   Health System Guidance; Support System Enhancement; Health Education

## Expected Outcomes

The client will:
1. Identify an understanding of factors contributing to current situation by her next clinic visit.
2. Adopt lifestyle changes necessary to support her health goals by her next clinic visit.

## Planning/Interventions/Rationales

1. Assess knowledge level regarding health status. *Provides an accurate baseline of information regarding the client.*
2. Assist client in identifying areas of health behavior that need to be changed (e.g., exercise routine, healthy eating habits). *Equips client with behaviors that will positively affect health maintenance.*

## Evaluation

Client came to her second appointment in 2 weeks. She kept a journal of her activities and prioritized which behaviors were unhealthy and which behaviors needed to be changed. She has exercised twice and states she is "starting a new diet."

## Nursing Diagnosis #2

*Health-Seeking Behavior* related to concern of current health practices.
**NOC:** Health-Promoting Behavior; Health-Seeking Behavior; Adherence Behavior; Health Beliefs
**NIC:**   Health System Guidance; Support System Enhancement; Health Education

## Expected Outcome

The client will:
1. Express desire to change current lifestyle patterns to achieve or maintain optimal health by her second clinic visit.

## Planning/Intervention/Rationale

1. Provide instruction on appropriate wellness behaviors (e.g., breast self-examination, skin examinations, exercise, diet). *Increases adherence to health maintenance practices.*

## Evaluation

Client states that she has performed breast self-examinations twice, and has a greater motivation to develop healthy practices (e.g., diet, exercise, stress management).

# Key Concepts

- Health is a process through which the person seeks to maintain an equilibrium that promotes stability and comfort and varies depending on context and situation.
- Illness is the inability of an individual's adaptive responses to maintain physical and emotional balance and results in an impairment in functional ability.
- Wellness is the condition in which an individual functions at optimal levels and is a dynamic process that occurs in varying degrees.
- The various theoretical models of health, such as the clinical, health-belief, high-level wellness, social learning theory, the host-agent-environment, and health promotion models, help nurses to understand the relationship between the experience of health and illness and clients' behaviors in response to this process.
- The three approaches to health maintenance (health promotion, health protection, and disease prevention) are centered on the individual's and society's responsibility in promoting one's own health.
- Nurses play a role in helping clients to adopt healthy lifestyles and use approaches such as role modeling and formal teaching to motivate client change.
- Nurses must focus their efforts on improving the health status of vulnerable populations.
- The satisfaction of basic human needs, such as physiological, psychological, sociocultural, intellectual, and spiritual needs, is necessary for every person's survival.
- Lifestyle, locus of control, self-efficacy, health care attitudes, and self-concept are examples of variables that influence health-promoting behaviors.
- An impairment in meeting basic needs results in an altered health status.
- A holistic viewpoint helps nurses to recognize the body-mind connection and see the client as a whole person rather than fragmented parts.
- Health protection, disease prevention, and health promotion are centered on individual and societal responsibilities for health.
- Nurses must focus their efforts on supporting and creating policy, structural resources, and economic resources that are conducive to health promotion.

# Review Questions and Activities

1. What are the nursing implications of Maslow's hierarchy of basic needs?
2. Critique one article from your local newspaper about a sociopolitical or economic issue that currently affects the health of the citizens in your community.
3. Select a classmate to interview. Note any relationship between attitudes and physical symptoms. Does your partner feel better physically when mentally relaxed? Vice versa?
4. Interview five people in your community. Ask them how they know when they are healthy. Compare the answers, and develop a brief list of determinants of health.
5. Think about motivation and lifestyle changes. What motivates you to engage in healthy behaviors? How can you find incentives to "use" in teaching clients about the need to modify habits that affect health?
6. What do you think are the three most important issues that affect the health of Americans today? List in terms of priority.
7. What health-promotion activities or programs are currently available for vulnerable populations in your community?

# Web Resources

American Holistic Nurses Association
    http://www.ahna.org
American Psychological Association
    http://www.apa.org
The Center for the Advancement of Health
    http://www.cfah.org
Health Promotion
    http://www.healthfinder.gov
Healthy People 2010
    http://www.health.gov
The Rockerfeller Foundation: Health Equity Program
    http://www.rockfound.org

# References

American Holistic Nurses Association. (2003). http://www.ahna.org

Bandura, A. (1977). *A social learning theory*. Englewood Cliffs, NJ: Prentice Hall.

Bandura, A. (1986). *Social foundation of thought and action: A social, cognitive theory*. Englewood Cliffs, NJ: Prentice Hall.

Becker, M. H. (1974). The health belief model and sick role behavior. *Health Education Monogram, 2,* 409–419.

Borsody, J. M., Courtney, M., Taylor, K., & Jairath, N. (1999). Using self-efficacy to increase physical activity in patients with heart failure. *Home Healthcare Nurse, 17*(2), 113–118.

Choudhry, U. K., Jandu, S., Mahl, J., Singh, R., Sohi-Pabla, H., & Mutta, B. (2002). Health promotion and participatory action research with South Asian women. *Journal of Nursing Scholarship, 34*(1), 75–81.

Chrvala, C. A., & Bulger, R. J. (1999). *Leading health indicators for Healthy People 2010: Final report*. Division of Health Promotion and Disease Prevention, Institute of Medicine. Washington, DC: National Academy Press.

Collins, A. M., & Diego, L. (2000). Mental health promotion and protection. *Journal of Psychosocial Nursing, 38*(1), 27–32.

Covington, C., Cybulski, M., Davis, T., Duca, G., Farrel, E., Kasgorgis, M., Kator, C., & Sell, T. (2001), Kids on the move: Preventing obesity among urban children. *American Journal of Nursing, 101*(3), 73–75, 77, 79, 81–82.

Daniels, R. (2003). *Delmar's manual of laboratory and diagnostic tests.* Clifton Park, NY: Delmar Learning.

Dossey, B., & Dossey, L. (1998). Attending to holistic care. *American Journal of Nursing, 98*(8), 35–38.

Dunn, H. (1961). *High-level wellness.* Arlington, VA: R. W. Beatty.

Edelman, C., & Mandle, C. (2002). *Health promotion throughout the life span* (5th ed.). St. Louis: Mosby.

Edmands, M. E., Hoff, L. A., Kaylor, L., Mower, L., & Sorrel, S. (1999). Bridging gaps between mind, body, and spirit. *Journal of Psychosocial Nursing, 37*(10), 35–42.

Erickson, H., Tomlin, E., & Swain, M. (1983). *Modeling and role-modeling.* New Jersey: Prentice-Hall, Inc.

Estes, M. (2002). *Health assessment & physical examination* (2nd ed.). Clifton Park, NY: Delmar Learning.

Flynn, B. (1997). Partnerships in health cities and communities: A social commitment for advanced practice nurses. *Advanced practice nursing quarterly 2*(4) 1–6.

Goodman, H. (1997). Patients' perception of their education needs in the first six weeks following discharge after cardiac surgery. *Journal of Advanced Nursing, 25*(6), 1241–1251.

Gordon, M. (1997). *Manual of nursing diagnoses.* St. Louis: Mosby.

Hancock, T., & Duhl, L. (1988). Promoting health in the urban context. *WHO Healthy Cities Papers* series, (1), 24.

Hitchcock, J., Schubert, P., & Thomas, S. (2003). *Community health nursing: Caring in action.* Clifton Park, NY: Delmar Learning.

Idzikowski, C. (2000). *Learn to sleep well: A practical guide to getting a good night's rest.* San Francisco: Chronicle Books.

Kantrowitz, B., & Wingert, P. (2001, May 28). Unmarried with children. *Newsweek,* 46–55.

Leavell, H., & Clark, A. E. (1965). *Preventive medicine for doctors in the community.* New York: McGraw-Hill.

Leighton, C. (1998). A change of heart. *American Journal of Nursing, 98*(10), 33–37.

Littleton, L., & Engebretson, J. (2002). *Maternal, neonatal, and women's health nursing.* Clifton Park, NY: Delmar Learning.

Maslow, A. (1970). *Motivation and personality* (2nd ed.). New York: Harper & Row.

Moeller, M. D. (1999). Meeting spiritual needs on an inpatient unit. *Journal of Psychosocial Nursing, 37*(11), 5–10.

Mosher, R., Youngman, D, & Day, J. (1999). *Human development across the life span: Educational and psychological Applications.* Westport, CT: Praeger.

Murray, R., & Zentner, J. (2001). *Health promotion strategies through the life span* (5th ed.). Upper Saddle River, NJ: Prentice-Hall.

Muscari, M. E. (1998 a,b). Coping with chronic illness. *American Journal of Nursing, 98*(9), 20–22.

National Center for Health Statistics (2002). http://www.cdd.gov/nchs

Olds, D. L., Henderson, C. R., Kitzman, J., & Cole, R. (1995). Effects of prenatal and infancy nurse home visitation on surveillance of child maltreatment. *Pediatrics, 95*(3), 365–372.

Pender, N., Murdaugh, C., & Parsons, M. (2002). *Health promotion in nursing practice* (4th ed.). New Jersey: Prentice Hall.

Potts, N., & Mandleco, B. (2002). *Pediatric nursing: Caring for children and their families.* Clifton Park, NY: Delmar Learning.

Québec World Health Organization (WHO) (1998). http://www.ulaval.ca.

Rosenstock, I. (1974). Historical origin of the health belief model. In M. H. Becker (Ed.), *The health belief model and personal health behavior.* Thorofare, NJ: Charles B. Slack.

Roth, R., & Townsend, C. (2002). *Nutrition & diet therapy* (8th ed.). Clifton Park, NY: Delmar Learning.

Sontag, S. (1988). *Illness as metaphor.* New York: Farrar, Straus and Giroux.

United States Public Health Service (1990). *Healthy people 2000: National health promotion and disease prevention objective.* [Conference edition summary] Washington, DC: U.S. Government Printing Office.

Wilson, L. M. (1999). Healthy people—a new millennium: Progress and comparison on the Healthy People 2000 and Healthy People 2010 objectives. *JONAs Healthcare Law, Ethics, and Regulation, 1*(2), 29–32.

World Health Organization (2002). *World health report 2002: Reducing risks, promoting health lifestyles.* Geneva, Switzerland.

World Health Organization (1986). Ottawa charter for health promotion. *Health Promotion, 1*(4), 2–5.

# 33 CHAPTER

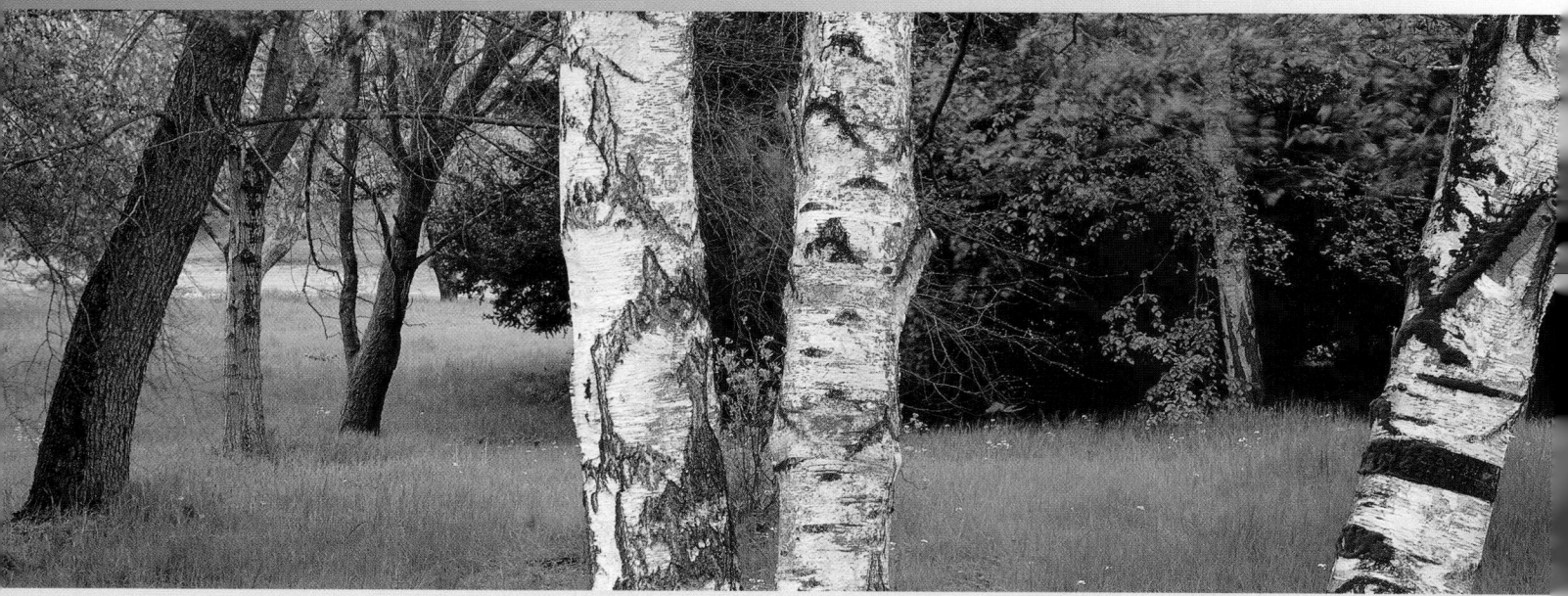

# Safety and Hygiene

Deborah L. Fell-Carlson, BSN, RN, COHN-S, HEM

*"The nurse owes the same duties to self as to others, including the responsibility to preserve integrity and safety, to maintain competence, and to continue personal and professional growth."*

(Code of Ethics for Nurses, *American Nurses Association, 2001*)

# Chapter Competencies

*Upon completion of this chapter, the reader should be able to:*

1. Discuss the importance of a positive safety culture in health care.
2. Describe factors affecting client safety.
3. Explain how factors related to environmental safety for the client relate to workplace safety for the caregiver.
4. Describe factors affecting the safety of the health care worker.
5. Discuss factors that influence a client's personal hygiene practices.
6. Explain the role of assessment in maintaining client safety.
7. Discuss nursing interventions that can be used to resolve environmental hazards and other safety concerns in institutional and home settings.
8. Describe nursing interventions that promote a client's personal hygiene.

# Key Terms

administrative controls
airborne precautions
body image
carcinogens
cavities
chemical restraints
client behavior incidents
contact precautions
corrosives
droplet precautions
engineering controls
equipment incidents
ergonomic stressors
gait belts
gingivitis
halitosis

hygiene
ingestion
inhalation
injection
laser plume
Material Safety Data Sheet (MSDS)
musculoskeletal disorders
N-95 particulate filtering respirator
percutaneous
perineal care
personal protective equipment
physical restraints
poison
pyorrhea

respirator
restraints
routes of exposure
sensitizer
sensory overload
skin absorption
skin contact
Standard Precautions
stomatitis
substitution
target organ chemicals
teratogens
therapeutic procedure incidents
transmission-based precautions

Excellent nursing care is professional, quality care—doing the right things right. Excellent nursing care, therefore, is safe for both the clients receiving the care *and* the workers involved in the health care delivery. Safety is a basic need and must always remain a priority for all. To provide excellent, safe care in any setting, the nurse consistently integrates infection control and safety principles into all activities. This chapter will focus on the nurse's role in safety and injury prevention for both client and health care worker, and will also cover the nurse's role in client hygiene assistance.

## Safety Culture

Health care delivery, especially in the hospital and long-term care setting, is potentially dangerous, for the client as well as for the health care worker. This culture can be changed. The nurse is in a key position to effect such change in the health care delivery system. As safe behaviors are learned and integrated into routine activities, the nurse sets a benchmark for excellence. Accountability is key—by holding themselves and their coworkers accountable to work safely and carefully, nurses establish safety as the accepted standard of care. By holding management accountable to provide a safe workplace, nurses allow safety to emerge as an organizational value. When clients are held accountable, safe behaviors are learned and are often transferred to the home and family environments.

An environment with safety as a core value is a caring and compassionate environment, but not all caring and compassionate environments are safe. Nurses should explore the organization's commitment to safety before accepting a position, and carefully weigh the risks of employment with an organization that does not invest sufficient and appropriate resources to train and equip them to function safely within their work environment. Health care organizations with safety integrated into the overall corporate strategy reap rewards in productivity, morale, and retention. These are great places to work, where staff recruitment is not a worry.

In their report "To Err Is Human" (Kohn, Corrigan, & Donaldson, 2000), the Institute of Medicine states that at least 44,000 Americans, and possibly as many as 98,000, die annually in hospitals due to medical errors. Motor vehicle accidents do not take as many lives as medical errors. It is estimated that 7,000 of these deaths are related to errors in medication delivery. Health care worker injury rates continue to climb, and are currently $2\frac{1}{2}$ times the rate of all other general industries.

The critical shortage of nurses and other caregivers exacerbates the safety problem. Long hours and heavy client loads take an intellectual, emotional, and physical toll on weary workers, decreasing morale and increasing risk of error and vulnerability to injury. The situation is emergent. Mandating staffing ratios is only part of the solution. Nurses must take the initiative to get involved in safety activities designed to improve working conditions.

Safety raises the bar in any setting, and it is essential in a client care environment. It can mean the difference between life and death for the client. For the nurse, it can mean the difference between continued employment and the personal suffering and financial challenges that often accompany temporary or permanent disability. Excellence cannot be achieved fully without safety. Safety is doing the right things right, and nurses have the responsibility to lead and teach by example.

## STOP AND THINK

### A Safe Environment

- If a health care facility does not support a safe environment for you as a nurse, what does that imply to clients about the safety of the care you are able to provide them?

- If your client observes that your work behaviors place you at increased risk for injury, how will she perceive the quality of your attentiveness to her safety?

# Factors Affecting Client Safety

Safety has a positive association with health promotion and illness prevention. A safe environment reduces the risk of accidents, subsequent alterations in health and lifestyle, and the cost of health care services. Many factors in the environment can threaten safety. Age, lifestyle, sensory and perceptual alterations, mobility, and emotional state are just a few of these factors.

## Age

Risk for injury varies with chronological age and developmental stage. Health education about preventive measures can facilitate injury prevention for various age groups (Figure 33-1).

As infants mature, their potential for injury increases. Infants, toddlers, and preschoolers are explorers of their environment. Most accidents involving these age groups, such as falls from bed, burns, electrical hazards, choking on small objects, and drowning, are preventable with careful adult supervision.

As school-aged children explore their environment outside the home, their risk for injury increases. Prevention measures during this stage focus on not accepting candy, food, gifts, or rides from strangers; bicycle, skating, and swimming safety; and substance abuse education.

Adolescents and young adults usually enjoy good physical health; however, their lifestyles put them at risk for injury. Since this age group spends much time away from home, collaborative educational efforts among parents, schools, and community health care providers need to focus on environmental safety. High-risk factors for injury and death are automobile accidents, substance abuse, violence, unwanted pregnancies, and sexually transmitted diseases.

Studies indicate that adolescents who initiate substance use in middle school and continue into high school are likely to become multisubstance users (tobacco, alcohol, and drugs). The progression from lighter to heavier use of illicit substances during adolescence may lead to more serious multisubstance use practices.

Adult risk for injury is generally related to lifestyle, work practices, and behaviors. Prevention measures during this period emphasize nutrition, exercise, and occupational safety. High-risk factors for this age group include fatigue, anxiety, sleep pattern disturbances, caregiver role strain, and altered health maintenance.

The older adult is prone to falls, especially in the bathroom, bedroom, and kitchen, because of a loss of agility and visual acuity, predisposition to dizziness and syncope, and side effects of medications. Prevention measures for this age group emphasize slow position changes, good lighting, hand rails, and skidproof strips in the bathtub or shower and under rugs and carpets.

Each year, approximately one-third of people over the age of 65 who live at home fall. Many falls cause serious

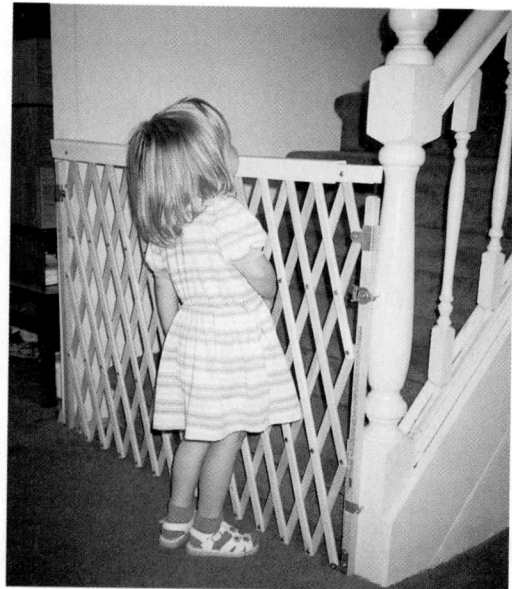

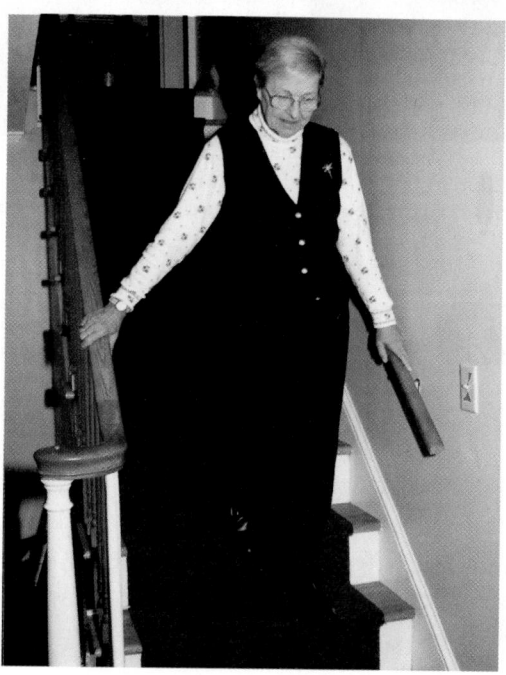

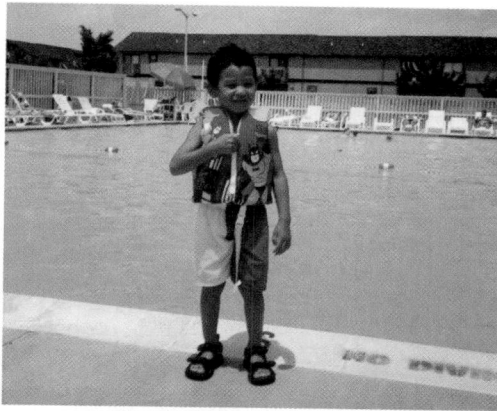

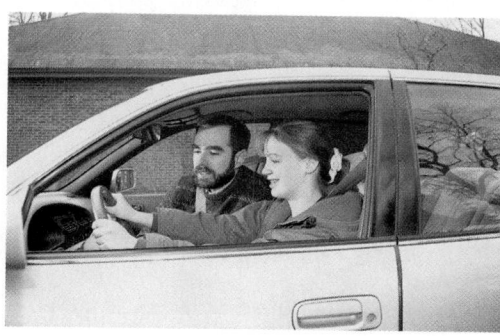

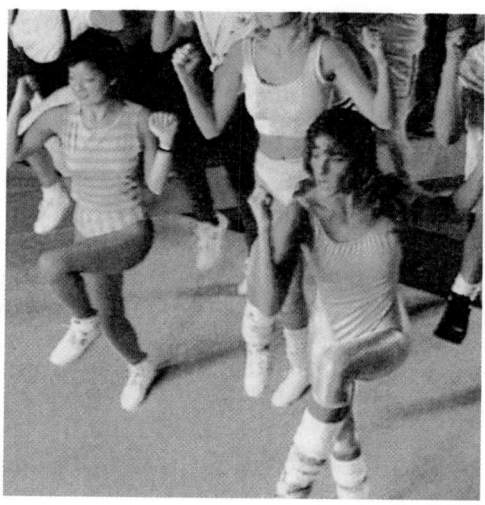

**Figure 33-1   Minimization of risks for injury. These photos show various methods by which people in different age groups can lessen or prevent their risk of injury. Can you identify other risks that may be more prevalent in certain age groups than others? What measures can be taken to prevent injury?**

injuries. Direct costs related to falls is expected to reach $32.4 billion by 2020. Two Maryland hospitals worked together to implement a fall precaution program in their medical-surgical units and within 1 year lowered their fall rates from 9.3 falls per 1,000 client days to 7.3 per 1,000 client days (Sullivan & Badros, 1999). See Chapter 19 for a complete discussion of the older adult.

## Lifestyle

Lifestyle practices can increase a person's risk for injury and potential for disease. Individuals who operate machin-

ery; experience stress, anxiety, and fatigue; use alcohol and drugs (prescription and nonprescription); and live in high-crime neighborhoods are at risk for injury. Risk-taking behaviors such as daredevil activities, driving vehicles at high speeds, and smoking are lifestyle factors associated with accidents (Figure 33-2).

## Sensory and Perceptual Alterations

Sensory functions are essential for accurate perception of environmental safety. If one of the senses is altered, then

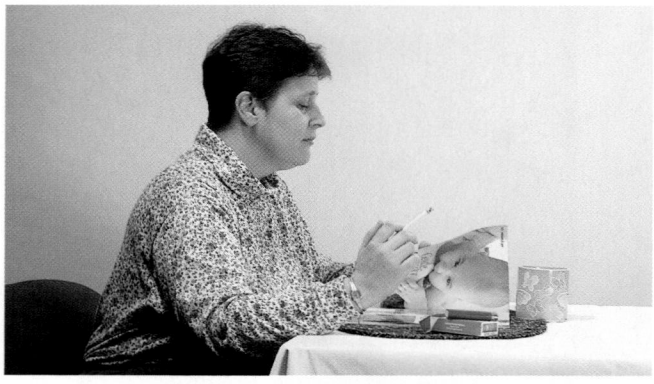

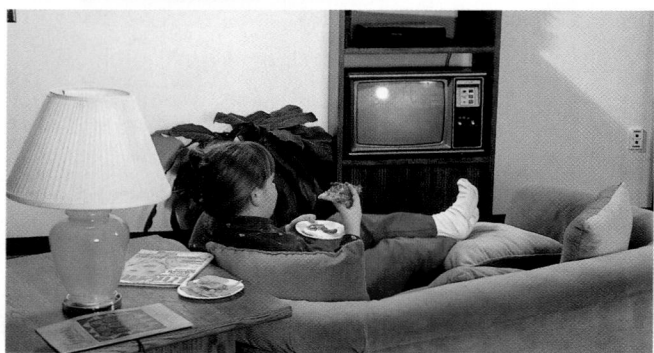

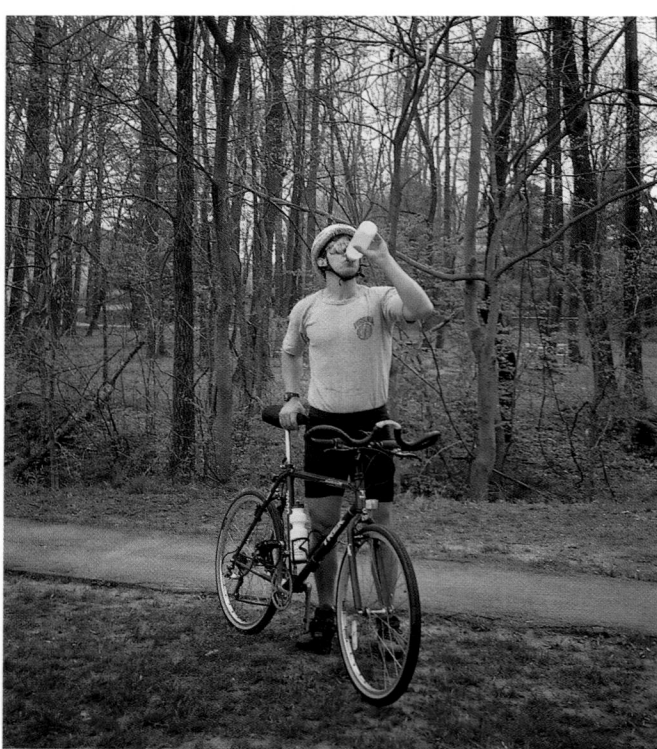

**Figure 33-2**    Lifestyle practices that can either increase or decrease a client's risk of injury. Can these practices be easily reversed, in terms of risky behavior, or adopted, in terms of promoting healthy approaches, by clients?

the other senses compensate to facilitate perception of the environment. For instance, a blind person usually will develop a keen sense of touch and hearing. Clients who have visual, hearing, taste, smell, communication, or touch perception impairments are at increased risk for injury. These clients are often not able to perceive a potential danger. See Chapter 41 for a complete discussion on sensory or perceptual alterations.

## Mobility

Clients who have impaired mobility are at increased risk for injury, especially falls. Mobility impairments may be a result of poor balance or coordination, muscle weakness, or paralysis. Immobility may also precipitate physiological and emotional complications such as decubitus and depression, respectively. See Chapter 38 for a complete discussion on mobility.

## Emotional State

Emotional states such as depression and anger affect a client's perception of environmental hazards and degree of risk-taking behavior. These emotional states alter a client's thinking patterns and reaction time. Usual safety precautions may be forgotten during periods of emotional stress. Self-confidence decreases when an older person falls; older people tend to limit their activities because they fear falling again (Winslow, 1998).

### COMMUNITY/HOME CARE

## Community Care in an Urban Environment: Pedestrian Safety Principles

All individuals, regardless of age, should learn the following pedestrian safety principles if they will be walking along roadways:

- Wear light-colored or reflective clothing to increase visibility, especially at night.

- Use a flashlight to help illuminate hazards in your path.

- Cross only in crosswalks, waiting until traffic is clear or has come to a stop.

- Always walk on the left, facing traffic, regardless of the time of day.

- Avoid roadways without an adequate shoulder.

## Types of Incidents

Mishaps in any health care setting have serious implications and should be investigated. By carefully planning care and anticipating the unexpected, the nurse provides an environment where such an incident is an unlikely occurrence. Incidents in the health care setting are categorized by their causative agent: client behaviors, therapeutic procedures, or equipment:

1. **Client behavior incidents** occur when the client's behavior or actions precipitate the incident—for example, poisonings, burns, and self-inflicted cuts and bruises.
2. **Therapeutic procedure incidents** occur during the delivery of medical or nursing interventions—for example, medication errors, client falls during transfers, contamination of sterile instruments or wounds, and improper performance of nursing activities.
3. **Equipment incidents** result from the malfunction or improper use of medical equipment—for example, electrocution and fire.

## Safety and the Environment of Care

Review the nursing responsibilities in providing a safe care environment outlined in Chapter 25. Table 25-2 and the sections on organizational safety and managing the "Environment of Care" provide information on the nurse's role in meeting these responsibilities. Each facility will have specific safety processes and procedures in place, derived from national and state directives, Joint Commission on Accreditation of Healthcare Organizations (JCAHO) guidelines, and best industry practices. Each nurse is responsible to know how safety issues are addressed in the facility, and to follow established policies and procedures. Often, simply doing a task according to established guidelines prevents a mishap. If a mishap does occur, the nurse is responsible to report promptly and document fully, according to facility guidelines (Hansen, 2000).

---

### CLIENT EDUCATION

#### Medication Safety

Clients should become familiar with the appearance of the medications they take. If, when they pick up their prescription, the medication looks different, the pharmacy should be contacted and the physician order confirmed before the medication is taken.

Reiss, B., Evans, M., & Broyles, B. (2002). *Pharmacological aspects of nursing care* (6th ed.). Clifton Park, NY: Delmar Learning.

---

## Potential Occupational Hazards Affecting the Safety of Health Care Workers

Nurses and other health care providers are at unnecessary risk for injury in today's health care environment. In 2000 alone, 281,400 health care workers suffered disabling work-related injuries, a rate much higher than most other industries and comprising 36% of the health care workforce. The Occupational Safety and Health Administration (OSHA), a division of the Department of Labor, has authority to cite and discipline employers who are not in compliance with worker safety and health standards. In addition, JCAHO (2001) has partnered with OSHA in a joint effort to improve health care worker safety, and are including health care worker safety issues in their survey. Even in such a highly regulated industry, health care worker injury and illness rates continue to climb as other industry injury and illness rates have been steadily declining.

Numerous potential hazard exposures exist in today's health care workplace. These include a variety of diseases and other biologic exposures, such as blood-borne pathogens and pulmonary tuberculosis. The nurse may be required to use a wide variety of chemical substances, such as chemotherapeutic agents, latex, ethylene oxide, nitrous oxide, and glutaraldehyde. Many of these are found in specialty areas. Physical exposures, such as lasers, ionizing radiation, and noise are potential hazards in selected areas such as the operating room and imaging departments. Psychosocial stressors, such as the shift work, overtime, and the threat of workplace violence or terrorism are potential risks to all nurses, and continued exposure to **ergonomic stressors**, such as lifting and moving clients, can cause work-related musculoskeletal disorders (Meier, 2002).

## Routes of Exposure

Chemical and biological substances are assimilated into the body much the same as medications through various **routes of exposure** (methods by which chemicals and other potentially hazardous substances are assimilated into the body; includes inhalation, ingestion, injection, skin contact, and skin absorption). Some substances are transmitted through the air, such as latex powder, **laser plume** (smoke from laser procedures), nitrous oxide, pulmonary tuberculosis, pneumonia, and other selected diseases. Exposure to these substances is via **inhalation** (exposure via respiratory tract). Some substances are **skin absorption** (route of exposure whereby exposure to chemical or biologic substance occurs via passage through the skin barrier) hazards, such as some chemotherapeutic agents and certain solvents. Some substances cause health effects upon **skin contact**, such as latex. Others are **ingestion** (route of exposure whereby exposure to chemical or microorganism is via gastrointestinal tract) hazards, such as lead and salmonella. Some are **injection** (route of exposure whereby exposure to chemical or microorganisms is via percutaneous exposure or compromised skin [e.g., cut, abrasion]) hazards, such as hepatitis B, causing health effects if **percutaneous** (through the skin) exposure occurs or if the substance enters through a cut on the skin or other skin compromise, such as chapping or dermatitis. Some substances are hazardous through more than one route, such as mercury. Knowing the route of exposure and the characteristics of a particular substance will assist the nurse to select the appropriate protective measures. The **Material Safety Data Sheets (MSDS)**, informational sheets that OSHA requires each employer to maintain at the worksite, will have information on routes of exposure for chemicals in use at the workplace. Information on routes of disease transmission and associated precautions can be found in guidelines published by the Centers for Disease Control (2002a) and in facility infection control policies.

## Exposure Prevention and Control

Nurses need not suffer ill effects from employment in a health care facility. As in any industry, the nurse attends training to identify potential hazards, evaluate them, and apply appropriate protective measures to reduce exposure. Protective measures include substitution, engineering controls, administrative controls, and personal protective equipment. Examples of these controls applied to a health care setting are depicted in Table 33-1. Table 33-2 provides information on **Standard Precautions** (protection required when handling blood; all body fluids secretions, and excretions except sweat, regardless of whether or not they contain visible blood; nonintact skin; and mucous membranes; designed to reduce the risk of transmission of microorganisms from both recognized and unrecognized sources of infection) used for all clients, and on additional **transmission-based precautions** (designed for clients documented or suspected to be infected with highly transmissible or epidemiologically important pathogens). Table 33-3 provides an excerpt from the CDC *Guideline for Isolation Precautions in Hospitals* (2002a), listing specific precautions associated with various diseases. Additional information on isolation guidelines and disease transmission is found in Chapter 26.

**Substitution** is simply replacing a particular substance with a less hazardous alternative. For example, many facilities have eliminated glutaraldehyde from their facilities, and are using similar products that are less likely to cause health problems. **Engineering controls** are strategies that eliminate or minimize the hazard exposure through substitution; mechanical devices, such as ventilators; or a process change. Engineering controls or substitution are always the preferred methods of hazard control when feasible. **Administrative controls** include strategies that minimize hazard exposure by altering work practices, such as training, labeling, and developing comprehensive policies and procedures. **Personal protective equipment** includes a variety of clothing and equipment worn to pro-

vide a barrier between the hazard and the nurse, and is used when engineering controls and administrative controls do not reduce the hazard to safe levels, or when engineering controls are infeasible. Examples are respirators and goggles.

**Respirators** are devices worn to protect the respiratory tract from exposure to inhalation hazards when the exposure exceeds safe levels. Different types of respirators are required for different types of exposures. Some respirators have hoods; some have a tight-fitting face-piece that offers eye protection as well. Some have cartridges and filters that can be changed based on the exposure. Some are self-contained, such as those used by firefighters, and others connect to a manifold or other air-generating device and deliver air through a hose (Plog & Quinlan, 2002).

Nurses may be fitted with many types of respirators, based on the exposure. For example, a nurse in the emergency room may be fitted with and trained on a respirator to use when decontaminating clients who are victims of a hazardous materials spill or terrorism event. The most common respirator in health care, however, is the **N-95 particulate filtering respirator**, which consists of a filtering face-piece that seals against the face to protect against diseases transmitted by tiny particles of virus or bacteria remaining suspended in the air for long periods of time. These diseases are transmitted by the airborne route and require the nurse to use airborne precautions to protect self, other clients, and visitors. **Airborne precautions** use a combination of controls: a private room with negative pressure ventilation or filtration (engineering controls), with the door closed (administrative control), and use of an N-95 respirator (personal protective equipment). The ventilation and closed door reduce the concentration of microorganisms in the room, and are designed to prevent the microorganisms from migrating into the hallway. Because the ventilation is insufficient to clear the room completely of microorganisms, the respirator is also worn to provide a barrier between the nurse's respiratory tract and the pathogenic microorganism. As depicted in Table 33-3, pulmonary tuberculosis and varicella are two examples of diseases requiring airborne precautions (Occupational Safety and Health Administration, 2002).

Respirators must go through a rigorous approval process by the National Institute of Occupational Safety and Health (NIOSH), a subagency of the Centers for Disease Control and Prevention (CDC) specializing in worker safety research. "NIOSH" will be stamped on the face-piece of approved particulate filtering respirators, as well as an alphanumeric designator indicating the respirator capabilities. The designator "N" on an N-95 respirator indicates the respirator is only appropriate in a nonoily environment. So it would not be appropriate in a machine shop or similar work area where oil mist may be generated, but it would be appropriate for health care. "P" designators indicate that the respirator is oil-proof, and safe for use in an oily environment, providing all other conditions of use

## TABLE 33-1　　TYPES OF HAZARD EXPOSURE CONTROLS AND APPLICATION TO HEALTH CARE

| Control Category | Example | How Hazard Is Controlled |
|---|---|---|
| Engineering Control | Ventilation in negative pressure isolation rooms | Removes airborne bacteria from the room and exhausts it outdoors through a special filter |
| | Lift equipment | Provides method of moving or transferring client that does not require manual patient handling |
| | Ventilation hoods and "scavengers" in pharmacy, laboratories, surgery | Removes biologic and chemical contaminants from the work area |
| | Adjustable carts | Reduces stress on arms and back; reduces tripping likelihood by increasing visibility |
| | Adjustable keyboard trays | Allows adjustability of computer workstation from worker to worker, reducing strain |
| | Safe needle devices | Covers contaminated needle after injection to reduce chance of needle stick |
| Administrative Control | Training | Attending routine safety training provided by employer and seeking additional training when needed ensures proficiency in protective measures. |
| | Labeling | Chemical identity and hazard warnings on label provide quick reference as to hazards of contents. |
| | Prompt reporting of injuries/unsafe conditions | Reporting an unsafe condition provides an opportunity to correct the hazard before an(other) injury occurs. |
| | Material Safety Data Sheets | Provides extensive reference information on safe handling and storage of chemical hazards in the work area. Available for injectable medications that require mixing. |
| | Good housekeeping | Prevents tripping or other hazard exposures associated with increased clutter. |
| | Checking and maintaining equipment | Ensures client and staff safety by identifying electrical and other hazards that could cause injury. |
| | Policies and procedures | Defines proper technique, including protective measures. Correct method is usually the safest method. |
| | Worker rotation | Divides stressor impact among several workers, allows time for tissue recovery (e.g., where there are several stations, such as health care laundry, workers rotate stations every 2 hours). |
| | Task variation | Changing activity throughout workday allows tissue recovery. |

*(continues)*

## TABLE 33-1    TYPES OF HAZARD EXPOSURE CONTROLS AND APPLICATION TO HEALTHCARE (continued)

| Control Category | Example | How Hazard Is Controlled |
|---|---|---|
| Personal Protective Equipment (PPE) | Gloves<br>Respirators<br>Shoe coverings<br>Gowns<br>Aprons<br>Surgical masks<br>Goggles<br>Safety glasses<br>Ear plugs<br>Other | PPE for protection against chemicals is selected based on chemical properties and route of exposure. Consulting MSDS ensures optimal protection.<br><br>PPE for protection against diseases is addressed under Infection Control. PPE will differ based on the disease.<br><br>Gloves appropriate to the hazard. If latex gloves are used, avoid petroleum products, including petroleum-based lotions.<br><br>Respirators are required for some chemicals and for some diseases (e.g., Pulmonary tuberculosis). Respirators must be fit-tested to ensure effectiveness. Selection is based on the hazard. An N-95 respirator is typically used for airborne precautions.<br><br>Hearing protection should be worn whenever noise exposure is such that two people standing 3 feet apart cannot have a conversation without raising their voice. |

## TABLE 33-2    ISOLATION PRECAUTIONS

| Type of Precautions | Definition | Required Measures |
|---|---|---|
| **Standard Precautions** | Standard Precautions apply to all clients, regardless of diagnosis infection status. Standard Precautions apply to (1) blood; (2) all body fluids, secretions, and excretions except sweat, regardless of whether or not they contain visible blood; (3) nonintact skin; and (4) mucous membranes. Standard Precautions are designed to reduce the risk of transmission of microorganisms from both recognized and unrecognized sources of infection. | Handwashing and gloves when contact with blood, non-intact skin, mucous membranes, and all other body fluids (except sweat)<br><br>Additional protective clothing and equipment based on exposure risk of task (e.g., goggles if splash to eye is likely, gown if splash to body is likely, mask if splash to nasal mucosa or mouth is likely) |

**Transmission-Based Precautions** are designed for clients documented or suspected to be infected with highly transmissible or epidemiologically important pathogens for which additional precautions beyond Standard Precautions are needed to interrupt transmission. They may be combined for diseases that have multiple routes of transmission, always used in addition to Standard Precautions.

(continues)

## TABLE 33-2   ISOLATION PRECAUTIONS (continued)

| Type of Precautions | Definition | Required Measures |
| --- | --- | --- |
| **Airborne Precautions** | Airborne precautions are designed to reduce the risk of airborne disease transmission on dust or microscopic moisture particles. Air currents carry these particles and can disperse them throughout the facility, where they may be inhaled by a susceptible host. Special ventilation and personal protective equipment is needed to prevent airborne transmission. Airborne precautions apply to clients who have known or suspected diseases transmitted via the airborne route. | Private room with negative air pressure or high-efficiency filtration—door *closed*! <br><br> N-95 respirator <br><br> Limit transport of client from room; if transport is necessary, apply surgical mask to client nose and mouth during transport. |
| **Droplet Precautions** | Droplet precautions are used for prevention of disease transmission via the droplet route of exposure. Droplet transmission occurs when the mucous membranes of a susceptible person contacts large droplets containing the infectious agent, usually generated from coughing, talking, sneezing, or invasive procedures of the respiratory tract, such as bronchoscopy. While droplet particles (at about 5 microns) are larger than airborne particles, they still are often invisible to the naked eye. Droplets do not remain suspended and usually travel less than 3 feet in air. Special ventilation is not required but a surgical mask is required if within 3 feet of the client. Droplet precautions apply to clients who have known or suspected diagnosis of disease that can be transmitted via the droplet route. | Private room preferred <br><br> Cohort if roommate is necessary, or maintain > 3-foot distance between clients <br><br> Surgical mask when required to be within 3-foot radius of client, or when entering room <br><br> Surgical mask on client if must transport from room |
| **Contact Precautions** | Contact precautions are used to prevent disease transmission by direct or indirect contact. Contact (skin to skin) can occur between clients, between caregivers, between client and caregiver, and between client or caregiver and contaminated objects. Contact precautions apply to clients who have known or suspected diagnosis of disease that can be transmitted via the contact route. These clients include clients who are colonized (presence of microorganism without clinical signs and symptoms of infection) with diseases that can be transmitted by direct or indirect contact. | Private room preferred <br><br> Gloves when entering room, remove before leaving room <br><br> Other protective garments as needed to prevent contact |

Adapted from Centers for Disease Control and Prevention (2001). http://www.cdc.gov

are met. The "95" indicates how efficiently the filter material removes particulate matter in the air—in this case, 95%. Because the respirators are used in conjunction with other controls, a 95% rate of filtration has been determined to be adequate for use with airborne precautions, although respirators with higher filtration rates are available. Health care facilities are mandated to follow OSHA (2002) guide-

lines for respirator use. For example, tight-fitting respirators, including filtering face-piece respirators such as the N-95 particulate filtering respirator, have requirements including medical clearance, fit-testing, and training.

Some diseases are inhalation hazards, but the virus or bacteria are carried on larger droplets and do not remain suspended in the air for long periods. Because of the size of

## TABLE 33-3    GUIDELINES FOR ISOLATION PRECAUTIONS IN HOSPITALS

| Infection/Condition | Precautions Type* | Duration† |
|---|---|---|
| Tuberculosis | | |
| Extrapulmonary, draining lesion (including scrofula) | S | |
| Extrapulmonary, meningitis° | S | |
| Pulmonary, confirmed or suspected or laryngeal disease | A | Fʷ |
| Skin-test positive with no evidence of current pulmonary disease | S | |
| Tularemia | | |
| Draining lesion | S | |
| Pulmonary | S | |
| Typhoid (*Salmonella typhi*) fever (see gastroenteritis) | | |
| Typhus, endemic and epidemic | S | |
| Urinary tract infection (including pyelonephritis), with or without urinary catheter | S | |
| Varicella (chickenpox) | A,C | Fᵉ |

* Type of Precautions: A, Airborne; C, Contact; D, Droplet; S, Standard; when A, C, and D are specified, also use S.

† Duration of precautions: CN, until off antibiotics and culture-negative; DI, duration of illness (with wound lesions, DI means until they stop draining); U, until time specified in hours (hrs) after initiation of effective therapy; F, see footnote.

ᵉ Maintain precautions until all lesions are crusted. The average incubation period for varicella is 10 to 16 days, with a range of 10 to 21 days. After exposure, use varicella-zoster immune globulin (VZIG) when appropriate, and discharge susceptible clients if possible. Place exposed susceptible patients on airborne precautions beginning 10 days after exposure and continuing until 21 days after last exposure (up to 28 days if VZIG has been given). Susceptible persons should not enter the room of clients on precautions if other immune caregivers are available.

° Client should be examined for evidence of current (active) pulmonary tuberculosis. If evidence exists, additional precautions are necessary (see tuberculosis).

ʷ Discontinue precautions *only* when TB client is on effective therapy, is improving clinically, and has three consecutive negative sputum smears collected on different days or TB is ruled out.

Adapted from Centers for Disease Control and Prevention (2002a). *Guidelines for Isolation Precautions in Hospitals.* http://www.cdc.gov/ncidod/hip/isolat/isoapp_a.htm

the particle, a surgical mask (Figure 33-3) is sufficient for diseases requiring **droplet precautions** (used for suspected or confirmed diagnosis of infectious disease transmitted via attachment to large droplets of moisture during exhalation), and is not required unless the nurse is within 3 feet of the client. **Contact precautions** (used for suspected or confirmed diagnosis of infectious disease transmitted via contact; includes handwashing and gloves while in room as minimum in addition to Standard Precautions) are used for clients with, for example, infectious exudates. Gloves are required upon entry into the room, and additional personal protective equipment (PPE) is added as needed for the task at hand. All transmission-based precautions are used in addition to Standard Precautions.

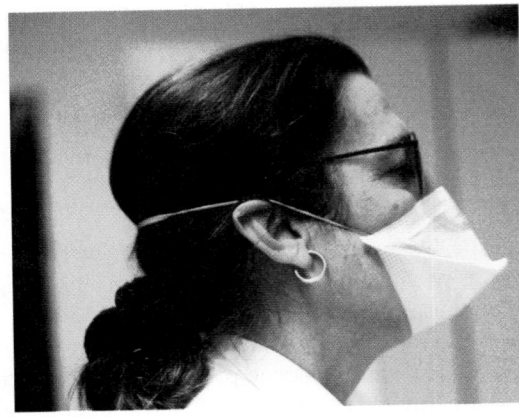

**Figure 33-3    A nurse wearing a surgical mask**

As described with airborne precautions, protective measures generally require a combination of controls, but will always be based on the route of exposure and characteristic of the substance. The MSDS will have detailed information on the necessary control measures for safe use of chemicals. Transmission-based precaution guidelines for infection control will provide control measures based on transmissibility and route of exposure for various diseases.

## Health Effects of Hazardous Substances

Just as nurses must be aware of adverse reactions of medications, the nurse must also be aware of health effects of chemicals and infectious diseases with which there may be contact. Chemicals are categorized by health effect, and some chemicals are in more than one category. The MSDS will provide this information. Examples are **corrosives**, which erode the skin on contact; **carcinogens**, which cause cancer; **teratogens**, which damage the developing fetus; and **target organ chemicals**, which provide stress on a particular organ, often the kidney or liver. **Sensitizers**, such as glutaraldehyde and latex, can generate mild to severe allergy symptoms, including anaphylaxis, in susceptible individuals (Environmental Protection Agency, 2002).

## Latex Allergy

NIOSH (1997) issued an Alert entitled *Preventing Allergic Reactions to Natural Rubber Latex in the Workplace*. Latex products are manufactured from a milky fluid derived from the Brazilian rubber tree, *Hevea brasiliensis*. The allergic response is attributed to the proteins contained in the milky fluid and to the chemicals that are added during the processing and manufacture of commercial latex. There are three types of latex reactions: irritant contact dermatitis; allergic contact dermatitis, the most common type of reaction; and immediate hypersensitivity, a systemic reaction also called type 1 IgE–mediated reaction.

Powdered latex gloves are an extreme exposure risk because the latex protein binds to the powder and becomes airborne, creating an inhalation hazard and increasing systemic exposure to the allergen. Latex is a sensitizing chemical, or sensitizer. When the latex proteins are inhaled, it can hasten development of a latex sensitivity, especially in atopic individuals, and can precipitate an anaphylactic reaction (Heumann, 2001).

## Hand Hygiene

Any dermatitis should be promptly reported to Employee Health, and should be carefully documented. Dermatitis related to latex sensitivity can be progressive and career-limiting, but any dermatitis on the hands of a caregiver increases exposure risk to both client and nurse. Barrier creams or special soaps may be needed to keep hands in good condition. Petroleum-based lotions and creams should be avoided if latex gloves are worn; petroleum degrades the latex, increasing exposure to latex and to the pathogens that the gloves were intended to protect against.

Many facilities are implementing hand-hygiene programs, often setting strict guidelines on nail care and nail coverings. Artificial nails, in particular, are banned by many facility hand-hygiene policies for direct care staff (Gershon, Karkashian, Grosch, Murphy, Escamilla-Cejudo, Flanagan, Bernacki, Kasting, & Martin, 2000).

Since 1992, when OSHA issued regulations requiring health care workers to wear gloves and other protective devices such as surgical masks and goggles as a safeguard against blood-borne pathogens, health care workers were placed at risk for developing latex allergy. Commercial latex is in many medical products (Burt, 1999) such as blood pressure cuffs, stethoscopes, catheters, and wound drains, to name a few, as well as many household items. The Food and Drug Administration requires labeling of latex-containing products. Reports indicate that 1% to 6% of the general population and about 8% to 12% of regularly exposed health care workers are sensitized to latex (NIOSH, 1997).

NIOSH (1997) recommends that employers and employees take a commonsense approach based on current knowledge to protect workers from latex exposure and allergy in the workplace; refer to Box 33-1 for NIOSH's recommendations. NIOSH recommends that if latex gloves are worn, they should be powder free and low allergen, because these gloves are less likely than powdered ones to produce allergic responses (Gritter, 1998).

## Work-Related Musculoskeletal Disorders

Two-thirds of all occupational injuries reported by private sector employers are work-related **musculoskeletal disorders (MSDs)**. Musculoskeletal disorders include a variety of soft tissue injuries, such as sprains, strains, and tendonitis. Private sector employers reported a total of 165,100 lost workday cases involving MSDs in 2000. A case is considered a lost workday case if the employee missed at least one day of work as a result of the injury or was on work restrictions for one day or more. As with any injury or illness, if work-relatedness is confirmed, the workers' compensation insurance carried by the employer will cover medical costs and wage reimbursement for the injured worker.

A work-related injury can be financially devastating for the nurse. Many of these cases involve surgery and months of recovery time away from the workplace, and while the nurse is reimbursed medical costs, the wage is often compensated at only a fraction of normal salary. A work-related injury can be financially devastating for an employer as well. All medical and wage-reimbursement costs associated with the injury are passed on to the employer as higher

## BOX 33-1  NIOSH'S RECOMMENDATIONS TO PREVENT LATEX EXPOSURE

### Employers

- Provide workers with nonlatex gloves.
- Provide appropriate barrier protection for workers handling infectious materials; if latex gloves are chosen, provide reduced protein, powder-free gloves to protect workers from infectious materials.
- Provide good housekeeping to remove latex-containing dust, and ensure that workers change ventilation filters and vacuum bags frequently in latex-contaminated areas.
- Provide education programs regarding latex allergy.
- Periodically screen high-risk workers for latex allergy symptoms.
- Evaluate current policies whenever a worker is diagnosed with latex allergy.

### Workers

- Use nonlatex gloves for contact with noninfectious materials.
- Use CDC-appropriate barrier protection when handling infectious materials; if latex gloves are chosen, use reduced protein, powder-free gloves to reduce exposure and reactions to latex chemical additives (allergic contact dermatitis).
- Use appropriate work practices when wearing latex gloves: avoid oil-based hand creams or lotions that can cause glove deterioration—unless they have been shown to reduce latex-related problems and maintain glove barrier protection; wash hands with a mild soap and dry thoroughly after removing latex gloves; use good housekeeping practices to remove latex-containing dust.
- Attend latex allergy educational programs to be knowledgeable of procedures and to recognize the symptoms of latex allergy: skin rashes; hives; flushing; itching; nasal, eye, or sinus symptoms; asthma; and shock.
- Avoid direct contact with latex gloves and other products if you develop symptoms, until you have been seen by a physician experienced in treating latex allergy.
- If you have latex allergy, consult your physician regarding exposure precautions, contact with gloves and other latex-containing products, and areas that contain latex powder from gloves worm by other workers; inform your employer and health care providers that you have latex allergy.
- Carefully follow your physician's instructions regarding allergic latex reactions.

Adapted from National Institute for Occupational Safety and Health Centers for Disease Control and Prevention (1997). *Preventing allergic reactions to natural rubber latex in the workplace* (DHHS [NIOSH] Publication No. 97-135).

premiums. The employer must also bear the cost of hiring and training staff to cover for the injured worker.

Nurses will be less likely to suffer a musculoskeletal injury if they stay in great physical condition; getting regular exercise is one of the most effective injury-prevention strategies. Learning and using proper techniques for client transfer is also important. In addition, nurses should make an effort to use lifting equipment, **gait belts** (devices placed snugly around the client's midsection, providing a firm handhold for client transfer and assisting with ambulation), and lift teams whenever possible (Croft, Hanssen, & Kuzma, 2001). Back injuries affect 38% of nurses, primarily because clients are lifted manually as much as 98% of the time. Client transfers using lift equipment and gait belts are safer and more comfortable for the client, and definitely lower injury risk to the nurse.

Facilities vary in their injury-prevention strategies. An injury-prevention strategy called "zero-lift" is gaining momentum in many parts of the country. This strategy incorporates a comprehensive approach to preventing injuries related to client handling, and early results of research suggest promising results. The facility must first determine the cause of most of the injuries. This is often done by forming a task force under the leadership of the safety committee to study injury reports and query staff about problem areas in their departments. The problem areas are then analyzed to determine the actual source of the injury. This can be done internally if expertise is available, or assistance can be obtained from the facility workers' compensation insurance carrier, the local OSHA consultation office, or a local ergonomic consultant. Lifting equipment is evaluated for adequacy and safety. The task force then examines each area and develops problem-solving solutions to the problem areas. A new policy will likely be needed, as well as focused training. In facilities where an injury prevention program has not yet been developed, and lift equipment and gait belts are unavailable, nurses should advocate for clients and for themselves by volunteering to participate on a task force or committee to develop a policy on safe client handling, perhaps using "zero-lift" principles (Gershon et al., 2000).

According to OSHA (2000), it is estimated that only 28% of all workplaces in general industry have voluntarily implemented ergonomics programs. In response to these workplace hazards, OSHA issued mandatory standards that required all employers to set up ergonomic programs to prevent work-related MSDs such as back injuries. These guidelines were declared to be an unreasonable burden to the employer and were rescinded, but alternative standards are being explored.

The ergonomic standards required that all employers provide workers the following information: common MSD hazards; signs and symptoms of MSDs, and the importance of reporting them early; how to report MSD signs and symptoms; and a summary of the requirement of the OSHA standard.

# Safety and Health Training

Health care worker injury rates and client safety concerns suggest that training currently provided to health care workers is insufficient to meet individual worker or client safety needs. Hazard exposures can be reduced through training, but training has traditionally been geared to meet compliance rather than injury prevention objectives, and may be insufficient to meet the needs of the nurse. Nurses should inquire as to what prevention training is available pertinent to the hazards encountered in their particular work area (e.g., chemotherapeutic pharmaceuticals, radiologicals, disinfectants). Injury prevention training programs should be upgraded as client and employee needs change (Gershon et al., 2000). In addition, blood-borne pathogen exposure plans are a critical aspect of safety in the health care setting (see Chapter 26 for blood-borne exposure information).

# Hygiene

**Hygiene** is the science of health. Hygienic care promotes cleanliness, provides for comfort and relaxation, improves self-image, and promotes healthy skin. Client hygiene is an extension of providing client safety and protecting the client's defense mechanisms. The health of the body's first line of defense (skin and mucous membranes) is promoted by client hygiene. Nurses are responsible for ensuring that the client's hygienic needs are met. The type of hygienic care provided depends on the client's ability, needs, and practices.

## Factors Influencing Hygienic Practices

Hygienic needs and practices are unique to each client; nurses should provide individualized care based on these needs and practices. Hygienic practices are influenced by several factors: body image, social and cultural practices, personal preferences, socioeconomic status, and knowledge.

### Body Image

**Body image** is the client's subjective belief about his or her own physical appearance. Body image is associated with the client's emotions, mood, attitude, and values. A client's body image directly affects the type of personal hygiene practiced; this may change if the client's body image is altered because of illness or surgical procedures. During this time, the nurse should help the client maintain hygienic practices in accordance with the client's pre-illness level of hygiene and personal preferences.

### Social and Cultural Practices

Social and cultural practices also directly influence hygienic practices. Clients are socialized to their hygienic practices by family practices in early childhood. As a person ages, hygienic practices are influenced by maturational development and socialization with people outside of the family. For example, teenagers are usually concerned with peer acceptance and follow the latest trends in personal hygiene. In later adulthood, hygienic practices may be influenced by coworkers and social networks.

Cultural practices and beliefs are derived from family, religious, and personal values developed during maturation. See Chapter 15 for a complete discussion of cultural diversity. Clients from diverse cultural backgrounds will have differing hygienic practices. For example, some cultures do not permit women to submerge their bodies in water during the time of menstruation, because there is fear that the woman may drown. In North America, people typically bathe daily and use numerous deodorant products. In Europe, people do not bathe daily and seldom use deodorant products. Europeans do not consider the smell of human perspiration as offensive as do North Americans. Nurses should have a nonjudgmental attitude when assessing or providing hygienic care to clients from different social or cultural backgrounds.

### Personal Preferences

Personal preferences influence when bathing occurs, what products are used, and what type of bath is performed. For example, some male clients may shave before bathing, while others prefer to wait until after the bath. Some clients prefer to bathe in the morning to facilitate waking, while others prefer to bathe before bedtime to encourage relaxation and sleep. Unless a client's health is affected, the nurse should permit clients to practice their usual routine and use the hygienic products that they prefer. Individualized nursing care should incorporate the client's personal hygiene preferences.

## STOP AND THINK

### A Client's Hygiene Habits

A client's hygiene habits can be influenced by personal values, knowledge, culture, and socioeconomic status. They can also be influenced by progressing disability.

- What can you do to assist in ensuring your client has safe bathing facilities and appropriate assistance with bathing and hygiene activities at home?

- How can you ask questions about personal hygiene habits that are easily accepted by the client?

## Socioeconomic Status

A client's hygienic practices may be influenced by socioeconomic status. Limited economic resources may affect the type, frequency, and extent of hygiene practiced. Assessment of socioeconomic status provides information about the availability of hygiene supplies. Some clients may not be able to afford deodorants, perfumes, soaps, shampoo, and toothpaste. The nurse can function as an advocate for the client by making referrals to community agencies that provide assistance to needy persons—for example, Catholic Charities or a local chapter of the AARP.

## Knowledge

Knowledge level influences the client's understanding about the relationship between hygiene and health. Thus, knowledge should influence a client's hygienic practices. In addition to being knowledgeable, before clients perform basic hygiene, they must be motivated and believe that they are capable of self-care.

Frequently, an illness or surgical procedure results in deficient knowledge about basic hygienic practices. In these situations, the client may not know the correct procedures or types of hygiene that can be performed. The nurse is responsible for providing the necessary education about hygiene during an illness. Sometimes, the nurse may have to perform all hygienic practices for a client during an illness until the client is able to regain this ability.

## Assessment to Identify At-Risk Clients

The nursing process facilitates an understanding of the scope of challenges inherent in the nursing care of clients at risk for injury, infections, or a self-care deficit. The assessment data should direct the prioritization of the client's problem and accompanying nursing diagnoses. Clients at risk for injury or infection require frequent reassessment of their status with appropriate changes in the plan of care and expected outcomes.

The assessment and physical examination data are correlated with the laboratory indicators to identify those clients who are at risk for problems relating to safety, infection, or hygiene. One of the assessment models should be used to provide structure to the assessment. See Chapter 11 for a complete discussion of assessment models. Appropriate risk appraisals may be incorporated into the nursing health history interview. These core elements of assessment are discussed in relation to clients in ambulatory, institutional, and home settings. Refer to Box 33-2 for a sample format for developing minimum safety standards applicable to all health care settings.

A comprehensive nursing assessment involves using specifically developed risk assessment tools and appraising the client's environment to detect potential hazards. The client's self-care abilities, used for determining the level of assistance needed in providing hygienic care, are appraised during the health history. The analysis of relevant risk factors alerts the nurse to actual or possible risks. Skin integrity is usually compromised when a person is placed on bed rest. A skin integrity risk appraisal should be completed to assist with planning care.

---

### BOX 33-2    STANDARD OF CARE: SAFETY

**Client Outcome**

The client will receive care in a safe health care environment and remain free of preventable injuries.

**Nursing Practice Standards**

1. Perform a client injury risk appraisal on admission and prior to therapeutic nursing interventions. Risk factors for injury include but are not limited to age, altered mental status, previous history of falls, impaired mobility, sensory deficits, perceptual deficits, and inability to communicate.

2. Eliminate or modify risk elements when possible, such as assisting with mobility and placing bed rails up with bed in the lowest position.

3. Implement environmental precautions such as hand rails, nonslip mats or rugs, and adequate lighting.

4. Use infection control practices that prevent or control the transmission of pathogens.

5. Maintain intravenous access according to intravenous protocols.

6. Implement emergency measures in accordance with American Heart Association guidelines for cardiopulmonary resuscitation (CPR) and advanced life support.

7. Know and comply with the institution's Environmental Health and Safety guidelines.

8. Implement emergency measures during fires and disasters.

9. Use mechanical, radiant, chemical, and thermal equipment according to the manufacturer's guidelines and institution's policy and procedures.

10. Use a multidisciplinary approach to enhance client safety as indicated.

# Health History

The nursing health history interview is the first part of assessment; it provides the client's subjective, specific health data. Key elements of relevant data regarding the client at risk for safety and infection are obtained in the health history. See Chapter 11 for a sample of a nursing health history tool.

The client is often asked to complete a health history questionnaire; however, depending on the client's status, the nurse may have to perform an interview to obtain these data. If the client is unable to provide the subjective data, the nurse must designate on the questionnaire or in the nursing progress notes who provided the information.

During the nursing health history interview, assess the client's general health perception and management status to determine how the client manages self-care. This information will provide data regarding the client's routine self-care and health promotion needs. Sample questions that relate specifically to habits that foster safe, healthy patterns of behavior are presented in Box 33-3. These questions are appropriate for home health and ambulatory care settings as well as inpatient settings.

---

**BOX 33-3   KEY INTERVIEW QUESTIONS ABOUT SAFETY, INFECTION CONTROL, AND HYGIENE**

- Describe the things you do to stay healthy.

- How do you typically spend a day (e.g., home or work)?

- What are your health care concerns?

- Do you need assistance with bathing and dressing?

- Do you regularly visit the dentist and eye doctor?

- Do you use dental floss on a regular basis?

- Have you recently come in contact with someone who has an infectious disease?

- Do you wash your hands when preparing food?

- Do you keep meats and dairy products refrigerated until ready to use?

- Is there a smoke detector or fire extinguisher in your home?

- Are emergency phone numbers readily available?

---

# Physical Examination

A complete health assessment includes a systematic physical examination, generally conducted from head to toe, in order to obtain objective data relative to the client's health status and presenting problems. See Chapter 27 for a complete discussion of a physical examination.

When assessing the client to determine the level of risk for injury or infection and hygienic deficits, focus the physical examination on the following areas and signs (Estes, 2002):

- Level of consciousness: Use the Glasgow Coma Scale to evaluate this attribute (see Chapter 41 for discussion of this tool).
- Range of motion or total immobilization of an extremity
- Localized infection: Redness, swelling, warmth, tenderness, pain, and loss of movement in a specific body part
- Systemic infection: Fever, with a corresponding increase in pulse and respirations; weakness; anorexia, with possible accompanying findings of nausea, vomiting, and diarrhea; enlarged and/or tender lymph nodes
- Secretions or exudate of the skin or mucous membranes and detection of crackles, rhonchi, or wheezes in the lungs on auscultation

The condition of the skin is a good indicator of a client's general health status. Assessment of skin integrity provides data concerning a client's nutritional and hydration status, continuity of intact skin, hygienic practices, and overall physical abilities. Similarly, a client with limited mobility is at risk for developing joint contractures, skin breakdown, and muscle atrophy.

# Diagnostic and Laboratory Data

Appraising the client's risk for injury should also include an evaluation of laboratory findings relative to an abnormal blood profile (e.g., altered clotting factors, anemic conditions, or leukocytosis). See Chapter 29 for a complete discussion of abnormal blood profiles. Malnourished clients are at risk for injury.

The laboratory indicators for an infection are (Daniels, 2003):

1. An elevated leukocyte (white blood cell [WBC]) and WBC differential:

   - Neutrophils: Increased in acute, severe inflammation
   - Lymphocytes: Increased in chronic bacterial and viral infections
   - Monocytes: Increased in some protozoan and rickettsial infections and tuberculosis
   - Eosinophils and basophils: Unaltered in an infectious process

2. An elevated erythrocyte sedimentation rate (ESR): Increased in the presence of inflammation
3. An elevated pH of involved body fluids (gastric, urine, or vaginal secretions): Indicates the presence of microorganisms

4. Positive cultures of involved body fluids (blood, sputum, urine, or other drainage): Indicates the growth of microorganisms

Refer to Chapter 29 for the age-related normal laboratory values for each of the preceding tests.

## Client in an Inpatient Setting

Inpatient clients should be assessed for fall and infection risk factors. The hospitalized or institutionalized client's risk for falls is identified after compiling specific assessment data that are correlated with contributing factors. Each of these indicators carries a specific weight to determine the client's risk. The inpatient client should be assessed for falls every shift or as designated by institutional policy. To minimize the chance of falls, make sure the client's environment is safe: the bed is kept in a low position, side rails are up, personal belongings are in easy reach, and assistive devices (e.g., walker) are nearby, as shown in Figure 33-4.

To determine risk for infection, review or listen to the client's response to the health history and interview questions related to "exposure to infectious diseases," "invasive procedures," and "behaviors you think you should change." An infection risk appraisal is based on the defining characteristics that place a client at risk for an infection. These factors are listed in the section entitled Nursing Diagnosis.

## Client in the Home

An injury risk appraisal will provide the nurse with assessment data to determine the client's level of safety knowledge as previously discussed in the standard of care for safety. Injuries in the home are primarily the result of falls, fires, electrical malfunctions, suffocation, weapons, and household and medication poisonings. Home health nurses may use a safety risk appraisal; refer to Box 33-4.

The safety risk data assessed in the home environment direct the nurse in planning for the client and caregiver's education. The home health nurse needs to prioritize these data when planning the client's care. Assessment, teaching, and outcome evaluation of all safety hazards can take several home visits.

## Nursing Diagnosis

After data collection and analysis, the nurse is able to formulate a nursing diagnosis. If Gordon's Functional Health Patterns model is used to conduct the assessment, the nurse can use the classification of nursing diagnoses by functional health patterns that relate to safety, infection, and hygienic deficits. For example:

I. Health perception–health management pattern
   - Risk for injury
   - Risk for infection

II. Activity-exercise pattern
   - Bathing/hygiene self-care deficit
   - Dressing/grooming self-care deficit
   - Toileting self-care deficit

## Risk for Injury

The primary nursing diagnosis *Risk for Injury* exists when the client is at risk of injury as a result of environmental conditions interacting with the individual's adaptive and defensive resources (NANDA, 2003). Although this diagnostic label does not have defining characteristics as set forth by NANDA, it is categorized as having either internal or external potential hazards. An internal biochemical risk factor for a client with impaired vision would be stated as *Risk for Injury* related to sensory dysfunction. In contrast, a home health nurse's assessment data that identify drugs on a nightstand with a toddler in the home as creating an external chemical risk factor for the toddler would be stated as *Risk for Injury* related to drugs (pharmaceutical agents).

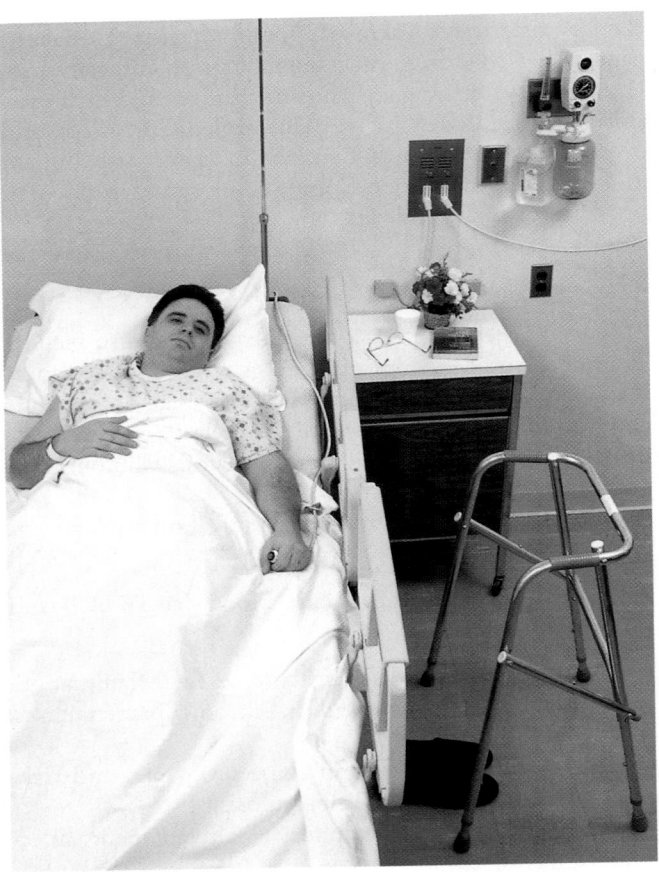

**Figure 33-4** This client's risk of falls has been assessed and responded to through the measures shown here. Do all clients within the hospital setting need to be assessed for the risk of falls, regardless of their health status or reason for hospitalization?

# BOX 33-4    HOME SAFETY RISK APPRAISAL

## Infant

- Crib has side rails that stay in the up position while infant is in the crib.
- Infants are not left unattended, especially on elevated surfaces or in the bath.
- Bath water temperature is 37.8°–40.6°C (100°–105°F). Check temperature for comfort with wrist.
- Environment is kept warm and draft-free at bath time.
- Bottles are sterilized and formula refrigerated.
- Toys are soft without detachable pieces.
- Car seat has restraint strap and is used consistently.
- Stroller and carry seat are sturdy with a restraint strap.
- Fire, police, and poison control numbers are posted by telephones.
- Caregivers know infant CPR.

## Toddler/Preschooler

- Sharp objects are placed out of reach and out of sight.
- Poisons are labeled and placed in a locked cabinet.
- Medications and other toxins have childproof lids and are stored in a locked cabinet.
- Small, hard food objects (peanuts, candy) are kept in locked cabinets.
- Stairs and floor furnaces have gates or barriers.
- Safety locks are on doors and windows.
- Electrical outlets are covered.
- Burners on the stove are not left on and unattended.
- Pots with hot liquids are placed on back burners with handles facing toward the back wall.
- Home and yard are free from poisonous plants.
- Play equipment is kept in proper functioning condition; toys have no small parts; crayons are nontoxic.
- Outdoor play is supervised in a fenced area with locks on gates.
- Car seat/belt is used consistently.
- Supervision is given child when crossing the street.
- Caregivers know child CPR and Heimlich maneuver.

## School-Aged Child

- Play and sports are supervised.
- Play equipment kept in proper functioning condition and free from hazards.
- Outdoor play limited to soft surfaces.
- Bicycle helmet worn consistently.
- Taught not to open the door or speak with strangers while at play.
- Firearms are kept unloaded in locked cabinets.
- Caregivers know child CPR and the Heimlich maneuver.
- Seat belt is worn at all times.

(continues)

## BOX 33-4    HOME SAFETY RISK APPRAISAL (*continued*)

### Adolescent

- Firearm safety is taught.
- Seat belt is worn at all times.
- Teenagers take drivers' education; cautioned about drinking and driving.
- Caregivers know adult CPR and the Heimlich maneuver.

### Adult

- Firearms have safety latches.
- Smoke detector and fire extinguisher installed in the home.
- Sharp-edged objects are safely stored.
- A nondrinking designated driver is chosen.
- Emergency phone numbers are readily available.
- Caregiver knows adult CPR and Heimlich maneuver.

### Older Adult

- Stairs have adequate lighting and nonskid surfaces, and rails are in good condition.
- Throw rugs are not present.
- Hallways are uncluttered.
- Carpets are free from frayed ends/pieces.
- Phone and other cords are behind furniture.
- Bathtub has rails and nonslip surface.
- Shower stall has seat.
- Bathroom is free from drafts.
- Shoes fit properly with nonskid soles.
- Home is adequately ventilated and heated.
- Home is free of space heaters.
- Pilot lights are functional for gas appliances.
- Electrical appliances are in good working condition.
- Food is properly refrigerated.
- Medications are kept in properly labeled containers with readable print.
- Emergency phone numbers are readily available.
- Fire and police departments are aware of older adult at home alone.
- Caregiver knows adult CPR and Heimlich maneuver.

NANDA (2003) has six defined subcategories of specific risk factors for this diagnostic labeling:

1. *Risk for Suffocation:* An accentuated risk of accidental suffocation
2. *Risk for Poisoning:* An accentuated risk of accidental exposure to, or ingestion of, drugs or dangerous products in doses sufficient to cause poisoning
3. *Risk for Trauma:* An accentuated risk of accidental tissue injury (e.g., wound, burn, fracture)
4. *Risk for Aspiration:* Risk for entry of gastrointestinal secretions, oropharyngeal secretions, or solids or fluids into the tracheobronchial passages
5. *Risk for Disuse Syndrome:* Risk for deterioration of body or body systems as the result of prescribed or unavoidable musculoskeletal inactivity

## STOP AND THINK

### Client with Self-Care Deficit

- When caring for a client with a self-care deficit, what are potential safety consequences if the nurse does not promptly respond to the call light?

- What should nurses communicate to other staff members when they suspect safety concerns for clients with self-care deficits?

- What should nurses tell family members of clients who have self-care deficits?

6. *Latex Allergy Response:* A response to natural latex rubber products

These six subcategories of nursing diagnoses provide the nurse with the opportunity to relate specific nursing interventions to the diagnosed problem. For example, the specific nursing diagnosis for the situation of a toddler in the home environment encountering medications on a nightstand would be *Risk for Poisoning* related to medicines not stored in locked cabinets and accessible to children. The level of risk would be increased if the medications on the client's nightstand were in open containers or the closed containers failed to have childproof caps. The subcategory diagnosis provides specific nursing interventions directed at the level of risk for the toddler and the need for client teaching.

## Risk for Infection

*Risk for Infection* is the state in which an individual is at increased risk for being invaded by pathogenic organisms (NANDA, 2003). The risk factors that increase the client's vulnerability to infections are:

- Inadequate primary defenses (broken skin, traumatized tissue, decrease in ciliary action, stasis of body fluids, change in pH of secretions, and altered peristalsis)
- Inadequate secondary defenses, acquired immunity, and immunosuppression
- Tissue destruction and increased environmental exposure
- Chronic diseases and malnutrition
- Invasive procedures and pharmaceutical agents
- Trauma
- Rupture of amniotic membranes
- Insufficient knowledge to avoid exposure to pathogens (NANDA, 2003)

## Self-Care Deficits

A *Self-Care Deficit* exists when the client is not able to perform one or more of the activities of daily living. NANDA

(2003) identifies three self-care deficits related to hygienic practices. These diagnostic labels, together with their defining characteristics and related factors, are presented in Table 33-4.

## Other Nursing Diagnoses

Clients who are at risk for injury and infection or have a self-care deficit may have other problems. These associated physiological and psychological problems are discussed in detail in other chapters in this unit. The common nursing diagnoses that often accompany diagnostic labels for risk or self-care deficits are:

- *Imbalanced Nutrition* (specify less than body requirements or more than body requirements)
- *Ineffective Protection*
- *Impaired Tissue Integrity*
- *Impaired Oral Mucous Membrane*
- *Impaired Skin Integrity*
- *Social Isolation*
- *Risk for Loneliness*
- *Ineffective Coping*
- *Impaired Physical Mobility*
- *Hopelessness*
- *Powerlessness*
- *Deficient Knowledge* (specify)
- *Acute Pain*
- *Anxiety*
- *Fear*

This list is not all-inclusive but gives an indication of the number of related problems that need to be considered when planning care.

## Outcome Identification and Planning

The primary nursing goal is to provide safe care through the identification of actual or potential hazards and the implementation of safety measures. The assessment data are reviewed with the client, and the nurse records the areas in which the client indicates a need for change and health teaching, for example—age-related exercise or maintaining a safe environment. These findings are incorporated into the plan of care, reflecting the individualized needs of each client.

During the planning phase, the nurse collaborates with the client and other health care providers to determine the goals, outcomes, and interventions and manipulates the external environment to reduce the risk of injury and infection. Identified outcomes provide direction for the nursing care that is implemented to reduce the risk of injury and infection.

Another critical element of the care plan is client/caregiver education related to the identification of potential hazards and health promotion practices. The nursing care plan should include safety measures that educate clients

## TABLE 33-4　　SELF-CARE DEFICITS

| Nursing Diagnosis and Definition | Defining Characteristics | Related Factors |
|---|---|---|
| *Bathing/Hygiene Self-Care Deficit:* A state in which the individual experiences an impaired ability to perform or complete bathing/hygiene activities for self | Inability to wash body or body parts, obtain or get water from a water source, or regulate the temperature or flow of water | Intolerance to activity; decreased strength and endurance; pain, discomfort; impairment of perception or cognition, neuromuscular activity, and musculoskeletal function; depression, severe anxiety |
| *Dressing/Grooming Self-Care Deficit:* A state in which the individual experiences an impaired ability to perform or complete dressing and grooming activities for self | Impaired ability to put on or take off necessary items of clothing, obtain or replace articles of clothing, fasten clothing, or maintain appearance at a satisfactory level | Intolerance to activity; decreased strength and endurance; pain, discomfort; impairment of perception or cognition, neuromuscular activity, and musculoskeletal function; depression, severe anxiety |
| *Toileting Self-Care Deficit:* A state in which an individual experiences an impaired ability to perform or complete toileting activities for self | Unable to get to toilet or commode, sit on or rise from toilet or commode, manipulate clothing for toileting, carry out proper toilet hygiene, or flush toilet or commode | Impaired transfer ability and mobility status; intolerance to activity; decreased strength and endurance; pain, discomfort; impairment of perception or cognition, neuromuscular activity, and musculoskeletal function; depression, severe anxiety |

From North American Nursing Diagnosis Association (2003). *Nursing diagnoses: Definitions and classification 2003–2004.* Philadelphia: Author.

about preventive actions and modification of an unsafe environment—for example, proper use of a call light or the side effects of medications.

Table 33-5 discusses the basic components of care planning and outcome measurements for clients at risk or with a self-care deficit. Sample statements of goals and expected outcomes are included in Table 33-5. The nursing interventions are statements taken from the Nursing Intervention Classification System. For each of these nursing interventions, specific actions are taken by the nurse to individualize the care for each client. The nurse could use Gordon's Functional Health Patterns to plan care. Gordon's Functional Health Patterns that may be used for clients at risk or with a self-care deficit are health perception–health management, activity-exercise pattern, and cognitive-perceptual pattern. Nursing actions are discussed in detail in the following section.

## Implementation

Nursing care implemented for clients with alterations in health perception–health management or activity and exercise involves continual assessment of client health risks and prioritization of risk reduction nursing interventions, such as:

- Administration of prescribed medications (refer to Chapter 30)

- Provision of balanced nutritional intake (refer to Chapter 35)
- Promotion of adequate rest and exercise (refer to Chapters 33 and 40)
- Decreasing the spread of infection

Implementation of safety measures may require an alteration in the physical environment as directed by a fall prevention protocol or Standard Precautions.

Nursing measures to counter common physical hazards that impair environmental safety are maintaining electric beds in the low position with side rails up and call light within easy reach, and keeping the bedroom and bathroom uncluttered to prevent falls. Some states consider side rails a form of restraint. Nurses must be knowledgeable about statutory provisions relative to health care in their state.

The implementation of Standard Precautions is the most effective nursing measure to prevent and control the spread of infections. Standard Precautions are discussed in detail later in this chapter.

## Raise Safety Awareness and Knowledge

Nurses in all settings must demonstrate an awareness of safety hazards and teach clients accordingly. Clients must be aware of and knowledgeable about safety precautions in

## TABLE 33-5    PLANNING THE CARE OF CLIENTS AT RISK FOR INJURY OR INFECTION AND/OR WITH A SELF-CARE DEFICIT

| Nursing Diagnosis and Definition | Goals | Expected Outcomes | Nursing Interventions |
|---|---|---|---|
| Risk for Injury | 1. The client will identify factors that increase the potential for injury. | 1. The client will identify internal and external factors that will increase the risk for injury. | Risk identification: Analysis of potential risk factors, determination of health risks, and prioritization of risk reduction strategies for an individual |
| | 2. The client will remain free of bodily injury. | 2. The client will identify and implement safety measures to decrease the risk for injury. | Fall prevention: Instituting special precautions with client at risk for injury |
| Risk for Infection | 1. The client will remain free of nosocomial infection. | 1. The client will remain afebrile during hospitalization. | Infection protection: Prevention and early detection of infection in a client at risk |
| | 2. The client will reduce exposure to known infectious agents. | 2. The client will not engage in unprotected sexual intercourse. | Infection control: Minimizing the acquisition and transmission of infectious agents |
| Bathing/Hygiene Self-Care Deficit | 1. The client will maintain an optimum functional level in hygienic practices in a safe and effective manner. | 1. The client will participate physically and/or verbally in bathing, dressing, and toileting activities. | Bathing: Cleaning of the body for the purpose of relaxation, cleanliness, and healing |
| | | | Dressing: choosing, putting on, and removing clothes for a person who cannot do this for self |
| | 2. The client's skin will remain clean and intact. | 2. The client's skin will be free from drainage or secretion, intact, and without redness. | Skin surveillance: Collection and analysis of client data to maintain skin and mucous membrane integrity |
| | | | Perineal care: Maintenance of perineal skin integrity and relief of perineal discomfort |
| Deficient Knowledge: related to health hazards | The client will not sustain injuries. | The client will verbalize feedback of instructions and willingness to comply. | Teaching individual: Planning, implementation, and evaluation of a teaching program designed to address a client's particular needs |

Adapted from Ackley, B., & Ladwig, G. (2002). *Nursing diagnosis handbook* (5th ed.). St. Louis: Mosby.

order to prevent injuries. Clients may also need specific safety information on oxygen, intravenous equipment, use of heating devices, and automatic bed controls. Clients must be carefully assessed to determine the best safety plan of care, especially when unsteady or confused.

## Bed Safety

Clients can become entrapped in beds with raised side rails. Figure 33-5 depicts common entrapment locations on the typical hospital bed, as identified by the Food and Drug Administration in a safety alert issued in 1995. Between 1985 and 1999, 228 bed entrapment deaths occurred, an additional 87 clients suffered injuries due to bed entrapment, and 56 were entrapped but had no injury due to close supervision and prompt intervention by staff members. The client may be strangled or suffocate when caught between the rails or between the rails and the mattress. The client may fall while attempting to climb over the rails. Skin tears, abrasions, and bruises occur when clients strike the bed rails. It has become apparent in recent years that the traditional client safety approach of

## CLIENT REFLECTIONS

### A Client's Perception of Side Rails

Mr. Parker, age 87, has been living independently at home. This past week, he fell from atop his woodpile, striking his head, and was admitted for observation. Mr. Parker states, "I do all right at home! Why can't you see that I can do all right here? Why do you keep putting those side rails up? I feel like I am in a crib! You are treating me like a child!"

As a nurse, how would you respond?

## LIFE SPAN CONSIDERATIONS

### Hazards in the Home Environment for Older Clients

As clients age, they may become less aware of hazards in their home environment. A conventional bathtub, for example, an accepted fixture in most homes, may pose a hazard to the older client who must frequently get in and out of the tub unassisted.

Hogstel, M. (2001). *Gerontology: Nursing care of the older adult.* Clifton Park, NY: Delmar Learning.

using soft restraints and bed rails may exacerbate agitated behavior in some clients. When bed rails impose a restriction on independence, they are viewed by some agencies as a restraint (Food and Drug Administration, 2000).

Raised side rails do have benefits. Clearly, they are needed to prevent the client from falling out of the bed during transport. They provide a place for the client to grasp when repositioning in bed and when getting in and out of bed. For some, they instill a sense of comfort. Having the rail up often increases access to bed controls, since they are often built into the rail. Clients can rest safely in bed with side rails. Anticipating client needs and frequent monitoring of at-risk clients are interventions critical to client safety.

In addition, beds should be adjustable to a level close to the floor for client safety, and up high enough for the nurse to deliver care without undue back strain, for the nurse's safety. Locked wheels provide safety for both the client and the nurse. In some settings, mats are placed on the floor beside the bed, with the bed in a very low position, to provide a soft surface should the client roll out of bed. This is not appropriate to all clients in all settings; however, as it can create additional hazards. This method is most commonly used in long-term care and similar facilities.

### Prevent Falls

Falls typically occur among clients who are weak, fatigued, uncoordinated, paralyzed, confused, or disoriented. The data obtained from the client's fall risk appraisal will identify which clients require special nursing measures to prevent falls. The risk for falls can be reduced by:

- Good supervision
- Orienting clients to the environment and call system
- Providing ambulatory aids (wheelchairs or walkers)
- Placing personal belongings on tables near the bed
- Keeping hospital beds in lowest position with side rails up
- Using nonslip mats and rugs
- Illuminating the environment

Although falls do not necessarily constitute malpractice, they are a major reason nurses are involved in lawsuits (Ignatavicius, 2000). Sullivan and Badros (1999) and Ignatavicius (2000) identify the need for registered nurses to assess clients' risk of falls and implement evidence-based interventions. The concept of Evidence-Based Practice (EBP) refers to health care based on research findings, expert consensus, or both (Davis & Madigan, 1999).

### Apply Restraints

**Restraints** are protective devices used to limit the physical activity of a client or to immobilize a client or extremity. Restraints are used to protect the client, allow for treatment in a safe environment, and reduce the risk of injury to others.

The use of restraints has become very controversial because of client injuries from restraints. The Omnibus

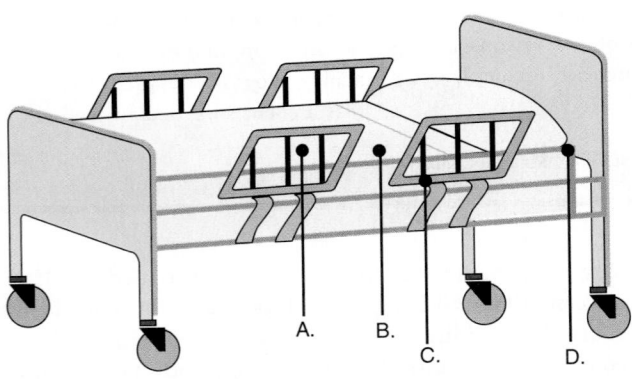

**Figure 33-5   Entrapment hazards with hospital bed side rails: A. Through the bars of an individual side rail B. Through the space between split side rail C. Between the side rail and mattress D. Between the headboard or footboard, side rail, and mattress** *From Food and Drug Administration, Safety Alert, August 23, 1995*

Budget Reconciliation Act (OBRA) of 1987 and the Health Care Financing Administration (now the Centers for Medicare and Medicaid Services) regulations of 1999 governing client's rights are forcing a reexamination of how clients are cared for in acute and critical care settings (Bower & McCullough, 2000). In response to more individualized care regarding the use of restraints, JCAHO revised their standards for restraint use with nonpsychiatric clients (see Box 33-5 for JCAHO revised standards).

Nurses must document, according to the institutional protocol, the application and care of the client in restraints (see Box 33-6). Refer to Chapter 8 for additional information regarding the use of restraints and their legal implications.

Restraints used to either limit physical activity or immobilize a client can be physical or chemical. **Physical restraints** reduce the client's movement through the application of a device. Most states require a physician's order for the application of physical restraints (Box 33-6). **Chemical restraints** are medications used to control the client's behavior. Commonly used chemical restraints are anxiolytics and sedatives.

---

## BOX 33-5    JCAHO RESTRAINT STANDARDS FOR NONPSYCHIATRIC CLIENTS

### Organizational Perspective

- Be individualized for each institution
- Demonstrate clinical justification
- Demonstrate the use of innovative alternatives
- Delineate preventive strategies
- Identify ways to reduce risks associated with restraint use

### Policies/Procedures/Protocols

- Be clearly stated
- Advocate use of least restrictive measures

### Preventive Strategies

- Identify potentially harmful client behaviors
- Identify effective and tried alternatives

### Plan of Care

- Be individualized and ensure client's assessed needs are met
- Preserve client's rights, dignity, and well-being

### Education

- Be ongoing for staff and client
- Be provided to families when appropriate

### Initiation and Monitoring of Restraint Use

- Based on state law

- Initiated based on individual orders or approved protocols with written physician order obtained within 12 hours
- Applied/monitored/assessed/reassessed by qualified staff
- Monitored at least every 2 hours
- Renewed every 24 hours when continuous restraint is used

### Special Conditions When Restraint Is Applied

- Based on significant change in the client's condition with the physician notified immediately and written orders obtained within 24 hours
- Initiated by a registered nurse
- Based on protocols established for situations where clients may harm themselves if staff initiate, maintain, and terminate restraint without an order from independent practitioner

### Documentation

- Include all restraint episodes according to organizational policies and procedures
- Occur, at a minimum, every 2 hours
- Indicate alternatives were tried before restraints were applied
- Be entered into the client's medical record

Adapted from the Joint Commission on Accreditation of Healthcare Organizations for Restraint Use (1999). *Introduction to the restraint standards in acute medical and surgical (nonpsychiatric) care. Comprehensive accreditation manual for hospitals.* Oakbrook Terrace, IL: Author.

## CLINICAL ALERT

### Restraints

Jacket or belt restraints should not restrict respiratory effort. Placing a restraint too tight on the diaphragm will inhibit the expansion of the lungs.

---

### BOX 33-6    KEY ELEMENTS OF RESTRAINT DOCUMENTATION

- Reason for the restraint
- Method of restraint
- Application: Date, time, and client's response
- Duration
- Frequency of observation and client's response
- Safety: Release from restraint with periodic, routine exercise and assessment for circulation and skin integrity
- Assessment of the continued need for restraint
- Client outcome

---

This chapter limits discussion to the common types of physical restraints (Figure 33-6):

- Jacket (body restraint): A sleeveless vest with straps that cross in front or back of the client and are tied to the bed frame or chair legs.
- Belt: Straps or belts applied across the client to secure him to the stretcher, bed, or wheelchair.
- Mitten or hand: Enclosed cloth material applied over the client's hand to prevent injury from scratching.
- Elbow: A combination of fabric and plastic or wooden tongue blades that immobilize the elbow to prevent flexion.
- Limb or extremity: Cloth devices that immobilize one or all limbs by securely tying the restraint to the bed frame or chair.
- Mummy: A blanket or sheet that is folded around the child to limit movement. Mummy restraints are used to perform procedures on children.

The nursing plan of care should include safety measures to reduce the potential for injury from restraints (Procedure 33-1). Additional safety measures to observe when using restraint devices are:

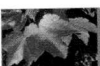

## RESEARCH FOCUS

**Title of Study:** Nursing outcome indicator: Preventing falls for elderly people

**Study Purpose:** To identify people at risk of falling and to mitigate that risk through established nursing interventions.

**Methods:** The study included 115 participants. Each participant received a comprehensive nursing assessment and a fall risk appraisal, which included the client's history of falling, episodes of confusion, diminished eyesight or hearing, and number and types of medications. Interventions were determined by each person's risk factors and included reducing medications or teaching about side effects, correcting vision and hearing, providing walkers and canes to persons who had previously fallen, and promoting improved strength and endurance through exercise. Homes were surveyed, and environmental changes were made: lighting was increased; loose carpet edges were taped; and grab rails were installed in showers, in tubs, and by toilets.

**Findings:** Only 4 (3%) of the 115 participants fell during the first year of the fall prevention program as opposed to 30 (or 26%) prior to the implementation of the program. Two of the four participants who fell where under the influence of alcohol, and the other two persons fell while they were away from their homes.

**Implications:** This study demonstrates that it is possible to prevent falls when the risk factors are identified and proper interventions are implemented to counter the risk factors.

Benzon, J., et al. (1999). Nursing outcome indicator: Preventing falls for elderly people. *Outcomes Management Nursing Practice, 3*(3), 132–137.

- Restraints can be changed and released easily, using only a clove hitch knot.
- Restraints should not interfere with any treatments (e.g., intravenous therapy) or aggravate the client's health problem.
- There should be enough slack on the straps so that the client can move both arms and legs and for range-of-motion exercises.
- At least once every 2 hours, the nurse must perform circulation and neurologic exams, assessing the color, sensation, temperature, motion, and capillary refill in the area distal to the restraint.
- There should be a provision for psychological support of client and significant others.

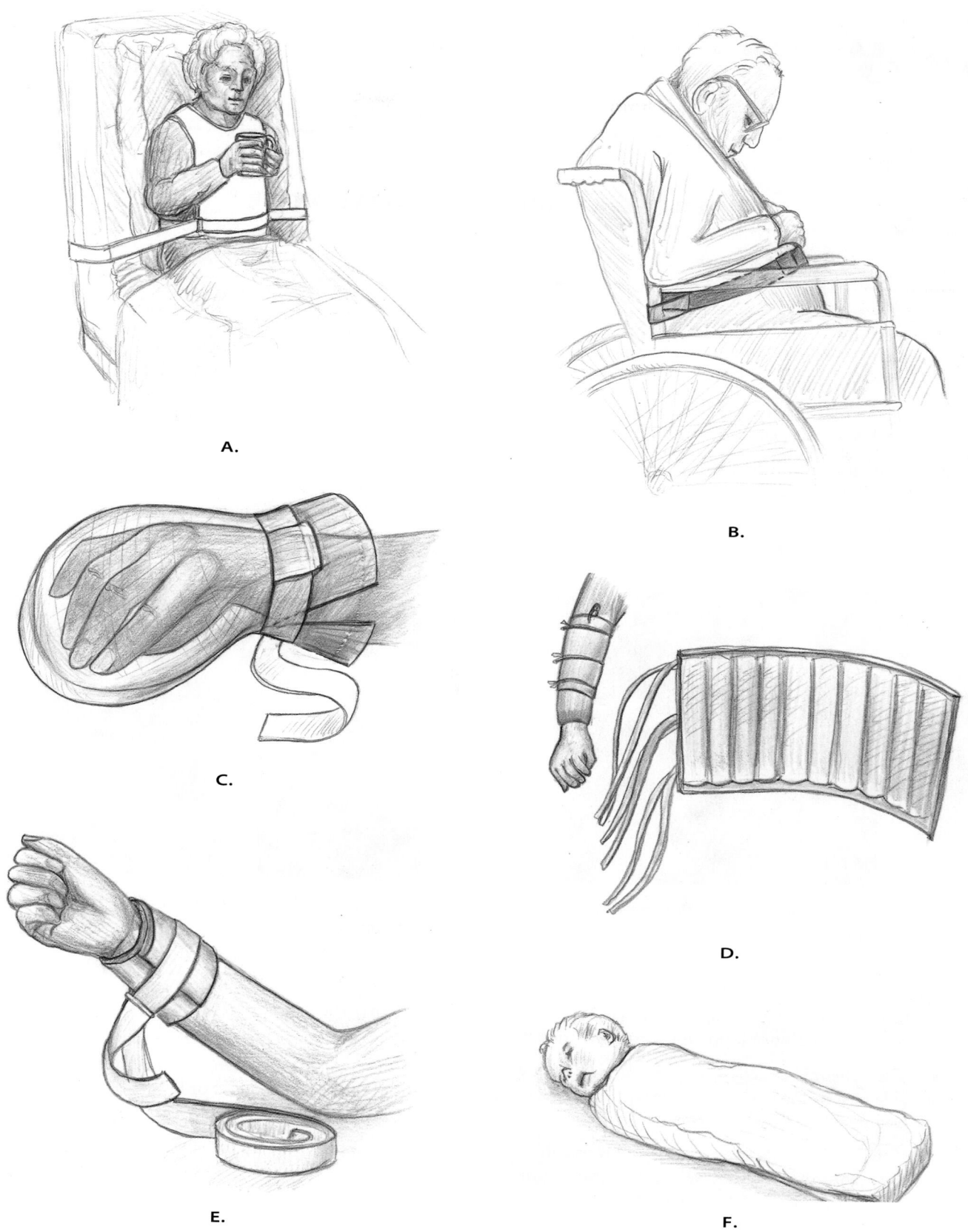

A.

B.

C.

D.

E.

F.

**Figure 33-6** Types of physical restraints: A. Jacket B. Belt C. Mitten or hand D. Elbow E. Limb or extremity, F. Mummy

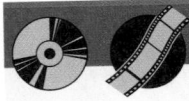

**PROCEDURE 33-1**    # Applying Restraints

## EQUIPMENT NEEDED

▪ Restraint

## IMPLEMENTATION—ACTION/RATIONALE

| ACTION | RATIONALE |
|---|---|

**Chest Restraint**

1. Ensure there is an order or urgent medical need to apply restraints of any kind on a client.

2. Explain that the client will be wearing a jacket attached to the bed. Explain that this is for safety.

3. Place the restraint over the client's hospital gown or clothing.

4. Place the restraint on the client with the opening in the front (Figure 33-7).

1. A physician's order is legally required.

2. Promotes client cooperation.

3. Provides for client privacy and prevents the restraint from rubbing the client's skin.

4. Allows movement but restricts freedom.

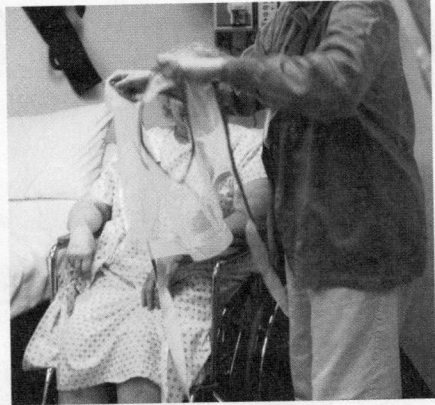

**Figure 33-7    Place the jacket restraint on the client. Make sure the restraint is the proper size for the client and has been applied correctly.**

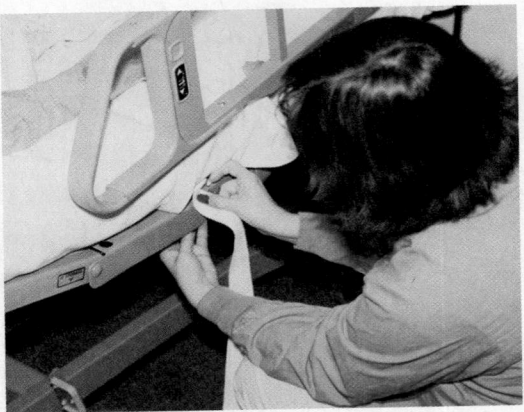

**Figure 33-8    Secure ties to the movable part of the frame.**

5. Overlap the front pieces, threading the ties through the slot or loop on the front of the vest.

6. If the client is in bed, secure the ties to the movable part of the mattress frame with a half-knot (Figure 33-8).

7. If the client is in a chair, cross the straps behind the seat of the chair and secure the straps to the chair's lower legs, out of the client's reach (Figure 33-9). If it is a wheelchair, be sure the straps will not get caught up in the wheels.

5. Secures the restraint.

6. Allows the restraint to move with the bed if the head of the bed is raised or lowered.

7. Provides support for the client to sit up while restricting freedom.

*(continues)*

## PROCEDURE 33-1 (continued)

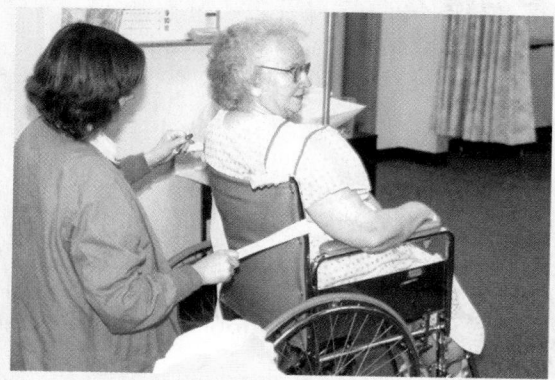

**Figure 33-9    Secure restraining straps out of the client's reach.**

8. Step back and assess the client's overall safety. Be sure the restraint is loose enough not to be a hazard to the client but tight enough to restrict the client from getting up and harming herself.

9. Wash your hands.

8. Looking at the overall picture can allow you to see dangers you might have missed.

9. Prevents the spread of microorganisms.

| ACTION | RATIONALE |
|---|---|

### Applying Wrist or Ankle Restraints

1. Explain to the client that you will be placing a wrist or ankle band that will restrict movement.

2. Place padding around the client's wrist or ankle.

3. Wrap the restraint around the client's wrist or ankle, pulling the tie through the loop in the restraint and tie a square knot (Figure 33-10).

4. Tie the restraint ties to the movable portion of the mattress frame.

5. Slip two fingers under the restraint to check for tightness. Be sure the restraint is tight enough that the client cannot slip it off, but loose enough that the neurovascular status of the client's extremity is not impaired.

6. Step back and assess the client's overall safety. Be sure the restraint is loose enough not to be a hazard to the client, but tight enough to restrict the client from getting up and harming himself (Figure 33-11).

7. Place the call light within the client's reach.

1. Promotes client cooperation.

2. Prevents the restraint from chafing the skin.

3. Secures the restraint, and prevents the restraint from overtightening at the wrist or ankle.

4. When the head or foot of the client's bed is moved, the restraint will move with it.

5. If the restraint is too tight, the client's neurovascular status may be impaired, causing injury to the client.

6. Looking at the overall picture can allow you to see dangers you might have missed.

7. Allows the client to contact the nurse to have any needs met. Provides the client with an increased sense of safety.

*(continues)*

## PROCEDURE 33-1 *(continued)*

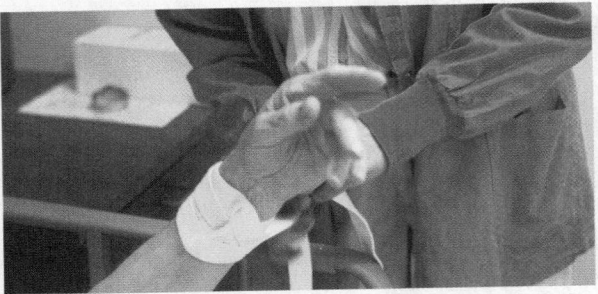

**Figure 33-10**    **Wrap restraint around the client's wrist.**

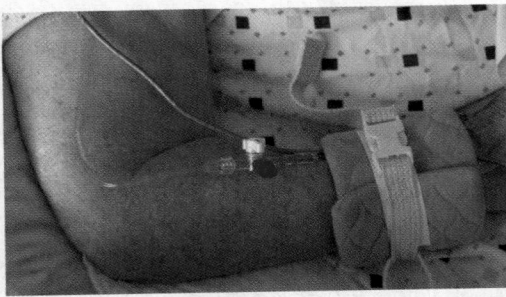

**Figure 33-11**    **Restraints should not be too tight or loose. Check frequently.**

8. Check on the client every half hour while restrained. Assess the safety of the restraint placement and the client's neurovascular status.

9. Assess circulatory status of restrained extremity every 2 hours and as needed. Release one restraint from each extremity for at least 15 minutes every two hours and record.

10. Wash your hands.

8. Assures that the client remains safe. Clients may try to escape from restraint and injure themselves in the attempt.

9. States and institutions may have regulations outlining the frequency of checks for whether the client is in restraint. Be aware of any regulations that apply.

10. Prevents the spread of microorganisms.

### Ensure Adequate Lighting

Adequate lighting assists in the visualization of environmental hazards. Rooms should be adequately lighted so that the client can safely perform activities of daily living (ADL) and health care providers can perform procedures. Lighting can be supplemented by lamps and night-lights. Lighting can also assist in protecting the home against crime.

### Remove Obstacles

Obstacles in heavily traveled areas of health care facilities or homes are a risk to the client's safety. Older adults or persons who are unfamiliar with the environment are at greatest risk of injury from obstacles. The risk that obstacles pose can be reduced by keeping hallways clear, removing excess furniture from heavily traveled areas, removing all electrical cords or taping cords securely to the floor, removing throw rugs, applying nonslip pads to rugs, cleaning up spills immediately, and removing objects that could fall from the tops of appliances.

## Reduce Bathroom Hazards

Bathrooms pose a threat to the client in the home because of the presence of water and storage of medication. Common bathroom accidents are falls, scalds or burns, and poisonings. Bathroom accidents can be reduced by the use of grab bars near the tub, shower, and toilet; nonslip mats in the tub and shower; and a secured bathroom rug near the tub or shower. Other safety measures include checking the temperature of the water before entering tub or shower, checking the thermostat setting on the water heater, and storing medications in a locked cabinet, out of reach of children or disoriented or confused adults.

## Prevent Fire

Fire is a potential danger to all people in an institutional or home environment. Immobilized or incapacitated clients are at increased risk during a fire. Common causes of fire are smoking in bed, discarding cigarette butts in trash cans, and faulty electrical equipment. Fire occurs with the interaction of three elements: sufficient heat to ignite the fire, combustible material, and oxygen to support the fire.

Nursing goals are fire prevention and protection of clients during a fire. Nursing interventions aimed at preventing or reducing the risk of fire include:

- Knowing safe areas for evacuation
- Clearly marking fire exits
- Knowing locations of fire extinguishers and their operation
- Practicing fire evacuation procedures
- Posting emergency phone numbers by all telephones

- Keeping open spaces and hallways clear of clutter
- Checking electrical cords and outlets for exposed or damaged wires
- Reporting identified electrical hazards
- Educating clients about fire hazards
- Maintaining minimum 18-inch clearance from ceiling for proper sprinkler operation

In the event of a fire, follow institutional policy and procedures for fire containment and evacuation. Nurses should be familiar with the location of fire alarm pull boxes. If a fire occurs, the nurse should use the nearest fire box for notification and move clients to safety.

Nurses should be familiar with the use of fire extinguishers and their locations. The fire extinguisher should be directed toward the base of the fire. The four types of fire extinguishers used are water, carbon dioxide, regular dry chemical, and multipurpose dry chemical. Each type of fire extinguisher is used for a specific class of fire, as listed in Table 33-6.

## Ensure Safe Operation of Electrical Equipment

Clients have contact with a variety of electrical equipment in the hospital environment, such as bed controls and intravenous and patient-controlled analgesia (PCA) pumps. All electrical equipment should have a three-pronged electrical plug that is grounded. A grounded plug transmits any stray electrical current from equipment to the ground. To protect the client from electrical injury, the nurse should read the warning labels on all equipment, use only grounded electrical equipment, check for frayed electrical cords, avoid overloading circuits, and report any shocks received from equipment to the biomedical department (see Figure 33-12).

If a client receives an electrical shock, the nurse should turn off or remove the electric source before touching the client. Then the client's pulse should be checked. If the client has no pulse, CPR should be initiated. If the client has a pulse, the nurse should assess vital signs, mental status, and skin integrity for burns. A physician and the biomedical department should be notified of the event. The

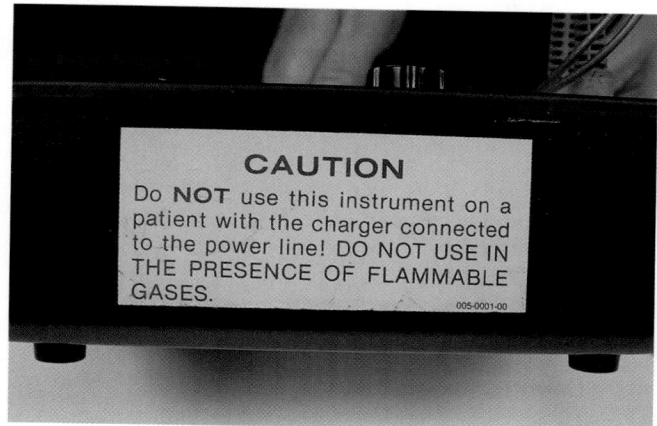

CAUTION
Do **NOT** use this instrument on a patient with the charger connected to the power line! DO NOT USE IN THE PRESENCE OF FLAMMABLE GASES.

005-0001-00

**Figure 33-12    Warning label on electrical equipment**

nurse should note points of entry and exit of electrical current to assess for potential complications.

## Reduce Exposure to Radiation

Clients are exposed to radiation during diagnostic testing and therapeutic interventions. Injury can occur from radiation if there is overexposure or exposure to untargeted tissues. Exposure to untargeted tissues can occur with radiation implants that become dislodged. General principles of radiation exposure and protection are based on time, distance, and shielding. Protection from radiation therapy includes:

- Minimizing time in contact with radiation source (implants or client)
- Maximizing distance from radiation source (implants or client)
- Using appropriate radiation shields
- Monitoring radiation exposure with a film badge
- Labeling all potentially radioactive material
- Never touching dislodged implants or body fluids of client

Both the client and the nurse are at risk for radiation injury. The client's risk for injury can be reduced by educating the client about radiation treatment and necessary precautions, placing the client in a private room, and providing a lead apron when necessary to protect nontargeted body tissues. The nurse's risk for injury can be reduced by observing all radioactive labels, wearing gloves when handling radioactive body discharges, washing hands, wearing lead aprons, disposing of radioactive substances in special containers, reducing time of client contact, and wearing badges that measure the amount of radiation exposure.

## Prevent Poisoning

A **poison** is any substance that causes an alteration in the client's health, such as injury or death, when inhaled, injected, ingested, or absorbed by the body. Antidotes and

| TABLE 33-6 | FIRE EXTINGUISHERS |
|---|---|
| Type | Class of Fire |
| Water (type A) | Paper, wood, draperies, upholstery, or rubbish |
| Carbon dioxide or dry chemical (types B and C) | Flammable liquids, flammable gases, or electrical fires |
| Multipurpose dry chemical (types A, B, and C) | Any type of fire |

treatments are available for some but not all types of poisonings. Direct and indirect causes of poisonings are:

- Inadequate supervision of children
- Ingestion of household plants
- Improper storage of toxic substances
- Insect or snake bites
- Accidental ingestion of a toxic substance or medication overdose

The poison control center should be notified when poisoning is suspected. The person reporting the poisoning should be prepared to state the amount and type of poison ingested, inhaled, or injected; client's age; and symptoms. Clients who have ingested poison should be turned on their side to prevent aspiration while awaiting further treatment. Client education about safety measures can

prevent some accidental poisonings. The accompanying Client Education box provides some safety measures to prevent accidental poisoning. Keep syrup of ipecac available at all times.

## Reduce Noise Pollution

Noise pollution, a situation that results when the noise level becomes uncomfortable for the client or staff, frequently occurs in the health care setting as a result of visitor traffic, medical equipment, and personnel. It can result in an unorganized environment, **sensory overload** (the condition in which sensory stimuli are received at a rate and intensity beyond the level that the client can handle—this stressful situation can lead to confusion, anxiety, mental distress, and panic), and in extreme cases, hearing loss. Sensory overload is an increased perception of the intensity of auditory and visual stimuli. Sensory overload can alter a client's recovery by increasing anxiety, paranoia, hallucinations, and depression. Safety measures include maintaining a quiet environment, traffic control, and providing earplugs. See Chapter 41 for a discussion of sensory overload.

## Provide for Client Bathing Needs

Bathing of clients is an essential component of nursing care. Whether the nurse performs the bath or delegates the activity to another health care provider, the nurse retains the responsibility for assuring that the hygienic needs of the client are met. The type of bath provided will depend on the purpose of the bath and the client's self-care ability. The two general categories of baths are cleaning and therapeutic.

### Cleaning Baths

Cleaning baths are provided as routine client care. The purpose of a cleaning bath is personal hygiene. The five types of cleaning baths are shower, tub, self-help, or assisted bed bath, complete bed bath, and partial bath.

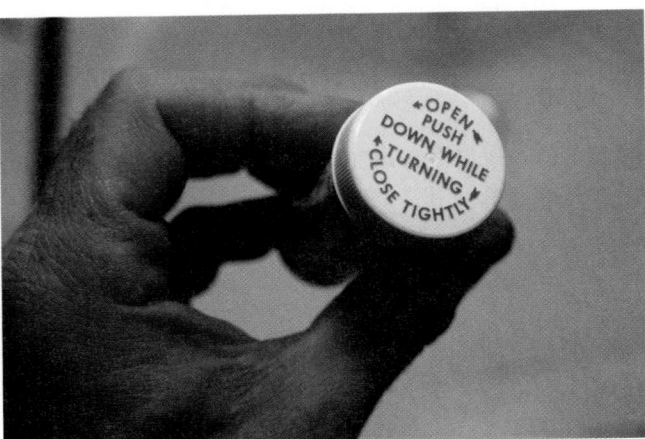

**Figure 33-13   Poison prevention measure: Medications stored in child-resistant containers**

## CLIENT EDUCATION

### Tub or Shower Bath

✓ Assemble necessary equipment.
✓ Place bath mat in tub or shower. Provide shower chair if necessary.
✓ Ensure privacy.
✓ Adjust room temperature and temperature of water.
✓ Half-fill tub with water. Do not allow client to soak longer than 20 minutes. Provide slip-resistant mat on floor outside tub or shower.
✓ Assist client with getting into and out of tub or shower. Provide with a call system.
✓ Assist with cleaning as necessary.
✓ Clean tub or shower after use.

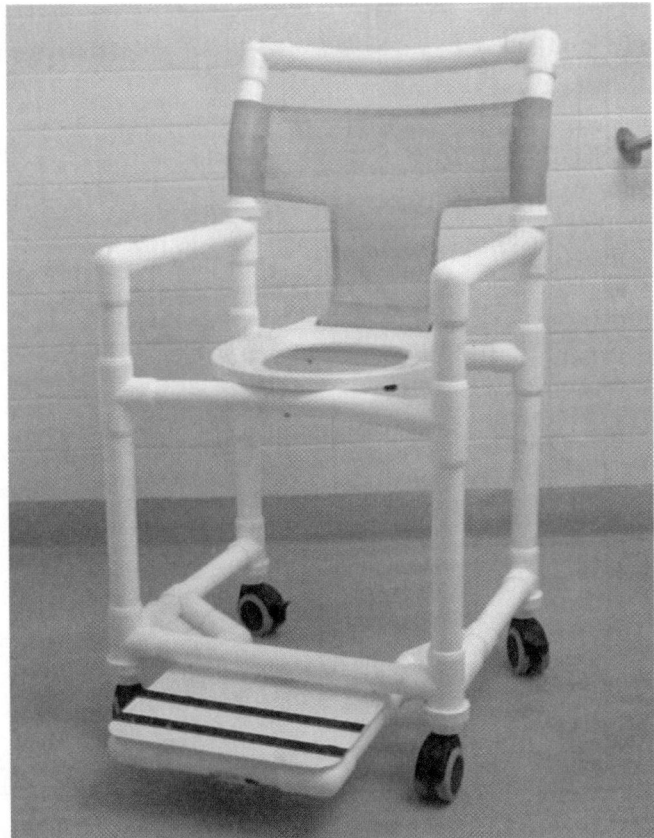

**Figure 33-14   Shower chair**

### Shower

Most ambulatory clients are capable of taking a shower. Clients with limited physical ability can be accommodated by placing a waterproof chair in the shower (Figure 33-14). The nurse provides minimal assistance with a shower. The Nursing Checklist discusses guidelines for helping clients with tub or shower baths.

### Tub Bath

Clients frequently prefer and enjoy tub baths. A tub bath permits washing and rinsing in the tub. Tub baths can also be therapeutic. Clients with limited physical ability should be assisted with entering and exiting the tub.

### Self-Help Bath

A self-help, or assisted, bed bath is used to provide hygienic care for clients who are confined to bed. In the self-help (assisted) bed bath, the nurse prepares bath equipment but provides minimal assistance. This assistance is usually limited to washing difficult-to-reach body areas such as the feet and back.

### Complete Bed Bath

A complete bed bath is provided to dependent clients confined to bed. The nurse washes the client's entire body during a complete bed bath. Procedure 33-2 outlines the actions involved in giving a complete bed bath.

### Partial Bath

A partial (or abbreviated) bath consists of cleaning only body areas that would cause discomfort or odor if not washed thoroughly. These areas are the face, axillae, hands, and perineal area. The nurse or client may perform a partial bath depending on the client's self-care ability. Partial baths may be performed with the client lying in bed or standing at the sink.

### Therapeutic Baths

Therapeutic baths require a physician's order stating the type of bath, temperature of water, body surface to be treated, and the type of medicated solutions to use. A therapeutic bath is usually performed in a tub and lasts about 20 to 31 minutes. Therapeutic baths are classified as hot or warm water, cool or tepid water, soak, sitz, oatmeal or Aveeno, cornstarch, or sodium bicarbonate, depending on the prescribed type of bath.

Hot- or warm-water tub baths are used to reduce muscle spasms, soreness, and tension. Hot- or warm-water baths, however, have the potential for causing skin burns. Cool or tepid baths are used to relieve tension or lower body temperature. The nurse needs to prevent chilling and rapid temperature fluctuations during a cool or tepid bath.

A soak can include the entire body or be limited to only one body part. A soak consists of applying water, with or without a medicated solution, to reduce pain, swelling, or irritation or to soften or remove dead tissue.

Sitz baths cleanse and reduce inflammation in the perineal and anal areas. Sitz baths are commonly used for hemorrhoids or anal fissures and after perineal or rectal surgery. Skin irritations can be soothed with oatmeal or Aveeno, cornstarch, or sodium bicarbonate baths.

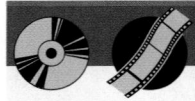

PROCEDURE 33-2     **Bathing a Client in Bed**

## EQUIPMENT NEEDED

- Bath towels (Figure 33-15)
- Washcloths
- Bath blanket
- Washbasin
- Soap
- Soap dish
- Lotion
- Deodorant
- Powder
- Clean gown
- Clean linen
- Disposable gloves

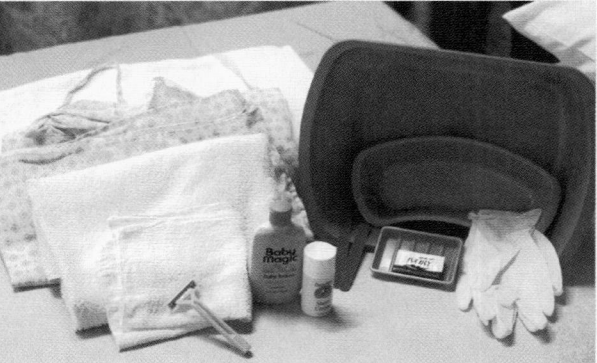

**Figure 33-15** Emesis and bath basins, soap, towels, and lotion are used to bathe the client. A razor and shaving cream are used to groom the male client.

## IMPLEMENTATION—ACTION/RATIONALE

| ACTION | RATIONALE |
|---|---|
| 1. Assess the client's preferences about bathing. | 1. Provides client opportunity to participate in care. |
| 2. Explain procedure to client. | 2. Enhances cooperation. |
| 3. Prepare environment. Close doors and windows, adjust temperature, provide time for elimination needs, and provide privacy (Figure 33-16). | 3. Protects from chills during bath and increases sense of privacy. |

**Figure 33-16** Close doors and/or curtains and provide privacy to begin the bath.

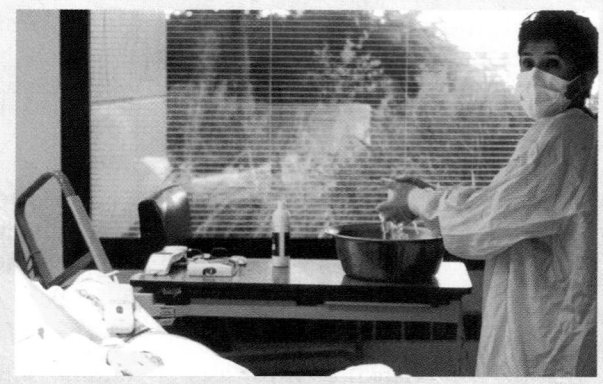

**Figure 33-17** Wet the washcloth and wring out the excess water. The nurse is wearing a mask because the client is in isolation.

*(continues)*

## PROCEDURE 33-2 (*continued*)

4. Wash hands. Apply gloves. Gloves should be changed when emptying water basin.

5. Lower side rail on the side close to you. Position client in a comfortable position close to the side near you.

6. If bath blankets are available, place bath blanket over top sheet. Remove top sheet from under bath blanket. Remove client's gown. Bath blanket should be folded to expose only the area being cleaned at that time (Top sheets or towels may also be used for bath blankets).

7. Fill washbasin two-thirds full. Permit client to test temperature of water with hand. Water should be changed when a soap film develops or water becomes soiled.

8. Wet the washcloth and wring it out (Figure 33-17).

9. Make a bath mitten with the washcloth. To make a mitten, grasp the edge of the washcloth with the thumb; fold a third over the palm of the hand; wrap remainder of cloth around hand and across palm, grasping the second edge under the thumb; fold the extended end of the washcloth onto the palm and tuck under the palmar surface of the cloth.

10. Wash the face (Figure 33-18). Ask the client about preference for using soap on the face. Use a separate corner of the washcloth for each eye, wiping from inner to outer canthus. Wash neck and ears. Rinse and pat dry. Male clients may want to shave at this time. Provide assistance with shaving as needed.

---

4. Reduces the transmission of microorganisms.

5. Prevents unnecessary reaching. Facilitates use of good body mechanics.

6. Prevents exposure of client. Promotes privacy. Protects from chills.

7. Prevents accidental burns or chills.

8. Prevents unnecessarily wetting of client.

9. Prevents ends of washcloth from dragging across skin. Promotes friction during bath.

10. Some clients may not use soap on their face. Using separate corners of washcloth reduces risk of transmitting microorganisms. Patting dry reduces skin irritation and drying.

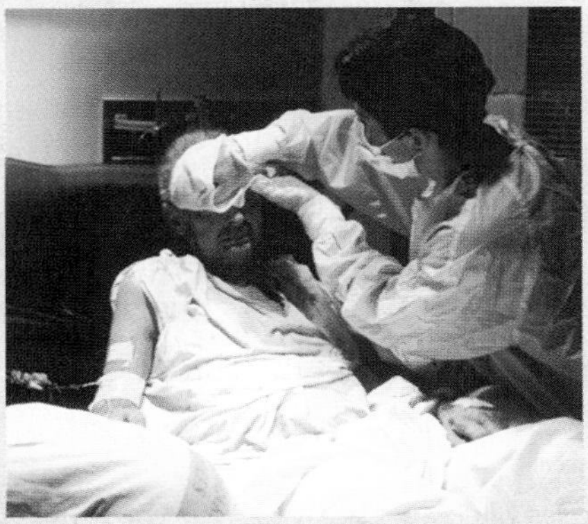

**Figure 33-18    Wash the client's face first.**

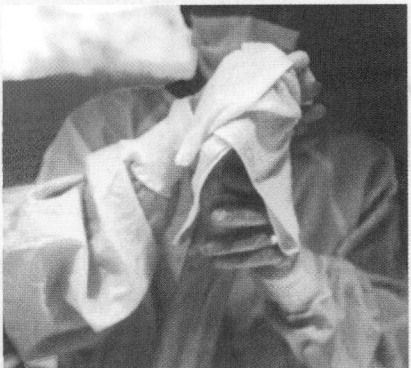

**Figure 33-19    Wash the hands and arms next.**

*(continues)*

## PROCEDURE 33-2 (continued)

11. Wash arms, forearms, and hands (Figure 33-19). Wash forearms and arms using long, firm strokes in the direction of distal to proximal (Figure 33-20). Arm may need to be supported while being washed. Wash axilla. Rinse and pat dry. Apply deodorant or powder if desired. Immerse client's hand into basin of water. Allow hand to soak about 3 to 5 minutes. Wash hands, interdigit area, fingers, and fingernails. Rinse and pat dry.

11. Long strokes promote circulation. Soaking hands softens nails and loosens soil from skin and nails. Strokes directed distal to proximal promote venous return.

12. Wash chest and abdomen. Fold bath blanket down to umbilicus. Wash chest using long, firm strokes. Wash skin fold under the female client's breast by lifting each breast. Rinse and pat dry. Fold bath blanket down to suprapubic area. Use another towel to cover chest area. Wash abdomen using long, firm strokes. Rinse and pat dry. Replace bath blanket over chest and abdomen. Cover chest or abdomen area in between washing, rinsing, and drying to prevent chilling.

12. Promotes privacy and prevents chills. Long strokes promote circulation. Perspiration and soil collect within skin folds.

13. Wash legs and feet. Expose leg farthest from you by folding bath blanket to midline. Bend the leg at the knee. Grasp the heel, elevate the leg from the bed, and cover bed with bath towel. Place washbasin on towel. Place client's foot into washbasin (Figure 33-21). Allow foot to soak while washing the leg with long, firm strokes in the direction of distal to proximal. Rinse and pat dry. Clean soles, interdigits, and toes. Rinse and pat dry. Perform same procedure with the other leg and foot.

13. Supports joints to prevent strain and fatigue. Soaking foot loosens dirt, softens nails, and promotes comfort.

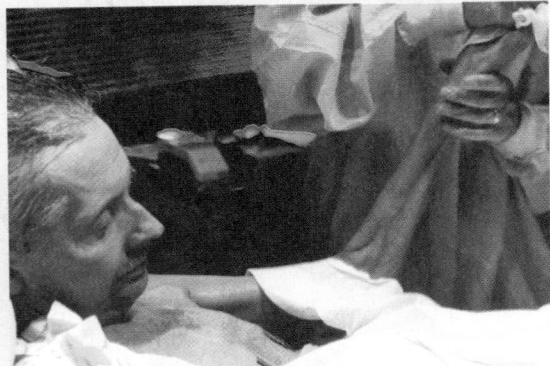

**Figure 33-20   Wash from distal to proximal—from hands to forearms to upper arms.**

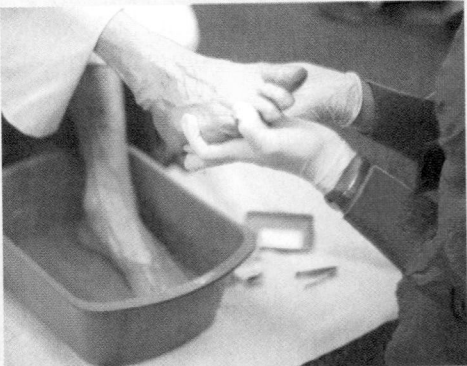

**Figure 33-21    Place feet in basin. Clean interdigits and soles of feet.**

14. Wash back. Assist client into prone or side-lying position facing away from you. Wash the back and buttocks using long, firm strokes. Rinse and pat dry. Give back rub and apply lotion.

14. Exposes back and buttocks for washing. Back rub promotes relaxation and circulation.

*(continues)*

**PROCEDURE 33-2** (*continued*)

15. Perineal care: Assist client to supine position. Perform perineal care (Figures 33-22 and 33-23).

15. Removes genital secretions and soil.

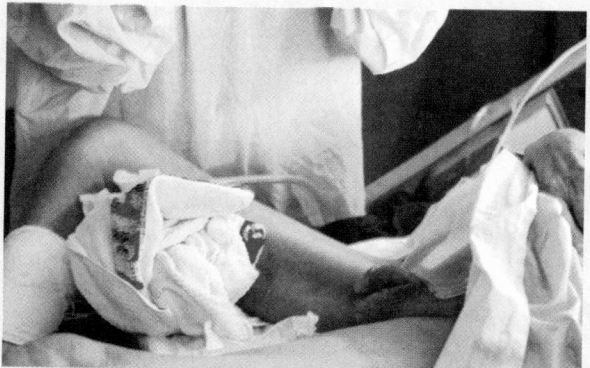

**Figure 33-22    Wash perineal area.**

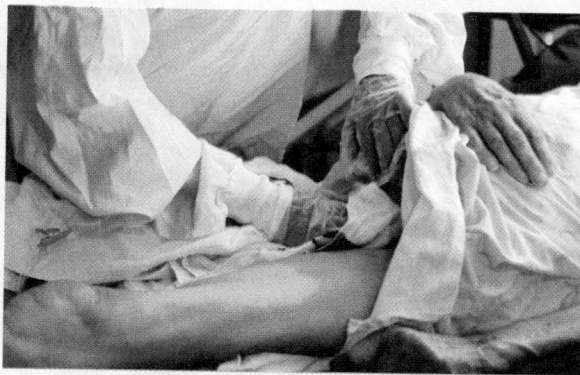

**Figure 33-23    Dry perineal area carefully to prevent moisture from contributing to skin irritation or skin breakdown.**

16. Apply lotion and powder as desired. Apply clean gown.

16. Lotion lubricates skin. Powder absorbs excess perspiration.

17. Document skin assessment, type of bath given, and client outcomes and responses.

17. Provides evidence of nursing care.

18. Wash hands.

18. Reduces the transmission of microorganisms.

## COMMUNITY/HOME CARE

### Bathing in the Home Care Setting

*Home Care Variations*

- Take extra care not to spill bathwater or soak the mattress in the home care setting. It may not be protected with a waterproof cover like those in the hospital. Bring along protective linens to protect the bed against accidental spills.

- In the more relaxed home care setting, the bath can be a perfect opportunity to do range-of-motion and gentle stretching exercises.

*Long-Term Care Variation*

- Focus on independence and autonomy in the bathing process as much as possible to help clients avoid developing unnecessary dependence on caretakers. A feeling of being overly dependent on others for basic care can lead to lowered self-esteem and possibly depression.

## LIFE SPAN CONSIDERATIONS

### Safety Considerations During Bathing

**Pediatric Variations**

- Children are easily embarrassed about strangers seeing and touching their bodies. Be sure to explain everything you are doing and why. Be sure to preserve the child's modesty as much as possible.

- With the heightened awareness regarding inappropriate touching, be aware of how you touch children while caring for them. If possible, have an appropriate family member present when you bathe a child.

- Make bath time play therapy if possible. A smaller child may enjoy playing with the slippery soap or hearing a nursery rhyme or song that changes with each part of the bath.

- Adolescents may be especially concerned over body image. The focus on the body during the bath draws attention to changes in body image due to illness or surgery. Be sensitive and practice active listening to help adolescents communicate their concerns.

**Geriatric Variations**

- Older clients often have very thin skin. Handle the skin carefully to avoid tearing or shearing the delicate tissue.

- The bath is an excellent opportunity to scan the skin for possible skin cancers. Review photos of the basic appearance of skin cancers in a dermatology test or website so they are recognizable to you.

- Make sure to check for hearing aids, and remove them prior to bathing the head and neck area. Water can damage many hearing aids.

- Be sure to replace necessary items such as eyeglasses, call light, bedside lighting, and hearing aids after the bath to help the older client remain independent.

## Provide Clean Bed Linen

After a bath, clean linens are placed on the bed to promote comfort. If the client is able to get out of the bed, assist the client to a chair and proceed with making the bed. Procedure 33-3 describes the steps involved with making an unoccupied bed. After surgery, the client should be returned to a clean bed with the linens folded to the foot of the bed to promote easy client transfer.

If the client is unable to get out of the bed, refer to Procedure 33-4 for a description of the steps involved in making an occupied bed. Assistance will be needed if the client is in traction or cannot be turned. Care must be taken to avoid disturbing the traction weights. If the client cannot be turned, change the linen from head to toe. Place a waterproof draw sheet on the beds of clients who are incontinent or have profuse drainage.

## Provide Skin Care

The skin functions as a protective barrier between the internal and external environments. In addition, the skin functions to regulate body temperature, secrete sebum, excrete sweat, transmit sensations, and facilitate absorption of vitamin D.

Skin care provides cleansing and conditioning to promote the optimal functioning of the skin. It consists of providing adequate nutrition, baths, perineal care, and back rubs. Excessive or abrasive skin care can damage skin and result in loss of function. Performing skin care provides an excellent opportunity for the nurse to assess skin integrity.

## Provide Perineal Care

**Perineal care** is cleansing of the external genitalia, perineum, and surrounding area. Perineal care is also referred to as "peri-care" or "perineal-genital" care. The purposes of perineal care are to prevent or eliminate infection and odor, promote healing, remove secretions, and provide comfort. Perineal care can be provided alone or as part of the bed bath.

Perineal care may be an embarrassing procedure for both the client and the nurse, especially if the client is of the opposite sex. Clients who are embarrassed may elect to perform their own perineal care. In this situation, the nurse should provide the client with warm water, moistened washcloth, soap, a dry towel, and privacy. If the client is unable to perform perineal care, the nurse is responsible for providing this care in a professional and private manner (see Procedure 33-5).

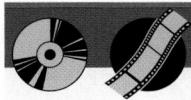

## PROCEDURE 33-3    Changing Linens in an Unoccupied Bed

### EQUIPMENT NEEDED

■ Bottom sheet (fitted, if available) (Figure 33-24)
■ Draw sheet (regular top sheet may be used)
■ Mattress pad
■ Linen bag hamper outside the room
■ Top sheet
■ Pillowcase (each pillow on the bed)
■ Antiseptic solution, washcloth, and towel
■ Nonsterile gloves

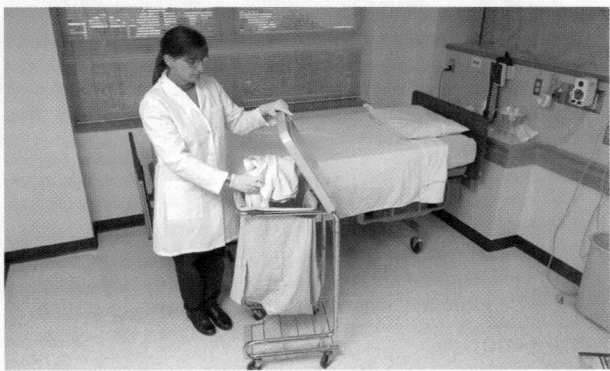

**Figure 33-24    Clean linens and a laundry hamper for used linens are brought to the bedside to make the unoccupied bed. Gloves help reduce the transmission of microorganisms.**

## IMPLEMENTATION—ACTION/RATIONALE

| ACTION | RATIONALE |
|---|---|
| 1. Place hamper by client's door if linen bags are not available. Explain procedure to client. Assess condition of blanket and/or bedspread. | 1. Provides for proper disposal of soiled linens. Encourages client cooperation. Allows for organization of supplies. |
| 2. Gather linens and gloves. Place linens on a clean, dry surface in reverse order of usage at the client's bedside (pillowcases, top sheet, draw sheet, bottom sheet). | 2. Provides easy access to items. |
| 3. Apply gloves. | 3. Reduces risk of infection from soiled, contaminated linens. |
| 4. Inquire about the client's toileting needs and attend as necessary. | 4. Provides for client comfort and prevents interruptions during bed making. |
| 5. Assist client to a safe, comfortable chair. | 5. Increases client's comfort and decreases risk of falls. |
| 6. Position bed: flat, side rails down, adjust height to waist level. | 6. Promotes good body mechanics and decreases back strain. |
| 7. Remove and fold blanket and/or bedspread. If clean and reusable, place on clean work area. | 7. Keeps reusable bed linens clean. |
| 8. Remove soiled pillowcases by grasping the closed end with one hand and slipping the pillow out with the other. Place the soiled cases on top of the soiled sheet, and place the pillows on clean work area. | 8. Allows easy removal of the pillowcases without contamination of uniform by soiled linens and keeps pillows clean. |

*(continues)*

9. Remove soiled linens: Start on the side of the bed closest to you; free the bottom sheet and mattress pad by lifting the mattress and rolling soiled linens to the middle of the bed. Go to the other side of the bed, repeat action.

9. Prevents tearing and fanning of linens. Linens are folded from cleanest area to most soiled to prevent contamination.

10. Fold soiled linens: head of bed to middle, foot of bed to middle. Place in linen bag or hamper, keeping soiled linens away from uniform.

10. Fanning linens increases the number of microorganisms in the air. Folding linens reduces the risk of transmission of infection to others.

11. Check mattress. If the mattress is soiled, clean it with an antiseptic solution and dry it thoroughly.

11. Reduces the transmission of microorganisms.

12. Remove gloves, wash hands, and apply a second pair of clean gloves.

12. Reduces the transmission of microorganisms to clean linens.

13. Open the clean mattress pad lengthwise onto the bed with the seamed side of the sheet toward the mattress. Unfold half of the pad's width to the center crease and smooth the pad flat. If there are elastic bands to hold the pad in place, slide them under the corners of the mattress.

13. Facilitates making bed in an organized, time-saving manner by not having to go from one side of the bed to the other.

14. Proceed with placing the bottom sheet onto the mattress. Linens differ from facility to facility. Bottom sheets may be fitted or they may be flat. Proceed to the appropriate Action for the linen available.

14. Use linen available at the facility.

**Fitted Bottom Sheet**

15. Position yourself diagonally toward the head of the bed.

15. Ensures good body mechanics and efficient procedure.

16. Start at the head with seamed side of the fitted sheet toward the mattress.

16. Placement of seamed side toward mattress prevents irritation to the client's skin.

17. Lift the mattress corner with your hand closest to the bed; with your other hand, pull and tuck the fitted sheet over the mattress corner; secure at the head of the bed.

17. Prevents straining of back muscles; decreases the chance that the sheet will pull out from under the mattress.

18. Pull and tuck the fitted sheet over the mattress corners at the foot of the bed.

18. Prevents straining of back muscles; decreases the chance that the sheet will pull out from under the mattress.

**Flat Regular Sheet**

19. Unfold the bottom sheet with the seamed side toward the mattress. Align the bottom edge of the sheet with the edge of the mattress at the foot of the bed.

19. Placement of the seamed side toward the mattress prevents irritation to the client's skin. Ensure proper placement of the sheet so that it can be tightly secured at the top and on both sides of the bed.

20. Allow the sheet to hang 10 inches (25 cm) over the mattress on the side and at the top of the bed.

20. Proper placement of linens ensures adequate sheeting for all sides of the bed.

*(continues)*

## PROCEDURE 33-3 (*continued*)

21. Position yourself diagonally toward the head of the bed. Lift the top of the mattress corner with the hand closest to the bed and smoothly tuck the sheet under the mattress.

22. Miter the corner at the head of the bed using the following technique.

23. Face the side of bed and lift and lay the top edge of the sheet onto the bed to form a triangular fold.

24. With your palms down, tuck the lower edge of sheet (hanging free at the side of the mattress) under the mattress.

25. Grasp the triangular fold and bring it down over the side of the mattress. Allow the sheet to hang free at the side of the mattress.

26. Place the draw sheet on the bottom sheet and unfold it to the middle crease.

27. Face the side of the bed, palms of hands down. Tuck both the bottom and draw sheets under the mattress. Ensure that the bottom sheet is tucked smoothly under the mattress all the way to the foot of the bed.

28. Go to the other side of the bed, unfold the bottom sheet, and repeat the actions used to apply the mattress pad and bottom sheet.

29. Unfold the draw sheet, if used, and grasp the free-hanging sides of both the bottom and draw sheets (Figure 33-25). Pull toward you, keeping your back straight, and with a firm grasp (sheets taut) tuck both sheets under the mattress. Use your arms and open palms to extend the linen under the mattress. Place the protective pad on the bottom sheet.

21. Prevents straining of back muscles; decreases the chance that the sheet will pull out from under the mattress.

22. Secures sheet tightly to the mattress, with the triangular fold providing a smooth tuck to keep the linen in place.

23. Forms the base for the tuck.

24. Forms the first half of the tuck.

25. Will form the final portion of the mitered corner when tucked in.

26. Provides a sheet to lift and move the client in bed without having to use the bottom sheet and remake the bed. Helps to keep the bottom sheet clean.

27. Keeps sheet taut, in place, and wrinkle-free, decreasing the risk of skin irritation.

28. Unfolding decreases air current; air currents can spread microorganisms.

29. Uses your body's weight in pulling the sheet taut and prevents strain on your back muscles.

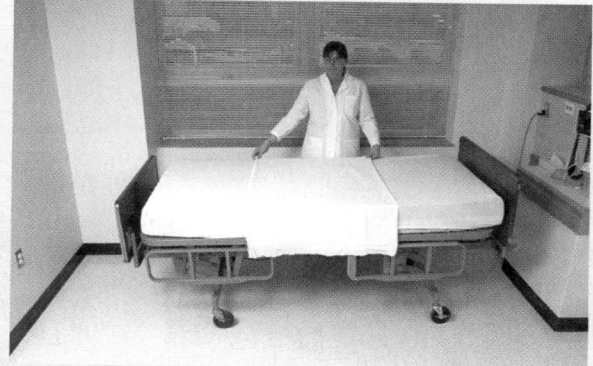

**Figure 33-25** The clean draw sheet is placed on top of the bottom sheet.

(continues)

30. Place the top sheet on the bed and unfold lengthwise, placing the center crease (width) of the sheet in the middle of the bed. Place the top edge of the sheet (seam up) even with the top of the mattress at the head of the bed. Pull the remaining length toward the bottom of the bed.

31. Unfold and apply the blanket or spread. Follow the same technique as used in applying the top sheet (Figure 33-26).

30. Saves time and movement, making one side of the bed at a time. Seam will be folded down to prevent contact with the client's skin, which can result in irritation.

31. Provides warmth.

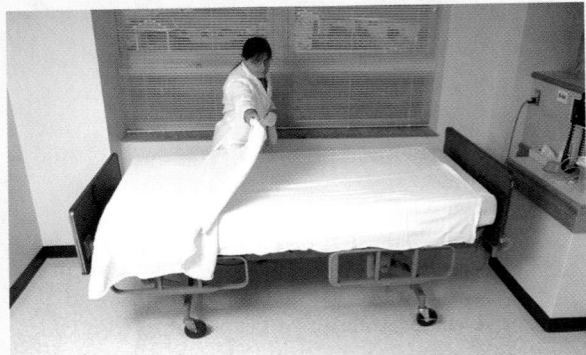

**Figure 33-26**   **Place the blanket or spread over the top sheet.**

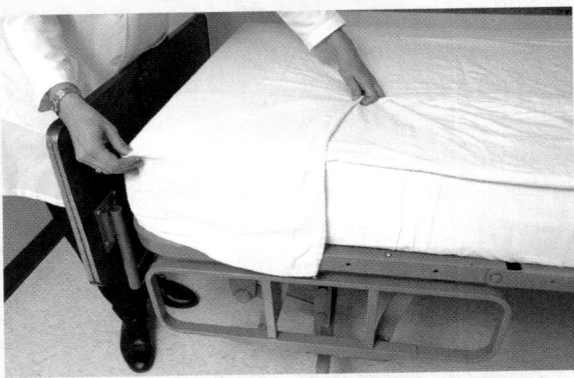

**Figure 33-27**   **Lift and lay the hem of the sheet and blanket onto the bed to form a triangular fold.**

32. Miter the bottom corners. With your palms down, tuck the lower edge of the sheet under the mattress. Grasp the triangular fold and bring it down over the side of the mattress. Allow the sheet to hang free at the side of the mattress (Figures 33-27, 33-28, and 33-29).

33. Face the head of the bed and fold the top sheet and blanket over 6 inches (15 cm). Fan-fold the sheet and blanket (from the foot to the middle of the bed) (Figure 33-30).

34. Apply clean pillowcase on each pillow (Figure 33-31). With one hand, grasp the closed end of the pillowcase. Gather case and turn it inside out over hand. With same hand, grasp the middle of one end of the pillow. With the other hand, pull the case over the length of the pillow. The corners of the pillow should fit snugly into the corners of the case.

35. Return the bed to the lowest position and elevate the head of the bed 30 to 45 degrees. Put side rails up on side, farthest from client.

32. Secures linen at the foot of the bed.

33. Allows the client easy access to the bed.

34. Keeps clean pillowcase away from your uniform.

35. Provides for client safety.

*(continues)*

## PROCEDURE 33-3 (continued)

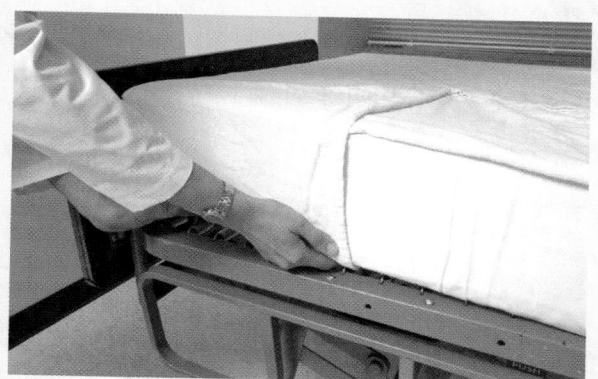

**Figure 33-28**    Tuck the lower edge of the sheet and blanket under the mattress.

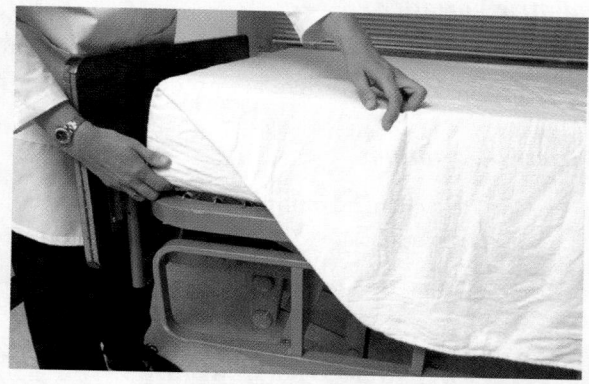

**Figure 33-29**    Bring the triangular fold down and let it hang freely at the side of the mattress.

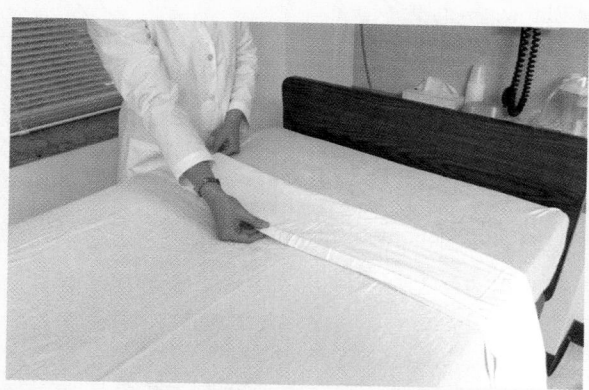

**Figure 33-30**    Fold the top sheet and blanket over 6 inches.

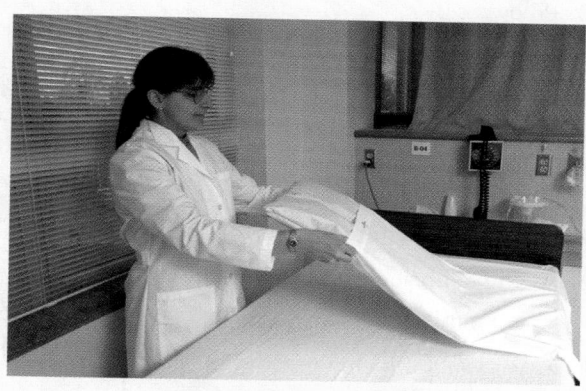

**Figure 33-31**    Place a clean pillowcase on each pillow, keeping the clean pillowcase away from your uniform.

36. Inquire about toileting needs of the client; assist as necessary.

37. Assist the client back into the bed and pull up the side rails; place call light in reach; take vital signs.

38. Remove gloves and wash hands.

39. Document your actions and the client's response during the procedure and to being up in a chair.

36. Saves client energy and provides time to care for the client's needs.

37. Promotes client safety and a means to call for assistance. Sitting up in a chair and movement may cause changes in the client's vital signs.

38. Reduces the transmission of microorganisms.

39. Documents completion of procedure and assessment findings of client's tolerance.

## LIFE SPAN CONSIDERATIONS

### Safety Considerations in Changing Linens

**Pediatric Variations**

- Be aware that children put things in their mouths, and only use linens that a child could safely chew on. Also be sure that there are no decorations or patches that a child could chew off and swallow.

**Geriatric Variations**

- Geriatric clients often have thin, easily damaged skin. Be sure to use linen that doesn't have jagged tags or rough edges.

---

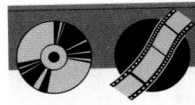 **PROCEDURE 33-4**    Changing Linens in an Occupied Bed

### EQUIPMENT NEEDED

- Linen hamper
- Pillowcase
- Bath blanket

- Top sheet, draw sheet, bottom sheet (Figure 33-32)
- Blanket

### IMPLEMENTATION—ACTION/RATIONALE

| ACTION | RATIONALE |
|---|---|
| 1. Explain procedure to client. | 1. Promotes client cooperation. |
| 2. Bring equipment to the bedside (Figure 33-33). | 2. Facilitates a smooth procedure. |

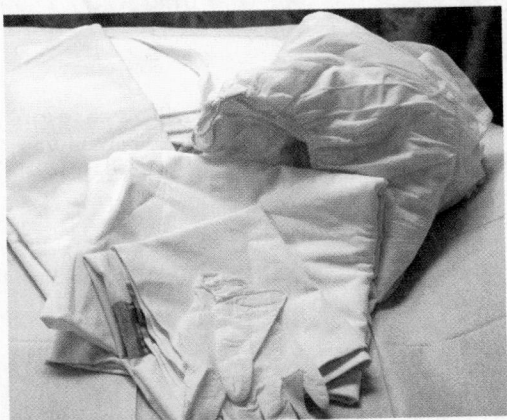

**Figure 33-32    Top and bottom sheets, draw sheet, and pillowcase are used to make the occupied bed. Gloves reduce the transmission of microorganisms.**

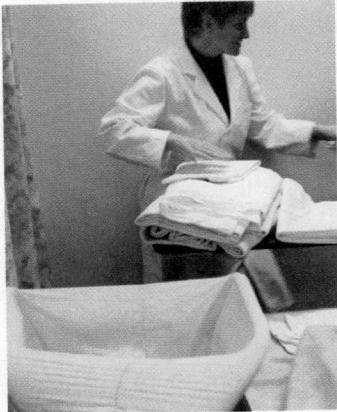

**Figure 33-33    Bring clean linen and empty linen hamper to the bedside.**

| | |
|---|---|
| 3. Remove top sheet and blanket. Loosen bottom sheet at foot and sides of bed. Lower side rail nearest to you if necessary for access. Client may be covered with a bath blanket (Figure 33-34). | 3. Facilitates easy removal of linens. Lowering only side rail close to you reduces client's risk of falls. Bath blanket prevents exposure and chills. |

*(continues)*

**PROCEDURE 33-4 (continued)**

4.  Position client on side, facing away from you. Reposition pillow under head.

5.  Fan-fold or roll bottom linens close to client toward the center of the bed.

6.  Smooth wrinkles out of mattress. Place clean bottom linens with the center fold nearest the client. Fan-fold or roll clean bottom linens nearest client and tuck under soiled linen (Figure 33-35). Maintain an adequate amount of sheet at head and foot of bed for tucking.

4.  Provides space to place clean linens.

5.  Keeps soiled linen together. Promotes comfort when client later rolls to other side.

6.  Provides for maximum fit of sheets and decreases chance of wrinkles.

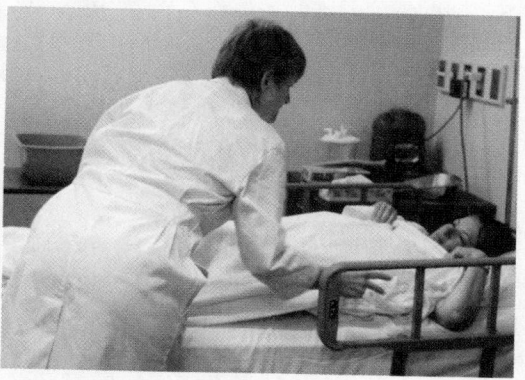

**Figure 33-34    Client may be covered with a bath blanket for warmth and modesty while top sheet and blanket are removed.**

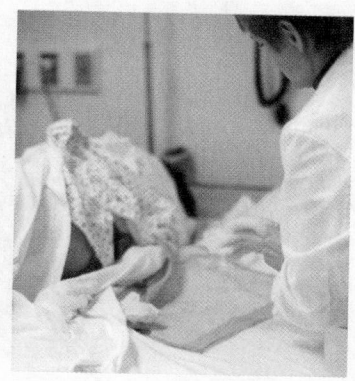

**Figure 33-35    Place clean linens and protective pad on mattress. Tuck clean linen nearest client under soiled linen. Change gloves, if soiled, before handling clean linen.**

7.  Miter bottom sheet at head of bed, then at foot of bed. To miter, lift the mattress and tuck the sheet over the edge of the mattress, lift edge of sheet that is hanging to form a triangle, and lay upper part of sheet back onto bed; tuck the lower hanging section under the mattress. Repeat for each corner. Tuck the sides of the sheet under the mattress.

8.  Fold the draw sheet in half. Identify the center of the draw sheet and place it close to the client. Fan-fold or roll draw sheet closest to client and tuck under soiled linen. Smooth linen. Add protective padding if needed. Tuck draw sheet under mattress, working from the center to the edges (Figure 33-36). Draw sheet should be positioned under the lower back and buttocks.

9.  Logroll client over onto side facing you. Raise side rail.

10. Move to other side of bed. Remove soiled linens by rolling into a bundle and place in linen hamper without touching uniform.

7.  Holds linens firmly in place.

8.  Draw sheet facilitates moving and lifting clients while in bed.

9.  Positions client off soiled linen. Protects client from falling.

10. Prevents cross-contamination.

*(continues)*

## PROCEDURE 33-4 (continued)

11. Unfold/unroll bottom sheet, then draw sheet. Look for objects left in the bed. Grasp each sheet with knuckles up and over the sheet and pull tightly while leaning back with your body weight. Client may be positioned supine.

12. Place top sheet over client with center of sheet in middle of bed. Unfold top of sheet over client. Remove bath blankets left on client to prevent exposure during bed making. Place top blanket over client, same as the top sheet (Figure 33-37).

11. Tight sheets keep linens wrinkle-free and decrease the risk of skin irritation. Leaning back uses body weight for good body mechanics.

12. Provides client with top sheet and blanket to prevent chilling.

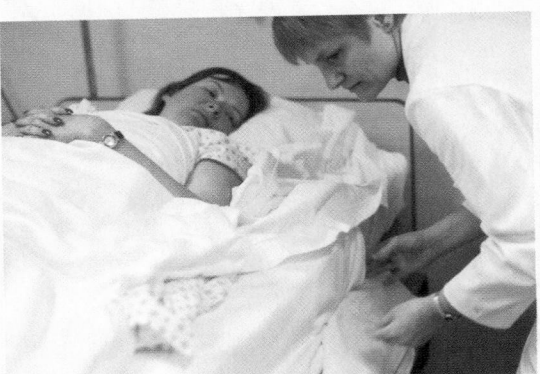

**Figure 33-36    Tuck the sides of sheet and draw sheet under the mattress.**

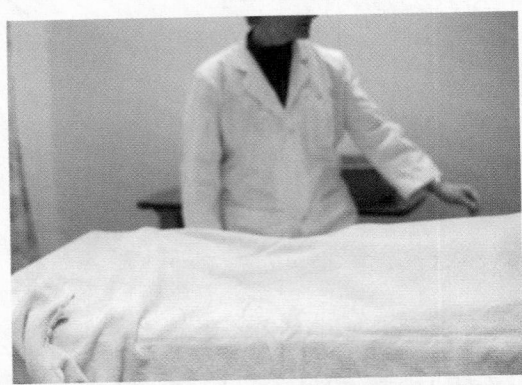

**Figure 33-37    Place the top blanket over the client.**

13. Raise foot of mattress and tuck the corner of the top sheet and blanket under. Miter the corner. Repeat with other side of mattress (Figure 33-38).

13. Secures top sheet and blanket in place.

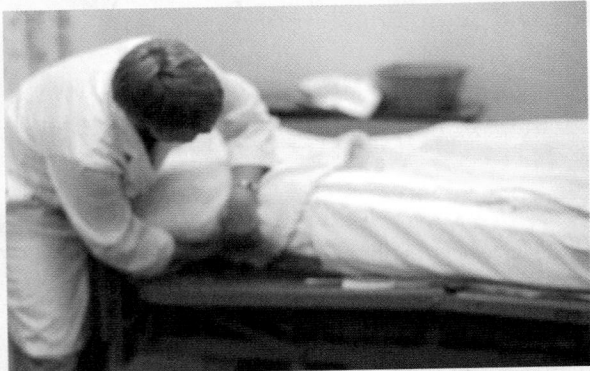

**Figure 33-38    Raise the foot of the mattress and tuck in the corner of the top sheet and blanket.**

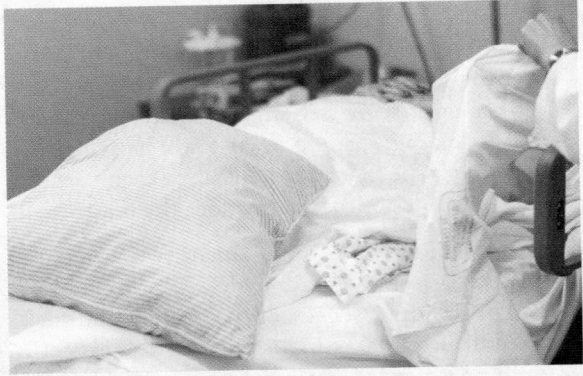

**Figure 33-39    Changing the pillowcase is the final step in making the occupied bed.**

14. Grasp top sheet and blanket over client's toes and pull upward, then make a small fan-fold in the sheet.

15. Remove soiled pillowcase. Grasp center of clean pillowcase and invert pillowcase over hand or arm. Maintain grasp of pillowcase while grasping center of pillow. Use other hand to pull pillowcase down over pillow (Figure 33-39). Place pillow under client's head. While changing pillowcase, client can

14. Permits client to move feet under the sheets. Provides room under the tight top sheet and blanket.

15. Provides clean pillowcase without shaking pillow or pillowcase. Promotes comfort.

*(continues)*

## PROCEDURE 33-4 (*continued*)

be instructed to rest head on bed, or place a blanket under client's head.

| | |
|---|---|
| 16. Document procedure used to change linens and client's condition during the procedure. | 16. Provides documentation of nursing care and assessment of client's status. |
| 17. Wash hands. | 17. Reduces the transmission of microorganisms. |

# LIFE SPAN CONSIDERATIONS

## Safety Concerns

### Pediatric Variations

- Small children can be moved physically from one side of the bed to another to avoid pulling linens underneath them.

- Children may be most comfortable with a familiar blanket or cover brought from home for the bed. Don't forget to put it back on when you have finished changing the linen.

### Geriatric Variations

- Geriatric clients often have thin, tender skin. Be careful not to tear it while pulling linens underneath the client.

- Be aware of wrinkles in the bed linens under the client to prevent damage to thin, tender skin.

- Provide towels, tissues, or washcloths within reach of clients to help them catch spills and keep their own linen clean.

- Older clients may have a certain way they "like" the bed linen to be most comfortable, such as untucked at the bottom, top sheet at the chin or at the armpits, or with an extra blanket. Give choices and seek advice on how to make them most comfortable whenever possible.

# COMMUNITY/HOME CARE

## Safety Concerns

### Home Care Variations

- You may be called upon to teach a caregiver how to change the linens in an occupied bed.

- If a hospital bed is not in use, enlist the aid of a caregiver, neighbor, or friend to improvise side rails to use at night or when making an occupied bed. An L-shaped device of wood or PVC tubing could be anchored under the mattress for support, then come up the side of the bed for safety. Make sure rough surfaces are smoothed or padded.

### Long-Term Care Variations

- Long-term care clients often have special padding in the bed for increased comfort. Be aware whether they have a sheepskin or egg-crate mattress and adjust your bed-making technique accordingly. Wash and replace special padding regularly.

- Remember to mark a client's personal linens, blankets, sheets, or protective padding so they can be returned if lost in the laundry. A family member may take these items home to launder.

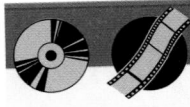

PROCEDURE 33-5    **Perineal and Genital Care**

## EQUIPMENT NEEDED

- Personal protective equipment (gloves, gown) (Figure 33-40)
- Toilet paper/washcloths
- Waterproof pads
- Cleansing solution if needed
- Perineal wash bottle (fill with plain, warm water)
- Water receptacle (bedpan or toilet if client is ambulatory)
- Dry towels
- Perineal treatment (i.e., ointment or lotions) if necessary
- Linen receptacle
- Room deodorizer

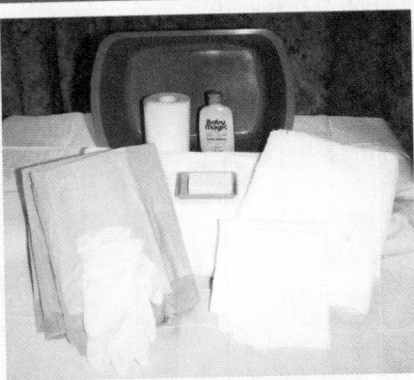

**Figure 33-40    Toilet paper, soap, lotion, towels, gloves, and a basin are all used to provide perineal care.**

## IMPLEMENTATION—ACTION/RATIONALE

| ACTION | RATIONALE |
| --- | --- |
| 1. Wash hands and wear gloves. If appropriate and if splashing is likely, wear gown and goggles. | 1. Reduces the transmission of microorganisms. |
| 2. Close privacy curtain or door. | 2. Provides privacy. |
| 3. Position client. | 3. If client is ambulatory, perineal care may be done either with client on or standing at the toilet. If perineal care is to be performed in the bed, place the client on her side or over a deep bedpan. |
| 4. Place waterproof pads under the client in the bed or under bedpan if used (Figure 33-41). | 4. Protects bed linen. |

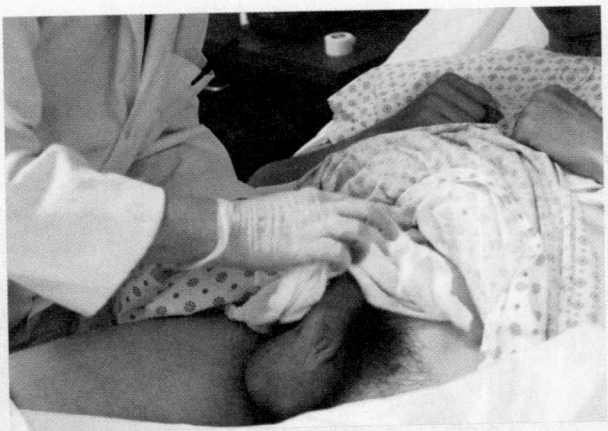

**Figure 33-41    Use waterproof pads to protect mattress and linen from getting wet.**

**Figure 33-42    Cleanse the penis with a warm, wet washcloth.**

*(continues)*

## PROCEDURE 33-5 (*continued*)

5. Remove fecal debris with disposable paper and dispose in toilet.

6. Spray perineum with washing solution if indicated. Alternatively, plain water may be used.

7. • Cleanse perineum with wet washcloths (front to back on females), changing to clean area on washcloth with each wipe.
   • Cleanse the penis on the male (Figure 33-42).

8. Carefully examine gluteal folds and scrotal folds for debris. Gently visualize vulva for debris.

9. If soap is used, spray area with clean water from the peri-bottle.

10. Change gloves.

11. Dry perineum carefully with towel.

12. If indicated, apply barrier lotion or ointment.

13. Reposition or dress client as appropriate.

14. Dispose of linens and garbage according to hospital policy.

15. Wash hands.

16. Deodorize room if appropriate.

---

5. May require several attempts. If performing at the bedside, may collect paper in disposable pad or linens until end of procedure.

6. Several perineal solutions are available, which may or may not require rinsing. Carefully evaluate this requirement. Solutions that require rinsing may cause skin breakdown if left on the skin.

7. • Maximizes cleaning; prevents spread of rectal flora to vagina.

8. Fecal material causes irritation and skin breakdown when left in contact with skin.

9. Rinses soap, which can irritate the skin, from the area.

10. Reduces the transmission of microorganisms.

11. Residual moisture provides an ideal environment for the growth of microorganisms.

12. Barrier ointments may be used if client is incontinent or skin folds tend to harbor moisture.

13. Promotes client comfort.

14. Prevents spread of disease or bacteria.

15. Reduces the transmission of microorganisms.

16. Promotes client comfort. This may also be done at the beginning of the procedure.

---

### Offer Back Rubs

Back rubs and massages stimulate the client's circulation, relax muscles, and relieve muscle tension as well as provide the nurse with an opportunity for skin assessment. Emollient creams and lotions are used to facilitate the rubbing and lubrication of the skin during a back rub or massage.

The client is positioned prone or side-lying. Nurses create friction and pressure by rubbing their hands on the client's skin. The friction creates heat, which dilates the peripheral circulation and increases the blood supply to the skin. The pressure provides manual stimulation to muscle fibers, which relaxes the muscles.

Prior to performing a back rub or massage, the nurse must assess for contraindications. Caution should be exercised when massaging limbs. Massaging limbs, especially the lower limbs, could dislodge a thrombus (blood clot), creating an embolus (circulating blood clot). Bony prominences should be massaged lightly to avoid damaging underlying tissue.

## CLINICAL ALERT

### Massage

Do not massage red, tender areas since this may increase risk of skin breakdown or dislodge a thrombus.

### Provide Foot and Nail Care

Proper foot and nail care are essential for ambulation and standing. Foot and nail care are often ignored until problems exist. Common problems with feet and nails may be

## LIFE SPAN CONSIDERATIONS

### Incontinence Issues

#### Pediatric Variations

- Encourage parents to change the child's diapers frequently to minimize skin contact with urine and feces.

- Be sensitive to cultural concerns, particularly in regard to genital care for female children. Some societies have strict cultural taboos. Some societies have deep concerns regarding inappropriate touching. A same-sex caregiver is more appropriate in this situation. If there are concerns regarding touch, it may be appropriate to have two caregivers provide peri-care or perhaps have a same-sex family member present during care.

- Be aware that the child might revert to bed-wetting because of the stress of hospitalization.

- Teach children to wipe from front to back when cleaning themselves.

#### Geriatric Variations

- Incontinence in older clients is a major influence in decisions to seek long-term care.

- Loss of ability to perform perineal self-care may be a source of embarrassment and a serious threat to ego integrity. Be sensitive to the emotional and self-image needs of the older client in need of perineal care.

- Some older clients, whether due to disease or as a way to compensate for poor self-image, may behave inappropriately during perineal care. Gently but firmly discourage the client from inappropriate touching or comments. If the behavior continues, a same-sex caregiver might be appropriate.

a direct result of abuse and neglect, such as from inadequate foot and nail hygiene, fingernail and cuticle biting, incorrect nail trimming, poorly fitted shoes, and exposure to harsh chemicals. These problems result in alterations of skin integrity with the potential for infection.

The first signs of foot and nail problems are usually pain or tenderness. These symptoms affect a client's posture and may result in limping with subsequent strain on certain muscle groups. Clients with illnesses such as diabetes mellitus need special foot and nail care. Clients with diabetes mellitus experience alterations in circulation that predispose them to foot problems.

The purposes of foot and nail care are to prevent infection and soft tissue trauma from ingrown or jagged nails and to eliminate odor. Hygienic care of feet and nails consists of regular trimming of nails; cleaning under nails; cleaning, rinsing, and drying feet and nails; and wearing properly fitted shoes. The Nursing Strategy box discusses the specific interventions that should be taken in providing foot and nail care.

Soaking nails assists with their cleaning if nails are dirty or thickened. An orangewood stick is used to clean under nails since a metal instrument can roughen the nail and cause it to harbor dirt. The safest instrument to trim nails is the nail clipper; however, some clients feel that cutting the nails makes them brittle. If the client chooses not to cut the nails, the nails should be filed straight across. Special attention should be given to drying the areas between the toes. An emollient, such as cold cream, helps to keep nails and cuticles soft.

Callused areas should never be cut. Repeated soaking usually facilitates the removal of calluses. Lotion should be applied to the foot to maintain moisture and soften callused areas. If the client's feet maintain excessive moisture (sweat), water-absorbent powder should be applied between the toes.

The client should wear clean, properly fitted shoes. The fit should not be extremely tight but should be snug

## NURSING STRATEGY

### Foot and Nail Care

- Soak feet in warm water and a detergent or in warm oil.

- Use an orangewood stick to clean the nails and release the cuticle growth from the nail.

- File or cut the nails straight across to prevent ingrown nails.

- Trim the cuticles as necessary.

- Pat all areas dry with a clean towel.

- Apply an emollient.

enough to provide support to the foot. An arch support should be in each shoe. Shoe size should be large enough so that the shoe is one-half inch longer than the longest toe. Common foot problems can often be alleviated by assessing footwear and providing proper education on footwear and foot and nail care.

### Provide Oral Care

The oral cavity functions in mastication, secretion of mucus to moisten and lubricate the digestive system, secretion of digestive enzymes, and absorption of essential nutrients. Common problems occurring in the oral cavity are:

- Bad breath (**halitosis**)
- Dental caries (**cavities**)
- Plaque
- Periodontal disease (**pyorrhea**)
- Inflammation of the gums (**gingivitis**)
- Inflammation of the oral mucosa (**stomatitis**)

Poor oral hygiene and loss of teeth may affect a client's social interaction and body image as well as nutritional intake. Daily oral care is essential to maintain the integrity of the mucous membranes, teeth, gums, and lips (see Procedure 33-6). Through preventive measures, the oral cavity and teeth can be preserved. Preventive oral care consists of fluoride rinsing, flossing, and brushing.

### Fluoride

Researchers have determined that fluoride can prevent dental caries. This finding has led to the fluoridation of water supplies in many communities. Fluoride is a common component of mouthwashes and toothpastes. However, persons with excessive dryness or irritated mucous membranes should avoid commercial mouthwashes because of the alcohol content, which causes drying of mucous membranes.

Fluoride supplements are available without a prescription. Infants can be given fluoride drops as early as 2 weeks of age to prevent dental caries. Nurses should educate clients about fluoride being an excellent preventive measure against dental caries. However, excessive fluoride usage can affect the color of tooth enamel. To prevent discoloration of the tooth enamel, fluoride should be administered with a dropper directed toward the back of the throat.

### Flossing

Flossing should be performed daily in conjunction with brushing of teeth. Flossing prevents the formation of plaque, removes plaque between the teeth, and removes food debris. Dental caries and periodontal disease can be prevented by regular flossing. Flossing is best performed after toothpaste is applied to the teeth but before brushing (see Procedure 33-6). This order permits the fluoride in the toothpaste to have direct contact with the tooth surfaces, thus preventing dental caries. Flossing can also be performed after brushing, but brushing first does not maximize the fluoride's contact with the tooth surfaces.

### Brushing

Brushing of teeth should follow flossing. Teeth should be brushed after each meal. Brushing should be performed

---

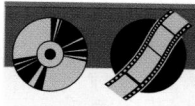 **PROCEDURE 33-6** **Oral Care**

## EQUIPMENT NEEDED

**Brushing and Flossing (Figure 33-43)**
- Toothbrush
- Toothpaste
- Emesis basin
- Towel
- Cup of water
- Nonsterile gloves
- Dental floss
- Dental-floss holder
- Mirror
- Lip moisturizer

**Denture Care (Figure 33-44)**
- Denture brush
- Denture cleaner
- Emesis basin
- Towel
- Cup of water
- Nonsterile gloves
- Tissue
- Denture cup

### Special Care Items for Clients with Impaired Physical Mobility or Who Are Unconscious (comatose)

- Soft toothbrush or toothette
- Tongue blade
- 3 × 3 gauze sponges
- Suction machine and catheter

- Prescribed solution and/or milk of magnesia
- Cotton-tip applicators
- Plastic Asepto syringe

*(continues)*

**PROCEDURE 33-6** (*continued*)

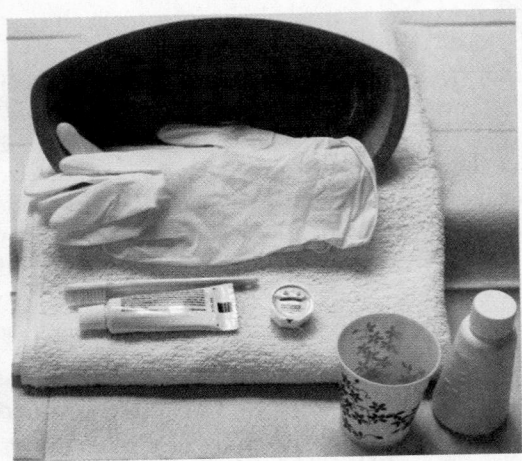

**Figure 33-43**    Toothbrush, dental floss, mouthwash, and emesis basin are all used in providing oral care.

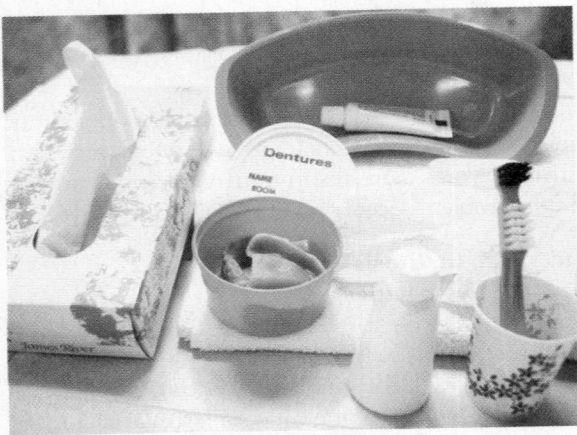

**Figure 33-44**    Denture brush and denture cup are added to oral care equipment when the client has full or partial dentures.

## IMPLEMENTATION—ACTION/RATIONALE

| ACTION | RATIONALE |
|---|---|
| **Self-Care Client: Flossing and Brushing** | |
| 1. Assemble articles for flossing and brushing. | 1. Promotes efficiency. |
| 2. Provide privacy. | 2. Relaxes the client. |
| 3. Place client in a high-Fowler's position (Figure 33-45). | 3. Decreases risk of aspiration. |
| 4. Wash hands and apply gloves. | 4. Reduces the transmission of microorganisms. |
| 5. Arrange articles within client's reach. | 5. Facilitates self-care. |
| 6. Assist client with flossing and brushing as necessary. Position mirror, emesis basin, and water with straw near the client and a towel across the chest (Figure 33-46). | 6. Flossing and brushing decrease microorganism growth in the mouth. Use of mirror permits cleaning back and sides of teeth. |

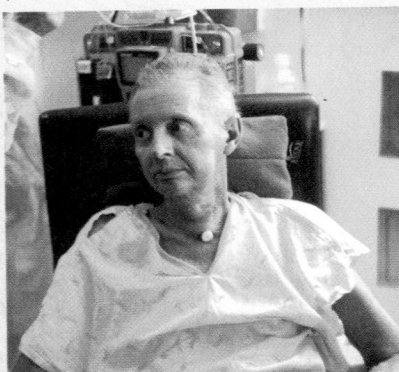

**Figure 33-45**    Place client in sitting position in a chair or in bed if possible.

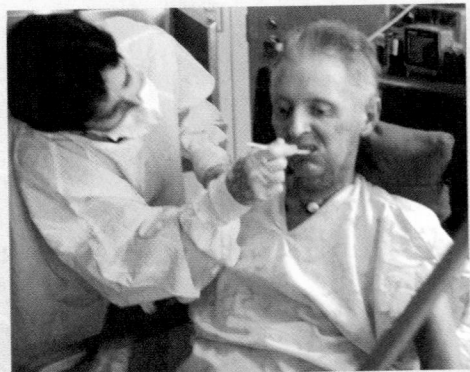

**Figure 33-46**    Promote independence, but assist with flossing or brushing as necessary.

(*continues*)

**PROCEDURE 33-6** (*continued*)

7. Assist client with rinsing mouth.

8. Reposition client, raise side rails, and place call button within reach.

9. Rinse, dry, and return articles to proper place.

10. Remove gloves, wash hands, and document care.

### Self-Care Client: Denture Care

11. Assemble articles for denture cleaning.

12. Provide privacy.

13. Assist client to a high-Fowler's position.

14. Wash hands and apply gloves.

15. Assist client with denture removal:
    a. Top denture:
       - With tissue, grasp the denture with thumb and forefinger and pull downward.
       - Place in denture cup.
    b. Bottom denture:
       - Place thumbs on the gums and release the denture. Grasp denture with thumb and forefinger and pull upward.
       - Place in denture cup.

16. Apply toothpaste to brush, and brush dentures either with cool water in the emesis basin or under running water in the sink. Pad sink with towel to protect dentures in case they are dropped.

17. Rinse thoroughly.

18. Assist client with rinsing mouth and replacing dentures.

19. Reposition client, with side rails up and call button within reach.

20. Rinse, dry, and return articles to proper place.

21. Remove gloves, wash hands, and document care.

### Full-Care Client: Brushing and Flossing

22. Assemble articles for flossing and brushing.

23. Provide privacy.

24. Wash hands and apply gloves.

---

7. Removes toothpaste and oral secretions.

8. Promotes comfort, safety, and communication.

9. Promotes a clean environment.

10. Reduces the transmission of microorganisms and documents nursing care.

11. Promotes efficiency.

12. Relaxes the client.

13. Facilitates removal of dentures.

14. Reduces the transmission of microorganisms and exposure to body fluids.

15. Breaks seal created with dentures without causing pressure and injury to oral membranes. Prevents breaking of dentures.

16. Facilitates removal of microorganisms.

17. Removes toothpaste.

18. Freshens mouth and facilitates intake of solid food.

19. Promotes comfort, safety, and communication.

20. Maintains a clean environment.

21. Reduces the transmission of microorganisms and documents nursing care.

22. Promotes efficiency.

23. Relaxes client.

24. Reduces the transmission of microorganisms and exposure to body fluids.

*(continues)*

## PROCEDURE 33-6 (*continued*)

25. Position client as condition allows: high-Fowler's; semi-Fowler's; or lateral position, head turned toward side (Figure 33-47).

25. Decreases risk of aspiration.

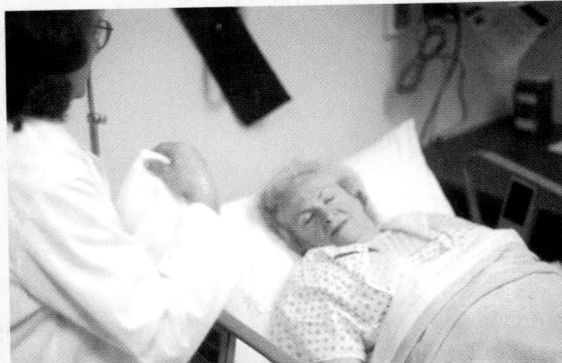

**Figure 33-47   If client is unable to sit up, turn head to the side.**

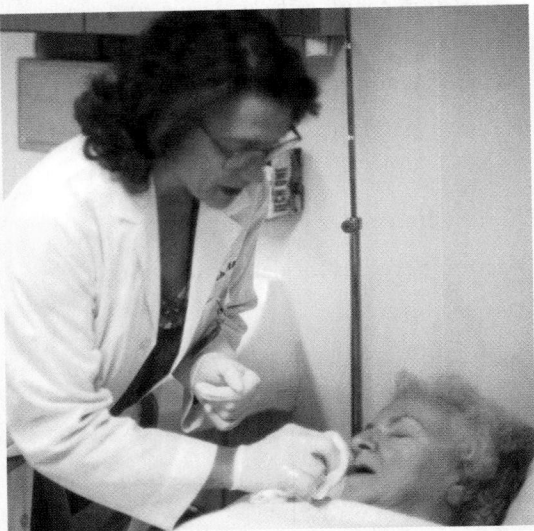

**Figure 33-48   After completing oral care, dry the lips and face gently and carefully.**

26. Place towel across client's chest or under face and mouth if head is turned to one side.

26. Catches secretions.

27. Moisten toothbrush, apply small amount of toothpaste, and brush teeth and gums.

27. Moistens mouth and facilitates plaque removal.

28. Grasp the dental floss in both hands or use a floss holder and floss between all teeth, holding floss against tooth while moving floss up and down sides of teeth.

28. Removes plaque and prevents gum disease.

29. Assist the client in rinsing mouth.

29. Removes toothpaste and oral secretions.

30. Reapply toothpaste and brush the teeth and gums using friction in a vertical or circular motion. On inner and outer surfaces of teeth, hold brush at 45-degree angle against teeth and brush from sulcus to crowns of teeth. On biting surfaces, move brush back and forth in short strokes. All surfaces of teeth should be brushed from every angle.

30. Permits cleaning of back and sides of teeth and decreases microorganism growth in mouth.

31. Assist the client in rinsing and drying mouth (Figure 33-48).

31. Removes toothpaste and oral secretions.

32. Apply lip moisturizer, if appropriate.

32. Maintains skin integrity of lips.

33. Reposition client, raise side rails, and place call button within reach.

33. Promotes comfort, safety, and communication.

34. Rinse, dry, and return articles to proper place.

34. Provides an orderly environment.

35. Remove gloves, wash hands, and document care.

35. Reduces the transmission of microorganisms and documents nursing care.

*(continues)*

**PROCEDURE 33-6** (*continued*)

**Clients at Risk for or with an Alteration of the Oral Cavity**

36. Assemble articles for flossing and brushing.

37. Provide privacy.

38. Wash hands and apply gloves.

39. Bleeding:
    a. Assess oral cavity with a padded tongue blade and flashlight for signs of bleeding.
    b. Proceed with the actions for oral care for a full-care client except:
       - Do not floss.

       - Use a soft toothbrush, toothette, or a tongue blade padded with 3 × 3 gauze sponges to gently swab teeth and gums.
       - Dispose of padded tongue blade into a biohazard bag according to institutional policy.
       - Rinse with tepid water.

40. Infection:
    a. Assess oral cavity with a tongue blade and flashlight for signs of infection.
    b. Culture lesions as ordered.
    c. Proceed with the actions for oral care for a full-care client except:
       - Do not floss.
       - Use prescribed antiseptic solution.

       - Use a tongue blade padded with 3 × 3 gauze sponges to gently swab the teeth and gums.
       - Dispose of padded tongue blade into a bio-hazard bag according to institutional policy.
       - Rinse mouth with tepid water.
       - Apply additional solution as prescribed.

41. Ulceration:
    a. Assess oral cavity with a tongue blade and flashlight for signs of ulceration.
    b. Culture lesions as ordered.
    c. Proceed with actions for oral care for a full-care client except:
       - Do not floss.
       - Use prescribed antiseptic solution.

       - Use a tongue blade padded with 3 × 3 gauze sponges to gently swab the teeth and gums.

36. Promotes efficiency.

37. Relaxes client.

38. Reduces the transmission of microorganisms and exposure to body fluids.

39.
    a. Determines whether bleeding is present, amount, and specific areas.
    b.

       - Decreases risk of bleeding and trauma to gums.
       - Decreases risk of bleeding and trauma to gums.

       - Promotes proper disposal of contaminated waste.

       - Cleanses mouth.

40.
    a. Determines appearance, integrity, and general condition.
    b. Identifies growth of specific microorganisms.
    c.

       - Prevents irritation, pain, and bleeding.
       - Antiseptic solutions decrease growth of microorganisms.

       - Promotes proper disposal of contaminated materials.
       - Cleanses mouth.
       - Provides a coating that promotes healing of the tissue.

41.
    a. Determines appearance, integrity, and general condition.
    b. Identifies growth of specific microorganisms.
    c.

       - Prevents irritation, pain, and bleeding.
       - Antiseptic solutions decrease growth of microorganisms.

*(continues)*

## PROCEDURE 33-6 (*continued*)

- Dispose of padded tongue blade into a biohazard bag according to institutional policy.
- Rinse mouth with tepid water.
- Apply additional solution as prescribed.

- Promotes proper disposal of contaminated materials.

- Cleanses mouth.
- Provides a coating that promotes healing of the tissue.

### Unconscious (Comatose) Client

42. Assemble articles for flossing and brushing.

43. Provide privacy.

44. Wash hands and apply gloves.

45. Explain the procedure to the client.

46. Place the client in a lateral position, head turned toward the side.

47. Use a floss holder and floss between all teeth.

48. Moisten toothbrush, and brush the teeth and gums using friction in a vertical or circular motion. Do not use toothpaste. On inner and outer surfaces of teeth, hold brush at 45-degree angle against teeth and brush from sulcus to crowns of teeth. On biting surfaces, move brush back and forth in short strokes. All surfaces of teeth should be brushed from every angle.

49. After flossing and brushing, rinse mouth with an Asepto syringe (do not force water into the mouth) and perform oral suction.

50. Dry the client's mouth.

51. Apply lip moisturizer.

52. Leave the client in a lateral position with head turned toward side for 30 to 60 minutes after oral hygiene care. Suction one more time. Remove the towel from under the client's mouth and face.

53. Dispose of any contaminated items in a biohazard bag, and clean, dry, and return all articles to the appropriate place.

54. Remove gloves, wash hands, and document care.

---

42. Promotes efficiency.

43. Relaxes client.

44. Reduces the transmission of microorganisms and exposure to body fluids.

45. Demonstrates respect for the client.

46. Prevents aspiration.

47. Prevents transfer of microorganisms from a client bite.

48. Permits cleaning of back and sides of teeth and decreases microorganism growth in mouth. Toothpaste may foam and cause aspiration.

49. Promotes cleansing and removal of secretions and prevents aspiration.

50. Prevents skin irritation.

51. Maintains skin integrity of lips.

52. Prevents pooling of secretions and aspiration.

53. Promotes proper disposal of contaminated materials.

54. Reduces the transmission of microorganisms and documents nursing care.

## LIFE SPAN CONSIDERATIONS

### Tooth Care

#### Pediatric Variations

- Children who don't have teeth yet should have their gums massaged and cleaned with a soft gauze.

- Be aware that children might bite. Keep your fingers out of harm's way.

- Use a pea-sized amount of toothpaste on child's toothbrush as the child often swallows toothpaste. Ingesting too much toothpaste causes excess fluoride consumption, which can affect tooth coloration.

- Braces or orthodontic appliances may require special handling. A child with appliances may need more thorough oral care to clean all surfaces of the appliance as well as the teeth. Ask the client or the client's parents about any special oral care needs the child may have and how to remove orthodontic devices, if applicable.

- Infants may benefit from fluoride drops given as a supplement.

- Children might be more comfortable using their own toothbrush or toothbrush brand. Parents can bring in these items.

#### Geriatric Variations

- Older clients often wear dentures. Wet dentures are slippery; take care not to drop them in the sink and possibly break them. Broken dentures cause undue stress, extra expenses, lack of nutrition, and possibly mouth sores from adjusting to new dentures. Fill the sink halfway with water or pad the bottom of the sink with a towel to break the fall of the dentures if dropped.

- Assess an older denture wearer's mouth carefully for ulceration or inflammation caused by poorly fitting dentures.

---

using a dentifrice (toothpaste) that contains fluoride to aid in preventing dental caries. An effective homemade dentifrice is the combination of two parts salt with one part baking soda. Brushing removes plaque and food debris and promotes blood circulation of the gums. Dentures should be brushed using the same brushing motion as that used for brushing teeth.

### Oral Care for the Unconscious Client

Oral care for the unconscious client maintains a clean oral cavity and intact mucous membranes. Special care should be exercised when performing oral care to unconscious clients to prevent client aspiration or injury to the nurse (client biting because of gag reflex). The Nursing Strategy box provides essential safety guidelines for providing oral care to unconscious clients.

### Provide Hair Care

Hair affects a client's personal appearance and body image. Hair functions to maintain the body temperature and as a receptor for the sense of touch. Assessment of hair texture, growth, and distribution provides information on a client's general health status.

## NURSING STRATEGY

### Oral Care for the Comatose Client

- Never place your fingers in the client's mouth. A bite block or padded tongue blade can be used to hold the client's mouth open. Assess for gag reflex.

- Client's head should be turned to one side with a basin placed under the mouth. Oral suctioning facilitates the removal of secretions. Only a small amount of liquids should be used.

- Flossing and brushing of teeth and tongue can be performed in the usual manner. Caution should be exercised to prevent aspiration.

## COMMUNITY/HOME CARE

### Oral Hygiene in the Home

*Home Care Variations*

- Oral care is especially important for clients who are receiving oxygen. Oxygen is drying to the mucous membranes. Teach home care clients the importance of diligent oral care.

- If clients have dentures, teach them or their caregivers to remove the upper dentures first and then the lower dentures.

- When replacing dentures in the mouth, the upper dentures should be placed first.

- When storing dentures in water, a few drops of white vinegar or mouthwash in the water can help prevent odor from clinging to the dentures.

*Long-Term Care Variations*

- Clients with nasogastric tubes or feeding tubes require diligent oral care. Their mouths are at a higher risk of dehydration, leading to cracking, bleeding, and infections.

- Don't use oral care products that contain lemon juice, which can etch the teeth, or glycerin, which actually absorbs moisture from the tissues.

- In unconscious clients, an oral cleansing solution of hydrogen peroxide and water (half and half; or one part peroxide to three parts water; or one-third water, one-third peroxide, and one-third mouthwash) may be used. If the stronger solution causes discomfort, use a weaker solution by increasing the percentage of water.

- In some facilities, milk of magnesia or buttermilk has been used in the oral care of unconscious clients. Both of these products can cause caries, so a noncarious solution, such as peroxide and water, is now preferred.

Common hair problems are dandruff, hair loss, tangled or matted hair, and infestations such as pediculosis and lice. Hair problems can be reduced by daily hair care, which helps to promote hair growth, prevent hair loss, prevent infections or infestations, promote circulation of the scalp, evenly distribute oils along hair shafts, and maintain the client's physical appearance. Hair care consists of brushing and combing, shampooing, shaving, and mustache and beard care.

### Brushing and Combing

Hair should be brushed or combed daily according to the client's preferred hairstyle. Brushing and combing stimulate circulation to the scalp, distribute oils along hair shafts, and arrange the placement of hair. A clean brush or comb should be used. Hair should be brushed from the scalp toward the hair ends. Sensitive scalps should be brushed or combed gently. Wetting the hair with water before brushing or combing can prevent damage to the hair and painful pulling of the scalp.

Clients who are immobilized may have tangled or matted hair. Care should be taken to prevent pain when combing tangled or matted hair by holding the tangled hair near the scalp while combing. If the client permits, the hair can be braided to avoid tangling or matting, but braiding the hair tightly should be avoided since tight braids may cause pain and hair loss. A nurse must receive written informed consent to cut a client's hair.

### Shampooing

When soiled, hair should be shampooed according to the client's usual routine. The purposes of shampooing are to stimulate scalp circulation, remove soil from hair, and facilitate brushing and combing. Hair can be shampooed in the tub, in the shower, at the sink, or in the bed depending on the client's abilities and preferences.

Clients confined to bed can have their hair shampooed with water or with shampoos that do not require water. Hair is shampooed by thoroughly wetting all hair, applying about a teaspoon of shampoo, lathering shampoo, and gently massaging the scalp with the pads of the fingertips. Hair should be rinsed thoroughly after shampooing. Hair should be dried with an absorbent towel, then brushed or combed in the preferred hairstyle.

## NURSING STRATEGY

### Shampooing Hair in Bed

- Remove pillow. Position client with head and shoulders near edge of bed. Cotton may be placed in the external ear canal.

- Place a linen protector or plastic head-washing tray under the head to protect the bed from becoming wet and to facilitate the draining off of water and shampoo.

- Offer the client a towel to cover eyes, if desired (Figure 33-49).

- Shampoo hair beginning at the hair line and working toward the back of the head.

- Rinse thoroughly to remove all residue from the scalp. Repeat washing and rinsing until hair squeaks when fingers move through hair.

- Squeeze excess water from hair. Wrap a towel around client's head and rub hair and scalp with towel. Remove linen protector or plastic tray and complete drying of hair.

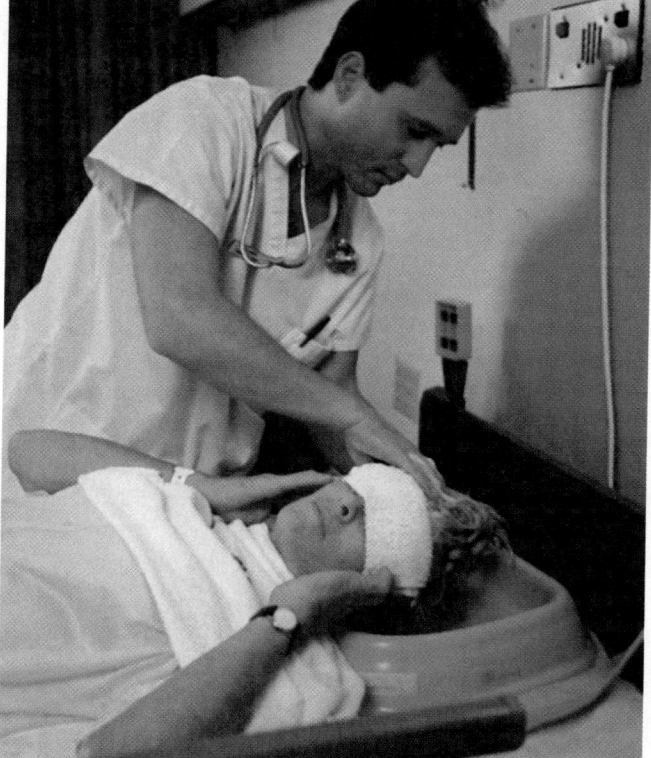

**Figure 33-49    Shampooing hair in bed**

### Shaving

Shaving is the removal of hair from the skin surface. Males often shave to remove facial hair, and women may shave to remove leg and/or axillary hair. Operative procedures may also require skin preparation that requires shaving of an area of the body.

Shaving may be performed before, during, or after the bath. Care should be used to avoid cutting the skin. Prior to shaving, the area should be washed with soap and warm water to soften the hair. A warm washcloth may be placed over the area for a few minutes to assist with softening the hair. A shaving cream or mild soap is applied to the area to ease hair removal. To shave, the skin should be pulled taut. The razor is held at a 45-degree angle and moved over the skin in short, firm strokes in the direction of hair growth. After the skin is shaved, it should be washed, rinsed, and patted dry.

### Mustache and Beard Care

Mustaches and beards require daily care. Mustache and beard care consists of keeping the hair clean, trimmed, and combed. Mustaches and beards can be washed with soap or a shampoo. Frequently, mustaches and beards require only gentle wiping with a moist washcloth. A mustache or beard should never be shaved by the nurse without written informed consent.

### Provide Eye, Ear, and Nose Care

Eye, ear, and nose care should be included in routine hygienic care.

### Eyes

Eyes are continually cleansed by the production of tears and movement of eyelids over the eyes. Eyelids should be washed daily with a warm washcloth from the inner to outer canthus. Eyelashes function to prevent foreign material from entering the eyes and conjunctival sacs. Eyelashes and eyebrows should be washed as necessary.

A client's artificial eye (prosthetic) may require daily cleaning, which requires that the eye be removed from the eye socket and washed (see Procedure 33-7). Some artificial eyes are permanently implanted.

## CLINICAL ALERT

### Shaving

Review the client's medical record and the facility's policy regarding the use of razors for shaving. Clients prone to bleeding, such as those on anticoagulants, should be instructed to use only electrical razors for shaving.

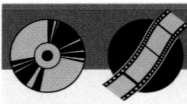

## PROCEDURE 33-7    Eye Care

### EQUIPMENT NEEDED

**Artificial Eye**

- Storage container
- Mild soap
- 3 × 3 gauze sponges
- Cotton balls
- Towel
- Emesis basins
- Eye irrigation syringe (optional)
- Running water
- Nonsterile gloves
- Biohazardous bag
- Saline solution

**Contact Lenses**

- Lens container
- Soaking solution (type used by client; Figure 33-50)
- Towel
- Suction cup (optional)
- Scotch tape (optional)
- Nonsterile gloves

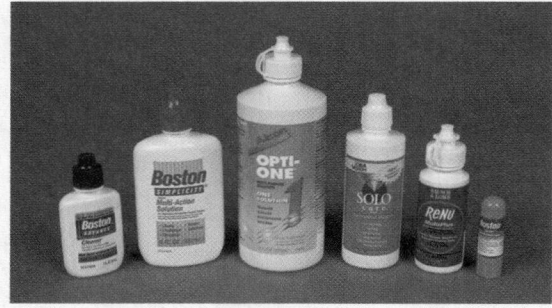

**Figure 33-50**    Commercial soaking and eye care solutions. Many types of soaking solutions are available. Select the type normally used by the client when possible.

### IMPLEMENTATION—ACTION/RATIONALE

| ACTION | RATIONALE |
|---|---|
| **Artificial Eye Removal** | |
| 1. Inquire about client's care regimen and gather equipment accordingly. | 1. Promotes continuity of care. |
| 2. Provide privacy. | 2. Relaxes the client. |
| 3. Wash hands; apply gloves. | 3. Reduces the transmission of microorganisms. |
| 4. Place client in a semi-Fowler's position. | 4. Facilitates procedure and client participation. |
| 5. Place the cotton balls in emesis basin filled halfway with warm tap water. | 5. Dry cotton balls could cause irritation. |
| 6. Place 3 × 3 gauze sponges in bottom of second emesis basin, and fill halfway with mild soap and tepid water. | 6. Gauze serves as padding to prevent breakage of the prosthesis. |
| 7. Grasp and squeeze excess water from a cotton ball. Cleanse the eyelid with the moistened cotton ball, starting at the inner canthus and moving outward toward the outer canthus. After each use, dispose of cotton ball in biohazard bag. Repeat | 7. Eliminating the excess water prevents water from running down the client's face. Cleansing the eyelid prevents contamination of the lacrimal system (inner canthus area). Disposal of cotton balls |

*(continues)*

**PROCEDURE 33-7** (*continued*)

procedure until eyelid is clean (without dried secretions).

8. Remove the artificial eye:
   a. Using dominant hand, raise the client's upper eyelid with index finger and depress the lower eyelid with thumb.
   b. Cup nondominant hand under the client's lower eyelid.
   c. Apply slight pressure with index finger between the brow and the artificial eye and remove it. Place it in an emesis basin filled with warm, soapy water.

9. Grasp a moistened cotton ball and cleanse around the edge of the eye socket. Dispose of the soiled cotton ball into biohazard bag.

10. Inspect the eye socket for any signs of irritation, drainage, or crusting.
    Note: If the client's usual care regimen or physician order requires irrigation of the socket, proceed with Action 11; otherwise, go to Action 12.

11. Eye socket irrigation:
    a. Lower the head of the bed and place the client in a supine position. Place protector pad on bed; turn head toward socket side and slightly extend neck.
    b. Fill the irrigation syringe with the prescribed amount and type of irrigating solution (warm tap water or normal saline).
    c. With nondominant hand, separate the eyelids with your forefinger and thumb, resting fingers on the brow and cheekbone.
    d. Hold the irrigating syringe in dominant hand several inches above the inner canthus; with thumb, gently apply pressure on the plunger, directing the flow of solution from the inner canthus along the conjunctival sac.
    e. Irrigate until the prescribed amount of solution has been used.
    f. Wipe the eyelids with a moistened cotton ball after irrigating. Dispose of soiled cotton ball in biohazard bag.
    g. Pat the skin dry with the towel.
    h. Return the client to a semi-Fowler's position.
    i. Remove gloves, wash hands, and apply clean gloves.

12. Rub the artificial eye between index finger and thumb in the basin of warm, soapy water.

reduces transmission of microorganisms to other health care workers.

8. Cleanses the artificial eye.
   a. Promotes removal of artificial eye.

   b. Cupping reduces dropping and possible breaking of the eye.
   c. Applying pressure will help the prosthesis to slip out.

9. Cleanses the eye socket. Disposal of cotton ball reduces transmission of microorganisms to other health care workers.

10. Indicates an infection.

11. Cleanses the eye socket and removes secretions.
    a. Positioning of client facilitates ease in performing the procedure and client comfort.

    b. Ensures compliance with client's regimen or prescribed orders.

    c. Keeps the eyelid open and the socket visible.

    d. Prevents injury to the client.

    e. Ensures compliance with client's regimen of prescribed orders.
    f. Reduces the transmission of microorganisms to prosthesis.

    g. Prevents maceration of the skin.
    h. Promotes client comfort.
    i. Reduces the transmission of microorganisms.

12. Creates cleaning with friction and prevents breakage of the prosthesis.

(continues)

## PROCEDURE 33-7 (continued)

13. Rinse the prosthesis under running water or place in the clean basin of tepid water. Do not dry the prosthesis.
    Note: Either reinsert the prosthesis (Action 14) or store in a container (Action 15).

13. Removes soap and secretions. Keeping the artificial eye wet prevents irritation from lint or other particles that might adhere to it and facilitates reinsertion.

14. Reinsert the prosthesis:
    a. With the thumb of the nondominant hand, raise and hold the upper eyelid open.
    b. With the dominant hand, grasp the artificial eye so that the indented part is facing toward the client's nose and slide it under the upper eyelid as far as possible.
    c. Depress the lower lid.
    d. Pull the lower lid forward to cover the edge of the prosthesis.

14. Allows for client comfort.
    a. Facilitates reinsertion of the prosthesis without discomfort to the client.
    b. Positions the prosthesis for insertion.

    c. Allows the prosthesis to slide into place.
    d. Holds the prosthesis in place.

15. Place the cleaned artificial eye in a labeled container with saline or tap water solution.

15. Protects the prosthesis from scratches and keeps it clean.

16. Grasp a moistened cotton ball and squeeze out excessive moisture. Wipe the eyelid from the inner to the outer canthus. Dispose of the soiled cotton ball in a biohazard bag.

16. Squeezing the cotton ball removes moisture. Cleansing the eyelid prevents contamination of lacrimal system. Disposal of cotton ball reduces the transmission of microorganisms to other health care workers.

17. Clean, dry, and replace equipment.

17. Promotes a clean environment.

18. Reposition the client, raise side rails, and place call light in reach.

18. Promotes client's comfort, safety, and communication.

19. Dispose of biohazard bag according to institutional policy.

19. Reduces the transmission of microorganisms to other health care workers.

20. Remove gloves and wash hands.

20. Same as Rationale 19.

21. Document procedure, client's response and participation, and client teaching and level of understanding.

21. Demonstrates that the procedure was done and the level of client participation and learning.

### Contact Lens Removal

22. Assemble equipment for lens removal.

22. Promotes efficiency.

23. Assess level of assistance needed, provide privacy, and explain the procedure to the client.

23. Level of assistance determines level of intervention. Privacy reduces anxiety. Explanation of procedure promotes cooperation.

24. Wash hands (Figure 33-51).

24. Reduces the transmission of microorganisms.

25. Assist the client to a semi-Fowler's position if needed.

25. Facilitates removal of lens.

*(continues)*

**PROCEDURE 33-7** (*continued*)

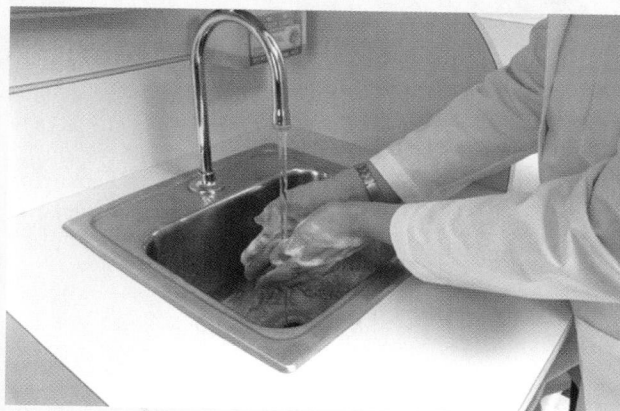

**Figure 33-51**    Wash hands prior to performing eye care. Have client wash hands if he will be performing his own eye care.

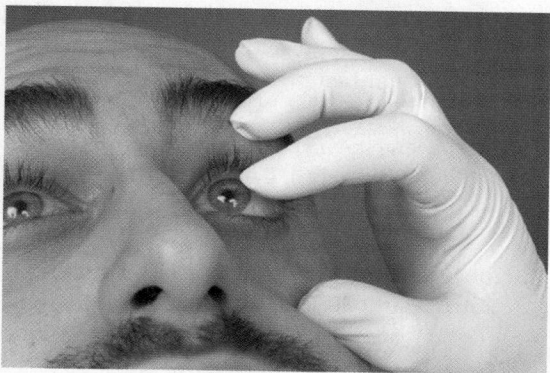

**Figure 33-52**    If the lens is not on the cornea, gently move it toward the cornea with the pad of the index finger

26.    Drape a clean towel over the client's chest.

27.    Prepare the lens storage case with the prescribed solution.

28.    Instruct the client to look straight ahead. Assess the location of the lens. If it is not on the cornea, either you or the client should gently move the lens toward the cornea with pad of index finger (Figure 33-52).

29.    Remove the lens.
    a.    Hard lens:
        • Cup nondominant hand under the eye.

        • Gently place index finger on the outside corner of the eye and pull toward the temple and ask client to blink. Catch the lens in your nondominant hand.
    b.    Soft lens:
        • With nondominant hand, separate the eyelid with your thumb and middle finger.
        • With the index finger of the dominant hand gently placed on the lower edge of the lens, slide the lens downward onto the sclera and gently squeeze the lens.
        • Release the top eyelid (continue holding the lower lid down) and remove the lens with your index finger and thumb.

26.    Provides a clean surface and facilitates the location of a lens if it falls during removal.

27.    Hard lenses can be stored dry or in a special soaking solution. Soft lenses are stored in sterile normal saline without a preservative.

28.    Client's position promotes easy removal of lens. Positioning lens on the cornea aids removal. Use of the fingerpad of the index finger prevents damage to cornea and lens.

29.    Provides for cleaning and storage of the lens.
    a.
        • Cupping the hand under eye helps to catch the lens and prevent breakage.
        • Pulling the corner of the eye tightens the eyelid against the eyeball. Pressure on the upper edge of lens causes the lens to tip forward.
    b.
        • Separating the eyelid exposes the lower edge of lens.
        • Positions lens for easy grasping with the pad of the index finger, which prevents injury to the cornea and lens. Squeezing the lens allows air to enter and release the suction.
        • Ensures control of the lens.

*(continues)*

## PROCEDURE 33-7 (*continued*)

Note: If Action 29 is unsuccessful, secure a suction cup to remove the contact lens. If you are unable to remove the lens, notify the physician or qualified practitioner.

- Suction cup is used to remove a lens from an unconscious or dependent client.

30. Store the lens in the correct compartment of the case ("right" or "left"). Label with the client's name.

30. Storage prevents damage to the lenses and ensures that each lens will be reinserted into the correct eye.

31. Remove and store the other lens by repeating Actions 29 and 30.

31. Refer to Rationales 29 and 30.

32. Assess eyes for irritation or redness.

32. Signs of corneal irritation.

33. Store the lens case in a safe place.

33. Prevents damage or loss.

34. Dispose of soiled articles and clean and return reusable articles to proper location.

34. Reduces the transmission of infection.

35. Reposition the client, raise side rails, and place call light in reach.

35. Promotes client comfort, safety, and communication.

36. Remove gloves and wash hands.

36. Reduces the transmission of infection.

37. Document procedure, client's response and assessment findings, and the storage place of the lenses.

37. Documents the removal of lenses, condition of the cornea, and where the lenses are stored.

---

## COMMUNITY/HOME CARE

### Eye Care in the Home

**Home Care Variations**

- Home care clients can become careless about the proper cleaning and storage of their contacts or prosthesis. Reinforce the proper techniques for cleaning and storage and the reasons proper technique is important.

- Bring a magnifying mirror on your home care visit to help clients do their own eye care when bedridden.

**Long-Term Care Variations**

- Long-term care clients may keep contacts or a prosthesis beyond the point of effectiveness. Examine the prosthesis or contacts to be sure they are not worn or ragged.

- Make sure eyewear prescriptions are kept up-to-date.

- Keep contacts in carefully labeled containers at the bedside to prevent damage or loss.

## LIFE SPAN CONSIDERATIONS

### Eye Care

**Pediatric Variations**

- Children grow quickly and can outgrow an ocular prosthesis. When caring for a child with an ocular prosthesis, be sure to note the fit.

- If a child needs glasses to see, make sure they are within reach. A colorful cord or cloth may be attached to the glasses to help keep them around the neck and to help locate them in the bed. Do not fasten any cord too tightly to avoid the risk of strangulation.

- Young children may not be able to tell you if they have injured or scratched their eye. Carefully examine the eye for signs of infection or injury if a discharge, redness, or irritation is present.

  To remove contacts in a child, an additional staff member or parent may be needed to help hold and support the child.

**Geriatric Variations**

- Make sure eyewear is within reach. Clients could become more confused and less able to communicate if they cannot see clearly.

- If your client is an older person with limited income or restricted social contact, verify that the client's eyeglass prescription is up-to-date.

- If the older person is wearing or caring for contacts, mark the containers clearly with a large *L* and *R* for left and right eye. This will help keep the lenses in the right place.

---

Comatose clients have special eye care needs since they lack a blink reflex. These clients require frequent instillations of lubricants or eyedrops to prevent corneal abrasions. The Nursing Strategy box describes eye care for the comatose client.

## NURSING STRATEGY

### Eye Care for the Comatose Client

- Cleanse eyelids, eyelashes, and eyebrows with warm washcloth at least every 4 hours. Clean from inner to outer canthus.

- If eyes remain open and blink reflex is absent, liquid tear solutions should be applied to prevent corneal drying and ulcerations.

- Eyes can be closed and covered with an eye patch or protective shield. The eye patch or protective shield should be removed at least every 4 hours to assess eyes and provide eye care.

**Contact Lenses**   The nursing history should indicate if the client wears contact lenses, and the routine care and level of assistance should be recorded on the client's care plan. Clients who can insert, remove, and manage the care of their lenses will require minimal assistance from the nurse. If the client is unable to assist with lens care and also has corrective eyeglasses, suggest to the client that he wear the eyeglasses during hospitalization. There are two types of contact lenses: hard and soft. Each type requires different cleaning and care (see Procedure 33-7). During emergency situations, the nurse should remove the lenses and place them in the appropriate solution.

### Ears

Hearing can be affected by foreign material or wax in the external ear canal. Cleaning of the ears involves cleaning of the external ear canal and auricles. Objects should not be inserted into the ear canal. Excess wax or foreign material should be removed by gently washing the external ear and auricles with a warm washcloth while pulling the ear downward in the adult client. Irrigation of the ear may be necessary to remove dried wax. The physician should be notified prior to irrigation of the ear.

**Hearing Aids**   Hearing aids amplify sound. The health history should indicate if the client is wearing a hearing aid and the plan of care should discuss the cleaning schedule of this aid. Clients with hearing aids should clean the ear mold regularly to ensure proper functioning. There are four types of hearing aids:

- Body-worn
- Eyeglass
- Behind the ear
- In the ear

Some hearing aids have a telephone switch that can be turned on and off.

If the hearing aid is not functioning properly, check the on-off switch and volume control, battery (replace as necessary), plastic tubing for cracks and loose connections, and telephone switch, which should be in the off position unless the client is using the phone. Hearing aids should be handled carefully since dropping or bumping the hearing aid can damage its delicate mechanisms. When not in use, the hearing aid should be stored in a container because dust and dirt can damage the mechanism.

When communicating with a client who has a hearing aid, you should address the client by name and then wait for the client to face you before speaking further. Always face the client and speak in a slow, natural voice. Shouting causes distortion of sound and usually makes the client feel uncomfortable.

### Nose

The nose provides the sense of smell, prevents entrance of foreign material into the respiratory tract, humidifies inhaled air, and facilitates breathing. Excessive or dried secretions may impair nasal function. Excessive nasal secretions are removed by inserting a cotton-tipped applicator moistened with water or saline into the nostrils. The applicator should not be inserted beyond the cotton tip. Infants may have excessive nasal secretions removed by a suction bulb. Clients with a nasogastric tube should receive meticulous skin care to the nose area to prevent skin breakdown.

## Evaluation

Evaluation is based on the achievement of goals and client-expected outcomes, regardless of the setting. Clients with alterations in health perception–health management pattern or activity-exercise pattern are at risk for injury, infection, and self-care deficits. Keeping the client free from injury and infection requires frequent reassessment,

### CLINICAL ALERT

#### Intervention

The use of restraints or other protective devices on confused clients usually increases their confusion, placing them at a greater risk for injury. Implementation of the fall protocol with frequent reassessment and visual observations, and special beds with alarms that notify the staff when the client is trying to get out of the bed are actions that support client safety. Restraints should be used only when all other nursing measures are ineffective in providing client safety.

through the use of risk appraisals, with timely adjustments made in the plan of care in order for nursing interventions to be effective.

It is imperative that the client not only be free of injury during hospitalization but also develop a true awareness of the internal and external factors that increase the risk for injury. Achievement of this outcome measure is directly related to the behaviors the client observes while in the hospital and through client teaching. Modification of a home to a safe environment is evidence for the home health nurse that learning has taken place.

Adherence to barrier precautions is critical in preventing the spread of infectious agents, especially nosocomial infections to clients, self, and other health care workers. The nurse needs to correlate the client's diagnostic laboratory results and temperature in evaluating the expected outcome of remaining free of signs and symptoms of infection. If the nurse is caring for a client with an infection, the evaluation should indicate the stage of the inflammatory process.

The therapeutic value of hygiene is maximized when the client can participate and is kept free from infection and alterations in skin integrity. Evaluation should identify the client's level of functioning in self-care activities.

At the time of discharge from the hospital, appropriate referrals should be made to home health care agencies to assist the client in achieving optimum functioning levels for safety and hygienic practices. Clients at risk for infection should have follow-up visits by the home health nurse to measure the effectiveness of client teaching and resources in the home to prevent the transmission of infections.

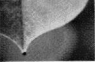 ## CASE STUDY/NURSING CARE PLAN

Mr. Corbett, age 75, is admitted to the hospital with coronary heart disease (CHD). His father died many years ago, and two brothers have died in recent years, all three from heart-related conditions. Mr. Corbett smokes two packs of cigarettes a day, suffers from diabetes mellitus, and is obese. Mr. Corbett has gained

*(continues)*

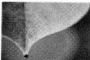

# CASE STUDY/NURSING CARE PLAN (continued)

an additional 7 pounds over the last month, has elevated blood pressure, has decreased bladder tone, and has diminished visual acuity. He is somewhat unstable when ambulating. Recently he has been slightly confused and occasionally attempts to walk by himself. The nurses are very concerned for Mr. Corbett's safety and are implementing a fall prevention protocol for his benefit.

## Assessment

Client is a 75-year-old male with CHD, who smokes two packs of cigarettes per day and has gained 7 pounds in a month. He has a cholesterol level of 320 mg/dl, high-density lipoproteins (HDL) of 28 mg/dl, and BP of 186/116. In addition, his visual acuity is decreased and he is somewhat confused, with generalized weakness. He is at risk for safety and requires close nursing supervision.

## Nursing Diagnosis

*Risk for Injury* related to sensory dysfunction and altered level of consciousness.
**NOC:** Risk Control; Safety Behavior: Personal: Safety Status: Fall Occurrence; Safety Status: Physical Injury
**NIC:**  Health Education; Behavior Modification; Patient Contracting; Self-Modification Assistance

## Expected Outcome

The client will:

1. Be protected from injury throughout the hospitalization.

## Planning/Interventions/Rationales

1. Initiate the fall prevention protocol. *Identifies and reduces risk for injury.*
2. Reassess the client's injury status every 4 hours. *Identifies changes and highlights need to modify plan of care.*
3. Place the client in a room as close as possible to the nurses' station. *Facilitates faster response time to client's needs.*
4. Place fall alert signs on the client's door and head of bed. *Alerts other health care workers to client's risk status.*
5. Put the bed alarm on. *Helps monitor client status and facilitates prompt response if client tries to get out of bed unassisted.*
6. Monitor the client and the environment every 2 hours and whenever a caregiver goes by the client's room. *Provides information on status, progress, and needs of client; encourages team approach to client care.*
7. Instruct all caregivers to respond promptly to call light. *Ensures rapid response to client's needs.*
8. Teach the client to use the call light; reinforce teaching each time before leaving the client alone. *Ensures that client has means and knowledge to call for assistance if necessary.*

## Evaluation

Fall prevention protocol implemented; client discharged on third day of hospitalization free from injury.

# Key Concepts

- Factors influencing client safety are age, lifestyle, sensory and perceptual alterations, mobility, and emotional state.
- Types of accidents that can occur in the health care setting are client behavior, therapeutic procedure, and equipment accidents.
- Assessment of a safe environment consists of performing an injury risk appraisal.
- Nurses can help clients in maintaining a safe environment by resolving or alleviating hazards related to falls, lighting, obstacles, bathroom hazards, fire, electricity, radiation, poisoning, and noise pollution.
- Nurses are in a key role to improve health care safety and health for both the client and the health care worker, by learning safe work practices and integrating them into client care routines.

- Protective measures to reduce exposures include a combination of controls. These controls include substitution, such as using nitrile instead of latex gloves; engineering controls, such as ventilation; administrative controls, such as keeping the door closed; and personal protective equipment, such as respirators.
- Hygienic care promotes cleanliness, provides for comfort and relaxation, improves self-image, and promotes healthy skin. Hygienic needs and practices are unique to each client; nurses should provide individualized care based on those needs and practices.
- The nursing process facilitates an understanding of the scope of challenges inherent in the nursing care of clients at risk for injury, infections, or a self-care deficit. The assessment data should direct the prioritization of the client's problem and the accompanying nursing diagnosis.

- A nursing diagnosis is formulated after data collection and analysis. The nurse can use the classification of nursing diagnoses by functional health patterns that relate to safety, infection, and hygienic deficits.
- The primary nursing goal is to provide safe care through the identification of actual or potential hazards and the implementation of safety measures.
- Nursing care implemented for clients with alterations in health perception–health management or activity and exercise involves continual assessment of client health risks and prioritization of risk reduction nursing interventions.
- Hygienic practices are influenced by body image, social and cultural practices, personal preference, socioeconomic status, and knowledge.
- Basic hygienic practices include bathing, skin care, perineal care, back rubs, foot and nail care, oral care, hair care, and eye, ear, and nose care.

## Review Questions and Activities

1. Write a description of a typical hospital room. From this description, describe what nursing interventions should be implemented to provide a safe client environment. Underline the interventions that also improve safety for visitors and staff.
2. Facilities have varying strategies for preventing musculoskeletal injuries among staff. Visit a local hospital or long-term care facility and inquire as to what measures are in place to prevent such injuries. Record the information. Do these strategies also improve safety for the client? How?
3. Develop a safety plan for a 65-year-old client who is confused and has severe arthritic contractures of the hands.
4. Several factors are known to affect a client's personal hygiene practices. List these factors. Describe how these factors may influence a client's personal hygiene practices.
5. A client has been admitted with symptoms of night sweats; chronic, persistent cough; and weight loss. The client reports he is always tired, and he appears very ill. The doctor did not provide specifics as far as room assignment for this client. The admitting diagnosis is pneumonia. What are your main admitting considerations for this client in order to provide optimal safety for staff and other clients?

## Multimedia Links

Altman *Basic Care DVD: Applying Restraints*
Altman *Basic Care II Video: Bed-Making*
Altman *Basic Care DVD: Bathing a Patient in Bed*

Altman *Basic Care III Video: Infection Control & Bathing*
Altman *Basic Care DVD: Warm Soaks & Sitz Baths*
Altman *Basic Care DVD: Changing Linens in an Unoccupied Bed*
Altman *Basic Care DVD: Changing Linens in an Occupied Bed*
Altman *Basic Care DVD: Perineal and Genital Care*
Altman *Basic Care DVD: Giving a Back Rub*
Altman *Basic Care DVD: Hand and Foot Care*
Altman *Basic Care DVD: Oral Care*
Altman *Basic Care DVD: Hair and Scalp Care*
Altman *Basic Care I Video: Personal Care*
Altman *Basic Care DVD: Shaving a Client*
Altman *Basic Care DVD: Eye Care*

## Web Resources

Agency for Healthcare Research and Quality (AHRQ)
    http://www.ahcpr.gov
American Association of Occupational Health Nurses,
    http://www.aaohn.org
American Industrial Hygiene Association
    http://www.aiha.org
Association of Occupational Health Professionals in Healthcare
    http://www.aohp.org
Association of Professionals in Infection Control
    http://www.apic.org
Environmental Protection Agency
    http://www.epa.gov
Occupational Safety and Health Administration
    http://www.osha.gov
Public Health Emergency Preparedness and Response: Centers for Disease Control and Prevention,
    http://www.bt.cdc.gov

## References

Ackley, B., & Ladwig, G. (2002). *Nursing diagnosis handbook* (5th ed.) St. Louis: Mosby.

Altman, G., Buchsel, P., & Coxon, V. (2000). *Delmar's fundamental & advanced nursing skills.* Clifton Park, NY: Delmar Learning.

American Nurses Association (2001). *Code of ethics.* Washington, DC: Author.

Benzon, J., et al. (1999). Nursing outcome indicator: Preventing falls for elderly people. *Outcomes Management Nursing Practice, 3*(3), 132–137.

Bower, F. L., & McCullough, C. S. (2000). Restraint use in acute care settings. *Journal of Nursing Administration, 30*(12): 592–598.

Burt, S. (1999). What you need to know about latex. *Nursing Management, 30*(8), 20–26.

Centers for Disease Control and Prevention (2002a). *Guideline for Isolation Precautions in Hospitals.* http://www.cdc.gov/ncidod/hip/isolat/isoapp_a.htm

Centers for Disease Control and Prevention, National Center for Injury Prevention and Control (2002b). *Costs of fall injuries among older adults: A fact sheet.* http://www.cdc.gov

Centers for Disease Control and Prevention (2001). Updated U.S. public health guidelines for the management of occupational exposures to HBV, HCV, and HIV and recommendations for postexposure prophylaxis. *Morbidity and Mortality Weekly Report, Recommendations and Reports, 50(*RR-11). http://www.cdc.gov

Croft, J., Hanssen, M., & Kuzma, T. (2001, September). *The zero lift challenge in health care facilities.* Paper presented at SAIF Corporation Safety Seminar, Salem, OR.

Daniels, R. (2003). *Delmar's manual of laboratory and diagnostic tests.* Clifton Park, NY: Delmar Learning.

Davis, P. L., & Madigan, E. A. (1999). Evidence-based practice and the home care nurse's bag. *Home Healthcare Nurse, 17*(5), 295–299.

Environmental Protection Agency (2002). Medical waste definition. http://www.epa.gov/epaoswer/other/medical/

Estes, M. (2002). *Health assessment & physical examination* (2nd ed.). Clifton Park, NY: Delmar Learning.

Food and Drug Administration (1995, August 23). *Safety Alert.*

Food and Drug Administration (2000). *A guide to bed safety: Bedrails in hospitals, nursing homes and home health care: The facts.* (Brochure). http://www.fda.gov/cdrh/beds/bedrail.pdf

Gershon, R., Karkashian, C., Grosch, J., Murphy, L., Escamilla-Cejudo, A., Flanagan, P., Bernacki, E., Kasting, C., & Martin, L. (2000). Hospital safety climate and its relationship with safe work practices and workplace exposure incidents. *American Journal of Infection Control, 26*(3), 211–221.

Gritter, M. (1998). The latex threat. *American Journal of Nursing, 98*(9), 26–32.

Hansen, L. (2000). The architecture of safety excellence. *Professional Safety.* http://www.asse.org/psmay0500.pdf

Heumann, M. (2001, March). *Latex glove allergy: Issues & solutions.* Paper presented at the Oregon Governor's Occupational Safety & Health Conference, Portland, OR.

Hogstel, M. (2001). *Gerontology: Nursing care of the older adult.* Clifton Park, NY: Delmar Learning.

Ignatavicius, D. (2000). Do you help staff rise to the fall-prevention challenge? *Nursing Management, 31*(1), 27–30.

Joint Commission of Accreditation of Healthcare Organizations for Restraint Use (1999). Introduction to the restraint standards in acute medical and surgical (nonpsychiatric) care. *Comprehensive accreditation manual for hospitals.* Oakbrook Terrace, IL: Author.

Joint Commission on Accreditation of Healthcare Organizations (2001). *Facts about patient safety.* http://www.jcaho.org

Kohn, L., Corrigan, J., & Donaldson, M. (Eds.) (2000). *To err is human: Building a safer health system.* Washington, DC: National Academy Press. http://www.nap.edu/catalog/9728.html

Meier, E. (2002). Ergonomic standards and implications for nursing. *Nursing economics, 19*(1), 31–32.

National Institute for Occupational Safety and Health (1997). *NIOSH alert: Preventing allergic reactions to natural rubber latex in the workplace.* (DHHS [NIOSH] Publication 97-135).

North American Nursing Diagnosis Association (2003). *Nursing diagnoses: Definitions and classification 2003–2004.* Philadelphia: Author.

Occupational Safety and Health Administration (2000). *OSHA's proposed ergonomics program standards.* http://www.osha-slc.gov/html/ subject-index.html

Occupational Safety and Health Administration (2002, July). OSHA announces national emphasis program for nursing and personal care facilities. (News release). http://www.osha-slc.gov/html/subject-index.html

Plog, B., & Quinlan, P. (2002). *Fundamentals of industrial hygiene* (5th ed.). National Safety Council.

Reiss, B., Evans, M., & Broyles, B. (2002). *Pharmacological aspects of nursing care* (6th ed.). Clifton Park, NY: Delmar Learning.

Sullivan, R. P., & Badros, K. K. (1999). Recognize risk factors to prevent patient falls. *Nursing Management, 30*(5), 37–40.

Winslow, E. H. (1998). Reducing falls in older patients. *American Journal of Nursing, 98*(10), 22.

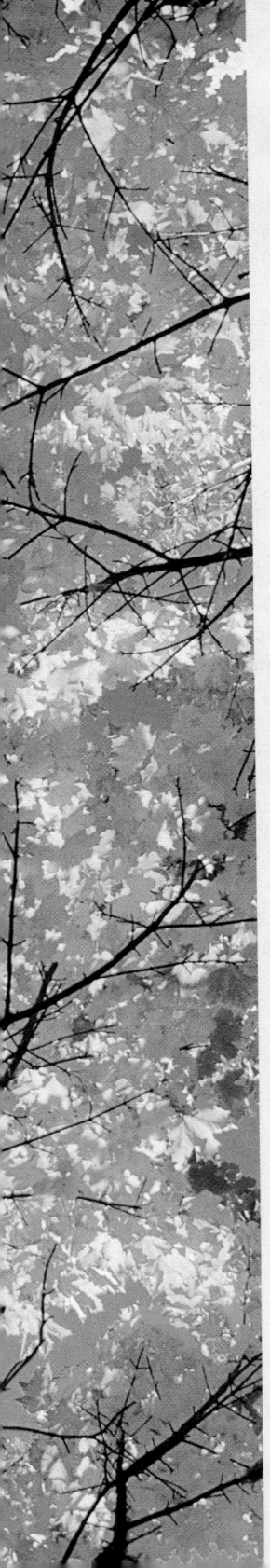

# UNIT VIII

# Nutritional-Metabolic

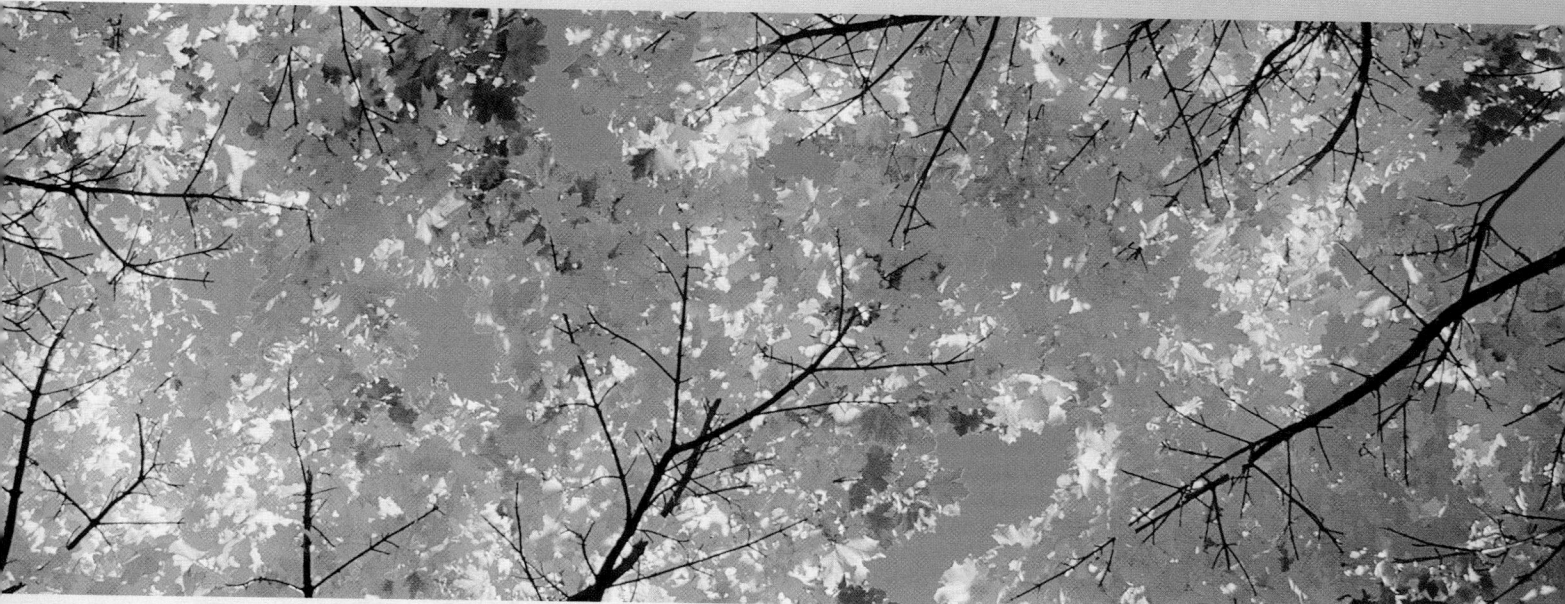

# CHAPTER 34

# Fluid, Electrolyte, and Acid-Base Balance

Milena Segatore, RN, BsN, MsN, MNI-PG, CNRN

*"The most important practical lesson that can be given to nurses is to teach them what to observe—how to observe—what are of importance."*

(Florence Nightingale [in Skretkowicz, 1992])

# Chapter Competencies

*Upon completion of this chapter, the reader should be able to:*

1. Review the physiological processes and core concepts related to body fluid and acid-base balance and imbalances.
2. Describe the clinical manifestations and nursing interventions related to common disturbances in fluid, electrolyte, and acid-base imbalances.
3. Identify the key assessment elements associated with body fluid and acid-base alterations.
4. Describe the nursing data that supports the common nursing diagnosis and goals for clients with body fluid and acid-base disturbances.
5. Describe the common nursing interventions for clients with alterations in body fluid and acid-base balance.
6. Identify the key indicators to evaluate client achievement of expected outcomes to restore and to maintain body fluid and acid-base balance.

# Key Terms

acid
acid-base balance
acid-base buffer systems
acidosis
alkalosis
angiocatheter
arterial blood gases (ABGs)
base
butterfly needles
colloid
crystalloid
cytomegalovirus (CMV)
diffusion
edema
electrochemical gradient
electrolyte
flashback
flow rate

homeostasis
hydrostatic pressure
hypercalcemia
hyperchloremia
hyperkalemia
hypermagnesemia
hypernatremia
hyperphosphatemia
hypertonic
hypervolemia
hypocalcemia
hypochloremia
hypokalemia
hypomagnesemia
hyponatremia
hypophosphatemia
hypotonic
hypoxemia

implantable port
infiltration
intracath
intravenous (IV) therapy
isotonic
osmolality
osmolarity
osmole
osmosis
osmotic pressure
permeability
phlebitis
piggybacked
semipermeable
skin turgor
solute
solvent
vesicant

The physiological functions and alterations of body fluid and acid-base balance are presented in this chapter. The term *body fluid* is used to denote both water and electrolytes, whereas the term *body water* refers to water alone. **Homeostasis** is the maintenance of a constant internal milieu in response to changes in the internal and external environments (McCance & Huether, 2002).

## Physiology of Fluid and Acid-Base Balance

The body normally maintains a balance between the amount of fluid taken in and the amount excreted.

## Fluid Compartments

The body's fluid is contained within three compartments: cells, blood vessels, and the tissue or interstitial space (space between the cells and blood vessels). To understand this concept, visualize cars on a freeway. The cars represent cells; the lanes represent the blood vessels, and the space between the cars in the lanes represents the tissue or interstitial space. The freeway itself is the body.

Just as traffic is ongoing and continuous, fluids move constantly from one compartment to another to accommodate the cell's metabolic needs (Figure 34-1). Specific terms are used to describe the location of compartmentalized body fluid, as demonstrated by Box 34-1 and the following terms:

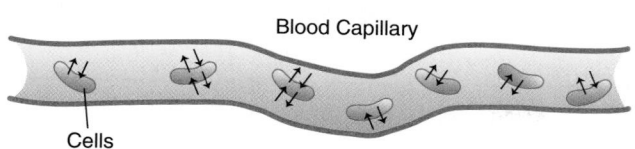

**Figure 34-1    The movement of fluid between the intracellular and extracellular compartments**

- *Intracellular fluid: within* the cell
- *Intravascular fluid: within* blood vessels
- *Interstitial fluid: between* cells; fluid that surrounds cells

There are two types of body fluid: intracellular (ICF) and extracellular (ECF). Because intravascular and interstitial fluid are outside the cells, these fluids are extracellular. Key terms used in the discussion of water and particle movement include:

- **Solute:** Substance dissolved in a solution
- **Solvent:** Liquid that contains a substance in solution
- **Permeability:** Capability of a substance, molecule, or ion to move across a membrane (covering of tissue over a surface, organ, or separating spaces)
- **Semipermeable:** Selectively permeable (All membranes in the body allow some solutes to pass through the membrane without restriction but will prevent the passage of other solutes.)

Cells have semipermeable membranes that allow fluid and solutes to pass into and out of the cell. This quality allows the cell to acquire the nutrients it needs from extracellular fluid to carry on metabolism and to eliminate metabolic waste products.

Blood vessels have semipermeable membranes that bathe and feed the cells. The intravascular fluid of arterioles carries oxygen and nutrients to the cells. The venules transport waste products from the cells' metabolic activity.

Cells and capillaries form a meshlike structure that creates a tissue space between cells and the vascular system to allow cellular access to the vascular system.

## Body Water Distribution

Water is the largest single constituent of the body, representing 45% to 75% of the body's total weight. About two-thirds of the body fluid is intracellular. The remaining one-third is extracellular, with one-fourth of this fluid being intravascular and three-fourths being interstitial

fluid. Bones are made up of nearly one-third water, while the muscles and brain cells contain 70% water. Body fat is essentially water-free; therefore, the ratio of water to body weight is greater in leaner people than in obese people (White & Duncan, 2002).

Water serves two main functions: to act as a solvent for the essential nutrients so that they can be used by the body, and to transport nutrients and oxygen from the blood to the cells and to remove waste material and other substances from the cells back to the blood so they can be excreted by the body. Water is also needed by the body to:

- Give shape and form to the cells
- Regulate body temperature
- Act as a lubricant in joints
- Cushion body organs

Water loss has a negative effect on the body's ability to function, because every 2% to 5% of water loss results in a 30% decrease in work performance (Kleiner, 1999).

## Electrolytes

An **electrolyte** is a compound that, when dissolved in water or another solvent, forms or dissociates into ions (electrically charged particles) (Figure 34-2). The electrolytes participate in cellular reactions and control mechanisms. Electrolytes have special physiological functions in the body that promote normal neuromuscular excitability, maintain body fluid osmolarity, regulate acid-base balance, and distribute body fluids between the fluid compartments.

Electrolytes produce either positively charged ions (cations) or negatively charged ions (anions). They are measured in terms of their electrical combining power. The quantity of cations and anions in solution is expressed as milliequivalents per liter (mEq/L) (White & Duncan, 2002).

The main electrolytes in body fluid are sodium ($Na^+$), potassium ($K^+$), calcium ($Ca^{2+}$), and magnesium ($Mg^{2+}$).

Table 34-1 discusses the distribution of electrolytes in body fluid, their regulatory functions, and dietary sources.

| BOX 34-1    PREFIXES | |
|---|---|
| *Inter-* | Between |
| *Intra-* | Within |
| *Extra-* | Outside |
| *Hypo-* | Under, beneath, deficient |
| *Hyper-* | Above, beyond, excessive |

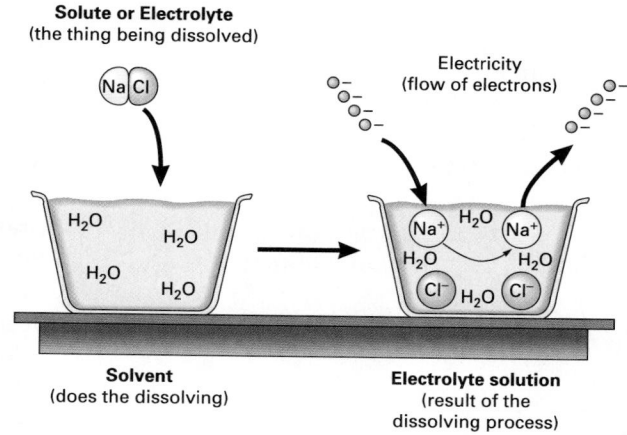

**Figure 34-2    Dissolution of electrolytes**

## TABLE 34-1 COMMON ELECTROLYTES

| Electrolyte Ion | Distribution in Body Fluid | | Basic Functions | Dietary Sources |
|---|---|---|---|---|
| | Extracellular (mEq/L) | Intracellular (mEq/L) | | |
| Sodium (Na+) | 135–154 | 15–20 | Regulates fluid volume within extracellular fluid (ECF) compartment. Regulates vascular osmotic pressure. Controls water distribution between ECF and intracellular fluid (ICF) compartments. Participates in conduction of nerve impulses. Maintains neuromuscular excitability. | Table salt (NaCl), 40% of which is sodium; cheese, milk, processed meat, poultry, shellfish, fish, eggs, and foods preserved with salt (e.g., ham and bacon) |
| Potassium (K+) | 3.5–5 | 150–155 | Regulates osmolality of ICF. Participates in transmission of nerve impulses. Promotes contraction of skeletal and smooth muscles. Promotes enzymatic action for cellular energy production by transforming carbohydrates into energy and restructuring amino acids into proteins. Regulates acid-base balance by cellular exchange of hydrogen ions. | Fruits, especially bananas, oranges, and dried fruits; vegetables, meats, and nuts |
| Calcium (Ca2+) | 4.5–5.5 | 1–2 | Provides strength and durability to bones and teeth. Establishes thickness and strength of cell membranes. Promotes transmission of nerve impulses. Maintains neuromuscular excitability. Is essential for blood coagulation. Promotes absorption and use of vitamin $B_{12}$. Activates enzyme reactions and hormone secretions. | Dairy products (milk, cheese, and yogurt), sardines, whole grains, and green leafy vegetables |
| Magnesium (Mg2+) | 4.5–5.5 | 27–29 | Activates enzyme systems, mainly those associated with vitamin B metabolism and the use of potassium, calcium, and protein. Promotes regulation of serum calcium, phosphorus, and potassium levels. Promotes neuromuscular activity. | Green leafy vegetables, whole grains, fish, and nuts |

## FOCUS ON WELLNESS

### Methods to Avoid Dehydration When Running

You can lose between 6 and 12 ounces of fluid for every 20 minutes of running. Therefore, it is important to pre-hydrate (10–15 ounces of fluid 10 to 15 minutes prior to running) and drink fluids every 20 to 30 minutes along the running route. To determine if you are hydrating properly, weigh yourself before and after running. You should have drunk 1 pint of fluid for every pound you're missing. Indicators that you are running dehydrated are a persistent elevated pulse rate after finishing your run and dark yellow urine. Keep in mind that thirst is not an adequate indicator of dehydration.

Road Runner's Club of America (2003). http://www.rrca.org

The extracellular fluid contains the largest quantities of sodium, chloride, and bicarbonate ions, but only small quantities of potassium, calcium, magnesium, phosphate, sulfate, and organic acid ions. The intracellular fluid contains only small quantities of sodium and chloride ions and almost no calcium ions. Large quantities of potassium and phosphate ions with moderate quantities of magnesium and sulfate ions are contained within intracellular fluid (see Table 34-2).

## Movement of Body Fluids

The physiological forces that affect the movement of body fluids through cell walls and capillaries can be perceived as a mass-transportation system that carries traffic between the compartments. These forces transport molecules of water, foods, gases, wastes, and ions to maintain a physiological balance between extracellular and intracellular compartments. These transport processes account for fluid shifts between the compartments (Table 34-3).

## Regulators of Fluid Balance

Numerous regulators act to maintain normal fluid balance. They include fluid and food intake, skin, lungs, gastrointestinal tract, and kidney function. When all organs are functioning normally, the body is able to maintain homeostasis.

## Fluid and Food Intake and Loss

There are three natural sources by which water enters the body: oral liquids, water in foods, and water formed by oxidation of foods (see Table 34-4). Body fluid is replenished by the ingestion of liquids and food products such as meats and vegetables, which contain 65% to 97% water. The third source of body fluid is the metabolism of foods, which yields water of oxidation. The kidneys excrete the largest quantity of fluid; other avenues for water loss are the lungs, skin, and gastrointestinal tract.

### Skin

An estimated water loss of 300–400 ml per day occurs by diffusion through the skin of an adult. Because the person is not aware of this water loss, it is called *insensible loss*. Water is also lost through the skin by perspiration; however, the total amount of water lost by perspiration can vary from 1.5–3.5 L per hour, depending on environmental factors, body temperature, and muscular exertion.

### Lungs

An estimated insensible water loss of 300–400 ml per day occurs in an adult through expired air, which is saturated with water vapor. This amount may vary with the rate and depth of respirations.

### Gastrointestinal Tract

Although a large amount of fluid—about 8,000 ml per day in the adult—is secreted into the gastrointestinal tract, almost all of this fluid is reabsorbed by the body. In adults, about 200 ml of water is lost per day in feces. Severe diarrhea can cause fluid and electrolyte deficits because the gastrointestinal fluids contain a large amount of electrolytes.

### Kidneys

The kidneys play a major role in maintaining fluid balance by excreting 1,200–1,500 ml/day in the adult. The excretion of water by healthy kidneys is proportional to the fluid ingested and the amount of waste or solutes excreted.

When an extracellular fluid volume deficit occurs, hormones play a key role in restoring the extracellular fluid volume. The release of the following hormones into circulation causes the kidneys to conserve water:

- Antidiuretic hormone (ADH) from the posterior pituitary gland acts on the distal tubules of the kidneys to reabsorb water.
- Aldosterone (produced in the adrenal cortex) causes the reabsorption of sodium from the renal tubules. The increased reabsorption of sodium causes water retention in the extracellular fluid, increasing its volume.
- Renin, which is released from the juxtaglomerular cells of the kidneys, promotes vasoconstriction and the release of aldosterone, which promotes sodium retention.

The interaction of these hormones serves as the body's compensatory mechanism to maintain homeostasis.

Sodium is the main electrolyte that promotes the retention of water. An intravascular water deficit causes the renal tubules to reabsorb more sodium into circulation.

## TABLE 34-2    DISTRIBUTION OF CHLORIDE, BICARBONATE, PHOSPHATE, AND SULFATE IN BODY FLUID

| Electrolyte | Extracellular (m/Eq/L) | Intracellular (mEq/L) |
|---|---|---|
| Chloride ($Cl^-$) | 98–106 | 1–4 |
| Bicarbonate ($HCO_3^-$) | 25–27 | 10–12 |
| Phosphate ($HPO_4^-$) | 1.7–4.6 | 100–104 |
| Sulfate ($SO_4^-$) | 1 | 2 |

Adapted from Daniels, R. (2003). Delmar's guide to laboratory and diagnostic tests. Clifton Park, NY: Delmar Learning.

Because water molecules go with the sodium ions, the intravascular water deficit is corrected by this action of the renal tubules.

## Acid-Base Balance

**Acid-base balance** refers to the homeostasis of the hydrogen ion concentration in extracellular fluid. The slightest variation in the hydrogen ion concentration causes marked alterations in the rate of cellular chemical reactions. The pH symbol is used to indicate the hydrogen ion concentration of body fluids; 7.35 to 7.45 is the normal pH range of extracellular fluid. Hydrogen ions ($H^+$) are protons and carry a positive charge. Depending on the number of hydrogen ions present, a solution can be acidic, neutral, or alkaline.

As the number of hydrogen ions increases, the fluid becomes acidic. *Acidity of a solution increases as the pH value decreases.* An **acid** is a substance that donates hydrogen ions. For example, hydrochloric acid (HCl) ionizes in water to hydrogen and chloride ions. HCl, which is found in gastric juices, has a strong tendency to form ions, discharging hydrogen ions into the solution. Carbonic and acetic acids are considered weak acids because they have a weaker tendency to dissociate.

As the number of hydrogen ions decreases, the fluid becomes alkaline. *Alkalinity of a solution increases as the pH value increases.* A **base** is a substance that accepts hydrogen ions (proton acceptor).

A neutral solution has a pH of 7. In such a solution there are equal numbers of hydrogen ions ($H^+$) and hydroxyl ions ($OH^-$), which can combine to form water ($H_2O$). When the number of hydrogen ions is increased, the solution becomes acidic (pH value below 7); a decrease in the number of hydrogen ions causes the solution to become alkaline (pH value above 7). When the number of free hydrogen ions in a solution increases to the point that the pH value becomes less than 7.35, the solution is acidic. The opposite occurs with **alkalosis**, in which a pH value higher than 7.45 reflects a low hydrogen ion concentration.

## Regulators of Acid-Base Balance

Three main control systems regulate acid-base balance, resisting **acidosis** or alkalosis: the buffer systems, respiratory systems, and renal control of hydrogen ion concentration. These systems vary in their reaction time in regulating and restoring balance to the hydrogen ion concentration of a solution.

### Buffer Systems

All body fluids contain **acid-base buffer systems**, two or more chemical compounds that prevent marked changes in hydrogen ion concentration when either an acid or a base is added to a solution. The buffer system reacts within a fraction of a second to prevent excessive changes in the hydrogen ion concentration.

*Chemical* buffer systems are activated under different conditions. The bicarbonate-carbonic acid system (carbonate system) is the body's primary buffer system. It consists of a mixture of carbonic acid ($H_2CO_3$) and sodium bicarbonate ($NaHCO_3$). The pH of the extracellular fluid can be returned to normal limits by this system because carbonic acid is a weak acid, which ionizes to a limited extent, and bicarbonate is a weak base, which yields the hydroxyl ion.

Bicarbonate helps to stabilize pH by combining reversibly with hydrogen ions. Most of the body's bicarbonate is produced in red blood cells, where the enzyme carbonic anhydrase accelerates the conversion of carbon dioxide to carbonic acid. The production of bicarbonate is illustrated in the following reversible equation:

$$CO_2 + H_2O \rightleftarrows H_2CO_3 \rightleftarrows H^+ + HCO_3^-$$

When the hydrogen ion concentration increases in the extracellular space, the reaction shifts toward the left. A decreased concentration of hydrogen ion drives the reaction to the right.

### Respiratory Regulation of Acid-Base Balance

The respiratory buffering system helps to maintain acid-base balance by controlling the amount of carbon dioxide in extracellular fluid. The *rate of metabolism* determines the formation of carbon dioxide. Carbon dioxide is continually being formed in the body by different intracellular metabolic processes. Carbon in foods is oxidized by oxygen to form carbon dioxide.

It takes the respiratory regulatory mechanism several minutes to respond to changes in carbon dioxide concentration. When carbon dioxide in extracellular fluids increases, respirations are increased in rate and depth so that more carbon dioxide is exhaled. As the respiratory system removes carbon dioxide, less carbon dioxide is in the blood to combine with water to form carbonic acid.

## TABLE 34-3    MOVEMENT OF BODY FLUID

| Physiological Force | Process | Related Factors |
|---|---|---|
| **Diffusion** | | |
| The rate of **diffusion** (continual movement of molecules in a solution or a gas) is influenced by:<br>• The size of the molecule. Smaller molecules diffuse faster than larger molecules.<br>• The concentration of the molecules. Molecules move from an area of greater concentration to an area of lesser concentration.<br>• The temperature of the solution. Higher temperatures increase the rate of diffusion. | Particles move across a permeable membrane and disperse in all directions through a solution or a gas (Figure 34-3). | The particle's electrical charge can also affect the process of diffusion because ions with opposite charges are pulled toward each other. |
| **Osmosis** | | |
| **Osmosis**, the movement of a solvent from an area of lesser concentration to an area of greater concentration, is influenced by:<br>• The net movement of water<br>• The semipermeability of the membrane | Solvent molecules ($H_2O$) move across a membrane to an area where there is a higher concentration of solute that cannot pass through the membrane (Figure 34-4). | **Osmotic pressure** is force created when two solutions of different concentrations are separated by a selectively permeable membrane. An **osmole** is the unit of measure of osmotic pressure. |
| **Active Transport** | | |
| An **electrochemical gradient** (sum of all the diffusion forces acting on the membrane, from either a concentration gradient or an electrical or pressure gradient) exists when there is active transport. | Occurs when energy is expended to move molecules or ions against an electrochemical gradient from an area of lesser concentration to an area of greater concentration. | In order for active transport to occur, there must be a carrier and adenosine triphosphate (ATP) molecules inside the cell membrane (Figure 34-5). |
| **Hydrostatic Pressure** | | |
| **Hydrostatic pressure** is the force exerted by a liquid against the sides of the container that holds it. It is governed by:<br>• Myocardial contractility<br>• The rate of blood flow<br>• The arterial blood pressure<br>• The venous blood pressure | The force of fluid exerts outward against the blood vessel wall. | The hydrostatic pressure is twice as great at the arterial end than at the venous end, causing fluid and solutes to go from the arterial end of the capillary into the interstitial space. |
| **Filtration** | | |
| **Filtration** is governed by the presence of a greater hydrostatic pressure in the arterial end capillaries than in the interstitial spaces. | The movement of fluid through a semipermeable membrane from an area with higher hydrostatic pressure to an area with lower hydrostatic pressure creates an outward gain of fluid in the interstitial space. | The body achieves total fluid balance when the excess fluid and solutes remaining in the interstitial spaces are returned to the intravascular compartment by the lymphatic system. |
| **Colloid Osmotic Pressure** | | |
| Created by solutes or **colloids** (proteins or nondiffusible substances) in the plasma | There is a movement of fluid between the intravascular and interstitial compartments, based on the number of solute particles on the concentrated side and the presence of a semipermeable membrane. | The protein content of intravascular fluid is 16 times as great as that of interstitial fluid. Thus, fluid tends to move into the capillary or intravascular compartment. |

| TABLE 34-4 | NORMAL DAILY BODY FLUID INTAKE FOR AN ADULT |
| --- | --- |
| Ingested liquids | 1,500 ml |
| Water in foods | 700 ml |
| Water from oxidation | 200 ml |
| TOTAL | 2,400 ml |

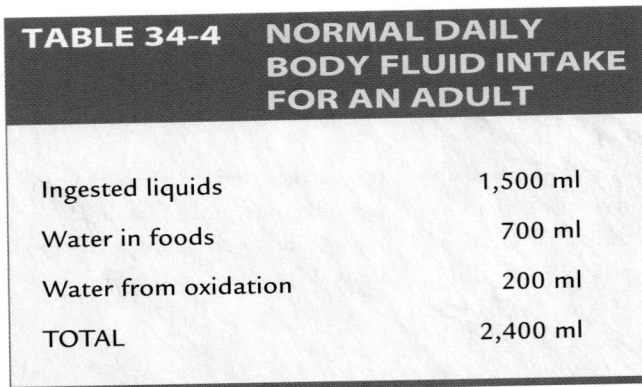

A.    B.    C.    D.

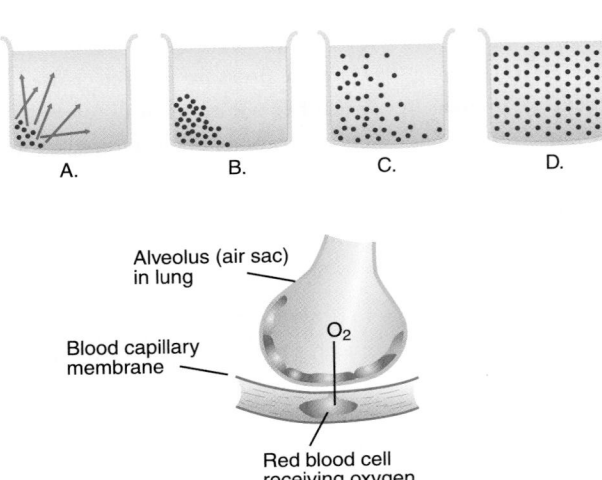

**Figure 34-3    The process of diffusion. A. A small lump of sugar is placed in a beaker of water; its molecules dissolve and begin to diffuse outward. B. and C. The sugar molecules continue to diffuse through the water from an area of greater concentration to an area of lesser concentration. D. Over a long period of time, the sugar molecules are evenly distributed throughout the water, reaching a state of equilibrium. Example of diffusion in the human body: Oxygen diffuses from an alveolus in a lung, where it is in greater concentration, across the capillary membrane and into a red blood cell, where it is in lesser concentration.**

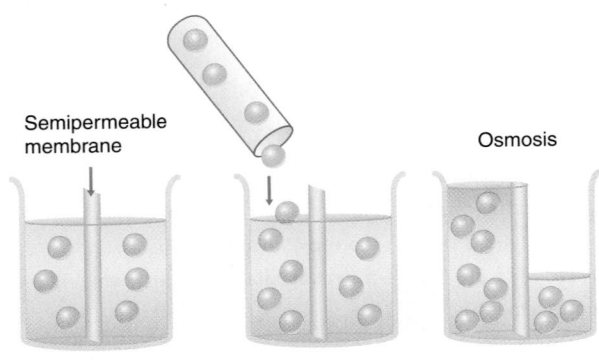

**Figure 34-4    The process of osmosis**

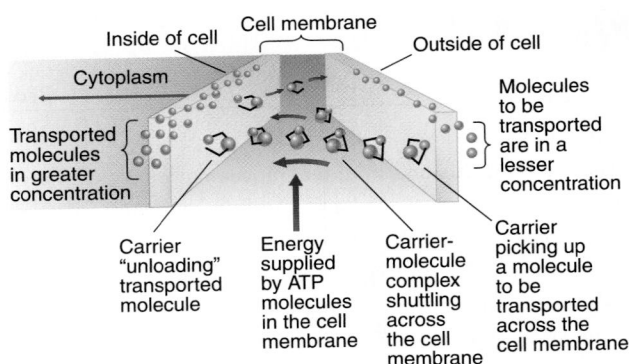

**Figure 34-5    The active transport of molecules from an area of lesser concentration to an area of greater concentration**

Likewise, if the blood level of carbon dioxide is low, respirations are depressed to maintain a normal ratio between carbonic acid and bicarbonate.

### Renal Control of Hydrogen Ion Concentration

The kidneys control extracellular fluid pH by removing hydrogen or bicarbonate ions from body fluids. If the bicarbonate concentration in the extracellular fluid is greater than normal, the kidneys excrete more bicarbonate ions, making the urine more alkaline. Conversely, if more hydrogen ions are excreted in the urine, the urine becomes more acidic. The renal mechanism for regulating acid-base balance cannot readjust the pH within seconds, as can the extracellular fluid buffer system, nor within minutes, as can the respiratory compensatory mechanism. Rather, it corrects acid-base imbalances over hours to days.

## Factors Affecting Fluid and Electrolyte Balance

The balance of fluids and electrolytes in the body also varies depending on age and lifestyle.

### Age

Body water distribution is relative to body size. The smaller the body, the larger the fluid content:

- Adult, 60% water
- Child, 60% to 77% water
- Infant, 77% water
- Embryo, 97% water

In older clients, body water diminishes because of tissue loss; the percentage of total body weight that is fluid may be reduced to 45% to 50% in persons over age 65. Caution must be used when administering diuretics to the elderly to prevent diuretic-induced electrolyte disturbances.

## Lifestyle

Loss of body fluids can result from stress, exercise, or a warm or humid environment. Stress leads to increased blood volume and decreased urine production, with a subsequent intensification of antidiuretic hormone levels. Sweating and exercise cause the body to lose water and sodium, thus necessitating electrolyte replacement and intensifying the thirst response. Warm climates can exert a similar effect. Dehydration is one of the most common and most serious fluid imbalances. One nursing goal is to ensure that all clients understand the critical role that water plays in health, and establish that clients know how to maintain adequate hydration.

An individual's diet will also determine fluid and electrolyte levels. Adequate intake of fluids, carbohydrates, potassium, calcium, sodium, fats, and protein is essential in helping the body maintain homeostatis and function properly.

## Disturbances in Electrolyte and Acid-Base Balance

The clinical management of clients experiencing disturbances in sodium, potassium, calcium, magnesium, and phosphate is presented using the functional health pattern model. Because chloride has several characteristics similar to other ions, a brief discussion of chloride imbalance is also presented. Acid-base imbalances caused by a disturbance in the level of either carbonic acid or bicarbonate are also presented. The causes, clinical manifestations, and nursing interventions for these common diagnoses are summarized in Table 34-5. Definitive corrective therapy is medical. Nursing responsibilities include protecting client safety, monitoring clinical sta-

tus and laboratory data, client and family education, and participating in the medical plan of care (Carpenito, 2002).

## Electrolyte Disturbances

In health, normal homeostatic mechanisms function to maintain electrolyte and acid-base balance. In illness, one or more of the regulating mechanisms may be affected, or the imbalance may become too great for the body to correct without treatment.

### Sodium

Sodium is the primary determinant of extracellular fluid concentration because of its high concentration and inability to cross the cell membrane easily. As discussed in Table 34-5, alterations in sodium concentration can produce profound central nervous system effects on cognition and sensory perception and on the circulating blood volume. When the kidneys reabsorb sodium ions, chloride and water are reabsorbed with the sodium to maintain the body's fluid volume.

### Hyponatremia

**Hyponatremia** is a deficit in the extracellular level of sodium. With hyponatremia, there is either a sodium deficit or a water excess. A hypo-osmolar state exists because the ratio of water to sodium is too high. Water moves out of the vascular space into the interstitial space and then into the intracellular space, causing edema. In the brain, water enters the cells and interstitial space, causing cerebral edema. This shift produces clinical changes in consciousness, cognition, and sensory function (Table 34-5).

## TABLE 34-5    THE CLINICAL MANAGEMENT OF CLIENTS EXPERIENCING COMMON ELECTROLYTE DISTURBANCES

| Disturbance/Causes | Clinical Manifestations | Nursing Interventions |
|---|---|---|
| **Hyponatremia**<br>Operational definition:<br>    Serum Na < 135 mEq/L<br>    Serum osmolality < 280 mOsm/kg<br><br>Nutrition and metabolism<br>• Low sodium intake<br>• High water intake<br>• Anorexia nervosa<br>• Loss of GI secretions (vomiting, diarrhea, bulimia, suctioning or drainage, tap-water enemas)<br>• Loss of ECF sodium (peritonitis, burns)<br>• Excessive ingestion of water or administration of IV solutions ($D_5W$)<br>• ECF sodium dilution (congestive heart failure [CHF], cirrhosis, nephrosis)<br><br>Elimination<br>• Advanced renal disorders<br>• Diuretics<br>• Syndrome of inappropriate antidiuretic hormone (SIADH) | 1. Cognitive and consciousness<br>• Headaches<br>• Apprehension<br>• Lethargy<br>• Confusion<br>• Depression<br>• Convulsion<br><br>2. Activity/mobility<br>• Muscular weakness<br><br>3. Skin and mucous membranes<br>• Dry, pale skin<br>• Dry mucous membranes<br><br>4. Oxygenation and ECG<br>• Tachycardia<br>• Hypotension/hypertension<br><br>5. Nutrition and metabolism<br>• Nausea<br>• Vomiting<br>• Diarrhea<br>• Abdominal cramps | Monitor level of consciousness.<br>Institute safety measures for seizures.<br><br><br>Administer IV isotonic solution (e.g., 0.9% NaCl) per order.<br>Restrict free water intake (e.g., 1.2 L/24 hr).<br><br>Monitor hourly vital signs and I&O (ECF excess, restrict fluids and administer diuretics).<br><br>Monitor daily intake of sodium & watch for water intoxication with SIADH (headaches and behavioral changes).<br><br>Monitor serum sodium levels.<br>Teach client about adequate intake of sodium, side effects of diuretics, and other causes for hyponatremia. |
| **Hypernatremia**<br>Operational definition:<br>    Serum Na > 145 mEq/L<br>    Serum osmolality > 295 mOsm/kg<br>    Urine Na < 40 mEq/L<br><br>Nutrition and metabolism<br>• High sodium intake<br>• Low water intake<br>• Severe GI loss (diarrhea and vomiting)<br>• Excessive insensible loss (perspiration)<br>• Salt-water drowning<br>• Administration of IV solutions (hypertonic or isotonic saline, sodium bicarbonate)<br>• Hypertonic saline abortions<br>• Bladder irrigation | 1. Cognitive and sensory<br>• Restlessness<br>• Agitation<br>• Delirium<br>• Twitching<br>• Convulsions<br>• Coma<br><br>2. Activity/mobility<br>• ↑ Muscle tone<br>• Hyperreflexia<br><br>3. Skin and mucous membranes<br>• Flushed, dry skin<br>• Red, dry tongue<br>• Sticky mucous membranes | Monitor level of consciousness.<br><br>Institute safety measures for seizures.<br><br><br>Maintain body alignment and assist with movement.<br><br><br>Administer oral hygiene hourly. |

*(continues)*

## TABLE 34-5   THE CLINICAL MANAGEMENT OF CLIENTS EXPERIENCING COMMON ELECTROLYTE DISTURBANCES (*continued*)

| Disturbance/Causes | Clinical Manifestations | Nursing Interventions |
|---|---|---|
| **Elimination**<br>• Renal dysfunction<br>• Peritoneal dialysis with glucose solution<br>• Uncompensated diabetes insipidus | 4. Oxygenation and ECG<br>• Tachycardia | Monitor vital signs. |
| **Hemostatic dysfunction**<br>• CHF ($\downarrow$ cardiac output, $\downarrow$ renal flow, $\uparrow$ sodium retention)<br>• Nephrotic syndrome and cirrhosis ($\uparrow$ aldosterone leading to $\uparrow$ sodium retention) | 5. Nutrition and metabolism<br>• Nausea<br>• Vomiting<br>• Anorexia<br><br>6. Elimination<br>• Polyuria (nephritis and uncompensated diabetes insipidus) | Administer oral fluids or a parenteral hypotonic solution (e.g., 0.3% NaCl or $D_5W$) as ordered.<br><br>Monitor I&O.<br>Monitor daily weights.<br>Monitor laboratory findings.<br>Teach client about foods high in sodium and about sodium-retaining drugs (cough medicines, cortisone, and laxatives with sodium). |
| **Hypokalemia**<br>Operational definition:<br>    Serum K < 3.5 mEq/L<br><br>**Nutrition and metabolism**<br>• Malnutrition<br>• Starvation<br>• Crash diets<br>• Alcoholism<br>• Anorexia nervosa<br>• Stress<br>• Licorice abuse<br>• GI loss (vomiting, diarrhea, gastric or intestinal suctioning, intestinal fistula)<br>• NPO and potassium-free IV fluids<br>• Diabetic ketoacidosis<br>• Hyperaldosteronism<br>• Adrenal tumor, cirrhosis, CHF | 1. Nutrition and metabolism<br>• $\downarrow$ Motility (hypoactive $\rightarrow$ absent bowel sounds)<br>• Abdominal distention<br>• Paralytic ileus<br>• Nausea<br>• Vomiting<br><br>2. Cognitive and sensory<br>• Malaise<br>• Disorientation<br>• Coma<br>• Loss of tactile discrimination | Administer potassium replacement therapy as ordered:<br>• Oral potassium should be diluted in 4–8 oz of water or juice ($\downarrow$ gastric mucosa irritation).<br>• Dilute IV potassium 20–40 mEq in 1 L of IV fluids (irritating to blood vessels and myocardium).<br>• Never administer bolus IV potassium.<br>Monitor IV site for phlebitis and infiltration. |
|  | 3. Activity/mobility<br>• Muscle weakness<br>• Hyporeflexia | Protect from injury. |
| **Elimination**<br>• Laxative abuse<br>• Bulimia<br>• Enemas<br>• Potassium-depleting diuretics (thiazide and furosemide)<br>• Diuretic phase of acute renal failure<br>• Dialysis<br>• Steroids<br>• Cushing's syndrome | 4. Elimination<br>• Constipation<br>• Polyuria<br><br>5. Oxygenation and ECG<br>• Shallow, rapid, ineffective respirations<br>• Tachycardia<br>• $\uparrow$ Sensitivity to digitalis<br>• ST depression<br>• T wave inverted | Monitor I&O hourly.<br><br>Monitor vital signs.<br>Monitor heart rate and rhythm.<br>Monitor client closely for signs of digitalis toxicity (premature atrial and ventricular beats). |

*(continues)*

## TABLE 34-5     THE CLINICAL MANAGEMENT OF CLIENTS EXPERIENCING COMMON ELECTROLYTE DISTURBANCES (continued)

| Disturbance/Causes | Clinical Manifestations | Nursing Interventions |
|---|---|---|
| **Skin and cellular integrity**<br>• Trauma<br>• Tissue injury<br>• Surgery<br><br>**Redistribution of potassium**<br>• Insulin<br>• Alkalotic state<br>• Healing phase of burns | • U wave prominent<br>• Heart block<br>• Cardiac arrest (severe hypokalemia) | Teach client about potassium-rich foods and how to prevent excessive loss (abuse of laxatives and diuretics). |
| **Hyperkalemia**<br>Operational definition:<br>  Serum K > 5.3 mEq/L<br><br>**Nutrition and metabolism**<br>• Oral potassium supplement<br>• IV potassium supplement<br><br>**Elimination**<br>• Acute and chronic renal failure<br>• Potassium-sparing diuretics<br>• Addison's disease<br><br>**Skin and cellular integrity**<br>• Massive trauma and crushing injuries<br>• Hemolysis<br>• Tourniquet application<br>• Phlebotomy<br>• Burns | 1. Nutrition and metabolism<br>• Abdominal cramps (intermittent GI pain)<br>• Nausea<br>• Diarrhea<br><br>2. Activity/mobility<br>• Muscular weakness<br>• Paresthesia<br>• Muscle cramps and pain<br><br>3. Elimination<br>• Oliguria or anuria<br><br>4. Oxygenation and ECG<br>• Bradycardia → arrest<br>• T wave tented<br>• P wave small → nonvisible<br>• QRS complex widened<br>• Life-threatening dysrhythmias (supraventricular and/or ventricular tachycardia, premature ventricular beats, and ventricular fibrillation → arrest) | Restrict oral and parenteral potassium intake as ordered.<br>Administer cation-exchange resins (Kayexalate) to reduce serum potassium.<br>Administer glucose and insulin parenteral solutions to facilitate movement of potassium into the cells as ordered.<br><br>Assess for pain and provide comfort measures as indicated.<br><br>Monitor I&O.<br><br>Monitor client closely if receiving diuretics.<br><br>Monitor vital signs and heart rhythm hourly for ECG changes.<br><br>Institute safety measures when drawing blood:<br>• Leave tourniquet on for 1 to 2 minutes.<br>• Draw blood from vein away from all infusions.<br><br>If the client is to receive whole blood, indicate on the blood bank requisition the potassium level (blood 10 days or older has an elevated serum potassium due to hemolysis of aging blood).<br>Teach client about potassium-rich foods, potassium-containing salt substitutes, and potassium-conserving diuretics. |

(continues)

## TABLE 34-5    THE CLINICAL MANAGEMENT OF CLIENTS EXPERIENCING COMMON ELECTROLYTE DISTURBANCES (continued)

| Disturbance/Causes | Clinical Manifestations | Nursing Interventions |
|---|---|---|
| **Hypocalcemia**<br>Operational definition:<br>    Serum Ca < 4.5 mEq/L (total)<br>    Elevated serum phosphorus<br>    Prolonged prothrombin time | 1. Cognitive and sensory<br>• Anxiety, irritability<br>• Tingling and numbness of fingers<br>• Tetany<br>• Convulsions | Monitor level of consciousness and breathing for laryngeal stridor. |
| Nutrition and metabolism<br>• Inadequate dietary intake of calcium-rich foods (e.g., during pregnancy and lactation, when calcium requirements are high)<br>• Poor vitamin D intake and absorption<br>• Associated disorders: hypoparathyroidism, pancreatitis, acute metabolic acidosis, and accidental surgical removal of parathyroid glands during a thyroidectomy | 2. Activity/mobility<br>• Abdominal and muscle cramps<br>• Positive Trousseau's sign—carpopedal spasm<br>• Positive Chvostek's sign—contraction of facial muscles when facial nerve is tapped<br>• Pathologic fractures | Administer 10% IV solution of calcium gluconate; observe IV solutions with calcium for infiltration.<br><br>Teach a diet high in calcium with vitamin D supplement.<br><br>Administer calcium carbonate orally. |
| Elimination<br>• Diarrhea<br>• Wound drainage<br>• Steroid therapy | 3. Oxygenation and ECG<br>• ↓ Stroke volume<br>• ECG changes:<br>ST segment lengthened and prolonged PR interval | Monitor ECG for changes. |
| **Hypercalcemia**<br>Operational definition:<br>    Serum Ca > 5.5 mEq/L (total) | 1. Cognitive and sensory<br>• Depression and lethargy | Monitor level of consciousness for safety. |
| Activity/mobility<br>• Excessive movement of calcium out of bones:<br>multiple fractures, bone tumors, immobility | 2. Activity/mobility<br>• ↓ Muscle tone and deep tendon reflexes<br>• Osteoporosis<br>• Osteomalacia<br>• Pathologic fractures<br>• Deep bone pain | Encourage client movement and exercise.<br><br>Assist client with movement to ↓ pain. |
| Nutrition and metabolism<br>• Overconsumption of milk or dietary salts<br>• Overactivity of parathyroid glands | 3. Oxygenation and ECG<br>• Heart block<br>• Arrest (hypercalcemia crisis) | Monitor for ECG changes. |
| Elimination<br>• Renal impairment<br>• Thiazide diuretics<br>• Steroid therapy | 4. Nutrition and metabolism<br>• Nausea, vomiting, anorexia<br>• Constipation | Teach client to ↓ calcium intake and ↑ fiber.<br>Encourage oral intake of acid-ash fluids to ↓ deposit of calcium salts. |
| | 5. Elimination<br>• Flank pain from calculi<br>• Polyuria | Monitor for symptoms of digitalis toxicity; calcium enhances the action of digitalis. |

*(continues)*

## TABLE 34-5    THE CLINICAL MANAGEMENT OF CLIENTS EXPERIENCING COMMON ELECTROLYTE DISTURBANCES (continued)

| Disturbance/Causes | Clinical Manifestations | Nursing Interventions |
|---|---|---|
| **Hypomagnesemia**<br>Operational definition:<br>　Serum Mg < 1.5 mEq/L | 1. Cognitive and sensory<br>　• Disorientation, confusion<br>　• Vertigo<br>　• Irritability, tremors | Monitor the client for seizure activity and laryngeal stridor.<br><br>Administer N magnesium sulphate. |
| Nutrition and metabolism<br>• Prolonged inadequate dietary intake of magnesium (e.g., malnutrition and alcoholism)<br>• Excessive losses of magnesium (e.g., vomiting, gastric suction)<br>• Prolonged administration of IV solutions without magnesium additives | 2. Activity/mobility<br>　• ↑ Tendon reflexes<br>　• Positive Chvostek's & Trousseau's signs<br><br>3. Oxygenation and ECG<br>　• ↑ BP<br>　• Tachycardia | Monitor for ECG changes and assess the client for digitalis toxicity. |
| Elimination<br>• Severe renal disease<br>• Thiazide diuretics<br>• Aldosterone excess<br>• Polyuria | 　• Dysrhythmias<br>　• T wave flat or inverted<br>　• ST segment depressed | Teach client to eat magnesium-rich foods and to avoid excessive use of laxatives and diuretics. |
| **Hypermagnesemia**<br>Operational definition:<br>　Serum Mg > 2.5 mEq/L | 1. Cognitive and sensory<br>　• Lethargy, drowsiness<br>　• Coma | Monitor level of consciousness. |
| Nutrition and metabolism<br>• Excessive treatment of magnesium deficit | 2. Activity/mobility<br>　• Muscle weakness, paralysis<br>　• ↓ Deep-tendon reflexes | Assess patellar reflexes; if absent notify practitioner. |
| Elimination<br>• Renal failure | 3. Oxygenation and ECG<br>　• ↓ respirations, 10 to 12 per minute<br>　• ↓ BP<br>　• Bradycardia<br>　• AV block<br>　• Respiratory and cardiac arrest (severe hypermagnesemia)<br>　• QRS complex widening<br>　• QT interval prolonged | Monitor vital signs q15–30 minutes until stable and for ECG changes.<br><br>Encourage fluids unless contraindicated to dilute the serum level of magnesium.<br><br>Teach client about over-the-counter drugs with magnesium content. |
| **Hypophosphatemia**<br>Operational definition:<br>　Serum phosphate < 1.7 mEq/L<br>　Reduced WBC; platelets<br>　Elevated cardiac isoenzymes | 1. Cognitive and sensory<br>　• Confusion, seizures, coma<br>　• Fatigue, memory loss | Monitor client's level of consciousness. Institute safety measures for seizures. |
| Nutrition and metabolism<br>• Inadequate intake: malnutrition, chronic alcoholism | 2. Activity/mobility<br>　• Muscle pain, weakness<br>　• Paresthesia<br>　• Hyporeflexia | Administer pain medications and other comfort measures.<br>Assist the client in maintaining proper body alignment. |

(continues)

## TABLE 34-5   THE CLINICAL MANAGEMENT OF CLIENTS EXPERIENCING COMMON ELECTROLYTE DISTURBANCES (*continued*)

| Disturbance/Causes | Clinical Manifestations | Nursing Interventions |
|---|---|---|
| • Prolonged administration of IV solutions that are phosphorus-poor or phosphorus-free<br>• Acid-base imbalances (e.g., diabetic ketoacidosis and respiratory alkalosis)<br>• Increased secretion of parathyroid hormone<br>• Overuse of aluminum-containing antacids | • Bone pain<br>• Joint stiffness<br><br>3. Oxygenation and ECG<br>• Tissue hypoxia<br>• Hyperventilation<br>• Possible bleeding<br>• Weak pulse | Monitor for bleeding and respiratory failure. |
| | 4. Safety<br>• Possible infection | Institute precautions to prevent infection. |
| | 5. Nutrition and metabolism<br>• Anorexia<br>• Dysphagia | Teach client about phosphorus-rich foods and over-the-counter drugs that contain aluminum hydroxide. |
| | | Administer IV phosphate with caution: dilute and infuse slowly to avoid phlebitis; infiltration at the IV site may cause tissue sloughing; do not infuse with calcium. |
| **Hyperphosphatemia**<br>Operational definition:<br>   Serum phosphate > 2.6 mEq/L<br>   Reduced serum calcium | 1. Activity/mobility<br>• Tetany<br>• Muscle weakness<br>• Flaccid paralysis<br>• Circumoral paraesthesia<br>• Hyperreflexia | Monitor for tetany and other signs of hypocalcemia. |
| Nutrition and metabolism<br>• Excessive administration of oral and IV solutions containing phosphate substances<br>• Hypoparathyroidism<br>• Laxatives containing phosphate | 2. Oxygenation and ECG<br>• Tachycardia<br>• ST segment shortened<br>• QT interval shortened | Monitor heart rate and assess for ECG changes. |
| Elimination<br>• Renal insufficiency | 3. Nutrition and metabolism<br>• Nausea, anorexia, vomiting, diarrhea | Administer calcium replacement. Monitor urinary output; < 25 ml/hour will increase serum phosphorus level. |
| | | Teach client to avoid foods high in phosphorus (to read the labels on canned foods) and excessive use of phosphorus-containing laxatives and enemas. |

Daniels, R. (2003). *Delmar's manual of laboratory and diagnostic tests.* Clifton Park, NY: Delmar Learning.

## Hypernatremia

**Hypernatremia** is an excess in the extracellular level of sodium. With an excess of sodium or a loss of water, a hyperosmolar state exists because the ratio of sodium to water is too high. This ratio causes an increase in the extracellular osmotic pressure, which pulls fluid out of the cells into the extracellular space. The symptoms of this increase depend on the cause and the location of the edema (Table 34-5).

## Potassium

The normal range of extracellular potassium is narrow (3.5–5.0 mEq/L). Small deviations can cause serious or life-threatening effects on physiological functions. A reciprocal relationship exists between sodium and potassium; large sodium intake results in an increased loss of potassium, and vice versa. When potassium is lost from the cells, sodium enters the cells. There are two main categories of diuretics that can alter electrolyte balance:

1. *Potassium-wasting diuretics* excrete potassium and other electrolytes, such as sodium and chloride.
2. *Potassium-sparing diuretics* retain potassium but excrete sodium and chloride.

### Hypokalemia

**Hypokalemia** is a decrease in the extracellular level of potassium. Gastrointestinal-tract disturbances and the use of diuretics can place the client at risk for hypokalemia and an acid-base imbalance (metabolic alkalosis). Potassium-wasting diuretics can cause hypokalemia. Besides diuretics, other major drug groups that can cause hypokalemia are laxatives, corticosteroids, and antibiotics.

### Hyperkalemia

**Hyperkalemia** is an increase in the extracellular level of potassium. Three major drug groups may cause hyperkalemia:

- Potassium-sparing diuretics
- Central nervous system agents
- Oral and intravenous replacement potassium salts

Hyperkalemia can also inhibit the action of digitalis.

## Calcium

Most of the body's calcium (99%) is deposited in bone as phosphate and carbonate salts. The remaining 1% is in

---

## CLINICAL ALERT

### Potassium Chloride

Never administer more than 10 mEq of intravenous potassium chloride (KCl) per hour; the normal dose of intravenous KCl is 20–40 mEq/L to infuse over an 8-hour period.

---

## CLINICAL ALERT

### Hypokalemia

Hypokalemia can cause a cardiac arrest when:

1. The potassium level is less than 2.5 mEq/L.
2. The client is taking digitalis (a drug that strengthens the contraction of the myocardium and slows down the rate of the heart). *Hypokalemia enhances the action of the drug, causing toxicity.*

---

the blood plasma (serum). Normally, 50% of the serum calcium is ionized and physiologically active. The remaining 50% is bound to protein. Free, ionized calcium is physiologically active. Calcium that is bound to plasma protein cannot pass through the capillary wall or leave the intravascular compartment. Calcium is essential for normal bone and teeth formation. It is also a critical factor in normal blood clotting and required for the maintenance of normal nerve and muscle excitability (Daniels, 2003).

A stable blood level of calcium is maintained by a negative-feedback system controlled by vitamin D, parathyroid hormone, calcitonin (thyrocalcitonin), and the serum concentrations of calcium and phosphate ions. Absorption and use of dietary calcium requires adequate quantities of protein and vitamin D. Absorption from the gastrointestinal tract, even with optimal intake, is never complete (Roth & Townsend, 2002). A decreased blood level stimulates the parathyroid gland to secrete parathyroid hormone, which in turn mobilizes the release of calcium from the bone, increases the renal reabsorption, and increases intestinal absorption in the presence of vitamin D. Calcitonin, secreted by the thyroid gland, reduces excess blood calcium.

### Hypocalcemia

**Hypocalcemia** is a decrease in the extracellular level of calcium. The rapid administration of citrated blood, alkalosis, and elevated levels of serum albumin increase the activity of calcium binders, thereby decreasing the amount of free calcium.

### Hypercalcemia

**Hypercalcemia** is an increase in the extracellular level of calcium. The clinical symptoms result from a decrease in neuromuscular activity, reabsorption of calcium from bone, and the kidney's response to a high serum calcium concentration.

## Magnesium

Magnesium plays an important role as a coenzyme in the metabolism of carbohydrates and proteins and as a mediator in neuromuscular activity. Magnesium has the unique characteristic of being the only cation that has a

## CLINICAL ALERT

### Hypercalcemic Crisis

A rapid increase in the extracellular level of calcium (above 8–9 mEq/L) can trigger a hypercalcemic crisis. To prevent a hypercalcemic crisis, provide adequate hydration and administer diuretics or phosphate or both as prescribed.

## STOP AND THINK

### Calcium and Phosphorous Intake

- What foods are high in calcium?

- What foods are high in phosphorus?

- How would you counsel clients who cannot have an adequate daily intake of milk to meet their necessary calcium and phosphorus intake?

higher concentration in cerebrospinal fluid than in extracellular fluid.

### Hypomagnesemia

**Hypomagnesemia** is a decrease in the extracellular level of magnesium and usually occurs with hypokalemia and hypocalcemia. It is probably the most undiagnosed electrolyte deficit because it is asymptomatic until the serum level approaches 1.0 mEq/L; the normal range is 4.5–5.5 mEq/L (Kee & Paulanka, 2000).

Drugs that may cause hypomagnesemia include digitalis, potassium-wasting diuretics, cortisone, aminoglycosides, and amphotericin B; the chronic use of laxatives may also cause the condition. Clinical manifestations are related to the neuromuscular, neurologic, or cardiovascular system (Table 34-5).

### Hypermagnesemia

**Hypermagnesemia** refers to an increase in the extracellular level of magnesium. It rarely occurs from excessive dietary ingestion. However, overuse of magnesium-containing drugs (e.g., antacids, laxatives, and intravenous magnesium sulfate) can cause hypermagnesemia. The clinical manifestations of hypermagnesemia are nonspecific (refer to Table 34-5).

### Phosphate

Phosphate is the main intracellular anion; it appears as phosphorus in the serum. Phosphorus is similar to calcium in that vitamin D is needed for its reabsorption from the renal tubules.

### Hypophosphatemia

**Hypophosphatemia** is a decreased extracellular level of phosphorus. An increase in parathyroid hormone causes decreased renal reabsorption and increased excretion of phosphates.

## CLINICAL ALERT

### Hyperalimentation

The continuous use of total parenteral nutrition (TPN, hyperalimentation) without a magnesium supplement can cause hypomagnesemia.

### Hyperphosphatemia

**Hyperphosphatemia** is an increased extracellular level of phosphorus. Excessive administration (oral or intravenous) of phosphate-containing substances can cause hyperphosphatemia. Other causes of hyperphosphatemia are hypoparathyroidism, renal insufficiency, and laxatives containing phosphate.

### Chloride

As previously stated, chloride and water move in the same direction as sodium ions, influencing the osmolality of extracellular fluid. Although chloride losses usually follow sodium losses, the proportion will differ because a loss of chloride can be compensated for by an increase in bicarbonate. Therefore, signs and symptoms of a chloride imbalance will be similar to those of a metabolic acid-base imbalance, discussed later in this chapter. A deficit of either chloride or potassium will lead to a deficiency of the other electrolyte.

### Hypochloremia

**Hypochloremia** is a decrease in the extracellular level of chloride. Gastrointestinal tract losses may cause a decrease in chloride because of the acid content of gastric juices, mainly hydrogen chloride. Because the bicarbonate ion compensates for the loss of chloride, the client is at risk for developing metabolic alkalosis. The signs and symptoms of hypochloremia are muscle twitching and slow, shallow breathing. With a severe loss of chloride and extracellular fluid volume, there may be a drop in blood pressure.

### Hyperchloremia

Hyperchloremia is an increase in the extracellular level of chloride. It usually occurs with dehydration, hypernatremia, and metabolic acidosis. The signs and symptoms of hyperchloremia are muscle weakness; deep, rapid breathing; and lethargy progressing to unconsciousness if untreated.

## Acid-Base Disturbances

The common types of acid-base imbalances are respiratory acidosis and alkalosis and metabolic acidosis and alkalosis (Figure 34-6).

Related to Respiratory Function       Related to Metabolism of the Body

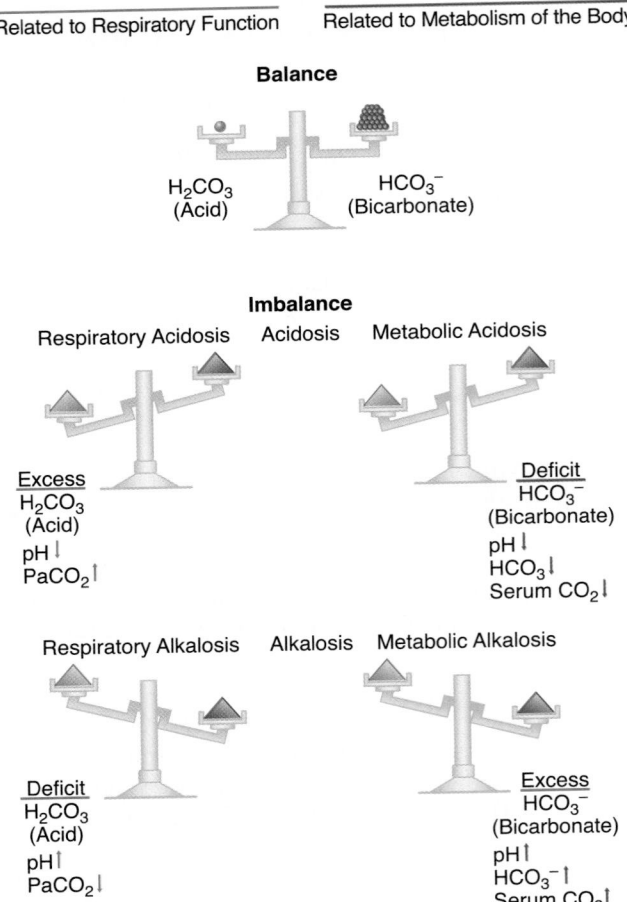

**Figure 34-6    Acid-base balance and imbalance**

| TABLE 34-6 | COMMON CAUSES OF ACUTE AND CHRONIC RESPIRATORY ACIDOSIS |
|---|---|
| **Acute** | **Chronic** |
| Drug-induced CNS depression | Asthma |
| Pneumonia and atelectasis | Cystic fibrosis |
| Pulmonary edema | Emphysema |
| Respiratory distress syndrome | Chronic Obstructive Pulmonary Disease |
| Pneumothorax | |
| Hypoventilation | |
| Poliomyelitis | |
| Chest trauma | |
| Brain and spinal cord injury | |

## Laboratory Data

The biochemical indicators of acid-base imbalance are assessed by measurement of arterial blood gases (ABGs). **Arterial blood gases** measure the levels of oxygen and carbon dioxide. Blood pH, bicarbonate ion concentration, sodium, potassium, and chloride levels are also important in the assessment of acid-base imbalance.

## Respiratory Acidosis (Carbonic Acid Excess)

Respiratory acidosis is characterized by an increased hydrogen ion concentration (a blood pH below 7.35), an increased arterial carbon dioxide pressure (greater than 45 mm Hg), and an excess of carbonic acid. Respiratory acidosis is caused by hypoventilation or any condition that depresses ventilation (Table 34-6).

Hypoventilation can have respiratory system causes, such as respiratory failure, or other system causes, such as drug overdose. Common central nervous system depressants include narcotics, barbiturates, and anesthetic agents.

Clients with respiratory acidosis experience neurologic changes resulting from the acidity of the cerebrospinal fluid and brain cells. Hypoventilation can

cause **hypoxemia** (decreased oxygen levels), which causes further neurologic impairments. Refer to Chapter 39 for a complete discussion of hypoxemia. Hyperkalemia may accompany acidosis. See Table 34-7 for the clinical manifestations and nursing interventions used to treat respiratory acidosis.

## Respiratory Alkalosis (Carbonic Acid Deficit)

Respiratory acidosis is characterized by a decreased hydrogen ion concentration (a blood pH above 7.45) and a decreased arterial carbon dioxide pressure (less than 35 mm Hg). Respiratory alkalosis is caused by hyperventilation (excessive exhalation of carbon dioxide) resulting in hypocapnia (decreased arterial carbon dioxide concentration). Hyperventilation can be triggered by hypoxia at high altitudes, anxiety, fear, pain, fever, and rapid mechanical ventilation. Other causes of hyperventilation, which involve overstimulation of the respiratory center, include salicylate poisoning, hyperthyroidism, pneumonia, atelectasis, asthma, adult respiratory distress syndrome, congestive heart failure, pulmonary edema and embolus, brain tumors, meningitis, and encephalitis; refer to Table 34-7 for the clinical manifestations and treatment.

## Metabolic Acidosis (Bicarbonate Deficit)

Metabolic acidosis is characterized by an increase in hydrogen ion concentration (blood pH below 7.35) or a decrease in bicarbonate concentration. Causes of metabolic acidosis can be divided into two categories: loss of base

**TABLE 34-7    RESPIRATORY AND METABOLIC ACIDOSIS AND ALKALOSIS**

| Imbalance/Causes | Clinical Manifestations | Nursing Interventions |
|---|---|---|
| **Respiratory Acidosis (Retention of Carbon Dioxide)** | | |
| Operational definition:<br>pH < 7.35<br>$PaCO_2$ > 45 mmHg<br>$HCO_3$ > 28 mEq/L (suggestive of renal compensation)<br><br>• CNS disorders<br>• Drug overdose<br>• Pneumonia<br>• Pulmonary edema<br>• Pneumothorax<br>• Restrictive lung disease | 1. Cognitive and sensory<br>• Disorientation<br>• Depression<br>• Weakness → stupor<br><br>2. Skin and mucous membranes<br>• Flushed and warm<br><br>3. Oxygenation and ECG<br>• Dyspnea<br>• Tachycardia<br>• Dysrhythmia | 1. Institute safety measures. Assist with positioning.<br><br>2. Monitor I&O and administer fluids as ordered.<br><br>3. Administer oxygen and medications per order; monitor hourly vital signs and respiratory status (may require mechanical ventilation).<br><br>4. Monitor arterial blood gases (ABGs), pH, $PaCO_2$, $HCO_3^-$. |
| **Respiratory Alkalosis (Hyperventilation)** | | |
| Operational definition:<br>pH > 7.45<br>$PaCO_2$ < 35 mmHg<br><br>• Anxiety, fear<br>• CNS disorders<br>• Pain<br>• Fever<br>• Pneumonia, atelectasis<br>• Asthma<br>• Adult respiratory distress syndrome (ARDS)<br>• Congestive heart failure, pulmonary edema<br>• Pulmonary embolus | 1. Cognitive and sensory<br>• Hyperactive reflexes<br>• Tetany<br>• Positive Chvostek's sign<br>• Positive Trousseau's sign<br>• Vertigo<br>• Unconsciousness<br><br>2. Skin and mucous membranes<br>• Sweating (may occur)<br><br>3. Oxygenation and ECG<br>• Rapid, shallow breathing<br>• Palpitations | 1. Institute safety measures for the client with vertigo or the unconscious client. Encourage the anxious client to verbalize fears. Administer sedation as ordered to relax the client.<br><br>2. Keep the client warm and dry.<br><br>3. Encourage the client to take deep, slow breaths or breathe into a brown paper bag (inspire $CO_2$). Monitor vital signs.<br><br>4. Monitor ABGs, primarily $PaCO_2$; a value ↓ 35 mm Hg indicates too little $CO_2$ (e.g., carbonic acid) |
| **Metabolic Acidosis (Gain of Metabolic Acids or Loss of Base)** | | |
| Operational definition:<br>pH < 7.35<br>$HCO_3$ < 24 mEq/L<br>BE < 2 mEq/L<br>Serum $CO_2$ < 22 mEq/L | 1. Cognitive and sensory<br>• Restlessness, disorientation<br>• Stupor, coma<br><br>2. Activity/mobility<br>• Weakness, lethargy | 1. Institute safety measures. Monitor client's sensorium; report alteration in level of consciousness.<br><br>2. Assist the client with positioning and proper body alignment. |

*(continues)*

## TABLE 34-7    RESPIRATORY AND METABOLIC ACIDOSIS AND ALKALOSIS (continued)

Increased acids:
- Renal failure
- Diabetic ketoacidosis
- Anaerobic metabolism
- Drug overdose (salicylates, methanol)

Loss of base:
- Diarrhea

3. Skin and mucous membranes
- Warm, flushed skin

4. Oxygenation and ECG
- Kussmaul breathing (deep, rapid respirations)
- Bradycardia, decreased cardiac output
- Dysrhythmias

5. Nutrition and metabolism
- Nausea, vomiting
- Abdominal pain

3. Keep the client comfortable.

4. Monitor vital signs and I&O. Monitor and report cardiac dysrhythmias. Administer sodium bicarbonate and fluid replacement as ordered.

5. Provide comfort measures. Correct metabolic problem as ordered.

6. Monitor ABGs and evaluate the metabolic indicators ($HCO_3^-$ & BE).

**Metabolic Alkalosis (Gain of Base or Loss of Metabolic Acids)**

Operation definition:
  pH > 7.45
  $HCO_3$ > 28 mEq/L
  BE > 2 mEq/L
  Reduced serum potassium and chloride

Gain of base:
- Excess ingestion of antacids
- Excess administration of sodium bicarbonate

Loss of metabolic acids:
- Vomiting
- Nasogastric suctioning or lavage
- Low potassium or chloride
- Increased aldosterone
- Administration of steroids or diuretics

1. Cognitive and sensory
- Irritability, confusion

2. Activity/mobility
- Tetany
- Hypertonic muscles
- Hypertonic reflexes

3. Oxygenation and ECG
- Depressed rate and depth of respirations

4. Nutrition and metabolism
- Vomiting

1. Monitor the client's sensorium and report increasing mental confusion.

2. Institute safety and comfort measures. Report symptoms of tetany.

3. Monitor vital signs and report changes in the client's respiratory status.

4. Monitor I&O, recording amount of fluid loss from vomiting and gastric suctioning. Administer intravenous fluid ± replacement as ordered.

5. Monitor ABGs and evaluate the metabolic indicators ($HCO_3^-$ and BE).

From Hartshorn, J., Sole, M. L., Lamborn, M., & Cullen, B. N. (1997). *Introduction to critical care nursing* (2nd ed.). Philadelphia: Saunders; Kee, J. L., & Paulanka, B. J. (2000). *Fluids and electrolytes with clinical applications* (6th ed.). Clifton Park, NY: Delmar Learning.

and gain in metabolic acids. Chronic diarrhea causes an excessive loss of bicarbonate and sodium ions from the small intestines. With the loss of sodium ions, chloride ions are in excess and combine with hydrogen to produce a strong acid (hydrochloric acid).

Clients with certain medical diagnoses are at risk for metabolic acidosis. Such conditions include:

1. Diabetic ketoacidosis: Cells are deprived of glucose (decrease or absence of insulin) for metabolism. The liver, in response to the needs of the cells, increases the metab-olism of fatty acids, which causes an increase in ketone bodies. These make the extracellular fluid more acidic.
2. Renal failure: The normal mechanism of the kidneys to conserve sodium and water and excrete hydrogen is compromised.
3. Anaerobic metabolism: Cellular catabolism and acid accumulation occur with starvation, severe malnutrition, infection, fever, trauma, shock, and excessive exercise.
4. Drug overdose: Acid accumulation (lactic acidosis) results from excessive ingestion of salicylate, paralde-hyde, and methanol.

In response to metabolic acidosis, the respiratory center is stimulated, causing an increase in the rate and depth of respirations (Kussmaul breathing), to lower the acid concentration in extracellular fluid by increasing the exhalation of carbon dioxide. The respiratory compensatory mechanism is usually ineffective in decreasing acids, especially if the client has chronic obstructive pulmonary disease or is in ketoacidosis. Refer to Chapter 39 for additional information on these diagnoses. The renal compensatory mechanism tries to increase the pH by exchanging sodium ions with hydrogen ions to increase the excretion of hydrogen; refer to Table 34-7 for the clinical manifestations and treatment of metabolic acidosis (Horne & Derrico, 1999).

## Metabolic Alkalosis (Bicarbonate Excess)

Metabolic alkalosis is characterized by an increased loss of acid from the body or a gain in base (increased levels of bicarbonate). The blood pH is above 7.45. A gain in base may result from excessive ingestion of antacids. These substances neutralize acids, producing alkalosis and hypercalcemia. Excessive oral or parenteral administration of sodium bicarbonate or other alkaline salts (e.g., sodium or potassium acetate, lactate, or citrate) increases the amount of base in extracellular fluids.

The following clinical conditions can place clients at risk for metabolic alkalosis:

1. Vomiting and nasogastric suctioning or lavage cause a loss in hydrochloric acid and chloride; with the loss of the hydrogen and chloride ions, bicarbonate ions are absorbed, unneutralized, into the bloodstream and the pH of the extracellular fluid rises (alkalosis).
2. Diarrhea, and steroid or diuretic therapy, can cause the excessive loss of potassium, chloride, and other electrolytes; the potassium deficit causes the kidneys to exchange hydrogen ions (instead of potassium ions) for sodium ions, which promotes the loss of hydrogen, thereby increasing bicarbonate level. Hydrochlorothiazide, a thiazide diuretic, blocks the reabsorption of sodium in the cortex in the distal tubule, causing sodium to be excreted in greater amounts than water (hyponatremia). Thiazides also cause hypokalemia

because of the loss of urinary potassium. The secondary effects of thiazides lead to metabolic alkalosis because of a depletion in volume, chloride, potassium, and hydrogen ions (DeJong, 1998).

Respiratory and renal compensatory mechanisms respond to an increased bicarbonate–carbonic acid ratio. The rate and depth of respirations are decreased in an effort to retain carbon dioxide. The arterial carbon dioxide concentration rises to counter the pH imbalance of metabolic alkalosis.

A normal serum potassium level is a prerequisite to renal compensation. In alkalosis, potassium ions enter the cells in exchange for hydrogen ions, causing hypokalemia. Hypokalemia further potentiates metabolic alkalosis because the kidneys conserve hydrogen ions by excreting potassium ions in exchange for sodium ions. When hypokalemia is present, the kidneys cannot function as a compensatory mechanism; therefore, they continue to excrete hydrogen, and bicarbonate excess continues. Refer to Table 34-7 for the clinical manifestations and treatment of metabolic alkalosis (Wong, 1999).

# Assessment

Assessment data are used to identify clients who have potential or actual alterations in fluid volume. Clients receiving certain treatments, such as medications and IV therapy, are at risk for developing imbalances. The key nursing assessment indicators that suggest possible imbalances are daily weights, vital signs, intake and output, and the physical findings of the skin, oral cavity, eyes, venous filling, and neuromuscular system. Laboratory data is confirmatory.

## Health History

The nursing history should elicit data specific to fluids (see Box 34-2 for sample topics to direct the interview).

## Physical Examination

The nurse performs a complete physical examination and identifies all abnormalities because fluid alterations may affect any body system. The physical assessment of clients with altered fluid status is discussed in this section: refer to Chapter 27 for procedures on weight and vital sign measurement.

### Daily Weight

Changes in the body's total fluid volume are indicated by weight; for instance, each kilogram (2.2 lb) of weight gained or lost is equivalent to one liter (1,000 ml) of fluid gained or lost. Accurate measurement of daily weight requires the control of certain variables. For example, the nurse should obtain the measurement at the same time each day, using the same scale.

## CLINICAL ALERT

### Electrolyte Shift

Metabolic acidosis causes an electrolyte shift: Hydrogen and sodium ions move into the cell, and potassium moves into the extracellular fluid. Hyperkalemia may cause ventricular fibrillation and death.

## BOX 34-2    HEALTH HISTORY

- Lifestyle—sociocultural and economic factors, stress, exercise

- Dietary intake—recent changes in the amount and types of fluid and food, increased thirst

- Religion—whether illness has had an effect on beliefs or religion (e.g., fasting, salt intake)

- Weight—sudden gain or loss

- Fluid output—recent changes in the frequency or amount of urine output

- Gastrointestinal disturbances—prolonged vomiting, diarrhea, anorexia, ulcers, hemorrhage

- Fever and diaphoresis

- Draining wounds, burns, trauma

- Disease conditions that could upset homeostasis—renal disease, endocrine disorders, neural malfunction, pulmonary disease

- Therapeutic programs that can produce imbalances—special diets, medications, chemotherapy, administration of intravenous fluid or total parenteral nutrition, gastric or intestinal suction

### Vital Signs

Measurement of vital signs allows the nurse to make inferences regarding the client's fluid, electrolyte, and acid-base status and the body's compensatory response for maintaining balance. For example, an elevated temperature places the client at risk for dehydration caused by an increased loss of body fluid.

Changes in the pulse rate, strength, and rhythm are suggestive of fluid alterations. Fluid volume alterations may cause the following pulse changes:

- Fluid volume deficit (FVD): increased pulse rate and weak pulse volume
- Fluid volume excess (FVE): increased pulse volume and third heart sound

Respiratory changes are assessed by inspecting the movement of the chest wall, counting the rate, and auscultating the lungs. Changes in respiratory rate and depth may cause respiratory acid-base imbalances or may be indicative of a compensatory response to metabolic acidosis or alkalosis.

Blood pressure measurements can be used to reflect extracellular fluid status and the degree of FVD. FVD can lower the blood pressure with or without orthostatic hypotension. A narrow pulse pressure (less than 20 mm Hg) may indicate FVD that occurs with severe hypovolemia.

### Intake and Output

Measuring and recording the client's intake and output for a 24-hour period documents actual or potential imbalance: A minimum intake of 1,500 ml is essential to balance urinary output and the body's insensible water loss. Intake includes all liquids (e.g., ice cream, soup, gelatin, juice, and water) taken by mouth and liquids administered through tube feedings (nasogastric or jejunostomy) and parenterally (IV fluids and blood or its components). Output includes urine, diarrhea, vomitus, and drainage from tubes such as through gastric suction. The recording of intake and output data is usually referred to as the I&O.

### Thirst

The most common indicator of FVD is thirst. With a decrease in extracellular fluid volume or an increase in the plasma osmolality, the hypothalamus triggers a thirst response.

### Food Intake

The intake of food also contributes to maintaining extracellular fluid volume. One-third of the body's fluid needs are met by ingested food. Food also provides the body with necessary nutrients. See Chapter 35 for a complete discussion of metabolism.

### Edema

**Edema** (the detectable accumulation of increased interstitial fluid) is the main symptom of FVE. Edema may be localized (confined to a specific area) or generalized (occurring throughout the body's tissue). Localized edema is characterized by taut, smooth, shiny, pale skin. The body may retain 5 to 10 pounds of fluid before

 **LIFE SPAN CONSIDERATIONS**

### Dehydration in Older Clients

There are a number of concerns specific to older clients as related to intake and output issues. For example, older clients are prone to a fluid volume deficit (dehydration), because the thirst mechanism in the hypothalamus becomes less responsive with aging. In addition, there are fewer elastic fibers in the skin, which results in reduced skin turgor. The older person's tongue should be assessed for creases or furrows to monitor dehydration.

Hogstel, M. O. (2001). *Gerontology: Nursing care of the older adult.* Clifton Park, NY: Delmar Learning.

edema is noticeable (Bulechek & McCloskey, 2000). Inspect the dependent body parts—sacrum, back, and legs—to assess peripheral edema. Pitting edema is rated on a four-point scale:

- +0" no pitting
- +1, 0"–1/4" pitting (mild)
- +2, 1/4"–1/2" pitting (moderate)
- +3, 1/2"–1" pitting (severe)
- +4, greater than 1" pitting (severe)

### Skin Turgor

**Skin turgor** is the normal resiliency of the skin. When the skin is pinched and released, it springs back to a normal position because of the outward pressure exerted by the cells and interstitial fluid. To measure the client's skin turgor, grasp and raise the skin with two fingers as follows:

- Adults: over the sternum, forehead, or inner aspect of the thigh; over lower arm by wrist
- Children: over the abdominal area or medial aspect of the thigh

With dehydration there is a decreased skin turgor, as manifested by lax skin that returns slowly to the normal position. Increased skin turgor, which occurs with edema, is manifested by smooth, taut, shiny skin that cannot be grasped and raised (Woods, 1998).

### Buccal (Oral) Cavity

Inspect the buccal cavity. With FVD, there is a decrease in saliva, which causes sticky, dry mucous membranes and dry, cracked lips. The tongue has longitudinal furrows.

### Eyes

Inspect the eyes. FVD causes sunken eyes, dry conjunctiva, and decreased or absent tearing. Puffy eyelids (periorbital edema, or papilledema) are characteristic of FVE.

### Jugular and Hand Veins

Circulatory volume is assessed by observing the venous filling of the jugular and hand veins. Place the client in a low Fowler's position. Then:

1. Palpate the jugular (neck) veins: FVE causes a distention in the jugular veins (Figure 34-7).
2. Place the client's hand below the heart level and palpate the jugular veins; with FVD there is decreased venous filling (flat neck veins).

### Neuromuscular System

Fluid and electrolyte imbalances may cause neuromuscular alterations: The muscles lose their tone and, possibly, strength. Reflexes are diminished. Calcium and magnesium imbalances cause an increase in neuromuscular irritability. To assess for neuromuscular irritability, perform the following tests:

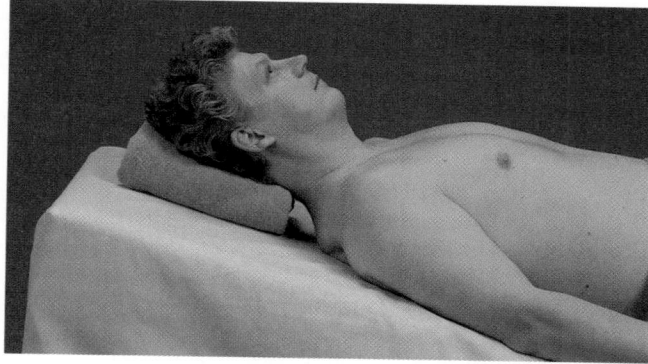

**Figure 34-7    Positioning the client to assess jugular vein distention**

1. Chvostek's sign: Tap the facial nerve 2 cm anterior to the earlobe. Ipsilateral twitching of the facial muscles (inclusive of the eyelids and lips) indicates a positive response (Figure 34-8).
2. Trousseau's sign: Place a blood pressure cuff on the arm, inflate the cuff slightly above the systolic pressure, leave the cuff inflated 2 to 3 minutes, and deflate; carpal spasm or tetany indicates a positive response.

A positive Chvostek's sign and Trousseau's sign may occur with hypocalcemia and hypomagnesemia.

Other neurologic clinical manifestations include changes in consciousness, cognition (e.g., inability to concentrate), and emotional liability (Tables 34-5 and 34-7).

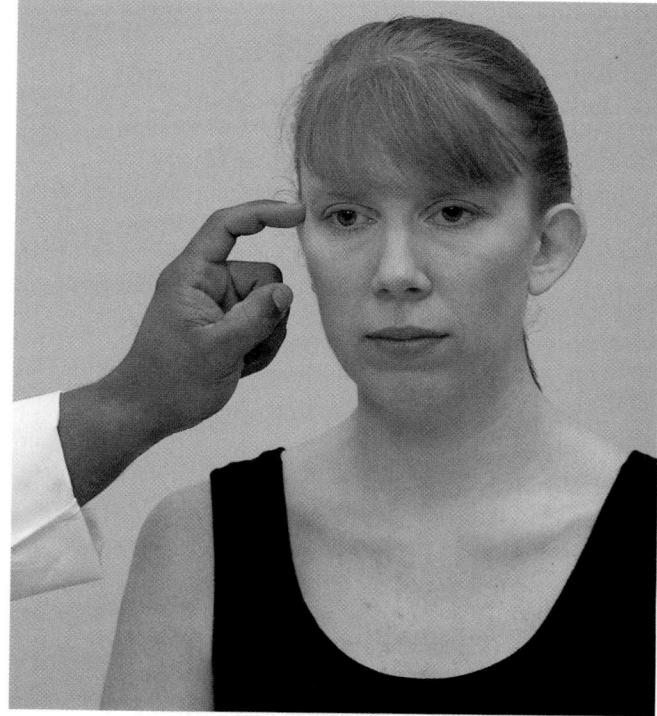

**Figure 34-8    Assessing for Chvostek's sign**

# Diagnostic and Laboratory Data

Laboratory data is diagnostic and an essential source of objective information. They may detect imbalances before clinical symptoms are assessed in the physical examination. Laboratory tests used in assessing clients with common alterations in extracellular fluid volume are discussed next; refer to Chapter 29 for the normal values presented in this section.

## Hemoglobin and Hematocrit Indices

The hematocrit is affected by changes in plasma volume. For instance, with severe dehydration and hypovolemic shock, the hematocrit is increased. Overhydration reduces hematocrit by dilution. Hemoglobin levels are decreased with severe hemorrhage.

## Osmolality

**Osmolality** is a measurement of the total concentration of dissolved particles (solutes) per kilogram of water. Osmolality can be measured in both serum and urine to determine alterations in fluid and electrolyte balance. Specific gravity expresses the weight of the solution when compared with an equal volume of distilled water. Osmolality of a solution can be roughly estimated by the specific gravity.

### Serum Osmolality

Serum osmolality is a measurement of the total concentration of dissolved particles per kilogram of water in serum. It is expressed as milliosmoles per kilogram (mOsm/kg). The particles measured in serum osmolality include ions, such as sodium and potassium, and electrically inactive substances, such as glucose and urea. Water and sodium are the main entities that control the osmolality of body fluids. Serum sodium is responsible for 85% to 90% of the serum osmolality.

The normal serum osmolality is 275 to 295 mOsm/kg (Daniels, 2003). It can increase with dehydration and loss of body water and decrease with water excess.

In clinical practice, the terms *osmolality* and **osmolarity** (the concentration of solutes per liter of cellular fluid) are often used interchangeably to refer to the concentration of body fluid. However, these terms are actually different: osmolality refers to the concentration of solutes in the total body water (solutes per kilogram of body weight) rather than in cellular fluid.

Figure 34-9 relates osmosis to the osmolality of a solution. The appropriate term to use in intravenous fluid therapy is *osmolarity* (Bulechek & McCloskey, 2000). An osmolaritic solution is described as:

- **Hypotonic** (hypo-osmolar) when there are less solutes in proportion to the volume of water than is the case in the body
- **Isotonic** (iso-osmolar) when body water and solutes (sodium) are in amounts equal to those in the body
- **Hypertonic** (hyperosmolar) when there are more solutes in proportion to the volume of water than is the case in the body

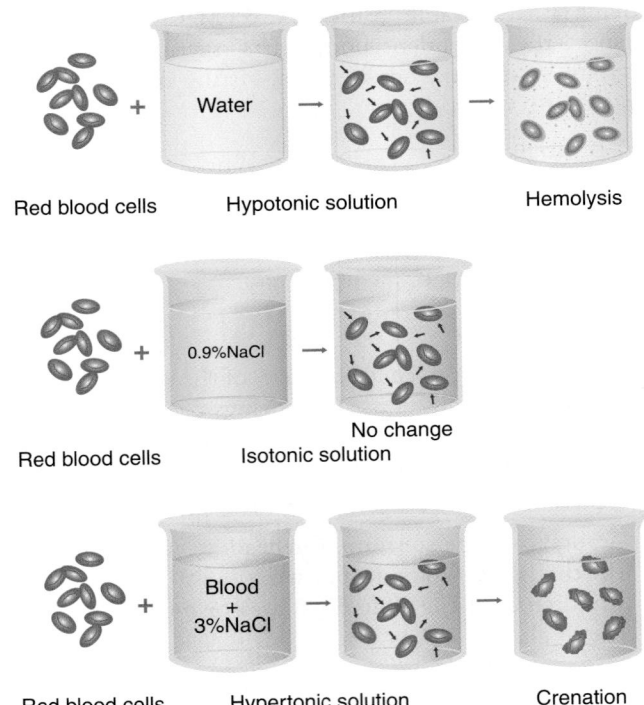

**Figure 34-9    Osmosis as it relates to the osmolarity of a solution. The movement of water through a membrane from an area of a lower solute concentration to a higher concentration is called osmosis. In a hypotonic solution, water moves into the cells, causing them to swell and burst. In an isotonic solution, cells are normal in size and shape because the same amount of water is entering and leaving the cells. Cells in the hypertonic solution are losing water because water moves from a weaker concentration inside the cell to a greater concentration outside the cell membrane.**

### Urine Osmolality

Urine osmolality is a measurement of the total concentration of dissolved particles per kilogram of water in urine, recorded in milliosmoles per kilogram (mOsm/kg). The particles measured in urine osmolality are nitrogenous waste—creatinine, urea, and uric acid. Urea contributes most. Urine osmolality varies greatly with diet and fluid intake and reflects the ability of the kidney to adjust the

## CLINICAL ALERT

### Urine Osmolality

Urine osmolality is a more accurate indicator of hydration than is the specific gravity of urine. Some medications and the presence of protein and glucose solutes in the urine can give a false high specific gravity reading.

concentration of urine in order to maintain fluid balance. With normal kidney function, a dehydrated client will have an elevated urine osmolality. Clients with shock, hyperglycemia, hemoconcentration, and acidosis will have elevations in urine and serum osmolality.

## Urine pH

The measurement of the pH of urine reveals the hydrogen ion concentration of the urine. When the kidney buffering system is compensating for either metabolic acidosis or alkalosis, the pH of the urine should be within normal range (4.6–8.0). When renal compensatory function fails to respond to the pH of the blood, the urine pH will increase with acidosis and decrease in alkalosis.

## Serum Albumin

Albumin is synthesized in the liver from amino acids. Serum albumin plays an important role in fluid and electrolyte balance by maintaining the colloid osmotic pressure of blood, which prevents the accumulation of fluid (edema) in the tissues. It has a half-life of 21 days and fluctuates according to the level of hydration. As such, it is not a good indicator of acute alterations in protein depletion. Clinically, this blood test is used to measure prolonged protein depletion, which occurs in chronic malnutrition.

# Nursing Diagnosis

In order to make a nursing diagnosis, the nurse must be able to interpret assessment and biochemical data and draw conclusions relative to the client's imbalance. The primary nursing diagnoses for clients with fluid imbalances are presented in Box 34-3.

## Excess Fluid Volume

Excess fluid volume (EFV) exists when the client has increased interstitial and intravascular fluid retention and edema. EFV is related to the excess fluid either in tissues of the extremities (peripheral edema) or in lung tissues (pulmonary edema). Factors that put the client at risk for EFV are:

- Excessive intake of fluids (e.g., intravenous therapy, sodium)
- Increased loss or decreased intake of protein (chronic diarrhea, burns, kidney disease, malnutrition)
- Compromised regulatory mechanisms (kidney failure)
- Decreased intravascular movement (impaired myocardial contractility)
- Lymphatic obstruction (cancer, surgical removal of lymph nodes, obesity)
- Medications (steroid excess)
- Allergic reaction

---

### BOX 34-3   NURSING DIAGNOSES FOR FLUID ALTERATIONS

***Excess Fluid Volume* related to:**

- Excessive fluid intake secondary to excess sodium intake
- Compromised regulatory mechanism (renal and cardiac dysfunction)
- Inaccurate intravenous infusion rate

***Deficient Fluid Volume* related to:**

- Excessive fluid loss secondary to vomiting, blood loss, surgical drains and tubes, diarrhea, and diuretics

***Risk for Deficient Fluid Volume* related to:**

- Extremes of age (very young or old) and weight
- NPO and fluid restrictions
- Increased fluid output from normal routes: vomiting, diarrhea, urine
- Increased fluid losses from drainage or suction routes: wounds, drains, indwelling tubes (e.g., urine catheter, nasogastric suction)
- Loss of plasma associated with severe trauma and burns
- Disorders that impair fluid intake or absorption (immobility, unconsciousness)
- Chronic disorders: congestive heart failure, pulmonary edema, chronic obstructive lung disease, renal failure, diabetes, cancer, transplant candidates
- Deficient knowledge related to factors influencing fluid requirements (hypermetabolic states, hyperthermia, and dry, hot environment)
- Medications (e.g., diuretics)

---

Assessment findings in the client with FEV include acute weight gain; decreased serum osmolality (less than 275 mOsm/kg), protein and albumin, BUN, Hgb, Hct; increased central venous pressure (greater than 12–15 cm $H_2O$); and signs and symptoms of edema. The clinical manifestations of edema are relative to the area of involvement, either pulmonary or peripheral (see Box 34-4).

## BOX 34-4    CLINICAL MANIFESTATIONS OF EDEMA

| Pulmonary Edema | Peripheral Edema |
|---|---|
| Constant cough | Pitting edema in extremities |
| Dyspnea | |
| Engorged neck and hand veins | Edematous area: tight, smooth, shiny, pale, cool skin |
| Moist crackles in lungs | Puffy eyelids |
| Bounding pulse | Weight gain |

## Deficient Fluid Volume

Deficient fluid volume (DFV) exists when the client experiences vascular, interstitial, or intracellular dehydration. The degree of dehydration is classified as mild, marked, severe, or fatal on the basis of the percentage of body weight lost.

The three types of dehydration differ in their respective proportions of fluid and particles in the intracellular and extracellular spaces (see Box 34-5).

Kleiner (1999) reports that a portion of the general population may be chronically mildly dehydrated based on

## BOX 34-5    TYPES OF DEHYDRATION

*Isotonic dehydration* (hypovolemia) refers to the loss of both fluid and particles in the vascular space that occurs with vomiting, diarrhea, and bleeding; it is the most common form of dehydration, especially in infants and children.

*Hypertonic dehydration* refers to a greater loss of fluid than particles in the vascular space when the body tries to maintain a normalized isotonic state by pulling fluids from the intracellular space into the vascular space; it occurs in diabetic ketoacidosis, renal insufficiency, and with the administration of hypertonic solutions.

*Hypotonic dehydration* refers to a greater loss of particles than fluid in the vascular space when the body tries to maintain a normal isotonic state by pushing fluids from the vascular space into the intracellular space, causing the cells to swell; it occurs in chronic disease states and with the administration of hypotonic solutions.

Adapted from Woods, A. (1998). Understanding types of dehydration. *The Nurse Practitioner, 23*(12), 62.

the Nationwide Food Consumption Surveys. According to Sansevero (1997), approximately 1 million older people a year are admitted to hospitals with isotonic dehydration, and 19% of emergency room admissions were prompted by dehydration, frequent falling, or failure to care for self. Mild dehydration, as little as 2% loss of body weight, results in impaired physiological and performance responses, and may be misinterpreted as a sign of aging and not hydration status (Kleiner, 1999).

Assessment findings in the client with DFV include thirst and weight loss, with the amount varying with the degree of dehydration. With marked dehydration, the mucous membranes and skin are dry. There is poor skin turgor; low-grade temperature elevation; tachycardia; respirations 28 or greater; a decrease (10–15 mm Hg) in systolic blood pressure; slowing in venous filling; a decrease in urine (less than 25 ml per hour); concentrated urine; elevated Hct, Hgb, BUN, and an acid blood pH (less than 7.4).

Severe dehydration is characterized by the symptoms of marked dehydration. Also, the skin becomes flushed. The systolic blood pressure continues to drop (60 mm Hg or below). There are behavioral changes (restlessness, irritability, disorientation, and delirium). The signs of fatal dehydration are anuria and coma that leads to death.

## Risk for Deficient Fluid Volume

Risk for fluid volume deficit exists when the client is at high risk of developing vascular, interstitial, or intracellular dehydration resulting from active or regulatory losses of body water in excess of needs. The multiple factors that can place the client at risk for FDV are listed in Box 34-5.

## Other Nursing Diagnoses

The relationship between the primary nursing diagnoses just discussed and the secondary diagnoses in clients with fluid imbalances are reciprocal: The primary diagnoses influence and are influenced by the secondary diagnoses. Holistic nursing requires that all diagnoses relative to clients be considered when developing their plan of care.

### Impaired Gas Exchange

Impaired gas exchange related to a ventilation perfusion imbalance occurs when clients experience a decreased passage of oxygen or carbon dioxide between the alveoli of the lungs and the vascular system. This alteration is assessed by measuring the oxygen and carbon dioxide content through arterial blood gas analysis or pulse oximetry or both. Refer to Chapter 39 for further discussion of oxygenation.

### Decreased Cardiac Output

Decreased cardiac output occurs when the blood pumped by a client's heart is reduced so much that it is inadequate to meet the needs of the body's tissue. This alteration may be caused by heart failure and various types of shock.

Assessment findings may include low blood pressure; cool, clammy skin; weak, thready pulses; decreased urinary output; and a diminished level of consciousness.

### Risk for Infection

Many disorders may place the client at risk for invasion by pathogenic organisms. Clients receiving IV therapy are at risk for an infection because their primary defense, the skin, is broken at the puncture site. Assessment findings indicative of IV site infection are client complaints of soreness around site, erythema, swelling at site, and foul-smelling discharge.

### Impaired Oral Mucous Membrane

Impaired oral mucous membrane occurs when a client experiences disruption in the tissue layers of the oral cavity. It is frequently related to dehydration. Assessment findings may include oral pain or discomfort, stomatitis, and decreased salivation.

## Deficient Knowledge

A knowledge deficit may exist to varying degrees in clients with fluid imbalances. Information obtained from a client's health history may indicate the client's level of understanding and perception of these alterations. Clients ought to be offered information appropriate to their level of education and interest.

## Planning and Outcome Identification

Holistic nursing care for clients experiencing fluid imbalances requires that the nurse, in collaboration with each client, identify specific goals. These goals should be appropriate to the assessment data and diagnosis and individualized to reflect specific client capabilities. Multiple goals ought to be prioritized by severity or risk to the client.

During the planning phase, the nurse also selects and prioritizes nursing interventions to support the client's achievement of expected outcomes (goals). That is, nursing interventions are linked to specific client outcomes. For example, if vomiting and diarrhea, with a weight loss

of 5% and dry mucous membranes, led to a diagnosis of *Deficient Fluid Volume*, then goals might include relief from vomiting and diarrhea and achievement of the proper fluid balance of intake and output.

Expected outcomes for clients with fluid imbalances include outcomes relative to interventions. An expected outcome for clients receiving IV therapy might read: *IV site remains free from erythema, edema, and purulent drainage, because these clients are at risk for infection.* Achievement of the goals and the client's expected outcomes indicates resolution of the problem.

## Implementation

Bulechek and McCloskey (2000) address the importance of the nursing interventions relative to fluid therapy by identifying the nurse's responsibilities to:

- Understand the client's metabolic needs and to make judgments concerning the outcomes of therapy
- Perform frequent assessment and monitoring to recognize the adverse effects of fluid and electrolyte therapy and prevent complications
- Prevent the rapid depletion of the body's protein and energy reserves

The nursing activities relative to assessment and implementation often require the same measurements: for example, weight and vital signs. Common interventions that promote attainment of expected outcomes to restore and maintain homeostasis are discussed next.

Nurses collaborate with and advocate for clients to ensure that care is safe, ethical, appropriate, and consistent with best practice standards. Historical data is used to develop nursing interventions. These, in turn, are linked to specific client outcomes. The goal of every intervention related to disturbances of fluids, electrolytes, and acid-base balance are to restore homeostasis. The selection of nursing interventions should reflect and consider client preferences and strengths.

### Monitor Daily Weight

Daily weight is one of the main indicators of water balance. The nurse is responsible for the accurate measurement and recording of daily weights. This data is used with other clinical findings to determine the client's fluid therapy.

### Measure Vital Signs

The frequency of measuring the vital signs is dependent upon the client's acuity level and clinical situation. For example, the vital signs of the typical postoperative client might be taken every 15 minutes until stable, whereas a client experiencing shock or hemorrhage should have vital signs monitored continuously. Vital sign measurements and other clinical data are used to determine the type and amount of fluid therapy.

# Measure Intake and Output

Intake and output measurements monitor the client's fluid status over a 24-hour period (see Procedure 34-1 for information on how to measure the I&O). Agency policy relative to I&O may vary with regard to:

- The time frames for charting (e.g., every 8 hours versus every 12 hours)
- The time at which the 24-hour totals are calculated
- The definition of "strict" I&O

"Strict" I&O measurement usually involves accounting for incontinent urine, emesis, and diaphoresis and might require weighing soiled bed linens. *Don gloves before handling soiled linen.*

The nurse reviews the client's 24-hour I&O calculations to evaluate fluid status. Intake may exceed the output by 500 ml to account for insensible body losses. I&O and daily weights are critical components of intervention because these measurements are also used to evaluate the effectiveness of diuretic or rehydration therapy. Clients who receive diuretics may have large negative fluid balances.

Securing an accurate I&O requires the full support of the client and his family. The client and family members should be taught how to measure and record the intake.

# Provide Oral Hygiene

The nurse is responsible for providing oral hygiene to promote client comfort and integrity of the buccal cavity. Refer to Chapter 35 for the procedure on oral hygiene. The frequency of oral hygiene depends on the condition of the client's buccal cavity and the type of fluid imbalance. A client who is dehydrated or NPO for more than 24 hours may have decreased or absent salivation, coated tongue, and furrows on the tongue. These clients are at risk for developing oral diseases such as stomatitis, oral lesions or ulcers, and gingivitis.

# Initiate Oral Fluid Therapy

Oral fluids may be totally restricted—a situation commonly referred to as *nothing by mouth* (NPO, which is from the Latin *non per os*)—or they may be restricted or forced, depending on the client's clinical situation. For example,

oral replacement therapy is often used for clients with mild dehydration. According to Hugger, Harkless, and Rentschler (1998), oral rehydration therapy has a very high success rate in the treatment of childhood diarrhea with mild to moderate dehydration, and it has fewer complications when compared to intravenous replacement therapy. However, severe dehydration in children is a medical emergency and must be treated with intravenous replacement therapy.

# Nothing by Mouth

Clients are placed NPO status as prescribed by the health care practitioner. On the basis of agency policy and clarification with the health care practitioner, the client may be allowed small amounts of ice chips or medications with a sip of water when NPO. Common clinical situations that may require NPO status include the need to:

- Avoid aspiration in unconscious, perioperative, and preprocedural clients who will receive anesthesia or conscious sedation
- Rest and heal the gastrointestinal (GI) tract in clients with severe vomiting or diarrhea or when the client has a GI disorder (inflammation or obstruction)
- Prevent the further loss of gastric juices in clients with nasogastric suctioning

NPO clients should receive oral hygiene every 1 to 2 hours or as needed for comfort and to prevent alterations of the mucous membranes.

# Restricted Fluids

Intake may be restricted to 200 ml over a 24-hour period; intake is commonly restricted in the treatment of EFV related to heart and renal failure. Client and family teaching and collaboration are the main nursing interventions in implementing this measure.

How the nurse limits the fluids should be determined in collaboration with the client. For example:

- 50% of the allowed fluids might be taken at breakfast and lunch.
- The remaining 50% might be taken with the evening meal, before bedtime, unless the client has to be awakened during the night for a medication.

---

## CLINICAL ALERT

### Remove Gloves Before Charting

Remove gloves and wash hands before recording the amount of drainage on the I&O form, to prevent the transfer of microorganisms when the form is removed from the client's room.

---

## CLIENT EDUCATION

### Mouthwashes

Avoid the use of alcohol and glycerin mouthwashes and glycerin swabs. These ingredients may feel refreshing, but they have a drying effect on the mucous membranes.

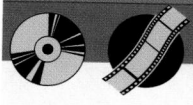

## PROCEDURE 34-1

# Measuring Intake and Output

## EQUIPMENT NEEDED

▪ I&O form at bedside (Figure 34-10)
▪ I&O graphic record in chart
▪ Glass or cup
▪ Bedpan or urinal bedside commode
▪ Graduated container for output
▪ Nonsterile gloves
▪ Sign at bedside stating patient is on I&O

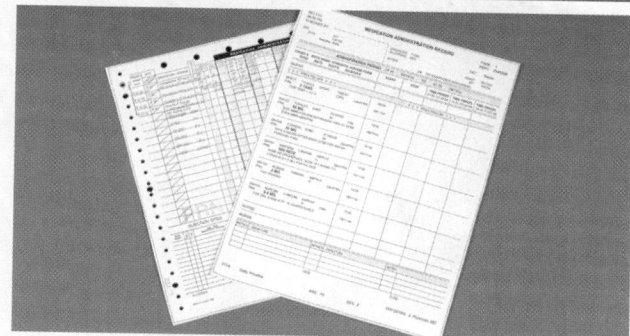

**Figure 34-10    Intake and output forms**

## IMPLEMENTATION—ACTION/RATIONALE

| ACTION | RATIONALE |
|---|---|
| **Intake** | |
| 1.  Wash hands. | 1.  Reduces transmission of microorganisms. |
| 2.  Explain rules of I&O record. All fluids taken orally must be recorded on the client's intake and output form (sometimes called a fluid balance flow sheet). | 2.  Elicits patient support. |
| •  Client must void into bedpan or urinal, not into toilet (Figures 34-11 and 34-12). | •  Fluid voided into the toilet cannot be measured. |
| •  Toilet tissue should be disposed of in plastic-lined container, not in bedpan. | •  Liquids absorbed into toilet tissue cannot be measured by volume. |

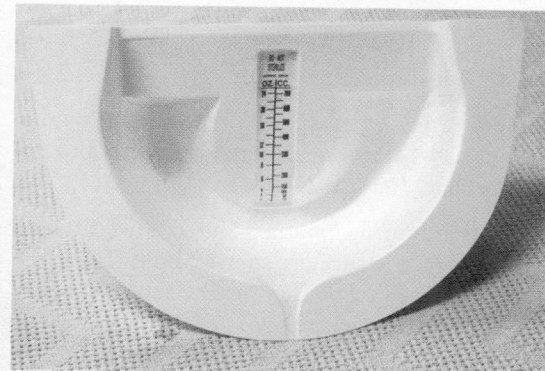

**Figure 34-11    Bedpan and urinal, protective pad, and graduated specimen container**

**Figure 34-12    Graduated specimen container is used to measure urine, drainage, or other output.**

| | |
|---|---|
| 3.  Measure all oral fluids in accord with agency policy (e.g., cup = 150 ml, glass = 240 ml). | 3.  Provides for consistency of measurement. |

*(continues)*

## PROCEDURE 34-1 (continued)

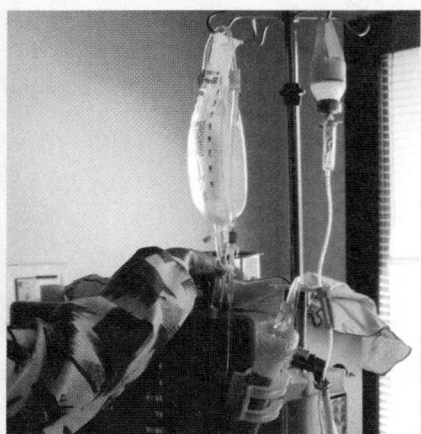

**Figure 34-13    All IV-infused fluids must be measured.**

- Record all IV fluids as they are infused (Figure 34-13).

4. Record time and amount of all fluid intake in the designated space on bedside form (oral, tube feedings, IV fluids).

4. Documents fluids.

5. Transfer 8-hour total fluid intake from bedside I&O record to graphic sheet or 24-hour I&O record on client's chart.

5. Provides for data analysis of client's fluid status.

6. Record all forms of intake, except blood and blood products, in the appropriate column of the 24-hour record.

6. Documents intake by type and amount.

7. Complete 24-hour intake record by adding all 8-hour totals.

7. Provides consistent data for analysis of client's fluid status over a 24-hour period.

### Output

8. Apply nonsterile gloves.

8. Reduces potential for transmission of pathogens.

9. Empty urinal, bedpan, or Foley drainage bag (Figure 34-14) into graduated container or commode "hat" (Figure 34-15).

9. Provides accurate measurement of urine.

- Other output may also be recorded, including nasogastric suction, suction bulb (i.e., Jackson-Pratt or Hemovac) or chest tubes. Refer to agency policy.

10. Remove gloves and wash hands.

10. Prevents cross-contamination.

11. Record time and amount of output (urine, drainage from nasogastric tube, drainage tube) on bedside I&O record.

11. Documents output.

12. Transfer 8-hour output totals to graphic sheet or 24-hour I&O record on the client's chart.

12. Provides for data analysis of client's fluid status.

*(continues)*

**PROCEDURE 34-1 (continued)**

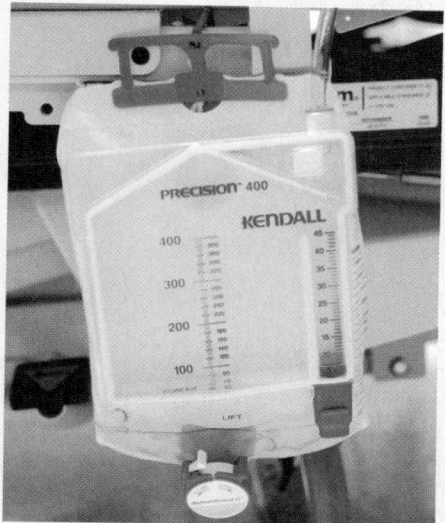

**Figure 34-14    Urine in Foley drainage bag must be measured.**

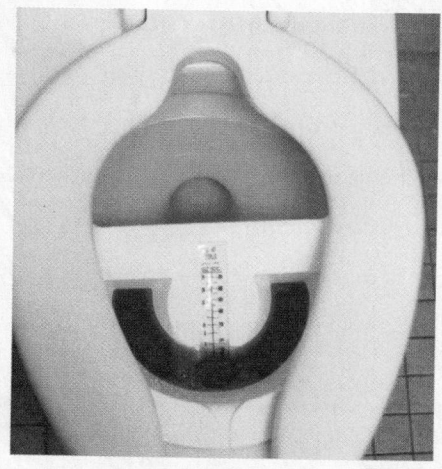

**Figure 34-15    Empty urine into a graduated container to measure.**

13. Complete 24-hour output record by totaling all 8-hour totals.

14. Wash hands.

13. Provides consistent data for analysis of client's fluid status over a 24-hour period.

14. Reduces transmission of microorganisms.

 ## LIFE SPAN CONSIDERATIONS

### Monitoring Intake and Output

**Pediatric Variations**

- The amount of fluid loss a child can tolerate is much smaller than that of an adult because of the proportionately smaller size of the child. Small amounts of fluid loss can be serious or fatal for small children.

- Infants and young children are at risk for fluid and electrolyte imbalances from prolonged fever or gastroenteritis.

**Geriatric Variations**

- Older clients are sometimes incontinent. Measuring output in an incontinent client can be challenging. Weighing the client's linen or incontinence pad prior to use and then weighing it again after it has been soiled can help the caregiver keep track of the amount of fluid output the client is generating.

- Older clients need a caregiver to monitor their fluid intake, especially when they are taking diuretics, supplemental potassium, and cardiac medication.

- Older clients are at risk for fluid and electrolyte imbalances from prolonged fever or gastroenteritis.

## Forced Fluids

Forcing or encouraging the intake of oral fluids, mainly water, may be done when treating older clients who are at risk for dehydration and clients with renal and urinary problems—for example, kidney stones. Compliance is obtained by client education and preference relative to timing and the type of liquids.

A client might, for example, be requested to consume 2,000 ml over a 24-hour period. If the client is intimidated on hearing this amount, which may sound very large, explain that the number of glasses to which this volume equates is only eight. Follow a similar time frame as set forth for restricted fluids, with the largest quantity of fluids administered with meals. Ice, gelatin, and ice cream count as liquid intake.

## Maintain Tube Feeding

When the client cannot ingest oral fluids and has a normal GI tract, fluids and nutrients can be administered through a feeding tube as prescribed by a health care practitioner. Refer to Chapter 37 for a complete discussion of feeding tubes.

## Monitor Intravenous Therapy

When fluid losses are severe or the client cannot tolerate oral or tube feedings, fluid volume is replaced parenterally through the intravenous route. **Intravenous (IV) therapy** is the administration of fluids, electrolytes, nutrients, or medications by the venous route. IV therapy is used to treat or prevent fluid and electrolyte or nutritional imbalances. The nurse has specific responsibilities relative to IV therapy (see the Nursing Strategy box).

The Intravenous Nurses Society (INS) is the professional organization that establishes standards of practice to promote excellence in intravenous nursing to ensure the highest quality, cost-effective care for all individuals requiring infusion therapies (INS, 2000). INS standards of practice direct the development of agency policy/protocols in accordance with state and federal regulations and should complement the manufacturer's direction for usage. The nurse should review the agency's protocols before gathering the equipment. IV therapy requires parenteral fluids (solutions) and special equipment: administration set, IV pole, filter, regulators to control IV flow rate, and an established venous route.

## Parenteral Fluids

The nurse confirms the type and amount of IV solution by reading prescription in the medical record. IV solutions

## NURSING STRATEGY

### Implementation of IV Therapy

- Know why the therapy is prescribed.

- Document client understanding.

- Select the appropriate equipment in accordance to agency policy.

- Obtain the correct solution as prescribed.

- Assess the client for allergies: tape, iodine, ointment, or antibiotic preparations to be used for skin preparation of the venipuncture site.

- Administer the fluid at the prescribed rate.

- Observe for signs of **infiltration** (the seepage of substances into the interstitial tissue that occurs as the results of accidental dislodgment of the needle from the vein) and other complications that are fluid-specific.

- Document implementation of prescribed IV therapy in the client's medical record.

---

are sterile, and those that are incompatible with plastic are dispensed in glass containers.

Plastic IV solution bags collapse under atmospheric pressure to allow the solution to enter the infusion set. Plastic solution bags are packaged with an outer plastic bag, which should remain intact until the nurse prepares the solution for administration. When the plastic solution bag is removed from its outer wrapper, the solution bag should be dry. If the solution bag is wet, the solution should not be used. The moisture on the bag indicates that the integrity of the bag has been compromised and that the solution cannot be considered sterile. The bag should be returned to the dispensing department that issued the solution. Glass containers are discussed in the section on equipment.

IV solutions are usually packaged in quantities ranging from 50 to 1,000 ml. The nurse should select a container that has the prescribed amount of solution or select several containers that together contain the prescribed volume. *At no time should the nurse select a container whose volume is greater than that prescribed.* For example, if the client is to receive 600 ml of normal (0.9%) saline, the nurse must not select a 1,000 ml container, but rather two containers, 100 ml and 500 ml (containers are not prepared in volumes of 600 ml). **Crystalloids** (electrolyte solutions with the potential to form crystals) are used to replace concurrent losses of water and electrolytes. Sodium chloride and Ringer's lactate are commonly used crystalloid solutions.

Parenteral fluids are classified in accord with the tonicity of the fluid relative to normal blood plasma. As previously discussed, an osmolar solution can be hypotonic, isotonic, or hypertonic. The type of solution is prescribed on the basis of the client's diagnosis and the goal of therapy. The normal osmolarity of blood is between 280 and 295 mOsm/L, so the desired effect of the tonicity of the fluid is determined as follows:

1. Hypotonic fluid (hypo-osmolar, less than 290 mOsm/L) lowers the osmotic pressure and causes fluid to move into the cells. If fluid is infused beyond the client's tolerance, water intoxication may result.
2. Isotonic fluid (iso-osmolar, 290 mOsm/L) increases extracellular fluid volume. If fluid is infused beyond the client's tolerance, cardiac overload may result.
3. Hypertonic fluid (hyperosmolar, greater than 290 mOsm/L) increases the osmotic pressure of the blood plasma, drawing fluid from the cells. If fluid is infused beyond the client's tolerance, cellular dehydration (Bulechek & McCloskey, 2000) and EC volume overload may result.

Table 34-8 discusses the common types of intravenous solutions in terms of their tonicity, contents, and clinical usage.

Crystalloid solutions can be isotonic (equal to the sodium chloride concentration of blood, 0.9% NaCL); hypotonic (less than the sodium chloride concentration of blood, 0.45% NaCL); and hypertonic (greater than the sodium chloride concentration of blood, 0.3% NS) (Kee & Paulanka, 2000).

Colloids (nondiffusable substances) function like plasma proteins in blood by exerting a colloidal pressure to expand intravascular volume. Examples of colloidal solutions are albumin, dextran, Plasmanate, and hetastarch (artificial blood substitute). During the administration of these solutions, the nurse should monitor the client for hypotension and allergic reactions (Bulechek & McCloskey, 2000; Kee & Paulanka, 2000). Blood transfusions are discussed later in this chapter.

### Equipment

IV equipment is sterile, disposable, and prepackaged with user instructions. The user instructions are usually placed on the outside of the package, with a schematic that labels the parts, allowing the user to read the package prior to opening. The following discussion regarding intravenous equipment, inclusive of the frequency of when to change disposal intravenous therapy equipment, is based on the revised *2000 Infusion Nursing Standards of Practice* developed by INS. All intravenous equipment must be inspected by the nurse to determine the integrity of the IV product before, during, and after use. Product integrity refers to the sterility of the equipment. Products are assessed for integrity by visual examination of the product and checking the expiration date on the equipment. All products identified with a defect must be returned to the appropriate

## TABLE 34-8    COMMON INTRAVENOUS SOLUTIONS

| Tonicity | Solution | Contents (MEq/L) | Clinical Implications |
|----------|----------|------------------|----------------------|
| Hypotonic | Sodium chloride 0.45% | 77 $Na^+$, 77 $Cl^-$ | Daily maintenance of body fluid and establishment of renal function |
| Isotonic | Dextrose 2.5% in 0.45% saline | 77 $Na^+$, 77 $Cl^-$ | Promotes renal function and urine output |
| | Dextrose 5% in 0.2% saline | 38 $Na^+$, 38 $Cl^-$ | Daily maintenance of body fluids when less $Na^+$ and $Cl^-$ are required |
| | Dextrose 5% in water ($D_5W$) | | Promotes rehydration and elimination; may cause urinary $Na^+$ loss; good vehicle for $K^+$ |
| | Ringer's lactate | 130 $Na^+$, 4 $K^+$, $Ca^{2+}$, 109 $Cl^-$, 28 lactate | Resembles the normal composition of blood serum and plasma; $K^+$ level below body's daily requirement |
| | Normal saline (NS), 0.9% | 154 $Na^+$, 154 $Cl^-$ | Restores sodium chloride deficit and extracellular fluid volume |
| | Dextran 40 10% in NS (0.9%) or $D_5W$ | | A colloidal solution used to increase plasma volume of clients in early shock. *It should not be given to* severely dehydrated clients and clients with renal disease, thrombocytopenia, or active hemorrhaging. |
| | Dextran 70% in NS | | A long-lived (20 hours) plasma volume expander. Used to treat shock or impending shock due to hemorrhage, surgery, or burns. *It can prolong bleeding and coats the RBCs (draw type and cross-match prior to administering).* |
| Hypertonic | Dextrose 5% in 0.45% saline | 77 $Na^+$, 77 $Cl^-$ | Daily maintenance of body fluid and nutrition; treatment of FVD |
| | Dextrose 5% in saline 0.9% | 154 $Na^+$, 154 $Cl^-$ | Fluid replacement of sodium, chloride, and calories (170) |
| | Dextrose 10% in saline 0.9% | 154 $Na^+$, 154 $Cl^-$ | Fluid replacement of sodium, chloride, and calories (340) |
| | Dextrose 5% in lactated Ringer's | 130 $Na^+$, 4 $K^+$, 3 $Ca^{2+}$, 109 $Cl^-$, 28 lactate | Resembles the normal composition of blood serum and plasma; $K^+$ level below body's daily requirement; caloric value 180 |
| | Hyperosmolar saline 3% and 5% NaCl | 856 $Na^+$, 865 $Cl^-$ | Treatment of hyponatremia; raises the $Na^+$ osmolarity of the blood, and reduces intracellular fluid excess |
| | Ionosol B with dextrose 5% | 57 $Na^+$, 25 $K^+$, 49 $Cl^-$, 25 lactate, 5 $Mg^{2+}$, 7 $PO_4^-$ | Treatment of polyionic parenteral replacement caused by vomiting-induced alkalosis, diabetic acidosis, fluid loss from burns, and postoperative FVD |

*(continues)*

| TABLE 34-8 | COMMON INTRAVENOUS SOLUTIONS (*continued*) | | |
|---|---|---|---|
| Hypertonic (*continued*) | Ionosol D-CM with dextrose 5% | 138 $Na^+$, 12 $K^+$, 5 $Ca^{2+}$, 108 $Cl^-$, 50 lactate, 3 $Mg^{2+}$ | Treatment of electrolyte losses of duodenal fluids caused by intestinal suction or biliary or pancreatic drainage; treatment of mild acidosis. |
| | Aminosyn RF 5.2% | 5.4 $K^+$ | Restores fluid and protein and promotes wound healing. |
| | Aminosyn II 3.5% | 18 $Na^+$ | Treatment of malnourished older clients and hypoproteinemia; *it is not to be given to clients with severe liver damage.* |

From Kee, J. L., & Paulanka, B. J. (2000). *Fluids and electrolytes with clinical applications* (6th ed.). Clifton Park, NY: Delmar Learning.

department within the agency with a written report identifying the defect.

Since intravenous therapy provides a direct access into the vascular system, the nurse must understand the basic epidemiology principles and common organisms that may cause an infection and observe infection control measures to minimize the potential for infectious complications. The nurse uses aseptic technique and Standard Precautions when assembling and changing intravenous equipment. To decrease the risk of pathogen transmission, handwashing is required before and immediately after all IV procedures and upon removal of gloves. The frequency of changing sterile intravenous equipment not only reflects the national standards of practice but the agency's established infection control policies. Infection control data may allow the agency to increase the time interval beyond the recommended standard provided the data verifies low infection rates. INS (2000) recommends that an organization that exhibits an increased rate of catheter-related bloodstream infection with the practice of 72-hour administration set changes should return to a 48-hour administration set change interval.

### Administration Set

The administration set (infusion set) refers to the plastic disposal tubing that provides for the infusion of a solution. There are several types of infusion sets to accommodate the solution and the mode of administration: primary continuous, secondary, primary intermittent, and special tubing for certain solutions such as blood/blood components. There are several add-on devices, such as extension sets, filters, stopcocks, PRN adaptor, and needleless devices that are used in conjunction with the administration set and changed whenever the set is changed. Administration sets are changed at established time intervals and immediately upon suspected contamination or when the integrity of the set has been compromised. The administration set contains an insertion spike with a protective cap, a drip chamber, tubing with a slide clamp and

regulating (roller) clamp, a rubber injection port, and a protective cap over the needle adapter. The protective caps keep both ends of the infusion set sterile and are removed only just before usage. The insertion spike is inserted into the port of the IV solution container.

Infusion sets can be vented or nonvented. The nonvented type is used with plastic bags of IV solutions and vented bottles. The vented set is used for glass containers that are not vented.

Glass containers require an air vent so that air can displace fluid from the container into the IV tubing. Some glass bottles are vented with an inside tube that exits the bottle into a rubber stopper in the neck of the bottle; if the bottle is not vented, then the nurse needs to select a vented infusion set.

The drip chamber is calibrated to allow a predictable amount of fluid to be delivered. There are two types of drip chambers: a macrodrip, which delivers 10 to 20 drops per milliliter of solution, and a microdrip, which delivers 60 drops per milliliter. The drip rate varies with the manufacturer as indicated on the package.

The administration set has a manual flow-control device such as a slide clamp (Figure 34-16), a roller clamp, or a screw to regulate a prescribed infusion rate. Follow the manufacturer's guidelines when using the manual flow-control device to regulate the prescribed infusion rate. The end of the IV tubing contains a needle adapter that attaches to the sterile device inserted in the client's vein. Extension tubing may be used to lengthen the primary tubing. A primary continuous administration set is used to administer routine solutions prescribed to infuse continuously over a 24-hour period. The primary administration set, inclusive of the add-on devices, is changed every 48 to 72 hours in conjunction with the peripheral cannula change. A bag of intravenous solution should not hang longer than 24 hours. Secondary administration sets are often referred to as "piggyback" administration sets. The secondary tubing is connected into the primary tubing at an injection site (Figure 34-17) and allows for the administration of a second solution such as medication.

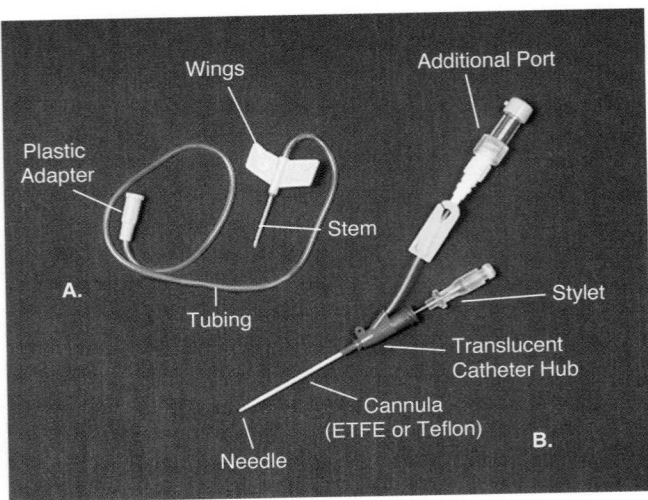

**Figure 34-16**   **Peripheral IV devices: A. Butterfly B. Angiocatheter**

Secondary administration sets are also changed every 48 to 72 hours.

Primary intermittent administration sets are used to deliver medications at prescribed intervals through an injection/access port and are changed every 48 to 72 hours; all add-on devices such as extension sets, filters, PRN adapters, and stopcocks are changed with the intermittent administration set. A sterile needle/needleless device should be aseptically attached to the intermittent administration set prior to administering the medication and removed immediately after each use.

### Health Hazard

A *Health Alert* from Health Care Without Harm (HCWH) (1999) cautioned the public about the potential risks of exposure to diethylhexyl phthalates (DEHP) from medical products such as IV bags and tubing. More than 500 million IV bags are used in the United States every year to deliver blood, medication, and other essential solutions to clients (HCWH, 1999). Eighty percent of the IV bags are made with polyvinyl chloride (PVC), which requires a plasticizer to make the bags soft and flexible. DEHP is the softener used in PVC products. DEHP has been shown to leach from IV bags into the solutions they contain and directly into the client's bloodstream.

The Environmental Protection Agency has classified DEHP as a probable human carcinogen, and HCWH claims that studies have shown that DEHP can damage

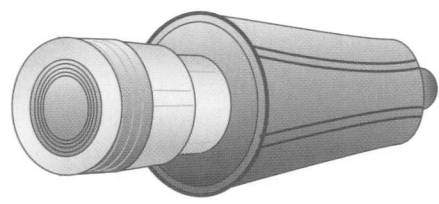

**Figure 34-17**   **Luer lock injection site**

the heart, liver, testes, and kidneys and interfere with sperm production. Certain drugs such as Taxol (used to treat breast cancer) and Taxotere (used to treat ovarian and breast cancer and AIDS-related Kaposi's sarcoma) have been shown to increase the leaching of DEHP from PVC plastics into the solution (Stewart, 1999); see Box 34-6 for additional drugs that can increase leaching of DEHP from PVC IV products. Although one leading producer of intravenous vinyl IV bags containing DEHP plans to develop an alternative to PVC for its products, no time frames were given to totally remove these products from the market.

A second health hazard is inherent in the use of DEHP. The disposal of medical products containing DEHP releases highly toxic and endocrine-disrupting dioxins. PVC is the only plastic linked both to phthalate chemical leaching and to the production of dioxin (Health Care Without Harm, 1999).

### Intravenous Filters

Intravenous filters prevent the passage of undesirable substances such as particulate matter and air from entering the vascular system. Particulate matter filters are used when preparing infusion medications for administration to prevent obstruction in the vascular/pulmonary systems, irritation, and **phlebitis** (inflammation of a vein). Air-eliminating filters are used for the delivery of infusion therapy to decrease the potential of air emboli; the filter should be located as close as possible to the cannula site. IV filters come in various sizes; the finer the filter, the greater is the degree of solution filtration. Although studies have shown that IV filters reduce the risk of bacteremia and phlebitis as much as 40%, some agencies do not use IV filters because of cost. Many IV catheters contain an in-line filter; if the catheter has an in-line filter, it is not necessary to add a filter to the tubing.

---

**BOX 34-6    DRUGS THAT INCREASE LEACHING OF DEHP FROM PVC PLASTICS**

- Chemotherapeutic agents: Etoposide (VePesid) and Teniposide (Vumon)

- Antianxiety agents: Chlordiazepoxide HCl (Librium)

- Antifungal agents: Miconazole (Monistat IV)

- Immunosuppressive agents: Cyclosporine (Sandimmune) and Tacrolimus (Prograf)

- Nutritional solutions: Fat emulsions and vitamin A

Adapted from Stewart, M. (1999, March/April). IV bags pose patient risk. *The American Nurse*, 12.

## LIFE SPAN CONSIDERATIONS

### Age Considerations for Choosing IVs and Equipment

Neonates, infants, and children are often suscepti-ble to *Excess Fluid Volume* related to overhydration because of the risk for administering too much IV fluid administration. IV tubing with a microdrip and special volume control chambers is used to regulate the amount of fluid to be administered over a specific time interval. Armboards and soft restraints are used to stabilize peripheral infusions by immobilizing the extremity to prevent accidental removal of infusion devices.

## CLINICAL ALERT

### Preventing Needle-Stick Injuries in Health Care Settings

Health care workers should take the following steps to protect themselves and their fellow work-ers from needle-stick injuries:

- Avoid the use of needles where safe and effec-tive alternatives are available.

- Help your employer select and evaluate devices with safety features.

- Use devices with safety features provided by your employer.

- Avoid recapping needles.

- Plan for safe handling and disposal before beginning any procedure using needles.

- Dispose of used needles promptly in sharps disposal containers.

- Report all needle-stick and other sharps-relat-ed injuries promptly to ensure that you receive appropriate follow-up care.

- Tell your employer about hazards from needles that you observe in your work environment.

- Participate in blood-borne pathogen training, and follow recommended infection prevention practices, including hepatitis B vaccination.

Centers for Disease Control. (2003). http://www.cdc.gov

### Needles and Venous Peripheral-Short Catheters

Needles and peripheral-short catheters provide access to the venous system. A variety of devices are available in different sizes to complement the age of the client, the type and duration of the therapy, and to protect the user from injury.

As with any gauge needle, the larger the number, the smaller the lumen. The nurse considers the client's age, body size, and the type of solution to be administered when selecting the gauge of the needle or catheter:

- Infants and small children, 24 gauge
- Preschool through preteen, 24 or 22 gauge
- Teenagers and adults, 22 or 20 gauge
- Geriatric, 22 or 24 gauge

**Butterfly** (scalp vein or wing-tipped) **needles** are short, beveled needles with plastic flaps attached to the shaft. The flaps (which are flexible) are held tightly togeth-er to facilitate ease of insertion and then flattened against the skin to prevent dislodgment during infusion. These needles are commonly used for short-term or intermittent therapy and for infants and children.

Several types of short catheters are used to access peripheral veins. Short peripheral venous catheters vary in length from ¾ to 1¼ inches. During insertion, some of these catheters are threaded over a needle, and others are threaded inside a needle. **Intracath** is a term used to refer to a plastic tube inserted into a vein. An **angiocatheter** is a type of intracath with a metal stylet to pierce the skin and vein, after which the plastic catheter is threaded into the vein and the metal stylet is removed, leaving only the plas-tic catheter in the vein. Short venous catheters can have safety devices to reduce the risk of accidental needlesticks. These devices are designed to allow for easy insertion of the catheter while providing a built-in safety feature for the user. As the catheter is threaded over the needle and advanced into the vein, the built-in needle guard advances forward toward the tip of the needle; when the catheter hub is removed from the device, the entire needle is encased within the needle guard.

### Peripheral Intravenous (PI) and Heparin Locks

Peripheral intravenous (PI) and heparin locks (i.e., inter-mittent venous locks) are devices that establish a venous route as a precautionary measure for clients whose condi-tion may change rapidly or who may require intermittent infusion therapy. A butterfly needle or peripheral catheter is inserted into a vein and the hub is capped with a lock port, also called a Luer lock (Figure 34-17).

### Needle-Free System

Safety is a concern associated with IV therapy. Accidental needle-stick injuries and puncture wounds with contami-nated devices increase the employee's risk for infectious diseases such as HIV, hepatitis (B and C), and other viral, rickettsial, bacterial, fungal, and parasitic infections. Most health care agencies now use totally needle-free IV systems (Figure 34-18) to decrease the risk of employee injuries.

## Vascular Access Devices

Vascular access devices (VAD) include various catheters, cannulas, and infusion ports that allow for long-term IV therapy or repeated access to the central venous system. The kind of VAD used depends on the client's diagnosis and the type and length of treatment (see Table 34-9). Site selection and insertion of central catheters, other than peripherally inserted central catheters, is a medical act. Although there are many types of catheter materials, insertion techniques, and kinds of central catheters, *all central catheters must be radiopaque to allow for radiographic verification of placement of the catheter and its tip prior to the administration of any solution.*

Central catheters are usually inserted into the internal jugular and subclavian veins with the distal tip located in the superior vena cava to minimize vessel irritation and sclerosis. The femoral vein can be used for central venous access when there is thrombosis of the internal jugular or subclavian veins; correct tip location is the inferior vena cava. Insertion of a central catheter can be performed either percutaneously or surgically. Surgically, a central catheter is either placed entirely under the skin (implanted), or the catheter partially exits the skin (tunneled).

A tunneled catheter is inserted through the subcutaneous tissue, usually between the nipple and clavicle, with the catheter tip inserted through the cephalic or external jugular vein and threaded to the right atrium.

An **implantable port** is a device made of a radiopaque silicone catheter and a plastic or stainless steel injection port with a self-sealing silicone-rubber septum. The device is inserted into a subcutaneous pocket, usually over the third or fourth rib, lateral to the sternum. The distal tip of the catheter is surgically tunneled in the cephalic or external jugular vein, with the proximal end of the catheter tunneled through the subcutaneous tissue into the injection port of the device.

Implanted ports and pumps are vascular access devices that provide for the delivery of prescribed parenteral therapies. Accessing these devices requires the use of aseptic

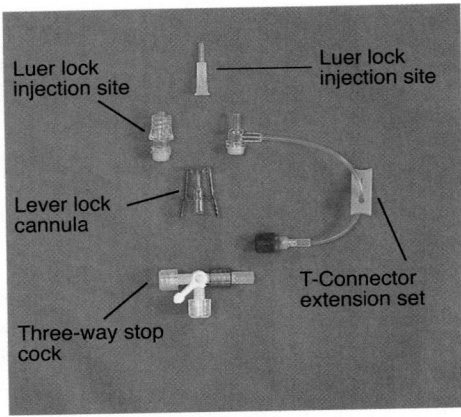

**Figure 34-18    Needle-free system**

## CLINICAL ALERT

### Inserting a CVC

When assisting with the insertion of a long-line central catheter, observe the client for symptoms of a pneumothorax: sudden shortness of breath or sharp chest pain; increased anxiety; a weak, rapid pulse; hypotension; pallor or cyanosis. These symptoms indicate accidental puncture of the pleural membrane.

technique. Noncoring needles such as a Huber needle are used to access an implanted port or pump and should be changed at least every 7 days. The smallest gauge noncoring needle that can deliver the prescribed therapy should be used when accessing the port or pump. Nurses caring for clients with implanted ports or pumps must have a thorough knowledge of the design features of the device, as explained in the manufacturer's guidelines, to ensure correct access and administration techniques, maintenance, and potential complications.

Implanted pumps have a reservoir designed to continuously infuse a specific volume of solution over a preset period of time; the pump must be routinely emptied and refilled at established intervals. Some pumps have an additional feature—a side port designed for administration of intermittent medication. The flow rate of some pumps is sensitive to changes in atmospheric pressure, body temperature, blood pressure, and the viscosity of the medications. Clients are instructed to report changes in their lifestyle and physical condition that may affect the pump's flow rate. *Only nurses who have been specially trained are allowed to access an implanted port or pump because of the risk of infiltration into the tissue if needle placement is incorrect.*

A peripherally inserted central catheter (PICC) is a silicone or polyurethane catheter inserted into one of the major veins in the antecubital fossa. Although the length of the catheter varies, on average a PICC is 52 cm long, and its tip resides in the lower-third section of the superior vena cava. A PICC can be trimmed at the time of insertion to a specific length that is determined by the approximate distance between the insertion site and the superior vena cava. The majority of state boards of registered nurses allow specially trained nurses to insert the PICC. Placement of the catheter's tip is confirmed by x-ray prior to the administration of any solution. The registered nurse who inserts the PICC must document the type of PICC inserted and the total length of the inserted catheter, and record if the length of the catheter was trimmed prior to insertion.

## Preparing an Intravenous Solution

To prepare an IV solution, read the agency's protocol and gather the necessary equipment. Because IV equipment and solutions are sterile, check the expiration date on the

## TABLE 34-9    VASCULAR ACCESS DEVICES

| Type | Brand Names | Use |
| --- | --- | --- |
| Nontunneled central venous catheter (single, double, triple lumen) | Hohn, Deseret | Short-term fluid or blood administration, obtaining blood specimens, and administering medications |
| Tunneled central venous catheter (single or double lumen) | Hickman, Broviac, Groshong | Long-term (months to years) fluid replacement therapy, medication administration, nutritional supplement, and blood specimen withdrawal |
| Implanted infusion port | Chemo-Port, Infuse-a-Port, Mediport, Port-a-Cath | Long-term (months to years) fluid replacement therapy, medication administration (especially chemotherapy), blood or blood product administration, and blood specimen withdrawal |
| Peripherally inserted central catheter (PICC) | C-PICC, Groshong PICC, SoloPICC | Long-term fluid replacement therapy, medication administration (chemotherapy, antibiotics, controlled narcotics), blood or blood product administration, and blood specimen withdrawal |

package prior to usage. The solution can be prepared at the nurses' work area or in the client's room (Procedure 34-2).

The nurse prepares and applies a time strip to the IV solution bag to facilitate monitoring of the infusion rate as prescribed by the health care practitioner. The IV tubing is tagged with the date and time to indicate when the tubing replacement is necessary. IV tubing is changed every 48 to 72 hours in accord with the agency's protocol. The nurse initials the time strip and IV tubing tag.

### Initiating IV Therapy

When initiating IV therapy, the nurse should assess for a venipuncture site. When assessing clients for potential sites, consider their age, body size, clinical status and impairments, and the skin condition (see the Nursing Strategy box for contraindications when selecting a site).

## CLINICAL ALERT

### Marking an IV Bag

Do not use a felt-tip pen to mark an IV bag; the ink from the pen can leak through the plastic and contaminate the solution. Do not label bag with time strip made of adhesive/silk/paper tape, as the adhesive will leach into the bag. Use only labels appropriate for IV bags.

Lower-extremity veins are used for IV therapy only when so prescribed by the health care practitioner; circulating blood in the lower extremities is likely to pool and clot, which may result in an embolism. Because contact with blood is likely, venipuncture requires the implementation of Standard Precautions. Refer to Chapter 24 for a complete discussion of Standard Precautions.

Select a vein for puncture at its most distal end to maintain the integrity of the vein, because venous blood flows with an upward movement toward the heart. When a vein is punctured with an instrument, such as a needle, fluids can infiltrate (leak from the vein into the tissue at the site of puncture). If IV therapy has to be discontinued for any reason, such as infiltration, it can be restarted above the initial puncture site only.

### Vein Finder

A vein finder is a device used to locate hard-to-find veins. It is helpful, for example, in working with obese clients whose superficial veins are difficult to locate. A Venoscope is a type of vein finder with adjustable fiber-optic arms that reveal veins. The room is dimmed, and the disposable skids are placed flush against the skin. The nurse slowly moves the Venoscope along the extremity until a dark, shadowy line is seen between the fiber-optic arms.

Once the vein is identified, it can also be checked to determine whether it is sclerotic. To assess for sclerotic veins, apply a downward pressure over the fiberoptic arms and observe the vein when pressure is applied and then released. A nonsclerotic vein will disappear with pressure and reappear when pressure is released.

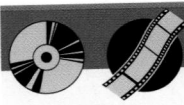

| PROCEDURE 34-2 | **Preparing an IV Solution** |

## EQUIPMENT NEEDED

■ IV solution in a bag or bottle (Figure 34-19)
■ Medication administration record (MAR)
■ IV flow sheet
■ IV tubing, if needed

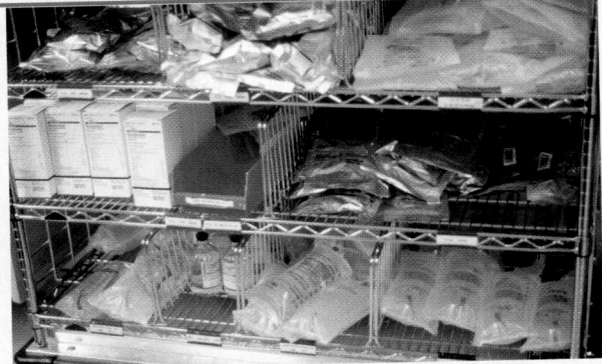

**Figure 34-19    Many types of prepackaged IV solutions are available.**

## IMPLEMENTATION—ACTION/RATIONALE

| ACTION | RATIONALE |
|---|---|
| 1. Check physician's or qualified practitioner's order for the IV solution. | 1. Ensures accurate administration of the solution. |
| 2. Wash hands. Apply gloves if required by institutional policy. | 2. Reduces transmission of microorganisms. |
| 3. Prepare new bag by removing protective cover from bag or bottle. | 3. Allows for access to the solution container. |
| 4. Inspect the bag or bottle for leaks, tears, or cracks. Inspect the fluid for clarity, particulate matter, and color. Check expiration date. | 4. Prevents infusing contaminated or outdated solution. |
| 5. Prepare a label for the IV bag or bottle: | 5. |
| • On the label, note date, time, and your initials. | • Communicates when the bag was opened. |
| • Attach the label to the bag or bottle. Keep in mind the bag or bottle will be inverted when it is hanging. Make sure the label can be read when the IV is hanging. | • Labeling the bag or bottle upside-down makes identification easier when the bottle is hanging. |
| 6. Store the prepared IV solution in the area assigned by the institution. | 6. Keeps the prepared solution readily available for when it is needed. |
| 7. Remove gloves and dispose of gloves with all used materials. | 7. Reduces transmission of microorganisms. |
| 8. Wash hands. | 8. Reduces transmission of microorganisms. |
| 9. Document the preparation of the IV solution. | 9. Provides a record to ensure continuity of care. |

*(continues)*

## PROCEDURE 34-2 (continued)

### Hanging the Prepared IV

10. Wash hands.

11. Obtain the IV solution for the client as ordered. Check the label on the IV bag to see that it matches the order.

12. Inspect the bag or bottle for leaks, tears, or cracks and inspect the fluid for clarity, particulate matter, and color.

13. Check client's identification bracelet.

14. Prepare an IV time tape for the IV bag or bottle:

    • On the time tape, note the rate at which the solution is to infuse.

    • Mark the approximate infusion intervals.

    • Attach the time tape to the bag or bottle. Keep in mind the bag or bottle will be inverted when it is hanging. Make sure the time tape can be read when the IV is hanging.

15. Make sure the clamp on the tubing is closed. Grasp the port of the IV bag with your nondominant hand, remove the plastic tab covering the port (Figure 34-20), and insert the full length of the spike into the bag's port (Figure 34-21).

10. Reduces transmission of microorganisms.

11. Ensures the ordered medication is administered.

12. Prevents infusing contaminated solution.

13. Ensures IV solution is given to the correct patient.

14. 

    • Communicates how long before the next IV should be hung.

    • Gives a rough estimate of the accuracy of the infusion rate.

    • Placing the time tape on the bag or bottle upside-down makes identification easier when the bottle is hanging.

15. Promotes rapid flow of solution through new tubing without air bubbles.

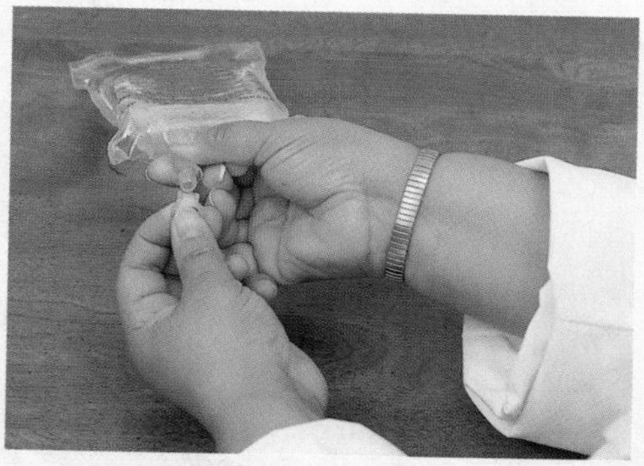

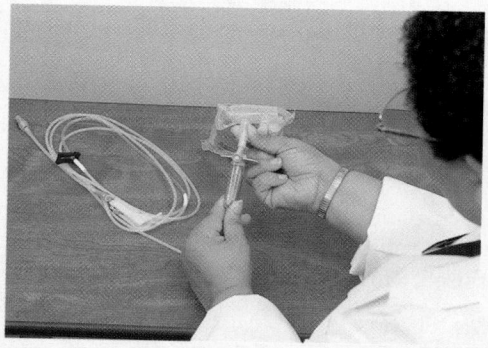

**Figure 34-20** Open the IV plastic bag and pull down the plastic tab covering the port with one hand while pinching the port with the other hand.

**Figure 34-21** Remove the cap from the spike and spike the IV port.

16. Compress drip chamber to fill halfway.

16. Filling chamber halfway allows the chamber to provide a clear measurement of drip rate when the IV is flowing.

*(continues)*

## PROCEDURE 34-2 *(continued)*

17. Loosen protective cap from the needle or end of the IV tubing, open roller clamp, and flush tubing with solution (Figure 34-22 A and B).

17. Removes air from tubing.

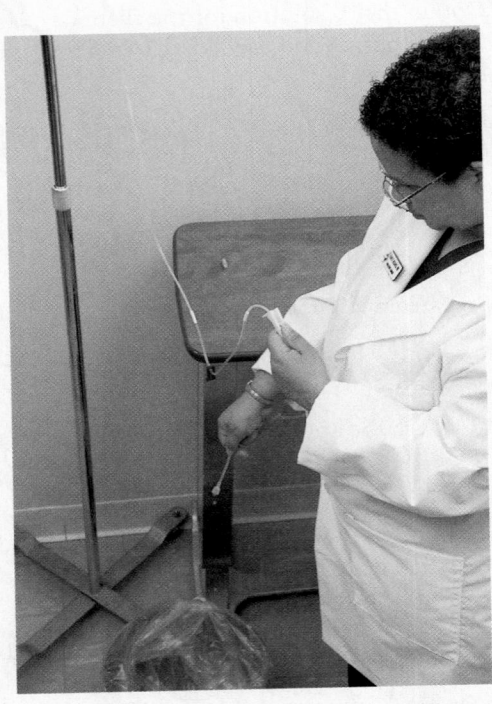

**Figure 34-22 A, B**　**A. Priming the IV tubing B. Open the roller clamp on the tubing to allow the fluid to enter the tube and expel the air.**

18. Close roller clamp and replace cap protector.

18. Prevents fluid from leaking and maintains sterility of needle.

19. When ready to initiate infusion, remove the cap protector from the tubing. Attach the IV tubing to venipuncture catheter.

19. Initiates infusion.

20. Open clamp and regulate flow or, if applicable, attach tubing to infusion device or rate controller if used. Turn on pump and set flow rate.

20. Allows flow rate to be regulated.

21. Wash hands.

21. Reduces transmission of microorganisms.

## Administering IV Therapy

Once the solution is prepared for administration, the nurse calculates the rate and explains the procedure to the client (see Procedure 34-3 for the administration of IV therapy). There are three ways to administer solutions:

1. Initiate the infusion by performing a venipuncture.
2. Use an existing IV system: catheter, heparin or PI lock, central line, or implanted port.
3. Add a solution to a continuous-infusion line.

Fluid administration can be continuous, ongoing over a 24-hour period, or intermittent, 1,000 ml ordered once in a 24-hour period. Although fluids may be continuous, the type of fluids can alternate over a 24-hour period; for example, an order might be *add 40 mEq of KCl to first bag of 1,000 ml of normal saline.*

IV medications may be **piggybacked**, added to an existing intravenous solution to infuse concurrently. IV solutions and medications that have been refrigerated should

## LIFE SPAN CONSIDERATIONS

### Fluid Administration

**Pediatric Variations**

- Small children require smaller volumes of fluid.

- Special effort needs to be taken to keep an IV site clean, dry, and intact in very young clients.

**Geriatric Variations**

- Older clients may be at higher risk of fluid overload. IV solutions containing sodium may increase fluid retention in older clients.

---

be warmed to room temperature before administration (usually 30 minutes) to increase client's comfort.

## Flushing

Flushing refers to the instillation of a solution into an intravenous cannula. Flushing is performed to assess and maintain cannula patency and prevent the mixing of incompatible medications and/or solutions, following the conversion of continuous IV therapy to intermittent IV therapy, and to maintain intermittent cannula patency following IV medication administration and blood sampling.

The type of solution and frequency of flushing an intermittent intravenous cannula is determined by the agency's policy/protocol. According to the INS (2000), flushing a cannula at established intervals with saline (0.9% sodium chloride injection) is the accepted solution to ensure and maintain patency of an intermittent PI cannula, while a heparin flush solution is the accepted solution to maintain patency of an intermittent central venous

devices. The volume of flush is equal to the volume capacity of the cannula and add-on devices times two (INS, 2000). Consideration is also given to the volume and frequency of heparin flush in order to prevent an alteration in the client's clotting factors.

When flushing a cannula, positive pressure within the lumen of the catheter must be maintained to prevent the reflex of blood into the cannula lumen. Use the manufacturer's recommended maximum pressure limits (pounds per square inch) when selecting the size of the syringe to

## CLINICAL ALERT

### Prepping Skin for Venipuncture

When prepping the client's skin for a venipuncture, cleanse the skin with Betadine and wait for it to dry. Do not apply alcohol after the skin has been prepped with Betadine. If these substances are combined, they form a toxic material that may be absorbed through the skin.

## NURSING STRATEGY

### Contraindications for Fluid Administration

The nurse should observe the venipuncture sites for the following contraindications:

- Signs of infection, infiltration, or thrombosis

- Affected arm of a postmastectomy client

- Arm with a functioning arteriovenous fistula

- Affected arm of a paralyzed client

- Any arm that has circulatory or neurologic impairments.

## LIFE SPAN CONSIDERATIONS

### Age Considerations for Initiating IV Therapy

The aging process causes physiological changes in the skin, muscles, and veins. The skin loses its durability, making it prone to tears and abrasions. Decrease in muscle mass may cause the vein to roll during puncture. The veins themselves are also more fragile in older clients. When first infusing fluid into the vein, administer it slowly and observe carefully for any sign of infiltration.

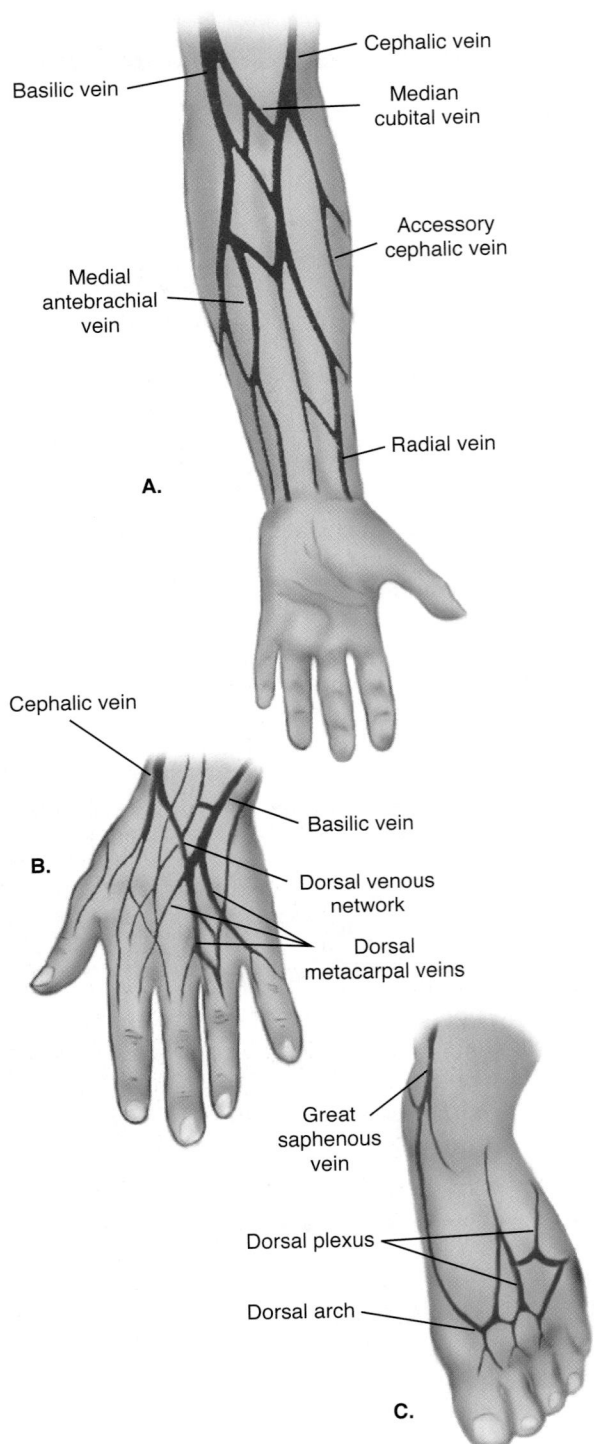

A.

Basilic vein
Cephalic vein
Median cubital vein
Accessory cephalic vein
Medial antebrachial vein
Radial vein

B.

Cephalic vein
Basilic vein
Dorsal venous network
Dorsal metacarpal veins

C.

Great saphenous vein
Dorsal plexus
Dorsal arch

**Figure 34-23    Peripheral veins used in intravenous therapy. A. Arm and forearm B. Dorsum of the hand C. Dorsal plexus of the foot**

use for flushing, since the smaller the syringe, the greater the pressure generated; excessive internal pressures in the device increase the potential for cannula damage and/or progressive internal cannula weakening over the life of the device (INS, 2000). If resistance is met when flushing a cannula, do not exert pressure in an attempt to restore

## CLINICAL ALERT

### Implementation

Instead of setting the total volume to be infused (e.g., 1,000 ml), set the volume slightly lower (e.g., 950 ml) so that the alarm will go off before the fluids are absorbed completely. This method will give you time to have the next bag of fluids ready when all 1,000 ml have been absorbed. This is especially helpful when dealing with refrigerated fluids that must be warmed to room temperature before administering. If you will be off duty when the volume will be absorbed and you have set the alarm to go off early, tell the oncoming nurse during report.

## RESEARCH FOCUS

**Title of Study:** The use of heparin and normal saline flushes in neonatal intravenous catheters

**Study Purpose:** To compare the use of heparin versus normal saline flush solutions on maintaining the patency of peripheral IV catheters in neonates.

**Methods:** This quasi-experimental study compared the outcomes in 87 infants with 159 IV starts who were 32 weeks or older gestation at birth; 32 received heparin, and 54 received normal saline.

**Findings:** There were no statistically significant differences in the duration of patency between the groups receiving heparin and normal saline; however, the duration of patency was significantly longer for term than pre-term infants and for insertion in the scalp, arm, or hand veins rather than the leg or foot veins.

**Implications:** Although this study found no difference in the duration of patency relative to the type of flush solution, two other variables were identified for duration of patency for IV catheters: gestational age and site of insertion. Results of this study also demonstrated the cost-saving benefit to the agency when using saline as a flush solution rather than heparin.

Paisley, M. K., Stamper, M., Brown, J., Brown, N., & Ganong, L. H. (1997). The use of heparin and normal saline flushes in neonatal intravenous catheters. *Pediatric Nursing, 23*(5), 521–524, 527.

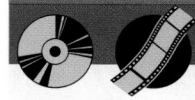

**PROCEDURE 34-3**     **Adding Medications to an IV Solution**

## EQUIPMENT NEEDED

▰ Prescribed medication in vial or ampoule
   (Figure 34-24)
▰ Prescribed diluent for medication
▰ Sterile syringe of appropriate size (5–20 ml)
▰ Sterile needle (1–1½ inches, 19–21 gauge)
▰ Sterile IV bag (500–100 ml)
▰ Antiseptic swab
▰ Label for IV bag
▰ Medication administration record

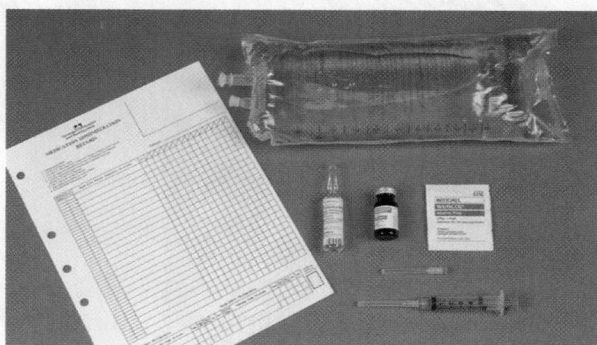

**Figure 34-24    Medications may be ordered to be added to IV solutions for administration.**

## IMPLEMENTATION—ACTION/RATIONALE

| ACTION | RATIONALE |
|---|---|
| 1. Check physician's or qualified practitioner's order for the IV solution and additives ordered. | 1. Ensures accurate administration of the solution and additives. |
| 2. Determine whether the ordered additives are compatible with the IV solution and with each other. | 2. Multiple additives increase the possibility of incompatibility. Some medications can only be mixed in saline. |
| 3. Wash hands. Apply gloves if required by institutional policy. | 3. Reduces transmission of microorganisms. |
| 4. Using the appropriate technique, draw up any additives ordered by the physician or qualified practitioner (Figure 34-25). | 4. Ordered additives may come in vials, ampoules, or bags. |

### Adding Medication to a New Solution

| ACTION | RATIONALE |
|---|---|
| 5. Prepare new bag by removing protective cover from bag or bottle. | 5. Allows for access to the injection port. |
| 6. Inspect the bag or bottle for leaks, tears, or cracks. Inspect the fluid for clarity, particulate matter, and color. Check expiration date. | 6. Prevents infusing contaminated or outdated solution. |
| 7. Add medication to IV solution: | 7. |
| • For plastic IV bag, locate port with rubber stopper. | • Avoids use of port of the IV tubing or the air vent. |
| • For IV bottle, locate the X, circle, or triangle indicating the IV injection site. | • Ensures the medication enters the bottle. |
| • Wipe off port or site with antiseptic swab. | • Reduces transmission of microorganisms. |
| • Insert needle into center of port or site. | • Facilitates adding medication to bag. |

*(continues)*

**PROCEDURE 34-3** *(continued)*

- Inject medication into bag (Figure 34-26).
- Remove needle from bag.

- Facilitates adding medication to bag.
- Injection ports are self-sealing.

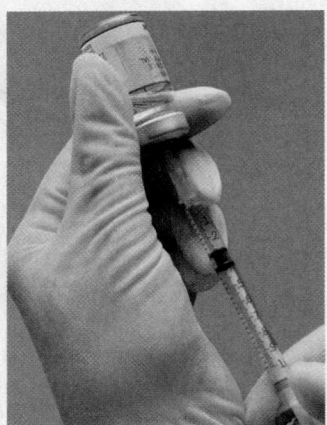

**Figure 34-25**    Draw the medication into the syringe.

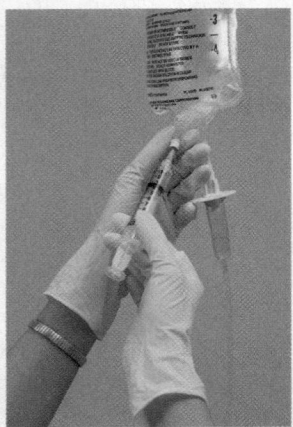

**Figure 34-26**    Inject the medication into the bag.

8. Mix medication into IV solution by gently turning the bag from end to end.

9. Label the bag:
   - Write the name and dose of medication. Write date, time, and nurse's initials.
   - Apply to bag upside-down.

10. Store the prepared IV solution in the area assigned by the institution.

8. Ensures even distribution of medication throughout the solution.

9.
   - Informs nurses and doctors regarding medications added to the solution.
   - Allows easy visualization when bag is hanging.

10. Keeps the prepared solution readily available for when it is needed.

## Adding Medication to an Existing Solution

11. Identify client using armband and calling name.

12. Explain the purpose of the medication and how it will be given.

13. Clamp the IV tubing and remove bag from IV pole.

14. Add medication to IV solution:
   - For plastic IV bag, locate port with rubber stopper.
   - For IV bottle, locate the X, circle, or triangle indicating the IV injection site.
   - Wipe off port or site with antiseptic swab.
   - Insert needle into center of port or site.
   - Inject medication into bag.
   - Remove needle from bag.

11. Ensures correct client received the medication.

12. Information reduces anxiety.

13. Prevents medication from being infused rapidly.

14.
   - Avoids use of port of the IV tubing or the air vent.
   - Ensures the medication enters the bottle.
   - Reduces transmission of microorganisms.
   - Facilitates adding medication to bag.
   - Facilitates adding medication to bag.
   - Injection ports are self-sealing.

*(continues)*

**PROCEDURE 34-3** *(continued)*

| | |
|---|---|
| 15. Mix medication into IV solution by gently turning the bag from end to end. | 15. Ensures even distribution of medication throughout the solution. |
| 16. Apply a new label: | 16. |
| • Write the name and dose of medication. Write date, time, and nurse's initials. | • Informs nurses and doctors regarding medications added to the solution. |
| • Apply to bag upside-down. | • Allows easy visualization when bag is hanging. |
| 17. Unclamp the tubing and regulate the flow. | 17. Prevents rapid infusion of the medication. |
| 18. Remove gloves and dispose of all used materials appropriately. | 18. Reduces transmission of organisms. |
| 19. Wash hands. | 19. Reduces transmission of organisms. |
| 20. Document the preparation of the IV solution. | 20. Provides a record to ensure continuity of care. |

# LIFE SPAN CONSIDERATIONS

## Fluid Administration Considerations

### Pediatric Variations

- Giving a medication to a child through an established IV may be less traumatic than an IM or subcutaneous injection.

- Special effort needs to be taken to keep an IV site clean, dry, and intact in very young clients.

- Remember that there is even less room for fluid and electrolyte and fluid volume administration errors in infants and children. Double-check all orders to make sure the additives and the infusion amounts are appropriate for the age of the child.

- Play therapy can be used with a child to help her understand the IV therapy. Play with the child as the child tapes and maintains an IV (without needles) on a doll or teddy bear. As you do, explain what is happening in simple terms appropriate for the child's age. Remind the child that this is one of the things nurses do to help sick people get better.

### Geriatric Variations

- Older clients may react more slowly to IV medications due to impaired circulation.

- Older clients may have more fragile veins and skin, which will be very sensitive to irritating additives.

- Older adults may have decreased renal and liver function, which can affect how IV additives and medications affect them.

- Older clients have more fragile veins and need extra-careful assessment for signs of infiltration.

- Veins in older clients tend to "blow" much easier than those of younger clients.

- When you tape an IV on an older person, try not to use too much tape. Use the least abrasive tape you have available to reduce the irritation to the skin.

- Be careful when removing tape as you may pull the skin off.

## COMMUNITY/HOME CARE

### Fluid Administration Considerations

#### Home Care Variations

- Medications should be added to IV solutions by the pharmacist before dispensing them for home use.

- Make sure the caregiver can clearly read and understand the labels on the IV bag and any additive labels.

- Assess that the client or caregiver can determine if an additive has been added to an IV bag.

- Educate the caregiver to recognize signs and symptoms of infiltration or phlebitis in any IV therapy. Make sure they know who to call, day and night, for assistance and that they are comfortable calling as soon as symptoms appear.

- Make sure the caregiver can see well enough to recognize subtle skin changes. You may wish to enroll a second caregiver to specifically check the IV site.

#### Long-Term Care Variations

- Clients receiving IV additives over the long-term need to be assessed regularly for continued need of those additives. For example, if the client is receiving a potassium supplement, regular laboratory tests should be performed to track the client's blood potassium level.

- A peripheral IV insertion site is not frequently chosen for long-term IV therapy.

- In clients who must have short-term IV infusions repeated over many months or years, assess for anticipatory anxiety, fear, or body image disturbances. Be especially aware of how these psychosocial factors develop over time secondary to pain, anxiety, and restricted mobility from IV therapy.

patency of an occluded cannula since this action may result in the dislodgment of a clot into the vascular system and/or rupture of the catheter.

### Regulating IV Solution Flow Rates

Infusion sets with macrodrip chambers are often used for adult clients, whereas microdrip chambers are used for volume-sensitive clients, such as geriatric or pediatric clients. Pediatric and geriatric clients usually require some type of device to regulate the fluids as a safety factor to prevent overload. Devices such as controllers and pumps are commonly used to regulate the rate of infusion.

### Calculation of Flow Rates

The **flow rate** is the volume of fluid to infuse over a set period of time as prescribed by the health care practitioner. The health care practitioner will identify either the amount to infuse per hour (such as 125 ml per hour or 1,000 ml over an 8-hour period). Calculate the hourly infusion rate as follows:

$$\frac{\text{Total volume}}{\text{Number of hours to infuse}} = \text{ml/hour infusion rate}$$

For example, if 1,000 ml is to infuse over 8 hours:

$$\frac{1,000}{8} = 125 \text{ ml/hour}$$

Calculate the actual infusion rate (drops per minute) as follows:

$$\frac{\text{Total fluid volume}}{\text{Total time (minutes)}} \times \text{drop factor} = \text{drops per minute}$$

For example, if 1,000 ml is to infuse over 8 hours with a tubing drop factor of 10 drops per milliliter:

$$\frac{1,000 \text{ ml}}{8(60) \text{ min}} \times 10 \text{ drops/ml} = \frac{10,000 \text{ drop}}{480 \text{ min}} = \frac{20.8 \text{ or } 21}{\text{drops/min}}$$

Another way to calculate the actual infusion rate is to use the hourly infusion rate. For the example just given:

$$\frac{125 \text{ ml} \times 10 \text{ drops/ml}}{60 \text{ min}} = 20.8 \text{ or } 21 \text{ drops/min}$$

### Flow-Control Devices

Flow-control devices are used to regulate the infusion at the prescribed administration rate. Safety factors such as the client's age and condition, prescribed therapy, and setting are considered when selecting a flow-control device. There are two basic types of flow-control devices: manual flow-control devices and electronic infusion devices. Manual flow-control devices include roller, screw, and slide clamps and may include volume-control devices such as Buretrol. These devices are used routinely to regulate the accurate delivery of most prescribed IV therapy.

Electronic infusion devices are operated either by electricity or battery and are used to administer IV fluids and medications, and should be considered on all central access devices (INS, 2000). Electronic infusion pumps have audible alarms that sound when the solution has infused, the infusion tubing contains air or is kinked, or the cannula is clotted. There are two types of electronic infusion devices: controllers and pumps. Controller infusion devices generate flow by gravity and are capable of maintaining a constant preset flow rate either by drop counting or volumetric delivery. The nurse sets the flow rate, and the specific gravity of the solution and the height of the bag determine the maximum delivery pressure. Fluids with low-viscosity are usually infused by electronic controllers.

Infusion pumps maintain the flow rate under positive pressure. Pumps counter the effects of resistance in the delivery system and pressure fluctuations at the infusion site (McConnell, 1999). Positive pressure infusion devices are classified as either volumetric or syringe pumps, and are used to deliver viscous fluids or large volumes of fluids. Volumetric pumps use either a peristaltic pumping action or a pumping cassette or chamber to delivery a fixed volume over a specified period of time. Syringe infusion pumps rely on a syringe or cartridge to deliver the fluid at a specific set rate.

## Managing IV Therapy

IV therapy requires frequent client monitoring by the nurse to ensure an accurate flow rate and other critical nursing actions; refer to Procedure 34-4. These other actions include ensuring client comfort and positioning; checking IV solution for correct solution, amount, and timing; monitoring expiration dates of the IV system (tubing, venipuncture site, dressing) and changing as necessary; and being aware of safety factors.

Coordinate client care with the maintenance of IV lines. Clients with IV therapy usually require assistance with hygienic measures, such as changing a gown. Change IV tubing when doing site care to decrease the number of times the access device is manipulated, thereby decreasing the risk for infiltration and phlebitis. PI devices are changed every 72 hours as directed by the Centers for Disease Control and Prevention (CDC) guidelines.

### Hypervolemia

**Hypervolemia** (increased circulating fluid volume) may result from rapid IV infusion of solutions. This causes cardiac overload, which may lead to pulmonary edema and cardiac failure. Monitor the infusion rate hourly.

If a solution infuses at a rate greater than prescribed, decrease the rate to *keep vein open* (KVO) and immediately notify the health care practitioner. Report the amount and type of solution that infused over the exact time period and the client's response.

### Infiltration

Infiltration may be caused by inserting the wrong type of device, using the wrong-gauge needle, or dislodgment of the device from the vein. When a drug or solution is administered under high pressure by a pump, it may also cause infiltration or vein irritation.

Infiltration results in the leaking of fluids or medications into the surrounding tissue. The client usually complains of discomfort at the IV site. Inspect the site by palpating for swelling, and feel the temperature of the skin (coolness and paleness of skin are indications of infiltration).

The nurse confirms that the needle is still in the vein by pinching the IV tubing; this action should cause a **flashback** (blood should rush into the tubing if the needle is still in the vein). If a flashback does not occur, aspirate the injection port nearest the device. Discontinue the needle or catheter if it cannot be aspirated, and apply a sterile dressing to the puncture site.

After the IV has been removed, the puncture site may ooze or bleed (especially in clients receiving anticoagulants). If oozing or bleeding occurs, apply pressure and reapply a sterile dressing until it stops. Accurately assess and document the degree of edema.

Clients may be injured by infiltration. If the IV site becomes grossly infiltrated, the edema in the soft tissue may cause a nerve compression injury with permanent loss of function to the extremity. If a **vesicant** (medication that causes blistering and tissue injury when it escapes into surrounding tissue) infiltrates, it may cause significant tissue loss with permanent disfigurement and loss of function.

### Phlebitis

Phlebitis may result from either mechanical or chemical trauma. Mechanical trauma may be caused by inserting a device with too large a gauge, using a vein that is too small or fragile, or leaving the device in place for too long. Chemical trauma may result from infusing too rapidly, or from an acidic solution, hypertonic solution, a solution that contains electrolytes (especially potassium and magnesium), or other medications (e.g., phenytoin).

## CLINICAL ALERT

### Catheter Sepsis

If client complains of chills and fever, check length of time that this IV solution has been hanging and the needle or catheter has been in place; assess client's vital signs, and assess for other symptoms of pyrogenic reactions, such as backache, headache, malaise, nausea, and vomiting. Unexplained fever may be related to catheter sepsis. Pulse rate increases and temperature is usually above 100°F if IV-related sepsis occurs. Stop infusion, notify health care practitioner, and obtain blood specimens if prescribed.

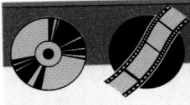

## PROCEDURE 34-4    Assessing and Maintaining an IV Insertion Site

### EQUIPMENT NEEDED

▪ Clean gloves (Figure 34-27)
▪ Gauze dressing
▪ Tape
▪ Nursing documentation record

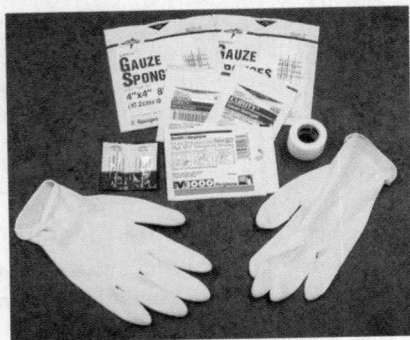

**Figure 34-27**    Transparent dressing, nonsterile gloves, tape, gauze sponges, and topical iodine ointment

### IMPLEMENTATION—ACTION/RATIONALE

| ACTION | RATIONALE |
|---|---|
| 1. Review physician's or qualified practitioner's order for IV therapy. | 1. Ensures accuracy in the administration of IV therapy. |
| 2. Review client's history for medical conditions or allergies. | 2. Decreases risk of fluid overload and allergic reactions. |
| 3. Review client's IV site record and intake and output record. | 3. Assesses for potential problems with fragile IV sites and fluid balance. |
| 4. Wash hands. | 4. Decreases transmission of microorganisms. |
| 5. Obtain client's vital signs. | 5. Assesses for changes in cardiovascular system. |
| 6. Check IV fluid for correct fluid, additives, rate, and volume at the beginning of your shift (Figure 34-28). | 6. Ensures client is receiving correct therapy. |
| 7. Check IV tubing for tight connections every 4 hours. | 7. Ensures that no fluid leaks from tubing and connections. |

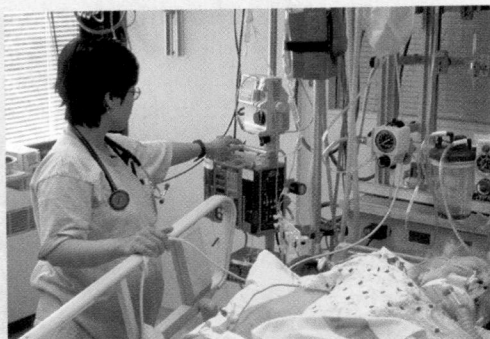

**Figure 34-28**    Check the IV fluid rate, volume, tubing, and additives at the beginning of the shift.

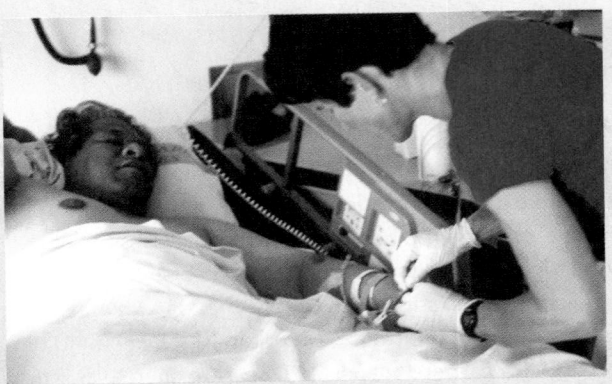

**Figure 34-29**    Check the IV dressing site every hour.

*(continues)*

## PROCEDURE 34-4 (continued)

8. Check gauze IV dressing hourly to be sure it is dry and intact (Figure 34-29).

9. If the gauze is not dry and intact, remove the dressing and observe site for redness, swelling, or drainage.

10. If an occlusive dressing is used, do not remove the dressing when assessing the site.

11. Observe vein track for redness, swelling, warmth, or pain hourly.

12. Document IV site findings in the nursing record or IV flow sheet.

13. Wash hands.

8. Ensures there is no sign of infiltration or infection at IV insertion site.

9. Ensures there is no sign of inflammation or infection at IV site.

10. Ensures there is no sign of inflammation or infection at IV site.

11. These are early signs of phlebitis or infiltration.

12. Provides documentation of frequent IV site observation.

13. Decreases transmission of microorganisms.

---

Phlebitis may be aseptic or a precursor of infection. Listen for client complaints of tenderness, the first indication of an inflammation. Inspect the IV site for changes in skin color and temperature (a reddened area or pink or red stripe along the vein, warmth, and swelling are indications of phlebitis).

If phlebitis is present, discontinue the IV infusion. Before removing and discarding the venous device, check the agency's protocol to see whether the tip of the device needs to be cultured and sent to the laboratory for a culture and sensitivity. After removing the device, apply a sterile dressing to the site and wet warm compresses to the affected area. Document in the nurses' notes the time, symptoms, and nursing interventions.

Hypertonic solutions may cause irritation necessitating frequent IV site changes. Observe site for symptoms of postinfusion phlebitis following IV removal. This may occur in response to either chemical or mechanical factors of the preexisting IV. Postinfusion phlebitis is treated with hot compresses to the site and elevation of the extremity.

### Intravenous Dressing Change

IV dressing changes require the use of Standard Precautions and aseptic technique. Institutional protocol and the type of intravenous access device and dressing determine the frequency of care:

1. Nontransparent (gauze) dressing may be used for a PI. It is changed every 24 hours.
2. Transparent dressings (Bioclusive, OpSite, Tega-derm) allow visualization of the IV site; these dressings are changed every 48 hours.

Persistent drainage at the IV site may require dressing changes more frequently or necessitate changing the IV site.

### Discontinuation of Intravenous Therapy

Intravenous therapy is discontinued on health care practitioner order as determined by the client's need or response to therapy. The removal of a short peripheral catheter is a nursing intervention. Peripheral catheters are removed every 48 hours and immediately upon suspected contamination or complications. Pressure and a dry sterile dressing are applied to the site upon removal of the catheter. The integrity of the catheter and insertion site should be assessed with observations and actions documented to the client's medical record.

The removal of a PICC is usually a simple procedure; however, research suggests that in 7% to 12% of PICC removals, difficulties can arise (Macklin, 2000). Only nurs-

---

## CLINICAL ALERT

### IVs and the Critically Ill

Never remove a functioning intravenous device from a critically ill client until another successful venipuncture has been performed. An established intravenous route may be needed for the administration of solutions, medications, or blood components.

---

## CLINICAL ALERT

### Infiltrated Vesicant

Notify pharmacist and physician immediately if a vesicant has infiltrated.

es who have been trained in the insertion of a PICC line should remove the catheter. Since the catheter is completely inserted in the vascular system and invisible, the nurse must feel for resistance during removal. If resistance is felt, the nurse stops and assesses for certain complicating factors: venous spasm, vagal reaction, phlebitis, thrombosis, and knotting of the catheter. Prior to removal, the nurse must verify in the client's medical record the type and the specific length of the inserted PICC.

## Blood Transfusion

The purpose of a blood transfusion is to replace blood loss (deficit) with whole blood or blood components. On the basis of the client's unique needs, the health care practitioner determines the type of transfusion to administer, either whole blood or a component of whole blood, such as packed red blood cells.

## Whole Blood and Blood Products

Clients with a demonstrated deficiency in either whole blood or a specific component of blood are given a blood transfusion. Whole blood contains red blood cells (RBCs) and plasma components of blood. It is used when the client needs all the components of blood to restore blood volume after severe hemorrhage and to restore the capacity of the blood to carry oxygen. Various types of blood components are used in the clinical setting (Table 34-10). Packed RBCs are more commonly prescribed than whole blood.

Plasma or fresh frozen plasma is separated and frozen within 8 hours after blood collection. Albumin (protein colloid) is a volume expander that maintains the colloid osmotic pressure of the blood. Albumin, heta-starch, and dextran (nonprotein colloids) are agents that increase intravascular volume in order to maintain hemodynamic stability and to provide adequate tissue perfusion. Cryoprecipitate is the most expensive of all blood components because it is constituted from many donor units.

When the health care practitioner prescribes the administration of whole blood or a blood product, the client's blood is typed and cross-matched. The blood is stored in the blood bank after typing and cross-matching until the nurse is ready to administer.

Although whole blood has a refrigerated shelf life of 35 days, platelets must be administered within 3 days after they have been extracted from whole blood. If the RBCs and plasma are frozen, their shelf life can be extended up to 3 years (Kee & Paulanka, 2000).

## Initial Assessment and Preparation

The nurse must perform an initial assessment before administering blood (see Box 34-7). The viscosity of whole blood usually requires the use of a 19- or 20-gauge needle or catheter to prevent damage to the red cells.

Scheduled IV medications should be infused before blood administration. This sequence prevents a reaction to a medication while blood is infusing; if a reaction were to

## TABLE 34-10    VASCULAR ACCESS DEVICES

| Type | Use | Special Considerations |
| --- | --- | --- |
| Fresh or frozen plasma | Replaces deficient coagulation factors. Increases intravascular compartment. | Use within 6 hours with any straight-line administration set. Client is at risk for blood-borne diseases (e.g., hepatitis). |
| Platelet special | Corrects bleeding disorders (e.g., thrombocytopenia). Replaces platelets. | Infuse at rate of 10 minutes a unit with platelet administration set. |
| Albumin | Restores intravascular volume. Treats shock and hypoproteinemia. | Available in 5% and 25% solution. Infuse slowly with special tubing that accompanies solution. |
| Granulocyte (white blood cell) | Restores the leukocyte count, usually depressed in clients receiving radiation or chemotherapy. | Infuse slowly, over 2- to 4-hour interval with Y-type blood filters, and prime with normal saline. |
| Cryoprecipitate | Restores factor VIII and fibrinogen in treating hemophilia A. | Infuse with a straight-line administration set. Observe for febrile reactions. |

## BOX 34-7   BLOOD TRANSFUSION, INITIAL ASSESSMENT

- Verify that client has signed a blood administration consent form and that this consent matches what the health care practitioner has prescribed.

- Verify whether the client has an 18- or 19-gauge needle or catheter in the vein; if the blood is to be infused quickly, a 14- or 15-gauge device must be used. Pediatric and older clients may require a 23-gauge device because of smaller or thin-walled veins.

- Ensure patency of the existing IV site.

- Establish baseline data for vital signs, especially temperature, and assess skin for eruptions or rashes.

- Check client's blood type against the label on the whole blood or blood component prior to administration to ensure compatibility.

- Assess client's age. If the client is at risk for circulatory overload (pediatric, geriatric, or malnourished clients), notify the blood bank to divide the 500 ml bag of blood into two 250 ml bags or discuss with the health care practitioner other alternatives, such as packed RBCs rather than whole blood.

occur, the nurse would not be able to discern which infusate was causing the reaction.

### Administering Whole Blood or a Blood Component

The agency's blood protocol may require that a licensed person sign a form to release the blood from the blood bank and that a blood product be checked by two licensed personnel prior to infusion. The following information must be on the blood bag label and verified for accuracy:

the client's name and identification number, ABO group and Rh factor, donor number, type of product ordered by the practitioner, and the expiration date.

Observe the blood bag for any signs of puncture, gas bubbles, color, and consistency (RBCs clumping). When the information has been verified, both licensed personnel sign the appropriate form. If any of the information does not match exactly or if the product has expired, return the product immediately to the blood bank.

Blood should be administered within 30 minutes after it has been received from the bank to maintain RBC integrity and to decrease the chance of infection. Whole blood should not go unrefrigerated for more than 4 hours. Room temperature will cause RBC lysis, releasing potassium and causing hyperkalemia (Procedure 34-5). Blood may only be stored in a special refrigerator.

### Safety Measures

As discussed in Procedure 34-5, the client should be observed for the initial 15 minutes for a transfusion reaction. Vital signs are usually taken every 15 minutes for the first hour, then every hour while the blood is transfusing.

To prevent blood contamination, change the blood tubing and filter every 4 hours or per policy. Transfuse each unit of blood over a 2- to 4-hour interval.

As a precaution against a blood transfusion reaction, prepare a bag of normal saline, as directed by protocol. The normal saline is prepared as a secondary infusion system; it should not be connected to the Y-set tubing that is transfusing blood. If the client has a reaction and the blood is discontinued, the secondary bag of normal saline should be connected and infused. This action prevents the client from receiving all the blood that is in the Y-set tubing, approximately 20–30 ml. Even though the procedure for infusing packed cells, and sometimes whole blood, requires a Y-set for coadministering normal saline, the secondary bag of normal saline is a precautionary measure for transfusion reactions.

There are three basic types of transfusion reactions: allergic, febrile, and hemolytic. Other complications include sepsis, hypervolemia, and hypothermia. An allergic reaction may be mild or severe, depending on the cause. Hemolytic reactions may be immediate or delayed up to 96 hours, depending on the cause of the reaction. The classic symptoms of a reaction are fever and chills.

## CLINICAL ALERT

### Transfusion Reaction

The severity of a transfusion reaction is relative to its onset. Severe reactions may occur shortly after the blood starts to infuse. At the first sign of a reaction, stop the blood infusion immediately.

## CLINICAL ALERT

### Blood Transfusion Incompatibility

Use only normal saline with a blood product. Blood transfusions are incompatible with dextrose and with Ringer's solution. Together, they cause hemolysis, clumping of RBCs.

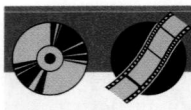

## PROCEDURE 34-5    Administering a Blood Transfusion

### EQUIPMENT NEEDED

- Blood administration set and filter (Figure 34-30)
- Intravenous solution of 0.9% sodium chloride (normal saline)
- Disposable gloves
- Infusion pump if compatible with the specific blood product
- Tape
- Leukocyte-depleting filter, if ordered
- Pressure bag, if needed
- Blood warmer, if needed

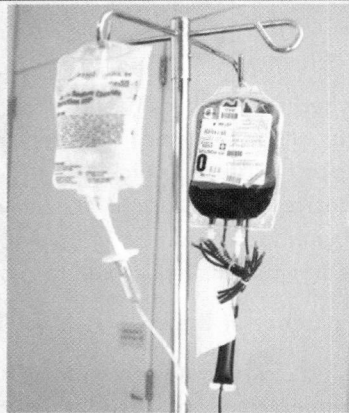

**Figure 34-30    Blood and 0.9% sodium chloride**

### IMPLEMENTATION—ACTION/RATIONALE

| ACTION | RATIONALE |
|---|---|
| 1. Verify the physician's or qualified practitioner's order for the transfusion. | 1. Blood must be ordered by a physician or qualified practitioner. |
| 2. If a venipuncture is necessary, refer to Procedure 34-2. | 2. Ensures a patent and adequate IV for infusion of blood. |
| 3. Explain procedure to the client. | 3. Ensures that client understands procedure and decreases anxiety. |
| 4. Review side effects (dyspnea, chills, headache, chest pain, itching) with client and ask client to report these to the nurse. | 4. Prompt reporting of a side effect will lead to earlier discontinuation of transfusion and minimize the reaction. |
| 5. Have the client sign consent forms. | 5. Some hospitals or agencies require the client to sign a consent form. |
| 6. Obtain baseline vital signs. | 6. Allows detection of a reaction by any change in vital signs during the transfusion. |
| 7. Obtain the blood product from the blood bank within 30 minutes of initiation. | 7. Prevents bacterial growth and destruction of red blood cells. |
| 8. Verify and record the blood product and identify the client with another nurse (Figure 34-31):<br>• Client's name, blood group, Rh type<br>• Cross-match compatibility<br>• Donor blood group and Rh type<br>• Unit and hospital number | 8. Strict verification procedures will reduce the risk of administering blood products to the wrong client. If there is an error during this procedure, notify the blood blank and do not administer the product. |

*(continues)*

**PROCEDURE 34-5** *(continued)*

- Expiration date and time on blood bag

- Type of blood product compared with physician's or qualified practitioner's order

- Presence of clots in blood

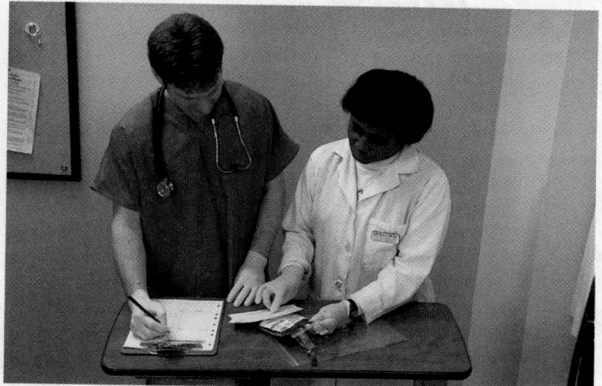

**Figure 34-31    Verify the blood product with another nurse.**

9.  Instruct client to empty the bladder.

10. Wash hands and put on gloves.

11. Open blood administration kit and move roller clamps to "off" position.

12. For Y-tubing set:

- Spike the normal saline bag and open the roller clamp on the Y-tubing connected to the bag and the roller clamp on the unused inlet tube until tubing from the normal saline bag is filled. Close clamp on unused tubing.

- Squeeze sides of drip chamber and allow filter to partially fill (see Figure 34-32).

- Open lower roller clamp and allow tubing to fill with normal saline to the hub.

- Close lower clamp.

- Invert blood bag once or twice. Spike blood bag, open clamps on inlet tube to allow blood to cover the filter completely (Figure 34-33).

9.  A urine specimen after initiation of the transfusion will be needed if a transfusion reaction occurs.

10. Reduces risk of transmission of human immunodeficiency virus (HIV), hepatitis, or blood-borne bacteria.

11. Closed roller clamps prevent accidental spilling of blood.

12.

- The Y-tubing allows the nurse to switch from infusing normal saline to blood. This is especially helpful when multiple transfusions are given. Follow institutional guidelines for the number of units that can be given before tubing needs to be changed. Dextrose solutions are not used with blood transfusions since they can clot the donor blood.

- A correctly filled drip chamber enables an accurate drip count.

- Removes all air from tubing system.

- Prevents waste of IV fluid.

- Equal distribution of cells prevents clumping, which can lead to clotting of cells. Fragile blood cells may be damaged if they drop on an uncovered filter.

*(continues)*

## PROCEDURE 34-5 (continued)

- Close lower clamp.

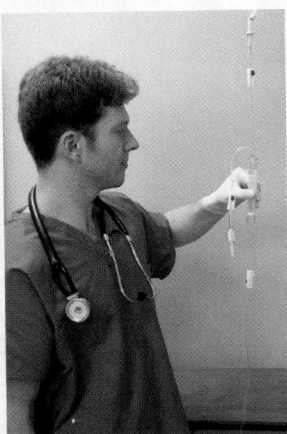

**Figure 34-32** Close the roller clamp on the administration set and priming drop chamber.

13. For single-tubing set:

- Spike blood unit.
- Squeeze drip chamber and allow the filter to fill with blood (see Figure 34-34).

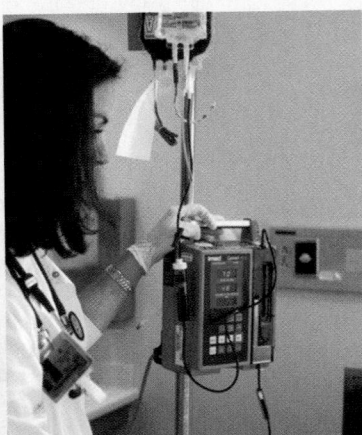

**Figure 34-34** Allow the filter to fill with blood.

- Open roller clamp and allow tubing to fill with blood to the hub.
- Prime another IV tubing with normal saline and piggyback it to the blood administration set with a needle and secure all connections with tape.

- Prevents blood from flowing until tubing is attached to venous catheter.

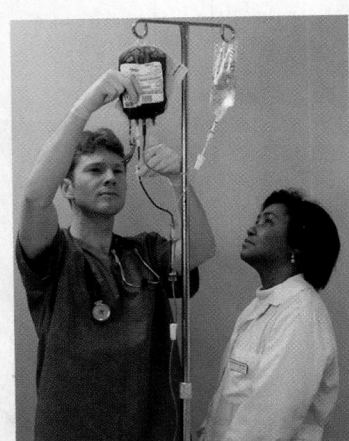

**Figure 34-33** Close the saline roller clamp and open the blood roller clamp.

13.

- Attaches tubing to blood unit.
- A correctly filled drip chamber enables an accurate drip count.

- Prevents air from being forced into the vein.

- The blood product should not be piggybacked into the normal saline line to avoid forcing blood cells through both a needle and a venous catheter.

*(continues)*

**PROCEDURE 34-5** *(continued)*

14. Attach tubing to venous catheter using sterile precautions and open lower clamp.

14. Allows the blood product to be infused into the client's vein.

15. Infuse the blood at a rate of 2–5 ml/min according to the physician's or qualified practitioner's order.

15. Packed red blood cells usually run over $1\frac{1}{2}$ to 2 hours; whole blood runs over 2 to 3 hours.

16. Remain with client for first 15 to 30 minutes, monitoring vital signs every 5 minutes for 15 minutes, then every 15 minutes for 1 hour, then hourly until 1 hour after the infusion is completed.

16. If a reaction occurs, it generally happens during the first 15 to 30 minutes. Changes in vital signs can warn of a transfusion reaction.

17. After blood has infused, allow the tubing to clear with normal saline.

17. The client will receive all of the blood that is left in the tubing.

18. Appropriately dispose of bag, tubing, and gloves. Wash hands.

18. Reduces transmission of microorganisms.

19. Document the procedure.

19. Ensures accurate records.

---

## COMMUNITY/HOME CARE

### Administration of Blood in the Home

*Home Care Variations*

- The blood component should be transported in an insulated container with ice according to the blood bank guidelines. The transfusion should be started as quickly as possible after leaving the blood bank.

- If the nurse is alone, she should be meticulous in cross-checking the unit of blood with the client to ensure correct administration of the product.

- The nurse must plan to have trained personnel available to monitor the client during the entire transfusion and for 1 hour after the transfusion in order to assess for a transfusion reaction.

- Assessing a client's eligibility to have a transfusion administered at home should include no previous transfusion reactions, no angina or congestive heart failure, and being alert and oriented in order to report any symptoms of a reaction.

- Policies of the home health agency regarding administration of blood products in the home include preparation of the nurse, client eligibility, location of client in relation to the blood bank, blood transport and storage, disposal of biohazardous materials, and emergency procedures.

- Blood component transfusions may be carried out in a home setting. Nurses in this setting should be knowledgeable and prepared to treat acute transfusion reactions with standing orders to avoid the delay of contacting a physician or qualified practitioner or transporting the client for treatment.

*Long-Term Care Variations*

- Personnel working in long-term care settings where blood is not frequently administered may need to review blood transfusion policies and procedures prior to the transfusion.

The immediate nursing actions for all types of reactions and complications are stop the transfusion, keep the vein open with normal saline, and notify the health care practitioner. Other measures include sending the IV tubing and bag of blood back to the blood bank, obtaining a blood and urine specimen, labeling the specimen "Blood Transfusion Reaction," processing a transfusion reaction report, monitoring vital signs every 15 minutes for 4 hours or until stable, and monitoring the intake and output.

A delayed hemolytic reaction results when the donor and client's anti-A or anti-B agglutinins are mismatched or when there has been improper storage of the blood unit. This reaction causes the cells to clump and form plugs in small blood vessels. Within a few hours or days, the phagocytic WBCs and the reticuloendothelial system destroy agglutinated cells, releasing hemoglobin into the plasma. The client is monitored for jaundice, persistent anemia or fever, oliguria, flank pain, and abnormal bleeding.

An immediate hemolytic reaction is a rare occurrence. It results from a mismatch of donor and client's blood, causing immediate hemolysis of RBCs. The antibodies cause lysis of RBCs, which release proteolytic enzymes that rupture the cell membranes. The clinical manifestations are headache, dyspnea, cyanosis, chest pain, and tachycardia.

Febrile reactions are common and result from the client's sensitivity to WBCs, platelets, or plasma proteins. Warm, flushed skin, headache, muscle pain, and anxiety are the symptoms of a febrile reaction. It is treated with antipyretic medication.

To help prevent febrile reactions, the client may be premedicated with acetaminophen and an antihistamine. The client should be kept warm during the transfusion. Policy may recommend the use of a leukocyte-reduction filter. These filters also reduce the risk of transmitting **cytomegalovirus (CMV)** (a DNA virus that causes intranuclear and intracytoplasmic changes in infected cells). Approximately 10% of seropositive donors are capable of transmitting CMV infection.

Mild allergic reactions are common, resulting from a sensitivity to infusing plasma proteins. Allergic reactions cause a rash, itching, hives (urticaria), and wheezing. Clients with these symptoms should be monitored for anaphylactic shock. Antihistamines or steroids may be prescribed to counter the allergic response.

Severe allergic reaction results from an antibody-antigen response as demonstrated by shortness of breath and chest pain; if untreated, it may cause circulatory collapse and cardiac arrest. If this occurs, begin CPR and discontinue the blood.

Sepsis results from the administration of contaminated blood (containing gram-negative bacteria). It is a serious complication. Clinical manifestations include chills and fever, vomiting, abdominal cramping, diarrhea, shock, and renal failure. It is treated with broad-spectrum antibiotics and steroids. Nursing measures are directed toward maintaining hydration and monitoring intake and output to evaluate renal function.

Hypervolemia from fluid overload is a preventable complication. Clients at risk for FVE are placed in a sitting position. The blood is transfused at a reduced flow rate; request the blood laboratory to divide the unit into 2 containers of blood so that none of it is unrefrigerated for more than 2 hours during transfusion. Clinical manifestations of hypervolemia are similar to those of FVE (dyspnea, cough and rales, distended neck veins, hypertension, tachycardia, and pulmonary edema). Administer oxygen and IV diuretics as prescribed to treat circulatory overload.

Clients needing rapid transfusions are at risk for transfusion-induced hypothermia. Such clients may include neonates needing exchange-transfusions and trauma victims who require large volumes of whole blood. A blood-warming device may be prescribed to prevent transfusion-induced hypothermia. The symptoms of transfusion-induced hypothermia result from the rapid transfusion of large amounts of cold blood. If the infusing blood temperature is below 30°C (86°F), the myocardial temperature decreases, causing hypotension

## NURSING STRATEGY

### Considerations for Using Herbal Therapies with Traditional Medications

To use complementary therapies (in the forms of herbs and natural products) and medication therapies, the nurse should:

- Perform a comprehensive admission history, particularly a focused review of medications, including any over-the-counter and herbal preparations

- Document preexisting abnormalities, by history or laboratory exam

- Consult the pharmacist promptly to assess the potential risk of interactions among medications and complementary products

- Recognize that gingko and anticonvulsants may increase the risk of seizures

- Consider that licorice and cardiac glycosides may increase the risk of digitalis toxicity and hypokalemia

National Center for Complementary and Alternative Medicine. (2003). http://nccam.nih.gov

and myocardial irritability that may progress to ventricular fibrillation and cardiac arrest. Nursing interventions are directed toward warming the client with temperature-regulating blankets after the transfusion has been stopped. Obtain an ECG to assess for cardiac arrhythmias.

## Complementary Therapy

Herbs and certain foods are used to maintain health and prevent the onset of chronic debilitating diseases such as diabetes mellitus and renal failure. Naturopathic health care practitioners (NDs) use herbs as medicine, and although herbs are the main ingredient of some of the drugs used in conventional medicine, NDs use herbs differently than MDs. MDs prescribe drugs to treat symptoms. For example, in hypertension, the prescribed drug controls the blood pressure but does not correct the reason why the body has increased the pressure in the first place; an ND uses herbs to correct the underlying problem (Morton & Morton, 1996). The following discussion will explain how herbs and foods can be used to treat certain conditions that create disturbances in body fluids and pH.

Traditional Chinese medicine relies on nutrition and dietetic principles to treat certain illnesses and/or imbalances. Foods are recommended based on their energetic properties such as toxifying, dispersing, heating, cooling, moistening, and drying, and by eating in tune with seasonal changes. Cooling foods such as watermelon, celery, and cucumber are recommended during the warmer months of spring and summer because they contain a higher percent of water than warming foods such as meats, garlic, and spices, which are eaten during the cooler months of autumn and winter (National Center for Complementary and Alternative Medicine, 2003).

Many plants have a hypoglycemic action; they lower blood sugar levels. Such plants include dandelion root, garlic, ginseng, and nettles. Other plants have also been identified as possessing hypoglycemic action, such as allspice, artichoke, banana, barley, bugleweed, lettuce, oats, onion, and spinach, to name a few. When herbs and diet are used in a tailor-made combination for the individual, the amount of glucose entering the blood is kept at a constant level (Hoffmann, 1998). Tierra (1998) recommends dandelion root in combination with other tonic herbs such as ginseng and a little ginger for maximum benefit, along with a balanced diet for hypoglycemia.

Herbs such as dandelion and cleavers, which aid the kidneys, are not only useful for renal problems but may aid the cleansing mechanism in treating the whole body, no matter what the problem (Hoffmann, 1998). The main benefits of dandelion are exerted upon the functions of the liver by clearing obstructions and stimulating and aiding the liver to eliminate toxins from the blood. Dandelion root is helpful in treating hypertension, thus aiding the action of the heart. Dandelion (root and leaf) acts as a diuretic and can be taken for fluid retention, cystitis, and nephritis. Dandelion also contains a high percentage of potassium and actually increases the potassium level, thereby avoiding the loss of potassium caused by synthetic diuretics.

Caution should be used when taking licorice since this herb contains a variety of active ingredients. Glycyrrhizin, an active ingredient of licorice, can produce effects similar to aldosterone. Due to the aldosterone-like effects, whole licorice can cause fluid retention, high blood pressure, and potassium loss in doses that exceed 3 g daily for more than 6 weeks. Clients who take digitalis or a thiazide diuretic or who have hypertension, heart disease, diabetes, or kidney disease should avoid the use of licorice.

## Evaluation

Focus on the client's responses when evaluating whether the time frames and expected outcomes are realistic (such as whether the intake and output are within 200–300 ml of each other). The client's vital signs should be within normal limits. The IV infusion rate is accurately calculated and reassessed throughout therapy to maintain the client's hydration. The IV site should remain free from erythema, edema, and purulent drainage. The nursing care plan is modified as necessary to support the client's expected outcomes.

# CONCEPT MAPPING CASE STUDY

Nancy Sherwin has been hospitalized for treatment of dehydration and electrolyte imbalances as the result of vomiting, diarrhea, and influenza-like symptoms for the past 3 days. Nancy, who is 47, had a Koch, or continent, ileostomy 4 years ago. Nancy lives with her sister in a third-floor apartment in a suburb of the city. She works part-time as a librarian. Nancy does most of the housework and meal preparation. Her sister's consultant work requires out-of-town traveling at least two to three times a month.

*(continues)*

# CONCEPT MAPPING CASE STUDY (continued)

Nancy's admission assessment findings included muscle weakness, dry mucous membranes and lips, tachy-cardia, oliguria (less than 30 ml per hour), and a temperature of 101.2°F. The laboratory diagnostic results reported in SI, or International System Units, indicated the following electrolyte imbalances for an adult: sodium, 125 mmol/L; potassium, 2.5 mmol/L; calcium 3.0, mmol/L; magnesium, 1 mmol/L; bicarbonate, 20 mmol/L; chloride, 90 mmol/L; phosphorus, 0.9 mmol/L; and proteins, 14 g/L. Intravenous replacement fluids and electrolytes have been ordered.

After reading your texts, you understand that the output from an ileostomy is a caustic, enzyme-rich liquid that can be yellow, green, or brown in color, and the amount of liquid output is dependent upon where the stoma is located in the ileum. After a time, the stool can have a paste-like consistency. A major complication for the individual with an ileostomy is the potential for fluid and electrolyte imbalances. Dehydration, deficiencies in potassium and sodium, and acidosis from the loss of bicarbonate can result very rapidly from diarrhea whether from antibiotics, illness, or changes in diet.

You will be Nancy's nurse on her second hospital day. She tells you that she is feeling much better, although she still tires easily and prefers to remain on bed rest. The diarrhea has subsided and her electrolytes and acid/base balance are within the normal ranges. A dietician and discharge planning coordinator are scheduled to meet with Nancy today.

This scenario was designed to include an appropriate assessment of fluid and electrolyte imbalances.

Refer back to the concept map example for areas to include in your map. Add concepts from the case study into the areas where you believe they belong. (Some concepts may belong in more than one area.) Cluster related concepts together. Draw connecting lines to indicate relationships among the clusters and with the client.

1. What are the normal values for the electrolytes and acid-base balance? What do the diagnostic study results indicate?
2. What symptoms in your assessment would be related to the hypokalemia, hyponatremia, and fluid volume deficit?
3. What additional information would you like to have to help you prepare a client-centered plan of care? How will you obtain this information?
4. Provide the information you would expect to see included in discharge planning and home care related to:
   a. Introduction of new foods into Nancy's diet
   b. Types of food that would help to thicken her stool
   c. How to monitor the symptoms of dehydration and electrolyte imbalances
   d. Prevention of fluid and electrolyte imbalances, and type of fluid for rapid electrolyte replacement
5. State the other precautions Nancy should take to prevent:
   a. Vitamin and mineral deficiencies
   b. Infections
   c. Skin excoriation
6. What instructions would you give her regarding side effects of antibiotics and problems encountered due to dietary changes (related to the ileostomy)?

***Suggested References:***
Refer back to the discussion of fluid and electrolytes in this chapter.
Review content in a current medical-surgical text related to care of the person with an ileostomy.
Current diagnostic studies text
Nursing diagnosis and intervention text

# CASE STUDY/NURSING CARE PLAN

Mrs. Holmes, a 46-year-old white female, underwent a total thyroidectomy for a large (4 × 7 cm) midline neck mass. A biopsy in the operating room revealed that is was cancerous. After a short stay in the postanesthetic care unit, she was transferred to the surgical ward. An initial assessment revealed stable vital signs, with pain that was well controlled. Mrs. Holmes complained of hoarseness, a sore throat, and difficulty swallowing (dysphagia). She was able to suction her own saliva with a Yankauer suction. The anesthetic record indicated that arterial blood gases sent prior to the arterial line removal were normal. Her neck dressing was dry and intact; two Jackson Pratt drains exited the surgical site. Neurologically, the client was drowsy but roused quickly to name. A sensorimotor exam was grossly normal, and she had absent Chvostek and Trousseau's signs. A calcium level before skin closure was reported as low normal.

## Assessment

Mrs. Holmes has cancer of the thyroid, which was treated with a thyroidectomy. She has been recovering normally in the postsurgical unit. Her neurologic status is stable, and she has clinical manisfestations of a low calcium level.

## Nursing Diagnosis #1

*Ineffective Airway Clearance* related to the thyroidectomy.
**NOC:** Respiratory Status: Ventilation; Respiratory Status: Airway Patency; Aspiration Control
**NIC:** Airway Management; Airway Suctioning

## Expected Outcomes

The client will:

1. Maintain a patent airway without airway difficulties at all times.
2. Demonstrate clear breath sounds and be free of cyanosis and dyspnea.

## Planning/Interventions/Rationales

1. Elevate the head of bed and place in a neutral body position. *Increases potential for stable airway.*
2. Monitor respiratory rate, effort, and assess for the presence of dyspnea q1h until stable. *Detects the presence of early airway difficulties.*

## Evaluation

Client's airway was maintained and patent throughout her admission. In addition, the client did not have any swallowing difficulties within 3 days of admission.

## Nursing Diagnosis #2

*Impaired Swallowing* related to recent thyroidectomy.
**NOC:** Swallowing Status
**NIC:** Aspiration Procedures; Swallowing Therapy

## Expected Outcomes

The client will:

1. Demonstrate effective swallowing without coughing or choking within 1 week.
2. Remain free from aspiration.

## Planning/Interventions/Rationales

1. Keep emergency equipment (e.g., tracheostomy set, suctioning equipment) at the bedside. *Allows emergency nursing response.*

*(continues)*

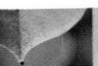

# CASE STUDY/NURSING CARE PLAN (continued)

2. Observe for signs associated with swallowing difficulties. *Early detection prevents serious problems with impairment of swallowing.*

**Evaluation**

Client experienced continued control of saliva and required less suctioning each day. Within 72 hours, client did not require suctioning and did not have further swallowing difficulties.

## Key Concepts

- Health promotion requires a maintenance of body fluid and acid-base balance.
- There are two types of body fluid: intracellular and extracellular. Because intravascular and interstitial fluid are outside the cells, these fluids are called extracellular fluids.
- Water is the largest single constituent of the body, representing 45% to 75% of the body's total weight.
- Electrolytes have special physiological functions in the body that promote neuromuscular irritability, maintain body fluid osmolarity, regulate acid-base balance, and distribute body fluids between the fluid compartments. The body has many regulators that maintain fluid balance: fluid and food intake, skin, lungs, gastrointestinal tract, and kidneys.
- Hormones play a key role in restoring the extracellular fluid volume.
- Sodium is the main electrolyte that promotes the retention of water.
- Acid-base balance refers to the homeostasis of the hydrogen ion concentration in body fluids.
- When the number of free hydrogen ions in a solution increases to lower the pH value below 7.35, the body is in a state of acidosis. The opposite occurs with alkalosis; a pH value higher than 7.45 results from a low hydrogen ion concentration.
- The body has three main control systems to regulate acid-base balance: buffer systems, respiratory regulation, and renal control of hydrogen ion concentration.
- In health, normal homeostatic mechanisms function to maintain electrolyte and acid-base balance; in illness, one or more of the regulating mechanisms may be affected, or the imbalance may become too great for the body to correct without treatment.
- Disturbances in one of the body's electrolytes usually cause changes in other electrolytes and can alter the pH of the blood.
- The slightest decrease or increase in extracellular potassium can cause serious, adverse, or life-threatening effects on physiological functions.

- The client's health history, physical assessment, and biochemical data are used by the nurse in formulating nursing goals, expected outcomes, diagnoses, and interventions.
- Nursing interventions that promote the resolution of alterations in fluid balance are based on the principles of client safety and standards of care.
- Following institutional protocol and established procedures for IV therapy helps ensure client safety.
- Hospitalized clients, especially older clients, are at risk for developing dehydration.
- Clients receiving intravenous therapy and blood transfusions require constant monitoring for complications.
- Evaluation of the achievement of client-expected outcomes requires the interrelational analysis of weight, intake and output, vital signs, and biochemical results.

## Review Questions and Activities

1. What are the three sources of body water replacement?
2. Which electrolyte regulates the osmotic pressure of extracellular fluid?
3. Which electrolyte deficit are clients with draining wounds prone to develop?
4. Given that half of serum calcium is bound to another solute in the blood, which other serum level do you have to evaluate when monitoring the serum level of calcium?
5. What is the most common indication of a fluid volume deficit?
6. What effect does an acid-base imbalance have on the body's cells?
7. Jennifer has been vomiting for 3 days and is unable to keep any food or water in her stomach. Besides having a fluid volume deficit, what other alterations would you expect from the excessive loss of gastric juices?
8. Besides potassium-wasting diuretics, what other drugs can cause hypokalemia?

9. What effect does potassium have on digitalis?

10. What is the maximum amount of intravenous potassium chloride (KCl) that can be infused per hour?

11. What is the first sign of phlebitis?

12. Why is a peripheral intravenous (PI) or heparin lock established?

13. Gloria is receiving a blood transfusion. The nurse is about to take the first set of 15-minute vital signs. Gloria states, "I am cold. I think I am having chills, and my chest hurts." What should the nurse do?

## Multimedia Links

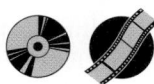

Altman *Basic Care DVD: Measuring Intake and Output*

Altman *Basic Care Video: Specimen Collection*

Altman *Advanced Care DVD: Assessing and Maintaining an IV Insertion Site*

Altman *Advanced Care Video: Circulatory II: Maintaining IV Therapy*

Altman *Intermediate Care DVD: Preparing an IV Solution*

Altman *Intermediate Care Video: Medication Administration IV: Intravenous Medication*

Altman *Intermediate Care DVD: Adding Medications to an IV Solution*

Altman *Advanced Care DVD: Starting an IV*

Altman *Advanced Care Video: Circulatory I: Venipuncture and Starting IV Therapy*

Altman *Advanced Care DVD: Inserting a Butterfly Needle*

Altman *Advanced Care DVD: Preparing the IV Bag and Tubing*

Altman *Advanced Care DVD: Changing the IV Solution*

Altman *Advanced Care DVD: Discontinuing the IV and Changing to a Saline Lock*

Altman *Advanced Care DVD: Administering a Blood Transfusion*

Altman *Advanced Care DVD: Assessing and Responding to Transfusion Reactions*

Altman *Advanced Care Video: Circulatory III: Blood Transfusions*

Altman *Advanced Care DVD: Setting the IV Flow Rate*

## Web Resources

American Heart Association
    http://www.americanheart.org
Infusion Nurses Society
    http://www.ins1.org
League of Intravenous Therapy Education
    http://www.lite.org

National Center for Complementary and Alternative Medicine
    http://nccam.nih.gov

## References

Altman, G., Buchsel, P., & Coxon, V. (2000). *Delmar's fundamental & advanced nursing skills.* Clifton Park, NY: Delmar Learning.

American Heart Association. (2003). http://www.american heart.org

Bulechek, G. M., & McCloskey, J. C. (2000). *Nursing interventions: Effective nursing treatments* (3rd ed.). Philadelphia: Saunders.

Carpenito, L. J. (2002). *Nursing diagnosis: Application to clinical practice* (9th ed.). Philadelphia: Lippincott.

Centers for Disease Control. (2003). http://www.cdc.gov

Daniels, R. (2003). *Delmar's manual of laboratory and diagnostic tests.* Clifton Park, NY: Delmar Learning.

DeJong, M. J. (1998). Hyponatremia: A life-threatening complication of the widely used thiazide diuretic. *American Journal of Nursing, 98*(12), 36.

Godin, G., Naccache, H., Morel, S., & Ebacher, M. (2000). Determinants of nurses' adherence to Universal Precautions for venipunctures. *American Journal of Infection Control, 28*(5), 359–364.

Hartshorn, J., Sole, M. L., Lamborn, M., & Cullen, B. N. (1997). *Introduction to critical care nursing* (2nd ed.). Philadelphia: Saunders.

Health Care Without Harm. (1999, February 22). *Vinyl IV bags leach toxic chemicals.* http://www.noharm.org.

Hoffmann, D. (1998). *The holistic herbal.* Boston: Element.

Hogstel, M. O. (2001). *Gerontology: Nursing care of the older adult.* Clifton Park, NY: Delmar Learning.

Horne, C., & Derrico, D. (1999). Mastering ABGs. *American Journal of Nursing, 99*(8), 26–32.

Hospice Foundation of America. (2003). http://www.hospicefoundation.org

Hugger, J., Harkless, G., & Rentschler, D. (1998). Oral rehydration therapy for children with acute diarrhea. *The Nurse Practitioner, 23*(12), 52, 57–64.

Intravenous Nurses Society (2000). Intravenous nursing standards of practice. *Journal of Intravenous Nursing, 23*(65), S13–S75.

Kee, J. L., & Paulanka, B. J. (2000). *Fluids and electrolytes with clinical applications* (6th ed.). Clifton Park, NY: Delmar Learning.

Kleiner, S. M. (1999). Water: An essential but overlooked nutrient. *Journal of the American Dietetic Association, 99,* 200–206.

Kloss, J. (1995). *Back to Eden.* Loma Linda, CA: Back To Eden Books Publishing Co.

Macklin, D. (2000). Removing PICC. *American Journal of Nursing, 100*(1), 52–54.

McCance, K., & Huether, S. (2002). Pathophysiology: The biologic basis for disease in adults & children. St. Louis: Mosby Co.

McConnell, E. A. (1999). Pump primer: How to choose the right infusion device. *Nursing Management, 30*(8), 49, 52.

Morton, M., & Morton, M. (1996). *Five steps to selecting the best alternative medicine.* Novato, CA: New World Library.

National Center for Complementary and Alternative Medicine. (2003). http://nccam.nih.gov

Paisley, M. K., Stamper, M., Brown, J., Brown, N., & Ganong, L. H. (1997). The use of heparin and normal saline flushes in neonatal intravenous catheters. *Pediatric Nursing, 23*(5), 521–524, 527.

Road Runner's Club of America. (2003). http://www.rrca.org

Roth, R., & Townsend, C. (2002). *Nutrition & diet therapy* (8th ed.). Clifton Park, NY: Delmar Learning.

Sansevero, A. C. (1997). Dehydration in the elderly: Strategies for prevention and management. *Nurse Practitioner, 22*(4), 41–55.

Skretkowicz, V. (Ed.) (1992). *Florence Nightingale's notes on nursing.* London: Scutari Press.

Stewart, M. (1999, March/April). IV bags pose patient risk. *The American Nurse,* 12.

Tierra, M. (1998). *The way of herbs.* New York: Pocket Books.

White, L., & Duncan, G. (2002). *Medical-surgical nursing: An integrated approach* (2nd ed.). Clifton Park, NY: Delmar Learning.

Wong, F. (1999). A new approach to ABG interpretation. *American Journal of Nursing, 99*(8), 34–36.

Woods, A. (1998). Understanding types of dehydration. *Nurse Practitioner, 23*(12), 62.

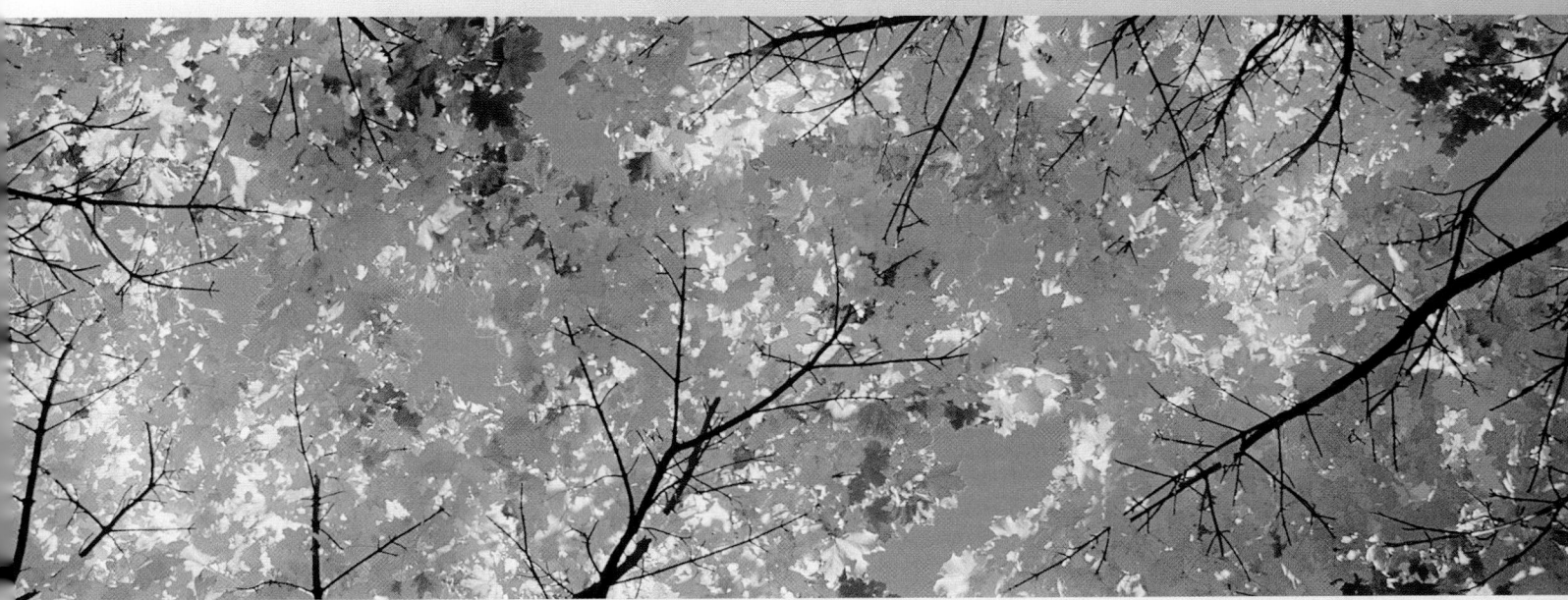

# CHAPTER 35

# Nutrition

Melissa Halas, RD, MA, CNSD

*"The human body is a complex organism with the ability to heal itself—if only you listen to it and respond with proper nourishment and care."*

(Balch and Balch, 1997)

# Chapter Competencies

*Upon completion of this chapter, the reader should be able to:*

1. Describe the physiology involved in the processes of nutrition (e.g., digestion, absorption, metabolism).
2. Explain the role of the following basic nutrients: water, vitamins, minerals, carbohydrates, proteins, and lipids.
3. Identify how diet guidelines and menu planning promote nutrition and health.
4. Analyze the effects of age, lifestyle, ethnicity, culture, religion, and various other factors on nutrition.
5. Evaluate the process of assessing a client's nutritional status.
6. Identify diagnostic and laboratory data appropriate for evaluating nutritional disorders.
7. Describe typical nursing diagnoses for imbalances in nutrition.
8. Define the expected outcomes of nursing interventions that promote optimum nutritional status.
9. Analyze the evaluative measures employed when treating nutritional imbalances.

# Key Terms

absorption
aerobic metabolism
anabolism
anaerobic metabolism
anorexia nervosa
anthropometric measurements
antioxidants
appetite
atherosclerosis
basal metabolic rate (BMR)
body mass index (BMI)
bulimia nervosa
calorie
carbohydrate
catabolism
cholesterol
chylomicrons
deamination
dietary fiber
digestion
disaccharides
enteral nutrition
essential amino acids
fat-soluble vitamins

fatty acids
free radicals
gluconeogenesis
glycolysis
high-biological-value proteins (complete proteins)
hyperglycemia
hypoglycemia
insulin
ketogenesis
ketones
kilocalorie
lipids
low-biological-value proteins (incomplete proteins)
malnutrition
mastication
metabolic rate
metabolism
mid-upper-arm circumference
minerals
monosaccharides
monounsaturated fatty acids
negative nitrogen balance

nitrogen balance
nonessential amino acids
nutrition
obligatory loss of proteins
parenteral nutrition
peristalsis
phospholipids
polysaccharides
polyunsaturated fatty acids
positive nitrogen balance
pre-albumin
proteins
recommended dietary allowances (RDAs)
saccharides
satiety
saturated fatty acids
skinfold measurement
total parenteral nutrition (TPN)
transferrin (nonheme iron)
triglycerides
unsaturated fatty acids
vitamins
water-soluble vitamins

The body requires the consumption of nutrients to support physiological activities of digestion, absorption, and metabolism to maintain homeostasis. The metabolism of nutrients (carbohydrates, proteins, fats, vitamins, and minerals) plays an essential role in providing the body with the necessary substances to maintain internal homeostasis.

## Physiology of Nutrition

**Nutrition** is the process by which the body metabolizes and uses the nutrients from food. Proteins, polysaccharides, lipids, DNA, and RNA are organic compounds. Polysaccharides (carbohydrates), lipids (fats), and proteins are further classified into macronutrients. Macronutrients are the energy-providing nutrients. Vitamins and minerals are considered micronutrients and do not provide energy. Water, an essential nutrient, is not classified as either a macronutrient or a micronutrient (Pentz, 2001).

In the body, all carbohydrates are broken up by the body into their simplest sugars and converted to glucose, which supplies energy to every cell in the body. Proteins are disassembled into amino acids and then reformulated into other polypeptides that the body needs. Fats are broken down into fatty acids. These nutrients are digested, absorbed by the blood or lymphatic system, and transported to the body's cells. Inside the cells' mitochondria, the nutrients react chemically with oxygen and various enzymes to produce energy.

### Digestion

**Digestion** is a process by which ingested foods are broken down in the gastrointestinal (GI) tract (digestive tract) into smaller segments in preparation for absorption. The GI tract is the largest immune system organ whose primary functions include the digestion and absorption of ingested nutrients and the protection of the body from ingested microorganisms and noxious substances (White & Duncan, 2002). Figure 35-1 shows the anatomical structures of the GI tract. Figure 35-2 explains the physiological mechanisms that support the digestive process in each anatomical structure.

The mouth prepares foodstuffs for digestion by **mastication** (chewing, tearing, or grinding of food by the teeth into fine particles and the mixing with enzymes in saliva). The food mixes with saliva, which contains enzymes that begin the breakdown of food.

**Peristalsis** is the coordinated, rhythmic, serial contraction of the smooth muscle lining of the intestines that pushes food contents down through the GI tract. This process begins at the top of the esophagus and promotes the absorption of vitamins, minerals, and water (White & Duncan, 2002). Relaxation of the lower esophageal sphincter (gastroesophageal constrictor muscle) allows food to enter the stomach; contraction of this

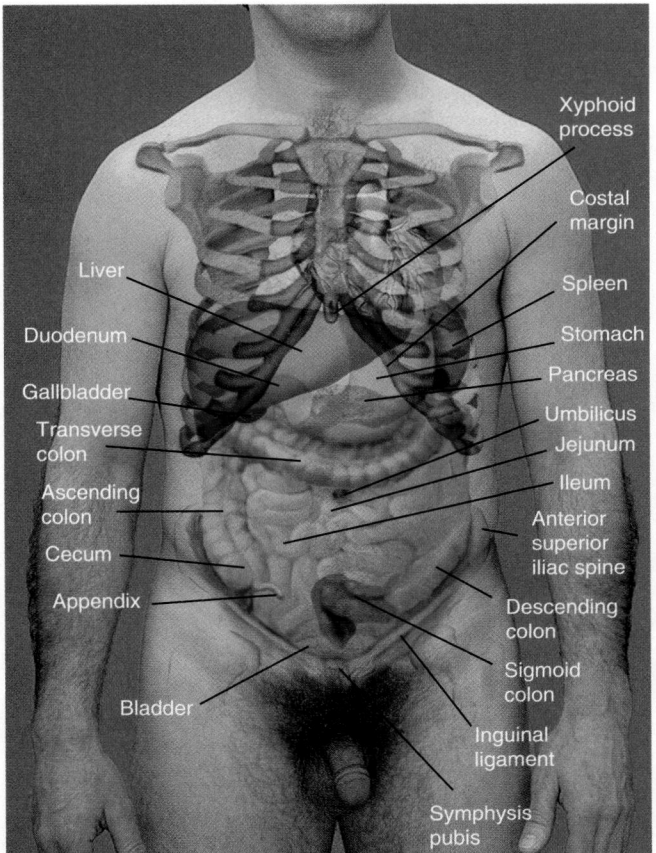

**Figure 35-1   Gastrointestinal tract**

sphincter muscle prevents regurgitation (reflux) of stomach contents.

Digestion continues in the stomach and is completed in the small intestines. This is accomplished by specific substances entering the duodenum: pancreatic enzymes through the pancreatic duct, bile through the common bile duct, and intestinal enzymes produced in the jejunum. Carbohydrates, proteins, and fats require chemical digestion by enzymatic activity for absorption.

### Absorption

**Absorption** is the process by which the end products of digestion—**monosaccharides** (simple sugars), amino acids, glycerol, fatty acid chains, vitamins, minerals, and water—pass through the epithelial membranes in the small and large intestines into the blood or lymph systems. Most absorption occurs in the small intestines through the processes of osmosis, diffusion, and active transport (Figure 35-3). Water absorption occurs throughout the digestive tract.

The main functions of the large intestines are to absorb water and collect food residue (dietary fiber). **Dietary fiber** is the part of food that body enzymes cannot digest and absorb. Fiber is found in all varieties of fruits, vegetables, and whole grains. There are two types of fiber, soluble and insoluble. Soluble fiber dissolves in the watery

## A. Carbohydrates

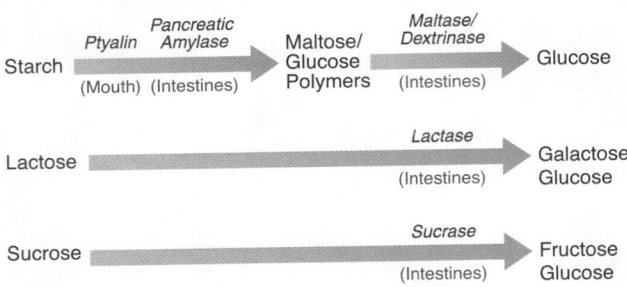

## B. Proteins

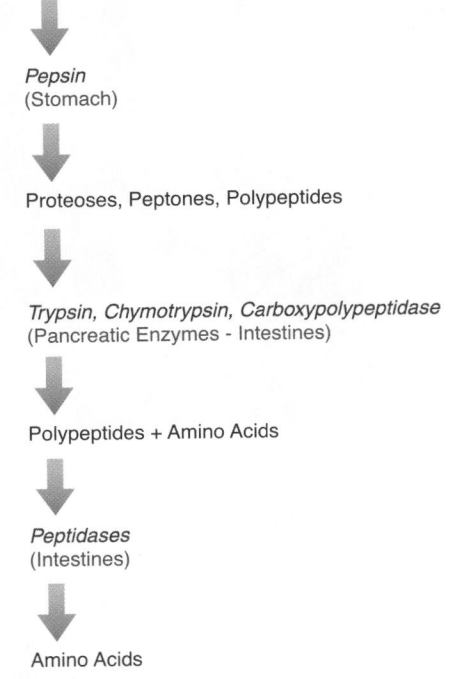

## C. Fats

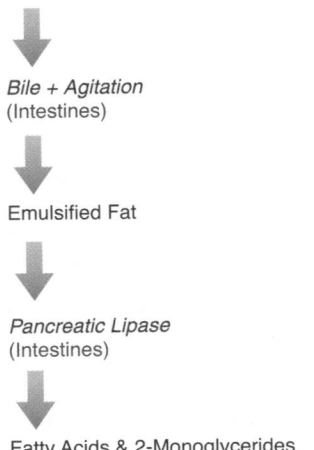

**Figure 35-2    Digestion of proteins, carbohydrates, and fats**

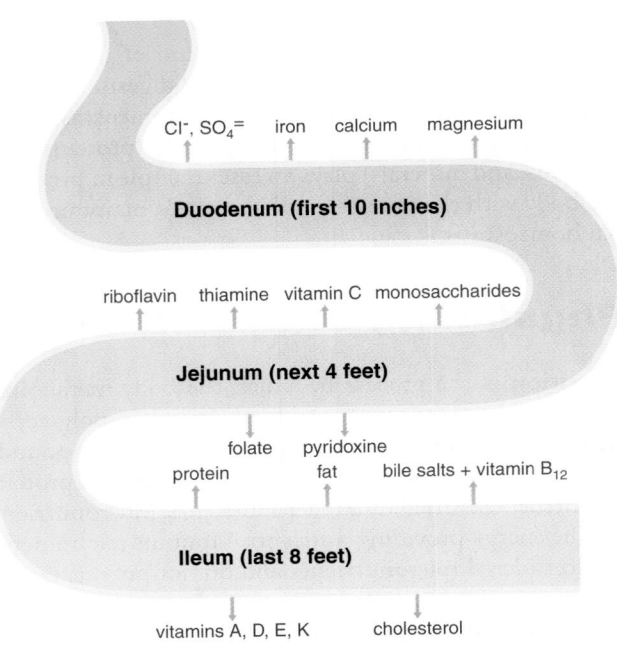

**Figure 35-3    Nutrient absorption in the small intestines**

## FOCUS ON WELLNESS

### Promoting Fiber Intake

A variety of disorders are prevented with adequate fiber intake, and health promotion is increased with adherence to high fiber diet patterns. The nurse must remember that many typical diet patterns in the American culture do not include an adequate fiber intake, and needs to assess the clients in this regard. Clients must be educated concerning what types of foods are high in fiber and be encouraged to increase their fiber.

Roth, R., & Townsend, C. (2002). Nutrition & Diet Therapy (8th ed.). Clifton Park, NY: Delmar Learning.

contents of the GI tract to form a gel that binds to substances like carcinogens and bile acids, which carry cholesterol. Insoluble fiber does not dissolve and absorbs in the large intestine, promoting the formation of a soft, bulky stool that is eliminated more quickly. A high-fiber diet has been effective in preventing diverticular disease, hypercholesterolemia, and colon rectal cancer (Meerschaert, 2001).

## Metabolism

**Metabolism** is the aggregate of all chemical reactions and processes in every body cell, such as growth, generation of energy, elimination of wastes, and other bodily functions as they relate to the distribution of nutrients in the blood after digestion.

The liver prepares nutrients for their role in energy production. The liver converts all monosaccharides to glucose and excess amino acids to urea, carbohydrates, or fats. Excess fats are converted in the liver to glycerol and fatty acids, then to acetyl coenzyme A (acetyl-CoA).

**Glycolysis** refers to the breakdown of glucose by enzymes located inside the cell's cytoplasm. This process produces adenosine triphosphate (ATP) and pyruvate, which provide the cell with energy. Pyruvate may be used in two different metabolic functions. In **aerobic metabolism**, pyruvate enters the cell's mitochondria and in the presence of oxygen is converted to acetyl-CoA. In **anaerobic metabolism** (metabolism without the presence of oxygen) lactate is produced in the cytoplasm by an enzyme (lactate dehydrogenase); this type of metabolism takes place when the oxygen supply is limited, as in the muscles and red blood cells, which lack mitochondria.

When pyruvic acid is formed by glycolysis, it is then converted into acetyl-CoA. This conversion begins a cyclic metabolic pathway called the Krebs cycle (citric acid cycle or tricarboxylic acid cycle). The Krebs cycle extracts energy through oxidation of acetyl-CoA within the mitochondria of body cells. The Krebs cycle is a pathway common to all energy nutrients because acetyl-CoA may be formed from carbohydrates, proteins, and fats (Figure 35-4).

Built into the inner mitochondrial membrane is a series of molecules that assist in electron transport during aerobic metabolism. The electron transport system converts energy released from the Krebs cycle into ATP for use by cells in anabolism and catabolism. **Anabolism** refers to the constructive phase of metabolism, in which smaller molecules, such as amino acids, are converted to larger molecules, such as proteins. **Catabolism** is the destructive phase in which larger molecules, such as glycogen, are converted to smaller molecules, such as pyruvic acid.

## Energy

**Metabolic rate** refers to the rate of heat liberation during chemical reactions; it is expressed in units called calories. A **calorie** is the quantity of heat required to raise the temperature of 1 gram of water 1°C; it is used to express the quantity of energy released from the different foods or expended by the different functional processes of the body. Because a large quantity of energy is released during metabolism, the energy is expressed in terms of **kilocalories** (kcal), each of which is equivalent to 1,000 calories. The **basal metabolic rate (BMR)** represents energy needed to maintain essential physiological functions, such as respiration, circulation, and muscle tone, when a person is at complete rest both physically and mentally.

## Excretion

Digestive and metabolic waste products are excreted through the intestines and rectum. Other excretory organs are the kidneys, sweat glands, skin, and lungs; refer to Chapter 37 for a complete discussion of elimination. The skin and sweat glands remove water, toxins, salts, and nitrogen wastes; the lungs remove carbon dioxide and water.

# Nutrients

Understanding the role of basic nutrients provides the foundation for selecting foods that promote health. Choosing the healthiest forms of macronutrients and the right amount of micronutrients and water enables the body to function at its optimal level of health (Roth & Townsend, 2002). Nutrients work synergistically; for example, there is a cooperative action between certain vitamins and minerals, which work as catalysts, promoting the absorption and assimilation of other vitamins and minerals.

## Water

Water is the most abundant nutrient in the body and accounts for 60% to 70% of an adult's total body weight and 77% of an infant's weight. It is a major component of body fluids, secretions, and excretions. Body water decreases as body fat increases and with aging.

Water and electrolytes are substances that must be acquired from the diet. In the United States, much of water consumption is in the form of beverages (milk, coffee, tea, and soft drinks). The water and electrolyte requirements for infants correspond to the water-to-energy ratio and the electrolyte composition in human milk and common formulas. Although pregnancy and lactation increase bodily demands for water and electrolytes, these demands are usually met with normal ingested amounts; the one exception is in a lactating woman, who requires, on average, an

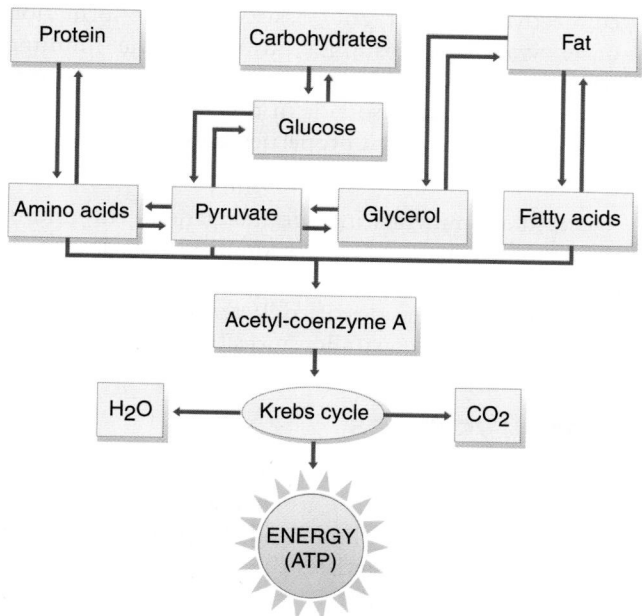

**Figure 35-4    Energy nutrients and the Krebs cycle**

additional 750 ml/day of water during the first 6 months to match the amount of milk secreted.

Normally, the body maintains a balance between the amount of fluid taken in and the amount excreted. The requirements for body water are met through the consumption of liquids and foods and the oxidation of food. Solid foods, especially fruits and vegetables, contain 85% to 95% water. The normal daily turnover of water is 4% of an adult's total body weight and 15% of an infant's total body weight; refer to Chapter 34 for a complete discussion of water's role in maintaining homeostasis.

## Vitamins

**Vitamins** are organic compounds that aid in the regulation of cellular metabolism and assist in the biochemical processes that release energy from digested food (White & Duncan, 2002). Vitamins are called micronutrients because they are needed in small quantities when compared with other nutrients (water, carbohydrates, proteins, and fats). Vitamin requirements are dependent on many factors, such as body size, amount of exercise, rate of growth, and pregnancy; refer to Appendix C for the recommended dietary allowances (RDAs) of vitamins.

Vitamins are classified into fat-soluble or water-soluble. **Fat-soluble vitamins** (vitamins A, D, E, and K) require the presence of fats for their absorption from the GI tract and for cellular metabolism and can be stored for longer periods of time in the body's fatty tissue and the liver. Fat-soluble vitamins have a higher propensity for toxicity than water-soluble vitamins. **Water-soluble vitamins** (vitamin C and B-complex vitamins) require daily ingestion in normal quantities because these vitamins are not stored in the body.

Certain vitamins, mineral, and enzymes are classified as **antioxidants**, a substance that blocks or inhibits destructive oxidative reactions. Oxidation is a continual process, which occurs in the body because every cell needs oxygen to generate energy. During oxidation, a by-product is formed called a **free radical**, which is an unstable atom that is missing an electron and can cause damage. This oxidation process creates a chain reaction unless antioxidants are there to provide protection. Antioxidants include vitamins C and E, beta-carotene, selenium, germanium, coenzyme

---

### CLINICAL ALERT

#### Vitamin Toxicity

Megadoses of both types of vitamins (fat- and water-soluble) can cause toxicity. Once the catalytic demands have been met by these vitamins, the remaining vitamins act as free chemicals that may be toxic to the body.

---

$Q_{10}$, and some amino acids. Plant foods also contain substances call phytochemicals that can provide antioxidant protection (Pawlak, 1998). Free radicals can impair the immune system and lead to infections and certain degenerative diseases such as heart disease and cancer. Certain herbs also act as antioxidants, such as bilberry, ginkgo, grape seed extract, green tea, and flavonoids. The functions, clinical significance, and dietary sources of fat-soluble and water-soluble vitamins are presented in Table 35-1.

## Minerals

**Minerals** (inorganic elements) serve as catalysts in biochemical reactions. Minerals are classified according to their daily requirement: macrominerals (quantities of 100 mg or greater) and microminerals (trace elements, quantities less than 100 mg). The major macrominerals required by the body are calcium, phosphorus, and magnesium; refer to Chapter 34 for a complete discussion of these minerals (electrolytes).

Microminerals such as copper, fluoride, iodine, iron, selenium, and zinc play an essential role in metabolism. For example:

- Copper and iron are needed for hemoglobin formation.
- Copper is needed for the synthesis of phospholipids and prostaglandin and for the formation of some enzymes.
- Iron is needed for the synthesis of vitamins, purines, and antibodies.
- Fluoride is required for teeth formation and the prevention of dental caries.
- Iodine is the basic component of thyroid hormones.
- Selenium enhances vitamin E absorption and stimulates antibody response to infection.
- Zinc plays a major role in wound healing, maintains connective tissue integrity, assists with the formation of enzymes and insulin, and boosts the immune response and maintains normal blood concentrations of vitamin E. Zinc also aids in the absorption of vitamin A, has antioxidant properties, and is a constituent of the antioxidant enzyme superoxide dismutase.

Other microminerals include manganese, chromium, molybdenum, cobalt, arsenic, cadmium, nickel, silicon, tin, and vanadium. Some of their specific roles in metabolism have not yet been identified. Refer to Appendix C for the recommended dietary allowances (RDAs) of minerals.

## Carbohydrates

**Carbohydrates** are organic compounds composed of carbon, hydrogen, and oxygen. Carbohydrates are the primary source of energy for the brain and the preferred fuel for the body. Table 35-2 identifies the functions of carbohydrates and the problems that result from insufficient intake.

## TABLE 35-1    FAT-SOLUBLE AND WATER-SOLUBLE VITAMINS

| Vitamin | Functions | Clinical Deficiency | Major Food Sources |
|---|---|---|---|
| **Fat-Soluble** | | | |
| Vitamin A (retinol, retinal, retinoic acid) | Epithelial tissue proliferation<br><br>Retinal pigmentation<br><br>Immune system (antigen recognition)<br><br>Antioxidant | Scaly skin, dry mucous membranes<br><br>Night blindness<br><br>Increased risk for infections<br><br>Cancer and other diseases | Milk and milk products, eggs, fruits and vegetables that contain beta-carotene, liver, and fish oil<br><br>*Caution:* Do not exceed a daily dose of over 10,000 international units if pregnant or history of liver disease |
| Vitamin D (cholecalciferol, ergosterol) | Bone and tooth development<br><br>May enhance immune function in older clients | Children: rickets and delayed dentition<br><br>Adults: osteomalacia | Fortified milk, margarine, eggs, fish, cod liver oil, oatmeal, sweet potatoes, vegetable oils |
| Vitamin E (tocopherol) | Aids in the formation of red blood cells and the use of vitamin K<br><br>Antioxidant; prevents oxidation of polyunsaturated fatty acids and of vitamins A and C | Premature infants: macrocytic anemia and hemolysis of RBCs<br><br>Damage to red blood cells, destruction to nerves | Vegetable oils, dark green leafy vegetables, asparagus, nuts, seeds, wheat germ, and olives |
| Vitamin K | Formation of prothrombin, blood clotting<br><br>Bone formation and repair<br><br>Synthesis of osteocalcin | Newborn: hemorrhagic disease<br><br>Adults: prolonged clotting times<br><br>Osteoporosis | Dark green leafy vegetables, asparagus, broccoli, Brussels sprouts, cabbage, cauliflower, egg yolks, safflower oil<br><br>Most of the vitamin K needed by the body is produced by intestinal bacteria. |
| **Water-Soluble** | | | |
| Vitamin C (ascorbic acid) | Aids in non-heme iron absorption<br><br>Helps in healing wounds<br><br>Production of collagen (capillary wall integrity) enzyme<br><br>Metabolism of amino acids<br><br>Prevention of oxidation of vitamins | Bleeding gums, bruising<br><br>Poor wound healing, retardation of bone growth, fragile blood vessel walls, gum lesions (referred to as scurvy) | Citrus fruits, strawberries, cantaloupe, potatoes, cabbage, broccoli, peppers (especially red), kale, cauliflower, and Brussels sprouts |
| Vitamin $B_1$ (thiamine) | Metabolism of carbohydrates and some amino acids (energy), production of hydrochloric acid, enhances circulation and assists in blood formation | Degeneration of myelin sheath in CNS (paralysis) and in peripheral nerves (polyneuritis)<br><br>Weakness of cardiac muscle: heart failure, peripheral vasodilation, and edema | Whole grains, enriched grain products, beans, meats, liver, wheat germ, nuts, fish |

*(continues)*

## TABLE 35-1　FAT-SOLUBLE AND WATER-SOLUBLE VITAMINS (continued)

| Vitamin | Functions | Clinical Deficiency | Major Food Sources |
| --- | --- | --- | --- |
| Vitamin $B_1$ (thiamine) (continued) | | GI: indigestion, severe constipation, anorexia, gastric atony, hypochlorhydria (referred to as beriberi—all above systems involved) | |
| Niacin ($B_3$) | Coenzyme in energy metabolism | Muscular weakness, CNS lesions, dementia<br><br>Skin: cracked, pigmented scaliness<br><br>Irritation and inflammation of the mucous membranes of GI tract, producing GI hemorrhage (referred to as pellagra) | Meats, dairy products, whole grains, cereals, tuna, broccoli, carrots, cheese, corn flour |
| Vitamin $B_2$ (riboflavin) | Oxidation and reduction of carbohydrates, fats, protein<br><br>Red blood cell formation, antibody production | Digestive disturbances, burning sensations in eyes and skin, headaches, mental depression, forgetfulness (frequently occurs with thiamine or niacin deficiency), skin lesions, eye disorders (cataracts) | Milk, whole grains, green vegetables, liver, cheese, egg yolks, fish, legumes, meat, poultry, yogurt |
| Vitamin $B_{12}$ (cobalamin compounds) | Metabolic functions as a coenzyme: hydrogen acceptor and replication of genes | Demyelination of large spinal cord nerves: loss of peripheral sensation and paralysis (usually the result of intrinsic factor deficiency) | Milk, eggs, cheese, yogurt, shellfish, meat, fish, poultry, fortified grains, fortified soy products |
| Folate (pteroylglutamic acid) | Synthesis of purines and thymine (DNA formation)<br><br>Maturation of RBCs<br><br>Functions as coenzyme in DNA and RNA synthesis | Retarded growth<br><br>Sore red tongue<br><br>Macrocytic anemia | Wheat germ, green leafy vegetables, whole grains, barley, beans, liver, citrus fruits |
| Vitamin $B_6$ (pyridoxine) | Functions as coenzyme to protein and amino acid metabolism, absorption of fats and protein | Convulsions, dermatitis, nausea, vomiting, anemia, and flaky skin | Whole grains, liver, fish, poultry, green beans, bananas, meats, nuts, potatoes, eggs, brewer's yeast |
| Pantothenic acid ($B_5$) | Metabolism of carbohydrates and fats | None known | Meat, whole grain cereals, legumes, milk, eggs |
| Biotin (a B vitamin) | Synthesis of fatty acids<br><br>Protein metabolism<br><br>Utilization of glucose | Infants: seborrheic dermatitis (cradle cap)<br><br>Adults: rare | Liver, kidneys, dark green vegetables, egg yolk, green beans, brewer's yeast, milk, poultry, saltwater fish, whole grains |

Adapted from Roth, R., & Townsend, C. (2002). *Nutrition and diet therapy.* (8th ed.). Clifton Park, NY: Delmar Learning.

Carbohydrates are classified according to the number of **saccharides** (sugar units):

- Monosaccharides (simple sugars: one or two sugars linked together) include glucose, galactose, and maltose.
- **Disaccharides** (double sugars) include sucrose, lactose, and maltose.
- **Polysaccharides** (complex sugars: many sugars linked together) include glycogen, cellulose (fiber), and starch.

Glucose supplies the major source of energy needed for cellular activity, such as muscle contractions and nerve impulse transmission. When metabolized, every gram of glucose yields 4 kcal. Glucose is also needed for the synthesis of fatty acids and amino acids.

Carbohydrates have a protein-sparing action, based on a minimum daily ingestion of 50–100 grams (200–400 kcal) to spare the metabolism of protein. When dietary intake is below minimum requirement, **triglycerides** (lipid

## TABLE 35-2    NORMAL FUNCTION AND DEFICIENCIES OF SELECTED NUTRIENTS

| Nutrient | Functions | Deficiencies |
|---|---|---|
| Proteins | Growth and replacement: clotting factor production, collagen synthesis, epithelial cell proliferation, fibroblast proliferation | Increased risk of bruising and hemorrhage<br>Muscular wasting<br>Depigmentation of hair and skin<br>Poor wound healing |
| | Immunity: antibodies, white blood cell production and migration, cell-mediated phagocytosis | Decreased enzyme production<br>Lymphopenia<br>Impaired cellular immunity |
| | Fluid balance: intracellular osmotic pressure, albumin, maintenance of blood volume | Edema<br>Hypoalbuminemia |
| | Sodium and potassium balance | Impaired nerve impulse transmission and muscle function |
| | Buffer action | pH imbalances |
| | Energy source | Negative nitrogen balance |
| Carbohydrates | Primary source of energy | Impaired brain functions |
| | Sparing of protein | Increased ketone bodies, producing acidosis |
| | | Poor wound healing |
| Fats | Source of concentrated energy and essential fatty acids | Inhibited tissue repair |
| | Cell membrane integrity | Irritated and reddened skin |
| | Promotes absorption of fat-soluble vitamins | Deficit in fat-soluble vitamins |
| | Maintains body temperature | Impaired fat digestion |
| | Synthesis of bile salts, steroid hormones, and vitamin D | Electrolyte depletion |
| Vitamin A | Collagen synthesis | Poor wound healing |
| | Epithelialization | Dry, scaly skin |

*(continues)*

**TABLE 35-2 NORMAL FUNCTION AND DEFICIENCIES OF SELECTED NUTRIENTS (continued)**

| Nutrient | Functions | Deficiencies |
|---|---|---|
| Vitamin C | Collagen synthesis | Poor wound healing |
| | Maintains capillary integrity | Increased risk of bruising and hemorrhage |
| Vitamin K | Coagulation | Increased risk of bruising and hemorrhage |
| Pyridoxine, riboflavin, and thiamine | Cofactors in cellular development | Irritated and reddened skin |
| | Red blood cell formation | Nerve and muscular weakness |
| | Immunity: antibodies and white blood cell formation | Anemia |
| | | Increased risk of infection |
| Copper | Red blood cell and connective tissue formation | Decreased collagen synthesis |
| | | Poor wound healing from local tissue ischemia (anemia) |
| Iron | Collagen synthesis | Impaired collagen cross-linkage |
| | Enhancement of leukocytic activity | Increased risk of infection |
| | Hemoglobin synthesis | Anemia |
| Zinc | Cell proliferation | Poor wound healing |
| | Cofactor in enzymes | Increased risk of infection |
| | | Alteration in taste |

Adapted from Roth, R., & Townsend, C. (2002). *Nutrition and diet therapy* (8th ed.). Clifton Park, NY: Delmar Learning.

compounds consisting of three fatty acids and a glycerol molecule) and proteins are metabolized to produce energy.

The three major sources of dietary carbohydrates in the American diet are starches (nonanimal foods, primary grains), lactose (milk), and sucrose (cane sugar). Fruits and vegetables are also considered carbohydrates, although nonstarchy vegetables are considered a low source of carbohydrates.

Cells are unable to store large quantities of carbohydrates. The liver converts excess galactose and fructose into glucose and stores it in the form of glycogen. **Insulin** (pancreatic hormone) aids in the diffusion of glucose into the liver and muscle cells and in the synthesis of glycogen. Glucose metabolism is dependent on the availability of insulin, as shown in Figure 35-5.

An increase in blood glucose levels can cause **hyperglycemia**. This can occur in impaired fasting glucose (fasting blood glucose > 110 and < 126) or in type 2 diabetes (fasting blood glucoses ≥ 126). This syndrome or disease occurs when the pancreas fails to secrete adequate levels of insulin to maintain normal blood glucose levels. When significant hyperglycemia occurs, ketones (the end prod-

uct of incomplete fat metabolism) can build up in the bloodstream, causing metabolic acidosis (Franz, Kulkarni, Polansky, Yarborough, & Zamudio, 2001). When hyperglycemia occurs, **ketones** (the end product of incomplete fat metabolism) build up in the bloodstream, causing metabolic acidosis.

In **hypoglycemia**, the blood glucose level is below normal (less than 70 mg/dl). Because brain tissue requires a constant source of glucose for energy, hypoglycemia can alter the normal functions of the brain.

Glucose (dextrose) is a common substance in intravenous therapy (dextrose-5%-water) because it is readily absorbed into the body's cells. This solution provides 170 kcal/L or 3.4 calories per gram of dextrose.

## Proteins

**Proteins** are organic compounds that contain carbon, hydrogen, oxygen, and nitrogen atoms; some proteins also contain sulfur.

After water, proteins are the most abundant intracellular substance. Proteins are essential for almost every bodi-

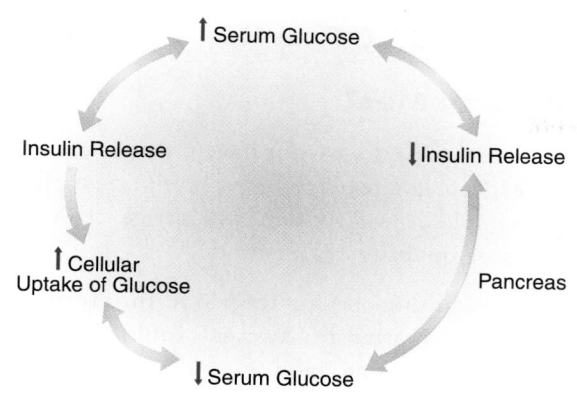

**Figure 35-5    Serum glucose-insulin feedback system**

ly function, beginning with the genetic control of protein synthesis, cell function, and cell reproduction (Table 35-2). The end products of protein digestion are amino acids.

The normal blood concentration of amino acids is between 35 and 65 mg/dl. There are 20 identified amino acids, which are categorized as either essential or nonessential:

- **Nonessential amino acids** can be synthesized (manufactured) in the cells; see Box 35-1.
- **Essential amino acids** must be ingested in the diet because they cannot be synthesized in the body; see Box 35-1.

Proteins are also classified as complete or incomplete. **High-biological-value proteins (complete proteins)** contain all of the essential amino acids. Complete proteins are primarily animal proteins, such as those in meats, poultry, fish, dairy products, eggs, and soy.

**Low-biological-value proteins (incomplete proteins)** lack one or more of the essential amino acids, usually lysine, methionine, and tryptophan. Most vegetables are incomplete proteins. In the course of a day, low-

**CLINICAL ALERT**

**Protein Ingestion**

A person must ingest a minimum of 20 to 30 grams of protein each day to prevent a net loss of body proteins.

biological-value proteins can provide the essential amino acids needed.

All essential amino acids are needed by cells for anabolism and repair. The surplus amino acids are sent back to the liver, where they are degraded (nitrogen is split from the amino acid); the remaining parts are used for energy or converted to carbohydrate or fat and stored as glycogen or adipose tissue. Carbon dioxide, water, and nitrogen are the end products of amino acid metabolism.

The degradation of amino acids begins the process of **deamination**, the removal of the amino groups from the amino acids. During protein deamination, several other physiological processes of clinical significance occur:

1. **Gluconeogenesis**, the conversion of amino acids into glucose or glycogen
2. **Ketogenesis**, the conversion of amino acids into keto acids or fatty acids
3. **Nitrogen balance**, the net result of intake and loss of nitrogen that measures protein anabolism and catabolism
4. **Positive nitrogen balance**, the condition that exists when nitrogen intake exceeds output (protein anabolism exceeds catabolism)
5. **Negative nitrogen balance**, the condition that exists when nitrogen output exceeds intake (protein catabolism exceeds anabolism)
6. **Obligatory loss of proteins**, the degrading of the body's own proteins into amino acids, which are then deaminated and oxidized (occurs when a person fails to ingest adequate amounts of proteins)

Nitrogen balance measures protein equilibrium and is used to evaluate the client's nutritional status. Clients on bed rest or with a fever are in a catabolic state that produces a negative nitrogen balance. The muscle wasting that occurs with immobility causes negative nitrogen balance. Massive trauma and burns are other common examples of catabolic states that produce a negative nitrogen balance initially upon injury. Diet therapy is directed toward providing adequate amounts of proteins and kilocalories so that the body does not use its own protein as an energy source (Roth & Townsend, 2002).

## Lipids

**Lipids** (fats) are organic compounds. They are the only essential nutrients that cannot mix with water; therefore, they must be emulsified by molecules to be absorbed.

**BOX 35-1    AMINO ACIDS**

**Nonessential Amino Acids**

| | | |
|---|---|---|
| glycine | cysteine | glutamine |
| alanine | aspartic acid | tyrosine |
| serine | glutamic acid | proline |
| asparagine | | |

**Essential Amino Acids**

| | | |
|---|---|---|
| threonine | methionine | valine |
| leucine | isoleucine | lysine |
| arginine | phenylalanine | tryptophan |
| histidine | | |

Lipids are composed of the same elements as carbohydrates (carbon, hydrogen, and oxygen) but have a higher hydrogen concentration. Refer to Table 35-2 for a discussion of the normal functions of fats and the problems that arise from insufficient intake.

**Fatty acids** are the simplest form of lipids and the basic components of more complex lipids. They contain carbon chains and hydrogen. **Saturated fatty acids** form fats, glycerol esters of organic acids whose carbon atoms are joined by single bonds (all the carbon atoms are saturated with hydrogen). Diets high in saturated fat are associated with a high incidence of coronary artery disease. Saturated fat, more than any other dietary fat, raises low-density lipoprotein (LDL). Foods high in such fats are animal meats (especially beef), whole-milk products, butter, most cheeses, and some plant fats, such as chocolate, coconut, and palm oils.

**Unsaturated fatty acids** form glycerol esters of organic acids whose carbon atoms are joined by double or triple bonds (at least two carbon atoms in the fatty acid chains in the esters are unattached to hydrogen atoms). **Monounsaturated fatty acids** are formed esters with one double or triple bond; foods high in this category are canola oil, olive oil, peanut oil, olives, most nuts, and avocado. Monounsaturated fatty acids can lower total cholesterol and increase the high-density lipoproteins (HDL). **Polyunsaturated fatty acids** form esters that have many carbons unbonded to hydrogen atoms. Food sources of polyunsaturated fatty acids include corn oil, safflower oil, soybean oil, cottonseed oil, tub margarine, salad dressing, many fried foods and chips, crackers and cookies, fish oils, and flaxseed oil. Polyunsaturated fatty acid can lower LDL, but it also lowers HDL. Hydrogenated or trans fatty acids are another category of fat that are not naturally occurring but man-made. These foods act like saturated fats and raise LDL cholesterol and contribute to heart disease. Hydrogenated fats are found in many snack foods, muffins, crackers, and pies.

---

## STOP AND THINK

### A Fatty Meal

- What impact would it have on a person, especially a teenager, if he could see a blood sample drawn 30 minutes after eating a large quantity of fast food?

- Do you think seeing the blood turn turbid or yellowish after a fatty meal would alter the person's eating habits?

---

## CLINICAL ALERT

### Decreasing High Blood Cholesterol

To decrease a high blood cholesterol level, the client needs to follow a diet high in fiber and low in saturated fat until the cholesterol level is decreased and within an acceptable range. The client needs to be educated that this process may be slow and adherence to the dietary plan will be vital. In addition, the client should be instructed that other factors also increase cholesterol (e.g., familial history, stress).

Adapted from Roth, R., & Townsend, C. (2002). *Nutrition and diet therapy* (8th ed.). Clifton Park, NY: Delmar Learning

---

The most important lipids follow:

- **Triglycerides** are lipid compounds composed of three fatty acid molecules attached to a glycerol molecule.
- **Phospholipids** are composed of one or more fatty acid molecules and one phosphoric acid radical, and usually contain a nitrogenous base.
- **Cholesterol** (a lipid that is produced by the body and used in the synthesis of steroid hormones and excreted in bile) is considered a fat and is found in whole milk and egg yolk.

Phospholipids and cholesterol lipids constitute 2% of the total cell mass; they are basically insoluble in water and are used to form membranous barriers that separate the different intracellular compartments. The cell membrane is composed almost entirely of proteins and lipids (phospholipids and cholesterol).

Besides phospholipids and cholesterol, some cells contain triglycerides, which account for 95% of the fat cell mass. Triglycerides are the body's main storehouse of energy-giving nutrients; when dissolved, they can be used for energy as needed.

Most dietary fats are triglycerides, found primarily in animal food. Most plant foods contain trace elements of triglycerides. Other than butter fat, which is digested by gastric lipase (tributyrase), essentially all fat digestion occurs in the small intestines in the presence of pancreatic juices, as shown in Figure 35-2C.

When free fatty acids, monoglycerides, free cholesterol, and phospholipids are absorbed by the blood and lymph system, they are resynthesized into minute molecules called **chylomicrons** (lipoproteins, synthesized in the intestines, that transport triglycerides to the liver).

Low-density lipoproteins are responsible for the formation of **atherosclerosis** (a disease of the arteries in which fatty lesions called atheromatous plaques develop inside the wall of the arteries). A diet high in saturated fats and cholesterol causes the formation of atherosclerosis. Almost half the deaths in the United States and Europe are attributed to atherosclerosis. These deaths are usually the result of coronary artery thrombosis.

# Promoting Proper Nutrition

When a person has not eaten for hours, the stomach undergoes intense rhythmic contractions called hunger contractions. These contractions sometimes cause pain, in the form of *hunger pangs*. Hunger is not only a physiological response; it also involves psychological sensations. For instance, with a total gastrectomy (surgical removal of the stomach) clients still report a feeling of hunger.

**Appetite** means the desire for specific types of food instead of food in general. A person's appetite determines the type of foods she eats. **Satiety** means a feeling of fulfillment from food. It is the opposite of hunger and occurs when the person's nutritional stores have been replenished and psychological cravings have been met.

Daily food guides have been developed by various organizations to establish standards that promote nutrition and health. These guides assist healthy persons in meal planning; however, the guides do not take into account the nutritional needs arising from metabolic and other medical disorders. Besides the American food guides, there are guidelines developed by other countries—for instance, Canada's *Food Guide to Healthy Eating*—and by the World Health Organization (Roth & Townsend, 2002).

## Dietary Reference Intakes and Recommended Dietary Allowances

The **recommended dietary allowances (RDAs)** are recommended allowances of essential nutrients (protein, fat-soluble and water-soluble vitamins, and minerals) by age category, inclusive of weight and height. RDAs are established by the National Nutrition Board of the National Academy of Sciences–National Research Council. See Appendix C. RDAs represent the normal nutritional needs of 97% to 98% of the people in each specific category; the RDAs do not take into consideration an individual's specific needs or physiological disorders.

There has been an increased awareness of the impact of nutrition on chronic diseases, which has brought together the teamwork of U.S. and Canadian scientists to develop a broader approach than the RDAs on nutrient guidelines known as the Dietary Reference Intakes. The Dietary Reference Intake (DRI) is a generic term that refers to at least three types of reference values: Estimated Average Requirement (EAR), RDA, and Tolerable Upper Intake Level (UL). EAR is the intake value that is estimated to meet the requirement defined by a specific indicator of adequacy in 50% of an age-specific and gender-specific group. UL is the maximum level of daily nutrient intake that is unlikely to pose risks of adverse health effects to almost all of the individuals in the group for whom it is designed. The goal of DRI is to set nutrient reference values for all the nutrients; see Box 35-2 for the first seven nutrient groups studied.

## The Food Guide Pyramid

The food guide pyramid outlines in graphic presentation six groups of food and the number of servings based on the dietary guidelines and the basic four food groups, as shown in Figure 35-6. The pyramid suggests a variety of foods with the right amount of calories and nutrients to maintain a healthy weight.

## Societal Concerns

The Leading Health Indicators for Healthy People 2010 report recognizes that one-third of the U.S. population is considered overweight, while undernutrition is a specific problem for older people and for people with eating disorders. Although "weight" is one of the 10 indicators in the Health Determinants and Health Outcome Set, diet and nutrition were excluded from the proposed set of

---

**STOP AND THINK**

### Satiety

- How does a person know when he has eaten enough food? What role do the *oral factors* of chewing, salivation, swallowing, and tasting play in satiety?

- How true is the saying that healthy eating habits require three meals a day and that each of those meals should be filling?

- How are lifelong eating habits developed in early childhood?

---

**BOX 35-2    EVALUATION OF DIETARY REFERENCE INTAKES**

The seven nutrient groups are as follows:

1. Calcium, vitamin D, phosphorus, magnesium, and fluoride

2. Folate and other B vitamins

3. Antioxidants (e.g., vitamins C and E, and selenium)

4. Macronutrients (e.g., protein, fat, carbohydrates)

5. Trace elements (e.g., iron, zinc)

6. Electrolytes and water

7. Other food components (e.g., fiber, phytoestrogens)

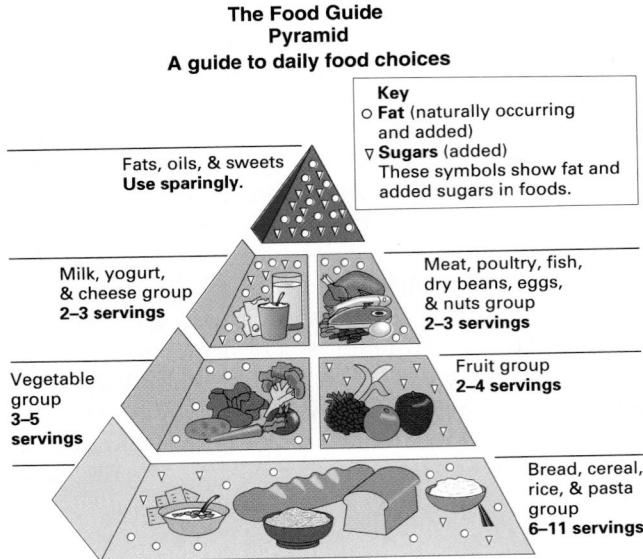

**The Food Guide Pyramid**
**A guide to daily food choices**

Key
○ **Fat** (naturally occurring and added)
▽ **Sugars** (added)
These symbols show fat and added sugars in foods.

Fats, oils, & sweets **Use sparingly.**

Milk, yogurt, & cheese group **2–3 servings**

Meat, poultry, fish, dry beans, eggs, & nuts group **2–3 servings**

Vegetable group **3–5 servings**

Fruit group **2–4 servings**

Bread, cereal, rice, & pasta group **6–11 servings**

**Figure 35-6**    Food guide pyramid. *Courtesy of the U.S. Departments of Agriculture and Health and Human Services, Revised 1996*

indicators because of measurement challenges inherent in this indicator. The committee based this decision on the fact "that the state-of-art of dietary measurement has not yet achieved a level that would provide regular, timely, valid and reliable measurement for each indicator, for diverse population groups, and at multiple jurisdictional levels" (Chrvala & Bulger, 1999).

Modern society has turned from a diet of whole grains, fruits, vegetables, and smaller portions of animal foods to a diet of processed foods, fast foods, additives, preservatives, and hydrogenated oils that can have a damaging effect on a person's health (Roth & Townsend, 2002). Processed foods usually contain excessive amounts of sodium that can cause fluid retention and lead to hypertension, aggravating many medical disorders such as congested heart failure, certain forms of kidney disorders, and premenstrual syndrome (PMS). Additives are placed in foods for one or more of the following reasons: to lengthen shelf life; to make a food more appealing by enhancing color, texture, or flavor; to facilitate food preparation; or to otherwise make the product more marketable. Some additives are derived from natural sources such as sugar, while other additives are made synthetically like aspartame (NutraSweet).

Genetic altering of the world's food has caused many persons to question the essential ingredients of nutrients and the role of the U.S. Food and Drug Administration (FDA) in regulating safe, healthy food products. Although the FDA in 1993 approved the use of rBGH, a genetically engineered bovine growth hormone that makes dairy cows produce 100% more milk than normal, Canadian health officials rejected a major U.S. corporation's request for approval of rBGH because the product label acknowledges that it can cause udder infections; painful, debilitating

foot disorders; and reduced life span in treated cows. Humans who drink the milk from cows treated with rBGH may be at increased risk for breast or prostate cancer as well as other reproductive disorders or diseases.

The European Union's Scientific Committee on Veterinary Measures reported that 17 beta-oestradiol, one of the six growth hormones that are used in 90% of all nonorganic beef raised in the United States, is "a complete carcinogen." American beef is banned in Europe because these hormones "may cause a variety of health problems, including cancer, developmental problems, harm to the immune system and brain disease" (Campaign for Food Safety, 1999).

In 1995, no genetically modified crops were grown for commercial sale. However, these statistics have changed rapidly in the past 3 years: by 1998, 73 million acres of genetically modified crops were grown worldwide, more than 50 million acres of them in the United States; in 1999 an estimated 30,000 genetically modified products were in U.S. grocery stores; and in 2000, 100% of a major U.S. corporation's soybeans (60 million acres) were genetically modified (Rachel's Environment and Health Weekly, 1999). The FDA's position is that genetically modified foods do not need to be labeled; therefore, the consumer is deprived the opportunity to make an informed choice in the grocery store.

"Consumers are increasingly choosing organic products out of concern for the purity of their food and the health of the environment" (Long, p. 44, 1999). In 2000, new organic certification rules were passed in the United States. These new regulations prohibit organic farmers from using toxic synthetic pesticides and fertilizers, genetically engineered seeds or other materials, irradiation, and sewage sludge. Organic farmers must adhere to strict standards regarding the use of fresh manure, animal confinement, and antibiotics and hormones. For a product to be labeled "certified organic" on the front of the package, 95% or more of the ingredients must be organically grown. To indicate on the label "made with organic ingredients," the product must contain at least 50% organic ingredients.

## Weight Management

Maintaining homeostasis requires a balance between intake of nutrients and energy expenditure. Average weight is relative to energy balance, the situation in which energy intake equals energy output.

### Overweight

Overweight is an energy imbalance in which more food is consumed than is needed, causing a storage of fat. Overweight indicates a positive energy balance. In the United States, obesity is becoming an epidemic that will soon rival cigarette smoking as the leading cause of preventable deaths. According to the 1999 statistics from the Centers for Disease Control and Prevention (CDC), 61% of adults in the United States are considered overweight. Overweight is defined as a **body mass index (BMI)** of 25 to 30, while obesity is defined

## STOP AND THINK

### Vulnerability to Obesity

Cultural practices may encourage a calorie-dense diet. Some ethnic groups consider overweight and obesity acceptable or even desirable. An individual's emotional status affects eating. What implications do these factors have in teaching clients about weight in relation to health?

## CLIENT EDUCATION

### Eating Heart Healthy

✓ Read nutritional labels for total fat, saturated fat content, and fiber content before buying products.

✓ Limit foods with hydrogenated, partially hydrogenated, or trans fatty acids, which will be listed in the ingredient section on the food label.

✓ Choose plant-based meals at lunch or dinner at least five times a week.

✓ Use low-fat dairy or dairy substitutes, such as skim milk, 1% milk, low-fat fortified soymilk, low-fat yogurt, or low-fat sour cream.

✓ Limit eggs to three a week, choose egg substitutes, or use three egg whites to replace one egg.

✓ Choose lean meats and trim fats from meats and skin from poultry before cooking; then drain fat from meat after cooking.

✓ Cook foods by baking, broiling, boiling, roasting, or microwaving to avoid additional fat from frying.

✓ Use vegetable oil sprays instead of shortening, lard, or butter when cooking.

✓ Substitute margarine without hydrogenated oils, or use olive or canola oil with herbs on whole grain breads instead of butter.

✓ Use low-fat salad dressings, and add balsamic vinegar to decrease calories and enhance taste.

✓ Include more fish and less red meat in your diet. Choose fish rich in omega-3 fatty acids, like salmon, albacore tuna, or lake trout at least once a week.

✓ Eat fresh fruits with low-fat yogurt as dessert instead of high-fat desserts.

Adapted from Roth, R., & Townsend, C. (2002). *Nutrition and diet therapy* (8th ed.). Clifton Park, NY: Delmar Learning.

as a BMI of more than 30. BMI is a way to evaluate weight in relation to height and is used as a predictor of chronic disease. Overweight may result from one or more factors: genetic, psychological, social, cultural, economic, or physiological. Genetically linked factors, such as a low BMR, excess fat distribution, and obese parents, place the person at risk for obesity. Sociocultural norms influence eating habits; some cultures place a high value on excess weight. Food availability, food abundance, convenience stores, fast-food choices, larger portion sizes, and vending machines have provided a challenging environment for weight management. Some people overeat in response to emotional stress or eat whenever food is available rather than in response to hunger. Longer workweeks and less leisure time can increase overeating in response to emotional stress. Technological advances such as drive-through dining, e-mail, cable channels, snowblowers, elevators, and escalators contribute to less energy expenditure (Brownell, 2002). Hormonal imbalances, such as decreased thyroxin levels, can lower the BMR, causing weight gain if food intake remains constant.

### Underweight

An underweight person expends more calories than are consumed. Underweight is a negative energy balance defined as a BMI of less than 18. Being underweight decreases the individual's resistance to infection and increases susceptibility to fatigue and sensitivity to cold environments.

Family dynamics and a fear of fatness are psychological conditions that can contribute to eating disorders. **Anorexia nervosa** (self-starvation) disrupts metabolism because of inadequate calorie intake and results in hair loss, low blood pressure, weakness, amenorrhea, brain damage, and even death (Roth & Townsend, 2002). **Bulimia nervosa** refers to food-gorging binges followed by purging of food, usually through self-induced vomiting or laxative abuse.

Underweight can also be caused by long-term conditions that deplete the body's resources, such as fever, infection, and cancer, or that prevent nutrient absorption, as occurs with diarrhea, metabolic or GI disorders, and laxative abuse. Other causes of underweight are hyperthyroidism and poverty.

## Factors Affecting Nutrition

Understanding the factors that may influence nutrition is essential in eliciting client and family cooperation in providing optimal nutritional care.

### Age

Infants and children vary in weight and energy requirements; refer to RDA, Appendix B. The infant's physiological development has implications for fluid, electrolyte, and food intake that can predispose this age group to various imbalances. These factors are directly related to the infant's total body surface area, immature physiological development, and the rate of growth and development during the first year of life; refer to Chapter 17 for a complete discussion on growth and development.

From ages 1 to 6 years, nutritional intake varies in relation to growth rate, making the child's eating habits erratic. The child will usually select foods based on developmental nutritional needs in accord with:

- High kilocalorie intake to maintain energy requirements
- Adequate levels of protein, vitamin D, calcium, and phosphate to complement teeth eruption and an increase in muscle mass and bone density

School-aged children can eat larger meals less frequently because of the digestive system's maturation and the presence of permanent teeth. A diet that supplies the RDAs will promote optimal development and health and at the same time avoid weight gains during the preadolescent period.

Adolescence, a period of rapid growth and sexual maturation, requires guidance in dietary choices. Hormonal changes associated with menstruation make girls prone to fluid imbalance. Teenagers eat many of their meals away from home—for example, in fast-food restaurants.

Peer groups influence a teenager's choices, such as what, when, and where to eat. At the same time, body image is of critical importance for teenagers. The social pressures and other emotional stressors of adolescence may have a negative effect on eating habits, leading to obesity, use of fad diets, and eating disorders such as anorexia nervosa and bulimia. See the Life Span Considerations box for some points about food-related behaviors.

During adulthood, growth stops and metabolism declines, thereby decreasing the need for kilocalorie intake. With pregnancy and lactation, the nutritional needs once again increase. During pregnancy, changes occur that may

result in fluid retention (dependent edema)—for example, hormonal changes, pressure of the fetus on the inferior vena cava, vascular congestion, and increased capillary filtration pressure.

The aging process brings about structural and functional changes that may put older adults at risk. The older population cannot be classified as a homogeneous group, because people do not age physically at the same rate as they do chronologically (Hogstel, 2001); refer to the Life Span Considerations box for dietary guidelines for older adults.

Socioeconomic factors, access to a grocery store, and lifestyle may affect the nutritional status of older adults. Having to prepare their own food and eat alone are other challenges older people face. Refer to Chapter 19 for additional information on older clients.

## Lifestyle

Eating is a social activity in most cultures. A person's lifestyle may have a major impact on food-related behaviors. Families with both parents working or with children involved in sports and other activities might find it difficult to sit down at the dinner table together for a home-cooked meal. When meals are eaten on the run, they tend to be high in fat and carbohydrate content, and the family misses the opportunity to be together and share important events of the day.

Food preferences are usually developed in childhood and modified throughout the life span. Lifestyle nutritional behaviors often come from traditional family practices. These practices affect not only food-related behaviors but also the individual's beliefs regarding health and wellness. If a person gets sufficient rest, has the self-awareness to recognize stress, exercises regularly, and avoids addictive behaviors, such as smoking and alcohol abuse, he will usually make healthy nutritional decisions.

## Ethnicity, Culture, and Religious Practices

Dietary customs reflect the socialization and cultural patterns of ethnic groups. Culture is evidenced by patterns of values and behaviors that are characteristics of a particular group. Religious beliefs often dictate what types of foods may be eaten and how they should be prepared.

Although it is not possible to learn the nutritional behaviors for all ethnic groups, recognize the need to comply with the client's routine patterns (see Box 35-3 for nutritional behaviors of some ethnic groups). Refer to Chapter 5 for additional cultural factors that are evidenced in food behaviors.

## Other Factors

Other factors influence the types of foods selected and their nutritional value. Economics exert a major influence on food selection; fresh fruits and vegetables and lean

---

### 🌰 LIFE SPAN CONSIDERATIONS

## Preventing Eating Disorders in Adolescents

- Encourage healthy dietary habits and adequate exercise.

- Emphasize a healthy lifestyle over physical appearance and weight loss.

- Encourage increased self-esteem and stress a positive self-worth.

- Avoid pressuring children to achieve perfection or to perform beyond their abilities.

- Recognize signs and symptoms of eating disorders, and seek professional help when suspected.

Estes, M. E. (2002). *Health assessment & physical examination* (2nd ed.). Clifton Park, NY: Delmar Learning.

## BOX 35-3  NUTRITIONAL BEHAVIORS OF SELECTED ETHNIC GROUPS

- Asians' main food types are rice, green tea, vegetables, and fish. A rice-and-water soup is often fed to the sick.

- The Islamic (Muslim) law does not permit the consumption of pork or alcohol or of meat that has not been slaughtered according to the Islamic code. The main meal is at midday.

- Orthodox Jews are not allowed to eat pig, rabbit, and shellfish; milk and meat are not taken at the same meal. A vegetarian diet is acceptable when kosher meat is not available. Strict guidelines dictate food preparation.

meats can be expensive and are often substituted with products that tend to be low in protein and high in starch. High-calorie, low-nutrient snack foods and soda are often consumed at higher rates in lower-income households, contributing to obesity.

Food preferences are an expression of an individual's likes and dislikes. They may be related to the texture of food, how it is prepared, or what was served to the individual during childhood. However, preferences can also be an expression of the person's economic, ecological, ethical, or religious beliefs. Vegetarians, for example, follow a diet of plant foods and may include eggs or milk, depending on preference. A vegetarian diet is healthy when it includes a wide variety of foods that supply adequate amounts of protein, vitamins, and minerals.

## CLIENT REFLECTIONS

### Dietary Practices in Orthodox Judaism

Mrs. Jakinowski is a 53-year-old woman who practices Orthodox Judaism. She makes the following statements to the nurse in a clinic setting: "I often have great difficulty ordering foods that I can eat when I go to restaurants. In fact, even when friends have me over to their home, they usually forget my dietary restrictions and don't have foods that I can eat. But I don't really blame them. I just try to reassure them that I am not upset, and I usually use the opportunity to teach them about the practices of my beliefs."

What would you say to this client?

## LIFE SPAN CONSIDERATIONS

### Special Dietary Considerations for Older Clients

- Special attention must be given to water needs, regardless of physical activity, because the thirst mechanism is less responsive than in younger people.

- Decrease the kilocaloric requirements in relation to activity: 10% for ages 51 to 75 and 20% to 25% for ages 75 and older. Bedridden and immobilized persons need a further reduction in kilocalories. Limit the quantities of empty kilocalorie foods (sugars, sweets, fats, oils, and alcohol).

- Maintain protein requirements, with 12% to 14% of the kilocalories being derived from protein food (lean meat, fish, eggs, lean poultry, low-fat dairy, and soy).

- Select carbohydrates as follows: limit concentrated sweets and simple sugars (candy, sugar, jellies, and syrups); the main source should be from whole grains, fruits, vegetables, and beans.

- Limit foods high in sodium, like canned foods and salted or cured meats.

- Ensure adequate consumption of fats, especially unsaturated fats, to provide a source of energy, provide the essential amino acids, use the fat-soluble vitamins, and serve as a lubricating agent.

- Ensure adequate amounts of vitamin D, calcium, and phosphorus to maintain bone integrity (fortified milk is a good source).

- Ensure high-fiber foods (dried fruits, whole grain cereals, nuts, fresh fruit, and vegetables) to increase satiety and maintain intestinal mobility to avoid constipation.

- Include foods from the food guide pyramid in the amounts that meet the RDAs for ages 51 and older.

Gender may play a role in food selection, owing mainly to stereotyping (for example, the idea that males eat meat and potatoes and females eat salads). Peer pressures often dictate what teenagers eat. Stress, depression, and alcohol abuse alter the appetite. Medications can alter food absorption and excretion and affect the taste of food. GI disorders can cause anorexia, nausea, vomiting, diarrhea,

## STOP AND THINK

### Food-Related Behaviors

How are food *fads* developed? What lasting impact do these fads have on health? What role does the media play in forming an individual's food beliefs? Is the statement "Yogurt and vitamin E retard aging" related to a fad or a misconception, or is it a fact based on research? To answer this last question, refer to Table 35-1.

constipation, discomfort, and pain, all of which may alter eating habits and food preferences.

## Assessment

The goals of a nursing assessment are to collect subjective and objective data regarding the client's nutritional status and to determine what type of nutritional support is needed. Nurses are in a unique position to recognize **malnutrition**, or alterations related to inadequate intake, disorders of digestion or absorption, and overeating. Assessment must be performed in a logical fashion and should include three basic components: nutritional history, physical examination with anthropometric measurements, and diagnostic and laboratory data.

### Nutritional History

The nutritional history of clients experiencing alterations in nutrition and metabolism is of critical importance in the development of the plan of care. Several methods can be used in collecting these subjective data: 24-hour recall, food frequency questionnaire, food record, and diet history; refer to Table 35-3 for an example of a nutritional history. Begin the history with a thorough exploration of the client's presenting problems as they relate to onset, duration, nature, pattern, severity, associated symptoms, and efforts taken to relieve the symptoms.

#### 24-Hour Recall

The 24-hour recall requires client identification of everything consumed in the previous 24 hours. It is performed easily and quickly by asking pertinent questions. However, clients may be unable to recall their intake accurately or anything atypical for their diet. Family members can often assist with these data, if necessary.

#### Food-Frequency Questionnaire

The food-frequency method gathers data relative to the number of times per day, week, or month the client eats particular foods. The nurse can tailor the questions to particular nutrients, such as cholesterol and saturated fat. This

method helps to validate the accuracy of the 24-hour recall and provides a more complete picture of foods consumed.

### Food Record

The food record provides quantitative information regarding all foods consumed, with portions weighed and measured for three consecutive days. This method requires full client or family member cooperation.

### Diet History

The diet history elicits detailed information regarding the client's nutritional status, general health pattern, socioeconomic status, and cultural factors, as presented in Table 35-3. This method incorporates information similar to that collected by the 24-hour recall and food-frequency questionnaire. Inform the client that the history might require more than one interview because of the amount of data to be collected.

Although the history data may indicate adequate nutrition, clients must be reassessed periodically to prevent nutritional problems from occurring. Fear, anxiety, or depression before or during hospitalization may lead to poor food intake, which is the leading cause of malnutrition.

## Physical Examination

A physical assessment requires decision making, problem solving, and organization; refer to Chapter 27 for a complete discussion of physical assessment. This section presents the physical assessment findings that suggest nutrient imbalance. "The nurse should be aware of rapidly proliferating tissues such as hair, skin, eyes, lips, and tongue that usually show nutrient deficiencies sooner than other tissues" (Hammond, 1999, p. 355). Refer to Table 35-4. Essential components of anthropometric measurements (height, weight, and skinfolds) are also discussed.

### Intake and Output (I&O)

Intake and output measurements and daily weights are critical components of a nutritional assessment; refer to Chapter 34 for intake and output measurements, and Chapter 27 for a complete discussion on weight measurements.

### Anthropometric Measurements

**Anthropometric measurements** (measurement of the size, weight, and proportions of the body) evaluate the client's calorie-energy expenditure balance, muscle mass, body fat, and protein reserves based on height, weight, skinfolds, and limb and girth circumferences. Chapter 27 discusses the assessment of height and weight; refer to Chapter 34 for additional nursing measures relative to daily weights. BMI can also be used to determine whether a person's weight is appropriate for her height.

### Skinfold Measurements

**Skinfold measurement** indicates the amount of body fat. This information is beneficial in promoting health and

## TABLE 35-3    HEALTH HISTORY RELATED TO NUTRITION AND METABOLISM

| Environment and Lifestyle | Possible Findings |
|---|---|
| Employment | Exposure to heat, toxic chemicals<br>Extent of physical exertion<br>Degree of stress |
| Home environment | Central air/heat; lives alone or with other family members; ability to shop/cook |
| Tobacco use | Use of smokeless tobacco; cigarettes: number of years; packs per day; if quit, how long |
| Nutritional status | Weight changes: loss or gain<br>Fluid consumption for 24 hours: number of glasses of water, cups of coffee or tea, soft drinks; amount of alcohol consumed<br>Food preferences and restrictions<br>Dietary restrictions (sodium)<br>Use of supplements: vitamins, minerals, commercial liquids, herbs |

| Presenting Problem | Possible Findings |
|---|---|
| Weight loss | Onset: sudden or gradual, duration<br>Pattern: decreased intake, increased activity<br>Severity: how much, specific time frame<br>Associated symptoms: anorexia, nausea, vomiting, diarrhea, chewing difficulty (poor dentition), dysphagia (difficulty in swallowing), odynophagia (pain in swallowing), polyuria (passage of excessive urine), fatigue, dyspnea, depression, cognitive impairment, motor weakness or paralysis<br>Efforts to relieve weight loss: increased intake, decreased activity |
| Anorexia | Onset: sudden, gradual, duration<br>Pattern: continuous, occasional, related to food intake—specific foods, time of day, activity, drugs, radiation or chemotherapy<br>Severity: intake for 24 hours<br>Associated symptoms: weight loss, nausea, vomiting, diarrhea, dysgeusia (distortion of sense of taste), fatigue, depression<br>Efforts to relieve anorexia: dietary changes—types of foods and preparation, time of day, eating with others or alone |
| Nausea and vomiting | Onset: sudden, gradual, duration<br>Nature of emesis: color, consistency, amount<br>Pattern: continuous, occasional, related to food intake—specific foods, time of day, position or activity<br>Severity: specific amount in a 24-hour period<br>Associated symptoms: weight loss, anorexia, dysphagia, diarrhea, fatigue, motor weakness, pain<br>Efforts to relieve nausea and vomiting: eliminating odors, certain foods, medications, changing position or activity after meals |
| Diarrhea | Onset: sudden or gradual, duration<br>Nature of feces: color, consistency, amount<br>Pattern: frequency, related to food intake<br>Severity: number of times in 24 hours<br>Associated symptoms: nausea, vomiting, pain, fatigue, motor weakness, weight loss<br>Efforts to relieve: decrease fluid intake with meals, identify foods, medications, and other stressors that trigger diarrhea |

*(continues)*

## TABLE 35-3    HEALTH HISTORY RELATED TO NUTRITION AND METABOLISM (continued)

| Past Health History | Possible Findings |
| --- | --- |
| Previous or chronic illnesses | Allergies, anorexia, malnutrition, gastroenteritis, cancer, diabetes mellitus<br>History of: heart disease, hypertension, renal disease, pulmonary disease<br>History of trauma: head or crushing injuries |
| Medications and therapies | Diuretics, steroids, antacids, antihypertensives, digoxin IV therapy, total parenteral nutrition, chemotherapy |
| **Family History** | **Possible Findings** |
| Illnesses in family members | Allergies, cancer, anorexia, diabetes mellitus, cardiovascular disease |
| **Knowledge Level** | **Possible Findings** |
| Client's knowledge of disease process | Ability to name illness<br>Ability to identify current treatments (e.g., medications) |
| **Coping Ability** | **Possible Findings** |
| Client and family coping strategies | Client's and family's perception of impact of illness on lifestyle<br>Presence of social support systems |

## TABLE 35-4    ADULT PHYSICAL ASSESSMENT FINDINGS: NUTRIENT IMBALANCE

| Assessment Findings | Nutrient Deficiencies and Excesses | Assessment Findings | Nutrient Deficiencies and Excesses |
| --- | --- | --- | --- |
| Hair: | | Nails: | |
| Dull, dry, brittle | Protein deficiency | Koilonychia (spoon-shaped nails) | Iron deficiency |
| Hair loss | Protein, zinc, and biotin deficiency or vit A excess | Brittle, fragile | Protein deficiency |
| Loss of pigment in strips around hair line | Protein and copper deficiency | Heart: | |
| | | Tachycardia | Vit $B_1$ deficiency |
| Head and neck: | | Hypertension | Calcium and potassium deficiency or sodium excess |
| Headache | Vit A and D excess | | |
| Epistaxis (nosebleed) | Vit K deficiency | Abdomen: | |
| Thyroid enlargement | Iodine deficiency | Ascites | Protein deficiency |
| Eyes: | | Musculoskeletal: | |
| Pale conjunctiva | Iron deficiency | Muscle wasting | |
| Blue sclerae | Iron deficiency | Edema | Protein and vit $B_1$ deficiency |
| Conjunctival and corneal dryness | Vit A deficiency | Calf tenderness | Vit $B_1$ and C, biotin, selenium deficiency |
| Corneal vascularization | Vit $B_2$ deficiency | Bone tenderness | Vit D, calcium, and phosphorus deficiency or vit A excess |
| Mouth: | | Knock knees, bowed legs, and fragile bones | Vit D, calcium, phosphorus, and copper deficiency |
| Lesions at corners of mouth | Vit $B_2$ deficiency | | |

*(continues)*

## TABLE 35-4 ADULT PHYSICAL ASSESSMENT FINDINGS: NUTRIENT IMBALANCE (*continued*)

| Assessment Findings | Nutrient Deficiencies and Excesses | Assessment Findings | Nutrient Deficiencies and Excesses |
|---|---|---|---|
| Mouth: (*continued*) | | | |
| Glossitis (red, sore tongue) | Niacin, folate, vit $B_{12}$, and other vit B deficiencies | Neurologic: | |
| Gingivitis (inflamed gums) | Vit C deficiency | Paresthesia | Vit $B_1$, $B_6$, $B_{12}$, and biotin deficiency |
| Hypogeusia (poor sense of taste) | Zinc deficiency | Weakness | Vit C, $B_1$, $B_6$, and $B_{12}$ deficiency |
| | | Ataxia | Vit $B_1$ and $B_{12}$ deficiency |
| Dysgeusia (bad taste) | Zinc deficiency | Tremor | Magnesium deficiency |
| Dental caries | Fluoride deficiency | Decreased tendon reflexes | Vit $B_1$ deficiency |
| Mottling of teeth | Fluoride excess | Disorientation | Vit $B_1$ deficiency |
| Atrophy of papillae on tongue | Iron and vit B deficiency | Drowsiness, lethargy | Vit $B_1$ deficiency or vit A and D excess |
| | | Depression | Vit $B_1$ and biotin deficiency |
| Skin: | | | |
| Dry, scaly | Vit A, zinc, and essential fatty acids deficiency or vit A excess | | |
| Eczematous lesions | Zinc deficiency | | |
| Petechiae and ecchymoses | Vit C and vit K deficiency | | |
| Darkening and peeling of sun-exposed areas | Niacin deficiency | | |
| Poor wound healing | Protein, zinc, and vit C deficiency | | |

determining risks and treatment modalities associated with chronic illness and surgery. This assessment is usually performed in an outpatient setting when the nurse develops a client's profile.

A special caliper is used to measure skinfolds. The caliper should grasp only the subcutaneous tissue, not the underlying muscle. Measurements can be taken of the triceps, subscapular, biceps, and suprailiac skinfolds.

1. To measure the triceps fold, locate the midpoint of the upper arm. Grasping the skin on the back of the upper arm, place the caliper 1 cm below your fingers (Figure 35-7), and measure the thickness to the nearest millimeter.
2. For a subscapular skinfold measurement, grasp the skin below the scapula with three fingers, angle the fold about 45 degrees laterally to the scapula (Figure 35-8), place the caliper 1 cm above your fingers, and read the measurement.

It is essential to document the skinfold sites, the type of caliper used, and the measurement in millimeters.

### Mid-Upper-Arm Circumference

The measurement of **mid-upper-arm circumference (MAC)** serves as an index for skeletal muscle mass and protein reserve. Instruct the client to relax and flex the forearm; with a measuring tape, measure the circumference at the midpoint of the upper arm (Figure 35-9).

### Abdominal-Girth Measurement

When made repeatedly over a span of time, an abdominal girth measurement serves as an index as to whether abdominal distention is increasing, decreasing, or remaining the same. With an indelible pen, place an X on the client's abdomen at the point of greatest distention. Using a measuring tape, measure the abdomen's circumference. This measurement should be performed at the same time each day and consistently recorded in either inches or centimeters.

# Diagnostic and Laboratory Data

Biochemical data assessment is another essential source of objective data. Trends revealed in laboratory results can be used to detect alterations in nutrition and metabolism before clinical symptoms are assessed in the examination. Refer to Chapter 29 for a detailed discussion of laboratory testing. No single laboratory test is diagnostic of malnutrition.

## Protein Indices

Several tests that reflect protein synthesis can also reflect nutritional status. Serum levels of albumin and transferrin are used to identify protein-calorie malnutrition.

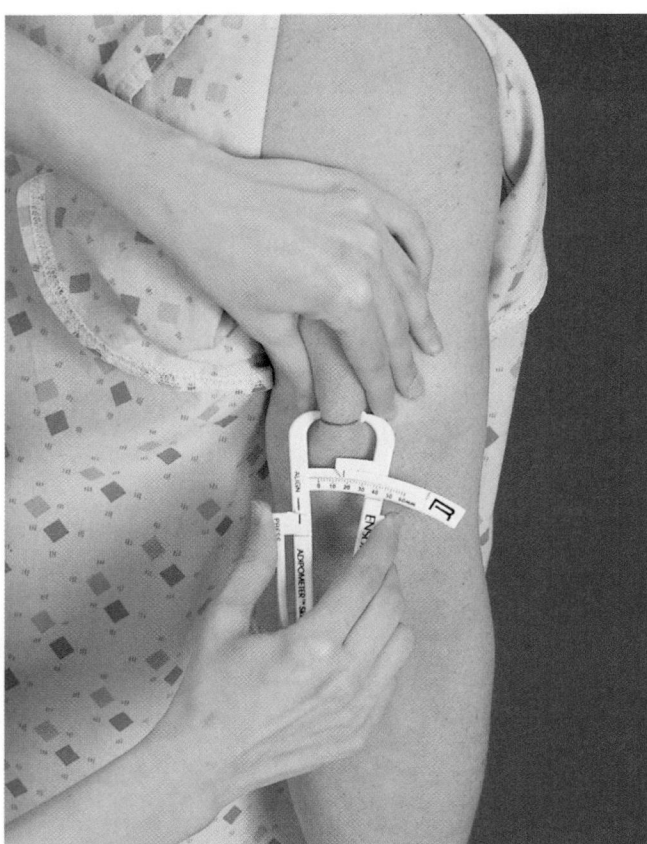

**Figure 35-7    Measuring triceps skinfold, at mid-point of the upper arm**

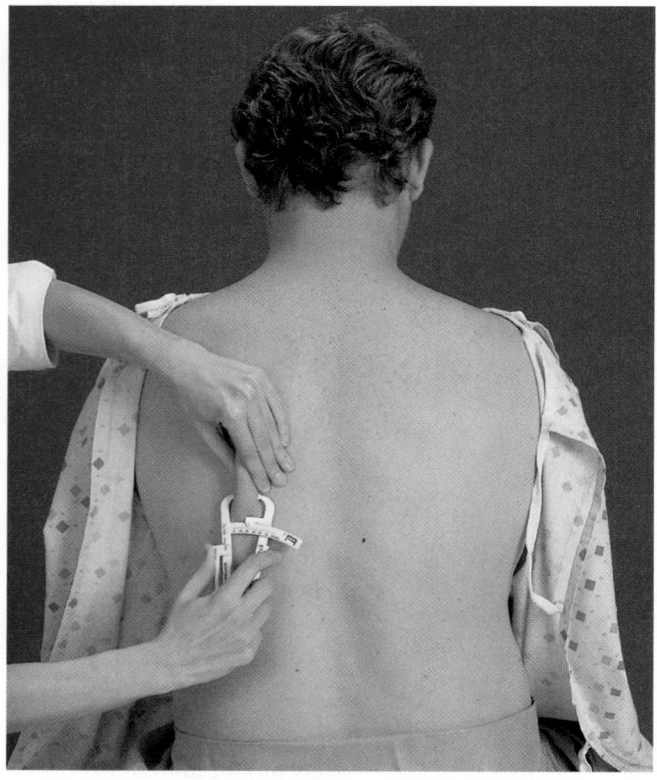

**Figure 35-8    Measuring the subscapular skinfold**

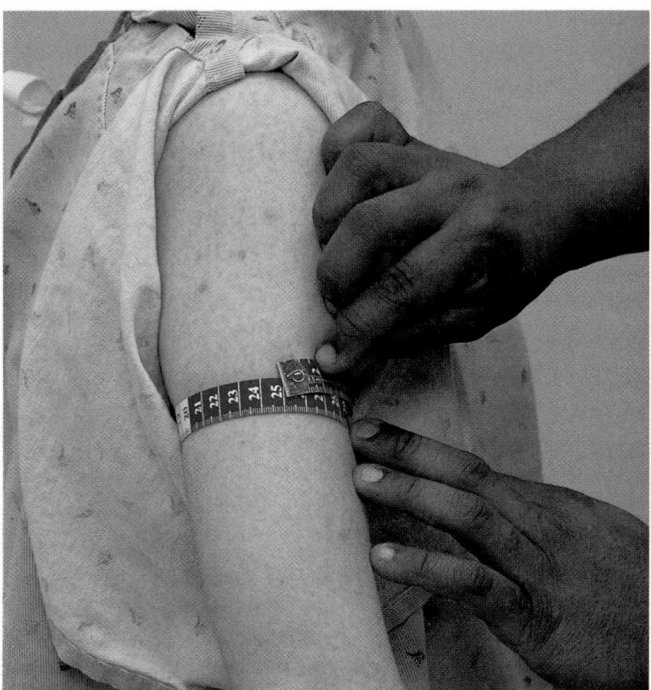

**Figure 35-9    Measuring    the    mid-upper-arm circumference**

### Serum Albumin

Albumin is synthesized in the liver from amino acids. Serum albumin plays an important role in fluid and electrolyte balance and the transport of nutrients, hormones, and drugs. However, serum albumin has a half-life of 18 to 21 days and fluctuates according to the level of hydration. Surgery, acute stress, and hepatic and renal diseases also affect albumin levels. Therefore, it is not a good indicator of acute alterations in protein status (American Society for Parental and Enteral Nutrition [ASPEN], 2002a). Clinically, this blood test is used to measure prolonged protein depletion that occurs in chronic malnutrition, liver disease, and nephrosis. Albumin levels below 3.5 g/dl may indicate some degree of malnutrition.

### Pre-Albumin

Research has provided a newer, more accurate test to evaluate protein status. **Pre-albumin** (a precursor of albumin) has a half-life of 2 to 3 days; it is used to determine protein depletion in acute conditions, such as trauma and inflammation, and serves as a guide for nutritional therapy. Renal failure can falsely elevate pre-albumin. In liver failure, pre-albumin is a poor indicator of nutrition status, as the liver does not manufacture acute phase proteins effectively. Pre-albumin levels between 8 mg/dL and 18 mg/dL reflect mild to moderate protein depletion, while levels below 8 mg/dL indicate severe protein depletion (ASPEN, 2002b).

### Serum Transferrin

**Transferrin** (non-heme iron) is a blood protein in combination with iron; it is used to transport iron throughout the body to all cells. It is responsive to iron stores, increas-

## NURSING STRATEGY

### Creatinine Excretion

Record the client's height and sex on the laboratory request for a creatinine excretion test because the normal values are standardized on the basis of these variables.

ing when iron stores are low and decreasing when iron stores are high. This test is considered a sensitive indicator of protein deficiency because it responds promptly to changes in protein intake. Levels below 200 mg/dl may indicate mild to moderate protein depletion and below 100 mg/dl may indicate severe depletion (Daniels, 2003).

### Hemoglobin Level

The hemoglobin test measures the oxygen- and iron-carrying capacity of the blood; the normal level is 12–15 g/100 ml. A decreased hemoglobin may indicate some form of anemia, such as microcytic iron deficiency anemia, or blood loss.

### Total Lymphocyte Count

Another test that may be used to measure protein depletion is total lymphocyte count. Protein deficiency may cause a depression in the immune system, with a resultant decrease in the total lymphocyte count; this can occur with severe debilitating diseases, such as cancer or renal disease.

### Nitrogen Balance

Nitrogen balance studies indicate the degree to which protein is being depleted or replaced in the body. The *blood urea nitrogen (BUN)* is increased with severe dehydration, malnutrition, starvation, excessive protein intake, and most commonly in kidney disease (the kidneys fail to excrete urea). A decreased BUN may result from a diet low in protein-rich foods.

### Urine Creatinine Excretion

During skeletal muscle metabolism, creatinine is released at a rate in proportion to the total body mass. A 24-hour urine test is done to measure the total amount of creatinine excreted by the kidneys. In malnutrition, the creatinine level is decreased as a result of muscle atrophy.

## Nursing Diagnosis

In order to make a nursing diagnosis, the nurse must interpret the subjective and objective data and draw conclusions from the client's assessment data obtained during a comprehensive health history and physical examination. The approved nursing diagnoses are discussed to assist with appropriate selection of primary and secondary nursing diagnoses for clients with nutritional alterations.

## Imbalanced Nutrition: Less Than Body Requirements

An estimated 30% to 50% of hospitalized clients are at risk for malnutrition; increased morbidity and mortality rates are associated with malnutrition (McCloskey & Bulechek, 1999). The diagnosis *Imbalanced Nutrition: Less Than Body Requirements* exists when the client fails to ingest or digest food or absorb nutrients.

Such clients may experience a weight loss of 20% or more from their ideal weight. The dietary history may reveal inadequate food intake based on the RDAs, a lack of interest in or an aversion to eating, perceived inability to ingest food, and a reduced energy level. Clients have poor muscle tone, with skinfolds less than 60% of standard measurement, and may experience difficulty in swallowing or masticating food because of muscular weakness. The conjunctive and mucous membranes are usually pale, and the buccal cavity is sore and inflamed.

## Imbalanced Nutrition: More Than Body Requirements or Risk for More Than Body Requirements

*Imbalanced Nutrition: More Than Body Requirements* exists when clients experience or are at risk for an intake of nutrients that exceeds metabolic needs. Clients may be at risk because of one or more of the following factors: hereditary predisposition or obesity in one or both parents; dysfunctional psychological conditioning in relationship to food, such as using food as a reward or comfort measure; and age-related factors, most notably early infancy, adolescence, and aging.

Clients with more than body requirements experience a weight gain of 10% to 20% over the ideal for height and frame and triceps skinfolds greater than 15 mm in men and 23 mm in women. The client's dietary history may reveal a sedentary activity level and one or more dysfunctional eating patterns: pairing food with other activities, such as watching TV; concentrating the intake of food at night; eating in response to internal cues (anxiety) or external cues (such as a social event) instead of in response to hunger.

## Other Nursing Diagnoses

The client who is protein-depleted may also experience deficiencies in vitamins (especially A and C) and minerals (especially zinc, magnesium, and iron). Refer to Box 35-4 for a listing of common secondary nursing diagnoses related to nutritional and metabolic problems. Because the secondary diagnosis is related to the nutritional/metabolic problem, it is written in terms of the etiology of the primary diagnosis—for example, *High Risk for Impaired Skin Integrity: related to inadequate intake of proteins, vitamins, and minerals.*

## BOX 35-4    SECONDARY NURSING DIAGNOSES FOR CLIENTS WITH NUTRITIONAL PROBLEMS

*Activity Intolerance:* related to insufficient energy from calorie/protein depletion

*Acute Pain:* related to lactose intolerance

*Ineffective Health Maintenance:* related to excessive intake of nutrients

*Impaired Oral Mucous Membrane:* related to dehydration

*Ineffective Breathing Pattern:* related to decreased energy and fatigue from protein depletion

*Constipation:* related to inadequate dietary and fiber intake and decreased activity.

*Ineffective Health Maintenance:* related to inadequate financial resources to purchase nutritious foods

*Risk for Infection:* related to nutrient replacement therapy

*Deficient Knowledge:* related to information of normal nutrition

*Ineffective Therapeutic Regimen Management (individual):* related to cultural influences on the client's food preferences

*Impaired Swallowing:* related to decreased strength of muscles involved in mastication

*Chronic Low Self-Esteem:* related to obesity

*Risk for Impaired Skin Integrity:* related to inadequate intake of proteins, vitamins, and minerals

North American Nursing Diagnosis Association (NANDA) (2003). *Nursing diagnosis: Definitions & classifications (2003–2004).* Philadelphia: Author.

## BOX 35-5    EXPECTED OUTCOMES FOR CLIENTS WITH IMBALANCED NUTRITION

- Client maintains intake and output balance.
- Client consumes the proper amounts of foods from the four food groups, as evidenced by the food-frequency record.
- Client complies with diet therapy, avoiding saturated fats.
- Client tolerates tube feeding without experiencing any vomiting and diarrhea.
- Client remains infection-free while receiving parenteral nutrition and is transitioned to enteral route as soon as stomach is available.

## Outcome Identification and Planning

The nurse relies heavily on the data obtained from the nutritional history and collaborates with the client and other health team members in formulating goals and expected outcomes to promote optimal nutritional care. Nursing diagnoses of life-threatening conditions, such as *Impaired Swallowing related to decreased or absent gag reflex,* are given first priority. Other diagnoses that are actual problems take priority over high-risk problems.

In the planning phase, the nurse identifies and explains to the client the need for and basis of the therapy. The nurse takes into consideration the client's dietary habits, likes, dislikes, needs, and nutritional assessment data in defining goals and developing outcomes in collaboration with the client. Refer to Box 35-5 for a sample list of expected outcomes for clients with imbalanced nutrition.

The nurse selects appropriate nursing interventions to match the client's routine patterns, as obtained in the health history, and to support achievement of the goals and outcomes. Proceeding in this fashion facilitates the client's adaptive capabilities through skillful interventions.

## Implementation

The nurse is responsible for understanding the client's nutritional needs and for making clinical judgments relative to outcomes of therapy. This responsibility includes intervening to prevent the rapid depletion of the body's protein and energy reserves. Performance of nursing interventions to accomplish goals and outcomes includes monitoring the client's weight and intake, diet therapy, and feeding. Client teaching occurs with each intervention to maximize the effectiveness of nutritional therapy.

### Monitoring Weight and Intake

Weight and intake measurements are used to assess the client's nutritional status and to monitor the effectiveness of therapy. Refer to Chapters 27 and 34 for nursing actions relative to daily weights and intake and output considerations.

### Initiating Diet Therapy

Nutritional problems often require dietary modification. Therapeutic nutrition requires consideration of the client's total needs: cultural, socioeconomic, psychological, and physiological. Modified diets should promote effective nutrition within the client's lifestyle; this often requires client teaching regarding the avoidance of certain foods or adding food items to the diet, given the client's sociocultural context, economic restraints, and religious beliefs.

## Nothing by Mouth

Placing the client on NPO (nothing by mouth) status is a type of diet modification as well as a fluid restriction; refer to Chapter 34 for a complete discussion of fluid restrictions. This intervention is prescribed prior to surgery and certain diagnostic procedures, to rest the GI tract (and prevent diarrhea or vomiting), or when the client's nutritional problem has not been identified. If a client remains NPO for longer than 3 to 4 days, he may be at nutritional risk if previously malnourished or acutely stressed. Notify the dietitian if the diet is not anticipated to increase in 1 to 2 days (White & Duncan, 2002).

## Clear-Liquid Diet

Dairy products are not allowed on a clear-liquid diet. The client is allowed to ingest only liquids that keep the GI tract empty (no residue), such as water, apple juice, and gelatin. A clear-liquid diet is prescribed primarily for surgical clients.

## Liquid Diet

A liquid (or full liquid diet) consisting of various types of liquids is prescribed mainly for postoperative clients because of calorie and nutrient considerations. If the client tolerates a liquid diet without nausea or vomiting and has normal bowel sounds, the diet is progressed to *as tolerated* (client eats whatever foods cause no problems).

## Soft Diet

A soft diet promotes the mechanical digestion of foods. It is prescribed for clients experiencing difficulty in chewing and swallowing. A soft diet may also be therapeutic for clients with impaired digestion and/or absorption, due to conditions such as ulcerative colitis and Crohn's disease. Foods to be avoided on this diet include nuts, seeds (tomatoes and berries with seeds), raw fruits and vegetables, fried foods, and whole grains.

## Mechanical Soft Diet

A mechanical soft diet is similar to a soft diet. It is prescribed for clients experiencing difficulty chewing or who are unable to chew food thoroughly, as may occur with poorly fitted dentures.

## Pureed Diet

A pureed diet provides food that has been blenderized to a smooth consistency. It is prescribed for clients with dysphagia, or difficulty in swallowing. Special consideration needs to be given to meal preparation; when food has the same consistency, it is difficult to distinguish the taste of different foods.

## Low-Residue Diet

A low-residue diet has reduced fiber and cellulose. It is prescribed to decrease GI mucosal irritation in clients with diverticulitis, ulcerative colitis, and Crohn's disease. Foods to be avoided are raw fruits, raw vegetables, seeds, plant fiber, and whole grains. Dairy products are limited to two servings a day.

## High-Fiber Diet

High-fiber-diet foods are the opposite of low-residue foods. A high-fiber diet is an integral part of the treatment regimen for diverticulosis because it increases the forward motion of the indigestible wastes through the colon.

## Liberal Bland Diet

A liberal bland diet eliminates chemical and mechanical food irritants, such as fried foods, alcohol, and caffeine. This diet is prescribed for clients with gastritis and ulcers because it reduces GI irritation.

## Fat-Controlled Diet

Fat-controlled diets reduce the amount of total fat ingested. Fat-controlled diets also substitute saturated fats for monounsaturated fats and polyunsaturated fats while decreasing cholesterol intake. They are prescribed for clients with atherosclerosis, heart disease, and obesity. Saturated foods to be avoided include animal fats, gravies, sauces, chocolate, and whole-milk products.

## Sodium-Restricted Diet

Sodium intake may be restricted as follows: mild, 2–3 g; moderate, 1,000 mg; strict, 500 mg; severe, 250 mg. A sodium-restricted diet is prescribed for clients with excess fluid volume, hypertension, heart failure, myocardial infarction, and renal failure. The Dietary Approach to Stop Hypertension (DASH) is a well-documented diet that emphasizes low sodium intake while increasing fruits, vegetables, and whole grains. This diet has been effective in lowering blood pressure. For information on the DASH diet, go to the website http://www.dash.bwh.harvard.edu.

## Lactose Intolerance Diet

A lactose intolerance diet eliminates milk and all dairy products except yogurt. **Lactose** is a sugar found in milk and aids the body absorption of calcium. Lactose intolerance is caused by a lack or deficiency of lactase, an enzyme normally made in the small intestines that splits lactose into glucose and galactose. Incomplete digestion of lactose results in diarrhea, gas, and abdominal cramps between 30 minutes and 2 hours after consumption of diary foods. Lactaid tablets and lactose-free milk can be used in clients with lactose intolerance. Many clients with lactose intolerance can tolerate yogurt or small amounts of milk and cheese.

## Assistance with Feeding

Assessment data provide direction regarding how to assist the client with eating (Figure 35-10). Clients with difficulty in self-feeding, chewing, or swallowing will require assistance to promote safety and adequate intake of nutrients; see the Nursing Strategy box.

Because eating is a social activity (Figure 35-11), it is important to encourage a family member or friend to be present at meals. If this is not possible, assess the availability of other resources to provide social stimulation during meals, such as watching TV, listening to music, or having a staff member remain with the client.

## Providing Nutrition Support

Proper nutrition in hospitalized clients is necessary for wound healing, recovery, reduction in morbidity, and consequent reductions in length of stay and mortality. The most common nutritional deficiency in hospitalized clients is protein-energy malnutrition. This type of malnutrition depletes body cell mass and impairs tissue and organ function. When protein-energy malnutrition is left untreated, the following client negative outcomes may occur:

- Weakness
- Compromised immunity
- Decreased wound healing
- Increased risk for complications

Nutrition support is prescribed for those clients at risk for protein-energy malnutrition.

There are two routes for delivery of nutrition support (NS) in adult clients: enteral nutrition (EN) and parenteral nutrition (PN). **Enteral nutrition** includes both the ingestion of food orally and the delivery of nutrients through a feeding tube. **Parenteral nutrition** refers to nutrients

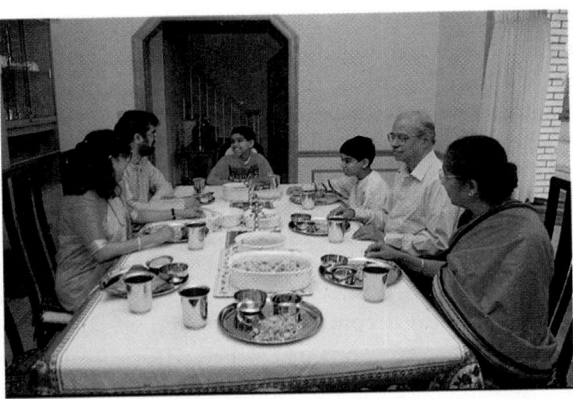

**Figure 35-11    Eating is often a very social time and can depict the cultural values of family and friends.**

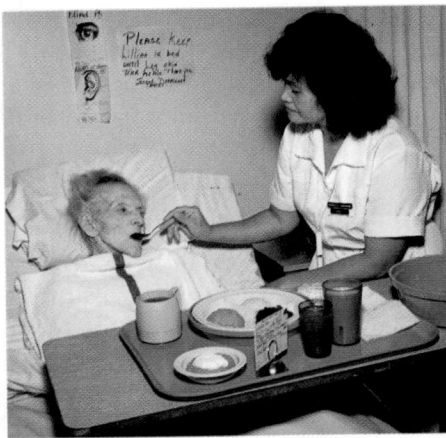

**Figure 35-10    Older adults may have health problems that affect their ability to self-feed.**

## NURSING STRATEGY

### Nursing Measures That Promote Client Feeding

- Before bringing the meal tray into the room, ask whether the client needs to void or have a bowel movement.

- Provide hygiene measures before serving the meal tray.

- Position the client in a comfortable position, preferably in a chair, if not contraindicated.

- Ask about the client's eating habits, and as to the foods she prefers to eat first. Ask what help is needed. For instance, older people may want scrambled eggs placed in a sandwich to make them easier to handle.

- Make sure the foods are being served at the correct temperature.

- Provide assistance if the client is unable to handle eating utensils or open containers and packages.

- Provide adequate time for the client who has difficulty in chewing or swallowing. Make sure that someone is in the room while the client is eating.

- Document the type and amount of food taken at each meal.

- Remove the tray after the meal and provide hygiene measures.

bypassing the small intestine and entering the blood directly through a peripheral or central line. EN is preferred over PN because of decreased bacterial translocation, decreased line sepsis, and reduced expense (ASPEN, 2002) (Figure 35-12).

Critical indicators for determining the feeding route and nutrition support formula include GI function, expected duration of therapy, aspiration risk, and the potential for or the actual development of organ dysfunction. For example, the decision to initiate PN or EN support is based on the availability of the gut, the client's ability to meet his nutritional needs, and the client's current level of nutrition status and metabolic stress. The client's nutrition support may be determined by a nutrition support team (NST) in accord with the American Society for Parenteral and Enteral Nutrition (ASPEN) guidelines.

## Nutrition Support Teams

Since the early 1980s, nutrition support teams (NSTs) were established to reduce the complications of PN. To achieve the expertise required for a consulting service, the teams have become multidisciplinary.

The nurse is seen as the vital link between the client and other team members to include a physician, nurse, pharmacist, and dietitian; see Box 35-6 for the functions of NSTs. The nurse's role is critical, both for the implementation of nutritional support and for ongoing assessment, because the nurse administers and monitors nutritional therapies.

The nurse is also responsible for eliciting the client's or family's continued consent and collaboration with the therapy. The physician obtains the client's informed consent for starting the therapy. The nurse teaches the client and family about the nutritional support to restore a sense of independence and self-esteem. Many staff nurses are board-certified in nutrition support by ASPEN.

## Providing Enteral Nutrition

Candidates for enteral tube feeding are clients who have a functional GI tract and will not, should not, or cannot eat. Therefore, tube feedings are used for clients who are (or may become) malnourished and in whom oral feedings are insufficient to maintain adequate nutritional status (Hamilton, 2000).

Enteral tube feedings maintain the structural and functional integrity of the GI tract, enhance the use of nutrients, and provide a safe and economical method of feeding. Enteral tube feedings are contraindicated in clients with the following:

- Diffused peritonitis
- Intestinal obstruction that prohibits normal bowel functioning
- Intractable vomiting; paralytic ileus
- Severe diarrhea

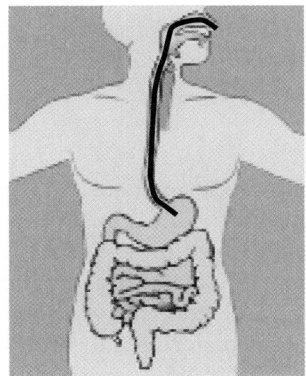
Nasogastric Route

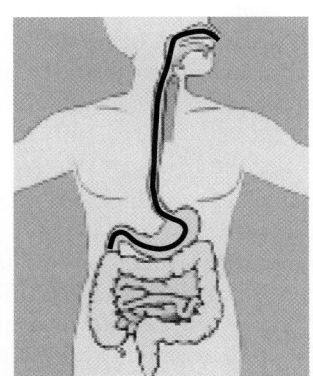
Nasoduodenal Route

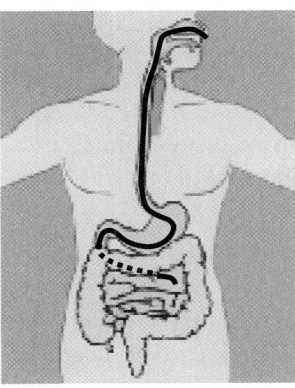
Nasojejunal Route

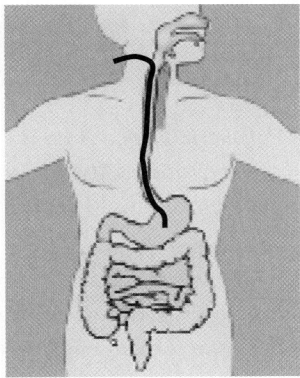
Esophagostomy Route

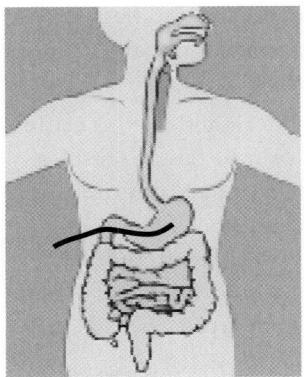
Gastrostomy Route

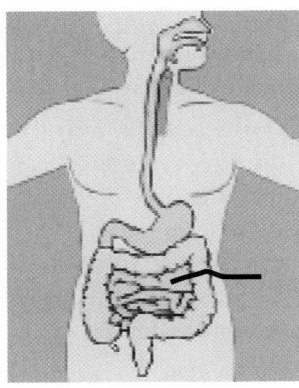
Jejunostomy Route

**Figure 35-12   Enteral feeding routes**

| BOX 35-6 | CLINICAL FUNCTIONS OF NUTRITION SUPPORT TEAMS |
|---|---|

- Identification of clients who are nutrition-impaired or at risk for malnutrition

- Performance of a nutritional assessment to guide nutritional therapy

- Provision of nutritional support that is safe and effective

## NURSING STRATEGY

### Facilitating Feeding for the Client with Impaired Vision

Clients with impaired vision need established routines that facilitate feeding. For example, foods are usually placed on the plate in a clockwise order: bread at the 12 o'clock position, meat at 3 o'clock, starches at 6 o'clock, and vegetables at 9 o'clock. The plate should have a raised edge so that the food can be scooped to the outside of the plate. Serving liquids in either a glass or a cup with a plastic lid and straw may be helpful to avoid spills.

## Feeding Tubes

Most feeding tubes are made of silicone or polyurethane, which are durable and biocompatible with formulas. They vary in diameter (8 to 12 French) and length in accord with the route and formula. The physician selects the route and type of feeding tube on the basis of the anticipated duration of feeding, client comfort, the condition of the GI tract, and the potential for aspiration.

## Insertion of Enteral Feeding Tubes

Nasoenteral insertion of a gastric feeding tube is the simplest and most often used method of tube feeding. It is used as a temporary measure for clients who are expected to resume oral feeding. Nasogastric intubation refers to insertion of a tube through the nostril into the stomach; refer to Procedure 35-1. Nasoduodenal or nasojejunal intubation allows nasal access to the duodenum and jejunum; it is done with a longer tube and decreases the client's risk of vomiting and aspiration (Penrod, Morse, & Wilson, 1999). Radiographic visualization is used to confirm tube placement prior to feeding.

Enterostomy is the surgical creation of an artificial fistula (gastrostomy, jejunostomy) in the intestines by incision through the abdominal wall. Tube enterostomies can be placed at various points along the GI tract and are performed when long-term tube feeding is anticipated or when obstruction makes nasal intubation impossible.

## CLINICAL ALERT

### Small-Bore Feeding Tube

When inserting a small-bore feeding tube with the guidewire or stylet, never attempt to reinsert the guidewire or stylet while the tube is in the client. The guidewire or stylet may perforate the GI mucosa, especially the esophagus, and injure the client.

## CLINICAL ALERT

### Allergies

Before administering a tube feeding, determine whether the client has any food allergies. Clients may be lactose-intolerant or have an allergy to the formula.

Percutaneous endoscopic gastrostomy (PEG) tube placement is usually performed by the physician at the bedside or in the endoscopy room; *insertion of a PEG tube does not require surgery.* Endoscopy nurses are often trained to assist with PEG placement. PEG has become an accepted technique to provide enteral access for both children and adults (Wilson, 2000).

## Enteral Formulas

Nutrients administered through tubes are liquefied so they can be easily digested and absorbed. Commercially prepared formulas are available and used in most health care settings. Formulas differ in osmolality, digestibility, kilocalories, electrolyte content, fiber content, viscosity, fat content, and lactose content. The majority of formulas are lactose free (ASPEN, 2002b). See Box 35-7 for a listing of basic types of formulas.

### BOX 35-7    BASIC TYPES OF FORMULAS

*Polymeric formulas* contain whole protein, fats, and carbohydrates for use with normal or near normal gastrointestinal function.

*Monomeric formulas* (elemental, semi-elemental, or hydrolyzed) contain predigested nutrients; most are low in fat or contain a significant source of medium chain triglycerides. They can be used in clients with minimally functional digestive and absorptive capabilities.

*Fiber-containing formulas* are polymeric diets containing fiber; beneficial for prevention and treatment of constipation and diarrhea.

*Disease-specific formulas* are designed for specific disease states such as renal or liver failure, respiratory disease, diabetes, and immune compromise. Well-designed clinical trials are lacking for many disease-specific formulas. Fluid-restricted (1.5–2 cal/cc) and electrolyte-restricted formulas often fall under disease-specific formulas.

ASPEN (2002). *The science and practice of nutrition support: A case-based core curriculum.* Dubuque: Kendall/Hunt Publishing Co., p. 148.

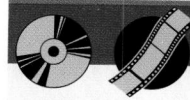

**PROCEDURE 35-1**

# Inserting and Maintaining a Nasogastric Tube

## EQUIPMENT NEEDED

- Nasogastric tube: adult, 14 to 18 French; child/infant, 5 to 10 French; single lumen (Levin's sump): feeding; double lumen (Salem sump tube): feeding, suction, irrigation (Figure 35-13)
- Water-soluble lubricant
- Syringe with catheter tip or adapter, 20–50 ml
- Glass of tap water with straw, or ice
- Towel or tissue
- Emesis basin with ice chips
- Tongue blade
- pH chemstrip
- Stethoscope
- Disposable gloves (nonsterile), goggles, gown
- Hypoallergenic tape, rubber band, and safety pin
- Penlight or flashlight
- Disposable irrigation set (if needed)
- Wall mount or portable suction equipment (if needed)
- Administration set with pump or controller for feeding tube

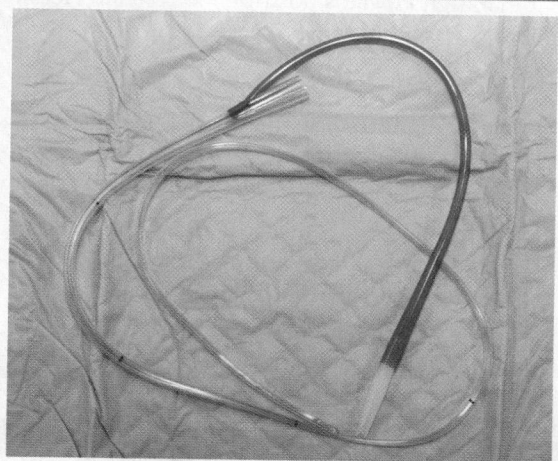

**Figure 35-13    Double-lumen nasogastric tube**

## IMPLEMENTATION—ACTION/RATIONALE

### ACTION

1. Review client's medical history.

2. Assess client's consciousness and ability to understand. Explain the procedure and develop a hand signal (Figure 35-14).

3. Prepare the equipment, putting tissues, a cup of water, and an emesis basin nearby (Figure 35-15).

### RATIONALE

1. To assess for any nostril surgery and abnormal bleeding.

2. Decreases anxiety and promotes cooperation.

3. Facilitates an efficient procedure.

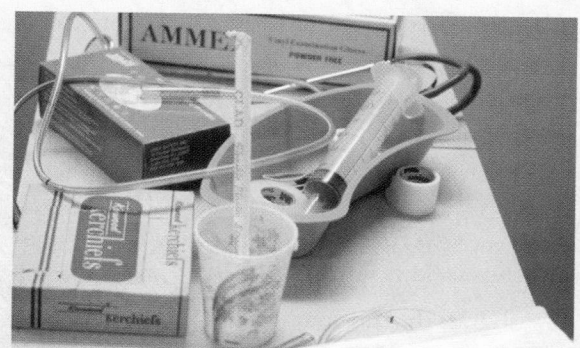

**Figure 35-14    Explain the procedure; demonstrate head position and tube.**

**Figure 35-15    Put an emesis basin, cup with straw, and tissues nearby.**

*(continues)*

## PROCEDURE 35-1 (continued)

4. Prepare the environment; raise the bed and place it in a high Fowler's position (45 to 60 degrees). Cover the chest with a towel.

5. Wash hands and then put on gloves.

6. Use a penlight to view the client's nostrils. Assess client's nostrils with penlight and have the client blow her nose one nostril at a time (Figure 35-16).

7. Using the NG tube, measure the distance from the bridge of the nose to the earlobe and then to the xiphoid process of the sternum and mark this distance on the tube with a piece of tape (Figure 35-17).

4. Facilitates insertion and prevents back strain.

5. Practices clean technique.

6. Choosing the more patent nostril for insertion decreases discomfort and unnecessary trauma.

7. Determines the approximate amount of tube needed to reach the stomach.

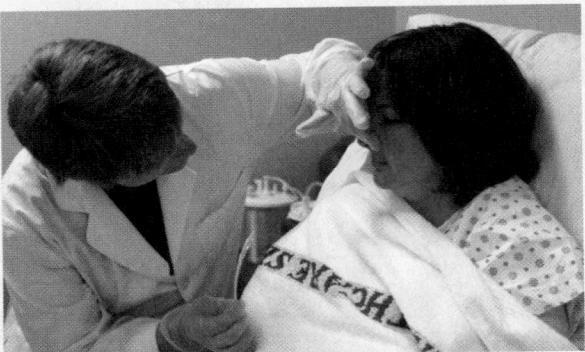

**Figure 35-16** Assess the client's nostrils before introducing the nasogastric tube.

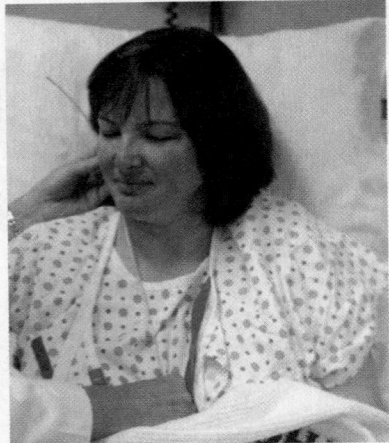

**Figure 35-17** Measure the distance from nose to earlobe to the xiphoid process to determine how much tube will need to be inserted to reach the stomach.

8. Lubricate first 4 inches of the tube with water-soluble lubricant.

9. Ask the client to slightly flex the neck backward.

10. Gently insert the tube into a naris (Figure 35-18).

11. Ask the client to tip the head forward once the tube reaches the nasopharynx. If the client continues to gag, stop a moment.

12. Advance the tube several inches at a time as the client swallows water or ice chips (Figure 35-19).

13. Withdraw the tube immediately if there are signs of respiratory distress.

14. Advance the tube until the taped mark is reached (Figure 35-20).

8. Facilitates passage into the naris.

9. Makes insertion easier.

10. Promotes passage of tube with minimal trauma to mucosa.

11. Tipping the head forward facilitates passage of the tube into the esophagus instead of the trachea. Tube may stimulate gag reflex. Allows the client to rest, reduces anxiety, and prevents vomiting.

12. Assists in pushing the tube past the oropharynx.

13. Prevents trauma to bronchus or lung.

14. Enables the tube to reach the stomach.

*(continues)*

## PROCEDURE 35-1 (continued)

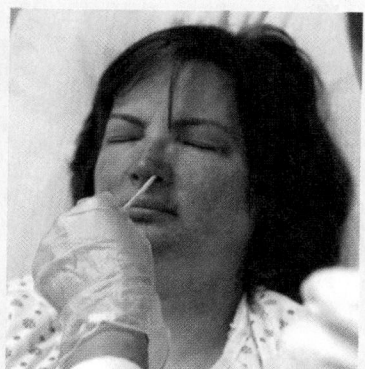

**Figure 35-18   Gently insert the tube into the naris.**

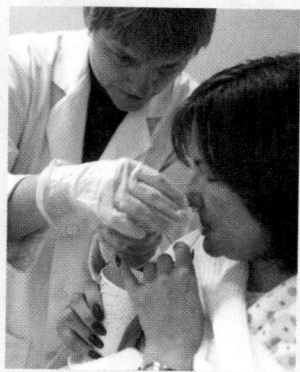

**Figure 35-19   Advance the tube slowly. The client swallows small sips of water to assist in pushing the tube past the oropharnyx.**

15. Split a 4-inch strip of tape lengthwise 2 inches. Secure the tube with the tape by placing the wide portion of the tape on the bridge of the nose and wrapping the split ends around the tube (Figure 35-21). Tape to cheek as well if desired (Figure 35-22).

15. Prevents tube displacement.

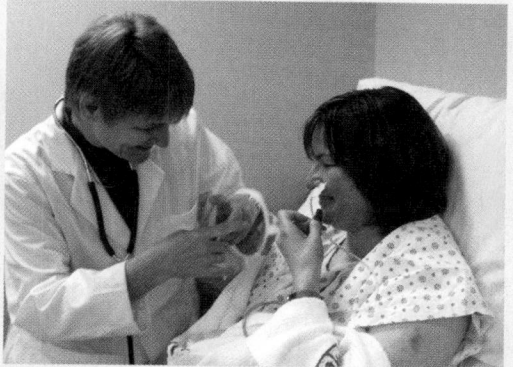

**Figure 35-20   Advance the tube until the taped mark is at the opening of the naris.**

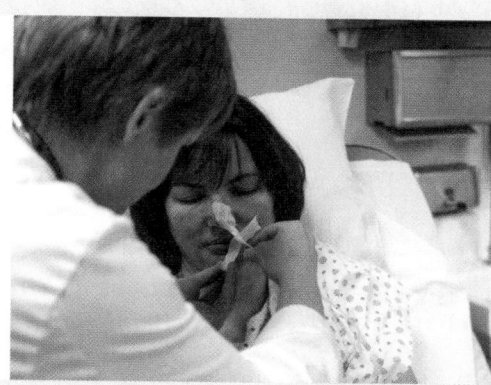

**Figure 35-21   Secure the tube to the nose.**

16. Check the placement of the tube:
    • Attach the syringe to the end of the tube for injecting 10 cc of air and auscultate over the epigastric area (upper left quadrant); Figure 35-23.
    • Aspirate sample gastric content and measure with chemstrip pH (Figure 35-24).
    • Prepare the client for x-ray check-up, if prescribed.

16. Ensures correct placement. (A pH below 4 indicates the tube is in the stomach; a pH range of 6–7 indicates intestinal sites.)

17. Connect the distal end of the tube to suction, draining bag, or adapter (Figure 35-25).

17. Establishes an appropriate pathway for intervention.

*(continues)*

**PROCEDURE 35-1** (*continued*)

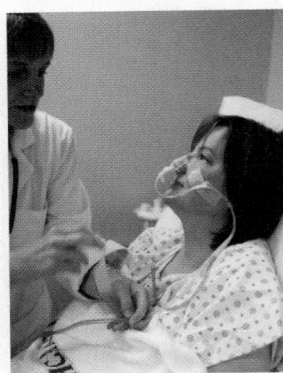

**Figure 35-22** Tape the tube to the cheek as well, if desired, to provide extra support.

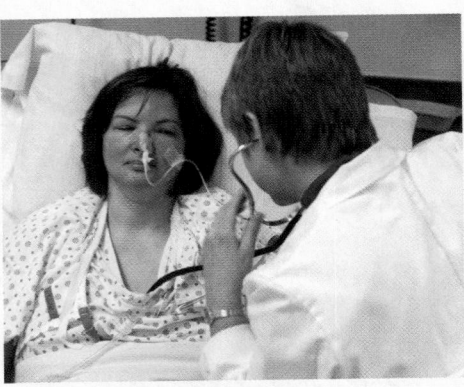

**Figure 35-23** Auscultate over the epigastric area.

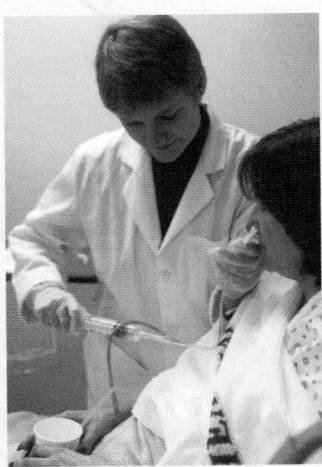

**Figure 35-24** Aspirate a sample of gastric content to check for pH.

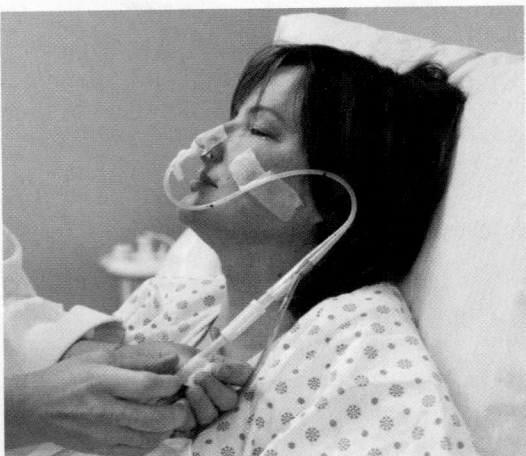

**Figure 35-25** Connect the distal end of the tube to suction or drainage to complete the procedure.

18. Secure the tube with rubber band and safety pin to client's gown or bed sheet.

19. Remove gloves, dispose of contaminated materials in proper container, and wash hands.

20. Position client comfortably and place the call light in easy reach.

21. Document procedure.

### Maintaining a Nasogastric Tube

22. Wash hands and apply gloves.

23. Follow the steps in Action 16 to check the proper tubing position before instilling anything per NG tube or at least every 8 hours.

18. Enhances the level of comfort and secures the tubing system.

19. Implements the principles of infection control.

20. Decreases client's anxiety and provides access to help if needed.

21. Records implementation of intervention and promotes continuity of care.

22. Reduces transmission of microorganisms.

23. Prevents complications from dislocation of the tube.

*(continues)*

## PROCEDURE 35-1 *(continued)*

24. Assess for signs that the tube has become blocked, including epigastric pain and vomiting, and/or the inability to pass medications or feedings through the tube.

24. Prevents complications from the loss of beneficial effects from the tube.

25. Remember never to irrigate or rotate a tube that has been placed by the physician or qualified practitioner during gastric or esophageal surgery.

25. Rotation or irrigation may disturb incisions.

26. Provide oral hygiene and assist client to clean nares daily.

26. Enhances client's comfort and the integrity of skin and nose mucosa.

27. Remove gloves, dispose of contaminated materials in proper container, and wash hands.

27. Reduces transmission of microorganisms.

---

### LIFE SPAN CONSIDERATIONS

#### Inserting an NG Tube

**Pediatric Variations**

- Dispose of or securely tape any small parts, such as plastic connectors or plugs, to prevent small children from accidentally aspirating or swallowing them.

**Geriatric Variations**

- For older clients who wear dentures, oral hygiene and denture care should not be overlooked simply because an NG tube is in place.

### COMMUNITY/HOME CARE

#### Nasogastric Tube

**Home Care Variations**

- Periodically assess the family member's ability to check the placement of the tube, check residual gastric contents, administer tube feedings, or connect the tube properly with suction.

**Long-Term Care Variations**

- Teach family members or caregivers to assess client's nutritional status and assess for any sign of complications related to the NG tube.

---

### Administration of Enteral Feedings

Once the feeding tube's position has been radiographically verified, the formula can be administered as prescribed; refer to Procedure 35-2. Most clients with a small-bore tube receive continuous feeding with a formula pump to regulate the rate. One of the advantages of continuous feeding is that it keeps gastric volume small, minimizing residual volume and reducing the risk of aspiration pneumonia; the client is less likely to experience bloating, nausea, abdominal distention, and diarrhea.

### Safety Considerations

Clients receiving EN through a feeding tube are at risk for aspiration. The prevalence of tube placement errors, as reported in the literature, varies from 1.3% to 50% in adults (Cirgin & Marsha, 1997). Tube feeding aspiration can result from several factors: displacement of the tube into the esophagus, large amounts of gastric residual, and lowered intestinal motility and delayed gastric emptying, which may occur in clients who are on bed rest or receiving narcotics for pain relief (Altman, 2004). Auscultate for bowel sounds to determine gastric motility. If the bowel sounds are hypoactive or absent, stop or withhold additional feeding and notify the physician.

Always assess placement of the feeding tube before administering any liquids. Clients who are receiving continuous gastric feeding should be assessed every 4 to 6 hours for tube placement and residual gastric contents. Aspirate gastric contents with a syringe. This is done more easily with a large-bore tube than a small-bore tube. The lumen of a small-bore tube collapses easily, making aspiration difficult and sometimes impossible. Observe and check the pH of the aspirate as explained in Procedure 35-1; refer to the Research Focus. Replace stomach contents after checking the residual to prevent fluid and electrolyte imbalance.

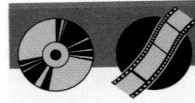

## PROCEDURE 35-2

# Assessing Placement of a Large-Bore Feeding Tube

## EQUIPMENT NEEDED

- Catheter tip syringe, 60 ml (Figure 35-26)
- Stethoscope
- Gloves
- pH indicator strip
- Emesis basin
- Towel

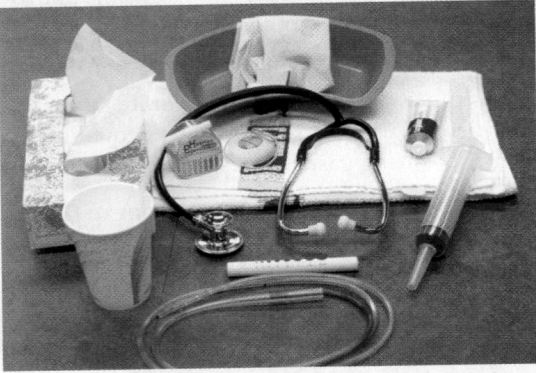

**Figure 35-26    Stethoscope, syringe, and pH strips are used to assess placement of the tube.**

## IMPLEMENTATION—ACTION/RATIONALE

| ACTION | RATIONALE |
|---|---|
| 1. Check physician's or qualified practitioner's order for the feeding tube. | 1. Ensures accurate placement of the tube. |
| 2. Wash hands (Figure 35-27). Apply gloves. | 2. Reduces the transmission of microorganisms. |
| 3. Assess placement of the tube by auscultation: | 3. This method is less reliable than checking for gastric contents, but it is the simplest way to assess for placement of the feeding tubes.<br>• Allows nurse to hear sound of air. |
| • Place stethoscope over left upper quadrant of the abdomen.<br>• Quickly inject 10–20 ml air with the 60 ml syringe (Figure 35-28).<br>• Assess for resistance. | |
| • Listen for sound. | • If resistance is felt, tells nurse to attempt to aspirate GI contents.<br>• A whooshing or gurgling sound can be heard as air enters the stomach. |

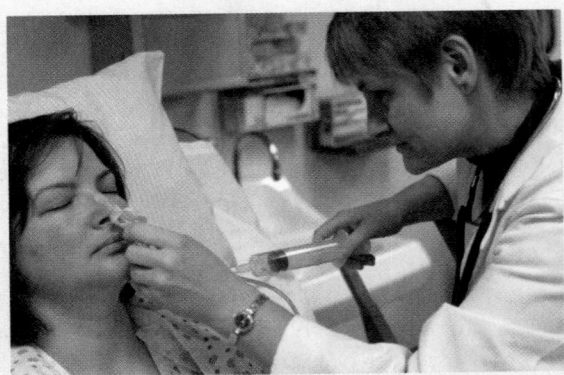

**Figure 35-27    Wash hands prior to beginning procedure.**

**Figure 35-28    Inject 10–20 ml of air.**

*(continues)*

**PROCEDURE 35-2 (*continued*)**

4. Measure pH of GI contents:

   - Aspirate 10 cc of GI contents with 60 cc syringe (Figure 35-29).
   - If unable to aspirate, reposition client on side and try again.
   - Measure pH of GI contents with pH indicator strip.

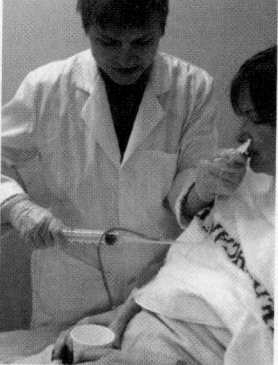

**Figure 35-29    Aspirate 10 cc of gastric contents to check pH.**

5. Proceed with feeding and medication (Figures 35-30 and 35-31). Continue to monitor the client for discomfort.

6. Recheck tube placement following the tube feeding.

   - Flush tube with 30 cc warm water after medication or tube feeding (Figure 35-32).
   - Wait 1 hour before testing pH.

   - Flush tube with 30 cc air and auscultate for sound as in Action 3.
   - Aspirate 10 cc of GI contents and check for pH as in Action 4.

7. Remove gloves and wash hands.

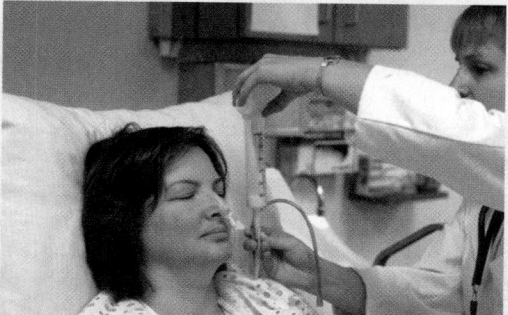

**Figure 35-31    Proceed with administering medications.**

4. Gastric contents have pH of 1–4. Intestinal contents have pH of 6–7.
   - Measure the pH of the gastric aspirate before instilling anything through the feeding tube.
   - The tube opening may be lying against the gastric wall.
   - To obtain accurate results.

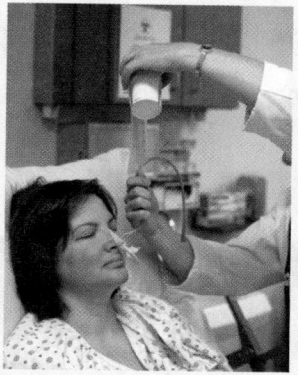

**Figure 35-30    After verifying placement of the tube, proceed with feeding.**

5. To provide the client with nutrition and treatment. Continuing to assess for signs of tube displacement ensures client safety.

6. Continuing to assess for signs of tube displacement ensures client safety.
   - Flushes out residual formula or medication.

   - Allows for digestion of the formula or assimilation of the medication.
   - Assesses placement of the feeding tube.

   - Assesses placement of the feeding tube.

7. Reduces transmission of microorganisms.

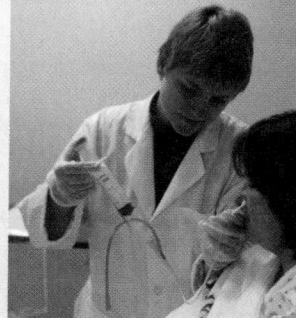

**Figure 35-32    After feeding or administering medications, flush the tube with 30 cc of warm water to rinse out residue.**

## LIFE SPAN CONSIDERATIONS

### Feeding Tube Concerns

**Pediatric Variations**

- Inject only 0.5–1.0 ml of air into a pediatric feeding tube.

- Be sure the child is quiet and calm while checking for placement so you can hear the air being injected.

**Geriatric Variations**

- Older clients may have more fragile tissue that could be damaged with a large-bore feeding tube.

- Older clients with other respiratory conditions are at increased risk for respiratory complications if the feeding tube migrates to the pulmonary tree.

## COMMUNITY/HOME CARE

### Feeding Tubes

**Home Care Variations**

- Assess the sanitation of the home to determine the client's risk for infection.

- The caregiver should be taught the normal range of pH for GI contents.

- The caregiver should be taught the signs and symptoms of feeding tube displacement and what to do if displacement is suspected.

**Long-Term Care Variations**

- The staff should be taught the normal range of pH for GI contents.

- Equipment for verifying tube placement should be at the client's bedside at all times.

- Staff members should be taught the signs and symptoms of tube displacement and to whom to report the symptoms.

- Staff members should be taught how to discontinue a feeding if they suspect tube displacement.

Another way of determining tube placement is to visually examine the aspirate (see Box 35-8). If the pleural aspirates contain blood, they will fail to show their normal characteristics.

Client safety and comfort require daily cleansing of the feeding tube's exit site. Cleanse the skin with a clean washcloth, soap, and water. Nasal feeding tubes require daily removal of the tape from the nose, cleansing, and inspection of the skin for irritation, inflammation, and infection and the nares for erosions, ulcers, or abscesses.

Enterostomy tubes require surgical asepsis of the exit site until the incision heals; rotate the tubes within the stoma to promote healing. Report any observations of redness, irritation, or gastric leakage at the site. Once the stoma has healed, the tube can be removed and reinserted for each feeding. Between feedings, a prosthetic device may be used to cover the ostomy opening.

PEG tubes require daily rotation to relieve pressure on the skin. Notify the physician if you are unable to rotate the PEG; it may be an indication of internal embedding of the tube into the gastric wall. When the tube is internally embedded, it can cause gastric acid reflux, which results in skin breakdown, sepsis, and cellulitis. Care must be taken to avoid dislodgment of the tube. Keep it

## BOX 35-8   CHARACTERISTICS OF ASPIRATES

*Gastric Aspirates*

Cloudy and green, tan or off-white, or bloody or brown (fresh or old blood)

*Intestinal Aspirates*

Basically clear and yellow to bile-colored

*Pleural Aspirates*

Tan or off-white mucus, may be pale yellow and serous (indicating blood)

## COMMUNITY/HOME CARE

### A Feeding Tube in the Home

Clients with feeding tubes may be discharged to the home. The NST evaluates these clients to determine:

- Ability to meet nutrient requirements orally
- Clinical status relative to home discharge
- Tolerance of prescribed nutritional therapy
- Willingness and ability to perform the necessary tasks of tube feeding
- Benefits of continuing therapy at home

The NST works with the client and caregiver to secure the necessary supplies prior to discharge from the hospital. If a client is discharged home with a nasogastric tube, a small-bore feeding tube (8 or 10 French) should be considered for comfort and safety. Clients on home feedings require monitoring by nurses and nutritional support specialists who are familiar with the procedure and complications of enteral tube feeding.

secured to the client's abdomen with tape, being careful not to use excessive tension. PEG tubes require frequent flushing to prevent clogging. These tubes have small lumens. If a tube becomes clogged, flush it with 60 ml of lukewarm tap water.

### Potential Complications

Clients receiving EN need to be monitored closely to prevent complications. The nurse should perform the following actions:

1. Assess the client for signs of gastric retention: nausea, vomiting, and cramping. Palpate the abdomen for distention, auscultate for bowel sounds with a stethoscope, and aspirate the gastric contents every 4 hours. If the aspirate exceeds 100 ml in a 4-hour period or if bowel sounds are absent (indicating an ileus), discontinue the feeding and notify the physician. *Do not remove the feeding tube.* Some clinicians believe that bowel sounds must be present to start enteral feeding. The absence of bowel sounds does not preclude safe EN. Paralytic ileus (absence of bowel sounds or flatus) has been considered in the past to be a contraindication to enteral feedings. However, it is now known that an ileus has different effects on different areas of the intestine. The presence of a soft, nontender abdomen, adequate perfusion, and hemodynamic stability are all indicators of the potential for the safe initiation of EN (ASPEN, 2002a).
2. Monitor the feeding tube placement every 4 hours by checking for any coils or kinks in the back of the throat and measuring the length of tubing outside the body.

## CLINICAL ALERT

### Gastric Resection

Never insert, manipulate, or remove a nasogastric tube on gastric resection clients; *the suture line could easily be interrupted, causing hemorrhage.*

In high-aspiration-risk clients, maintain head of bed above 35% while EN infusing.

3. Assess the client for pulmonary aspiration by checking the gag reflex. If the reflex is absent, suction the client. Discontinue the feeding and remove the tube if signs of respiratory distress are present, and notify the physician.
4. Keep the client in a high Fowler's position to prevent aspiration if vomiting should occur. If vomiting does occur, suction client immediately and assess the formula amount and rate at which it was given.
5. Dilute feedings to half strength and slow the feeding time to prevent diarrhea.
6. To maintain or achieve patency of gastric and/or jejunostomy feeding tubes, a medical device called a DeClogger may be used as prescribed by the client's physician to maintain the patency of these tubes (see Box 35-9).

Teach the client and caregiver how to monitor for complications prior to discharge for home treatment. The client and caregiver should be given the opportunity to practice these assessment measures and demonstrate competency in performing the actual procedures.

### Removal of a Nasogastric Tube

When the physician determines that the client's nutritional status no longer warrants EN therapy or the need to provide decompression of the gastric contents, the nasogastric tube is removed (see Box 35-10). If the client

## BOX 35-9    USE OF A DECLOGGER

1. Gather equipment: towel, receptacle for used items, nonsterile gloves, and appropriate size DeClogger that corresponds to the size of the feeding tube as prescribed by the physician.

2. Verify the health care practitioner's prescription.

3. Review the agency's policy.

4. Check the client's armband, and explain the procedure.

5. Provide for privacy.

6. Wash hands.

7. Turn the enteral feeding pump to the PAUSE mode; if feeding to gravity, clamp the tubing.

8. Don nonsterile gloves.

9. Place the clean towel under the tube to protect the bed linens.

10. Disconnect tubing, and place cap on delivery tube to prevent contamination.

11. Attempt to flush tube with 30–60 cc of water.

12. Gently insert the appropriate size DeClogger into the opening of the tube.

13. Slowly rotate the DeClogger in a clockwise fashion until the stop disc meets the opening of the tube.

14. To remove, slowly rotate the DeClogger in a counterclockwise fashion as you pull back on the device.

15. Flush the feeding tube with 30–60 cc of water.

16. Reconnect the delivery tube, and restart enteral feedings.

17. Discard the DeClogger into the receptacle, remove gloves, place in receptacle, and dispose of receptacle in accord with agency policy.

18. Wash hands, and document procedure in the client's medical record.

## BOX 35-10    REMOVAL OF A NASOGASTRIC TUBE

1. Gather equipment: tube plug or clamp, towel, washcloth, paper towel, receptacle for contaminated items, and nonsterile gloves.

2. Verify the physician's prescription.

3. Check the client's armband and explain the procedure.

4. Provide for privacy.

5. Wash hands and don gloves.

6. Place the client in a high Fowler's position and adjust the height of the bed to a comfortable working position.

7. Place the towel across the client's chest.

8. Clamp or plug the tube and unpin the tube from client's gown.

9. Remove the tape securing the tube from the client's nose.

10. Hold the paper towel open in your nondominant hand under the client's chin; with your dominant hand, grasp and pinch the tube near the nostril, and remove the tube with a steady, continuous pull, allowing the tube to fall into the paper towel.

11. Dispose of the tube and paper towel in the receptacle.

12. Clean the client's nares and provide oral hygiene.

13. Position the client comfortably, place call light in easy reach, and return bed to a low position.

14. Remove gloves, place in receptacle, and dispose of receptacle in accord with agency policy.

15. Wash hands and document procedure in the client's medical record.

is connected to suction for decompression, the physician may prescribe clamping the tubing for several hours prior to removal, to ensure a functioning GI tract.

## Providing Parenteral Nutrition

Parenteral nutrition is the infusion of a solution directly into a vein to meet the client's daily nutritional requirements. Formerly called hyperalimentation, it is frequently

## RESEARCH FOCUS

**Title of Study:** pH and concentration of bilirubin in feeding tube aspirates as predictors of tube placement

**Study Purpose:** This is a descriptive study to correctly predict feeding tube placement based on pH and the concentration of bilirubin in feeding tube aspirates.

**Methods:** Over a 3-year period, a total of 587 samples were collected and analyzed for concurrent pH and bilirubin from adult clients in a variety of acute care settings. A total of 437 gastrointestinal samples were obtained for pH and bilirubin testing from newly inserted small-bore feeding tubes; 125 tracheobronchial secretions were obtained by suctioning clients with artificial airways, and 24 pleural fluid samples were obtained at the time of thoracenteses to provide additional respiratory samples. Certain clients were excluded from the study based on previous gastric surgery or trauma, oral or tube-administered medications prior to sample collection, and samples that were grossly bloody. Data from the pH and bilirubin tests were compared with tube location as determined by radiography.

**Findings:** Samples from concurrent pH and bilirubin testing could significantly decrease the number of x-rays needed to exclude respiratory placement and to distinguish between gastric and intestinal placement.

**Implications:** The professional nurse needs quantifiable methods at the bedside to determine placement of feeding tubes. Although the pH is measurable at the bedside, research needs to address a clinical laboratory testing product for measuring bilirubin content in gastrointestinal and respiratory aspirates at the bedside.

Metheny, N. A., Stewart, B. J., Smith, L., Yan, H., Diebold, M., & Clouse, R. E. (1999). pH and concentration of bilirubin in feeding tube aspirates as predictors of tube placement. *Nursing Research, 48*(4), 189–197.

referred to as parenteral nutrition (PN), the intravenous infusion of a solution containing dextrose, amino acids, fats, essential fatty acids, vitamins, and minerals. Other terms used interchangeably with *PN* are *3 in 1* (dextrose, amino acids, and fats) and *total nutrient admixtures* (TNA).

PN is used to treat malnourished clients or clients who have the potential for becoming malnourished and who are not candidates for enteral support. PN can be prescribed for either short-term or long-term use.

The type of device used for the PN therapy is determined by the duration of the therapy and the osmolality of the solution. Peripheral parenteral nutrition (PPN) is used for short-term treatment to deliver isotonic or mildly hypertonic solutions into a peripheral vein; the volume is usually limited to between 2,000 and 3,000 ml/day, providing a caloric value of about 2,000 kcal/day.

**Total parenteral nutrition (TPN)** is used for long-term therapy to infuse highly hypertonic solutions directly into a central line. The delivery of highly hypertonic solutions into peripheral veins can cause sclerosis, phlebitis, or swelling; refer to Chapter 34 for a complete discussion of intravenous therapy complications. Specific client populations that benefit from PPN or TPN are described in Box 35-11 (Hamilton, 2000).

## Components of Parenteral Nutrition

PN solutions are chemically prepared nutrients that can be administered singly or as admixtures. The basic components of PN are as follows:

1. Carbohydrates in PN are found primarily in the form of dextrose. Dextrose is available in concentrations ranging from 2.5% to 70%. In PPN formulations, the total dextrose concentration is less than 10%. Dextrose provides 3.4 cal/gram and usually provides 50% to 60% of total calories.
2. Amino acids, in the form of crystalline amino acids, provide 4 cal/gram. Most hospital pharmacies stock 3% to 15% amino acid concentrations. Amino acids provide 10% to 20% of total calories.
3. Lipids (fat emulsions) are typically soybean oil or a combination of safflower and soybean oils. Other

## NURSING STRATEGY

### Implementation

Malnourished clients are prone to infections because their immune systems have been compromised. EN and PN provide a positive medium for potential growth of microorganisms. To decrease the risk of infection, institute the following nursing measures:

1. Verify placement of feeding line prior to administration of liquids.
2. Administer nutrients in accordance with the prescribed time interval.
3. Add small quantities of enteral formula to the bag.
4. Wash reusable EN feeding bag with warm water and soap after each use, at least every 24 hours.
5. Keep PN refrigerated; remove from refrigerator 30 minutes prior to administration.
6. Change EN and PN tubing every 24 hours.

## BOX 35-11 CANDIDATES FOR PN: TPN OR PN

1. In critically ill clients, PN is indicated if EN is not possible and hypermetabolism is expected to last more than 4 to 5 days

2. Preoperative PN should be administered to moderately or severely malnourished clients undergoing major gastrointestinal surgery for 7 to 14 days if operation can be safely postponed when enteral route is not available.

3. Postoperative PN should be administered to clients who will be unable to meet their nutritional needs enterally for a period of 7 to 10 days.

4. PN has been shown to benefit allogeneic bone marrow transplantation, severe acute necrotizing pancreatitis, and enterocutaneous or high-output fistula.

5. PN should be reserved for those clients with inflammatory bowel disease in whom EN is not tolerated first. In the malnourished client, PN may be indicated with inflamed or ulcerated bowel, causing the client to need 1 or more weeks of rest and colitis, radiation enteritis. In acute exacerbations of Crohn's disease or in fistulas associated with Crohn's disease, a brief course of bowel rest and PN may be indicated.

6. PN is appropriate in clients receiving active anticancer treatment who are malnourished and who are anticipated to be unable to use the enteral route to absorb adequate nutrients for a prolonged period of time (Cozzaglio, Balzola, Cosentino, DeCicco, Fellagara, & Gaggiotti, 1997).

7. PN is required in clients with intractable diarrhea that does not respond to medication or an elemental formula.

8. PN is indicated if the intestinal tract has severely diminished function due to underlying disease such as mesenteric ischemia, small bowel obstruction, congenital anomalies, or in short bowel syndrome to control diarrhea and prevent dehydration and malnutrition.

9. PPN may be used in selected clients to provide partial or total nutrition support for up to 2 weeks in clients who cannot ingest or absorb oral- or enteral-tube-delivered nutrients, or when central-vein parenteral nutrition is not feasible.

ASPEN (2002b).

components of lipid emulsions include egg yolk phospholipid as an emulsifier and glycerin to render the formulation isotonic. Lipids are used to provide energy as well as essential fatty acids. 10% lipids provide 1.1 cal/cc, and 20% lipids provide 2 cal/cc. Lipids usually provide up to 30% of total calories (ASPEN, 2002b).

Other ingredients, called admixtures, provide for the client's biochemical needs (electrolytes, vitamins, and trace elements such as zinc, selenium, chromium, magnesium, iodine, copper, iron, and molybdenum).

Medications, such as heparin, may also be added to the TPN solution. Heparin is commonly added to reduce the buildup of a fibrinous clot at the catheter's tip. When the TPN catheter is the only available venous access, TPN may be used to deliver antibiotics. The TPN solution should be prepared only by a pharmacist using sterile technique and a laminar flow hood to reduce the risk of contamination.

## Administering Medication Through a Feeding Tube

Refer to agency protocol regarding medication administration and contraindications. Feeding tubes with a double lumen have two separate ports; read the manufacturer's instructions to determine which port to use to administer the medication. Administering medications through the wrong port may cause the tube to clog.

Check for tube placement, clear the tubing of formula, and check the patency of the tube by flushing it with water before administering the medication. It is advisable to use the liquid form of any medications when possible. After administering each medication, flush the port to prevent clogging. Measure the aspirates removed, all liquids instilled into the tube, and the water used for flushing and medications, and record them on the client's intake and output record. Refer to Chapter 30 for additional information on administering medication through a feeding tube.

## Nutritional Support for Terminal Clients

Many clients who are in the last stages of physical life face difficult decisions regarding their end-of-life care interventions. Among these decisions is whether or not to continue nutritional support, and then to determine which type or level of nutritional support to administer. An advanced directive assists in clarifying the solution for the health care team if nutritional support is specified. However, if there is no advanced directive, the decision to withhold or withdraw nutritional support must be made by the closest family members if possible. If no family is available, the health care team must make the decision. The options are many and complex and vary from no nutritional support on one end of the continuum to total parenteral nutrition on the other (Mahoney, Riley, Fry, & Feild, 1999).

## NURSING STRATEGY

### Interventions for Client Receiving PN

1. Monitor weight: baseline and daily weight for 1 week and twice a week thereafter. Rapid weight gain may be indicative of fluid overload; monitor such a client for peripheral and pulmonary edema.

2. Monitor I&O: record daily intake and output and compare these data with the client's weight. Closely monitor the infusion rate with an infusion pump (preferably a volumetric pump for the greatest accuracy).

3. Monitor biochemical lab values:

   • Electrolytes, especially magnesium, phosphorus, and potassium should be monitored on days 1 to 3, and twice a week thereafter until stable. With severely malnourished clients, observe for "refeeding syndrome." Refeeding syndrome can be life-threatening if not treated promptly. Rapid reintroduction of large amounts of carbohydrate feedings can cause a drop in the above electrolytes. Severe hypophosphatemia is associated with the hematologic, neuromuscular, cardiac, and respiratory dysfunction. It can also cause fluid retention and lead to cardiac decompensation in severely marasmic clients.

   • In clients with hyperglycemia or diabetes, dextrose should be limited to between 100 and 150 grams on day 1 and slowly increased. Check blood glucose every 6 hours the first week, and weekly once glucose values are at goal, for all clients. Maintain blood glucose at less than 180 mg/dL initially. Once stable, maintain blood glucose between 100 and 150 mg/dL.

   • Check Na, BUN, creatinine, Cl, $CO_2$ on days 1 to 3.

   • Pre-albumin serum levels: check on day 1 and once a week while on PN. In clients who are severely dehydrated, the albumin levels may drop initially as treatment restores hydration.

   • Bleeding indices (PT) on day 1 and once a week while on PN; indicated for clients receiving heparin therapy.

4. Administer solution with an IV tubing filter to remove crystals from the solution, vent air, and trap microorganisms.

5. Change IV tubing, using aseptic technique, as indicated by the agency's protocol; most infection control guidelines recommend changing the tubing every 24 hours.

6. Use a volumetric pump to ensure accurate infusion rates.

7. Monitor for common complications of PN therapy:

   • Phlebitis or thrombosis at the IV site, as indicated by tenderness and redness

   • Catheter tip sepsis, as indicated by fever and other signs and symptoms of sepsis

   • Liver, renal, and metabolic complications (as discussed in monitoring the biochemical laboratory values)

8. Wean the client from PN, documenting the dietary intake of total calories and protein.

9. Teach the client and the caregiver about the management of PN therapy and arrange for a home health care consult; if possible, have the home health nurse consult with the client while the client is still in the hospital, to promote continuity of care.

## Complementary Therapy

Holistic nursing recognizes wellness as a state of harmony among mind, body, and spirit. To nourish means to provide that which is necessary for life, health, and growth; to nourish also means to cherish, to strengthen, and to promote (Jackson, 2000). Nourishment encourages expansion

### CLINICAL ALERT

#### Egg Allergy

Clients with a known egg allergy should not receive TPN with lipid emulsions.

## LEGAL AND ETHICAL ISSUES

### Advanced Directives and Nutritional Support

Obtaining advanced directives that delineate nutritional support is critical for all clients, particularly those with serious disorders. In the absence of advanced directives, family members may not have an agreed-upon decision. In this event, nurses must use techniques of conflict resolution and therapeutic communication to strive for a successful plan of action. In addition, an ethics committee may be an excellent group to consult, and coordinating a "team meeting" with the family members and health care team members may be necessary.

## COMMUNITY/HOME CARE

### Home Parenteral Nutrition (HPN)

Client assessment for home parenteral nutrition (HPN) should consider the physical, psychosocial, and financial resources of the client and the caregiver. Maintaining a client on HPN is challenging because of the expense, technology, and required changes in lifestyle. When the PN is prescribed daily, it is usually administered overnight to minimize disruption to the client's lifestyle. Home health nurses should visit the client daily until the client and caregiver demonstrate proficiency in handling the equipment and maintaining aseptic technique.

Clients receiving PN in the home environment require close monitoring to prevent catheter sepsis and cardiac overload. The PN solution should be administered with a volumetric infusion pump. If the home does not have air conditioning to maintain the proper temperature of the solution during infusion, the solution can be divided into two bags. The second bag can be refrigerated while the first bag is infusing. The same schedule is followed for monitoring the biochemical effectiveness of PN, as discussed above for the hospitalized client.

and growth, supporting each being as unique, whole, and individual. The following discussion provides a broad perspective regarding the use of nutrients in complementary therapies and how herbal medicine incorporates certain plants for their specific properties in order to treat digestive symptoms/diseases.

Although there are numerous types of complementary therapies, they all integrate, to some degree, nutrition as part of their therapeutic regimen. Diet and nutrition are used by many alternative modalities for the prevention and treatment of chronic diseases:

1. *Ayurvedic medicine*, India's ancient system of healing, treats the whole person with diet, nutrition, and lifestyle recommendations to promote health and spiritual development.
2. *Traditional Chinese medicine*, one of the oldest systems of healing, incorporates acupuncture, Chinese herbs, massage, food therapy, exercise, and lifestyle changes into prevention and treatment.
3. *Chiropractic medicine*, an American heritage, relies on a sound nutritional program as adjunct therapy to support the body's inherent ability to heal itself by reestablishing an unobstructed flow of nerve impulses between the brain and the rest of the body.
4. *Naturopathic medicine*, an ancient form of healing that was formalized in America into a system of preventive and restorative treatments around the early 1900s, uses clinical nutrition as a main cornerstone of therapy to achieve and maintain health.
5. *Osteopathic medicine*, founded by Dr. Andrew Taylor Still, a medical surgeon for the Union Army during the Civil War, integrates into conventional medicine nutritional recommendations for prevention. For example, to prevent coronary heart disease, a diet low in saturated fats is combined with antioxidants (vitamins C, A, and E) to help prevent free radical formation, thus preventing tissue breakdown as well as the accumulation of plaque in the arteries.
6. *Herbal medicine* recognizes food as medicine, ensuring that the unique healing properties of specific herbs have a direct effect upon tissue. The healing effect is through direct contact with the tissue and the effects caused by the metabolism and absorption of the chemicals present in the various plants. Based on a holistic context, herbal medicine recognizes that true healing must involve all dimensions of the person to change whatever dietary indiscretions exist as well as to make other adjustments in one's lifestyle.

Americans have increased their use of herbal preparations fourfold in the past decade. The Food and Drug Administration (FDA) does not monitor the herbal industry. The FDA has to prove an herbal product is dangerous before taking it off the shelf, and the manufacturer does not have to prove it safe. An herbal supplement is not usually taken off the market until a number of cases of adverse health events, reported deaths, and evidence have been gathered. There is no assurance that a product contains the amount of herb stated on the supplement, as manufacturers are not required to adhere to any standards of potency, purity, or efficacy (Tufts University Health and Nutrition Letter, 2002). Independent analysis has shown that often a supplement does not contain the dosage listed and it may contain other substances that can be harmful. Although some herbal supplements can be beneficial, the supplement manufacturers often capitalize on the public's anxieties and make claims that have not been scientifically researched. Some supplements purport "advanced memory enhancing," "burn fat while you sleep," or various other false statements.

Clients must be educated to always check for drug-herbal interactions and avoid taking unnecessary herbal products when pregnant or nursing. In addition, the client must communicate with the health care provider when taking any herbal supplements. The following discussion addresses the digestive and nondigestive actions of certain herbs: chamomile, dandelion, and peppermint.

Chamomile's oils contain anti-inflammatory properties and may aid in digestion. Chamomile does contain varying amounts of allergens as well as pollen, and tea made from it may cause contact dermatitis, anaphylaxis, or other hypersensitivity reactions in allergic individuals. Persons known to be allergic to ragweed, asters, or chrysanthemums should be cautious with this herb.

Dandelion root has no significant therapeutic benefits but appears to be essentially free of significant toxicity or side effects. The roots may mildly stimulate the appetite and aid in digestion. Leaves of the plant may also have a transient diuretic action as well as a slight laxative effect. They are a good source of vitamin A. The culinary application likely outweighs any medicinal uses.

Peppermint is primarily used for its stimulating and carminative properties in treating indigestion. It contains a volatile oil, which may reduce the tone of the lower esophageal sphincter and can facilitate belching. It is generally recognized as safe.

## Evaluation

Evaluation of nutritional therapy is ongoing. The nurse uses current data to measure the achievement of goals and outcomes; once they are achieved, the plan of care is revised accordingly. If goals are not met, the nurse should determine whether the nursing diagnosis was accurate or whether the nursing interventions were appropriate and the outcomes achievable.

The plan of care should be modified to maximize the client's response to therapy. For example, if the home health client states compliance with diet therapy to maintain the HDL, LDL, and cholesterol levels within normal limits, but the values are not within normal limits, institute a food record to monitor cholesterol and fat intake for 3 consecutive days. Visit the client on the fourth day and review the record. Provide teaching as necessary to assist the client in changing eating patterns.

 # CASE STUDY/NURSING CARE PLAN

Mr. Turnbeau, age 46, has been HIV positive for 6 years. He is in the physician's clinic complaining of non-bloody diarrhea and abdominal cramping for 3 weeks. In addition, he has a small burn wound on his right forearm, which he states has not been healing well. He has lost 10% of his body weight in the past 3 weeks. He says, "I do not have the energy to eat or get dressed." Upon questioning, he has eaten primarily bread, cereal, milk, and potatoes.

Mr. Turnbeau's vital signs are B/P = 138/72, P = 82, R = 18, and T = 98.6°F. While at the clinic, Mr. Turnbeau produces a stool specimen, and testing is performed for ova parasites, bacterial pathogens, C. *difficile*, leukocytes, fecal fat, and D-xylose. Mr. Turnbeau is educated as to appropriate nutritional habits and evaluated for dehydration symptomatology.

### Assessment

Mr. Turnbeau is a 46-year-old client with diarrhea, abdominal cramping, and a recent weight loss of 10% of his body weight. He has dry, scaly skin; pale conjuctiva; decreased hemoglobin, hematocrit, and MCV; decreased Na, K, Fe, Zn; decreased serum albumin, transferrin; and a specific gravity of 1.028.

### Nursing Diagnosis #1

*Imbalanced Nutrition: Less Than Body Requirements*, related to inability to absorb nutrients because of HIV enteropathy.

**NOC:** Nutritional Status; Nutritional Status: Food and Fluid Intake; Nutritional Status: Nutrient Intake

**NIC:** Nutrition Management; Electrolyte Management; Enteral Tube Feeding; Nutrition Therapy; Nutritional Counseling; Nutritional Monitoring; Weight Gain Assistance

*(continues)*

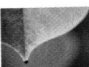

# CASE STUDY/NURSING CARE PLAN (continued)

## Expected Outcomes

The client will:

1. Receive adequate nutrients to meet metabolic needs.
2. Stabilize weight within 48 hours after initiation of nutrition support.
3. Gain 0.25–0.5 kg/wk.
4. Select a diet high in calcium, iron, protein, and calories.

## Planning/Interventions/Rationales

1. Weigh daily; record hourly I&O; monitor q h BP, P, R rate, breath sounds, edema. *Monitors overall health status for changes, balance of fluid intake and output, and signs of deterioration.*
2. Use a nocturnal tube feeding to deliver formula. *Antidiarrheal agents (antimotility drugs) can be very effective in reducing most diarrhea within 24 to 48 hours when administered correctly.*
3. Obtain food preferences from client, and offer smaller frequent meals. *Facilitates digestion and improves energy levels.*
4. Record percentage of meals consumed. *Monitors accurate consumption of nutrients.*
5. Coordinate administration of medication with their absorptive characteristics. *To decrease malabsorption.*

## Evaluation

Fluid intake and output balanced; diarrhea subsided in 24 hours; afebrile.

Laboratory values with normal limits 48 hours postadmission.

Weight stabilized within 48 hours, and client is tolerating small, frequent meals.

The client was able to select food items as prescribed by the nutritional support team and gained 0.45 kg in 8 days.

## Nursing Diagnosis #2

*Diarrhea* related to opportunistic enteric pathogens secondary to HIV
**NOC:** Bowel Elimination; Electrolyte and Acid-Base Balance; Fluid Balance; Hydration
**NIC:** Diarrhea Management

## Expected Outcomes

The client will:

1. Report less diarrhea within 24 to 48 hours.
2. Describe contributing factors to the diarrhea episodes.
3. Increase signs of rehydration within 24 to 48 hours (e.g., moist mucous membranes, skin turgor).

## Planning/Interventions/Rationales

1. Monitor vital signs very 4 hours. *Severe dehydration causes a febrile response, and decreased fluids can cause hypotension.*
2. Increase oral intake to maintain a normal urine specific gravity or to approximate volume of diarrhea losses. *Good indicator of renal function and severity of dehydration.*
3. Encourage liquids (water, apple juice, flat ginger ale), and discontinue solids.
4. Gradually add semisolids and solids (crackers, yogurt, rice, bananas, applesauce) as diarrhea improves. *Absorption increases as diarrhea subsides.*

## Evaluation

Client will begin to show increased signs of hydration as diarrhea episodes decrease.

## Key Concepts

- The metabolism of nutrients (carbohydrates, proteins, fats, vitamins, and minerals) plays an essential role in providing the body with the substances necessary for maintaining homeostasis.

- Most nutrients are absorbed in the small intestines through the processes of osmosis, diffusion, and active transport.
- The intracellular productions of energy from carbohydrates, proteins, and fats are interrelated and depend on other physiological processes, such as conversions

that take place in the liver, glycolysis, Krebs cycle, and electron transport system.

- A calorie is the quantity of heat required to raise the temperature of 1 gram of water 1 °C.
- There are six categories of nutrients: water, carbohydrates, proteins, fats, vitamins, and minerals.
- Carbohydrates have a protein-sparing action, based on a minimum daily ingestion of 50 to 100 grams (200–400 kcal).
- Proteins are essential for almost every bodily function, beginning with the genetic control of protein synthesis, cell function, and cell reproduction.
- Diets high in saturated fats are associated with an increased incidence of coronary heart disease.
- Low-density lipoproteins are responsible for the formation of atherosclerosis, which develops from a high blood plasma level of cholesterol and usually results from a diet high in saturated fats.
- Daily food guides assist healthy persons in meal planning.
- The recommended dietary allowance represents the dietary intake of essential nutrients by age category, inclusive of weight and height.
- The Food Guide Pyramid outlines the number of servings in each of the six foods groups needed to maintain a healthy weight.
- Peer-group influence, social pressures, and other emotional stressors of adolescence may have a negative effect on eating habits, leading to obesity, fad diets, anorexia nervosa, and bulimia.
- Food preferences are usually developed in childhood, are modified throughout the life span, and are an expression of an individual's likes and dislikes.
- Malnutrition refers to alterations relative to inadequate intake, disorders of digestion or absorption, and overeating.
- Assessment includes three basic components: nutritional history, physical examination with anthropometric measurements, and diagnostic and laboratory data.
- Anthropometric measurements evaluate the client's calorie-energy expenditure balance, muscle mass, body fat, and protein reserves, based on height, weight, skinfold, and limb and girth circumferences.
- The blood urea nitrogen (BUN) is increased with severe dehydration, malnutrition, starvation, excessive protein intake, and, most commonly, in kidney disease.
- The nurse is responsible for understanding the client's metabolic needs and for making clinical judgments relative to nutritional outcomes.
- Therapeutic nutrition requires consideration of the client's total needs: cultural, socioeconomic, psychological, and physiological.
- Protein-energy malnutrition is the most common nutritional deficiency in hospitalized clients.
- Enteral and parenteral nutrition are two methods of delivering nutrition support in adult clients.
- Clients receiving PN in the home environment require close monitoring to prevent catheter sepsis and cardiac overload.

# Review Questions and Activities

1. Which mineral is important in the formation of collagen?
2. Why does the body need dietary fiber?
3. Atherosclerosis may result from an excessive ingestion of which nutrient?
4. What conditions cause a client to develop a negative nitrogen balance?
5. What are several nursing interventions for assisting a client to change eating behaviors?
6. What is the best method for determining whether a client is overweight or obese?
7. How frequently should you assess a client who is receiving a continuous tube feeding? What nursing measures are included in such an assessment?
8. Which outcomes are desired in a client receiving nasoenteral tube feeding?
9. Which nursing actions should be instituted when a client with a continuous-feed nasoenteral tube vomits?
10. What is the main advantage of CPN over PPN?

# Multimedia Links

Christensen *Core Concept Videos: Nutrition and Diet Therapy I, II, & III*
Altman *Intermediate Care DVD: Inserting and Maintaining a Nasogastric Tube*
Altman *Intermediate Care Video: Nutrition and Elimination I*
Altman *Intermediate Care DVD: Assessing Placement of a Large-Bore Feeding Tube*
Altman *Intermediate Care DVD: Assessing Placement of a Small-Bore Feeding Tube*

# Web Resources

American Association of Diabetes Educators
    http://www.aadenet.org
American Liver Foundation
    http://www.liverfoundation.org
HerbalDave's Notebook
    http://www.herbaldave.com
The Holistic Haven
    http://www.holistichaven.com
National Academy Press
    http://www4.nationalacademies.org

# References

Altman, G., (2004). *Delmar's fundamental & advanced nursing skills* (2nd ed.). Clifton Park, NY: Delmar Learning.

American Society for Parenteral and Enteral Nutrition (ASPEN), Board of Directors and the Clinical Guidelines Task Force (2002a). Guidelines for the use of parenteral and enteral nutrition in adult and pediatric patients. *Journal of Parenteral and Enteral Nutrition, 26*(1), 34–42.

ASPEN (2002b). *The science and practice of nutrition support: A case-based core curriculum.* Dubuque: Kendall/Hunt Publishing Co., 148.

Balch, J., & Balch, P. (1997). *Prescription for nutritional healing* (2nd ed.). Garden City Park, NY: Avery Publishing Group.

Brownell, K. D. (2002). *The LEARN program for weight management.* Dallas: American Health Publishing Company.

Campaign for Food Safety. (1999). *Campaign for food safety news.* http://www.purefood.org.

Chrvala, C., & Bulger, R. (Eds.) (1999). *Leading health indicators for healthy people 2010, Final report.* Committee on Leading Health Indicators for Healthy People 2010, Division of Health Promotion and Disease Prevention, Institute of Medicine. Washington, DC: National Academy Press.

Cirgin, E., & Marsha, L. (1997). What is the prevalence of feeding tube placement errors and what are the associated risk factors? [Abstract]. *Online Journal of Knowledge Synthesis for Nursing, 4*(5). http://www.stti.iupui.edu/library/ojksn/abstracts/040005. htm.

Cozzaglio, L., Balzola, F., Cosentino F., DeCicco, M., Fellagara, P., & Gaggiotti, G. (1997). Outcome of cancer patients receiving home parenteral nutrition. *Journal of Parenteral and Enteral Nutrition, 21,* 339.

Daniels, R. (2003). *Delmar's manual of laboratory and diagnostic tests.* Clifton Park, NY: Delmar Learning.

Dietary Approach to Stop Hypertension (2001). http://www.dash.bwh.harvard.edu

Estes, M. E. (2002) *Health assessment & physical examination* (2nd ed.). Clifton Park, NY: Delmar Learning.

Franz, M., Kulkarni, K., Polansky, W., Yarborough, P., & Zamudio, V. (2001). A core curriculum for diabetes educators (4th ed.). Chicago: American Association of Diabetes Educators, 6–7.

Hamilton, H. (Ed.) (2000). *Total parenteral nutrition: a practical guide for nurses.* Philadelphia: Churchill Livingstone.

Hogstel, M. O. (2001). *Nursing care of the older adult* (4th ed.). Clifton Park, NY: Delmar Learning.

Jackson, V. (2000). *The holistic haven.* http://www.holistic haven.com.

Long, C. (1999). Certified organic. *Organic Gardening, 46*(6), 44–45.

Mahoney, M., Riley, J., Fry, S., & Feild, L. (1999). Factors related to providers' decisions for and against withholding or withdrawing nutrition and/or hydration in adult patient care [Abstract]. *Online Journal of Knowledge Synthesis for Nursing, 6*(4). http://www.stti.iupui.edu/library/ojksn/abstracts/060004. htm

McCloskey, J. C., & Bulechek, G. M. (1999). *Iowa intervention project: Nursing interventions classification (NIC)* (3rd ed.). St. Louis: Mosby.

Meerschaert, C. (2001) Fiber talk. *Today's Dietitian, 3*(10), 23–24.

Metheny, N. A., Stewart, B. J., Smith, L., Yan, H., Diebold, M., & Clouse, R. E. (1999). PH and concentration of bilirubin in feeding tube aspirates as predictors of tube placement. *Nursing Research, 48*(4), 189–197.

North American Nursing Diagnosis Association (NANDA) (2003). *Nursing diagnoses: Definitions and classification. 2003–2004.* Philadelphia: Author.

Pawlak, L. (1998). *A perfect 10: Phyto "new-trients" against cancers.* Emeryville, CA: Biomed General Corporation.

Penrod, J., Morse, J., & Wilson, S. (1999). Comforting strategies used during nasogastric tube insertion. *Journal of Clinical Nursing, 8*(1), 31–38.

Pentz, J. (2001). *Nutrition specialist manual* (6th ed.). West Roxbury, MA: LMA Publishing.

Pratt, J. C., & Tolbert, C. G. (1996). Tube feeding aspiration. *American Journal of Nursing, 96*(5), 37.

Rachel's Environment and Health Weekly (1999, February 25). *#639—Genetically Altering The World's Food.* http://erf@rachel.org.

Roth, R., & Townsend, C. (2002). *Nutrition & diet therapy* (8th ed.). Clifton Park, NY: Delmar Learning.

Tufts University Health and Nutrition Letter (2002, May). Vol. 20, Number 3.

U.S. Departments of Agriculture and Health and Human Services. *The food guide pyramid: A guide to daily food choices.* Leaflet no. 572. Washington, DC: Author.

White, L., & Duncan, G. (2002). *Medical-surgical nursing: An integrated approach* (2nd ed.). Clifton Park: Delmar Learning.

Wilson, L. (2000). Nurse-assisted PEG in pediatric patients. *Gastroenterology Nursing, 23*(3), 121–24.

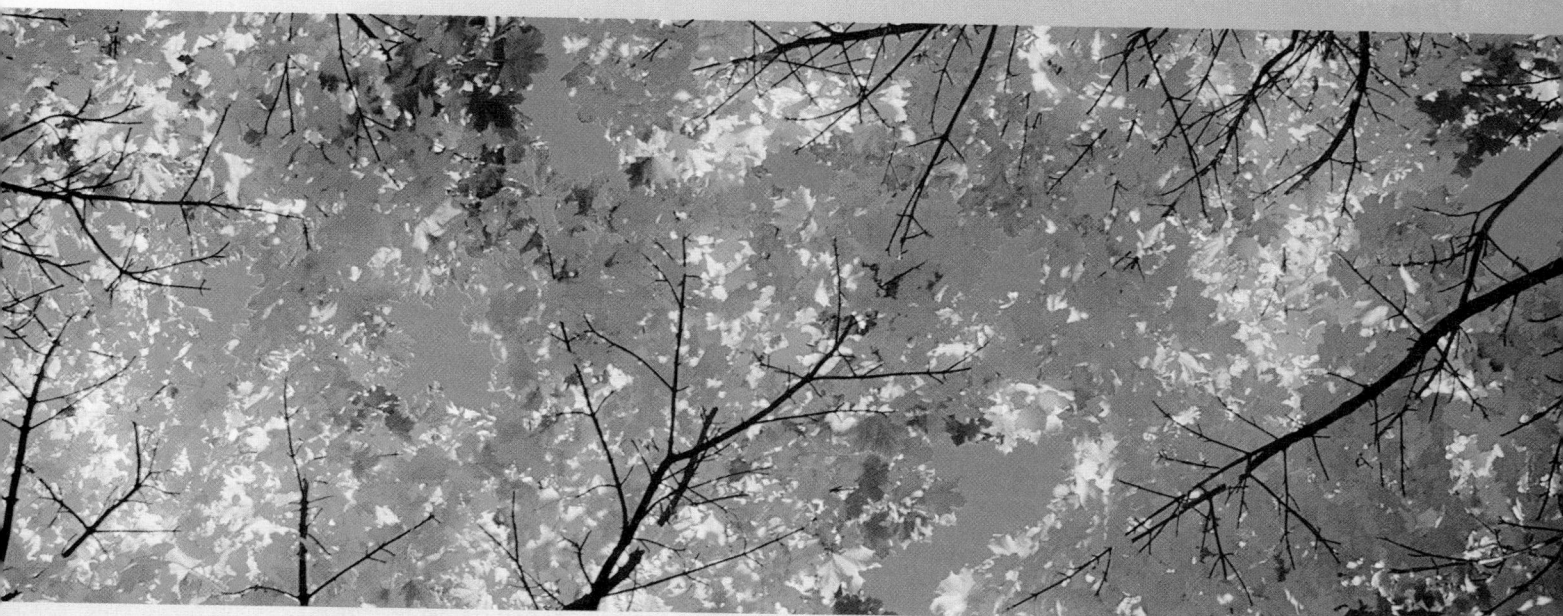

# CHAPTER 36

# Skin Integrity and Wound Healing

## Dorothy B. Doughty, MN, RN, FNP, CWOCN, FAAN

*"Healing . . . is a complex process that requires the interaction of many factors for normal repair . . . Nursing interventions can either enhance or delay the wound-healing process."*

*(Nancy Stotts, 1999)*

# Chapter Competencies

*Upon completion of this chapter, the reader should be able to:*

1. Identify key structures within the skin and soft tissues.
2. Describe strategies that contribute to skin health and tissue integrity across the life span.
3. Explain pressure ulcer prevention, the importance of risk assessment tools, and prevention protocols.
4. Describe the characteristics of wound healing.
5. Discuss the key parameters of the nursing process to be included in wound management.
6. Use assessment data and understanding of wound care to make appropriate recommendations for a specific wound.
7. Discuss the management guidelines for contusions, strains, and sprains.
8. Describe the administration of heat and cold therapies.

# Key Terms

| | | |
|---|---|---|
| abrasion | fascia | partial-thickness wound |
| acute wound | fibroblasts | Penrose drain |
| arterial ulcer | friction | pressure/shear force |
| burns | full-thickness wound | pressure ulcer |
| chronic wound | granulation tissue | primary intention healing |
| closed suction drainage system | growth factors | proliferative phase |
| collagen synthesis | humectants | regeneration |
| contraction | hypodermis | scar formation |
| contusion | inflammatory phase | secondary intention healing |
| debridement | keloid | shear force |
| dehiscence | laceration | skin tear |
| dermal-epidermal junction | maceration | slough |
| dermis | macrophages | sprain |
| emollients | maturation phase | strain |
| epidermis | melanocyte | tertiary intention healing |
| epithelialization | muscle layer | tunneling |
| eschar | necrotizing fasciitis | vasoconstriction |
| evisceration | neuropathic ulcer | vasodilation |
| exudate | nonblanching erythema | venous ulcers |

Maintenance of skin integrity and promotion of wound healing are important aspects of nursing care in all health care settings. Many clients are admitted with traumatic injuries or require surgical intervention; in these situations, nursing interventions are designed to optimize the healing process and prevent complications. Other clients are admitted with skin breakdown due to friction, pressure, shear, or maceration; in these cases, nursing care is focused on measures to correct the causative factors as well as on strategies to promote wound healing. In addition, nurses in all settings are expected to maintain skin integrity in the great number of clients admitted with problems that place them at risk for skin and soft tissue breakdown. Nurses must identify these "at risk" individuals and promptly implement strategies to prevent skin breakdown and maintain intact skin. Effective skin and wound care is based on an understanding of normal skin structures and functions, the physiology of wound healing, and products available for protection of existing skin or support for wound healing.

# Normal Structures and Function of Healthy Skin

The skin is the body's largest organ and its primary defense against pathogenic invasion. The skin also contributes to temperature regulation, prevents loss of internal fluids, and provides sensory awareness of touch, pressure, heat and cold, and pain. Normal skin is dry but supple with an acidic pH resulting from the production of skin oils that are acidic. This "acid mantle" provides an environment that is hostile to bacterial growth (Ehrlich, 1998).

## Epidermis

The **epidermis** is the outermost layer of the skin, and its primary function is to maintain a barrier against loss of internal fluids and against pathogenic invasion (Figure 36-1). The basal layer of the epidermis is the only mitotically active layer. New epidermal cells are produced in the epidermis and then migrate to the skin surface. By the time the epidermal cells arrive at the surface, they are prepared to act as waterproof barrier cells. The epidermis also contains (1) **melanocytes**, the cells that produce pigment and provide each individual with a unique skin color, and (2) immunologically active cells known as Langerhans' cells (Estes, 2002).

## Dermal-Epidermal Junction

The **dermal-epidermal junction** is the anatomical point at which the epidermis connects with the dermis. This junction is characterized by interdigitating connections, which provide resistance to superficial skin injury because the two layers move jointly as opposed to separately. This interlocking configuration is lost late in life, which contributes to the increased incidence of **skin tears** among older adults. In addition, skin tears occur when the superficial layers of the skin "tear away" from the underlying tissues.

## Dermis

The **dermis** is the innermost layer of the skin (Figure 36-2). Its primary functions are to nourish the basal layer of the epidermis, provide sensory awareness, and contribute to temperature regulation through the processes of vasodilation or vasoconstriction as well as through sweating and evaporation. The dermis is composed primarily of collagen and elastin fibers, which give the skin its strength and elasticity. The dermal layer also contains blood vessels, cutaneous nerves, sweat glands, sebaceous glands, and hair follicles just above the junction between the dermis and the subcutaneous tissue.

Key cells found in the dermal layer include **fibroblasts**, which are responsible for collagen synthesis, and **macrophages**, immunologically active cells that phagocytize any invading pathogens (White & Duncan, 2002). The fibroblasts and macrophages are critical to the process of healing by scar formation, as will be discussed later in this chapter.

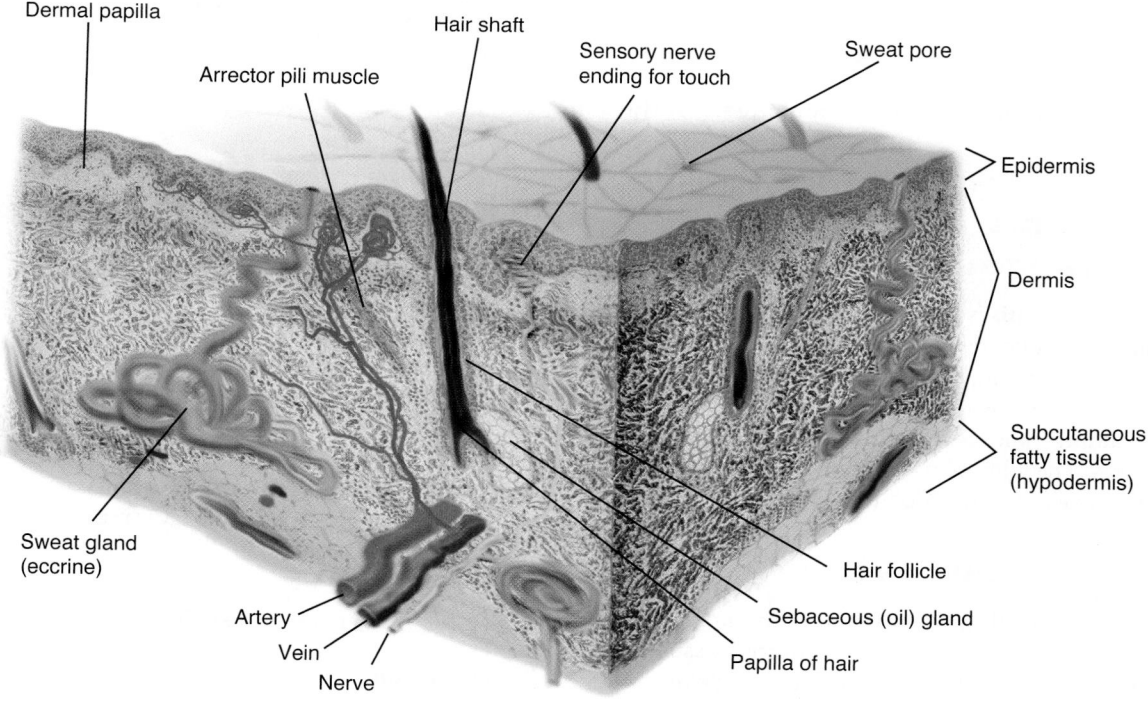

Dermal papilla

Hair shaft

Sensory nerve
ending for touch

Sweat pore

Arrector pili muscle

Epidermis

Dermis

Subcutaneous
fatty tissue
(hypodermis)

Sweat gland
(eccrine)

Hair follicle

Artery

Sebaceous (oil) gland

Vein

Papilla of hair

Nerve

**Figure 36-1    Structures of the skin**

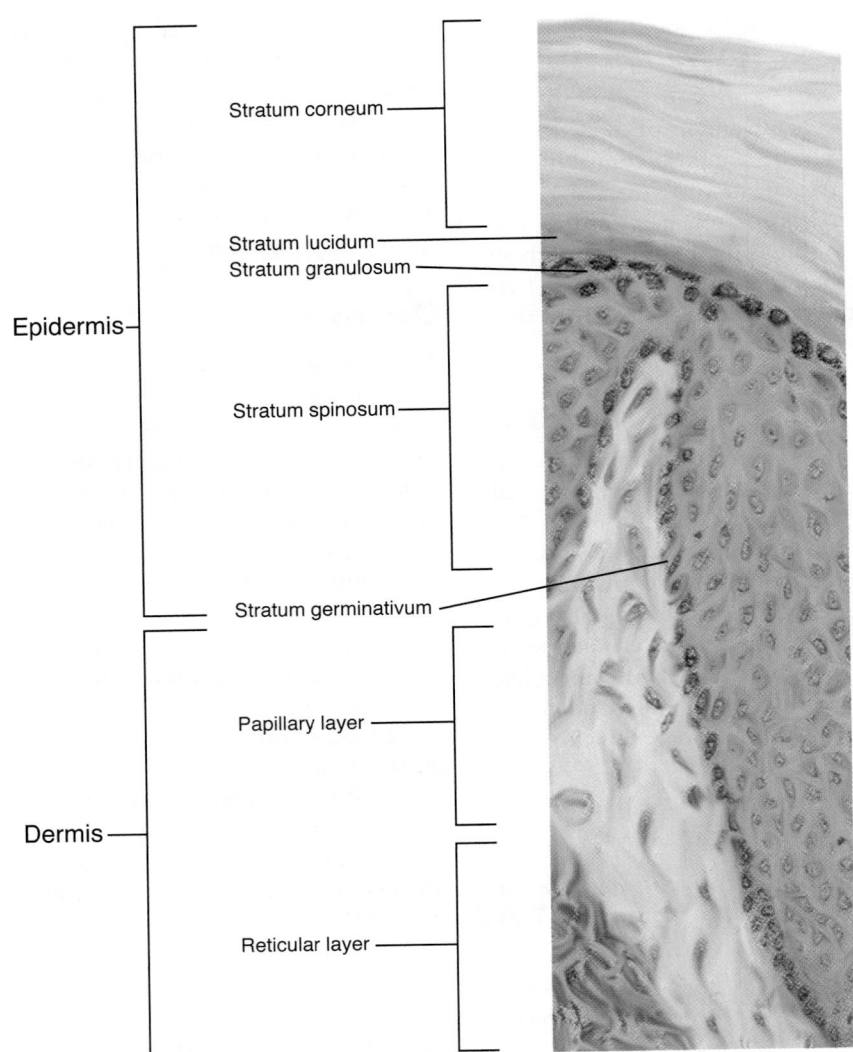

**Figure 36-2    Epidermal and dermal layers of the skin**

## Hypodermis (Subcutaneous Layer)

The term **hypodermis** is sometimes used to refer to the subcutaneous tissue underlying the dermis. The subcutaneous tissue consists primarily of adipose tissue and connective tissue. The subcutaneous tissue plays the critical role of providing "padding" and even weight distribution over bony prominences. The adipose tissue layer is relatively avascular and is incapable of regeneration (Rodeheaver, 2001).

## Fascia/Muscle Layer

Underlying the subcutaneous tissue is the fascia/muscle layer. The **fascia** is a thin layer of connective tissue covering the muscle. Recently, the facia layer has gained additional attention due to the increased incidence of a severe and rapidly progressing infectious process known as **necrotizing fasciitis**. This infection spreads along the fascial planes and is typically caused by beta-hemolytic strep, which is frequently in combination with other microorganisms. The **muscle layer** is composed of contractile fibers that control position and movement. The muscle layer is the most metabolically active layer of the skin and soft tissues and is therefore the tissue layer most vulnerable to ischemic damage. Pressure ulcers typically begin at the muscle-bone interface. The fascia-muscle layer also contains tendons, which attach the muscles to the bones. Tendons, fascia, and muscles do not regenerate, and any lesions extending to this tissue layer must heal by scar formation (Baharestani, 1999).

## Changes Across the Life Span

There are unique characteristics in the structures and functions of the skin that occur across the life span. Nurses must consider these developmental changes when providing skin care to a neonate, infant, or geriatric client.

## Neonates and Infants

The primary differences in neonatal skin include increased permeability and reduced cohesion between the epidermal and dermal layers. This means that topical agents are readily absorbed into the bloodstream and the skin is easily damaged or disrupted by tape removal or aggressive cleansing. Infant skin is managed similarly to neonatal skin, although the risk of systemic absorption of topical agents is significantly reduced by 2 weeks of age. In infants, the epidermal layer remains thin and the problem with reduced cohesion between the epidermal and dermal layers persists. Thus, the guidelines for bathing and adhesive use outlined for neonates should be followed with infants as well.

## Older Adults

The skin and soft tissue layers undergo significant changes with aging. Older adults typically have reduced subcutaneous tissue, which places them at increased risk for **pressure/shear force** injuries (deep wounds caused by prolonged pressure or exposure to sliding force) (Figure 36-3). In addition, the sebaceous glands become less active, so the acid mantle is compromised and the skin becomes dry and possibly pruritic. This places the individual at risk for altered skin integrity due to spontaneous "cracking" or to scratching. Skin tears occur more commonly because epidermal-dermal cohesion is lost, and any traction against the skin surface moves the epidermal layer in opposition to the dermal layer (or the epidermis and dermis in opposition to the subcutaneous tissue). There is reduced

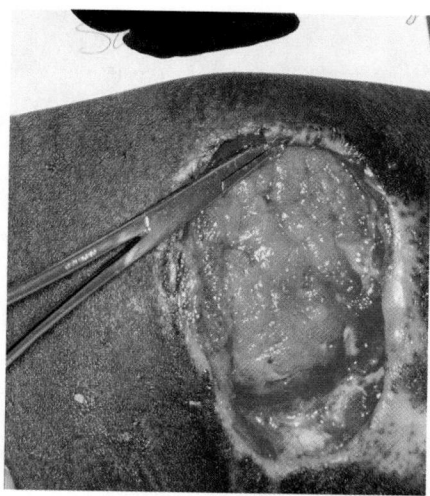

**Figure 36-3    Pressure-shear injury with evidence of tunneling.** *With permission from Emory University Wound Ostomy Continence Nursing Education Center*

immunologic activity within the skin layers, which increases the risk of cutaneous malignancies and infections. Finally, there is diminished blood flow and reduced rate of epidermal regeneration, which results in prolonged time for healing (McGough-Csarny & Kopac, 1998).

# Strategies to Maintain Healthy Skin

Nursing care for individuals across the life span should include measures to keep the skin healthy and to prevent damage to the skin and soft tissues. The skin and soft tissues can be affected by both internal and external factors. Thus, any program to maximize skin health must include attention to both.

## Nutrition and Hydration

Internal factors affecting skin and soft tissue health primarily include the individual's nutritional and hydration status. Malnutrition causes loss of subcutaneous tissue and thinning of the epidermal layer due to inability to produce new epidermal cells at the normal rate. These changes place the individual at increased risk for pressure/shear injuries and for epidermal injury caused by surface trauma, such as sliding in bed or repeated episodes of incontinence. Optimal skin and soft tissue health therefore requires normal nutritional status, as evidenced by stable weight or controlled weight loss coupled with adequate protein intake. Hydration status is also important to skin health. Inadequate fluid intake results in dry skin that is prone to cracking. In assuring adequate intake, the usual goal is 30 cc per kilogram of body weight a day. In addition, preventive measures should be taken to maintain the health promotion of the skin, particularly avoiding sun exposure.

 **LIFE SPAN CONSIDERATIONS**

### Skin Care for the Pediatric Client

- Limit use of topical agents to those that are proven safe for neonatal skin.

- Avoid use of alcohol-based products, antiseptics, and other agents that could be absorbed through the skin.

- Use gentle technique for bathing and skin care.

- Avoid the application of tape and adhesives directly onto the skin; if it is necessary to use tape to secure a device or dressing, apply a protective hydrocolloid dressing first and then apply the tape over the protective dressing.

Adapted from Dolynchuk, K., Keast, D., Campbell, K., Houghton, P., Orsted, H., Sibbald, G., & Atkinson, A. (2000). Best practices for the prevention and treatment of pressure ulcers. *Ostomy/Wound Management, 46*(11), 38–51; Garcia-Gonzalez, E., & Rivera-Rueda, M. (1998). Neonatal dermatology: Skin care guidelines. *Dermatology Nursing, 10*(4), 274–281.

## Impact of Chronic Steroid Intake

Another intrinsic factor that can alter skin integrity is steroid dependence. These individuals experience significant thinning of the epidermis and tremendous risk for skin damage resulting from minimal trauma. Protective care includes measures to minimize trauma to the skin, such as very gentle bathing and avoidance of tape application directly to the skin.

## Bathing and Lubrication

Routine hygienic measures are the external factors most likely to affect skin status. Excessive bathing frequency or use of alkaline cleansing agents may result in stripping of the skin oils that help to maintain an intact epidermal barrier. Bathing frequency should therefore be individualized based on the individual's age and skin status. Infants, older adults, and individuals with dry or fragile skin generally should be bathed less frequently (e.g., every other day and as needed). It is equally important to select appropriate cleansing agents. The ideal skin cleanser is slightly acidic, requires no rinsing, and leaves no soap residue. Finally, lubricating agents such as lotions and creams should be applied correctly. Most lubricating agents contain a combination of **emollients** and **humectants**. Emollients include products that penetrate the epidermis to restore lost skin oils and to keep the skin soft and supple (e.g., various oils and lanolin), and humectants include products that attract and hold water in the epidermal layer (e.g., urea). Lubricants are most effective when applied to clean, slightly damp skin. The emollients readily penetrate the epidermis, and the humectants "seal" the water into the epidermal layer and significantly reduce evaporative loss (Robeson, 1999).

## Managing Pruritic Skin

Chronic pruritis may result from dry skin or from systemic conditions such as renal failure or liver failure. The chronic itching and secondary scratching may result in skin ulcerations as well as significant client discomfort. Management strategies include routine use of emollients to keep the skin soft and supple, and use of soothing agents such as oatmeal baths during episodes of itching. Itching that does not respond to simple strategies mandates a dermatologic referral and may require treatment with anti-inflammatory agents or antihistamines.

## Common Skin Lesions

The skin is constantly exposed to a variety of pathogens and irritants. Clients who have altered skin integrity or a compromised immune system are at risk for developing common skin lesions, such as skin infections, inflammatory conditions, and cutaneous malignancies.

## Skin Infections

Most skin infections are caused by organisms that normally exist on the skin surface. Infection occurs when these organisms invade the skin structures, and ranges from mild to severe. Skin infections can be caused by bacterial, fungal, or viral organisms (Baranoski, 2000).

## Bacterial Infections

Bacterial skin infections are usually caused by staphylococcal or streptococcal organisms. Most commonly these infections are relatively mild and easily managed. For example, folliculitis (infection/inflammation of the hair follicle) may occur when the hair follicles are damaged by recurrent friction or traction (e.g., razor burn). The typical presentation is a pustular lesion surrounding the hair follicle, and management involves elimination of irritants (e.g., modification of shaving technique to eliminate traction and trauma to the hair follicle), use of warm soaks and gentle cleansing, and possibly topical or systemic antibiotics. Impetigo is another bacterial infection commonly seen in children and typically caused by staphylococcal aureus. Impetigo lesions are superficial pustules that form a yellow-tan crust. Management involves gentle cleansing and topical or systemic antibiotics. Skin infections extending into the dermis and subcutaneous tissue are known as cellulitis. These infections produce significant symptomatology (pain, edema, erythema, induration, vesicle formation, lymph node enlargement, and fever) and require systemic antibiotic therapy (Nishijima, Kurokawa, & Nakaya, 2002).

## Fungal Infections

Fungus is an umbrella term that includes both candida and dermatophyte pathogens. Candida organisms such as candida albicans are responsible for yeast rashes, which are common in areas exposed to moisture and among clients on antibiotic therapy. In fair-skinned clients, these infections present as an erythematous rash with pustules and papules. The rash is usually solid in the center but thins toward the periphery, with distinct individual lesions. In dark-skinned clients, the rash may appear lighter or darker than the individual's normal skin color. Clients usually report both itching and tenderness. Nursing measures involve elimination of moisture and the application of a topical anti-yeast product (e.g., nystatin, ketoconazole). Dermatophyte organisms produce tinea infections (tinea pedis [athlete's foot], tinea cruris [jock itch], or tinea corporis [ringworm]). Tinea rashes differ from yeast rashes in that the rash is most intense at the periphery, with thinning toward the center (hence the term *ringworm*). The focus of the nursing treatment involves moisture control and the application of an antifungal agent (Fishman, 2002).

## Viral Infections

Common viral infections include herpes simplex and herpes zoster. These lesions present as clusters of small painful vesicles (blisters) that rupture to reveal a red or pale yellow ulcer bed. Herpes simplex lesions are typically clustered around the lips and mouth, or in the genital region, while herpes zoster lesions (shingles) extend along the path of a single dermatome (Colgan, Michocki, Greisman, & Moore, 2003). Viral lesions are typically treated with systemic antiviral agents. The nurse applies topical treatments, which may include use of a thick, zinc oxide paste or a foam dressing to absorb the exudate and occlude the exposed nerve endings.

## Inflammatory Conditions

Inflammatory conditions range from a localized contact dermatitis to a severe generalized response resulting in sloughing of the epidermis. The most common inflammatory lesion is contact dermatitis, an inflammation of the epidermis and dermis in response to an environmental irritant or allergen (e.g., "poison ivy"). The client presents with edema, erythema, itching, and blistering in the area corresponding to contact with the offending agent. Treatment involves elimination of the allergen or irritant and use of topical or systemic antihistamines and corticosteroids (Blauvelt, Hwang, & Udey, 2003).

## Cutaneous Malignancies

As noted earlier, the major risk factor for skin cancer is sun exposure. The most common skin cancers are basal cell carcinoma, squamous cell carcinoma, and malignant melanoma. Malignant melanoma is the least common but the most virulent, and accounts for the majority of skin cancer deaths. Basal cell cancers may appear as pearl-colored nodules with rolled edges, while squamous cell lesions are typically papules with scaly and friable surfaces. Classic indicators for melanoma are captured in the acronym *ABCD*—Asymmetry, Border irregularity, Color variegation, and Diameter greater than 6 mm. The nurse should refer any client with a suspicious skin lesion to the dermatologist (Jamora, Wainwright, Meehan, & Bystryn, 2003).

# Pressure Ulcer Formation

Pressure ulcer formation resulting in skin breakdown is an increasingly common problem among clients in all health care settings. The increased prevalence of skin breakdown is related to the aging process and to the increased number of individuals who are debilitated and immobile. Effective nursing management of any compromised client includes measures to prevent skin breakdown.

## Pathology of Pressure Ulcers

In the narrowest sense of the word, a **pressure ulcer** is an area of skin and tissue loss caused by prolonged or excessive soft tissue pressure. The unrelieved pressure results in blood vessel compression and loss of blood flow to the involved area. Areas at risk for pressure ulcer formation include the bony prominences. At these points the soft tissue may be compressed between the underlying bone and

## LEGAL AND ETHICAL ISSUES

### Prevention of Skin Breakdown

Prevention of skin breakdown is primarily a nursing responsibility, and the incidence of pressure ulcer development within an agency is considered to be a quality-of-care indicator. While most clinicians agree that some pressure ulcers are unavoidable, most can be avoided through prompt identification of individuals at risk and aggressive preventive measures. Health care agencies are now benchmarking their own performance in the area of preventive skin care by conducting periodic studies to measure the incidence of skin breakdown within their facility and comparing their rates to national averages (average incidence in acute care facilities is 7%). Regulatory agencies, consumers, and malpractice attorneys are also acutely aware of the role played by nursing in the prevention of skin breakdown, as reflected by the increased focus on skin integrity during regulatory agency review, and by the tremendous increase in lawsuits related to pressure ulcer development.

Allman, R., Goode, P., Burst, N., Bartolucci, A., & Thomas, D. (1999). Pressure ulcers, hospital complications, and disease severity: Impact on hospital costs and length of stay. *Advances in Wound Care, 12*(1), 22–30; Soloway, D. (1998). Civil claims relating to pressure ulcers: A claimant's lawyer's perspective. *Ostomy/Wound Management, 44*(92), 20–26.

or stool); overhydration of the skin reduces its tensile strength and makes it more vulnerable to damage from other forces, such as friction (Haalboom, den Boer, & Buskens, 1999).

## Assessment

Prevention of skin breakdown must begin on admission, with accurate identification of clients who are at risk. The most effective way to identify at-risk clients is to use a research-based risk assessment tool to screen all nonambulatory clients. These tools provide a systematic and objective approach to quantification of an individual's risk. The tools most commonly used include the Braden scale and the Norton scale (Note: cutoff scores for "at-risk" status are ≤ = 18 [Braden] and ≤ = 16 [Norton]). Any client found to be at risk for skin breakdown must be placed on an individualized prevention protocol immediately (see Box 36-1).

The first sign of a pressure ulceration is **nonblanching erythema**, which is redness that cannot be dissipated with direct pressure. Then deeper tissue damage is indicated when there is induration with palpation. Finally, if

---

### BOX 36-1    TURNING AND REPOSITIONING PROTOCOL

1. Clients should be repositioned at least every 2 hours.
2. If possible, clients should be turned only onto intact surfaces. For example, a client with sacral breakdown but no trochanteric breakdown should be turned right to left but not to the supine position. Clients who have breakdown on more than one turning surface must be repositioned side to side to back and should be placed on a high-level support surface.
3. A 30-degree lateral tilt should be used when turning clients to the side-lying position; this maximizes pressure distribution and avoids high pressures over the trochanters.
4. Clients who get up in the chair should be repositioned or returned to bed within 1 to 2 hours. Individuals who have ischial or coccygeal breakdown should not be up in the chair except for meals.
5. Pillows, towels, and positioning aids should be used to keep body surfaces and bony prominences from rubbing against each other.

Calliano, C. (2000). Assessing and preventing pressure ulcers. *Advances in Skin and Wound Care, 13*(5), 244–246.

---

the resting surface (bed or chair) or rigid device (such as cast or splint). In actual use, the term *pressure ulcer* is used to refer to skin and soft tissue damage caused by external mechanical forces. These external forces primarily include pressure, shear, and friction, though maceration may render the skin more vulnerable to damage from these forces. Ulceration caused by prolonged or excessive pressure typically presents as a round or oval lesion extending to the muscle layer. **Shear forces** occur when tissue layers slide against one another (e.g., when clients "slide down" in bed). These shear forces are usually dispersed unevenly in the tissues, causing angulation or disruption of blood vessels in the involved area. When the ulcer is caused by a combination of pressure and shear, the ulcer usually presents as an irregular lesion and frequently exhibits areas of **tunneling** (areas of soft tissue destruction under intact skin that extend in one direction from the primary area of ulceration). **Friction** forces can best be described as repetitive "rubbing" against the epidermal surface, which has a "sanding" effect. **Maceration** occurs when the skin becomes overhydrated, either due to diaphoresis or to prolonged exposure to moisture (e.g., wound drainage, urine,

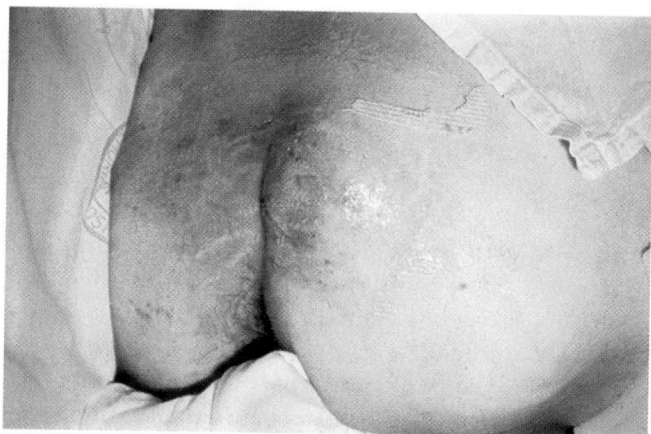

**Figure 36-4** **Skin breakdown with extension into dermis.** *With permission from Emory University Wound Ostomy Continence Nursing Education Center*

there is extensive tissue damage, an open ulcer results (Figure 36-4). These ulcers usually extend to the deep tissue layers (bone, muscle) and are not reversible with treatment (Bowler, 1998).

## Etiologic Risk Factors

The primary etiologic risk factors for true pressure ulcers include prolonged or high-intensity pressure and shear force. The nurse must also consider the impact of tissue tolerance (ability of tissues to resist damage) on an individual's risk for breakdown. In addition, there are many risk factors for the development of pressure ulcers (see Box 36-2).

## Prolonged or High-Intensity Pressure

Prolonged or high-intensity pressure reduces or eliminates blood flow to the involved tissues, which results in ischemic injury and eventual necrosis. High pressures, which cause total occlusion of the capillaries, are tolerated for relatively short periods of time, whereas lower pressures, which cause only partial occlusion of the capillary beds, are tolerated for longer periods of time (Calliano, 2000).

## Shear Force

Shear force is thought to be a major contributor to pressure ulcer development. Materials such as standard mattress covers and bed linens create moderate frictional forces. The amount of gravitational force is dependent on the individual's weight and the degree of incline, or head elevation. Heavier clients and those positioned with greater degrees of head elevation experience greater gravitational force. When tissue is exposed to friction and gravity, there is significant potential for damage because the superficial layers (epidermis and dermis) respond primarily to the frictional forces and remain "locked into place," while the deep tissue layers (muscles and bone) respond primarily to gravitational forces and move downward. The subcutaneous tissue layer is literally "caught in the mid-

---

**BOX 36-2     RISK FACTORS FOR DEVELOPING PRESSURE ULCERS**

The conditions most commonly identified as risk factors for pressure ulcer development are:

- Altered sensory function or level of consciousness (i.e., inability to recognize or respond to ischemic signals)

- Altered activity and mobility (e.g., client who is bed-bound or chair-bound and who lacks the ability to respond to ischemic signals with appropriate repositioning)

- Excessive moisture (e.g., the client who is diaphoretic or incontinent and therefore at greater risk for superficial skin damage)

- Malnutrition (possibly due to soft tissue wasting and reduced ability to distribute weight evenly, as well as compromised immune system function)

- Exposure to shear and friction (a common problem with any client who is unable to reposition effectively, since such individuals are at increased risk for "dragging" or "sliding" injuries)

- General debilitation (e.g., hypovolemic conditions, hyperthermic conditions, and other conditions that compromise tissue perfusion or increase the tissues' metabolic demands)

Adapted from Bergstrom, N., Braden, B., Kemp, M., Champagne, M., & Ruby, E. (1998). Predicting pressure ulcer risk—A multisite study of the predictive validity of the Braden scale. *Nursing Research, 47*(5), 261–269; Doughty, D., Waldrop, J., & Ramundo, J. (2000). Lower extremity ulcers of vascular etiology. In R. Bryant, (Ed.), *Acute and chronic wounds: Nursing management* (2nd ed., pp. 265–300). St. Louis: Mosby.

---

dle," with disruption of the blood vessels and resultant necrosis (Wywialowski, 1999) (Figure 36-5).

## Compromised Tissue Tolerance

Compromised tissue tolerance can also lead to pressure ulcer development. For example, an individual with adequate amounts of well-perfused subcutaneous tissue will be more resistant to breakdown than a malnourished and debilitated individual who is hypovolemic. Conditions that compromise a client's "tissue tolerance" are (1) chronic tissue ischemia (e.g., hypovolemia, vascular disease, or tobacco use), (2) increased pressure over bony prominences, and (3) increased tissue demands for oxygen (e.g., fever).

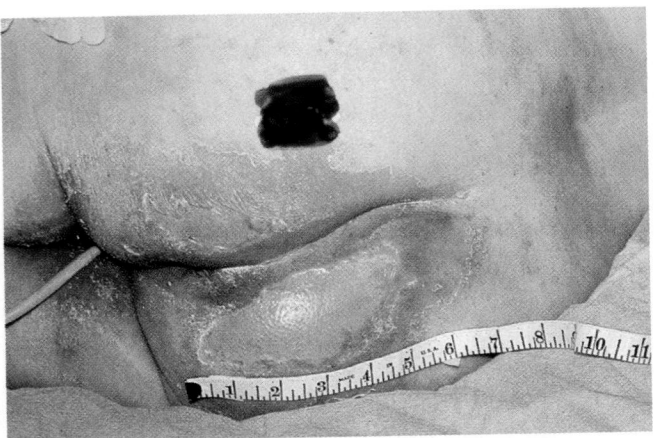

**Figure 36-5**   Friction injury: Note that lesions are superficial. Lesions occurred as a result of aggressive perineal cleansing and friction between skin and incontinence pads. *With permission from Emory University Wound Ostomy Continence Nursing Education Center*

## Nursing Diagnosis

Nursing diagnosis for clients with pressure ulcers will be similar to those for clients with wounds because the type of injury and its consequences are similar. The emphasis is on gentle client care and client teaching to promote healing of the ulcer and to prevent its recurrence. Identifying the client's psychological needs as well, in terms of diagnoses such as *Disturbed Body Image* and *Anxiety*, will ensure that the client's symptoms are addressed holistically.

## Outcome Identification and Planning

As with nursing diagnoses, the outcome identification and planning phase of the nursing process is similar to that for clients with wounds. Individualized outcomes based on the client's overall physical condition, the stage of the wound, and the client's risk factors will help in identifying priority interventions. Client teaching should be included as an integral part of the planning process; if the client desires, family and support persons should be brought into the learning cycle as well.

## Implementation

Pressure ulcers can be prevented through a variety of measures. Early identification of high-risk individuals and contributing risk factors, and an ongoing assessment of risk factors and skin integrity should be done to decrease the possibility of pressure ulcer formation. Other areas of focus in the prevention of pressure ulcers include hygiene and skin care, positioning, and the use of support surface therapy. However, once the pressure is developed, effective management begins with an aggressive focus on preventive strategies such as repositioning, therapeutic support

 **CLIENT REFLECTIONS**

### A Pressure Ulcer

An 84-year-old male with prostatic cancer and bone metastases is referred to the hospice agency for terminal care; he has been cared for at home by his wife until this time. On admission, the nurse discovers a pressure-shear injury on the client's sacrum. When she asks the client's wife how long he has had the ulcer, the wife becomes tearful and says: "I feel so bad about this. I have always heard that people only get these sores when they get poor care. I tried to do everything to take good care of him. What did I do wrong?"

What would you say to this client's wife?

surfaces, measures to reduce exposure to shear and friction, and interventions to control moisture. Once the causative factors have been addressed, the nurse can focus on systemic support measures and provision of appropriate topical therapy. Chronic wounds are particularly prone to become refractory to treatment. The following section will present interventions that may be used as guidelines in caring for clients with pressure ulcer development.

### Appropriate Use and Selection of Support Surfaces

Therapeutic support surfaces should be used for all bedbound and chair-bound clients to help prevent pressure ulcer development. A wide variety of support surfaces are available for both bed and chair; therapeutic features vary among the many devices, but all are designed either to reduce interface pressures or to constantly change the pressure points. Some devices place a comfortable layer next to the client and provide an alternating pressure pad as the base layer. Additional therapeutic options include low-friction and air support surfaces that provide low-volume airflow against the skin to control moisture and prevent maceration.

In selecting a support surface for an individual client, the nurse must consider the client's level of risk, specific risk factors, and number of intact turning surfaces. For example, a high-risk client who is diaphoretic and who has breakdown on two turning surfaces needs a high-level pressure reduction device with a low-friction surface and a low-volume airflow feature. In contrast, a client at moderate risk who is not diaphoretic or incontinent and who has at least two intact turning surfaces can be managed effectively and appropriately with a moderate-level pressure reduction device (Calliano, 2000).

### Monitoring Support Surfaces

It is critical to monitor the support devices for proper function. Static air devices should be checked frequently to ensure that the proper level of inflation is being maintained.

In addition, support devices can also be evaluated for the client's bony prominences not being adequately protected.

## Measures to Control Moisture and Maceration

The first measure to control maceration from moisture is to create a barrier to the source of the moisture. If the source is internal, as in perspiration, management should focus on measures to increase evaporative loss or to provide absorption. If the source is external, the focus is on creating a barrier between the skin and the moisture (e.g., plasticizing films, moisture barrier creams, ointments) (Alvarez, Fernandez-Obregon, Rogers, & Bergano, 2000). In addition to providing a barrier between the skin and the moisture, the source of the moisture should be addressed. For example, a male client with urinary incontinence should be evaluated for a toileting program or an external catheter; a female should be evaluated for a toileting program or absorptive products. If absorptive products are used to contain urine, they should be placed under the client but not closed around the client; closing an absorptive product around the client creates an occlusive environment that increases skin permeability and penetration of irritants and pathogens. Any client being managed with an absorptive product should be checked at least every 2 hours and changed promptly when incontinence has occurred.

## Nutritional and Fluid Support

Any client found to be at risk for skin breakdown should be evaluated in terms of nutritional and fluid status and adequacy of current nutrient and fluid intake. Any client whose intake is assessed as inadequate or who has indicators of compromised nutritional status should be evaluated by the nutritionist or nutritional support nurse (Roth & Townsend, 2002).

## Routine Skin Assessment

All clients at risk for breakdown should have routine periodic inspection of all "at-risk" areas to ensure the efficacy of the current prevention program and to promptly detect any evidence of threatened skin breakdown. Any evidence of threatened breakdown (e.g., persistent or nonblanching erythema) should prompt a thorough review of the existing prevention program with modifications as indicated (e.g., the repositioning program should be adjusted to keep the client off the threatened area, and the support surface should be changed) (Haalboom, den Boer, & Buskens, 1999).

## Management for Shear Force

Strategies to reduce shear and friction include gentle skin care, measures to reduce sliding, and measures to reduce skin and tissue "drag" if sliding occurs.

## Avoidance of Massage to Tissue at Risk

Avoiding the use of massage for at-risk tissue bears special mention because it represents a major change in thinking. For many years, nurses were taught to massage all pressure points and any reddened areas to "enhance circulation." More recent research suggests that massage to at-risk areas may actually cause additional tissue

---

### CLINICAL ALERT

#### Heels High Risk for Pressure Ulcer Formation

The incidence of heel ulcers has increased significantly in all care settings; the heels are a high-risk area because they have very little soft tissue to provide pressure distribution. Current studies indicate unacceptably high levels of tissue pressures exerted against the heels, even when clients are being managed on high-level air support surfaces. To prevent heel ulcers, be sure to follow these guidelines:

- Elevate the heels slightly when the client is in the supine position, using heel elevation devices or pillows placed lengthwise under the client's legs.

- Monitor the heels closely for any evidence of impending breakdown.

Calliano, C. (2000). Assessing and preventing pressure ulcers. *Advances in Skin and Wound Care, 13*(5), 244–246.

---

### NURSING STRATEGY

#### Measures to Prevent Shear/Friction Damage

- Use lift sheets to reposition clients.

- Limit head-of-bed elevation; raise knees slightly when head of bed is elevated to reduce gravitational force.

- Position clients who are up in a chair with their feet flat on the floor; consider using a "wedged" cushion that is elevated in front to hold the client securely in place.

- Select a support surface with a low-friction cover such as Goretex (to reduce frictional forces and the resultant "drag.")

- Apply transparent adhesive to protect skin surfaces exposed to repetitive "rubbing."

Baranoski, S. (2000). Skin tears: The enemy of frail skin. *Advances in Skin and Wound Care, 13*(3), 123–126.

damage. Current guidelines therefore stress the importance of avoiding massage to areas of threatened breakdown (Baranoski, 2000).

## Evaluation

When evaluating the plan of care for a client with a pressure ulcer, consider the physical signs of healing and the status of the pressure ulcer, as well as the client's adaptation to the altered skin integrity. Each intervention should be evaluated for its effectiveness, and the plan of care revised to reflect those actions that have proven the most beneficial in realizing the expected outcomes of care.

## Wound Healing

The ability to repair damage to the skin and soft tissues is obviously critical to long-term survival and health for any organism. Recent research has provided many new insights into the physiology of human wound repair. As a result, nursing has changed its approach to wound care and wound management.

## Definitions and Classifications of Wounds

Wounds can be classified by onset and duration, by tissue layers involved, and by mechanisms of healing. For example, the term **acute wound** usually refers to wounds that are incurred suddenly (e.g., traumatic injuries or surgical incisions) and that heal in an orderly and predictable cascade of overlapping events. In contrast, the term **chronic wound** is used to describe wounds that are caused by a chronic condition or that fail to heal in an orderly manner.

**Partial-thickness wounds** involve partial loss of the skin layers but do not involve the deeper tissues, while full-thickness wounds involve total loss of the epidermis and dermis with extension into the subcutaneous tissue and possibly the muscle.

Wounds are said to heal by **primary intention healing** when the wound edges are closed surgically, and by **secondary intention healing** when they are left open to heal through the processes of granulation, contraction, and epithelialization (Figure 36-6). Wounds that are initially left open and are subsequently closed surgically are said to heal by **tertiary intention healing**.

Humans heal wounds in one of two ways. The ideal approach to repair is **regeneration**. The lost tissue is replaced with "more of the same" so there is no cosmetic or functional deficit. However, this approach to repair is limited to wounds involving epidermal and partial dermal loss. The deep dermal structures (hair follicles, sebaceous glands, and sweat glands), subcutaneous tissue, and muscle are all incapable of regeneration. Therefore, any wound extending into the deep dermis or beyond is forced to heal by scar formation (Ehrlich, 1998).

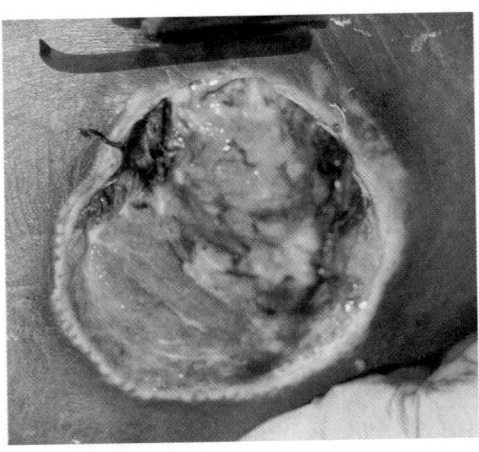

**Figure 36-6    Wound bed that is 60% clean but not yet granulating.** *With permission from Emory University Wound Ostomy Continence Nursing Education Center*

## Partial-Thickness Wound Repair

Everyone who has ever had a scraped knee or a heel blister has experienced partial-thickness repair. These wounds are typically very superficial and very painful, because they expose nerve endings and they usually heal quickly. The key steps in partial-thickness repair are seen in Box 36-3.

## Full-Thickness Wound Repair

Full-thickness wounds by definition involve total loss of the skin layers and extend into the "nonregenerative" tissue layers (i.e., the subcutaneous tissue and possibly the muscle, joint, or bone). These wounds are forced to heal by scar formation, which is a complex process involving three distinct though overlapping phases: the inflammatory phase, the proliferative phase, and the maturation phase.

### Inflammatory Phase

During the **inflammatory phase**, the focus is on controlling any bleeding and establishing a clean wound bed. Once the bleeding is controlled, the clot is gradually broken down, and the process of clot dissolution is accompanied by the release of **growth factors** (i.e., powerful polypeptides that regulate the repair process).

The second key event in the inflammatory phase is the inflammatory response itself. It occurs in response to tissue injury and is augmented tremendously by the chemoattractant role played by growth factors. Cellular damage causes the release of vasoactive substances such as histamine that cause dilatation of the vessels in the area. This causes increased blood flow to the area, and the dilatation of area vessels produces the redness and warmth typically observed during the inflammatory phase. At the same time, the white blood cells migrate to the area of injury. Polymorphonuclear leukocytes (PMNs) are the first to arrive, followed by the macrophages. The inflammatory phase is fairly brief (e.g., 1 to 4 days). However, in a chronic

## BOX 36-3   PARTIAL-THICKNESS WOUND REPAIR

The key steps in partial-thickness wound repair are:

- Brief inflammatory phase, during which white blood cells migrate to the area of injury to engulf bacteria and break down any avascular tissue. The clinical indicators of inflammation include mild erythema and edema and production of a serous exudate. The inflammatory phase usually subsides within 24 hours.

- Epithelial cell proliferation and migration to reestablish a closed skin surface. The new epidermis is very fragile and should be protected until vertical migration restores normal epithelial thickness.

- Vertical migration to restore normal epidermal thickness and function. Once the defect has been resurfaced, the epithelial cells resume their usual "upward" migration, which gradually reestablishes the normal thickness of the epidermis.

- **Collagen synthesis**, the formation of new connective tissue, begins 1 to 3 days postinjury and continues until about day 15.

Ehrlich, P. (1998). The physiology of wound healing—a summary of normal and abnormal wound healing processes. *Advances in Wound Care, 11*(7), 326–328.

months. The strength of the "replacement" tissue is never as good as the "original" tissue (note: optimal wound strength is about 80% of the original tissue). In addition, newly healed wounds are extremely vulnerable during the first few months following "surface healing" and will need continued protection. For example, a bed-bound client with a newly healed trochanteric pressure ulcer should be maintained on a support surface that provides pressure reduction and shear reduction, in addition to a routine repositioning schedule. One complication that may arise during the maturation phase is hypertrophic scarring or even **keloid** formation (scar tissue that extends beyond the boundaries of the original wound) (Rodeheaver, 2001).

# Wound Management

To provide appropriate comprehensive wound care, the nurse must identify and address etiologic factors, establish appropriate goals, and provide systemic support and topical therapy that is consistent with the established goals. Previous sections have addressed causative factors and systemic support. This section will focus on establishment of goals and provision of topical therapy.

## Assessment

When it comes to wound care, the nurse is confronted with wounds that are extremely diverse. The wound may have occurred traumatically just before the client presents to the emergency room, or the wound may be a slow-healing chronic ulcer. Despite all this diversity, the nurse should assess the wound in a systematic manner, evaluating the wound's stage in the healing process. The nurse also needs to show sensitivity to the client's pain and tolerance levels during assessment and must always follow Standard Precautions to prevent transfer of pathogens.

A thorough assessment of wound characteristics and wound status is essential in assessing wounds. The nurse must carefully document the findings from the wound assessment. The following parameters are essential factors to include when assessing the wound:

- Location of the wound
- Dimensions and depth of the wound
- Stage of the wound (the tissue layers involved in the wound)
- Status of wound bed (e.g, **eschar** [brown-black tissue that is usually dry]; see Figure 36-7); **slough** (gray or yellow-white tissue that is usually soft; tissue that is clean but not granulating).
- Exudate: The nurse should describe the **exudate** (fluid released as a result of inflammation) in terms of estimated volume (none, minimal, moderate, large), color, and odor.
- Status of wound edges: Wound edges are carefully evaluated to determine whether they are open and proliferative

wound complicated by necrosis and infection, the inflammatory phase is prolonged (Eaglestein & Falanga, 1998).

### Proliferative Phase

The **proliferative phase** can be conceptualized as the "rebuilding" phase. During this phase, the tissue defect is filled with **granulation tissue** (tissue consisting of newly formed blood vessels and newly synthesized connective tissue), and the new tissue is then "covered" with skin through the process of **epithelialization**. In an open wound such as a pressure ulcer, the phenomenon known as **contraction** can also contribute to the repair process. **Contraction** involves mobilization of the wound edges to reduce the size of the tissue defect so that less granulation tissue is required to repair the wound (Ehrlich, 1998).

### Maturation Phase

The final phase of full-thickness wound repair is the **maturation phase**, also known as the "remodeling" phase. The remodeling process may continue for up to 2 years, though wound strength is typically acquired within 3

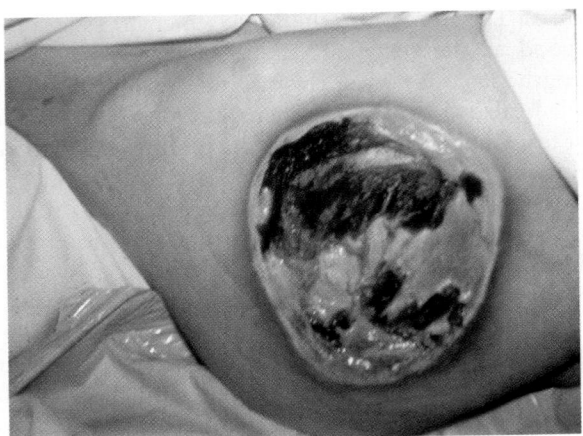

**Figure 36-7** Extensive skin breakdown with exposed muscle and large amount of eschar. *With permission from Emory University Wound Ostomy Continence Nursing Education Center*

(flat, red, and moist), or closed (covered with skin and appearing dry and possibly raised or "curled").

- Status of surrounding skin: In assessing the surrounding skin, the nurse looks for problems that require intervention (e.g., signs of infection, maceration, edema, or additional tissue damage).
- Pain associated with wound or wound care: Pain is a common complication of wounds and wound care and must be carefully assessed and aggressively managed.

## Factors Affecting Wound Healing

Wound repair is clearly a complex phenomenon that is significantly affected by many factors. These factors are

---

## RESEARCH FOCUS

**Title of Study:** Painful venous ulcers: Themes and stories about living with the pain and suffering

**Study Purpose:** To describe and explore the meaning of the experience of living with painful venous ulcers

**Methods:** A descriptive qualitative approach was used; semistructured interviews were audiotaped, transcribed, and analyzed using Martin Qualitative Analysis Software.

**Findings:** Four of the eight most compelling themes identified by the clients were expecting pain with the ulcer, swelling equals pain, not standing, and starting the pain all over again (painful debridements).

**Implications:** The identified pain descriptors and the concept of "carrying on despite the pain" have important implications for nursing practice. Nurses must assess clients for procedural and nonprocedural pain and must intervene appropriately. Nurses must be aware of whether they should premedicate the client before debriding the wound or applying substances to the wound area.

Krasner, D. (1998). Painful venous ulcers: Themes and stories about living with the pain and suffering. *Journal of Wound Ostomy Continence Nursing, 25*(3), 158–168.

---

## COMMUNITY/HOME CARE

### Wound Assessment and Documentation

Accurate wound assessment is of particular importance in home health, since wound status is one of the factors affecting reimbursement for care, and established parameters are used in documenting wound status. Specifically, open wounds must be classified as "nonhealing," "early/partial granulation," or "fully granulating." It is critical to differentiate between wounds that are clean but not granulating and wounds that have moved into the proliferative phase as evidenced by the presence of granulation tissue.

Colburn, L. (2001). Prevention of chronic wounds. In D. Krasner, G. Rodeheaver, & R. G. Sibbald (Eds.), *Chronic wound care* (3rd ed., pp. 67–78). Wayne, PA: HMP Communications.

---

perfusion and oxygenation, nutritional status, diabetes mellitus, corticosteriods, and aging.

### Perfusion and Oxygenation

Adequate levels of oxygen are essential for fibroblast proliferation and collagen synthesis, leukocyte activity and phagocytosis, and reepithelialization. Adequate tissue perfusion is essential for delivery of oxygen and nutrients to the wound bed. It is therefore critical to assess the client for any condition that adversely affects perfusion and oxygenation (e.g., unrelieved pressure, edema, hypovolemia, smoking, or advanced vascular disease), and to initiate measures to optimize oxygenation at the wound site (Colburn, 2001).

### Nutritional Status

The ability to synthesize connective tissue depends on availability of the raw ingredients, such as amino acids, vitamins, and minerals. Malnutrition is a common cause of delayed healing. In addition, malnutrition compromises immune system function, increases the client's risk of infection, and can be a very serious condition.

## CLINICAL ALERT

### The Importance of a Dietitian Consult

The dietitian is a critical member of the health care team, and dietary consults should be the "standard of care" for any client with a wound or at risk for skin breakdown who has indicators of nutritional compromise. Dietitians can perform a comprehensive nutritional assessment and can direct the team in providing appropriate nutritional support.

Roth, R., & Townsend, C. (2002). *Nutrition & diet therapy* (8th ed.). Clifton Park, NY: Delmar Learning.

### Diabetes Mellitus

Diabetes is widely recognized as a profound inhibitor of normal repair. Elevated glucose levels interfere with leukocytosis and predispose the client to infection. In addition, diabetes is associated with reduced levels of growth factors, impaired collagen synthesis, and reduced tensile strength, for reasons not totally understood. It is therefore critical to closely monitor blood glucose levels and to maintain normoglycemia. Client education plays an essential role in promoting repair for the diabetic client (Inlow, Orsted, & Sibbald, 2000).

### Corticosteroids

Corticosteroids significantly inhibit multiple components of the repair process. These adverse effects are most profound at doses of 40 mg/day or greater, but are seen to a lesser extent at doses of 20 to 40 mg per day. Low-dose steroids (i.e., less than 20 mg/day) are not thought to have a significant effect on repair (Rodeheaver, 2001).

### Aging

Aging is known to affect multiple aspects of the repair process. Therefore the client's age must be taken into consideration when evaluating progress in wound repair. Older individuals will heal at a slower rate than children and younger adults.

### Laboratory Data

Cultures of the wound drainage are used to determine the presence of infection and to identify the causative organism. The sensitivity results list the antibiotics that will effectively treat the infection. An elevated white blood cell count is indicative of an infectious process. A decreased leukocyte count may indicate that the client is at increased risk for developing an infection related to decreased defense mechanisms. Albumin is a measure of the client's protein reserves; if decreased, there are decreased resources of protein for wound healing

(Daniels, 2003). Procedure 36-1 outlines the correct techniques for culturing a wound.

## Nursing Diagnosis

Nursing diagnoses for clients with wounds focus on prevention of complications and promotion of the healing process through proper wound care and client teaching. Following are the North American Nursing Diagnosis Association-approved nursing diagnoses with a partial list of related factors:

1. *Impaired Tissue Integrity* related to surgical incision, pressure shearing forces, decreased blood flow, immobility, mechanical (pressure, shear, friction), radiation, nutritional deficit or excess, thermal irritants, including body excretions, secretions, and medications
2. *Risk for Infection* related to malnutrition, decreased defense mechanisms
3. *Pain* related to inflammation, infection
4. *Disturbed Body Image* related to changes in body appearance secondary to scars, drains, removal of body parts
5. *Deficient Knowledge (wound care)* related to lack of exposure to information, misinterpretation, lack of interest in learning

## Outcome Identification and Planning

After identifying the nursing diagnoses, the nurse establishes targeted outcomes for wound healing. When formulating outcomes, keep in mind that they should be based on the client's identified needs and should be individualized on the basis of the client's condition. Changes in the health care delivery system have brought about early discharge from the hospital, so clients are often sent home with wounds that need continued care. The goals for clients with wounds generally focus on promoting wound healing, preventing infection, and educating the client. An example of a goal for debilitated clients would be demonstrating no signs of infection and preventing pressure to certain skin areas for extended periods of time.

## Implementation

Nursing interventions to promote wound healing and prevent infection include a variety of therapies. The nurse implements such therapies as cleansing the wound, dressing the wound, debriding the necrotic tissue, and monitoring the wound drainage.

### Systemic Support Measures

Systemic support is of critical importance whenever the goal is wound repair. Specific aspects of systemic support

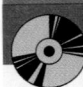

**PROCEDURE 36-1**

## Obtaining a Wound Drainage Specimen for Culturing

### EQUIPMENT NEEDED

- Disposable gloves
- Sterile gloves and dressing supplies
- Normal saline and irrigation tray

- Culture tube and swab (Figure 36-8)
- Moisture-proof container or bag

## IMPLEMENTATION—ACTION/RATIONALE

| ACTION | RATIONALE |
|---|---|
| 1. Wash hands, apply disposable gloves, and remove old dressing. Place old dressing in moisture-proof container, and remove and discard gloves. Wash hands again. | 1. Reduces the transmission of microorganisms. Makes the wound accessible for obtaining the culture. |
| 2. Open the dressing supplies using sterile technique, and apply gloves. | 2. Maintains sterile environment. |
| 3. Assess the wound's appearance; note quality, quantity, color, and odor of discharge. | 3. Provides assessment of the amount and character of the wound's drainage prior to irrigation. Reddened areas and heavy drainage suggest infection. |
| 4. Irrigate the wound with normal saline prior to culturing the wound; do not irrigate with antiseptic. | 4. Irrigation decreases the risk of culturing normal flora and other exudates such as protein; irrigating with an antiseptic prior to culturing may destroy the bacteria. |
| 5. Using a sterile gauze pad, absorb the excess saline, then discard the pad. | 5. Removal of excess irrigant prevents maceration of tissue due to excess moisture. |
| 6. Remove the culture tube from the packaging (Figure 36-9). Remove the culture swab from the culture tube and gently roll the swab over the granulation tissue. Avoid eschar and wound edges (Figure 36-10). | 6. Decreases the chance of collecting superficial skin microorganisms. |

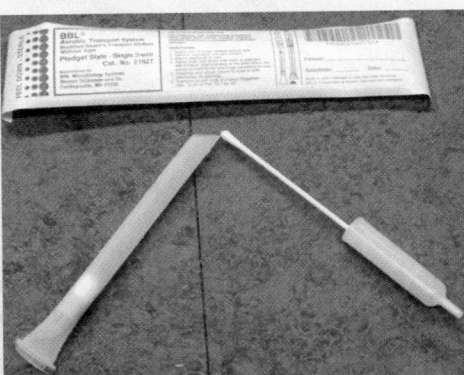

**Figure 36-8    Sterile culture tube and swab**

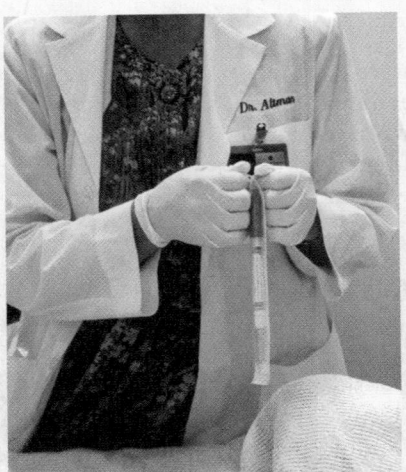

**Figure 36-9    Remove the culture tube from the packaging.**

*(continues)*

**PROCEDURE 36-1 (*continued*)**

7. Replace the swab into the culture tube, being careful not to touch the swab to the outside of the tube. Recap the tube. Crush the ampoule of medium located in the bottom or cap of the tube (Figure 36-11).

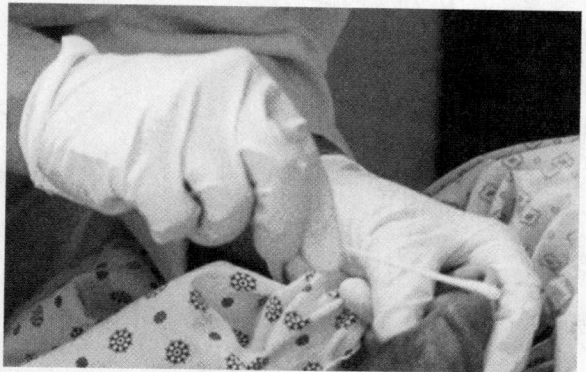

**Figure 36-10    Role the swab over the area to be cultured.**

8. Remove gloves, wash hands, and apply sterile gloves. Dress the wound with sterile dressing.

9. Label the specimen and arrange to transport the specimen to the laboratory according to agency policy.

10. Remove gloves and wash hands.

11. Document all assessment findings and actions taken. Document that a specimen was obtained.

7. Avoids contamination with microorganisms. Releases the medium to surround the swab.

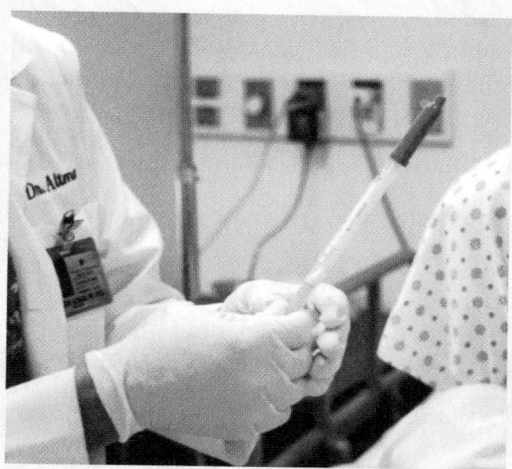

**Figure 36-11    Crush the ampoule to release the medium inside the culture tube.**

8. Prevents contamination of the wound.

9. Ensures proper handling of specimen.

10. Reduces the transmission of microorganisms.

11. Records information for evaluation and promotes continuity of care.

 **LIFE SPAN CONSIDERATIONS**

### Preparation for Obtaining a Culture

*Pediatric Variations*

- Explain to the child in age-appropriate terms what the culture procedure is for.

- Allow older children to assist in positioning and watch the procedure if they wish.

- Answer questions and reassure the child that the procedure will not hurt any more than the normal dressing change.

*Geriatric Variations*

- Explain the procedure step-by-step to clients who cannot hear or see well so they know what you are doing.

- Enlist help if needed to hold an older or debilitated client in position so you can obtain a proper culture.

## COMMUNITY/HOME CARE

### Obtaining a Culture

#### Home Care Variations

- When conducting a home care visit, make sure you know where to send the culture after you have collected it. Will it be picked up by the lab? Will you or a caregiver be responsible for delivery to a location? Will the lab be open, or do you need to make special arrangements?

- Make sure you bring the correct equipment to the visit. A cotton-tip applicator and a sandwich bag will not provide the appropriate sterile culture receptacle.

- Make sure that the culture can be sent without excessive delay.

#### Long-Term Care Variations

- If the long-term facility does not stock the necessary equipment, make sure you know where to obtain the culture tubes and where to deliver the specimen before you approach the client.

- A culture order must be written by the attending physician or qualified practitioner of the facility.

have been addressed in detail in the previous section and are highlighted in Table 36-1.

## Topical Therapy

A key nursing responsibility in management of any wound is the provision of topical therapy. In providing topical therapy, the nurse must consider the following: the goals of local wound care (establishment of a clean, moist, and insulated wound bed), the characteristics of the wound itself, and the goals of care for this client.

## Wound Cleansing

Wound cleansing should be designed to rid the wound surface of impediments to repair (e.g., bacteria and exu-

| TABLE 36-1 | SYSTEMIC SUPPORT FOR WOUND REPAIR |
|---|---|
| Key Elements of Support | Nursing Implications |
| Tissue Perfusion and Oxygenation | • Maintain warmth and hydration<br>• Control pain and edema<br>• Supplemental oxygen if needed<br>• Vascular consult for client with inadequate blood flow |
| Nutritional Support | • Monitor weight, nutrient intake, and laboratory indices for protein status<br>• Encourage food and fluid intake<br>• Obtain nutritional consult for any client with wound who is nutritionally compromised |
| Glucose Levels Within Normal Limits | • Monitor glucose levels<br>• Maintain glucose levels within normoglycemic range or as close to that as possible |
| Compensation for Chronic Steroid Intake | • Consult primary care provider regarding topical vitamin A for wound client receiving more than 40 mg of Prednisone a day |

date), while minimizing interference with the repair process and damage to "good cells" (white blood cells, fibroblasts, and epithelial cells). Cleansing agents and procedures are varied and require specific instructions for irrigating the individual wound (see Procedure 36-2).

## Dressing Selection

The principles of dressing selection are based on the goals of topical wound care. The primary functions of wound dressings are (1) absorption of wound exudate, (2) maintenance of a moist wound surface, (3) protection of the

---

 **PROCEDURE 36-2**   **Irrigating a Wound**

### EQUIPMENT NEEDED

- Sterile gloves (Figure 36-12)
- Disposable gloves
- Sterile irrigation kit (basin, piston irrigation syringe, solution container)
- Irrigation solution (per physician's or qualified practitioner's order)

- Waterproof pad
- Sterile dressing material to redress the wound
- Moisture-proof container or bag for use after the irrigation procedure

### IMPLEMENTATION—ACTION/RATIONALE

| ACTION | RATIONALE |
|---|---|
| 1. Confirm the physician's or qualified practitioner's order for wound irrigation and note the type and strength of the ordered irrigation solution. | 1. Wound irrigation is a dependent nursing action that requires a medical order stating the type of solution to be used. |
| 2. Assess the client's pain level and medicate if needed with an analgesic 30 minutes before procedure if the medication is to be given p.o. or I.M. | 2. Allows time for medication to be absorbed to increase the analgesic effect. |
| 3. Explain the procedure to the client. | 3. Helps to decrease the client's anxiety and increase the client's cooperation. |
| 4. Place a waterproof pad on the bed. Assist the client onto the pad. Then assist the client into a position that will allow the irrigant to flow through the wound and into the basin from the cleanest to dirtiest area of the wound. | 4. Positioning of the client and placement of a waterproof pad will decrease contamination of bed linen. |
| 5. Wash hands and apply the disposable gloves; remove and discard the old dressing. | 5. Reduces transmission of microorganisms. |
| 6. Assess the wound's appearance and note quality, quantity, color, and odor of drainage. | 6. Provides assessment of the status of the wound. |
| 7. Remove and discard the disposable gloves, and wash hands. | 7. Reduces transmission of microorganisms. |
| 8. Prepare the sterile irrigation tray and dressing supplies. Pour the room-temperature irrigation solution into the solution container. | 8. Aseptic technique is used to prevent introduction of microorganisms into the wound. Room-temperature solution reduces client discomfort. |
| 9. Apply sterile gloves (and goggles if needed). | 9. Promotes sterile environment. |
| 10. Position the sterile basin below the wound so the irrigant will flow from the cleanest area to the dirtiest area and into the basin. | 10. Decreases possibility of wound contamination. |

*(continues)*

## PROCEDURE 36-2 (continued)

11. Fill the piston or bulb syringe with irrigant and gently flush the wound. Hold the syringe approximately 1 inch above the wound bed to irrigate. Refill the syringe and continue to flush the wound until the solution returns clear and no exudate is noted or until the prescribed amount of fluid has been used (Figures 36-13 and 36-14).

11. Gently irrigating the wound decreases trauma to granulation tissue. This provides the ideal pressure for cleansing and removal of debris.

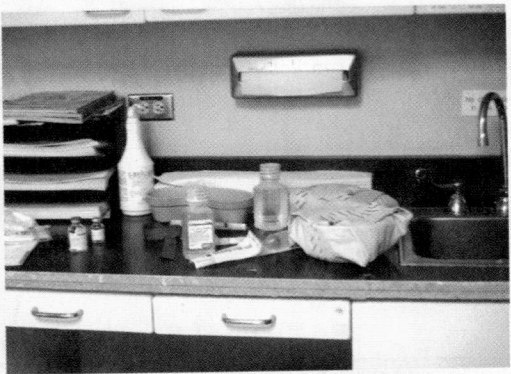

**Figure 36-12** Sterile basin, sterile irrigating solution, and sterile syringes are used to irrigate a wound.

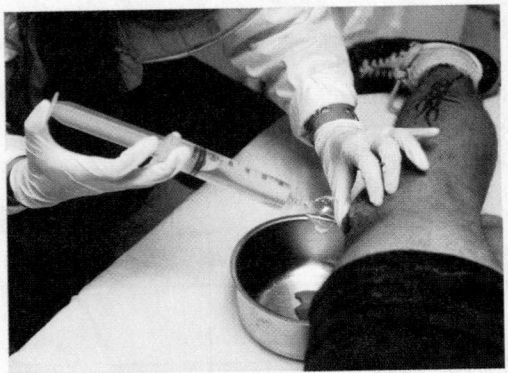

**Figure 36-13** Gently flush the wound.

12. Dry the edges of the wound with sterile gauze (Figure 36-15).

12. Drying the edges of the wound prevents maceration of tissues due to excess moisture.

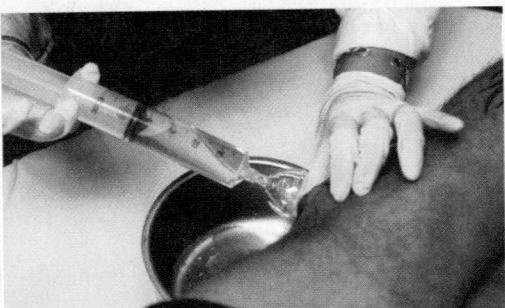

**Figure 36-14** Hold the syringe close to the wound, but be careful not to touch the wound with the syringe.

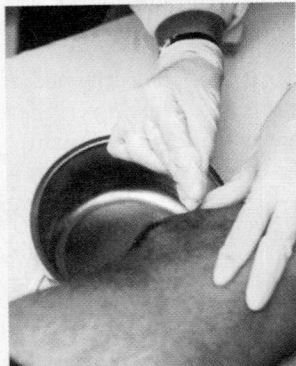

**Figure 36-15** Dry the edges of the wound with sterile gauze.

13. Assess the wound's appearance and drainage.

13. Provides indication of change in wound status.

14. Apply a sterile dressing. Remove sterile gloves and dispose of properly. Wash hands.

14. Application of a sterile dressing protects the wound from microorganisms.

15. Document all assessment findings and actions taken.

15. Records information for evaluation.

---

## COMMUNITY/HOME CARE

### Wound Care

**Home Care Variations**

- Clients with slow-healing wounds are often sent home to be cared for. The nurse is often in the position of teaching the client or a caregiver how to perform the irrigation and dressing change. She should periodically assess the irrigation and dressing change to ensure it is still being done correctly.

**Long-Term Care Variations**

- Clients with long-term wounds need to plan a regular schedule of wound care and a clear method to document the progress of healing and signs of infection.

- An irrigation order and dressing change order will need to be written by the attending physician or qualified practitioner of the facility.

---

healing wound from trauma or bacterial invasion, and (4) insulation. Nurses must also be aware of the limitations of certain wound coverings. See Procedures 36-3 and 36-4 for descriptions of dry dressings and wet-to-damp dressings. In addition, the wound dressings are generally classified as one of four types:

1. Exudative wounds that have depth, undermining, or tunnels (deep, wet wounds)
2. Wounds with depth, undermining, or tunnels that have minimal or no exudate (deep, dry wounds)
3. Exudative wounds that have minimal depth and no tunneled or undermined areas (shallow, wet wounds)
4. Wounds with minimal depth, no tunneled or undermined areas, and minimal or no exudate (shallow, dry wounds)

### Debridement of Necrotic Tissue

Necrotic tissue delays the repair process because it prolongs the inflammatory phase; in addition, necrotic tissue can contribute to infection by providing a medium for bacterial growth. Therefore, **debridement** (removal of necrotic tissue) is an important component of topical therapy for necrotic wounds whenever the goal is wound healing and anytime the wound is infected (Alvarez, Fernandez-Obregon, Rogers, & Bergano, 2000).

### Monitor Drainage of Wounds

During the inflammatory response, exudates develop within a wound. When excessive drainage accumulates in the wound bed, tissue healing is delayed. If the outer surface is allowed to heal while the drainage remains entrapped within the wound, an abscess formation may occur. To facilitate drainage of any excess fluid, the physician may insert a tube or drain. When the drain is inserted by the surgeon at the time of surgery, one end of the drain is placed in the operative site and the other end is usually passed through a separate, small stab wound near the main incision. Various types

of drains exist on the market. Some flexible drains such as **Penrose drains** function by gravity and have an open end that drains onto dressings. **Closed suction drainage systems** commonly have a reservoir that is capable of creating negative pressure or a vacuum. The gentle suction that is

---

### CLINICAL ALERT

#### Application of Gauze Dressings

Gauze is the most commonly ordered wound dressing, but several potential problems are associated with its use, and incorrect use can delay wound healing and cause the client pain. When dressing a wound with gauze, remember the following:

- Moisten the gauze before you place it into the wound, and "remoisten" if necessary before removing it. This minimizes the client's discomfort and prevents traumatic disruption of newly formed tissue.

- When using gauze as a filler dressing, "fluff" the gauze and pack the wound lightly. Tight packing interferes with blood flow to the wound and with wound closure.

- When selecting gauze to be placed into a wound, avoid gauze with loose fibers or cotton fillers, since these can act as foreign bodies if retained in the wound.

Ovington, L., & Peirce, B. (2001). Wound dressings: Form, function, feasibility, and facts. In D. Krasner, G. Rodeheaver, & R. Sibbald (Eds.), *Chronic wound care* (3rd ed., pp. 311–320). Wayne, PA: HMP Communications.

**PROCEDURE 36-3**    **Applying a Dry Dressing**

## EQUIPMENT NEEDED

■ Clean exam gloves (Figure 36-16)
■ Container for proper disposal of soiled dressing
■ Sterile 4 × 4 gauze pads
■ Washcloth (optional)
■ ABD pads (optional)
■ 2-inch tape (foam or paper)

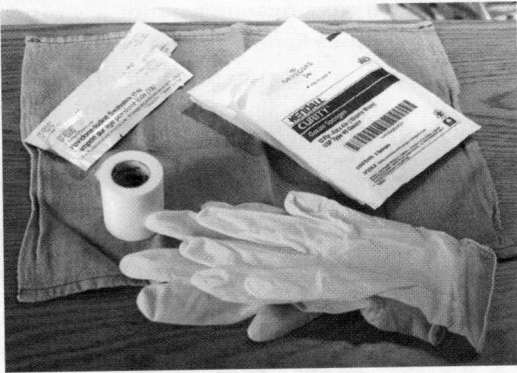

**Figure 36-16** Gauze sponges, clean gloves, tape, and povidone-iodine are used to change a dry dressing.

## IMPLEMENTATION—ACTION/RATIONALE

| ACTION | RATIONALE |
|---|---|
| 1. Gather supplies. | 1. Promotes a smooth work flow. |
| 2. Provide privacy; draw curtains; close door. | 2. Maintains client comfort and privacy while body is exposed during procedure. |
| 3. Explain procedure to client. | 3. Provides information about the procedure. |
| 4. Wash hands. | 4. Reduces transmission of microorganisms. |
| 5. Apply clean exam gloves. | 5. Infection control and protection from body fluids. |
| 6. Remove dressing and place in appropriate receptacle. Remove soiled gloves with contaminated surfaces inward and discard in appropriate receptacle and apply clean gloves. | 6. Dressings and gloves soiled with body fluids are considered contaminated and subject to biohazard disposal in the correct manner per institution protocol.<br><br>   It is often standard for the surgeon to do the first postoperative dressing change. The initial dressing is maintained for 24 to 48 hours postoperatively, unless conditions of the dressing call for contacting the physician or qualified practitioner for a dressing change order. Until the removal of the initial dressing, the nurse will reinforce the dressing as needed.<br><br>   The frequency of the dressing change is dependent upon the needs of the wound and the preference of the physician or qualified practitioner. This will usually be specified in the orders. |
| 7. Assess the appearance of the undressed wound bed for healing. | 7. Assess for signs of redness, foul odor, swelling, irritation, drainage, dehiscence, bleeding, or skin breakdown. |

*(continues)*

## PROCEDURE 36-3 (*continued*)

8. Cleanse the skin around the incision if necessary with a clean, warm, wet washcloth.
   - If the suture line requires cleansing, it should be done gently. Use normal saline, half-strength hydrogen peroxide, or Betadine swab (consult orders of physician or qualified practitioner and/or hospital policy regarding antiseptic agents) and cotton-tip applicators using a rolling motion.
   - Used applicators should not be reintroduced into the sterile solution (Figure 36-17).

8. Dried blood or drainage on the surrounding skin can be an irritant and a medium for microbes.
   - The suture line itself should not be disturbed unnecessarily.



   - Reintroduction of the soiled applicator into sterile solution will contaminate the solution.

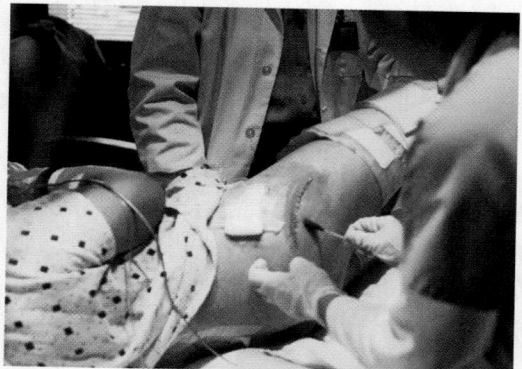

**Figure 36-17** Clean the suture lines gently, if necessary.

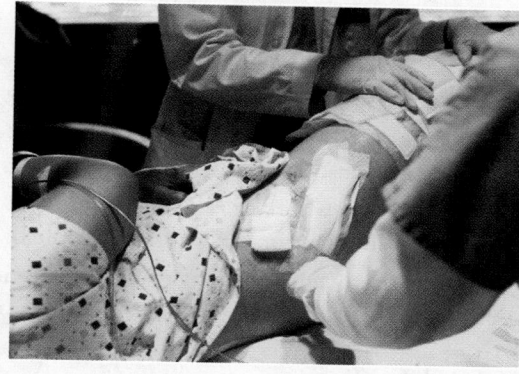

**Figure 36-18** Apply 4 x 4 gauze pads, folded in half. Tape the gauze in place.

9. Remove used exam gloves.

9. Exam gloves used to remove the old dressing are considered dirty and should be removed and discarded appropriately.

10. Wash hands.

10. Hands should be washed prior to setting up dressing supplies to reduce transmission of microorganisms.

11. Set up supplies.

11. Following removal of the dressing, you will have a better idea of what supplies are needed and in what amount.

12. Apply a new pair of clean exam gloves.

12. This is considered to be a clean procedure after the initial dressing is removed if the skin margins are approximated with the skin closures.

13. Grasping just the edges, apply a new dressing using 4 × 4 gauze pads folded in half to the 2 × 4 size. Place the folded gauze pad lengthwise on wound and tape lightly or apply tubular mesh for those with sensitive skin (Figure 36-18). Initial the dressing, date, and time it was changed.

    **Optional:** An ABD pad may be applied on top of the dressing for added protection over sutures or for client comfort.

13. A light dressing of 4 × 4 pads may be the only dressing that is needed to protect the incision from clothing or to collect a small amount of tissue drainage. This maintains a record of the dressing change for the next nurse.

(*continues*)

**PROCEDURE 36-3 (continued)**

14. Remove gloves and dispose of appropriately, then wash hands.

14. Reduces the transmission of microorganisms.

15. Conduct client and family education about the dressing, which may include teaching the dressing technique to the client and family.

15. Educates the client and family and prepares for discharge.

## LIFE SPAN CONSIDERATIONS

### Wound Care in the Elderly and Children

**Pediatric Variations**

- Remind all children who are old enough to understand not to touch the dressing site or play with the drainage tubes. Make sure that the dressing is secure and the small child cannot easily pull or dislodge a drain.
- Demonstration of wound care on a doll or stuffed animal may be appropriate for younger children.
- Young children will require explanation that their wound will heal and does not mean that their body part is missing or that their insides will leak out of the wound.
- Older children can be taught to participate in self-care of dressings. Special bright stickers, bright Band-Aids, or brightly colored wrap (Coban) are options for securing and decorating children's wound dressings.

**Geriatric Variations**

- Older people have thin skin, which can be sensitive to tape and solutions. Special attention should be given to the skin when removing the dressing.
- Older clients often live alone and may need home health care to assist with dressings.

## COMMUNITY/HOME CARE

### Dressing Care

**Home Care Variations**

- Where and how to obtain additional supplies should be reviewed with the client and family.
- Review proper disposal of contaminated dressings.
- Discharge instructions need to include how to care for the dressing at home and when and who to call if the client experiences problems with the dressing change or wound care.
- Problems that might occur should be reviewed with the client and family and include fever, bleeding, infected wound, and pain management during dressing changes.

**Long-Term Care Variations**

- Special supplies are most likely not going to be needed for the clean, closed surgical wound other than gauze 4 × 4 or 2 × 2 pads and tape.
- Review with the long-term care facility the physician's or qualified practitioner's preference for wound care, as the facility may have to special-order or replace with equivalent supplies. If necessary, provide the client with a 3-day supply until supplies can be obtained by the facility.

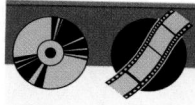

## PROCEDURE 36-4

# Applying a Wet to Damp Dressing (Wet to Dry to Moist Dressing)

## EQUIPMENT NEEDED

- Clean exam gloves (Figure 36-19)
- Container for proper disposal of soiled dressing
- Sterile gloves
- Moisture-proof gown (optional)
- Sterile towel
- Normal saline or ordered solution
- Sterile bowl
- Sterile 4 × 4 gauze pads, multiple
- Cover sponges or fluffs (optional)
- ABD dressing pads
- 2-inch tape (foam or paper)
- Tubular mesh (optional)
- Montgomery straps (optional)

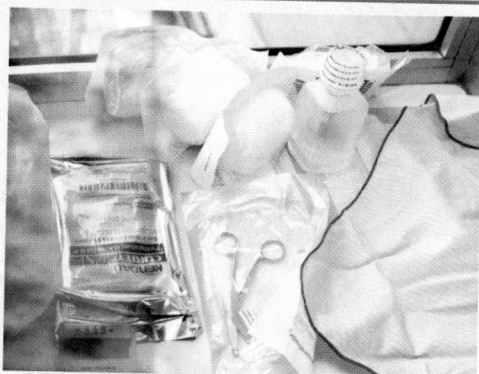

**Figure 36-19** Sterile bandages, sterile saline, sterile field, and sterile scissors are used to create a wet to damp or moist dressing.

## IMPLEMENTATION—ACTION/RATIONALE

| ACTION | RATIONALE |
|---|---|
| 1. Review order of physician or qualified practitioner for wound care and gather supplies. | 1. Promotes a smooth work flow. |
| 2. Provide privacy; draw curtains; close door. | 2. Maintains client comfort and privacy while body is exposed during procedure. |
| 3. Explain procedure to client. | 3. Provides information about the procedure. |
| 4. Wash hands. | 4. Reduces transmission of microorganisms. |
| 5. Apply clean exam gloves, a moisture-proof gown, mask, and eye protection, if needed. | 5. Provides infection control and protection from body fluids. If there is copious drainage or the wound is infected, a gown, a mask, and eye protection should be worn. A mask will also help the nurse if the drainage is foul smelling. |
| 6. Assess need for pain medication. Pain is rated on a scale from 0 (lowest) to 10 (greatest). Assess need based on quality, pain pattern, location, and last pain medication received. | 6. Removal of a wet to damp or moist dressing may be painful to the client, so careful assessment of pain medication needs prior to the dressing change is important. |
| 7. Inform client that the dressing is going to be removed. | 7. This helps prepare client and alleviates anxiety. |
| 8. Remove wet to damp dressing, noting number of gauze pads used, and place in appropriate receptacle (Figure 36-20). | 8. The dressing should be removed slowly yet deliberately. It is not recommended to moisten the dressing with saline because this defeats the purpose of the debriding and cleaning action. If it is found that the dressing is extremely dry and removal will result in injury, a small amount of saline to loosen |

*(continues)*

## PROCEDURE 36-4 (continued)

that portion of the dressing is indicated (Figure 36-21). To counteract the problem of an extremely dry dressing, increase the wetness of the dressing or increase the frequency of the dressing change. Count the number of gauze pads so you know how many to use when replacing the dressing.

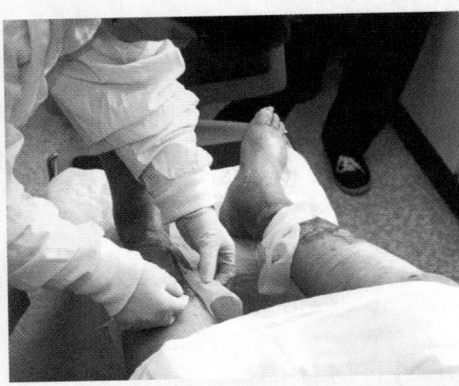

**Figure 36-20    Carefully remove the old dressing, allowing the old dressing to debride the wound as you pull it away.**

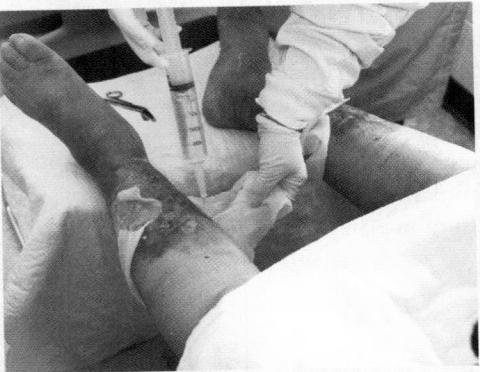

**Figure 36-21    If the dressing is too dry and removing it will cause injury, use a small amount of saline to loosen the portion of the dressing that adheres too tightly to the wound.**

9. Observe the undressed wound for healing (granulation and approximation of edges), signs of infection (inflammation, edema, warmth, pain), and drainage.

9. Allows for evaluation of effectiveness of treatment.

10. Cleanse the skin around the incision if necessary with a clean, warm, wet washcloth.

10. Dried blood or drainage on the surrounding skin can be an irritant and a medium for microbes.

11. Remove used exam gloves.

11. Exam gloves used to remove the old dressing are considered dirty and should be removed and discarded appropriately.

12. Wash hands.

12. Reduces transmission of microorganisms.

13. Set up supplies in a sterile field, including pouring ordered solutions into appropriate containers if indicated for the dressing change.

13. Following removal of the dressing, you will have a better idea of what supplies are needed and in what amount.

14. Apply sterile gloves.

14. This is a sterile dressing change.

15. Place gauze or packing material to be moistened in the bowl with the normal saline or other solution.

15. If a solution is not specified, then normal saline is used. Wounds that are considered dirty or contaminated may have special solutions ordered by the physician or qualified practitioner to moisten the wound packing. Alternate solutions are a dilute povidone-iodine solution and a dilute acetic acid solution. Follow institutional guidelines.

*(continues)*

**PROCEDURE 36-4** (*continued*)

- Wring gauze or packing of saline until damp.

- Gently place damp gauze over the area (Figure 36-22).

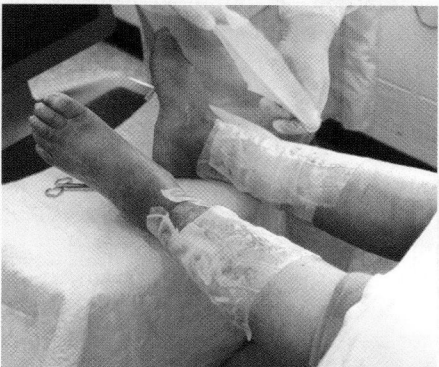

**Figure 36-22    Place the gauze on the wound.**

16. Apply external dressing of dry 4 × 4 gauze pads, cover sponges, fluffs, or ABD pads.
    - Secure dressing in place with tape, Montgomery straps, or tubular mesh (Figure 36-23).

17. Remove gloves and wash hands.

18. Mark the dressing with the date and time it was changed. Initial the dressing.

19. Conduct client and family education about the dressing, which may include teaching the dressing technique to the client and family.

- Avoid overwringing of the dressing to prevent excessive drying. The dressing should be wet to damp depending upon the depth and size of the wound and the interval of the dressing change.
- Dresses the wound.

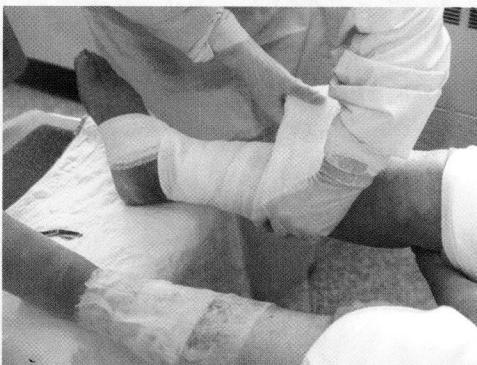

**Figure 36-23    Wrap the wet gauze with an external dressing of dry gauze bandages.**

16. The external dressing is determined by the size and shape of the wound.
    - Tape for short-term dressings in clients who are not sensitive to adhesives is the method of choice for securing dressings. For long-term dressings or for those who are sensitive to tape, use Montgomery straps or tubular mesh.
      Tubular mesh is a nice alternative to hold the dressing in place because tape is not involved—the mesh is simply pulled up or down to accommodate the dressing change.

17. Reduces transmission of microorganisms. Be sure to discard gloves in appropriate receptacle.

18. This maintains a record of the dressing change for the next nurse and provides for continuity of care.

19. Educates the client and family and prepares for discharge.

created draws exudate from the wound into the reservoir. As fluid enters the reservoir, suction is lost; therefore, the nurse must empty the reservoir when it is half-full. Hemovac and Jackson-Pratt drains are examples of closed suction drainage systems (Figure 36-24).

Nurses are responsible for maintaining the patency of the system and for assessing the amount, type, and color of the drainage. It is important for the nurse to be cau-

tious when changing wound dressings to prevent accidental removal or dislodgment of drains.

### Maintenance of Open Proliferative Wound Edges

As explained previously, epithelialization cannot occur if the surrounding wound edges are closed. Therefore, one aspect of comprehensive wound care is ongoing assessment

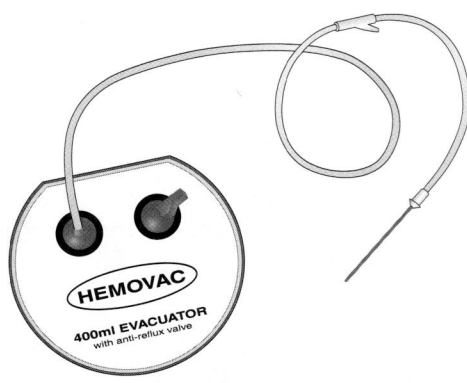

**A. Closed system (Hemovac)**

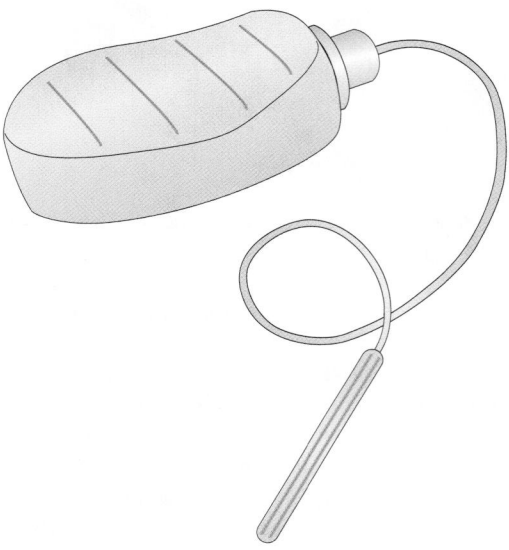

**B. Tube and reservoir system (Jackson-Pratt)**

**Figure 36-24    Drainage systems**

of the wound edges; if the wound edges are closed and the wound is approaching the epithelialization phase, the nurse should intervene by requesting chemical cauterization or a surgical consult.

## Evaluation

The nurse needs to evaluate the client's achievement of the goals established during the planning phase to achieve or maintain skin integrity. Goals for clients with wounds generally focus on wound healing, prevention of infection, and client education. If the goals are not achieved, the nurse will need to examine the nursing interventions and strategies that were employed and revise the nursing care plan accordingly. Reviewing techniques and procedures, especially those performed by the

client or other caregivers in the client's support system, is especially important.

# Management Guidelines for Specific Wounds

In addition to providing systemic and local support for wound healing, the nurse must consider the etiology of the particular wound and must incorporate additional interventions as required, based on the cause of the wound. Commonly encountered wounds include abrasions and lacerations (Figure 36-25), surgical incisions, skin tears, pressure ulcers, leg ulcers, and burns.

## Abrasions and Lacerations

**Abrasions** are surface wounds involving loss of the epidermis and possibly partial dermal loss. They are most commonly incurred during accidents that cause "dragging" of the skin surface against pavement, dirt, or gravel. In assessing and managing abrasions, it is critical to palpate the area carefully to rule out any retained foreign bodies and to remove all debris from the wound surface. Removing the debris often requires application of a topical anesthetic, followed by thorough irrigation and possibly gentle scrubbing with a nonabrasive sponge and cleanser. These wounds are typically exudative and best managed with nonadherent but absorptive surface dressings.

    **Lacerations** involve cuts to the skin and soft tissues. The initial goal in management of these lesions is usually hemostasis, followed by thorough assessment to rule out

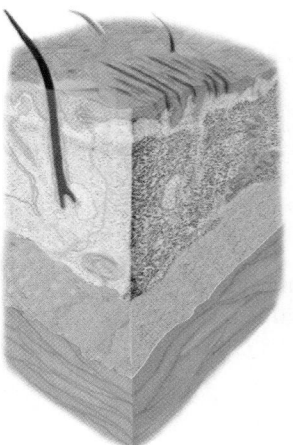
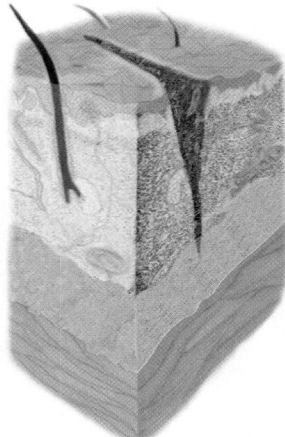

A. **Abrasion**, also known as a scrape or rug burn, results when the outer layer of skin is scraped or rubbed away. Exposure of nerve endings makes this type of wound painful, and the presence of debris from the scraped surface (rug fibers, gravel, sand) makes abrasions highly susceptible to infection.

B. **Laceration**, cut or incision, is caused by sharp objects such as knives or glass; or from trauma due to a strike from a blunt object that opens the skin, such as a baseball bat. If the wound is deep, the cut may bleed profusely; if nerve endings are exposed, it may also be painful.

**Figure 36-25    Types of wounds**

foreign bodies and to determine the extent of injury. Clean lacerations are usually closed primarily, while contaminated wounds are frequently left open to heal by secondary intention, or closed at a later date following control of infection. Management of closed lacerations is essentially the same as management of a closed surgical incision. Management of lacerations healing by secondary intention is based on the depth and volume of exudate (Dickerson, Purdue, & Hunt, 1999).

## Surgical Incisions

Surgical incisions are acute wounds sustained under sterile conditions and closed by sutures or staples that heal quickly. Preoperative measures to optimize postoperative wound healing include elimination of aspirin and aspirin products (to reduce bleeding), client education (to reduce anxiety), and interventions to improve and optimize nutritional status. Postoperative care includes pain control, maintenance of warmth, hydration, and control of edema. These measures all improve perfusion to the wound bed. In addition, clients with cardiorespiratory conditions resulting in low blood oxygen levels may benefit from supplemental oxygen.

In assessing a surgical incision, the nurse should be alert to any evidence of delayed healing and any signs of infection. Normal healing is evidenced by presence of a "healing ridge" (palpable just underneath the incision) by days 5 to 9 postoperatively. Absence of a healing ridge is indicative of delayed healing and increased risk of wound **dehiscence** (partial or complete separation of the wound edges and the layers below the skin) or **evisceration** (protrusion of the internal viscera through a disrupted wound). These clients may benefit from supportive dressings or binders to minimize tension on the incision, in addition to the measures already listed to optimize healing. Signs of infection include purulent drainage, acute inflammation, and incisional separation. Infection usually mandates reopening of the suture line to permit free drainage, in addition to systemic antibiotic therapy (White & Duncan, 2002).

## Skin Tears

Skin tears occur when the superficial skin layers slide against each other, causing separation between the epidermis and dermis or between the dermis and subcutaneous tissue. Skin tears are much more common in older people due to the reduced cohesion between the epidermal, dermal, and subcutaneous tissue layers.

In assessing a skin tear, the nurse should note whether or not there is a viable "flap" of skin. If there is, the best way to manage the skin tear is to use the skin flap as a physiological dressing. The wound should be gently cleansed, and the flap should be rolled back into place and secured with adhesive strips. If there is no viable flap, the wound should be cleansed and managed as a surface wound with minimal to moderate amounts of exudate (Baranoski, 2000).

## Lower Extremity Ulcers

Lower extremity ulcers are common among older adults due to the increased prevalence of chronic venous insufficiency, peripheral arterial disease, and diabetic neuropathy. Effective management of lower extremity ulcers depends primarily on accurate identification and aggressive management of the causative factors, coupled with appropriate systemic support and topical therapy (Boulton, Meneses, & Ennis, 1999). Accurate identification of the causative and contributing factors requires a careful history and focused physical exam.

### Venous Ulcers

**Venous ulcers** are caused by chronic venous insufficiency (i.e., *Chronic Venous Congestion* related to poor venous return). Contributing conditions include deep vein thrombosis, which damages the one-way valves that normally support venous return. Venous ulcers typically occur around the ankles, and physical findings usually include edema, a dark red ulcer bed, and moderate to large volumes

---

### NURSING STRATEGY

#### Assessment of Factors That Cause Lower Extremity Ulcers

The nurse should assess for the following factors that can cause lower extremity ulcers:

- History of medical conditions associated with vascular disease or neuropathy (e.g., deep vein thrombosis, atherosclerotic disease, tobacco use, diabetes)

- Onset, duration, and past management of the ulcer

- Vascular assessment involving the presence and quality of the dorsalis pedis and posterior tibialis pulses, and the presence of edema

- Sensorimotor assessment as evidenced by sensory loss in the feet

- Ulcer characteristics, with particular attention to location, appearance of the wound bed, and volume of exudate

Adapted from Broussard, C., Mendez-Eastman, S., & Frantz, R. (2000). Adjuvant wound therapies. In R. Bryant (Ed.), *Acute and chronic wounds: Nursing management* (2nd ed., pp. 431–454). St. Louis: Mosby; Colburn, L. (2001). Prevention of chronic wounds. In D. Krasner, G. Rodeheaver, and R. G. Sibbald (Eds.), *Chronic wound care* (3rd ed., pp. 67–78). Wayne, PA: HMP Communications.

of exudate. Strategies include such measures as the application of compression wraps (Kunimoto, Cooling, Gulliver, Houghton, Orsted, & Sibbald, 2001).

### Arterial Ulcers

**Arterial ulcers** are caused by chronic arterial insufficiency, or the inability to adequately perfuse the peripheral tissues. The resulting ischemia renders the tissues very vulnerable to minor trauma and may even result in spontaneous necrosis of the toes. Arterial ulcers are usually seen in clients with a history of atherosclerotic disease, smoking, and diabetes. They commonly occur on the toes or in areas exposed to pressure or trauma. Effective management is dependent on strategies to improve tissue perfusion and oxygenation (e.g., surgical revascularization procedures, medications that reduce platelet aggregation and thus improve blood flow through narrow vessels, and lifestyle changes such as elimination of tobacco use, and avoidance of cold and constriction). Topical therapy is determined by the severity of the perfusion deficit and the status of the wound (Goldstein, Vogel, Mureebe, & Kerstein, 1998).

### Neuropathic Ulcers

**Neuropathic ulcers** are usually caused by painless trauma. Clients at risk are those with nerve damage secondary to diabetes mellitus or a neurologic lesion. Neuropathic ulcers typically occur on the plantar surface or other areas of the foot that are exposed to repetitive trauma. Effective management includes elimination of any trauma to the wound surface, close glucose control for the diabetic, and meticulous foot care.

### Atypical Ulcers

While most leg ulcers are caused by venous insufficiency, arterial insufficiency, or neuropathy, the nurse must be aware that some ulcers represent combination pathology and that some ulcers are caused by other disease processes. Any client whose ulcer appears atypical or who fails to respond to initial therapy should be referred to a specialist for further evaluation. For example, clients with autoimmune disorders such as rheumatoid arthritis may develop vasculitic ulcers. These ulcers are caused by the deposition of immune complexes on the walls of the blood vessels, which triggers acute inflammation and necrosis of the vessels and ulceration of the overlying skin. The ulcers are typically seen on the distal leg close to the ankle, are painful, and may be difficult to distinguish from arterial or venous ulcers. Accurate diagnosis is critical and usually involves biopsy of the initial lesions and the skin around the lesions (Goldstein et al., 1998). Treatment involves control of the underlying autoimmune disorder, usually with immunosuppressive agents, in addition to topical therapy as explained earlier in this chapter.

## Burns

**Burns** are tissue injuries resulting from thermal, chemical, or electrical injury. Major burns and burns involving the joints, face, hands or feet, or perineum typically require treatment in a burn facility. Additional factors mandating

---

### NURSING STRATEGY

#### Application of Compression Wrap

- If possible, schedule application of wrap when edema has been minimized by elevation.

- Always wrap from distal to proximal.

- Instruct the client or caregiver to keep the leg elevated to heart level as much as possible.

- Instruct the client or caregiver to monitor the involved extremity for color changes, numbness, or pain (signs of circulatory impairment) and to remove the wrap if these signs occur.

Altman, G. (2004). *Delmar's fundamental & advanced nursing skills* (2nd ed.). Clifton Park, NY: Delmar Learning.

---

### CLIENT EDUCATION

#### Foot Care for Client with Diabetes Mellitus or Neuropathy

Client education to protect the feet are:

- ✓ Never go barefoot, even at home.
- ✓ Always shake out shoes before putting them on the feet.
- ✓ Make sure that your shoes fit you correctly and have the shoes professionally "fit."
- ✓ Always wear clean cotton socks.
- ✓ Bathe feet in warm water every day, and dry well between the toes. Apply lotion or cream to the skin on your feet to keep it soft. Do not put cream between the toes.
- ✓ Inspect the feet every day, and report any injury or problem to the health care provider.
- ✓ Check the temperature of the bath or shower water with the hand to be sure the water is not too hot.
- ✓ Never use heating pads on the feet, and do not prop the feet on heaters.

Catanzariti, A., Haverstock, B., Grossman, J., & Mendicino, R. (1999). Off-loading techniques in the treatment of diabetic plantar neuropathic foot ulcerations. *Advances in Wound Care, 12*(9), 452–458.

burn center management include client age, related injuries, and comorbidities. Classification of a burn as major or minor is determined by assessment of burn depth and extent of the burn injury.

In the past, burn depth was classified as first-degree, second-degree, or third degree burns. The trend now is to use the terms *epidermal (superficial epidermal)*, *superficial partial-thickness, deep partial-thickness*, and *full-thickness* (Figure 36-26). Epidermal burns involve only an acute inflammation of the epidermis. The epidermis remains intact, though later it peels away to reveal healthy skin underneath. These burns are not included in calculation of total burn surface area. Superficial partial-thickness burns involve loss of the epidermis and partial penetration into the dermis. They are exudative and painful, but they usually heal fairly rapidly by the process of epithelialization. Deep partial-thickness burns extend into the deep dermis. They are relatively dry and typically less painful than superficial partial-thickness burns. Deep partial-thickness burns are also slower to heal and more likely to "convert" to full-thickness burns as a result of tissue dehydration, infection, or trauma. Deep partial-thickness burns may require excision and grafting if they fail to epithelialize on their own. Full-thickness burns extend through the dermis into the underlying soft tissues. Full-thickness burns are associated with eschar formation and routinely require debridement and grafting.

Burns are considered to be major and to require burn center management if the total burn surface area (TBSA), including both partial- and full-thickness burns, equals more than 20% (more than 10% in children under 10 or adults over 50), or if the area of full thickness burns is greater than 5%. Management of major burns is initially focused on fluid resuscitation, management of associated injuries, incision of any constricting eschar, nutritional support, pain control, and topical burn care (e.g., daily cleansing followed by application of a topical antimicrobial agent such as silver sulfadiazine). Once the client is stable, the focus shifts to management of the burn itself (e.g., debridement and grafting) as indicated. Long-term care includes measures to control itching, maintain range of motion, and minimize scarring. Specific forms of treatment are range-of-motion exercises, scar stretching, splinting, and the use of pressure dressings and pressure garments (Helvig, 2000).

Minor burns can be managed in the outpatient setting using the principles of wound management as discussed earlier in the chapter. Deep partial-thickness burns may develop hypertrophic tissue as they heal. This hypertrophic tissue is characterized by excess vasculature and poorly organized collagen, and is best managed with support garments until the scars soften and fade, which may take as long as 2 years. Itching is another common problem and can be managed with moisturizing products, support garments, and systemic antihistamines. Avoidance of sun exposure is critical for at least 1 to 2 years following healing.

# Contusions, Strains, and Sprains: Management Guidelines

Contusions, strains, and sprains are commonly encountered injuries involving the skin and connective tissues. Contusions and strains involve limited tissue damage and

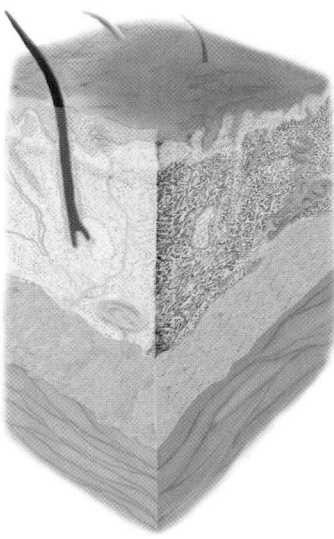 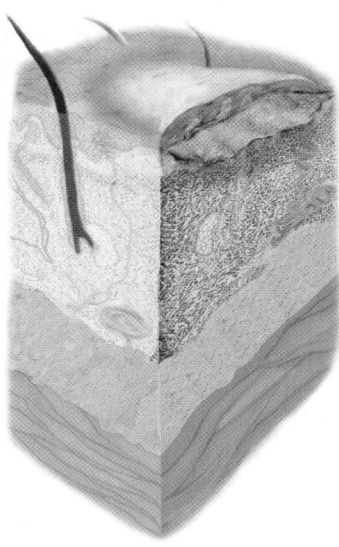 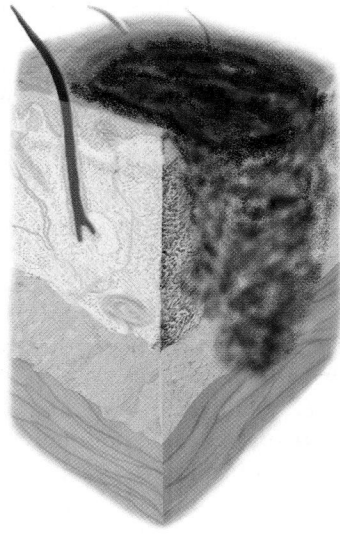

A. **Superficial epidermal** (first-degree burn): Injury to the epidermis; skin is red, dry, and painful.

B. **Deep** (second-degree burn): Injury to the epidermis and upper layers of the dermis; skin is red, moist or dry blisters, and extremely painful; exudate and swelling usually occur.

C. **Full-thickness** (third-degree burn): Injury is to the epidermis, dermis, and subcutaneous tissue; skin is dry, pearly white to charred, inelastic, and leathery.

**Figure 36-26   Types of burns**

can be managed symptomatically. Sprains may be minor or severe, and their management varies accordingly. Full return of function is the expected outcome of effective management.

## Contusions

**Contusions** are bruises of the soft tissues with no break in the skin surface; they occur when sudden pressure or shear force applied to the skin and soft tissues causes disruption of blood vessels in the subcutaneous tissue. Bleeding into the tissues from the damaged vessels produces the classic blue-toned "bruise" and possibly edema. Contusions resolve spontaneously and require no active management, though the application of ice for 24 hours following injury can reduce the amount of edema and bruising.

## Strains

**Strains** represent "stretch" injuries of muscles, tendons, or ligaments. This type of injury is fairly common among athletes. The injury causes temporary weakness and numbness. Bleeding may occur if vessels are also stretched. The numbness usually resolves within a few hours, and the weakness usually resolves within 2 to 3 days. Management is conservative and involves the application of ice for 24 hours to reduce swelling and bleeding, elevation to reduce swelling (if the injury involves an extremity), use of an elastic wrap or sling, and aspirin or acetaminophen as needed. The client can resume weight bearing and exercise when symptoms have resolved.

## Sprains

**Sprains** involve trauma to the ligaments, tendons, or bones around a joint. Sprains are caused by twisting or pulling forces and most commonly occur during sports activities. First- and second-degree sprains involve damage to the fibers within the tendons and ligaments, and variable amounts of bleeding, swelling, and pain. These clients usually require routine administration of non-steroidal anti-inflammatory drugs, in addition to ice for 24 to 72 hours, use of an elastic wrap or sling, and restricted activity to include crutch use until symptoms have resolved. A third-degree sprain represents a much more serious injury, characterized by separation of the tendons and ligaments from their bony attachments (possibly with bone attached). These injuries produce severe bleeding, swelling, pain, and loss of function, and require careful management to minimize complications. Initial management involves the standard interventions for trauma to the musculoskeletal system: rest (e.g., restricted activity and crutch to prevent weight bearing) during ambulation, ice for 24 to 72 hours, compression with an elastic wrap, soft cast or sling, and elevation. Clients may require narcotic analgesics for severe pain and may have restricted mobility for up to 3 weeks. Surgery may be

---

## CLIENT EDUCATION

### Management of Strains and Sprains

#### Strains

✓ A strain is a stretch injury involving the muscles, tendons, or ligaments. The stretched fibers cause temporary weakness, numbness, and soreness, but these symptoms will resolve within 72 hours and full return of function is expected.

✓ To speed recovery and prevent additional damage:

- Use ice during the first 24 hours to reduce the swelling and minimize bleeding and bruising (cover ice pack with dry cloth and limit application to 20 minutes at a time).
- Use an elastic wrap (such as an Ace Bandage) if the strain involves the arm or leg.
- If the strain involves an arm or leg, elevate that extremity to heart level to reduce swelling.
- Limit use of the involved muscles and tendons until the soreness and weakness resolve (2 to 3 days).
- Take aspirin or acetaminophen as directed by the physician or nurse.

#### Sprains

✓ A sprain involves tearing of muscle fibers, tendons, or ligaments around a joint, resulting in weakness, numbness, bruising, swelling, and pain. A sprain can be minor or severe. Most sprains heal completely with simple measures. Severe sprains may require surgery to maintain full function of the involved area.

- To maximize healing and prevent additional injury, follow these guidelines:
- Use ice until the swelling has begun to resolve (at least 24 hours), cover the ice pack with a dry cloth, and limit application to 20 minutes at a time.
- Use an elastic wrap (such as an Ace Bandage) or support device prescribed by the health care provider to reduce swelling and pain.
- Elevate the involved extremity to heart level to reduce swelling.
- Avoid weight bearing and use of involved joint until the pain and swelling have resolved (usually 1 to 3 weeks).
- Take pain medicines as prescribed.

required for reattachment of the torn tendons and ligaments or, in the case of severe damage, for removal of torn tendons or ligaments. While most clients recover full mobility, there is the potential for individuals with severe sprains to develop post-traumatic arthritis in the future (Weber & Maleski, 2002).

# Administer Heat and Cold Therapy

Cells in the hypothalamus act as a thermostat to regulate body temperature. When the hypothalamic thermostat detects that the body temperature is either too high or too low, it responds systemically by instituting appropriate temperature-decreasing (vasodilation, sweating) or temperature-increasing (vasoconstriction, shivering) mechanisms to restore body temperature to the normal level.

Local responses to heat and cold occur through stimulation of temperature-sensitive receptors in the skin. Impulses travel from the periphery to the hypothalamus and the cerebral cortex. The hypothalamus then initiates heat-producing or heat-reducing reactions of the body. The conscious sensations of temperature are aroused in the cerebral cortex.

Heat and cold receptors adapt to changes in temperature. On initial exposure, receptors are strongly stimulated by extremes in temperature, but within a short time this response declines as the receptors adapt to the new temperature variations. This adaptive ability of the body to temperature variations can be dangerous to clients insensitive to heat and cold extremes and may predispose them to serious injury. Nurses and clients need to understand this adaptive response when applying heat and cold.

Heat is one of the oldest nursing measures used to reduce pain and promote healing. Heat causes **vasodilation** and increases blood flow to the affected area, producing skin redness and warmth. Heat produces maximum vasodilation in 20 to 30 minutes; after this period, reflex vasoconstriction occurs along with tissue congestion. Periodic removal and reapplication of heat will restore vasodilation. Prolonged exposure to heat damages epithelial cells and results in redness, tenderness, and even blister formation.

The application of cold lowers the temperature of the skin and underlying tissues and causes **vasoconstriction**. Vasoconstriction reduces blood flow to the affected area and produces skin pallor or a bluish discoloration and coolness. Maximum vasoconstriction is achieved at 15°C (60°F); at temperatures below 15°C, the vessels begin to dilate. Prolonged exposure to cold results in a reflex vasodilation. Initially the skin is reddened, but later it takes on a bluish purple mottled appearance with numbness and pain because of impaired circulation and tissue ischemia. Vasodilation and vasoconstriction of the blood vessels in the skin result primarily from increased sensitivity of the vessels to nerve stimulation, but also from a protective reflex response that passes to the spinal cord and then back to the vessels. The therapeutic effects of heat and cold applications are outlined in Table 36-2.

| TABLE 36-2    THERAPEUTIC EFFECTS OF HEAT AND COLD APPLICATIONS | |
|---|---|
| **Physiological Responses** | **Therapeutic Benefits** |
| **Heat Therapy** | |
| Promotes vasodilation. | Improves blood flow. |
| Decreases blood viscosity. | Increases delivery of oxygen and nutrients, leukocytes, antibodies |
| Increases tissue metabolism. | to facilitate the inflammatory process. |
| Increases capillary permeability. | Facilitates removal of wastes and toxins. |
| Reduces muscle tension. | Produces a local warming effect. |
| | Decreases venous congestion in injured tissues. |
| | Increases absorption of fluid by capillaries and promotes removal of excess fluid from interstitial spaces, thereby reducing edema. |
| | Promotes muscle relaxation and decreases pain from spasm or stiffness. |
| **Cold Therapy** | |
| Promotes vasoconstriction. | Decreases blood flow to site of injury, thereby decreasing |
| Increases blood viscosity. | inflammation and edema formation. |
| Decreases tissue metabolism. | Decreases blood flow, facilitating clotting and control of bleeding. |
| Has a local anesthetic effect. | Reduces the tissues' oxygen consumption. |
| Decreases muscle tension. | Raises the threshold of pain receptors, thereby decreasing pain. |

The body's response to the application of heat and cold is influenced by a number of factors. See Box 36-4 for a discussion of the factors that affect tolerance to heat and cold.

The following conditions necessitate precautions in the use of heat and cold applications:

- Neurosensory impairment: Clients with reduced perception of sensory or painful stimuli (e.g., spinal cord injuries) are at an increased risk for tissue injury.
- Impaired mental status: Clients who are confused or unconscious need to be monitored and assessed frequently to ensure safety.
- Impaired circulation: Clients with cardiovascular and peripheral vascular problems or diabetes may not have the ability to dissipate heat through dilation of blood vessels and are at an increased risk for tissue injury.
- Skin and tissue integrity (open wounds, broken skin, scar formation, edema): Subcutaneous tissues are more

---

### BOX 36-4    FACTORS AFFECTING HEAT AND COLD TOLERANCE

- **Body part:** Certain areas of the skin have a sensitivity to temperature variations. The inner aspect of the wrist and forearm, the neck, and the perineal area are temperature-sensitive, while the back of the hand and the foot are not as sensitive.

- **Duration of application:** Therapeutic benefits of heat and cold applications are achieved with short periods of exposure to temperature variations. Tolerance increases as the length of exposure increases.

- **Area of body exposed:** The larger the area exposed to heat and cold, the lower the tolerance to temperature changes.

- **Damage to body surface area:** Injured skin areas are more sensitive than intact areas to temperature variations.

- **Individual tolerance:** Tolerance to temperature variations is affected by age and physical condition. The young and the aged are especially susceptible to heat and cold. Neurosensory impairments may interfere with the reception and perception of stimuli, increasing the risk of injury.

- **Age:** Thinner skin layers in children and older people increase the risk for burns from the heat and cold applications. Older adults have a decreased sensitivity to pain.

---

### NURSING STRATEGY

#### Heat and Cold Applications

General guidelines to follow when using heat and cold applications include:

1. Obtain a physician's order that details the site to be treated, the type of therapy, and the frequency and duration of application.

2. Select temperature on the basis of client status and agency policy.

3. Thoroughly explain procedure and expected benefits to client.

4. Assess client's status before, during, and after treatment is performed to prevent injury.

5. Document effects of therapy.

---

sensitive to temperature variations than are superficial tissues (e.g., cold can decrease blood flow to an open wound, thereby inhibiting healing).

Heat and cold can be applied in dry and moist forms (Figure 36-27). The type of wound or injury, location, and presence of drainage or inflammation are considered when selecting moist or dry applications.

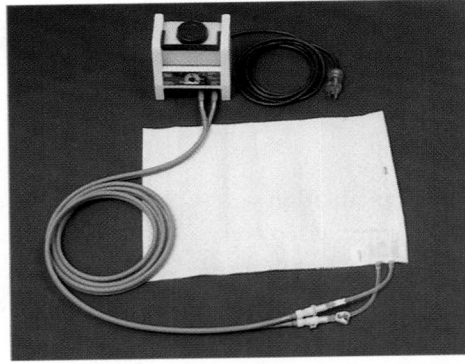

A.

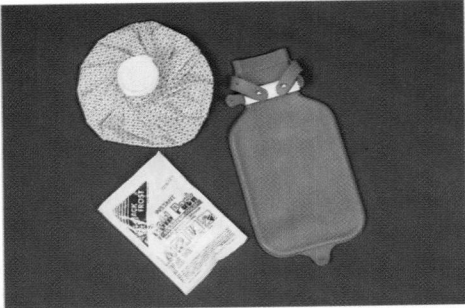

B.

**Figure 36-27    Types of heat and cold applications: A. Aquathermal heating unit B. Cold packs**

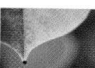

# CASE STUDY/NURSING CARE PLAN

Ms. Johnson is a 78-year-old female who is admitted to a long-term care facility for wound care and rehabilitation following a stroke. She has hypertension now controlled by medications, type 2 diabetes mellitus, and a resolving urinary tract infection. She had an indwelling catheter that has now been removed; she has occasional episodes of urinary incontinence but no bowel incontinence. She lost 15 pounds over 3 weeks in the hospital and now weighs 140. She is able to assist with turning but cannot turn independently and is bedbound or chair-bound. She has a deep ulcer over the sacral area. The ulcer is stage 4, 5 cm $\times$ 4 cm $\times$ 2 cm, has tunneling at 9 o'clock and 3 o'clock, and extends 2 cm from wound edge. Ms. Johnson's vital signs are temperature = 98.8° F, pulse = 88, respirations = 22, and BP = 136/78. The lab tests are albumin = 20, a random serum glucose = 195, and a WBC count = 6,200.

## Assessment

A 78-year-old female living in long-term care who has recently lost weight, is incontinent of urine, and is bedbound or chair-bound. The client has a decubital sacral ulcer with a wound base that is 80% clean (no granulation tissue). In addition, 20% of the ulcer is covered with thin layer of yellow slough. The wound has a moderate amount of serous drainage, the wound edges are open, and the surrounding skin is intact with no redness. The client is afebrile and has vital signs within normal limits. In addition, the serum lab tests drawn reveal hyperglycemia.

## Nursing Diagnosis #1

*Impaired Skin Integrity* related to pressure/shear injury.
**NOC:** Tissue Integrity: Skin and Mucous Membrane; Wound Healing
**NIC:** Pressure Ulcer Care; Skin Care; Skin Surveillance Wound Care

## Expected Outcomes

The client will:
1. Be free of necrotic tissue as evidenced by a wound bed that has no slough and is 100% clean and red.
2. Be free of infection as evidenced by progress in wound healing and the absence of erythema, tenderness, and induration in the surrounding tissues.
3. Exhibit signs of healing as evidenced by the presence of granulation tissue and remain free of any additional skin breakdown.

## Planning/Interventions/Rationales

1. Change dressing daily as follows: irrigate wound with normal saline, lightly pack wound and tunnels with alginate dressing, and cover with foam dressing that is adhesive and waterproof. *Irrigation removes debris from wound surface; alginate dressing absorbs exudate and maintains moist wound environment, which facilitates autolytic debridement; waterproof foam cover dressing prevents contamination.*
2. Complete comprehensive documentation of wound status on weekly basis, to include dimensions, status of wound bed, status of wound edges, and status of surrounding tissue. *Ongoing assessment is critical to determination of progress in wound repair; progress in repair is reflected by reduction in necrotic tissue, absence of infection, increase in granulation tissue, and reduction in exudate volume.*
3. Maintain clean technique when providing wound care. *Prevents bacterial invasion of wound.*
4. Place client on air support surface; turn side to side q 2 hrs; limit time in chair to 1 hour at meals, and assure appropriate positioning while in chair; place pressure-reducing cushion in chair; use lift sheet to reposition. *Provides even pressure distribution to reduce the interference to blood flow; keeps client off back to prevent any compromise to blood flow; minimizes the risk of additional injury/impaired healing.*

## Evaluation

Within 1 week, the wound was free of slough and the wound bed was not infected. Within 2 weeks, the wound was actively granulating and the client's general condition and mobility were improving.

*(continues)*

# CASE STUDY/NURSING CARE PLAN (continued)

### Nursing Diagnosis #2
*Imbalanced Nutrition: Less Than Body Requirements* related to rehabilitation from stroke process.
**NOC:** Nutritional Status; Nutritional Status: Food and Fluid Intake; Nutritional Status: Nutrient Intake
**NIC:** Nutrition Management; Nutrition Therapy; Nutritional Monitoring; Nutritional Counseling

### Expected Outcomes
The client will:
1. Ingest daily nutritional requirements in accordance with activity level and metabolic needs within 72 hours.
2. Acknowledge the importance of good nutrition within 1 week.
3. Gain weight at a rate of 2 to 4 pounds per week until within normal weight range for body build and muscle mass.

### Planning/Interventions/Rationale
1. Obtain dietary consult to evaluate client's current nutrient intake and to ensure adequate calorie and protein intake. *Adequate nutrient intake is critical for the formation of granulation tissue.*
2. Explain the need for adequate consumption of carbohydrates, fats, proteins, vitamins, minerals, and fluids. *Educates the client in nutritional needs, and increases compliance with the nutrition regimen.*
3. Take steps to promote appetite (e.g., encourage client's family to bring foods from home, provide a relaxed atmosphere), and determine food preferences. *Increases nutritional intake to meet body requirements.*

### Evaluation
Client gained 3 pounds and had a balanced nutritional intake within 1 week. In addition, the client verbalized an understanding of why she should eat a balanced diet within 1 week.

## Key Concepts

- The skin and soft tissues play a critical role in protection against pathogenic invasion, as well as sensory awareness and temperature regulation. Maintenance of healthy skin is a critical nursing function.
- Healthy skin is dry, supple, and acidic; routine hygienic care should focus on maintaining these properties through use of pH-balanced cleansing agents and appropriate use of emollients and humectants.
- Pressure ulcers occur as a result of prolonged pressure, shear force, and compromised tissue tolerance. Individuals at greatest risk are those with reduced mobility and/or reduced sensory awareness.
- Pressure ulcer prevention is a key nursing responsibility; the two critical elements include prompt identification of individuals at risk and prompt implementation of prevention protocols (e.g., appropriate use of support surfaces; measures to reduce shear, friction, and maceration; attention to nutritional status).
- Wounds involving only partial loss of the skin layers normally heal quickly by regeneration. Wounds involving total loss of the skin layers heal by a complex sequence of events resulting in scar formation.
- Wound healing is primarily a systemic phenomenon, and wound repair requires continual focus on perfusion and oxygenation, maintenance of nutritional status, and control of comorbidities such as diabetes mellitus.
- Topical wound care should focus on measures such as wound cleansing, appropriate dressing selection, elimination of necrotic tissue, and the monitoring of wound drainage.
- Most dressings provide passive support for wound healing (e.g., absorption of exudate, maintenance of a moist wound surface, and insulation).
- Comprehensive wound management must always include attention to the unique issues in the management of skin tears, surgical incisions, leg ulcers, burns, lacerations, and abrasions.
- Contusions, strains, and sprains are commonly encountered injuries of the skin and connective tissue that require specific management methods.
- Heat and cold therapies require nursing care that assesses both the vasoconstriction and vasodilation of an individual.

## Review Questions and Activities

1. Explain why older adults are at increased risk for skin breakdown.

2. Explain the statement that "Most true pressure ulcers are stage 4 wounds."

3. What strategies should a nurse use to ensure that a comatose client will not develop a pressure ulcer?

4. Explain the differences between partial-thickness and full-thickness wound repair and the implications for nursing management.

5. Why do dehisced surgical incisions usually heal much more rapidly than pressure ulcers, even when the pressure ulcer is a smaller wound?

6. Describe measures the nurse and client can take to promote wound healing and to prevent complications that could hinder the repair process.

7. Identify one aspect of care that is a unique consideration for each of the following wounds:
   a. Lacerations and abrasions
   b. Skin tears
   c. Leg ulcers
   d. Burns
   e. Contusions, strains, or sprains
   f. Heat and cold injuries

## Multimedia Links

Altman *Intermediate Care DVD: Obtaining a Wound Drainage Specimen for Culturing*
Altman *Intermediate Care DVD: Irrigating a Wound*
Altman *Intermediate Care DVD: Applying a Dry Dressing*
Altman *Intermediate Care DVD: Applying a Wet to Damp Dressing*
Altman *Basic Care DVD: Preventing and Managing the Pressure Ulcer*
Altman *Basic Care IV Video: Aiding Client Movement*
Altman *Intermediate Care DVD: Maintaining a Closed Wound Drainage System*
Altman *Intermediate Care Video: Wound Care*
Altman *Intermediate Care DVD: Care of the Jackson-Pratt (JP) Drain Site and Emptying the Drain Bulb*
Altman *Basic Care DVD: Applying Dry Heat*
Altman *Basic Care DVD: Applying Cold Treatment*

## Web Resources

Agency for Healthcare Research and Quality
   http://www.ahrq.gov
Mayo Clinic Cancer Center
   http://www.mayohealth.org
National Pressure Ulcer Advisory Panel
   http://www.npuap.org
Wound Care Communication Network
   http://www.woundcarenet.com
Wound Care Institute
   http://www.woundcare.org

Wound Healing Society
   http://www.woundheal.org
Wound, Ostomy and Continence Nurses Society
   http://www.wocn.org

## References

Allman, R., Goode, P., Burst, N., Bartolucci, A., & Thomas, D. (1999). Pressure ulcers, hospital complications, and disease severity: Impact on hospital costs and length of stay. *Advances in Wound Care, 12*(1), 22–30.

Altman, G. (2004). *Delmar's fundamental & advanced nursing skills* (2nd ed.). Clifton Park, NY: Delmar Learning.

Alvarez, O., Fernandez-Obregon, A., Rogers, R., & Bergano, L. (2000). Chemical debridement of pressure ulcers: A prospective, randomized, comparative trial of collagenase and papain/urea formulations. *Wounds, 12*(2), 15–25.

Baharestani, M. (1999). Pressure ulcers in an age of managed care: A nursing perspective. *Ostomy/Wound Management, 45*(5), 18–40.

Baranoski, S. (2000). Skin tears: The enemy of frail skin. *Advances in Skin and Wound Care, 13*(3), 123–126.

Bergstrom, N., Braden, B., Kemp, M., Champagne, M., & Ruby, E. (1998). Predicting pressure ulcer risk—A multisite study of the predictive validity of the Braden scale. *Nursing Research, 47*(5), 261–269.

Blauvelt, A., Hwang, S. T., & Udey, M. C. (2003). Allergic and immunologic diseases of the skin. *Journal of Allergy & Clinical Immunology, 111*(Suppl. 2), 560–570.

Boulton, A., Meneses, P., and Ennis, W. (1999). Diabetic foot ulcers: A framework for prevention and care. *Wound Repair and Regeneration, 7*(1), 7–16.

Bowler, P. (1998). The anaerobic and aerobic microbiology of wounds: A review. *Wounds, 10*(6), 170–178.

Broussard, C., Mendez-Eastman, S., and Frantz, R. (2000). Adjuvant wound therapies. In R. Bryant (Ed.), *Acute and chronic wounds: Nursing management* (2nd ed., pp. 431–454). St. Louis: Mosby.

Calliano, C. (2000). Assessing and preventing pressure ulcers. *Advances in Skin and Wound Care, 13*(5), 244–246.

Catanzariti, A., Haverstock, B., Grossman, J., & Mendicino, R. (1999). Off-loading techniques in the treatment of diabetic plantar neuropathic foot ulcerations. *Advances in Wound Care, 12*(9), 452–458.

Colburn, L. (2001). Prevention of chronic wounds. In D. Krasner, G. Rodeheaver, & R. G. Sibbald (Eds.), *Chronic wound care* (3rd ed., pp. 67–78). Wayne, PA: HMP Communications.

Colgan, R., Michocki, R., Greisman, L., & Moore, T. A. (2003). Antiviral drugs in the immunocompetent host: Part I. Treatment of hepatitis, cytomegalovirus, and herpes infections. *American Family Physician, 67*(4), 757–762, 675.

Daniels, R. (2003). *Delmar's manual of laboratory and diagnostic tests.* Clifton Park, NY: Delmar Learning.

Dickerson, P., Purdue, G., & Hunt, J. (1999). Traumatic wound care. *Dermatology Nursing, 11*(1), 53–80.

Dolynchuk, K., Keast, D., Campbell, K., Houghton, P., Orsted, H. Sibbald, G., & Atkinson, A. (2000). Best practices for the prevention and treatment of pressure ulcers. *Ostomy/Wound Management, 46*(11), 38–51.

Doughty, D., Waldrop, J., & Ramundo, J. (2000). Lower extremity ulcers of vascular etiology. In R. Bryant (Ed.), *Acute and chronic wounds: Nursing management* (2nd ed., pp. 265–300). St. Louis: Mosby.

Eaglestein, W., & Falanga, V. (1998). Tissue engineering and the development of Apligraf, a human skin equivalent. *Advances in Wound Care, 11*(Suppl. 4), 1–8.

Ehrlich, P. (1998). The physiology of wound healing—a summary of normal and abnormal wound healing processes. *Advances in Wound Care, 11*(7), 326–328.

Estes, M. (2002). *Health assessment & physical examination* (2nd ed.). Clifton Park, NY: Delmar Learning.

Fishman, J. A. (2002). Summary: future directions in antifungal therapy. *Transplant Infectious Disease, 4*(Suppl. 3), 67–68.

Garcia-Gonzalez, E., & Rivera-Rueda, M. (1998). Neonatal dermatology: Skin care guidelines. *Dermatology Nursing, 10*(4), 274–281.

Goebel, R., & Goebel, M. (1999), Clinical practice guidelines for pressure ulcer prevention can prevent malpractice lawsuits in older patients. *Journal of Wound Ostomy Continence Nursing, 26*(4), 175–184.

Goldstein, D., Vogel, K., Mureebe, L., & Kerstein, M. (1998). Differential diagnosis of the lower extremity ulcer—is it arterial, venous, neuropathic? *Wounds, 10*(4), 125–131.

Haalboom, J., den Boer, J., & Buskens, E. (1999). Risk assessment tools in the prevention of pressure ulcers. *Ostomy/Wound Management, 45*(2), 20–34.

Helvig, B. (2000). The role of the WOC nurse in burn management. *Journal of Wound Ostomy Continence Nursing, 12*(4), 14–16.

Inlow, S., Orsted, H., and Sibbald, R. (2000). Best practices for the prevention, diagnosis, and treatment of diabetic foot ulcers. *Ostomy/Wound Management, 46*(11), 55–68.

Jamora, M. J., Wainwright, B. D., Meehan, S. A., & Bystryn, J. C. (2003). Improved identification of potentially dangerous pigmented skin lesions by computerized image analysis. *Archives of Dermatology, 139*(2), 195–198.

Krasner, D. (1998). Painful venous ulcers: Themes and stories about living with the pain and suffering. *Journal of Wound Ostomy Continence Nursing, 25*(3), 158–168.

Kunimoto, B., Cooling, M., Gulliver, W., Houghton, P., Orsted, H., & Sibbald, R. (2001). Best practices for the prevention and management of venous leg ulcers. *Ostomy/Wound Management, 47*(2), 34–50.

Mayo Clinic Cancer Center. (2003). Retrieved from http://*www.mayohealth.org*

McGough-Csarny, J., & Kopac, C. (1998). Skin tears in institutionalized elderly: An epidemiologic study. *Ostomy/Wound Management, 44*(Suppl. 3A): 14S–25S.

Nishijima, S., Kurokawa, I., & Nakaya H. (2002). Susceptibility change to antibiotics of *Staphylococcus aureus* strains isolated from skin infections between July 1994 and November 2000. *Journal of Infection & Chemotherapy, 8*(2), 187–189.

Ovington, L., & Peirce, B. (2001). Wound dressings: form, function, feasibility, and facts. In D. Krasner, G. Rodeheaver, & R. G. Sibbald (Eds.), *Chronic wound care* (3rd ed., pp. 311–320). Wayne, PA: HMP Communications.

Robeson, M. (1999). Lessons gleaned from the sport of wound-watching. *Wound Repair and Regeneration, 7*(1), 2–6.

Rodeheaver, G. (2001). Wound cleansing, wound irrigation, wound disinfection. In D. Krasner, G. Rodeheaver, & R. G. Sibbald (Eds.), *Chronic wound care* (3rd ed., pp. 369–384). Wayne, PA: HMP Communications.

Roth, R., & Townsend, C. (2002). *Nutrition & diet therapy* (8th ed.). Clifton Park, NY: Delmar Learning.

Soloway, D. (1998). Civil claims relating to pressure ulcers: A claimant's lawyer's perspective. *Ostomy/Wound Management, 44*(92), 20–26.

Stotts, N. (1999). Risk of pressure ulcer development in surgical patients: A review of the literature. *Advances in Wound Care, 12*(3), 127–136.

Weber, J. M., & Maleski, R. M. (2002). Conservative treatment of acute lateral ankle sprains. *Clinics in Podiatric Medicine & Surgery, 19*(2), 309–318.

White, L., & Duncan, G. (2002). *Medical-surgical nursing: An integrated approach* (2nd ed.). Clifton Park, NY: Delmar Learning.

Wywialowski, E. (1999). Tissue perfusion as a key underlying concept of pressure ulcer development and treatment. *Journal of Vascular Nursing, 17*(1), 12–16.

# UNIT IX

# Elimination

Chapter 37  Urinary and Bowel Elimination

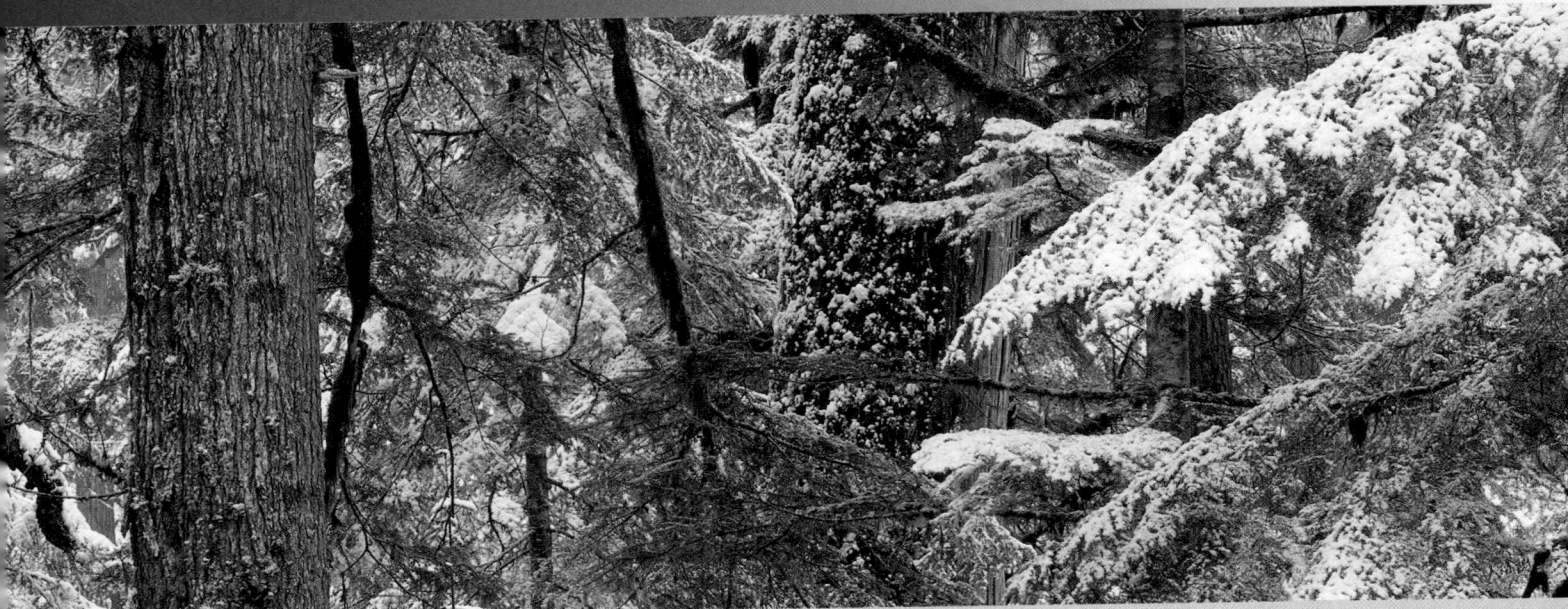

# Urinary and Bowel Elimination

Katherine Moore, RN, PhD

*"The person also knows what will make him or her well, optimize his or her effectiveness or fulfillment (given circumstances), or promote his or her growth."*

*(Erickson, Tomlin, and Swain, 1983)*

# Chapter Competencies

## Upon completion of this chapter, the reader should be able to:

1. Describe the normal urinary elimination process.
2. Assess the critical elements of urinary structures.
3. Explain various factors that affect elimination.
4. Evaluate common nursing diagnoses associated with alterations in urinary and bowel alterations.
5. Discuss normal bowel elimination.
6. Assess the critical elements of bowel function.
7. Describe the expected outcomes of nursing interventions that promote normal elimination.
8. Discuss nursing interventions for selected alterations in bowel function.
9. Synthesize the evaluative process for alterations in elimination.

# Key Terms

bacteriuria

bladder training

constipation

defecation

detrusor muscle

diarrhea

dysuria

extraurethral incontinence

fecal incontinence

functional incontinence

hematuria

hemorrhoids

impaction

nocturia

peristalsis

pyuria

specific gravity

stoma

stool

stress urinary incontinence

urge urinary incontinence

urinalysis

urinary incontinence

urinary retention

urodynamics

void

Elimination patterns are essential to maintain health. The urinary and gastrointestinal systems together provide for the elimination of body wastes. The urinary system filters and excretes urine from the body, thereby maintaining fluid, electrolyte, and acid-base balance. Normal bowel function provides for the regular elimination of solid wastes.

During periods of stress and illness, clients experience alterations in elimination patterns. Nurses assess for changes, identify problems, and intervene to assist clients with maintaining proper elimination patterns. The nurse's role encompasses teaching clients self-care activities to promote independence and health.

## Physiology of Elimination

The urinary system is composed of the kidneys, ureters, bladder, and urethra. The kidneys form the urine, the ureters carry urine to the bladder, the bladder acts as a reservoir for the urine, and the urethra is the passageway for the urine to exit the body.

The gastrointestinal tract is composed of the stomach, small intestine, large intestine, and rectum. The small intestine absorbs nutrients, the large intestine absorbs fluids and the remaining nutrients, and the distal portion of the large intestine collects and stores the remaining solid waste until elimination occurs.

## Urinary Elimination

The physiological mechanisms that govern urinary elimination are complex and not yet completely understood. Continence in the adult requires anatomical integrity of the urinary system, nervous control of the detrusor muscle, and a competent sphincter mechanism. **Urinary incontinence** occurs when abnormalities of one or more of these factors causes an uncontrolled loss of urine that produces social, physiological, or hygienic difficulties for the client.

## Structures of the Urinary Tract

The urinary system is typically divided into upper and lower tracts. The upper urinary tract includes the kidneys, renal pelvis, and ureters; the lower urinary tract includes the urinary bladder, urethra, and pelvic muscles (Figure 37-1).

## Upper Urinary Tract

The kidneys are a pair of reddish brown, bean-shaped organs located in the retroperitoneal space, adjacent to vertebral bones T-12 to L-2. The right kidney lies slightly lower than the left because of the presence of the liver. The periphery of the kidney contains approximately 1 million nephrons; collectively this aspect of the organ is called the parenchyma. The hilus of the kidney (its convex surface) contains the renal pelvis and the ureters, which connect the kidneys and the bladder. The primary function of the kidney is to maintain internal homeostasis through filtration of the blood and production of urine. In addition, the kidney is an endocrine organ (producing erythropoietin, a hormone that aids in the production of red blood cells), and it plays a role in vitamin D synthesis.

After production within the nephron, urine passes through the calyceal system of the kidneys into the renal pelvis. The renal pelvis is shaped like a funnel, holds approximately 15 ml of urine, and serves as a temporary storage area for urine before transport to the lower urinary tract. The ureter is a long tube, shaped like an inverted S, that begins at the renal pelvis, passes under the psoas muscle of the back, and enters the pelvis near the sacroiliac junction. When entering the pelvis, the ureters curve medially to end in the base of the bladder. The union between bladder and ureter is called the ureterovesical junction.

Both the renal pelvis and ureters consist primarily of smooth muscle, and they move urine from the upper to the lower urinary tract by muscular contraction. This process is called **peristalsis**, and it is similar to the peristaltic waves of the gastrointestinal system used to digest food and produce fecal waste. The process of peristalsis occurs during the prolonged phases of bladder filling and storage, but it is temporarily interrupted during micturition.

## Lower Urinary Tract

The bladder is a hollow, muscular organ located in the pelvis. It has a fixed base and a distensile upper portion composed of multiple bundles of smooth muscle. Collectively, the smooth muscle bundles are called the detrusor muscle.

The urethra is a tube that is a conduit for urinary elimination. The urethra differs significantly in women and men. In women, the urethra exits the bladder base and travels at a 16-degree angle to the external meatus located at the vestibule. The female urethra is approximately 3.5–5.5 cm long, and the distal third is histologically fused with the vaginal wall (Figure 37-1). The entire length of the urethra forms a sphincter mechanism with elements of compression and elements of tension.

In men, the urethra is approximately 23 cm long. It begins at the bladder base, pierces the anterior portion of the prostate, and turns to exit the body through the penis. The proximal third of the male urethra forms a sphincter mechanism comparable to the female urethra. The distal two-thirds is a conduit for the expulsion of urine or semen.

The pelvic muscles connect the anterior and posterior aspects of the bony pelvis, support the organs of the true pelvis, and contribute to the urethral sphincter mechanism in both women and men. The pelvic muscles contain primarily slow-twitch fibers that are physiologically suited for prolonged periods of time. In addition, fast-twitch fibers within the pelvic muscles respond rapidly to sudden increases in

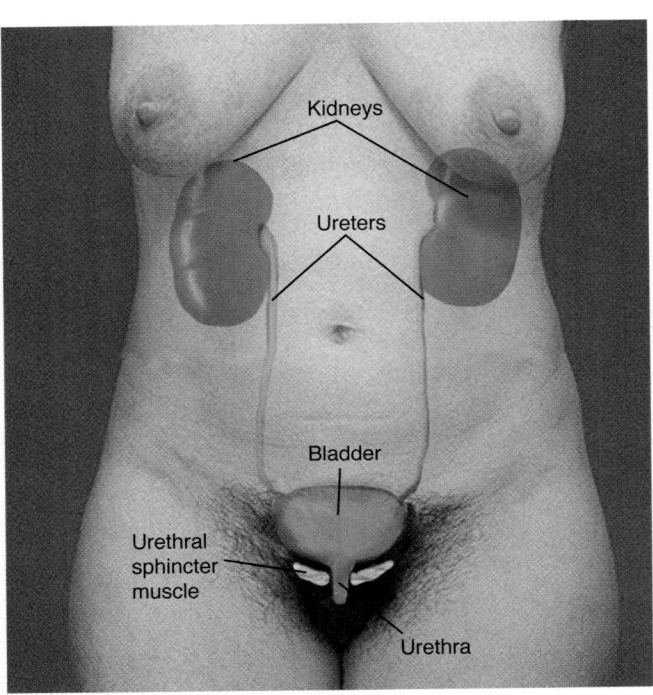

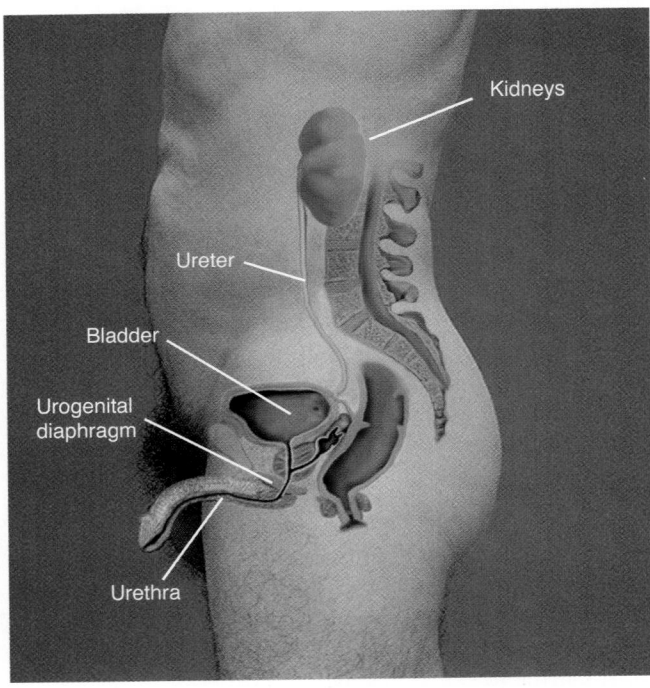

**Figure 37-1    Urinary tract: A. Female B. Male**

abdominal pressure such as sneezing or coughing, although they soon fatigue. Fibers from the pelvic muscles surround the membranous urethra of the male and the proximal two-thirds of the female urethra. In both sexes, the urethra pierces the muscular diaphragm of the pelvic muscles.

## Nervous Control of the Detrusor Muscle

The **detrusor muscle**, the smooth muscle of the bladder, is under indirect voluntary control, allowing the continent adult to postpone urination until "socially appropriate." Specific areas of the brain, spinal cord, and peripheral nervous system modulate the reflex activity of the detrusor muscle.

Central nervous control of the bladder begins in several centers in the brain. The primary areas in the brain that modulate the detrusor muscle are located in the frontal lobes, the thalamus, hypothalamus, basal ganglia, and cerebellum. The limbic system, which controls many aspects of autonomic nervous function, also influences continence. A neurologic lesion affecting one or more of these areas causes hyperactive detrusor contractions and a loss of bladder control.

A micturition center, located near the base of the brain, has two groups of neurons that mark the origin of the urination (micturition). In the infant, urinary elimination is controlled entirely by the micturition center, which evacuates the bladder when a specific "threshold" volume is reached or when the bladder is stimulated in another way. In the adult, voiding is controlled by the multiple centers of the brain, and urination usually occurs when the individual wishes to empty the bladder.

Reticulospinal tracts in the spinal cord transmit messages from the brain and brain stem to the peripheral nerves of the bladder. Bladder filling and urinary storage are promoted by excitation of the sympathetic nervous system via efferent, sympathetic spinal nuclei at spinal segments T-10 to L-2. Excitation of these neurons relaxes the detrusor muscle and contracts the muscular elements of the sphincter mechanism. Voiding is accomplished through the parasympathetic nervous system. Excitation of neurons located at segments S-2 to S-4 causes **voiding** (urination) by contraction of the detrusor muscle and relaxation of muscular elements of the sphincter mechanism.

Two peripheral nerves transmit messages from the central nervous system to the detrusor muscle. The pelvic plexus transmits parasympathetic impulses to the smooth muscle of the detrusor. Nervous excitation of the parasympathetic nerves causes release of a neurotransmitter, acetylcholine, which produces contraction of detrusor muscle cells. Other substances also affect contraction of the detrusor muscle, but all act under the influence of the central nervous system.

The inferior hypogastric nerves provide the majority of sympathetic tone to the bladder wall and sphincter mechanism. In the detrusor muscle, excitation of β-adrenergic receptors causes release of norepinephrine, which inhibits detrusor muscle contraction. In addition, stimulation of α-adrenergic (excitatory) receptors at the bladder neck, proximal urethra, and in the prostatic urethra in men causes contraction of muscular components of the sphincter mechanism, promoting urethral closure and continence.

## Urethral Sphincter Mechanism

The urethral sphincter is traditionally divided into two muscles, an internal (smooth muscle) and external (striated) sphincter. Unfortunately, this schema leads to more confusion than it addresses, and it should be discarded for a conceptualization of the sphincter as a single mechanism, comprising elements of compression and elements of tone, with essential supportive structures.

Urethral compression relies on three components: urethral mucosa softness, mucus secretions, and a vascular cushion. During bladder filling and urinary storage, the epithelium must fill in the gaps of the collapsed (closed) urethral lumen, creating a watertight seal through which no urine can escape. Coaptation requires a pliable, soft, and nonscarred urethra, with adequate mucus secretions to reduce surface tension and to fill in the microscopic gaps left by the epithelium. These elements of compression are supplemented by a rich network of vascular connections in the submucosal space. This vascular network promotes urethral closure by nourishing the epithelium and mucous production cells and by serving as a cushion for the transmission of force exerted by the muscular elements of the sphincter mechanism. In women, all the elements of compression are directly influenced by the presence of estrogens.

Urethral tension protects the individual from urinary leakage during physical exercise or exertion. Smooth muscle bundles at the bladder neck and proximal urethra (and prostatic urethra of the male) close the urethra during bladder filling and urinary storage. The urethral wall also contains a set of highly specialized, triple-innervated striated muscle fibers that form a rhabdosphincter. It is crucial for maintaining continence during normal exertion. Striated muscle fibers from the pelvic muscle surround the urethra and contribute to the sphincter. These muscles are particularly needed when abdominal pressure changes from sneezing, coughing, or lifting a heavy object.

The muscular elements of the urethra rely on supportive structures to provide an optimal configuration allowing them to contract and relax efficiently. Loss of support interferes with efficient urethral sphincter function.

## Bowel Elimination

The process of normal fecal elimination is not completely understood. Continence primarily relies on the consistency of the **stool** (fecal material), intestinal motility, compliance and contractility of the rectum, and competence of the anal sphincters.

## Structures of the Gastrointestinal Tract

The gastrointestinal system (alimentary canal) begins at the mouth and ends at the anus. The small intestine in the adult is approximately 22 feet long. The small intestine is primarily responsible for the digestion and absorption of nutrients, vitamins, minerals, fluids, and electrolytes. The digestive chyme (mixture of partially digested food and secretions) travels through the small bowel by a combination of segmental contractions and peristaltic waves. Substances that are well tolerated move through the bowel relatively slowly; foods or drugs that are toxic or irritable to the small bowel are evacuated rapidly. The small intestine joins the large bowel (colon) at the ileocecal valve. This valve works in conjunction with the ileocecal sphincter to control emptying of contents from the small intestine into the colon and to prevent regurgitation of digestive chyme from the large to small bowel (Figure 37-2).

The colon is approximately 5 to 6 feet long in adults. It is divided into six segments: the cecum, ascending colon, transverse colon, descending colon, sigmoid colon, and anal canal. The primary functions of the colon are to collect, concentrate, transport, and eliminate waste materials (feces). The anal sphincter consists of smooth and striated muscles that line the distal portion of the anal canal. It works with the anus to store and to eliminate feces under voluntary control.

## Intestinal Motility and Rectal Accommodation

Fecal continence relies on regular delivery of small boluses of stool that are stored in the rectum before elimination. The transit time from ingestion of food to passage of stool from the bowels varies. Typically, at least 80% of intake that is not absorbed by the body is excreted from the bowel within 5 days following ingestion.

Transit time is significantly affected by the type of foods ingested, subsequent dietary intake, exercise, and stress-related factors.

Rectal filling causes an awareness of the presence of stool, which is stored until an appropriate opportunity for **defecation** (evacuation of stool from the rectum) is identified. In the continent individual, an initial awareness of stool in the rectum is identified at 150 ml. The desire to defecate is typically transient, diminishing as the rectum accommodates larger volumes of stool. When 400 ml or more of stool is collected in the rectum, this urge becomes strong, and the call to defecate becomes more persistent. Failure to heed the call to defecate may lead to overdistension of the rectum with hardening of the stool and subsequent constipation.

## Anal Sphincter Mechanism

The anal sphincter is divided into two mechanisms, called the internal and external sphincters (Figure 37-3). An internal anal sphincter is primarily made up of smooth muscle bundles that are connected to the smooth muscle of the rectum. It begins in the distal portion of the rectum and extends approximately 3 cm into the anal canal. The internal sphincter mechanism is primarily innervated by sympathetic nerves that promote smooth muscle contraction and by parasympathetic nerves that cause sphincter relaxation.

The external sphincter is composed of striated muscle fibers that are divided into deep and superficial components. The deep portion of the external anal sphincter comprises muscle fibers that encircle the proximal aspect of the anal canal and attach to the symphysis pubis, forming a U shape. The superficial portion of the anal sphincter also encircles the anal canal, forming a U shape; however, it

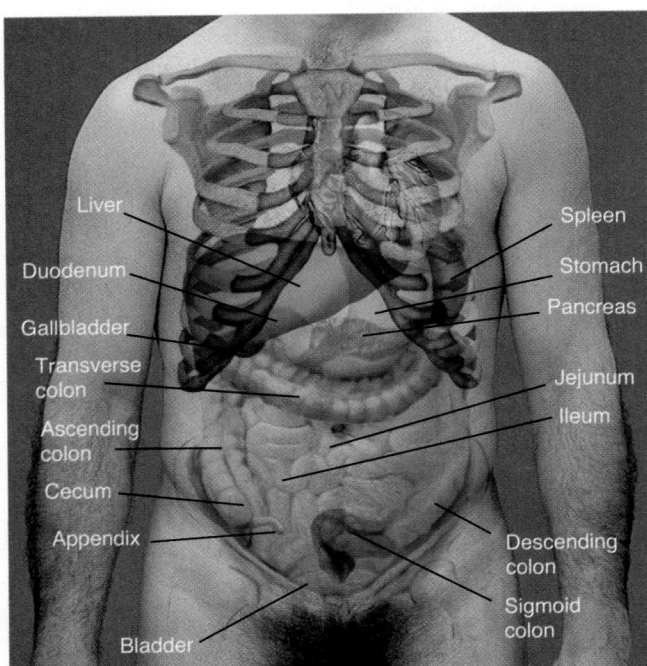

**Figure 37-2    Gastrointestinal tract**

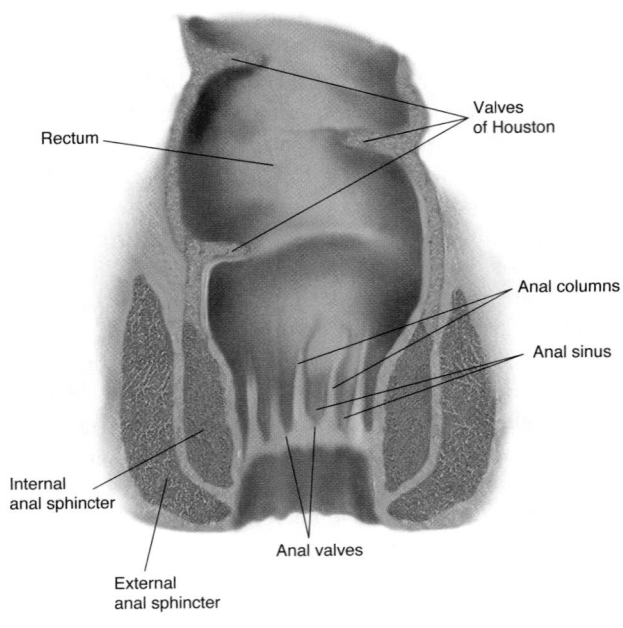

**Figure 37-3    Anal sphincter**

attaches to the coccyx and postanal plate rather than to the anterior aspect of the pelvis. Like the periurethral muscles, the striated component of the external anal sphincter contains both fast- and slow-twitch fibers that allow sustained tone over a period of time before voluntary defecation.

Distension of the rectum causes a reflex inhibition of the internal anal sphincter and contraction of the external sphincter. Sensory receptors located at the proximal anal canal affect anal function. These specialized sensory receptors are able to "sample" fecal contents, allowing the individual to differentiate among solid stool, liquid stool, and gas. If the person postpones defecation, rectal accommodation occurs and the desire to defecate is postponed. If the desire to defecate is heeded, the person voluntarily relaxes the external anal sphincter and evacuates the bowel of feces.

The significance of rectal contractions during defecation remains unclear. Many persons strain to defecate, and abdominal force is readily transmitted to the rectum, creating an effective expulsive force. The continent individual is able to simultaneously increase abdominal pressure by straining and maintain external anal sphincter relaxation, allowing effective evacuation of feces from the bowel.

## Factors Affecting Elimination

### Age

Age or developmental level affects urinary and bowel control. Infants initially lack a pattern to their elimination. Control over bladder and bowel movements can begin as early as 18 months of age but is not usually mastered until age 4. Nighttime control usually takes longer to achieve, and boys typically take longer than girls.

Control of elimination is generally constant throughout the adult years, with the exception of illness and pregnancy, when temporary loss of control, urgency, or retention may develop. With increasing age comes loss of muscle tone and therefore a risk of loss of bladder control. Incontinence is not a normal aspect of aging and should always be treated.

### Diet

Adequate fluid and fiber intake are critical factors to urinary and bowel health. Inadequate fluid intake is a primary cause of constipation.

### Exercise

Exercise enhances muscle tone, which leads to better bladder and sphincter control. Peristalsis is also aided by activity, thus promoting healthy bowel elimination patterns.

### Medications

Medications can have an impact on a client's elimination health and patterns and should be assessed during the

## LIFE SPAN CONSIDERATIONS

### Elimination Habits in Older Clients

Elimination habits can be something that the older person focuses on with great concern. Often, an older person will adhere to very specific dietary considerations in preventing constipation and encouraging regular bowel movements (e.g., prune juice, oat bran). In addition, older people can become very stressed from not being able to participate in their "normal elimination diet." Consequently, the nurse must be astute in the assessment of an older client's elimination habits.

Hogstel, M. (2001). *Gerontology: Nursing care of the older adult.* Clifton Park, NY: Delmar Learning.

health history interview. Diuretics increase urine production. Antidepressants, antihypertensives, and some antihistamines and over-the-counter (OTC) cold medications may lead to urinary retention (Nelson, Furner, & Jesudason, 2001). It is part of the nursing assessment to inquire about all medications being taken in order to provide proper care for a client experiencing alterations in elimination patterns. Table 37-1 provides details on medications used for bladder control.

## Common Alterations in Elimination

### Urinary Elimination

Urinary incontinence and urinary retention are the most common causes of altered urinary elimination patterns. Urinary incontinence is the uncontrolled loss of urine that constitutes a social or hygienic problem. **Urinary retention** is the inability to completely evacuate urine from the bladder during micturition. Incontinence can be acute or chronic. It is important to determine the type of incontinence before subjecting the client to the expense, potential risks, and rigors of a treatment program (Palmer, 2002).

### Acute Urinary Incontinence

Acute urinary incontinence is a transient and reversible loss of urine, occuring during an acute illness or after an injury. Common causes include urinary tract infection, atrophic vaginitis, polyuria related to diabetes, acute confusion, immobility, and sedation. Medications that increase or decrease bladder or urethral sphincter tone also may contribute to acute incontinence. Box 37-1 shows transient causes of acute incontinence.

## TABLE 37-1    MEDICATIONS COMMONLY PRESCRIBED FOR THE TREATMENT OF URINARY INCONTINENCE (UI)

| Classification | Generic Name | Mechanism of Action | Dose | Side Effects | Contraindications |
|---|---|---|---|---|---|
| **Drugs That Decrease Activity of Overactive Bladder (Urge UI)** | | | | | |
| Anticholinergics/ Antimuscarinics | Oxybutynin | Antispasmodic and slight analgesic effect on smooth muscle; inhibits acetylcholine on smooth muscle | 2.5–5 mg OD to QID | Side effects: constipation, dry mucosal (mouth, vagina, eyes); in older clients confusion, decreased cognition (crosses blood-brain barrier); blurred vision; may result in urinary retention—at-risk patients should be monitored for residual urine. NB: Gradual increase of oral dose increases tolerability, especially in older adults; doses as low as 2.5 mg at HS are effective for some older patients. | As per all anticholinergic medications: narrow angle glaucoma; GI obstruction or atony; ulcerative colitis, myasthenia gravis; urinary retention or residual urine (can be used in conjunction with intermittent catheterization) |
| | Oxybutynin XL | All are metabolized primarily by liver. | Oxybutynin XL available in 5 & 10 mg | **Warn client that empty capsule from oxybutynin LA will be excreted in the feces. | |
| | Tolterodine | More selective on muscarinic (M3) receptors than oxybutynin, resulting in fewer anticholinergic side effects | 1–2 mg bid; may take up to 8 weeks to reach optimum benefit; LA 4 mg | As above but less severe because of selectivity of M3 bladder receptors over salivary receptors | As above; adjust dosage if concurrent use of cytochrome P-450 3A4 inhibitors (fluoxetine increases concentration by 4.8 times). |
| | Tolterodine LA | | | | |
| | Propantheline bromide | Nonselective anticholinergic and antispasmodic | 15–30 mg PO q 6h, daily if necessary | As above | As above |
| Tricyclic Antidepressants | Imipramine, doxepin, desipramine, nortriptyline | | 25 mg at HS up to 25 mg tid | As above; occasional orthostatic hypotension | Decrease in nocturnal UI; side effects common |

(continues)

## TABLE 37-1    MEDICATIONS COMMONLY PRESCRIBED FOR THE TREATMENT OF URINARY INCONTINENCE (UI) (continued)

| Classification | Generic Name | Mechanism of Action | Dose | Side Effects | Contraindications |
|---|---|---|---|---|---|
| *Drugs That Increase Urethral Sphincter Tone (Stress UI)* | | | | | |
| Alpha Adrenergic Agent | Pseudoephedrine | Stimulates alpha fibers at bladder neck and sphincter causing increased tone | 75 mg Q 12h | Hypertension, insomnia, tremor, agitation | Clients on MAO-inhibitors, those with hypertension, with narrow angle glaucoma, and older clients |
| Hormone Replacement Therapy | Premarin vaginal cream Slow-release estradiol ring | Reduces irritation from atrophic vaginitis NB: Dose is too low to provide systemic benefits of estrogen therapy. | Cream: 1–2 g qHS x 2 weeks, then twice per week at HS Estradiol ring: change q 3 months | May cause sore breasts; spotting; must be applied intravaginally and not on the labia | Generally contraindicated in women with history of endometrial, ovarian, or breast cancer |
| *Drugs That Decrease Urethral Sphincter Tone (Benign Prostatic Hyperplasia)* | | | | | |
| Alpha Adrenergic Blockers (Agonists) | Terazosin, prazosin, doxazosin | Blocks alpha 1A fibers at the bladder neck and sphincter, causing decreased tone and improving voiding in men with mild obstruction | Varies with medication; for all alpha blockers, start at a very low dose and gradually increase until therapeutic effect is achieved. | Postural hypotension, syncope, fainting (especially with first dose) | Clients on antihypertensive medications will need to have doses titrated. |
| 5-Alpha-Reductase Inhibitors | Finasteride | Inhibits the conversion of testosterone to dihydrotestosterone; this causes a reduction on prostate size and improves voiding symptoms from prostatic enlargement. | 5 mg per day | Medication is taken on a long-term basis; when it is stopped, the prostate will gradually increase in size again. | Food may delay the rate and extent of oral absorption; not indicated in clients with urinary obstruction unless they are being carefully monitored by a urologist. |

Adapted from Reiss, B., Evans, M., & Broyles, B. (2002). *Pharmacological aspects of nursing care* (6th ed.). Clifton Park, NY: Delmar Learning.

## BOX 37-1 TRANSIENT CAUSES OF URINARY INCONTINENCE

- Delirium
- Infection-urinary (symptomatic)
- Atrophic urethritis and vaginitis
- Pharmaceuticals
- Psychological disorders, especially depression
- Excessive urine output
- Restricted mobility
- Stool impaction

Palmer, M. H. (2002). Urinary incontinence in nursing homes. *Journal of Wound, Ostomy, and Continence Nursing, 29*(1), 4–5.

## TABLE 37-2 COMMON CAUSES OF STRESS URINARY INCONTINENCE

| Urethral hypermobility | Multiple vaginal deliveries |
|---|---|
| | • Forceps-assisted deliveries |
| | • Pelvic muscle denervation |
| | • Estrogen deficiency |
| | • Obesity (exacerbating factor) |
| Intrinsic sphincter deficiency | Iatrogenic |
| | • Multiple bladder suspensions (women) |
| | • Radical prostatectomy (men) |
| | • Transurethral resection of prostate (rare in men) |
| | • Y-V plasty surgery (both genders) |
| | Neuropathic |
| | • Lesion of lumbosacral spine |
| | • Cauda equina syndrome |
| | • Pelvic fracture |

## Chronic Urinary Incontinence

The four predominant types of chronic urine loss are stress urinary incontinence, overactive bladder (urge incontinence), overflow incontinence, and extraurethral incontinence. The term **functional incontinence** may be applied if the individual has difficulty accessing the toilet.

### Stress Urinary Incontinence

**Stress urinary incontinence (SUI)** is the uncontrolled loss of urine caused by physical exertion in the absence of a detrusor muscle contraction. SUI is associated with urethral hypermobility or with intrinsic sphincter deficiency. It occurs with coughing, jumping, sneezing, or other activities that increase the abdominal pressure on the bladder.

Urethral hypermobility is the abnormal movement of the bladder base and urethra during physical exertion. The relationship between urethral hypermobility and SUI is not entirely understood, although several mechanisms have been proposed. Descent of the urethra into the lower portion of the pelvis may cause a loss of abdominal pressure transmission when compared with forces that affect the bladder. In addition, muscular contraction is compromised in the hypermobile urethra. Loss of the normal anatomical relationships between the urethral sphincter and related structures also may contribute to SUI by reducing the efficiency of the muscular elements of the sphincter. The contribution of estrogen deficiency, which compromises the elements of urethral coaptation in the woman, remains unclear. Table 37-2 identifies common factors that contribute to SUI.

Intrinsic sphincter deficiency is a disorder of the muscular components of the urethral sphincter. Sphincter closure is compromised, and urinary leakage is often severe. Severe urine loss caused by intrinsic sphincter deficiency is defined as *Total Urinary Incontinence* by the North American

Nursing Diagnosis Association (NANDA) system. Unlike urethral hypermobility, which is a women's health concern, intrinsic sphincter deficiency occurs in both genders and is related primarily to iatrogenic or neuropathic causes. Table 37-2 identifies common causes of intrinsic sphincter deficiency. Intrinsic sphincter deficiency and urethral hypermobility frequently coexist in women.

### Urgency and Urge Urinary Incontinence

**Urge urinary incontinence** (overactive bladder) is the complaint of involuntary leakage accompanied by or immediately preceded by an urge to void. It may also be referred to as *overactive bladder syndrome*. In the person with normal sensations of the lower urinary tract, detrusor overactivity incontinence causes a precipitous desire to urinate, followed by urinary leakage unless a toilet is immediately available. In those without normal sensation of bladder filling and impending urination, the contraction is followed by urinary incontinence that is often described as unpredictable. The NANDA classification schema divides this type of incontinence into two forms: *Urge Urinary Incontinence* and *Reflex Urinary Incontinence* (NANDA, 2003). This distinction is clinically relevant because reflex incontinence is commonly associated with detrusor sphincter dyssynergia. Dyssynergia, or a loss of coordination between the bladder and sphincter mechanism, causes a functional obstruction of the bladder outlet and urinary retention. Table 37-3 outlines common causes of urge incontinence of urine.

| TABLE 37-3 | COMMON CAUSES OF URGE INCONTINENCE |
|---|---|
| Urge urinary incontinence (overactive bladder) | **Neuropathic (sensations preserved)**<br>• Cerebrovascular accident<br>• Brain tumor<br>• Hydrocephalus<br>• Organic brain syndrome (also associated with functional urinary incontinence)<br>• Incomplete spinal lesions (when sensations of bladder filling are preserved)<br><br>**Bladder inflammation**<br>• Bladder calculi<br>• Bladder tumor (particularly carcinoma in situ)<br>• Cystitis (may exacerbate subclinical instability)<br>• Atrophic vaginitis<br><br>**SUI** (39% of women with SUI experience instability and urge incontinence; cause of relationship unclear)<br><br>**Bladder outlet obstruction**<br><br>**Idiopathic** (may represent subtle neuropathy or other undiagnosed disorder) |
| Reflex incontinence | **Spinal lesions above neurologic level S-2**<br>• Complete cord injury<br>• Transverse myelitis<br>• Multiple sclerosis |

## Functional Urinary Incontinence

Factors that can contribute to incontinence are altered mobility, manual dexterity, ability to easily access the toilet, or cognitive changes. Altered mobility and dexterity produce incontinence when the individual is unable to reach the toilet within a reasonable time after the onset of the urge to urinate. These conditions are worsened in an unfamiliar environment, such as a hospital, where side rails are raised on beds and sedatives are used to enhance sleep. Difficulty in reaching the toilet due to environmental factors, such as stairs, poor lighting, toilet height, and narrow doors that are impassable to wheelchairs or walkers, can also affect continence.

Acute confusion or dementia causes urinary incontinence when the signals to toilet become unclear. Functional incontinence exists as a separate entity from stress or instability urinary leakage. Nonetheless, it is important to remember that functional limitations also exacerbate these forms of urine loss.

### Extraurethral Incontinence

**Extraurethral incontinence** is the uncontrolled loss of urine that exists when the sphincter mechanism has been bypassed. According to the NANDA classification system, extraurethral leakage is termed *Total Urinary Incontinence*, although that term is also applied to severe SUI. The three causes of extraurethral incontinence are ectopia (a congenital defect in which leaks occur from a source outside the urethra), a fistula (acquired passage allowing urinary leakage), or a surgical bypass of the urinary bladder (such as the ileal conduit). The severity of extraurethral incontinence varies from a dribbling leakage superimposed on an otherwise normal voiding pattern to a continuous urine loss that replaces any recognizable voiding pattern.

## Urinary Retention

Urinary retention is caused by two conditions: bladder outlet obstruction and deficient detrusor muscle contraction strength. Bladder outlet obstruction causes incomplete bladder evacuation by blocking the outflow of urine. Deficient detrusor muscle contraction strength occurs when contractions are insufficient to maintain urethral opening long enough for complete bladder emptying. Because the management of each condition is different, it is important to differentiate between these disorders during evaluation. Table 37-4 describes common causes of urinary retention.

## Bowel Retention

Many diseases and conditions affect bowel function. Although many alterations in bowel elimination patterns may be observed, this discussion is limited to three common alterations: constipation, diarrhea, and fecal incontinence.

### Constipation

Colonic **constipation** is the infrequent and difficult passage of hardened stool (perceived constipation, influenced by psychological and emotional stress, is not included in this discussion).

Dietary factors may contribute to constipation. Dehydration causes drying of the stool as water and sodium are absorbed from the bowel. Inadequate dietary bulk also dehydrates the stool. Diverticular disease, a common problem in older adults, also reduces colonic transit, further increasing the risk of constipation.

Neuropathic conditions promote constipation by diminishing the efficiency of gastric motility. Stroke and spinal disorders, disc problems, or spinal stenosis contribute to

| TABLE 37-4 | COMMON CAUSES OF URINARY RETENTION |
|---|---|
| Bladder outlet obstruction | **Prostatic enlargement**<br>• Benign prostatic hyperplasia<br>• Prostate cancer<br>• Prostatitis<br><br>**Bladder neck dyssynergia (dyssynergia of the smooth muscle of the sphincter mechanism)**<br><br>**Detrusor sphincter dyssynergia (dyssynergia between detrusor and striated muscle of sphincter)**<br><br>**Urethral stricture**<br><br>**Urethral tumor (rare)**<br><br>**Constipation**<br><br>**Pelvic organ prolapse**<br>• Cystocele<br>• Uterine prolapse |
| Deficient detrusor contraction strength | **Transient conditions**<br>• Fecal impaction<br>• Acute immobility<br>• Side effect of drugs including anticholinergics, tricyclic antidepressants<br>• Side effect of recreational drugs including hallucinogens<br>• Herpes zoster of sacral dermatomes<br>• $B_{12}$ deficiency<br><br>**Established conditions**<br>• Lesions of sacral spine<br>• Cauda equina syndrome<br>• Diabetes mellitus (late stages)<br>• Tabes dorsalis<br>• Poliomyelitis<br>• Chronic alcoholism |

Adapted from Nelson, R., Furner, S., & Jesudason, V. (2001). Urinary incontinence in Wisconsin skilled nursing facilities: Prevalence and associations in common with fecal incontinence. *Journal of Aging & Health, 13*(4), 539–547.

constipation by reducing mobility, weakening the abdominal muscles, and diminishing the motility of the smooth muscle of the colon and rectum. Functional limitations, particularly impaired mobility, predispose older clients to constipation; they perceive a diminished desire to defecate and have prolonged colonic transit time. Multiple medications, particularly narcotics, sedatives, anticholinergics, antidepressants, antiparkinsonian drugs, and iron, also contribute to constipation.

In women, pelvic organ prolapse may exacerbate constipation. A rectocele is the herniation of the rectum and surrounding tissues into the potential space of the vagina. A significant rectocele causes a mechanical obstruction to defecation. Both women and men may experience constipation because of incomplete control of the anal sphincter. In this case, failure of complete relaxation of the anal sphincter causes fecal retention, drying of stool, and constipation.

In severe cases, the hardened stool may consolidate into an **impaction**. This bolus of stool serves as a nidus for bacterial overgrowth and produces an obstruction that further slows colonic transit time and the passage of further fecal contents (Robinson, Fritch, Hullett, Petersen, Sikkema, Theuninck, & Timmer, 2000).

Dietary fiber and fluid intake can be increased to promote the passage of soft, hydrated stool. The client who is unable or unwilling to obtain adequate fiber from the diet may be given a bulk laxative (such as Metamucil) or a bran mixture as a specific dietary supplement. The nurse should present options for taking this supplement, honoring the client's preferences whenever feasible. Initially, 3 to 6 grams of the supplement are administered, and the dosage is gradually increased until a soft, well-formed stool is obtained.

## CLIENT REFLECTIONS

### Bowel Training in a Person with a Spinal Cord Injury

Mr. Potter had a spinal cord injury 2 years ago in a diving accident. He is permanently paralyzed from the waist down and comes into the rehabilitation unit once a month for physiotherapy. He reflects on his condition with the following comments: "I remember the first time I was assisted onto one of those bedside commodes to have a bowel movement. The nurse had to use her hand with gloves on to 'dig out' my stool. I was so embarrassed, and yet there was nothing I could do. Now, I am used to the bowel training procedure and the digital method of cleaning out my rectum. But for the first couple of months that was the most difficult thing I dealt with. It was almost worse than not being able to walk."

## NURSING STRATEGY

### Managing Constipation

- Remove hardened or impacted stool by mechanical means, cleansing enema, stimulant or laxative, or pulsed irrigation evacuation (PIEE).

- Increase dietary fiber and fluid until soft, formed stool is obtained.

- Administer supplemental bulk laxative for client intolerant of dietary fiber.

- Encourage light exercise to stimulate defecation.

- Encourage regular pattern of defecation.

- Teach client to stimulate defecation by mini-enema, oral laxative or stimulant, or digital stimulation as needed.

McKenna, S., Wallis, M., Brannelly, A., & Cawood, J. (2001). The nursing management of diarrhea and constipation before and after the implementation of a bowel management protocol. *Australian Critical Care, 14*(1),10–16.

Constipation is initially managed by assisting the individual to pass hardened stool or by removing any impacted feces. Bowel evacuation is encouraged by an oral laxative, such as psyllium, a bulk-forming agent. Constipation resulting in an impaction requires mechanical disruption and removal, followed by a cleansing enema or an oral laxative. As an alternative, a pulsed irrigation enhanced evacuation (PIEE) system can be used to remove severe impaction. The PIEE uses gravity to deliver intermittent pulses of warmed saline to break up and remove hardened and impacting fecal material.

### Diarrhea

**Diarrhea** is the passage of liquefied stool that, because of its increased frequency and consistency, represents a change in the person's bowel habits. The primary causes of diarrhea include infectious agents, malabsorption disorders, inflammatory bowel disease, short bowel syndrome, side effects of drugs, and laxative or enema misuse.

Infectious diarrhea occurs when overgrowth of a pathogen produces osmotic diarrhea via toxins or reduced absorptive ability due to mucosal damage. Common pathogens include *Clostridium difficile*, enterotoxigenic *Escherichia coli*, *Salmonella*, *Shigella*, *Entamoeba histolytica*, and *Giardia*.

Malabsorption syndromes produce diarrhea when non-absorbed substances in the diet create an osmotic imbalance and liquefaction of the stool. Lactose intolerance, sorbitol intolerance, and celiac sprue syndrome are exam-ples of common malabsorption syndromes that predispose clients to diarrhea. Persons with inflammatory bowel disease or short bowel syndrome are predisposed toward diarrhea because of a reduced surface area for reabsorption.

Medications may cause diarrhea as a side effect. Administration of multiple antimicrobial agents may indirectly predispose the client to diarrhea by promoting an overgrowth of *C. difficile* in the bowel. Cholinergic drugs increase motility and reduce reabsorption of water and electrolytes from the stool. Other drugs produce osmotic diarrhea, primarily because of the vehicle for delivery, which frequently contains sorbitol and a high osmolality.

Enteral feedings contain a relatively high osmolality that frequently predisposes the client to diarrhea. These formulas may contain lactose, which causes intolerance in some people. The risk of diarrhea is further enhanced in the critically ill who have highly catabolic states and decreased absorptive ability and among those receiving bolus administration of intravenous fluids.

The misuse of laxatives and enemas is frequently associated with diarrhea among clients living at home. Overuse of saline cathartics may produce osmotic diarrhea, and the chronic misuse of laxatives may alter motility patterns and cause an osmotic shift in the bowel.

Secretory diarrhea occurs when the normal mechanisms that produce intestinal fluid are hyperactivated, causing excessive production and movement of food through the intestinal system. Zollinger-Ellison syndrome, pancreatic cholera, carcinoid syndrome, and villous adenoma may produce severe, chronic diarrhea.

The initial management of diarrhea involves the removal of factors that predispose the individual to the condition and the maintenance of adequate fluid and electrolyte balance. The nurse collaborates with the client, physician, and dietitian to determine foods that contribute to diarrhea by malabsorption or inflammation of the gastrointestinal tract. These foods are then eliminated from the diet or given with a substance (such as Lactaid) that renders them tolerable to the client. Persons with infectious diarrhea are given antimicrobials to destroy the pathogens that produce diarrhea. Anti-inflammatory drugs are administered as directed for diarrhea caused by inflammatory disorders of the bowel. Bulking agents may be used for clients with watery diarrhea. These agents absorb water in the stool and improve the consistency of feces. Antidiarrheal drugs, including diphenoxylate and loperamide, may be administered to reduce intestinal motility and increase absorption of water from the stool. However, these drugs are contraindicated in clients with infectious diarrhea because the diminished motility would enhance overgrowth of pathogens in the gastrointestinal tract.

Clients who have significant diarrhea may experience mild to severe dehydration and electrolyte imbalances. Oral fluids are given as tolerated; beverages containing glucose and electrolytes are encouraged. In contrast, beverages that contain caffeine are avoided because they stimulate colonic motility. Individuals with severe fluid volume deficits and

## NURSING STRATEGY

### Managing Diarrhea

- Eliminate from the diet foods and beverages that contain malabsorbed substances.

- Administer antimicrobials for infectious diarrhea.

- Administer anti-inflammatory agents for irritative disorders of the bowel.

- Administer bulking agents for watery stools.

- Provide oral fluids as tolerated; offer fluids rich in electrolytes.

- Administer intravenous fluids and electrolytes as directed for clients unable to tolerate oral fluids.

- Monitor perianal skin for integrity.

- Apply skin barriers for altered integrity.

- Apply a rectal pouch or insert a rectal tube for severe, large-volume diarrhea.

McKenna, S., Wallis, M., Brannelly, A., & Cawood, J. (2001). The nursing management of diarrhea and constipation before and after the implementation of a bowel management protocol. *Australian Critical Care, 14*(1),10–16.

## RESEARCH FOCUS

**Title of Study:** Fecal incontinence in hospitalized patients who are acutely ill

**Study Purpose:** To determine the incidence of fecal incontinence in acutely ill hospitalized clients, and to ascertain the relationship between fecal incontinence and stool consistency, and between diarrhea and two well-known nosocomial or iatrogenic etiologies of diarrhea: *Clostridium difficile* and tube feeding.

**Methods:** Rectal swabs and stool specimens were obtained weekly from 152 patients on acute or critical care units; information regarding tube feeding and medications, severity of illness, and nutritional data were prospectively recorded on each client.

**Findings:** A total of 33% of the clients had fecal incontinence. Although a greater percentage of clients with diarrhea had fecal incontinence than clients without diarrhea, the condition was not associated with any specific cause of diarrhea.

**Implications:** Even though treatments may be beneficial in managing fecal incontinence, treatments that slow intestinal transit should be avoided in clients with *Clostridium difficile*–associated diarrhea.

Bliss, D. Z., Johnson, S., Savik, K., Clabots, C. R., & Gerding, D. N. (2000). Fecal incontinence in hospitalized patients who are acutely ill. *Nursing Research, 49*(2), 101.

large-volume diarrhea may require intravenous fluid and electrolyte support until the diarrhea subsides.

### Fecal Incontinence

**Fecal incontinence** is an even more devastating health problem than urinary incontinence. The primary mechanisms that predispose the adult to incontinence of stool are dysfunction of the anal sphincter, disorders of the delivery of stool to the rectum, disorders of rectal storage, and anatomical defects.

A disorder of stool volume and consistency is typically not enough to produce fecal incontinence in the otherwise normal individual. Instead, the person is likely to perceive a precipitous urgency to defecate, an impulse that is heeded rapidly. However, if the volume of stool is sufficient and the storage capacity of the rectum is compromised, or sphincter function is suboptimal, fecal incontinence may result. When severe constipation leads to an impaction of stool, bacteria in the rectum overgrow, producing a liquefied medium. The toxins produced by this liquefied stool are likely to stimulate the bowel and may produce transient seepage of stool in the normally continent client.

Low compliance of the rectum also predisposes the client to fecal incontinence. In the normal individual, the rectum is able to accommodate 400 ml of feces at low pressure. However, clients with radiation proctitis, rectal wall fibrosis due to inflammatory disorders, infectious proctitis, chronic obstruction, or malignancies store lower volumes of stool at higher pressures. Low rectal compliance diminishes storage capacity and causes greater than normal urgency to defecate when stool enters the rectum. When a large volume of stool enters the rectum rapidly, the urgency to defecate is likely to be overwhelming, and the risk of incontinence is significant.

Anal sphincter dysfunction is likely to cause incontinence when both the internal and external mechanisms are compromised. Neurologic lesions are the most common cause of anal sphincter dysfunction. Typically, the client is able to compensate for sphincter weakness, provided the rectum is presented with a normal delivery of solid stool. However, in the presence of diarrhea, significant fecal incontinence may occur.

Sensory disorders also predispose the client to fecal incontinence. Loss of the sensitive epithelium in the proximal anal canal interferes with the client's ability to differentiate gas and solid and liquid contents in the rectum. In addition, loss of proprioception in the rectum disturbs the client's ability to detect rectal fullness. These individuals are particularly prone to incontinence when a large bolus of stool enters the rectum rapidly or when an impaction occurs.

Anatomical disorders also may compromise sphincter function and predispose the individual to fecal incontinence. Among women, the most common risk factor is obstetric trauma. Vaginal deliveries, particularly those requiring the use of forceps and those complicated by third-degree tearing, are likely to damage the anal sphincter mechanism.

## Assessment

The nursing assessment of elimination is based on a client interview, evaluation of an objective log or record of urinary or fecal elimination patterns, focused physical examination, and review of diagnostic laboratory data. When altered patterns of elimination indicate a significant health problem, additional diagnostic information is used to formulate a plan of care.

### Health History

Because issues of urinary and fecal elimination may produce feelings of embarrassment, anxiety, guilt, or shame among clients, the interview must be instigated by the nurse and conducted in a setting that provides adequate privacy. Clients are asked to describe their usual elimination habits. Table 37-5 presents the typical questions asked when assessing urinary and fecal elimination patterns.

When screening questions concerning altered patterns of elimination reveal significant findings, the interview should be expanded to include specific questions about the nature of the elimination disorder. These questions explore the type of incontinence, complicating factors, and bladder and bowel management strategies currently used by the client.

---

### STOP AND THINK

#### Assessment of Elimination Patterns

Consider the feelings of clients who have lost control of their bowels or bladder:

- Why would these clients want health care providers to consider this a significant problem worthy of aggressive treatment?

- Why might clients feel embarrassed about raising this problem with a nurse or physician?

- Why would clients wait to bring up this topic with their family members or health care providers?

---

### CLINICAL ALERT

#### Spotting Sexual Abuse

Suspect abuse if you note any of the following during inspection of a client's genital area: bruises, cuts, tears, or bleeding, especially around the genitals, anus, buttocks, hips, and thighs. Emotional signs such as refusing a rectal examination, lack of eye contact during the examination, or extreme anxiety or guarding of body parts during the assessment may all be indicators of abuse. Document all signs of suspected abuse, and know your state's and institution's policies regarding reporting abuse. Remember that no client, regardless of age or gender, should be excluded from evaluation for sexual abuse.

---

### Physical Examination

The physical examination for elimination patterns focuses on functional issues associated with urinary or fecal incontinence and assesses the perineal and perianal areas. Functional evaluation begins with the interview and continues throughout the physical examination. Mental status can be evaluated by listening to the client's responses to questions and by observing interactions with others. When mental assessment reveals changes from normal or

---

### NURSING STRATEGY

#### Sensitivity During the Genital Exam

- Assessment of the genital area can produce feelings of anxiety and embarrassment in both clients and nurses.

- Before beginning the genital examination, consider your client's cultural background and what beliefs or attitudes she may have about having the examination.

- Remember to assess whether the client's culture prohibit a female nurse from examining a male client—or whether the client's culture prohibit a male nurse from examining a male client.

- Remember to be sensitive during the examination and that you are assessing a person and not just a "body part."

Estes, M. (2002). *Health assessment & physical examination* (2nd ed.). Clifton Park, NY: Delmar Learning.

## TABLE 37-5    HEALTH HISTORY QUESTIONS FOR CLIENTS WITH ALTERED ELIMINATION

| Area of Inquiry | Sample Question | Significant Findings |
| --- | --- | --- |
| Determine duration of problem. | How long have you been bothered with problems controlling your bladder or bowels? | Association of onset of urinary or fecal incontinence with injury; disorder of central nervous system, brain, or spine; pelvic trauma; vaginal delivery; onset of climacteric |
| Elicit client's description of the problem. | Tell me about your bladder (or bowel) function. | Client description may reveal more than one problem; this helps prioritize issues as client sees them. |
| Determine type of urinary incontinence. | What activities make you leak?<br><br>Do you leak when you cough, sneeze, laugh, exercise, or walk?<br><br>Do you leak with a strong urge to urinate?<br><br>Do you leak with no sensation or warning?<br><br>How much do you typically leak?<br><br>Is the leak enough to dampen your underclothing?<br><br>Do you wear a pad? Size? Number per day? | Leakage with physical exertion is related to SUI.<br><br>Leakage associated with a sudden urge to urinate is related to detrusor hyperactivity (urge incontinence).<br><br>Leakage associated with no sensation or warning is generally associated with bypassing of sphincter (extraurethral incontinence).<br><br>SUI is typically associated with smaller volumes of leakage with each episode.<br><br>Urge incontinence often produces larger-volume leakage. |
| Ask client about previous treatment and success thereof. | Have you had any treatment for the bladder (bowels)?<br><br>By whom? What was it? Did it help? | Client may undergo many and varied treatment protocols. |
| Determine type of fecal incontinence. | Do you have trouble controlling gas or liquid stool? | Fecal incontinence associated with motility disorders (dietary intolerance), low compliance of the rectal vault, or rectal urgency is associated with diarrhea. Intermittent fecal incontinence associated with mild anal sphincter intolerance may cause loss of control only when coping with liquid stool or gas. Regular loss of solid stool is typically associated with central nervous system disorders or significant dysfunction of the anal sphincter mechanism. |

*(continues)*

## TABLE 37-5    HEALTH HISTORY QUESTIONS FOR CLIENTS WITH ALTERED ELIMINATION (*continued*)

| Area of Inquiry | Sample Question | Significant Findings |
|---|---|---|
| Identify complicating factors of urinary incontinence. | Do you ever experience bladder (urine or urinary tract) infections?<br><br>Do you feel you completely empty your bladder?<br><br>Do you ever lose control of your bowels?<br><br>Do you ever leak or ooze stool? | Urinary tract infections are commonly associated with incontinence complicated by obstruction or urinary retention.<br><br>Combined fecal and urinary incontinence typically implies neurologic disorders, including altered mentation. |
| Identify complicating factors of fecal incontinence. | Are there any foods that routinely cause you to experience nausea, vomiting, or diarrhea?<br><br>Do you experience constipation?<br><br>Do you pass hardened stool?<br><br>How frequently do *you* move your bowels? | Intolerance of specific dietary elements (such as lactose) increases small bowel motility and the subsequent risk of incontinence.<br><br>The infrequent, difficult passage of hardened stool (constipation) increases the bacterial load within the rectum, creating a liquid stool around the hardened stool. This bacteria-laden, liquefied stool increases both rectal urgency and the risk of fecal incontinence. |
| Identify bladder management program. | How do you manage your leakage? | Clients often experience complications of urinary incontinence (including altered skin integrity, shame, and humiliation). These can be prevented by using better containment devices. |
| Identify the bowel management program. | How often do you evacuate (move) your bowels?<br><br>Do you regularly use laxatives, suppositories or other stool softeners, or an enema to assist with a bowel movement? | The normal individual may move the bowels as frequently as once each day or as little as once every 2 to 3 days. Clients with perceived or organic constipation frequently use laxatives, stool softeners, or enemas to assist with bowel movements.<br><br>Clients with paralyzing neurologic lesions often must use a digital stimulation, an enema, or a suppository to stimulate a bowel movement. |

Adapted from Annells, M., & Koch, T. (2002). Fecal impaction: Older people's experiences and nursing practice. *British Journal of Community Nursing, 7*(3), 118–126.; Koch T., & Hudson, S. (2000). Older people and laxative use: Literature review and pilot study report. *Journal of Clinical Nursing, 9*(4), 516–525.; Palmer, M. H. (2002). Urinary incontinence in nursing homes. *Journal of Wound, Ostomy, and Continence Nursing, 29*(1), 4–5.

expected function, a more specific tool such as the Mini-Mental Status Examination may be administered.

Mobility and dexterity are evaluated by observing the client undress or move onto a table, chair, or bed. Dexterity is assessed by observing the client remove clothing; particular attention is paid to the manipulation of zippers, buttons, shoestrings, and snaps.

The perineum is initially inspected for skin integrity. Among clients with severe urinary leakage, the characteristic odor of urine may be present, and the skin may show signs of a monilial rash (maculopapular, red rash with satellite lesions) or an ammonia contact dermatitis (papular rash with saturated, macerated skin). Among clients with severe fecal incontinence, the skin is frequently denuded, red, and painful to touch, particularly if it has been exposed to liquid stool. The integrity of the skin typically remains intact with mild to moderate fecal or urinary incontinence, although a monilial rash may be present. This monilial rash may involve the inner aspect of the thighs, and it frequently extends throughout the skin surface covered by a containment device.

The vaginal vault of the woman is inspected for signs of atrophic vaginitis and for bladder and urethral support. The atrophic vagina has a dry, thin, friable mucosa with a loss of rugae (regular folds of tissue observed in the nor-mal vagina). It is tender to touch, pale, and cracks or bleeds easily. The vaginal introitus and vault may be quite small, and the client may be intolerant of even gentle efforts to distend the vagina for examination. Atrophic vaginal changes are associated with SUI, irritative voiding symptoms, and urge incontinence.

Pelvic support is assessed in the woman because it is associated with pelvic muscle weakness. Loss of pelvic muscle tone is associated with pelvic descent, increasing the risk of urethral hypermobility or intrinsic sphincter deficiency. Both can lead to SUI or defects of the anal sphincter or rectocele, causing chronic constipation and incomplete evacuation of stool with defecation. Paravaginal support is assessed using a gloved hand or speculum. The posterior vaginal wall is supported using either a Sims' speculum or a gloved finger gently inserted into the vagina. The woman is asked to cough or strain down, and movement of the posterior vaginal wall is evaluated. Bulging of the anterior wall indicates a cystocele or loss of support of the bladder base. This maneuver is repeated, and the posterior vaginal wall is evaluated for the presence of a rectocele. Uterine prolapse is noted when the uterus or cervix migrates toward the vaginal introitus in response to physical exertion.

Perineal sensation is assessed, using a small needle to evaluate sharp versus dull stimuli and using two probes to determine one- versus two-point discrimination. The bulbocavernosus reflex (BCR) is evaluated by gently tapping on the clitoris while observing the anal sphincter. A positive reflex will produce an anal "wink" or contraction of the perianal muscle. A weaker response is assessed by placing a gloved finger at the anus or by pelvic muscle electromyogram using patch or needle electrodes. Loss of sensations or absence of the BCR indicates neurologic damage.

Careful inspection of the perianal area and a digital rectal examination are important for both men and women. The cheeks of the buttocks should be pulled apart and the anus and surrounding area visually inspected. The client may be asked to bear down and the anus inspected for pro-

---

## CLIENT EDUCATION

### Questions the Nurse Can Ask Clients Who Have Altered Patterns of Urinary Elimination

#### Diurnal Voiding Habits

✓ How long can you postpone urination?
✓ Can you postpone urination for 2 hours?

#### Nocturia (Awakening from Sleep to Urinate)

✓ How many times do you wake up at night and urinate?
✓ Does the urge to urinate interrupt your sleep?

#### Urinary Incontinence

✓ Do you leak urine or lose bladder control?
✓ Does this leakage cause any problems for you?

#### Urinary Retention

✓ Do you feel you completely empty your bladder?
✓ Have you ever been unable to urinate at all?
✓ Do you strain to start your stream?
✓ Does your stream start and stop?

---

 ## STOP AND THINK

### Professionalism During the Rectal Assessment

The rectal examination may cause the client to feel uncomfortable or embarrassed. How would you handle the following situations if they were to occur during the rectal assessment?

● The client has an erection.

● The client loses bowel control.

● The client passes flatus.

lapse or for gaping, indicating significant weakness of the anal sphincter. The anal sphincter is assessed for tone and symmetry. The gloved, lubricated finger is gently inserted into the anal sphincter. The finger is rotated 360 degrees and the tone of the external sphincter is assessed. In addition, the rectum is palpated for evidence of stool or the hardened, large mass of feces characteristic of fecal impaction. **Hemorrhoids** (perianal varicosities of the hemorrhoidal veins) may also be identified. The prostate is examined for size, consistency, and induration. Benign prostatic hyperplasia, a common cause of urinary retention in older men, produces a uniform enlargement of the prostate. In contrast, prostate cancer causes asymmetric enlargement or discrete, hard nodules.

When altered patterns of urinary or fecal elimination are suspected from the health history, a log or diary should be completed. The bladder diary is kept over 1 to 7 days to determine voiding and fluid intake patterns of incontinence. A log allows the nurse to evaluate client responses to prompted toileting, functional bladder capacity, and the estimated volume of an incontinent episode. Table 37-6 shows a typical bladder diary.

## Diagnostic and Laboratory Data

A dipstick **urinalysis** is obtained and evaluated for nitrites, leukocytes, hemoglobin, glucose, and specific gravity. When nitrites or leukocytes are present, a microscopic analysis is completed to determine the presence of white blood cells in the urine (**pyuria**) and bacteria in the urine (**bacteriuria**). Urine culture and sensitivity testing are completed and the client is treated for a urinary tract infection. If glucose is noted in the urine, the client may undergo further evaluation for diabetes mellitus, or methods of glucose control may be reviewed and adjusted in the client with known diabetes. If the **specific gravity** (weight of urine compared with weight of distilled water) of the urine is abnormally low (below 1.010), the volume of fluid consumed by the client over a 24-hour period is evaluated further. **Hematuria** (blood in the urine) may be noted (see Table 37-7).

More detailed diagnostic testing of urinary tract function may also be obtained, including ultrasound, renal scan, and urodynamics. **Urodynamics** is a set of tests that measure bladder and surrounding abdominal pressures. Pressure data are combined with electromyography of the pelvic

| TABLE 37-6 | FLUID VOLUME CHART | | | |
|---|---|---|---|---|

**Date:** _____    **Name:** _____

| Time | Amount Urinated | Leakage? (Yes or No) | Liquid Intake | Comments |
|---|---|---|---|---|
| 6–8 A.M. | | | | |
| 8–10 A.M. | | | | |
| 10–12 A.M. | | | | |
| 12–2 P.M. | | | | |
| 2–4 P.M. | | | | |
| 4–6 P.M. | | | | |
| 6–8 P.M. | | | | |
| 8–10 P.M. | | | | |
| 10–12 P.M. | | | | |
| Overnight | | | | |
| Total in 24 hours | *Voids* | *Wet pads* | *Fluid Intake* | |

**TABLE 37-7    BUN AND CREATININE LEVELS**

| BUN (blood urea nitrogen) | Normal in adult 5–20 mg/dL; older adult 8–21 mg/dL; child 5–18 mg/dL | BUN measures the nitrogen fraction of urea, the chief end product of protein metabolism. It is formed by the liver from ammonia and excreted by the kidney. BUN reflects protein intake, the liver's ability to metabolize, and the renal excretory ability. BUN exists in a normal ratio with serum creatinine, and they often arise together in pathological conditions of the renal system. |
| Creatinine | Normal in adult 0.4–1.5 mg/dL (blood)  Range depends on age and gender: from as low as 52 in older females to as high as 146 in young men. | Creatinine clearance (mL/min/1.73 m$^2$) Creatinine is a catabolic by-product of muscle energy metabolism and is excreted by the kidneys. It is dependent on muscle mass. Kidney disorders hinder creatinine excretion; creatinine clearance is the rate at which the kidneys are able to clear creatinine from the blood. |

Daniels, R. (2002). *Delmar's guide to laboratory and diagnostic tests.* Clifton Park, NY: Delmar Learning.

muscles and urinary flow rate to determine lower urinary tract function during bladder filling and micturition.

Laboratory tests also may be obtained for select cases of fecal incontinence. A stool culture may be analyzed for ova and parasites, electrolytes, or culture when dietary intolerance or a gastrointestinal infection is thought to be causing diarrhea and related incontinence. When anal sphincter weakness is suspected as a cause of fecal incontinence, anorectal manometry may be completed to further evaluate anal sphincter and rectal vault function. When pelvic muscle weakness and descent are thought to cause fecal incontinence, defecography (x-ray images of the rectal vault and anal sphincter obtained during defecation) or anorectal ultrasonography may be completed.

## Nursing Diagnoses

The following nursing diagnoses are frequently encountered in clients experiencing changes in urinary and bowel habits.

## Impaired Urinary Elimination

*Impaired Urinary Elimination* is the state in which the individual experiences a disturbance in urine elimination. Defining characteristics include **dysuria** (painful urination), frequency, hesitancy, incontinence, nocturia, retention, and urgency. Altered urinary elimination patterns can result from multiple causes, including anatomical obstruction, sensory motor impairment, and urinary tract infection.

## Stress Urinary Incontinence

Stress urinary incontinence is the state in which an individual experiences a loss of urine less than 50 ml occurring with increased abdominal pressure. Major characteristics include reported or observed dribbling with increased abdominal pressure. Minor characteristics may include urinary urgency and urinary frequency (more often than every 2 hours). The client may also be experiencing related factors such as degenerative changes in pelvic muscles and structural supports associated with increased age, high intra-abdominal pressure (e.g., obesity, gravid uterus), incompetent bladder outlet, overdistension between voidings, or weak pelvic muscles and structural supports.

## Reflex Urinary Incontinence

The state in which an individual experiences an involuntary loss of urine, occurring at somewhat predictable intervals when a specific bladder volume is reached, is known as *Reflex Urinary Incontinence*. Major characteristics include no awareness of bladder filling, no urge to void or feelings of bladder fullness, and uninhibited bladder contraction or spasm at regular intervals. Related factors include a neurologic impairment (e.g., spinal cord lesion that interferes with conduction of cerebral messages above the level of the reflex arc).

## Urge Urinary Incontinence

*Urge Urinary Incontinence* is the state in which an individual experiences involuntary passage of urine occurring soon after a strong sense of urgency to void. Major characteristics include urinary urgency, frequency (voiding more often than every 2 hours), and bladder contracture or spasm. Minor characteristics include nocturia (more than two times per night), voiding small amounts (less than 100 ml) or large amounts (more than 550 ml), and inability to reach the toilet in time. Urge incontinence may be related to decreased bladder capacity (e.g., history of pelvic inflammatory disease, abdominal surgeries, indwelling urinary catheter), irritation of bladder stretch receptors causing spasm (e.g., bladder infection), alcohol, caffeine, increased fluids, increased urine concentration, or overdistension of the bladder.

## Functional Urinary Incontinence

The state in which an individual experiences an involuntary, unpredictable passage of urine is called *Functional Urinary Incontinence*. Major characteristics include urge to void or bladder contractions sufficiently strong to result in loss of urine before reaching an appropriate receptacle. Altered environment, sensory, cognitive, or mobility deficits may contribute to functional incontinence.

## Total Urinary Incontinence

*Total Urinary Incontinence* is the state in which an individual experiences a continuous and unpredictable loss of urine. Major characteristics include constant flow of urine occurring at unpredictable times without distension, uninhibited bladder contractions or spasms, unsuccessful incontinence refractory treatments, and nocturia. Related factors include neuropathy that prevents transmission of the reflex that indicates bladder fullness, neurologic dysfunction causing triggering of micturition at unpredictable times, independent contraction of the detrusor reflex owing to surgery, trauma, or disease that affects spinal cord nerves, or anatomy (fistula).

## Urinary Retention

The state in which the individual experiences incomplete emptying of the bladder is known as *Urinary Retention*. Major characteristics for urinary retention include bladder distension and small, frequent voiding or absence of urine output. Minor characteristics include sensation of bladder fullness, dribbling, residual urine, dysuria, and overflow incontinence. High urethral pressure caused by weak detrusor, inhibition of reflex arc, strong sphincter, and blockage are related factors for urinary retention.

## Constipation

A state in which an individual experiences a change in normal bowel habits characterized by a decrease in frequency or passage of hard, dry stools is called *Constipation*.

Defining characteristics include decreased activity level, frequency less than usual pattern, hard-formed stools, palpable mass, reported feeling of pressure and fullness in rectum, and straining at stool. Other possible characteristics include abdominal pain, appetite impairment, back pain, headache, interference with daily living, and use of laxatives. Related factors for constipation are still under development by NANDA; some possible considerations may be change in daily routine and less than adequate fluid and dietary intake.

## Perceived Constipation

*Perceived Constipation* is the state in which an individual makes a self-diagnosis of constipation and ensures a daily bowel movement through abuse of laxatives, enemas, and suppositories. Major characteristics include expectation of daily bowel movement, with the resulting overuse of laxatives, enemas, and suppositories, and expected passage of stool at the same time every day. Related factors may include cultural or family health beliefs, faulty appraisal, or impaired thought processes.

## Diarrhea

*Diarrhea* is the state in which an individual experiences a change in normal bowel habits characterized by the frequent passage of loose, fluid, unformed stools. Defining characteristics include abdominal pain, cramping, increased frequency, increased frequency of bowel sounds, loose or liquid stools, and urgency. Other possible characteristics include change in color of stools. Gastrointestinal, metabolic, nutritional, or endocrine disorders; infectious processes; tube feedings; fecal impaction; change in dietary intake; adverse affects of medications; and high stress levels may all contribute to diarrhea.

## Bowel Incontinence

A state in which an individual experiences a change in normal bowel habits characterized by involuntary passage of stool is called *Bowel Incontinence*. Related factors may include gastrointestinal and neuromuscular disorders, colostomy, loss of rectal sphincter control, and impaired cognition.

## Other Diagnoses

Other nursing diagnoses that may be important for clients experiencing alterations in elimination patterns include *Situational Low Self-Esteem, Deficient Knowledge, Risk for Infection, Risk for Impaired Skin Integrity*, and *Toileting Self-Care Deficit*. Nursing diagnoses and the resulting plan of care need to be developed to ensure delivery of thoughtful nursing care for both the physical and psychosocial aspects of altered elimination patterns that may affect a client's well-being.

## Outcome Identification and Planning

The targeted outcomes for clients with alterations in elimination patterns center around restoring and maintaining regular elimination habits and preventing potential associated complications such as infections and altered skin integrity. Interventions to respond to the client's physical and psychosocial needs need to be developed, such as countering deficient knowledge, enhancing self-esteem, and reducing or controlling anxiety.

Teaching is a critical factor in planning care for clients with urinary and fecal complications, including education about proper diet and exercise regimens to maintain urinary and fecal health. When ostomies are involved, clients and their families will need instruction and demonstration on proper care and the warning signs of infection.

## Implementation

### Maintain Elimination Health

The nursing management of altered patterns of urinary and bowel elimination begins with an understanding of the principles for general bladder and bowel health and by primary prevention of problems whenever feasible. All clients should be taught basic principles of fluid intake and urinary output, regular bowel evacuation, stool consistency, and altered patterns of elimination. The Client Education boxes offer suggestions for maintaining urinary and bowel elimination patterns.

### Fluid Intake

Teach clients about the importance of drinking an adequate volume of fluid each day. The recommended daily allowance (RDA) for fluids is 30 ml/kg body weight, or roughly ½ oz/lb body weight. In the average-sized adult, this equals 1,500 to 2,000 ml/d, although obese and thin individuals will vary from this range. A person who experiences altered patterns of urinary elimination, particularly incontinence, is likely to reduce fluid intake in an

---

**CLIENT EDUCATION**

**Managing Altered Fecal Elimination**

✓ Understand the relationship between dietary and fluid intake and stool consistency.
✓ Understand the relationship between altered stool consistency and altered patterns of bowel elimination, including incontinence.
✓ Ensure adequate daily fluid intake (15 ml/lb body weight).
✓ Ensure adequate intake of dietary fiber.
✓ Establish regular schedule of defecation.
✓ Heed the urge to defecate.

---

attempt to manage the problem. Many clients reason that curtailing fluid intake will reduce urinary output and the risk of incontinence. Unfortunately, it will not. Systematic dehydration may increase rather than diminish the risk of urinary incontinence by promoting bacteriuria and by concentrating the urine, thereby enhancing its irritative properties. Dehydration also causes the body to compensate for a shortage of available fluids by reabsorbing fluids and sodium from the bowel, causing drying of the stool and constipation (Figure 37-4).

### Diet

Potential bladder irritants may make urinary symptoms worse. Foods and beverages that may irritate the bladder and produce frequent urination and bladder discomfort in certain persons are (Table 37-8):

- Caffeinated beverages, carbonated drinks, and acidic fluids (including coffee and tea)
- Aspartame, particularly when added to a caffeinated or carbonated beverage

---

**CLIENT EDUCATION**

**Managing Altered Urinary Elimination**

✓ Ensure adequate daily fluid intake (15 ml/lb body weight).
✓ Reduce or avoid bladder irritants.
✓ Reduce alcohol consumption.
✓ Stop smoking.
✓ Teach pelvic muscle exercises to women (Kegel exercises).

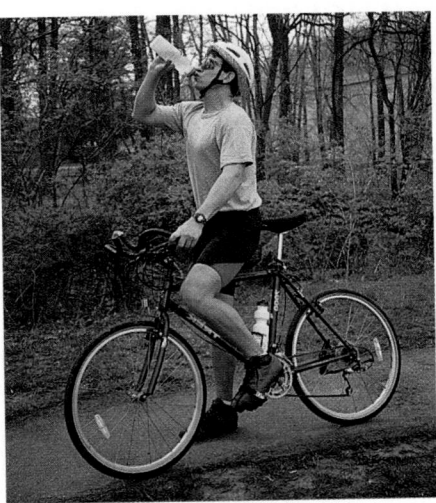

**Figure 37-4    Preventing dehydration is an important element of proper nutrition.**

| TABLE 37-8 | COMMON DIETARY FIBER SOURCES |
|---|---|

(Recommended: 30 grams of fiber per day)

| Whole grains | **Higher (> 4 grams/serving)**<br>All bran cereal<br><br>**Medium (2–4 grams/serving)**<br>Wheat, rye, oat, millet, buckwheat<br>Shredded wheat cereal<br>Popcorn<br><br>**Lower (1–2 grams/serving)**<br>Brown rice |
|---|---|
| Fruits | **Higher (> 4 grams/serving)**<br>Blackberries<br>Raspberries<br>Pear<br><br>**Medium (2–4 grams/serving)**<br>Apple<br>Strawberries<br><br>**Lower (1–2 grams/serving)**<br>Apricot<br>Bananas<br>Peach |
| Vegetables | **Higher (>4 grams/serving)**<br>Beans<br>Lentils<br><br>**Medium (2-4 grams/serving)**<br>Broccoli<br>Brussels sprouts<br>Carrots<br><br>**Lower (1-2 grams/serving)**<br>Asparagus<br>Garlic<br>Acorn squash<br>Zucchini squash |

Adapted from Jaffe, M. (1998). *Geriatric nutrition & diet* (3rd ed.). Clifton Park, NY: Delmar Learning.

- Citrus fruits or juices
- Foods containing tomatoes or tomato-based sauces
- Chocolate
- Greasy or spicy foods

Dietary fiber and adequate fluids may prevent constipation and increase the desire to defecate.

## Lifestyle and Prevention

For many clients, lifestyle and habits affect normal elimination patterns. Individual, social, family, and cultural variables play an important role in elimination. Proper nutrition, adequate rest and sleep, and regular exercise help maintain healthy elimination patterns. Clients with elimination problems can take measures to correct or alter the problem by modifying their lifestyle.

### Alcohol and Tobacco Use

Consumption of alcohol exerts significant effects on the bladder. Alcohol suppresses antidiuretic hormone (ADH) excretion by the hypothalamus, causing polyuria and increasing the risk of urinary leakage. In addition, the sedative effects of alcohol increase the risk of urinary incontinence, both while awake and during sleep. Alcohol irritates the intestines and bowels, causing inflammation. The irritant effect causes increased elimination of fluid in the stool, resulting in diarrhea. With chronic use of alcohol, inflammation results, causing enteritis or colitis.

Cigarette smoking also may irritate the bladder. Cigarette smoke may increase the risk of SUI because of its association with a chronic cough, and smoking is a significant risk factor for the development of bladder cancer. Smoking stimulates the bowel through the action of nicotine, present in tobacco, causing increased bowel tone and motility. The result is diarrhea.

### Stress Management

Managing stress promotes healthy bowel and urinary patterns. Acute and chronic stress affect both elimination systems. The bowel responds by increasing activity when the parasympathetic nervous system is stimulated. However, the longer-lasting effect of norepinephrine causes slowing of the gastrointestinal tract. In response to the effect of ADH,

## FOCUS ON WELLNESS

### Wellness Practices and Elimination

Many facets to wellness are often overlooked. The health care provider must remember that elimination patterns are one such aspect of the wellness focus. Many preventive measures for healthy elimination habits are available. For example, urinary patterns may be improved simply by drinking 6–8 glasses of water per day. This prevents urinary tract infections and assists in increasing the efficiency of the renal system in its detoxification capabilities. In addition, wellness practices for bowel elimination can include such measures as eating a high-fiber diet, avoiding dehydration, and ingesting regular portions of fruits and vegetables.

the kidneys retain fluid. The effect of ADH in combination with the effect of norepinephrine and epinephrine elevates blood pressure. Using education and support, nurses can help clients manage stress. See Chapter 47.

## Obesity

Obesity is a known risk factor for UI in women and is independent of obstetric history, surgery, smoking, and family history. Morbid obesity is defined as greater than 120% of the average weight for height and age; women who are obese are more likely to have SUI and/or urge incontinence than women who are not obese. Women with profound weight loss after gastric bypass surgery report a marked improvement in SUI (Goldberg, Rivers, Smith, & Homan, 2000).

## Elimination Habits

The client is urged to establish a regular schedule of bowel elimination and to answer the desire to defecate. In the normal individual, the desire to move the bowel is transient and lost when avoided or ignored. Although occasional avoidance of the urge to defecate is a useful tool for continence, routine avoidance may predispose the client to constipation and reduce the efficiency of bowel evacuation. The urge to defecate is typically greatest after a meal, and it may be enhanced by dietary stimulants such as fiber or a caffeinated beverage or by light exercise. In an unfamiliar setting, such as the hospital, it is important to provide adequate privacy so that the client can heed the urge to defecate without undue interruption or embarrassment.

Encourage the client to establish a regular elimination pattern to prevent urinary incontinence. This can be successfully accomplished by using techniques such as relaxation and timing. The client, with the assistance of the nurse, establishes a voiding schedule. Once the client has met the goal of staying continent for the established time period, the interval between voidings can be lengthened. Within the interval between urinations, the client can use relaxation exercises to help manage the feelings of urgency.

## Positioning

Sitting with the feet flat on the floor is the usual position for both men and women for bowel elimination. Sitting is also the usual position for women to urinate; standing is the position preferred by some men. Clients unable to use the toilet require assistance in accomplishing elimination. Devices such as the bedpan, commode, or urinal can be substituted.

Clients who use a bedpan need as comfortable a setting as possible. After placement of the bedpan the head of the bed should be elevated to a 45-degree angle, unless contraindicated. The nurse may need to assist the client to cross the legs in order to create somewhat of a sitting position. Male clients who are unable to stand should have the head of the bed elevated to a 45-degree angle, unless contraindicated, while using the urinal. Procedure 37-1 outlines the steps in positioning and removing a bedpan.

Clients who are able to get out of bed but are unable to ambulate to the toilet can use a bedside commode, which resembles a toilet but is portable. The feet must touch the floor or be placed on a footstool.

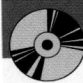

**PROCEDURE 37-1** **Assisting with a Bedpan or Urinal**

### EQUIPMENT NEEDED

- Bedpan (regular or fracture) or urinal (Figure 37-5)
- Disposable gloves
- Bedpan cover
- Toilet paper
- Washcloth and towel

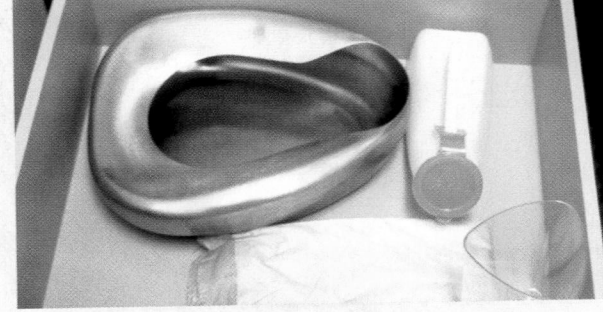

**Figure 37-5** **The bedpan and urinal are used for elimination when clients are confined to bed. A graduated container measures urine for intake and output records.**

*(continues)*

**PROCEDURE 37-1** (*continued*)

## IMPLEMENTATION—ACTION/RATIONALE

| ACTION | RATIONALE |
|---|---|
| **Positioning a Bedpan** | |
| 1. Close curtain or door. | 1. Provides for privacy. |
| 2. Wash hands; apply gloves. | 2. Reduces transmission of microorganisms. |
| 3. Lower head of bed so client is in supine position. | 3. The supine position will increase ability of client to move to side-lying position. |
| 4. Elevate bed. | 4. Ensures proper body mechanics. |
| 5. Assist client to side-lying position using side rail for support. | 5. Provides for best position for proper placement of bedpan. |
| 6. Warm bedpan under warm water if needed; powder if necessary (see Figure 37-6). | 6. For comfort; prevents bedpan from sticking to the skin. |
| 7. Place bedpan under buttocks. Place a fracture pan with the lower end near the client's lower back region. Place large bedpans with the opening near the client's thighs. | 7. Ensures proper placement of the bedpan before client rolls on top of bedpan. |
| 8. While holding the bedpan with one hand, help the client roll onto the back, while pushing against the bedpan (toward the center of the bed) to hold it in place. | 8. Prevents dislocation or alignment of bedpan. |
| 9. Alternate: Help the client raise the hips using the overbed trapeze, and slide the pan in place. Alternate: If the client is unable to turn or raise hips, use a fracture pan instead of a bedpan. With a fracture pan, the flat side is placed toward the client's head (see Figure 37-7). | 9. Provides an alternate way to position the pan. Fracture pan reduces the amount of movement and lift required to place the pan. |

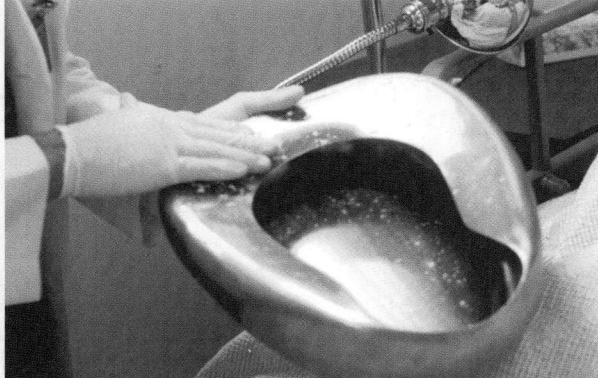

**Figure 37-6    Applying powder to the bedpan prevents it from sticking to the skin.**

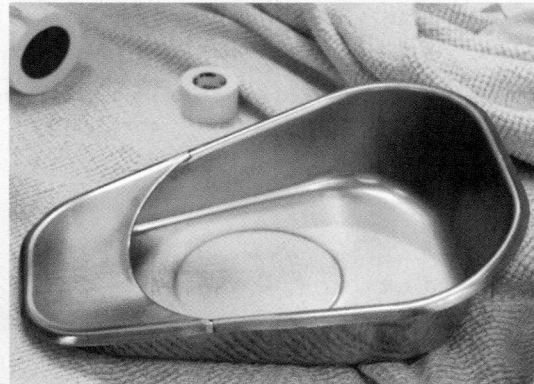

**Figure 37-7    A fracture pan is used when the client is unable to turn or raise the hips.**

*(continues)*

10. Check placement of bedpan by looking between client's legs.

11. If indicated, elevate head of bed to 45-degree angle or higher for comfort.

12. Place call light within reach of client; place side rails in upright position, lower bed, and provide privacy.

13. Remove gloves; wash hands.

### Positioning a Urinal

14. Repeat Actions 1 and 2.

15. Lift the covers and place the urinal so the client may grasp the handle and position it. If the client cannot do this, you must position the urinal and place the penis into the opening (see Figures 37-8 and 37-9).

10. May prevent spillage due to misalignment of bedpan.

11. Check order of physician or qualified practitioner; bed remains flat if client has a spinal cord injury or spinal surgery. Elevating the head of bed creates a more normal elimination position.

12. Privacy allows for a more comfortable elimination environment; elevated side rails provide for safety.

13. Reduces transmission of microorganisms.

14. See Rationales 1 and 2.

15. Ensures proper placement of the urinal and reduces the risk of spillage.

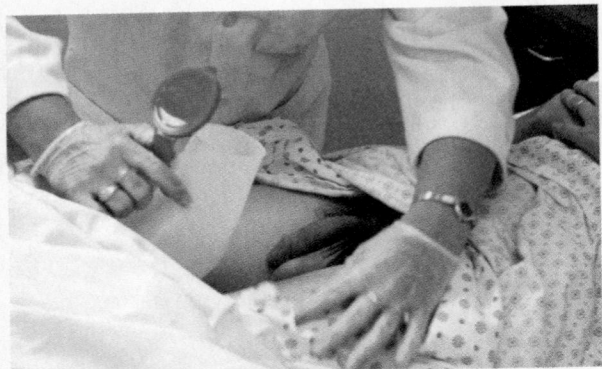

**Figure 37-8** **Lift the covers and place the urinal. Allow the client to adjust the position.**

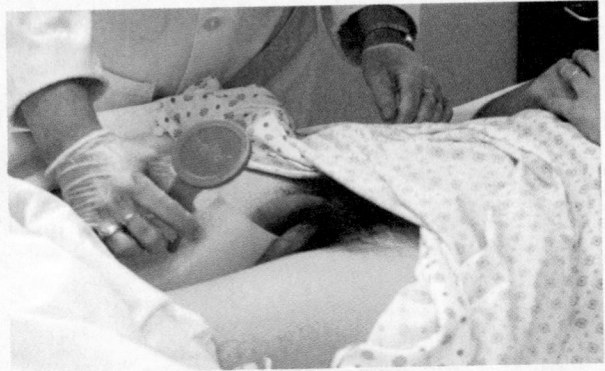

**Figure 37-9** **If the client is unable to assist, place the penis into the opening of the urinal.**

16. Remove gloves; wash hands.

### Removing a Bedpan

17. Wash hands; apply gloves.

18. Gather toilet paper and washing supplies.

19. Lower head of bed to supine position.

16. Reduces transmission of microorganisms.

17. Reduces transmission of microorganisms.

18. Having supplies at the bedside allows smooth and safe completion of the procedure.

19. Increases client's ability to move to side-lying position.

*(continues)*

**PROCEDURE 37-1** (*continued*)

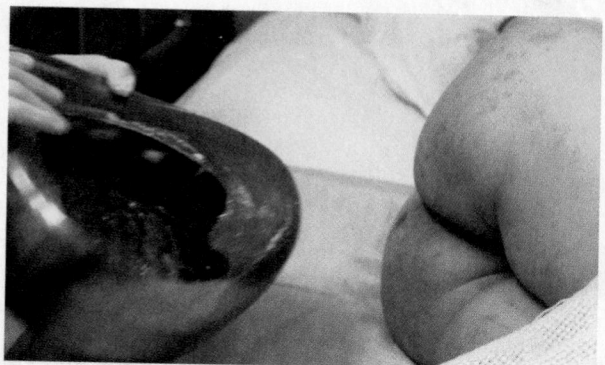

**Figure 37-10** Roll the client to one side and remove the pan.

| | |
|---|---|
| **20.** While holding bedpan with one hand, roll client to side and remove the pan, being careful not to pull or shear skin sticking to the pan and being careful not to spill contents (see Figure 37-10). | **20.** Prevents possible spillage of bedpan contents. |
| **21.** Assist with cleaning or wiping; always wipe with a front-to-back motion. | **21.** Client may not be able to clean herself; wiping from front to back decreases chances of cross-contamination from anus to urethra. |
| **22.** Empty bedpan (measure urine output if ordered), clean bedpan, and store it in proper place; if bedpan is to be emptied outside client's room, cover it during transport. | **22.** Promotes privacy and decreases the chance of spilling contents. |
| **23.** Remove soiled gloves. Wash hands. | **23.** Reduces transmission of microorganisms. |
| **24.** Allow client to wash hands. | **24.** Provides for physical hygiene and comfort. |
| **25.** Place call light within reach; recheck that side rails are in the upright position; lower bed. | **25.** Ensures client safety and comfort. |
| **26.** Wash hands. | **26.** Reduces transmission of microorganisms. |

**Removing a Urinal**

| | |
|---|---|
| **27.** Wash hands and apply gloves. | **27.** Reduces transmission of microorganisms. |
| **28.** Empty the urinal, measuring urine output if ordered; rinse the urinal and replace it within the client's reach. | **28.** Provides a way to measure the client's output. Keeping the urinal within reach promotes client autonomy. |
| **29.** Remove soiled gloves. Wash hands. | **29.** Reduces transmission of microorganisms. |
| **30.** Allow client to wash hands. | **30.** Provides for physical hygiene and comfort. |
| **31.** Place call light within reach; recheck that side rails are in the upright position. | **31.** Ensures client safety and comfort. |
| **32.** Wash hands. | **32.** Reduces transmission of microorganisms. |

## LIFE SPAN CONSIDERATIONS

### Bedpan or Urinal Use

**Pediatric Variations**

- Children may be more comfortable with assistance from a parent.

- Adolescents may need extra privacy and control over their toileting time.

**Geriatric Variations**

- Geriatric clients may have more difficulty with incontinence of urine or stool because of reduced muscle tone.

- The use of diuretics may increase the risk of incontinence.

- Reduced mobility in an older client may increase both the risk of constipation and the risk of incontinence because the client may not be able to "make it to the bathroom" in time. Clients may benefit by having a bedpan placed within reach.

## COMMUNITY/HOME CARE

### Bedpan or Urinal Use

**Home Care Variations**

- In the home care setting, the client does not have a call button. Make sure the client can summon you when needed.

- A pillowcase can be used as a bedpan cover in the home setting.

- A client who would be able to use a bedside commode in the hospital, but doesn't have one at home, can use a bedpan while sitting on the edge of the bed, or on a bedside chair. Make sure there is adequate support and handholds. Assess for the potential risk of falling.

**Long-Term Care Variations**

- If the client is very thin, a folded towel placed on the bedpan to pad the bony sacrum area will increase comfort.

### Initiate Pelvic Muscle Exercise Regimen

Regular exercise leads to good muscle tone and body metabolism. Exercise also stimulates the bowels to move regularly and leads to good urine production. Poor muscle tone can lead to impaired bladder muscle contraction and poor urination control. Pelvic muscle exercises are taught to manage SUI, and a strength training program is begun using principles of exercise physiology. Clients are taught to identify, isolate, and contract the pelvic muscles and to avoid contraction of distant muscles groups such as the thigh or abdominal muscles. Because clients frequently have difficulty isolating the pelvic muscles, biofeedback may be helpful. The nurse teaches the client to perform a single exercise that combines maximal strength and endurance. The client is asked to perform a maximal strength contrac-

tion of the muscles "surrounding the urethra and vagina or rectum" for a count of 10, or approximately 6 seconds, followed by a rest period of equal length. The program begins with a few contractions (typically 10 or fewer), and the number of repetitions is increased to a maximum of 35 to 50. The exercise regimen must be integrated into activities of daily living for maximal effectiveness. Pelvic muscle exercises, particularly when combined with biofeedback techniques, are typically taught by a specialist physiotherapist or advanced practice nurse with specific education in the management of the client with incontinence.

### Bladder Training for Urge Incontinence

For clients with urge incontinence, **bladder training** may be helpful. The purpose of bladder training is to teach the client to suppress the urge to void, thereby gradually increasing the intervals between voiding. Successful bladder training depends on a cognitively able, motivated client and a supportive health care professional. It may take several weeks to significantly improve urge symptoms. Box 37-2 provides an outline of a schedule of instructions for a specific bladder-training regimen.

### Management of Urinary Retention

Urinary retention is managed by several methods, depending on the severity and cause of the urinary problem. Mild urinary retention caused by poor detrusor contractility or obstruction may be managed by timed voiding or by double voiding. Timed voiding is a strategy to reduce overdistension and loss of muscle tone in clients with diminished sensations of urinary urgency. The client is taught to urinate at specific intervals, typically every 3 to 4 hours or to *double void* in an attempt to improve bladder emptying. The client is taught to void, rest on the toilet for 2 to 5 minutes, and void again. Medications such as alpha-blockers may be effective.

Clean, intermittent catheterization is used for moderate to severe urinary retention, when the residual urine volume is 50% or more of the total bladder capacity. Intermittent self-catheterization is taught using a clean technique. The client is taught to wash his hands and to locate and catheterize the urethra using a water-based soluble lubricant. Catheters may be cleaned with soap and water and reused many times, and the client or significant other may catheterize without applying sterile gloves.

The advanced practice or specialty practice nurse administers other management techniques for incontinence. These include transvaginal or transrectal electrical stimulation and placement of a vaginal pessary (a supportive device). Inadequate tone in the abdominal muscles, diaphragm, and the perineal muscles can cause difficulty in defecating. If a client is suffering from constipation, a regimen of walking or light recreational exercise should be recommended to promote peristalsis and defecation (Gray, 2000a; Gray, 2000b).

### Management of Functional Urinary Incontinence

*Functional Urinary Incontinence* related to dementia may also be managed by a prompted voiding technique. Prompted voiding provides the opportunity to toilet on the basis of an individualized urge response toileting program (PURT) or using a routine schedule. A PURT program is based on knowledge of the individual's typical voiding pattern. The client's voiding pattern is assessed by the use of a bladder diary or by routine assessment of containment devices for wetness. The client is then placed on a prompted voiding schedule requiring the nurse or other caregiver to approach the client, offer the opportunity to urinate, and assist with toileting. Voiding is praised, as is dryness during the period before voiding. PURT is limited to clients with adequate cognitive awareness to respond to the prompted voiding and to those with caregivers willing to comply with the demands of this ongoing program. Prompted voiding programs also may be instituted using a more arbitrary schedule for toileting, usually every 2 to 3 hours (see Table 37-9 for a summarization of the types of incontinence and the usual management strategies).

### Suggest Environmental Modifications

Incontinence can be managed by removing the barriers to toileting. The environment is manipulated to maximize opportunities for toileting, to minimize the impact of poor mobility, and to remove any environmental barriers. Clothing is carefully evaluated, and buttons, zippers, and

---

> ## BOX 37-2  SCHEDULED (TIMED) VOIDING FOR BLADDER TRAINING
>
> 1. **Establish a voiding pattern** by using a bladder diary (frequency/volume chart) to record volume of voids, incontinence episodes, and fluid intake.
>
> 2. **Determine a voiding interval** based on the voiding pattern. If frequency is more than every 60 minutes, void every 60 minutes; if less than 60 minutes, start with a 30-minute interval. After 2 days without urinary incontinence, increase the time between voids by 30 minutes. Continue this process until voiding every 3 to 4 hours.
>
> 3. **Teach urge suppression.** Pelvic muscle exercises and distraction techniques may help dissipate the urge to void when it is felt.
>
>    To control the urge, take a deep breath and relax. Stand still or sit down. Contract your pelvic floor muscles 5 or 6 times. Count backward from 100. Concentrate on having the urge decrease. Wait until it passes, and then resume your activities. If it is longer than 2 hours since you last used the toilet, proceed slowly to the toilet to empty your bladder. Rushing to the toilet will make the symptoms of urgency much worse.
>
> 4. **Gradually increase the length of time** between voids as continence is achieved.
>
> 5. **Record progress by bladder diary.** A daily or weekly bladder diary helps to track progress.
>
> 6. **Follow up regularly.** Bladder retraining requires a lot of work and commitment. Encouragement is important for success. Successful bladder retraining can take several weeks.
>
> Wyman, J. F. (2000). Management of urinary incontinence in adult ambulatory care populations. *Annual Review of Nursing Research, 18,* 171–194.

## TABLE 37-9 SYMPTOM PRESENTATION AND USUAL TREATMENT STRATEGIES FOR URINARY INCONTINENCE

| Presumed Etiology | Description | Treatment Options at the Primary Care Level |
|---|---|---|
| *Overactive Bladder (OAB)* *(Urge Incontinence)* | Loss of urine associated with a strong desire to void; may be accompanied by frequency and nocturia; nocturia is typically described by patients with overactive bladder but not by those with stress urinary incontinence. | Bladder training, timed toileting, fluid management, medication review Constipation management Pelvic muscle exercises (PFME) PFME + biofeedback Electrical stimulation (10–20 Hz) Estrogen therapy Anticholinergic/antimuscarinic medications Incontinence pads Environmental modifications such as bedside commodes, night lights and clearly marked toilets |
| *Stress Urinary Incontinence* *(SUI)* | Loss of urine on physical exertion or increases in abdominal pressure due to laughing, coughing, sneezing, etc., due to sphincter deficiency; patients with stress incontinence are usually dry at night and do not complain of nocturia. | Weight loss, Fluid increase/decrease Smoking cessation Constipation management PFME PFME + biofeedback Pessary (occasionally) ; penile compression device (occasionally) Alpha agonists Incontinence pads |
| *Mixed Incontinence* *(OAB + SUI)* | Loss of urine with both urge and increases in abdominal stress; symptoms are mixed with urgency, frequency, nocturia, leaking with increased abdominal pressures | Combination of above conservative measures, with an initial focus on the dominant symptom |
| *Overflow* | Leakage associated with bladder distension/urinary retention; leak with increased abdominal pressure; may be confused with stress incontinence; due to acontractile or poorly contractile detrusor or outlet obstruction; chronic retention is usually painless. | Refer Clean, intermittent catheterization Relief of obstruction (in females—cystocoele, uterine, prolapse, tumor; males—prostatic enlargement hyperplasia, urethral stricture, bladder tumor) Medication review Alpha blockers Last resort: indwelling catheter |

Jervis, L. L. (2001). The pollution of incontinence and the dirty work of caregiving in a U.S. nursing home. *Medical Anthropology Quarterly,* 15(1), 84–99.

multiple layers of clothing are exchanged for items that are simpler to remove. Mobility is maximized by selection of shoes with nonskid soles, and Velcro straps are preferred over strings when dexterity is compromised. The accompanying Community/Home Care box shows the effectiveness of environmental modifications for someone with functional incontinence.

The nursing management of fecal incontinence begins with measures to normalize stool consistency because constipation and diarrhea increase the risk of incontinent episodes. The environment is also manipulated to minimize functional limitations to bowel elimination. Mobility is enhanced by assistive devices (canes, walkers) as needed, and by altering seating and toilets to a height that allows optimal ease when transferring. Clothing is altered to minimize the time required for removal in preparation for defecation. Environmental barriers including poor light-ing, narrow doorways, and slippery flooring are removed, or portable toileting facilities are made available.

### Initiate Behavioral Interventions

A scheduled defecation program is used for clients with either a diminished ability to sense rectal distension or altered cognition who are unable to adequately respond to the presence of a bolus of stool in the rectum. The colon is cleansed of any excess stool, using an oral laxative or enema. The diet is altered to enhance the formation of a soft, solid stool, and supplemental bulk is added if indicated. Patterns of bowel elimination are evaluated, and the client is encouraged to defecate on this schedule if feasible. Otherwise, bowel elimination is scheduled after either a meal or another stimulant, such as a caffeinated beverage or a pharmacological agent. The importance of heeding the urge to defecate is emphasized, and the client with altered cognition is prompted to defecate.

Clients with significant sensory and motor deficits of the rectum and anus typically require a scheduled defecation program combined with vigorous stimulation of defecation. Persons with a paralyzing neurologic disorder have significant loss of anal sphincter control, poor abdominal muscle control, and altered colonic mobility. As a result, defecation must be scheduled and vigorously stimulated to avoid impaction and fecal incontinence. The colon is cleansed and stool consistency is normalized at the outset of the program. A timetable for bowel elimination is identified. Because of the need for an extensive process for effective defecation, this program must consider the schedule of the client and significant others, as well as premorbid defecation patterns. The bowel is stimulated by a medication, such as bisacodyl or a mini-enema.

### Monitor Skin Integrity

Because problems with elimination may result in disturbances in hydration and excretion of body wastes, the skin should be carefully assessed for color, texture, turgor, and the excretion of any wastes. The integrity of the skin in the perineal area also should be assessed. Problems with incontinence may result in severe excoriation.

When monitoring a client with diarrhea, the nurse should assess the perineal skin for altered integrity. After each defecation, the skin is routinely cleansed with tap water or a gentle cleanser specifically designed for incontinence. Avoid soap and water and abrasive cleaning techniques because they increase discomfort and the risk of altered skin integrity. Protect skin by application of a sealant or moisture barrier. Denuded skin is first treated with a pectin-based powder, followed by a skin sealant or moisture barrier.

### Apply a Containment Device

**Condom Catheter**  The condom catheter is a device that resembles a condom with a large-caliber connector at its distal end. This is connected to a drainage bag via a leg bag or bedside container for urinary containment. Procedure 37-2

## CLIENT EDUCATION

### Elimination and Skin Integrity

Skin integrity is a very real problem associated with elimination disorders. The following are interventions that the client may be taught as related to alterations in skin integrity:

✓ Regularly clean and thoroughly dry the skin after a bowel movement.

✓ Clients with fragile skin can be advised to use a skin cleanser.

✓ Use soap and water for normal skin conditions.

✓ After cleansing, the skin should be dried thoroughly.

✓ A hair dryer set on the low (cool) setting may be recommended.

Jervis, L. L. (2001). The pollution of incontinence and the dirty work of caregiving in a U.S. nursing home. *Medical Anthropology Quarterly, 15*(1), 84–99.

discusses the application of a condom catheter. Several types of condom catheters are available. The ideal device adheres to the penile skin without producing irritation and has sufficient elasticity to maintain its watertight seal whether the penis is in an erect or a flaccid state. Because of the potential for altered skin integrity, the condom catheter is reserved for severe SUI. Men without adequate upper extremity dexterity may benefit the most from the use of a condom catheter (see Procedure 37-2). The bladder outlet resistance caused by detrusor sphincter dyssynergia must be managed by pharmacotherapy or by transurethral or laser sphincterotomy. A special device, the urethral stent, also may be inserted. This device consists of a wire mesh that is inserted into the urethra via a special cystoscopic device and expanded at the membranous urethra. The wire mesh gently holds the sphincter open, promoting urine evacuation and preventing the deleterious effects of sphincter dyssynergia.

**Incontinence and Dribble Pads**  Many women attempt to contain urine with feminine hygiene pads. Although these pads effectively contain menstrual flow, they are not designed for urine loss. As a result, they must be changed frequently, and the risk of odor and soiling outer clothing

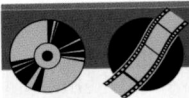

### PROCEDURE 37-2        Applying a Condom Catheter

#### EQUIPMENT NEEDED

- Condom catheter kit with adhesive strip (Figure 37-11)
- Urinary drainage bag
- Clean gloves
- Basin with warm water and soap
- Towel and washcloth

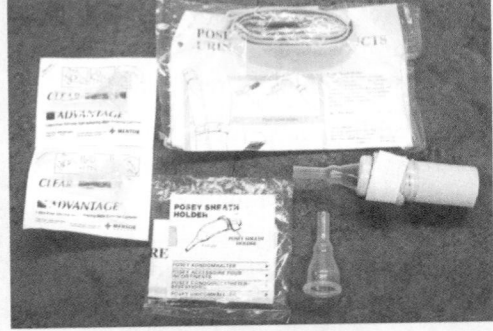

Figure 37-11    Condom catheters

### IMPLEMENTATION—ACTION/RATIONALE

| ACTION | RATIONALE |
|---|---|
| 1.  Wash hands. | 1.  Reduces transmission of microorganisms. |
| 2.  Protect the client's privacy by closing the door and pulling curtains around the bed. | 2.  Allows privacy for the client. |
| 3.  Position the client in a comfortable position, preferably in a supine position, if tolerated by the client. Raise the bed to a comfortable height for the nurse. | 3.  The client will be more comfortable and better tolerate the procedure; a supine position facilitates the cleaning and application of the catheter. Raising the bed to a comfortable height promotes good body mechanics. |

*(continues)*

**PROCEDURE 37-2 (continued)**

4. Apply gloves.

5. Fold the client's gown across the abdomen and pull the sheet up over the client's legs.

6. Assess the client's penis for any signs of redness, irritation, or skin breakdown.

7. Clean the client's penis with warm soapy water. Retract the foreskin on the uncircumcised male and clean thoroughly in folds.

8. Return the client's foreskin to its normal position (Figure 37-12).

9. Shave any excess hair around the base of the penis if required by institutional policy.

10. Rinse and dry the area.

11. If a condom kit is used, open the package containing the skin preparation (Figure 37-13). Wipe and apply skin preparation solution to the shaft of the penis. If the client has an erection, wait for termination of erection before applying the catheter.

4. Gloves should be worn to prevent the possible transmission of microorganisms when there is a chance of coming into contact with any body fluid.

5. Provides minimal exposure of the client, reducing the client's embarrassment.

6. The client may require an indwelling catheter if there is a significant amount of skin breakdown. Assessment will give baseline data for comparison with future assessments.

7. Removes microorganisms present in any drainage or feces that could enter the urinary meatus and cause a urinary tract infection. Avoids trapping microorganisms in folds around the meatus.

8. Failure to return the foreskin to a normal position can lead to swelling of the penis and possible constriction.

9. Prevents additional discomfort from the adhesive strip when the condom catheter is removed. Also prevents hair from catching onto the adhesive strip, causing discomfort.

10. Moist, warm environment can lead to the growth of microorganisms.

11. Preparation solutions protect the client's skin from irritation. An erection may occur due to manipulation of the penis while cleaning the area. This is a normal reaction and will terminate in a few minutes.

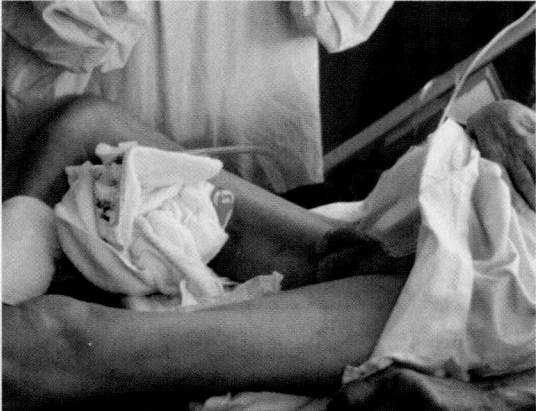

**Figure 37-12**    After cleaning the client's penis, return the foreskin to its normal position.

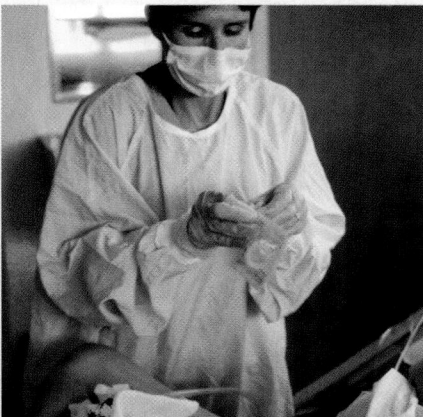

**Figure 37-13**    After preparing the penis, open the condom kit. Apply the skin preparation solution.

*(continues)*

**PROCEDURE 37-2 (*continued*)**

12. Apply the double-sided adhesive strip around the base of the client's penis in a spiral fashion. The strip is applied 1 inch from the proximal end of the penis. Do not completely encircle the penis or tightly encompass penis.

12. Applying the adhesive in a spiral fashion does not compromise circulation of the penis. Encircling the penis can constrict the penis, impair circulation, and cause edema.

13. Position the rolled condom at the distal portion of the penis and unroll it, covering the penis and the double-sided strip of adhesive. Leave a 1- to 2-inch space between the tip of the penis and the end of the condom (see Figure 37-14).

13. The condom sticks to the adhesive and remains in place. The extra spacing prevents pressure and erosion of the tip of the penis.

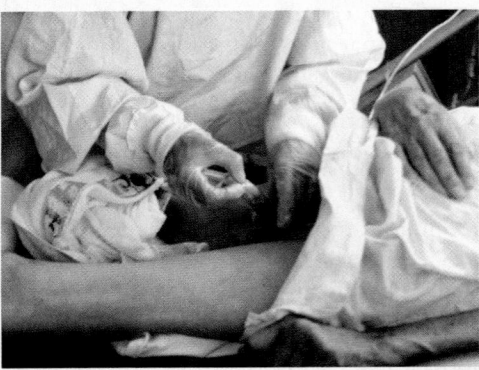

**Figure 37-14    Unroll the condom from the distal portion of the penis upward to the base.**

14. Gently press the condom to the adhesive strip.

14. Enables the condom to adhere evenly to the adhesive strip.

15. Attach the drainage bag tubing to the catheter tubing. Make sure the tubing lays over the client's legs, not under. Secure the drainage bag to the side of the bed below the level of the client's bladder or to the drainage bag attached to the leg (see Figures 37-15 and 37-16).

15. The drainage bag is positioned below the level of the client's bladder to prevent reflux of the urine onto the penis and microorganisms from entering the penis. The tubing is placed over the leg to promote urine flow away from the client. Constant exposure to urine and moisture can irritate the penis.

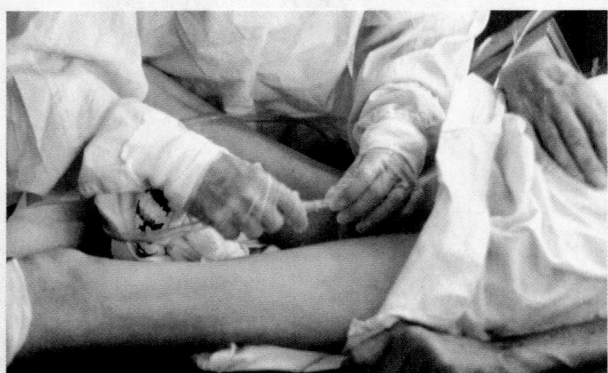

**Figure 37-15    Attach the drainage bag tubing to the catheter tubing.**

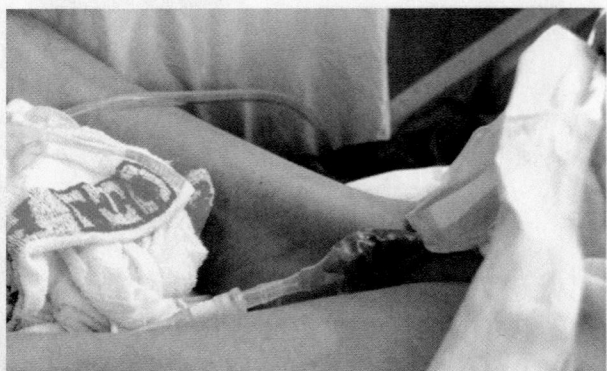

**Figure 37-16    Make sure the drainage bag tubing lays over the client's leg.**

*(continues)*

## PROCEDURE 37-2 (continued)

16. Determine that the condom and tubing are not twisted.

17. Cover the client.

18. Dispose of the used equipment in appropriate receptacle and wash hands.

19. Return the client's bed to the lowest position and reposition client to comfortable or appropriate position.

20. Empty the bag, measure the client's urinary output, and record every 4 hours.

21. Remove the condom once a day to clean the area and assess the skin for signs of impaired skin integrity.

16. If the condom or tubing is twisted, the urine cannot flow out and the condom will leak or fall off.

17. Maintains privacy of the client.

18. Reduces transmission of microorganisms.

19. Reduces potential injury from falls.

20. Records output and prevents bag from becoming overfull and/or too heavy.

21. Promotes hygiene and reduces the possibility of skin breakdown.

---

# LIFE SPAN CONSIDERATIONS

## Condom Catheter

### Pediatric Variations

- Use a condom size appropriate to the child.

- Other means such as diapers can be used for younger children; however, if output measurements are needed, a condom catheter may be necessary.

- This procedure can be extremely embarrassing to children. If the use of a condom catheter is absolutely necessary, the procedure may be best performed by a male staff member.

- If the child has an erection, inform him that this can naturally occur.

---

# COMMUNITY/HOME CARE

## Condom Catheter

### Home Care Variations

- Change the catheter often since the adhesive and the condom can lead to skin breakdown. Diapers, blue pads, or Attends may be more useful or may be used periodically to give the skin on the penis a chance to heal.

- Instruct the home caregiver on how to clean, use, apply, and remove the condom catheter.

- Discuss signs and symptoms of irritation or skin breakdown.

- Discuss alternatives to the condom should it need to be removed.

### Long-Term Care Variations

- If irritation occurs, remove the condom and clean the area more frequently, three times a day if possible.

is high. Women with mild SUI typically benefit from a small incontinent pad that adheres to the undergarments. Unlike the feminine hygiene pad, the ideal incontinent pad contains Superabsorbents® that increase the product's absorptive ability. Women with more severe SUI also may use a device that adheres to the undergarments. However, larger pads that are capable of absorbing up to 500 ml are recommended. Only women with very severe leakage are advised to use an incontinent brief. It is important to remember that containment devices are considered temporary, and the ultimate goal is reduction or ablation of urinary leakage so that pads are not needed.

Men with mild SUI may use a "dribble pad," a device that adheres to the undergarments and holds the penis in a specially designed pouch. More absorptive pads or incontinent briefs are reserved for severe cases. Two additional devices, the penile clamp and condom catheter, are also used for men with SUI. The penile compression device is a constrictive device that mechanically closes the pendulous urethra. The device is worn for a brief period and removed to prevent ischemia to local tissues. Because of the risk of necrosis and discomfort associated with the clamp, its use is limited.

**Rectal Pouch and Rectal Tube** Severe diarrhea may justify the use of a rectal pouch or rectal tube to contain leakage and to protect the surrounding skin. The rectal pouch is a drainable pouch attached to an adhesive skin barrier that conforms to the perianal region. The pouch is attached to the perianal area and any exposed skin surfaces are carefully protected with a skin sealant. Attachment to intact skin is relatively straightforward; however, application to denuded skin is difficult, and consultation with an enterostomal therapist or incontinence nurse specialist is recommended.

The rectal tube is an alternative to the rectal pouch. A larger catheter (30 French) is passed into the rectum and attached to a large bedside drainage bag. Although the rectal tube is effective for short-term use, its safety when used over longer periods of time is uncertain.

### Administer Medications

The medical management of SUI includes both OTC and prescription drugs. OTC medications such as Dexatrim without caffeine and Sudafed contain the α-adrenergic agonists phenylpropanolamine and pseudoephedrine, respectively, which increase urethral sphincter tone and relieve urinary leakage. Nurses teach the client the specific purpose of these medications, and they advise clients to ignore the dosage and scheduling recommendations on the medication container. Instead, the client is taught to take the medication only during waking hours rather than around the clock to reduce the risk of associated insomnia. Potential side effects associated with these medications, such as restlessness and hypertension, are discussed with the client, and blood pressure is monitored regularly.

Stress urinary incontinence also may be managed by prescription medications including imipramine (Tofranil)

and topical estrogens, often administered in combination. The client is taught the dosage and administration of each of these agents. Because imipramine has anticholinergic as well as α-adrenergic effects, clients are advised of additional side effects including dry mouth, the potential for constipation, and mydriasis. Women who are placed on topical or systemic estrogens are advised to seek ongoing care from their gynecologist, including routine vaginal examinations and Papanicolaou (Pap) smears.

Medications are often prescribed for urge urinary incontinence. Anticholinergics or antispasmodics relax detrusor muscle contractions by blocking the action of acetylcholine, by a local anesthetic effect, or by a direct effect on the detrusor muscle. None of these agents will be effective unless the client is taught to adhere to a timed voiding schedule and to identify and limit the intake of bladder irritants.

Several pharmacological agents may be used in the management of urinary retention. Finasteride, a 5-α-reductase inhibitor, is used to reduce prostatic size and related urinary retention. Men who take finasteride are taught the dosage and administration of the drug and its potential side effects, including impotence and loss of libido. Caregivers are cautioned to refrain from handling the drug without gloves, because transdermal absorption and irritation of the skin have been reported.

Alpha-adrenergic blocking agents also may be used to manage urinary retention caused by prostatic hyperplasia, bladder neck dyssynergia, or detrusor striated sphincter dyssynergia. Because of the risk of postural hypotension when the medication reaches a peak plasma level, the client is taught to take these drugs before bedtime. Clients are also taught to monitor for medication side effects, including postural dizziness during waking hours, fatigue, and headache. The significance of titrating the dosage of an α-blocking agent is emphasized, and the client is reminded that the dosage must be retitrated if the medication is inadvertently stopped for a period of more than 72 hours.

### Perform Catheterization

Occasionally, an indwelling urethral or suprapubic catheter may be used to provide continuous drainage. An indwelling catheter may be inserted for an acute episode of urinary retention or when other strategies to manage retention are ineffective. A catheter is chosen that minimizes urethral irritation and maximizes drainage from the bladder. A silicone or other inert-material catheter is preferred over a Silastic catheter coated with Teflon. A Lubricious-coated catheter (Bard Urological, Covington, Georgia) also may be used because of its hydrophilic nature and its low friction coefficient. The client is provided with a drainage bag with adequate storage capacity for overnight use (typically 2,000 ml) and a leg bag with nonlatex straps when indicated.

Procedures 37-3 and 37-4 discuss catheterizations in males and females. Procedures 37-5 and 37-6 discuss irrigation of catheters.

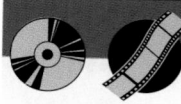

PROCEDURE 37-3  **Inserting an Indwelling Catheter: Male**

## EQUIPMENT NEEDED

- Indwelling or straight catheter with drainage system
- Sterile catheterization kit (Figure 38-17)
- Adequate lighting source
- Disposable gloves
- Blanket or drape
- Soap and washcloth
- Warm water
- Towel
- Forceps

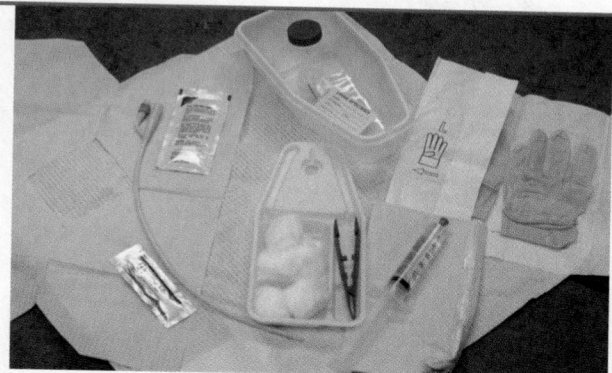

**Figure 37-17** **Catheterization kit**

## IMPLEMENTATION—ACTION/RATIONALE

| ACTION | RATIONALE |
|---|---|
| **Performing Urinary Catheterization** | |
| 1. Gather the equipment needed. Read the label on the catheterization kit. Note if the catheter is included in the kit and, if so, what type it is. Gather any supplies you will need that are not in the prepackaged kit. | 1. Promotes efficiency in the procedure. Kits from various manufacturers come with different equipment. The catheter may or may not be packaged in the kit. Sterile gloves and the urine drainage bag may also need to be gathered separately. |
| 2. Provide for privacy and explain procedure to client. | 2. Promotes cooperation and client dignity. |
| 3. Set the bed to a comfortable height to work, and raise the side rail on the side opposite you. | 3. Promotes proper body mechanics and ensures client safety. |
| 4. Assist the client to a supine position with legs slightly spread (Figure 37-18). | 4. Relaxes muscle and allows visualization of the area to facilitate insertion of the catheter. |
| 5. Drape the client's abdomen and thighs if needed. | 5. Promotes client comfort and warmth. |
| 6. Ensure adequate lighting of the penis and perineal area. | 6. Facilitates proper execution of technique. |
| 7. Wash hands, apply disposable gloves, and wash perineal area. | 7. Reduces transfer of microorganisms. |
| 8. Remove gloves and wash hands. | 8. Reduces transfer of microorganisms. |
| 9. Open the catheterization kit, using aseptic technique. Use the wrapper to establish a sterile field (Figure 37-19). | 9. Provides an area for the sterile equipment to be laid out and assembled. Establish the sterile field close to the client. If the client is able to cooperate, the sterile field can sometimes be established in the open area between the client's legs. |
| 10. If the catheter is not included in the kit, carefully drop the sterile catheter onto the field using aseptic technique. Add any other items needed. | 10. Prevents contamination of the sterile equipment and the sterile field. |

*(continues)*

**PROCEDURE 37-3 (continued)**

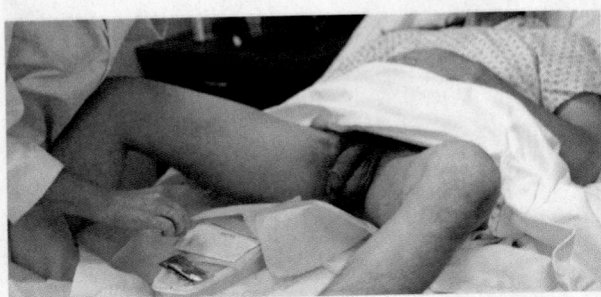

**Figure 37-18    Assist the client to a supine position with legs spread. This allows visualization of the area and relaxes muscles.**

11. Apply sterile gloves. These may be included in the kit.

12. Place the fenestrated drape from the catheterization kit over the client's perineal area with the penis extending through the opening.

13. If inserting a retention catheter, attach the syringe filled with sterile water to the Luer-Lok tail of the catheter. Inflate and deflate the retention balloon. Detach the water-filled syringe (Figure 37-20).

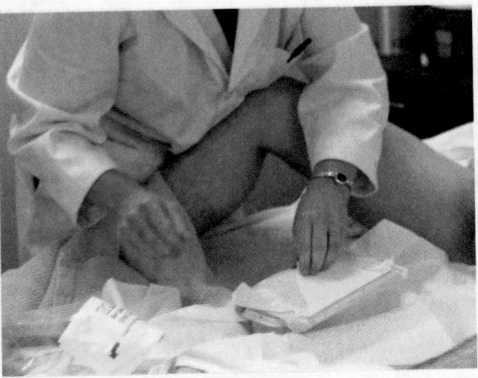

**Figure 37-19    Open the catheterization kit, using the wrapper to establish a sterile field between the client's legs.**

11. Prevents contamination of the sterile equipment and the sterile field.

12. Provides a sterile field at the procedural site. Prevents accidental contamination from adjacent areas.

13. Tests the patency of the retention balloon. Detaching the syringe prevents accidental inflation during catheter insertion.

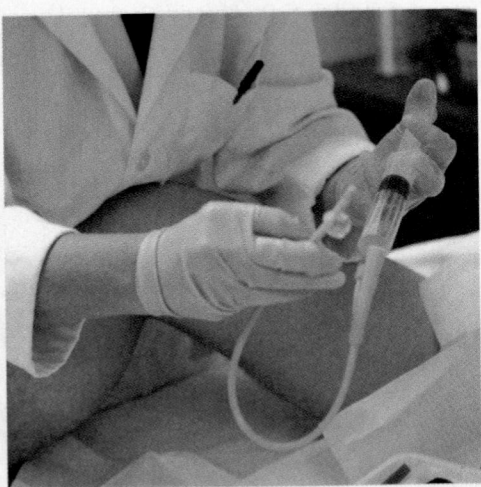

**Figure 37-20    Inflate and deflate the retention balloon to test its patency.**

14. Attach the catheter to the urine drainage bag if it is not preconnected.

14. The catheter and drainage system may be preconnected; otherwise it is connected before catheterization to avoid exposing the client to ascending infection from an open-ended catheter.

*(continues)*

**PROCEDURE 37-3** (*continued*)

15. Generously coat the distal portion of the catheter with water-soluble, sterile lubricant and place it nearby on the sterile field.

15. Facilitates catheter insertion.

16. With your nondominant hand, gently grasp the penis and retract the foreskin (if present). With your dominant hand, cleanse the glans penis with a povidone-iodine solution or other antimicrobial cleanser (Figure 37-21).

16. Removes dirt and minimizes the risk of urinary tract infection by removing surface pathogens.

17. Hold the penis perpendicular to the body and gently pull up.

17. Facilitates catheter insertion by straightening urethra.

18. Inject 10 ml sterile, water-soluble lubricant (use a 2% Xylocaine lubricant whenever feasible) into the urethra.

18. Avoids urethral trauma and discomfort during catheter insertion and facilitates insertion.

19. Holding the catheter in the dominant hand, steadily insert the catheter about 8 inches, until urine is noted in the drainage bag or tubing (Figure 37-22).

19. Provides a visual confirmation that the catheter tip is in the bladder.

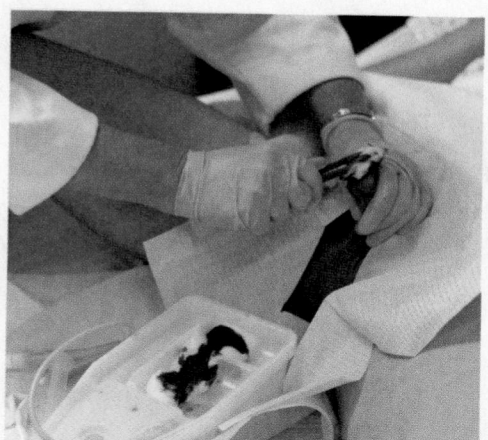

**Figure 37-21    Cleanse the glans penis with a povidone-iodine solution.**

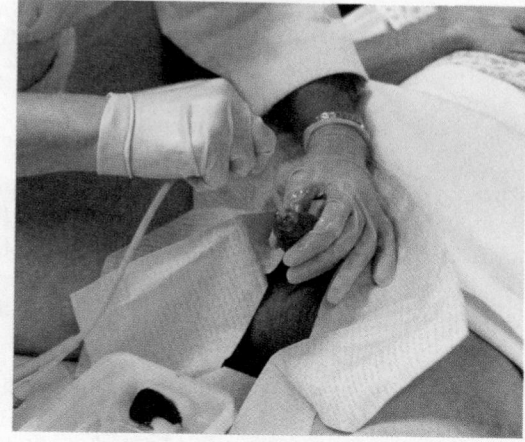

**Figure 37-22    Steadily insert the catheter.**

20. If the catheter will be removed as soon as the client's bladder is empty, insert the catheter another inch, place the penis in a comfortable position, and hold the catheter in place as the bladder drains into a sterile receptacle.

20. The catheter needs to be inserted far enough to allow complete bladder drainage, but not so far as to possibly irritate the bladder, causing spasms.

21. If the catheter will be indwelling with a retention balloon, continue inserting until the hub of the catheter (bifurcation between drainage port and retention balloon arm) is met (Figure 37-23).

21. Ensures adequate catheter insertion before retention balloon is inflated.

22. Reattach the water-filled syringe to the inflation port.

22. Provides a sterile method of inflating the retention balloon.

(*continues*)

**PROCEDURE 37-3 (*continued*)**

23. Inflate the retention balloon with sterile water per manufacturer's recommendations or the physician's or qualified practitioner's orders (Figure 37-24).

23. Ensures retention of the balloon. Retention catheters are available with a variety of balloon sizes. Use a catheter with the appropriate size balloon.

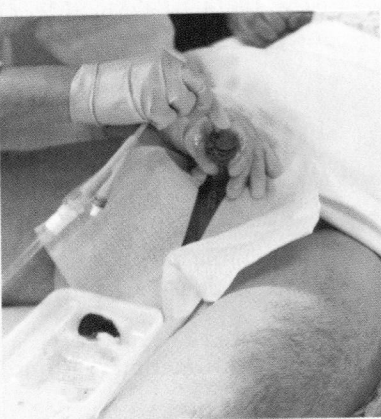

**Figure 37-23** Continue inserting the catheter until the bifurcation between the drainage port and the retention balloon reaches the end of the penis. This ensures the retention balloon will be fully in the bladder prior to inflation.

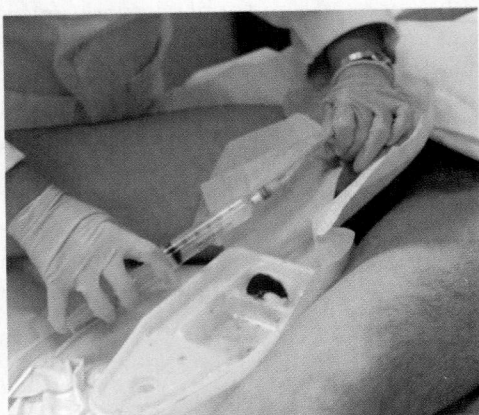

**Figure 37-24** Inflate the retention balloon.

24. Instruct the client to immediately report discomfort or pressure during balloon inflation; if pain occurs, discontinue the procedure, deflate the balloon, and insert the catheter farther into the bladder. If the client continues to complain of pain with balloon inflation, remove the catheter and notify the client's qualified practitioner.

24. Pain or pressure indicates inflation of the balloon in the urethra; further insertion will prevent misplacement and further pain or bleeding.

25. Once the balloon has been inflated, gently pull the catheter until the retention balloon is resting snug against the bladder neck (resistance will be felt when the balloon is properly seated).

25. Maximizes continuous bladder drainage and prevents urine leakage around the catheter.

26. Secure the catheter according to institutional policy. Securing it to either the client's thigh or abdomen is generally acceptable.

26. Prevents excessive traction from the balloon rubbing against the bladder neck, inadvertent catheter removal, or urethral erosion.

27. Place the drainage bag below the level of the bladder. Do not let it rest on the floor (Figures 37-25 and 37-26). Secure the drainage tubing to prevent pulling on the tubing and the catheter.

27. Maximizes continuous drainage of urine from the bladder (drainage is prevented when the drainage bag is placed above the abdomen).

28. Remove gloves, dispose of equipment, and wash hands.

28. Prevents transfer of microorganisms.

29. Help client adjust position. Lower the bed.

29. Promotes client comfort and safety.

30. Assess and document the amount, color, odor, and quality of urine.

30. Monitors urinary status.

*(continues)*

**PROCEDURE 37-3** (*continued*)

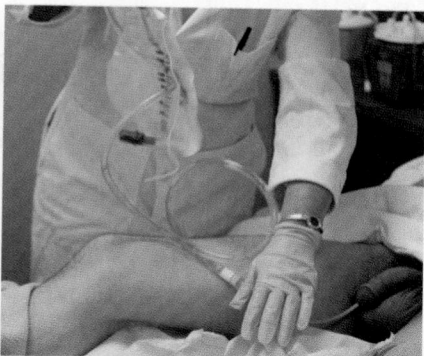

**Figure 37-25**   Place the drainage bag tubing over the leg.

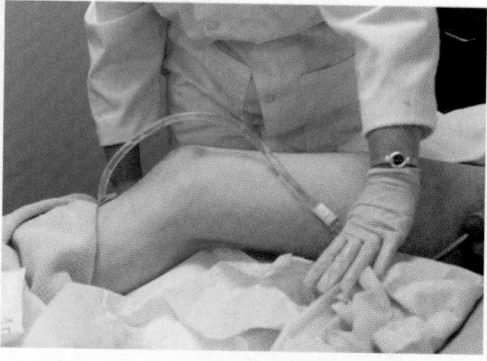

**Figure 37-26**   Place the drainage bag below the level of the bladder, but do not rest it on the floor.

 ## LIFE SPAN CONSIDERATIONS

### Indwelling Catheter: Male

**Pediatric Variations**

- Children need the support of a parent, who can also help the child hold the position and provide distraction during the procedure.

**Geriatric Variations**

- Geriatric clients may need help holding the correct position.
- Anatomical landmarks may be more difficult to visualize in an older client.

## COMMUNITY/HOME CARE

### Indwelling Catheter: Male

**Home Care Variations**

- If the client will be catheterized at home, go over the catheterization technique step by step to determine how it will be accomplished in the home setting. For example, will the procedure be done in bed, on a couch, or in the bathroom? Where will clean supplies be obtained and stored? How will the procedure be assessed and documented. Is urine testing needed?
- Emphasize the need for good handwashing, cleaning of the catheter, and adequate lubrication of the catheter to reduce the frequency of infection and urethral trauma.

**Long-Term Care Variations**

- Clients who practice long-term self-catheterization may use clean, instead of sterile, technique to catheterize themselves. Reinforce the need for good handwashing and cleaning of the catheter and adequate lubrication of the catheter to reduce the frequency of infection and urethral trauma.

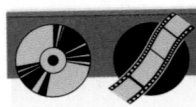

**PROCEDURE 37-4**    **Inserting an Indwelling Catheter: Female**

## EQUIPMENT NEEDED

- Indwelling or straight catheter with drainage system
- Sterile catheterization kit (Figure 37-27)
- Adequate lighting source
- Disposable clean gloves
- Blanket or drape
- Soap and washcloth
- Warm water
- Towel

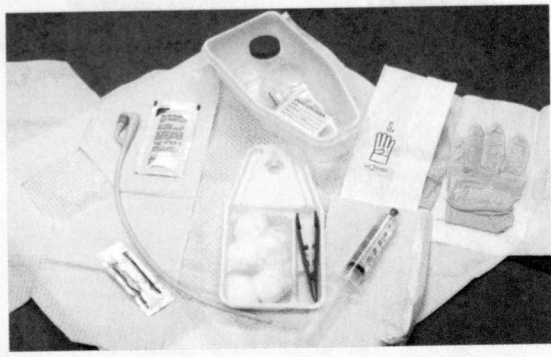

Figure 37-27    **Catheterization kit**

## IMPLEMENTATION—ACTION/RATIONALE

| ACTION | RATIONALE |
|---|---|
| **Performing Urinary Catheterization** | |
| 1. Gather the equipment needed. Read the label on the catheterization kit. Note if the catheter is included in the kit and, if so, what type it is. Gather any supplies you will need that are not in the prepackaged kit. | 1. Promotes efficiency in the procedure. Kits from various manufacturers come with different equipment. The catheter may or may not be packaged in the kit. Sterile gloves and the urine drainage bag may also need to be gathered separately. |
| 2. Provide for privacy and explain procedure to client. Assess for allergy to povidone-iodine. | 2. Promotes cooperation and client dignity. |
| 3. Set the bed to a comfortable height to work, and raise the side rail on the side opposite you. | 3. Promotes proper body mechanics and ensures client safety. |
| 4. Assist the client to a supine position with legs spread and feet together or to a side-lying position with upper leg flexed (Figure 37-28). | 4. Relaxes muscles and allows visualization of the area to facilitate insertion of the catheter. |

Figure 37-28    **Position the client supine with legs spread.**

| | |
|---|---|
| 5. Drape the client's abdomen and thighs for warmth if needed. | 5. Promotes client comfort and warmth. |

*(continues)*

**PROCEDURE 37-4 (continued)**

6.  Ensure adequate lighting of the perineal area.

7.  Wash hands and apply disposable gloves.

8.  Wash perineal area.

9.  Remove gloves and wash hands.

10. Open the catheterization kit, using aseptic technique. Use the wrapper to establish a sterile field (Figure 37-29).

11. If the catheter is not included in the kit, drop the sterile catheter onto the field using aseptic technique. Add any other items needed.

12. Apply sterile gloves. These may be included in the kit.

13. If inserting a retention catheter, attach the syringe filled with sterile water to the Luer-Lok tail of the catheter. Inflate and deflate the retention balloon. Detach the water-filled syringe.

14. Attach the catheter to the urine drainage bag if it is not preconnected.

15. Generously coat the distal portion of the catheter with water-soluble, sterile lubricant and place it nearby on the sterile field (Figure 37-30).

6.  Facilitates proper execution of technique.

7.  Reduces transfer of microorganisms.

8.  Reduces transfer of microorganisms.

9.  Reduces transfer of microorganisms.

10. Provides an area for the sterile equipment to be laid out and assembled. Establish the sterile field close to the client. If the client is able to cooperate, the sterile field can sometimes be established in the open area between the client's legs.

11. Prevents contamination of the sterile equipment and the sterile field.

12. Prevents contamination of the sterile equipment and the sterile field.

13. Tests the patency of the retention balloon. Detaching the syringe prevents accidental inflation during catheter insertion.

14. The catheter and drainage system may be preconnected; otherwise connect it before catheterization to avoid exposing the client to ascending infection from an open-ended catheter.

15. Facilitates catheter insertion.

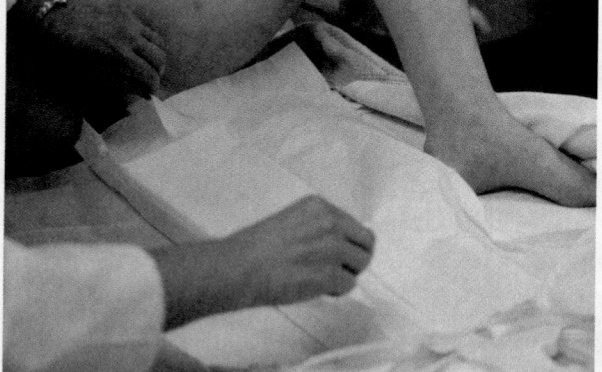

**Figure 37-29   Open the catheterization kit, using the wrapper to establish a sterile field between the client's legs.**

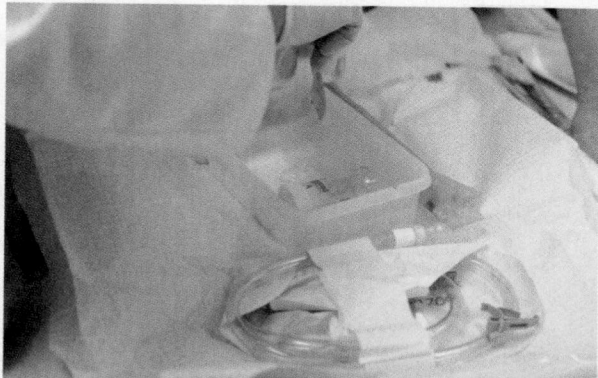

**Figure 37-30    Open the lubrication package and squeeze lubricant onto the sterile field where it will be used to lubricate the catheter.**

16. Place the fenestrated drape from the catheterization kit over the client's perineal area with the labia visible through the opening.

16. Provides a sterile field at the procedural site. Prevents accidental contamination from adjacent areas.

*(continues)*

## PROCEDURE 37-4 (*continued*)

17. Gently spread the labia minora with the fingers of your nondominant hand and visualize the urinary meatus (Figure 37-31).

18. Holding the labia apart with your nondominant hand, use the forceps to pick up a cotton ball soaked in povidone-iodine, and cleanse the peri-urethral mucosa. Use one downward stroke for each cotton ball and dispose. Keep the labia separated with your nondominant hand until you insert the catheter (Figure 37-32).

17. Helps locate the meatus, so the catheter can be placed in the correct spot.

18. Cleans the area and minimizes the risk of urinary tract infection by removing surface pathogens.

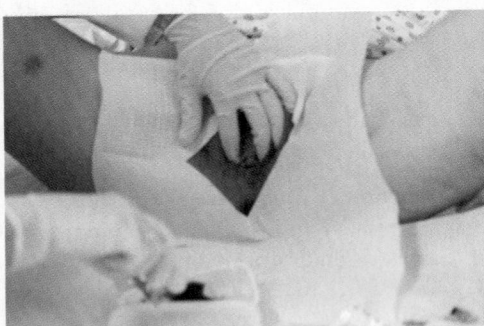

**Figure 37-31    Spread the labia minora and visualize the urinary meatus.**

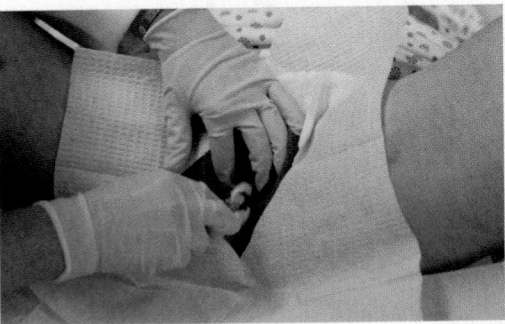

**Figure 37-32    Using forceps, pick up a cotton ball soaked in povidone-iodine. Cleanse the peri-urethral mucosa.**

19. Holding the catheter in the dominant hand, steadily insert the catheter into the meatus until urine is noted in the drainage bag or tubing (Figure 37-33).

20. If the catheter will be removed as soon as the client's bladder is empty, insert the catheter another inch and hold the catheter in place as the bladder drains into a sterile receptacle.

21. If the catheter will be indwelling with a retention balloon, continue inserting another 1 to 3 inches.

22. Reattach the water-filled syringe to the inflation port.

23. Inflate the retention balloon using manufacturer's recommendations or according to the physician's or qualified practitioner's orders (Figure 37-34).

24. Instruct the client to immediately report discomfort or pressure during balloon inflation; if pain occurs, discontinue the procedure, deflate the balloon, and insert the catheter farther into the bladder. If the client continues to complain of pain with balloon inflation, remove the catheter and notify the client's qualified practitioner.

19. Provides a visual confirmation that the catheter tip is in the bladder.

20. The catheter needs to be inserted far enough to allow complete bladder drainage, but not so far as to possibly irritate the bladder, causing spasms.

21. Ensures adequate catheter insertion before retention balloon is inflated.

22. Provides a sterile method of inflating the retention balloon.

23. Ensures retention of the balloon. Retention catheters are available with a variety of balloon sizes. Use a catheter with the appropriate size balloon.

24. Pain or pressure indicates inflation of the balloon in the urethra; further insertion will prevent misplacement and further pain or bleeding.

*(continues)*

**PROCEDURE 37-4** (*continued*)

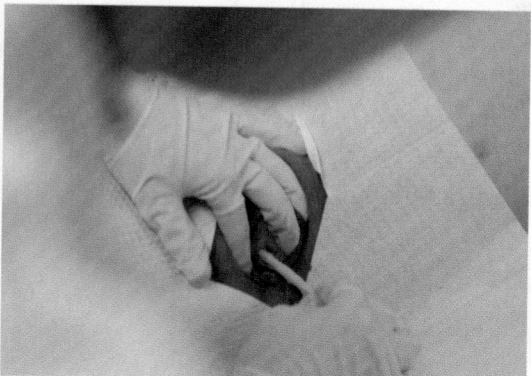

**Figure 37-33**   Steadily insert the catheter into the meatus.

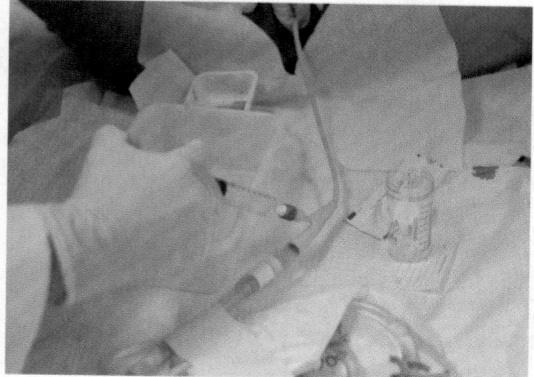

**Figure 37-34**   Inflate the retention balloon.

25. Once the balloon has been inflated, gently pull the catheter until the retention balloon is resting snug against the bladder neck (resistance will be felt when the balloon is properly seated).

26. Tape the catheter to the abdomen or thigh snugly, yet with enough slack so it will not pull on the bladder (Figure 37-35).

27. Place the drainage bag below the level of the bladder. Do not let it rest on the floor. Make sure the tubing lies over, not under, the leg.

28. Remove gloves, dispose of equipment, and wash hands.

29. Help client adjust position. Lower the bed.

30. Assess and document the amount, color, odor, and quality of urine (Figure 37-36).

31. Wash hands.

25. Maximizes continuous bladder drainage and prevents urine leakage around the catheter.

26. Prevents excessive traction from the balloon rubbing against the bladder neck, inadvertent catheter removal, or urethral erosion.

27. Maximizes continuous drainage of urine from the bladder (drainage is prevented when the drainage bag is placed above the abdomen).

28. Prevents transfer of microorganisms.

29. Promotes client comfort and safety.

30. Monitors urinary status.

31. Reduces transmission of microorganisms.

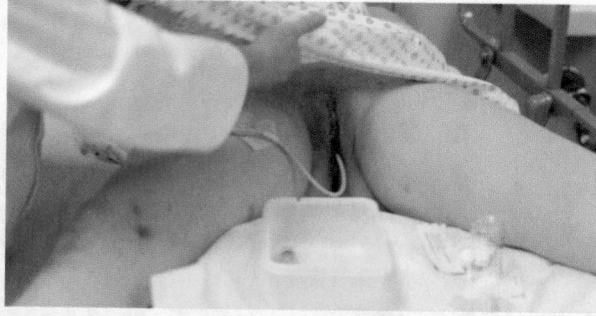

**Figure 37-35**   Tape the catheter to the client's thigh.

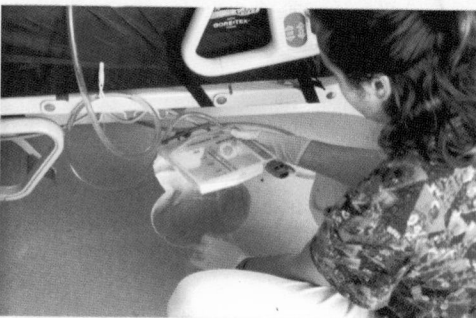

**Figure 37-36**   Monitor the urinary status. Assess and document the amount, color, and quality of urine.

## LIFE SPAN CONSIDERATIONS

### Indwelling Catheter: Female

#### Pediatric Variations

- When a catheter is used with a child or adolescent, provide simple explanations.
- Allow for privacy and respect the child's or adolescent's wishes regarding the presence of a parent during catheter insertion and care.
- Children or adolescents may be more tempted to pull or tug on the catheter. Children and adolescents may be more active in or out of bed, so the catheter must be taped securely to the thigh to prevent it from being pulled out.

#### Geriatric Variations

- Geriatric clients may need help holding the position.
- Anatomical landmarks may be more difficult to visualize.
- It is important to clearly explain the procedure and check that client understands.

## COMMUNITY/HOME CARE

### Indwelling Catheter: Female

#### Home Care Variations

- Clients who practice long-term self-catheterization may use clean, instead of sterile, technique to catheterize themselves. Reinforce the need for good handwashing, cleaning of the catheter, and adequate lubrication of the catheter to reduce the frequency of infection and urethral trauma.

#### Long-Term Care Variations

- Follow institutional policy regarding the long-term use and replacement schedule for an indwelling catheter.

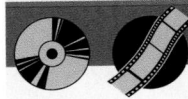 **PROCEDURE 37-5**    ## Irrigating a Urinary Catheter

### EQUIPMENT NEEDED

- Sterile gloves (Figure 37-37)
- Sterile cover for the end of the drainage tubing
- Disposable, water-resistant drape or towel
- Sterile asepto or Toomey syringe with container for irrigant
- Sterile antiseptic swabs
- Sterile irrigating solution (labeled with date and time of opening, if opened)

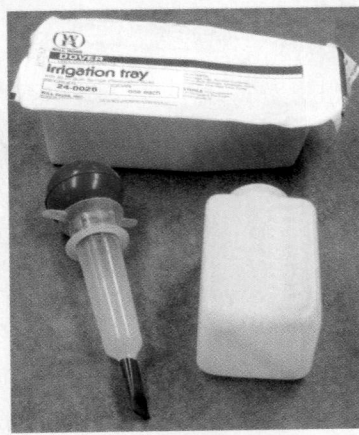

**Figure 37-37    Irrigation kit**

*(continues)*

**PROCEDURE 37-5 (continued)**

## IMPLEMENTATION—ACTION/RATIONALE

| ACTION | RATIONALE |
|---|---|
| 1. Verify the need for bladder or catheter irrigation. | 1. Ensures that procedure is being applied correctly, to reduce unnecessary opening of the system and risk of infection. |
| 2. For prn catheter irrigation, palpate for full bladder and check current output against previous totals. | 2. If irrigation is on a prn basis, may not be needed currently. |
| 3. Verify physician's or qualified practitioner's orders for type of irrigation and irrigant as well as amount. | 3. Ensures accuracy in the provision of treatment. |
| 4. If repeat procedure, read previous documentation in the record. | 4. Establishes prior client responses to prior teaching done by staff. |
| 5. Assemble all supplies. | 5. Having all supplies in room enables the nurse to maintain sterility of supplies once they are opened and laid out. |
| 6. Premedicate client if ordered or needed. | 6. Increases comfort for the procedure. |
| 7. Provide teaching to the client as needed, based on what client already knows. | 7. Knowledge will increase patient cooperation and decrease anxiety. |
| 8. Assist the client to a dorsal recumbent position. | 8. Facilitates the flow of irrigant into the bladder. |
| 9. Wash your hands. | 9. Decreases transmission of microorganisms. |
| 10. Provide for client privacy with a closed door or curtain. | 10. Decreases patient anxiety. |
| 11. Empty the collection bag of urine. | 11. Starting with an empty collection bag makes it easier to identify clots or sediment passed as a result of irrigation. |
| 12. Expose the retention catheter, and place the water-resistant drape underneath it (Figures 37-38 and 37-39). | 12. Protects the bedclothes and client from urine and body fluids. |

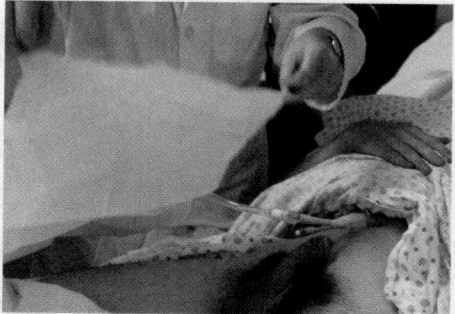

**Figure 37-38    Expose the retention catheter.**

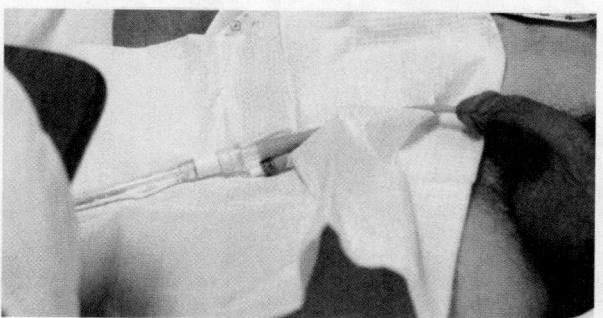

**Figure 37-39    Place a water-resistant drape under the retention catheter.**

*(continues)*

## PROCEDURE 37-5 (*continued*)

13. Open the sterile syringe and container. Stand it up carefully in or on the wrapper and add 100–200 cc sterile diluent without touching or contaminating the tip of the syringe or the inside of the receptacle.

13. Enables nurse to maintain sterility of gloves once they are applied.

14. Open the end of the antiseptic swab package, exposing the swab sticks.

14. Enables nurse to maintain sterility of gloves once they are applied.

15. Open the sterile cover for drainage tube.

15. Enables nurse to maintain sterility of gloves once they are applied.

16. Apply the sterile gloves.

16. Maintains sterility of the procedure.

17. Disinfect the connection between the catheter and the drainage tubing.

17. Minimizes risk of contaminating the system.

18. After the disinfectant dries, loosen the ends of the connection.

18. Enables the nurse to open the connection without accidently contaminating either end.

19. Grasp the catheter and tubing 1 to 2 inches from their ends, catheter in the nondominant hand.

19. Maintains sterility of the procedure and allows the nurse to be positioned to use the dominant hand for the syringe.

20. Fold the catheter to pinch it closed between the palm and last three fingers; use the thumb and first finger to hold the sterile cap for the drainage tube.

20. Allows for a single nurse to handle all equipment simultaneously, maintaining sterility.

21. Separate the catheter and tube, covering the tube tightly with the sterile cap.

21. Maintains sterility of equipment.

22. Fill the syringe with 30 cc for catheter irrigation, 60 cc for bladder irrigation. Insert the tip of the syringe into the catheter and gently instill the solution into the catheter (Figures 37-40 and 37-41).

22. Catheter can be irrigated with 30 cc of solution, minimizing bladder discomfort, while irrigating a bladder would take 60 cc.

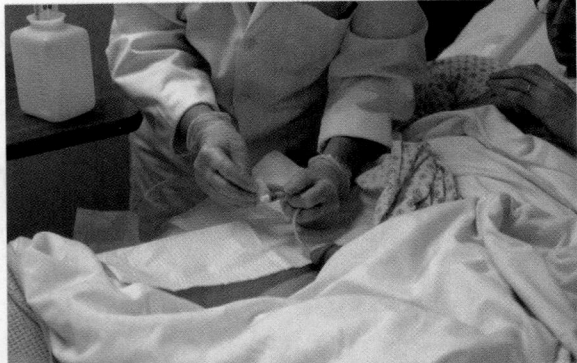

**Figure 37-40    Separate the catheter and tube.**

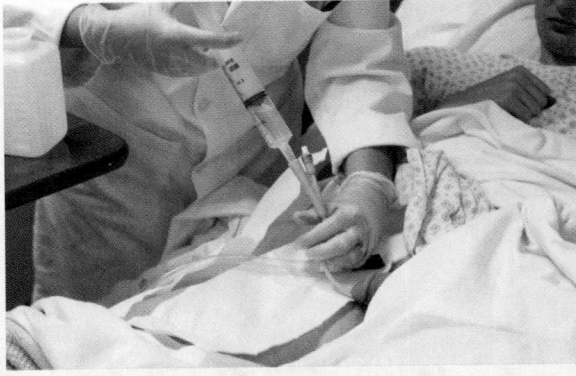

**Figure 37-41    Insert the tip of the syringe into the catheter and gently instill the solution.**

23. Clamp catheter if ordered (medicated solution). If not clamped, irrigant may be released into a collection container or aspirated back into the syringe (Figure 37-42).

23. Fine sediment or clear irrigant with medication can run freely; material with more solids (sediment or clots) may need gentle aspiration.

*(continues)*

**PROCEDURE 37-5 (*continued*)**

24. If the bladder or catheter is being irrigated to clear solid material, repeat irrigation until return is clear.

24. Clearing the catheter completely in this irrigation means a lower total number of irrigations and less opening of the system, decreasing the risk of infection.

25. Reconnect system and remove sterile gloves. Wash your hands (Figure 37-43).

25. Maintains sterility of system and reduces transmission of microorganisms.

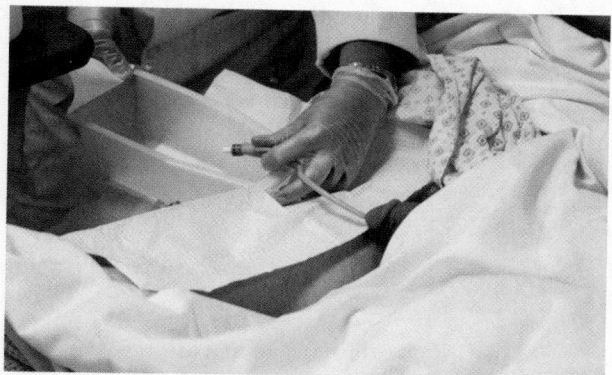

**Figure 37-42**   **Irrigant is released into a collection container.**

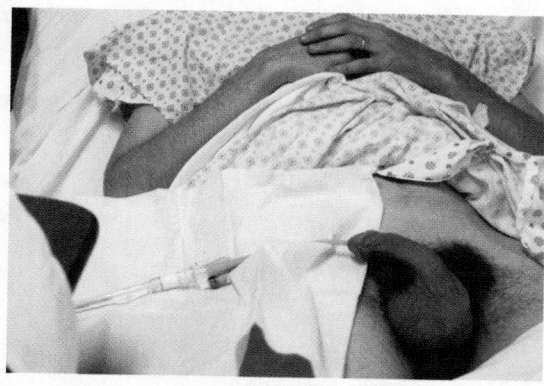

**Figure 37-43**   **Reconnect the tubing to the catheter.**

26. When irrigation is finished, chart type of returns and total amount of irrigation fluid used.

26. This information can be compared to evaluate status of the urinary tract and catheter. A catheter that is being frequently irrigated for sediment, for instance, may need to be changed, or medications may need to be adjusted.

27. Monitor client for pain, urine color and clarity, any solid material passed, and total intake and output.

27. Monitoring output after irrigation evaluates the efficacy of the treatment.

 **LIFE SPAN CONSIDERATIONS**

### Irrigating Urinary Catheters

#### *Pediatric Variations*

- Use very small volumes, as children's bladders are smaller than adults.
- Use plain language that young children can understand ("pee," not *urinate*, for instance). A demonstration doll is useful to explain the procedure to younger children.

#### *Geriatric Variations*

- Geriatric clients are most likely to have poor oral intakes; assess intake and output (I&O) carefully, especially if the bladder is not palpable, before deciding to irrigate.
- Be very slow and clear about discussing the procedure with older clients to facilitate their understanding of what will be done. Take another nurse if the older client is demented or confused.
- Use smaller volumes to irrigate as bladder capacity and sphincter tone are decreased.

## COMMUNITY/HOME CARE

### Irrigation of a Urinary Catheter

**Home Care Variations**

- Irrigation setups (syringes and containers) can be washed in very hot water and boiled for 20 minutes if sterility is desired, to reduce costs for the home care client.

- The person performing the irrigation must notify the nurse if there are any changes in the amount or character of returns when irrigating, as it can indicate bladder or systemic changes.

- Caretakers must be able to use whatever thermometer at hand to correctly take a temperature and should call the home care nurse for temperatures over 100.5°F, as infection may be beginning.

- Any severe lower back pain should be reported, as it may indicate a kidney infection.

**Long-Term Care Variations**

- Agitation in an older clients can be associated with bladder pressure, so irrigation may help open the catheter.

- Another possible cause of agitation in an older client can be infection, which may have resulted from poor technique.

- Remember to offer fluids that the client likes to facilitate proper intake; do not use irrigation for a substitute for proper hydration.

---

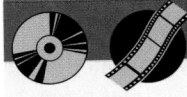 **PROCEDURE 37-6**

### Irrigating the Bladder Using a Closed-System Catheter

#### EQUIPMENT NEEDED

- Three-way indwelling catheter or Y adapter (Figure 37-44)
- IV pole
- Ordered irrigating solution
- Sterile gloves
- Closed-irrigation tubing
- Large urine drainage bag
- Antiseptic swabs

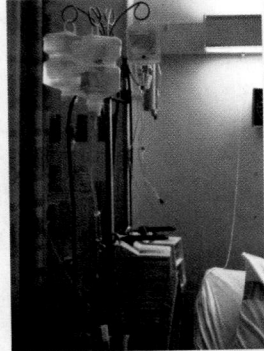

**Figure 37-44** IV pole, irrigating solution, and irrigation tubing are used to irrigate the bladder using a closed-system catheter.

#### IMPLEMENTATION—ACTION/RATIONALE

| ACTION | RATIONALE |
|---|---|
| **Intermittent Bladder Irrigation Using a Standard Retention Catheter and a Y Adapter** | |
| 1. Close privacy curtain or door. | 1. Provides privacy. |

*(continues)*

## PROCEDURE 37-6 (*continued*)

2. Wash hands.

3. Hang the prescribed irrigation solution from an IV pole.

4. Insert the clamped irrigation tubing into the bottle of irrigant and prime the tubing with fluid, expelling all air and reclamping the tube.

5. Prepare sterile antiseptic swabs and sterile Y connector if one will be used.

6. Apply sterile gloves.

7. Clamp the urinary catheter.

8. Unhook the drainage bag from the retention catheter.

9. While holding the drainage tubing and the drainage port of the catheter in your nondominant hand, cleanse both the tubing and the port with antiseptic swabs.

10. Connect one port of the Y adapter to the drainage port of the retention catheter.

11. Connect another port of the Y adapter to the drainage tubing and bag.

12. Attach the third port of the Y adapter to the irrigant tubing.

13. Unclamp the urinary catheter and establish that urine is draining through the catheter into the drainage bag.

14. To irrigate the catheter and bladder, clamp the drainage tubing distal to the Y adapter.

15. Infuse the prescribed amount of irrigant.

16. Clamp the irrigant tubing (Figure 37-45).

2. Prevents the spread of microorganisms.

3. Different solutions may be ordered depending on the results the physician or qualified practitioner desires. Bladder irrigant is generally packaged in 2,000- to 4,000-ml bottles.

4. Prevents introduction of air into the bladder.

5. Prevents contamination of sterile gloves and field.

6. Minimizes the client's risk of infection when connecting the irrigant to the catheter and drainage system.

7. Prevents urine leakage onto the bed linens.

8. Allows the Y adapter to be inserted into the system.

9. Prevents contamination and infection.

10. Provides a bifurcation for irrigant to infuse as well as urine to drain.

11. Collects the urine and drained irrigant. This may be the established urine drainage bag or a new, sterile bag that is large enough to hold the increased volume of drainage.

12. Infuses the irrigant into the closed system.

13. If the urine does not flow freely after unclamping, the catheter may have become clogged with a clot or debris. Notify the client's physician or qualified practitioner of the lack of urine drainage.

14. Prevents the irrigant from bypassing the bladder and flowing directly into the drainage bag.

15. The bladder normally feels full when it contains approximately 300 cc of urine. If a prescribed amount of irrigant was not ordered, do not infuse more than 150 cc of irrigant. If the client has undergone bladder surgery, do not infuse irrigant without knowing the specific amount ordered.

16. Prevents further infusion of irrigant.

*(continues)*

## PROCEDURE 37-6 *(continued)*

17. If the physician or qualified practitioner has ordered the irrigant to remain in the bladder for a measured length of time, wait the prescribed length of time.

17. Some irrigation solutions contain medication and are meant to remain in contact with the bladder wall for a prescribed length of time.

18. Unclamp the drainage tubing and monitor the drainage as it flows into the drainage bag.

18. Assess the drainage for volume, color, clarity, and the presence of any clots or debris.

### Closed Bladder Irrigation Using a Three-Way Catheter

19. Close privacy curtain or door.

19. Provides privacy.

20. Wash hands.

20. Reduces transmission of microorganisms.

21. Explain the procedure to the client. Answer questions and provide support.

21. Reduces anxiety and uncertainty associated with the procedure.

22. Hang the prescribed irrigation solution from an IV pole.

22. Different solutions may be ordered depending on the results desired. Bladder irrigant is generally packaged in 2,000- to 4,000-ml bottles.

23. Insert the clamped irrigation tubing into the bottle of irrigant and prime the tubing with fluid, expelling all air and reclamping the tube (Figure 37-46).

23. Prevents introduction of air into the bladder.

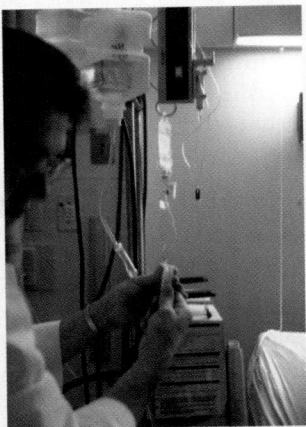

**Figure 37-45    Clamp the irrigant tubing.**

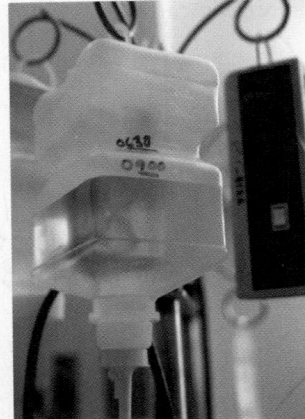

**Figure 37-46    Insert the clamped irrigation tubing into the bottle of irrigant.**

24. Prepare sterile antiseptic swabs and any other sterile equipment needed.

24. Prevents contamination of sterile gloves and field.

25. Apply sterile gloves (Figure 37-47).

25. Minimizes the client's risk of infection when connecting the irrigant to the catheter and drainage system.

26. Clamp the urinary catheter.

26. Prevents leakage of urine onto the bedclothes.

27. Remove the cap from the irrigation port of the three-way catheter (Figure 37-48).

27. Allows access for the irrigant tubing.

*(continues)*

**PROCEDURE 37-6 (continued)**

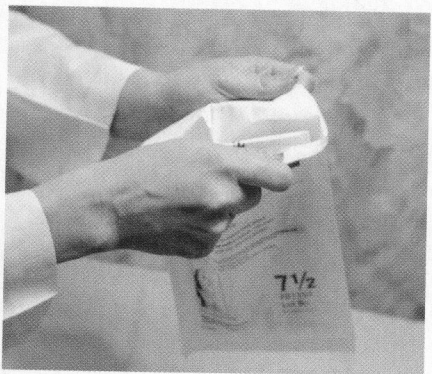

Figure 37-47　**Apply sterile gloves.**

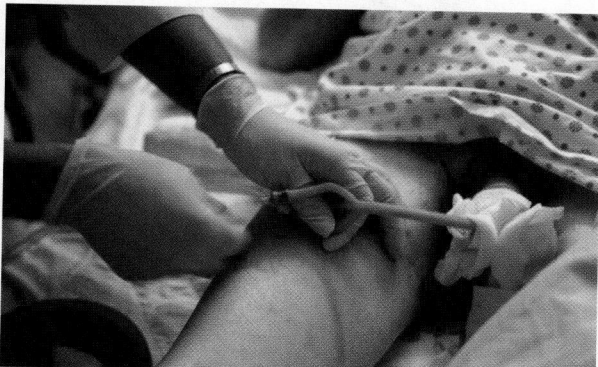

Figure 37-48　**Remove the cap from the irrigation port of the three-way catheter.**

28. Cleanse the irrigation port with the sterile antiseptic swabs.

29. Attach the irrigation tubing to the irrigation port of the three-way catheter.

30. Remove the clamp from the catheter and observe for urine drainage (Figure 37-49).

28. Minimizes the risk of infection.

29. Introduces the irrigant into the system.

30. Ensures catheter remains patent after being clamped. Some surgical procedures can cause bleeding and clotting of the catheter.

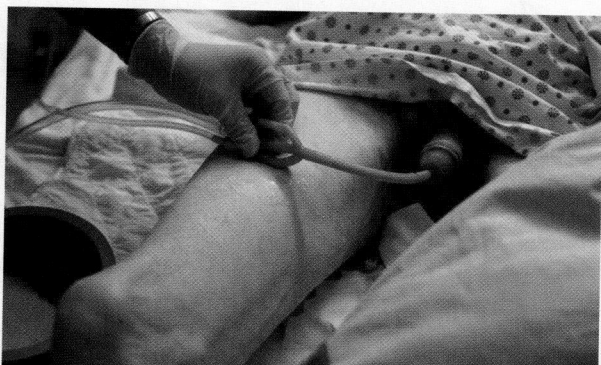

Figure 37-49　**Attach the irrigation tubing, remove the clamp from the catheter, and observe for urine drainage. Carefully observe the drainage for color, clarity, and the presence of debris.**

*If intermittent irrigation has been ordered:*

31. Infuse the prescribed amount of irrigant.

31. The bladder normally feels full when it contains approximately 300 cc of urine. If a prescribed amount of irrigant was not ordered, do not infuse more than 150 cc of irrigant. If the client has undergone bladder surgery, do not infuse irrigant without knowing the specific amount ordered.

32. Clamp the irrigant tubing.

32. Prevents further infusion of irrigant.

*(continues)*

## PROCEDURE 37-6 (*continued*)

33. If the physician or qualified practitioner has ordered the irrigant to remain in the bladder for a measured length of time, clamp the drainage tube prior to infusing the irrigant and wait the prescribed length of time.

34. Monitor the drainage as it flows into the drainage bag.

*If continuous bladder irrigation has been ordered:*

35. Adjust the clamp on the irrigation tubing to allow the prescribed rate of irrigant to flow into the catheter and bladder.

36. Monitor the drainage for color, clarity, debris, and volume as it flows back into the drainage bag.

37. Tape the catheter securely to the thigh (Figure 37-50).

33. Some irrigation solutions contain medication and are meant to remain in contact with the bladder wall for a prescribed length of time.

34. Assesses the drainage for volume, color, clarity, and the presence of any clots or debris.

35. Regulates the amount of irrigant flowing in and out of the bladder to prevent distention or damage to any surgical site.

36. Assesses for bleeding, clotting, and blockage of urine drainage or other complications.

37. Prevents the catheter from becoming dislodged.

**Figure 37-50** **Securely tape the catheter to the thigh to prevent it from becoming dislodged.**

38. Wash hands.

38. Reduces transmission of microorganisms.

## LIFE SPAN CONSIDERATIONS

### Bladder Irrigation Considerations

**Pediatric Variations**

- Children have much smaller bladders and require smaller amounts of irrigant.
- Children have smaller bladders and a catheter is more prone to plug with mucus or clots. The patency of the catheter and the first signs of bladder distention must be carefully watched for.
- Children may be very embarrassed regarding bladder irrigation and monitoring for clots or distention. Be sure to provide privacy and explanations to allay their fears and embarrassment.

**Geriatric Variations**

- Older clients may have a larger amount of debris in their urine. Their urine/irrigant output must be monitored closely for potential blockages or retention.

## Intermittent Self-Catheterization

Women with reflex incontinence have more-limited options for management because no effective condom device has been designed for women. Intermittent self-catheterization is chosen whenever feasible. This option is typically used in combination with pharmacotherapy for detrusor hyper-reflexia. Indwelling catheterization is used only when other means of bladder management are not feasible.

Of the bladder management programs available for the client with a spinal injury, multiple sclerosis, or reflex incontinence, intermittent self-catheterization is preferred when feasible. The nurse teaches the client with adequate upper extremity dexterity to perform self-catheterization, and the skill is also taught to significant others. Pharmacotherapy, consisting of an anticholinergic agent, imipramine, or (rarely) a calcium channel blocker, is frequently required to control hyperreflexic detrusor contractions.

## Administer Enemas

Enema administration is a procedure used to introduce fluid into the lower bowel. The purpose of an enema is to cleanse the lower bowel, to assist in the evacuation of stool or flatus, or to instill medication. Table 37-10 outlines four types of enemas, along with the solutions and the indications for use of each.

Enemas can be large or small depending on their purpose. Large-volume enemas, which typically contain 500–1,000 ml fluid, are administered to cleanse the bowel. Small-volume enemas are used for the purpose of evacuating stool or instilling medications in the lower bowel. These are usually found as prepackaged solutions, which contain 150–240 ml fluid. Refer to Procedure 37-7 for guidelines on enema administration.

Caution should be used when administering large-volume enemas, because fluid and electrolyte imbalance

can occur. This is related to the volume, frequency, and type of solution used. Table 37-11 lists the types of enema solutions and their effects.

## Initiate Rectal Stimulation

As an alternative to a scheduled defecation program, digital rectal stimulation may be used to regulate fecal elimination

---

### COMMUNITY/HOME CARE

#### Administering an Enema in the Home Environment

Clients in home settings often self-administer small-volume enemas. These clients should be taught that these small enemas come premixed in their own receptacles containing about 150–240 ml solution. In addition, the home care client should be informed that mini-enemas usually contain 4–10 ml liquid. The clients should be instructed to call for assistance immediately if light-headedness, dizziness, or faint feelings occur.

Altman, G. (2004). *Delmar's fundamental & advanced nursing skills* (2nd ed.). Clifton Park, NY: Delmar Learning.

---

### TABLE 37-10    TYPES OF ENEMAS

| Type | Solution | Indication |
| --- | --- | --- |
| Cleansing | Tap water<br>Soap suds<br>Normal saline | Evacuate lower bowel before diagnostic studies or surgery |
| Retention (should be retained for at least 30 min) | Emollient (oil) | Soften and lubricate stool for easy evacuation |
| Carminative (return flow) | Tap water<br>Normal saline | Relief of distension due to flatus |
| Medication | Normal saline<br>Sterile water mixed with prescribed medication | Will depend on what medication is introduced |

---

### TABLE 37-11    SOLUTIONS USED FOR ENEMAS

| Solution | Action | Class |
| --- | --- | --- |
| Tap water | Stimulates, dilates bowel | Hypotonic |
| Soap suds | Dilates, stimulates, and irritates bowel | Hypotonic |
| Normal saline | Dilates, simulates, irritates bowel | 0.9% (isotonic)<br>< 0.9% (hypotonic)<br>> 0.9% (hypertonic) |
| Oil | Lubricates, softens | |
| Sodium polystyrene sulfonate (Kayexalate) | Medication reduces serum potassium | Hypertonic |
| Antibiotic | Cleansing | Antibacterial, may be hypertonic or hypotonic |

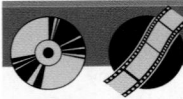

## PROCEDURE 37-7    Administering an Enema

### EQUIPMENT NEEDED

*Large Volume, Cleansing Enema*

- Absorbent pad for the bed (Figure 37-51)
- Disposable gloves
- Bedside commode or bedpan if client will not be able to ambulate to bathroom (Figure 38-52)
- Lubricant
- Enema container
- Tubing with clamp and nozzle
- Thermometer for enema solution
- Toilet tissue
- IV pole
- Washcloth, towel, and basin

*Small-Volume, Prepackaged Enema*

- Prescribed prepackaged enema (Figure 37-53)
- Lubricant if the tip is not prelubricated
- Toilet tissue
- Bedpan or commode if the client cannot use the bathroom
- Absorbent pad for bed
- Gloves

*Return-Flow Enema*

- Absorbent pad for the bed
- Disposable gloves
- Bedside commode or bedpan if client will not be able to ambulate to bathroom
- Prescribed solution
- Lubricant
- Enema container
- Tubing with clamp and nozzle
- Thermometer
- Toilet tissue

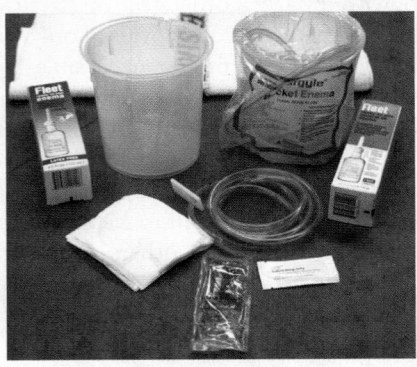

**Figure 37-51**  Various types of enema equipment and solutions

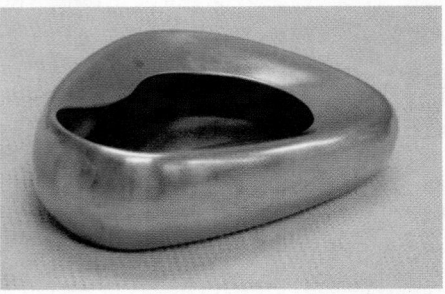

**Figure 37-52**  Bedpans are used when administering an enema if the client cannot ambulate to the bathroom or use a bedside commode.

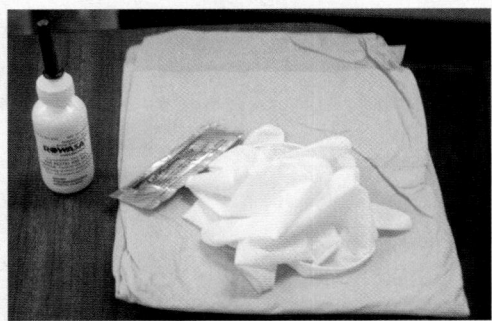

**Figure 37-53**  Small-volume prepackaged enema, gloves, protective pad, and lubricant

### IMPLEMENTATION—ACTION/RATIONALE

| ACTION | RATIONALE |
|---|---|
| **Large-Volume, Cleansing Enema** | |
| 1. Wash hands. | 1. Reduces transmission of microorganisms. |
| 2. Assess client's understanding of procedure and provide privacy. | 2. Prepares client for procedure. |

*(continues)*

PROCEDURE 37-7 (*continued*)

3. Apply gloves.

4. Prepare equipment (Figure 37-54).

5. Place absorbent pad on bed under client. Assist client in attaining left lateral position with right leg flexed as sharply as possible. If there is a question regarding the client's ability to hold the solution, place a bedpan on the bed nearby (Figure 37-55).

3. Prevents contact with feces.

4. Ensures a smooth procedure.

5. Facilitates flow of solution into the rectum and colon. The flexed leg provides the best exposure of the anus.

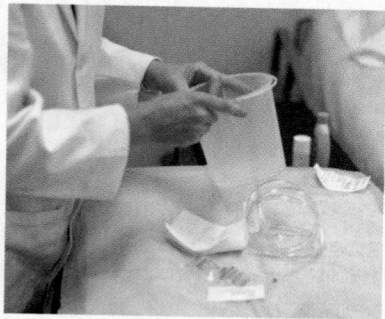

**Figure 37-54    Assemble equipment at the bedside.**

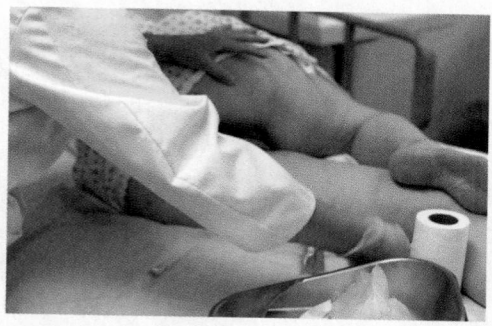

**Figure 37-55    Position the client in the left lateral position with the right leg sharply flexed.**

6. If specified, heat solution to desired temperature, using thermometer to measure. Enemas administered to adults are usually given at 105°–110°F (40.5°–43°C), and those administered to children are usually administered at 100°F (37.7°C). Solution should be at least body temperature to prevent cramping and discomfort.

7. Pour solution into the bag or bucket; add water if needed (Figure 37-56). Open clamp and allow solution to prime tubing. Clamp tubing when primed.

8. Lubricate 5 cm (2 inches) of the rectal tube unless the tube is part of a prelubricated enema set (Figure 37-57).

6. Enemas work best when solution is warm. If enemas are too hot, damage can be done to the bowel mucosa. If enemas are too cold, spasms may occur.

7. Expels air from the tubing, which could cause intestinal distention and discomfort.

8. Minimizes trauma to the anal sphincter during insertion of the rectal tube.

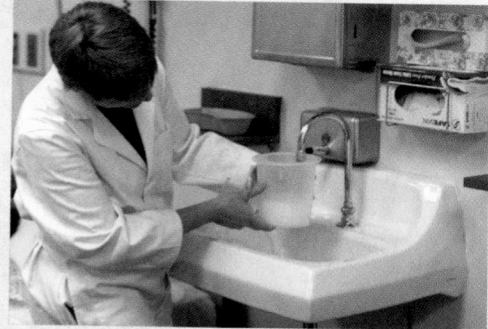

**Figure 37-56    Place the solution into the bucket and add water as needed.**

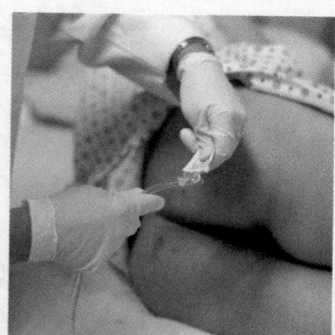

**Figure 37-57    Lubricate 2 inches of the rectal tube with lubricant.**

*(continues)*

**PROCEDURE 37-7 (continued)**

9. Holding the enema container level with the rectum, have the client take a deep breath. Slowly and smoothly insert rectal tube into rectum approximately 7–10 cm in an adult. The rectum of an adult is usually 10–20 cm (4–6 inches). The tube should be inserted beyond the internal sphincter. Aim the rectal tube toward the client's umbilicus (Figure 37-58).

9. A deep breath helps to relax the sphincter. Insertion of rectal tube toward the umbilicus guides tube along rectum.

10. Raise the container holding the solution and open clamp. (If using an enema set, squeeze the container holding solution). The solution should be 30–45 cm (12–18 inches) above the rectum for an adult, and 7.5 cm (3 inches) above the rectum for an infant. The solution may be placed on an IV pole at the proper height.

10. Solution should be at a height above rectum that allows gravity flow of solution into the rectum, but does not cause damage to the rectal lining due to a too rapid increase in rectal pressure.

11. Slowly administer the fluid.

11. Administering enema slowly with momentary pauses decreases the incidence of intestinal spasms and cramps.

12. When solution has been completely administered or when the client cannot hold any more fluid, clamp the tubing and remove the rectal tube, disposing of it properly.

12. The urge to defecate indicates that a sufficient amount of fluid has been administered.

13. Clean lubricant, any solution, and any feces from the anus with toilet tissue (Figure 37-59).

13. Minimizes skin irritation.

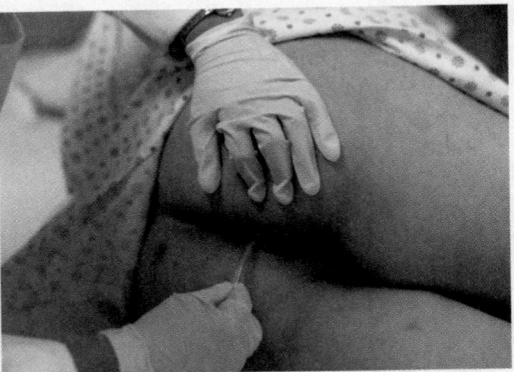

**Figure 37-58** Gently and smoothly insert the rectal tube into the rectum.

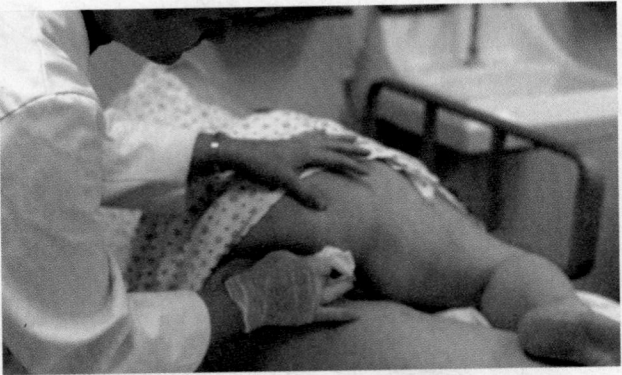

**Figure 37-59** Clean the anal area to remove excess lubricant.

14. Have the client continue to lie on the left side for the prescribed length of time.

14. Certain types of enemas are more effective when retained for a specified amount of time. It is easier for the client to retain the enema in a lying position, where gravity can be resisted.

15. When the client has retained the enema for the prescribed amount of time, assist to the bedside commode or toilet or onto the bedpan. If the client is using the bathroom, instruct not to flush the toilet when finished.

15. Client will be prepared to expel fluid and feces.

*(continues)*

16. When the client is finished expelling the enema, assist to clean the perineal area if needed.

17. Return the client to a comfortable position. Place a clean, dry protective pad under the client to catch any solution or feces that may continue to be expelled.

18. Observe feces.

19. Remove gloves and wash hands.

20. Document the procedure and results.

### Small-Volume, Prepackaged Enema

21. Wash hands.

22. Remove prepackaged enema from packaging. Be familiar with any special instructions included with the enema. The packaged enema may be stood in a basin of warm water to warm the fluid prior to use (Figure 37-60).

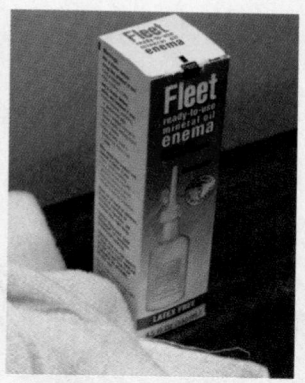

**Figure 37-60    A commercial enema**

23. Apply gloves.

24. Place absorbent pad on bed under client. Assist client in attaining left lateral position with right leg flexed as sharply as possible (Figure 37-61). Or you may use the knee-chest position (Figure 37-62). If there is a question regarding the client's ability to hold the solution, place a bedpan on the bed nearby.

25. Remove the protective cap from the nozzle and inspect the nozzle for lubrication. If the lubrication is not adequate, add more.

16. Prevents skin breakdown and excoriation.

17. Provides comfort for the client and protects the linen from potential soiling.

18. Provides a record of the results.

19. Reduces transmission of microorganisms.

20. To document results and maintain continuity of care.

21. Reduces transmission of microorganisms.

22. Prepares the enema for use.

23. Protects hands from exposure to feces.

24. Facilitates flow of solution into the rectum and colon. The flexed leg provides the best exposure of the anus. The knee-chest position provides good exposure and allows gravity to aid in retention of the enema.

25. Prevents trauma to the rectal mucosa.

(*continues*)

**PROCEDURE 37-7 (continued)**

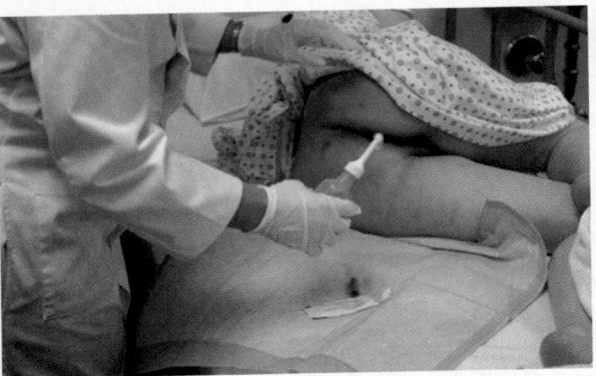

**Figure 37-61** Position the client in the left lateral position with the right leg sharply flexed.

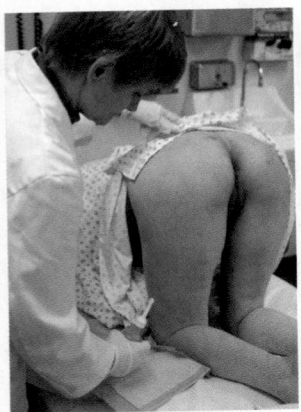

**Figure 37-62** Alternately, you may position the client in the knee-chest position.

26. Squeeze the container gently to remove any air and prime the nozzle.

27. Have the client take a deep breath. Simultaneously gently insert the enema nozzle into the anus, pointing the nozzle toward the umbilicus.

28. Squeeze the container until all the solution is instilled (Figure 37-63).

29. Remove the nozzle from the anus and dispose of the empty container in a trash receptacle (Figure 37-64).

26. Reduces introduction of air into the rectum.

27. Relaxes the rectal sphincter. Pointing the nozzle toward the umbilicus positions the nozzle away from the rectal walls.

28. Allows the client to get the full benefit of the solution.

29. Prevents the spread of microorganisms.

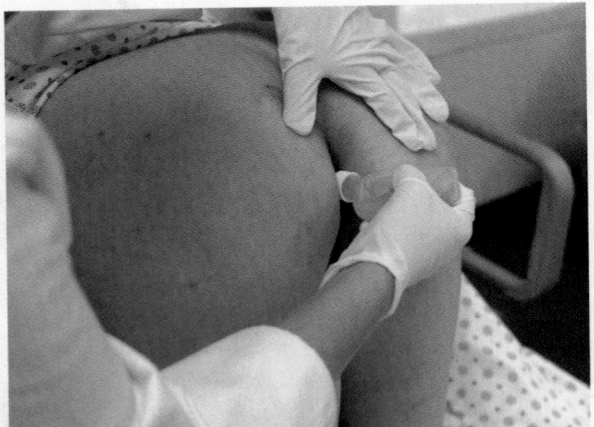

**Figure 37-63** After inserting the nozzle into the anus, squeeze the container until all of the solution is instilled.

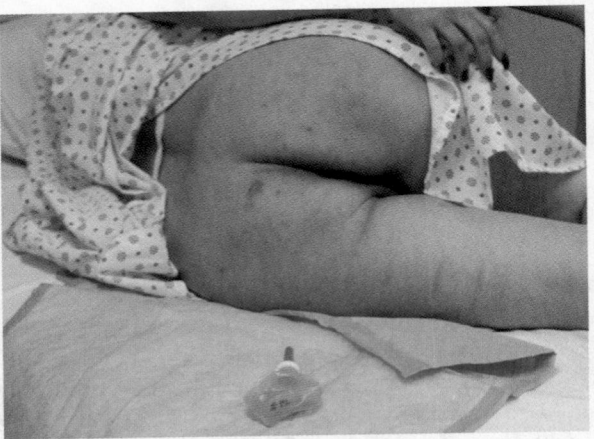

**Figure 37-64** Remove the nozzle and container and have the client continue to lie on the left side for the prescribed length of time. Dispose of the empty container in a trash receptacle.

*(continues)*

## PROCEDURE 37-7 (*continued*)

30. Clean lubricant, any solution, and any feces from the anus with toilet tissue.

31. Have the client continue to lie on the left side for the prescribed length of time.

32. When the client has retained the enema for the prescribed amount of time, assist to the bedside commode or toilet or onto the bedpan. If the client is using the bathroom, instruct not to flush the toilet when finished.

33. When the client is finished expelling the enema, assist to clean the perineal area if needed.

34. Return the client to a comfortable position. Place a clean, dry protective pad under the client to catch any solution or feces that may continue to be expelled (Figure 37-65).

30. Minimizes skin irritation.

31. Certain types of enemas are more effective when retained for a specified amount of time. It is easier for the client to retain the enema in a lying position, where gravity can be resisted.

32. Client will be prepared to expel fluid and feces.

33. Prevents skin breakdown and excoriation.

34. Provides comfort for the client and protects the linen from potential soiling.

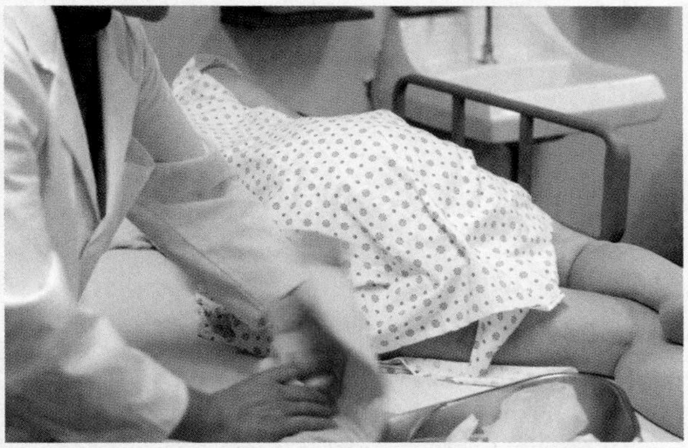

**Figure 37-65    Clean up equipment. Place a protective pad under the client and keep a bedpan nearby if needed to catch any solution that may continue to be expelled.**

35. Observe feces and document data.

36. Remove gloves and wash hands.

37. Document procedure and record results.

35. Provides a record of the results.

36. Reduces transmission of microorganisms.

37. To record results of procedure and maintain continuity of care.

### Return-Flow Enema

38. Wash hands.

39. Assess if client understands procedure.

38. Practices clean technique.

39. Prepares client for procedure.

*(continues)*

## PROCEDURE 37-7 (continued)

40. Apply gloves.

41. Place absorbent pad on bed under client. Assist client in attaining left lateral position with right leg flexed as sharply as possible.

42. If specified, heat solution to desired temperature using thermometer to measure. Enemas administered to adults are usually given at 105°–110°F (40.5°–43°C) and those administered to children are usually administered at 100°F (37.7°C). Solution should be at least body temperature to prevent cramping and discomfort.

43. Pour solution into the bag or bucket, open clamp, and allow solution to prime tubing. Clamp tubing when primed.

44. Lubricate 5 cm (2 inches) of the rectal tube unless the tube is part of a prelubricated enema set.

45. Holding the enema container level with the rectum, have the client take a deep breath. Simultaneously, slowly and smoothly insert rectal tube into rectum approximately 7–10 cm in an adult. Insertion of rectal tube toward the umbilicus guides tube along rectum. Rectum of an adult is usually 10–20 cm (4–6 inches). The tube should be inserted beyond the internal sphincter. Aim the rectal tube toward the client's umbilicus.

46. Raise the container holding the solution and open clamp. The solution should be 30–45 cm (12–18 inches) above the rectum for an adult and 7.5 cm (3 inches) above the rectum for an infant (Figure 37-66).

47. Slowly administer approximately 200 cc of solution.

48. Clamp the tubing and lower the enema container 12–18 inches below the client's rectum. Open the clamp (Figure 37-67).

49. Observe the solution container for air bubbles as the solution returns. Note any fecal particles that may be returned.

40. Prevents contact with feces.

41. Facilitates flow of solution into the rectum and colon. The flexed leg provides the best exposure of the anus.

42. Enemas work best when solution is warm. If enemas are too hot, damage can be done to the bowel mucosa. If enemas are too cold, spasms may occur.

43. Expels air from the tubing that could cause intestinal distention and discomfort.

44. Minimizes trauma to the anal sphincter during insertion of the rectal tube.

45. A deep breath helps to relax the sphincter.

46. Solution should be at a height that allows gravity flow of solution into the rectum, but does not cause damage to the rectal lining due to a too rapid increase in rectal pressure.

47. Administering enema slowly with momentary pauses decreases the incidence of intestinal spasms and cramps.

48. Allows the solution to flow back out of the rectum.

49. Assesses the effectiveness of the procedure. Air bubbles in the container indicate flatus being passed from the rectum.

*(continues)*

**PROCEDURE 37-7 (continued)**

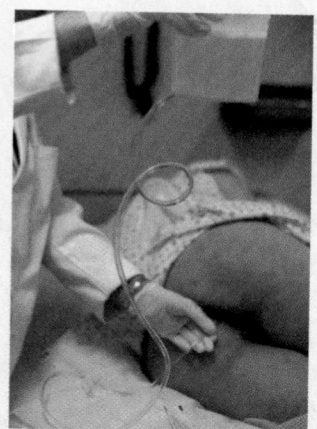

**Figure 37-66    Raise the container 12–18 inches above the rectum and instill 200 cc of solution.**

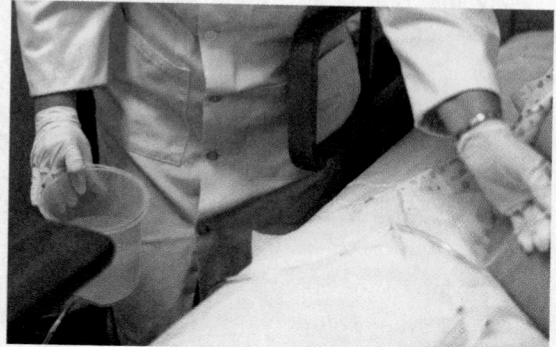

**Figure 37-67    Lower the container 12–18 inches below the client's rectum. Observe for air bubbles as the solution returns.**

50. When no further solution is returned to the container, clamp the tubing and raise the enema container 12–18 inches above the client's rectum. Open the clamp and instill approximately 200 cc of fluid.

50. Continues to stimulate peristalsis and remove flatus.

51. Repeat raising and lowering the solution container until no further flatus is seen. Most institutions have guidelines regarding the number of returns to perform. A good rule of thumb is not more than three times.

51. Limiting the number of returns prevents unduly tiring or stressing the client.

52. After the final return of fluid, clamp the tubing and gently remove it from the client's anus. Clean the anus with tissue to remove any lubricant or solution.

52. Prevents skin irritation.

53. If the client feels the need to empty his rectum, assist him onto the bedpan or up to the bathroom or commode.

53. Allows any retained solution to be expelled. Stimulates peristalsis.

54. When the client is finished expelling any retained solution, assist him to clean the perineal area if needed.

54. Prevents skin breakdown and excoriation.

55. Return the client to a comfortable position. Place a clean, dry protective pad under the client to catch any solution or feces that may continue to be expelled.

55. Provides comfort for the client and protects the linen from potential soiling.

56. Observe any expelled solution.

56. Provides a record of the results.

57. Remove gloves and wash hands.

57. Reduces transmission of microorganisms.

58. Document the results of the enema.

58. Provides continuity of care.

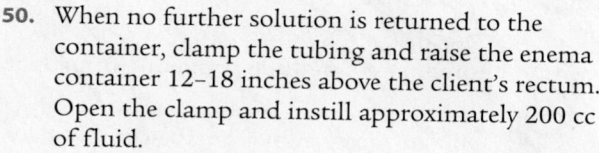

# LIFE SPAN CONSIDERATIONS

## Enemas

### Pediatric Variations

- The child may be too young to understand why an enema is being administered, which may cause increased anxiety on the child's part.
- Have a parent administer the enema if reasonable, or have the parent present to comfort the child and facilitate cooperation.
- Care must be taken to ensure that the temperature of the solution is maintained to prevent damaging the child or make the child uncomfortable.
- It is important that the enema nozzle be well lubricated and that it is inserted only 7.5 cm (2–3 inches) in children and 2.5–3.75 cm (1–1.5 inches) in infants.
- Be aware of the volumes required for different body sizes in infants and children.
- Only isotonic solutions should be used in infants and children.
- Children who are not toilet trained will not be able to retain the enema solution. Give the enema on an absorbent pad or while the child is on the bedpan.

### Geriatric Variations

- Older clients may have impaired mobility, thus having difficulty maintaining an acutely flexed right leg as well as having difficulty quickly walking to the bathroom.
- The client may need encouragement to maintain the position desired, and a bedside commode or bedpan may be required.
- Older clients may not be able to hear instructions well, especially if you are facing away from the client or have a soft voice. Make sure to communicate at eye level and allow the client to see your lips as you speak. Establish hand signals prior to the procedure to use if the client cannot hear you while you are administering the enema.
- Take extra precautions to protect privacy and dignity if you must speak in a loud voice to communicate with the client.

# COMMUNITY/HOME CARE

## Enemas

### Home Care Variations

- Clients can be taught to administer the enemas to themselves if needed.
- Enema kits are easily available and may be easier for the client to use without assistance.
- Clients may find that lying on their backs with their knees flexed and legs raised or using the knee-chest position are easier positions for self-administration of the enema.
- Clients should be instructed not to use the same nozzle for douching and enemas. Douche bags often come with an enema tip and the bag can be used for either purpose, but the tips are not interchangeable.
- Clients should not use enema/douche bags that hold the solution under pressure and forcefully expel the fluid into the rectum.

### Long-Term Care Variations

- Constipation is a common concern in the long-term setting. Clients at risk must be monitored regarding their bowel habits.
- Long-term care clients may develop rituals regarding their bowel habits. As long as the rituals are not unhealthy, a client should be allowed to perform any ritual that will help maintain bowel regularity.

## CLINICAL ALERT

### Enema Administration

If "enema till clear" is ordered, no more than 3 L of fluid should be administered in any one series of enemas. Repeated enemas produce irritation of bowel mucosa and perianal area, as well as electrolyte loss and exhaustion. If returns are not clear, consult physician for further instructions.

## CLINICAL ALERT

### Effects of Enemas

Large-volume enemas disrupt the normal flora of the bowel, predisposing the client to diarrhea as the bowels recover from this traumatic event. Provide yogurt with active cultures or buttermilk to help the client restore normal flora. Antibiotic enemas may disrupt vitamin K synthesis by intestinal flora. Supplemental vitamin K may be required until normal intestinal flora is restored.

patterns. This process requires circular palpation of the anal sphincter and distal anus for 2 to 3 minutes. This process is repeated in 20 minutes if defecation does not occur. Deep breathing is encouraged during defecation because it drops the diaphragm and partially compensates for the client's inability to effectively strain.

Persons with chronic fecal incontinence due to anal sphincter incompetence may be managed with biofeedback techniques. These techniques are typically taught by a specialty or advanced practice nurse with specific training in the field of gastrointestinal disorders and biofeedback techniques.

### Monitor Elimination Diversions

**Urinary Diversions** Surgically created extraurethral incontinence is managed by a pouch. The ileal conduit is, by design, an incontinent stoma constructed from a 10-cm segment of ileum. The ileum is isolated from the fecal stream and connected to the ureters using a refluxing end-to-end anastomosis. A small incision is made in the abdominal wall, and a stoma is constructed from the distal portion of the ileal segment. An enterostomal nurse is consulted to advise the surgeon on stoma site selection and to assist the client to adapt to and learn to manage the stoma.

The continent urinary diversion is an alternative to the ileal conduit. It contains a reservoir for urinary storage and gains continence from various mechanisms. The urinary reservoir may be created from small or large bowel. The Kock Indiana and Florida pouches are types of pouch-es created from intestinal material. Continence is obtained by forming an abdominal reservoir. Continence also may be preserved by the Mitrofanoff technique, which uses a segment of appendix or ureter to create a continent stoma. Evacuation of urine from the reservoir relies on intermittent catheterization of these continent mechanisms. Orthotopic urinary diversions have been described in which the neo-bladder is attached to the urethra, and its sphincter mechanism is relied on for continence. Urine may be evacuated from the urinary reservoir by catheterization of the urethra or by strain voiding.

**Bowel Diversions** The fecal stream is diverted when tissue damage from trauma or inflammation necessitates the temporary bypassing of a segment of bowel or when permanent resection of malignant or irreversibly damaged tissue is necessary. Several techniques are used to create a fecal diversion; some require a pouch to contain fecal contents, whereas others maintain continence. Continent diversions rely on catheterization of an abdominal stoma or evacuation of stool from a pouch reservoir reattached to the anal sphincter.

Virtually any portion of the large and small intestine can be diverted or used to form a fecal reservoir. Some diversions rely on a **stoma** (surgically created opening) for the evacuation of fecal contents. Stomas are primarily constructed in three ways. An *end stoma* is created by dividing the bowel and bringing the proximal segment to the abdominal wall. The end is rolled and attached to the skin of the abdomen, creating a red rosette of intestinal mucosa. A *double-barrel stoma* is constructed by dividing the bowel and bringing both the proximal and distal ends to the abdominal wall. The proximal end is used to evacuate stool. The distal stoma is typically referred to as a mucous fistula. The double-barrel stoma is designed for temporary diversion of the fecal stream. A *loop stoma* is created by opening the anterior aspect of the bowel either longitudinally or transversely. The resulting stoma has both proximal and distal openings that are separated by the posterior wall of the bowel loop. It is designed for temporary fecal diversion (O'Brien, 1999).

The fecal stream is diverted at the most distal point possible to maximize the absorption of food, fluid, and electrolytes and to preserve continence. The *ileostomy* (diversion of the bowel at the level of the ileum) is more uncommon than it was during earlier decades. A permanent ileostomy is typically reserved for clients with severe Crohn's colitis, familial adenomatous polyposis, or chronic ulcerative colitis. A loop (temporary) ileostomy may be created as one stage in an ileoanal reservoir procedure or as a staged procedure for the relief of obstruction of the ascending colon.

The colostomy is created as a permanent or temporary fecal diversion (Figure 37-68). Among adults, it may be created in cases of severe diverticulitis or trauma. The most common indication for a permanent colostomy among adults is an abdominoperineal resection for lower rectal

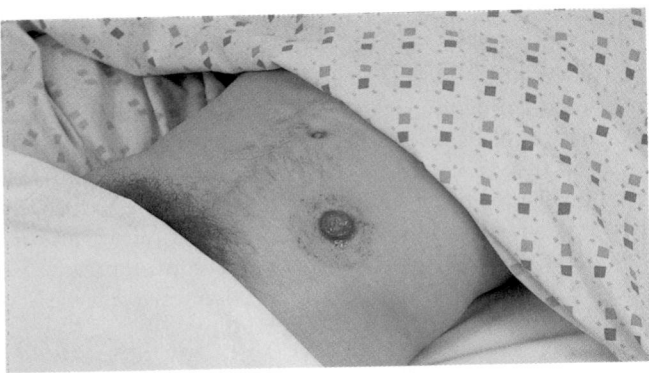

**Figure 37-68    Colostomy: What are some major nursing implications when caring for this client?**

cancer. A temporary colostomy may be created from the transverse colon or (rarely) from the cecum. The descending or sigmoid colon may be temporarily diverted because of radiation proctitis or low rectal carcinoma. Procedure 37-8 outlines steps for changing a colostomy pouch.

Continent diversions of the bowel may incorporate the anus and sphincter or may be constructed with an abdominal stoma. The ileoanal reservoir is created in a staged approach. In the first stage an abdominal colectomy is completed, followed by a rectal mucosectomy, creation of a J- or S-shaped pouch comprising anus and ileum, and a temporary end or loop ileostomy. In the second stage the temporary ileostomy is taken down and the ileoanal reservoir is reattached to the rectal stream.

The Kock continent ileostomy is performed as a single procedure. A colectomy and proctectomy are performed, and the distal 45 cm of the ileum is used to form the reservoir for the ileostomy and the abdominal stoma. The abdominal stoma is rendered continent by intussusception of the bowel that is stabilized to the abdominal wall by stapling or suturing the nipple valve. A polyglycolic acid mesh may be incorporated to provide further support if necessary. Effluent gathered in the reservoir is evacuated by catheterization through the abdominal stoma.

## Surgical Management

The surgical management for SUI differs for urethral hypermobility as compared with intrinsic sphincter deficiency. Urethral hypermobility is managed by a bladder suspension designed to prevent descent of the bladder base and urine loss during physical exertion.

Clients with adequate urethral support and intrinsic sphincter deficiency may be managed with a urethral bulking agent, such as Contigen (Bard Urological, Covington, Georgia), a product that may improve continence by enhancing compressive elements of the urethral sphincter mechanism. It is injected transurethrally, and local anesthesia with systemic sedation is often used in preference to general anesthesia. Women with a combination of urethral hypermobility and intrinsic sphincter deficiency may undergo a suburethral sling procedure, in which the proximal third of the urethra is supported with fascia or a synthetic material (tension-free vaginal tape).

Rarely, an artificial urinary sphincter device may be used to manage intrinsic sphincter deficiency. This mechanical device allows the client to mechanically inflate and deflate a cuff that compresses underlying urethral tissues. Each of these procedures requires specific nursing care and instruction. See a urologic nursing text for a detailed discussion of the nursing care for urologic surgery.

Surgery plays only a limited role in the management of urge incontinence. Surgical procedures designed to denervate the bladder (severed nerves needed for contraction of the detrusor muscle) have had little success because of significant complications, including fecal incontinence and impotence among men. A surgically implanted device designed to deliver electrical stimulation to the lower urinary tract has been approved for use in the United States. Refer to a urologic nursing text for management of these clients.

The management of reflex incontinence is complicated by the combination of urine leakage and urinary retention caused by detrusor sphincter dyssynergia. A bladder management program is chosen that both protects the upper urinary tracts from serious damage and maximizes continence.

Surgical reconstruction is sometimes used in the long-term management of reflex incontinence. An augmentation enterocystoplasty enlarges bladder capacity and alleviates reflex incontinence by converting the hyper-reflexic bladder into a large, atonic bladder with improved storage ability. Unfortunately, the augmented bladder rarely empties efficiently, and clients are advised that life-long intermittent self-catheterization will be necessary after augmentation surgery. A continent or incontinent urinary diversion is occasionally used to manage urine elimination in the patient with reflex incontinence. However, urinary diversion is completed only when bladder function threatens the normal function of the upper urinary tracts.

Fistulae and ectopia are managed by surgical closure whenever possible. When surgery is not feasible, a fistula may be treated by careful application of a sclerosing agent, such as tetracycline or doxycycline in suspension. The solution is applied monthly, and a skin barrier is used on the area surrounding the fistula to prevent scarring. The fistula that cannot be closed surgically or by sclerosing therapy must be managed by application of a urinary containment device and a preventive skin program.

Surgery or endoscopic procedures alleviate urinary retention caused by bladder outlet obstruction. Transurethral resection of the prostate, open prostatectomy, visual ablation of the prostate, and other procedures are used to alleviate obstruction caused by benign prostatic hyperplasia. Transurethral incision of the bladder neck or transurethral sphincterotomy may be used for bladder neck or striated sphincter dyssynergia. Refer to a textbook

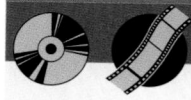

**PROCEDURE 37-8**

# Changing a Bowel Diversion Ostomy Appliance: Pouching a Stoma

## EQUIPMENT NEEDED

- Clean washcloth or 4 × 4 gauze pads (Figures 37-69 to 37-71)
- Warm tap water
- Appropriate drainable ostomy appliance
- Scissors
- Pen or pencil
- Clean gloves

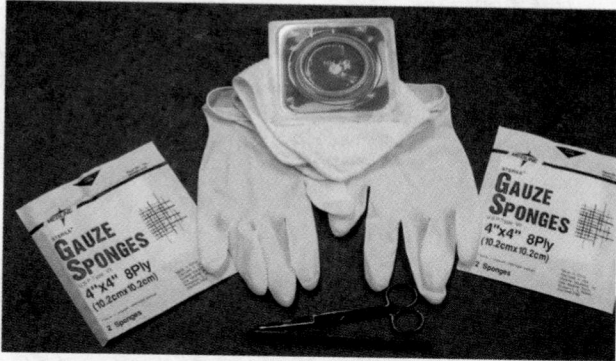

**Figure 37-69** Ostomy wafer, gloves, scissors, pen or pencil, and sponges are used when pouching a stoma.

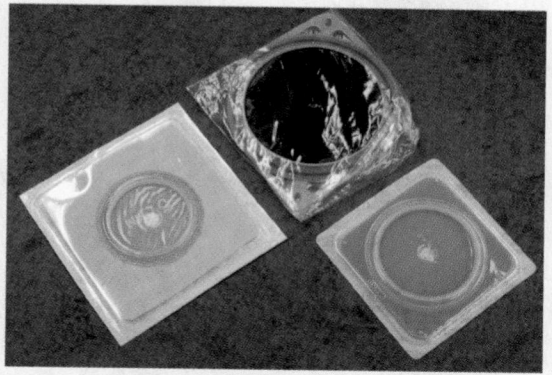

**Figure 37-70** Ostomy skin barriers, also called wafers

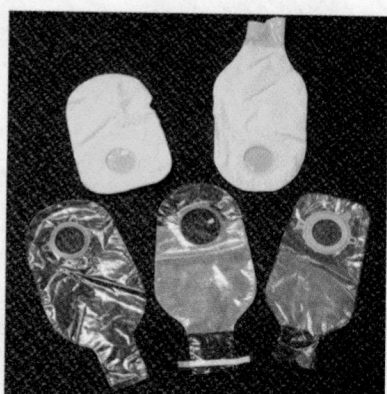

**Figure 37-71** Ostomy drainage bags

## IMPLEMENTATION—ACTION/RATIONALE

| ACTION | RATIONALE |
|---|---|
| 1. Wash hands. | 1. Practices aseptic technique. |
| 2. Assemble drainable pouch and wafer. | 2. Assures that all equipment is ready to use. |
| 3. Apply clean gloves. | 3. Practices clean technique. |
| 4. Remove current ostomy appliance after emptying pouch of stool, if present. | 4. Prevents contamination of surrounding environment if stool accidentally leaks from appliance when removed from client's skin. |
| 5. Dispose of appliance in appropriate waste container. | 5. Practices infection control. |

*(continues)*

## PROCEDURE 37-8 (*continued*)

6. Remove gloves and wash hands.

7. Apply clean gloves.

8. Cleanse stoma and skin with warm tap water. Pat dry (Figure 37-72).

9. Measure stoma using a measuring guide for appropriate length and width of stoma at base (where skin meets stoma).

10. Place gauze pad over orifice of stoma to wick stool while you are preparing the wafer and pouch for application (Figure 37-73).

6. Practices aseptic technique.

7. Practices clean technique.

8. Gentle care of the stoma prevents injury to the mucosa, which has no nerve endings and is very friable.

9. Correct measurement of the stoma's dimensions ensures a good fit of the ostomy appliance without excess skin at the base of the stoma exposed to stool.

10. Using something to wick stool away from the skin ensures a good seal of the wafer to the client's skin.

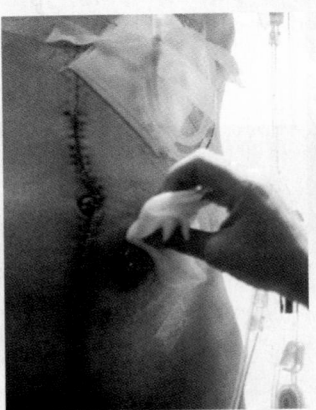

**Figure 37-72    Cleanse the stoma and surrounding skin with warm tap water.**

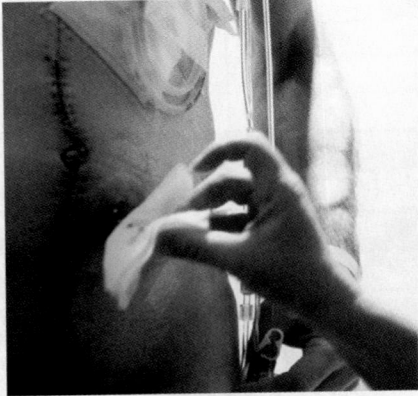

**Figure 37-73    Place gauze over the stoma to absorb stool while the wafer and pouch are being prepared.**

11. Trace pattern onto paper backing of wafer.

12. Cut wafer as traced.

13. Attach clean pouch to wafer. Make sure port closure is closed.

14. Remove gauze pad from orifice of stoma.

11. It is important to trace the measurements of the stoma and not "eye ball" the stoma measurements. Inaccurate pattern size results in either laceration of the stoma by the wafer or maceration of peristomal skin from constant contact with stool.

12. Accurately cutting the traced pattern ensures a snug fit.

13. Preattaching the pouch to the wafer saves time and prevents stool from leaking underneath the wafer during application process.

14. It is easier to visualize the stoma.

*(continues)*

**PROCEDURE 37-8 (continued)**

15. Remove paper backing from wafer (Figure 37-74) and place on skin with stoma centered in cutout opening of wafer (Figures 37-75 and 37-76).

15. Paper backing needs to be removed from wafer in order for wafer to become adherent to skin.

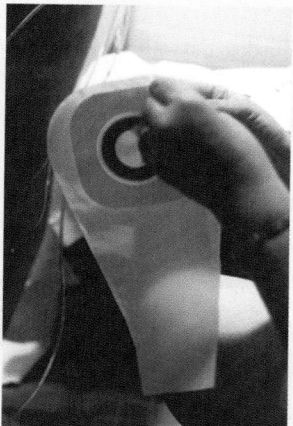

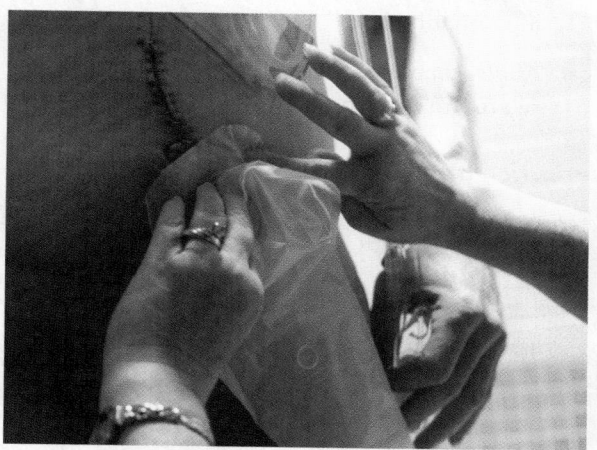

**Figure 37-74**    Remove the paper backing from the wafer. Many pouching systems are available. This pouch is a one-piece system and has a skin barrier already attached. Others are two-piece systems where the skin barrier is attached first and the pouch is attached to the skin barrier.

**Figure 37-75**    Place the wafer and pouch with the stoma centered in the cutout opening of the wafer.

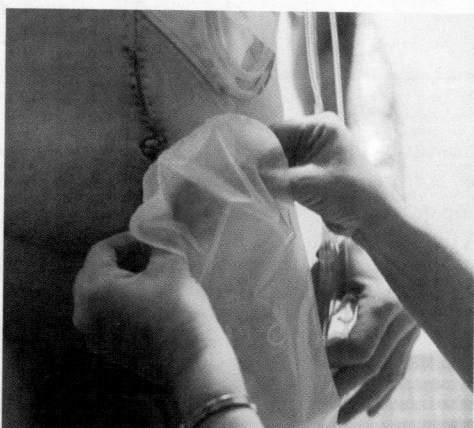

**Figure 37-76**    Check to make sure the stoma fits the hole so only a minimum of the surrounding skin is exposed to contact with stool.

16. Tape the wafer edges down with hypoallergenic tape (optional).

16. Ensures that the edges of the wafer will not adhere to client's clothing.

17. Wash hands.

17. Reduces transmission of microorganisms.

## LIFE SPAN CONSIDERATIONS

### Ostomy Appliance Variations

**Pediatric Variations**

- A child's ostomy bag needs to be very flexible so it can bend with the client's movement without becoming nonadherent.

- Adolescents need careful assessment and intervention to help them adjust to changes in body images related to the stoma and appliance.

**Geriatric Variations**

- If a client has arthritic hands, it is best to use either a one-piece appliance that is precut or a two-piece appliance that is adaptive to decreases in hand dexterity.

## COMMUNITY/HOME CARE

### Ostomy Considerations

**Home Care Variations**

- Assess the client's home for an appropriate setting in which to change the ostomy appliance and proper means to dispose of the contaminated items.

**Long-Term Care Variations**

- Consider the ongoing stress of a slowly healing colostomy and the potential changes to body image large scars and marks will cause even after they have healed. Connect the client with support groups or further assessment if needed.

---

of urologic nursing for the care following these specialized procedures

## Complementary Therapies

When the body fails to eliminate waste, other systems are compromised and the person becomes prone to illness. Herbalists view the role of the kidneys and the intestines in a holistic manner. The proper function of any part of the body is dependent on the effective elimination of waste products and toxins.

Herbs that may aid the functions of the urinary system are:

- *Diuretics:* Dandelion root and leaf and cleavers
- *Antiseptics:* bearberry, birch, boldo, buchu, celery seed, couchgrass, juniper, and yarrow
- *Antimicrobials:* Echinacea root and wild indigo root
- *Demulcents:* corn silk, couchgrass, and marshmallow leaf

Herbs that possess other properties may also be used, such as urinary astringents (beth root, horsetail, and plantain tormentil), to treat blood in the urine caused by minor problems and to aid the healing of lesions, and antilithics (gravel root, hydrangea, and stone root), to prevent the formation of or aid in the removal of calculi (stones or gravel) in the urinary system.

Both urinary and fecal elimination rely upon sufficient amounts of fiber and fluids in the diet. The following herbs are helpful in relieving constipation: *Cascara sagrada* bark, senna, ginger root, butternut root bark, and burdock root. Milk thistle, a cholagogue, may be used to aid liver function and to enhance bile flow to soften stools.

*Cascara sagrada* bark is an old Indian remedy to encourage peristalsis and tone relaxed muscles of the digestive tract. Senna is a widely used stimulant laxative when compared to synthetic drugs. *Cascara* and senna should be combined with aromatics and carminatives such as licorice and ginger root to increase palatability and reduce gripping. Ginger root aids in digestion and enhances bile flow from the liver. Burdock root is a mild laxative and an effective diuretic; its cleansing effect goes beyond its diuretic and laxative properties as it promotes perspiration and strengthens the liver.

Psyllium seed and flaxseed are also helpful for constipation. Psyllium seed must be taken with a full glass of water.

Mineral oil should not be taken on a regular basis because, if inhaled, it can damage the lungs, and it reduces the absorption of fat-soluble vitamins (Balch & Balch, 2001).

## Evaluation

Evaluating the effectiveness of the nursing interventions is an ongoing process. The client's level of maintenance or restoration of elimination patterns and return to an appropriate level of independence are indicators of success. When evaluating these aspects, it is important for the nurse to reassess how realistic the original identified outcomes were, especially for goals that were not met, and to modify the target outcomes accordingly. Prevention of skin breakdown and infection can also be used to determine the appropriateness of the plan of care. Client understanding of procedures and self-care should be evaluated to determine the effectiveness of teaching plans, and modifications should be made to address deficiencies and ongoing learning needs. If support persons are included in the teaching process, their understanding of skills and competence with procedures should also be measured. If additional care or teaching is deemed necessary, clients should be given referrals for community and other resources to support their continuing learning needs.

# CASE STUDY/NURSING CARE PLAN

Mrs. Price is a 30-year-old woman who sustained a complete spinal cord injury of the seventh cervical vertebra 2 years before this hospital admission. She is currently admitted to an inpatient rehabilitative unit. She currently manages her bowels by administering enemas every 5 to 7 days when she notes pressure and distention of her abdomen. She has frequent episodes of fecal incontinence, described as passage of moderate amounts of black, watery stool. Mrs. Price manages these episodes by administering one or two enemas, followed by passage of a large volume of odorous, dark feces. She denies having had problems with her bowel control before her spinal injury. She states that she moved her bowels every other day, typically after breakfast. Currently, Mrs. Price reports fluid intake of 3 to 4 glasses per day. She eats primarily meats, white breads, some pastas, and one portion of vegetables per day. Mrs. Price does not routinely eat cereals or fruits or supplement her diet with bulk laxatives. It is determined that Mrs. Price is constipated and needs a "workup" to intervene with her condition.

## Assessment

Mrs. Price is a 30-year-old woman with a spinal cord injury who is constipated and has developed an impaction in her colon or rectal areas. She does not take in adequate fluids, nor does she ingest enough fiber.

## Nursing Diagnosis #1

*Constipation* related to spinal cord injury and neurogenic bowel.
**NOC:** Bowel Elimination; Medication Response; Self-Care Toileting
**NIC:**  Constipation/Impaction Management; Bowel Training; Teaching; Prescribed Medication

## Expected Outcome

The client will:
1. Have a rectum that is cleansed of the current impaction within 24 hours.

## Planning/Interventions/Rationales

1. Administer PIEE until impaction is disrupted. *Bowel is clear of impacted stool as assessed by digital examination.*
2. Encourage dietary intake of fiber-rich foods, including one serving of cereal per day, one serving of fruit, and two servings of vegetables. *Fiber encourages a pressure-free movement of stool through the lower GI tract.*
3. Increase fluid intake to 30 ml/kg body weight; encourage water intake to equal at least 50% of fluids. *Fluids assist the stool to become more liquid and easier to evacuate.*
4. Administer supplemental bulk laxatives (Metamucil) if client is unable to alter diet to meet needs for fiber. *Stool will be soft, formed, without impacted or dry, hardened material.*

## Evaluation

Client had a regular bowel movement of a soft, formed consistency in 24 hours.

*(continues)*

# CASE STUDY/NURSING CARE PLAN (continued)

## Nursing Diagnosis #2

*Diarrhea* related to fecal impaction, and neurogenic bowel.

**NOC:** Bowel Continence; Self-Care Toileting

**NIC:** Bowel Incontinence Care; Bowel Management; Bowel Training; Self-Care Assistance; Toileting

### Expected Outcomes

The client will:

1. Maintain a bowel management program that will cause completed elimination of feces from rectum within 24 hours.
2. Not have any fecal incontinent episodes within 24 hours.

### Planning/Interventions/Rationales

1. Begin a bowel program every other day by determining time for evacuation with client; encourage defecation after breakfast, based on premorbid bowel elimination pattern; encourage bowel evacuation program after meal if premorbid schedule is not feasible with current activities. *Bowel evacuation will occur every other day after a meal, based on client's activities of daily living, preferences, and premorbid bowel elimination patterns.*
2. Teach client relationship among stool consistency, regularity of evacuation, fecal impaction, and fecal continence. *Increase knowledge level.*
3. Advise client to consult nurse specialist or gastroenterologist if fecal incontinent episodes persist despite regulation of bowel management program. *Prevents uncontrolled crisis.*
4. Warn client that occurrence of diarrhea may predispose to acute transient fecal incontinence. *Fecal incontinent episodes will be reduced by greater than 50%.*

### Evaluation

Client did not have any fecal incontinent episodes within 24 hours.

## Key Concepts

- Normal urination requires anatomical integrity of the lower urinary tract, nervous control of the detrusor muscle, and competence of the urethral sphincter mechanism.
- Normal bowel evacuation relies on motility factors, the storage abilities of the rectum, and competence of the internal and external sphincter mechanisms.
- Common alterations in urinary elimination include SUI, urge and reflex incontinence, extraurethral incontinence, and urinary retention.
- Constipation and diarrhea are common alterations in stool consistency that cause changes in fecal elimination patterns and predispose clients to fecal incontinence.
- Clients with altered patterns of urinary and bowel elimination are evaluated with a detailed history, focused physical examination, record of bladder and bowel elimination patterns, and review of laboratory values.
- Altered stool consistency is prevented or alleviated by managing malabsorption syndromes, maintaining a regular pattern of elimination, ensuring adequate fluid and fiber intake, and heeding the urge to defecate.
- Multiple options, including behavioral management strategies, pharmacotherapy, and surgical interventions are used to manage clients with altered patterns of elimination.
- Fecal incontinence is managed by normalization of stool consistency, maximization of rectal storage abilities, and management of anal sphincter incompetence.

## Review Questions and Activities

1. Which central nervous system structures regulate detrusor muscle contractions?
2. How do urethral support mechanisms help prevent stress urinary incontinence?
3. What are the causes of stress urinary incontinence?
4. How do urge and reflex incontinence differ? Why are clients with reflex incontinence at greater risk for urinary retention than those with urge incontinence?
5. What functional limitation may contribute to incontinence?
6. What are the general principles of bladder health? What is the RDA for fluid intake in an adult? Calculate the RDA for fluids for yourself, for a 110-lb client, for a 379-lb client.

7. What is the primary behavioral intervention for the management of stress urinary incontinence? Teach yourself to perform a pelvic muscle contraction. Test yourself by performing 10, 20, or 35 repetitions. Can you detect fatigue of the muscles as you exercise? Do you find yourself using distant muscle groups, such as the abdominal or thigh muscles?

8. What is the primary behavioral intervention for urge incontinence? Teach yourself to perform a quick flick contraction of the pelvic muscles.

9. Identify at least six strategies to reduce environmental barriers to toileting. Develop a checklist when assessing the client with urinary incontinence.

10. What are the two elements of the anal sphincter?

11. What are the primary causes of diarrhea? Differentiate the treatment of secretory, malabsorptive, and inflammatory diarrhea. Determine which forms of diarrhea are likely to respond to antidiarrheal agents. Determine which forms of diarrhea are likely to be exacerbated by antidiarrheal agents.

12. What are the indications for consultation with the enterostomal technician for a client experiencing diarrhea? Identify and introduce yourself to the enterostomal nurses in your health care facility.

13. What is the purpose of regulating fluid and fiber intake when managing constipation? Determine your daily intake of fluids using a record. Determine the servings of fiber-rich foods in your diet and observe the consistency (and pattern) of your bowel elimination. Slowly add fluids and fiber to your diet and note changes in your bowel elimination patterns.

14. Why does diarrhea or constipation increase the risk of fecal incontinence?

15. What are the indications for referral for a client with bowel elimination problems?

## Multimedia Links

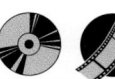

Altman *Basic Care DVD: Assisting with a Bedpan or Urinal*
Altman *Intermediate Care DVD: Applying a Condom Catheter*
Altman *Intermediate Care DVD: Inserting an Indwelling Catheter: Male*
Altman *Intermediate Care DVD: Inserting an Indwelling Catheter: Female*
Altman *Intermediate Care DVD: Irrigating a Urinary Catheter*
Altman *Intermediate Care DVD: Irrigating the Bladder Using a Closed-System Catheter*
Altman *Intermediate Care DVD: Changing a Bowel Diversion Ostomy Appliance—Pouching a Stoma*
Altman *Intermediate Care DVD: Administering an Enema*
Altman *Intermediate Care Video: Nutrition and Elimination II: Catheter Care*
Altman *Intermediate Care Video: Nutrition and Elimination III*

## Web Resources

Canadian Association for Enterostomal Therapy
    http://www.caet.ca
Canadian Continence Foundation
    http://www.continence-fdn.ca
Continent Ostomy Center
    http://www.ostomy.com
International Continence Society
    http://www.icsoffice.org
Society of Urologic Nurses and Associates
    http://www.suna.org
United Ostomy Association
    http://www.ostomy.evansville.net
United Ostomy Association of Canada, Inc.
    http://www3.ns.sympatico.ca/canada.ostomy
Wound, Ostomy, and Continence Nurses Society
    http://www.wocn.org

## References

Altman, G. (2004). *Delmar's fundamental & advanced nursing skills* (2nd ed.). Clifton Park, NY: Delmar Learning.

Annells, M., & Koch, T. (2002). Fecal impaction: Older people's experiences and nursing practice. *British Journal of Community Nursing, 7(3)*, 118–126.

Balch, J., & Balch, P. (2001). Prescription for nutritional healing (3rd ed.). New York: Garden City Park.

Bliss, D. Z., Johnson, S., Savik, K, Clabots, C. R., & Gerding, D. N. (2000). Fecal incontinence in hospitalized patients who are acutely ill. *Nursing Research, 49(2)*, 101.

Daniels, R. (2002). *Delmar's guide to laboratory and diagnostic tests.* Clifton Park, NY: Delmar Learning.

Erickson, H., Tomlin, E., & Swain, M. (1983). *Modeling and role-modeling: A theory and paradigm for nursing.* Englewood Cliffs, NJ: Appleton & Lange.

Estes, M. (2002). *Health assessment & physical examination* (2nd ed.). Clifton Park, NY: Delmar Learning

Goldberg, S., Rivers, P., Smith, K., & Homan, W. (2000). Vertical banded gastroplasty: a treatment for morbid obesity. *AORN Journal, 72(6)*, 988, 991–1010.

Gray, M. (2000a). Urinary retention: Management in the acute care setting. Part I. *American Journal of Nursing, 100(7)*, 41–48.

Gray, M. (2000b). Urinary retention: Management in the acute care setting. Part II. *American Journal of Nursing, 100(8)*, 41–48.

Hogstel, M. (2001). *Gerontology: Nursing care of the older adult.* Clifton Park, NY: Delmar Learning

Jaffe, M. (1998). *Geriatric nutrition & diet* (3rd ed.). Clifton Park, NY: Delmar Learning

Jervis, L. L. (2001). The pollution of incontinence and the dirty work of caregiving in a U.S. nursing home. *Medical Anthropology Quarterly, 15(1)*, 84–99.

Koch, T., & Hudson, S. (2000). Older people and laxative use: Literature review and pilot study report. *Journal of Clinical Nursing, 9*(4), 516–525.

McKenna, S., Wallis, M., Brannelly, A., & Cawood, J. (2001). The nursing management of diarrhea and constipation before and after the implementation of a bowel management protocol. *Australian Critical Care, 14*(1),10–16.

Nelson, R., Furner, S., & Jesudason, V. (2001). Urinary incontinence in Wisconsin skilled nursing facilities: Prevalence and associations in common with fecal incontinence. *Journal of Aging & Health, 13*(4), 539–547.

North American Nursing Diagnosis Association (NANDA) (2003). *Nursing diagnosis: Definitions and classification, 2003–2004.* Philadelphia: Author.

O'Brien, B. K. (1999). Coming of age with an ostomy. *American Journal of Nursing, 99*(8), 71–75.

Palmer, M. H. (2002). Urinary incontinence in nursing homes. *Journal of Wound, Ostomy, and Continence Nursing, 29*(1), 4–5.

Reiss, B., Evans, M., & Broyles, B. (2002). *Pharmacological aspects of nursing care* (6th ed.). Clifton Park, NY: Delmar Learning.

Robinson, C. B., Fritch, M., Hullett, L., Petersen, M. A., Sikkema, S., Theuninck, L., & Timmer, K. (2000). Development of a protocol to prevent opioid-induced constipation in patients with cancer: A research utilization project. *Clinical Journal of Oncology Nursing, 4*(2), 79–84.

Wyman, J. F. (2000). Management of urinary incontinence in adult ambulatory care populations. *Annual Review of Nursing Research, 18,* 171–194.

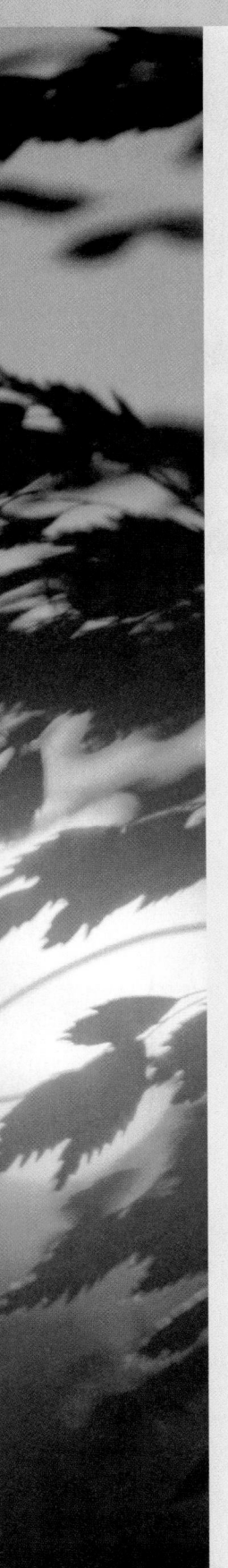

# X UNIT

# Activity-Exercise

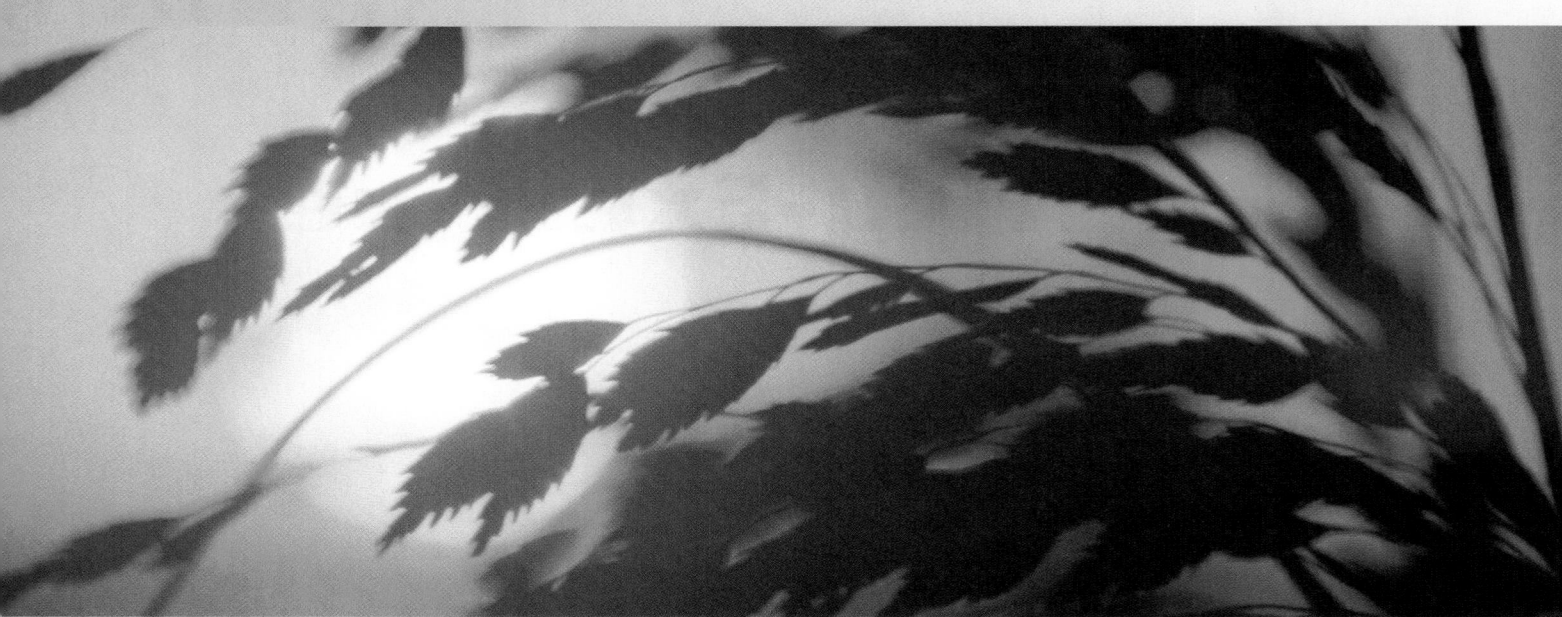

# Mobility and Biomechanics

Annemarie Day, RN, MSN, FNP-C

*"Worms will not eat living wood where the vital sap is flowing; rust will not hinder the opening of a gate when the hinges are used each day. Movement gives health and life. Stagnation brings disease and death."*

*(Ancient proverb in traditional Chinese medicine)*

# Chapter Competencies

*Upon completion of this chapter, the reader should be able to:*

1. Explain the physiology of mobility and the basic elements of body mechanics.
2. Identify various types of exercise and its benefits.
3. Discuss factors that affect mobility.
4. Describe the physiological effects of mobility and immobility.
5. Identify the process of assessing mobility.
6. Discuss nursing diagnoses relevant to clients experiencing mobility impairments.
7. Develop client goals for activity and mobility.
8. Describe specific nursing interventions that promote mobility and prevent complications due to immobility.
9. Identify evaluation procedures for client activity and mobility status.

# Key Terms

active range of motion (ROM)
ambulation
atrophy
balance
base of support
body alignment
body mechanics

functional assessment
hypertrophy
hypotonicity
incontinence
line of gravity
logrolling
mobility
muscle tone

myoneuronal junction
orthostatic hypotension
passive range of motion
proprioception
range of motion
skin shear
spasticity
thrombus

Movement is an activity most people take for granted. The ability to move and be active benefits health status, whereas immobility presents a threat to one's physical, mental, and social well-being. This chapter explores nursing responses to individuals with impaired ability to move.

## Overview of Mobility

**Mobility** refers to the ability to engage in activity and free movement, which includes walking, running, sitting, standing, lifting, pushing, pulling, and performing activities of daily living (ADLs). Mobility is often considered an indicator of health status because it influences the correct functioning of many body systems, especially the respiratory, gastrointestinal, and urinary systems. Mobility enhances muscle tone, increases energy levels, and is associated with psychological benefits such as independence and freedom. Mobility also influences self-esteem and body image, which are major components of self-concept.

## Body Alignment

**Body alignment** refers to the position of body parts in relation to each other. Proper body alignment (also called posture) results in **balance**, which is an individual's ability to maintain equilibrium. When the body is in good posture, the center of gravity (the center point of an object's mass) is evenly distributed over the foundation points. Good posture promotes balance, reduces strain and injury to support structures, facilitates respiratory effort, enhances gastrointestinal processes, and gives an appearance of confidence and health. A correct postural stance is maintained by a well-functioning musculoskeletal system. The normal alignment of the spine has a cervical concavity, a thoracic convexity, and a lumbar concavity; see Figure 38-1.

Proper standing body alignment (as noted in Figure 38-2) is characterized by the following:

- Head upright
- Face forward
- Shoulders squared
- Back straight

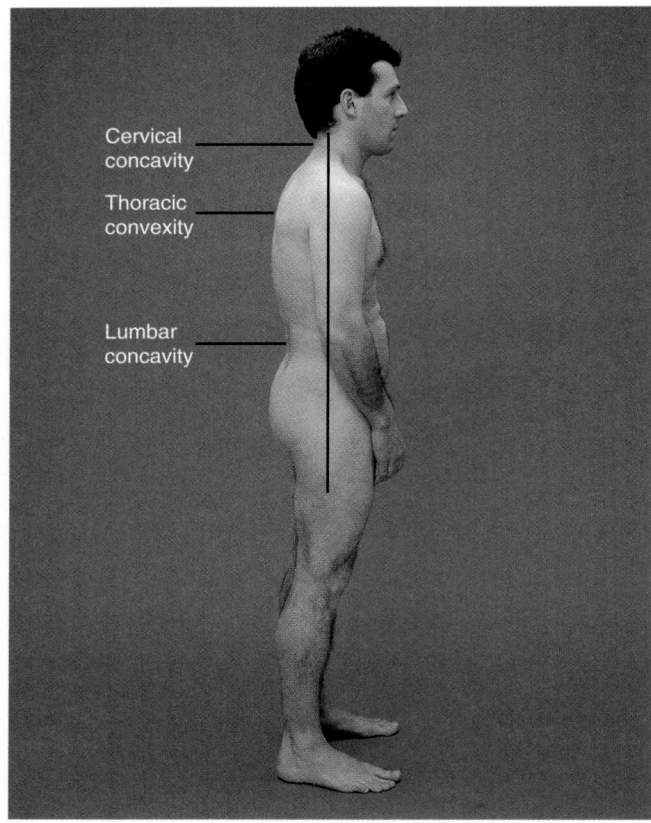
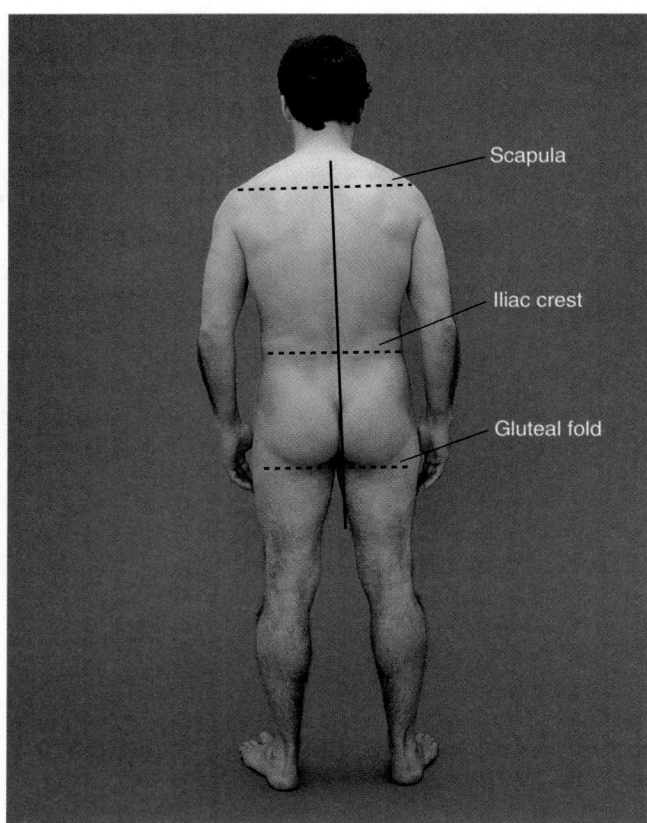

**Figure 38-1    Normal spinal concavity: A. Lateral view B. Posterior view**

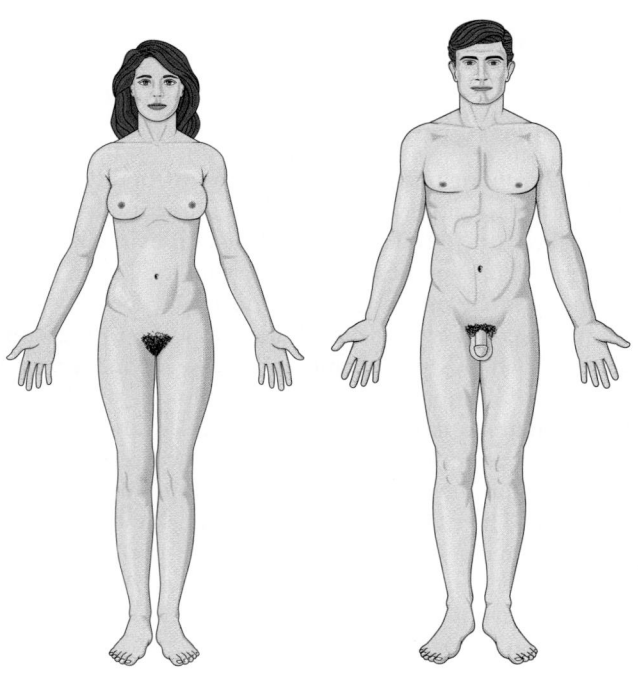

**Figure 38-2    Proper alignment and posture: Standing male and female**

- Abdominal muscles tucked in
- Arms straight at side
- Hands palm forward
- Legs straight
- Feet forward

The sitting position in proper alignment has similar characteristics; however, the hips and knees are flexed. Figure 38-3 shows proper alignment and posture for the sitting position.

Proper alignment and posture of the client lying in bed appear similar to the standing position; however, the client is supine, as shown in Figure 38-4.

The benefits of proper alignment and posture include (1) client comfort; (2) prevention of contractures; (3) promotion of circulation; (4) less stress on muscle, tendons, nerves, and joints; and (5) prevention of foot drop (plantar flexion). Proper body alignment promotes efficient circulatory, renal, pulmonary, and gastrointestinal functions (Estes, 2002).

In a person standing upright, the center of gravity is located in the middle of the pelvis about halfway between the umbilicus and the symphysis pubis. The **line of gravity** (vertical line passing through the center of gravity) is shown in Figures 38-3 and 38-4. The **base of support** is the foundation on which a person or object rests. Stability of one's balance is promoted by a steady base of support and a low center of gravity.

Muscle tone and bone strength allow a person to maintain an erect posture. Muscle contour is affected by the

and neurologic systems and reduces the body's exposure to strain or injury during movement.

Body mechanics involve three basic elements: (1) body alignment (posture), (2) balance (stability), and (3) coordinated movement. Proper body mechanics are as important to the nurse as to the client. The purpose of proper body mechanics is prevention of strain and injury to the muscles, joints, and tendons.

**Range of motion** reflects the extent to which a joint can move. The ranges vary with each joint and are affected by several factors, including age, physical condition, and heredity. Parameters for range of motion are outlined in Tables 38-1 and 38-2.

The clinical application of body mechanics is described later in the implementation section of this chapter.

## Physiology of Mobility

Mobility is regulated by the coordinated effort of the musculoskeletal and neurologic systems. The major functions of the musculoskeletal system are to maintain body alignment and to facilitate mobility. The musculoskeletal system consists of a framework of bones, muscles, joints, tendons, ligaments, bursae, and cartilage.

### Musculoskeletal System

The musculoskeletal system (comprised of bones, cartilage, joints, tendons, ligaments, bursa, and muscles) serves several functions as described in Table 38-1.

Bone is the foundation of the musculoskeletal system. Mobility and weight-bearing capacity are directly related to the bone's size and shape. Joints work with muscles to provide motion and flexibility. Skeletal muscles overlying the joint exert opposing forces and, therefore, cause movement.

Muscles are basically machines that convert energy into mechanical work. Contractility is the common property among the three types of muscles: smooth, cardiac, and skeletal. Skeletal muscle fibers are innervated by somatic nerves and, therefore, are generally under voluntary control.

The muscles work in cooperation with the nervous system to maintain body alignment and cause movement. Muscles act in pairs to perform work. One muscle of the pair produces movement in a single direction. The other muscle of the pair produces movement in the opposite direction. When one muscle of the pair is contracted, the other is relaxed. The opposing actions of contraction and relaxation make motion possible. The position of the tendons upon the bones and the articulation of the bones make possible types of motion such as flexion, extension, circumduction, rotation, and gliding.

Muscles that maintain body alignment work together to stabilize surrounding body parts and to support the body's weight. Posture is maintained primarily by the muscles in the back, neck, trunk, and lower extremities.

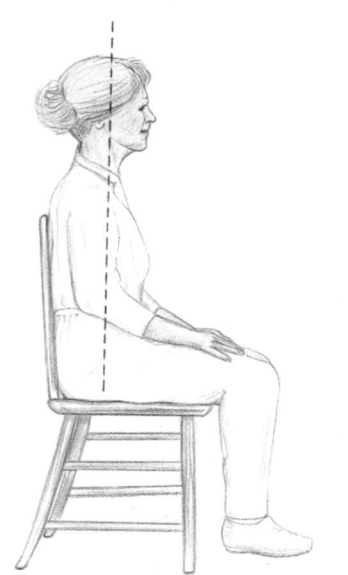

**Figure 38-3    Proper sitting posture and line of gravity**

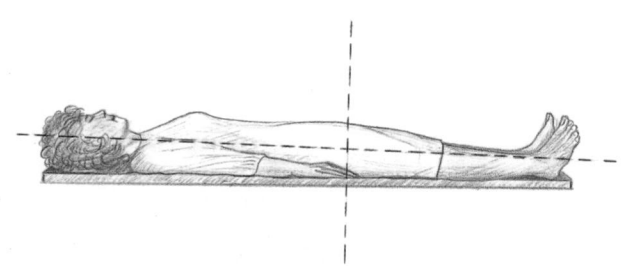

**Figure 38-4    Proper supine posture and line of gravity**

individual's exercise and activity patterns. **Muscle tone** is the normal state of balanced tension present in the body; it allows a muscle to respond quickly to stimuli. Two aberrations of muscle tone include **hypotonicity** (flaccidity), which is a decrease in muscle tone, and **spasticity**, which is an increase in muscle tension and is often noted with extreme flexion or extension.

Muscle shape should be symmetrical. There may be **hypertrophy** (increased muscle size and shape due to an increase in muscle fibers) or **atrophy** (a reduction in muscle size and shape which manifests as thin, flabby muscles with indistinct contour). Atrophy is usually a result of disuse, whereas hypertrophy occurs when the muscle is overworked.

### Body Mechanics

Functional mobility is governed by **body mechanics**, the purposeful and coordinated use of body parts and positions during activity. Use of proper body mechanics maximizes the effectiveness of the efforts of the musculoskeletal

## TABLE 38-1    MUSCULOSKELETAL SYSTEM COMPONENTS

| Anatomical Structure | Description | Function |
|---|---|---|
| Bone | Ossified connective tissue | Facilitates mobility<br>Protects body structures (e.g., brain, spinal cord)<br>Produces blood cells |
| Joint | Site of a union between two bones | Facilitates motion<br>Allows flexibility |
| Tendon | Cord or band of inelastic connective tissue | Causes movement of muscles |
| Ligament | Band of fibrous tissue connecting bones or cartilages | Supports and strengthens joints<br>Facilitates mobility<br>Protects structures (e.g., knee, hip) |
| Bursa | Fluid-filled sac or cavity | Prevents friction between bones and cartilage<br>Facilitates gliding of muscles or tendons over bony surfaces |
| Cartilage | Dense connective tissue | Facilitates mobility |

## TABLE 38-2    REFLEXES THAT MAINTAIN POSTURAL TONUS

| Reflex | Description |
|---|---|
| Labyrinthine sense | Sensory organs in the inner ear activate impulses when the head is turned; impulses are transmitted to cerebellum |
| Tonic neck-righting reflexes | Affected by movement of head from side to side; neck muscle tonus is affected most when neck is hyperextended |
| Optic reflexes | Visual sensations affect posture by helping the person establish spatial relationships to surrounding objects |
| Proprioceptor or kinesthetic sense | Activated when nerve endings in muscles and tendons are stimulated by movements of the joints; informs the brain of the location of a body part |
| Antigravity (extensor) reflexes | When extensor muscles are stretched beyond a certain point, their stimulation causes a reflex contraction that counteracts the gravitational pull |
| Plantar reflexes | Reflexive contraction of the extensor muscles of the lower legs in response to pressure against the sole of the foot by the floor or ground |

## Nervous System

Muscle contraction is controlled by the central nervous system (CNS) and is influenced by the transport of nutrients and oxygen and by the removal of waste products. An intact CNS is essential for coordinated movement to occur. Nerve impulses stimulate the muscles to contract. The **myoneuronal junction** is the point at which nerve endings come into contact with muscle cells. The afferent pathway conveys information from sensory receptors to the CNS; these neurons conduct impulses throughout the body. The CNS processes the sensory input and determines a response. The efferent pathway transmits the desired response to skeletal muscles via the somatic nervous system. If the nerve impulses are interrupted, the muscle is paralyzed and cannot contract.

## Proprioception

**Proprioception** is the awareness of posture, movement, and changes in equilibrium and the knowledge of position, weight, and resistance of objects in relation to the body. Nerve endings in muscles, tendons, and joints (proprioceptors) continuously provide input to the brain, which, in turn, regulates smooth, coordinated involuntary movement. Proprioception tells a person where her body is in space relative to other objects. An example of this is walking downstairs while looking straight ahead and not down at the feet.

## Postural Reflexes

Postural tonus is maintained by postural or righting reflexes. Table 38-2 describes the major reflexes involved in maintaining posture.

# Exercise

Exercise is any physical activity involving muscles that elevates the heart rate above resting levels. Exercise reduces joint pain and stiffness, and increases flexibility, muscle strength, and endurance. It also helps with weight reduction and contributes to an improved sense of well-being. Americans have become less active in recent years (Edelman & Mandle, 2002).

The U.S. Surgeon General's Report on Physical Health and Activity (Centers for Disease Control and Prevention, 1999) lists the following facts about exercise:

- People who are usually inactive can improve their health and well-being by becoming even moderately active on a regular basis.
- Physical activity need not be strenuous to achieve health benefits.
- Greater health benefits can be achieved by increasing the amount (duration, frequency, or intensity) of physical activity.

Vigorous exercise stimulates an increased production of endorphins, which promote a sense of well-being. However, it is important to caution people not to overdo the exercise, especially when first starting a new regimen. The following may be signs of too much exercise: unusual or persistent fatigue, increased weakness, decreased range

## CLINICAL ALERT

### Cautions for Isometric Exercise

Individuals with cardiovascular problems should be cautioned to exhale when performing isometric exercises, to avoid increasing blood pressure.

of motion, joint swelling, or continuing pain (pain that lasts more than 1 hour after exercising). Instruct clients, especially those with sedentary lifestyles, to consult their nurse practitioner or physician before beginning an exercise program (Pender, Murdaugh, & Parsons, 2002).

## Types of Exercise

Several types of exercise promote physical and psychological health; see Table 38-3.

### Range-of-Motion Exercise

**Active range-of-motion (ROM)** activities are performed independently by the client. During active ROM exercises, the client moves various muscle groups. **Passive range-of-motion (ROM)** exercises are done by the nurse to help maintain or restore a client's mobility by achieving several outcomes; see Box 38-1.

## TABLE 38-3   TYPES OF EXERCISE

| Exercise Type | Function | Examples |
|---|---|---|
| Aerobic | Improve cardiovascular fitness<br>Assist with weight control<br>Improve general functional ability | Rowing<br>Jumping rope<br>Walking<br>Running<br>Kickboxing<br>Swimming |
| Strengthening | Maintain or increase muscle strength | Weight training<br>Calisthenics<br>Physical labor<br>Tai chi<br>Yoga |
| Isometric | Maintain muscle tone and strength | Quadriceps setting<br>Gluteal setting<br>Triceps setting |
| Isotonic | Increase and maintain muscle tone and strength<br>Shape muscles<br>Maintain joint mobility<br>Improve cardiovascular fitness | Weight lifting<br>Working with pulleys<br>Range-of-motion exercises<br>Performance of activities of daily living (ADL) |
| Isokinetic | Condition muscle groups | Exercise equipment<br>Resistive water exercises |
| Range-of-Motion (ROM) | Maintain joint movement<br>Maintain or increase flexibility | Adduction and abduction<br>Flexion and contraction |

## BOX 38-1    OUTCOMES OF PASSIVE RANGE-OF-MOTION EXERCISES

Prevention of contractures

Improves muscle strength and tone

Increases circulation

Decreases vascular complications of immobility

Facilitates client comfort

## BOX 38-2    BENEFITS OF EXERCISE

Normalizes glucose tolerance

Improves gait and balance

Improves cardiovascular function

Increases energy

Promotes bone density

Improves mobility

Promotes weight loss

Reduces blood pressure

Lowers cholesterol

Promotes rest and relaxation

Improves sleep

Data from Fleming, J. M. (2001). Successful aging. In M. O. Hogstel (Ed.), *Gerontology: Nursing care of the older adult* (p. 145), Clifton Park, NY: Delmar Learning.

## Physical Fitness

The ultimate outcome of regular physical activity is physical fitness, which affects an individual's functional ability. There are four components of physical fitness: endurance and strength, joint flexibility, cardiorespiratory fitness, and body composition.

### Endurance and Strength

Endurance is the ability to withstand movement in terms of duration and absence of fatigue. A physically fit individual has adequate muscular strength and endurance to accomplish her goals.

Muscle strength is the amount of force exerted by the muscles against resistance. Good muscle strength allows an individual to lift more safely.

### Joint Flexibility

The ability to use a muscle through its complete range of motion is referred to as flexibility; see Table 38-4 for a complete description of joint movement. People with limited flexibility are likely to experience shortened muscles and tendons with resultant imbalance in muscle strength and joint injury. Flexibility can be improved by stretching exercises such as yoga, tai chi, and dancing. Performance of ADLs also helps maintain flexibility.

##  LIFE SPAN CONSIDERATIONS

### Fitness in Older Adults

Approximately 33% of those aged 65 and older fall each year (Lamb & Cummings, 2000). "No one is too old to enjoy the benefits of regular physical activity. Of special interest to older adults is evidence that muscle-strengthening exercises can reduce the risk of fall and fracturing bones and improve the ability to live independently" (Centers for Disease Control & Prevention, 1999, p. 5). Box 38-2 lists benefits of physical exercise in older adults.

Walking, stooping, and lifting activities can promote and maintain flexibility.

### Cardiorespiratory Fitness

Exercises that improve cardiorespiratory fitness are discussed in Table 38-3. To improve cardiorespiratory function, physical activity must be maintained for at least 20 minutes in order to raise the heart rate to the target level.

### Body Composition

The recommended proportion of fat to lean body tissue is referred to as body composition. Having a body that falls within the normal range of body weight and percentage of body fat depends on balancing caloric intake and expenditure. Any type of physical activity can be useful in developing and maintaining physical fitness (see Chapter 35 for information on calculating body mass index [BMI]).

## Factors Affecting Mobility

Mobility and activity level can be influenced by many factors, including overall health status, developmental stage, environment, attitudes, beliefs, and lifestyle.

### Health Status

An individual's general health status will influence desire for exercise and activity tolerance. Compromised status of any of the body systems may affect an individual's mobility

## TABLE 38-4    JOINT RANGE OF MOTION

| Joint Movement | Range | Muscle Group(s) |
|---|---|---|
| **1. Temporomandibular Joint (TMJ) (Synovial Joint)** | | |
| a. Open mouth. | 1–2.5 in. | |
| b. Close mouth. | Complete closure | Masseter, temporalis |
| c. *Protrusion:* Push out lower jaw. | 0.5 in. | Pterygoideus lateralis |
| d. *Retrusion:* Tuck in lower jaw. | 0.5 in. | |
| e. *Lateral motion:* Slide jaw from side to side. | 0.5 in. | Pterygoideus lateralis, pterygoideus medialis |
| **2. Cervical Spine (Pivot Joint)** | | |
| a. *Flexion:* Rest chin on chest. | 45 degrees each side | Sternocleidomastoid |
| b. *Extension:* Return head to midline. | 45 degrees | Trapezius |
| c. *Hyperextension:* Tilt head back. | 10 degrees | Trapezius |
| d. *Lateral flexion:* Move head to touch ear to shoulder. | 40 degrees each side | Sternocleidomastoid |
| e. *Rotation:* Turn head to look to side. | 90 degrees each side | Sternocleidomastoid, trapezius |
| **3. Shoulder (Ball-and-Socket Joint)** | | |
| a. *Flexion:* Raise straight arm forward to a position above the head. | 180 degrees | Pectoralis major, coracobrachialis, deltoid, biceps brachii |
| b. *Extension:* Return straight arm forward and down to side of body. | 180 degrees | Latissimus dorsi, deltoid, triceps brachii, teres major |
| c. *Hyperextension:* Move straight arm behind body. | 50 degrees | Latissimus dorsi, deltoid, teres major |

*(continues)*

## TABLE 38-4    JOINT RANGE OF MOTION (*continued*)

| Joint Movement | Range | Muscle Group(s) |
|---|---|---|
| d. *Abduction:* Move straight arm laterally from side to a position above the head, palm facing away from head. | 180 degrees | Deltoid, supraspinatus |
| e. *Adduction:* Move straight arm downward laterally and across front of body as far as possible. | 230 degrees | Pectoralis major, teres major |
| f. *Circumduction:* Move straight arm in a full circle. | 360 degrees | Deltoid, coracobrachialis, latissimus dorsi, teres major |
| g. *External rotation:* Bent arm lateral, parallel to floor, palm down, rotate shoulder so fingers point up. | 90 degrees | Infraspinatus, teres minor, deltoid |
| h. *Internal rotation:* Bent arm lateral, parallel to floor, rotate shoulder so fingers point down. | 90 degrees | Subscapularis, pectoralis major, latissimus dorsi, teres major |
| **4. Elbow (Hinge Joint)** | | |
| a. *Flexion:* Bend elbow, move lower arm toward shoulder, palm facing shoulder. | 150 degrees | Biceps brachii, brachialis, brachioradialis |
| b. *Extension:* Straighten lower arm forward and downward. | 150 degrees | Triceps brachii |
| c. *Rotation for supination:* Elbow bent, turn hand and forearm so palm is facing upward. | 70 degrees to 90 degrees | Biceps brachii, supinator |
| d. *Rotation for pronation:* Elbow bent, turn hand and forearm so palm is facing downward. | 70 degrees to 90 degrees | Pronator teres, pronator quadratus |

*(continues)*

## TABLE 38-4   JOINT RANGE OF MOTION (*continued*)

| Joint Movement | Range | Muscle Group(s) |
|---|---|---|
| **5. Wrist (Condyloid Joint)** | | |
| a. *Flexion:* Bend wrist so fingers move toward inner aspect of forearm. | 80 degrees to 90 degrees | Flexor carpi radialis, flexor carpi ulnaris |
| b. *Extension:* Straighten hand to same plane as arm. | 80 degrees to 90 degrees | Extensor carpi radialis longus, extensor carpi radialis brevis, extensor carpi ulnaris |
| c. *Hyperextension:* Bend wrist so fingers move back as far as possible. | 80 degrees to 90 degrees | Extensor carpi radialis longus, extensor carpi radialis brevis, extensor carpi ulnaris |
| d. *Radial flexion: abduction*—Bend wrist laterally toward thumb. | Up to 20 degrees | Extensor carpi radialis longus, extensor carpi radialis brevis, flexor carpi radialis |
| e. *Ulnar flexion: adduction*—Bend wrist laterally away from thumb. | 30 degrees to 50 degrees | Extensor carpi ulnaris, flexor carpi ulnaris |
| **6. Hand and Fingers (Condyloid and Hinge Joints)** | | |
| a. *Flexion:* Make a fist. | 90 degrees | Interosseus dorsalis manus, flexor digitorum superficialis |
| b. *Extension:* Straighten fingers. | 90 degrees | Extensor indicis, extensor digiti minimi |
| c. *Hyperextension:* Bend fingers back as far as possible. | 30 degrees to 50 degrees | Extensor indicis, extensor digiti minimi |
| d. *Abduction:* Spread fingers apart. | 25 degrees | Interosseus dorsalis manus |
| e. *Adduction:* Bring fingers together. | 25 degrees | Interrosseus palmares |
| **7. Thumb (Saddle Joint)** | | |
| a. *Flexion:* Move thumb across palmar surface of hand. | 90 degrees | Flexor pollicis brevis, opponens pollicis |
| b. *Extension:* Move thumb away from hand. | 90 degrees | Extensor pollicis brevis, extensor pollicis longus |
| c. *Abduction:* Move thumb laterally. | 30 degrees | Abductor pollicis brevis, abductor pollicis longus |
| d. *Adduction:* Move thumb back to hand. | 30 degrees | Adductor pollicis transversus, adductor pollicis obliquus |
| e. *Opposition:* Touch thumb to tip of each finger of same hand. | Touching | Opponens pollicis, flexor pollicis brevis |

*(continues)*

## TABLE 38-4    JOINT RANGE OF MOTION (*continued*)

| Joint Movement | Range | Muscle Group(s) |
|---|---|---|
| **8. Hip (Ball-and-Socket Joint)** | | |
| a. *Flexion:* Move straight leg forward and upward. | 90 degrees to 120 degrees | Psoas major, iliacus, iliopsoas |
| b. *Extension:* Move leg back beside the other leg. | 90 degrees to 120 degrees | Gluteus maximus, adductor magnus, semitendinosus, semimembranosus |
| c. *Hyperextension:* Move leg behind body. | 30 degrees to 50 degrees | Gluteus maximus, semitendinosus, semimembranosus |
| d. *Abduction:* Move leg laterally from midline. | 40 degrees to 50 degrees | Gluteus medius, gluteus minimus |
| e. *Adduction:* Move leg back past midline. | 20 degrees to 30 degrees past midline | Adductor magnus, adductor brevis, adductor longus |
| f. *Circumduction:* Move leg backward in a circle. | 360 degrees | Psoas major, gluteus maximus, gluteus medius, adductor magnus |
| g. *Internal rotation:* Turn foot and leg inward, pointing toes toward other leg. | 90 degrees | Gluteus minimus, gluteus medius, tensor fasciae latae |
| h. *External rotation:* Turn foot and leg outward, pointing toes away from other leg. | 90 degrees | Obturator externus, obturator internus, quadratus femoris |
| **9. Knee (Hinge Joint)** | | |
| a. *Flexion:* Bend knee to bring heel back toward thigh. | 120 degrees to 130 degrees | Biceps femoris, semitendinosus, semimembranosus |
| b. *Extension:* Straighten each leg, place foot beside other foot. | 120 degrees to 130 degrees | Rectus femoris, vastus lateralis, vastus medialis, vastus intermedius |
| **10. Ankle (Hinge Joint)** | | |
| a. *Plantar flexion:* Point toes downward. | 45 degrees to 50 degrees | Gastrocnemius, soleus |
| b. *Dorsiflexion:* Point toes upward. | 20 degrees | Peroneus tertius, tibialis anterior |

*(continues)*

## TABLE 38-4   JOINT RANGE OF MOTION (continued)

| Joint Movement | Range | Muscle Group(s) |
|---|---|---|
| **11. Foot (Gliding Joint)** | | |
| a. *Eversion:* Turn sole of foot laterally. | 5 degrees | Peroneus longus, peroneus brevis |
| b. *Inversion:* Turn sole of foot medially. | 5 degrees | Tibialis posterior, tibialis anterior |
| **12. Toes (Condyloid)** | | |
| a. *Flexion:* Curve toes downward. | 35 degrees to 60 degrees | Flexor hallucis brevis, lumbricales pedis, flexor digitorum brevis |
| b. *Extension:* Straighten toes. | 35 degrees to 60 degrees | Extensor digitorum longus, extensor digitorum brevis, extensor hallucis longus |
| c. *Abduction:* Spread toes apart. | Up to 15 degrees | Interosseus dorsales pedis, abductor hallucis |
| d. *Adduction:* Bring toes together. | Up to 15 degrees | Adductor hallucis, interosseus plantares |

and may, in turn, be affected by a lack of activity. Physical conditioning will also influence mobility and stamina. Physical factors interfering with mobility or exercise include fatigue, muscle cramping, dyspnea, neuromuscular or perceptual deficits, and chest pain (World Health Organization, 2002).

Mental status is often manifested as changes in mobility or appearance. For instance, a client who shuffles into the room, slumps down into a chair, and avoids eye contact may be sending a message of depression through low activity levels, poor posture, and a flattened affect.

## Developmental Stage

An individual's developmental stage will affect the parameters of targeted mobility levels. Developmental stages are also related to broader topics of nursing concerns, such as participation in health-promotive activities.

See Table 38-5 for examples of common age-related musculoskeletal trauma.

### Children

Developmental norms related to mobility have been established for the infant and toddler. Childhood development is monitored through achievement of milestones such as sitting, crawling, walking, running, and hopping. For *infants,* the mobility focus is on gross motor behavior such as posture, head balance, grasping, sitting, creeping, and standing. *Toddlers* are more active, with walking, running, jumping, kicking, and going up and down stairs. Activity and mobility parameters for the toddler encompass gross and fine motor behaviors, manual dexterity, and exploration within environmental safety parameters. The *pre-*

*schooler* increases strength and refines skills by walking, running, and jumping. During *middle childhood* (from 6 to 12 years of age), children have improved posture and locomotion abilities and increased muscle efficiency of the extremities and trunk; these children also have an increase

## TABLE 38-5   COMMON AGE-RELATED MUSCULOSKELETAL TRAUMA

| Age Range | Common Trauma |
|---|---|
| 0 to 18 months | Falls |
| 18 months to 6 years | Falls |
| 6 to 20 years | Sports-related injuries<br>Motorcycle accidents<br>High-impact falls (e.g., cycling, skiing) |
| 20 to 50 years | Sports-related injuries<br>Stress or overuse injuries (e.g., tendonitis)<br>Pedestrian injuries |
| 50 to 65+ years | Recreation-related injuries<br>Falls<br>Pathological fractures<br>Pedestrian injuries |

## FOCUS ON WELLNESS

### Self-Esteem and Mobility

Any change in mobility changes a client's self-esteem, through loss of a body part, physiological function, or a psychological attribute. The degree to which the losses affect a person's self-esteem largely depends on the integrity of the client's body image as well as the client's developmental stage. Knowledge of developmental stages will help the nurse recognize factors that influence the concept of a client's self-esteem by understanding his needs and responses. The nurse can then work with the client in moving toward health-promotive behaviors and attitudes.

Adapted from Pender, J., Murdaugh, C., & Parsons, M. A. (2002). *Health promotion in nursing practice* (4th ed.). Upper Saddle River, NJ: Prentice-Hall.

---

in muscle tissue with a decrease of fat. For both preschool and middle childhood, activity and mobility expectations are centered on development of strength, coordination, and physical capacities (Covington, Cybulski, Davis, Duca, Farrel, Kasgorgis, Kator, & Sell, 2001).

### Adolescents

The *adolescent* years (approximately ages 12 to 18) begin with onset of puberty and end with cessation of somatic growth. Changes are dramatic at this stage, with physical growth and development of secondary sex characteristics. Activity and mobility landmarks are development of muscles plus cardiac, respiratory, and metabolic functions through physical conditioning.

### Adults

Adulthood is divided into young, middle, and older age groups. The *young adult* has well-developed myoskeletal and nervous systems that ideally function at peak efficiency. The *middle-aged adult* has a gradual decrease in muscle mass, strength, and agility. The focus of activity and mobility for both these groups is on maintaining or developing tone, strength, and coordination of the musculoskeletal system.

*Older adults* often have progressive changes in the physiological systems. The rate of bone reabsorption (which affects bone density) increases with aging. Bone density loss accelerates in postmenopausal females due to estrogen deficiency. Decreased bone density makes a person more vulnerable to fractures, kyphosis, and a reduction in height.

Aging also negatively impacts muscles and connective tissue. The development of muscle atrophy is a gradual

process in which muscle fibers deteriorate and are replaced by fibrous connective tissue. Muscle atrophy is accompanied by reduced muscle mass, a loss of muscle strength, and a reduction in overall body mass. The degree of muscle atrophy will be affected by the person's activity level. Staying physically active helps prevent disuse muscle atrophy and helps maximize muscle strength.

Cartilage ages better than bone or muscle; however, some changes occur that do affect joint flexibility. Aging leads to a loss of water content of hyaline cartilage and a reduction in the ability of cartilage to regenerate following trauma. Articulating cartilage may slightly deteriorate as a result of lifetime wear and tear.

Aging also affects the health of intervertebral disks. For example, the water content of the disks decreases, which leads to less vertebral flexibility. Thinning of the disks causes older individuals to be more vulnerable to back pain and injury.

As a result of the age-related physical changes, older people often experience some functional alterations in mobility. Ambulation may be altered as a result of joint inflexibility and decreased muscle strength; such alterations are noticed as a reduction in step height and length as demonstrated in a shuffling gait. Vertebral inflexibility and reduced muscle strength may cause difficulty with client transfers in and out of a sitting position. The older client may need assistance in rising from a chair, ambulating, or climbing stairs. Table 38-6 provides an overview of age-related effects on mobility. Aging also affects the cardiovascular and respiratory systems, which directly affect endurance and stamina. Activity and mobility goals focus on maintenance of functional status and safety (Bonder & Wagner, 2001).

| TABLE 38-6 | EFFECTS OF AGING ON MUSCULOSKELETAL SYSTEM | |
|---|---|
| **Physiological Changes** | **Results** |
| Muscle cells replaced by fibrous connective tissue | Decreased muscle mass, tone, and strength |
| Decreased elasticity of ligaments, tendons, and cartilage | Weaker bones |
| Decreased bone mass | Weaker bones |
| Dehydration of intervertebral disks | Possible loss of height |
| Flattening of convex curvature of spine | Posture becomes more flexed Center of gravity shifts |

Data from Lamb, K. V. D., & Cummings, M. (2000). Musculoskeletal function. In A. G. Lueckenotte, (Ed.), *Gerontologic nursing* (2nd ed.). St. Louis: Mosby.

## Environment

Environment can influence activity level in several ways. Home environments, for instance, can be considered safe and "mobility friendly" if they are free of hazards that can disrupt or endanger mobility and activity. Work environments can also affect mobility; repetitive handwork, such as keystroking or sewing, can impair mobility and worsen arthritis. A sedentary lifestyle can lead to muscle atrophy, weakened bones, and a lack of motivation and energy to engage in physical activity.

## Attitudes and Beliefs

Influential factors related to exercise are one's attitudes and beliefs, which are greatly affected by culture and family. Leisure activities provide a clue to the person's value system. Individuals who engage in hiking, bicycle riding, or swimming for recreation value an active lifestyle. On the other hand, individuals who consider work to be the dominant area of life may view exercise as "a waste of time." Does the individual go everywhere in a car, or is walking a part of normal transportation? Are elevators routinely used instead of climbing stairs? Activities enjoyed by the individual are less likely to produce fatigue than are activities that hold no interest for the person. Thus, preferences should be matched with capabilities when planning an exercise program.

## Lifestyle

Modern lifestyles require little physical activity; thus, few adults in America are naturally fit. The use of many convenience items (e.g., fast food, remote controls) encourage little physical exertion. The sedentary lifestyles of many Americans result in loss of muscle strength, decreased endurance, inadequate cardiorespiratory function, and obesity. Individuals with active lifestyles value exercise and, therefore, are more likely to experience its therapeutic outcomes.

# Physiological Effects of Mobility and immobility

Maintaining functional mobility and desired activity levels is important for both psychological and physiological reasons. Mobility and lack thereof will each affect the various systems of the body. Table 38-7 summarizes the major complications associated with immobility.

## Neurologic Effects/Mental Status

As for mental status, mobility and activity can increase an individual's energy levels and sense of well-being. Activity and exercise are excellent means to relieve tension and reduce stress, which result in better sleep patterns and an enhanced sense of well-being.

Client inactivity and immobility are stressors that can lead to frustration, lower self-esteem, anxiety, helplessness, depression, general dissatisfaction, restlessness, unhappiness, and

| TABLE 38-7 | NEGATIVE OUTCOMES OF IMMOBILITY | |
|---|---|
| **Neurologic** | **Gastrointestinal** |
| Sensory deprivation | Decreased appetite |
| | Stress ulcers |
| | Constipation |
| | Fecal impaction |
| **Cardiovascular** | **Urinary** |
| Increased cardiac workload | Urinary stasis |
| Orthostatic hypotension | Urinary tract infection |
| Formation of thrombus | Calculi |
| **Respiratory** | **Integumentary** |
| Increased respiratory effort | Pressure ulcers |
| Hypostatic pneumonia | Skin shearing |
| Altered gas exchange | Prolonged healing process |
| **Musculoskeletal** | **Psychological** |
| Decreased bone density (increased risk of fracture) | Anxiety |
| | Depression |
| Contractures | Helplessness, |
| Muscle atrophy | hopelessness |
| Increased pain | Increased dependency |

decreased competency self-rating. Immobility impacts cognitive abilities, affect, lifestyle, and social and family responsibilities. The fear of falls, pain, and sensory deficits such as visual problems, fatigue, and weakness are compounding factors that increase inactivity and immobility.

## Cardiovascular Effects

The cardiovascular system reaps many benefits from mobility and exercise. The heart becomes more efficient as it adapts to increased demands for oxygen, and cardiac output increases. A healthy heart muscle leads to a decreased resting heart rate and decreased resting blood pressure, which means that the heart does not have to work as hard in an individual who exercises regularly as it does in an individual who leads a sedentary lifestyle. Activity increases the oxygen supply to the heart and muscles and thereby benefits overall health.

Immobility increases the workload on the heart as the supine position increases the volume of blood circulating to the heart. This fluid shift increases central venous pressure along with left ventricular diastolic volume and stroke volume, and the cardiac workload increases. The cardiovascular system is prone to form **thrombi**, or blood clots, due to venous stasis related to lack of muscle contractions of the legs and pressure on veins, especially the popliteal areas (Figure 38-5). Thrombi are caused by increased coagulation of the blood due to free calcium from bone demineralization, stasis of venous blood, and intimal damage to veins (as from venipuncture).

Another cardiovascular problem related to immobility is **orthostatic hypotension**, or a decrease in blood pressure resulting from sudden position changes, caused by decreased vessel tone. In orthostatic hypotension, the blood pressure parameters drop at least 25 mm systolic and 10 mm diastolic with the postural changes. Orthostatic hypotension is a result of several factors associated with immobility, including:

- Decreased circulating fluid volume
- Decreased autonomic nervous system response
- Blood pooling in lower extremities

These factors lead to decreased venous return, which negatively affects cardiac output. Thus, the blood pressure is lowered. Orthostatic hypotension is an indication that the heart is working harder and less efficiently.

Clients who have experienced immobility (such as with bed rest) need to have blood pressure checked lying down, sitting, then standing. This is done to establish baseline parameters to assist in determining the presence of postural-related changes in blood pressure.

## Respiratory Effects

The respiratory system response to activity and mobility is increased intake of oxygen, which results in increased overall respiratory capacity and an easing in the work of breathing. The effects of oxygenation to the tissues are enhanced and pooling of secretions in the bronchioles is less likely.

Immobility from sitting or lying limits chest expansion, which is compounded by the effects of respiratory muscle atrophy and ineffective cough (Figure 38-6). Stasis of respiratory secretions can be worsened by the use of CNS-depressant medications and dehydration, and can lead to hypostatic pneumonia and atelectasis.

## Musculoskeletal Effects

Musculoskeletal responses to activity are numerous, including stronger and better-defined muscles, stronger bones, and increased mobility and range of motion of the joints. Exercise can enhance endurance and tolerance of the muscle groups. Weight-bearing exercises such as walking (as opposed to swimming) are especially beneficial in preventing osteoporosis, or loss of strength and minerals in the bones.

Decreased physical mobility results in gross musculoskeletal impairment, especially when muscular atrophy occurs. Decreased mobilization alters muscle structure by reducing muscle mass and decreasing muscle cell diameter and the actual number of muscle cells. Clients experience rapid fatigue, decreased muscle strength and tone, decreased endurance, decreased mobility of joints, muscle stiffness, joint contracture, and negative nitrogen balance due to protein catabolism. Loss of calcium is a response to immobility and indicates an imbalance between bone formation and breakdown. The lack of pressure (e.g., weight bearing) on bones triggers calcium loss. Bone demineralization occurs as early as 2 or 3 days after onset of immobility and may lead to pathological fractures, renal calculi, and osteoporosis (White & Duncan, 2002).

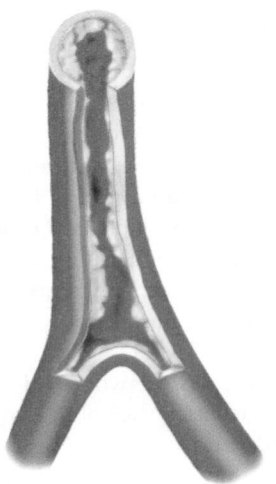

**Figure 38-5**    Effect of immobility on the cardiovascular system

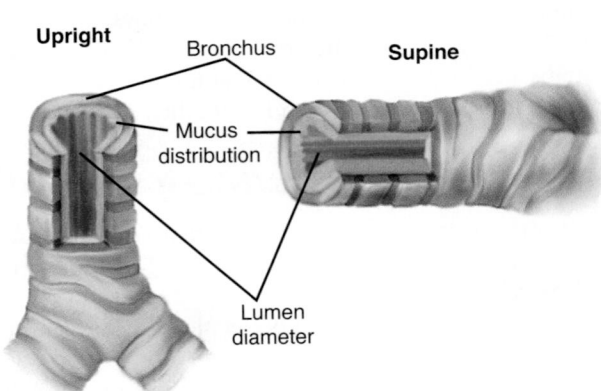

**Figure 38-6**    Effect of immobility on the respiratory system

## Digestive Effects

Digestive responses to activity include increased appetite and thirst, which indicate that the body's rate of processing nutritional intake is increased.

Loss of appetite is commonly related to lack of activity, negative nitrogen balance, and altered elimination patterns. Negative nitrogen balance occurs when the nitrogen output exceeds nitrogen intake. The causes of negative nitrogen balance include the increased need for protein in situations of extensive tissue damage, such as following surgery, and extended immobility. Extended periods of immobility cause muscle atrophy or muscle wasting; thus, there is a need for extra protein intake to provide for muscle repair.

## Elimination Effects

Elimination patterns are facilitated by mobility in that retention of wastes is usually prevented and the risk of constipation is reduced or avoided. The muscles become stronger and more efficient, thus enhancing the overall efficiency of elimination.

Constipation and fecal impaction are frequent complications of immobility. Variables contributing to these elimination problems are shown in the Client Education box.

Urinary stasis and urinary infections are related to the recumbent position of the immobile person. Decreased peristalsis of the ureters leads to stasis of urine, which is the etiology of urinary calculi (stones) and infection. Bladder distention occurs due to difficult relaxation of the external sphincter and decreased intra-abdominal pressure, thus causing overflow **incontinence** (loss of bladder control) and infection. The combination of increased urinary calcium, urinary stasis, and urinary infection leads to calculi formation (Palmer, 2002).

## Integumentary Effects

The integumentary system benefits from activity and exercise in that increased circulation and blood flow enhance

---

### CLIENT EDUCATION

#### Variables That Affect Elimination

The nurse should teach the client with constipation to remember the following variables that contribute to elimination problems:

- ✓ Lack of activity (which decreases peristalsis)
- ✓ Lack of privacy
- ✓ Inability to sit upright
- ✓ Improper diet
- ✓ Inadequate fluid intake
- ✓ Some medications, particularly narcotics
- ✓ Overuse of laxatives

McKenna, S., Wallis, M., Brannelly, A., & Cawood, J. (2001). The nursing management of diarrhea and constipation before and after the implementation of a bowel management protocol. *Australian Critical Care, 14*(1),10–16.

---

oxygenation of tissues, maintaining the turgor and luster of the skin and hair.

Pressure ulcers are serious problems related to immobility. Prolonged pressure, shearing force, friction (rubbing), and moisture lead to tissue ischemia (impaired blood circulation), causing skin breakdown and decubiti. Moisture in the form of urine, feces, perspiration, and wound drainage can also lead to skin softening, which increases decubiti risk. Secondary factors contributing to pressure sore development are decreased nutrition, decreased arterial pressure, increased age, and edema.

## Assessment

During the assessment phase of the nursing process, data regarding activity and mobility of the client are gathered. Assessment data are used to initiate, individualize, plan, evaluate, and modify care on the basis of the client's strengths and limitations. Assessment of mobility status includes a health history and physical examination.

### Health History

Taking a client's health history is the first step in determining the mobility needs and concerns of a client. Basic information about ADL, exercise patterns (type, frequency), lifestyle (active, sedentary), activity tolerance, and use of medications should be discussed. If an alteration or recent change in status is noted, then a detailed health history is in order. The nurse should ask what impact the mobility impairment has had on the client's ADL and should have the client describe the exact nature of the problem (onset, duration, associated factors, aggravating factors, alleviating factors). The nurse should ask clients about the use (past

---

 ### CLIENT REFLECTIONS

#### Immobility and Its Effects on Digestion

Mr. Arego, age 82, is heard discussing the following with his home health nurse: "I hate it when I get sick—even when I get a little cold (virus). It makes me not feel like going for my (daily) walk, and that always makes me constipated. Then I don't feel like eating anything, and my energy level goes down. That adds to my not wanting to exercise, and it becomes a vicious cycle."

What would you say to this client?

and current) of medications, both prescription and over-the-counter, with the explanation that many drugs negatively affect the musculoskeletal system; see Table 38-8. It is also important to ask about the use of calcium supplements and estrogen replacement medication.

## Physical Examination

The physical examination of mobility status typically covers three basic areas: musculoskeletal assessment, neurologic assessment, and functional assessment.

### Musculoskeletal Assessment

The nurse observes musculoskeletal functioning during every interaction with the client. Specific factors for objective assessment include the following:

- Body alignment
- Body mechanics
- Posture (sitting and standing)
- Range of motion of joints
- Strength of muscles
- Endurance
- Muscle tone
- Size and contour of joints
- Inspection of the skin
- Palpation of skin, muscles, and joints

Subjective data include assessment of client's pain, joint stiffness, muscle cramping, fatigue, weakness, exercise habits, and environmental variables. Children should be evaluated by comparing physical development and abilities with normal values for the age. Older clients should be evaluated on functional abilities, strengths, weaknesses, joint limitations, and use of assistive devices such as canes or walkers to assist the client in ADLs.

A complete musculoskeletal assessment needs to include data related to client weakness, stiffness, and pain related to movement. A 0 to 10 intensity scale can be used to assess these subjective factors. When assessing weakness, 0 represents complete absence of weakness and 10 represents weakness requiring complete bed rest. For determining stiffness, 0 represents complete absence of stiffness and 10 represents total inflexibility.

### Movement and Gait

Gait, the way that one walks, is assessed to determine a baseline. Normal gait is characterized by a smooth rhythmic movement of muscles when walking. Step height and length are symmetrical for each foot and the arms swing freely at each side of the torso in opposite movement of the legs. Normally, the lower limbs are able to bear full body weight during standing and ambulation. Gait is described in terms of smoothness, balance, arm movement, effectiveness, and the length and width of the step.

### Alignment

When assessing body alignment, the nurse seeks to determine whether the movement results in fatigue, muscle stress, or strain. Structural deformities may interfere with body alignment and functional ability; see Table 38-9.

### Endurance

When assessing a client's endurance during physical activity, look for reactions such as mood changes, indicators of pain, presence of fatigue, and changes in respiratory and circulatory status. Oxygen consumption increases during muscle activity; thus, assessment of vital signs is essential. The time required for vital signs to return to the normal (baseline) resting values is a significant factor to include in the assessment of mobility.

### Pathological Alterations

Assessment to determine the presence of pathological alterations—such as bone disorders, joint impairment, impaired muscle development, postural abnormalities, musculoskeletal trauma, and neurologic damage—can offer important data for the determination of mobility limitations.

**Muscle Impairments**    Overuse injuries are a common type of musculoskeletal problem, especially in people who exercise too much and/or incorrectly. Common overuse injuries are listed in Table 38-10.

**Postural Abnormalities**    In addition to the postural abnormalities described in Table 38-10, contractures may also affect body alignment.

**Contractures**    A contracture develops when the muscle fibers become unable to flex. Each muscle has an antagonist that works in the opposite direction. If a muscle

| TABLE 38-8 | MUSCULOSKELETAL SIDE EFFECTS OF MEDICATIONS/ SUBSTANCES |
|---|---|
| **Medication** | **Musculoskeletal Effect** |
| Amphetamines | Muscle hyperactivity |
| Anticoagulants | Bleeding into the joints |
| Antipsychotics | Dystonic movements, altered gait |
| Caffeine | Muscle hyperactivity |
| Corticosteroids | Necrosis of femur head |
| Diuretics | Muscle weakness and cramping |
| Phenothiazines | Gait disturbances |

Data from Davison, M. A. (1998). Antipsychotic medications. In M. E. Kuhn (Ed.), *Pharmacotherapeutics: A nursing process approach* (4th ed. p. 393). Philadelphia: F. A. Davis; O'Hanlon-Nichols, T. (1998). A review of the adult musculoskeletal system. *American Journal of Nursing, 98*(6), 49.

## TABLE 38-9   SPINAL MISALIGNMENT

| Anomaly | Description | Clinical Implications |
| --- | --- | --- |
| **Scoliosis**<br><br>• *Postural scoliosis:* no fixed rotation of vertebrae; can be corrected with exercise<br>• *Structural scoliosis:* fixed rotation of the vertebrae in the direction of the convexity of the curve<br><br>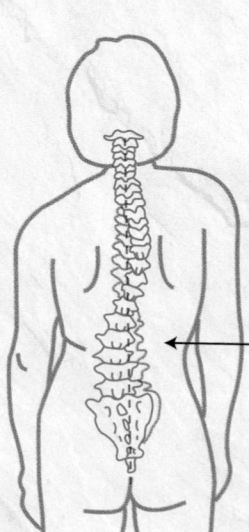 | • Lateral deviation in the normally straight vertical line of the spine<br>• More common in females, especially during adolescence<br>• Some indicators:<br>  • One side higher than the other or one shoulder blade more prominent<br>  • Abnormal waistline tilt with more indentation on one side<br>  • Tilting of the hips with one hip more prominent<br>  • A prominence of the posterior chest or the shoulder when bending over. | • Can progress to a severe curvature in a short period of time if untreated. |
| **Kyphosis**<br><br>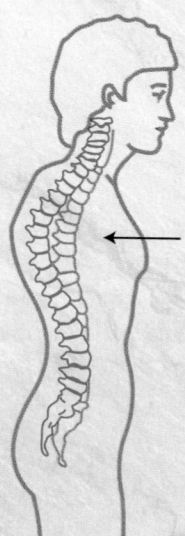 | • Abnormally increased convexity in the curvature of the spine<br>• Chin tilts downward onto chest with abdominal protrusion<br>• Decreased interval between lower rib cage and iliac crests | • In advanced stages, can interfere with lung expansion<br>• Commonly seen:<br>  — older clients<br>  — osteoporosis<br>• Paget's disease |

*(continues)*

## TABLE 38-9    SPINAL MISALIGNMENT (continued)

| Anomaly | Description | Clinical Implications |
|---|---|---|
| **Lordosis** | • Forward curvature of the lumbar spine | • More pronounced in obesity and pregnancy (due to change in center of gravity) |
| **List** | • Lateral lean of the spine<br>• Iliac crests are unequal in height<br>• Decreased ROM, usually accompanied by pain | • Commonly present in:<br>—back injury<br>—osteoarthritis<br>—herniated vertebral disk |

## TABLE 38-10    MUSCULOSKELETAL TRAUMA, COMMON OVERUSE INJURIES

| | |
|---|---|
| Strain | Commonly referred to as "pulled muscles"<br>Caused by overstretching, tearing, or ripping of a muscle and/or its tendon |
| Tendonitis | Inflammation of a tendon caused by chronic, low-grade strain of a muscle-tendon unit |
| Bursitis | Inflammation of the bursa (lubricating sac surrounding a joint)<br>Caused by repeated low-grade strains of the joint's supporting tissues |
| Sprain | Overstretching or tearing of ligaments |

group is not moved for a period of time or if proper body alignment is not maintained, the stronger muscle will predominate, causing contracture deformities.

Once a contracture occurs, the only corrective action is surgery to release the fibrous tissue. Prevention of contractures is a major nursing focus with immobile clients. Nursing interventions to prevent a muscle contracture include:

- Encouraging clients to be as active as possible
- Performing ROM exercises
- Positioning to maintain proper body alignment
- Repositioning every 2 hours or more often as needed

### Musculoskeletal Trauma

Trauma to musculoskeletal tissues can result in many types of impairments (such as those described in the display on overuse disorders). Another common type of musculoskeletal trauma is a fracture (broken bone). The second type of trauma discussed below is surgical amputation.

***Fractures*** According to Lamb and Cummings (2000), hip fractures are the most disabling for older people. Hip fractures are usually a result of falls and approximately 24% of those with hip fracture die from complications within 1 year after the injury. Hip fracture complications result from immobility and include pressure ulcers, pneumonia, and sepsis from urinary tract infections (Salkeld, Cameron, & Cumming, 2000).

When a fracture is suspected, the nurse should assess the area for mobility, pain, color, temperature, pulse, and sensation.

***Amputation*** Any condition in which circulation is inadequate to maintain cellular function can necessitate amputation. For example, lower limb amputations are often required as a result of infection, peripheral vascular disease (PVD), neoplasm, and trauma. Pressure ulcers, if inadequately treated, can also lead to the loss of a limb. When the decubiti do not heal, infection and gangrene develop. Gangrene first manifests as a blackened area and is often accompanied by pain.

Lower limb amputation is either above the knee or below the knee; the level of amputation depends on the extent of the disease process. Below-the-knee amputation is the most commonly performed type. The goal of the surgery is to preserve the length of the extremity in order to assist with prosthetic fitting. Therefore, as much limb as possible is salvaged.

### Central Nervous System Damage

As movement is a result of coordination between muscles and nerves, an intact central nervous system (CNS) is necessary for mobility. Any disruption in the CNS, such as those occurring with spinal cord injury, can impair mobility. Spinal cord injury can lead to partial paralysis or complete loss of mobility.

***Spinal Cord Injury*** There are 15,000 to 20,000 traumatic spinal cord injuries each year in the United States (Huston,

1998). Damage to the spinal cord can be a result of hyperextension and/or compression. With hyperextension, the spinal cord is overstretched, leading to dislocation of the vertebrae or disks and possible compression of the spinal cord. Hyperextension can also completely dissect the spinal cord. In a complete spinal cord injury, voluntary motor activity, sensory function, and proprioception below the level of the injury are lacking.

Compression injuries occur when the force of impact fractures the vertebrae or ruptures the disks, forcing bony fragments or disks into the spinal canal. These particles can lacerate or compress the spinal cord, resulting in paralysis below the level of the injury. Prevention of spinal cord injuries is a major concern of nurses and may be addressed through educating the public on safety precautions related to driving, participation in sports, and leisure activities.

### Neurologic Assessment

An intact neurologic system is essential for activity and mobility. Objective neurologic assessment includes (1) cranial nerves, (2) motor system, (3) sensory system, and (4) reflexes. The nurse assesses the motor system for the following variables:

- Size, strength, and tone of muscles
- Presence of involuntary movements
- Balance
- Gait
- Coordination
- Proprioception
- Fine motor function
- Gross motor function

## CLINICAL ALERT

### Autonomic Dysreflexia

Autonomic dysreflexia is an emergent physiological condition most commonly seen in clients with upper spinal cord injury. It is caused by massive sympathetic discharge of stimuli from the autonomic nervous system and may be triggered by distention of the bladder or colon. Symptoms include sudden hypertension, bradycardia, sweating, severe headache, and gooseflesh. Nursing interventions include having client sit upright, draining bladder, and checking catheter for blockage. Remove any other stimuli that may be triggering response; monitor vital signs, especially blood pressure; and administer any antihypertensives ordered.

Guin, P. R. (2001). Advances in spinal cord injury care. *Critical Care Nursing Clinics of North America, 13*(3), 399–409.

The sensory system is assessed for integrity of peripheral nerves, pain, tactile discrimination (fine touch), and sensation of vibration. Assessment of deep tendon or stretch reflexes focuses on the biceps, triceps, brachioradialis, quadriceps, and Achilles reflexes.

### Functional Assessment

**Functional assessment** focuses on the client's abilities to perform ADL. The client's functional status is assessed in terms of the ability to feed, dress, toilet, move, transfer, and ambulate self independently or with some degree of required assistance (Figure 38-7). Functional assessment data are used for initial planning, for discharge planning, for planning continuity of care in a nursing home or private home, and to provide baseline and ongoing data for rehabilitation.

Clients at high-risk for falls include those with prolonged hospitalization, those taking sedatives or tranquilizers, confused clients, or those with a history of physical restraint use. A great majority of falls:

- Occur in the evening
- Occur in the client's room
- Involve wheelchairs
- Involve unattended clients
- Involve clients with poor footwear
- Occur with poor lighting
- Involve clients with poor vision
- Occur with clients experiencing neuromuscular impairment

Awareness of these risk factors for falls allows the nurse to prevent many client injuries (Gillespie, Gillespie, & Cumming, 2000).

The nurse continually evaluates the client's strength and endurance during the entire ambulation process. The Risk Assessment Tool (RAT) for falls was developed to identify clients at high risk for falls and to individualize

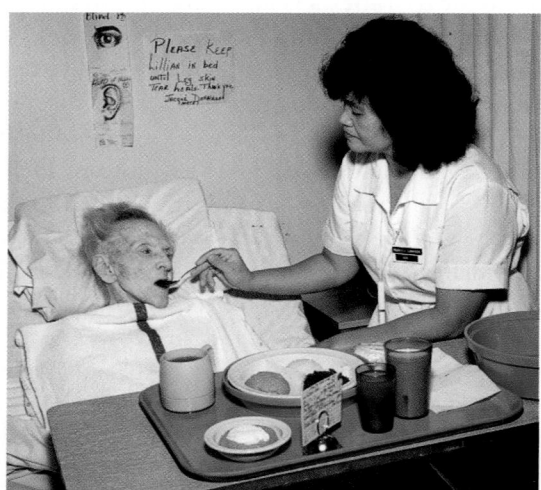

**Figure 38-7** Some mobility impairments significantly limit a person's ability to perform ADLs.

care (Brians, Alexander, Grota, Chen, & Dumas, 1991; Feder, Cryer, Donovan, & Carter, 2000).

## Nursing Diagnosis

Nursing diagnoses related to mobility focus primarily on activity and mobility levels, and the psychosocial impact that alterations in mobility can have on a client and the client's family. Common NANDA nursing diagnoses related to the physical adaptations or risks resulting from altered mobility include (NANDA, 2003):

- *Activity Intolerance* related to bed rest and immobility, generalized weakness, sedentary lifestyle, and imbalance between oxygen supply and demand.
- *Impaired Physical Mobility* related to intolerance to activity or decreased strength and endurance, pain, perceptual or cognitive impairment, neuromuscular impairment, musculoskeletal impairment, and depression or severe anxiety.
- *Risk for Disuse Syndrome* per risk factors of paralysis, mechanical immobilization, prescribed immobilization, and severe pain
- *Self-Care Deficits* related to inability to wash body or body parts, inability to obtain or get to water source, activity intolerance, decreased strength and endurance, pain, and impaired transfer ability
- *Ineffective Health Maintenance* related to lack of or significant alteration in communication skills (written, nonverbal)
- *Risk for Falls* related to impaired mobility

Alterations in family and social processes may also result from immobility and inactivity. Disruption in activity and mobility leads to impairment of the ability to perform one's usual social, vocational, educational, and family roles. There are often changes in the client's perception of role. *Disturbed Body Image* and *Situational Low Self-Esteem* can result from:

1. Changes in physical abilities
2. Changes in family responsibilities
3. Lack of knowledge regarding rehabilitation
4. Denial of abilities and strengths
5. Social insecurity
6. Feelings of worthlessness, hopelessness, or depression

## Planning and Outcome Identification

In the development of outcomes for clients with mobility needs, client involvement is essential. Realistic outcomes can be targeted by considering the client's (1) understanding of mobility status; (2) values, thoughts, and concerns regarding mobility problems; (3) general health status; and (4) ability to solve problems.

The goal of the interdisciplinary health team during acute hospitalization and rehabilitation is to restore function, thus maximizing the level of the client's independ-

## STOP AND THINK

### Intervening After a Client Falls

While charting at the nurses' station you hear a loud noise in a client's room. As you enter the room, you find the client has fallen while attempting to ambulate to the bathroom unassisted and is unable to get up on his own.

● What do you plan to do first upon entering the client's room?

● How will you safely assist the client back to bed and begin to assess for injuries?

● How will you protect yourself and be "safe" when assisting the client?

ence. Maximal independence includes the ability to function in ADL (eating, dressing, bathing, and moving). Independence in these activities contributes to self-reliance, self-care, self-determination, self-direction, and personal control. Personal client variables determining the maximal level of independence include extent of disability, competence, age, self-confidence, cognitive ability, knowledge level, and mood state. It is important to develop short-term goals that encourage clients to gain a sense of accomplishment. The nurse should recognize and praise the client's accomplishments that increase mobility.

The level of independence and ability for performance of ADL is enhanced or inhibited by the physical environment. Collaboration of the client, family, caregivers, nurses, physical therapists, and occupational therapists is essential for individualizing the physical environment to permit optimal activity and mobilization. Adaptive devices, such as those that follow, enhance independence for personal activities:

- Eating (e.g., plate guards and hand splints to hold utensils)
- Bathing (e.g., shower chairs and long-handled sponges)
- Dressing (e.g., Velcro closures and zipper pulls)
- Toileting (e.g., elevated toilet seats)
- Mobility (e.g., walkers)

Continued practice in self-care activities with adaptive devices promotes confidence. Interdisciplinary cooperation can be used to plan modifications for the home for activity and mobility, especially in the bathroom and kitchen. Physical modifications with adaptive equipment in home environments maximize client activity and mobility (Derstine & Hargrove, 2001).

## Bed Rest

Bed rest is a therapeutic intervention that achieves several objectives, including the following:

- Provide rest for clients who are exhausted.
- Decrease the body's oxygen consumption.
- Reduce pain and discomfort.

The planned duration of bed rest depends on the client's physical condition and ability to move.

Even though implemented for therapeutic reasons, bed rest can be counterproductive to a client's recovery. The inactivity imposed by bed rest causes structural changes in joints and shortens muscles. Such changes, which may lead to decreased range of motion and contractures, can occur within 48 hours of bed rest (Lamb & Cummings, 2000). To prevent such complications, bed rest should be avoided as much as possible. For clients whose medical condition necessitates bed rest, range-of-motion exercises must be implemented. When planning care, it is important to "prevent immobility if possible; approximately 7 days are needed for the client to regain the function lost during 1 day of bedrest" (Eliopoulos, 1999, p. 278).

## Restorative Nursing Care

Being able to move about independently is an important part of the recovery process and can determine whether the client is cared for at home or in a health care facility. Environmental evaluation is particularly important, with the focus on ease and safety of mobility. Promotion of activity through environmental modification increases the quality of life for the client whether injured, ill, or aging. Efforts by the client and the rehabilitation team to promote activity and mobility can be negated quickly by environmental barriers such as stairs and narrow passageways.

Clients who have limited mobility may be at risk for falls. To decrease the probability of falls at home, client

## COMMUNITY/HOME CARE

### Promoting Safety at Home

1. Avoid unsecured rugs or loose rugs.
2. Use banisters on stairways.
3. Install bright lights near steps and stairways.
4. Avoid wearing shoes that are ill-fitting, unlaced, or high-heeled, or have slippery soles.
5. Keep all walkways unobstructed (remove clutter).
6. Use caution with telephone lines; use a cordless phone if available to avoid tripping danger.
7. Do not walk on wet or waxed floors.
8. Use nonskid mats in shower/bathtub.
9. Use grab bars near toilet and shower/bathtub.
10. Keep commonly used objects within easy reach.
11. Keep neighbor's phone number by phone.

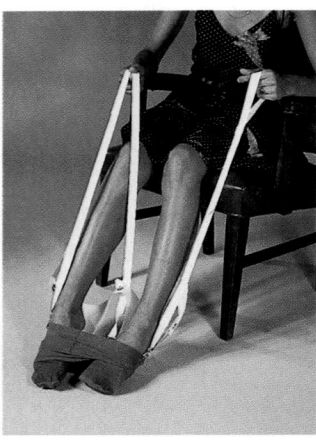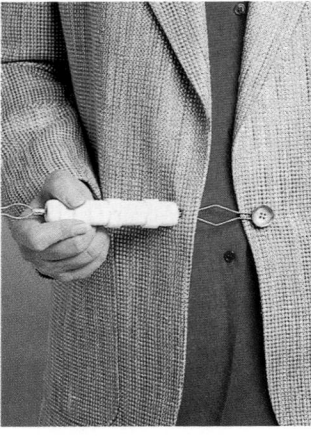

**Figure 38-8**   Assistive devices, such as those shown here, help clients dress independently.

education should focus on creating a safe environment for ambulation. The accompanying Community/Home Care boxes list some assistive devices for clients receiving care in the home setting. Other types of assistive devices are available to help clients perform ADL (Figure 38-8).

## Health Promotion and Fitness

The client's long-term goals include the promotion of activity, mobility, and fitness. Therapeutic exercises maintain flexibility, strength of muscles, range of motion, and energy and increase endurance and sense of well-being. Health promotion models stress the importance of cognitive and perceptual factors on exercise participation. Factors affecting targeted health promotion outcomes include perceived health status, perceived benefits of exercise, perceived barriers to exercise, and attitudes toward exercise. Perceived benefits of exercise and exercise attitudes held by the client have been identified as critical in goal setting for a program of health promotion and fitness.

## Implementation

Interventions for clients with impaired mobility include meeting psychosocial needs, using body mechanics, maintaining body alignment, performing ROM exercises, transferring clients, assisting with ambulation, promoting wellness, using complementary treatment approaches, and documentation.

## Meeting Psychosocial Needs

Nursing interventions for role change due to deficits in activity and mobility include (1) fostering open family communication, (2) providing opportunities for family role resumption, (3) prioritizing family roles and responsibilities, and (4) modifying family roles and responsibilities.

---

### COMMUNITY/HOME CARE

#### Assistive Devices in the Home

The following devices may be rented and may qualify for reimbursement from Medicare or private insurance.

- Electric hospital bed with overhead trapeze (gives client more control of environment)

- Portable commode (extends client's independence in elimination)

- Lifting device (assists with transferring dependent client from bed to chair)

- Portable telephone (for client safety and convenience)

- Shower chair and handheld shower for bathtub (promote client independence and safety)

- Special mattresses for bed and cushions for chairs (promote comfort and help maintain skin integrity)

- Overbed table for eating or hand activities (promotes client's ability to perform ADL)

- Comfortable chairs close to the bed (promote socialization by facilitating visits of family and friends)

- Remote control for client who enjoys television (provides leisure/diversion activity)

---

### COMMUNITY/HOME CARE

#### Home Modifications

Increased accessibility and mobility can be achieved through planning home modifications such as:

1. Ramps (paths to freedom)
2. Wide doorways
3. Open-ended door handles replacing doorknobs
4. Remote-controlled lighting
5. Spacious room arrangements
6. Bare floor or low-level pile carpeting
7. Grab bars for bathrooms

## Body Mechanics

Think ahead to eliminate hazards and injuries.

- Consider the weight and bulk of a client or object before lifting.

- Take your time and lift properly.

- Watch your footing.

- Teach proper body mechanics to others.

- Ask for help as needed.

## Application of Body Mechanics

- When lifting objects from the floor, bend at the hips and knees while keeping the back straight and maintaining a wide base of support.

- Avoid bending from the waist as this will strain muscles of the lower back.

- Adjust the height of the client's bed to avoid back strain.

- Carry objects close to the midline of the body.

- Avoid stretching to reach objects.

## Applying Principles of Body Mechanics

Often nurses are required to have physical strength in order to assist clients in achieving mobility. Carrying, pulling, pushing, or lifting clients and/or equipment are all activities involved in the delivery of nursing care. Nurses' implementation of correct body mechanics helps minimize the following:

- Client injury
- Nurse work-related musculoskeletal injury
- Nurse fatigue

"Back injury is mainly caused by lifting unreasonable loads . . . the most stressful tasks involve the transferring of patients (from a bed to a chair, for example)" (Owen, 1999, p. 76). The following variables can increase the risk of nurse injury:

- Client weight
- Client weight-bearing ability

- Client combativeness and unpredictability
- Height of bed
- Confined work space
- Wheelchairs without adjustable arms

Educating staff about the use of proper body mechanics is essential in preventing injury; see Procedure 38-1. The U.S. Department of Labor Occupational Safety & Health Administration (OSHA) has implemented new standards for the prevention of musculoskeletal injuries. OSHA (2000) defines musculoskeletal disorders (MSDs) as injuries and disorders of the muscles, nerves, tendons, ligaments, joints, cartilage, and spinal disks. Examples of MSDs include carpal tunnel syndrome, tendonitis, sciatica, herniated disk, and low back pain. Work-related MSDs account for more than one-third of all occupational injuries and illnesses that are serious enough to result in days away from work (OSHA, 2000).

**PROCEDURE 38-1**  **Proper Body Mechanics and Safe Lifting**

### EQUIPMENT NEEDED

- Wheelchair equipped with working locks
- Transfer board
- Draw or lift sheet

- Nonslip shoes or slippers
- Safety or gait belt
- Stretcher equipped with working locks

### IMPLEMENTATION—ACTION/RATIONALE

| ACTION | RATIONALE |
|---|---|
| 1. Wash hands. | 1. Reduces the transmission of microorganisms. |

*(continues)*

## PROCEDURE 38-1 (*continued*)

2. Assess the situation for obstacles, heavy clients, poor handholds, or equipment or objects in the way. Reduce or remove safety hazards prior to lifting the client or object.

2. Good planning helps prevent accidental injury.

3. Assess the situation for slippery surfaces, including wet floors; slippery shoes on client, helper, or nurse; and towels, linen, or paper on the floor. Resolve the slippery surface prior to lifting the client or object.

3. Removes the cause of many falls and slips.

4. Assess the situation for hidden risks, including client confusion, combativeness, orthostatic hypotension, drug effects, pain, or fear (Figure 38-9).

4. Allows the nurse to anticipate and plan for unexpected events.

5. Maintain low center of gravity by bending at the hips and knees, not the waist. Squat down rather than bend over to lift and lower (Figure 38-10).

5. Provides for the equal distribution of body weight and assists in maintaining safe balance.

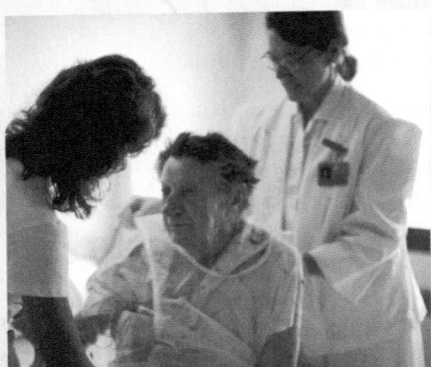

**Figure 38-9    Assess the client and the setting for safety risks before moving, lifting, or transferring the client.**

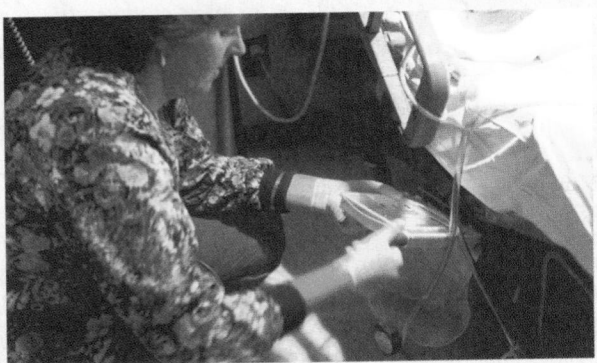

**Figure 38-10    Squat, rather than bend, to maintain good posture.**

6. Establish a wide support base with feet spread apart (Figure 38-11).

6. Provides stability and lowers the center of gravity.

7. Use feet to move, not a twisting or bending motion from the waist.

7. Assists in maintaining correct body alignment, which increases strength to lift, push, pull, and carry.

8. When pushing or pulling, stand near the object and stagger one foot partially ahead of the other.

8. Provides a safety net for avoiding potential back injuries.

9. When pushing a client or an object, lean into the client or object and apply continuous light pressure (Figure 38-12). When pulling a client or an object, lean away and grasp with light pressure. Never jerk or twist your body to force a weight to move.

9. Firm pressure will provide continuous movement of the object and will avoid abrupt movements that require the expenditure of increased energy.

10. When stooping to move an object, maintain a wide base of support with feet, flex knees to lower, and maintain straight upper body.

10. Provides the appropriate mechanics for the strength and endurance to achieve the task and to stand up straight upon completion.

(continues)

**PROCEDURE 38-1 (*continued*)**

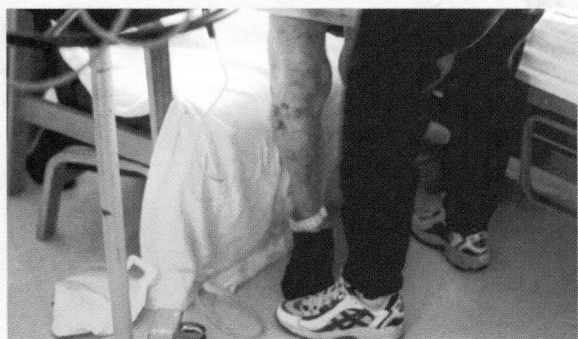

**Figure 38-11   Spread feet apart to establish a wide base of support.**

11. When lifting or carrying an object, bend the knees in front of the object, take a firm hold, and assume a standing position by using the leg muscles and keeping the back straight.

12. When raising up from a squatting position, arch your back slightly. Keep the buttocks and abdomen tucked in and raise up with your head first.

13. When lifting or carrying heavy objects, keep the weight as close to your center of gravity as possible (Figure 38-13).

14. When reaching for a client or an object, keep the back straight (Figure 38-14). If the client or object is heavy, do not try to lift the client or object without repositioning yourself closer to the weight.

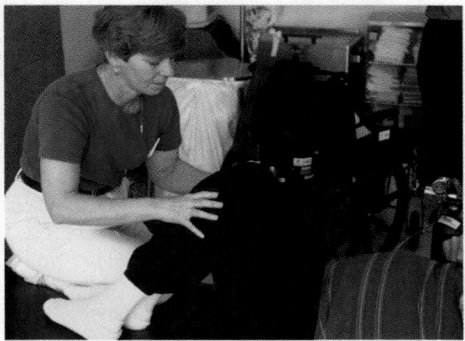

**Figure 38-12   Lean into the client or object being pushed.**

11. This stance will avoid the use of the back, diminish the potential for spinal twisting, and provide the lifter with a firm center of gravity and strength to lift the required weight.

12. Keeps the back from bowing and increasing the strain on the back muscles.

13. Reduces the strain on arm, leg, and back muscles.

14. Avoids straining the back and arm muscles.

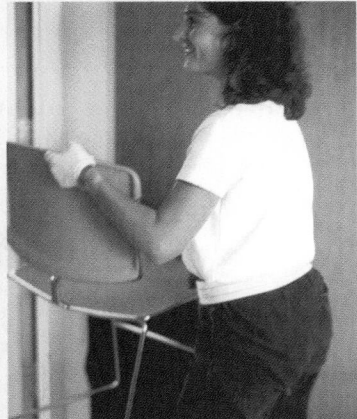

**Figure 38-13   Hold weight close to your center of gravity.**

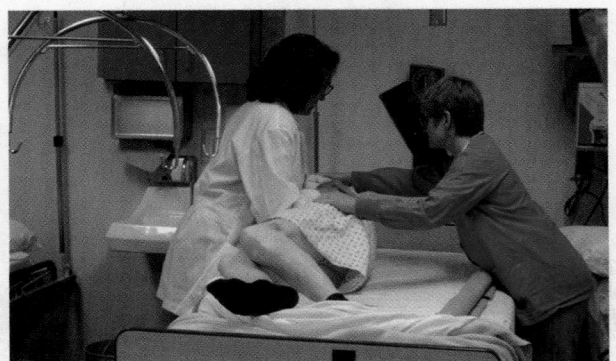

**Figure 38-14   Keep your back straight when reaching.**

15. Use safety aids and equipment. Use gait belts (Figure 38-15), lifts (Figure 38-16), drawsheets, and other transfer assistance devices (Figure 38-17).

15. Reduces the strain on the nurse and improves the safety for the client.

*(continues)*

### PROCEDURE 38-1 (continued)

Encourage clients to use handrails and grab bars (Figure 38-18). Wheelchair, cart, and stretcher wheels should be locked when they are not actually being moved.

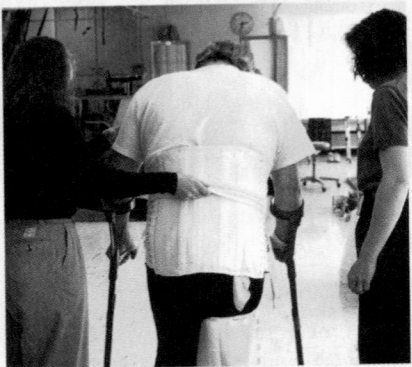

**Figure 38-15** Use gait belts for better grip and control.

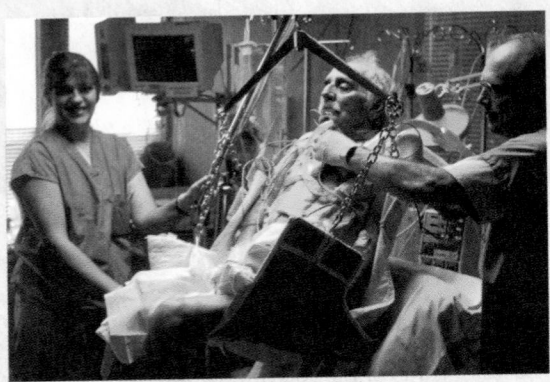

**Figure 38-16** Use lifts to carry the weight of the client. Monitor equipment, lines, tubes, and drains, and adjust as needed to prevent them from being dislodged.

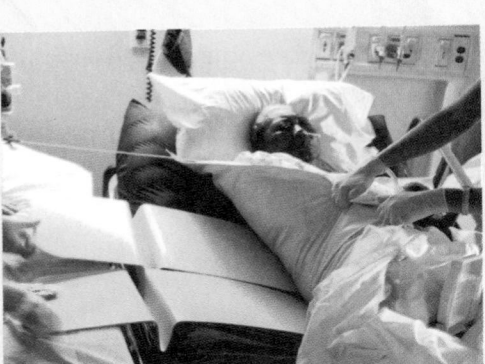

**Figure 38-17** Use transfer boards to reduce shearing forces and to reduce the effort needed to slide the client.

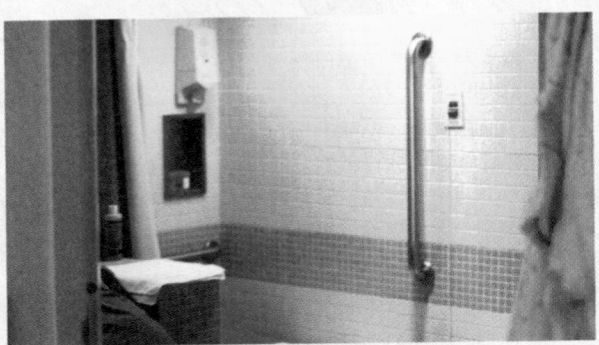

**Figure 38-18** Encourage the client to use handrails and grab bars to reduce the risk of slipping or falling.

## LIFE SPAN CONSIDERATIONS

### Muscle Strength

*Geriatric Variations*

- Older clients often have reduced flexibility and muscle strength.
- While frail-looking older clients are assumed to have lower muscle strength, obesity may hide poor muscle tone as well.
- Older clients often live alone and are very independent. They know what their bodies can and cannot do. When assessing an older client, ask her about her normal routine. Assist older clients, but follow their lead when possible to promote independence, control, and exercise.

MSDs are preventable by educating the workers and modifying the work environment. The following recommendations are made by OSHA (2000) to prevent MSDs:

- Adjust the height of working surfaces to reduce long reaches and awkward postures.
- Reduce the weight and size of items that workers must lift.
- Provide mechanical lifting equipment.

## Maintaining Body Alignment: Positioning

Clients cannot always move independently and reposition themselves in bed. In such instances, nurses must use proper turning and positioning techniques in order to achieve the following outcomes:

- Increase client comfort
- Prevent contractures
- Prevent decubiti (pressure sores)
- Make portions of the client's body accessible for procedures
- Help clients access their environment

Clients who cannot move independently must be repositioned every 2 hours. Repositioning must be done more often for clients who are uncomfortable or incontinent, or who have fragile skin, poor circulation, fragile skin, decreased sensation, poor nutritional status, or impaired mental status.

Nurses need to be aware of three essential concepts when positioning clients: pressure, friction, and skin shear. A pressure site is any skin surface area on which the client is lying or sitting. The force of the pressure can compromise circulation and lead to skin breakdown and ulceration. Tissue areas over bony prominences are more likely to experience impaired skin integrity. It is important to always inspect the skin and tissue areas under increased pressure for signs of irritation (e.g., redness).

Friction is caused when the skin is dragged across a rough surface such as bedsheets or stretcher surfaces. Friction causes heat, which damages the skin and may lead to decreased skin integrity with resultant infection and/or skin breakdown.

**Skin shear** is the result of dragging skin across a hard surface. The force of resistance to being dragged tears the deep layers of skin, which can lead to skin ulceration (see Chapter 36).

For clients in bed, limit the number of pillows under the head in order to avoid neck flexion. Arms should be abducted from the body and straight with slight flexion. Hands should rest comfortably in a flat position with fingers open. The knees and hips should be aligned; use sandbags or pillows to prevent external hip rotation. Avoid flexing the knees by the use of pillows placed behind the knees. Ankles should be flexed at 90 degrees; use pillows or footboard if necessary.

## CLINICAL ALERT

### Client Positioning

To prevent the development of contractures and decubiti, change the client's position every 2 hours.

# TABLE 38-11    POSITIONING

| Position | Description | Indications | Potential Complications | Corrective Measures |
|---|---|---|---|---|
| Fowler's | Semi-sitting position<br>Head of bed elevated to 45 to 60 degrees<br>Knees slightly elevated | Promotes comfort<br>Improves respiratory problems (i.e., dyspnea, pneumonia)<br>Encourages postoperative drainage | Flexion contracture of cervical spine | Rest head directly on mattress or support with small pillow only |
| | | | Exaggerated flexion of lumbar spine | Firm support to back<br>Pillow to support lower back |
| | | | Dislocation of shoulder | Elevate forearms on pillows to avoid tension on shoulders<br>Support hands on pillows to maintain natural alignment |
| | | | Flexion contracture of wrist | Hand-wrist splints |
| | | | Finger contractures and thumb abduction | Trochanter roll |
| | | | External hip rotation | |
| | | | Hyperextension of knees | Flex knees with small pillow under the thighs |
| | | | Footdrop (plantar flexion) | Maintain dorsal flexion with footboard or high-top tennis shoes |
| Dorsal recumbent (Supine) | Back-lying position<br>Head and shoulders may be slightly raised. | Promotes comfort<br>NOTE: Head and shoulders are kept flat after procedures involving spinal anesthetics | Cervical hyperextension | Maintain correct alignment with pillows under upper shoulders, neck, and head |
| | | | Posterior flexion of lumbar spine | Small pillow or roll under lumbar curvature |
| | | | Clawhand deformities (extension of fingers and abduction of thumbs) | Hand-wrist splints |
| | | | Hyperextension of knees | Pillow under lower legs from below the knees to ankles or small pillow under thighs to slightly flex knees |
| | | | Footdrop (plantar flexion) | Maintain dorsal flexion with footboard or high-top tennis shoes |

*(continues)*

## TABLE 38-11 POSITIONING (continued)

| Position | Description | Indications | Potential Complications | Corrective Measures |
|---|---|---|---|---|
| Prone | Facedown position<br>Head is turned to one side. | Helps prevent contractures of hips and knees<br>Promotes drainage from mouth | Cervical spine flexion<br>Hyperextension of spine; respiratory impairment<br>Footdrop | Small pillow under head<br>Small pillow just below the diaphragm<br>Allow feet to dangle over end of mattress<br>Place lower legs on pillow to keep toes from resting on bed |
| Lateral | Side-lying position<br>Lateral aspects of lower scapula and lower ilium support most of body weight. | Promotes comfort<br>Relieves pressure on sacrum and heels | Lateral flexion of neck<br>Internal rotation of arm; limited chest expansion leading to respiratory impairment<br>Extension of fingers and abduction of thumbs<br>Internal rotation and abduction of femur<br>Twisting of spine | Pillow under head and neck<br>Maintain alignment of upper arm with pillow underneath<br>Slightly flex lower arm<br>Hand-wrist splints<br>Pillows to support leg from groin to foot<br>Align both shoulders with both hips |
| Sims' | Semiprone position<br>Upper arm is flexed at shoulder and elbow; lower arm is positioned behind client<br>Both legs flexed in front of client with more flexion in upper leg<br>Promotes comfort especially in pregnant clients | Promotes drainage from mouth<br>Prevents aspiration<br>Reduces pressure on sacrum and greater trochanter of hip | Lateral flexion of cervical spine<br>Damaged nerves and blood vessels of lower arm axillae<br>Internal shoulder rotation and abduction<br>Internal rotation and adduction of hip and leg; lumbar lordosis<br>Footdrop | Support head with pillow unless drainage from mouth is necessary<br>Position lower arm behind and away from the back<br>Pillow between chest and upper arm<br>Pillow under upper flexed leg from groin to foot<br>Sandbag to dorsiflex lower foot |

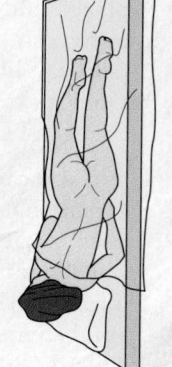

To maintain proper positioning for a client seated in a chair, be sure the head is straight without bending the neck or head dangling. The trunk should be upright without bending or curving. Arms and hands are to be supported on armrests or the tabletop; avoid dangling the arms. The hands should be in a flat position with the fingers open. Hips and knees should be flexed. The feet are to be flat on the floor or footrest with the ankles at a 90-degree angle. If the legs are supported on leg rests and are straight, keep the ankles flexed at a 90-degree angle.

Table 38-11 provides a description of the most commonly used positions: Fowler's (elevated head and trunk), dorsal recumbent (back-lying with slight elevation of head and shoulders), prone (face down), lateral (side-lying), and Sims' (semi-prone).

Assisting clients to comfortable therapeutic positions requires much skill; see Procedure 38-2. Often the client is unable to assist in repositioning; in such cases, it is best to use two or more staff members to reposition the client in order to prevent injury.

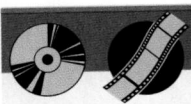

## PROCEDURE 38-2

## Turning and Positioning a Client

### EQUIPMENT NEEDED

- Pillows
- Rolled blankets or towels
- Footboard
- Heel protectors
- Hand rolls

### IMPLEMENTATION—ACTION/RATIONALE

| ACTION | RATIONALE |
|---|---|
| 1. Wash hands. | 1. Reduces transmission of microorganisms. |
| 2. Explain procedure to client. Elicit client cooperation and participation. | 2. Decreases anxiety. Improves client compliance and cooperation. |
| 3. Gather all necessary equipment. Provide for client privacy. | 3. Ensures client dignity and allows for a smooth procedure. |
| 4. Secure adequate assistance to safely complete task. | 4. Prevents caregiver back and muscle strain as well as provides for client safety. |
| 5. Adjust bed to comfortable working height. Lower side rail on side of bed from which you are assisting client. | 5. Prevents caregiver back and muscle strain. |
| 6. Follow proper body mechanics guidelines: | 6. Prevents caregiver back injury and muscle strain and promotes client safety. Spreading feet to create a wide base helps prevent loss of balance. |

6. When moving a client in bed, position the bed so that your legs are slightly bent at the knees and hips. Maintain the natural curves in your back while lifting. Position one foot slightly in front of the other and spread feet apart to create a wide base for balance. When your arms are placed under the client, slowly lean backward onto your back leg using your body weight to help you lift the client to one side of the bed. Do not extend or rotate your back to move a client in bed.

If you cannot move the client easily, always ask for and obtain assistance for both your and the client's safety (Figure 38-19). Be sure the floor is not slippery and that the bed is locked. Always use a turning sheet when rolling a client if this gives you better support and control of the client (Figure 38-20).

*(continues)*

**PROCEDURE 38-2** (*continued*)

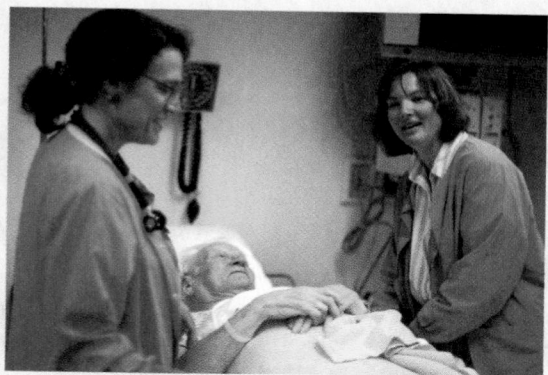

**Figure 38-19    If the client is heavy or hard to move, always obtain assistance for both the client's and your safety.**

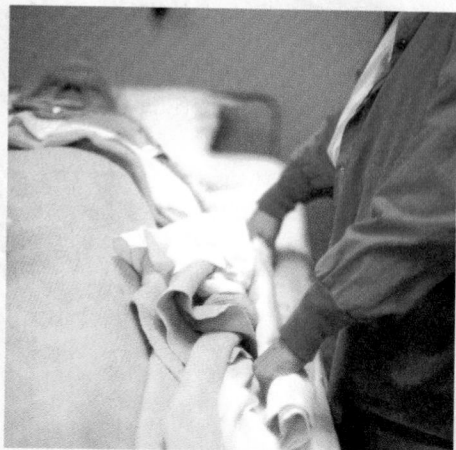

**Figure 38-20    When rolling a client, use a turning sheet for better support and control.**

7. Position drains, tubes, and IVs to accommodate new client position.

8. Place or assist client into appropriate starting position. Monitor client status, providing adequate rest breaks or support as necessary.

### Moving from Supine to Side-Lying Position

9. Slide your hands underneath the client. Move the client to one side of the bed by lifting the client's body toward you in stages—first the upper trunk, then the lower trunk, and finally the legs. Lift the client's body; do not drag the client across the sheets.

   Roll the client to side-lying position by placing the client's inside arm next to the client's body with the palm of the hand against the hip. Cross the client's outside arm and leg toward midline and logroll the client toward you using the client's outside shoulder and hip for leverage while maintaining stability and control of top arm and leg.

### Maintaining Side-Lying Position

10. Repeat Actions 1 to 8.

11. Pillows may be placed to support the client's head and arms (Figure 38-21). An additional pillow may be used to support the topside leg, fully and equally supporting the thigh, knee, ankle, and foot (Figure 38-22). Move the lower arm forward slightly

7. Prevents accidental dislodgment and/or discomfort from movement by reduced mechanical tension.

8. Prevents client injury.

9. Prevents shearing of skin tissue. Maintains client body alignment. Protects caregiver's back and prevents muscle strain. Prevents client injury and shearing of skin tissue.

10. See Rationales 1 to 8.

11. Provide support and comfort.

*(continues)*

**PROCEDURE 38-2** (*continued*)

at the shoulder and bend the elbow for comfort. If the client is unstable, a pillow placed against the back will provide additional support and keep the client from rolling supine (Figure 38-23).

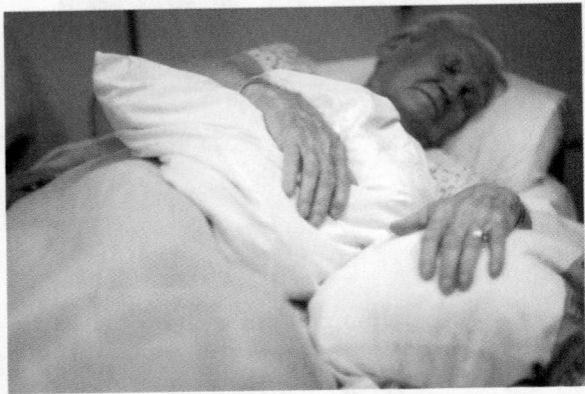

**Figure 38-21**    Place pillows to support the head and arms.

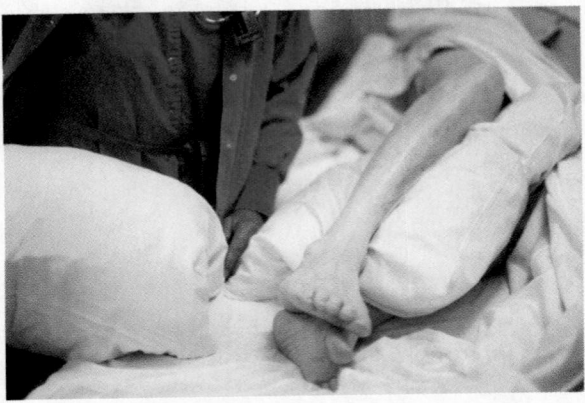

**Figure 38-22**    Place pillows to support the leg, ankle, and foot.

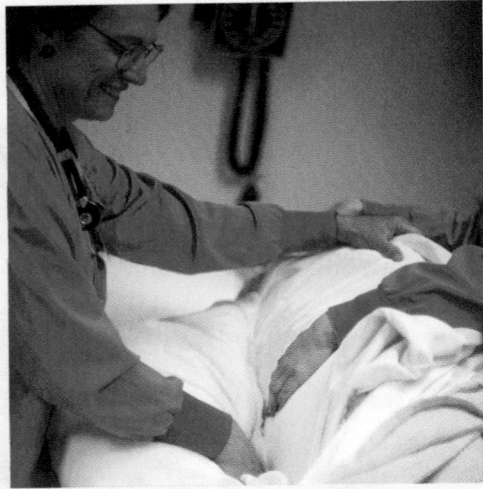

**Figure 38-23**    A pillow against the back will prevent a side-lying client from rolling into a supine position.

### Moving from Side-Lying to Prone Position

**12.** Repeat Actions 1 to 8.

**13.** Remove positioning towels, pillows, or other support devices. Assess whether the client's position in bed needs to be adjusted to accommodate the continued movement into prone. Move the

**12.** See Rationales 1 to 8.

**13.** Ensures comfort and safety in movement.

(*continues*)

client's inside arm next to the client's body with palm against hip. Roll the client onto the stomach using the shoulder and hip as key points of control. The head must be placed in a comfortable position to one side without excessive pressure to sensitive areas. Pillows under the trunk are placed as needed to relieve pressure and increase comfort. The client's arms are placed comfortably at the client's side and the legs are uncrossed with the feet approximately a foot apart.

### Maintaining Prone Position

14. A shallow pillow or a folded towel may be used to support the client's head comfortably as well as a pillow placed under the abdomen to support the back. An additional pillow may be placed under the lower leg to reduce the pressure of the toes and forefoot against the bed.

14. Provides support and comfort.

### Moving from Prone to Supine Position

15. Repeat Actions 1 to 8.

15. See Rationales 1 to 8.

16. Remove positioning towels, pillows, or other supporting devices. Slide your hands underneath the client. Move the client segmentally to one side of the bed to accommodate the new position. Position the inside arm next to the client's body with the client's palm next to the hip. Roll the client to supine by logrolling the client toward you using the client's outside shoulder and hip for leverage. Have the client's face positioned away from the direction of the roll to prevent undue pressure to the face or neck. When the client reaches supine, uncross the client's arms and legs and place them comfortably into anatomical positions.

16. Provides support and comfort.

### Maintaining Supine Position

17. A footboard may be used to support the foot as well as heel protectors or a pillow placed between the heel and gastrocnemius muscle to reduce the pressure on the heels (Figures 38-24 and 38-25). To prevent excessive external rotation of the lower extremity, a trochanter roll may be used. For comfort, additional pillows may be used to support the client's head, arms, or lower back.

17. Provides support and comfort.

18. Be sure to replace side rails to upright position as well as lower bed to beginning position.

18. Provides for client safety.

*(continues)*

## PROCEDURE 38-2 (*continued*)

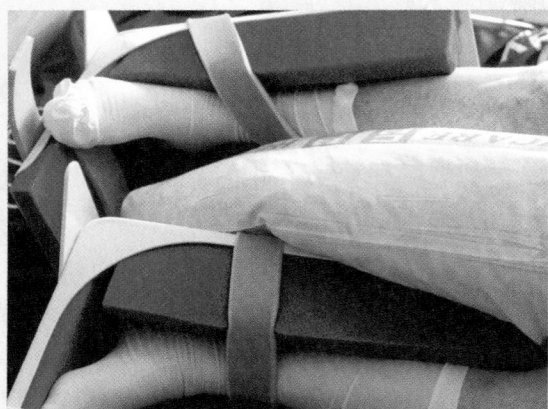

**Figure 38-24** Heel protectors are placed on the foot to provide support and comfort.

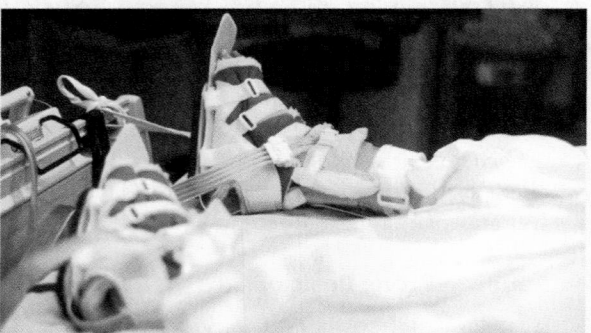

**Figure 38-25** Heel protectors also provide padding to reduce the risk of skin breakdown where the heel rests on the mattress.

19. Place call light within reach of the client.

20. Move bedside table close to bed and place items of frequent use within reach of the client.

21. Wash hands.

19. Provides for client safety.

20. Provides for client safety.

21. Reduces transmission of microorganisms.

---

## COMMUNITY/HOME CARE

### Turning and Positioning

*Home Care Variations*

- Assess the ability of the primary caregiver to adequately turn and position the client in the home care setting. Does the caregiver know proper body alignment technique, as well as basic information on the prevention and detection of pressure sores?

- Assess if the home caregiver has enough support and help (friends, neighbors, or family) to turn the client as often as needed to avoid prolonged pressure over bony prominences.

- Examine the bed or chair where the client spends most of the day and night. Can the sheets be tucked tight? Is the upholstery on the chair a rough fabric, or plastic? Could the fabric on the bed or the chair contribute to friction or shearing forces when the client is moved?

*Long-Term Care Variations*

- Long-term clients may have a "favorite" position and may shift back to this position, even if turned at regular intervals. Such a client needs to be assessed more frequently than every 2 hours.

## LIFE SPAN CONSIDERATIONS

### Positioning

**Pediatric Variations**

- Take care not to place babies in the prone position to sleep because this may contribute to sudden infant death. Infants should be propped in a side-lying position to sleep.

**Geriatric Variations**

- Older clients may have more compromised body systems such as delicate skin, a more brittle skeletal system, cardiovascular shifts, more difficulty with balance, and less muscle strength to assist during positioning.

Specialized equipment used for client positioning includes pillows, foam wedges, trochanter rolls, footboards, bed boards, hand-wrist splints, traction, side rails, restraints, and trapeze bars. Table 38-12 describes devices used to help maintain proper positioning.

Hand-wrist splints can facilitate extension of the wrist-hand-fingers, prevent contracture, and reduce spasticity. The goal for splint use is to maintain a functional hand for the client. Clients must be taught the correct way to put on the device, as incorrect use of a splint or brace can cause joint damage, stiffness, or pain.

Falls are common types of injuries in hospitals and long-term care facilities. For clients who are at risk for falls, side rails should always be considered; however, they should not give nurses a sense of security. Beds must still be placed in the lowest position to reduce the force of a possible fall, should one occur. Also, clients identified as being at-risk for falls should be closely monitored.

Restraints are protective devices used to limit physical activity or to immobilize a client or body part. Restraints are used for the following purposes: to protect the client from falls, to protect a body part, to prevent the client from interfering with therapies (e.g., pulling out tubes or catheters), and to reduce the risk of injury to others.

Traction may be used to maintain alignment, especially following injury or surgery. There are several traction techniques, including manual, skin, and skeletal (Figure 38-26). See Table 38-13 for a listing of key assessment data for clients using skeletal and skin traction. In addition to assessing, the nurse also documents the findings.

## Performing Range-of-Motion Exercises

Range-of-motion exercises are performed several times a day by placing each joint through its full functional motion. The purposes of ROM exercises are to maintain full flexibility,

## TABLE 38-12    MAINTAINING PROPER POSITION: ASSISTIVE DEVICES

| | |
|---|---|
| Bed board | Plywood board placed under entire mattress; improves spinal alignment by providing support |
| Footboard | Board placed at end of bed to provide support for feet to maintain dorsiflexion |
| Hand-wrist splint | Individually contoured for each client; maintains thumb adduction and opposition to fingers |
| Pillow | Available in various thicknesses; provides support; elevates body parts |
| Restraint | Variety of types available (jacket or vest, wrist belt, ankle belt, waist belt); provides immobilization |
| Side rails | Bars attached to the sides of the bed. Assists with mobility and prevents falls |
| Trochanter roll | Folded blanket placed under client's buttocks and rolled inward toward client to place thigh in a neutral position; used when client is supine to avoid external rotation of hips and legs |
| Traction | Used for immobilization and to promote healing of fractures |
| Trapeze bar | Triangular device hanging from above-bed bar that is secured to bed frame; used by clients with upper extremity function to assist in repositioning and transferring |

**Figure 38-26    Traction techniques: A. Manual B. Skin C. Skeletal**

| TABLE 38-13 | SKELETAL AND SKIN TRACTION: ASSESSMENT FACTORS |
| --- | --- |
| **Skeletal Traction** | **Skin Traction** |
| Location of traction | Location of traction |
| Amount of traction being applied | Type of traction (e.g., cervical, Buck's, Russell's) |
| Countertraction applied | Amount of traction weight being applied to the affected body part |
| Body position to be maintained | Body position to be maintained |
| Duration of application (continuous, intermittent, or as-needed basis) | Duration of application (continuous, intermittent, or as-needed basis) |
| Traction weights free-falling | Traction weights free-falling |
| Traction rope intact, taut, and unobstructed through the pulley | Traction rope intact, taut, and unobstructed through the pulley |
| Immobilized body part in alignment with rest of body | Immobilized body part in alignment with rest of body |
| Appearance of the skeletal pin or wire sites (e.g., dry, encrusted, reddened, edematous) | |
| Presence of drainage from the skeletal pin or wire sites | |
| Evidence of skin breakdown | |

maintain muscle tone and strength, prevent contractures, and improve circulation. Refer to Procedure 38-3.

## Transfer Techniques

Planning plays a major role in safe effective client transfers; the nurse must determine to what extent the client is able to

help with the transfer. If the client is totally dependent or is heavy, the nurse will need other staff members to help. Table 38-14 lists potential hazards involved in client transfers with corresponding nursing interventions to promote safety.

### Moving Clients

Prolonged immobility can cause discomfort, muscle wasting, clot formation, and skin breakdown. Also, the client who slides down toward the foot of the bed while the head is elevated can experience reduced lung capacity and impaired respiratory effort. Nurses often must move clients up in the bed or reposition them. Moving a client may sometimes be done by one person, but often requires two staff members to ensure safe transfer; see Procedure 38-4.

---

**CLINICAL ALERT**

**Restraints**

Restraints are never to be used for staff convenience but instead to prevent injury to clients or others.

## STOP AND THINK

### Restraint Use with Confused Clients

- What are noninvasive alternatives to restraints for confused clients?

- What can the family be encouraged to do for the client to avoid unnecessary use of restraints?

- What advantages can you think of for maintaining a restraint-free environment?

Hogstel, M. (2001). *Gerontology: Nursing care of the older adult.* Clifton Park, NY: Delmar Learning.

 ## NURSING STRATEGY

### ROM Exercises

- Assess the motion of joints for every client.

- Do not flex, extend, rotate, abduct, or adduct a joint if the client complains of discomfort or stiffness.

- Encourage the client to perform range-of-motion exercises with as much independence as possible.

- Teach family members or caregivers to perform range-of-motion exercises with the client.

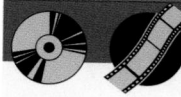 **PROCEDURE 38-3**

## Administering Passive Range-of-Motion (ROM) Exercises

### EQUIPMENT NEEDED

■ No special equipment is needed, except gloves when contact with body fluids is possible

### IMPLEMENTATION—ACTION/RATIONALE

| ACTION | RATIONALE |
|---|---|
| 1. Wash hands, wear gloves if contact with body fluids is possible. | 1. Reduces transmission of microorganisms. |
| 2. Explain procedure to client, including estimated duration. | 2. Decreases anxiety, encourages compliance and participation. |
| 3. Provide for privacy, including exposing only the extremity to be exercised. | 3. Decreases embarrassment. |
| 4. Adjust bed to comfortable height for performing ROM. | 4. Prevents muscle strain and discomfort for nurse. |
| 5. Lower bed rail only on the side you are working. | 5. Prevents falls. |
| 6. Describe the passive ROM exercises you are performing, or verbally cue client to perform ROM exercises with your assistance. Include all applicable exercises (Refer to Table 38-14). | 6. Exercises all joint areas. |
| 7. Start at the client's head and perform ROM exercises down each side of the body. | 7. Provides a systematic method to ensure that all body parts are exercised. |
| 8. Repeat each ROM exercise as the client tolerates, to a maximum of 5 times. Perform each motion in a slow, firm manner. Encourage full joint movement, but do not go beyond the point of pain, resistance, or fatigue. | 8. Provides exercise to the client's tolerance or to a level that will maintain the joint function. |

*(continues)*

## PROCEDURE 38-3 (continued)

9. Head

   Perform these movements with the client in a sitting position, if possible.

   • Rotation: Turn the head from side to side.

   • Flexion and extension: Tilt the head toward the chest and then tilt slightly upward.

   • Lateral flexion: Tilt the head on each side so as to almost touch the ear to the shoulder.

10. Neck

    Perform these movements with the client in a sitting position, if possible.

    • Rotation: Rotate the neck in a semicircle while supporting the head.

11. Trunk

    Perform these movements with the client in a sitting position, if possible.

    • Flexion and extension: Bend the trunk forward, straighten the trunk, and then extend slightly backward.

    • Rotation: Turn the shoulders forward and return to normal position.

    • Lateral flexion: Tip trunk to the left side, straighten trunk, and tip to the right side.

12. Arm

    • Flexion and extension: Extend the arm in a straight position upward toward the head, and then downward along the side.

    • Adduction and abduction: Extend the arm in a straight position toward the midline (adduction) and away from the midline (abduction).

13. Shoulder

    • Internal and external rotation: Bend the elbow at a 90-degree angle with the upper arm parallel to the shoulder; rotate the shoulder by moving the lower arm upward and downward.

14. Elbow

    • Flexion and extension: Supporting the arm, flex and extend the elbow.

    • Pronation and supination: Flex elbow, move the hand in palm-up and palm-down position.

9.

To optimize the performance of the movements.

   • To preserve muscle tone and joint flexibility.

10.

To optimize the performance of the movements.

   • To preserve muscle tone and joint flexibility.

11.

To optimize the performance of the movements.

   • To preserve muscle tone and joint flexibility.

12.

   • To preserve muscle tone and joint flexibility.

13.

   • To preserve muscle tone and joint flexibility.

14.

   • To preserve muscle tone and joint flexibility.

(continues)

**PROCEDURE 38-3 (*continued*)**

15. Wrist

    • Flexion and extension: Supporting the wrist, flex and extend the wrist (Figure 38-27).

    • Adduction and abduction: Supporting the lower arm, turn wrist right to left, left to right, and then rotate the wrist in a circular motion.

16. Hand

    • Flexion and extension: Supporting the wrist, flex and extend the fingers (Figure 38-28).

15.

    • To preserve muscle tone and joint flexibility.

16.

    • To preserve muscle tone and joint flexibility.

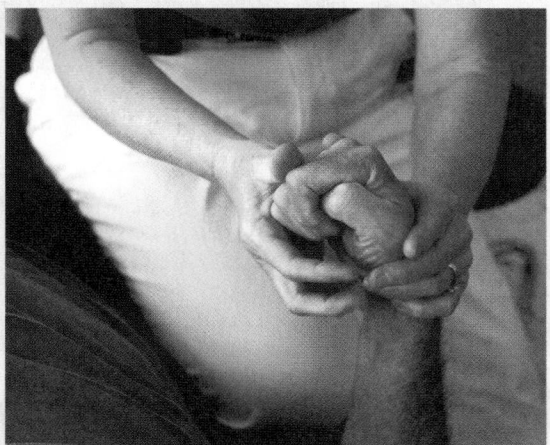

**Figure 38-27    Flex and extend the wrist.**

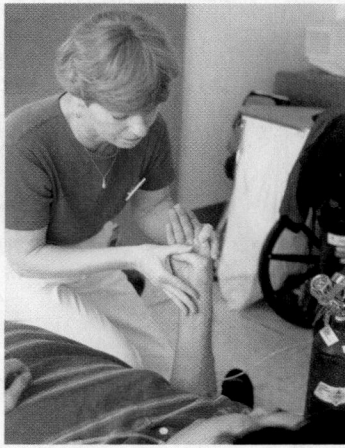

**Figure 38-28    Flex and extend the fingers.**

    • Adduction and abduction: Supporting the wrist, spread fingers apart and then bring them close together.

    • Opposition: Supporting the wrist, touch each finger with the tip of the thumb.

    • Thumb rotation: Supporting the wrist, rotate the thumb in a circular manner.

17. Hip and leg

    Perform these movements with the client in a supine position, if possible.

    • Flexion and extension: Supporting the lower leg, flex the leg toward the chest and then extend the leg.

    • Internal and external rotation: Supporting the lower leg, angle the foot inward and outward.

    • Adduction and abduction: Slide the leg away from the client's midline and then back to the midline (Figure 38-29).

17.

    To optimize the performance of the movements.

    • To preserve muscle tone and joint flexibility.

*(continues)*

**PROCEDURE 38-3 (*continued*)**

18. Knee

- Flexion and extension: Supporting the lower leg, flex and extend the knee (Figure 38-30).

18.

- To preserve muscle tone and joint flexibility.

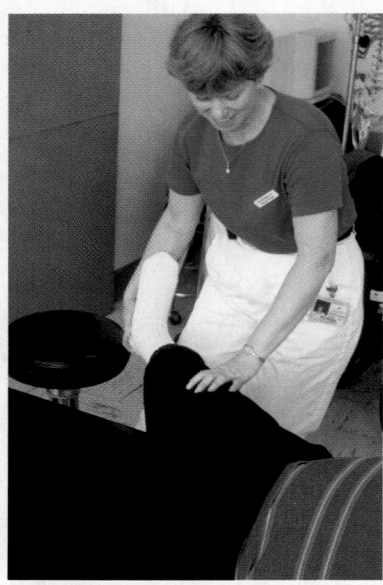

**Figure 38-29**    Slide the leg away from the client's midline and then return.

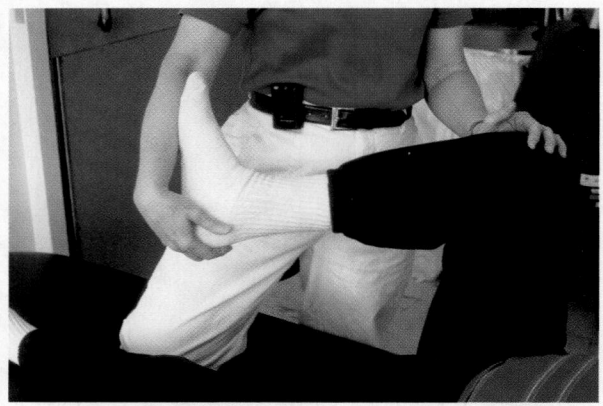

**Figure 38-30**    Flex and extend the knee.

19. Ankle

- Flexion and extension: Supporting the lower leg, flex and extend the ankle.

20. Foot

- Adduction and abduction: Supporting the ankle, spread the toes apart and then bring them close together.

- Flexion and extension: Supporting the ankle, extend the toes upward and then flex the toes downward.

21. Observe client's joints and face for signs of exertion, pain, or fatigue during movement.

22. Replace covers and position client in proper body alignment.

23. Place side rails in original position.

24. Place call light within reach.

25. Wash hands.

19.

- To preserve muscle tone and joint flexibility.

20.

- To preserve muscle tone and joint flexibility.

21. Alerts nurse to discontinue exercise.

22. Promotes comfort.

23. Prevents falls.

24. Facilitates communication.

25. Reduces transmission of microorganisms.

## LIFE SPAN CONSIDERATIONS

### ROM

**Pediatric Variations**

- For a child of appropriate age, demonstrate each movement to be performed either on yourself, a doll, or some other nonthreatening surrogate.

**Geriatric Variations**

- The ultimate goal of ROM exercise is client independence; so encourage as much participation as possible.

- Arrange for ROM to be performed at the same time each day, at the client's convenience.

- Various chronic conditions (COPD, hypertension, etc.) require extra caution and careful observation for fatigue, pain, and respiratory difficulty.

## COMMUNITY/HOME CARE

### ROM

**Home Care Variations**

- Instruct family members and caregivers to perform ROM between scheduled visits. Lower extremity ROM is best performed on a flat, raised surface, while upper extremity ROM can be executed in a seated position.

### Logrolling the Client

**Logrolling** is a technique for moving a client whose body must remain in straight alignment. Situations requiring total alignment of the spine include spinal injury or recovery from spinal surgery. Logrolling is accomplished by two or three nurses working in a coordinated fashion; see Procedure 38-5.

### Transferring from Bed to Chair

A client may need to be moved from the bed to a chair, commode, or wheelchair. Procedure 38-6 describes the steps involved in safely assisting a client from bed to wheelchair, commode, or chair.

A wheelchair is a means of transportation for clients unable to support their weight while standing. Safety instructions for use of a wheelchair include the need to keep the wheels locked when not deliberately moving and to move the footrests out of the way when getting in and out of the wheelchair; see the Nursing Strategy box for other recommendations for wheelchair usage.

### Transferring from Bed to Stretcher

Some clients (e.g., those who are too weak to sit upright, those who are unconscious, or those with injuries prohibiting the erect position) must lie flat during transfers. In such situations, a stretcher (gurney) is used to facilitate client transfer. Stretchers have several safety features, including side rails, safety belts/straps, and locking wheels. The nurse should caution clients to move carefully while on the

## CLINICAL ALERT

### Safety During Logrolling

For a very weak or immobile client, use extra personnel for logrolling. Two nurses should stand on each side of the client.

## CLINICAL ALERT

### Wheelchair Safety

Caution client to avoid leaning forward in the wheelchair because leaning forward can cause tipping and falling. Use a seat belt in impulsive clients who may not display good judgment or balance, such as those who have suffered spinal cord injury or stroke.

## TABLE 38-14    CLIENT TRANSFER: HAZARDS AND SAFETY MEASURES

| Potential Hazard | Preventive Measures |
|---|---|
| Falling | • Assess client's size and ability to assist.<br>• Ask for help from other staff members if needed.<br>• If client starts to fall, lower gently to the floor while protecting the head.<br>• If client has fallen, assess thoroughly for signs of injury. |
| Skin damage | • Use a transfer board or draw sheet.<br>• Lift client instead of sliding across surfaces.<br>• Pad surfaces that may cause injury (e.g., bed rails). |
| Foot injury | • Place nonskid slippers on client.<br>• Do not tuck sheets/blankets tightly over feet.<br>• Ensure that feet do not become tangled in side rails, chair legs, or other equipment. |
| Dislodging client care equipment | • Assess for presence of all tubes and lines (e.g., catheters, IV lines).<br>• Determine if equipment must be temporarily disconnected during the transfer.<br>• Reconnect equipment promptly when transfer is completed.<br>• Keep the urinary drainage bag at a level lower than the bladder. |

## NURSING STRATEGY

### Wheelchair Technique

● When pushing a wheelchair, back into and out of elevators.

● Back slowly down wheelchair ramps.

● Push the wheelchair ahead of you when going up ramps.

● If going through a self-closing door, back the wheelchair out of the room. You can keep the door open by backing against the door. The wheelchair can then be guided out of the room.

● Lock brakes when the wheelchair is standing still.

● Intravenous infusion bags can be placed on portable IV poles attached to the wheelchair during transport.

● Urinary drainage bags can be placed on the lower body of the wheelchair during transport. Coil the drainage tubing so the catheter is not tugged during transport. Empty urinary drainage bag prior to wheelchair transfer. Keep the urinary drainage bag below the level of the client's urinary bladder.

stretcher as it is more narrow than the bed. Reassure the client that side rails will be used to prevent falls. Refer to Procedure 38-7 for instructions on moving clients who need minimal and maximal assistance.

### Assistive Devices

Several devices are available for helping with client transfers. Slide boards or transfer boards assist the bed-wheelchair transfer by bridging the same level space between the bed and the wheelchair. Note that specialized wheelchairs with removable armrests are used with slide boards. As the client becomes more independent, the slide board can be used to transfer from wheelchair to car.

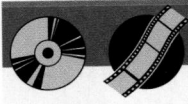

PROCEDURE 38-4    **Moving a Client in Bed**

### EQUIPMENT NEEDED

■ Hospital bed with side rails
■ Trapeze if required

■ Turn sheet or draw sheet

*(continues)*

**PROCEDURE 38-4** (*continued*)

## IMPLEMENTATION—ACTION/RATIONALE

| ACTION | RATIONALE |
|---|---|

### Moving a Client Up in Bed with One Nurse

1. Wash hands.

2. Inform client of reason for the move and how to assist (if able).

3. Elevate bed to just below waist height. Lower head of bed if tolerated by client. Lower side rails on the side where you are standing.

4. Remove the pillow and place it against the headboard.

5. Have the client fold arms across the chest.

6. Have client hold on to the overhead trapeze, if available (Figure 38-31).

7. Have the client bend the knees and place the feet flat on the bed if able (Figure 38-32).

1. Reduces transmission of microorganisms.

2. Reduces anxiety; helps increase comprehension and cooperation; promotes client autonomy.

3. Lessens strain on nurse's back muscles.

4. Prevents having to move against the pillow. Provides padding of the headboard if the client should be moved too high in the bed.

5. Prevents getting the client's arms trapped or injured during the move.

6. Promotes client autonomy by allowing the client to assist with the move.

7. Allows the client to assist in the move; promotes client autonomy.

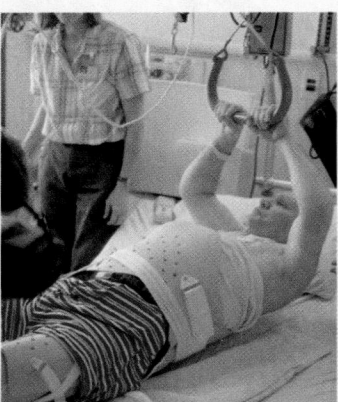

**Figure 38-31    Have client hold on to the overhead trapeze, if one is available to assist in the move.**

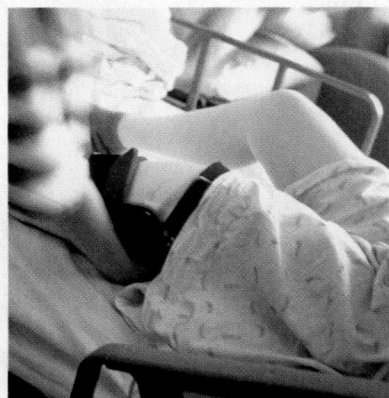

**Figure 38-32    Have the client bend the knees and place feet flat on the bed.**

8. Stand at an angle to the head of the bed, feet apart, knees bent, feet toward the head of the bed.

9. Slide one hand and arm under the client's shoulder, the other under the client's thigh.

10. Rock forward toward the head of the bed, lifting the client with you. Simultaneously have the client push with the legs.

11. If the client has a trapeze, have the client pull up holding on to the trapeze as you move the client upward in bed.

8. Promotes good body mechanics.

9. Distributes the client's weight more evenly. Promotes good lifting technique.

10. Allows a smooth motion to lift the client. Client assistance lessens strain on nurse's back muscles; promotes client autonomy.

11. Client assistance lessens strain on nurse's back muscles; promotes client autonomy.

*(continues)*

## PROCEDURE 38-4 (*continued*)

| | |
|---|---|
| **12.** Repeat these steps until the client is high enough in bed. | **12.** Large or very immobile clients are often not moved far enough in one step. |
| **13.** Return the client's pillow under the head. | **13.** Promotes client comfort. |
| **14.** Elevate head of bed, if tolerated by client. | **14.** Promotes comfort; facilitates eating and drinking; facilitates communication. |
| **15.** Assess client for comfort. | **15.** Comfort is subjective. |
| **16.** Adjust the client's bedclothes as needed for comfort. | **16.** Comfort is subjective. |
| **17.** Lower bed and elevate side rails. | **17.** Promotes client safety. |
| **18.** Wash hands. | **18.** Reduces transmission of microorganisms. |

### Moving a Client Up in Bed with Two or More Nurses

| | |
|---|---|
| **19.** Wash hands and apply gloves if needed (Figure 38-33). | **19.** Reduces transmission of microorganisms. |
| **20.** Inform client of reason for the move and how to assist (if able). | **20.** Reduces anxiety; helps increase comprehension and cooperation; promotes client autonomy. |
| **21.** Elevate bed to just below waist height. Lower head of bed if tolerated by client. Lower side rails (Figure 38-34). | **21.** Lessens strain on nurse's back muscles. |

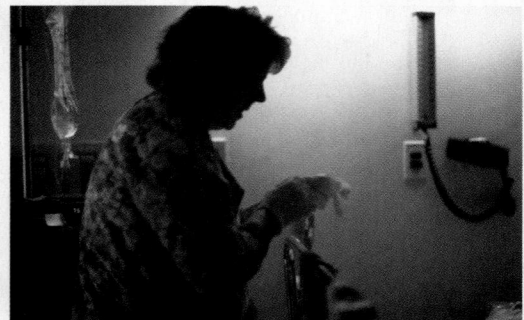

**Figure 38-33    Apply gloves before repositioning the client, if needed.**

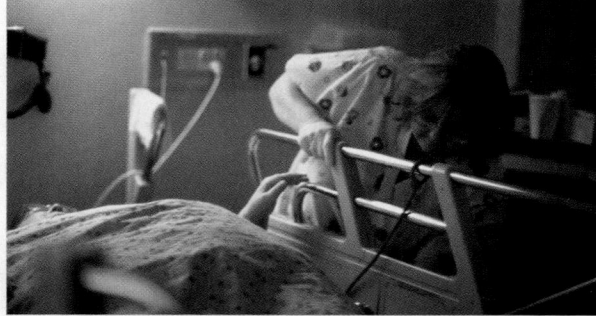

**Figure 38-34    Lower the side rails to allow the nurse to use good body mechanics.**

| | |
|---|---|
| **22.** With two nurses, place turn/draw sheet under client's back and head. | **22.** Reduces shearing force, which can precipitate skin breakdown. |
| **23.** Roll up the draw sheet on each side until it is next to the client (Figures 38-35 and 38-36). | **23.** Provides support under the heavy parts of the body and places the nurse's hands close to the weight to be moved. |
| **24.** Follow Actions 4 to 7. | **24.** See Rationales 4 to 7. |
| **25.** The nurses stand on either side of the bed, at an angle to the head of the bed. They stand with knees flexed, feet apart in a wide stance. | **25.** Promotes good body mechanics. |

*(continues)*

## PROCEDURE 38-4 (continued)

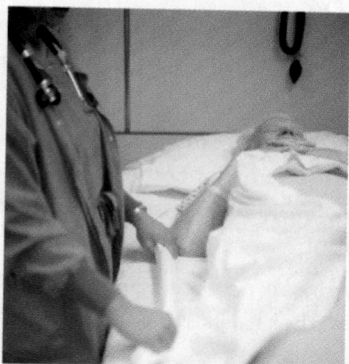

**Figure 38-35**    Roll up the draw sheet tightly on each side of the client.

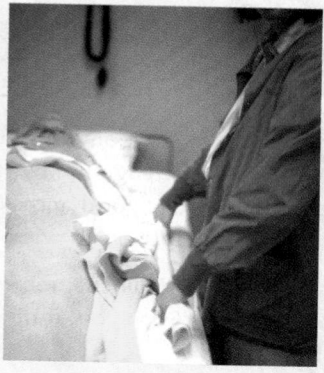

**Figure 38-36**    Rolling the draw sheet up tightly next to the client places the nurse's hands close to the weight of the client.

26.  The nurses hold their elbows as close as possible to their bodies.

27.  The lead nurse will give the signal to move: 1-2-3, go. The nurses will lift up (off the bed) on the turn/draw sheet and forward (toward the head of the bed) in one smooth motion (Figure 38-37). The move is coordinated to transfer the client toward the head of the bed. Simultaneously, have the client push with the legs or pull using the trapeze.

26.  Allows the muscles of the torso to assist the arm muscles in bearing and moving the weight of the client.

27.  Allows a smooth motion to lift the client. Client assistance lessens strain on the nurse's back muscles; promotes client autonomy.

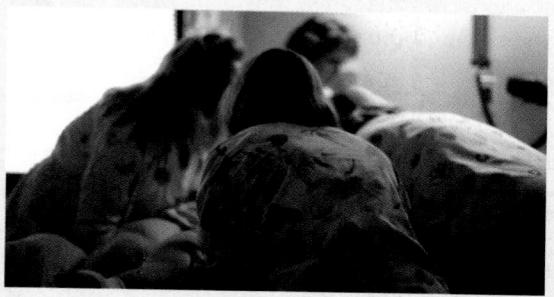

**Figure 38-37**    At the signal from the lead nurse, lift and pull in one smooth motion.

28.  Repeat until the client is high enough in bed to be comfortable.

29.  Return the client's pillow under the head.

30.  Elevate head of bed, if tolerated by client.

31.  Assess client for comfort.

32.  Adjust the client's bedclothes for comfort.

33.  Lower bed and elevate side rails.

34.  Wash hands.

28.  Large or very immobile clients are often not moved far enough in one step.

29.  Promotes client comfort.

30.  Promotes comfort; facilitates eating and drinking; facilitates communication.

31.  Promotes comfort.

32.  Promotes comfort.

33.  Promotes client safety.

34.  Reduces transmission of microorganisms.

## COMMUNITY/HOME CARE

### Moving a Client in Bed

#### Home Care Variations

- Often a family member is caring for the home care client. The family member should be taught proper body mechanics to prevent injury to the caregiver.

- Very often, beds in the home care setting, even rented hospital beds, are in small rooms, positioned against the wall, or wedged in by furniture. Enlist the assistance of a family member or caregiver to assess whether the nurse has good access to the bed or if the care area should be rearranged. Consider moving the sick room to another part of the home such as the dining room.

- When using the home linens, remember they are often old and worn or not as strong as hospital linen. Bring a draw sheet with you, if needed. Check the linen to see whether it is strong enough to hold and pull without tearing.

- The family member should be encouraged to demonstrate and use proper lifting skills to become more comfortable with them.

- If the home bed is a regular double, queen, or king-size bed, think how you will modify the moving technique to maintain good body alignment. For example, extra care and thought will be needed to move a client in a waterbed.

#### Long-Term Care Variations

- Long-term care clients are pulled up in bed fairly often. They are at increased risk for pressure ulcers on their coccyx and heels. Check these areas often, and be sure they aren't dragged across the sheets during the move. Make sure heels have protectors on them prior to moving the client. Use draw sheets as much as possible to avoid shearing fragile skin.

- Encourage independence as much as possible. Give clients "something to grab on to" to help them move up in bed. A trapeze, a cloth tied to the headboard, or something to brace against may help. Make sure clients are able to move themselves without tearing or shearing the skin and that they are able to assess this.

---

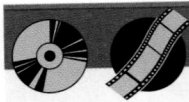 **PROCEDURE 38-5**   **Logrolling a Client**

### EQUIPMENT NEEDED

▇ Hospital bed with side rails
▇ Pillows

▇ Turn sheet or draw sheet

### IMPLEMENTATION—ACTION/RATIONALE

| ACTION | RATIONALE |
|---|---|
| 1. Inform client of reason for the move and how to assist (if able). | 1. Reduces anxiety; helps increase comprehension and cooperation; promotes client autonomy. |
| 2. Elevate hospital bed to high position. | 2. Avoids strain on nurse's back muscles. |
| 3. Using one or more staff members, place a turn/draw sheet under the client's back and head. | 3. Reduces shearing force, which can precipitate pressure ulcer formation. |

*(continues)*

## PROCEDURE 38-5 (continued)

4. The lead nurse tells the client and other personnel the direction of the move.

5. One person stands on each side of bed. The lead nurse gives the signal for the move. The staff member on side of the bed in the direction of the move holds the turn/draw sheet to guide the move. The second staff member applies gentle pressure on client's back toward the direction of the move, assisting client to roll (Figure 38-38).

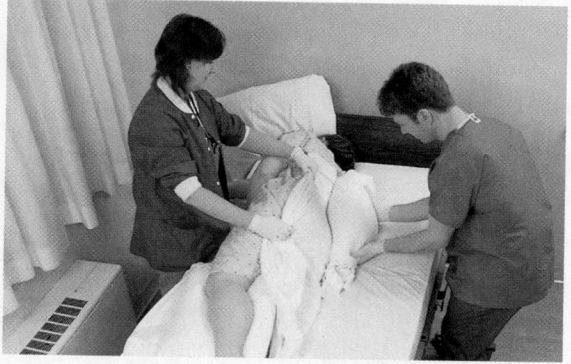

**Figure 38-38    Logrolling: two-person move**

6. Tuck pillows at client's back and abdomen.

7. Assess the client for comfort and proper alignment.

8. Elevate side rails and lower the bed height.

9. This procedure can be reversed to reposition clients on their backs.

4. Cooperation and coordination place less strain on client and personnel.

5. Two persons give more support to client than one person could and are better able to maintain proper alignment of client's spine and neck.

6. Maintains side-lying position.

7. Comfort is subjective.

8. Promotes client safety.

9. Repositioning can prevent development of pressure sores and promote circulation.

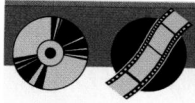 **PROCEDURE 38-6**

## Assisting from Bed to Wheelchair, Commode, or Chair

### EQUIPMENT NEEDED

- Bed
- Wheelchair, chair, or commode
- Any splints, braces, or supportive equipment specific to the client

- Shoes or slippers with nonskid soles
- Gait belt
- Transfer board (if necessary)

### IMPLEMENTATION—ACTION/RATIONALE

| ACTION | RATIONALE |
|---|---|
| 1. Inform client about desired purpose and destination. | 1. Reduces client anxiety and increases cooperation. |

*(continues)*

## PROCEDURE 38-6 (*continued*)

2. Assess client for ability to assist with the transfer and for presence of cognitive or sensory deficits.

3. Lock the bed in position.

4. Place any splints, braces, or other devices on the client.

5. Place the client's shoes or slippers on the client's feet.

6. Lower the height of the bed to lowest possible position.

7. Slowly raise the head of the bed if this is not contraindicated by the client's condition.

8. Place one arm under the client's legs and one arm behind the client's back. Slowly pivot the client so the client's legs are dangling over the edge of the bed and he is in a sitting position on the edge of the bed (Figure 38-39).

9. Allow client to dangle for 2 to 5 minutes. Help support client if necessary (Figure 38-40).

2. Allows planning regarding the amount of assistance and cooperation to expect from the client.

3. Prevents the bed from rolling during the procedure.

4. Provides support and prevents injury to the client.

5. Provides a nonslip surface for stability.

6. Reduces distance client has to step down, thus decreasing risk of injury.

7. Minimizes lifting.

8. Supports the client while sitting him upright.

9. Allows time for assessing client's response to sitting; reduces possibility of orthostatic hypotension.

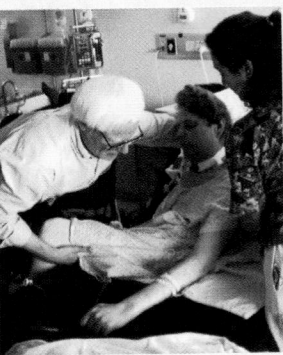

**Figure 38-39    Pivot the client to a sitting position on the edge of the bed.**

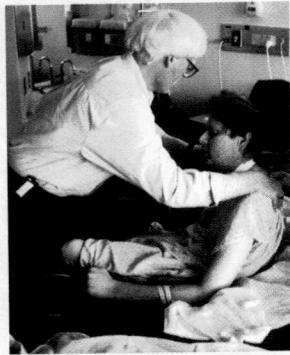

**Figure 38-40    Support the client, if needed, while the client adjusts to the sitting position.**

10. Bring the chair or wheelchair close to the side of the bed. Place it at a 45-degree angle to the bed. If the client has a weaker side, place the chair or wheelchair on the client's strong side.

11. Lock wheelchair brakes and elevate the foot pedals. For chairs, lock brakes if available.

12. If you will be using a gait belt to assist the client, place it around the client's waist.

13. Assist client to side of bed until feet are firmly on the floor and slightly apart.

14. Grasp the sides of the gait belt or place your hands just below the client's axilla. Using a wide stance, bend your knees and assist the client to a standing position (Figure 38-41).

10. Minimizes transfer distance. Allows the client to pivot on the stronger leg.

11. Provides stability.

12. Provides a secure handhold for the nurse during the transfer.

13. Moves client into proper position for transfer. Provides stable footing for client.

14. Wide stance increases nurse stability and minimizes strain on the back. Avoids putting pressure directly on the axilla, risking nerve damage or shoulder subluxation.

*(continues)*

## PROCEDURE 38-6 (continued)

15. Standing close to the client, pivot until the client's back is toward the chair.

16. Instruct the client to place hands on the arm supports, or place the client's hands on the arm supports of the chair.

17. Bend at the knees, easing the client into a sitting position.

18. Assist client to maintain proper posture (Figure 38-42). Support weak side with pillow if needed.

15. Moves client into proper position to be seated.

16. Allows client to gain balance and judge distance to seat.

17. Increases stability and minimizes strain on back.

18. Increases client comfort.

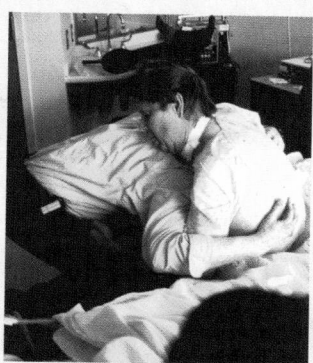

**Figure 38-41**    Bend your knees, grasp the client firmly, and help him into a standing position.

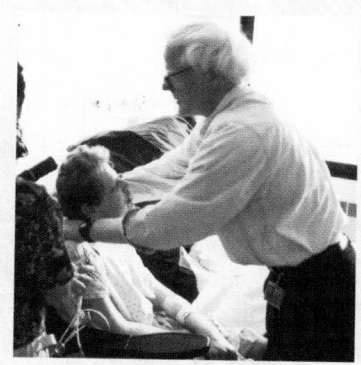

**Figure 38-42**    Assist client to maintain proper position.

19. Secure the safety belt, place client's feet on feet pedals, and release brakes if you will be moving the client immediately. Make sure tubes and lines, arms, and hands are not pinched or caught between the client and the chair (Figure 38-43). If the client is sitting in a chair, offer a footstool if available (Figure 38-44).

20. Wash hands.

19. Ensures client safety; prepares client for movement.

20. Reduces transmission of microorganisms.

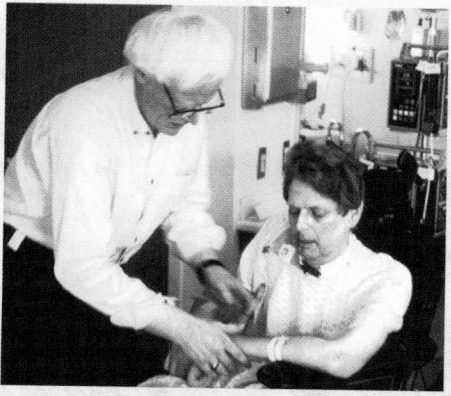

**Figure 38-43**    Once the client is moved, make sure skin, tubing, or equipment is not pinched between the client and the chair.

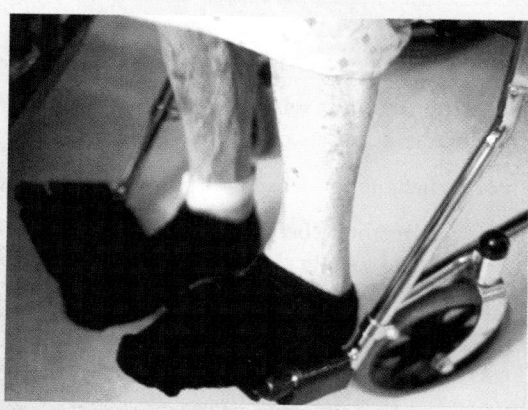

**Figure 38-44**    Position the wheelchair footrests or use a footstool if the client is sitting in a chair.

## COMMUNITY/HOME CARE

### Moving a Client

**Home Care Variations**

● The bed of a home care client may be at a poor height for safe transfer from bed to wheelchair. If the bed is too low, the nurse may be required to lift the client farther than is safe. If the bed is too high, the risk of a client fall is increased. Advise the client or caregiver of the proper height for bed-to-wheelchair transfers and the reason it is important. Problem-solve with the caregiver to outline ways to use proper body mechanics, adjust the height of the bed, or acquire an adjustable bed.

● Assess the wheelchair of home care clients. Home care clients may have modified their equipment or failed to maintain it for safe use. Check for sharp, exposed edges; frayed or damaged material; and other damage or modification that might be unsafe for the client.

**Long-Term Care Variations**

● Long-term care clients may have contractures or pressure ulcers that will affect their ability to transfer safely and their ability to sit in a wheelchair comfortably. Be sure to assess for these possibilities prior to transferring a client.

---

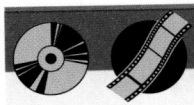

**PROCEDURE 38-7**   **Assisting from Bed to Stretcher**

### EQUIPMENT NEEDED

**Transferring a Client with Minimum Assistance**

■ Bed
■ Stretcher

**Transferring a Client with Maximum Assistance**

■ Bed
■ Stretcher
■ Pillows
■ Transfer/slider boards
■ Lift sheet
■ Other qualified personnel to assist

### IMPLEMENTATION—ACTION/RATIONALE

| ACTION | RATIONALE |
|---|---|
| **Transferring a Client with Minimum Assistance** | |
| 1. Inform client about desired purpose and destination. | 1. Reduces client anxiety and increases cooperation. |
| 2. Raise the height of bed to 1 inch higher than the stretcher and lock brakes of bed. | 2. Reduces distance nurse must bend, thus preventing back strain; prevents bed from moving. |
| 3. Instruct client to move to side of bed close to stretcher. Lower side rails of bed and stretcher. Leave side rails on opposite side up (Figure 38-45). | 3. Decreases risk of client falling. |
| 4. Stand at outer side of stretcher and push it toward bed. | 4. Diminishes the gap between bed and stretcher; secures the stretcher position. |

*(continues)*

## PROCEDURE 38-7 (continued)

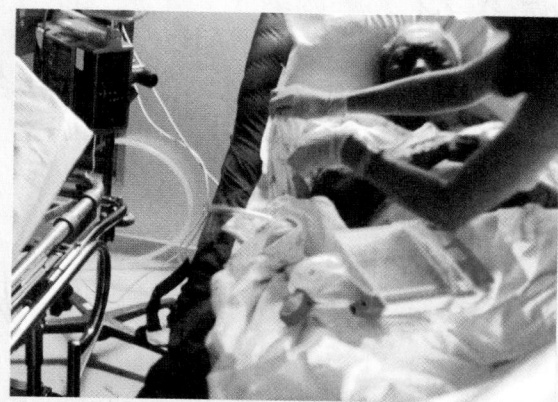

**Figure 38-45    Lower side rails of bed and stretcher.**

5.  Instruct client to move onto stretcher with assistance as needed.

6.  Cover client with sheet or bath blanket.

7.  Elevate side rails on stretcher and secure safety belts about client. Release brakes of stretcher.

8.  Stand at head of stretcher to guide it when pushing.

9.  Wash hands.

### Transferring a Client with Maximum Assistance

10.  Repeat Actions 1 and 2.

11.  Assess amount of assistance required for transfer. Usually two to four staff members are required for the maximum-assisted transfer.

12.  Lock wheels of bed and stretcher.

13.  Have one nurse stand close to client's head.

14.  Logroll the client and place a lift sheet under the client's back, trunk, and upper legs. The lift sheet can extend under the head if client lacks head control abilities.

15.  Empty all drainage bags (e.g., T-tube, Hemovac, Jackson-Pratt). Record amounts. Secure drainage system to client's gown prior to transfer.

16.  Move client to edge of bed near stretcher. Lift up and over to avoid dragging.

17.  Because the client is now on the side of the bed, without the side rail up, the nurse on nonstretcher side of bed holds the stretcher side of the lift

5.  Promotes client independence.

6.  Promotes comfort; protects privacy.

7.  Prevents falls.

8.  Pushing, not pulling, ensures proper body mechanics.

9.  Reduces transmission of microorganisms.

10.  See Rationales 1 and 2.

11.  Promotes client independence; ensures that enough staff are present before beginning transfer.

12.  Prevents falls.

13.  Supports client's head during the move.

14.  Prevents flexion and rotation of client's hips and spine; maintains correct body alignment.

15.  Decreases possibility of spills; prevents dislodging of tubes.

16.  Prevents dragging, which causes shearing force.

17.  Protects the client from falling.

*(continues)*

**PROCEDURE 38-7 (continued)**

sheet up (by reaching across the client's chest) to prevent the client from falling onto the stretcher or off the bed.

18. Place pillow or slider board overlapping the bed and stretcher (Figure 38-46).

19. Have staff members grasp edges of lift sheet. Be sure to use good body mechanics (Figure 38-47).

18. Protects head from injury. Slider board eases movement of the client.

19. Provides surface for client to slide on. Prevents dragging and shearing.

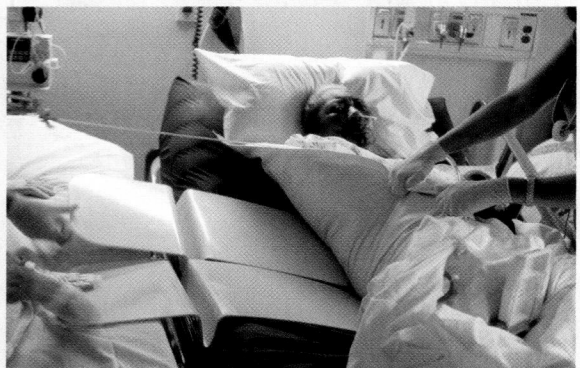

**Figure 38-46    Place pillow or slider board over-lapping the bed and stretcher.**

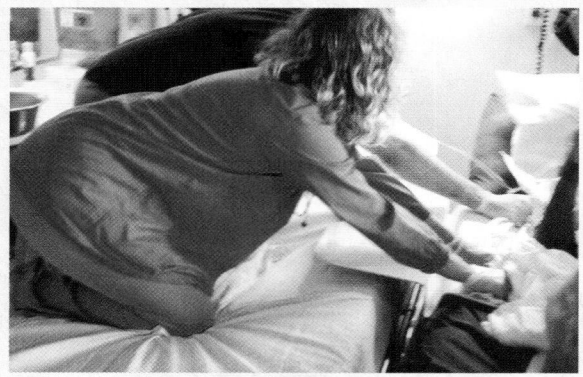

**Figure 38-47    Firmly grasp edges of lift sheet.**

20. On the count of three, have staff members pull lift sheet and the client onto the stretcher.

21. Position client on stretcher, place pillow under head, and cover with a sheet or bath blanket (Figure 38-48).

20. Working in unison makes the overall job easier and prevents staff injury.

21. Promotes comfort and provides for privacy.

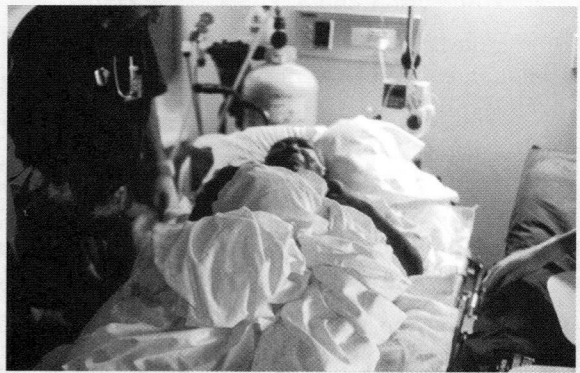

**Figure 38-48    Place pillow under head and cover client with blanket.**

22. Secure safety belts and elevate side rails of stretcher.

23. If IV pole is present, move it from bed IV pole to stretcher IV pole after client transfer.

24. Wash hands.

22. Prevents falls.

23. Prevents tubing from being pulled and IV from being dislodged.

24. Reduces transmission of microorganisms.

## LIFE SPAN CONSIDERATIONS

### Transfer Techniques

#### Pediatric Variations

- A child may be small enough to lift onto a stretcher. If the parent is lifting, make sure the parent can hold the weight of the child. Give brief instructions on proper body mechanics prior to the lifting of the child.

- Children may be small enough to slip through the side rails on a gurney. Be sure to fasten any safety straps or restrain the child some other way.

#### Geriatric Variations

- Geriatric clients may have contractures or other disabilities that impair their ability to lie flat. Be aware that your transfer technique may need to be altered to accommodate this.

- Older clients may have thin, fragile skin. Care should be taken during the transfer not to tear or damage their skin.

---

Other transfer appliances include stretchers (gurneys) and hydraulic lifts. The hydraulic (Hoyer, mechanical) lift is used for moving immobile clients who are obese; see Procedure 38-8. A client may be transferred to a chair, wheelchair, bedside commode, stretcher, or scale using a hydraulic lift. The manufacturer's equipment instructions should be followed and the weight limits must not exceed the manufacturer's specifications. Two staff members are needed to safely operate a hydraulic lift. Hydraulic lifts are not for use with clients who have spinal cord injury as spinal alignment is not maintained during use of the lift (Altman, 2004).

## NURSING STRATEGY

### Transferring from Bed to Chair

- Do not allow client to grab onto or around nurse's neck.

- Remove stethoscope before transfer.

- Avoid pulling on client's arms, always have a firm grip on the gait belt or client's torso in case client loses balance during the transfer.

- Downward placement of thumbs prevents potential wrist injury as the nurse lifts.

- Place wheelchair parallel to the bed and as close to the bed as possible.

- Placement of nurse's feet should mirror that of the client's.

## Assisting with Ambulation

Client **ambulation** (assisted or unassisted walking) is encouraged soon after the onset of illness or surgery to prevent the complications of immobility. In planning ambulation, the nurse assesses the client's strength, endurance, and mobility status. Can the client walk alone, or is assistance needed? The presence of equipment (e.g., urinary catheters, IV infusions, drainage tubes) requires assistance.

In order to maintain client safety, ambulation must occur in progressive stages. First the client should be able to tolerate sitting on the bedside and dangling the feet. The next step is client tolerance of standing at the side of the bed. Then progressive ambulation can be initiated; see Procedure 38-9.

As ambulation activities are initiated, it is important to assess the client's blood pressure, respiratory rate, pulse, skin color and moisture, and subjective responses. While the client is walking, observe for signs of exertion, including diaphoresis, shortness of breath, or weakness. It is also important to assess for the presence of orthostatic hypotension in order to prevent falls. Depending on the client's physical conditioning and the effects of orthostatic hypotension, the client may need to slowly progress to independent ambulation. Once the activity is completed,

## CLINICAL ALERT

### Transfers and Closed Chest Drainage System

The closed chest drainage system must remain vertical at all times, including during transfers, to maintain the water seal.

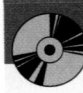

**PROCEDURE 38-8**    ## Using a Hydraulic Lift

## EQUIPMENT NEEDED

- Mechanical lift, such as hydraulic or Hoyer lift
- Equipment should include lift, plus canvas or mesh sheet and bars to slide into sheet
- Protective disposable cover or disinfectant to clean canvas
- Gloves (when applicable)

## IMPLEMENTATION—ACTION/RATIONALE

| ACTION | RATIONALE |
|---|---|
| 1. Wash hands. | 1. Reduces transmission of microorganisms. |
| 2. Check the physician's or qualified practitioner's order to determine the length of time the client may sit. | 2. The physician or qualified practitioner may want the client to sit only for a specified length of time or for as long as possible. |
| 3. Check the client's medical diagnosis and any other medical problems. | 3. Assists you in determining any problems that sitting may cause or any restrictions needed. |
| 4. Ask the client how long ago she last sat. | 4. If the client has been in the bed several days, she may complain of dizziness or faintness. |
| 5. Lock the wheels of the bed. | 5. Prevents the bed from rolling when the client is moved. |
| 6. Position the chair close to the bed. | 6. Always transfer the client the shortest possible distance. |
| 7. Position urine drainage, NG, and IV tubing on the side of the bed where the chair will be placed. Ensure slack in the tubing. | 7. Prevents the tubing from being dislodged when the client is moved. |
| 8. Clamp and disconnect any tubing if permitted. | 8. NG suction tubing and tube-feeding tubing are often allowed to be clamped. This will make moving the client easier. |
| 9. Roll the client on her side and position the sling on the bed behind the client (Figure 38-49). | 9. The sling is positioned behind the client so that she can be turned in the opposite direction and the sling can be pulled through. |

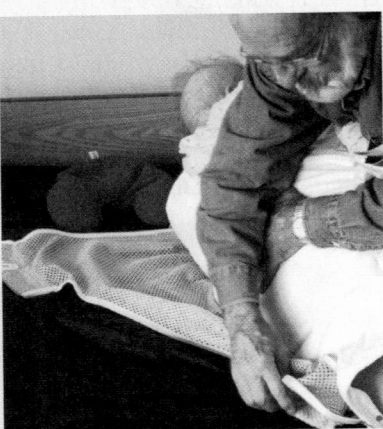

**Figure 38-49    Adjust the sling so it is smooth and flat under the client.**

*(continues)*

10. Roll the client on her opposite side, pull the sling through, and position the sling smoothly on the bed.

11. Roll the client back onto the sling and fold her arms over her chest (Figure 38-50).

12. Make sure the sling is centered.

13. Lower the side rail and position the lift on the side of the bed with the chair. Be sure to spread the base of the hydraulic lift as indicated in manufacturer's instructions to provide stability (Figure 38-51). Protect the client from falls while the side rail is down.

10. Prevents skin breakdown.

11. Prevents injury to the client's arms during the transfer.

12. Evenly distributes the client's weight.

13. The side rail must be down to use the lift. Always transfer the client the shortest possible distance. The wheels and base of the lift should be spread to provide a wide, stable base to prevent the lift from tipping.

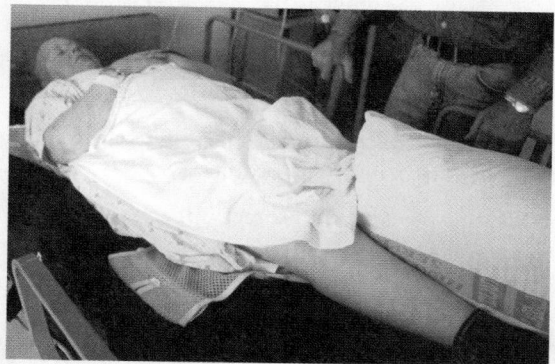

**Figure 38-50    Roll the client back onto the sling. Position the client's arms across her chest.**

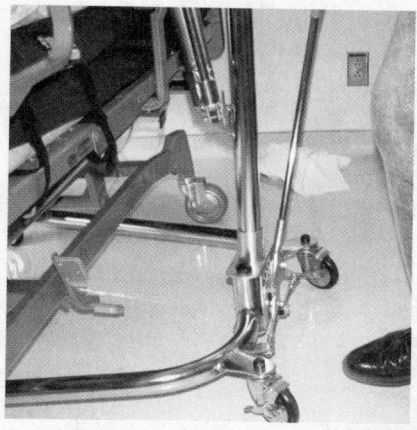

**Figure 38-51    Spread the base of the hydraulic lift to provide stability.**

14. Lift the frame and pass it over the client. Carefully lower the frame and attach the hooks to the sling (Figures 38-52 and 38-53).

14. Safely attaches sling to frame.

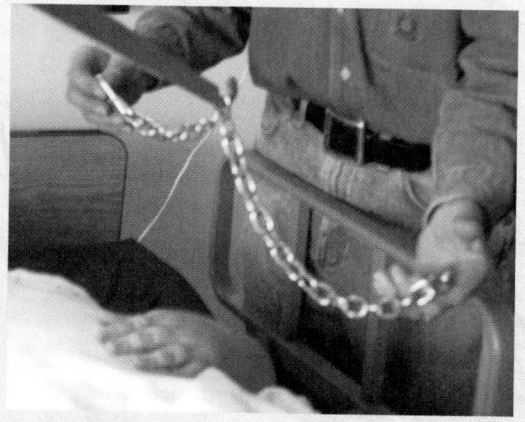

**Figure 38-52    Locate the correct hook for each corner of the sling.**

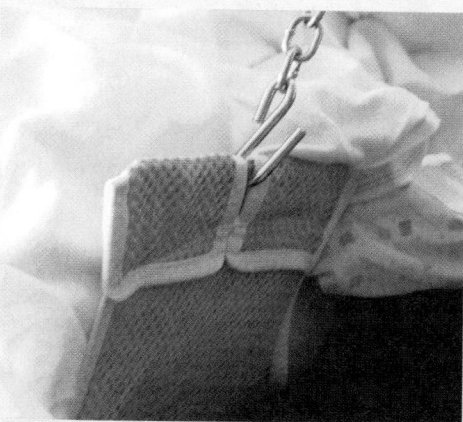

**Figure 38-53    Attach the hooks to the sling.**

*(continues)*

## PROCEDURE 38-8 (*continued*)

15. Raise the client from the bed by pumping the handle.

15. Read the manufacturer's directions to determine the mechanism for raising the particular lift you are using. The various models do not operate in the same manner.

16. Secure the client with a safety belt and cover the client with a blanket.

16. Provides safety and comfort.

17. Steer the client away from the bed and slide a chair through the base of the lift.

17. It is safer to slide the chair through the base than to slide the base around the chair.

18. The sling can be disconnected and the lift can be moved out of the way while the client is sitting in the chair. If the lift will be used to return the client to bed, the sling may be left in place beneath the client.

18. The sling can be disconnected and the lift can be moved out of the way while the client is sitting in the chair.

19. Reposition and reconnect any tubing necessary.

19. Tubing should not be left disconnected. The client may sit for a while and will need all the equipment to function properly.

20. Assess how well the client tolerated the move and whether any dizziness was experienced.

20. The data is necessary for charting whether the client experienced any problems.

21. Place call light, appropriate covers, and padding as needed after transfer. Place protective restraints as needed. Cover feet with slippers if in sitting position.

21. Ensures privacy and protection.

22. Reverse the procedure to return the client to the bed.

22. Transfers client safely and comfortably.

23. Wash hands.

23. Reduces transmission of microorganisms.

## LIFE SPAN CONSIDERATIONS

### Hydraulic Lift

#### Pediatric Variations

- Children may be fearful of the suspension above the bed and being moved to the chair.

- Explain the procedure and first demonstrate how the lift is locked in place and then released to allow the sling to lower. Smaller children can often just be picked up. The weight of a child who must be moved with a hydraulic lift may be determined by hospital policy.

#### Geriatric Variations

- Older clients may have difficulty with sudden moves; therefore, take time to explain procedures and move slowly.

- Make sure the client can see and hear what you are doing.

- Make sure eyeglasses and hearing aids are in place.

## COMMUNITY/HOME CARE

### Hydraulic Lift

*Home Care Variations*

- Check hydraulic fluid and functioning of the lift to ascertain that the equipment works.

- Have appropriate maintenance performed.

- Make sure any caregiver who is using the lift is trained in the procedure. The client can often instruct the caregiver and control the procedure in the home setting.

- Make sure there is enough space to maneuver the lift.

- Launder the sling periodically to keep it clean.

*Long-Term Care Variations*

- These are the same as home care variations. In the long-term setting, increase the independence and control the client has over the procedure as much as possible.

---

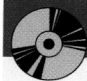 **PROCEDURE 38-9**    ## Assisting with Ambulation and Safe Falling

### EQUIPMENT NEEDED

- Gait belt as needed (prn)
- Assistive devices

- Shoes or nonslip footwear

## IMPLEMENTATION—ACTION/RATIONALE

| ACTION | RATIONALE |
|---|---|
| **Ambulation Safety** | |
| 1. When assisting a client with an IV infusion, place the IV pole with wheels at the head of the bed before having the client dangle the legs—then there is room to swing the legs from the bed to the floor. | 1. Prevents the client's legs from becoming tangled in the IV pole or tubing, causing a fall or causing the tubing to become dislodged. |
| 2. Transfer the IV infusion from the bed IV pole to the portable IV pole. The client or the nurse can guide the portable IV pole ahead during ambulation (Figure 38-54). | 2. Supports the IV while the client ambulates. |
| 3. When assisting the client with a urinary drainage bag, empty the drainage bag prior to ambulation. Have the client sit on the side of the bed with legs dangling. | 3. Emptying the bag reduces the weight of the bag. An empty bag kept below the level of the bladder reduces the risk of urine flowing back into the bladder. |
| Remove the urinary drainage bag from the bed. The nurse or client can hold the urinary drainage bag during ambulation. Make sure the drainage bag remains below the level of the bladder (Figure 38-55). | Having the nurse hold the drainage bag allows the client to concentrate on safe ambulation. |

*(continues)*

**PROCEDURE 38-9** (*continued*)

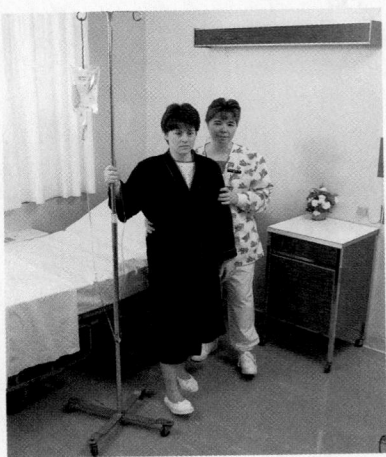

**Figure 38-54    Ambulating client with an IV**

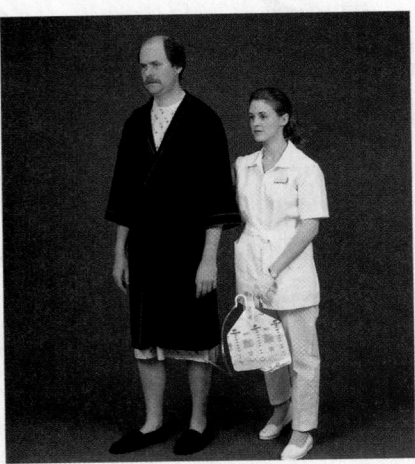

**Figure 38-55    Ambulating client with a urinary drainage bag**

4. When the client has a drainage tube such as a T-tube, Hemovac, or Jackson-Pratt drainage system, be sure to secure the drainage tube and bag prior to ambulation. Place a rubber band around the drainage tube near the drainage bag. Secure the drainage tube and bag with a safety pin through the rubber band. Allow slack. The safety pin can be secured to the client's gown or robe (Figure 38-56).

4. Prevents the tubing from becoming dislodged or tangled in clothing or other tubes.

5. Ambulating the client with a closed chest tube drainage system often requires two nurses, one assisting the client and one nurse managing the closed chest tube drainage system. While the client is sitting on the edge of the bed with feet dangling, remove the hangers from the drainage system. Hold the closed chest tube drainage system upright at all times to maintain the water seal. Do not pull or tug on the chest tubes; they may not be sutured into place.

5. Two nurses allows one to focus on the client's safety and ambulation while another focuses on maintaining the chest drainage system and keeping tubes from becoming dislodged.

6. Use a transfer belt or gait belt when ambulating a client who is weak (Figure 38-57).

6. The transfer belt is a 2-inch-wide webbed belt worn by the client for the purposes of stabilization during transfers and ambulation. It provides more support for the client by having the nurse hold the back of the belt.

7. If a client feels faint or dizzy during dangling, return the client to a supine position in bed and lower the head of the bed. Monitor the client's blood pressure and pulse.

7. Keeps the client from falling from the bed. Lowering the head of the bed will allow gravity to support blood flow to the brain in the hypotensive client.

(continues)

## PROCEDURE 38-9 (*continued*)

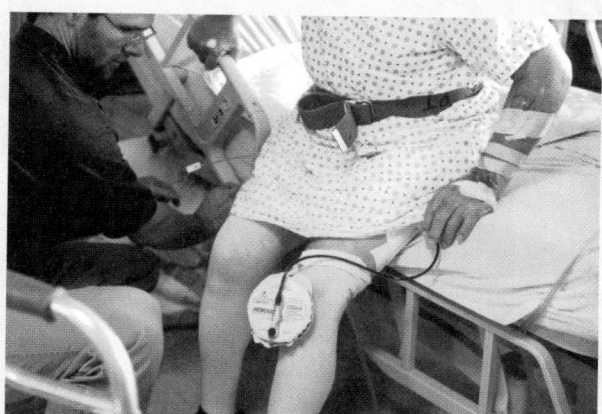

**Figure 38-56**   **Secure tubes and drainage bags prior to ambulation, so they do not become dislodged.**

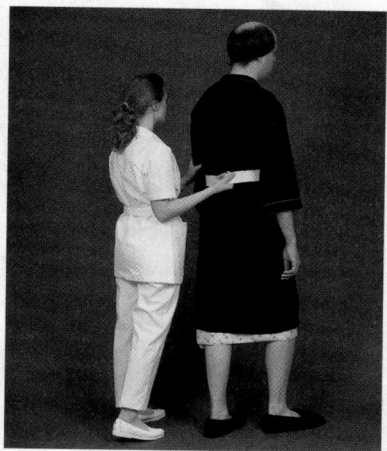

**Figure 38-57**   **Ambulating the client using a gait belt for better grip and control**

8. If the client feels faint or dizzy during ambulation, allow the client to sit in a chair. Stay with the client for safety. Request another nurse to secure a wheelchair to return the client to bed.

9. If the client feels faint or dizzy during the ambulation and starts to fall, ease the client to the floor while supporting and protecting the client's head. Position yourself next to and slightly behind the ambulating client, thus being able to step behind the client, and safely ease the client to the floor. Ask other personnel to assist you in returning the client to bed. Assess orthostatic blood pressures.

8. May stop the client from progressing to a full faint.

9. Easing the client to the floor prevents injury to the client.

### Safe Walking

10. Inform client of the purposes and distance of the walking exercise (Figure 38-58).

11. Elevate the head of the bed and wait several minutes.

12. Lower the bed height.

13. With one arm on the client's back and one arm under the client's upper legs, move the client into the dangling position.

14. Encourage client to dangle at side of bed for several minutes.

15. Place gait belt around client's waist; secure the buckle in front.

16. Stand in front of client with your knees touching client's knees.

10. Reduces client anxiety and increases cooperation.

11. Prevents orthostatic hypotension.

12. Reduces distance client has to step down, thus decreasing risk of injury.

13. Provides client support and reduces risk of fall.

14. Prevents orthostatic hypotension. Allows for assessing tolerance for the sitting position.

15. Provides handholds for the caregiver to support the client.

16. Prevents client from sliding forward if dizziness or faintness occurs.

*(continues)*

**PROCEDURE 38-9 (continued)**

17. Place arms under client's axilla.

18. Assist client to a standing position, allowing client time to balance (Figure 38-59).

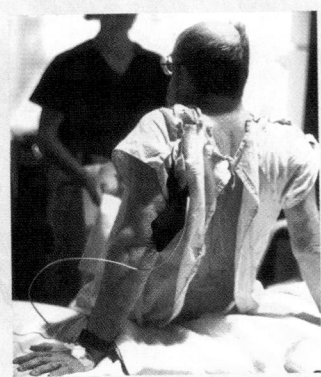

**Figure 38-58    Discuss the planned walking exercise with the client prior to ambulation.**

19. Help the client ambulate the desired distance or distance of tolerance by placing your hand under the client's forearm and ambulating close to the client. Alternatively, place a gait belt around the client's waist and walk to the client's side and slightly behind with one hand grasping the belt at the center back.

20. Help the client back to the bed or chair. Make the client comfortable, and make sure all lines and tubes are secure.

21. Document the activity.

22. Wash hands.

17. Supports client's trunk.

18. Reduces risk of fall.

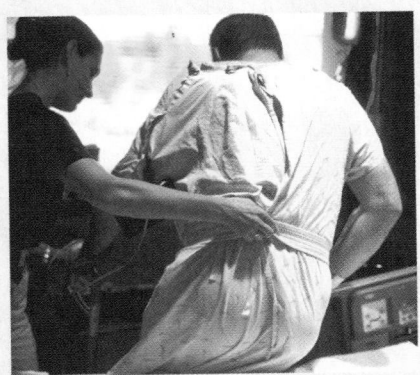

**Figure 38-59    Assist the client to stand.**

19. Provides assistance in achieving ambulatory goals.

20. Promotes safety and comfort.

21. Provides a record to measure progress.

22. Reduces transmission of microorganisms.

## COMMUNITY/HOME CARE

### Ambulation

*Home Care Variations*

- Home care environments vary widely. Be sure the environment is safe for the client to ambulate in.

- Do not let barriers keep the client from moving about. Think of creative ways to overcome obstacles. Being able to go outdoors or to move to the living room from the bedroom can offer an uplifting change of scenery and improve feelings of independence.

*Long-Term Care Variations*

- Clients with long-term ambulatory problems may become careless regarding their gait and their equipment. Be sure to check their equipment and reinforce proper gait.

## NURSING STRATEGY

### Stretcher Transport Safety

- Use hall ceiling mirrors at intersections before turning corners.

- Lock elevator door open when entering or exiting.

- Stand at head of stretcher to push stretcher up a ramp.

- Back down a steep ramp while positioned at head of stretcher.

- Lock stretcher brakes when standing still.

the nurse assesses the client evaluation focusing on progression of activity. Continuous evaluation of the client's strength and endurance is performed by the nurse.

### Preparing the Client to Walk

One of the best ways to encourage ambulation is to help the client become and remain as independent as possible while lying in bed. This includes urging clients to participate in ROM exercises and perform self-care activities as much as possible.

Independent mobility, the goal of most clients, is the ability to walk, run, sit, and turn without mechanical or personal aid. Progressive exercises and activities that promote independent mobility include:

1. *Turning.* The client can turn in bed using side rails for stabilization and leverage.
2. *Sitting.* The client can raise the head of the bed and lower the height of the bed. Then the client turns to the side of the bed and swings legs over the side of the bed to assume the dangling position. Arms held in the tripod position give balance to the sitting position.
3. *Standing.* The client dangles for a few minutes to assure balance and then bears weight with both feet at the side of the bed. For additional stability and balance, the client can perch on the edge of the bed for several minutes.
4. *Walking.* The client assesses strength and balance while walking, thus allowing a gradual progression of the duration of walking. Instruct clients to rest by sitting or standing still stabilized with a guide rail if fatigued.

### Client Education

Prior to ambulation, clients who have been immobile need to be prepared adequately in order to prevent injury. Listing the therapeutic outcomes of ambulation is one way to teach clients the importance of ambulation. Clients should also be taught to sit down or use side rails if dizziness occurs.

Teach clients the technique for safe falling in order to minimize risk of injury (Figure 38-60). Clients should be told that if they begin to feel faint they should fall toward the affected side of the body and to use the unaffected side to raise self from the floor or chair.

### Preambulatory Exercise

Helping immobile clients to prepare for ambulation includes instruction of preambulatory exercises in order to strengthen and tone muscles. The quadriceps femoris is the major muscle used for walking; thus, clients should be directed to gently contract and release the leg muscles several times a day. Clients who will be walking with the assistance of walkers and crutches need upper body strength. Instruction in the safe use of ambulatory assistive devices is also necessary for many clients with impaired mobility.

### Assistive Devices

Clients who are unable to ambulate independently can use devices designed to help them walk safely. Determination of which device to use is based on the following:

- Upper arm strength
- Endurance (stamina)
- Presence or absence of one-sided weakness
- Weight-bearing ability

See Table 38-15 for a comparison of the three most common devices used to assist in walking: canes, walkers, and crutches.

### Canes

A cane is to be used by clients who can bear weight on both legs but have some weakness in one leg or hip. The straight (standard) cane is used most often; canes with three or four legs are used with clients who need more stability

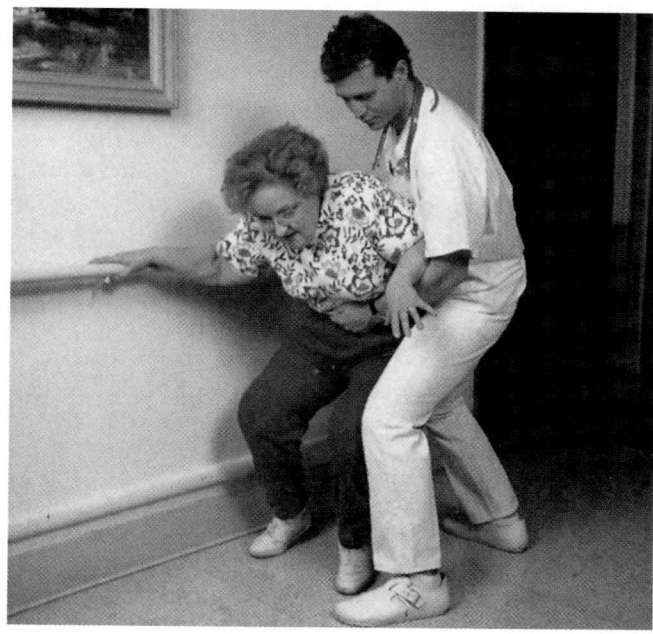

**Figure 38-60  Support for fainting client**

## TABLE 38-15    ASSISTIVE DEVICES FOR AMBULATION

| Equipment | Description | Directions for Use |
|---|---|---|
| Cane | Widens base of support | Use on unaffected side |
|  | Various styles: | Advance cane simultaneously with affected limb |
|  | (1) Regular (straight)—gives minimal support for balance | Hold close to body; do not move cane forward beyond toes of affected foot |
|  | (2) Three-point—provides broader base of support; more cumbersome |  |
|  | (3) Four-point (quad)—broader base of support; more cumbersome |  |
| Walker | Provides more stability than canes due to broader base of support | For clients with weight-bearing status: Advance walker and step normally |
|  | Various styles: | For partial or non-weight bearing on one limb: |
|  | (1) Pickup—assists with weight bearing; lifting may cause some strain for client | Thrust weight forward, then lift walker and replace all four legs on floor |
|  | (2) Rolling—pushed on wheels; thus reduces physical strain on client |  |
| Crutches | Less stable than canes and walkers | Use good posture |
|  | Requires upper body strength and ability to maintain balance | Maintain proper foot position on affected side (foot drop can result from walking on toes or ball of foot) |
|  |  | Eliminate obstacles in ambulatory path |

Data adapted from Eliopoulos, C. (1999). *Manual of gerontologic nursing* (2nd ed.). St. Louis: Mosby, pp. 286–287.

than provided by the straight cane. Quad canes provide more stability but are sometimes more awkward to use than the straight cane (Figure 38-61).

### Walkers

A walker is a waist-high metal tubular device with a hand-grip and four legs. Some walkers have rubber tips on all four legs, whereas others have wheels on the two front legs. The advantages of using a walker include provision of extra support, provision of a sense of security, and independence. The client first moves the walker forward and then takes a step while balancing her weight on the walker.

A walker is used by clients who need more support than that provided by a cane. Walkers are available with and without wheels. The walker without wheels provides more stability but also requires more client stamina in order to lift the walker. Walkers with wheels are intended for use by clients with limited upper body strength. The nurse should determine the following for clients using walkers:

1. Amount of weight bearing allowed on lower limb
2. Appropriateness for client's height
3. Type of walker (pick-up or rolling)
4. With pick-up walker: client's ability to grip, lift, and propel the walker forward

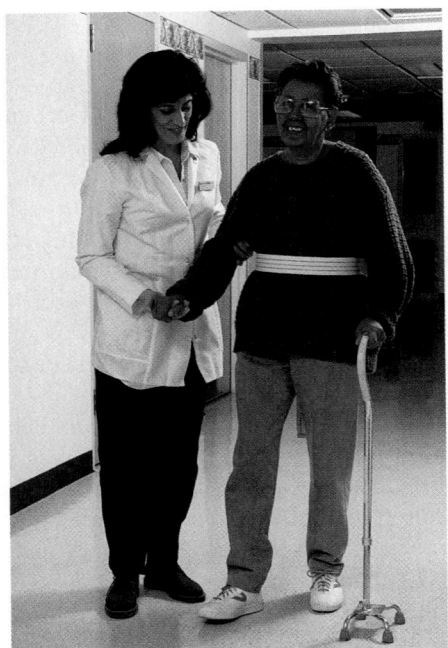

**Figure 38-61**  Nurse promotes safety of a client using a quad cane. Note the use of gait belt for added stability.

**5.** With rolling walker: client's ability to grip and propel the walker forward

When educating clients about the use of walkers, inform them that when transferring from chair or commode, they should back the walker to the toilet seat and use arms of chair or commode to assist in standing. Teach clients to always use both hands when using a walker to transfer from standing to sitting (Figure 38-62). Clients should always push off the surface with their hands wherever they are sitting, instead of pulling up on the walker to stand.

### Crutches

A crutch is a wooden or metal staff used to increase client mobility. There are two types of crutches: axillary and forearm. The most commonly used type, the axillary crutch, fits under the axilla with the weight being placed on the handgrips. The forearm crutch, which has a handgrip and a metal cuff that fits around the arm, is more convenient but provides less stability than the axillary crutch.

To prevent slipping, crutches have rubber tips, which must be kept dry. If the tips are worn or loose, they must be replaced. The crutch must be regularly inspected; if cracks or bends are present, the person's weight will not be properly supported.

Crutches can be used by clients who are unable to bear any weight on one leg, clients who can bear partial weight on one leg, and clients who have full weight bearing on both legs.

Several gaits are used with crutches: the four-point gait, three-point gait, two-point gait, and swing-through gait.

The *four-point gait* for weight bearing with both legs follows the pattern of right crutch forward, left foot forward, left crutch forward, then right foot forward. The four-point gait with crutches is very stable but slow. The *two-point gait* for weight bearing with both legs has the pattern of right crutch and left foot forward together, then left crutch and right foot forward together. The two-point gait requires more balance

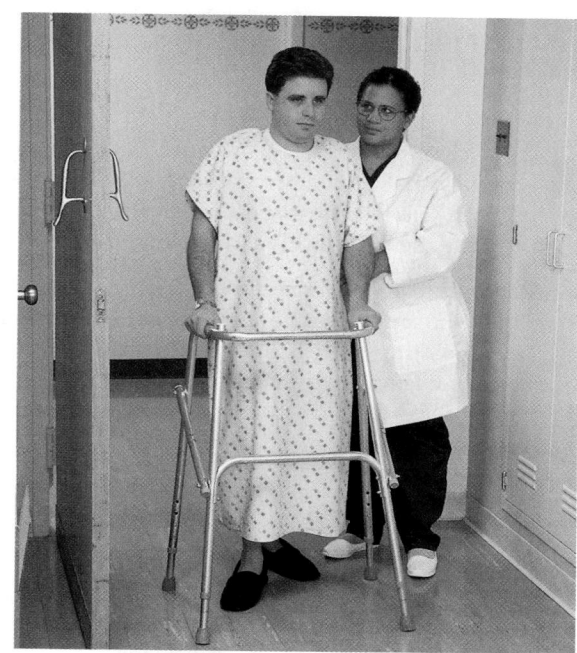

**Figure 38-62   Client using a walker**

but is a faster gait. The *three-point gait* for weight bearing with one leg has the pattern of crutches and weak leg forward together, then weight-bearing leg forward. The *swing-through gait* has the pattern of crutches forward, then legs swing forward together. The swing-through gait has the advantage of speed; however, it requires good balance. See Procedure 38-10 for a description of crutch-walking techniques.

## Wellness Promotion

Wellness promotion emphasizes the need for physical fitness, which increases well-being, increases sympathetic

---

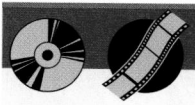 **PROCEDURE 38-10   Assisting with Crutches, Cane, or Walker**

### EQUIPMENT NEEDED

- Gait belt
- Assistive device: crutches, cane, or walker
- Tape measure
- Sturdy footwear, properly fitted

### IMPLEMENTATION—ACTION/RATIONALE

| ACTION | RATIONALE |
|---|---|
| **Crutch Walking** | |
| 1. Inform client that you will be assisting with ambulation using crutches. | 1. Reduces anxiety; helps increase comprehension and cooperation; promotes client autonomy. |

*(continues)*

## PROCEDURE 38-10 (*continued*)

2. Assess client for strength, mobility, range of motion, visual acuity, perceptual difficulties, and balance. *Note:* The nurse and physical therapist often collaborate on this assessment.

3. Adjust crutches to fit the client. With the client supine, measure from the heel to the axilla. With the client standing, set the crutch position at a point 4 to 5 inches lateral to the client and 4 to 6 inches in front of the client. The crutch pad should fit 1.5 to 2 inches below the axilla (3-finger width) (Figure 38-63). The hand grip should be adjusted to allow for the client to have elbows bent at 30-degree flexion.

2. Helps determine the client's capabilities and amount of assistance required.

3. Provides broad base of support for client. Space between the crutch pad and the axilla prevents pressure on radial nerves. The elbow flexion allows for space between the crutch pad and axilla.

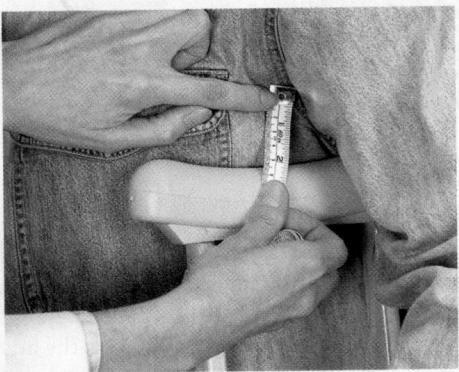

**Figure 38-63    Adjust the crutches to fit the client.**

4. Lower the height of the bed.

5. Dangle the client at the side of bed for several minutes. Assess for vertigo.

6. Instruct client on method to hold the crutches; that is, with elbows bent 30 degrees and pad 1.5 to 2 inches below the axilla. Instruct client to position crutches lateral to and forward of feet. Demonstrate correct positioning.

7. Apply the gait belt around the client's waist if balance and stability are unreliable.

8. Assist the client to a standing position with crutches. Stand close to the client to support as needed.

4. Allows client to sit with feet on floor for stability.

5. Allows for stabilization of blood pressure, thus preventing orthostatic hypotension.

6. Increases client comprehension and cooperation.

7. Provides support; promotes client safety.

8. Standing for a few minutes will assist in preventing orthostatic hypotension.

### Four-Point Gait (Figure 38-64)

9. Position the crutches 4.5 to 6 inches to the side and in front of each foot. Move the right crutch forward 4 to 6 inches and move the left foot forward, even with the left crutch. Move the left crutch forward 4 to 6 inches and move the right foot forward, even with the right crutch. Repeat the four-point gait.

9. The four-point gait (used for partial or full weight bearing) provides greater stability. Weight bearing is on three points (two crutches and one foot or two feet and one crutch) at all times. The client must be able to bear weight with both legs.

*(continues)*

**PROCEDURE 38-10** (*continued*)

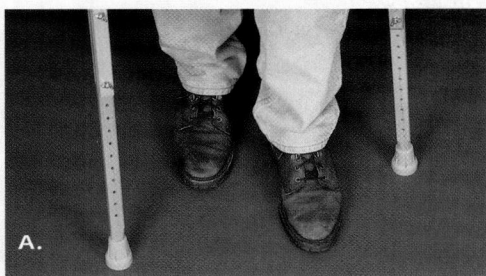
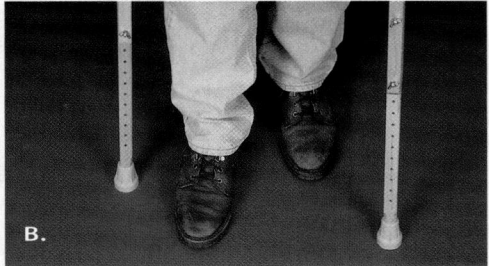

**Figure 38-64    Crutch walking, four-point gait: A. Moving right crutch forward and left foot forward B. Moving left crutch forward and right foot forward, even with right crutch**

### Three-Point Gait (Figure 38-65)

10. Advance both crutches and the weaker leg forward together 4 to 6 inches. Move the stronger leg forward, even with the crutches. Repeat the three-point gait.

### Two-Point Gait

11. Move the left crutch and right leg forward 4 to 6 inches. Move the right crutch and left leg forward 4 to 6 inches. Repeat the two-point gait.

### Swing-Through Gait (Figure 38-66)

12. Move both crutches forward together 4 to 6 inches. Move both legs forward together in a swinging motion, even with the crutches. Repeat the swing-through gait.

10. The three-point gait (used for partial or non-weight-bearing) provides a strong base of support. This gait can be used if the client has a weak or non-weight-bearing leg.

11. The two-point gait (used for partial weight bearing) provides a strong base of support. The client must be able to bear weight on both legs. This gait is faster than the four-point gait.

12. The swing-through gait (used for non-weight-bearing) permits a faster pace. This gait requires weight bearing on both legs, greater balance, and more strength.

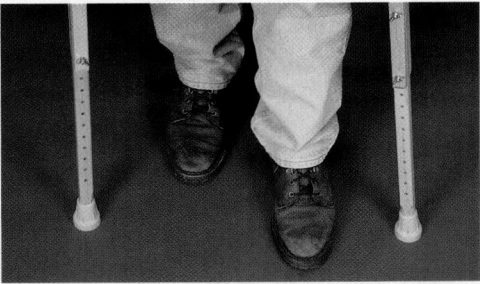

**Figure 38-65    Crutch walking, three-point gait: advancing both crutches and weaker leg forward together**

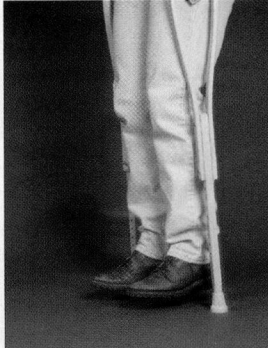

**Figure 38-66    Crutch walking; swing-through gait**

### Walking Up Stairs

13. Stand beside and slightly behind client. Instruct client to position the crutches as if walking. Place body weight on hands. Place the strong leg on the

13. Prevents weight bearing on the weaker leg.

*(continues)*

**PROCEDURE 38-10** (*continued*)

first step. Pull the weak leg up and move the crutches up to the first step. Repeat for all steps.

### Walking Down Stairs

14. Position the crutches as if walking. Place weight on the strong leg. Move the crutches down to the next lower step. Place partial weight on hands and crutches. Move the weak leg down to the step with the crutches. Put total weight on arms and crutches. Move strong leg to same step as weak leg and crutches. Repeat for all steps. A second caregiver standing behind the client holding on to the gait belt will further decrease the risk of falling.

15. Set realistic goals and opportunities for progressive ambulation using crutches.

16. Consult with a physical therapist for clients learning to walk with crutches.

17. Wash hands.

### Walking with a Cane

18. Inform client that you will be assisting with ambulation using a cane.

19. Lower the height of the bed.

20. Dangle the client at the side of bed for several minutes. Assess for vertigo.

21. Assess client for strength, mobility, range of motion, visual acuity, perceptual difficulties, and balance. *Note:* The nurse and physical therapist often collaborate on this assessment.

22. Apply the gait belt around the client's waist if balance and stability are unreliable.

23. Have the client hold the cane in the hand opposite the affected leg. Explain the safety and body mechanics underlying using the cane on the strong side.

24. Have the client push himself up from the sitting position while pushing down on the bed with his arms.

25. Have the client stand at the bedside for a few moments.

26. Assess the height of the cane. With the cane placed 6 inches ahead of the client's body, the top of the cane should be at wrist level with the arm bent 25% to 30% at the elbow.

14. Prevents weight bearing on the weaker leg.

15. Crutch walking takes up to 10 times the energy required for unassisted ambulation.

16. The physical therapist is the expert on the health care team for crutch-walking techniques.

17. Reduces transmission of microorganisms.

18. Reduces anxiety; helps increase comprehension and cooperation; promotes client autonomy.

19. Allows client to sit with feet on floor for stability.

20. Allows for stabilization of blood pressure, thus preventing orthostatic hypotension.

21. Helps determine the client's capabilities and amount of assistance required.

22. Provides support; promotes client safety.

23. Promotes safety and cooperation. Promotes client autonomy. By holding the cane on the stronger side the client has more control and strength for using it.

24. Increases upper body strength.

25. Allows the client to gain balance. The nurse can check for strength and balance.

26. A 25% to 30% bend at the elbow provides for better muscle strength and support than if the arm is straight.

(continues)

## PROCEDURE 38-10 (*continued*)

27. Walk to the side and slightly behind the client, holding the gait belt if needed for stability.

27. Allows the nurse to provide stability or assistance if the client needs it.

### The Cane Gait

28. Move the cane and the weaker leg forward at the same time for the same distance (Figure 38-67). Place weight on the weaker leg and the cane. Move the strong leg forward. Place weight on the strong leg.

28. The cane helps to provide a wide base of support for the body when the weight is on the weaker leg.

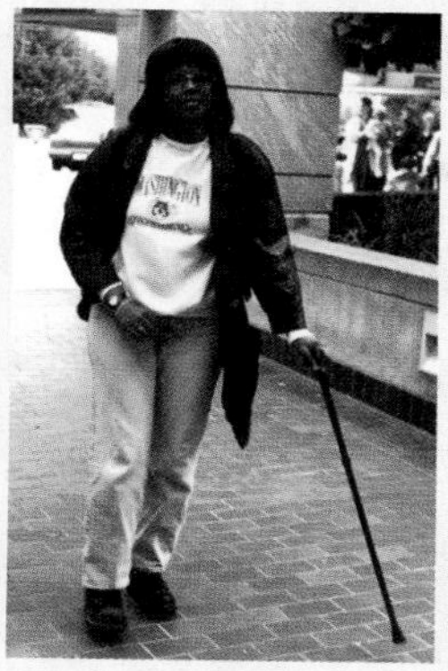

**Figure 38-67    Move the cane and the weaker leg forward.**

### Sitting with a Cane

29. Have client turn around and back up to the chair. Have her grasp the arm of the chair with the free hand and lower herself into the chair. Be sure to place the cane out of the way but within reach.

29. The cane provides additional support for the client as she lowers herself into the chair.

30. Set realistic goals and opportunities for progressive ambulation using a cane.

30. Walking with a cane takes practice.

31. Consult with a physical therapist for clients learning to walk with a cane.

31. The physical therapist is the expert on the health care team for cane-walking techniques.

32. Wash hands.

32. Reduces transmission of microorganisms.

### Walking with a Walker

33. Inform client that you will be assisting with ambulation using a walker.

33. Reduces anxiety; helps increase comprehension and cooperation; promotes client autonomy.

34. Lower the height of the bed.

34. Allows client to sit with feet on floor for stability.

35. Dangle the client at the side of bed for several minutes. Assess for vertigo.

35. Allows for stabilization of blood pressure, thus preventing orthostatic hypotension.

36. Provide a robe or other covering and shoes with firm, nonslip soles.

36. Provides for modesty and safety.

37. Assess client for strength, mobility, range of motion, visual acuity, perceptual difficulties,

37. Helps determine the client's capabilities and amount of assistance required.

*(continues)*

## PROCEDURE 38-10 (continued)

and balance. *Note:* The nurse and physical therapist often collaborate on this assessment.

38. Apply the gait belt around the client's waist if balance and stability are unreliable.

39. Place the walker in front of the client.

40. Have the client push himself up from the sitting
position while pushing down on the bed with
his arms.

41. Have the client transfer his hands to the walker
handgrips, one at a time.

42. Be sure the walker is adjusted so the handgrips are
just below waist level and the client's arms are
slightly bent at the elbow.

43. Walk to the side and slightly behind the client,
holding the gait belt if needed for stability.

### Walker Gait

44. Move the walker and the weaker leg forward at the
same time (Figure 38-68). Place as much weight as
possible or as allowed on the weaker leg, using the
arms for supporting the rest of the weight. Move
the strong leg forward and shift the weight to the
strong leg (Figure 38-69).

38. Provides support; promotes client safety.

39. Position the walker for use.

40. Increases upper body strength.

41. Allows the client to maintain balance while transferring his weight.

42. Provides maximum support from the arms while
ambulating.

43. Allows the nurse to provide stability or assistance
if the client needs it.

44. Provides support for a weak or non-weight-bearing leg by using arm and upper body strength.

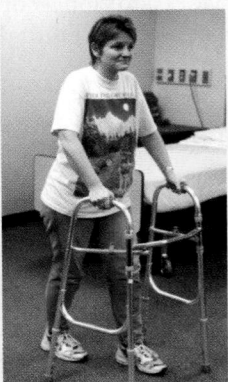

**Figure 38-68    Move the walker and the weaker
leg forward.**

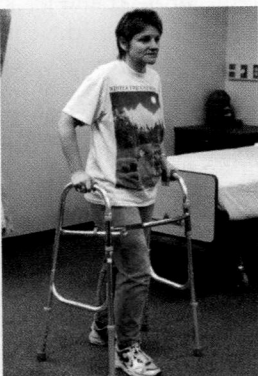

**Figure 38-69    Use the arms to support the rest
of the weight and move the strong leg forward.**

### Sitting with a Walker

45. Have the client turn around in front of the
chair and back up until the back of his legs
touch the chair. Have him place his hands on
the chair armrests, one hand at a time. He then
lowers himself into the chair using the armrests
for support.

45. Using the armrests of the chair is a more stable
support than using the walker.

*(continues)*

## PROCEDURE 38-10 (continued)

46. Set realistic goals and opportunities for progressive ambulation using a walker.

46. Walking with a walker takes practice.

47. Consult with a physical therapist for clients learning to walk with a walker.

47. The physical therapist is the expert on the health care team for walker techniques.

48. Wash hands.

48. Reduces transmission of microorganisms.

# LIFE SPAN CONSIDERATIONS

## Ambulation Aids

### Pediatric Variations

- Be sure to get the correct size device for a child. Children grow quickly and they will need to be assessed more often regarding the size of the device.

- If a child is very young, he may revert to crawling or creeping rather than try to use a device to assist with walking. Try to make using the device fun and a treat.

- Children may feel more comfortable with a walker they can "customize" with decals and decorations. Make sure these do not pose a safety hazard, however.

### Geriatric Variations

- Older clients may not have sufficient upper body strength to lift a walker prior to each step. They may need a rolling walker.

- If an older client tends to tire easily, walkers with fold-down seats built in are available so they can sit and rest whenever they need to.

- To foster independence, a basket or an apron with pockets on the front of a walker can help the client carry small items.

- Walkers outdoors pose special hazards to older clients. Wheels and tips can become stuck in the mud, grass, or cracks in the pavement.

# COMMUNITY/HOME CARE

## Ambulation Aids

### Home Care Variations

- Assess the home for narrow hallways, doorways, and steps. Advise the client regarding ways to negotiate narrow passages.

- Mark the front edge of steps with tape or paint so it is highly visible to clients walking with assistive devices.

- Advise clients to remove or fasten down throw rugs that might slide and cause the client to fall.

- Make sure handrails on stairs are securely fastened to the wall.

### Long-Term Care Variations

- Be sure to check the rubber tips on assistive devices for wear. With the rubber worn away, the client is at risk of slipping and falling.

- Clients who use an assistive device frequently may need hand protection such as gloves or padding on the handgrip.

## CLIENT EDUCATION

### Crutch Walking

#### Climbing Stairs

This method of climbing stairs provides a broad base of support and stability for the weaker leg:

✓ Climb stairs using the stronger leg first.
✓ Bring the crutches to the level of the stronger leg.
✓ Bring the weaker leg to the level of the crutches and the stronger leg.
✓ Repeat to climb stairs. *This requires time, balance, and strength.*

#### Descending Stairs

This method of descending stairs provides a broad base of support and stability for the weaker leg:

✓ Support the body with the stronger leg.
✓ Move the crutches down to the first descending step.
✓ Move the stronger leg to the first descending step.
✓ Repeat to descend the staircase. *This requires time, balance, and strength.*

#### Sitting in a Chair

The client has greater stability using the stronger leg and chair arm for support:

✓ Stand in front of a chair.
✓ Hold the crutches on the side with the weaker leg.
✓ Grasp the chair arm using the arm on the side of the stronger leg.
✓ Flex knees and hips to sit in chair.
✓ Reposition self in chair using arms and stronger leg while sitting.

#### Rising from the Chair

The client has greater strength using the stronger leg to rise. More stability is provided by the chair arm and crutches for support. Rising requires more strength than sitting:

✓ Move forward in chair, placing strongest leg on the floor.
✓ Grasp the chair arm on the same side of the stronger leg.
✓ Hold the crutches with the hand on the side of the weaker leg.
✓ Use the chair arm and crutches for support while rising.
✓ Once standing, place the crutches in the position for ambulation.
✓ Weak clients may need assistance. The gait belt is useful in such situations.

## RESEARCH FOCUS

**Title of Study:** Planning an osteoporosis education program for older adults in a residential setting.

**Study Purpose:** To develop and test an osteoporosis education program for older adults. The project was conducted to provide direction for developing a model program.

**Methods:** The study was conducted using a convenience sample of adults aged 65 and older living in a group residential setting. The pilot Osteoporosis Education Program (OEP) was advertised with mailed and posted flyers. A total of 26 residents participated in at least one session. The participants were tested for general knowledge of osteoporosis at the beginning of the program and at the end of the fourth session.

**Findings:** The OEP evaluation study suggests the use of the following in planning education for older adults:

- Sessions not to exceed 1 hour
- A minimum of four program sessions
- Use of prepared educational materials
- Use of an experiential activity (game) to reinforce learning
- Meeting time that does not conflict with other planned activities
- An informal teaching-learning environment

**Implications:** The pilot study provided direction for developing both the program format and content. The participants' interest in the program indicated that this type of intervention could be useful to help older adults, who are at greatest risk for osteoporosis, to adopt self-care behaviors. Such behaviors may help decrease the risk of fractures and help maintain the greatest possible level of independence.

Davis, G. C., & White, T. L. (2000). Planning an osteoporosis education program for older adults in a residential setting. *Journal of Gerontological Nursing*, 26(1), 16–23.

nervous system activity, improves cardiovascular functioning, and produces and maintains weight loss. "Increasing physical activity is beneficial for all ages and all groups" (Bray, 1998, p. 238). The nurse should identify activities enjoyed by the client and encourage increased participation. When planning an exercise program, the following elements should be considered:

- Health status (existing medical conditions)
- Physical condition
- Age
- Preferences for types of activities

# Complementary Treatment Modalities

Numerous complementary modalities help improve musculoskeletal health; see Box 38-3. Also, physical activity and relaxation exercises help reduce muscular tension and improve functional abilities.

# Evaluation

Family support for a client with activity or mobility deficits is a delicate balance between independence and dependence that is necessary for positive self-esteem and confidence. This healthy balance can be influenced by the client's family and friends. Healthy balance is fostered through support of the client as requested and needed, and through encouragement and positive acceptance and affection.

Family members are often unaware of the client's potential to improve. Thus, they give unnecessary assistance in activities and mobility rather than allow the client to function independently. The client then becomes resentful because there is a loss of self-control. Resentment can also occur with the family who has accepted the heavy responsibilities of caregiving.

For the client who overestimates her own cognitive and physical capabilities and energy level, safety becomes an important issue.

Actual long-term activity and mobility are the foci of evaluation as the client transfers skills and knowledge from the acute-care hospital or rehabilitation facility to home. Common areas of concern regarding activity include:

- Mobility status
- Activities of daily living capacity
- Use of appropriate adaptive devices
- Expansion of client activities
- Use of activities as a basis for building areas of competence and achievement

Measures of physical assessment, functional assessment, and performance of ADLs are used for follow-up evaluation of the client's status for activity and mobility.

## BOX 38-3   COMPLEMENTARY/ ALTERNATIVE THERAPY

- The herb *Ginkgo biloba* may be used to promote circulation (Eliopoulos, 1999).

- Yoga increases circulation as a result of postural changes on the endocrine glands and nerve plexus (Eliopoulos, 1999).

- Acupuncture is a traditional Chinese medicine (TCM) method of pain relief in which a qualified practitioner inserts needles in certain body sites to promote the release of endorphins (i.e., natural painkillers) (National Institute of Arthritis and Musculoskeletal and Skin Diseases, 1997).

- Acupressure is a technique similar to acupuncture; pressure instead of needles is applied to the acupuncture sites to relieve pain.

- Massage protects skin integrity by promoting circulation.

- Moist heat (warm towels, hot packs, bath/shower) promotes circulation.

- Cold (ice bag) helps reduce swelling.

- Transcutaneous electrical nerve stimulation (TENS) is used to decrease pain.

- Biofeedback is used to help clients decrease muscular tension.

Ongoing assessment of the client's activity and mobility is important because compliance with home exercise programs may lessen over time after discharge. When evaluating long-term activity and mobility goal achievement, the nurse should observe the client in the home setting to note the client's ability to function within her own environment.

 # CASE STUDY/NURSING CARE PLAN

Magda Constantin is a 15-year-old high school student who comes to your clinic for her regularly scheduled visit. She is recovering from a closed fracture of her right tibia suffered in a soccer game 4 weeks ago. She states that she is having trouble using crutches and getting around school, especially up and down the stairs. Upon questioning, she states that her arms are not strong enough to easily use the crutches. In addition, Magda is unhappy about not being able to play soccer and says, "People stare at me when I walk down the hall."

*(continues)*

# CASE STUDY/NURSING CARE PLAN (continued)

## Assessment

The client has a cast applied to her right leg and is walking with crutches. Her pedal pulses are strong and her right foot has good circulation, movement, and sensation. She states she is experiencing difficulty with ambulating up stairs on the crutches and that she is somewhat depressed. Her speech is soft, and she does not make eye contact well.

## Nursing Diagnosis

*Impaired Physical Mobility* related to inability to use legs normally and difficulty using crutches.
*Disturbed Body Image* related to change in lifestyle and appearance and fear of rejection by others.
**NOC:** Ambulation: Walking; Mobility Level; Self-Care: Activities of Daily Living; Joint Movement: Active
**NIC:**   Exercise Therapy; Ambulation; Exercise Therapy

## Expected Outcomes

The client will:
1. Understand and demonstrate proper crutch techniques (particularly on stairs) by end of her next clinic visit.
2. Verbalize persons with which she will discuss her feelings about her current condition by end of her next clinic visit.
3. State an increased positive self-image and acceptance of her temporary condition by her second clinic visit.

## Planning/Interventions/Rationales

1. Measure crutch height and fit for client. *Determines proper fit, which will relieve pressure, if any, and facilitate ambulation.*
2. Watch client as she walks across the room using the crutches. *Provides baseline assessment of crutch-walking skills.*
3. Demonstrate correct mechanics of crutch walking using three-point gait. *Allows for partial or non-weight-bearing ambulation.*
4. Ask client to return demonstrate crutch-walking technique. *Demonstrates client's understanding and ability to execute technique.*
5. Suggest ways that crutch walking can be facilitated, such as wearing soft-soled flat shoes, carrying a backpack strapped over both shoulders, wearing nonbulky shirts to minimize clothing under arms, and taking frequent rest stops while walking. *Tips on facilitating crutch gait will remove barriers to effective walking and increase client comfort and confidence in technique.*
6. Help client understand that cast and crutches are a temporary measure to promote proper healing and are not a reflection of overall body health. *Client should learn to view situation as temporary and keep in mind that the broken leg is only one part of the whole person and need not detract from other positive qualities.*

## Evaluation

Magda successfully demonstrates correct crutch-walking technique and decides to purchase a backpack to replace her shoulder bag. She is still somewhat shy about "people staring at me" but seems to be starting to accept the fact that the cast and crutches are temporary. She even jokes that "maybe this is an easy way to get noticed at school."

## Key Concepts

- There are many benefits to proper body alignment and applying effective body mechanics.
- The physiology of mobility primarily involves the musculoskeletal system and the nervous system.
- Clients should recognize several types of exercise that promote both physiological and psychological health.
- The nurse must be knowledgeable about the developmental considerations in understanding the factors that affect mobility.

- Many physiological effects of mobility and immobility affect multiple body systems (e.g., cardiovascular, respiratory, musculoskeletal).
- The nurse must assess the client on an ongoing basis for activity and mobility during acute hospitalization, rehabilitation, and postdischarge.
- Collaboration between client, family, and members of the interdisciplinary health care team is essential for establishing and modifying goals for activity and mobility.

- Nursing interventions are individualized to maximize activity, mobility, and independence for the client and family.
- The nurse should be aware of the home environment and lifestyle of the client as related to immobility issues.
- The family or caregivers should be included in educational sessions regarding activity and mobility. Practice sessions of activities and mobility by client, family, and caregivers under the direction of the nurse are essential.
- The need for adaptive equipment should be assessed and acquisition of equipment facilitated.
- The client, family, and caregiver should be provided instructions in many forms regarding immobility: demonstrations, videos, pamphlets, and handouts.
- The client and family should be informed of community resources to maximize activity, mobility, and independence.

## Review Questions and Activities

1. What various types of exercise promote physiological and psychological health? How do they benefit the client?

2. What factors would help the client ambulate independently 20 feet with the use of a walker within 2 days? What factors would hinder the client?

3. Think about persons of various age groups functioning normally in activities. Note the difference in the stages of growth and development.

4. Assess clients of various ages within the acute-care hospital setting. What are the alterations of activity and mobility of these clients as compared with normal expectations?

5. What are the negative outcomes of immobility, and what are the effects of immobility on the different body systems?

6. Evaluate your mobility and lifting habits. Do you have a backache or feel strained after work?

7. What equipment is available in your clinical setting to promote safe body mechanics?

## Multimedia Links

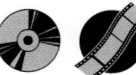

Altman *Basic Care DVD: Proper Body Mechanics and Safe Lifting/Transferring*
Altman *Basic Care DVD: Assisting with Ambulation and Safe Falling*
Altman *Basic Care DVD: Applying Restraints*
Altman *Basic Care DVD: Turning and Positioning a Client*
Altman *Basic Care DVD: Moving a Client in Bed*
Altman *Basic Care DVD: Assisting from Bed to Stretcher*
Altman *Basic Care DVD: Assisting from Bed to Wheelchair, Commode, or Chair*
Altman *Basic Care DVD: Assisting from Bed to Walking*
Altman *Basic Care DVD: Using a Hydraulic Lift*
Altman *Basic Care DVD: Administering Passive Range-of-Motion (ROM) Exercises*
Altman *Basic Care II Video: Bed Making*
Altman *Basic Care IV Video: Aiding Client Movement*
Altman *Basic Care V Video: Aiding Client Movement*

## Web Resources

American Association of Spinal Cord Injury Nurses
  http://www.aascin.org
Falls and Mobility
  http://www.sunnybrook.utoronto.ca:8080
National Easter Seal Society, Inc.
  http://www.easter-seals.org
National Institute of Arthritis and Musculoskeletal and Skin Diseases, National Institutes of Health
  http://www.niams.nih.gov
National Institutes of Health
  http://www.nih.gov
National Stroke Association
  http://www.stroke.org
Occupational Safety and Health Administration, U.S. Department of Labor
  http://www.osha.gov

## References

Altman, G. B. (2004). Using a hydraulic lift. In G. B., Altman (Ed.), *Delmar's fundamental and advanced nursing skills* (2nd ed.). Clifton Park, NY: Delmar Learning.

Bonder, B. R., & Wagner, M. B. (2001). Functional performance in older adults (2nd ed.). Philadelphia: F. A. Davis Co.

Brians, L. K., Alexander, K., Grota, P., Chen, R. W. H., & Dumas, V. (1991). The development of the RISK tool for fall prevention. *Rehabilitation Nursing, 16*(2), 67–69.

Bray, G. A. (1998). *Contemporary diagnosis and management of obesity.* Newtown, PA: Handbooks in Health Care Co.

Centers for Disease Control & Prevention. (1999). *A report of the Surgeon General: Physical activity and health.* http://www.cdc.gov/sgr/ ataglan.html

Covington, C., Cybulski, M., Davis, T., Duca, G., Farrel, E., Kasgorgis, M., Kator, C., & Sell, T. (2001). Kids on the move: Preventing obesity among urban children. *American Journal of Nursing, 101*(3), 73–75, 77, 79, 81–82.

Davis, G. D., & White, T. L. (2000). Planning an osteoporosis education program for older adults in a residential setting. *Journal of Gerontological Nursing, 26*(1), 16–23.

Davison, M. A. (1998). Antipsychotic medications. In M. E. Kuhn (Ed.), *Pharmacotherapeutics: A nursing process approach* (4th ed., pp. 388–399). Philadelphia: F. A. Davis.

Derstine, J. B., & Hargrove, S. D. (2001). *Comprehensive rehabilitation nursing.* Philadelphia: Saunders.

Edelman, C., & Mandle, C. (2002). *Health promotion throughout the life span* (5th ed.). St. Louis: Mosby.

Eliopoulos, C. (1999). *Manual of gerontologic nursing* (2nd ed.). St. Louis: Mosby.

Estes, M. E. Z. (2002). *Health assessment & physical examination* (2nd ed.). Clifton Park, NY: Delmar Learning.

Feder, G., Cryer, C., Donovan, S., & Carter, Y. (2000). Guidelines for the prevention of falls in people over 65. The Guidelines' Development Group. *British Medical Journal, 321*(1007).

Fleming, J. M. (2001) Successful aging. In M. O. Hogstel (Ed.), *Gerontology: Nursing care of the older adult* (p. 145). Clifton Park, NY: Delmar Learning.

Fontaine, K. L. (2000). *Healing practices: Alternative therapies for nursing.* Upper Saddle River, NJ: Prentice Hall.

Gillespie, L. D., Gillespie, W. J., & Cumming, R. (2000). Interventions for preventing falls in the elderly. *Cochrane Database of Systematic Reviews,* CD000340.

Guin, P. R. (2001). Advances in spinal cord injury care. *Critical Care Nursing Clinics of North America, 13*(3), 399–409.

Hogstel, M. (2001). *Gerontology: Nursing care of the older adult.* Clifton Park, NY: Delmar Learning.

Huston, C. J. (1998). Cervical spine injury. *American Journal of Nursing, 98*(6), 33.

Lamb, K. V. D., & Cummings, M. (2000). Musculoskeletal function. In A. G. Lueckenotte (Ed.), *Gerontologic nursing* (2nd ed.). St. Louis: Mosby.

McKenna, S., Wallis, M., Brannelly, A., Cawood, J. (2001). The nursing management of diarrhea and constipation before and after the implementation of a bowel management protocol. *Australian Critical Care, 14*(1), 10–16.

National Institute of Arthritis and Musculoskeletal and Skin Diseases (1997). *Questions and answers about arthritis and exercise.* http://www.niams.nih.gov/hi/topics/arthritis/arthexfs.htm

North American Nursing Diagnosis Association (2003). *Nursing diagnoses: Diagnoses and classification: 2003–2004.* Philadelphia: Author.

Occupational Safety and Health Administration (OSHA). (2000)....title...[On-line]. Retrieved from http://www.osha-slc.gov/ ergonomics-standard.html#Q1

O'Hanlon-Nichols, T. (1998). A review of the adult musculoskeletal system. *American Journal of Nursing, 98*(6), 48–52.

Owen, B. D. (1999). Preventing back injuries. *American Journal of Nursing, 99*(5), 76.

Palmer, M. H. (2002). Urinary incontinence in nursing homes. *Journal of WOCN, 29*(1), 4–5.

Pender, J., Murdaugh, C., & Parsons, M. A. (2002). *Health promotion in nursing practice* (4th ed.). Upper Saddle River, NJ: Prentice-Hall.

Salkeld, G., Cameron, I. D., & Cumming, R. G. (2000). Quality of life related to fear of falling and hip fracture in older women: A time trade-off study. *British Medical Journal, 320*(341).

White, L., & Duncan, G. (2002). *Medical-surgical nursing: An integrated approach* (2nd ed.). Clifton Park, NY: Delmar Learning.

World Health Organization (2002). *World health report 2002: Reducing risks, promoting healthy lifestyles.* Geneva, Switzerland.

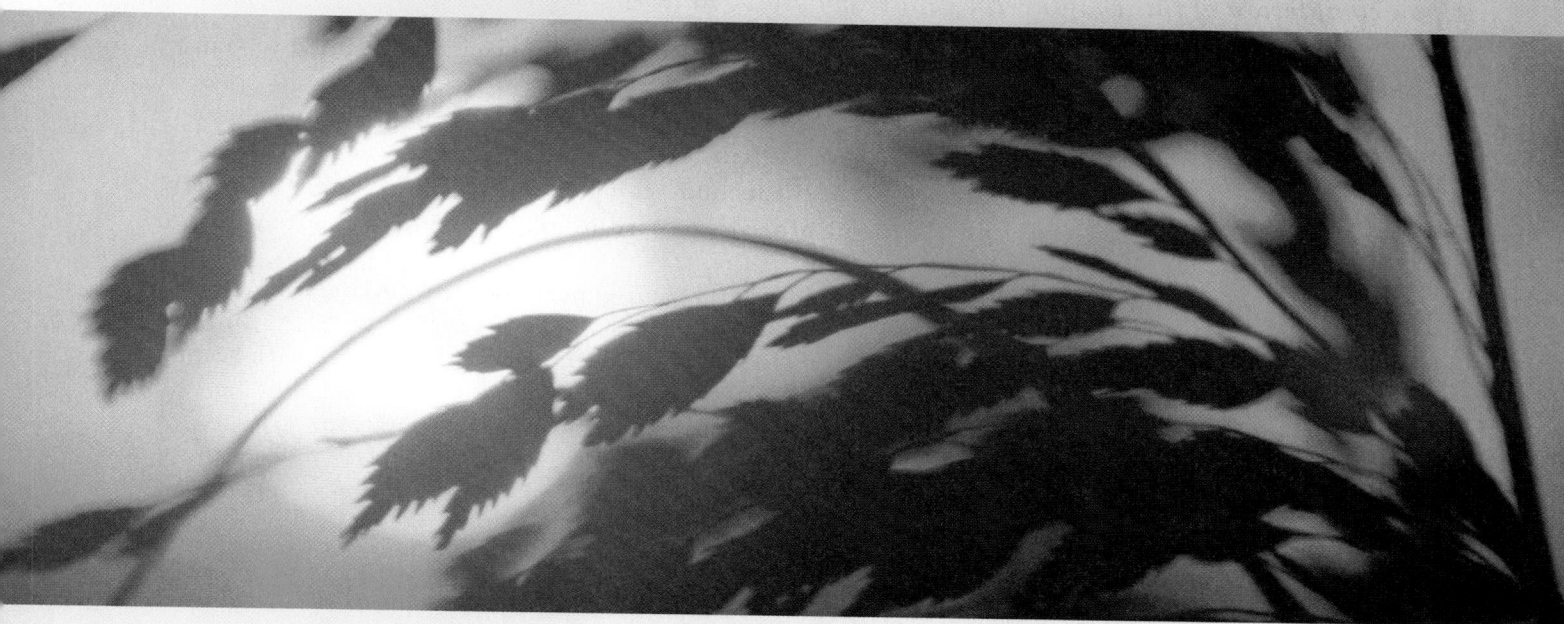

# CHAPTER 39

# Oxygenation

Ruth N. Grendell, DNSc, RN

*"The first canon of nursing . . . [and] the first essential to the patient . . . is this:* to keep the air he breathes as pure as the external air without chilling him. *Without cleanliness, within and without your house, ventilation is comparatively useless."*

(Florence Nightingale, 1860)

# Chapter Competencies

**Upon completion of this chapter, the reader should be able to:**

1. Describe the basic normal anatomical structures and physiological mechanisms related to ventilation, gas exchange, circulation (perfusion), and cellular respiration.
2. Discuss common developmental, social, and environmental factors affecting oxygenation function.
3. Identify essential information required for assessment of normal respiratory status.
4. Describe essential information for assessment of clients undergoing treatment of respiratory disorders.
5. Describe basic diagnostic tests and treatment procedures used in management of clients with respiratory dysfunction.
6. Describe primary and secondary nursing diagnoses and their expected client outcomes commonly used for clients during treatment of respiratory disorders.
7. Describe and provide rationales for commonly used nursing interventions for clients with respiratory disorders.
8. Discuss components of teaching self-care strategies to promote optimal oxygenation.

# Key Terms

aerobic metabolism
anaerobic metabolism
anemia
angina pectoris
atelectasis
atherosclerosis
autoregulation
cardiac conduction system
cardiac cycle
cardiac output
cardiopulmonary resuscitation (CPR)
chest physiotherapy (CPT)
chronic obstructive pulmonary disease (COPD)
cyanosis

deadspace
diastole
diffusion defect
external respiration
gallop
heart failure
Heimlich maneuver
hypercapnia
hypoxemia
hypoxia
infarction
intermittent claudication
internal respiration
ischemia
murmur
obstructive pulmonary disease

oxygen uptake
oxyhemoglobin dissociation curve
paroxysmal nocturnal dyspnea
postural drainage
precapillary sphincters
restrictive pulmonary disease
shunting
surfactant
systole
tachypnea
tracheotomy
ventilation
ventilation-perfusion (V/Q) mismatching
work of breathing

Normally a person is unaware of breathing processes, a physiological function that is essential to life itself. However, it is quickly recognized that even a slight disturbance of the respiratory system causes both psychological and physiological responses. Fear and anxiety are common reactions to difficult breathing, and the body attempts to gain control of its breathing. Several automatic, protective physiological responses are also in place to increase air conduction and to protect the airways from inhaled irritants and excess mucus when needed. Systemic mechanisms ensure gas exchange and circulation throughout the body.

Respiratory dysfunctions range from mild conditions such as colds, to life-threatening occurrences that include asthma, certain pneumonias, and chest trauma. The dysfunctions can be acute (short term) or chronic (long term) in nature. Impaired respiratory functions have many causes, including infection, inflammation, allergens, environmental factors, exposure to tobacco smoke, chest trauma, pulmonary vascular abnormalities, cardiovascular and neuromuscular disorders, chest abnormalities, and genetic and age-specific factors.

"Any compromise of oxygenation can be serious. Nurses can prevent some oxygenation problems and teach patients/clients how to prevent others" (Archibald, 1999, p. 1000). Respiratory function is complex and requires a comprehensive understanding of anatomy and physiology as the foundation for understanding nursing care management of persons with respiratory disorders. This chapter explores the elements of the oxygenation process, the common mechanisms that contribute to malfunction, and the interventions that are used to promote optimal respiratory function.

## Physiology of Oxygenation

The delivery of oxygen to the body's cells is a process that depends upon the interplay of the pulmonary, hematologic, and cardiovascular systems. Specifically, the processes involved include ventilation, alveolar gas exchange, oxygen transport and delivery, and cellular respiration. The basic anatomy of the lungs is shown in Figure 39-1. A summary of anatomy and physiology related to oxygenation and its functions and alterations is presented in Table 39-1.

### Ventilation

The first step in the process of oxygenation is **ventilation**, which is the movement of air into and out of the lungs for the purpose of delivering fresh air into the lung's alveoli (Figure 39-2). Ventilation is regulated by respiratory control centers in the pons and medulla oblongata, which are located in the brain stem. The rate and depth of ventilation are constantly adjusted in response to changes in the concentrations of hydrogen ion (pH) and carbon dioxide ($CO_2$) in the body's fluids. For instance, an increase in carbon dioxide in the blood or a decrease in pH in the body's fluids will stimulate faster and deeper ventilation. A decrease in blood oxygen concentration (**hypoxemia**) will also stimulate ventilation, but to a lesser degree.

Inhalation of air is initiated when the diaphragm contracts, pulling it downward and thus increasing the size of the intrathoracic space (Figure 39-3). This space is also increased by contraction of the external intercostal muscles, which elevate and separate the ribs and move the sternum forward. The effect of increasing the space inside the thorax is to decrease the intrathoracic pressure, so that air will be drawn in from the atmosphere. Stretch receptors in the lung tissue send signals back to the brain to cause cessation of inhalation, preventing overdistension of the lungs. Exhalation occurs when the respiratory muscles relax, thus reducing the size of the intrathoracic space, increasing the intrathoracic pressure, and forcing air to exit the lungs. Under normal conditions, exhalation is a passive process.

When the movement of air is impeded, additional muscles may be used to increase the ventilatory ability. These accessory muscles of ventilation include the sternocleidomastoid muscle, the abdominal muscles, and the internal intercostal muscles. In some disease states, exhalation is impaired, requiring that the individual actively force air out of the lungs rather than passively exhaling. Forced expiration is aided by the intercostal muscles and the abdominal recti. When additional muscular force is required for breathing, the **work of breathing** is said to be increased.

Several mechanisms exist to keep the airways clear of microorganisms and debris. As air is inhaled through the nose, the larger particles are filtered out through hairs lining the nasal passages. The mucous membranes of the nasopharynx and sinuses warm and humidify the inspired air, and the film of mucus lining these membranes traps smaller particles. Closure of the glottis protects the airway from aspiration of food and fluids during swallowing. In the trachea and larger bronchi, tiny hairlike cilia continually produce wavelike movements to propel mucus and particles upward, where they can be coughed out. If any invaders manage to reach the alveoli, specialized alveolar macrophages will engulf and destroy the offending organism. Disease processes can interfere with any of these protective mechanisms, increasing the individual's vulnerability to infection and injury (Carroll, 2001).

### Alveolar Gas Exchange

The major functions of the upper airway include (1) air conduction to the lower airway for gas exchange; (2) protection of the lower airway from foreign matter; and (3) warming, filtration, and humidification of inspired air (Cronin & Mirocle, 2001). Once fresh air reaches the lung's alveoli, the next step in the process of oxygenation begins. The exchange of oxygen from the alveolar space into the pulmonary capillary blood is referred to as **oxygen uptake**; it may also be called **external respiration**.

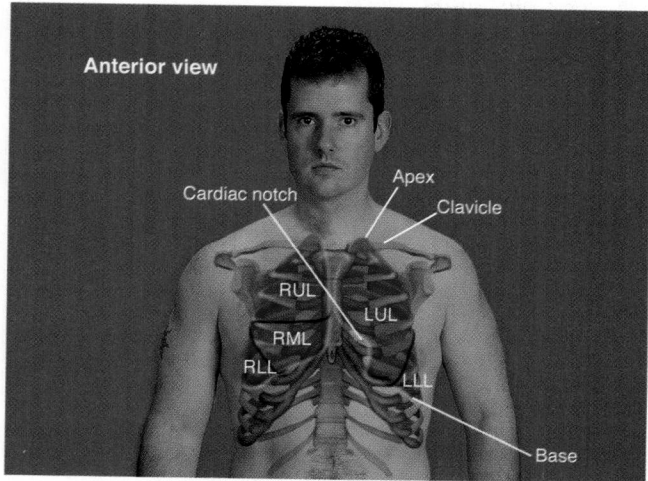

**Figure 39-1    Lungs: RUL = right upper lobe, RML = right middle lobe, RLL = right lower lobe, LUL = left upper lobe, LLL = left lower lobe**

## TABLE 39-1    OVERVIEW OF OXYGENATION PROCESS: ANATOMICAL STRUCTURES, FUNCTIONS, AND ALTERATIONS

| Ventilation Process | Functions | Examples of Alterations/Barriers |
| --- | --- | --- |
| **Ventilation Process** | | |
| *Upper Airways* | | |
| • Nasal cavity and nasal pharynx | • Passageways for inspiration and expiration<br>• Filter microorganisms and debris<br>• Warm and humidify air | • Anatomical defects that impede ventilation (deviated nasal septum, polyps; infections, edema, excess secretions; shallow breathing). |
| • Pharynx | • Passage for both air and food | • Potential for choking/aspirating on food particles. |
| • Glottis | • Closure protects airway from aspiration and foods and solids | • Aspiration most often in right bronchus due to short, straight structure. |
| *Lower Airways* | | |
| • Thoracic cage | • Protect chest contents. External and intercostals muscles elevate and separate ribs, move sternum forward to increase thoracic space | • Anatomical defects inhibit full expansion (barrel chest, diminished alveoli, traumatic injury—may cause atelectasis and shifting of chest contents). Obstructive and restrictive lung diseases, edema. Acute pulmonary failure. |
| • Trachea | • Continue to warm, humidify, and filter inspired air. Wavelike movements of cilia propel mucus and particles into trachea to be swallowed or expectorated. | • Infections, trauma, obstruction of trachea. |
| • Lung tissues | • Right lung = 3 lobes; left lung = 2 lobes. Houses bronchial tree, alveoli, capillary bed for gas exchange. | • Infections, pneumonia, tumors, asthma, obstructive and restrictive lung diseases (see above alterations). |
| • Cough reflex | • Forced expiration of aspirated particles, allergens or foreign objects. | • Loss of cough reflex. Damage to diaphragm, abdominal muscles, or intercostals muscles. |
| • Alveoli | • Capillary network for gas exchange. Immune system cells in alveoli areas (Macrophages destroy microorganisms.) | • Thickened capillary membrane inhibits gas exchange. Immune system compromised (due to changes related to immaturity, age, or disease). |
| • Diaphragm | • Changes size of thoracic space by expanding downward and constricting upward during respiration. | • Obesity, distended abdomen, pregnancy can interfere with diaphragm movement. |
| • Stress receptors (lung) | • Send message to brain to halt inhalation—prevent overexpansion of lung. | • Loss of lung tissue flexibility. Obstructive and restrictive disease. |
| • Pleura | • Help hold lungs in expanded condition. Allow lungs to follow movement of thorax. | • Puncture injury of pleura, infection, excess fluid in pleural space, cancer infiltration. |

*(continues)*

## TABLE 39-1    OVERVIEW OF OXYGENATION PROCESS: ANATOMICAL STRUCTURES, FUNCTIONS, AND ALTERATIONS (*continued*)

| Ventilation Process | Functions | Examples of Alterations/Barriers |
|---|---|---|
| **Gas Exchange** | | |
| • Alveoli space and capillary network | • Large expanse of thin membrane that permits exchange of air from higher pressure area to lower pressure area, and $CO_2$ from blood to alveolar space (external respiration). | • Thickened membrane and less gas exchange. Diseases causing air trapping (COPD). |
| • Blood plasma | • Hemoglobin molecules accept and release oxygen where needed. | • Anemia—low hemoglobin levels, degree of hemoglobin affinity for $O_2$, acidosis, hypoxia, hyperthermia. |
| • Peripheral capillary beds | • Portion of $O_2$ dissolved in plasma released to cells. This is dependent upon amount of dissolves $O_2$ ($PaO_2$) plasma and amount of hemoglobin available and tendency to bind with $O_2$ ($SaO_2$) | • Cell/tissue damage, ischemia, blood vessel damage. |
| **Perfusion/Circulation of Oxygen** | | |
| • Heart | • Cyclic filling (diastole) and emptying (systole) of atria and ventricles transports blood throughout the body. | • Heart failure (CHF), hemorrhage, anemia, sepsis, poisons (carbon monoxide and cyanide) impede blood flow. |
| • Blood vessels | • Arteries carry oxygenated blood to organs and tissues (priority is area of greatest need—auto-regulation). Vena cavae return unoxygenated blood to heart. | • Atherosclerosis, plaque deposits in vessel lumen, blood pressure changes. |
| • Cellular respiration | • Diffusion of $O_2$ from blood to tissues and $CO_2$ from tissues to blood (internal respiration). Some cells are capable of extracting additional $O_2$ from plasma when needed. | • Damage of cells—especially mitochondria by poisoning, sepsis, or low concentrations of $O_2$ in plasma. |
| • Anaerobic metabolism | • Use of glucose for cellular energy through changes in metabolic pathways. | • Can lead to metabolic acidosis. |
| **Neurologic Control** | | |
| • Respiratory centers in medulla and pons and at blood/brain barrier | • Receptors respond to $O_2$, $CO_2$, and pH serum levels and assist in changes as needed. | • Damage to respiratory centers in brain and or peripheral blood vessels; hypoxia changes, decreased perfusion; ischemia. |
| **Peripheral Control** | | |
| • Receptors in carotid arteries and aortic arch | • (See above.) Reciprocal interchange with neurologic control centers. | |

Adapted from Archibald, C. (1999). Oxygenation. In K. Berger & M. Williams (Eds.), *Fundamentals of nursing* (pp. 999–1086). Stamford, CT: Appleton & Lange; Clark A. (2002). Legal lessons: "But his $O_2$ Sat was normal!" *Clinical Nurse Specialist, 16*(3), 162–163; Carroll, R. (2001). Anatomy and physiology of the heart. In J. Black, J. Hawks, & A. Keene (Eds.), *Medical-surgical nursing: Clinical management for continuity of care.* Philadelphia: W. B. Saunders; Cronin, R., & Mirocle, K. (2001). Management of clients with lower airway and pulmonary vessels disorders. In J. Black, J. Hawks, & A. Keene (Eds.), *Medical-surgical nursing: Clinical management for continuity of care.* Philadelphia: W. B. Saunders; Stacy, K. (2000). Pulmonary disorders. In L. Urden & K. Stacy (Eds.), *Priorities in critical care nursing.* St. Louis: Mosby.

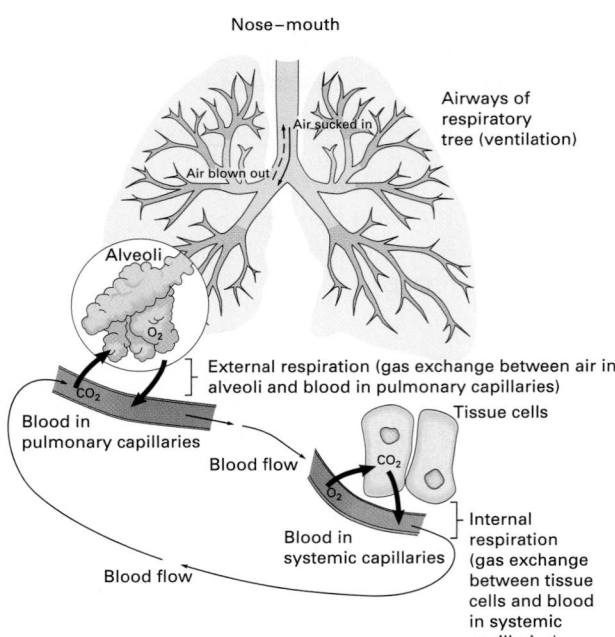

**Figure 39-2    Elements of oxygenation of the pulmonary and hematologic systems**

Oxygen diffuses across the alveolar membrane in response to a concentration gradient; that is, it moves from an area of higher concentration (the alveoli) to an area of lower concentration (the pulmonary capillary blood), seeking equilibrium. At the same time, carbon dioxide diffuses from the blood to the alveolar space, also in response to a concentration gradient (Figure 39-4) (Cronin & Mirocle, 2001; Stacy, 2000).

## Oxygen Transport and Delivery

### Oxygen Transport in the Blood

Once the diffusion of oxygen across the alveolar-capillary membrane occurs, the oxygen molecules are dissolved in the blood plasma. Three factors influence the capacity of the blood to carry oxygen: the amount of dissolved oxygen in the plasma, the amount of hemoglobin, and the tendency of the hemoglobin to bind with oxygen. However, the plasma is not able to carry nearly enough dissolved oxygen to meet the metabolic needs of the body. The oxygen-carrying capacity of the blood is greatly enhanced by the presence of hemoglobin in the erythrocytes.

The amount of oxygen carried in a sample of blood is measured in two ways. Oxygen dissolved in plasma is expressed as the partial pressure of oxygen ($PaO_2$). The normal $PaO_2$ in arterial blood is about 80–100 mm Hg. The oxygen dissolved in plasma, however, represents only about 1% to 5% of the total oxygen content of the blood. The vast majority of oxygen in the blood is carried bound to the hemoglobin molecule. The amount of oxygen bound to hemoglobin is expressed as the percentage of hemoglobin that is saturated with oxygen ($SaO_2$), with 100% being fully saturated. Since the $SaO_2$ is a percentage indicating the relationship between oxygen and hemoglobin, the nurse should interpret the client's $SaO_2$ measurement with the hemoglobin level. Normal saturation of arterial blood ($SaO_2$) is about 96% to 98% (Harrah, 1998).

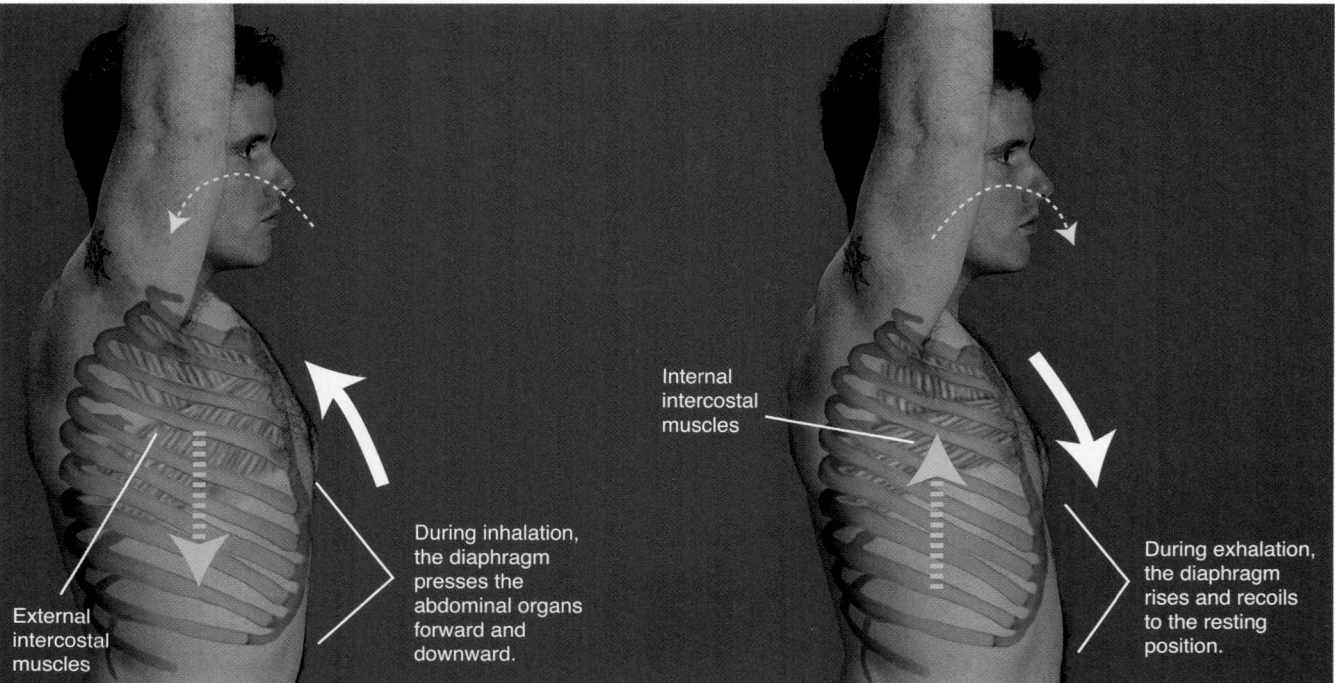

**Figure 39-3    Mechanics of breathing: Inhalation increases the volume of the thorax by diaphragmatic excursion and elevation of the sternum; exhalation is normally accomplished by passive elastic recoil.**

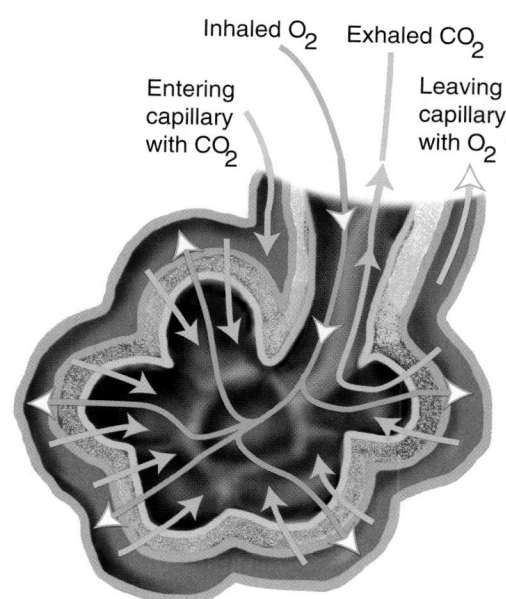

**Figure 39-4    Alveolar gas exchange**

Hemoglobin molecules have the ability to form a reversible bond with oxygen molecules. Thus, the hemoglobin readily takes up oxygen in the lungs, while it also readily releases oxygen to the body's cells in the systemic capillary beds. This seemingly paradoxical shift in hemoglobin's affinity for oxygen is represented by the **oxyhemoglobin dissociation curve**, which is a graphic representation of the relationship between the partial pressure of oxygen and oxygen saturation.

The affinity of hemoglobin for oxygen is highest when the $PaO_2$ (the measure of oxygen dissolved in the arterial blood plasma) is 70 mm Hg or higher; in this portion of the curve, further increases in $PaO_2$ result in very little change in $SaO_2$ (Figure 39-5A). This characteristic of the oxyhemoglobin dissociation curve accounts for the rapid

uptake of oxygen by hemoglobin in the pulmonary circulation and allows for some decrease in $PaO_2$ (such as might occur with disease or in high altitudes) without significantly sacrificing $SaO_2$.

As the oxygen-saturated blood is circulated to the peripheral capillary beds, dissolved oxygen diffuses out of blood. This decrease in dissolved oxygen causes hemoglobin to lose its affinity for oxygen, so the oxygen is then released to the body's cells. Once the partial pressure of oxygen in the blood drops below 60 mm Hg, hemoglobin releases oxygen very easily. This release is represented in the lower left portion of the curve, also known as the venous portion, and permits rapid unloading of oxygen to the cells (Figure 39-5B).

Several physiological factors may alter the affinity of hemoglobin for oxygen, and these shifts can be represented on the oxyhemoglobin dissociation curve. A shift to the left occurs when affinity is increased so that for a given $PaO_2$, the associated $SaO_2$ will be higher. This means that although the arterial blood may be carrying adequate oxygen, little of it is being released to the tissues. A shift to the left may be caused by increased pH (alkalosis), hypothermia, or a decrease in the red blood cell enzyme 2,3-diphosphoglycerate (2,3-DPG), which may occur after massive transfusions of banked blood.

A shift to the right of the oxyhemoglobin dissociation curve means that for a given $PaO_2$, the $SaO_2$ will be lower. This phenomenon represents a decreased affinity of hemoglobin for oxygen so that oxygen is more readily released to the tissues. This shift occurs in response to acidosis, hyperthermia, and hypoxia (which induces increased production of 2,3-DPG) and results in improved delivery of oxygen to the tissues (Stacy, 2000).

## Circulation/Perfusion

Once oxygen is bound to hemoglobin, the oxygen is delivered to the cells of the body by the process of circulation. The function of the heart is to pump oxygenated blood

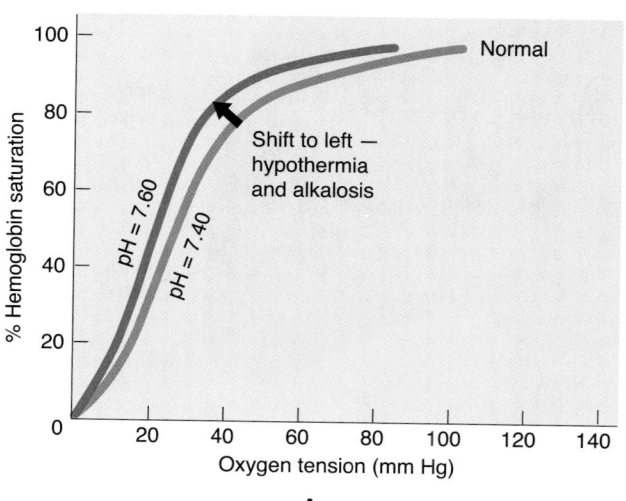

A.

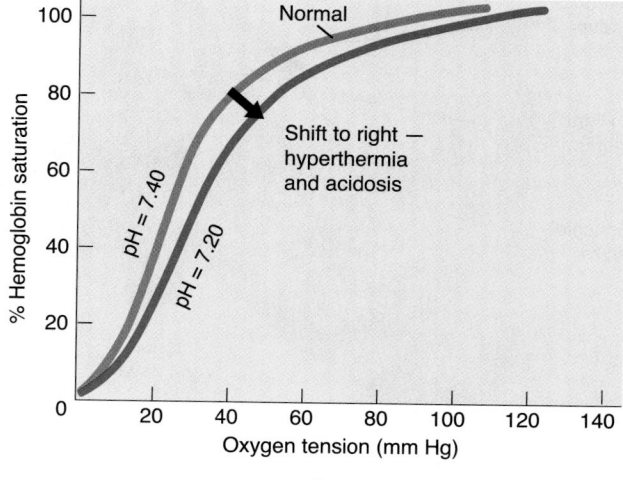

B.

**Figure 39-5    Oxyhemoglobin dissociation curve: A. Effect of increase in pH  B. Effect of decrease in pH**

into the arterial system, which carries it to the cells, and to collect deoxygenated blood from the venous system.

The heart is a muscular pump that is divided into four chambers: the right and left atria (blood-collecting chambers) and the right and left ventricles (the pumping chambers). A series of valves allows for unidirectional blood flow through the four chambers, which is controlled by the sequential relaxation and contraction of the heart muscle. The right and left sides of the heart are separated by the septum, a muscular wall. The heart is actually comprised of two pumps that work in unison (Figure 39-6).

A single cycle of atrial and ventricular contraction and relaxation is referred to as a **cardiac cycle**, which is the product of the interplay of electrical and mechanical events. The electrical activity of the heart involves the generation and transmission of electrical current by specialized cardiac cells known as the **cardiac conduction system** (Figure 39-7). A small mass of cells in the right atrium, the *sinoatrial node,* or *SA node,* normally controls the heart rate by rhythmically generating electrical impulses. For this reason, the SA node is often referred to as the heart's "pacemaker." The impulses created by the SA node travel along specialized internodal pathways to spread throughout the atria, resulting in mechanical muscular contraction. The electrical activity is then transmitted

down to the ventricles via the *atrioventricular (AV) node* and spreads through the ventricular tissue along the *bundle of His, right and left bundle branches,* and *Purkinje fibers.* Again, the result is muscular contraction. The sequential contraction and relaxation of the atria and ventricles is an essential factor in the cyclical filling and emptying of the chambers, which produce circulation.

The time period from the beginning of one heartbeat to the beginning of the next beat is the cardiac cycle. The process of chamber filling is referred to as **diastole** as the right and left atria relax. Deoxygenated blood flows from the systemic circulation through the inferior and superior venae cavae into the right atrium. At the same time, oxygenated blood flows from the pulmonary capillary bed via the four pulmonary veins into the left atrium. **Systole** is the process of chamber emptying. As pressure rises in the atria, the right triscuspid and left mitral atrioventricular valves open, thus permitting the blood to begin flowing into the ventricles. Ventricular filling is further augmented by contraction of the atrial muscle (atrial systole), sometimes referred to as "atrial kick."

Filling of the ventricles causes the intraventricular pressure to rise. When this pressure exceeds the pressure in the atria, the tricuspid and mitral valves close. (This prevents blood flowing back into the atria during ventricular emptying.) The ventricular muscle then begins to

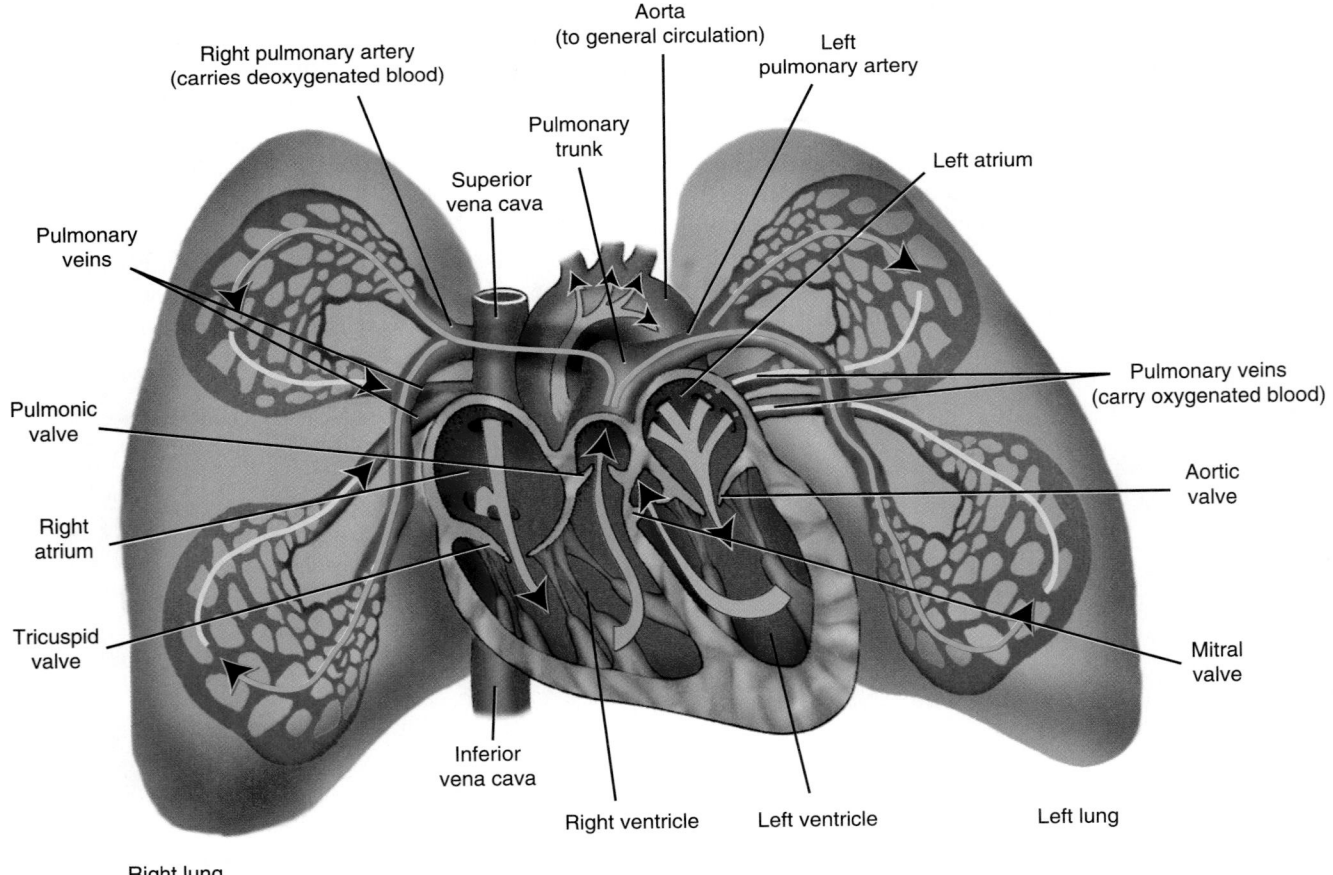

**Figure 39-6    Major structures of the heart and pulmonary circulation**

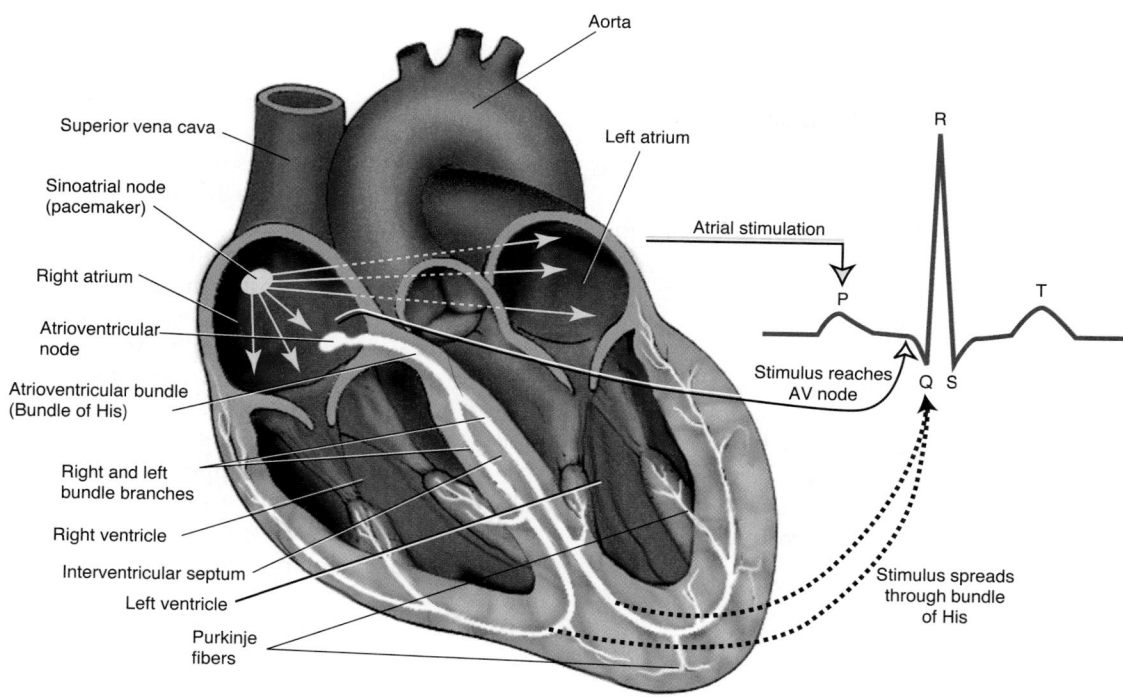

**Figure 39-7 Cardiac conduction system**

contract, further increasing the intraventricular pressure until it is sufficient to force open the two semilunar valves (the right pulmonic valve and the left aortic valve). As contraction of the ventricular walls proceeds, deoxygenated blood is forced out of the right ventricle via the pulmonary arteries to the capillary bed in the lungs, and oxygenated blood leaves the left ventricle via the aorta into the systemic circulation. This process is ventricular systole (Carroll, 2001).

Blood leaving the right ventricle is pumped into the pulmonary artery, which quickly branches into right and left pulmonary arteries. Further division of the pulmonary arterial tree culminates in the pulmonary capillary bed. Blood in the pulmonary capillaries is in very close contact with the alveolar air; it is here that alveolar-capillary gas exchanges take place. From the pulmonary capillaries, the freshly oxygenated blood flows into the pulmonary veins and to the left atrium, which delivers it to the left ventricle (Figure 39-8).

Blood leaving the left ventricle enters the aorta. The aorta serves as the "trunk" of the arterial tree, with branches leading to every organ and tissue group in the body. Blood flow through the arterial system is driven by the pressure generated during ventricular systole and is influenced by the volume and viscosity of the blood and the amount of resistance within the arterial system. Blood flow to specific organs and tissues may be increased or reduced by the relaxation or contraction of **precapillary sphincters**, which are rings of smooth muscle surrounding the arterioles. This mechanism allows for redistribution of blood flow to the areas of greatest need, a process known as **autoregulation**.

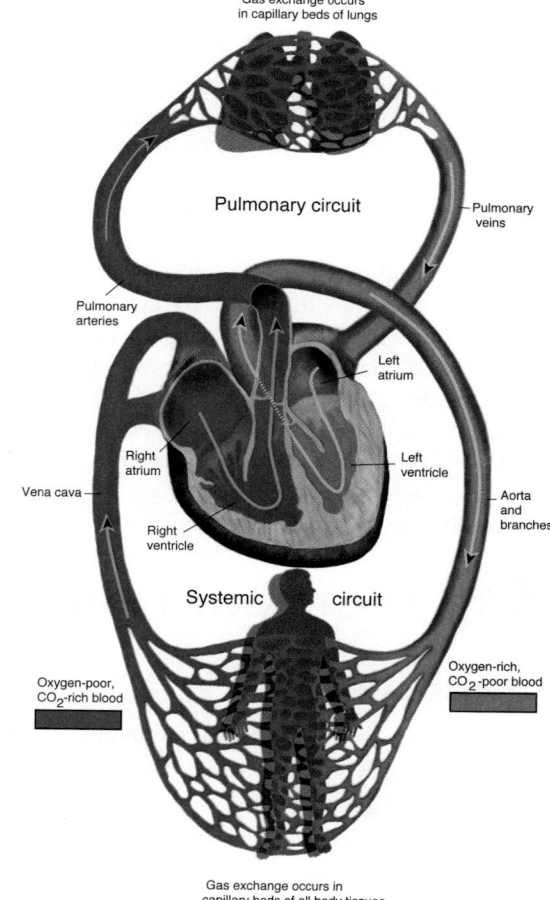

**Figure 39-8 Systemic and pulmonary circuits**

Blood return through the venous system is also driven by pressure gradients, although the venous system operates under lower pressure than the arterial system does. In order to boost venous return, many veins (particularly in the lower extremities) are equipped with valves that prevent backward flow of blood (regurgitation); as the veins are compressed by their surrounding skeletal muscles, blood is forced along toward the vena cava and ultimately to the right atrium (Carroll, 2001).

## Cellular Respiration

Gas exchange at the cellular level, like that at the alveolar level, takes place via diffusion in response to concentration gradients. Oxygen diffuses from the blood to the tissues, while carbon dioxide moves from the tissues to the blood; the blood is then reoxygenated by the heart. This process is referred to as **internal respiration**.

# Factors Affecting Oxygenation

Adequate oxygenation is influenced by many factors, including age, environmental and lifestyle factors, and disease processes.

## Development: Age Differences

Oxygenation status can be influenced by changes due to immaturity, development, and aging. The transition from fetal to pulmonary circulation can be affected by several factors, including insufficient or inactivated surfactant that is necessary to decrease surface tension and to prevent collapse of the alveoli, cardiovascular abnormalities such as ventricular septal defect (VSD), and congestive heart failure (CHF). Alterations in cardiovascular function may be the result of a congenital defect, acquired infection, or injury (Berger & Williams, 1999; Potts & Mandleco, 2002).

The child's upper airway is shorter and narrower than an adult's. Lymph tissues (tonsils and adenoids) enlarge during early childhood and atrophy after age 12. The tongue is large within a smaller oral cavity, the larynx and epiglottis are higher in the neck, the epiglottis is long and floppy and vulnerable to swelling, tracheal cartilages are immature and may easily collapse when the neck is flexed, and fewer muscles are functional in the airway. These changes lead to a greater potential for obstruction and airway resistance.

Lower airway differences in infants and young children include fewer alveoli at birth with increases in size and numbers at 12 years of age. Bronchial passages are narrower and children under 6 years rely heavily on diaphragmatic breathing. Intercostal muscles are immature and ribs consist primarily of flexible cartilage, permitting the chest wall to expand horizontally. At times of respiratory distress, the chest may be retracted inward during inspiration. The intercostal muscles are more effective by 6 years of age. These differences impact the oxygenation process. The differences in both upper and lower airways also adversely affect children's reactions to viral and bacterial infections, allergens, and other irritants.

The normal aging process includes the increase in the antero-posterior circumference of the thorax, which is referred to as "barrel chest." There is a loss of lung elasticity and deterioration in alveoli, even if there is no history of smoking. Cilia movement in the upper airway slows and is less effective, making the older client more vulnerable to infections (Keene, 2001). Normal $PaO_2$ also decreases with age. A normal $PaO_2$ level for each older person is considered on an individual basis; however, anything above 80 mm of Hg is considered acceptable. A low $PaO_2$ impacts cardiac workload and activity tolerance (Archibald, 1999). There is also an increase in cholesterol deposits in the arterial system and calcium deposits in the coronary arteries that narrow the vessel lumen. Some of the elasticity of the blood vessels is lost, and increases in blood pressure place the older person at greater risk of coronary artery disease and impaired circulation function.

## Environmental and Lifestyle Factors

Environmental and lifestyle factors can significantly affect a client's oxygenation status. Clients who are exposed to dust, animal dander, asbestos, or toxic chemicals in the home or workplace are at increased risk for alterations in oxygenation. Optimum oxygenation depends upon clean air. Pollution increases in stagnant air. Some noxious gases due to air pollution replace oxygen in the lungs and in the blood. Barometric pressure decreases at high altitudes and oxygen content is decreased. Additional red blood cells must be produced to carry more oxygen if the person remains at the higher altitude. Individuals with pulmonary or cardiac disease cannot adapt easily and can experience serious respiratory distress at higher altitudes due to falling $PaO_2$ levels. Extremes in weather conditions increase body needs for oxygen, and these individuals should take precautions to avoid detrimental effects of hot or cold weather (Berger & Williams, 1999).

## STOP AND THINK

### Tobacco Use

If you are a smoker, would you feel comfortable suggesting that your clients avoid smoking in order to maintain a healthy oxygenation status? Imagine that a client commented on smelling cigarette smoke on your breath when you returned from your break. How would you respond?

## NURSING STRATEGY

### Maintaining Healthy Oxygenation

Encourage clients to:

- Leave windows open for ventilation instead of using an air conditioner or humidifier.

- Change filters on furnaces, heaters, and range hoods as recommended by manufacturer.

- Wear a mask when working with hazardous materials, such as asbestos.

- Limit physical exertion if it causes shortness of breath.

- Refrain from smoking.

A sedentary lifestyle, shallow breathing, poor posture, thoracic changes, obesity, poor nutritional intake, and emotional stress all adversely affect oxygenation. Side effects of opiates (e.g. morphine and Demerol) contribute to shallow respirations, hypoxia, hypotension, and cardiac dysrhythmias. Detrimental effects of stimulants such as amphetamines and cocaine cause serious tachycardia, hypertension, and tachypnea, and place the individual at risk for cardiac arrest. Physical or emotional stress has detrimental effects as well. Smokers and persons exposed to secondhand smoke should be questioned as to the type and amount of tobacco and number of years of exposure. Secondhand smoke is particularly harmful for children and persons with compromised respiratory and cardiac systems (Berger & Williams, 1999; Holland & McCurren, 2001; 1999; Potts & Mandleco, 2002). Individuals who experience significant physical or emotional stress or who are obese or underweight are also subject to changes in oxygenation status. Smokers and those exposed to second-hand smoke should be questioned as to the type and amount of tobacco and number of years of exposure.

## Disease Processes

Oxygenation alterations can often be traced to disease states related to alterations in ventilation, alveolar gas exchange, oxygen uptake, or circulation. There are many disease states that may affect oxygenation, including obstructive pulmonary disease, restrictive pulmonary disease, diffusion defects, ventilation-perfusion mismatching, atherosclerosis, heart failure, anemia, and alterations in oxygen uptake.

### Obstructive Pulmonary Disease

Alterations in ventilation may be related to obstructive or restrictive pulmonary disease. **Obstructive pulmonary disease** occurs when the airways become partially or com-

pletely blocked, diminishing airflow, or the lungs lose some of their elastic recoil, trapping stale air, which should be exhaled. In both cases, the end result is impaired exhalation, air trapping, and difficulty bringing fresh air into the alveoli (Figure 39-9). The most common obstructive pulmonary diseases are asthma, emphysema, and chronic bronchitis, collectively known as **chronic obstructive pulmonary disease (COPD)** or *chronic airflow limitation*, a newer term preferred by some health care professionals (Cronin & Mirocle, 2001).

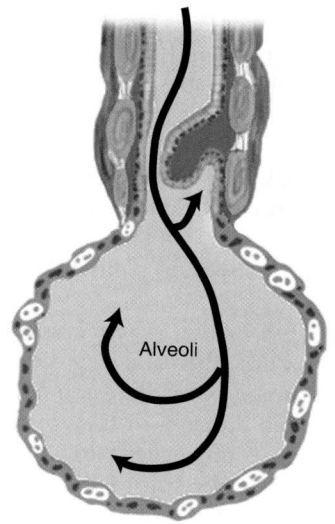

**Inspiration**

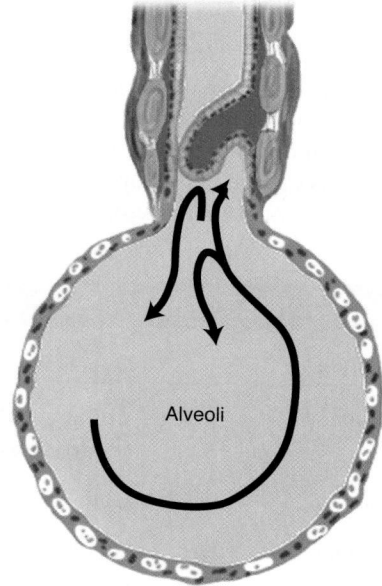

**Expiration**

**Figure 39-9**   One mechanism of air trapping in COPD: During inspiration, the airway widens and opens. During exhalation, the airway closes, trapping air distal to the obstruction and preventing fresh air from entering the alveoli.

## Restrictive Pulmonary Disease

**Restrictive pulmonary disease** represents pathologies that impair the ability of the chest wall and/or lungs to expand during the inspiratory phase of ventilation. This impairment increases the work of breathing and also reduces airflow to the alveoli. A wide variety of disorders cause restrictive lung disease, including pneumonia and pulmonary fibrosis (scarring).

Traumatic injury to the thorax or a break in the pleural membrane that surrounds the lungs may also produce restrictive pulmonary dysfunction. The stability of the chest depends upon the rib cage; multiple rib fractures may produce a type of paradoxical chest wall movement called "flail chest" that impedes normal airflow. The dual-layer pleural membrane also has an important structural function; it helps maintain a negative pressure between its two layers that keeps the lungs from collapsing upon themselves. A break in either layer of the membrane or an abnormal collection of fluid between them interferes with this function, permits alveoli to collapse, and increases the work of breathing. Common pleural defects are described in Table 39-2.

Alveolar collapse, known as **atelectasis**, can be caused by pleural defects as described above, by compression from a mass such as a tumor, or by occlusion of the small airways by secretions, which prevents air movement into the associated alveoli. Failure of a client to breathe deeply after abdominal surgery may result in atelectasis. Regardless of the cause, atelectasis results in restrictive pulmonary dysfunction and reduces the amount of alveolar-capillary surface area engaged in gas exchange (Cronin & Mirocle, 2001).

### Diffusion Defects

Another mechanism of oxygenation impairment is a decrease in the efficiency of gas diffusion from the alveolar space into the pulmonary capillary blood, known as a **diffusion defect**. This may be caused by thickening of the alveolar-capillary basement membrane or by marked increases

### CLINICAL ALERT

#### Risk Factors for Pneumonia

The following compromise a client's respiratory health, increasing the susceptibility to pneumonia:

- Smoking
- Emphysema
- Intoxication
- Weak cough reflex
- Immunosuppressed status
- Medicated or unconscious status

in the speed of blood flow through the pulmonary capillary beds, which reduce contact time with the alveoli. Fluid accumulation, or pulmonary edema, can result from failure in pumping capacity of the left heart ventricle. Blood then backs up into the pulmonary circulation, creating a layer of fluid between the pulmonary capillary bed and the alveoli. Diffusion of blood and carbon dioxide between the air and blood is compromised. Diffusion defects by themselves are uncommon but may coexist with obstructive or restrictive pulmonary diseases such as emphysema, fibrosis, and excess secretions caused by infections such as pneumonia (Cronin & Mirocle, 2001; Archibald, 1999).

### Ventilation-Perfusion Mismatching

Gas exchange across the alveolar-capillary membrane is also influenced by **ventilation-perfusion (V/Q) mismatching**, or the balance between ventilation and perfusion. The amount of fresh air entering the alveoli (alveolar ventilation) and the amount of blood flow to various

| TABLE 39-2 | COMMON PLEURAL DEFECTS |
|---|---|
| **Pleural Defect** | **Description** |
| Pleural effusion | Collection of fluid between the pleural layers. May consist of serous fluid (hydrothorax), purulent fluid (empyema), or chyle (chylothorax). |
| Hemothorax | Collection of blood between the pleural layers. |
| Pneumothorax | A collection of air between the pleural layers caused by a hole in one or both layers of the pleural membrane. May be classified as *open* (communicating with a chest wall wound) or *closed* (no exterior wound). |
| Tension pneumothorax | A pneumothorax that rapidly expands with each respiratory cycle, compressing the lungs and heart and pushing the great vessels and trachea toward the opposite side of the chest. *A tension pneumothorax is a medical emergency requiring immediate intervention.* |

regions of the pulmonary capillary network (perfusion) are not uniform throughout the lungs. Due to alterations in position and the effect of gravity, certain zones of lung tissue may have better ventilation or perfusion than others at any given time.

An important mechanism of compensation in healthy lung tissue is to produce vasoconstriction or bronchoconstriction as needed to better match ventilation to perfusion or vice versa. Many disease states, however, produce areas of ventilation-perfusion mismatching that cannot be overcome by compensatory responses. When mismatching occurs, some alveolar regions will be well ventilated but poorly perfused (a condition known as **deadspace**), while others may be well perfused but poorly ventilated (known as **shunting**). This phenomenon is illustrated in Figure 39-10.

Alterations in circulation may occur in either the pulmonary or the systemic vasculature and may be localized or generalized. Generalized decreases in pulmonary circulation may be caused by right-sided heart failure or by pathologies in the pulmonary vascular system such as pulmonary hypertension and the resultant pulmonary artery sclerosis. Normally, the pulmonary circulation is a low-pressure, low-resistance system (Cronin & Mirocle, 2001). Pulmonary hypertension (PH) may be due to primary or secondary causes. Primary, or idiopathic, PH is quite rare and affects mostly adults between 30 and 40 years of age. Ten percent of the cases have a genetic origin, and women are affected more than men. Even with aggressive treatment, the usual life expectancy is less than 3 years. A lung transplant may be the only option. Secondary HP results from various causes, such as chronic obstructive disease, sleep apnea, and long-term exposure to high altitudes. Increased pressure in the pulmonary artery and its many small branches in the lungs causes the right ventricle of the heart to work harder to pump blood back to the lungs. Other causes include blood clots in the pulmonary artery and its branches, weakness of the left ventricle with backup of blood into the lungs, and an eventual rise in pulmonary pressure, autoimmune disorders such as HIV, lupus, rheumatoid arthritis, and some forms of chronic liver disease (Rosenfeld, 2002; Cronin & Mirocle, 2001). Regional decreases in pulmonary circulation may be related to blockage of a pulmonary artery by an embolus or by regional vasoconstriction.

## Atherosclerosis

Alterations in systemic circulation may also be generalized or localized. A common cause of altered arterial circulation is **atherosclerosis**. This disease is characterized by narrowing and eventual occlusion of the lumen (opening of the arteries) by deposits of lipids, fibrin, and calcium on the

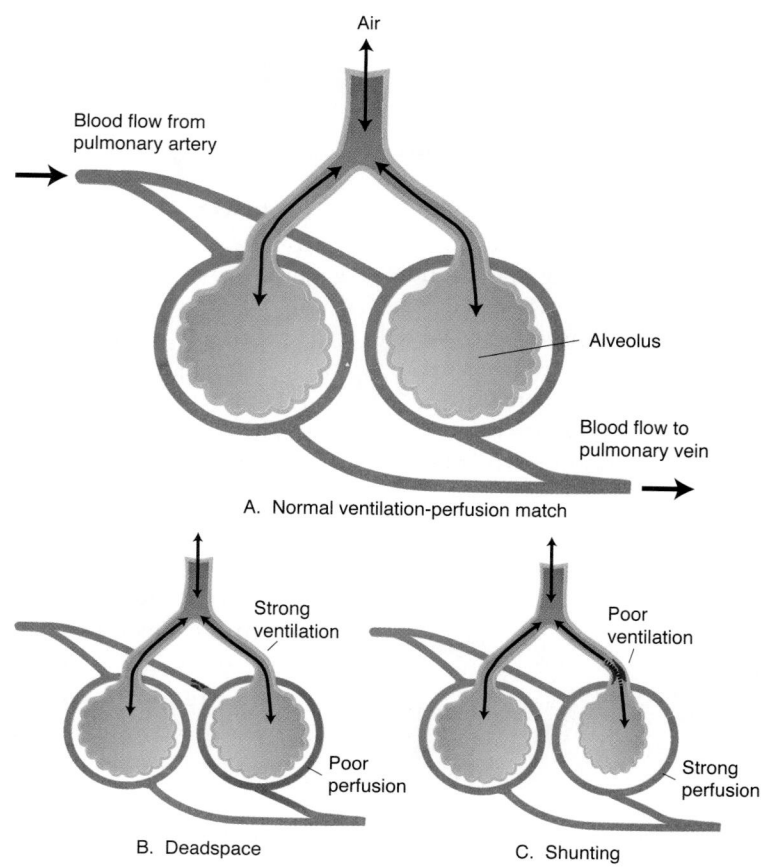

**Figure 39-10    Types of ventilation-perfusion abnormalities**

put (amount of blood pumped by the heart) may be mild, causing only vague symptoms, or may be profound enough to cause death. Causes of congestive heart failure include myocardial infarction, hypertensive heart disease, and valvular disorders, among others.

Loss of circulating blood volume (hypovolemia) may result from massive bleeding, loss of fluid through a wound (such as an extensive burn injury), or severe dehydration.

### Anemia

Another factor that influences oxygenation is the amount of hemoglobin in the blood available to bind with oxygen. A deficiency of hemoglobin **(anemia)** may decrease the oxygen-carrying capacity of the blood. A person who is anemic may have normal $SaO_2$ levels but still continue to experience inadequate tissue oxygenation at the cellular level. Certain poisoning syndromes, most notably carbon monoxide poisoning, mimic anemia in that they reduce oxygenation by competing with oxygen for binding sites on the hemoglobin molecule.

The use of a pulse oximeter to measure heart rate and blood oxygen saturation is currently a common practice in acute care and ambulatory care settings. The noninvasive oximeter uses light wavelengths to measure oxyhemoglobin saturation. However, the readings are not as accurate as the $SaO_2$ of arterial blood gases. The normal oxygen saturation is expected to be equal to or greater than 95%. Pulse oximetry is one measure of oxygenation status—the deliv-

---

## NURSING STRATEGY

### Reducing Risk for Atherosclerosis

Because accumulation of fats is a primary cause of atherosclerosis, encourage your clients to reduce their risk of this disease by:

- Monitoring cholesterol intake
- Lowering fat intake to less than 30% of daily calories
- Increasing intake of carbohydrates to compensate for loss of calories not consumed in fat
- Exercising according to a plan outlined by a health care provider

---

interior walls of the arteries (Figure 39-11). The reduction in blood flow with accompanying oxygen deprivation leads to **ischemia** (deprivation of blood flow) and eventual **infarction** (necrosis or death) of the affected tissue. Atherosclerosis in the coronary arteries (coronary heart disease) and the arteries of the brain (cerebral vascular disease) causes myocardial infarction and stroke, respectively, two of the leading causes of death in contemporary America.

### Heart Failure

Generalized decreases in tissue perfusion may be caused by left-sided heart failure or by loss of circulating blood volume as may occur with shock or hemorrhage. **Heart failure** is a condition in which the heart is unable to pump enough blood to meet the metabolic needs of the body; typically, this is accompanied by a backup of blood in the venous circuits (pulmonary and systemic veins), leading to the condition known as congestive heart failure. The increased pressure of the blood in the engorged veins causes fluid to leak out of the associated capillary beds, causing edema in the tissue, including the lungs (pulmonary edema).

Congestive heart failure results in poor arterial perfusion to the body's tissues. This reduction in **cardiac out-**

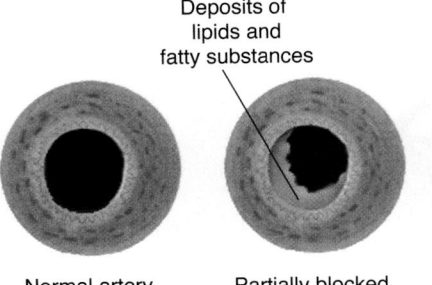
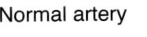
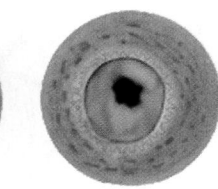

Deposits of lipids and fatty substances

Normal artery        Partially blocked artery        Occluded lumen

**Figure 39-11    Progression of atherosclerosis**

---

## CLIENT EDUCATION

### Sexuality

Clients who are recovering from acute cardiac compromise, such as congestive heart failure or myocardial infarction, will need sensitive nursing care and education regarding sexual activity. Help alleviate their concerns by sharing the following American Heart Association (AHA) recommendations:

✓ Check with your health care provider.
✓ Resume sexual activity when you feel ready; most cardiac-compromised clients can safely resume sexual activity within 2 to 4 weeks.
✓ Take it slowly and establish your comfort level; begin with lower energy forms of sexual expression, such as touching and holding.
✓ Continue taking prescribed cardiac medications; report to your health care provider any impact of these medications on sexual desire and performance.
✓ Experiencing an increased awareness of breathing, heartbeat, and muscle tightening during sexual activity is normal.

ery or transport of oxygen to the cells. It does not provide information about the amount of oxygen actually used by the client. Oximetry readings can also be affected by the amount of lighting in the environment. Bright light competes with the pulse oximetry sensor light source, which can cause an inaccurate reading. Anemia and low blood pressure, blood pH, $PCO_2$, and body temperature can also affect oximeter readings (Clark, 2002).

## Alterations in Oxygen Uptake

A final factor to consider in the process of oxygenation involves the uptake of oxygen by the body's cells. Certain conditions may impair the cells' ability to take up and use oxygen, particularly when the mitochondria are damaged. Cyanide poisoning and severe sepsis impair mitochondrial functioning, rendering the oxygen in arterial blood useless to the cells (Koschel, 2002).

# Physiological Responses to Reduced Oxygenation

When oxygen delivery is inadequate to meet the metabolic needs of the body, various responses to this deficit can be expected, including changes in metabolic pathways and efforts to increase the extraction of available oxygen. If these efforts fail, cells will be damaged and ultimately die.

## Increased Oxygen Extraction

Under normal conditions, the cells of the body do not extract all of the oxygen carried in the arterial blood. In fact, blood returning to the heart via the venous circulation is typically about 75% saturated with oxygen. In response to poor oxygen delivery or increased oxygen need, the cells can extract more oxygen from the arterial blood.

## Anaerobic Metabolism

The use of food (glucose) for cellular energy occurs via metabolic pathways that use oxygen; this is known as **aerobic metabolism**. Many cells are also capable of using alternate metabolic pathways in the absence of oxygen for short periods of time; this is referred to as **anaerobic metabolism**. Anaerobic metabolism is limited by several factors:

1. Not all cells are capable of significant anaerobic metabolism (most notably brain cells).
2. Anaerobic metabolism yields less energy per unit of fuel than does aerobic metabolism.
3. Anaerobic metabolism results in the accumulation of acid by-products, such as lactate, which upset the chemical environment of the cell and induce the release of cell-damaging (lysosomal) enzymes.

## Tissue Ischemia and Cell Death

Prolonged oxygen deprivation **(hypoxia)** will lead to a syndrome ending in cellular death. The decreased production of adenosine triphosphate (ATP) resulting from anaerobic

# LEGAL AND ETHICAL ISSUES

## Legal Issues with Using Pulse Oximetry

Nonuse or incorrect interpretation of pulse oximetry results has been the subject of numerous medical malpractice cases. Recommendations to avoid overdependence on technology include:

- Use oxygen saturation *trend data* for clients at risk for respiratory arrest by obtaining periodic arterial blood gases (ABG).

- Realize the limitations of pulse oximetry oxygen saturation compared to ABG findings. Consider the client's blood pressure in interpretation of pulse oximetry readings.

- Evaluate the amount of lighting in the environment of the pulse oximeter.

- Observe and document routine vital signs, level of consciousness, skin color, and breath sounds.

- Recognize that oxygen saturation values do not reflect oxygen consumption by the client.

- Know the client's hemoglobin level (often in malpractice cases, nurses have reported that in the present cost-containment era, no postoperative hemoglobin measures were taken).

- Know the relationship of oxygen saturation and arterial oxygen.

Adapted from Clark, A. (2002). Legal lessons: "But his $O_2$ Sat was normal!" *Clinical Nurse Specialist, 16*(3), 162–163.

# CLINICAL ALERT

## Cyanide Poisoning

Hydrogen cyanide is a common combustion by-product of fires at industrial sites where it is used in fumigation, metal treatment, paper manufacturing, photography, blueprinting, and engraving (note: in the case study at the end of the chapter, Mike Calloway works in a paper manufacturing plant). It is also a result from burning nylon, wool, silk, polyurethane, or rubber. Cyanide can be 20 times more toxic than carbon monoxide. Nurses should suspect concurrent cyanide poisoning in clients admitted from fires in enclosed spaces (Koschel, 2002).

metabolism reduces the amount of energy available for cellular metabolic functions and results in a breakdown in all cellular functions. The integrity of the cell membrane becomes impaired, and the cell begins to swell. Cellular organelles may become damaged and lysosomal enzymes released, killing the cell. The destruction of tissues or organs as a result of oxygen deprivation is known as an infarction. Widespread cellular death resulting from oxygenation disturbances is the underlying characteristic of a devastating syndrome known as *multiple-organ-system failure* (Carroll, 2001; Stacy, 2000).

## Carbon Dioxide Transport and Excretion

Carbon dioxide is a natural by-product of glucose metabolism. Like oxygen, it exists normally as a gas and can be dissolved in the plasma as well as loosely bound to the hemoglobin molecule (although carbon dioxide attaches to a different binding site on the hemoglobin molecule than does oxygen). In the lungs, carbon dioxide is released into the alveoli by diffusion, and when the individual exhales, the carbon dioxide exits to the atmosphere.

In the body fluids, carbon dioxide functions as an acid because, combined with water, it produces carbonic acid. The hydrogen ions that are liberated in this process stimulate the respiratory control centers in the pons and medulla to increase the rate and depth of breathing; more carbon dioxide is then released by the lungs and the pH of the body is brought back to normal. Likewise, increased production of carbon dioxide, as may be associated with fever or exercise, is often a cause of increased ventilatory rate **(tachypnea)** and depth. Elevated blood levels of carbon dioxide **(hypercapnia)** indicate inadequate alveolar ventilation (Carroll, 2001; Stacy, 2000).

# Assessment

## Health History

The health history of the individual experiencing oxygenation deficits is important in the development of the plan of care. The health history begins with a thorough exploration of the presenting problem (Table 39-3), including the events leading up to the problem, its duration, methods used to alleviate symptoms, and the problem's impact on activities of daily living. A past health history, psychosocial history, and family history are helpful in establishing priorities for intervention and to determine the client's understanding of the current health problem. In emergency or acute situations, questions are prioritized and limited to current symptoms. Additional data can be obtained when the patient is stable or from significant others. A comprehensive history provides valuable information for addressing the client's needs on an ongoing basis (Keene, 2001).

# Physical Examination

Inspection will begin when the nurse first encounters the client. This is a time to make general notes of the client's efforts at ventilation, especially anxious or distressed appearance, flaring of nostrils, position preferences, and general chest configuration (Figure 39-12). While counting the respiratory rate, also note the rhythm or pattern of the breathing for regularity or irregularity (Figure 39-13). Allow sufficient time when counting the respiratory rate to note whether the rhythm or pattern of the breathing is regular or irregular. The signs and symptoms of hypoxia are relative to the onset. Early clinical manifestations of hypoxia include restlessness, apprehension, anxiety, dizziness, inability to concentrate, confusion, agitation, increased pulse rate, increased rate and depth of respiration, and elevated blood pressure (unless the hypoxia is caused by shock). If the hypoxia goes untreated, the respiratory rate may decline and changes in the level of consciousness progress to stupor, or coma, indicating ischemia of neuronal cells resulting from oxygen deprivation.

Perfusion deficits resulting in poor circulation can be visually noted in mottled skin, **cyanosis** (bluish coloration of the skin), and edema. There may be excessive bruising or purpura (tiny purple spots). Skin of the feet and lower legs may be darkly discolored and thin, and there may be breaks in the skin or skin ulcers. Persons with insufficient arterial circulation may have no hair below their knees, the feet may feel cold to the touch, and edema is a common complication. The skin may appear ashen, pale, gray, or cyanotic—a bluish discoloration of the skin as the result of the presence of unsaturated hemoglobin in capillaries that may occur from either hypoxia or stagnant blood flow. Cyanosis occurs when more than one-third of hemoglobin is unsaturated with oxygen and may be generalized or localized to certain areas such as lips and nailbeds (Archibald, 1999). When cyanosis is observed in the tongue, soft palate, and

---

### CLINICAL ALERT

#### Cyanosis

Regardless of the mechanism behind it, it is important to remember that cyanosis is often a late development in clients with poor oxygenation and may be further delayed in those with dark skin pigmentation or low blood hemoglobin (anemia). *Therefore, the absence of cyanosis should not be taken as an assurance that oxygenation is adequate.* However, the presence of cyanosis, especially central cyanosis, should be considered to be an indicator of a hypoxic emergency.

## TABLE 39-3   HEALTH HISTORY RELATED TO OXYGENATION

| Presenting Problem | Qualifiers and Considerations |
|---|---|
| Cough | *Onset:* Sudden or gradual and when it began. |
| | *Nature:* Dry, moist, barking, hacking, wheezing, productive/nonproductive. |
| | *Pattern:* Continuous, occasional, related to time of day, position or activity, weather conditions, and severity of pattern. |
| | *Associated symptoms:* Pain, shortness of breath, wheezing. |
| | *Alleviating factors:* Type of medications/treatments used (vaporizers/nebulizers). |
| | Note if precautions were taken to prevent spread of infection (if present). |
| | Use the opportunity to educate client. |
| | Stress incontinence can occur, especially for women. This should clear once the coughing has subsided. |
| Sputum | Determine amount, color changes, consistency, odor. (*Normally 3 ounces of mucus are produced daily as part of the normal cleaning process.*) Ask if sputum was produced only after lying in a certain position. |
| | Hemoptysis (expectorated blood) may be from lungs, oral and nasopharyngeal area, or sinuses. Ask if hemoptysis was produced by forceful coughing, an estimate of the amount, and whether it is blood-tinged or frank bloody sputum. Identify color (bright red, dark red, or brown). Blood from lungs is usually bright red, but can turn dark over a period of time. |
| Shortness of breath (Dyspnea) | *Onset:* Sudden or gradual. |
| | *Nature:* Precipitated by choking or gagging. Client may define it as suffocation, tightness, being winded or breathless. |
| | *Pattern:* Associated with activity or position; continuous or intermittent. |
| | *Associated symptoms:* Pain, cough, diaphoresis. |
| | *Alleviated factors:* Determine what has been used to relieve symptoms. |
| Pain | *Onset:* Location/radiation. |
| | *Nature:* (Intensity) stabbing, dull, aching, burning, squeezing, crushing. Differentiation between pulmonary and cardiac symptoms is very important. Pleuritic chest pain is sharp/stabbing pain on one side of chest, especially during inspiration; coughing can cause pain; pain can originate in cartilage/bony parts of thorax; retrosternal pain is usually burning, constant, and aching; cardiac pain is usually an aching, heavy, squeezing sensation; angina can radiate into the neck and arms. |
| | *Associated symptoms:* Dizziness, nausea, diaphoresis, palpitations. Ask client what aggravates the pain. |
| | *Alleviating factors:* Determine what medications (nitroglycerin, analgesics) and actions (splinting the chest wall, use of heat, ointments, etc.). |

Adapted from Keene, A. (2001). Health history. In J. Black, J. Hawks, & A. Keene (Eds.), *Medical-surgical nursing: Clinical management for continuity of care*. Philadelphia: W. B. Saunders.

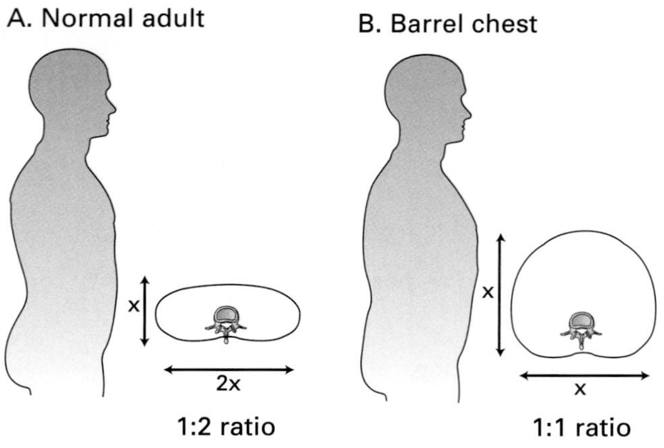

## A. Normal adult

## B. Barrel chest

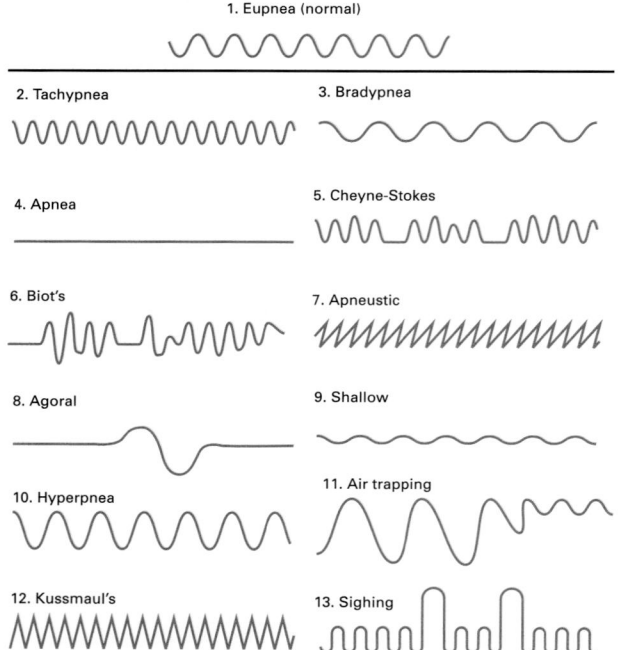

1:2 ratio     1:1 ratio

**Figure 39-12    Changes in chest configuration and posture:** The normal ratio of the anterior posterior diameter to the lateral diameter is 1:2. With a barrel chest, the ratio between the diameters is 1:1.

1. Eupnea (normal)

2. Tachypnea

3. Bradypnea

4. Apnea

5. Cheyne-Stokes

6. Biot's

7. Apneustic

8. Agoral

9. Shallow

10. Hyperpnea

11. Air trapping

12. Kussmaul's

13. Sighing

**Figure 39-13    Respiratory patterns**

conjunctiva of the eye, it indicates hypoxemia, whereas cyanosis of the extremities, nailbeds, and earlobes is often a result of vasoconstriction. Clubbing of the fingers, which manifests as a flattened angle of the nailbed and a rounding of the fingertips, is a sign of chronic hypoxia (Figure 39-14).

Common palpation findings related to compromised ventilation include vocal fremitus and displacement of the trachea. Perfusion deficits are noted in changes in pulse rate or character, clammy skin, and stasis ulcers in the lower extremities.

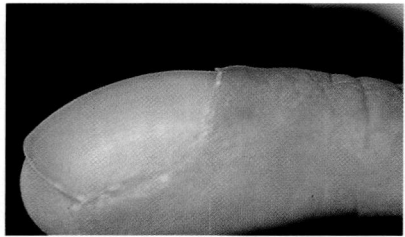

**Figure 39-14    Clubbing of the fingers,** as a result of chronic hypoxia *Courtesy of Robert A. Silverman, MD, Clinical Associate Professor, Department of Pediatrics, Georgetown University*

Percussion may reveal hyperresonance, dull percussion tone, or changes in the density of the lungs and surrounding tissues.

Auscultation may reveal adventitious breath sounds such as rales (crackles) or wheezes (rhonci), pleural friction rub, or stridor, all indicators or alterations in ventilation

## NURSING STRATEGY

### Assessment Strategies for Cyanosis

- Use favorable lighting conditions.

- Recognize changes that can be influenced by environmental factors (air conditioning), use of vasoconstricting medications, and smoking.

- Examine the least pigmented areas such as the nails, lips, mucous membrane, conjunctiva, and palms and soles. In brown-skinned individuals, cyanosis may appear as a yellow-brown tinge. In black-skinned individuals, it may appear ashen or gray; there is a gray hue in the lips and tongue and bluish hue in nails, palms, and soles. However, darker skin may mask the underlying cyanosis. Observe for other clinical signs of decreased oxygenation to the brain: changes in levels of consciousness, increased respiratory rate, use of accessory muscles of respiration, nasal flaring, positional changes, and other attempts to increase oxygenation.

Adapted from Carroll, R. (2001). Anatomy and physiology of the heart. In J. Black, J. Hawks, & A. Keene (Eds.), *Medical-surgical nursing: Clinical management for continuity of care.* Philadelphia: W. B. Saunders; Stapleton, M. (1998). Knowledge base for patients with respiratory dysfunction. In F. Monahan & M. Neighbors (Eds.), *Medical/surgical nursing: Foundations for practice.* Philadelphia: W. B. Saunders.

## NURSING STRATEGY

### Percussion Hint

Sound waves travel better through a solid medium than through an air-filled medium. Therefore:

- The more solid a structure, the higher its pitch, the softer its intensity, and the shorter its duration.

- The more air-filled a structure, the lower its pitch, the louder its intensity, and the longer its duration.

## NURSING STRATEGY

### Percussion Techniques

Percussion is a technique performed by tapping on the chest wall to assess the density of an area by the sound that is produced. Direct percussion is the use of one or two fingers to gently strike the body surface (e.g., over the sinuses). Indirect percussion requires dexterity and practice. It is done as follows:

1. Place the distal phalanx of the middle finger of the nondominant hand on the client's skin over soft tissue (the remaining fingers do not touch the skin).
2. Bend the distal phalanx of the middle finger of the dominant hand to create a "hammer."
3. Strike the finger resting on the client's skin sharply and quickly with the "hammer" finger (a light, quick blow delivers the clearest sound). Repeat two or three times to adequately assess the sound.

Estes, M. (2002). *Health assessment & physical examination* (2nd ed.). Clifton Park, NY: Delmar Learning.

(Table 39-4). Circulation deficits will be noted upon auscultation by **gallops**, or extra heart sounds, and **murmurs**, or sounds produced by blood flowing through a malfunctioning valve (Carroll, 2001).

## Diagnostic and Laboratory Data

There are many tests to measure oxygenation status. Pulse oximetry uses light waves to measure oxygen saturation ($SaO_2$) noninvasively (Figure 39-15). Arterial blood gases (ABGs) measure a number of indicators

## TABLE 39-4   CHARACTERISTICS OF ADVENTITIOUS BREATH SOUNDS

| Breath Sound | Respiratory Phase | Description | Conditions |
| --- | --- | --- | --- |
| Fine crackle | Predominantly inspiration | Dry, high-pitched crackling, popping; short duration; roll hair by ears between your fingers to simulate this sound | Chronic obstructive pulmonary disease, congestive heart failure, pneumonia, pulmonary fibrosis, atelectasis |
| Coarse crackle | Predominantly inspiration | Moist, low-pitched crackling, gurgling; long duration | Pneumonia, pulmonary edema, bronchitis, atelectasis |
| Sonorous wheeze | Predominantly expiration | Low-pitched; snoring | Asthma, bronchitis, airway edema, tumor, bronchiolar spasm, foreign body obstruction |
| Sibilant wheeze | Predominantly expiration | High-pitched; musical | Asthma, chronic bronchitis, emphysema, tumor, foreign body obstruction |
| Pleural friction rub | Inspiration and expiration | Creaking, grating | Pleurisy, tuberculosis, pulmonary infarction, pneumonia, lung abscess |
| Stridor | Predominantly inspiration | Crowing | Croup, foreign body obstruction, large airway tumor |

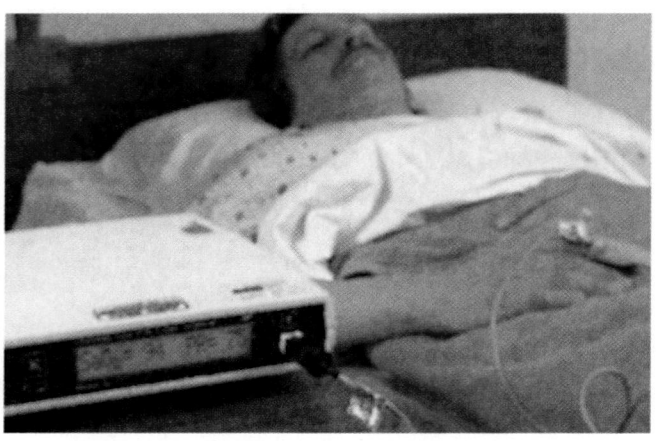

**Figure 39-15    Client with pulse oximeter**

that can affect oxygenation status; these factors and their values are listed in Table 39-5. Sputum collection is another valuable tool in assessing a client's oxygenation functioning; this procedure is outlined in Table 39-6, and common findings and their indications are listed in Table 39-7. Measurements of lactic acid, hemoglobin, and hematocrit are also useful in determining the effectiveness of the body's oxygen delivery to tissues.

Selected tests to determine oxygenation status are discussed in Table 39-8. (See also Figure 39-16 for ventilatory function.) Clients undergoing these tests are often apprehensive and need nursing care and education directed at their knowledge levels.

## TABLE 39-5    ARTERIAL BLOOD GASES: NORMAL VALUES

| Measurement | Normal Arterial Values | Clinical Significance |
|---|---|---|
| PH | 7.35–7.45 or SI 7.35–7.45 | Indicates acid-base balance |
| $PCO_2$ | 35–45 mm Hg or SI 4.7–7.45 | Partial pressure of carbon dioxide; indicates adequacy of alveolar ventilation; represents respiratory component of acid-base balance |
| $HCO_3$ | 21–28 mEq/L or SI 21–28 mmol/L | Bicarbonate level; indicates metabolic component of acid-base balance |
| $PaO_2$ | Adult: 80–100 mm Hg or SI 10.6–13.3 kPa Newborn: 60–70 mm Hg or SI 0–10.33 kPa | Partial pressure of oxygen; represents oxygen dissolved in plasma |
| $SaO_2$ | Adult > 95% or SI fraction saturated > 0.95 Newborn: 40%–90% or SI fraction saturated 0.40–0.90 | Saturation of hemoglobin with oxygen |

**Note:** *SI* indicates *System International Units,* a system that reports laboratory data in terms of standardized international measurements. It is used in several countries with the goal of worldwide use in the near future.

**Procedure:** Five ml of blood is commonly taken from the radial or femoral artery by puncture or from an inserted arterial line (the temporal artery is used in infants). Experienced nurses in specialized units may perform arterial punctures. Usually a physician, laboratory technician, or respiratory therapist performs the procedure.

**Nursing Considerations:**
1. The client's temperature affects the results because the ABG machines are calibrated at 37°C. Document the client's temperature on the requisition form at time blood is drawn.
2. Record on requisition form whether client was breathing room air or $O_2$ at time of blood draw.
3. Instruct the client that an arterial puncture is painful, and cooperation is necessary.
4. Encourage the client to breathe normally. Hyperventilation causes false reading due to blow off of $CO_2$.
5. ABG readings should not be obtained for 20 to 30 minutes after a procedure (e.g., suctioning) that would alter the client's current respiratory status.
6. Pressure is exerted on the arterial site for a minimum of 5 minutes afterward. If the client is taking anticoagulants, pressure should be maintained for at least 10 minutes or more.
7. Monitor closely. Arterial occlusion may result from a hematoma or thrombosis, bleeding, and infection.

Adapted from Daniels, R. (2003). *Delmar's manual of laboratory and diagnostic tests.* Clifton Park, NY: Delmar Learning.

## TABLE 39-6   PROTOCOL: ASSISTING A CLIENT WITH SPUTUM COLLECTION

| | |
|---|---|
| Purpose | To collect an adequate sample of sputum for laboratory analysis and/or culture. |
| | To minimize contamination of the sample with oral or other secretions. |
| Level | Independent |
| Supportive data | Increasing the client's knowledge promotes cooperation and increases the diagnostic value of the sample obtained. |
| Assessment | Verify the type of test to be performed (cytology studies should be collected into a cup containing a preservative solution; cultures must be collected into a sterile container). |
| | Assess the client's level of consciousness and ability to follow instructions. |
| | Assess the client's breath sounds; coarse rales indicate the presence of sputum in the airways. |
| Interventions | Obtain correct specimen container. |
| | Wash hands and don clean gloves. |
| | Assist the client to rinse the mouth with water (not mouthwash). |
| | Instruct client to raise sputum from the lungs, not the throat or nose. |
| | Instruct client to expectorate sputum into the cup without touching the inside of the container. |
| | Replace cap on container as soon as sample is obtained. Label container and wash the outside if indicated. |
| | Place in a bag with a biohazard label for transport. |
| | Provide mouth care for the client and assist to a comfortable position. |
| | Remove gloves and wash hands. Send specimen to lab immediately. |
| Documentation | Document amount, color, character, and odor of sputum obtained and time the specimen was sent to the lab. |

Adapted from Daniels, R. (2003). *Delmar's manual of laboratory and diagnostic tests.* Clifton Park, NY: Delmar Learning.

## TABLE 39-7   PATHOLOGIES ASSOCIATED WITH DIFFERENT COLORS OF SPUTUM

| Sputum Color | Suspected Pathology |
|---|---|
| Mucoid | Tracheobronchitis, asthma |
| Yellow or green | Bacterial infection |
| Rust or blood-tinged | Pneumonia, pulmonary infarction, tuberculosis |
| Black | Black lung disease |
| Pink | Pulmonary edema |

## TABLE 39-8    SELECTED TESTS FOR OXYGENATION STATUS

| Test | Indications/Possible Findings |
|---|---|
| Ventilatory function tests | • Volume of air in the lungs at various phases of the ventilatory cycle<br><br>• Speed and ease of airflow through the airways<br><br>• Strength of the respiratory muscles |
| Chest x-ray | • Areas of fluid accumulation (infiltrates)<br><br>• Solid masses (suggestive of tumors)<br><br>• Abnormal accumulations of calcium, areas of necrosis (as seen in tuberculosis)<br><br>• Excessive air trapping (suggestive of emphysema)<br><br>• Abnormal accumulations of air or fluid in the pleural space (suggestive of pleural effusion or pneumothorax)<br><br>• Gross abnormalities in size, shape, position of thoracic structures |
| Computerized tomography (CT) scan, magnetic resonance imaging (MRI) | • Detailed pictures of thoracic structures |
| Ventilation scan | • Areas of impaired airflow (suggestive of pulmonary emboli) |
| Bronchoscopy | • Sputum collection<br><br>• Examination of tissue |
| Thoracentesis | • Tissue sample collection |
| Echocardiography | • Size and motion of cardiac structures<br><br>• Accumulation of fluid in the pericardial sac (suggestive of pericardial effusion) |
| Electrocardiography | • Heart rate and rhythm<br><br>• Abnormal sites of impulse formation (ectopic pacemakers)<br><br>• Areas of blocked or delayed impulse transmission<br><br>• Chamber enlargement (as seen in heart failure)<br><br>• Areas of ischemia, injury or infarction |
| Stress test | • Changes in ECG tracings (may indicate ischemic heart disease) |

Daniels, R. (2003). *Delmar's manual of laboratory and diagnostic tests.* Clifton Park, NY: Delmar Learning.

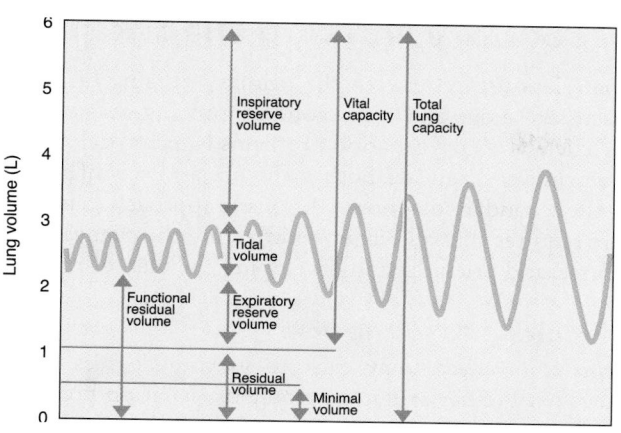

**Figure 39-16** Graphic representation of lung volumes and capacities

 **LIFE SPAN CONSIDERATIONS**

### Assessment and Treatment Guidelines for Children with Asthma

The diagnosis of asthma is confirmed by (1) frequency of daytime and nighttime symptoms of coughing, wheezing, shortness of breath, and chest tightness; (2) x-ray findings that indicate expanded lung or lungs with flattened diaphragm and air trapping; and (3) pulmonary function spirometry testing (forced expiratory volume in one second-$FEV_1$) or peak expiratory flow (PEF). Spirometry testing, the most sensitive measurement, represents a percentage of lung vital capacity. PEF measures how fast the lungs can exhale. PEF is measured by a small, handheld, peak flow meter, and can be performed by the client (or caregiver). PEF is commonly used as a tool to monitor a client's breathing patterns.

Symptom diaries are used to monitor and record symptoms over a period of time. These recordings are very useful in diagnosing the severity and frequency of symptoms and suggest triggering causes. The diaries are often continued after the client is placed on treatment, in order to document responses to the therapy. The diaries are particularly beneficial for children under 5 years to permit early intervention and prevention of permanent structural change to the airways or airway remodeling. Symptom diaries form the basis for the development of management plans for asthma and other childhood conditions, including allergies, otitis media, and other childhood conditions.

Childhood Asthma Management. (2002). http://www.better health4kids.com; Gallagher, C. (2002). Childhood asthma: Tools that help parents manage it. *American Journal of Nursing, 102*(8), 71–83.

# Nursing Diagnosis

Nursing care of the client experiencing oxygenation problems should be prioritized on the basis of the A-B-C format used in basic life support; that is, consider the *airway, breathing,* and *circulation* first and foremost. The primary nursing diagnoses are related to these priorities.

## Primary Diagnoses

### Ineffective Airway Clearance

*Ineffective airway clearance* exists when the client has difficulty maintaining a patent (open) airway at any point along the airway. This occlusion of the airway may be partial or complete. Causes of ineffective airway clearance include:

- Obstruction of the airway by the tongue that may occur in the comatose client, client with a cerebrovascular accident, or anesthetized client, particularly when lying in the supine position
- Obstruction of airway by secretion (as may occur with excessive sputum production, and ineffective or absent cough)
- Upper airway obstruction caused by edema of the larynx or glottis
- Obstruction of the trachea or a bronchus by foreign body aspiration
- Partial occlusion of the bronchi and bronchioles by infection (bronchitis, bronchiolitis), inflammation and smooth muscle spasm (asthma), or occlusion or compression by a tumor mass
- Occlusion of the more distal airways by the changes associated with emphysema

Assessment findings in the client with ineffective airway clearance include a complaint of feeling short of breath or suffocating, a condition sometimes referred to as "air hunger." The use of accessory muscles of ventilation may be noted, and the client may complain of fatigue. Shortness of breath may be noted on observation, and the client may have difficulty speaking because of it. A cough may be noted, and on auscultation rales and rhonchi may be heard. Poor aeration of the alveoli, as can occur with emphysema and severe asthma, will cause diminished breath sounds over the peripheral lung fields. Complete obstruction of a large or medium-sized airway will result in a loss of breath sounds over the affected lung segment (Doenges, Moorhouse, & Geissler-Murr, 2002).

### Ineffective Breathing Patterns

*Ineffective breathing pattern* is commonly a problem for clients with restrictive pulmonary disease or central nervous system disorders that affect breathing. Those with restrictive pulmonary disease, in an effort to decrease their work of breathing, tend to adopt a pattern of rapid, shallow respirations. This respiratory pattern does not deliver adequate fresh air to the alveoli, resulting in chronic air hunger while contributing to muscle fatigue. Central nervous system disorders, including the effects of anesthetics and narcotics, may reduce both the rate and the depth of ventilation. Lesions affecting the brain stem in particular may reduce ventilation to dangerous levels.

Another group of clients at risk for ineffective breathing patterns are those who have had major abdominal or thoracic surgery or whose mobility is restricted. These individuals have a tendency to take shallow breaths and to avoid sighing and coughing, both necessary to maintain airway integrity.

Neuromuscular diseases that weaken the respiratory muscles may also result in ineffective breathing patterns as well as impaired airway clearance. Examples of such disorders include Guillain-Barré syndrome and myasthenia gravis. Alterations in thoracic structures that interfere with breathing patterns include abnormal curvatures of the spine (scoliosis, kyphosis), chest wall injury, and pleural defects.

### Impaired Gas Exchange

*Impaired gas exchange* occurs when, despite the delivery of fresh air to the alveoli, adequate oxygen does not enter the arterial blood and/or carbon dioxide is not removed from the venous blood. Often this condition is the result of ventilation-perfusion mismatching or overall decreases in the amount of alveolar-capillary surface area available for gas exchange, a characteristic of emphysema. Another cause of impaired gas exchange is widespread shunting, as may occur with atelectasis (alveolar collapse) and pneumonia. Impaired gas exchange is assessed by measuring the oxygen and carbon dioxide content in the arterial blood via arterial blood gas analysis or pulse oximetry or both (Cronin & Mirocle, 2001).

### Decreased Cardiac Output

*Decreased cardiac output* impairs oxygen delivery to the tissues and may also be a factor in impaired gas exchange, as when congestive heart failure causes pulmonary edema. Causes of decreased cardiac output include heart failure and various types of shock. The assessment findings associated with decreased cardiac output may include low blood pressure; cool, clammy skin; weak, thready pulses; low urine output; and a diminished level of consciousness. If pulmonary edema is present, crackles will be heard over the lung bases and the client may produce frothy pink or white sputum.

### Ineffective Tissue Perfusion

*Ineffective (decreased) tissue perfusion* may be widespread, as in the case of decreased cardiac output, or it may be confined to one or more tissues or organs of the body. A common cause of regional decreases in tissue perfusion is atherosclerosis, which may impair perfusion to the heart, brain, kidneys, or extremities. Assessment findings depend upon the organ or tissue involved, but one common finding is pain. The tissue that is deprived of oxygen will in many cases be painful, as the accumulation of lactic acid and the chemical mediators of the inflammatory response stimulate local pain receptors (Carroll, 2001).

## Secondary Nursing Diagnoses

The relationship between the primary nursing diagnoses discussed above and the secondary nursing diagnoses in the client with oxygenation problems is reciprocal; that is, the primary diagnoses both influence and are influenced by the secondary diagnoses. A holistic approach to nursing care requires that all diagnoses affecting the client be considered and prioritized in developing the plan of care.

### Deficient Knowledge

*Deficient knowledge* may exist to varying degrees in the client with either acute or chronic oxygenation problems. Involving the client in the plan of care requires that the client be informed regarding the disease process, diagnostic procedures, and treatment modalities. Assessment for deficient knowledge involves questioning the client and family with regard to their understanding and perceptions of these subjects. It is a mistake to assume that a client with a long-standing chronic illness has a good understanding of that illness.

### Activity Intolerance

*Activity intolerance* reflects the impact of the illness on the client's ability to perform activities of daily living; the degree of this impairment may range from mild to severe, but it is important that this judgment be based on the client's, not the nurse's, perception of the activity intolerance. Activity restrictions that may be a mere annoyance for one individual can be viewed as catastrophic by another.

To assess activity intolerance, both interview and observation are useful. Ask the client to compare the current level of activity with the previous level and desired level. In addition, observe the client performing activities such as moving about in bed, ambulating, and performing personal care activities; note the point at which fatigue and/or dyspnea occurs and the amount of rest required. Objective tests of exercise tolerance, such as stress tests, may be performed in certain cases.

### Disturbed Sleep Pattern

*Disturbed sleep pattern* is common in people with both cardiac and pulmonary disease. As mentioned earlier, many people with restrictive and obstructive pulmonary diseases find that breathing is easiest in an upright position; this position is also more comfortable for those with congestive heart failure. Sudden attacks of dyspnea during sleep, called **paroxysmal nocturnal dyspnea**, may interrupt the sleep of these clients, resulting in chronic fatigue. Complaints of poor sleep, along with daytime sleepiness and fatigue, are common assessment findings. Severe sleep deprivation can result in personality changes, hallucinations, and delusions.

A particular sleep problem associated with airway obstruction is **sleep apnea**. It is often seen in males who are overweight and have short, thick necks and is commonly associated with loud, heavy snoring. The soft tissues of the upper airways collapse during sleep, resulting in periods of absence of breathing (apnea). The individual then rouses enough to resume breathing, interrupting the normal sleep cycle. These individuals may complain of persistent daytime fatigue despite what seems to be adequate nighttime sleep.

### Imbalanced Nutrition

Nutritional alterations are also commonly associated with both cardiac and pulmonary disease. The client with dyspnea may have difficulty consuming adequate food because of the effort involved; in turn, the malnutrition contributes to respiratory muscle weakness. The client with a productive cough may have an unpleasant taste in the mouth, interfering with appetite. Congestive heart failure may cause a poor appetite (anorexia) because of decreased perfusion to the gut. On the other hand, obesity can affect oxygenation by increasing the work of breathing as well as the cardiac workload.

### Acute Pain

*Acute pain* may be present in the client with ischemia to the heart or to the extremities due to inadequate perfusion; chest wall or pleuritic pain may also be a feature of many pulmonary disorders. Adequate pain control can influence the effectiveness of breathing patterns and coughing, making pain control a priority in these cases. Pain assessment should address the nature of the pain, its intensity, its location and radiation, factors that make it better or worse, and any associated symptoms. For instance, pain caused by myocardial ischemia is called **angina pectoris** and is often described as crushing or squeezing in nature; it may be confined to the chest or it may radiate to the neck, shoulder, jaw, arm, or hand. Ischemia to the extremities (most often the legs) produces a pain known as **intermittent claudication**, which is typically brought on by exercise and relieved by rest. See Chapter 42 for further discussion of pain assessment.

### Anxiety

*Anxiety* is often a prominent finding in individuals who are experiencing breathing difficulties or acute cardiac problems, such as chest pain. The anxious client may have difficulty answering questions and focusing on the instructions being given and may expend excessive amounts of precious energy in the process. Therefore, recognition and control of anxiety bring both psychological and physiological benefits (Stacy, 2000; Doenges et al., 2002).

## Outcome Identification and Planning

In identifying goals and planning nursing care for the client with oxygenation disorders, carefully consider individual objectives for each nursing diagnosis and each client; the goals should be individualized to reflect the client's capabilities and limitations. In many cases, identifying desired outcomes of care is best accomplished in small steps, progressing from one level of functioning to the next until the

ultimate objective is attained. Such an approach prevents the client from feeling overwhelmed with the magnitude of the task at hand while allowing for the satisfaction of reaching intermediate outcomes. Outcomes may be based on physiological parameters such as respiratory rate or arterial blood gas values, on activity tolerance and client comfort levels, or on identified learning needs.

The outcomes for a particular client should be based upon the assessment findings that led to the nursing diagnoses at hand. For example, if a respiratory rate of 30 breaths per minute with a shallow breathing pattern and suprasternal retraction led to a diagnosis of *ineffective breathing pattern*, then the desired outcome of intervention might be a respiratory rate of 20 breaths per minute or less and the absence of retractions. Achievement of the outcome indicates resolution of the problem.

## Implementation

## Interventions to Promote Airway Clearance

Interventions to promote airway clearance focus on clearing the airways of secretions, relieving bronchospasm, and, when necessary, bypassing the natural airway structures with an artificial airway. All of these procedures are facilitated when the client has been well informed of the purpose for the interventions and knows what to expect.

### Teach Effective Coughing

Effective coughing techniques may need to be taught to the client experiencing either short-term or chronic airway obstruction. Nurses, physical therapists, and respiratory therapists perform these therapies. Coughing is an important element of postoperative care in order to prevent pulmonary complications. Effective coughing should be preceded by a series of slow, deep breaths. One technique

## CLINICAL ALERT

### Sputum Collection

Proper collection of a sputum specimen is critical for quickly determining the causative factor of a pulmonary infection. Generally, a good specimen requires the cooperation of a sufficiently hydrated client. It may be necessary to use nebulized saline by itself or in combination with chest physiotherapy to help loosen the secretions (note: check with institutional guidelines). Sputum collection is best accomplished in the morning when there is a greater amount of secretions due to nighttime pooling.

Daniels, R. (2003). *Delmar's manual of laboratory and diagnostic tests.* Clifton Park, NY: Delmar Learning.

that may be useful is "huffing," or delivering a series of short, forceful exhalations, prior to actual coughing. The intent is to raise the sputum to the level where it can then be coughed out. If the client is recovering from thoracic or abdominal surgery, splinting the incision by holding a pillow firmly against it will reduce the pain caused by coughing. In most cases, assisting the client to a sitting position will increase the effectiveness of the cough.

Assess the sputum produced by coughing, noting the amount, color, and odor. Recognize that the client may become fatigued after coughing and need a rest period; also offer oral care such as a mouth rinse after sputum has been expectorated (Cronin & Mirocle, 2001).

### Initiate Postural Drainage and Chest Physiotherapy

**Postural drainage** and **chest physiotherapy (CPT)** are techniques intended to promote the drainage of secretions from the lungs. Positioning for drainage of each of the lung lobes is accompanied by percussion and/or vibration applied to the chest wall to loosen secretions (Figure 39-17). CPT percussion is clapping the chest wall with cupped hands (Archibald, 1999) (Note: This type of percussion is different from the percussion method used for assessment). Vibration is done using a special vibrator applied to the chest wall. Inhalation treatments containing bronchodilator or mucolytic drugs may be administered before chest physiotherapy and postural drainage. Clients are expected to cough up secretions in each position. When an individual is unable to cough effectively following the CPT, tracheobronchial suctioning may be used (Archibald, 1999).

Measures should be taken to minimize the client's anxiety and discomfort during these procedures. Pain medications, if indicated, should be timed so that their effectiveness peaks at the time of the treatment. Also, the nurse must recognize that some clients may be unable to tolerate certain postural drainage positions, and the treatment must be modified. Those with congestive heart failure or increased intracranial pressure particularly will not be able to tolerate a head-down position.

### Monitor Hydration

Hydration, that is, the provision of adequate fluid intake, is important in thinning the pulmonary secretions so that they may be more easily expectorated. This may be beneficial in cases of pneumonia, bronchitis, and asthma. Clients experiencing congestive heart failure, on the other hand, may require limitation of fluid intake to reduce pulmonary congestion due to fluid volume overload.

Each exhalation contains not only carbon dioxide and other gases but also water vapor. This "insensible fluid loss" will be increased in those who are tachypneic as well as in clients receiving supplemental oxygen if the oxygen is not adequately humidified. Artificial airways that bypass the natural humidification processes of the nose and oropharynx also contribute to increased insensible fluid losses. Drying and inflammation of the respiratory

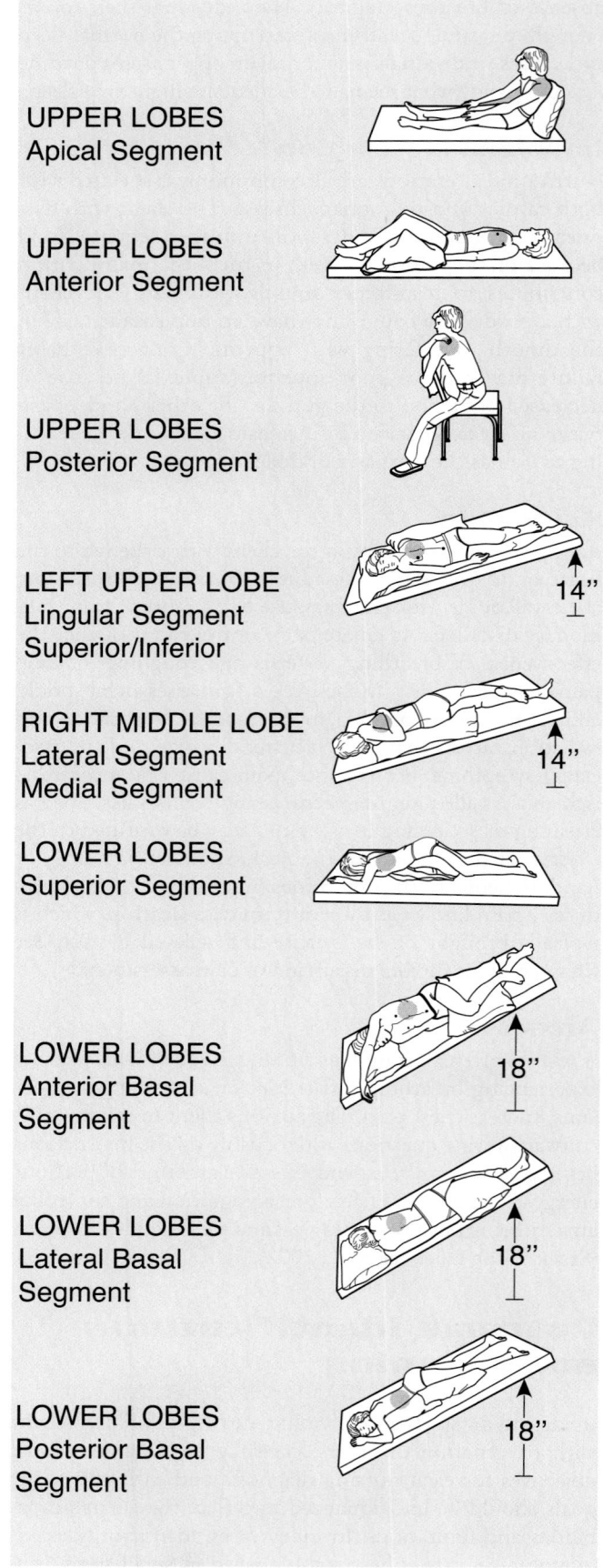

**UPPER LOBES**
Apical Segment

**UPPER LOBES**
Anterior Segment

**UPPER LOBES**
Posterior Segment

**LEFT UPPER LOBE**
Lingular Segment
Superior/Inferior          14"

**RIGHT MIDDLE LOBE**
Lateral Segment
Medial Segment             14"

**LOWER LOBES**
Superior Segment

**LOWER LOBES**
Anterior Basal
Segment                    18"

**LOWER LOBES**
Lateral Basal
Segment                    18"

**LOWER LOBES**
Posterior Basal
Segment                    18"

**Figure 39-17    Postural drainage positions**

mucosa may result. For this reason, humidification of inspired oxygen, especially that which is delivered through an artificial airway, is very important.

## Administer Medication

Medications that assist in airway clearance include expectorants, mucolytics, and bronchodilators. It may be beneficial to administer the medications before chest physiotherapy or postural drainage treatments in order to maximize the treatment's effectiveness. Clients must be taught the name of the medications they are receiving, the purpose of the medication, the dose, and how it is to be taken. The most common and/or most significant side effects should also be reviewed with the client (Kee & Hayes, 2000). A summary of medications for airway clearance is presented in Table 39-9.

## Monitor Environmental and Lifestyle Conditions

Environmental and lifestyle conditions may greatly influence the client's long-term recovery. Allergic conditions such as asthma may improve dramatically if the allergens to which the client is sensitive are identified and removed from the client's environment. Certain allergens such as animal dander or feather pillows may be relatively easy to eliminate; others, such as house dust and pollen, may be impossible to eliminate but can be reduced using devices such as air filters.

### CLINICAL ALERT

#### Women with Asthma

The number of women with asthma has increased, perhaps because women spend more time doing housework cleaning with strong chemicals and increased exposure to allergens. Women have narrower airways than men. Also, fluctuating hormones prior to menstrual period, during pregnancy, and during menopause may trigger asthmatic symptoms.

### CLINICAL ALERT

#### Cigarette Smoking

Cigarette smoking is the primary risk factor for chronic bronchitis, emphysema, and lung cancer. Lung cancer is the primary cause of cancer deaths among men and now surpasses breast cancer as the number one cancer killer in women.

## TABLE 39-9    MEDICATIONS USED FOR AIRWAY CLEARANCE

| Drug Type | Common Examples | Actions |
|---|---|---|
| Mucolytic/expectorant | Mucomyst (acetylcysteine) | Thins respiratory secretions by increasing the amount of fluid produced |
|  | Guaifenesin |  |
| Methylxanthine | Aminophylline | Dilates bronchi |
|  | Theophylline | Increases ciliary movement |
| Beta-adrenergic sympathomimetic | Epinephrine | Causes bronchial smooth muscle relaxation (dilates bronchi) |
|  | Isoproterenol |  |
|  | Albuterol |  |
|  | Metaproterenol |  |
|  | Terbutaline |  |
| Mast cell stabilizer | Cromolyn sodium | Prevents histamine release from mast cells |
| Corticosteroid | Beclomethasone | Anti-inflammatory action |
|  | Prednisone |  |
|  | Prednisolone |  |
|  | Hydrocortisone |  |

Smoking is a significant contributing factor in both heart and lung disease. Smoking cessation may not reverse advanced disease but will often reduce the client's symptoms and improve the quality of life. Smoking cessation programs and support groups, along with nicotine replacements such as transdermal patches, may help the client succeed in quitting smoking.

---

## FOCUS ON WELLNESS

### Allergies to Dust in the Home

The following are interventions the client can use to promote wellness in the home, as related to dust allergies:

- Use mask when exposed to dust and vacuuming.

- Keep allergies in check by eliminating dust from rooms, especially bedrooms. Use clean sheets. Cover mattress and pillows with protective vinyl encasements.

- Map out action plan with health care provider.
  - Use peak flow meter to measure how much air the lungs are expelling on a good day to use as a baseline. Use the meter daily to gauge the quality of your breathing compared to your personal best. If your peak flow is between 51% and 80% and remains there for 24 hours, call the health care provider, who may increase inhaled medications or add oral ones. If your peak flow is 50%, it is a red alert. Seek help immediately.
  - If you use more than 8 puffs of albuterol a day or more than your baseline dosage, it's time to contact the health care provider.
  - Trust your body. If it is sending messages to get help, do it. Stay psychologically and physically fit. Exercise can trigger an attack, but it also trains your cardiovascular and respiratory systems to do more work. A short-term beta-agonist, 15 to 20 minutes, may be prescribed to use prior to exercise.

Cronin, R., & Mirocle, K. (2001). Management of clients with lower airway and pulmonary vessels disorders. In J. Black, J. Hawks, & A. Keene (Eds.), *Medical-surgical nursing: Clinical management for continuity of care.* Philadelphia: W. B. Saunders; Gallagher, C. (2002). Childhood asthma: Tools that help parents manage it. *American Journal of Nursing, 102*(8), 71–83.

---

## Manage Artificial Airways

Artificial airways (Figure 39-18) may be used for clients with significant airway obstruction that cannot be relieved by more conservative means or who require mechanical ventilatory support. Nasal airways, also known as nasal trumpets, may be placed in conscious adults who have adequate breathing ability but require assistance in keeping their upper airways open. These airways are usually fairly well tolerated and can provide a conduit for frequent nasotracheal suctioning while minimizing trauma to the nasal mucosa.

The oral airway is used to maintain the tongue away from the posterior oropharynx in the unconscious client. It is essential to choose the correct size, since an airway that is too large may actually cause occlusion, while one that is too small may compress the tongue, stimulating the vomiting center. Oral airways are not well tolerated in conscious individuals, who may gag and vomit if an oral airway is in place.

Endotracheal tubes bypass the upper airway structures altogether; they may be inserted via the nose or mouth and are passed beyond the vocal cords into the trachea. An inflatable cuff near the distal end of the tube serves to seal off the airway, allowing for mechanical ventilatory assistance and protecting the airway from aspiration.

Since endotracheal tubes bypass the filtration and humidification normally provided by the nose and oropharynx, care must be taken to humidify the inspired air and to prevent introduction of pathogenic organisms into the lungs. Meticulous attention to aseptic technique when caring for clients with endotracheal tube and ventilator circuits is mandatory.

Mouth care must be provided for the client with an endotracheal tube. The tube prevents adequate swallowing, so the client will be unable to eat. Frequent cleansing and suctioning of the oral cavity (every 2 hours) reduces discomfort and the risk of breakdown and infection of the oral mucosa.

Nutritional needs for the client with an endotracheal tube must be addressed by providing enteral feeding (via nasogastric or gastrostomy tube) or total parenteral nutrition (hyperalimentation). Whatever the means, adequate nutrition is necessary to maintain and improve respiratory muscle strength.

---

## CLINICAL ALERT

### Artificial Airways

The cuff of an endotracheal tube or tracheostomy tube must be deflated before removing the tube; removal of a tube with an inflated cuff may cause laryngeal edema and damage to the vocal cords. For this reason, the tube must be taped securely in place, and confused or agitated clients may require sedation and/or wrist restraints to prevent them from pulling at the tube.

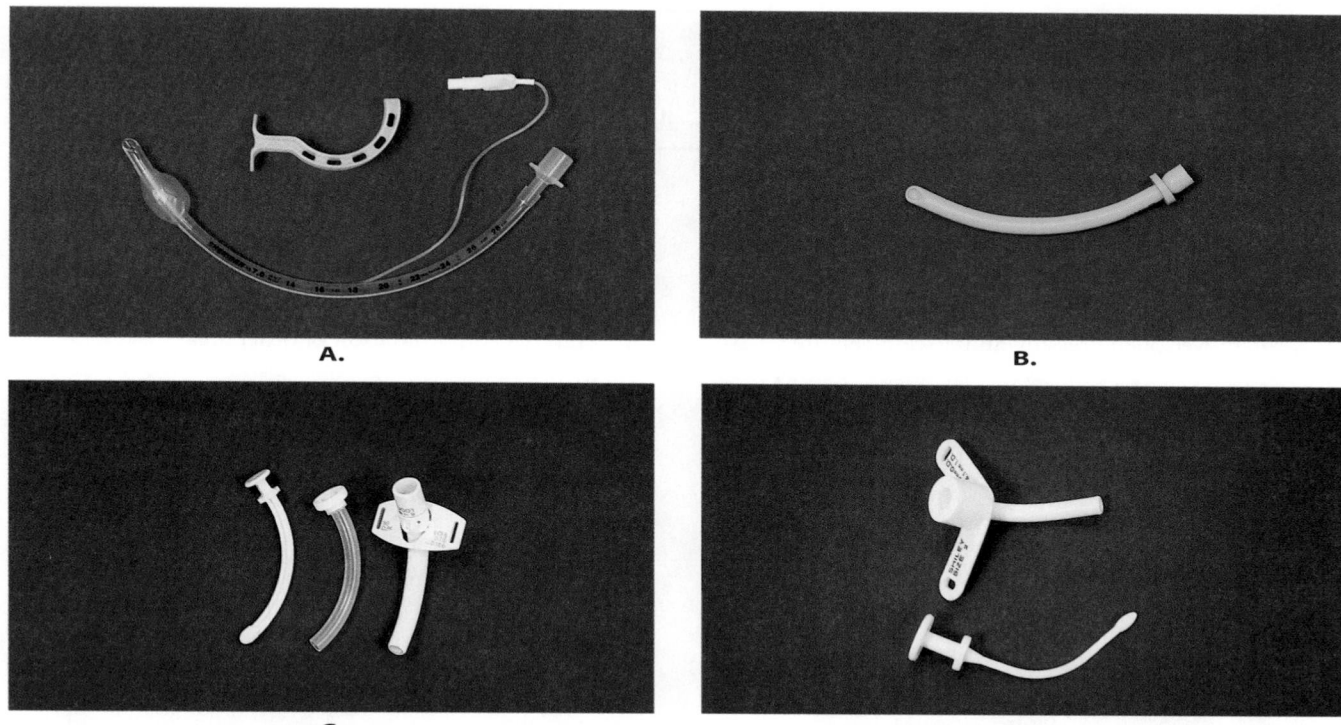

**Figure 39-18** Types of artificial airways: A. Oral airway and endotracheal tube B. Nasal trumpet C. Tracheostomy tube D. Pediatric tracheostomy tube

A **tracheotomy** is a surgical procedure done to provide long-term airway support or as an emergency procedure when an endotracheal tube cannot be passed successfully. An opening (stoma) is made in the trachea below the cricoid cartilage, and a semirigid plastic tube (tracheostomy tube) is passed through the opening and into the trachea. A cuff, similar to that in an endotracheal tube, is inflated near the distal airway.

Many tracheostomy tubes consist of two tubes or *cannulae:* an outer cannula that stays in place and an inner cannula that can be removed to be cleaned or replaced. This permits thorough removal of encrusted secretions to prevent occlusion of the airway. The outer cannula is connected to a flange that permits the tubes to be secured around the neck with twill tape or a cloth strap. See Procedure 39-1 for tracheostomy care.

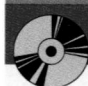

| PROCEDURE 39-1 | **Maintaining and Cleaning the Tracheostomy Tube** |

## EQUIPMENT NEEDED

- Gloves (Figure 39-19)
- Hydrogen peroxide
- Sterile water or saline
- Cotton-tip applicators
- Tracheostomy dressing (4 × 4 gauze *without* cotton lining)
- Tracheostomy ties (twill tape, intravenous tubing, or commercially available Velcro ties)

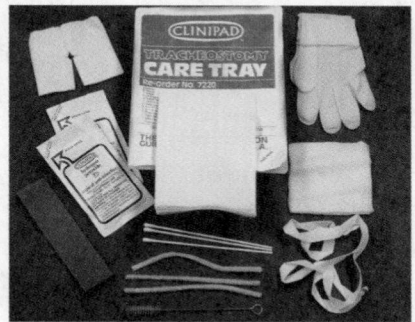

**Figure 39-19** Tracheostomy care tray, hydrogen peroxide, tape, dressing, and clean gloves

*(continues)*

**PROCEDURE 39-1** (*continued*)

## IMPLEMENTATION—ACTION/RATIONALE

| ACTION | RATIONALE |
|---|---|

### Cleaning Trach Tube Site

1. Wash hands and apply gloves.

2. Remove soiled dressing and discard (Figure 39-20).

3. Cleanse neck plate of tracheostomy tube with cotton applicators moistened with hydrogen peroxide.

4. Rinse neck plate of tracheostomy tube with applicators moistened with sterile water or saline.

5. Cleanse skin under neck plate of tube with cotton applicator moistened with hydrogen peroxide (Figure 39-21).

---

1. Reduces the transmission of microorganisms.

2. Prevents contamination of other areas.

3. Removes crusted secretions from neck plate of tracheostomy tube.

4. Removes hydrogen peroxide.

5. Removes dried and crusted secretions from under neck plate of tracheostomy tube.

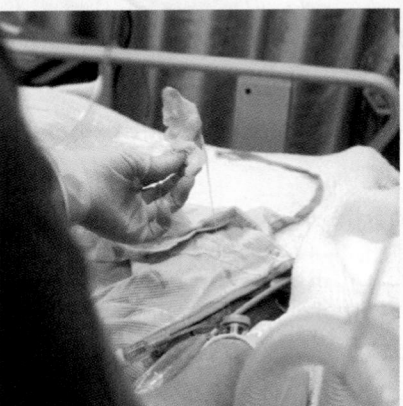

**Figure 39-20    Remove old dressings and discard.**

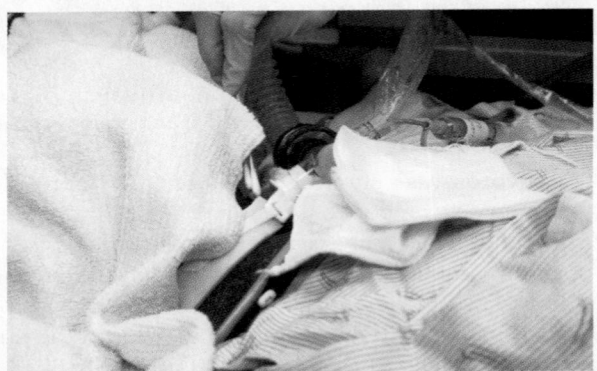

**Figure 39-21    Cleanse skin under the neck plate with a cotton applicator moistened with hydrogen peroxide.** *Note:* **The towel placed over the client's face is for privacy and is not required for the procedure.**

6. Rinse skin under neck plate with applicators moistened with sterile water or saline.

7. Dry skin under neck plate with cotton applicators.

### One-Person Technique of Changing Tracheostomy Ties

8. Prepare clean tracheostomy ties.

   • Cut a length of twill tape that will fit around the client's neck, plus 6 inches. Cut the ends of the twill tape on the diagonal.

   • Open Velcro ties on continuous neck band.

---

6. Removes hydrogen peroxide.

7. Removes moisture, which can result in skin irritation.

8. To have all equipment prepared prior to beginning procedure. A diagonal cut will make the tape easier to thread.

*(continues)*

**PROCEDURE 39-1** (*continued*)

9. Leaving the old tracheostomy ties in place, insert one end of the new tracheostomy tie through the hole in the tracheostomy neck plate from back to front. Pull the ends even, and slide both ends of the tape around the back of the head to the other side.

9. Maintains tube security while tapes are changed.

10. Insert one end of tape through the opening on the other side of the tracheostomy tube neck plate from back to front.

10. Secures tracheostomy tube.

11. Tie the two ends of the new tape with a square knot at side of neck. Keep two fingers under the tape as the knot is tied. Without putting pressure on the neck plate or the tape, pull on the knot to make sure it will stay tied.

11. Secures tracheostomy tube. Fingers under tape prevent the tape from being tied too tightly.

12. Cut and remove old tracheostomy tapes and discard. Hold the neck plate firmly with one hand while cutting the old tapes.

12. Old tapes can be removed once the tracheostomy tube has been secured. Holding the plate firmly prevents dislodgment if the new tie is accidentally cut.

13. Place one finger under tracheostomy ties.

13. Checks for tightness and security.

**Two-Person Technique of Changing Tracheostomy Ties**

14. Cut two pieces of twill tape about 12 to 14 inches in length.

14. Prepares equipment prior to beginning procedure.

15. Make a fold about 1 inch below the end of each piece of twill tape and cut a half-inch slit lengthwise in the center of the fold.

15. Prepares tape for insertion.

16. Have a second person gently hold the tracheostomy tube in place with fingers on both sides of the neck plate.

16. Prevents accidental movement of the tracheostomy tube resulting in coughing and accidental decannulation.

17. Cut old tracheostomy ties and discard.

17. Removes tracheostomy ties.

18. Insert the split end of the tracheostomy tape through the opening on one side of the tracheostomy tube neck plate. Pull the distal end of the tracheostomy tie through the cut end and pull tightly.

18. Secures tracheostomy tie within neck plate.

19. Repeat procedure with second piece of twill tape.

19. Secures tracheostomy tube.

20. Tie tracheostomy tapes with a double knot at the side of the neck.

20. Secures tracheostomy tube.

21. Insert one finger under tracheostomy tapes.

21. Ensures that tube has been tied securely.

22. Insert tracheostomy gauze under neck plate of tube (Figure 39-22).

22. Prevents irritation of skin from secretions and rubbing of tracheostomy tube.

*(continues)*

**PROCEDURE 39-1** (*continued*)

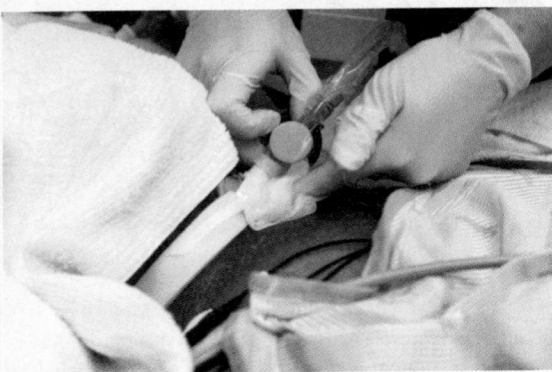

**Figure 39-22    Insert gauge under neck plate of the tracheostomy tube.**

23. Discard all used materials and wash hands.

23. Reduces transmission of microorganisms.

## COMMUNITY/HOME CARE

### Tracheostomy Care in the Home

*Home Care Variations*

- The procedure is a clean technique in a home care setting.

- Good handwashing technique should be stressed.

- Use tap water for rinsing the inner cannula.

- Inner cannula care should be performed on a routine basis.

- Normal saline can be made by adding 2 teaspoons of table salt to 1 quart of boiled water.

- Store normal saline in a quart or pint jar that has been sterilized.

*Long-Term Care Variations*

- Care of the tracheostomy tube may be done by the nursing personnel or the client.

- It is a "sterile" procedure if done by the nurse and a "clean" technique if done by the client.

Like an endotracheal tube, a tracheostomy tube bypasses the upper airways, so humidification and prevention of infection must be considered. Because both types of airways prevent the movement of air through the vocal cords, which produce speech, the client will not be able to talk while these tubes are in place (some long-term tracheostomy clients may be outfitted with a tracheostomy tube that has slits, or "fenestrations," that permit speech). If possible, reviewing an alternate method of communication prior to tube insertion can reduce the anxiety and isola-

tion that may be felt by the intubated client. Writing of messages and use of an alphabet board are two possible methods of communication. Significant others should also be advised that the intubated client will not be able to speak but can hear and understand what is being said.

### Suction the Airway

Suctioning of the airway, whether a natural or artificial airway, may be necessary to clear secretions the client cannot remove by coughing. Suctioning becomes especially important when an endotracheal tube or tracheostomy tube is present, because coughing is significantly impaired by these devices.

Nasotracheal suctioning involves passing a suction catheter or nasal trumpet through the nare, down the pharynx, through the larynx, and into the trachea. See Procedure 39-2 regarding suctioning. Once the tip is in the trachea, a strong cough reflex will often be elicited. At this time suction is applied to the catheter and it is withdrawn while a twisting motion is applied to the catheter.

Endotracheal suctioning involves passing the suction catheter through the endotracheal tube or tracheostomy into the trachea and applying suction as the catheter is withdrawn.

---

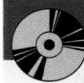 **PROCEDURE 39-2**   ## Suctioning Endotracheal and Tracheal Tubes

### EQUIPMENT NEEDED

- Sterile gloves (Figures 39-23 and 39-24)
- Mask, eye protection, and gown if appropriate
- Source of negative pressure (suction machine or wall suction)

- Sterile suction catheter
- Oxygen or Ambu bag
- Equipment for tracheostomy care or tracheostomy care tray

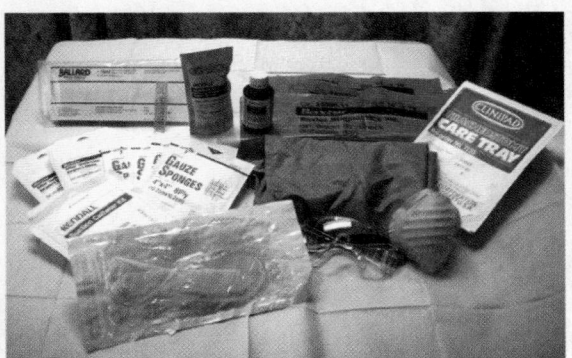

**Figure 39-23   Protective gear, dressing, and a tracheostomy care tray**

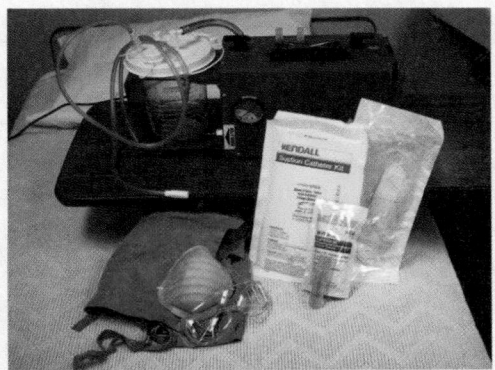

**Figure 39-24   Protective gear and suction equipment**

### IMPLEMENTATION—ACTION/RATIONALE

| ACTION | RATIONALE |
|---|---|
| **Suctioning Tracheal Tube** | |
| 1. Assess depth and rate of respirations; auscultate breath sounds (Figure 39-25). | 1. Determines need for suctioning. |
| 2. Assemble supplies on bedside table. | 2. Organizes work. |
| 3. Wash hands. | 3. Reduces transmission of microorganisms. |
| 4. Connect suction tube to source of negative pressure. | 4. Prepares for suctioning procedure. |
| 5. Administer oxygen or use Ambu bag before beginning procedure. | 5. Hyperoxygenates client and prevents hypoxia during suctioning. |
| 6. Remove inner cannula and place in basin of hydrogen peroxide to loosen secretions, if reusable, or set aside if disposable (Figure 39-26). Do not dispose of disposable cannula until new inner cannula is securely in place. | 6. Suctioning should be performed after inner cannula has been removed to allow easier passage of the suction catheter. Retain the old cannula until you are sure the new cannula fits correctly. |

*(continues)*

## PROCEDURE 39-2 (*continued*)

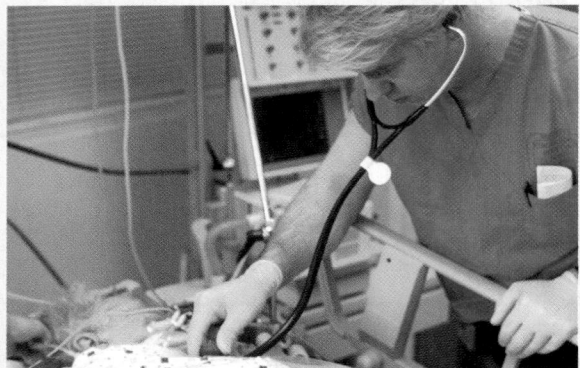

**Figure 39-25    Assess respirations and auscultate breath sounds.**

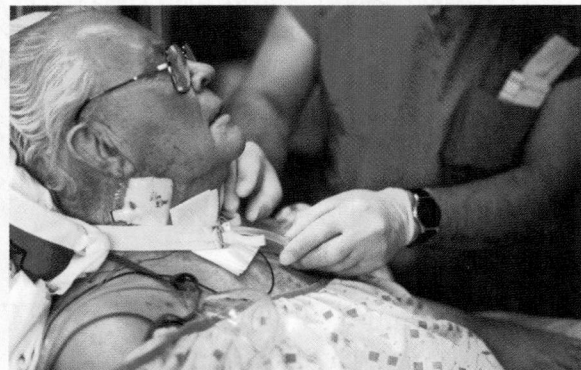

**Figure 39-26    Remove the inner cannula.**

7.  Apply sterile glove to your dominant hand.

8.  Open sterile suction catheter or use the reusable closed system catheter. The sterile suction catheter is removed from the package with your dominant, sterile hand. Wrap the catheter tubing around your hand from the tip of the catheter down to the port end. Attach catheter to suction.

9.  Insert the catheter into the trachea without suction.

10. Apply suction intermittently while gently rotating the catheter and removing it.

    • In a disposable catheter, suction is applied by placing the thumb of your dominant hand over the open port of the catheter connector.

    • In a closed system catheter, suction is applied by depressing the white button at the connector end of the catheter.

11. Wrap the disposable suction catheter around your sterile, dominant hand while withdrawing it from the endotracheal tube.

12. Suction for no more than 10 seconds.

13. Administer oxygen using the sigh function on the ventilator or using an Ambu bag.

14. Assess airway and repeat suctioning as necessary.

15. Clean inner cannula using tracheostomy brush and rinse well in sterile water or sterile saline. Dry (or open new disposable inner cannula).

16. Reinsert inner cannula and lock into place.

17. Apply humidified oxygen or compressed air (Figure 39-27).

7.  For sterile technique.

8.  This maintains catheter sterility and prevents accidental contamination.

9.  Minimizes removal of oxygen and trauma to the tracheal mucosa.

10. Increases removal of mucus while minimizing irritation to tracheal mucosa.

11. This prevents accidental contamination of the catheter.

12. Prevents hypoxia.

13. Reoxygenates the client.

14. Determines need to continue suctioning.

15. Removes secretions and maintains patent inner cannula.

16. Prevents secretions from obstructing outer cannula.

17. Thins secretions.

*(continues)*

## PROCEDURE 39-2 (*continued*)

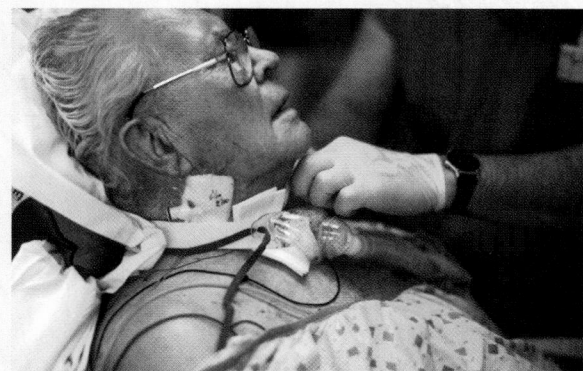

**Figure 39-27    Attach oxygen.**

18. Remove gloves and discard.

19. Wash hands.

20. Record the procedure and client's tolerance of the procedure, including amount and consistency of secretions.

### Suctioning an Endotracheal Tube

21. Repeat Actions 1 to 14 (Figures 39-28 and 39-29).

18. Prevents transmission of microorganisms to other clients.

19. Reduces transmission of microorganisms.

20. Provides documentation of the procedure.

21. See Rationales 1 to 14.

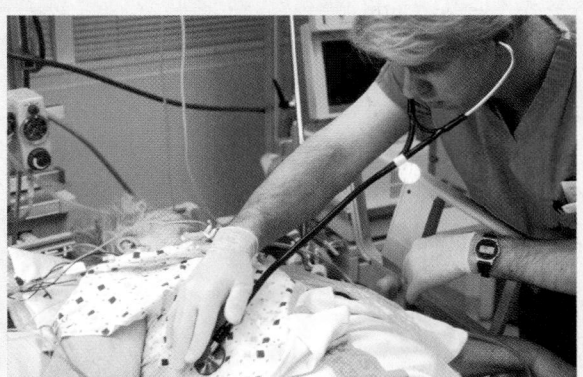

**Figure 39-28    Assess for respiratory rate and lung sounds. Repeat suctioning if needed.**

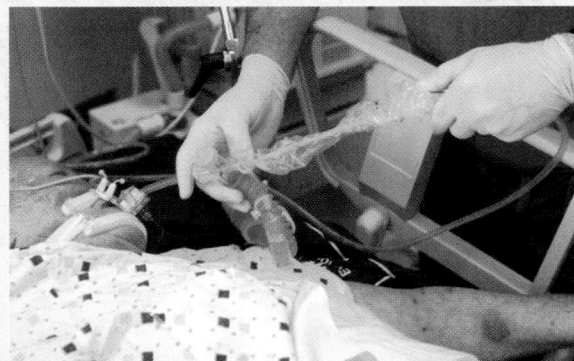

**Figure 39-29    Endotracheal suctioning: Apply suction while gently rotating the catheter and removing it. Do not suction for more than 10 seconds.**

22. Remove gloves and discard.

23. Wash hands.

24. Record the procedure and client's tolerance of the procedure, including amount and consistency of secretions.

22. Prevents transmission of microorganisms to other clients.

23. Reduces transmission of microorganisms.

24. Provides documentation of the procedure.

## LIFE SPAN CONSIDERATIONS

### Suctioning Tubes

*Pediatric Variations*

- In infants and young children, airways have smaller diameters, the glottis is higher, the thorax is smaller, and the diaphragm is higher. Be sure to use a suction catheter with the proper diameter, and be sure not to insert it too deeply.

- The amount of negative pressure necessary for suctioning an infant or child is much less than the pressure needed for an adult.

- The infant's or child's head should be turned to the right or left to facilitate bronchial suctioning on that side.

- The size of the suction catheter used depends upon the age of the client and size of the tracheostomy tube.

- The suction catheter should be of a diameter equal to or less than one-half the inside diameter of the tracheostomy tube.

*Geriatric Variations*

- The tissues of the trachea and bronchi may be more fragile and need special care when suctioning.

- Older clients with decreased levels of consciousness, impaired gag reflex, stroke, chronic obstructive pulmonary disease, congestive heart failure, and pulmonary edema may be at greater risk for retained secretions.

- Older clients may have lost some properties of elastic recoil and gas exchange.

## COMMUNITY/HOME CARE

### Suctioning Tubes

*Home Care Variations*

- All self-care instructions need to be reinforced before the client leaves the hospital.

- Durable medical equipment must be available in the home prior to hospital discharge.

- Specific instructions related to durable medical equipment need to be given to the client and/or family before and after discharge.

*Long-Term Care Variations*

- A source of humidity and oxygen is needed for clients in long-term care.

- Promoting adequate fluid intake may help decrease the client's risk for thick secretions.

# Interventions to Improve Breathing Patterns

## Position Client Properly

Client positioning to improve breathing patterns may begin by taking cues from the client. If the client finds that breathing is easier in an upright or sitting position, you should allow that position to be maintained. Supporting the client with elevation of the head of the bed or with pillows can reduce the client's workload and minimize fatigue. Maintaining proper body alignment and preventing slouching or slumping in the bed increase the efficiency of ventilatory efforts.

As previously stated, clients with obstructive respiratory disease may find that leaning forward, with the clavicles elevated, is most comfortable. Providing an overbed table

## NURSING STRATEGY

### General Guidelines for Tracheal Suctioning

1. Explain the procedure to the client, including the expected benefits.
2. Because suctioning removes air (and oxygen) from the client's airways as well as secretions, care must be taken to avoid excessive suctioning and prevent severe oxygen desaturation. In particular:

   a. Do not apply excessive negative pressure (suction) to the catheter; suction levels should not exceed 80–100 cm H2O. In addition to causing oxygen desaturation, excessive suction can damage the tracheal mucosa.

   b. Do not suction for more than 10 to 15 seconds. Apply intermittent suction only while the catheter is being withdrawn. Do not suction until the catheter is introduced and the cough reflex is stimulated.

   c. Provide supplemental oxygen before and after suctioning by increasing the oxygen flow or concentration (unless contraindicated) and encouraging the client to take several deep breaths. Clients with endotracheal or tracheostomy tubes may be hyperoxygenated using a manual resuscitation bag with high-flow oxygen attached.

3. Use sterile technique in handling the suction catheter, and observe standard precautions to prevent cross-contamination.
4. After suctioning, provide mouth care and suction the oropharynx if indicated. Assist the client to a comfortable position and allow for a rest period.

for the client on which to rest his elbows may facilitate this position, *provided the wheels are locked or removed to prevent the table from rolling away and placing the client at risk for a fall.*

### Teach Controlled Breathing Exercises

Controlled breathing exercises may also improve breathing efficiency for the client with obstructive respiratory disease. One technique that is especially useful is *pursed-lip breathing*. This technique involves forced exhalation against pursed (partially closed) lips, which maintains positive pressure in the lungs during the expiratory phase and prevents collapse of the smaller airways. This in turn reduces the amount of air trapping characteristic of obstructive disease (Collins et al., 2000).

## RESEARCH FOCUS

**Title of Study:** Breathing pattern retraining and exercise in persons with chronic obstructive pulmonary disease

**Study Purpose:** The primary purpose of this study was to explore the potential for integrating breathing retraining into pulmonary rehabilitation as a method to decrease symptoms of chronic lung disease, such as dyspnea, with physical activity.

**Methods:** The study examined several research reports describing the various techniques used in pulmonary rehabilitation programs to improve the capability of persons who had COPD to perform activities of daily living.

**Findings:** Most rehabilitation programs were structured to assist participants to establish the upper limits for activities at a tolerable level of breathlessness. However, persons with COPD take smaller breaths at a more frequent rate than people with normal lung capacity. "The smaller breaths conserve energy in the short-term but contribute to respiratory muscle fatigue and hyperinflation as the work of exercise increases or is prolonged." The efficiency of the breathing patterns was markedly deteriorated as the participants approached 80% of their peak aerobic capacity. A few studies emphasized pursed lip and diaphragmatic breathing and biofeedback techniques. Electromyography biofeedback was used in one study to teach relaxation to assist in managing the frequent anxiety and dyspnea experienced by persons with COPD.

**Implications:** It is very important that persons with COPD remain physically active to improve their quality of life. Nurses can reinforce rehabilitation techniques and help clients master the controlled breathing techniques during activities as well as at rest. The usefulness of controlled breathing should be evaluated on an individual basis. Further research is indicated to support these physical and psychological findings for individuals with COPD in performing different activities.

Collins, E., Langbein, W., Fehr, L., & Maloney, C. (2001). Breathing pattern retraining and exercise in persons with chronic obstructive pulmonary disease. *AACN Clinical Issues: Advanced Practice of Critical-Care Nurses, 12*(2), 202–209.

*Deep-breathing exercises* encourage the client to take slow, deep breaths instead of the rapid, shallow breathing pattern that may be present in restrictive lung disease and in

## CLINICAL ALERT

### Safety

Clients with oxygenation impairment may be confused or agitated, making safety a vital concern of the nurse.

those who are anxious or in pain. Abdominal breathing involves the use of the abdominal muscles to pull the diaphragm downward. Placing your hand on the client's abdomen and instructing the client to watch it rise give a visual aid to teaching the technique.

Apical and basal expansion exercises direct the client to focus on achieving maximal expansion of the upper lung lobes (apices) and lower lobes (bases), respectively. To perform these techniques, place your hands flat against the chest wall just below the clavicles for apical exercises or over the lower ribs along the midaxillary lines for basal exercise and apply gentle pressure. Instruct the client to push your hands away with the chest wall by breathing. These exercises should be repeated several times a day.

## NURSING STRATEGY

### Teaching Purse-Lipped Breathing

- Select a time that is convenient for you and when the client can be focused on learning and understanding the purpose for using the technique.

- Have client assume a sitting position (in chair or bed) to facilitate descent of the diaphragm.

- Instruct the client to inhale slowly through the nose with the lips closed (you may choose to count the numbers, 1-2, slowly).

- Ask the client to form the lips as to whistle and to exhale slowly (4 to 6 seconds) through the lips. Tell the client to listen for a "whooshing" sound as the air passes through the lips.

- Provide positive reinforcement. Encourage the client to practice the exercise and to use the technique frequently to relieve dyspnea at rest and during and after exercise.

Adapted from Archibald, C. (1999). Oxygenation. In K. Berger, & M. Williams (Eds.), *Fundamentals of nursing* (pp. 999–1086). Stamford, CT: Appleton & Lange; Collins, E., Langbein, W., Fehr, L., & Maloney, C. (2001). Breathing pattern retraining and exercise in persons with chronic obstructive pulmonary disease. *AACN Clinical Issues: Advanced Practice of Critical-Care Nurses, 12*(2), 202–209.

Incentive spirometry is another technique used to encourage deep breathing. The client draws air through the spirometry device, which measures the volume of air displaced by moving a float ball or similar device up a col-

## NURSING STRATEGY

### Strategies to Prevent Hypoventilation in Acute Care Setting

- Elevate head of bed at least 30 degrees to facilitate descent of the diaphragm and action of intercostal muscles.

- Change client's position at least every 2 hours. Maintain client's chest alignment.

- Encourage client to take a deep breath and hold at least 3 seconds every 1 to 2 hours while awake to expand alveoli.

- Encourage client to take 10 deep breaths using incentive spirometer every 1 to 2 hours while awake. (This provides client with a visual feedback regarding progress.)

- Auscultate the chest during inhalation (inflation) to determine that all dependent parts of the lungs are well ventilated.

- Be aware that postoperative chest surgery clients are encouraged to cough only to assist in mobilizing secretions for removal. For clients in respiratory failure, coughing is avoided unless secretions are present, because coughing promotes collapse of the smaller airways.

- Coughing is most effective with client sitting in upright position. If unable to do so, have client lie on side with hips and knees flexed to decrease abdominal tension.

- Teach client to splint incisions and painful areas when changing positions, coughing, or performing movements that cause discomfort.

- Provide comfort measures to reduce pain and anxiety prior to procedures or activities (analgesics are frequently prescribed prior to a painful procedure to assist the client).

Keene, A. (2001). Health history. In J. Black, J. Hawks, & A. Keene (Eds.), *Medical-surgical nursing: Clinical management for continuity of care.* Philadelphia: W. B. Saunders; Stacy, K. (2000). Pulmonary disorders. In L. Urden, & K. Stacy (Eds.), *Priorities in critical care nursing.* St. Louis: Mosby.

## CLIENT REFLECTIONS

### Cascade Coughing

Mr. Nottingham is 54 years old, has pneumonia related to a postoperative infection, and is hospitalized for continued respiratory insufficiency. The following comments were made by Mr. Nottingham while he was learning to perform cascade coughing methods: "I felt the need to cough, but it was so painful. Even holding a pillow tight against my chest didn't help very much, and I couldn't get rid of the mucus. My nurse raised the head of my bed and told me to take a slow deep breath and to hold it for 2 seconds. Then he told me to try to breathe out while contracting my diaphragm and stomach muscles, and to open my mouth, cover it with a tissue, and cough repeatedly without taking in another breath. Then I should breathe in slowly, rest for a short time, and repeat the same process about three times. He explained that the technique was called cascade coughing. I really felt like I breathed better after performing this coughing exercise."

What did this nurse do that worked well with this client?

umn. Goals (incentives) can be marked on the spirometer, and the client can compare her progress with the desired goal. Incentive spirometry is often performed in the care of postoperative clients and is usually done every 1 to 2 hours while awake.

Deep breathing may also be augmented using intermittent positive-pressure breathing (IPPB). An IPPB machine delivers a volume of air under pressure through a mouthpiece when the client draws air through the mouthpiece. IPPB requires the client's cooperation, so preparatory teaching is essential. IPPB may include the administration of aerosolized medications and may be followed by coughing exercise, CPT, and postural drainage (Cronin & Mirocle, 2001).

### Manage Chest Drainage Systems

Chest drainage systems (chest tubes) improve breathing patterns by removing accumulations of air and/or fluid from the pleural space, permitting the lungs to return to normal expansion. The tubes are inserted through the chest wall via a stab wound; multiple holes in the tip of the tube collect drainage from the pleural space. This drainage is then collected into a drainage system by either suction control or gravity. A special feature called a water seal prevents the reintroduction of air into the pleural space through the chest tube.

Chest tubes are inserted for clients following thoracic surgery, as emergency measures for immediate relief for air leak disorders (pneumothorax), and for hemothorax (presence of blood usually due to blunt or penetrating chest trauma) (Archibald, 1999; Thelan, Urden, Lough, & Stacy, 1998). (Note: a discussion of advanced nursing care of these seriously ill clients and for maintaining the chest tube system is beyond the scope of this text.)

## Interventions to Improve Oxygen Uptake and Delivery

### Administer Oxygen

Oxygen uptake in the pulmonary capillary beds can be improved by increasing the concentration of oxygen in the alveolar air; this increase in the partial pressure of oxygen in the alveoli ($PaO_2$) increases the driving pressure for gas diffusion across the alveolar-capillary membrane.

The percentage of oxygen in the inspired air is referred to as the fraction of inspired oxygen, or $FiO_2$, expressed as a percentage; normal atmospheric air has an $FiO_2$ of 21%. Supplemental oxygen delivery systems are capable of increasing the $FiO_2$ to anywhere from 24% to nearly 100% oxygen (see Procedure 39-3).

Low-flow oxygen delivery systems provide supplemental oxygen. These systems cannot regulate the exact amount of oxygen that a client takes in, because room air enters the device as the client breathes. Therefore, the client's respiratory rate and depth determines the mix of room air and oxygen taken in. Humidifiers attached to the oxygen delivery systems prevent drying and irritation of the respiratory tract, prevent loss of body water, and facilitate secretion removal (Archibald, 1999; Stacy, 2000).

Oxygen administration, like the administration of any drug, is not without hazards. Clients who have chronic pulmonary disease associated with carbon dioxide retention (hypercapnia) may become insensitive to carbon dioxide levels to drive their respiratory rate. Instead, these clients may depend upon a chronic low oxygen level in the blood (hypoxemia) to stimulate their respiratory drive.

## LIFE SPAN CONSIDERATIONS

### Monitoring Oxygen in Older Clients

The following are considerations for older clients when administering oxygen:

1. Maintain low-flow oxygen therapy. *Older clients are more susceptible to oxygen-induced respiratory depression.*
2. Use central nervous system depressants carefully. *Older clients are prone to respiratory depression.*

Hogstel, M. (2001). *Gerontology: Nursing care of the older adult.* Clifton Park, NY: Delmar Learning.

**PROCEDURE 39-3**    **Administering Oxygen Therapy**

## EQUIPMENT NEEDED

- Stethoscope (Figures 39-30, 39-31, and 39-32)
- Oxygen source—portable or in-line
- Oxygen flow meter
- Oxygen delivery device: nasal cannula, mask, tent, or T-tube with adapter for artificial airway
- Oxygen tubing
- Pulse oximetry (optional)
- Humidifier and distilled or sterile water (not needed with low flow rates per nasal cannula)

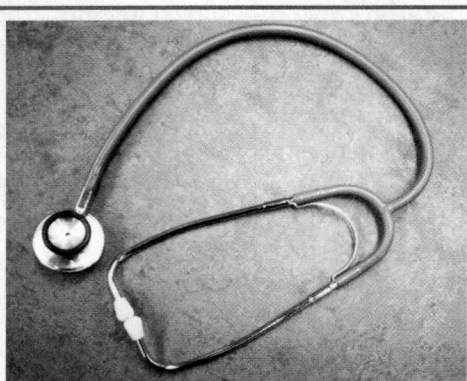

Figure 39-30    Stethoscope

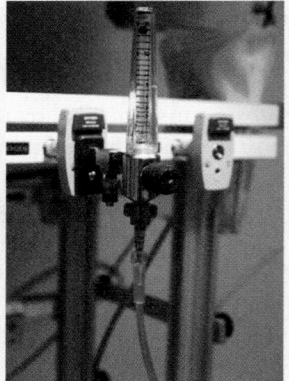

**Figure 39-31    In-line oxygen and flow meter**

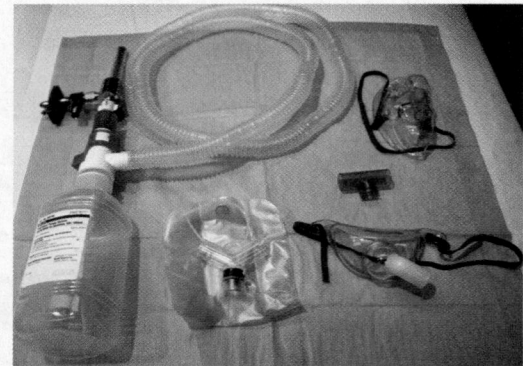

**Figure 39-32    Humidifier, reservoir bag, tracheostomy mask, T-tube, and a simple face mask are used when administering oxygen therapy.**

## IMPLEMENTATION—ACTION/RATIONALE

| ACTION | RATIONALE |
|---|---|
| **Nasal Cannula (Figure 39-33)** | |
| 1. Wash hands. | 1. Reduces transmission of microorganisms. |
| 2. Verify the physician's or qualified practitioner's order. | 2. Ensures correct dosage and route. |
| 3. Explain procedure and hazards to the client. Remind clients who smoke of the reasons for no smoking while $O_2$ is in use. | 3. Increases compliance with procedures. Oxygen supports combustion. |
| 4. If using humidity, fill humidifier to fill line with distilled water and close container. | 4. Prevents drying of the client's airway and thins any secretions. |
| 5. Attach humidifier to oxygen flow meter. | 5. Allows the oxygen to pass through the water and become humidified. |

*(continues)*

6. Insert humidifier and flow meter into oxygen source in wall or portable unit.

6. For access to oxygen. Many institutions also have compressed air available from outlets very similar in appearance to oxygen outlets. Green always stands for oxygen. Be sure to plug the flow meter into the green outlet.

7. Attach the oxygen tubing and nasal cannula to the flow meter and turn it on to the prescribed flow rate (1–5 liters/min). Use extension tubing for ambulatory clients so they can get up to go to the bathroom (Figure 39-34).

7. Rates above 6 liters/minute are not efficacious and can dry the nasal mucosa.

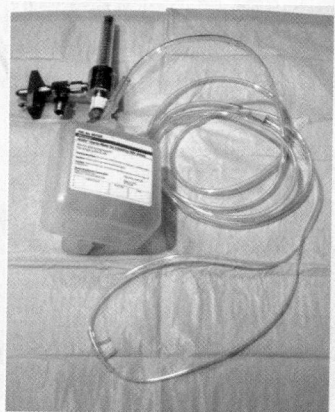

**Figure 39-33   Nasal cannula and oxygen tubing attached to a humidifier**

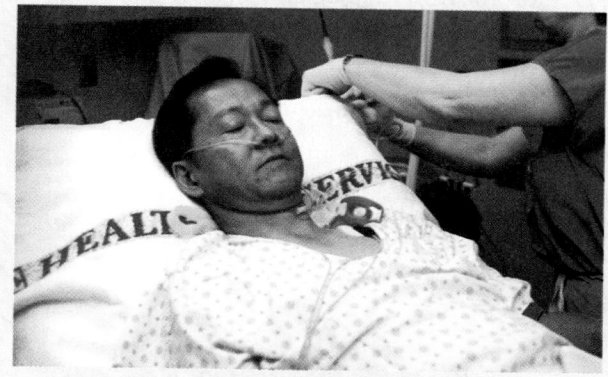

**Figure 39-34   Oxygen delivered via a nasal cannula**

8. Check for bubbling in the humidifier.

8. Ensures proper functioning.

9. Place the nasal prongs in the client's nostrils. Secure the cannula in place by adjusting the tubing around the client's ears and using the slip ring to stabilize it under the client's chin.

9. Keeps delivery system in place so client receives the amount of oxygen ordered.

10. Check for proper flow rate every 4 hours.

10. Ensures that client receives proper dose. The nasal cannula is a low flow system because it administers oxygen while the client also inspires room air. The actual dose of oxygen received by the client will vary depending on the client's respiratory pattern.

11. Assess client nostrils every 8 hours. If the client complains of dryness or has signs of irritation, use sterile lubricant to keep mucous membranes moist. Add humidifier if not already in place.

11. Dry membranes are more prone to breakdown by friction or pressure from nasal cannula.

12. Monitor vital signs, oxygen saturation, and client condition every 4 to 8 hours for signs and symptoms of hypoxia.

12. Detects any untoward effects from therapy.

13. Wean client from oxygen as soon as possible using standard protocols.

13. Oxygen is not without side effects and should be used only as long as needed. Problems with reimbursement may develop if criteria for therapy are not met.

(continues)

## PROCEDURE 39-3 (continued)

**Mask: Venturi (high flow device), simple mask (low flow), partial rebreather mask, nonrebreather mask, and face tent**

14. Wash hands.

15. Repeat Actions 2 to 6.

16. Attach appropriately sized mask (Figure 39-35) or face tent to oxygen tubing and turn on flow meter to prescribed flow rate. The Venturi mask will have color-coded inserts that list the flow rate necessary to obtain the desired percentage of oxygen. Allow the reservoir bag of the nonrebreathing or partial rebreathing mask to fill completely. Figure 39-36 shows several types of oxygen masks.

14. Reduces transmission of microorganisms.

15. See Rationales 2 to 6.

16. To ensure proper fit, determine the size needed based on the client's size. Checks the oxygen source and primes the tubing and mask or tent.

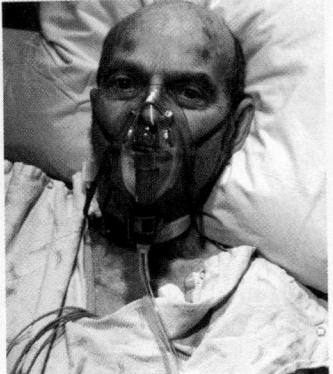

**Figure 39-35    Make sure the mask used is the appropriate size for the client.**

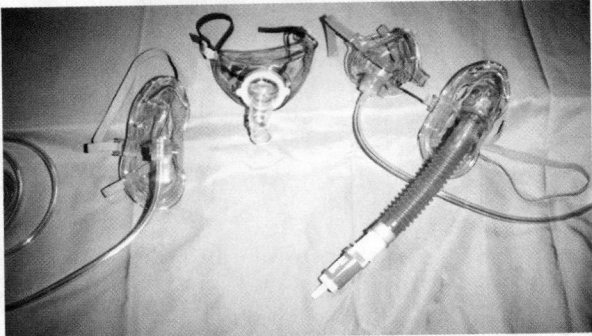

**Figure 39-36    Different types of oxygen masks: simple oxygen mask, tracheostomy mask, pediatric mask, and Venturi mask**

17. Check for bubbling in the humidifier.

18. Place the mask or tent on the client's face, fasten the elastic band around the client's ears, and tighten until the mask fits snugly.

19. Check for proper flow rate every 4 hours.

20. Ensure that the ports of the Venturi mask are not under covers or impeded by any other source.

21. Assess client's face and ears for pressure from the mask and use padding as needed.

22. Wean client to nasal cannula and then wean off oxygen per protocol.

17. Ensures proper functioning.

18. Prevents loss of oxygen from the sides of the mask.

19. Ensures that client is receiving the proper dose.

20. Air must be entrained to mix room air and oxygen coming from source to ensure proper oxygen percentage ($FIO_2$).

21. Provides client comfort and prevents skin breakdown.

22. Oxygen is not without side effects and should be used only as long as needed. The nasal cannula provides a lower $FIO_2$ than the mask. Problems with reimbursement may develop if criteria for therapy are not met.

*(continues)*

**PROCEDURE 39-3 (*continued*)**

### Oxygen via an Artificial Airway (tracheostomy or endotracheal tube)

23. Wash hands.

24. Verify the physician's or qualified practitioner's order.

25. Fill the humidifier with water and close the container.

26. Attach humidifier and warmer to the oxygen flow meter (Figure 39-37).

27. Attach the wide-bore oxygen tubing and T-tube adapter or tracheostomy mask to the flow meter and turn the meter to the flow rate needed to achieve the prescribed oxygen concentration. An oxygen analyzer may be used to check the actual oxygen percentage being delivered.

28. Check for bubbling in the humidifier and a fine mist from the adapter.

29. Attach the T-piece to the client's artificial airway or place the mask over the client's airway. Be sure the T-piece is firmly attached to the airway (Figure 39-38).

23. Reduces transmission of microorganisms.

24. Ensures correct dosage and time.

25. Avoids contamination of the water.

26. Humidification and warming of the air is essential with an artificial airway because the upper airway is bypassed by the tube.

27. Checks the oxygen source and primes the tubing and adapter.

28. Ensures proper functioning.

29. Ensures that client will not develop complications related to an interrupted oxygen supply.

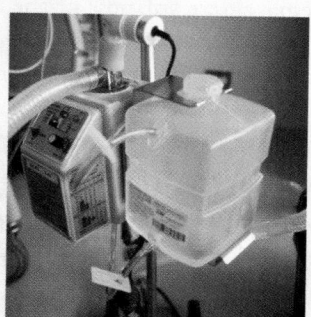

**Figure 39-37　Oxygen humidifier and warmer**

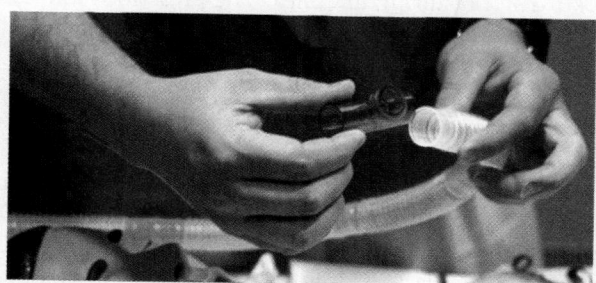

**Figure 39-38　Attach the T-piece to the oxygen tubing.**

30. Position tubing so that it is not pulling client's airway.

31. Check for proper flow rate and patency of the system every 1 to 2 hours depending on the acuity of the client. Suction as needed to maintain a patent airway.

32. Monitor airway patency, vital signs, oxygen saturation, and for signs and symptoms of hypoxia every 2 hours. Additionally, monitor breath sounds and tube position every 4 hours.

33. Wean client from therapy as ordered by physician or qualified practitioner. The client will probably receive oxygen via another route once the tube is removed. Some clients have tracheotomies permanently.

30. Provides for client comfort and prevents dislodgment of the artificial airway.

31. Ensures that client is receiving proper dose.

32. Detects response to or any untoward effects from therapy. Determines whether tube is in place.

33. Prevents untoward effects of oxygen.

## COMMUNITY/HOME CARE

### Oxygen Therapy

*Home Care Variations*

- Oxygen may be provided by a high-pressure cylinder, an oxygen concentrator, or a liquid oxygen system. Spare tanks and a backup power source are recommended. Compressed oxygen gas in a cylinder is available in sizes H or K for large stationary tanks and sizes D and E for travel and in the event there is power failure. Portable carts and carrying shoulder cases are also available. The company supplying the equipment will usually have personnel that will help with the setup and specific cleaning needs of the oxygen source.

- While any delivery system may be used in the home, nasal cannulas and tracheostomy tents/masks are the most commonly used. Home care clients may receive oxygen via a Spofford Christopher Oxygen Optimizing Prosthesis transtracheal system (SCOOP) catheter placed down into the trachea via a small stoma. It is held in place by a bead chain necklace and needs regular cleaning. Tubing, delivery system, and humidifier container should be washed regularly every 2 to 7 days with soap and water, disinfected, and dried before reuse, so an alternate setup should be available. Post safety precautions in the home. Oxygen sources should be kept from heating units, walls, drapes, and combustible substances such as hair spray.

*Long-Term Care Variations*

- Long-term clients are more likely to develop skin irritation and mucous membrane dryness from oxygen therapy. Padding may be needed at friction sites. Humidity may be needed to reduce dryness.

While low-flow oxygen may be beneficial to these clients, excessive oxygen administration may obliterate that hypoxic drive, resulting in apnea. The prescribed amount of supplemental oxygen should be maintained. Instruct all health care personnel, clients, and visitors not to adjust the volume. Oxygen administration can be dangerous due to the flammable nature of the oxygen. In addition, take precautions when administering oxygen to older clients.

Another possible hazard of oxygen administration is oxygen toxicity. Prolonged administration of high $FiO_2$ (greater than 50% for more than 24 hours) may actually damage lung tissue and produce severe respiratory difficulties. The mechanisms by which oxygen toxicity occurs are twofold. First, it should be understood that 78% of the inspired air consists of the gas nitrogen. Although nitrogen is (under normal conditions) physiologically inert, it does serve an important function in the lung: it keeps the alveoli open simply by occupying space. High concentrations of oxygen displace nitrogen from the alveoli; as this oxygen is absorbed by the alveolar capillary blood, the volume of gas in the alveolar space is reduced and the alveoli collapse. Once the alveoli have collapsed (atelectasis), no airflow occurs and the work of breathing increases dramatically.

Second, oxygen in high concentrations is toxic to the type II alveolar cells, which are responsible for the production of **surfactant**. Surfactant is a substance that assists in keeping the alveoli open by reducing the alveolar surface tension (the tendency of the alveolar walls to collapse upon themselves). Atelectasis results when surfactant is insufficient.

Widespread atelectasis due to oxygen toxicity may result in a syndrome known as the adult respiratory distress syndrome (ARDS), which is characterized by diffuse pulmonary edema, severe stiffness of the lung tissue, and profound hypoxemia (see Procedure 39-3).

## COMMUNITY/HOME CARE

### Using Oxygen in the Home

- Post "Oxygen in Use" signs at entry to home.

- Caution all family members and visitors to avoid lighting matches, cigarettes, or other substances in presence of oxygen equipment. (Oxygen increases the risk of fire. Although oxygen itself is not a flammable gas, it is a necessary catalyst for fire to occur, and fire will burn more vigorously in an oxygen-rich environment.)

- Inspect all electrical equipment prior to use to avoid possibility of electrical sparks.

- Backup oxygen tanks should always be available.

- Backup procedures for power outages should be in place.

Archibald, C. (1999). Oxygenation. In K. Berger & M. Williams (Eds.), *Fundamentals of nursing* (pp. 999–1086). Stamford, CT: Appleton & Lange.

## Administer Blood Components

Blood component administration is indicated when the client's oxygenation is impaired because of decreased circulating blood volume, decreased hemoglobin concentration in the blood (anemia), or hemorrhage. Red blood cells, plasma, clotting factors, proteins, or whole blood may be administered. Since a blood transfusion is really a type of tissue transplant, extreme care must be taken to decrease the possibility of an immune system rejection response known as a transfusion reaction.

# Interventions to Increase Cardiac Output and Tissue Perfusion

The client with impaired cardiac output and tissue perfusion is likely to be experiencing edema of the lower extremities and/or the lungs, fatigue, activity intolerance related to poor tissue oxygenation, and possibly angina and/or intermittent claudication. Interventions are aimed at reducing symptom severity while optimizing cardiac performance.

Additional supportive measures are the administration of supplemental oxygen and medications that improve cardiac function. Other multidisciplinary interventions to promote cardiac output include the application of antiembolism support hose, passive and active exercises, positioning, improving hydration, conducting chest physiotherapy, and using airway clearance measures. Sometimes, the modified Trendelenberg position is used. The foot of the bed is elevated 30 to 40 degrees, the body trunk remains flat, and the head of the bed is slightly elevated. This position promotes venous return without compressing the abdominal organs on the diaphragm. In some cases, counter-pulsation devices are applied to the legs. The legs are enclosed in tubular bags filled with air or water that are connected to a pumping unit. Pressure is applied during diastole and released during systole. Frequent monitoring of vital signs and results of arterial blood gases and hemodynamic monitoring via a central venous pressure (CVP) catheter helps to determine the client's response to the therapeutic procedures (Collins et al., 2001).

### Manage Fluid Balance

Management of fluid balance is a cornerstone in the care of the client with reduced cardiac output. If congestive heart failure is present, fluid intake may be restricted to prevent edema and circulatory overload. Often, sodium intake is also limited because sodium promotes fluid retention. Diuretics may also be given to increase fluid excretion by the kidneys.

Monitoring of fluid balance by the nurse may involve the measurement of fluid intake and output (I&O) and measurement of daily weights. I&O measurement involves teaching the client the importance of accounting for all I&O and providing a container for the measurement of urine. Daily weights should be performed at the same time each day (usually early in the morning) with the same amount of clothing on, and on the same scale, to maximize accuracy.

Clients receiving diuretics may also require monitoring for electrolyte imbalances. Potassium, particularly, may become depleted in the client receiving loop diuretics such as furosemide. Encouraging the consumption of potassium-rich foods such as bananas, and perhaps potassium supplementation, is often required.

### Encourage Activity Restrictions and Assistance with Activities of Daily Living

Activity restrictions and assistance with activities of daily living (ADL) should be based upon the client's activity tolerance. The purpose of activity assistance is to decrease the oxygen demands of the body. The client's activity tolerance may be gradually increased through a sequence of exercise protocols as part of a cardiac rehabilitation program. The client learns to set priorities and to pace self in performing activities. Such a program incorporates careful monitoring of the client as the exercise level increases over time.

### Position Client Properly

Positioning of the client with decreased cardiac output is done to decrease the fluid load to the heart and to decrease the development of pulmonary edema. The venous system is able to pool blood when aided by gravity; this "venous capacitance" is increased when the client's head and upper body are elevated and the legs are

## CLINICAL ALERT

### Blood Administration

To minimize the risk of a serious transfusion reaction when administering blood components, be sure to:

- Follow institutional policy regarding client identification for each transfusion.

- Assess and record client vital signs (temperature, pulse, blood pressure, respirations) before initiating the transfusion and within 1 hour of completing the transfusion.

- Instruct the client to report any unusual feelings, including flushing, itching, headache, or back pain.

- Reassess vital signs after the first 10 to 15 minutes of slowly infusing the blood component. Stop the transfusion immediately if fever, tachycardia, hypotension, dyspnea, or any reports of the above symptoms occur. Notify the client's physician and the blood bank for further instructions.

in a dependent position. Although it is customary in the hospital environment to place clients in a supine position, this position may be detrimental for the client with congestive heart failure, as evidenced by worsening dyspnea, tachycardia and tachypnea, and decreased arterial oxygen saturation.

## Administer Medications

Medications to improve cardiac output and perfusion include diuretics as mentioned above, cardiac glycosides, and other inotropic agents. Antihypertensives, nitrates, and vasodilators may also be given to increase cardiac oxygen supply and/or reduce the myocardium's demand for oxygen. Table 39-10 lists the drugs most commonly used.

## Emergency Interventions

Complete airway obstruction, cardiac arrest, and respiratory arrest are emergency situations that will result in death if not immediately rectified. Nurses receive regular training in the basic life support techniques described below; hands-on practice is an essential component of that training, and this text is not intended to serve as a substitute.

## Remove Airway Obstruction

Complete airway obstruction is often the result of aspiration of food or some other foreign object into the trachea. The presence of a complete airway obstruction is characterized by an inability to speak or cough; the victim may also raise his hands to the throat and will likely appear very anxious. The rescuer should verify that obstruction is present by asking the victim, "Are you choking?" Relief of the obstruction is attempted by way of the **Heimlich maneuver** (see Procedure 39-4).

## Initiate Cardiopulmonary Resuscitation

Cardiac and respiratory arrest require artificial support of circulation and ventilation if the victim is to survive. **Cardiopulmonary resuscitation (CPR)** is the accepted technique of basic life support (see Procedure 39-5).

| TABLE 39-10 | MEDICATIONS USED TO IMPROVE CARDIAC FUNCTION | |
|---|---|---|
| **Drug Type** | **Common Examples** | **Actions** |
| Diuretic | Furosemide (Lasix) Bumetanide (Bumex) Hydrochlorothiazide (Hydro-diuril, HCTZ) Spironolactone (Aldactone) | Affects renal tubules, resulting in increased excretion of water and certain electrolytes Lowers blood pressure and decreases cardiac workload |
| Cardiac glycoside | Digoxin (Lanoxin) | Increases force of cardiac contraction and slows heart rate |
| Inotropic agent | Dobutamine (Dobutrex) Amrinone (Inocor) Dopamine (Intropin) Isoproterenol (Isuprel) | Increases force of cardiac contraction |
| Antihypertensive | ACE inhibitors (captopril, enalapril) Beta-adrenergic blockers (labetolol, propanolol, atenolol) Calcium channel blockers (nicardipine, diltiazem) Centrally acting alpha-adrenergics (clonidine, methyldopa) Ganglionic blockers (trimethaphan) Peripherally acting anti-adrenergics (guanethidine, prazosin) Vasodilators (minoxidil, hydralazine) | Lowers blood pressure by various mechanisms, decreasing the heart's workload |
| Nitrate | Nitroglycerin Isosorbide dinitrate (Isordil) | Dilates the coronary arteries and peripheral vessels, increasing cardiac oxygen supply while decreasing cardiac workload |

Adapted from Kee, J., & Hayes, E. (2000). *Pharmacology: A nursing process approach.* Philadelphia: W. B. Saunders.

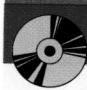

**PROCEDURE 39-4**   **Performing the Heimlich Maneuver**

## EQUIPMENT NEEDED

◾ An individual with the training to perform this procedure

## IMPLEMENTATION—ACTION/RATIONALE

| ACTION | RATIONALE |
|---|---|
| **Foreign Body Obstruction—All Clients** | |
| 1. Assess airway for complete or partial blockage (Figure 39-39). | 1. If there is good air exchange and the client is able to forcefully cough, you should not intervene or interfere with the client's attempts to expel the foreign body. Encourage attempts to cough and breathe, as attempts to cough will provide a more forceful effort. If complete airway obstruction is apparent, the Heimlich maneuver or alternative method of subdiaphragmatic thrust should be performed immediately. |
| 2. Activate emergency response assistance if respiratory distress or complete blockage (e.g., ask bystander to call 911). | 2. Provides follow-up care by professionally trained personnel. |
| **Conscious Adult Client—Sitting or Standing (Heimlich Maneuver)** | |
| 3. Stand behind the client (Figure 39-40). | 3. Proper positioning is necessary to provide an effective subdiaphragmatic thrust. |

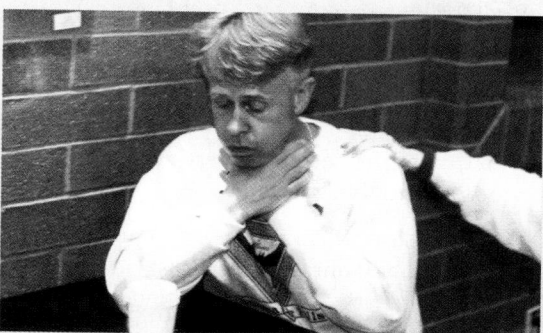

**Figure 39-39   Assess the client. Assess the airway for blockage.**

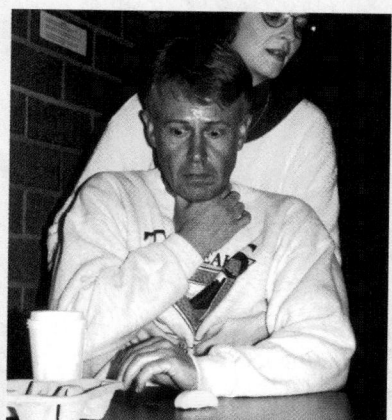

**Figure 39-40   Stand behind the client.**

| | |
|---|---|
| 4. Wrap your arms around the client's waist (Figure 39-41). | 4. Proper positioning is necessary to provide an effective subdiaphragmatic thrust. |

*(continues)*

## PROCEDURE 39-4 (continued)

5. Make a fist with one hand and grasp the fist with your other hand, placing the thumb side of the fist against the client's abdomen. The fist should be placed midline, below the xiphoid process and lower margins of the rib cage and above the navel (Figure 39-42).

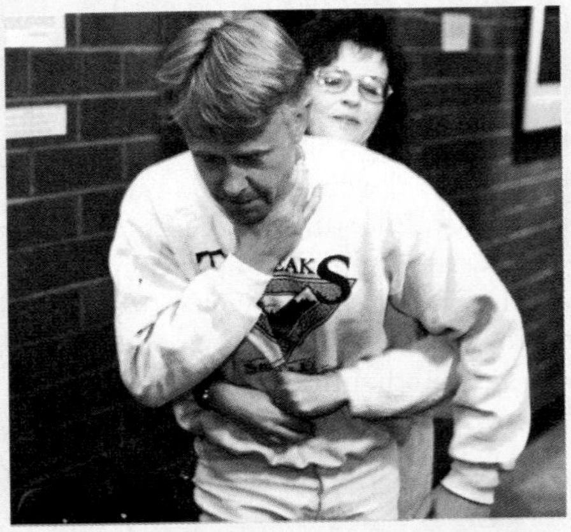

Figure 39-41  Wrap both arms around the client's waist.

5. Correct hand placement is important to prevent internal organ damage.

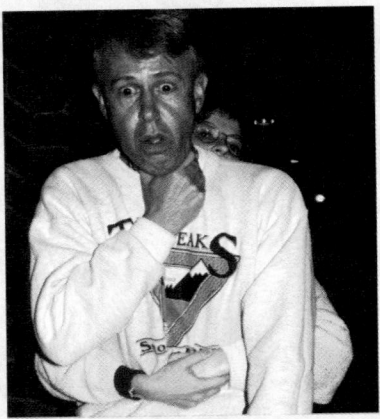

Figure 39-42  Make a fist. Place the fist below the xiphoid process, above the client's navel.

6. Perform a quick upward thrust into the client's abdomen; each thrust should be separate and distinct.

7. Repeat this process 6 to 10 times until the client either expels the foreign body or loses consciousness.

6. This subdiaphragmatic thrust can produce an artificial cough by forcing air from the lungs.

7. Attempts to dislodge food or a foreign body to relieve airway obstruction should be continued as long as necessary due to the serious consequences of hypoxia.

### Unconscious Adult Client or Adult Client Who Becomes Unconscious

8. Repeat Actions 1 and 2.

9. Position the client supine; kneel astride the client's abdomen.

10. Place the heel of one hand midline, below the xiphoid process and lower margin of the rib cage and above the navel. Place the second hand directly on top of the first hand.

11. Perform a quick upward thrust into the diaphragm, repeating 6 to 10 times.

8. Determines the need for intervention and summons essential help.

9. Proper positioning is necessary to provide an effective subdiaphragmatic thrust.

10. Proper positioning is necessary to provide an effective subdiaphragmatic thrust.

11. A client who becomes unconscious may become more relaxed so that the previously unsuccessful Heimlich maneuver may be successful.

*(continues)*

## PROCEDURE 39-4 (*continued*)

12. Perform a finger sweep:

    a. Use one hand to grasp the lower jaw and tongue between your thumb and fingers and lift. This will open the mouth and pull the tongue away from the back of the throat.

    b. Using the index finger of the other hand, insert the finger into the client's mouth next to the cheek and using a hooking motion dislodge any foreign body. Caution must be used to prevent pushing the foreign body farther down into the airway (Figure 39-43).

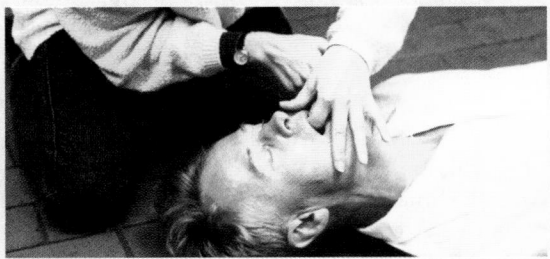

**Figure 39-43    Use a sweeping, hooking motion to dislodge and remove obstruction.**

13. Open the client's airway and attempt ventilation.

14. Continue sequence of Heimlich maneuver, finger sweep, and rescue breathing as long as necessary.

### Conscious Adult Sitting or Standing—Chest Thrusts

15. Repeat Actions 1 and 2.

16. Stand behind the client and encircle the chest with arms under the axilla.

17. Make a fist and place the thumb side of the fist on the middle of the client's sternum and grasp the fist with the second hand.

18. Perform backward thrusts until the client either becomes unconscious or the foreign body is expelled.

12. Should only be used on the unconscious client, who will not fight the action.

    a. Draw the tongue away from any foreign body lodged in the back of the throat.

13. The brain can suffer irreversible damage if it is without oxygen for over 4 to 6 minutes.

14. Life-saving efforts must continue until they are successful, or until the rescuer becomes exhausted and cannot go on.

    Chest thrusts should only be used for the very obese client or a woman in the late stages of pregnancy.

15. Determines the need for intervention and summons essential help.

16. Proper hand placement should avoid the xiphoid process and rib cage margins to minimize internal organ damage.

17. Proper hand placement should avoid the xiphoid process and rib cage margins to minimize internal organ damage.

18. Thrusts may not be effective on the first tries. Keep trying.

    Chest thrusts should be used only for the very obese or a woman in the late stages of pregnancy.

*(continues)*

## PROCEDURE 39-4 (*continued*)

### Unconscious Adult—Chest Thrusts

19. Repeat Actions 1 and 2.

20. Place client in the supine position and kneel at the client's side.

21. Place the heel of one hand on the lower half of the sternum—same position as with external cardiac compressions.

22. Perform each thrust in a slow, separate, and distinct manner.

23. Follow Actions 9 to 12 for the adult Heimlich maneuver, unconscious client.

### Airway Obstruction—Infants and Small Children

24. Differentiate between infection and airway obstruction.

### Infant Airway Obstruction

25. Straddle infant over forearm in the prone position with the head lower than the trunk. Support the infant's head, positioning a hand around the jaws and chest.

26. Deliver four back blows between the infant's shoulder blades.

27. Keeping the infant's head down, place the free hand on the infant's back and turn the infant over, supporting the back of the child with your hand and thigh.

28. With your free hand, deliver four thrusts in the same manner as infant external cardiac compressions.

29. Assess for a foreign body in the mouth of an unconscious infant and use the finger sweep only if a foreign body is visualized.

30. Open airway and assess for respiration. If respirations are absent, attempt rescue breathing. Assess for the rise and fall of the chest; if not seen, reposition infant and attempt rescue breathing again.

---

19. Determines the need for intervention and summons essential help.

20. Places the client and the rescuer in the most effective position to apply interventions.

21. This is the most effective position for thrust.

22. Each thrust should be delivered with the intention of relieving the airway obstruction.

23. Performs the life-saving procedure.

24. Infectious complications that lead to airway obstruction require immediate medical attention, establishment of a patent airway (intubation or emergency tracheotomy), and treatment of the underlying infection. Food or foreign body airway obstruction also needs immediate attention; however, airway management differs between each scenario.

25. Proper positioning is essential for success of the maneuver and prevention of other organ damage.

26. Technique for dislodging the obstruction.

27. Safely rotates the infant's position to continue life-saving procedures.

28. Technique for dislodging the obstruction.

29. A blind finger sweep is avoided in infants and children since a foreign object can be pushed back farther into the airway, increasing obstruction.

30. Many times some air can get around the foreign body causing the airway obstruction. This allows for some oxygenation of the client. Without oxygen, irreversible brain damage can occur within 4 to 6 minutes.

*(continues)*

31. Repeat the entire sequence again: four back blows, four chest thrusts, assessment for foreign body in oral cavity, and rescue breathing as long as necessary.

31. Life-saving efforts must continue until they are successful or until the rescuer becomes exhausted and cannot go on.

### Small Child—Airway Obstruction (Conscious, Standing or Sitting)

32. Assess air exchange and encourage coughing and breathing. Provide reassurance to the child that you are there to help.

32. Inability to breathe is a distressing event for anyone, especially a small child who may not fully understand the circumstance. Reassurance is important to gain the child's trust and cooperation with the maneuvers necessary to help him, especially if the child is conscious.

33. Ask the child if he is choking. If the response is affirmative, follow the steps outlined below. In addition, if the child has poor air exchange (and infection has been ruled out), initiate the following steps:

33. Many small children are capable of responding to simple questions such as "Are you choking?"

   a. Stand behind the child with your arms wrapped around his waist and administer 6 to 10 subdiaphragmatic abdominal thrusts.

   a. Proper positioning is essential for success of the maneuver and prevention of other organ damage.

   b. Continue until foreign object is expelled or the child becomes unconscious.

   b. Life-saving efforts must continue until they are successful or until the rescuer becomes exhausted and cannot go on.

### Small Child—Airway Obstruction (Conscious or Unconscious, Lying)

34. Position the child supine, kneel at the child's feet, and gently deliver 6 to 10 subdiaphragmatic abdominal thrusts. The subdiaphragmatic thrusts are delivered in the same manner as for an adult, but more gently.

34. This is the recommended position for small children; the astride position may be used for larger children. Proper positioning is essential for success of the maneuver and prevention of other organ damage.

35. Open airway by lifting the lower jaw and tongue forward. Perform a finger sweep only if a foreign body is visualized.

35. Opens the airway and allows visualization of the oral cavity. A blind finger sweep can cause increased obstruction by pushing a foreign object farther back into the airway.

36. If breathing is absent, begin rescue breathing. If the chest does not rise, reposition the child and attempt rescue breathing again.

36. Many times some air can get around the foreign body causing the airway obstruction. This allows for some oxygenation of the client. Without oxygen, irreversible brain damage can occur within 4 to 6 minutes.

37. Repeat this sequence as long as necessary.

37. Life-saving efforts must continue until they are successful or until the rescuer becomes exhausted and cannot go on.

38. Wash hands.

38. Reduces transmission of microorganisms.

## LIFE SPAN CONSIDERATIONS

### Heimlich Maneuver

*Pediatric Variations*

● All individuals in health care and day care settings should be educated in the hand placement and methods to remove food or foreign bodies from a child with an airway obstruction and in how they differ from treating an adult.

● In addition, how to access emergency medical assistance as well as prevention should be a key educational piece for all new parents and any facility that has infants and young children under its care.

● Infants and toddlers should not be given foods that they can choke on, especially children who do not have the ability to properly chew yet. These foods include peanuts, round hard candies, and cut-up hot dogs.

*Geriatric Variations*

● The older adult is at risk for rib or cartilage fractures, which may result from forceful thrusts or improper hand positioning.

● Age-related changes in the musculoskeletal system (e.g., osteoporosis) might limit positioning of the geriatric client.

● Many older adults may be at risk of choking due to dentures, and appropriate education should take place when such devices are fitted on an individual and reinforced by all other health care professionals working with the client.

## COMMUNITY/HOME CARE

### Heimlich Maneuver

*Home Care Variations*

● Both the caregivers and the clients requiring home care should be assessed for their educational level on interventions to take if someone is choking.

● Identify a working phone in the home; the client/caregiver should know how to access the emergency medical assistance available in the area.

● Referrals to community resources may be necessary (e.g., classes held at the local American Red Cross or the local hospital).

● Clients in the home care setting may have impaired swallowing abilities and are at higher risk of choking. They and their caregivers should be made aware of the proper feeding techniques to decrease the possibility of choking on food.

*Long-Term Care Variations*

● In a long-term care facility, all employees should be educated in emergency resuscitation measures.

● Special attention should be made for individuals wearing dentures and those at higher risk for choking—for example, stroke victims.

● Foods may have to be pureed and liquids may need to be thickened.

| PROCEDURE 39-5 | **Administering Cardiopulmonary Resuscitation (CPR)** |

## EQUIPMENT NEEDED

### *Hospital or Clinical Setting*

▪ Hard, flat surface (e.g., chest compression board) (Figures 39-44, 39-45, and 39-46)
▪ Body substance isolation items
  — Gloves
  — Face shield
  — Mask/CPR oral barrier device
▪ Ambu bag
▪ Oral airway
▪ Emergency resuscitation cart
▪ Documentation forms

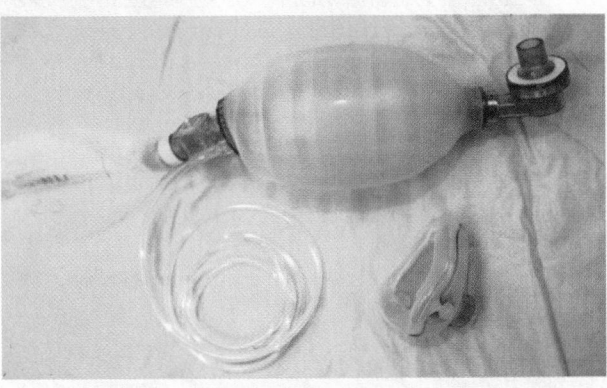

**Figure 39-44    Ambu bag**

### *Outside: Public Environment*

▪ Hard, flat surface (e.g., floor)
▪ Body substance isolation items, if available
  — Gloves
  — Face shield
  — Mask/CPR oral barrier device

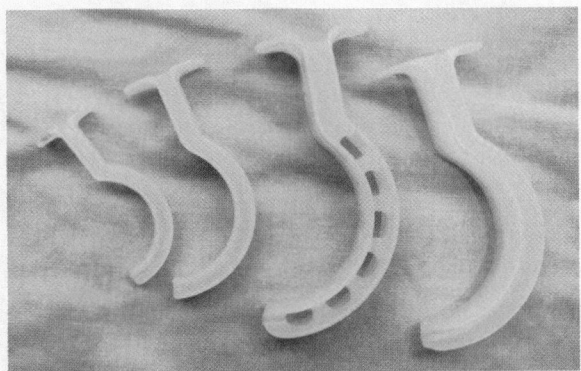

**Figure 39-45    Oropharyngeal airways**

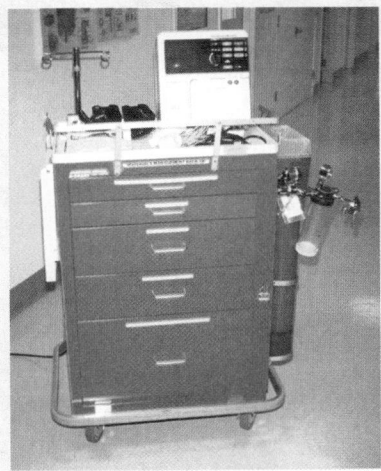

**Figure 39-46    Emergency resuscitation cart**

## IMPLEMENTATION—ACTION/RATIONALE

| ACTION | RATIONALE |
| --- | --- |

### CPR: One Rescuer—Adult, Adolescent

1. Assess responsiveness by tapping or gently shaking client while shouting, "Are you OK?" (Figure 39-47).

2. Activate emergency medical system. In the hospital or clinical setting, follow institutional protocol. In the community or home environment, activate the local emergency response system

1. Prevents injury to a client who is not experiencing cardiac or respiratory arrest. Also assists in assessing level of consciousness and possible etiology of crisis.

2. Activates assistance from personnel trained in advanced life support. Also, one person cannot perform CPR indefinitely. If the rescuer is alone, providing 1 minute of CPR before activating the

*(continues)*

**PROCEDURE 39-5 (*continued*)**

(e.g., 911). The one exception to this sequence is if the rescuer is alone with no other bystanders; the rescuer should position the client and assess for respirations and a pulse. If absent, initiate CPR for 1 full minute and then activate emergency medical assistance.

emergency response system helps reduce the risk of irreversible brain and tissue damage that can occur if a client is hypoxic for over 4 to 6 minutes.

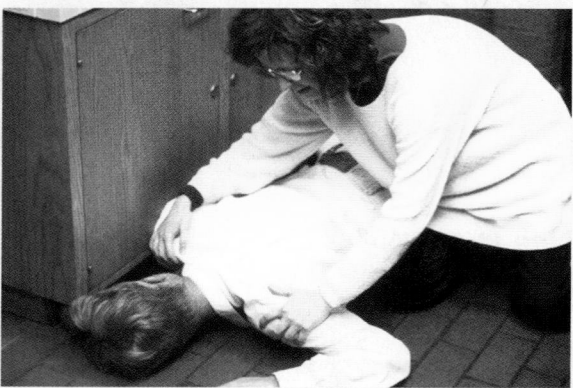

**Figure 39-47    Assess the client's responsiveness.**

3.  Position client in a supine position on a hard, flat surface (e.g., floor or cardiac board). Use caution when positioning a client with a possible head or neck injury.

3.  Proper positioning facilitates assessment of the cardiac and respiratory status and successful external cardiac massage. Care must be taken in positioning a client with a potential head or neck injury to prevent further damage.

4.  Apply appropriate body substance isolation items (e.g., gloves, face shield) if available.

4.  Prevents transmission of disease.

5.  Position self. Face the client on your knees parallel to the client, next to the head, to begin to assess the airway and breathing status.

5.  Proper positioning prevents rescuer fatigue and facilitates CPR by allowing the rescuer to move from chest compressions to artificial breathing with minimal movement.

6.  Open airway. The most commonly used method is the head-tilt/chin-lift method. This is accomplished by placing one hand on the client's forehead and applying a steady backward pressure to tilt the head back while placing the fingers of the other hand below the jaw at the location of the chin and lifting the chin (Figure 39-48). In the event of a suspected head or neck injury, this lift is modified and the jaw thrust is used. To perform the jaw thrust, place hands at the angles of the lower jaw and lift, displacing the mandible forward while tilting the head backward (Figure 39-49). Additionally, if available, insert oral airway.

6.  A patent airway is essential for successful artificial respirations. The head-tilt/chin-lift assists in preventing the tongue from obstructing the airway. The jaw thrust is used when a head or neck injury is suspected because it prevents extension of the neck and decreases the potential of further injury.

*(continues)*

**PROCEDURE 39-5 (*continued*)**

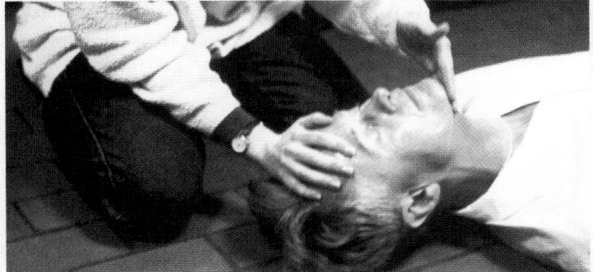

**Figure 39-48**   Use the head-tilt/chin-lift method to open airway.

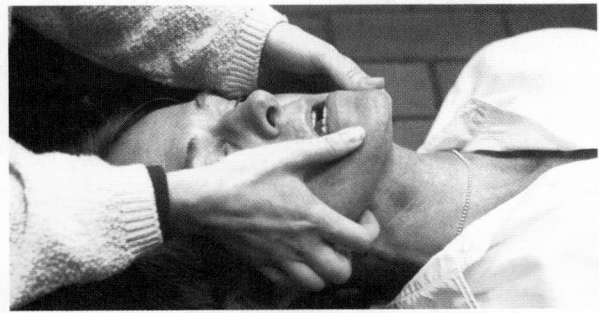

**Figure 39-49**   The jaw-thrust method is used to open the airway if a neck injury is suspected.

7. Assess for respirations. Look, listen, and feel for air movement.

8. If respirations are absent:
   - Occlude nostrils with the thumb and index finger of the hand on the forehead that is tilting the head back (Figure 39-50).
   - Form a seal over the client's mouth using either your mouth or the appropriate respiratory assist device (e.g., Ambu bag and mask) and give two full breaths of about 0.5 to 2 seconds, allowing time for both inspiration and expiration (Figure 39-51).

7. Cardiopulmonary resuscitation should not be administered to a client with spontaneous respirations or pulse due to the potential risk of injury.

8. Occluding the nostrils and forming a seal over the client's mouth will prevent air leakage and provide full inflation of the lungs. Excessive air volume and rapid inspiratory flow rates can create pharyngeal pressures that are greater than esophageal opening pressures. This will allow air into the stomach, resulting in gastric distention and increased risk of vomiting.

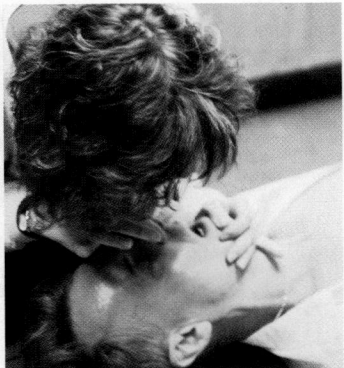

**Figure 39-50**   Occlude both nostrils with fingers.

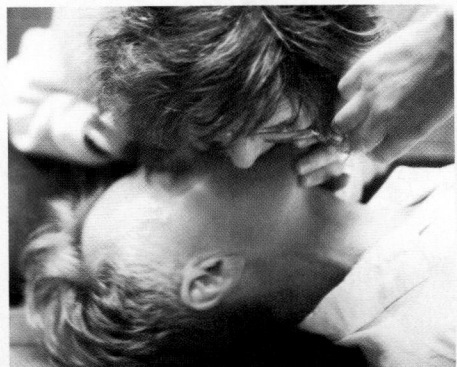

**Figure 39-51**   Give two full breaths.

- In the event of a serious mouth or jaw injury that prevents mouth-to-mouth ventilation, mouth-to-nose ventilation may be used by tilting the head as described earlier with one hand and using the other hand to lift the jaw and close the mouth.

*(continues)*

## PROCEDURE 39-5 (*continued*)

9. Assess for the rise and fall of the chest:

   • If the chest rises and falls, continue to Action 10.

   • If the chest does not move, assess for excessive oral secretions, vomit, airway obstruction, or improper positioning.

10. Palpate the carotid pulse (5 to 10 seconds) (Figure 39-52):

    • If present, continue rescue breathing, at the rate of 12 breaths/minute.

    • If absent, begin external cardiac compressions.

11. Cardiac compressions are performed as follows:

    • Maintain a position on knees parallel to sternum.

    • Position the hands for compressions:

    a. Using the hand nearest to the legs, use the index finger to locate the lower rib margin and quickly move the fingers up to the location where the ribs connect to the sternum.

    b. Place the middle finger of this hand on the notch where the ribs meet the sternum and the index finger next to it.

    c. Place the heel of the opposite hand next to the index finger on the sternum (Figure 39-53).

9. Visual assessment of chest movement helps confirm an open airway. A volume of 800–1200 ml is usually sufficient to make the chest rise in most adults.

10. Performing chest compressions on an individual with a pulse could result in injury. Additionally, the carotid pulse may persist when peripheral pulses are no longer palpable. Hyperventilation assists in maintaining blood oxygen levels. Additionally, a pulse may be present for about 6 minutes after respirations have ceased.

11. Irreversible brain and tissue damage can occur if a client is hypoxic for over 4 to 6 minutes. Proper positioning is essential for the following reasons:

    • Allows for maximum compression of the heart between the sternum and vertebrae.

    • Compressions over the xiphoid process can lacerate the liver.

    • Keeping fingers off the chest during compressions reduces the risk of rib fracture.

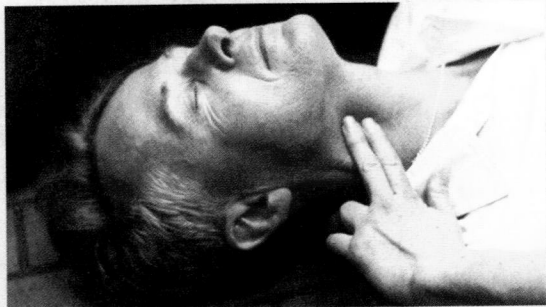

**Figure 39-52    Palpate for a carotid pulse.**

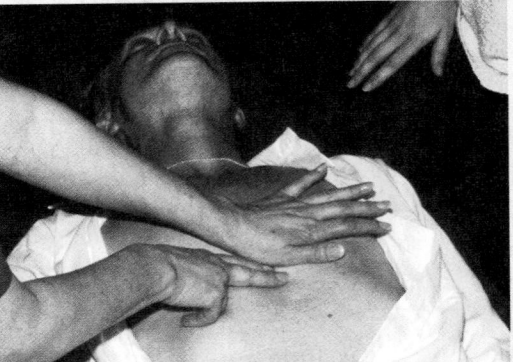

**Figure 39-53    Place the heel of one hand next to the index finger on the client's sternum.**

d. Remove the first hand from the notch and place it on top of the hand that is on the sternum so that they are on top of each other.

*(continues)*

## PROCEDURE 39-5 (*continued*)

e. Extend or interlace fingers and do not allow them to touch the chest (Figure 39-54).

f. Keep arms straight with shoulders directly over hands on sternum and lock elbows (Figure 39-55).

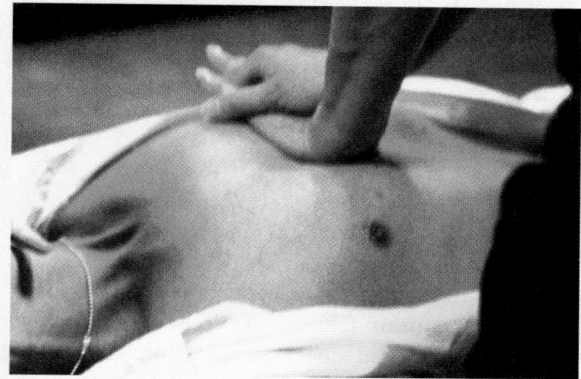

**Figure 39-54    Extend or interface the fingers.**

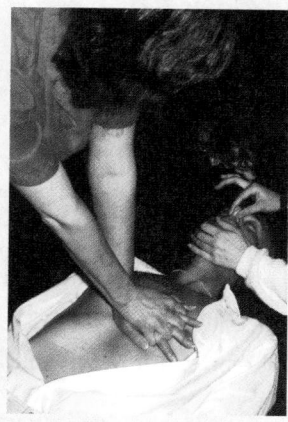

**Figure 39-55    Keep arms straight and lock elbows.**

g. Compress the adult chest 3.8–5.0 cm (1½–2 inches) at the rate of 80 to 100 compressions per minute.

h. The heel of the hand must completely release the pressure between compressions, but it should remain in constant contact with the client's skin.

i. Use the mnemonic "one and, two and, three and . . ." to keep rhythm and timing.

j. Ventilate client as described in Action 8.

12. Maintain the compression rate for 80–100 times/minute, interjecting ventilation after every 15 compressions.

13. Reassess the client after four cycles.

### CPR: Two Rescuers—Adult, Adolescent

14. Follow the steps above with the following changes:

- One rescuer is positioned facing the client parallel to the head while the other rescuer is positioned on the opposite side facing the client parallel to the sternum next to the trunk (Figure 39-56).

- The rescuer positioned at the client's trunk is responsible for performing cardiac compressions and maintaining the verbal mnemonic count. This is rescuer 1.

12. Faster rate increases blood flow to key organ tissues.

13. Determines return of spontaneous pulse and respirations and need to continue CPR.

14. Proper positioning allows one rescuer to perform artificial respirations while the other administers chest compressions without getting in each other's way. In addition, this facilitates ease in changing positions when one of the rescuers becomes fatigued. Palpating the carotid pulse with each chest compression during the first full minute ensures that adequate stroke volume is being delivered with each compression.

*(continues)*

## PROCEDURE 39-5 (*continued*)

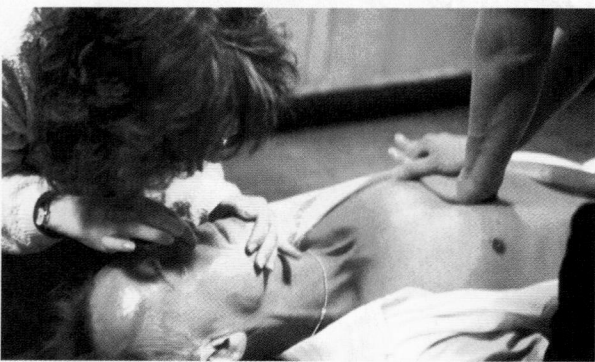

**Figure 39-56    Two-rescuer positioning: One person kneels on each side of the client.**

- The rescuer positioned at the client's head is responsible for monitoring respirations, assessing the carotid pulse, establishing an open airway, and performing rescue breathing. This is rescuer 2.

- The compression-to-ventilation rate changes to 5:1, pausing 1 to 1½ seconds for ventilation.

- Rescuer 2 palpates the carotid pulse with each chest compression during the first full minute.

- Rescuer 2 is responsible for calling for a change when fatigued, following this protocol.

- Rescuer 1 calls for a change and completes the five chest compressions.

- Rescuer 2 administers two breaths and then moves to a position parallel to the client's sternum and assumes the proper hand position.

- Rescuer 1 moves to the rescue breathing position and checks the carotid pulse for 5 seconds. If cardiac arrest persists, rescuer 1 says, "continue CPR" and delivers one breath. Rescuer 2 resumes cardiac compressions immediately after the breath.

### CPR: One Rescuer—Child (1 to 7 years)

15. Assess responsiveness, activate emergency medical system, position the child, apply appropriate body substance isolation, position self, open airway, and assess for respirations as described in Actions 1 to 7. Remember, respiratory arrest is more common in the pediatric population.

Two rescuers are needed because one person cannot maintain CPR indefinitely. When a rescuer becomes fatigued, chest compressions can become ineffective, decreasing the volume of oxygenated blood circulated to key organs and tissue.

15. See Rationales 1 to 7.

(continues)

**PROCEDURE 39-5** (*continued*)

16. If respirations are absent, begin rescue breathing:

    • Give two slow breaths (1–1½ seconds/breath), pausing to take a breath in between.

    • Use only the amount of air needed to make the chest rise. When you see the chest rise and fall, you are using the right volume of air.

17. Palpate the carotid pulse (5 to 10 seconds). If present, ventilate at a rate of once every 4 seconds or 15 times/minute. If absent, begin cardiac compressions.

18. Cardiac compressions (child 1 to 7 years):

    • Maintain a position on knees parallel to child's sternum.

    • Place a small towel or other support under the child's shoulders.

    • Position the hands for compressions:

      a. Locate the lower margin of the rib cage using the hand closest to the feet and find the notch where the ribs and sternum meet.

      b. Place the middle finger of this hand on the notch and then place the index finger next to the middle finger.

      c. Place the heel of the other hand next to the index finger of the first hand on the sternum with the heel parallel to the sternum (1 cm above the xiphoid process).

      d. Keeping the elbows locked and the shoulders over the child, compress the sternum 2.5–3.8 cm (1–1½ inches) at the rate of 80–100 times/minute.

      e. Keep the other hand on the child's forehead.

      f. At the end of every fifth compression administer a ventilation (1–1½ seconds).

      g. Reevaluate the child after 10 cycles.

16. Hypoxia can cause irreversible brain and tissue damage after 4 to 6 minutes.

    • The volume of air in a small child's lungs is less than an adult's. Excessive air volume and rapid inspiratory rates can increase pharyngeal pressures that exceed esophageal opening pressures. This allows air to enter the stomach, causing gastric distention, increasing the risk of vomiting, and further compromising the client's respiratory status.

17. Performing chest compressions on a child with a pulse could result in injury. Additionally, the carotid pulse may persist when peripheral pulses are no longer palpable. Hyperventilation assists in maintaining blood oxygen levels. Additionally, a pulse may be present for approximately 6 minutes after respirations have ceased.

18. Irreversible brain and tissue damage can occur if a client is hypoxic for over 4 to 6 minutes. Proper positioning is essential for the following reasons:

    • Allows for maximum compression of the heart between the sternum and vertebrae.

    • The backward tilt of the head lifts the back of small children and a small towel or some other type of support is necessary for effective cardiac compressions.

    • Compressions over the xiphoid process can lacerate the liver.

    • Keeping fingers off the chest during compressions reduces the risk of rib fracture.

    • Keeping one hand on the child's forehead helps maintain an open airway.

*(continues)*

**PROCEDURE 39-5** (*continued*)

### CPR: One Rescuer—Infant (1 to 12 months)

19. Assess responsiveness, activate emergency medical system, position the child, apply appropriate body substance isolation, position self, open airway, and assess for respirations as described in Actions 1 to 7. Remember, respiratory arrest is more common in the pediatric population.

19. See Rationales 1 to 7.

20. If respirations are absent, begin rescue breathing:

    • Avoid overextension of the infant's neck.

    • Place a small towel or diaper under the infant's shoulders or use a hand to support the neck.

    • Make a tight seal over both the infant's nose and mouth and gently administer artificial respirations.

    • Give two slow breaths (1–1½ seconds/breath), pausing to take a breath in between.

    • Use only the amount of air needed to make the chest rise.

20. Irreversible brain and tissue damage can occur if a client is hypoxic for over 4 to 6 minutes. Proper positioning is essential for the following reasons:

    • It is believed that overextension of an infant's head can cause a closing or narrowing of the airway.

    • Proper positioning with support allows maximum compression of the heart between the sternum and vertebrae.

    • Making a complete seal over the infant's mouth and nose prevents air leakage.

    • The volume of air in a small child's lungs is less than an adult's. Excessive air volume and rapid inspiratory rates can increase pharyngeal pressures that exceed esophageal opening pressures. This allows air to enter the stomach, causing gastric distention, increasing the risk of vomiting, and further compromising the client's respiratory status.

21. Assess circulatory status using the brachial pulse:

    • Locate the brachial pulse on the inside of the upper arm between the elbow and shoulder by placing your thumb on the outside of the arm and palpating the proximal side of the arm with the index finger and middle fingers.

    • If a pulse is palpated, continue rescue breathing 20 times/minute or once every 3 seconds.

    • If a pulse is absent, begin cardiac compressions.

21. The carotid pulse is often difficult to locate in the infant; therefore the brachial artery is the recommended site.

22. Cardiac compressions (infant 1 to 12 months):

    • Maintain a position parallel to the infant. Infants can easily be placed on a table or other hard surface.

22. Irreversible brain and tissue damage can occur if a client is hypoxic for over 4 to 6 minutes. Proper positioning is essential for the following reasons:

    • Allows for maximum compression of the heart between the sternum and vertebrae.

*(continues)*

**PROCEDURE 39-5 (*continued*)**

- Place a small towel or other support under the infant's shoulders/neck.

- Position the hands for compressions:

  a. Using the hand closest to the infant's feet, locate the intermammary line where it intersects the sternum.

  b. Place the index finger 1 cm below this location on the sternum and place the middle finger next to the index finger.

  c. Using these two fingers, compress in a downward motion 1.3–2.5 cm ($\frac{1}{2}$–1 inch) at the rate of 100 times/minute.

  d. Keep the other hand on the infant's forehead.

  e. At the end of every fifth compression, administer a ventilation (1–1$\frac{1}{2}$ seconds).

  f. Reevaluate infant after 10 cycles.

- A small towel, diaper roll, or some other type of support is necessary for effective cardiac compressions.

- Compressions over the xiphoid process can lacerate the liver.

- Keeping other fingers and hands off the chest during compressions reduces risk of rib fracture.

- Keeping one hand on the infant's forehead helps maintain an open airway.

**CPR: Two Rescuers—Child (1 to 7 years) and Infant (1 to 12 months)**

23. Follow Action 14 for two-rescuer CPR for adults with the following changes:

   - Use the child or infant procedure for chest compressions.

   - Change the ratio of compressions to ventilation to 3:1 (three chest compressions to one ventilation).

   - Deliver the ventilation on the upstroke of the third compression.

23. Improper hand placement can cause internal organ damage or other medical complications in infants or children. Increased rate of ventilation allows for maximum oxygen delivery to prevent tissue hypoxia. Delivering compressions during the upstroke phase allows for full lung expansion during inspiration.

**CPR—Neonate or Premature Infant**

24. Follow the infant guidelines with the following changes for chest compressions:

   - Encircle the chest with both hands.

   - Position thumbs over the midsternum.

   - Compress the midsternum with both thumbs.

   - Compress 1.3–1.8 cm ($\frac{1}{2}$–$\frac{1}{4}$ inch) at a rate of 100–120 times/minute.

24. Improper hand placement can cause internal organ damage or other medical complications in infants or children.

## LIFE SPAN CONSIDERATIONS

### CPR

**Pediatric Variations**

- Parents and caregivers should be taught the proper hand positions, ventilation-to-compression ratio, and breathing techniques for use in the pediatric population.

- It is important to reinforce that respiratory arrest is more common than a cardiopulmonary arrest in the pediatric population.

- Safety education with a focus on accident prevention should also be included in CPR instructional sessions. Refresher courses should be encouraged on an annual basis.

**Geriatric Variations**

- It is important to remember that the older adult is at risk for rib or cartilage fractures, which may result from improper hand positioning.

- Age-related changes in the musculoskeletal system (e.g., osteoporosis) might limit positioning of the geriatric client.

- Many older adults may be wearing dentures, which should be removed during emergency resuscitation.

## COMMUNITY/HOME CARE

### CPR

**Home Care Variations**

- Caregivers and family members of clients requiring home care should be assessed for their educational level and ability to learn and retain the principles of CPR.

- It is important to have a working phone in the home, and the client, family member, and caregiver should know how to assess the emergency medical response system in the community.

- The home care nurse is ideally in a position to assess the home environment and the ability of the caregiver or family members to return demonstrate CPR skills. Referrals to the community resources may be useful (e.g., the American Red Cross, the American Heart Association, or the local hospital).

**Long-Term Care Variations**

- In a long-term care facility, it should be expected that all health care providers have certification in CPR.

- Special attention should be made for individuals wearing dentures, those at risk for choking (e.g., stroke victims), and clients with impaired cognitive function who may be at risk for falls or accidents.

- A complete evaluation should be made on all clients, and care plans should include choking prevention measures as well as reinforcement of safety measures.

The technique described above is used for adult victims; different techniques are applied for children and infants and can be learned through courses such as those offered by the American Heart Association or the American Red Cross (check with school/institution policies for type of education required).

## Interventions to Address Associated Nursing Diagnoses

### Explore Lifestyle and Activity Adaptations

Lifestyle and activity adaptations may be necessary for the client with chronic alterations in oxygenation. Interventions related to lifestyle and activity have three general purposes:

1. To minimize energy and oxygen consumption
2. To reduce factors that contribute to the disease process
3. To systematically increase activity tolerance

Measures to reduce energy and oxygen consumption are chosen after a careful assessment of the client's activity tolerance. Clients may need assistance with activities of daily living, including hygiene and toileting; however, it should be noted that complete bedrest is not always the best option. Many clients find that using a bedside commode or toilet is less physically taxing than using a bedpan, especially for bowel movements.

Occupational roles may also need to be modified. If the client is not able to continue working in the old job, it may be possible to take on a new job that is less taxing or to reduce the number of hours worked. If such changes are not possible, the client may have to quit working altogether. All of these possibilities may cause much distress to the client and family, who must grapple with role issues, authority and autonomy issues, and possibly financial concerns. Signs of inadequate family coping, such as marital discord, anger or hostility, sleep disturbances, and depression, should be noted and appropriate interventions, such as a referral for counseling, should be instituted.

Lifestyle adaptations aimed at reducing factors that contribute to the disease process include removal of allergens from the environment, smoking cessation, and control of modifiable risk factors for heart disease. Allergen control

and smoking cessation were discussed in the section Interventions to Promote Airway Clearance. Modification of cardiac risk factors includes smoking cessation as well as dietary alterations and weight control, control of diabetes and hypertension if present, exercise, and stress management. A comprehensive cardiac rehabilitation program addresses all of these issues while monitoring the client's progress toward his individualized goals.

### Encourage Dietary and Nutritional Modifications

Dietary modifications for cardiovascular disease may include reduction of sodium intake and reduction of total fat, saturated fat, and cholesterol intake. Sodium

---

## COMMUNITY/HOME CARE

### Activity Adaptations

Activity adaptations in the home setting may involve alterations in the physical environment of the home, changes in family roles, or changes in work roles. The client who cannot climb stairs may need to have her sleeping quarters moved to the first floor of the house. Clients may also need to give up household chores that cause distress and perhaps take on other, less physically taxing roles. Changes such as these can be trying for the entire family, and they will need support during the period of transition. Home health nurses are a tremendous resource for families facing role changes related to illness.

---

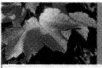

## RESEARCH FOCUS

**Title of Study:** Functional status from the patient's perspective: The challenge of preserving personal integrity

**Study Purpose:** The purpose of this qualitative research was to explore how clients with chronic obstructive pulmonary disease (COPD) cope with the changes in their ability to perform day-to-day activities.

**Methods:** Twelve clients from a pulmonary outpatient clinic in the southeast with varying sociodemographic backgrounds and moderate to severe emphysema, chronic bronchitis, asthma (with underlying chronic airways obstruction), or COPD participated in the study. During recorded interviews, the clients were asked to describe a typical day and were then encouraged to self-direct the content of the interview. The interviews were transcribed, and theme clusters were identified and findings validated for credibility.

**Findings:** Clients with COPD experienced ongoing challenges in preserving a sense of wholeness as they faced physical changes that interfered with their daily activities. They wanted to maintain personal integrity, which was described as having a sense of effectiveness and connectedness through their daily activities.

**Implications:** This study identifies the need for further research in order to define nursing interventions that focus on individual client needs, and support emotional expression, goal setting, and recollection.

Leidy, N. K., & Haase, J. E. (1999). Functional status from the patient's perspective: The challenge of preserving personal integrity. *Research in Nursing Health, 22*(2), 67–77.

consumption may be reduced by decreasing or eliminating salt used in cooking and added at the table, and avoiding highly processed foods such as prepared meats, canned meat or fish, and many prepared sauces. The client should be taught to examine food labels for sodium content per serving.

The client who is not receiving adequate nutrient intake because of poor appetite or severe dyspnea will need assistance in finding ways to increase intake of calories and essential nutrients. Eating small, frequent meals of high nutritional value and using dietary supplements are often helpful. Some studies have shown the anticlotting benefits from omega-3 oils and vitamin E, and the effectiveness of the mineral selenium in reduction of blood pressure. Foods rich in beta-carotene, such as deeply colored yellow, red, and orange fruits and vegetables, are also beneficial in treating heart disease. Soluble fiber from whole oats is one of the foods approved by the U.S. government to help in prevention of heart disease (Pelletier, 2000).

---

## CLIENT EDUCATION

### Following a Healthy Diet

Reduction of total dietary fat, saturated fat, and cholesterol can be a challenge and requires careful client teaching. Use food labels and reference charts to help clients follow these dietary outlines:

✓ Reduce fat intake to no more than 30% of the total caloric intake.

✓ Keep saturated fats down to no more than 10% of the total caloric intake. Saturated fats include those from animal sources such as milk and dairy products. Palm and coconut oils, although from a vegetable source, have the same effect as animal fats in terms of raising serum cholesterol.

✓ Limit cholesterol intake to less than 300 mg per day.

✓ Eat less meat and dairy products and more fresh fruits, vegetables, and whole grains.

✓ Avoid processed foods, especially those with sauces or fillings. When eating out, choose baked or grilled dishes rather than fried, sautéed, or stewed.

✓ Enjoy treats such as rich desserts only occasionally; choose low-fat desserts such as low-fat frozen yogurt, fruit sorbets, or angel food cake whenever possible.

American Heart Association (2003). http://www.american heart.org

---

### Promote Comfort Measures

Promoting comfort for the client with oxygenation disturbances can be a challenge but is extremely important. Comfort influences the client's ability to eat, sleep, learn, and cope with the illness and the care being provided.

Altered comfort related to pain is best approached by removing or modifying the cause of the pain if possible and administering analgesics if indicated. The use of analgesics in the postoperative client is particularly important in allowing the client to participate fully in deep-breathing and coughing exercises. Analgesics are most effective when combined with other pain-relief techniques such as meditation, biofeedback, and distractive measures such as music or a calm quiet environment. Allowing the client to express concerns, providing emotional support, and teaching the client self-management strategies are important comfort measures (National Center for Complementary and Alternative Medicine, 2003).

Pain related to tissue ischemia is best relieved by improving the oxygen delivery to the tissues while reducing the oxygen demand. The first response to ischemic pain should be to rest the affected tissue. If the pain is in the legs, for example, the client should sit down. Improving delivery of oxygen to the legs in the client with peripheral vascular disease may involve positioning the legs lower than heart level (elevating the legs will often make the pain worse).

Heart pain related to ischemia (angina pectoris) should also be dealt with first and foremost by resting. Resting will decrease the heart's workload and in some cases is sufficient to relieve the pain. Improving oxygen delivery to the heart may be accomplished by providing supplemental oxygen or by using medications, such as nitrates, that improve coronary blood flow. In some cases, narcotic analgesics such as morphine are necessary. However, narcotic analgesics also depress the cough reflex and ciliary activity and have direct depression on the respiratory center in the brain. Close monitoring is necessary. Encourage the client to take deep breaths periodically (Stacy, 2000).

### Complementary Therapies

Some complementary/alternative medical (CAM) practices have been accepted into conventional medicine, particularly in pain management, treatment of chronic illness, and the prevention of diseases such as allergies, asthma, hypertension, and cardiovascular problems and their associated factors of anxiety and depression. The primary focus of CAM is to restore a balance of the whole person. Many complementary therapies originated in the ancient healing traditions of the Orient. Therapies that enhance oxygenation include meditation, aroma therapy, tai chi, qi gong, and yoga. The psychological and physiological benefits of these stress-reduction therapies have been supported by scientific studies. The client is also encouraged to make lifestyle changes that include a low-fat diet and exercise as tolerated. Most authorities agree that these measures can reverse the adverse effects of coronary artery disease (CAD), hypertension, and other circulatory problems (National Center for Complementary and Alternative Medicine, 2003; Pelletier, 2000).

## Herbs

Herbs are often used with relaxation techniques, exercise, and diet to prevent diseases of the cardiovascular and respiratory systems; According to landmark national studies by Eisenberg et al. in 1993 and 1997, approximately 70% to 90% of adults in the United States used at least one alternative therapy. These included over-the-counter (OTC) drugs, vitamins, herbs, or nutritional supplements. These products are often used in conjunction with relaxation techniques, exercise, and diet to prevent or alleviate the effects of chronic respiratory and cardiovascular diseases, and other chronic health problems (Eisenberg et al., 1998).

Hawthorn is used to decrease angina symptoms and to increase exercise tolerance. Ginseng is used for reducing stress, and parsley, skullcap, hawthorn, and wild black cherry have antihypertensive properties. Angelica (a bronchodilator), ginger, rosemary, and cinnamon are used in aromatherapy. Salvia and garlic are beneficial in reducing cholesterol and lowering blood pressure. Lobelia (Indian tobacco) contains lobeine, a nonaddicting substance similar to nicotine, and is often used in antismoking therapy and as an antidepressant, antianxiety agent.

The participants in the Eisenberg study also reported using both traditional and alternative therapies with or without informing their medical care providers. More than one-quarter of herbs have plant origins. Different parts of a plant or tree may have different properties and different concentrations, and can be used for different purposes (Grendell, 2000). It is crucial that people understand that herb and drug interactions can be harmful. Guggul (used in Ayurvedic medicine) has shown some promise in reducing cholesterol, but should not be used by pregnant women. Excessive amounts of licorice over an extended period can cause sodium-potassium imbalances. Ephedra (ma huang) has amphetamine-like effects and is used for weight loss, to increase energy, and to promote expectoration of secretions. Warnings have recently been issued about the detrimental effects of ephedra for persons with hypertension, hyperthyroidism, and cardiovascular problems (National Center for Complementary and Alternative Medicine, 2003).

## Evaluation

Clients with compromised oxygenation status need careful nursing care to address both their physical and psychological needs. Evaluation will be based on the expected outcomes that the nurse and client have established together. In many instances, the evaluation of the success of the specific interventions will be a matter of degree—that is, the degree to which the client is or can be returned to a satisfactory state of respiratory functioning. It is important when evaluating progress to revisit the initial plan of care to determine if each expected outcome was within reasonable expectations, and then to revise the goals, interventions, and plan of care to reflect truly reasonable expectations.

# CASE STUDY/NURSING CARE PLAN

Mike Calloway, age 27, was admitted to the emergency department following a fire at a paper manufacturing plant where he worked. He had been exposed to the fumes from the burning paper and the fire's extreme heat and smoke. His face and surrounding hair, lower arms, and hands have first-, second-, and third-degree burns. His eyebrows and nasal hairs are singed, and his teeth have deposits of soot on them. To escape from the rear of the building, he had to make his way through the smoke and flames before reaching the outside. He rolled on the ground to extinguish the flames from his clothing. Mike is alert enough to answer questions.

One hundred percent oxygen is administered by mask. His neck is stabilized, and blood is drawn for baseline hematocrit, electrolyte, BUN, cyanide, and carboxyhemoglobin levels. Lactated Ringer's solution is started through a large-bore cannula in a peripheral vein. Pain medication is administered. The physician requests close monitoring of Mike for signs of impaired oxygenation (e.g., tachypnea, agitation or anxiety, and symptoms of upper airway obstruction such as hoarseness, wheezing, or stridor). She mentions that burns can result in multisystem damage; therefore, assessment of neurologic, cardiovascular changes, and symptoms of shock are also of prime importance. She comments that the first 24 to 36 hours are critical for burn clients and that early intubation may be necessary to avoid later difficulty due to edema of the larynx.

## Assessment

A 27-year-old suffering from first-, second-, and third-degree burns to approximately 27% of his body (according to the rule of nines assessment tool). The majority of the burns are superficial and first degree in nature,

*(continues)*

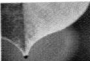

# CASE STUDY/NURSING CARE PLAN (continued)

but there is a potential of damage to the upper airway as evidenced by the nasal hairs and eyebrows being singed. In addition, the client's oxygen saturation level is 92%, which is somewhat low for a man of this client's age. The blood pressure = 138/86, pulse = 90, and respirations = 22. The client's breath sounds are clear to auscultation and not diminished in the bases.

## Nursing Diagnosis #1

*Impaired Gas Exchange* due to exposure to smoke poisoning and heat damage to lungs.

**NOC:** Respiratory Status: Gas Exchange; Respiratory Status: Ventilation; Tissue Perfusion: Pulmonary; Vital Signs Status

**NIC:** Airway Management; Oxygen Therapy; Respiratory Monitoring

### Expected Outcomes

The client will:

1. Demonstrate improved ventilation, adequate oxygenation as evidenced by an oxygen saturation level of at least 95% during his hospitalization.
2. Maintain clear lung fields and remain free of signs of respiratory distress during his hospitalization.

### Planning/Interventions/Rationales

1. Monitor respiratory rate, depth, and effort, including use of accessory muscles, nasal flaring, and abnormal breathing patterns. *These behaviors and a look of panic in the client's expression may be indicators of hypoxia.*
2. Auscultate breath sounds every hour, or more frequently as needed. *Crackles and wheezes may signify airway obstruction that can lead to or exacerbate existing hypoxia.*
3. Administer humidified oxygen through appropriate device; monitor client's behavior and mental status for onset of restlessness, agitation, or confusion. *Behavioral changes and mental status can be early signs of hypoventilation and impaired gas exchange.*
4. Monitor oxygen saturation continuously. Note blood gas results as available. $O_2$ *saturation of less than 90% or a partial pressure of $O_2$ of less than 80 indicates significant oxygenation problems.*
5. Position client in semi-Fowler's. Turn client every 2 hours. Observe client closely following position changes. *Turning critically ill clients with low hemoglobin levels or decreased cardiac output on either side can result in desaturation. Turn very carefully and watch closely.*

### Evaluation

Client's oxygen saturation levels increased to 94% within 24 hours and to 96% and above within 48 hours. In addition, the client's respiratory rate slowed to 16 to 20 breaths/minute within 24 hours and the lungs were clear upon auscultation throughout the acute hospitalization.

## Nursing Diagnosis #2

*Ineffective Breathing Pattern* due to compensatory tachypnea.

**NOC:** Respiratory Status: Ventilation; Vital Signs Status; Respiratory Status: Airway Patency

**NIC:** Airway Management; Respiratory Monitoring

### Expected Outcomes

The client will:

1. Return to a normal (regular) or effective breathing pattern.
2. Demonstrate an absence of cyanosis and other signs and symptoms of hypoxia.
3. Maintain ABGs within an acceptable range.
4. Demonstrate appropriate coping behaviors related to breath control.

### Planning/Interventions/Rationales

1. Observe rate and depth of respirations, breathing patterns, and signs of cyanosis. Auscultate chest for presence of breath sounds and secretions. Monitor diagnostic test results. *Ongoing assessment provides basis for interventions to aid in restoring adequate breathing patterns and oxygenation.*

*(continues)*

## CASE STUDY/NURSING CARE PLAN (continued)

2. Observe for changes in emotional responses. *Dyspnea can have physiological or psychogenic causes. Fear, anger, and anxiety adversely influence breathing patterns (hyperventilation) and loss of sense of control.*
3. Medicate with analgesics as appropriate. *Promotes deeper respiration and ability to cough if necessary to clear airway (pain may be cause of hyperventilation).*
4. Suction airway as needed. *Removes obstructing secretions, clears airway for clients who are unable to cough.*
5. Administer oxygen at lowest concentration prescribed. *Higher levels can inhibit client's respiratory drive.*

### Evaluation

Client maintained a respiratory rate of 16 to 20 per minute without any signs of cyanosis. He did not have any uncontrolled anxiety and was able to breathe in a controlled manner throughout this time of crisis. Analgesics were given periodically without affecting his rate and breathing pattern.

## Key Concepts

- Adequate tissue oxygenation is essential to survival and may be threatened by deficits in air movement through the lungs to deliver fresh air to the alveoli (ventilation), the exchange of oxygen and carbon dioxide across the alveolar-capillary membrane (diffusion or external respiration), oxygen transport in the blood, the delivery of oxygen to the tissues (circulation), or the uptake of oxygen by the cells (internal respiration).
- Oxygen status can be determined by a variety of diagnostic and laboratory data. Some of these tests are pulse oximetry, arterial blood gases, sputum analysis, chest radiography, ventilation scans, and computerized tomography.
- Client teaching related to oxygenation impairment involves teaching about the disease process, treatments, and lifestyle alterations that may be indicated; teaching should involve not only the client but also the family.
- Nursing care related to oxygenation focuses on maintaining a patent airway, promoting effective ventilation, promoting optimal circulation and perfusion, and meeting the client's learning, nutritional, activity, and sleep needs.
- A holistic approach to care recognizes that each of the problems experienced by the client with oxygenation deficits is interrelated.
- Emergency support of airway, ventilation, and circulation is achieved by instituting the Heimlich maneuver for airway obstruction and cardiopulmonary resuscitation for cardiopulmonary arrest.

## Review Questions and Activities

1. Which accounts for the greatest amount of oxygen carried in the arterial blood: the partial pressure of oxygen ($PaO_2$) or the hemoglobin saturation ($SaO_2$)?

2. Describe how positioning might affect the client with ineffective breathing patterns.
3. List two limitations of anaerobic metabolism.
4. What is the difference between intermittent positive-pressure breathing (IPPB) and incentive spirometry?
5. List two potential complications of oxygen administration.
6. Artificial airways such as endotracheal tubes and tracheostomies bypass the upper airways. What is the significance of this?
7. How does heart failure cause edema?
8. When experiencing pain related to peripheral atherosclerosis (claudication), the client should position the extremity below heart level. Why?

## Multimedia Links

Altman *Advanced Care DVD: Maintaining and Cleaning Endotracheal Tubes*
Altman *Advanced Care DVD: Suctioning Endotracheal and Tracheal Tubes*
Altman *Advanced Care DVD: Maintaining and Cleaning the Tracheostomy Tube*
Altman *Advanced Care DVD: Maintaining a Double Cannula Tracheostomy Tube*
Altman *Advanced Care DVD: Plugging the Tracheostomy Tube*
Altman *Advanced Care DVD: Administering Oxygen Therapy*
Altman *Advanced Care DVD: Assisting a Client with Controlled Coughing and Deep Breathing*
Altman *Advanced Care DVD: Assisting a Client with an Incentive Spirometer*
Altman *Advanced Care DVD: Administering Pulmonary Therapy and Postural Drainage*
Altman *Advanced Care DVD: Administering Pulse Oximetry*
Altman *Basic Care DVD: Performing the Heimlich Maneuver*
Altman *Basic Care DVD: Administering Cardiopulmonary Resuscitation (CPR)*
Altman *Advanced Care Video: Oxygenation*
Christensen *Core Concept Videos: Oxygenation*

# Web Resources

Agency for Health Care Policy and Research
  http://www.ahrq.gov
American Heart Association
  http://www.americanheart.org
American Holistic Nurses Association
  http://www.ahna.org
American Lung Association
  http://www.lungusa.org
American Stroke Association
  http://www.strokeassociation.org
Childhood Asthma Management
  http://www.betterhealth4kids.com
National Center for Complementary and Alternative
  Medicine (NCCAM)
  http://nccam.nih.gov
National Heart, Lung, and Blood Institute (Asthma
  Education and Prevention Program Guidelines)
  http://www.nhlbi.nih.gov

# References

Altman, G. (2004). *Delmar's fundamental & advanced nursing skills* (2nd ed.). Clifton Park, NY: Delmar Learning.

American Heart Association (2003) http://www.american heart.org

Archibald, C. (1999). Oxygenation. In K. Berger & M. Williams (Eds.), *Fundamentals of nursing* (pp. 999–1086). Stamford, CT: Appleton & Lange.

Berger, K., & Williams, M. (1999). *Fundamentals of nursing: Collaborating for optimal health.* Stamford, CT: Addison Wesley.

Carroll, R. (2001). Anatomy and physiology of the heart. In J. Black, J. Hawks, & A. Keene (Eds.), *Medical-surgical nursing: Clinical management for continuity of care.* Philadelphia: W. B. Saunders.

Childhood Asthma Management (2002). http://www. betterhealth4kids.com

Clark, A. (2002). Legal lessons: "But his $O_2$ Sat was normal!" *Clinical Nurse Specialist, 16*(3), 162–163.

Collins, E., Langbein, W., Fehr, L., & Maloney, C. (2001). Breathing pattern retraining and exercise in persons with chronic obstructive pulmonary disease. *AACN Clinical Issues: Advanced Practice of Critical-Care Nurses, 12*(2), 202–209.

Cronin, R., & Mirocle, K. (2001). Management of clients with lower airway and pulmonary vessels disorders. In J. Black, J. Hawks, & A. Keene (Eds.), *Medical-surgical nursing: Clinical management for continuity of care.* Philadelphia: W. B. Saunders.

Daniels, R. (2003). *Delmar's manual of laboratory and diagnostic tests.* Clifton Park, NY: Delmar Learning.

Doenges, M., Moorhouse, M., & Geissler-Murr, A. (2002). *Nurse's pocket guide: Diagnoses, interventions, and rationales* (8th ed.). Philadelphia: F. A. Davis.

Eisenberg, D., Davis, R., Etter, S., Appel, S., Wilkey, S., Van Rompay, M., & Kessler, R. (1998). Trends in alternative medicine use in the United States, 1990–1997. *Journal of the American Medical Association, 280*(18), 1569–1575.

Estes, M. (2002). *Health assessment & physical examination* (2nd ed.). Clifton Park, NY: Delmar Learning.

Gallagher, C. (2002). Childhood asthma: Tools that help parents manage it. *American Journal of Nursing, 102*(8), 71–83.

Grendell, R. (2000). Psychological aspects of physiologic illness. In K. Fortinash & P. Holoday-Worret (Eds.), *Psychiatric mental health nursing.* St. Louis: Mosby.

Harrah, B. (1998). Knowledge base for patients with cardiac dysfunction. In F. Monahan & M. Neighbors (Eds.), *Medical-surgical nursing: Foundation for clinical practice.* Philadelphia: W. B. Saunders.

Hogstel, M. (2001). *Gerontology: Nursing care of the older adult.* Clifton Park, NY: Delmar Learning.

Holland, B., & McCurren, C. (2001). Health promotion in older adults. In J. Black, J. Hawks, & A. Keene (Eds.), *Medical-surgical nursing: Clinical management for continuity of care.* Philadelphia: W. B. Saunders.

Kee, J., & Hayes, E. (2000). *Pharmacology: A nursing process approach.* Philadelphia: W. B. Saunders.

Keene, A. (2001). Health history. In J. Black, J. Hawks, & A. Keene (Eds.), *Medical-surgical nursing: Clinical management for continuity of care.* Philadelphia: W. B. Saunders.

Koschel, M. (2002). Where there's smoke, there may be cyanide. *American Journal of Nursing, 102*(8), 39–42.

Leidy, N. K., & Haase, J. E. (1999). Functional status from the patient's perspective: The challenge of preserving personal integrity. *Research in Nursing Health, 22*(2), 67–77.

National Center for Complementary and Alternative Medicine (NCCAM) (2003). http://nccam.nih.gov

Nightingale, F. (1860). *Notes on nursing: What it is and what it is not.* London: Pall Mall Bookseller to the Queen.

Pelletier, K. (2000). *The best of alternative medicine.* New York: Fireside Book, Simon & Schuster.

Potts, N., & Mandleco, B. (2002). *Pediatric nursing: Caring for children and their families.* Clifton Park, NY: Delmar Learning.

Stacy, K. (2000). Pulmonary disorders. In L. Urden & K. Stacy (Eds.), *Priorities in critical care nursing.* St. Louis: Mosby.

Stapleton, M. (1998). Knowledge base for patients with respiratory dysfunction. In F. Monahan & M. Neighbors (Eds.), *Medical/surgical nursing: Foundations for practice.* Philadelphia: W. B. Saunders.

Urden, L., Stacy, K., & Lough, M., (2002). *Thelan's critical care nursing: Diagnosis and management* (4th ed.). St. Louis: C. V. Mosby.

# Sleep-Rest

**Chapter 40**  Sleep and Rest

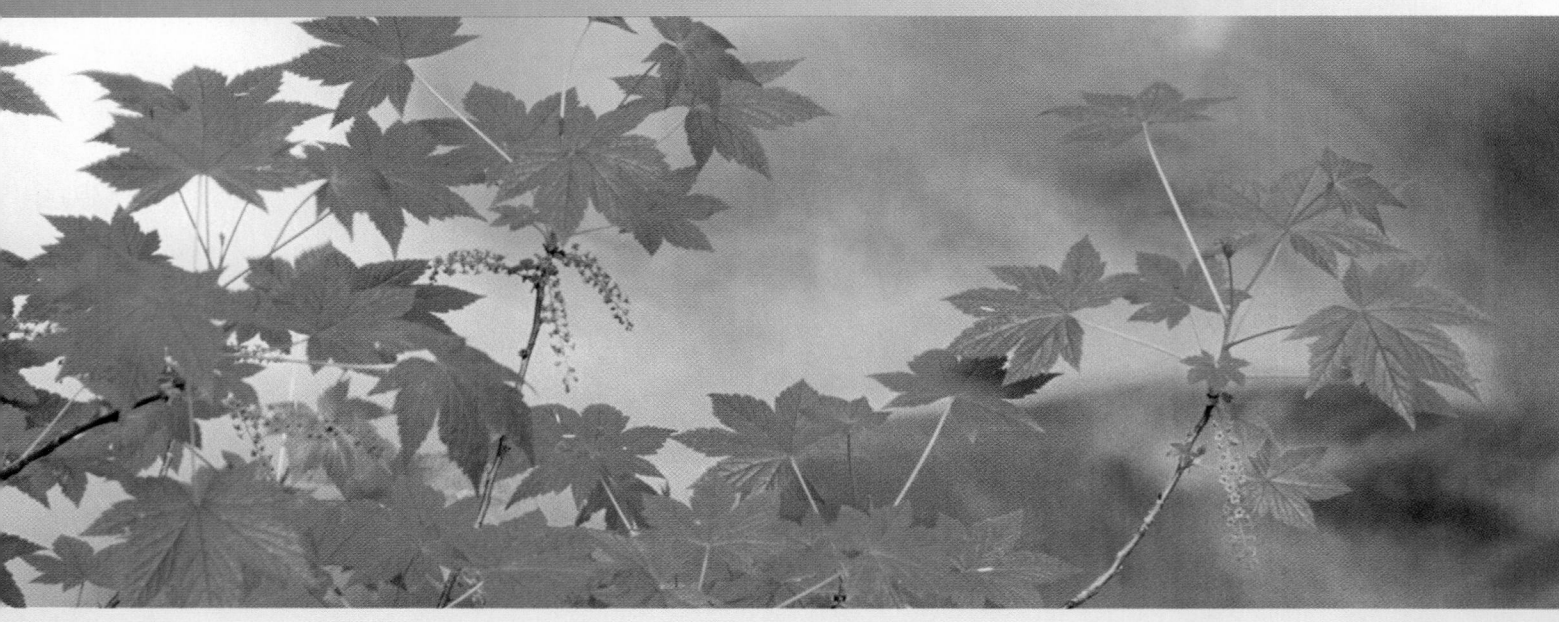

# Sleep and Rest

Debra L. Topham, PhD, RN, CNS, ACRN

*"Whatever our race, creed, or culture, we all sleep."*

(Idzikowski, 2000)

# Chapter Competencies

*Upon completion of this chapter, the reader should be able to:*

1. Describe the physiology of rest and sleep.
2. Identify the stages of sleep.
3. Define the factors that affect rest and sleep.
4. Evaluate the effects of hospitalization and illness on rest and sleep.
5. Identify alterations in sleep patterns.
6. Discuss the nursing process as it relates to rest and sleep.
7. Develop nursing interventions that promote rest and sleep.

# Key Terms

biological clock
bruxism
chronobiology
circadian rhythm
endorphin
hypersomnia
hypnagogic hallucinations

hypnagogic state
idiopathic insomnia
insomnia
narcolepsy
parasomnia
rest
sleep

sleep apnea
sleep cycle
sleep deprivation
sleep paralysis
somnambulism

Rest and sleep are fundamental to physiological and psychological well-being. All individuals require certain periods of calm and lesser activity so that their bodies can regain energy and rebuild stamina. The need for rest and sleep varies with age, developmental level, health status, and activity level.

**Rest** refers to a state of relaxation and calmness, both mental and physical. Activity during rest periods can range from lying down to reading a book to taking a meditative walk. When discussing a client's rest patterns, the nurse should try to understand what activities and environments the client defines as restful.

**Sleep** refers to a state of altered consciousness during which an individual experiences minimal physical activity and a general slowing of the body's physiological process-es. Sleep generally occurs in a periodic cycle and usually lasts for several hours at a time; disruptions in the usual sleep routine can be distressing to clients and will most likely impair sleep further. As a restorative function, sleep is necessary for physiological and psychological healing to occur. It is important for clients, their significant others, and health care providers to understand the normal sleep-wake cycle and how sleep affects mood and healing (National Sleep Foundation, 2003).

# Physiology of Rest and Sleep

The cycles of wakefulness and sleep are controlled by centers in the brain. The hormone melatonin, secreted from the pineal gland, regulates these sleep-wake centers (Hilton, 2002). Sleep is also influenced by routines, seasons, and environmental factors. Finally, an individual's biological clock helps determine the specific cycles that will be followed for wakefulness and sleep (Wyatt, 2001).

## Stages of Sleep

Electroencephalograph (EEG) patterns, eye movements, and muscle activity are used to identify stages of sleep. The five stages of sleep are classified in two categories: non-rapid eye movement (NREM) and rapid eye movement (REM) sleep.

## NREM Sleep

With the onset of sleep, the heart rate and respiratory rate slow slightly and remain regular. This first phase of sleep is referred to as non-rapid eye movement, or NREM, sleep. NREM sleep consists of four different stages. As the client enters *stage 1 sleep*, there is a general

## RESEARCH FOCUS

**Title of Study:** The relationship between chronically disrupted sleep and health care use

**Study Purpose:** The descriptive study sought to determine whether chronic sleep disorders were associated with increased health care use by persons in the general population.

**Methods:** This was a cross-sectional design that collected survey data from 6,440 participants in a heart health study. Chronic disease scores were computed using the modified Chronic Disease Score (CDS) instrument.

**Findings:** Chronic disease scores in healthy individuals with sleep apnea were similar to scores of persons with hypertension, chronic bronchitis, or asthma. An association was found between complaints of daytime sleepiness, inadequate sleep, and severity of apnea and health care use.

**Implications:** The authors assert that improving sleep would decrease health care use. Thus, the implications are that persons who have chronically disturbed sleep have more health problems. As a person's sleep improves, theoretically she would have fewer health problems.

Kapur, V. K., Redline, S., Nieto, F. J., Young, T. B., Newman, A. B., & Henderson, J. A. (2002). The relationship between chronically disrupted sleep and health care use. *Sleep, 25*(3), 289–296.

slowing of EEG frequency but an appearance of theta waves and spikes, the eyes tend to roll slowly from side to side, and muscle tension remains absent except in the facial and neck muscles. In adult clients with normal sleep patterns, stage 1 sleep usually lasts only 10 minutes or so. Stage 1 NREM sleep is of a very light quality, which means that during this stage a sleeper can be easily awakened. It is also during stage 1 that a person is in a hypnagogic state. The **hypnagogic state** is the condition experienced when a person is between sleep and wakefulness.

*Stage 2 sleep* is still fairly light sleep, with a further slowing of EEG patterns and loss of slow rolling eye movements. In stage 2 sleep, the person loses awareness of the outside world. Fifty percent of normal adult sleep may be spent in stage 2. After an initial 20 minutes or so of stage 2 sleep, a deep form of sleep called stage 3 to 4 is entered.

*Stage 3* and *stage 4* sleep are frequently discussed together because of the difficulty of identifying and separating the two. Stage 3 refers to medium-depth sleep, and stage 4 signals the deepest sleep. During these stages, all cortical brain cells appear to be firing at the same time, resulting in large slow waves on the EEG, known as delta waves. When roused from stage 3 to 4 sleep, an adult can take 15 seconds or so to become fully awake. This difficulty in awakening is even more pronounced in children. Stage 3 to 4 sleep is where most sleepwalking, sleeptalking, enuresis, and night terrors occur.

Stage 3 to 4 sleep is believed to have restorative value, necessary for physical recovery. After sleep deprivation, stage 3 to 4 sleep is the first to be regained. The majority of growth hormone is secreted at night, peaking during stage 3 to 4 sleep near the beginning of a sleep period. Growth hormone is required not only for growth but also for normal tissue repair in clients of all ages. Stage 3 to 4 sleep accounts for approximately 25% of sleep in children, declines slightly in young adulthood, then gradually declines in middle age and may be absent in older clients.

### REM Sleep

After the initial 90 minutes or so of NREM sleep in adults, the client enters rapid eye movement (REM) sleep, or stage 5 sleep. The EEG pattern, beta waves, resembles that of the awake state; there are rapid conjugate eye movements; heart rate and respiratory rate are irregular and often higher than when awake; and muscles, including those of the face and neck, are flaccid, leaving the body immobilized. REM sleep is essential to emotional well-being and emotional adaptation. REM sleep needs are greater after periods of increased stress and illness. Dreams occur 80% of the time clients are in REM sleep. Unlike stage 3 to 4 sleep, which is most abundant during the early portion of a sleep period, REM sleep periods become longer as the night progresses and the individual becomes more rested. An adult typically has four to six REM sleep periods through the night, accounting for 20% to 25% of sleep. REM sleep makes up 50% of sleep in the newborn, then gradually declines to 20% to 25% of sleep by early childhood, and remains fairly constant throughout the remainder of the life span (Wyatt, 2001).

### Sleep Cycle

A **sleep cycle** refers to the sequence of sleep that begins with the four stages of NREM sleep in order, with a return to stage 3, then 2, then passage into the first REM stage (Figure 40-1). The duration of a sleep cycle is generally between 70 and 100 minutes, and the typical sleeper will pass through four to six sleep cycles during an average sleep period of 7 to 9 hours.

The length of the NREM and REM periods of sleep will change as the overall sleep period progresses and the person becomes more relaxed and reenergized. There is less need for stage 3 to 4 sleep and more need for REM

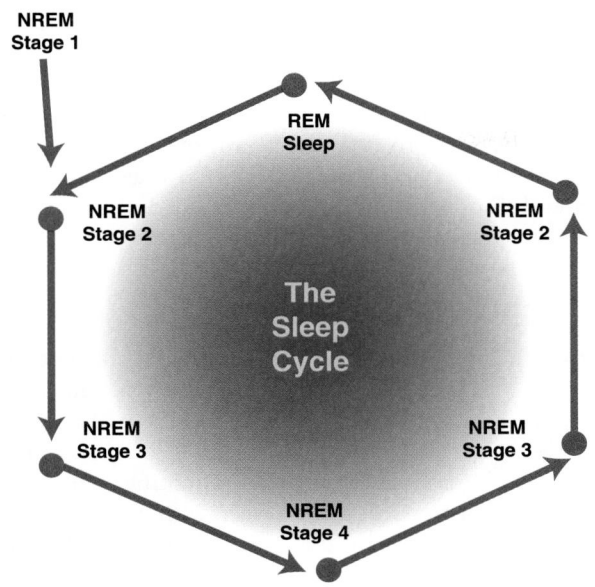

**Figure 40-1 The sleep cycle**

sleep as the sleep period progresses, and dreams during the REM phases of later sleep may become more vivid and intense. If the sleep cycle is broken at any point, a new sleep cycle will start, beginning again at stage 1 of NREM sleep and progressing through all the stages to REM sleep.

## Biological Clock

The **biological clock** (an endogenous mechanism that measures time) controls the daily fluctuations in hundreds of physiological processes, including body temperature, respiratory rate, performance, alertness, and hormone levels.

**Chronobiology** is a relatively new branch of science that studies these rhythms that are controlled by the biological clock. The most widely studied are the **circadian rhythms**, or those that cycle on a daily basis. Other biological rhythms include:

- Ultradian—those much shorter than a day
- Infradian—those lasting a month or more
- Circannual—those requiring about 1 year to complete the cycle

When external time cues such as day-night, change in time zones, sleep-wake, and mealtimes are inconsistent, a desynchronization, or mismatching, of the circadian biological rhythms occurs. This internal desynchronization disrupts the timing of physiological and behavioral activity, which in turn causes chronic fatigue, disrupts sleep patterns, and causes decreased performance and coping abilities. An example of desynchronization is that of the newborn, whose biological rhythms are not established until 3 to 4 months of age. At this point, infants will start to develop longer sleep periods at night and become more predictable in their waking and sleeping patterns. At this age, sleep patterns become learned behaviors.

## Factors Affecting Rest and Sleep

Several factors can influence the quality and quantity of both sleep and rest. These factors include comfort level, anxiety or stress, environment, lifestyle, hormones, diet and nutrition, medications and drugs, and developmental stage.

### Comfort Level

Comfort is a highly subjective experience. The nurse must assess the degree to which the client's physical and psychological needs have been met. Whenever basic needs are unmet, the person experiences discomfort, which leads to physiological tension, resultant anxiety, and potential impairments in sleep. Pain is a state of physiological discomfort that often results in muscular tension and difficulty sleeping. When pain is extreme, clients may not be able to sleep without prescription medications. Occasionally, clients must be reminded that taking mild sedatives can be very therapeutic.

### Anxiety/Stress

A restless body and mind interfere with the ability to sleep. When trying to go to sleep, many individuals often have intrusive thoughts, which interferes with rest and sleep. Anxiety related to work pressures, family demands, and other stressors does not automatically cease when an individual attempts to go to sleep. Anxiety and stress often result in difficulty falling or staying asleep.

### Environment

Environmental factors can either enhance or impair sleep. Lighting, temperature, odors, ventilation, and noise level can all interrupt the sleep process when they differ from the norms of the client's usual sleep environment.

### Lifestyle

A fast-paced life filled with multiple stressors can result in the person's inability to relax easily or to fall asleep quickly. Relaxation precedes healthy sleep.

Another lifestyle factor that interferes with sleep is having a work schedule that does not coincide with an individual's biological clock (e.g., working at times other than the day shift). Individuals who frequently change work shifts have a real challenge in trying to stabilize biological rhythms and rest comfortably. Persons who work a rotating shift are at greater risk for sleep disturbances than persons who work straight night shifts.

## CLIENT REFLECTIONS

### Taking Sedatives for Sleep

Mr. Bennett had back surgery last month, and his postoperative pain is making it difficult for him to sleep. At his first follow-up visit, Mr. Bennett states, "I know you (nurse practitioner) told me I could take that pill (sedative) to help me sleep, but I don't like taking drugs. I'm afraid I'll get used to taking the pill and then won't be able to sleep without it. And besides, I probably wouldn't be able to wake up very easily in the morning."

What would you say to this client?

## Hormones

Hormone levels are thought to affect sleep patterns and quality, especially in women. Hormone fluctuation during menses and the third trimester of pregnancy can cause sleeplessness in healthy women. Hormone shifts during perimenopause and menopause may also induce sleep problems.

## Diet/Nutrition

The type of food consumed has an impact on the quality and quantity of sleep. Foods high in caffeine, such as coffee, colas, and chocolate, serve as stimulants and often disrupt the normal sleep cycle. Also, consuming a large, heavy, or spicy meal just before bedtime may cause indigestion, which will likely interfere with sleep. Conversely, going to bed when hungry can also result in sleep problems because the individual may be preoccupied with food and hunger pangs instead of concentrating on sleep.

## Drugs/Medications

Alcohol and nicotine use can impair sleep. Small amounts of alcohol may help some people fall asleep; however, as effects of alcohol wear off, the person is susceptible to frequent wakening during the night, causing restless and nonrefreshing sleep. Nicotine, which is a stimulant, can also impair the sleep cycle by stimulating the body, resulting in difficulty falling and staying asleep. Many medications (both prescription and over-the-counter) cause fatigue, sleepiness, restlessness, agitation, or insomnia, thus affecting the quality and quantity of rest and sleep.

## Cultural Norms

Cultural and societal expectations also affect sleep. Some people perceive sleep as a luxury to be indulged in when they are not too busy with "important" activities. Others view sleep as an absolute necessity. The amount of sleep that a person considers to be necessary is partially determined by the attitudes of family and culture (see Box 40-1).

## NURSING STRATEGY

### Facilitating a Sleep Environment

- Sleep is best facilitated at a temperature of 62°F for adults and 65°F for children.

- Pleasant, white noise promotes sleep, while noxious noise interrupts sleep. For example, the sound of the ocean facilitates sleep while the sound of heavy road traffic disrupts sleep.

- Sleep is facilitated in dark environments. Use of heavy curtains, blackout shades, and blinds facilitates a more restful sleep.

- The sleep surface is key in facilitating sleep. The mattress should be firm and supportive of the back and spine. Mattresses should be replaced every 10 years or so.

Idzikowski, C. (2000). *Learn to sleep well: A practical guide to getting a good night's rest.* San Francisco: Chronicle Books.

## NURSING STRATEGY

### Interventions for Sleeplessness During Menopause

The following are suggestions for clients who have difficulty sleeping due to menopause:

1. Encourage herbal remedies such as herbal teas and drinks that induce relaxation.
2. Take such nature products as black cohash, which assist in reducing menopausal symptoms.
3. Exercise regularly to decrease stress and increase propensity to sleep in normal pattern.
4. Refer to family health practitioner with women's health specialty for evaluation.
5. Discuss frequency of "hot flashes" and encourage the use of a fan in the bedroom to decrease wakefulness.

Sleep Medicine Home Page (2002). http://www.users.cloud9.net

## BOX 40-1   CULTURAL CONSIDERATIONS

The practice of having children sleep alone or with parents is culturally determined. For instance, most Anglo-Americans have babies and children sleep separately from the parents. African Americans, Appalachians, and Japanese Americans encourage interdependent family links throughout life, and thus encourage children, up to age 6, to sleep with parents. Children who co-sleep with parents are found to have fewer nightmares and less sleepwalking (Idzikowski, 2000).

## Life Span Considerations

A person's need for sleep changes with age in a fairly predictable pattern. Although sleep and rest patterns are closely tied to lifestyle and other variables, there are some common variations (Potts & Mandleco, 2002):

- The *neonate* (birth to 1 month) sleeps in 3- to 4-hour intervals for a total of about 16 to 20 hours per day. The newborn usually is very passive, with little activity during sleep ("sleeping like a baby"), and typically sleeps very soundly. For the first few days or weeks of life, a baby's biological clock is not attuned to regular day-night patterns, so there is often no difference in sleep patterns between day and night.
- The *infant* averages about 12 to 18 hours of sleep per day. As the infant ages, the amount of sleep needed decreases. At approximately 2 months of age, infants can begin to sleep through the night and will typically nap two or three times during the day.
- During *toddlerhood* the daily average amount of sleep is 12 to 14 hours, which is usually broken down into 10 to 12 hours at night with one or two daytime naps. During this stage, bedtime rituals often develop and assume great importance in providing nighttime security. Repeated and predictable nighttime routines such as baths, brushing teeth, and reading books are helpful in establishing expectations and comfort.
- The *preschool* child sleeps approximately 10 to 12 hours per day. Daytime napping decreases or ceases, unless cultural norms dictate otherwise. Night sleep is often filled with vivid dreams and nightmares, which often awaken children several times during the night.
- A *school-age* child also averages about 10 to 12 hours of sleep daily. Resistance to bedtime and struggles for independence are hallmarks of the school-age child. During this time, the child may develop fear of the dark and will need reassurance and methods to handle this fear.
- *Adolescents* sleep about 8 to 10 hours per day and often decide themselves their bedtime routines and hours.

High activity levels often interfere with regular sleep patterns and irregular sleeping habits often become the norm at this stage. Despite the high activity level of adolescence, sleep needs remain high because of hormonal fluctuations and increased stress. It is typical for an adolescent to sleep less during the week and then catch up on sleep on the weekends.

- The *young adult* averages about 8 hours of sleep per day. During this stage, sleep is often interrupted by young children in the home or work responsibilities. Lifestyle patterns cause many young adults to experience difficulties falling or staying asleep.
- The *middle-aged adult* sleeps about 6 to 8 hours a day. Because of the decreased hours of sleep and the poorer quality of sleep that occurs with aging, persons in middle adulthood often use naps to enhance nighttime sleep.
- The sleep requirements for the *older adult* decrease to 5 to 7 hours per day, and often include a daytime nap. The quality of sleep often diminishes due to frequent waking, physical pain, and shortened REM sleep.

## LIFE SPAN CONSIDERATIONS

### Tips for Parents of Sleepless Infants

Infants' sleep patterns are often unpredictable and greatly affect their parents' sleep habits. The parents of new infants should be taught that they will need to take measures to cope with this situation. First, the parents need to do what they can to enhance the infant's sleep environment (e.g., quiet environment, warmth, good nutrition). Second, parents can "take turns getting up with their child" while the other parent sleeps. Third, parents can talk with each other, their support peers, and health care providers about their "sleeplessness." Communicating openly with others helps in the acceptance of their lack of sleep and "normalizes" this condition. Fourth, and last, parents must be objective about their sleeplessness and know "it will get better." Parents must work on anger issues (if appropriate) and not take out their frustrations on their family and others. Note: single-parent families may have more difficulty coping with the infant's sleeplessness and need encouragement and additional support networking to assist during this time.

Potts, N., & Mandleco, B. (2002). *Pediatric nursing: Caring for children and their families.* Clifton Park, NY: Delmar Learning.

# Illness or Hospitalization

The stress imposed by illness usually disrupts sleep. Sleep is especially disrupted when a person is hospitalized. Some factors associated with hospitalization that lead to sleep impairment include:

- Physical or emotional pain
- Loss of familiar surroundings
- Loss of routine
- Fear of the unknown
- Disruption of sleep because of procedures or treatments (Figure 40-2)
- Exposure to continuous light during nighttime
- Noise level (especially unfamiliar noises)
- Loss of privacy

# Alteration in Sleep Patterns

Sleep disturbances can take many forms and are quite common. According to Carpenito (2004), disturbed sleep pattern is defined as:

> The state in which an individual experiences or is at risk of experiencing a change in the quantity or quality of his or her rest pattern as related to the person's biological and emotional needs.

Alterations in sleep patterns are generally viewed as either primary sleep disorders (those in which the sleep alteration is the fundamental problem) or secondary sleep disorders (those in which the alteration has a medical or clinical cause that results in or contributes to the sleep alteration). The most common sleep alterations include insomnia, hypersomnia or narcolepsy, sleep apnea, sleep deprivation, and parasomnias.

Chronic insomnia is a widespread problem, affecting 10% to 20% of Americans; approximately 40% to 50% report

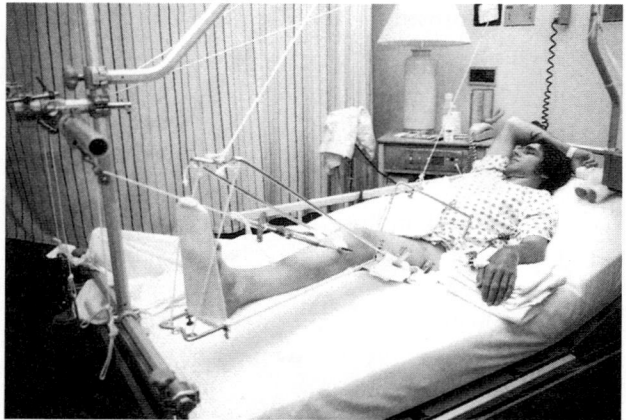

**Figure 40-2** This hospitalized client has difficulty sleeping because of the traction for his fractured femur.

## STOP AND THINK

### Sleeping in the Hospital

- What barriers to sleep have you observed in the hospital setting?

- How easy would it be for you to sleep in a hospital?

- What interventions would help decrease or remove these barriers?

occasional insomnia (Doghramji & Fredman, 1999). Listed below are problems associated with sleep disturbances:

- Decreased work productivity (more missed days of work)
- Increased use of health care services
- Greater risk of accidents
- Short-term memory problems
- Cognitive and motor performance impairments
- Irritability, short temper, anger

## Insomnia

**Insomnia** refers to the chronic inability to sleep or inadequate quality of sleep due to sleep prematurely ended or interrupted by periods of wakefulness. Insomnia is *not* a disease, but it may be a manifestation of many illnesses. The person experiencing insomnia often gets caught up in a vicious cycle of not being able to sleep, trying harder to fall asleep, increasing anxiety about not sleeping, which in turn increases the inability to fall asleep. There are three types of insomnia: psychophysiological, idiopathic, and sleep-state misinterpretation.

### Psychophysiological

Psychophysiological insomnia occurs when a physiological problem creates lack of sleep, which increases anxiety about sleep and leads to further lack of sleep. Because sleep is a learned behavior, behavioral interventions are effective in treating psychophysiological insomnia. The most important intervention is to have the client use the bed for sleep and sex only. The second most important intervention is to help the client's mind relearn a normal sleep pattern.

### Idiopathic

**Idiopathic insomnia** (sleeplessness with an unknown origin) is diagnosed with use of an EEG. In clients who do not have any other indicators for insomnia, sleep studies using EEGs are useful in diagnosing idiopathic insomnia. The EEG is abnormal, indicating disturbances of the sleep centers of the brain. This type of insomnia will not respond to behavioral interventions and often requires pharmacological interventions (Wyatt, 2001).

## CLIENT EDUCATION

### Treating Psychophysiological Insomnia

To treat psychophysiological insomnia, do the following:

✓ Go to bed only when you are sleepy.

✓ If you are not asleep within 20 minutes, get out of bed.

✓ Do something until you are sleepy, then return to bed.

✓ Set the alarm to rise at the same time each morning.

✓ Do not sleep in past the alarm.

✓ Do not take naps in the daytime.

Dement, W. C., and Vaughan, C. (1999). *The promise of sleep: A pioneer in sleep medicine explores the vital connection between health, happiness, and a good night's sleep.* New York: Dell Publishers.

### Sleep-State Misinterpretation

Sleep-state misinterpretation (a condition where the client is in a dreamlike state but not in a deeper level of sleep state) is also diagnosed by an EEG taking during sleep studies. The EEG will show the person is asleep, but the person will claim to be awake. This is an extremely debilitating type of insomnia, and is often disbelieved by health care workers. Pharmacological interventions are most effective, but not completely effective in treating sleep-state misinterpretations (National Sleep Foundation, 2003).

## Hypersomnia or Narcolepsy

**Hypersomnia** is an alteration in sleep pattern characterized by excessive sleep, especially in the daytime. Persons suffering from hypersomnia often feel that they cannot get enough sleep at night, and therefore they sleep very late into the morning and nap several times throughout the day. Causes of hypersomnia can be physical or psychological; treatment depends on addressing the underlying cause.

**Narcolepsy**, another sleep alteration, manifests as sudden uncontrollable urges to fall asleep during the daytime. Besides the amount of sleep, the quality of sleep in the person with narcolepsy is poor. This is because the person with narcolepsy starts with REM stage sleep and then moves into other sleep stages. A person with narcolepsy often gets enough hours of sleep at night, but because of the poor quality they are overwhelmed by sleepiness at unexpected and unpredictable periods during the day. Two hallmarks of narcolepsy include the experience of hypnagogic hallucinations and sleep paralysis. **Hypnagogic hallucinations** are lifelike dreams and hallucinations that often incorporate elements of the environment and are experienced during the hypnagogic state. **Sleep paralysis** is the experience of waking from sleep and being unable to move, speak, or cry out. Narcolepsy is a hereditary disorder, with 60% of those affected having relatives who are also affected. Effective treatments for narcolepsy include avoiding substances or activities that cause sleepiness, taking planned daytime naps, or taking prescribed stimulant medications.

## Sleep Apnea and Snoring

**Sleep apnea** refers to periods of sleep during which airflow stops for 10 seconds or more. Sleep apnea occurs because the tissue of the soft palate closes off the airway, resulting in the person not breathing. It then ends with a loud snore as the brain sends the message to breathe more forcefully. Persons at risk for sleep apnea are those who are overweight, who indulge in alcohol or tobacco, or who sleep on their backs. Sleep apnea gives rise to complications as a result of oxygen desaturation and carbon dioxide retention. Short-term consequences may include cognitive impairment (including memory changes), personality changes, and impotence. A major problem is daytime sleepiness, which may interfere with functional abilities such as driving and working. If untreated, sleep apnea can result in the following (Forth, 1998):

- Hypertension
- Cardiac arrhythmias
- Right-sided congestive heart failure
- Cerebral vascular accident (stroke)
- Cognitive dysfunction
- Death

The first line of defense against apnea is treating its cause. Use of a nasal continuous positive airway pressure (CPAP) device may also give relief. The CPAP machine provides continuous airway pressure, which prevents the soft palate from closing off the airway. In extreme cases, a uvulopalatoplasty is performed to revise the soft palate and prevent tissue from occluding the airway. This is a radical procedure and used only as a last resort.

Snoring is loud, noisy breathing during sleep. There are no periods of apnea for someone who snores. Persons with sleep apnea, however, often also snore. The snoring does not wake up the snorer, but sleep is disrupted. It is believed to be caused by weakness of the muscles in the back of the throat. As with sleep apnea, obesity, smoking, alcohol use, and sleeping on one's back are all thought to contribute to snoring. In children, tonsillitis can contribute to snoring. Snoring is rare among professional singers, because it is believed they have strong muscles in the back of the throat. In addition to changing risk behaviors, singing exercises have been found to be useful in decreasing the incidence of snoring (National Sleep Foundation, 2003).

## Sleep Deprivation

**Sleep deprivation** is a term used to describe prolonged inadequate quality and quantity of sleep, either of the REM or the NREM type. Sleep deprivation can result from age, prolonged hospitalization, drug and substance use, illness, and frequent changes in lifestyle patterns. Sleep and dreaming have a restorative value necessary for mental and emotional recovery, and enhance the ability to cope with emotional problems. Therefore, sleep deprivation can cause symptoms ranging from irritability, hypersensitivity, and confusion to apathy, sleepiness, and diminished reflexes. Treating or minimizing the factors that cause the sleep deprivation is the most effective resolution.

## Parasomnia

**Parasomnias** refer to sleep alterations resulting from "an activation of physiological systems at inappropriate times during the sleep-wake cycle" (American Psychiatric Association, 2001, p. 564). **Somnambulism** (sleepwalking), sleeptalking, bed-wetting, and **bruxism** (teeth grinding) are the most common parasomnias. Treatment for parasomnias varies, and care should be focused on helping the client and family understand the disorder and its potential safety risks.

Restless Leg Syndrome (RLM) and Periodic Limb Movement Syndrome (PLMS) are two types of involuntary leg movements that interfere with sleep. Restless Leg Syndrome is when the client has creepy, crawly sensations in one or both legs. This sensation makes it difficult to fall asleep and occurs in 8% of the general population to 30% of those with rheumatoid arthritis (Idzikowski, 2000). Periodic Limb Movement Syndrome involves uncontrolled movement of some or all extremities during sleep. This can cause frequent awakenings and poor quality of sleep (Ohayou & Roth, 2002).

## CLINICAL ALERT

### Acute Sleep Deprivation in Intensive Care Units

Intensive care units (ICUs) are often difficult areas in which to sleep. Consequently, clients may suffer from acute sleep deprivation, which can manifest as severe changes in cognitive functions of memory, judgment, and personality disorders. The ICU nurses must assess their clients for early clinical symptoms of sleep deprivation and then take measures to increase the likelihood of their obtaining adequate sleep and rest.

## Assessment

Discussion of sleep habits is included as part of the regular health history. Any client acknowledging a sleep disturbance should be thoroughly assessed to determine sleep routines, sleep alterations, type of disturbances, and impact of sleep problems. Typically the client is a reliable source for this information, but a spouse or partner who shares sleeping arrangements may be able to add valuable information to the client's report. Questions regarding the client's usual sleep patterns should include:

1. Nature of sleep (restful, uninterrupted)
2. Quality of sleep (usual sleep pattern, schedules, hours of sleep, feeling on waking)
3. Sleep environment (description of room, temperature, noise level)
4. Associated factors (bedtime routines, use of sleep medications or any other sleep inducers)
5. Opinion of sleep (adequate, restores energy adequately, inadequate, problematic)

Questions regarding altered sleep patterns are intended to discover such information as:

1. Nature of the problem (inability to fall asleep, difficulty remaining asleep, inability to fall asleep after awakening, restless sleep, daytime sleepiness)
2. Quality of the problem (number of hours of sleep versus number of hours spent trying to sleep, number of hours of sleep a night, duration and frequency of naps or other compensatory measures, number of wakings per sleep period)

## COMMUNITY/HOME CARE

### Sleep Issues for Home Care

When assessing the client in a home setting, the nurse must carefully examine the physical environment. The home health nurse must give attention to the location of the bedroom as related to outside noises (e.g., highways, close neighbors). The nurse must ask specific questions as to whether the client sees the home setting as a conducive location for sleep. Often the psychological influences among the persons living in the home create either a "good versus bad" location for sleep (e.g., family stress, financial problems). Initially, gathering the information is important; then the nurse can follow up with potential interventions.

Adapted from Kapur, V. K., Redline, S., Nieto, F. J., Young, T. B., Newman, A. B., & Henderson, J. A. (2002). The relationship between chronically disrupted sleep and health care use. *Sleep, 25*(3), 289–296.

3. Environmental factors (lighting, bed, noise level, surrounding stimulation, sleep partner)
4. Associated factors (relation to meals eaten, activity before retiring, life stressors, work stressors, anxiety level, pain, recent illness or surgery)
5. Alleviating factors (mild diet, warm drink before retiring, reading a book, listening to quiet music, taking a hot bath)
6. Effect of problem (fatigue, irritability, confusion)

For clients whose sleep problems do not seem to be well defined, a daily journal of sleep patterns may prove useful. A sleep journal should include the time of the last food or drink prior to going to bed, time of going to bed, time of falling asleep, time of awakenings and duration of awakenings, periods of interrupted or disturbed sleep, time of rising, and feeling of fatigue or drowsiness level upon morning awakening.

## Nursing Diagnosis

After information about the sleep impairment has been collected, data need to be analyzed to formulate appropriate nursing diagnoses. The primary diagnosis for individuals experiencing sleep problems is *Disturbed Sleep Pattern*.

According to NANDA (2003), *Disturbed Sleep Pattern* is defined as "time-limited disruption of sleep (natural, periodic suspension of consciousness) amount and quality" (p. 170). Alterations in sleep can manifest through verbal complaints of the client, physical signs such as yawning or dark circles under the eyes, or alterations in mood such as apathy or irritability.

If the client presents with problems in addition to the sleep disturbance, the nurse must be alert to the possibility that the sleep disturbance is the *cause* (not the effect) of another problem. For example, a client may be experiencing *Activity Intolerance* related to lack of sleep as evidenced by verbal complaint, extreme fatigue, disorientation, confusion, and lack of energy.

## Outcome Identification and Planning

The plan of care for the sleep-disordered client must be individualized. For the nursing care to be effective, client input should be incorporated when developing expected outcomes. It is important to tailor the outcomes and plan of care to the true cause related to the sleep disturbance or alteration. For example, if the client is experiencing *Disturbed Sleep Pattern* because of bed-wetting, then the bed-wetting should be targeted for intervention.

Effective outcome identification and planning will also consider the fact that many sleep disturbances will require extended periods of time (weeks or months) to correct.

Sleep patterns are by nature habitual and intertwined with lifestyle patterns, and these types of disturbances typically require interventions that have long-term goals. When planning care for the hospitalized client, the nurse should remember to perform procedures and treatments in a manner that disturbs sleep time and routines as little as possible.

## Implementation

Several interventions can promote rest and sleep in clients. The interventions range from simple (altering the environment) to complex (lifestyle modifications). Several interventions that facilitate sleep are discussed here.

### Create a Relaxing Environment

Arranging the immediate surroundings to promote sleep is important for the sleep-impaired client. A place to sleep should be inviting. Determine the type of environment the client finds relaxing, then provide this environment in the inpatient setting, or help the client establish this type of environment in the home setting.

Considerations for the sleep environment include noise level, lighting, temperature, and sleep surface. In general, cooler, darker, and quieter environments are most conducive to quality and uninterrupted sleep. Room color can also facilitate or impair sleep. Bright, stimulating colors such as oranges, reds, and yellows tend to impede sleep, while blues and greens facilitate sleep.

### Calm the Mind

Because stress, anxiety, and worry can lead to an active mind at bedtime, it is crucial to calm the mind to facilitate quality sleep. Techniques used to calm the mind include replacing negative thoughts with positive affirmations, meditation prior to bedtime, music therapy (Figure 40-3), visualization, and ceasing activity 30 minutes prior to bedtime. Ceasing activity includes not watching television, reading, or writing (Dement & Vaughan, 1999).

### Ensure Appropriate Nutrition

Certain foods can actually enhance sleep. Tryptophan, a substance in milk, promotes sleep by stimulating the brain's production of the neurotransmitter serotonin. Other dietary considerations include avoiding large or heavy meals close to bedtime. The last food ingested should be more than 3 hours before bedtime. Foods that cause indigestion or heartburn, such as spicy foods, should be avoided throughout the day. Lean meats and organic foods, because they lack additives, have also been found to promote sleep. B-complex vitamins, niacin, pantothenic acid, $B_6$, and $B_{12}$, as well as magnesium, all promote sleep. Avoidance of caffeine and alcohol will also promote a healthy sleep pattern.

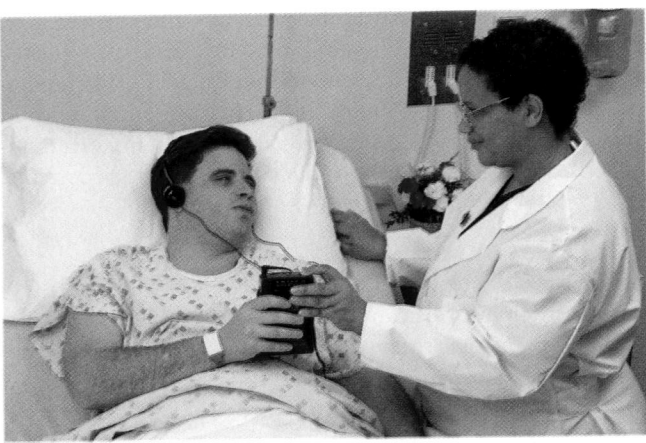

**Figure 40-3** Music therapy promotes client's sleep and rest.

## Promote Daytime Activity and Exercise

Daytime exercise increases metabolic rate and when completed by late afternoon, promotes relaxation at bedtime. The minimum amount of exercise to facilitate sleep is 3 times a week for 20 minutes. If a person cannot exercise, use of yoga or other stretching before bedtime can facilitate muscle relaxation, which then promotes sleep. A variety of alternative modalities promote sleep (Long, Huntley, & Ernst, 2001) (see Box 40-2).

## Manage Stress

Stress management is essential to quality sleep as it helps to slow down body processes. Progressive muscle relaxation, breathing exercises such as qi gong, or tai chi all have been found to be effective in stress management. Having the client evaluate work and living conditions for stressful relationships and situations can lead to elimination of situations that may be interfering with sleep and rest. Finally, warm baths prior to bedtime facilitate relaxation, especially if chamomile or lavender oils are added to the bathwater (Long, Huntley, & Ernst, 2001).

## Initiate Pharmacological Interventions

Pharmacological agents that may be therapeutic for clients with sleep disturbances include tricyclic antidepressants, antihistamines, and short-acting hypnotics (McCaffery & Pasero, 1999). The tricyclic antidepressants of choice are amitriptyline (Elavil®) or doxepin (Sinequan®). Amitriptyline improves the client's ability to fall asleep and stay asleep by causing sedation when given 1 to 3 hours before bedtime. Doses of amitriptyline for sleep disturbances are significantly lower than doses for treatment of depression, starting at 10–25 mg at bedtime and titrating up by 10–25 mg every 2 or 3 days until therapeutic effect is achieved.

---

### BOX 40-2   COMPLEMENTARY/ALTERNATIVE MODALITIES THAT PROMOTE SLEEP

- Acupressure
- Acupuncture
- Aromatherapy
  - Chamomile oil
  - Lavender oil
  - Guided Imagery/Visualization
- Herbs:
  - Chamomile
  - Hops
  - Lavender
  - Kava
  - Passion flower
  - Skullcap
  - Valerian root
- Homeopathy
- Massage
- Meditation
- Reflexology
- Reiki
- Therapeutic Touch

Adapted from Long, L., Huntley, A., & Ernst, E. (2001). Which complementary and alternative therapies benefit which conditions? A survey of the opinions of 223 professional organizations. *Complementary Therapies in Medicine, 9*(3), 178–185.

---

Antihistamines such as hydroxyzine (Vistaril®, Atarax®) and diphenhydramine (Benadryl®) have mild sedative effects that could promote sleep if given at bedtime. If anxiety throughout the day is of concern, low doses of these medications at regular intervals throughout the day may be effective.

The final group of pharmacological interventions for sleep disturbances are the short-acting benzodiazepines. These are *not* recommended for routine or long-term use, but they may be effective as a short-term intervention. When they are chosen, it is recommended that one with a short half-life be used. In addition, nurses must be careful to not misuse short-acting medications solely to induce sleep in clients experiencing mental health problems.

## CLINICAL ALERT

### Kava Ingestion

Ingestion of high levels of kava has been found to lead to liver failure, especially in clients who also use hepatotoxic medications. The nurse should assess the amount of kava used if a client reports that he uses kava.

Long, L., Huntley, A., & Ernst, E. (2001). Which complementary and alternative therapies benefit which conditions? A survey of the opinions of 223 professional organizations. *Complementary Therapies in Medicine, 9*(3), 178–185.

## LEGAL AND ETHICAL ISSUES

### Misuse of "Sleeper Medications" such as Benzodiazepines

Clients with mental health problems (in acute care settings) may have disruptive sleep patterns. During times of wakefulness, these clients may also require greater amounts of nursing care. The nurse must be careful to assess the client and differentiate between using medications for the purpose of inducing sleep versus using medications for decreasing staff workloads. As fundamental as this seems, high nurse-to-client ratios can be an ethical consideration that influences this "overmedication issue."

## FOCUS ON WELLNESS

### Wellness Behaviors That Promote Healthy Sleep

1. Abstain from caffeine, alcohol, and tobacco use.
2. Exercise 3 times a week for 20 minutes each.
3. Eat a nutritionally balanced diet.
4. Supplement diet with B-complex vitamins as needed.
5. Avoid eating less than 3 hours before bedtime.
6. Engage in stress management activities each day.
7. Buy a new mattress every 10 years, more frequently if it does not provide good back support.
8. Limit activity in bed to sleep and sex. Do reading, meditation, and other activities outside of bed.
9. Establish a routine time for sleep and awakening. Stick to the same schedule daily.

Adapted from Dement, W. C., and Vaughan, C. (1999). *The promise of sleep: A pioneer in sleep medicine explores the vital connection between health, happiness, and a good night's sleep.* New York: Dell Publishers.

## Promote Sleep in the Hospitalized Client

In addition to sleep disruption as a result of illness, hospitalization is disruptive to normal sleep because of the change of environment and client routine. As much as possible, the nurse should arrange for the client to engage in her normal bedtime rituals. The hospital room should be kept clean and neat. When possible, a private room or roommate who has similar sleep patterns should be provided. The client should be interrupted minimally during the night, from 2400 to 0600. Vital signs should be taken during this time only if necessary. Lab work and other procedures should not be completed during this sleep time. Noise levels should also be kept to a minimum by keeping the client's door closed, minimizing use of noisy machinery, or adding white noise to the room. Finally, the room should be kept as dark as possible, with the nurse using minimal light when having to enter the client's room at night (American Academy of Sleep Medicine, 2003).

## Evaluation

The plan of care must be individualized for and negotiated with the client. It must be updated on a regular schedule and additional interventions initiated as needed. One of the strongest supportive activities nurses can perform is to make sure clients understand that there is help for sleep problems and that they are not alone in having difficulty successfully managing their sleep patterns.

## CASE STUDY/NURSING CARE PLAN

Jackie Varner is a 45-year-old who has come to the clinic for her annual pelvic examination. In the process of doing her health history, Mrs. Varner shares that she feels irritable and moody. The client also states she experiences drowsiness in the early afternoon and has difficulty falling asleep at night. A detailed history reveals that Mrs. Varner goes to bed at variable times during the week, anywhere from 2100 to 2400, and

*(continues)*

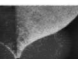

# CASE STUDY/NURSING CARE PLAN (continued)

wakes anywhere from 0600 to 0900. She drinks 6 cups of coffee a day, works at an office desk for 9 hours a day, is dissatisfied with her job, and has been fighting with her husband over money problems.

## Assessment

A 45-year-old client who has inconsistent sleep patterns and reports difficulty falling asleep. The client states she is drowsy in the daytime while at work and irritable with her family and coworkers. She has been "fighting a lot" with her spouse and is worried about their relationship. Further questioning reveals a high frequency of hot flashes associated with menopause, and she states that the hot flashes keep her awake. In addition, Mrs. Varner lives a sedentary lifestyle, drinks excessive amounts of caffeine, and does not like her job.

## Nursing Diagnosis

*Disturbed Sleep Pattern* related to menopause, caffeine use, sedentary lifestyle, and stress.
**NOC:** Anxiety Control; Sleep; Rest
**NIC:** Sleep Enhancement

## Expected Outcomes

The client will:
1. Obtain 8 to 9 hours of sleep each night.
2. Establish a consistent sleep pattern where she goes to bed no later than 2300.
3. Report staying awake during the daytime within 1 week.

## Planning/Interventions/Rationales

1. Have client keep a 2-week sleep diary, which records time to sleep, any disruptions, and waking. *Process of record keeping increases client awareness about sleep pattern and assists in determining consistent sleep times.*
2. Explore with client possible sleep and wake times that can be consistent for each day of the week. *Consistent sleep times allow the body to get into a routine, which is calming to the body and promotes sleep.*
3. Instruct client to decrease caffeine use, having the last ingestion of caffeine be noon. *Caffeine is a stimulant and interrupts sleep patterns. Stopping caffeine ingestion by noon minimizes sleep-altering effects.*
4. Explore with client possible areas for increasing exercise daily. This would include walking up and down stairs instead of using elevators, taking 15-minute walking breaks twice a day while at work. Three times a week, have client walk for at least 20 minutes at a brisk pace. *Exercise promotes relaxation, stress reduction, and sleepiness at the end of the day.*
5. Discuss with client possible stress-reducing interventions to handle anxiety and stress related to work and with her husband. *Stress management techniques help to calm the mind, which promotes sleep.*
6. Teach client how to do a 5-minute meditation prior to sleep. *Meditation calms the mind, which promotes sleep.*

## Evaluation

After 6 months, Mrs. Varner reported that her energy was better, she was sleeping better, and she was no longer drowsy in the daytime. She goes to bed at 1030 each night and is up at 0600, without an alarm clock. She walks 30 minutes each day and meditates 30 minutes prior to her sleep time. She reports that her irritability and moodiness are better, stating she is enjoying life more. She no longer fights with her husband. Although she reports a great deal of stress at work, she believes that her sleep helps prevent little things from bothering her so much.

# Key Concepts

- The physiology of rest and includes stages of NREM and REM.
- Individuals have different biological clocks, which control a variety of their physiological processes.
- Many factors affect rest and sleep, such as comfort level, stress, environment, and lifestyle.
- Hospitalization causes definite changes in rest and sleep.
- Alterations in sleep patterns include insomnia, sleep deprivation, and parasomnia.

- Assessing the client for sleep disturbances is an important aspect of the nursing process.
- Nonpharmacological interventions (stress management, meditation, music therapy) may be used in promoting sleep and rest.
- Pharmacological agents can be therapeutic for clients experiencing sleep pattern disturbances.

## Review Questions and Activities

1. Describe the stages of sleep and how they are related to the sleep cycle.
2. What age-related sleep variations would you need to consider when assessing the sleep habits of neonates, infants, toddlers, and older adults?
3. How do stress and the environment affect rest and sleep?
4. How does hospitalization affect the client's sleep pattern?
5. State the outcomes that sleep deprivation may have on an individual.
6. What are several nursing interventions that promote rest and sleep?
7. What pharmacological agents can assist the client to experience more restful sleep patterns?

## Web Resources

American Academy of Sleep Medicine
   http://www.aasmnet.org
American Sleep Disorders Association
   http://www.asda.org
National Center on Sleep Disorders Research of the
   National Heart, Lung, and Blood Institute
   http://www.nhlbi.nih.gov
National Institutes of Health
   http://www.nih.gov
National Sleep Foundation
   http://www.sleepfoundation.org
Sleep Medicine Home Page
   http://www.users.cloud9.net

## References

American Academy of Sleep Medicine (2003).
   http://www.aasmnet.org

American Psychiatric Association (2001) *Diagnostic and statistical manual* (5th ed., rev.). Washington, DC: Author.

Carpenito, L. J. (2004). *Handbook of nursing diagnosis* (10th ed.). Philadelphia: Lippincott.

Dement, W. C., and Vaughan, C. (1999). *The promise of sleep: A pioneer in sleep medicine explores the vital connection between health, happiness, and a good night's sleep.* NY: Dell Publishers.

Doghramji, K., & Fredman, S. (1999). *Clinical frontiers in the sleep/psychiatry interface: Satellite symposium of the 1999 American Psychiatric Association annual meeting.* http://www.medscape.com/ Medscape/psychiatry

Forth, R. (1998). Common questions about obstructive sleep apnea. *American Journal of Nursing, 98*(2), 60–64.

Hilton, G. (2002). Melatonin and the pineal gland. *Journal of Neuroscience Nursing, 34*(2), 74–81.

Hockenberry, M., Wilson, D., Winkelstein, M., & Kline, N. (2003). *Wong's nursing care of infants and children* (7th ed.). St. Louis: Mosby.

Idzikowski, C. (2000). *Learn to sleep well: A practical guide to getting a good night's rest.* San Francisco: Chronicle Books.

Kapur, V. K., Redline, S., Nieto, F. J., Young, T. B., Newman, A. B., & Henderson, J. A. (2002). The relationship between chronically disrupted sleep and health care use. *Sleep, 25*(3), 289–296.

Long, L., Huntley, A., & Ernst, E. (2001). Which complementary and alternative therapies benefit which conditions? A survey of the opinions of 223 professional organizations. *Complementary Therapies in Medicine, 9*(3), 178–185.

Lueckenotte, A. G. (2000). *Gerontologic nursing* (2nd ed.). St. Louis: Mosby.

McCaffery, M., & Pasero, C. (1999). *Pain: Clinical manual for nursing practice* (2nd ed.). St. Louis: Mosby.

National Sleep Foundation (2003). http://www.sleep foundation.org

North American Nursing Diagnosis Association (2003). *Nursing diagnoses: Definitions and classification, 2003–2004.* Philadelphia: Author.

Ohayou, M. N., & Roth, T. (2002). Prevalence of Restless Leg Syndrome and Periodic Limb Movement Disorder in the General Population. *Journal of Psychosomatic Research, 53*(1), 547–554.

Potts, N., & Mandleco, B. (2002). Pediatric nursing: Caring for children and their families. Clifton Park, NY: Delmar Learning.

Sleep Medicine Home Page (2002). http://www.users. cloud9.net

Wyatt, J. K. (2001). Sleep and circadian rhythms: Basic and clinical findings. *Nutrition Reviews 59*(1), S27–S29.

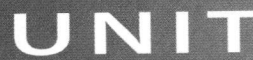

# XII UNIT

# Cognitive-Perceptual

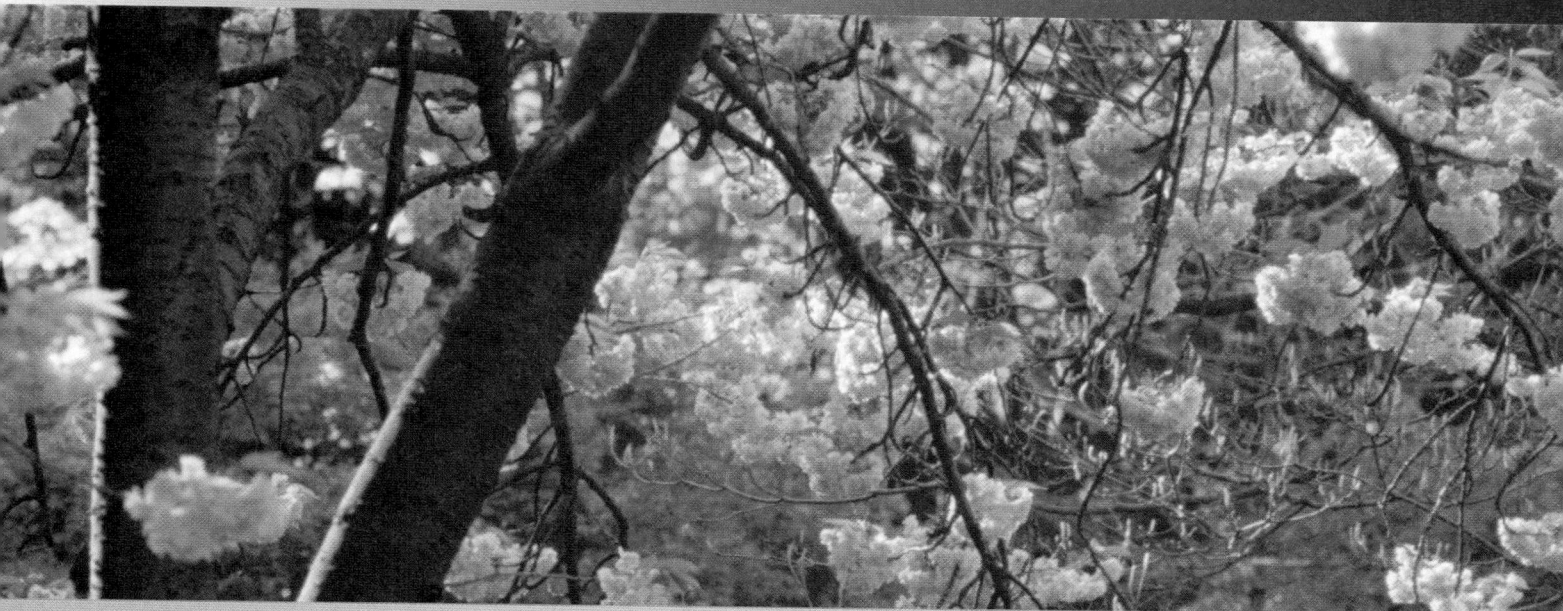

# CHAPTER 41

# Sensation, Perception, and Cognition

## Annemarie Day, RN, MSN, FNP-C

*"To use all senses, experiences, and intuition requires involvement and immersion in situations as whole, and to describe patterns of responses theoretically requires longer periods of engagement in situations where nursing phenomena occur."*

*(Afaf I. Meleis, 1997)*

# Chapter Competencies

*Upon completion of this chapter, the reader should be able to:*

1. Describe the physiology of sensation, perception, and cognition.
2. Enumerate various factors that affect sensation, perception, and cognition.
3. Assess the alterations that occur in sensation, perception, and cognition.
4. Identify the components of assessment used in sensation, perception, and cognition.
5. Develop nursing diagnoses and outcome criteria for clients with cognitive and sensory perception.
6. Identify interventions that help the client adapt to altered sensory functions and maximize existing abilities.
7. Describe the complementary/alternative therapies employed with cognitive and sensory perceptual alterations.
8. Evaluate methods of evaluating the nursing care of clients with cognitive and sensory perceptual difficulties.

# Key Terms

| | | |
|---|---|---|
| affect | expressive aphasia | recent memory |
| afferent nerve pathway | fluency | receptive aphasia |
| aphasia | fluid intelligence | remote memory |
| arousal | hallucination | sensation |
| awareness | illusion | sensory deficit |
| cognition | immediate memory | sensory deprivation |
| consciousness | judgment | sensory overload |
| crystallized intelligence | orientation | sensory perception |
| disorientation | perception | |
| efferent nerve pathway | prosody | |

**Sensation** is the ability to receive and process stimuli received through the sensory organs. There are two types of stimuli: external and internal. External stimuli are received and processed through the sight (visual), hearing (auditory), smell (olfactory), taste (gustatory), and touch (tactile) modes. Internal stimuli are received and processed through kinesthetic (an awareness of the position of the body) and visceral modes. Visceral refers to any large organ in the body that may produce stimuli, such as stomach fullness.

**Perception** is the ability to experience, recognize, organize, and interpret sensory stimuli. **Sensory perception** is the ability to receive sensory impressions and, through cortical association, translates to conscious organization of the stimulus or data into meaningful information.

Perception is closely associated with **cognition**, the intellectual ability to think. The processes of organizing and interpreting stimuli are dependent on a person's level of intellectual functioning. Cognition includes the elements of memory, judgment, and orientation. The well-being of an individual is dependent on the functions of sensation, perception, and cognition because it is through these mechanisms that the person fully experiences and interacts with her environment.

Sensory, perceptual, and cognitive alterations can be either temporary or progressive in their manifestations and can result from disease or trauma. Whatever the status or cause of the alterations, these conditions usually lead to social isolation and increased dependence on others. In addition, impairment in sensory, perceptual, and cognitive functions can place the individual at risk for injury to self or to others.

This chapter discusses the physiology of sensation, perception, and cognition and the common alterations in each functional area. Information on the nurse's role in caring for individuals with sensory, perceptual, or cognitive alterations is presented.

# Physiology of Sensation, Perception, and Cognition

Sensation, perception, and cognition are neurologic functions. The nervous system is composed of two major subsystems: the central nervous system (CNS) and the peripheral nervous system (PNS), which consists of the somatic and autonomic nervous systems (Figure 41-1).

The CNS and PNS act in unison to accomplish three purposes: collection of stimuli from the receptors at the end of the peripheral nerves, transport of the stimuli to the brain for integration and cognition processing, and conduction of responses to the stimuli from the brain to responsive motor centers in the body.

The CNS is composed of the brain and spinal cord, which are protected by the bony structures of the skull and vertebral column. The brain, the most complex of the body's organs, is composed of three basic structures: the cerebrum (which consists of the temporal, frontal, parietal, and occipital lobes), the cerebellum, and the brain stem (Figure 41-2). Table 41-1 describes each of these structures. The structures of the brain serve as both receptors and reactors by collecting stimuli and effecting responses to those stimuli. The spinal cord links the advanced neu-

rosensory mechanisms that occur in the brain to the rest of the body via a coordinated pathway of neurons.

Sensory perception involves the function of both the cranial and peripheral nerves. The cranial nerves arise from the three structures of the brain and govern the movement and function of various muscles and nerves throughout the body (Figure 41-3). The peripheral nerves connect the CNS to other parts of the body (Figure 41-4).

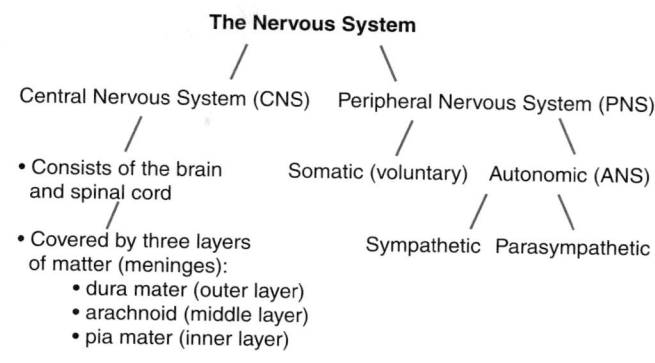

Figure 41-1    The nervous system

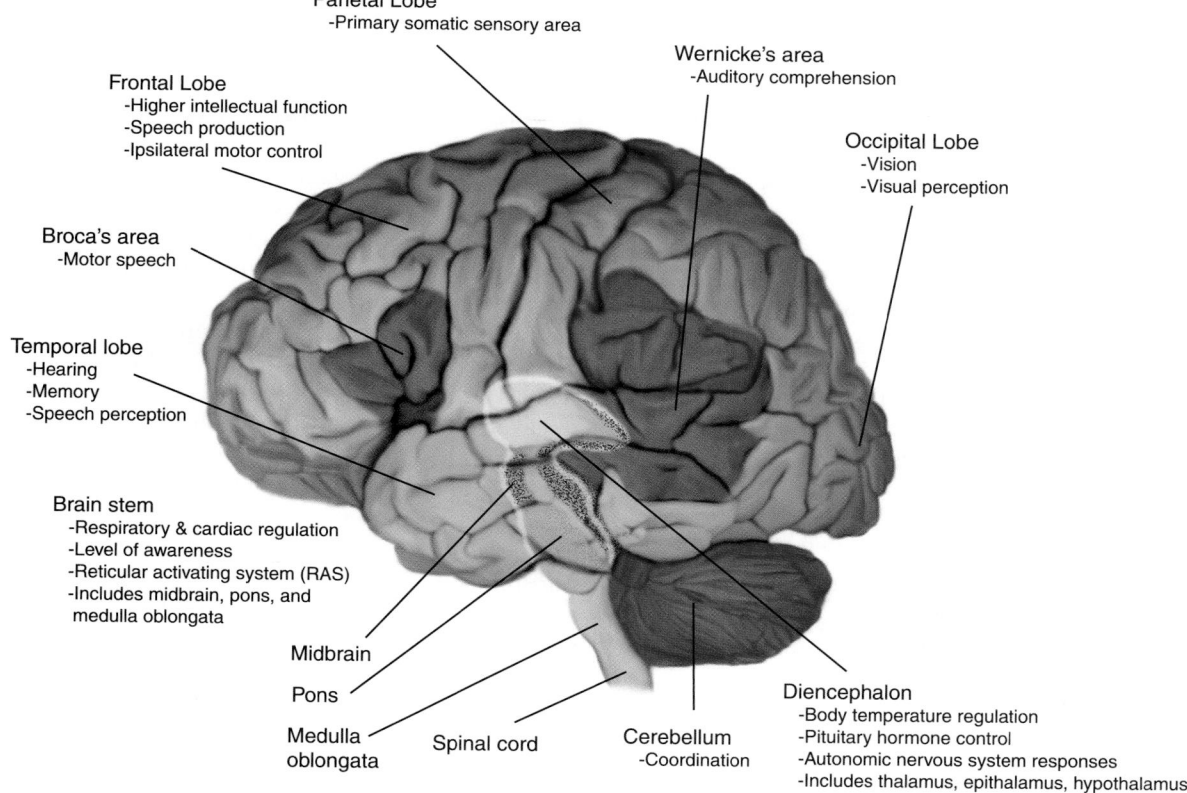

Figure 41-2    Cross-section of the brain

## TABLE 41-1   STRUCTURES AND FUNCTIONS OF THE BRAIN

| Structure | Description | Primary Functions |
|-----------|-------------|-------------------|
| Cerebrum | Composed of gray matter and white matter.<br><br>Basal ganglia (masses of gray matter) are part of the extrapyramidal system. | Is responsible for:<br>• Thinking<br>• Memory<br>• Learning<br>Receives and interprets sensory input (stimuli); responds to sensory stimuli.<br>Helps control motor function. |
| Cerebellum | Located behind and under the cerebrum.<br>Is a fissured mass consisting of a body that includes a narrow middle strip and two lateral lobes. | Is concerned with unconscious functions.<br>Is responsible for smooth-muscle functioning.<br>Maintains equilibrium. |
| Brain stem | Composed of three structures:<br>• The midbrain<br>• The pons<br>• The medulla oblongata | Influences visual and auditory senses.<br>Connects the upper and lower levels of the CNS.<br>Affects respiratory rate. Prevents coma by maintaining wakefulness.<br>Controls vital functions:<br>• Heart rate<br>• Respiratory rate<br>• Swallowing<br>• Coughing<br>Processes sensory input from spinal tract. |

From Guyton, A. C., & Hall, J. (2000). *Textbook of medical physiology* (10th ed.). Philadelphia: Saunders.

## Components of Sensation and Perception

The sensory system is a complex network that consists of **afferent nerve pathways** (ascending pathways that transmit sensory impulses to the brain), **efferent nerve pathways** (descending pathways that send sensory impulses from the brain), the spinal cord, the brain stem, and the higher cortex (cerebral lobes). Figure 41-5 shows the major sensory pathways.

## Components of Cognition

Cognition includes the cerebral functions of memory, judgment, and emotion. In order for higher functions (such as memory, affect, judgment, perception, and language to occur) consciousness must be present.

### Consciousness

**Consciousness** is a state of awareness of self, others, and the surrounding environment. It affects both cognitive (intellectual) and affective (emotional) functions. An alert individual (one who is aware of self and stimuli) is able to perceive reality accurately and to base behavior on those perceptions. The components of consciousness provide a foundation for behavior and emotional expression, thereby contributing to the uniqueness of each individual's personality.

Consciousness depends on the functioning of the reticular activating system (RAS), which is located in the brain stem. The activity level of the RAS depends largely on receiving sensory stimuli, such as pain. Pain increases the activity of the RAS, and these messages are passed along to the cerebral cortex, which stores and interprets these messages in an organized manner. The RAS controls activities such as sleep and wakefulness and monitors the selective transmission of stimuli to other parts of the neurosensory system. Consciousness may be altered by various metabolic, traumatic, or other factors, such as the pharmacological actions of drugs that affect mental status. The primary components of consciousness are arousal and awareness, both of which must be present before higher cognitive functioning occurs. "The reticular formation is the arousal or alerting system for the cerebral cortex; its functioning is crucial for maintaining consciousness" (Kuhn, Herlihy, & Herlihy, 1998, p. 208).

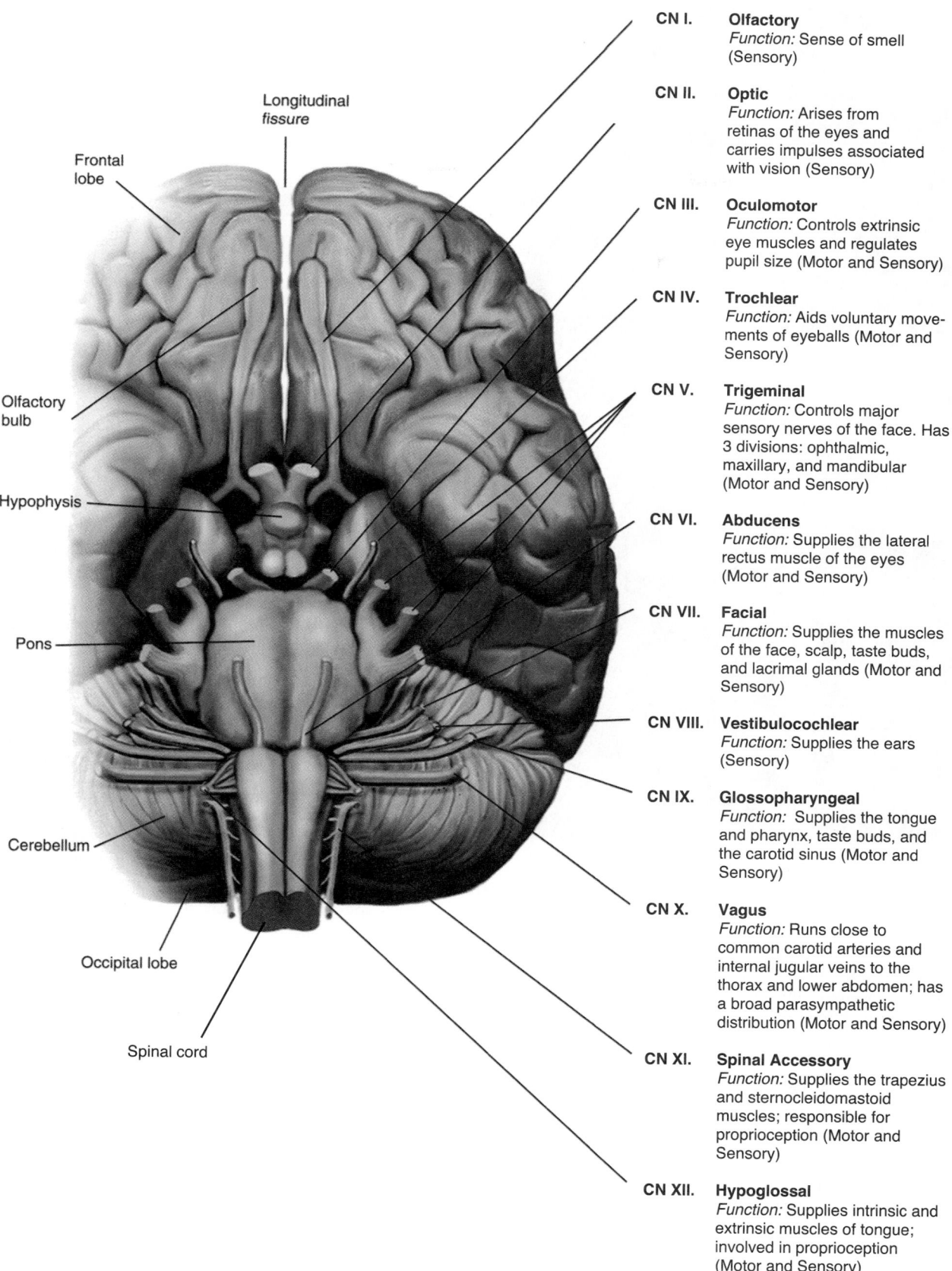

**CN I.**   **Olfactory**
*Function:* Sense of smell
(Sensory)

**CN II.**   **Optic**
*Function:* Arises from
retinas of the eyes and
carries impulses associated
with vision (Sensory)

**CN III.**   **Oculomotor**
*Function:* Controls extrinsic
eye muscles and regulates
pupil size (Motor and Sensory)

**CN IV.**   **Trochlear**
*Function:* Aids voluntary move-
ments of eyeballs (Motor and
Sensory)

**CN V.**   **Trigeminal**
*Function:* Controls major
sensory nerves of the face. Has
3 divisions: ophthalmic,
maxillary, and mandibular
(Motor and Sensory)

**CN VI.**   **Abducens**
*Function:* Supplies the lateral
rectus muscle of the eyes
(Motor and Sensory)

**CN VII.**   **Facial**
*Function:* Supplies the muscles
of the face, scalp, taste buds,
and lacrimal glands (Motor and
Sensory)

**CN VIII.**   **Vestibulocochlear**
*Function:* Supplies the ears
(Sensory)

**CN IX.**   **Glossopharyngeal**
*Function:* Supplies the tongue
and pharynx, taste buds, and
the carotid sinus (Motor and
Sensory)

**CN X.**   **Vagus**
*Function:* Runs close to
common carotid arteries and
internal jugular veins to the
thorax and lower abdomen; has
a broad parasympathetic
distribution (Motor and Sensory)

**CN XI.**   **Spinal Accessory**
*Function:* Supplies the trapezius
and sternocleidomastoid
muscles; responsible for
proprioception (Motor and
Sensory)

**CN XII.**   **Hypoglossal**
*Function:* Supplies intrinsic and
extrinsic muscles of tongue;
involved in proprioception
(Motor and Sensory)

Longitudinal *fissure*

Frontal lobe

Olfactory bulb

Hypophysis

Pons

Cerebellum

Occipital lobe

Spinal cord

**Figure 41-3    The cranial nerves**

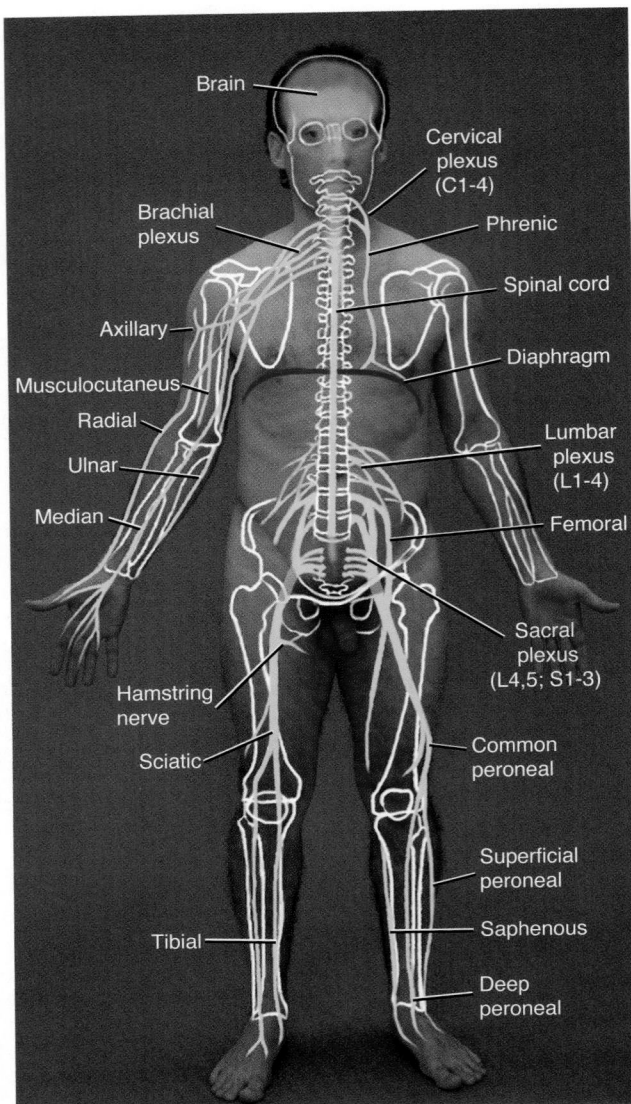

**Figure 41-4** **The peripheral nerves**

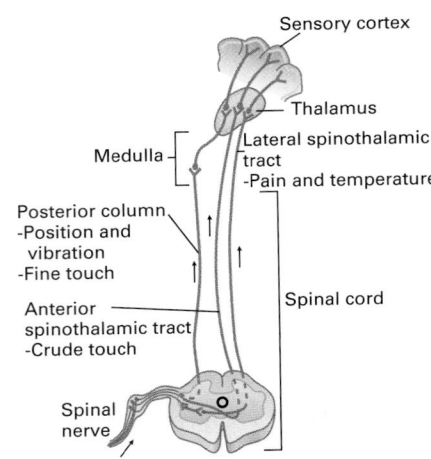

**Figure 41-5** **Major sensory pathways**

## Arousal

The degree of **arousal** (a component linked closely to the appearance of wakefulness and alertness) is indicated by a person's general response and reaction to the environment.

People exhibit arousal, the state of being prepared to act, by behaving in an alert and aware manner and by experiencing periods of wakefulness. The degree of an individual's arousal is indicated by the general response and reaction to the environment. Impaired arousal can exist when a sleep pattern deficit is experienced; there may be an inability to take advantage of opportunities for activity because of limited periods of rest.

## Awareness

**Awareness** is the capacity to perceive sensory impressions and react appropriately through thoughts and actions. An essential element in awareness is **orientation** (perception of self in relation to the surrounding environment). According to Roy (1988), orientation is a person's ability to be cognitively aroused, to attend to the environment, and to recognize patterns. When awareness is impaired, orientation to time is frequently the first area affected. The degree of disorientation is worse when the individual loses awareness of place and self (person). Changes in a client's orientation to time, place, and person are often early indicators of an altered level of consciousness. Several tools have been developed to measure level of consciousness, which includes a measure of orientation.

## Memory

There are three types of memory: immediate, recent, and remote. **Immediate memory** is the retention of information for a specified and usually short period of time. An example of this function is the recall of a telephone number long enough to dial it. **Recent memory** is the result of events that have occurred over the past 24 hours. An example of recent memory is the remembrance of foods eaten for dinner the previous night. **Remote memory** is the retention of experiences that occurred during earlier periods of life, such as an adult's memories of childhood or school days. The ability to learn is dependent on remote memory (McDougall, 2002).

---

### NURSING STRATEGY

#### Assessing Remote Memory

- Remote memory should be assessed only when the client responses can be validated, either by others or by written account.

- When assessing recent memory, be sure to ask questions for which you know the answers.

## STOP AND THINK

### Assessment of Memory

The following are questions to consider when assessing a client's memory:

- What events in the immediate memory are you likely to have knowledge about that verifies your questions?

- What are questions to avoid in assessing recent memory?

- With which persons might you verify information that the client gives to you?

- What are examples of questions you can ask to assess remote memory? What if you cannot verify the information that the client shares?

## Affect

**Affect** (mood or feeling) is an important component of cognition, in that variations of mood can affect one's thinking ability. For example, depression may affect the client's concentration and attention (Figure 41-6). Also, anxiety narrows the perceptual field and interferes with the ability to concentrate by decreasing attention span.

## Judgment

**Judgment**, the ability to compare or evaluate alternatives to life situations and arrive at an appropriate course of action, is closely related to reality testing and depends on effective cognitive functioning. When assessing logic and judgment, it is important to decide whether the client is answering questions appropriately. The goal is to determine the use of reasoning and decision-making ability. It may be assessed by asking a ques-

tion such as "What would you do if you were inside a burning building?" Answers that indicate impaired judgment may be given by clients experiencing frontal lobe damage, dementia, mental retardation, or psychosis. Behaviors indicative of impaired judgment include impulsiveness, unrealistic decision making, and inadequate problem-solving ability.

## Perception

Cognitive perceptions are considered in the context of the individual's awareness of reality. Misperceptions of reality can occur in the form of an **illusion** (an inaccurate perception or misinterpretation of sensory stimuli) or a **hallucination** (a sensory perception that occurs in the absence of external stimuli and is not based on reality).

Clients who are anxious and fearful or who are on therapeutic regimens involving the use of certain medications may experience misperceptions of environmental stimuli. For example, a postoperative client, after receiving analgesic medication for pain, sees a belt from his bathrobe lying on the floor and becomes terrified because he thinks there is a snake in the room. Once the nurse determines that the client is experiencing an illusion, appropriate reassurance and reality orientation can be implemented to reduce the client's anxiety.

## Language

Language is one of the most complex cognitive functions, involving not only the spoken word but also reading, writing, and comprehension. Each of these skills is controlled by specific areas located in the cerebral cortex (Figure 41-7).

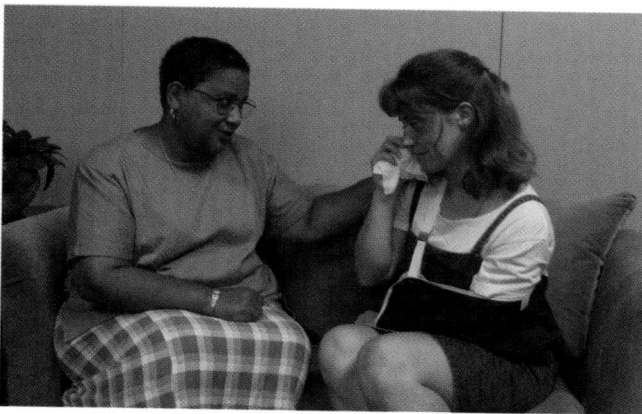

**Figure 41-6**    The mood of the client must be assessed by the health care provider.

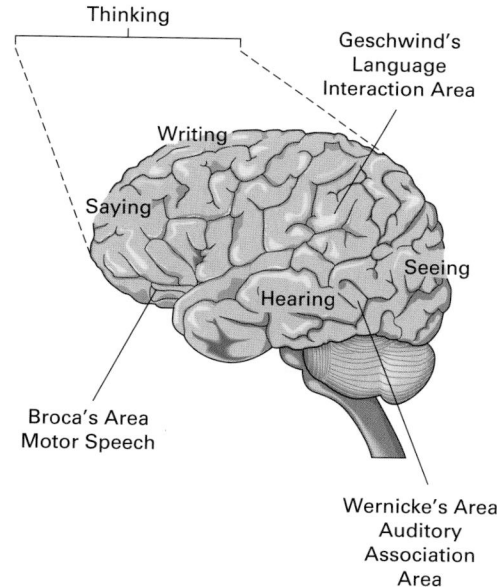

**Figure 41-7    Language perception areas of the brain:** Note Broca's motor speech area in the frontal lobe, Wenicke's auditory association area in the temporal lobe, and Geschwind's language interaction area in the parietal lobe.

## LIFE SPAN CONSIDERATIONS

### Receptive Aphasia

Older clients who have experienced cerebrovascular accidents (CVA) often have receptive aphasia. The nurse can address this condition by (1) speaking very clearly and enunciating well, (2) using short phrases in conversations, (3) choosing words that are easily understood, and (4) keeping "extra" communication to a minimum.

Characteristics of speech are **fluency** (ability to talk in a steady manner), **prosody** (melody of speech that conveys meaning through changes in the tempo, rhythm, and intonation), and content. Clients with alterations in their speech often experience motor dysfunctions and are unable to make proper intonations. The inability to speak is termed **aphasia**. There are two broad categories of aphasia. First is **expressive aphasia**, which is defined as the ability to understand communication but inability to speak clearly in response to the sender of a message. The second, **receptive aphasia**, refers to the ability to speak well but inability to understand the message that is spoken.

## Factors Affecting Sensation, Perception, and Cognition

The functions of sensation, perception, and cognition are influenced by many factors, including age, environment, lifestyle, stress, illness, and medications.

### Age

Neurosensory pathways in infants and children are immature and do not allow for sophisticated discrimination among stimuli. As children mature, they learn to apply their perceptions of the environment to different situations and can thus modify their behaviors accordingly. This process continues throughout the life cycle. For young adults, cognitive functioning is generally more advanced than during adolescence. According to Miller (1999):

> The young adult uses systematic and sophisticated problem-solving techniques and achieves new levels of creative thought with less egocentrism than is seen in younger individuals. Thinking is more reality based and mental activities are proficient. (p. 386)

Intelligence is difficult to measure; intelligence quotient (IQ) tests (which are intended to predict academic achievement) are not very reliable indicators of adult intelligence. The measurement of intelligence in middle-aged adults is affected by several variables, including motivation, cultural differences, risk-taking and/or caution, and anxiety. "Middle age is considered . . . to be the height of intellectual endowment, as memory and problem solving are maintained and learning continues" (Miller, 1999, p. 391).

Intellectual functioning is maintained in part by a stimulating environment. **Crystallized intelligence** (the application of life experiences and learned skills to solve problems; also called acquired knowledge) generally increases with age as **fluid intelligence** (ability to acquire new concepts and adapt to unfamiliar situations; mental activities based on organizing information) decreases over time (Miller, 1999).

Cognitive development in older adults shows no decline in intellectual function. Memory loss is an area of concern for many older adults. "The older person who is mentally active and well educated will not show the same problems with memory as will those adults without similar opportunities to use their minds" (Miller, 1999, p. 397). Memory impairments that occur in older clients are usually the result of pathophysiological processes and are not a part of normal aging. Strategies such as list making and posting reminder notes can be helpful in compensating for minor memory losses. Some activities that encourage cognitive development in older people are reading, studying a new topic (such as language or computer skills), solving mathematical problems, and working word puzzles (Davis, 2001).

### Environment

The amount and type of environmental stimuli affects sensation, perception, and cognition. Excessive stimuli in the form of visual impressions and noise can create feelings of anxiety and disorientation within clients. Too few relevant stimuli decrease the client's response to people and the environment, thus leading to isolation.

Crowded living conditions, traffic congestion, or living where sound levels are high are stressors associated with negative physical and psychological health outcomes. "Environmental noise has been associated with delayed healing and other physical effects, as well as cognitive effects, including a diminished efficiency of prefrontal cortical regions of the brain resulting in a decrease in the variety and speed of cognitive responses" (Holmberg & Coon, 1999, p. 117).

## LIFE SPAN CONSIDERATIONS

### Assessing Cognitive Function

When assessing an older client's cognitive functioning, remember that aging does not occur in the same way in every individual. Some older clients may have very intact memory recall. You will need to assess them for their uniqueness.

## Lifestyle

The amount and quality of sensory information that people feel comfortable in processing are based on their work and leisure habits. Some people may prefer quiet environments in which to think, whereas others derive energy and productivity from the activity around them.

## Stress

Stress and anxiety can have a negative influence on a person's behavior and thought patterns. Depending on the type and degree of stress, the person either finds ways to cope with the situation or becomes overwhelmed with the stimuli being received and can possibly become disoriented.

## Illness

Specific conditions, such as diabetes mellitus and atherosclerosis, can impair neurosensory pathways and result in deficits in sensation, perception, and cognition. Diseases of the CNS, such as stroke or multiple sclerosis, can result in loss of sensory function and paralysis (Bays, 2001).

## Medications

Certain medications have the potential to alter or depress the neurosensory system. For example, sedatives and narcotics can alter the perception of sensory stimuli. Medications such as analgesics can alter level of consciousness (see Box 41-1).

# Sensory, Perceptual, and Cognitive Alterations

An individual usually experiences discomfort and/or anxiety when subjected to a change in the type or amount of incoming stimuli. A person can become confused as a result of either overstimulation or understimulation. According to the individual's ability to process the stimuli, confusion (or disorientation) may occur. **Disorientation** is a mentally confused state in which the person's awareness of time, place, self, and/or situation is impaired; when awareness of these four factors is accurate, a person is said to be "oriented × 4."

Sensory overstimulation and sensory deprivation can lead to cognitive alterations in healthy adults. Such alterations include physical symptoms (e.g., nausea), altered time perceptions, paranoid ideation, and visual, auditory, and olfactory distortions (similar to hallucinations). A person admitted to a health care agency experiences stimuli that are different from those usually encountered. A change in environment can overwhelm one's ability to perceive and interpret sensory input. As a result, the treatment milieu itself can become a stressor that negatively affects sensory, perceptual, and cognitive functions. If one or more of the factors just discussed causes an alteration in sensation, perception, or cognition, the client may experience problems with perceiving and interpreting stimuli. These problems are manifested by three types of alterations: sensory deficits, sensory deprivation, and sensory overload.

## Sensory Deficits

A **sensory deficit** is a change in the perception of sensory stimuli. These deficits can affect all five senses. Examples of sensory deficits are vision and hearing losses such as those caused by cataracts, glaucoma, and nerve degeneration.

The client's response to these losses usually depends on the time of onset and severity of the condition. If the problem occurs suddenly and without warning, the client may have difficulty in adjusting to the loss of sensory and perceptual function. If these alterations occur gradually, the client may be able to accommodate the change and actually compensate for it by strengthening one or more of the other senses (Perkins & Rouanzoin, 2002).

The effects of hospitalization or intensive medical treatments can exacerbate the problems related to sensory deficits. For example, a client with acute hearing loss can feel alone and vulnerable when faced with an environment that does not provide an effective means (such as interpreters who sign) through which communication can occur. Because of these responses, clients with sensory deficits are at serious risk of experiencing either sensory deprivation or sensory overload.

## Sensory Deprivation

**Sensory deprivation** is a state of reduced sensory input from the internal or external environment, manifested by alterations in sensory perception. Individuals can experience sensory deprivation as a result of illness, trauma, or isolation. A person experiencing sensory deprivation misinterprets the limited stimuli with a resultant impairment of thoughts and feelings (Figure 41-8). Factors contributing to sensory deprivation are outlined in Box 41-2.

---

**BOX 41-1    MEDICATIONS THAT ALTER LEVEL OF CONSCIOUSNESS: A PARTIAL LIST**

- Analgesics
- Antidepressants
- Antidiuretics
- Antihypertensives
- Benzodiazepines (especially long-acting agents)
- Sedatives

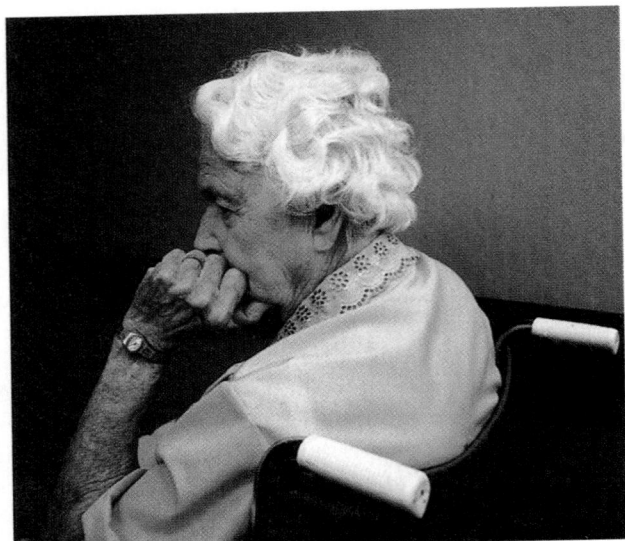

**Figure 41-8**    An older client with sensory deprivation is experiencing acute depression.

Some contributing factors (such as brain damage or blindness) result in chronic sensory deprivation, whereas others lead to acute, transient states of deprivation (e.g., an individual receiving analgesic medications).

Individuals who are sensory-deprived may exhibit any of the following characteristics:

• Inability to concentrate
• Poor memory
• Impaired problem-solving ability
• Confusion
• Irritability
• Emotional liability (mood swings)
• Depression
• Boredom and apathy
• Drowsiness
• Hallucinations (see Table 41-2)

## Sensory Overload

**Sensory overload** is a state of excessive and sustained multisensory stimulation manifested by behavior change and perceptual distortion. The individual experiencing this alteration is unable to process the amount or intensity of stimuli being received. Box 41-3 lists factors contributing to sensory overload and deprivation. Individuals experiencing sensory overload may exhibit any of the following characteristics:

• Anxiety and restlessness
• Irritability
• Disorientation
• Insomnia
• Fatigue
• Impaired problem-solving ability

| TABLE 41-2 | TYPES OF HALLUCINATIONS | |
| --- | --- | --- |
| Hallucination | Definition | Example |
| Visual | Perception of sights that are not actually present in the environment | "Do you see that little gray cat at the foot of my bed?" |
| Auditory | Perception of sounds that are not present in the environment | "I hear the police telling me that I'll be able to escape soon." |
| Tactile | Perception of being touched by things not actually present in the environment | "I feel bugs crawling underneath my skin." |
| Olfactory | Perception of odors not present in the environment | "I can smell old rubber tires burning all the time." |
| Gustatory | Perception of tastes that do not actually correspond to the foods being eaten | "That chlorine taste is in all the food." |

## BOX 41-3   FACTORS CONTRIBUTING TO SENSORY OVERLOAD

### Sensory Overload

1. Increased internal stimuli, such as pain or disease, that affects the CNS and maximizes the perception of stimuli
2. Invasive treatments, such as indwelling catheters, IVs, chest tubes, or endotracheal tubes
3. Increased external stimulus, such as noise from the nurses' station, frequent vital signs, alarms and monitors beeping
4. Presence of strangers (both health care professionals and others) who contribute to the quality of stimuli
5. Medications that stimulate the CNS

A common type of stimulus that clients often experience is excessive noise; exposure to high noise levels interferes with the following:

- Ability to shift attention
- Ability to perform complex tasks requiring sustained attention
- Verbal learning and memory
- Ability to make verbal associations

"Excessive sound affects cognitive processing activity in the prefrontal cortex" (Holmberg & Coon, 1999, p. 120).

## Assessment

When caring for clients with sensory, perceptual, and cognitive alterations, the nurse must conduct a thorough health history and perform a complete physical examination of the client in order to identify existing or potential problems in this area of functioning. See Table 41-3 for an overview of assessing cognition and sensory perception.

## TABLE 41-3   NEUROLOGIC SCREENING ASSESSMENT

| Assessment Parameter | Assessment Skill | Comments |
|---|---|---|
| Mental status/level of consciousness | Note general appearance, speech content, memory, logic, judgment, and speech patterns during history-taking. | If any abnormalities or inconsistencies are evident, perform full mental status assessment. |
| | Perform Glasgow Coma Scale (GCS) with motor assessment component and pupil assessment. | If GCS is < 15, perform full assessment of mental status and consciousness. If motor assessment is abnormal or asymmetrical, perform complete motor and sensory assessment. |
| Sensation | Assess pain and vibration in the hands and feet, light touch on the limbs. | If deficits are identified, perform a complete sensory assessment. |
| Cranial nerves | Assess CN II, III, IV, VI: visual acuity, gross visual fields, fundoscopic examination, pupillary reactions, and extraocular movements. | If any abnormalities exist, perform complete assessment of all 12 cranial nerves. |
| | Assess CN VII, VIII, IX, X, XII: facial expression, gross hearing, voice, and tongue. | |
| Cerebellar function | Observe the client's:<br>• Initial gait<br>• Ability to: (a) walk heel-to-toe, (b) walk on toes, (c) walk on heels, (d) hop in place, and (e) perform shallow knee bends | If any abnormalities exist, perform complete cerebellar assessment. |
| Reflexes | Assess the muscle stretch reflexes and the plantar response. | If an abnormal response is elicited, perform a complete reflex assessment. |

Adapted from Estes, M. E. Z. (2002). *Health assessment & physical examination* (2nd ed.). Clifton Park, NY: Delmar Learning.

## Health History

In order to collect data that are used to develop the plan of care, the nurse collects the health history of the client experiencing alterations in sensation, perception, and cognition. Elements of the health history include the client's usual level of functioning, current sensory problems, and potential alterations. The nurse should also explore issues such as the client's current occupation, home environment, and ability to perform both daily routines and self-care activities. Box 41-4 presents examples of questions that the nurse can ask the client during this part of the assessment process.

## Physical Examination

During the physical examination, the nurse evaluates the client's visual, auditory, gustatory, olfactory, and tactile status. Physical examination focuses specifically on the client's ability to see, hear, taste, smell, perceive heat and cold, and perceive pain. Table 41-4 provides some guidelines helpful in assessing sensory perceptual status.

### Assessment of Cranial Nerves

As stated earlier, there are 12 pairs of cranial nerves. Most of the cranial nerves have both sensory and motor functions (refer to Table 41-4). Assessment of the cranial nerves

---

### BOX 41-4     HEALTH HISTORY: SAMPLE QUESTIONS

- Are you experiencing any difficulty in seeing objects, either near or far from you?

- Do you currently wear eyeglasses, bifocals, or contacts?

- Have you recently experienced any changes in your vision—for example, blurred vision, pain, sensitivity to light, or eye fatigue?

- Are you experiencing any changes in your hearing?

- Do you currently wear a hearing aid?

- Have you experienced any unusual sensations in the ears, such as a buzzing or ringing noise?

- Has your appetite or preference for certain foods changed recently?

- Are you experiencing any difficulty in your ability to smell particular odors?

- Do you experience unusual heat or cold in any of your extremities?

- Are you having any problems performing activities such as eating, brushing your hair, bathing, or toileting?

- Have you been exposed to loud noises or chemicals in your work environment or neighborhood?

---

### TABLE 41-4     ASSESSING SENSORY PERCEPTUAL STATUS

| Sensation Being Assessed | Assessment Focus |
| --- | --- |
| Visual | Presence of visual problems, including:<br>• Blurred vision<br>• Double vision<br>• Blind spots<br>• Rainbows or halos around objects<br>• Photosensitivity<br>Difficulty seeing far or near<br>Family history of visual problems (such as glaucoma, cataracts)<br>Use of contact lenses or eyeglasses<br>Date of last eye examination |
| Auditory | Presence of hearing problems<br>Recent changes in hearing ability<br>Ability to distinguish sounds (tone and pitch)<br>Presence of buzzing or ringing noises<br>Use of a hearing aid |
| Gustatory | Changes in ability to taste<br>Difficulty in differentiating salty, sweet, sour, and bitter tastes<br>Changes in appetite |
| Olfactory | Changes in ability to smell<br>Ability to distinguish common smells (such as food, perfume, flowers) |
| Tactile | Difficulty in feeling temperature changes in extremities<br>Impairment of pain perception in extremities<br>Presence of unusual sensations in extremities (such as tingling or numbness) |

is done to determine the presence of any neurologic deficits (Figure 41-9). Chapter 27 provides a detailed discussion on assessing the cranial nerves.

## Mental-Status Assessment

A thorough mental-status examination includes a systematic assessment of all the emotional and cognitive functions. Mental status is usually assessed during the health history interview.

The Mini-Mental Status Examination I (MMSE) (Folstein, Folstein, & McHugh, 1975) was developed to determine one's baseline mental status; it includes several questions to assess orientation. The MMSE can be administered as a screening tool in acute, community-based, and long-term care settings. It is not intended to be used as a diagnostic tool but rather to screen clients for the cognitive aspects of mental functioning: orientation, registration, attention and recall, and language (Folstein, Folstein, & McHugh, 1975). The highest possible score is 30, with a score of 21 or less usually indicating cognitive impairment. A more detailed mental-status assessment is warranted if the client presents with any of the following: memory deficit, confusion, aphasia (impairment in language functioning), mood swings, irritability, excessive headaches, behavioral changes, or seizures.

### Levels of Consciousness

When assessing clients for sensory, perceptual, and cognitive alterations, the nurse should evaluate the level of consciousness (LOC). When describing assessment data relative to LOC, the nurse should include a brief description of the type of stimuli used to test LOC and the client's response. Box 41-5 gives a list of terms commonly used in describing LOC.

The Glasgow Coma Scale (GCS) was developed as a standardized tool to assess LOC objectively (Table 41-5). The tool may be used in a variety of clinical situations and is meant to be used in conjunction with a complete neurologic assessment.

### Functional Abilities

The nurse needs to have an understanding of the client's ability to conduct self-care activities (Peterson, 2000). Any sensory, perceptual, or cognitive impairments may interfere with the client's ability to perform activities of daily living (ADL). Also, such impairments can interfere with the client's ability to keep the home environment clean and safe. A thorough assessment of self-care abilities includes assessment of skills related to dressing, grooming, bathing, feeding, and toileting.

### Environment

A person's environment can affect sensory, perceptual, and cognitive status in a variety of ways. For example, a non-stimulating environment can lead to sensory deprivation, whereas an environment that is excessively stimulating can result in sensory overload.

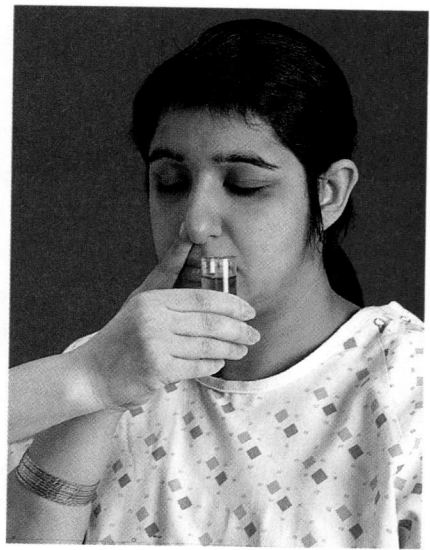

**Figure 41-9    Assessment of cranial nerve I**

## BOX 41-5  DESCRIPTIVE TERMS FOR LEVELS OF CONSCIOUSNESS

*Alert.* Oriented and aware of stimuli; responds appropriately.

*Lethargic.* Responds appropriately to stimuli but may be slow to respond; may be drowsy and may drift off to sleep when not stimulated.

*Obtunded.* Sleeps most of the time; difficult to arouse with minimal response; requires constant stimulation; inconsistently follows commands.

*Semicomatose.* Responds with purposeful movements when stimulated, but does not follow commands and is nonverbal.

*Comatose.* Unconscious with no meaningful response to stimuli. Light coma may include reflex motor response to painful stimuli (decorticate or decerebrate posturing); deep coma includes no motor response to any stimuli.

## TABLE 41-5  GLASGOW COMA SCALE

| Behavior | Response | Score |
|---|---|---|
| Eye opening response | Spontaneous | 4 |
| | To verbal command | 3 |
| | To pain | 2 |
| | No response | 1 |
| Best verbal response | Oriented, conversing | 5 |
| | Disoriented, conversing | 4 |
| | Use of inappropriate words | 3 |
| | Incomprehensible sounds | 2 |
| | No response | 1 |
| Best motor response | Obeys verbal commands | 6 |
| | Moves to localized pain | 5 |
| | Flexion withdrawal to pain | 4 |
| | Abnormal posturing—decorticate | 3 |
| | Abnormal posturing—decerebrate | 2 |
| | No response | 1 |
| Total | | 3 to 15 |

With the GCS, a score of 15 indicates a fully oriented person. A score of 7 or less is considered a state of coma. A score of 3 is the lowest possible score and is indicative of deep coma.

## NURSING STRATEGY

### Promoting Sensory Stimulation for Clients in a Long-Term Care Facility

1. Wear a readable name tag.
2. Introduce yourself by name.
3. On every shift, inform the client of the year, month, day, week, and name of the facility.
4. Keep a calendar or clock that can be easily read by the client's bed.
5. Explain all procedures prior to implementation.
6. Keep all necessary assistive devices (e.g., eyeglasses, dentures, hearing aid) accessible.
7. Encourage client and family to personalize immediate environment with items from home, such as photos and quilts.

People who are at increased risk for sensory perceptual deficits include:

- The older adult
- Those who live alone
- Those who are institutionalized
- The homebound
- Those with chronic illness or physical handicaps
- Those who are mentally ill
- Those who have a developmental delay

The nurse assesses the type and quantity of stimuli in the client's environment. See the Community/Home Care box for information on assessing the client's home environment.

People with sensory, perceptual, and cognitive alterations are at increased risk of injury. Impairment of sensory perceptual and cognitive abilities can present the following hazards:

- Visual: Risk of tripping, falling
- Auditory: Lack of awareness of warning sounds (such as automobile horns, sirens, smoke alarms)

## CLIENT REFLECTIONS

### Safety of the General Public versus Individual Liberty

Your 78-year-old neighbor, Mrs. Henke, confides in you one afternoon at her home that she is becoming "more deaf by the minute." She tells you, "Next week when I go in for my driver's license renewal, I am not going to tell them about my little problem." Your neighborhood has several small children who run into and out of the street playing. How do you respond to Mrs. Henke?

- Olfactory: Inability to perceive warning odors (such as burning food, escaping gas)
- Gustatory: Unawareness of spoiled or contaminated food or beverages
- Tactile: Lack of awareness of excessive pressure on a body part; at risk for exposure to extreme temperatures (frostbite, burns)

# Diagnosis

Several nursing diagnoses are applicable to clients experiencing sensory, perceptual, and cognitive alterations. The nurse needs to establish a diagnosis that is most closely related to the client's priority needs. The North American Nursing Diagnosis Association (NANDA) diagnostic label that is applicable for many clients experiencing altered sensory perception and cognition is *Disturbed Sensory Perception* (specify *visual, auditory, kinesthetic, gustatory, tactile, olfactory*). This condition is defined as "a state in which an individual experiences a change in the amount or patterning of incoming stimuli accompanied by a diminished, exaggerated, distorted, or impaired response to such stimuli" (NANDA, 2003, p. 70). See Table 41-6 for other relevant diagnoses, with defining characteristics and related factors.

# Planning and Outcome Identification

Nurses understand the importance of promoting optimal sensory stimulation for clients in every area of care. The following goals will promote supportive, restorative care for clients experiencing sensory, perceptual, or cognitive alterations:

The client will:

- Remain safe and free from injury
- Experience a level of arousal that promotes the meaningful perception of stimuli
- Remain oriented to time, place, person, and situation
- Demonstrate intact functioning of senses (using assistive devices if necessary)
- Perform self-care activities appropriate to own functional capability

The current trend is to provide care for individuals experiencing cognitive deficits at home. "The goal of using creative strategies to manage dementia is to slow the rate of deterioration in order to prevent institutionalization for as long as possible" (Cacchione, 2000, p. 631).

The American Psychiatric Association (1994) has identified the following as skills to be encouraged in order to promote cognitive functioning: stability, consistency, self-identification, and active participation. Table 41-7 lists nursing interventions that enhance the development of these four essential skills.

# Implementation

A major concern of nurses caring for clients with sensory, perceptual, and cognitive alterations is safety. Actions must be taken to ensure that the client's environment is hazard-free and, at the same time, that it provides adequate stimulation. This section describes nursing interventions that promote appropriate sensory, perceptual, and cognitive functioning. Care of clients with visual and hearing impairments is discussed. Also presented is information on communicating with a confused client and a client who is unconscious.

## Managing Sensory Deficits

Clients with sensory deficits, including tactile, auditory, and visual impairments, need sensitive nursing care to best adapt to their environments and specific challenges.

### Tactile Alterations

The client with impaired tactile sensation is placed at an increased risk for development of skin breakdown.

## TABLE 41-6   NURSING DIAGNOSES RELATED TO SENSORY, PERCEPTUAL, AND COGNITIVE IMPAIRMENTS

| Diagnosis | Defining Characteristics | Related Factors |
|---|---|---|
| Disturbed Sensory Perception (specify) | **Major**<br>• Inaccurate interpretation of environmental stimuli<br>• Negative change in amount or pattern of incoming stimuli<br>**Minor**<br>• Disoriented to time, place, or people<br>• Impaired problem-solving ability<br>• Changes in behavior or communication pattern<br>• Restlessness<br>• Disturbed sleep patterns<br>• Hallucinations<br>• Fear<br>• Anxiety | • Cerebrovascular accident<br>• Meningitis or encephalitis<br>• Fluid and electrolyte imbalance<br>• Decreased oxygen transport<br>• Medications<br>• Physical isolation<br>• Immobility<br>• Social isolation<br>• Stress |
| Disturbed Thought Processes | **Major**<br>• Inaccurate interpretation of stimuli, internal and/or external<br>**Minor**<br>• Cognitive deficits, including memory deficits<br>• Suspiciousness<br>• Delusions<br>• Hallucinations<br>• Distractibility<br>• Confusion, disorientation<br>• Impulsivity | • Mental disorders or personality changes resulting from biochemical changes<br>• Hormonal changes<br>• Depression<br>• Anxiety<br>• Fear<br>• Loss<br>• Isolation<br>• Ambiguous communication<br>• Abuse<br>• Social isolation |
| Social Isolation | **Major**<br>• Expressed feelings of aloneness and/or desire for more social contact<br>**Minor**<br>• Verbalization that time is passing slowly<br>• Inability to concentrate<br>• Impaired decision making<br>• Expressed feelings of uselessness<br>• Feelings of rejection<br>• Increased irritability<br>• Restlessness<br>• Failure to interact with others nearby<br>• Feelings of hopelessness | • Communicable disease<br>• Psychiatric illness<br>• Death of a significant other<br>• Divorce<br>• Terminal illness<br>• Hospitalization<br>• Institutionalization<br>• Loss of means of transportation<br>• Unemployment |
| Risk for Injury | **Major**<br>• Developmental age<br>• Altered mobility<br>• Confusion<br>• Disorientation<br>**Minor**<br>• Malnutrition | • Sensory dysfunction (decreased sensation, impaired vision, diminished sense of smell) |

From Carpenito, L. J. (2002). *Nursing diagnosis: Application to practice* (9th ed.). Philadelphia: Lippincott; North American Nursing Diagnosis Association (2003). *Nursing diagnoses: Definitions and classification. 2003–2004.* Philadelphia: Author.)

## TABLE 41-7  NURSING INTERVENTIONS TO PROMOTE COGNITIVE FUNCTION

| Intervention | Examples |
| --- | --- |
| Memory retraining | Reality orientation |
| Social skills therapy | Reinforcing behaviors to be used when interacting with others |
| Communication therapy | Improving speech patterns or words to complete a thought<br>Minimizing sensory deprivation |
| Stress management therapy | Identifying and using factors that minimize stress |
| Reminiscence therapy | Using storytelling and memory recall to identify with past experiences |
| Behavioral therapy | Maintaining consistency and stability to specify expected behaviors<br>Recognizing and controlling environmental stressors<br>Using written schedules and directions to assist with activities |
| Medication administration | Using pharmacological agents to manage disruptive behaviors |

From American Psychiatric Association. (1994). *Diagnostic and statistical manual of mental disorders* (4th ed., rev.). Washington, DC: Author.

Therefore, it is important to encourage a safe living environment and to educate the individual and significant others in injury prevention measures. For more information on preventing tissue and skin breakdown, refer to Chapter 36. The accompanying Client Education box describes therapeutic approaches for maintaining skin integrity of clients with altered touch sensation.

## Auditory Impairments

In addition to safety hazards, individuals with impaired hearing are also at risk for social isolation because of the difficulty in communicating with others. Nurses must ensure that they spend time with hearing-impaired clients, focus on nonverbal communication, and face the client when speaking. Check all assistive devices used by clients to ensure that they are working properly (Figure 41-10). Use an interpreter when one is available for signing; often the client's family can serve as interpreters. If an interpreter is

## CLIENT EDUCATION

### Client with a Tactile Deficit

Teach the client and family that burns can occur not only from heat but also from friction, chemicals, or tape. It is important for the client to inspect her skin daily and to avoid the following:

✓ Sun exposure (use sunblock)
✓ Hot bathwater (use a bath thermometer)
✓ Hot water bottles, heating pads
✓ Placing containers of hot food or liquids in lap
✓ Eating hot foods, such as pizza, or other items that maintain heat for extended periods, without first testing the temperature
✓ Sitting on objects that may be hot (heaters, concrete, or rocks in sunlight)
✓ Walking on hot surfaces (pavement or concrete) without shoes
✓ Contact with items in or on an automobile that are hot from exhaust or sunlight (for instance, tailpipe, heater vents directed at feet, seat belt buckles, steering wheel, or leather or vinyl upholstery)
✓ Overexposure to very low temperatures (cold weather or ice packs) without proper protection

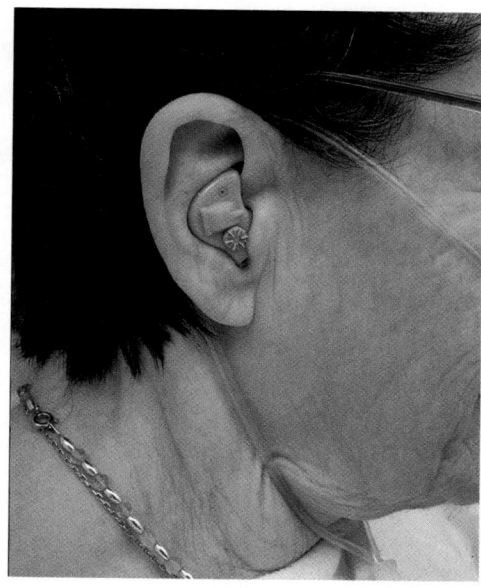

Figure 41-10  The use of hearing aids helps to compensate for hearing loss experienced by some clients.

available, the nurse must talk to the *client*, not to the interpreter; see the Nursing Strategy box for more information on communicating through an interpreter. Other communication aids include finger spelling, communication boards, and the use of paper and pen for writing messages. Refer to Chapter 4 for more information on communicating with clients who are hearing impaired.

## Visual Impairments

Clients with visual impairments often have developed the other senses to a high degree. The nurse can, therefore, use a variety of ways to enhance communication with such clients. For example, the nurse should do the following:

- Ask client to explain what is helpful (such as preferred means of communicating, usual routine).
- Look directly at the client while speaking.
- Encourage the client to handle items and objects; use objects that can be identified by other senses.
- Keep furniture and other items in their usual place; orient the client to the environment by using clock hours to indicate position of items in relation to the client.
- Use your normal tone, volume, and rate of speaking.
- Inform client when you are entering or leaving the room.
- Ask for permission before touching the client.

## Managing Sensory Deprivation

It is important to provide an adequate amount of sensory stimulation to those clients who are understimulated or at risk for developing sensory deprivation.

## Managing Sensory Overload

Caring for clients experiencing sensory overload can be very challenging for nurses, especially in critical care areas (such as the emergency department or intensive care unit). It is important to reduce environmental stimuli as much as possible. The Nursing Strategy box provides guidelines for nursing interventions for clients experiencing sensory overload.

## Assisting the Confused Client

Nurses need to be extra supportive when communicating with a client who is confused. Many clients are aware of their cognitive deficit and become frustrated about their inability to process environmental stimuli correctly. The nurse must ask about the client's preferred means of communication, and tailor the interaction accordingly (McDougall, 2001). Sensitive nursing care includes allowing additional time for the client to respond to questions, speaking directly to the client in uncomplicated language, repeating information as needed, and using visual clues and body language to reinforce verbal messages. It is also important to address only one topic at a time and to give simple directions in sequence. For example, "First, sit up in bed. Then slide your legs over the edge of the bed." Other interventions that are therapeutic for confused clients include the following:

- Written schedule of activities
- Written checklists for performing ADL
- Written directions for medication self-administration
- Active participation in activities
- Prevent social withdrawal

The following Client Education box provides information to share with significant others caring for a confused client.

## Caring for the Unconscious Client

Individuals who are unconscious can often hear what is spoken even though they are unable to respond. Thus, it is important for the nurse to be cautious of what is said in the presence of an unconscious client. Nurses should talk in a normal conversational tone while providing care. Also, remember the value of nonverbal communication, and touch the unconscious client. See the Nursing Strategy box for additional guidelines in communicating with a client who is unconscious. See Chapter 4 for additional information on communicating with unconscious clients.

---

### NURSING STRATEGY

#### Communicating Through an Interpreter

- Use short sentences and questions.

- Avoid the use of ambiguous statements and questions.

- Plan what you intend to say ahead of time; this avoids confusing the interpreter by having to back up, restate, or revise previous statements.

- Avoid the use of technical jargon.

Data from Kneisl, C. R. (1996). Therapeutic communication. In H. S. Wilson & C. R. Kneisl (Eds.), *Psychiatric Nursing* (5th ed., p. 129). Menlo Park, CA: Addison-Wesley.

---

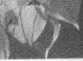

### NURSING STRATEGY

#### Consistency and Cognitive Deficits

When caring for clients with cognitive deficits such as stroke or head injury, it is important to maintain consistency of caregivers providing care, response time to client's needs, and the client's environment.

## NURSING STRATEGY

### Care of the Client Experiencing Sensory Overload

- Address the client by name.

- Provide explanations of all procedures prior to implementation.

- Modify environment to reduce excessive multisensory stimulation; reduce distractions, loud noise, excessive light.

- Use a calm, unhurried manner when communicating with the client.

- Provide a private room whenever feasible.

- Plan the delivery of care to allow for rest periods with no stimulation.

- Use soft background music.

- Keep the environment free of strong odors (including perfume or after-shave lotion).

- Limit the number and frequency of visitors.

## NURSING STRATEGY

### Communicating with an Unconscious Client

- Orient the client to self, situation, place, and time.

- Address the client by name and explain all procedures prior to implementation.

- Maintain a routine to increase the client's sense of security.

- Use touch deliberately.

- Actively listen to significant others.

- Encourage significant others to talk to and touch the client often.

- Treat the client with the same respect and dignity you display to all clients.

## CLIENT EDUCATION

### The Confused Client

✓ Keep clutter in traffic areas at a minimum; remove small rugs that can cause tripping.

✓ Make sure bed is low, and that there is proper lighting to help prevent falls.

✓ Keep dangerous objects from client's reach (including matches, firearms, knives).

✓ Keep medications out of client's reach.

✓ Lock doors to areas that could be potentially dangerous if client wanders there.

✓ Assist in dressing appropriately for the season.

✓ Do not allow the client to stay alone; have a responsible adult provide supervision.

✓ Try to keep daily activities as routine as possible.

✓ Keep activities simple and uncomplicated.

✓ Provide signs, posters, clocks, and calendars as memory aids.

✓ Encourage client to be independent while providing assistance as needed.

✓ Always treat the client with respect and dignity.

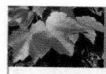

## RESEARCH FOCUS

**Title of Study:** Consequences of not recognizing delirium superimposed on dementia in hospitalized elderly individuals

**Study Purpose:** To describe the recognition and management of delirium in hospitalized clients with and without dementia

**Methods:** A descriptive, exploratory design was used with a convenience sample of 20 hospitalized older individuals. The clients were observed using qualitative interviews and observations by hospital staff and family members.

**Findings:** The prevalence of delirium in this study was 60%. The incidence (new onset) of delirium was 30%. The presence of delirium was associated with lower baseline MMSE scores, depression, incontinence, and weight loss. Delirium superimposed on dementia was less likely to be recognized by nurses and physicians.

**Implications:** Clients with dementia should be routinely assessed for signs of delirium in order to treat the reversible processes and avoid long-term sequelae. The small sample of 20 clients is a drawback to this study, which should be replicated with larger numbers of participants.

Fick, D., & Foreman, M. (2000). Consequences of not recognizing delirium superimposed on dementia in hospitalized elderly individuals. *Journal of Gerontological Nursing, 26*(1), 30–40.

## Using Restraints

Restraints, both physical and chemical, are sometimes used with clients experiencing cognitive and/or sensory perceptual alterations. Cognitively impaired residents of long-term care facilities are the most frequently restrained (Mayhew et al., 1999).

Many risks are associated with the use of restraints, including strangulation, impaired circulation, increased risk of falls, the stigma of being "tied down," and perception that one is being punished. Minimizing the use of restraints must be done in order to respect client dignity while at the same time promoting safety of clients and staff members. See Chapter 33 for guidelines on the safe use of restraints.

## Complementary/Alternative Therapies

Natural therapies can play an essential role in maintaining a healthy CNS. This section discusses the use of herbs

## CLINICAL ALERT

The only therapeutic rationale for the use of restraints is promotion of safety.

and aromatherapy as methods for enhancing mental well-being. Refer to Chapter 31 for a complete discussion of complementary/alternative treatment approaches.

### Herbals

Four groups of herbs especially benefit the nervous system: tonics, sedatives, demulcents, stimulants (Table 41-8).

### Aromatherapy

Aromatherapy can be used to relax or stimulate the CNS. Aromatic molecules give off signals that travel to the limbic system (the so-called "emotional switchboard" of the

| TABLE 41-8 | HERBS FOR THE NERVOUS SYSTEM | |
|---|---|---|
| **Classification** | **Functions** | **Herbs** |
| Nerve Tonics | • Feed, tone, and strengthen the nervous tissues and cells<br>• High in calcium, magnesium, B vitamins, and protein content<br>• To be most effective, should be taken over long period of time | Chamomile (*Anthemis nobilis*)<br>*Ginkgo (*Ginkgo biloba*)<br>Hops (*Humulus lupulus*)<br>Skullcap (*Scutellaria lactiflora*)<br><br>*NOTE: Ginkgo has vasoconstrictive properties that help improve cerebral blood flow (Tierra, 1998); is licensed in Germany for treatment of cerebral dysfunction (Goldberg, 1999). |
| Nerve Demulcents | • Soothe and heal irritated, inflamed nerve endings.<br>• Gel-like consistency coats and protects nerve endings. | Barley (*Hordeum vulgare*)<br>Flax seed<br>Marsh mallow root (*Althea officinalis*)<br>Oats (*Avena sativa*)<br>Slippery elm (*Ulmus rubra*) |
| Nerve Sedatives | • Relax the nervous<br>• Help reduce pain and tension<br>• Promote sleep<br>• Many exert antispasmodic effects. | Catnip (*Catnip cataria*)<br>Passion flower (*Passiflora incarnata*)<br>St. John's wort (*Hypericum perforatum*) |
| Nerve Stimulants | • Activate nerve endings by increasing circulation<br>• Provide nutrients<br>• Revitalize the nervous system | Cayenne (*Capsicum annuum*)<br>Ginger (*Zingiber officinalis*)<br>Ginseng (*Panax quinquefolius; Eleutherococcus senticosus*)<br>Lemon balm (*Melissa officinalis*)<br>Peppermint (*Mentha piperita*)<br>Rosemary (*Rosmarinus officinalis*)<br>Sage (*Salvia officinalis*) |

brain). "Because the limbic system is directly connected to those parts of the brain that control heart rate, blood pressure, breathing, memory, stress levels, and hormone balance, scientists have learned that oil fragrances may be one of the fastest ways to achieve physiological and psychological effects" (Goldberg, 1999, p. 54). Box 41-6 lists some essential oils used to promote a healthy CNS.

## Evaluation

Evaluating the care of the client with sensory, perceptual, and cognitive alterations depends on the specific expected outcomes for each client. Evaluation of outcome achievement is performed through the nurse's use of observation and communication skills. An important component of evaluation is determination of the client's need for continued assistance in meeting needs. Evaluation of the client's self-care abilities provides information for discharge planning, including follow-up care or placement in a long-term care facility, if necessary.

### BOX 41-6   ESSENTIAL OILS AND CNS HEALTH

| | |
|---|---|
| Chamomile (*Anthemis nobilis*) | Alleviates physical and mental stress |
| Lavender (*Lavandula angustifolia*) | Calming, sedative effect |
| Mandarin (*Citrus reticulata*) | Relieves anxiety |
| Peppermint (*Mentha piperita*) | Stimulant; strengthens adrenal cortex |
| Yarrow (*Achillea millefolium*) | Promotes sleep |

Data from Goldberg, B. (1999). *Alternative medicine: The definitive guide.* Tiburon, CA: Future Medicine Publishing; Tierra, M. (1998). *The way of herbs.* New York: Pocket Books; Walters, C. (1998). *Aromatherapy: A basic guide.* New York: Barnes & Noble.

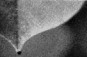

# CASE STUDY/NURSING CARE PLAN

Mr. Carter, a 53-year-old contract worker, arrives at the clinic with his son, who had found Mr. Carter wandering aimlessly along a road in his community. The son is worried that his father is becoming "more and more forgetful every day." This was first noticed one month ago, when Mr. Carter forgot his phone number when completing a job application. Since then, the memory lapses have become more frequent and are now interfering with daily routines (he forgets to take his blood pressure medicine and gets lost returning home). Mr. Carter is currently unemployed and has no health care insurance. He denies that there is any problem and reluctantly agreed to come in today after hearing on the radio about free blood-pressure screenings offered by the clinic.

The nurse takes Mr. Carter's blood pressure, and it has a reading of 184/106 mm/Hg. As the nurse continues to assess Mr. Carter, there is a pronounced bilateral deficit of hearing. In addition, as Mr. Carter is questioned, he is unable to remember with accuracy daily events that have occurred within the past week. He is able to remember things from his childhood, and his long-term memory seems intact.

### Nursing Diagnosis #1

*Acute Confusion* related to unknown etiology as evidenced by fluctuations in cognition and level of consciousness, and memory disturbances.

**NOC:** Cognitive orientation, decision making, distorted thoughts, safety behavior

**NIC:** Dementia management, environmental management, safety, family involvement promotion

### Expected Outcome

1. The client will maintain current level of consciousness with no demonstrated deterioration.

### Planning/Interventions/Rationales

1. Assess level of consciousness. *Establishes a baseline of data in order to intervene quickly if mental status changes.*
2. Tell Mr. Carter your name and why you are meeting with him. *Keeps client oriented to reality.*
3. Talk to Mr. Carter while providing care. *Maintains reality orientation.*
4. Whenever possible, avoid the use of drugs that may cause drowsiness or sedation. *Increased drowsiness or sedation will make it difficult to determine changes in neurologic function.*
5. Encourage physical and mental activity, daily exercise, and interaction (e.g., with family or friends, newspaper, TV, etc.) *Improves memory, attention, and orientation.*
6. Prepare the client for changes in activity or routines. *Reduces confusion and creates a routine to improve orientation.*

### Evaluation

Goal partially met. Mr. Carter maintained current level of consciousness.

*(continues)*

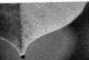

# CASE STUDY/NURSING CARE PLAN (continued)

### Nursing Diagnosis #2

*Risk for Injury* related to cognitive deficits.

**NOC:** Risk control, social safety, safety behavior, physical injury

**NIC:** Health education, behavior modification, patient contracting

### Expected Outcome

1. The client will remain free of injury.

### Planning/Interventions/Rationales

1. Assess environment and make alterations to enhance safety if necessary. *Alterations will lessen likelihood of injury.*
2. Provide support to significant others and/or supervision for tasks deemed potentially harmful to client, discouraging tasks as appropriate (e.g., cooking, smoking). *Prevents physical injury to client or danger to others.*
3. Provide a list of community resources and cost of services (e.g., day treatment centers, home health agencies) and encourage utilization of resources as appropriate. *A list will promote access to available resources that offer a safe environment through part- or full-time supervised care.*

### Evaluation

Goal partially met. Mr. Carter remained free of injury while at the clinic. He stated he was not interested in the list of community resources.

## Key Concepts

- The well-being of an individual depends upon the functions of sensation, perception, and cognition, which are controlled by the central nervous system.
- Primary components of consciousness include arousal and awareness.
- Cognitive and perceptual functioning is inferred through assessment of the client's behaviors (e.g., consciousness, orientation, speech, thought processes, and perceptions).
- The sensory system is made up of a complex network of afferent fibers within the peripheral nerves, afferent tracts located in the spinal cord and brain stem, and the higher cortex (cerebral lobes).
- Consciousness is a state of awareness of one's self, others, and the surrounding environment, and it affects intellect and emotions.
- Consciousness is controlled by the reticular activating system located within the midbrain and thalamus, as well as connective fibers between these structures and areas within the cerebral cortex.
- The degree of arousal (alertness) is indicated by a person's general response to the environment.
- Orientation refers to awareness of self in relation to the surrounding environment; an individual who is "oriented × 4" is aware of time, place, person, and situation.
- There are three distinct types of memory: immediate, recent, and remote.
- An individual's affect (mood or feeling tone) can affect thinking ability.
- Judgment is the ability to compare or evaluate alternatives to life situations and arrive at an appropriate course of action.

- There are two types of perceptual distortions, illusions and hallucinations.
- Language is one of the most complex of cognitive functions, involving the ability to speak, read, write, and comprehend.
- A person can become confused as a result of either overstimulation or understimulation.
- Sensory deprivation, a state of reduced sensory input, can occur as a result of illness, trauma, or isolation.
- Sensory overload is a state of excessive and sustained multisensory stimulation manifested by behavior change and perceptual distortion.

## Review Questions and Activities

1. What are the physiological components underlying sensation, perception, and cognition?
2. Compare and contrast the three types of memory.
3. Why might a drug such as morphine sulfate be contraindicated in a client who has an altered level of consciousness?
4. What are the characteristics of a client experiencing sensory overload?
5. What are important elements of a neurologic screening assessment?
6. What are examples of nursing diagnoses applicable to clients with sensory, perceptual, and cognitive alterations?
7. What are nursing interventions for clients with alterations in auditory function?

**8.** What are nursing strategies in providing care for unconscious clients?

**9.** Describe several types of complementary/alternative therapies.

## Web Resources

Alterations in cognition
   http://www.nursing.iupui.edu
American Association of Critical-Care Nurses
   http://www.aacn.org
American Association of Neuroscience Nurses
   http://www.aann.org
American Nurses Association
   http://www.ana.org
Canadian Association of Neuroscience Nurses
   http://www.cann.ca
Cognition and related topics
   http://www.nmap.ac.uk
Cognitive alterations in Alzheimer's disease
   http://www.alzheimersupport.com
National Institutes of Health
   http://www.nih.gov

## References

Alverzo, J. P. & Galski, T. (1999). Nurses' assessment of patients' cognitive orientation in a rehabilitation setting. *Rehabilitation Nursing, 24,* 7–23.

American Psychiatric Association. (1994). *Diagnostic and statistical manual of mental disorders* (4th ed., rev.). Washington, DC: Author.

Bays, C .L. (2001). Quality of life of stroke survivors: A research synthesis. *Journal of Neuroscience Nursing, 33*(6), 310-316.

Cacchione, P. Z. (2000). Cognitive and neurologic function. In A.G. Lueckenotte (Ed.), *Gerontologic nursing* (2nd ed.). St. Louis: Mosby.

Carpenito, L. J. (2002). *Nursing diagnosis: Application to practice* (9th ed.). Philadelphia: Lippincott.

Davis, L. L. (2001). Assessing functional ability in persons with dementia: Using family caregivers as informants. *Journal of Neuroscience Nursing, 33*(4): 194-195.

Estes, M. E. Z. (2002). *Health assessment & physical examination* (2nd ed.). Clifton Park, NY: Delmar Learning.

Fick, D., & Foreman, M. (2000). Consequences of not recognizing delirium, superimposed on dementia in hospitalized elderly individuals. *Journal of Gerontological Nursing, 26*(1), 30–40.

Folstein, M. F., Folstein, S. E., & McHugh, P. R. (1975). Mini-mental state: A practical method for grading the cognitive state of patients for the clinician. *Journal of Psychiatric Research, 12,* 189–198. Oxford, England: Elsevier Science, Pergamon Imprint.

Goldberg, B. (1999). *Alternative medicine: The definitive guide.* Tibruon, CA: Future Medicine Publishing.

Guyton, A. C., & Hall, J. (2000). *Textbook of medical physiology* (10th ed.). Philadelphia: Saunders.

Holmberg, S. K., & Coon, S. (1999). Ambient sound levels in a state psychiatric hospital. *Archives of Psychiatric Nursing, 13*(3), 117–126.

Kneisl, C. R. (1996). Therapeutic communication. In H. S. Wilson & C. R. Kneisl (Eds.), *Psychiatric Nursing* (5th ed., pp. 129). Menlo Park, CA: Addison-Wesley.

Kuhn, M. A., Herlihy, J. T., & Herlihy, B. L. (1998). Overview of the anatomy and physiology of the nervous system. In M. Kuhn (Ed.), *Pharmacotherapeutics: A nursing process approach* (4th ed.). Philadelphia: F. A. Davis.

Mayhew, P. A., Christy, K., Berkebile, J., Miller, C., & Farrish, A. (1999). Restraint reduction: Research utilization and case study with cognitive impairment. *Geriatric Nursing, 20*(6), 305–308.

McDougall, G. J. (2001). Rehabilitation of memory and memory self-efficacy in cognitively impaired nursing home residents. *Clinical Gerontologist, 23*(3/4), 127-139.

McDougall, G. J. (2002). Memory improvement in octogenarians. *Applied Nursing Research, 15*(1), 2-10.

Meleis, A. (1997). *Theoretical Nursing: Development and Progress* (3rd ed.). Philadelphia: Lippincott.

Miller, J. J. (1999). Care of young, middle, and older adults. In J. E. Hitchcock, P. E. Schubert, & S. A. Thomas (Eds.), *Community health nursing: Caring in action.* Clifton Park, NY: Delmar Learning.

North American Nursing Diagnosis Association. (2003). *Nursing diagnoses: Definitions and classification. 2003–2004.* Philadelphia: Author.

Perkins, B. R., & Rouanzoin, C. (2002). A critical evaluation of current views regarding eye movement desensitization and reprocessing (EMDR): clarifying points of confusion. *Journal of Clinical Psychology 58*(1), pp. 77–97.

Peterson, P. (2001). Why neuroscience nursing? *Journal of Neuroscience Nursing, 33*(3), 128-129.

Roy, S. C. (1988). Alterations in cognitive processing. In P. H. Mitchell, L. C. Hodges, M. Muwaswes, & C. A. Walleck (Eds.), *AANN's neuroscience nursing: Phenomena and practice—Human responses to neurological health problems* (pp. 185–211). Norwalk, CT: Appleton & Lange.

Tierra, M. (1998). *The way of herbs.* New York: Pocket Books.

Walters, C. (1998). *Aromatherapy: A basic guide.* New York: Barnes & Noble.

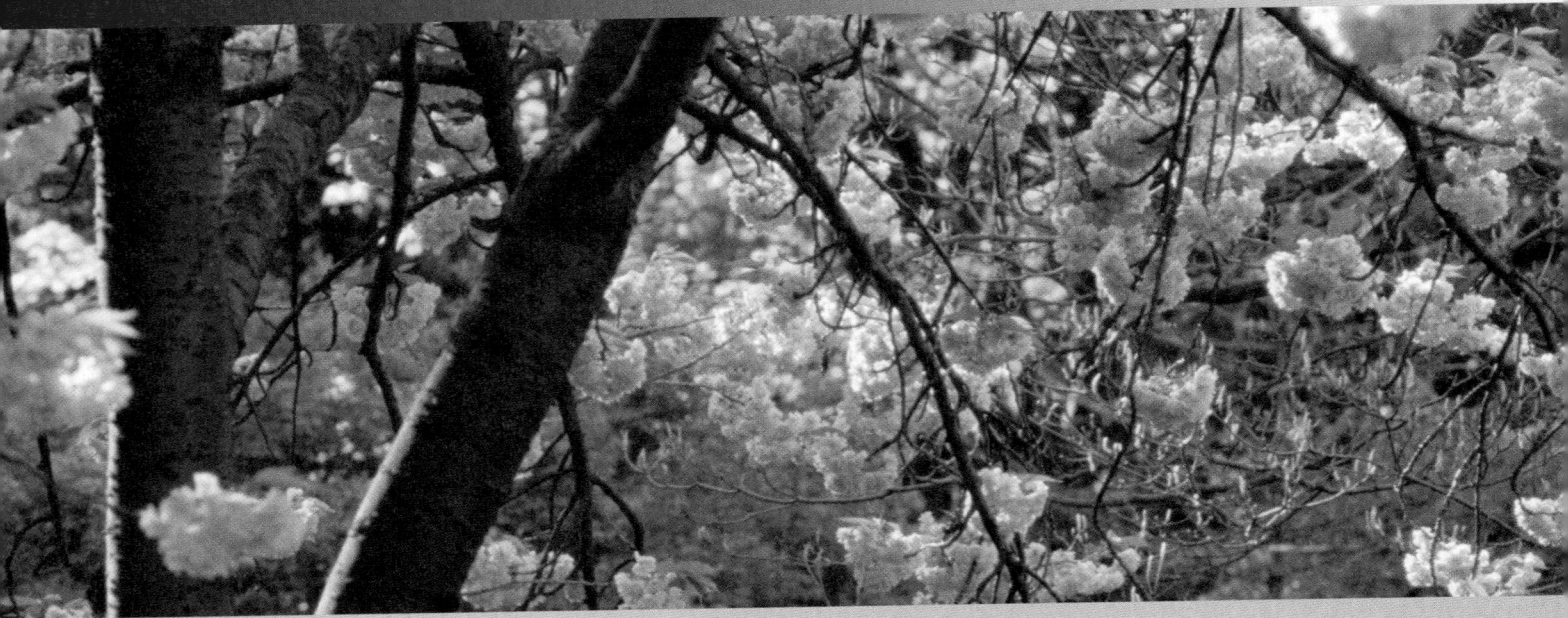

# Pain

## Debra L. Topham, PhD, RN, CNS, ACRN

*"In the past decade, pain has come into its own and with it the knowledge that pain, more than a mere physiologic response to a painful stimulus, is a biopsychosocial phenomenon."*

(Lasch, 2000)

# Chapter Competencies

*Upon completion of this chapter, the reader should be able to:*

1. Assess the nature of pain as it relates to onset, intensity, and duration.
2. Discuss the physiology of pain.
3. Compare and contrast factors that affect the pain experience.
4. Describe different pain assessment tools.
5. Evaluate the nursing process as it is implemented with pain control.
6. Describe nonpharmacological interventions implemented in the management of pain.
7. Discuss the use of pharmacological interventions used in pain control.

# Key Terms

| | | |
|---|---|---|
| acute pain | endorphin | pain tolerance |
| addiction | gate control pain theory | paresthesia |
| adjuvant medication | hyperalgesia | patient controlled-analgesia (PCA) |
| afferent pain pathway | hypnosis | |
| allodynia | imagery | phantom limb pain |
| biofeedback | intractable pain | physical dependence |
| ceiling effect | ischemic pain | progressive muscle relaxation |
| chronic acute pain | lancinating | recurrent acute pain |
| chronic malignant pain | mixed agonist-antagonist | referred pain |
| chronic nonmalignant pain | myofascial pain syndromes | reframing |
| chronic pain | neuralgia | relaxation techniques |
| colic | neuropathic pain | somatic pain |
| counterstimulation | nociception | tolerance |
| cutaneous pain | nociceptor | transcutaneous electrical nerve stimulation (TENS) |
| distraction | pain | trigger point |
| efferent pain pathway | pain threshold | visceral pain |

The experience of pain can have a significant impact on a client's health. Pain is a personal experience that can affect all other aspects of an individual's health, including physical well-being, mental status, and effectiveness of coping mechanisms. This chapter explores the nature of pain and nursing care to help clients maintain their optimal health when the presence of pain threatens to compromise their health status.

## Pain

**Pain** is a universal human experience; it is defined as "a state in which an individual experiences and reports the presence of severe discomfort or an uncomfortable sensa-tion" (Carpenito, 2002, p. 50). Pain is a subjective experience that is often difficult for clients to describe and nurses to understand, yet it is among the most common complaints that cause individuals to seek health care. McCaffery and Pasero (1999) recognize the subjective nature of pain by stating, "Pain is whatever the experiencing person says it is, existing whenever he says it does" (p. 17). Until recently, pain was viewed as a symptom that required diagnosis and treatment of the underlying cause. It is now clear that pain itself can be detrimental to the health and healing of clients. "Unrelieved pain is not only detrimental, it's avoidable" (Williams-Lee, 1999, p. 9). Pain is a stressor that can trigger both physiological and psychological discomfort. Untreated pain can lead to physical disorders related to undernutri-tion, immobility, and immune suppression.

# Nature of Pain

Pain, a response to noxious stimuli, can be a protective mechanism to prevent further injury, as is seen in clients who guard or protect an injured body part. The sensation of pain as the warning of potential tissue damage may be absent in people with nerve/spinal cord abnormalities, diabetic neuropathy, multiple sclerosis, nerve/spinal cord injury, or other neurologic disorders.

## Common Myths About Pain

Because pain is subjective (dependent on client's perception) and cannot be objectively measured by another individual through a laboratory test or diagnostic data, pain is often misunderstood and misjudged. A client's reports of level of pain will vary on the basis of cultural and experiential backgrounds, and the nurse's interpretations of a client's pain will be filtered through the nurse's own biases and expectations. "Pain doesn't go untreated (or under-treated) because of cruelty or apathy by the staff, but because of lack of knowledge. Just as [long-term care] residents have preconceived notions and concerns regarding pain and pain management, so do staff members" (Loeb, 1999, p. 49). Incongruence of the nurse's view and the client's perception of pain can often lead to undermedication and unnecessary suffering on the client's part. Table 42-1 outlines some of the common myths about pain, along with factual statements countering those beliefs.

## Types of Pain

Pain can be qualified or described in two basic ways: by its cause or origin and by its description or nature.

### Pain Origin

Pain categorized by its origin is either cutaneous, somatic, or visceral. **Cutaneous pain** is caused by stimulation of the cutaneous nerve endings in the skin and results in a well-localized "burning" or "prickling" sensation; getting a knot in the hair that is pulled out during combing may cause cutaneous pain. **Somatic pain** is nonlocalized and originates in support structures such as tendons, ligaments, and nerves; jamming a knee or finger will result in somatic pain. **Visceral pain** is discomfort in the internal organs and is less localized and more slowly transmitted than cutaneous pain. Visceral pain is often difficult to assess because the location may not be directly related to the cause. Pain originating from the abdominal organs is often called **referred pain** because the sensation of pain is not felt in the organ itself but instead is perceived at the spot where the organs were located during fetal development. Figure 42-1 shows the cutaneous areas where visceral pain is often referred.

    **Neuropathic pain** arises from damage to portions of the peripheral or central nervous system. This pain is *not* nociceptive pain, nor that which is due to ongoing tissue injury or inflammation. It is important to differentiate neuropathic pain from other types of pain because the treat-

| TABLE 42-1 | COMMON MYTHS ABOUT PAIN |
|---|---|
| **Myth** | **Fact** |
| • The nurse is the best judge of a client's pain. | • Pain is a subjective experience; only the client can judge the level and severity of pain. |
| • If pain is ignored, it will go away. | • Pain is a real experience that can be appropriately treated. |
| • Clients should not take any measures to relieve their pain until the pain is unbearable. | • Pain control and relief measures are effective in lowering pain levels, which will help clients function more normally and comfortably. |
| • Most complaints of pain are purely psychological (e.g., "it's all in your head"); only "real" pain will manifest in obvious physical signs such as moaning or grimacing. | • Most clients honestly report their perception of pain.<br>• Physical responses to pain vary greatly depending on experience and cultural norms.<br>• Visible expressions of pain are not always reliable indicators of its severity. |
| • Clients with severe tissue damage will experience significant pain; those with lesser damage will feel less pain. | • Individuals' perceptions of pain are subjective; the extent of tissue damage is not necessarily proportional to the extent of pain experienced. |
| • Clients taking pain medications will become addicted to the drug. | • Addiction is unlikely when analgesics are carefully administered and closely monitored. |

ment differs significantly. Table 42-2 identifies some of the differences between nociceptive and neuropathic pain.

    Neuropathic pain is a result of abnormal processing of sensory input by either the peripheral or central nervous system. Two types of neuropathic pain are **allodynia** (a nonpainful stimulus is felt as painful in spite of the tissue appearing normal) and **paresthesia** (abnormal sensation such as burning, prickling, or tingling).

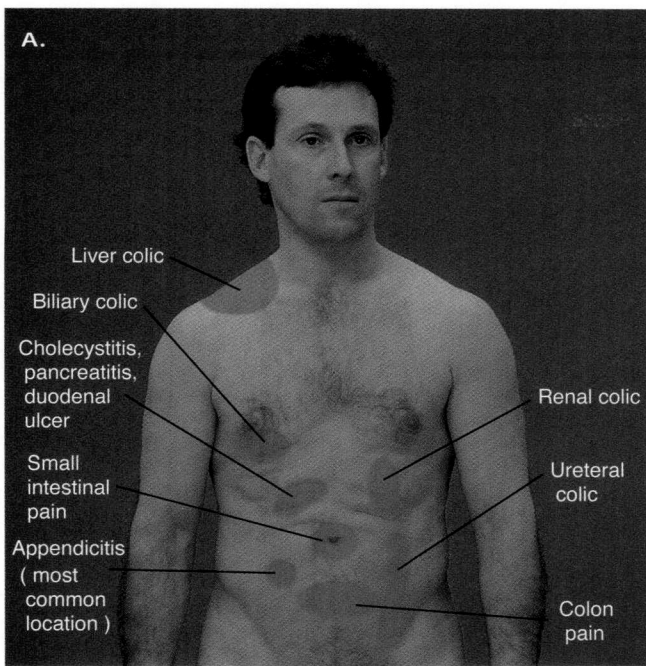 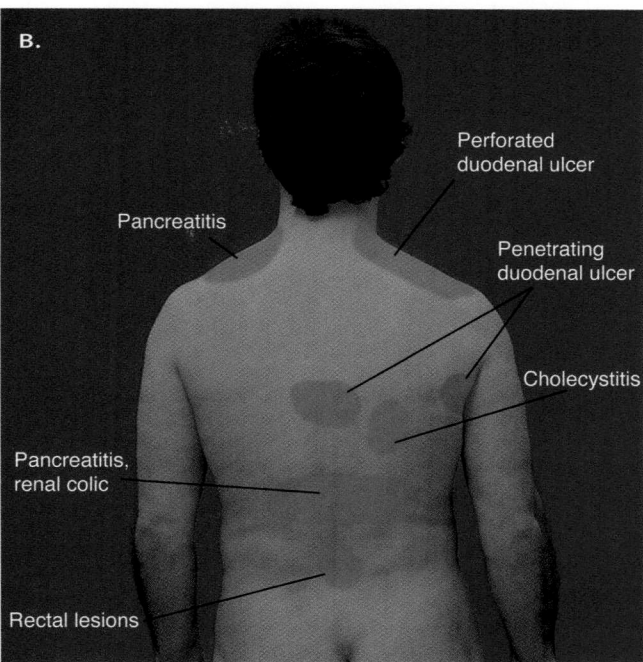

**Figure 42-1    Areas of referred pain: A. Anterior view B. Posterior view**

Myofascial pain was first described by Travell and Rinzler (1952) as pain that occurs as a result of a small, hypersensitive region in a muscle, ligament, fascia, or joint capsule called a **trigger point**. The trigger point is a hypersensitive point that, when stimulated, causes a local twitch or "jump" response. Myofascial pain is often accompanied by a localized deep ache that is surrounded by a referred area of **hyperalgesia**, or extreme sensitivity to pain.

## Pain Duration

Pain is most commonly described by its duration. Pain can be classified as acute or chronic.

**Acute pain** is most frequently identified by its sudden onset and relatively short duration, mild to severe intensity, and a steady decrease in intensity over a period of days to weeks. Some forms of acute pain may have a slower onset. Once the noxious stimulus is resolved, the pain usually decreases. Examples of noxious stimuli are needle sticks, surgical incisions, burns, and fractures.

**Recurrent acute pain** is identified by repetitive painful episodes that may recur over a prolonged period or throughout the client's lifetime. These painful episodes alternate with pain-free intervals. Examples of recurrent pain include migraine headaches, sickle cell pain crises, and the pain of angina pectoris due to myocardial hypoxia.

**Chronic pain** is identified as long-term (lasting 6 months or longer), persistent, nearly constant, or recurrent pain that produces significant negative changes in the client's life. Unlike acute pain, chronic pain may last long after the pathology is resolved.

**Chronic malignant pain** is pain that occurs as a result of progressive tissue injury. Persons with cancer or third-degree burns are examples of persons who suffer chronic malignant

pain. This pain can occur for months or years, but has a high probability of ending once tissue injury is stopped.

**Chronic nonmalignant pain** occurs in persons who do not have progressive tissue injury. Chronic malignant pain occurs almost daily and lasts for at least 6 months, with intensity ranging from mild to severe.

Chronic pain, a primary motivator for individuals to seek health care intervention, can greatly influence a client's quality of life, including emotional, social, vocational, and financial areas.

There is a relationship between chronic conditions (including pain) and depression. Thus, the client experiencing chronic pain should always be assessed for the presence of depression. "Not only do patients with CNP have a higher rate of depression, but suicide potential is also a serious concern for this population" (McCaffery & Pasero, 1999, p. 487). Examples of pathophysiology leading to chronic nonmalignant pain include:

- Many forms of **neuralgia** (paroxysmal pain that extends along the course of one or more nerves)
- Low back pain
- Rheumatoid arthritis
- Ankylosing spondylitis
- **Phantom limb pain** (a form of neuropathic pain that occurs after amputation with pain sensations referred to an area in the missing portion of the limb)
- **Myofascial pain syndromes** (a group of muscle disorders characterized by pain, muscle spasm, tenderness, stiffness, and limited motion)

CNP may be associated with several problems, including:

- Activity intolerance, which leads to physical deconditioning

- Functional impairment with resultant changes in role performance (parent, breadwinner)
- Social isolation, which alters relationships
- Sleep deprivation
- Frustration, anxiety, anger, and depression

When CNP is severe enough to disable the client, nurses understand that in order "To improve your patient's quality of life, pain management becomes a priority" (Bral, 1998, p. 27). The term **intractable pain** is used when pain is resistant to all therapies.

# Physiology of Pain

Noxious stimuli activate **nociceptors** (receptive neurons for painful sensations) that, together with the axons of neurons, convey information to the spinal cord where reflexes are activated. The information is simultaneously transmitted to the brain supraspinally (Cleland & Gebhart, 1997). Long-lasting changes in cells within the spinal cord **afferent** (ascending) and **efferent** (descending) **pain pathways** may occur after a brief noxious stimulus.

Physiological responses (such as elevated blood pressure, pulse rate, and respiratory rate; dilated pupils; pallor; and perspiration) to even a brief acute pain episode will begin showing adaptation within a short period, possibly minutes to a few hours. Physiologically, the body cannot sustain the extreme stress response for other than short periods of time. The body conserves its resources by physiological adaptation (returning to normal or near normal blood pressure, pulse rate, and respiratory rate; normal pupil size, and dry skin) even in the face of continuing pain of the same intensity. Pain can be categorized into two types according to its pathophysiology (see Table 42-2).

# Nociceptive Pain

The four fundamental processes involved in **nociception** (process by which individual becomes consciously aware of pain) are as follows (McCaffery & Pasero, 1999):

- **Transduction**—The changing of noxious stimuli in sensory nerve endings to energy impulses
- **Transmission**—Movement of impulses from site of origin to the brain
- **Perception**—Developing conscious awareness of pain
- **Modulation**—The changing of pain impulses

## Transduction of Pain

When noxious stimuli occur, tissues are damaged. Cell damage releases the following sensitizing substances:

- Prostaglandins (PG)
- Bradykinin (BK)
- Serotonin (5HT)
- Substance P (SP)
- Histamine (H)

Release of these substances alters the electrical charge on the neuronal membrane. This change in electrical charge is a result of movement of $Na^+$ and other ions into the cells. The impulse is then ready to be transmitted along the nociceptor fibers (McCaffery & Pasero, 1999).

## Transmission of Pain

The specific action of pain varies depending on the type of pain. In cutaneous pain, cutaneous nerve transmissions travel through a reflex arc from the nerve ending (point of pain) to the brain at a speed of approximately 300 feet per second, with a reflex response causing an almost immediate reaction. This explains why, when a hot stove is

---

## TABLE 42-2    PATHOLOGY-BASED PAIN CLASSIFICATION

| Nociceptive Pain | Neuropathic Pain |
|---|---|
| **Description:**<br>Normal processing of noxious stimuli<br>May damage tissue if prolonged | **Description:**<br>Abnormal processing of stimuli by peripheral nervous system (PNS) or central nervous system (CNS) |
| **Examples:**<br>Somatic pain<br>Visceral pain | **Examples:**<br>Centrally generated pain:<br>• Phantom pain<br>• Spinal cord injury<br>Peripherally generated pain:<br>• Diabetic neuropathy<br>• Trigeminal neuralgia |
| **Therapy:**<br>Nonsteroidal anti-inflammatory drugs (NSAIDs), opioids | **Therapy:**<br>NSAIDS, opioids, adjuvant analgesics |

Adapted from McCaffery, M., & Pasero, C. (1999). *Pain: Clinical manual* (2nd ed.). St. Louis: Mosby, p. 19.

touched, the person's hand jerks back *before* there is conscious awareness that damage is occurring (Figure 42-2). After a hot stove is touched, a sensory nerve ending in the skin of the finger initiates nerve transmission that travels through the dorsal root ganglion to the dorsal horn in the gray matter of the spinal cord. From there, the impulse travels though an interneuron that synapses with a motor neuron, which exits the spinal cord at the same level. This motor neuron, and the stimulation of the muscle it innervates, is responsible for the swift movement of the hand away from the hot stove.

In the case of the hot stove, the sensory neuron synapses not only with an interneuron but also with an afferent sensory neuron. The impulse travels up the spinal cord to the thalamus, where a final synapse conducts the impulse to the cortex of the brain. Efferent or descending motor neuron response is conducted from the brain through the spinal cord, where it synapses with a motor neuron that exits the spinal cord and innervates the muscle.

In visceral pain, transmission of pain impulses is slower and less localized than in cutaneous pain. The internal organs (including the gastrointestinal tract) have a minimal number of nociceptors, which explains why visceral pain is poorly localized and is felt as a dull aching or throbbing sensation. However, internal organs have extreme sensitivity to distension. The cramping pain of **colic** (acute abdominal pain), for example, results when:

- Flatus or constipation causes distension of the stomach or intestines
- There is hyperperistalsis, as in gastroenteritis
- Something tries to pass through a lumen (an opening) that is too small

The physiology of **ischemic pain**, or pain occurring when the blood supply of an area is restricted or cut off completely, also differs from that of cutaneous pain. The restriction of blood flow causes inadequate oxygenation of the tissue supplied by those vessels, as well as inadequate metabolic waste product removal. Ischemic pain has the most rapid onset in an active muscle and a much slower onset in a passive muscle. Examples of ischemic pain are muscle cramps, sickle cell pain crisis, angina pectoris, and myocardial infarction. When ischemic pain occurs in a muscle that continues to work, a muscle spasm (cramp) is the outcome. If the blood supply to the heart is severely restricted or completely cut off and is not restored quickly, a myocardial infarction will occur.

In acute pain episodes, substances released from injured tissue lead to stress hormone responses in the client. This causes an increased metabolic rate, enhanced

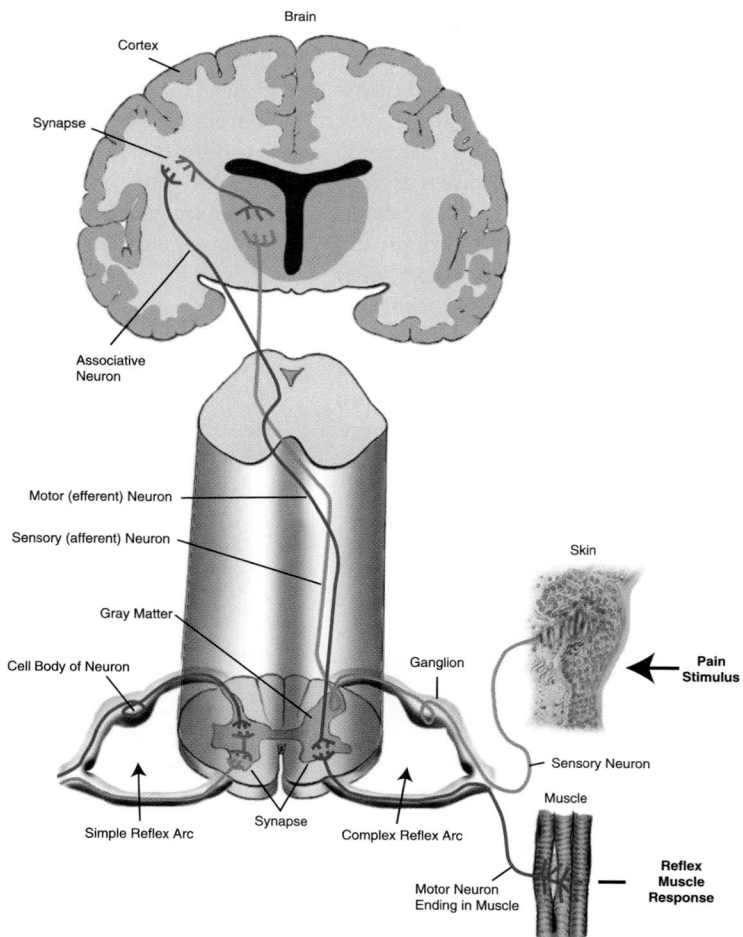

**Figure 42-2    Reflex arcs**

breakdown of body tissue, impaired immune function, and increased blood clotting and water retention, and it triggers the fight-or-flight reaction, leading to tachycardia and negative emotions.

## Gate Control Theory of Pain

Theories of pain transmission and interpretation attempt to describe and explain the pain experience. In 1965, Melzack and Wall proposed the **gate control pain theory**, which was the first to recognize that the psychological aspects of pain are as important as the physiological aspects. The gate control theory combines cognitive, sensory, and emotional components—in addition to the physiological aspects—and proposes that they can act on a gate control system to block the individual's perception of pain. Bezkor and Lee (1997, p. 181) describe gate control as "regulation of pain perception through a gating mechanism at the dorsal horn of the spinal cord. Vasoconstriction and decreased nerve conduction velocity result in reduced transmission of noxious stimuli to the 'gate.'" As a result, the level of conscious awareness of painful sensation is altered.

The gate control theory is based on the premise that pain impulses travel through either small-diameter nerve cells or large-diameter nerve cells, both of which pass through the same gate. The large-diameter cells have the ability, when properly stimulated, to "close the gate" and thus block transmission of the pain impulse to the brain (Figure 42-3). Stimulants such as cutaneous massage, opioid release, and excessive stimulation all activate the large-diameter cells to close the gate. Clinically, the effectiveness of several non-pharmacological modalities, such as massage, acupuncture, and acupressure, supports gate control theory.

## Pain Perception

When the impulse has been transmitted to the cortex and is interpreted by the brain, the information is available on a conscious level. It is then that the person becomes aware of the intensity, location, and quality of pain. This information is interpreted in light of previous experience, adding the affective component to the pain experience. **Pain threshold** is the level of intensity at which pain becomes appreciable or perceptible and will vary with each individual and type of pain. **Pain tolerance** is the level of intensity or duration of pain the client is willing or able to endure. A client's perceptions and attitudes about pain are dramatically influenced by many factors, including previous experiences and cultural background.

## Modulation

Modulation refers to activation of descending neural pathways that inhibit transmission of pain. "The pathways are described as descending because they involve neurons originating in the brain stem that descend to the dorsal horn of the spinal cord" (McCaffery & Pasero, 1999, p. 22). The descending fibers release substances that produce analgesia by blocking the transmission of noxious stimuli. Pain modulation is a result of the effects of endogenous opioids, also called enkephalins and endorphins. Endorphins are produced at various points in the central nervous system, often in response to pain or stress. When produced, they bind to opioid receptor sites, providing pain relief and a sense of euphoria. Enkephalins, believed to be less potent than endorphins, are found throughout the brain and parts of the spinal cord. Research into the role of endorphins and enkephalins in pain management shows new promise in the pain management field (Porth, 2002).

# Factors Affecting the Pain Experience

The subjective nature of pain varies from person to person and is influenced by several variables. Many factors account for the differences in a client's individual response

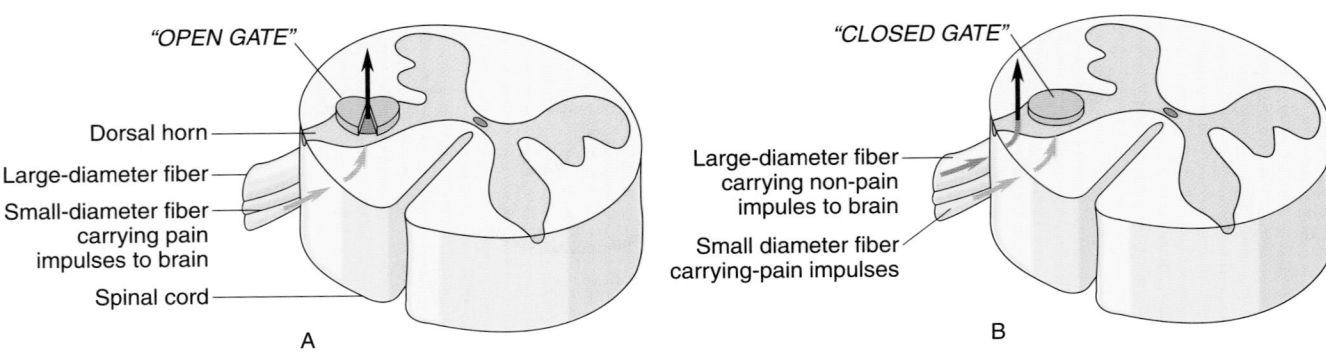

**Figure 42-3    Gate control theory: Blocking transmission of pain**

## FOCUS ON WELLNESS

### The Role of Endorphins and Enkephalins in Wellness

Endorphins and enkephalins are endogenous (produced within the body) opiates that respond to stress and painful stimuli. These substances may actually enhance the "mood" of an individual. For example, endorphins and enkephalins are thought to cause the so-called "high" in long-distance runners. Besides reducing the perception of pain, these substances may contribute to the positive attitude and wellness of individuals participating in activities that cause the release of endorphins and enkephalins.

American Pain Foundation (2002). http://www.painfoundation.org

## RESEARCH FOCUS

**Title of Study:** Pain assessment in the cognitively impaired and unimpaired elderly

**Study Purpose:** The purpose of the study was to evaluate self-report pain rating scales in older adults, comparing cognitively impaired and unimpaired older adults.

**Methods:** One hundred older subjects were assessed for cognitive function and ability to complete a variety of pain-rating scales. These scales were Memorial Pain Assessment Card verbal subscale, COOP pain subscale, numeric rating scale, McGill Pain Questionnaire's subscale of Present Pain Intensity, and the Wong/Baker Faces Rating Scale.

**Findings:** The authors found that most older adults could use self-report tools to rate their pain. Fewer of the severely cognitively impaired could use the tools, but some still could. The tools found to be most useful with the severely cognitively impaired were the Memorial Pain Assessment Card verbal subscale, McGill Pain Questionnaire's subscale of Present Pain Intensity, and the Wong/Baker Faces Rating Scale.

**Implications:** Nurses need to be aware of cognitive functioning levels of older clients when assessing pain. Numeric rating scales were found to be less reliable than other scales in this population.

Manz, B., Mosier, R., Nusser-Gerlach, M., Bergstrom, N., & Agrawal, S. (2000). Pain assessment in the cognitively impaired and unimpaired elderly. *Pain Management Nursing, 1*(4), 106–115.

to pain, including age and gender, previous experience with pain, and cultural factors.

## Age and Gender

Age can greatly influence a client's perception of the pain experience. Infants are sensitive to pain and typically exhibit discomfort through crying or physical movement. Toddlers also use crying and physical movement to indicate pain, and they begin to develop the skills needed to verbally describe pain or point to the area that is hurting. Children often do not understand why pain occurs and can therefore be frightened or resentful of the pain experience; in some cases, children revert to habits of their younger years (regression) as a coping mechanism when faced with pain they cannot otherwise manage.

Adolescents often sense great peer pressure and may be reluctant to admit having pain for fear of being called weak or sensitive. Adults may continue pain behaviors they learned as children and may also be reluctant to admit pain or seek medical care because of fear of the unknown or fear of the impact that treatment may have on their lifestyle.

Older adults may often ignore their pain, viewing it as an unavoidable consequence of aging; family and health care members may inadvertently support this stereotype and be less than responsive to an older client's complaints of pain. Pain related to chronic disease is prevalent among the older population. Up to 70% of noninstutionalized older adults report the occurrence of pain (Luggen, 2000, p. 281). Frequently, pain is under-treated in older people. Loeb (1999) states that three major factors contribute to inadequate pain management in older clients:

1. Pain is under-reported by older people who believe the myth that pain is a normal part of aging. Older adults

with such misconceptions believe nothing can be done to relieve the pain.

2. Under-detection of pain may be a result of the client's cognitive-perceptual deficits.

3. Under-treatment of pain is a result of under-reporting and under-detection.

Gender can also affect pain perception, intensity, and management. Vallerand and Polomano (2000) found that women tend to have "lower pain thresholds, a greater ability to discriminate painful sensations, higher pain ratings, and a lower tolerance for pain" (p. 8). They did, however, find inconsistent results in their study. While this is a new and promising field of study, more research is needed.

## Stress and Anxiety

Stress and anxiety tend to increase muscle tension and sensitize the nervous system to stimuli. A painful stimulus further excites the nervous system, creating a pain-anxiety-stress cycle. In a person who has a high level of stress or anxiety, the pain experience will be felt more intensely and acutely. Even in a person who is not stressed or anxious, a pain experience can create anxiety and stress, initiating the pain-anxiety-stress cycle. Additionally, the anxiety, pain, and stress can inhibit sleep and rest, leading to fatigue and insomnia. Because of the healing nature of sleep, lack of sleep further contributes to the pain experience. Keys to pain control then become helping the client to decrease stress and anxiety, and to promote sleep and rest.

## Previous Experience with Pain

Clients' previous exposures to pain will often influence their reactions. Coping mechanisms that were used in the past may affect clients' judgments as to how the pain will affect their lives and what measures they can use to successfully manage the pain on their own. Client teaching about pain expectations and management methods can often allay client fears and lead to more successful pain management, especially in those clients who do not have previous pain experience or who have memories of a previous devastating pain experience that they do not wish to repeat.

Pain is fatiguing as a significant amount of energy is used to deal with pain. The longer a person suffers from pain, the greater the level of fatigue. Although there is no conscious awareness of pain during sleep, there may be a dream-state awareness (McCaffery & Pasero, 1999). The stress response continues, and the body physiologically pays the price. Clients also wake up with considerably more pain than they had going to sleep, thereby requiring even more intervention (pharmacological and nonpharmacological) to reduce the pain.

## Cultural Norms and Attitudes

Cultural diversity in pain responses can easily lead to problems in pain management. There are no significant differences among groups in the level of intensity at which pain becomes appreciable or perceptible. However, the level of intensity or duration of pain the client is willing to endure is culturally determined.

Expression of pain is also governed by cultural values. In some cultures, tolerance to pain, and therefore "suffering in silence," is expected; in others, full expression of pain may include animated physical and emotional responses. The nurse must be careful not to equate the level of expression of pain with the level of actual pain experienced, but to instead consider cultural influences that affect the expression of pain.

Purnell and Paulanka (1998) describe various ethnic groups' responses to pain. For example, African Americans have a high tolerance for pain, Greek Americans are more demonstrative of their pain, and Mexican Americans report pain less often than other groups but tend to experience it more.

## Pain Assessment

Assessment of pain includes collection of subjective and objective data through the use of various assessment tools and construction of a database to use in developing a pain management plan. Pain assessment should be performed for every client. "In the normal course of doing business, pain should be nursing's fifth vital sign, as basic to practice as temperature, pulse, respiration, and blood pressure" (Joel, 1999, p. 9).

## Data Collection

Cheever (1999) emphasizes the need to prevent pain rather than treat it. Prevention calls for accurate assessment in order to alleviate pain before it escalates. "Even if a patient fails to report pain, you must make efforts to detect it" (Loeb, 1999, p. 52). Gathering subjective information regarding the client's pain is the first step in pain assessment. The client's perception of the pain should cover a description of several qualifiers, including:

- Intensity
- Location
- Quality (radiating, burning, diffuse)
- Associated manifestations (factors that often accompany the pain, such as nausea, constipation, or dizziness)
- Aggravating factors (variables that worsen the pain, such as exercise, certain foods, or stress)
- Alleviating factors (measures the client can take that lessen the effect of the pain, such as lying down, avoiding certain foods, or taking medication)

---

### NURSING STRATEGY

#### Pain Management

- Make pain the Fifth Vital Sign, assessing it every time you assess a client's blood pressure, pulse, respiration, and temperature.

- Counsel colleagues to take clients' complaints of pain seriously, especially in clients who utilize a lot of narcotic analgesics.

- Inform clients that they have a right to adequate pain relief.

- Select pain control measures appropriate to the client and setting.

- Provide interventions in a timely manner.

Adapted from Joel, L. (1999). The fifth vital sign: Pain. *American Journal of Nursing, 99*(2), 9.; Loeb, J. L. (1999). Pain management in long-term care. *American Journal of Nursing, 99*(2), 48–52.

## LEGAL AND ETHICAL ISSUES

### The Legalities of Assessing Pain

In January 2000, California law AB791 took effect, mandating that pain management be a part of medical school curriculum. It also mandated that inpatient facilities include pain as a fifth vital sign, to be documented in the client's medical record (Thomson, 2001). The Joint Commission on Accreditation of Healthcare Organizations (JCAHO) has followed suit, and most health care facilities now include pain assessment as part of clients' admission databases.

## STOP AND THINK

### Distractions in Pain Management

- What ways have you observed clients using to distract themselves from pain?

- Have you distracted yourself from pain? What methods have you used?

- How might these distractions be used intentionally in pain management?

- What other kinds of distraction might be useful in pain management?

Nurses must look for nonverbal signs of pain such as changes in motor activity or facial expression. It is also important to ask family members to share their observations; they may be the first ones to note subtle behavior changes indicative of pain. When assessing a client's report of pain, the nurse should also determine a client's pain threshold and pain tolerance level.

Clients' behavioral adaptation may yield no report of pain unless questioned specifically. **Distraction** (focusing attention on stimuli other than pain) may also be used by clients. McCaffery and Pasero (1999) recognize that clients often minimize the pain behaviors they are able to control for a number of reasons, including:

- To be a "good" client and avoid making demands
- To maintain a positive self-image by not becoming a "sissy"
- By using distraction as a method of making pain more bearable (young children are particularly adept at this)
- Exhaustion

Occasionally, there is a discrepancy between pain behaviors observed by the nurse and the client's self-report of pain. Client pain behaviors include splinting of the painful area, distorted posture, impaired mobility, insomnia, anxiety, attention seeking, and depression. Discrepancies between behaviors and the client's self-report can be due to good coping skills (e.g., relaxation techniques or distraction), stoicism, anxiety, or cultural differences in expected pain behaviors. Whenever these discrepancies occur, they should be addressed with the client. The nurse needs to remember that pain is a subjective experience, and that the most important indicator of pain is the client's self-report.

### Assessment Tools

Pain assessment tools are the single most effective method of identifying the presence and intensity of pain in clients. Tools used for assessing pain must be appropriate to the client's age and cultural context. "Make sure your assessments are culturally appropriate, keeping in mind that cultural mores and personal values can affect both the

patient's beliefs and pain and her responses to it" (Acello, 2000, p. 53). See Table 42-3 for sample questions used in pain assessment.

### Initial Pain Assessment Tool

An Initial Pain Assessment Tool was developed by McCaffery and Pasero (1999). This tool is particularly effective when clients have complex pain problems because it assesses location, intensity, quality, precipitating and alleviating factors, and how the pain affects function and quality of life. Once this tool is completed, another less detailed tool can be used for ongoing monitoring of the client's pain level.

### Pain Intensity Scales

Pain intensity scales are another quick, effective method for clients to rate the intensity of their pain. The verbal rating scale (VRS) and the numeric rating scale (NRS) are

## CLIENT REFLECTIONS

### A Client Hides Her Pain

Wilma is a 62-year-old Euro-American female hospitalized for treatment of her chronic leukemia. During her initial assessment, Wilma rates her pain a 9 on a scale of 1 to 10. She asks if she might have some more pain medication. The nurse challenges this because she observes Wilma lying calmly in bed with a relaxed-looking face, breathing evenly, and knitting a sweater. Wilma responds, "I am in terrible pain, and I knit to keep my mind off of it. If I wasn't knitting, I would be screaming and yelling about it."

What would you say to Wilma? What actions would you take?

## TABLE 42-3  PAIN ASSESSMENT QUESTIONS

| Characteristic | Question | Explanation |
|---|---|---|
| Quality | "How do you feel?" | Common descriptors:<br>• Aching<br>• Burning<br>• Dull<br>• Numb<br>• Sharp<br>• Throbbing |
| Intensity | "Using this scale, what number best describes your pain?" | Use the verbal rating scale (VRS) and the numeric rating scale (NRS) in combination. |
| | "Which picture best describes your pain?" | Use the Wong-Baker faces scale. |
| Location | "Where does it hurt?"<br>"What part of your body is painful?" | Encourage client to point to the affected area. On a printed body outline, have client shade in the areas that correspond to painful areas of his body. |
| Duration | "Is the pain constant?"<br>"Does the pain come and go?" | Instruct client to time painful episodes. |
| Aggravating Factors | "What makes the pain worse?"<br>"What lessens the pain?" | Have client focus on triggers such as positions, activities, or situations. |
| Alleviating Factors | "What have you done to treat the pain?" | Focus on over-the-counter medications, rest or immobilization, and use of ice or heat. |
| Effects | "How has the pain affected your life?" | Include effects on:<br>• Work/school<br>• Relationships<br>• Eating<br>• Sleep<br>• Energy level<br>• Recreation/leisure<br>• Moods |
| | "Do you have any symptoms in addition to pain?" | Ask client about presence of:<br>• Confusion<br>• Constipation<br>• Itching<br>• Nausea/vomiting<br>• Problems with urination<br>• Sleepiness/drowsiness |
| Knowledge Level | "What do you understand about your pain and its causes?"<br>"What have you been taught about your pain?"<br>"Have you taken any medicine for pain? If so, what?" | Document the client's responses. |

Adapted from Jacox, A., Carr, D., Payne, R., et al. (1994). *Pain assessment methodology* (Publication No. 94-0592). Rockville, MD: Agency for Health Care Policy and Research (AHCPR), U.S. Department of Health and Human Services.

often used together to collect more accurate client input. The VRS uses adjectives ranging from "no pain" to "excruciating pain" in order to describe intensity. Frequent use of these tools will increase understanding of the pain severity. When using the NRS, clients are asked to assign their pain a number, with 0 meaning no pain and 10 representing the worst possible pain. "On a scale of 0 to 10, with 0 being no pain at all and 10 being the worst pain you could ever have, how much do you hurt right now?" If there are multiple painful areas, this question can be asked regarding each area.

### Pain Diary

Client input is essential if accurate assessment data are to be collected. Self-monitoring of symptoms can be promoted by having clients complete a pain diary (see Box 42-1).

### Psychosocial Pain Assessment

Plaisance and Price (1999) state the following questions should be included on the psychosocial assessment of a client experiencing pain:

- Do the client and family/caregivers understand the diagnosis?
- How have previous experiences with pain affected the client and family?
- How does the client usually cope with pain and/or stress?
- What concerns do the client and family have about using certain medications such as opioids?
- Do the client and family understand the differences between tolerance, dependence, and addiction?

## Developmental Considerations

Because pain experiences and reports can be influenced by age and developmental level, special consideration should be used to factor in those influences.

### Children and Adolescents

Infants, children, and adolescents provide a special challenge in pain assessment because their pain behaviors often differ from those considered normal in the adult population. Certain myths hinder the accurate assessment and management of pain in children.

Two useful tools for assessing pain in children are the Wong/Baker Faces Rating Scale and the Poker Chip Tool. The Wong/Baker Faces Rating Scale can be used with children as young as 3 years, and it helps children express their level of pain by pointing to a cartoon face that most closely resembles how they are feeling. This tool has also been found to be useful for non-English-speaking clients and cognitively impaired, older clients.

The Poker Chip Tool consists of four red poker chips that can easily be carried in a pocket to be available when needed. The chips are aligned horizontally on a hard surface in front of the child, and they are described as "pieces of hurt." The chips are described from left to right as just a little bit of hurt, a little more hurt, more hurt, and the most hurt you could ever have. The child is then asked, "How many pieces of hurt do you have right now?" This tool can be used with children 4 to 13 years old.

The verbal 0 to 10 scale is also frequently used for school-age and adolescent clients in a number of settings.

---

### BOX 42-1   PAIN DIARY

- Date/Time
- Intensity
- Situation
  (What were you doing?)
- How did you feel?
- What were you thinking?
- What did you do to ease the pain?
- How effective was the pain control strategy?

---

 **LIFE SPAN CONSIDERATIONS**

#### Pain Management in Infants

Until just over a decade ago, myths regarding pain in neonates were pervasive in the NICU (neonate intensive care unit). Among the most common myths were (1) the central nervous system of the preterm neonate was too immature to perceive pain resulting from common neonatal therapies, coupled with (2) the myth that expounded the dangers of administering narcotics to neonates. Despite current evidence that neonates have the anatomical and functional capacity to perceive and respond to noxious stimuli, inadequate pain management practices continue to persist within the NICU.

Think about it. Would you want to have a chest tube inserted without local and systemic analgesic? Does it make sense when medical care providers say they do not use local anesthesia to perform circumcisions on male infants because the infant cries more when immobilized on the circumcision board than when the prepuce is cut away from the glans penis? The golden rule of pain management states that what is considered painful for older children and adults must also be considered painful for neonates (Figure 42-4).

Adapted from Anand, K., & McGrath, P. (1999). *Pain in neonates.* New York: Elsevier Science.

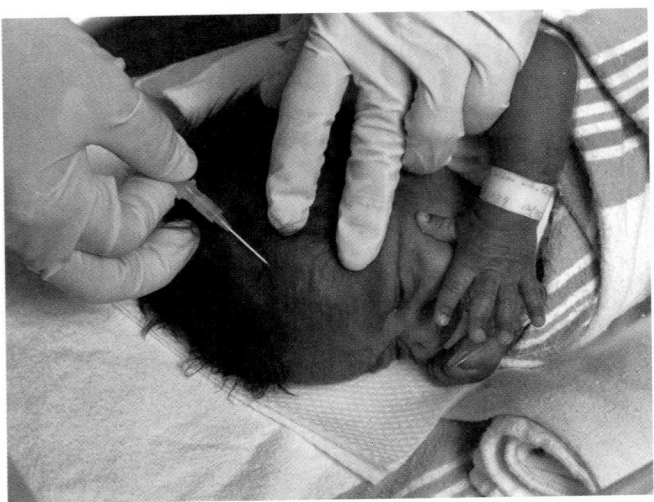

**Figure 42-4** Offering a pacifier during a painful procedure, such as venipuncture, can help calm and reassure the infant.

## LIFE SPAN CONSIDERATIONS

### Myths About Pain and Children

| Misconception | Fact |
|---|---|
| Infants do not feel pain. | Anatomical structures for pain processing reach adult maturity at 36 weeks after conception. |
| Children tolerate pain better than adults. | Even though children may not express pain as adults do, there are behavioral indicators of pain in children. Children as young as age 3 can use pain scales to communicate the level of pain experienced. |
| Children become accustomed to pain or painful procedures. | Some children show increased signs of discomfort with repeated painful procedures. Anxiety over impending procedures only exacerbates pain. |
| Narcotics are more dangerous for children than adults. | When used appropriately, opioids are not more dangerous for children than adults. |

Data adapted from McCaffery, M., & Pasero, C. L. (1999). *Pain clinical manual* (2nd ed.). St. Louis: Mosby, p. 627.

## STOP AND THINK

### Pain Assessment Tools

What type of pain assessment tool would you use for the following clients?

1. A 6-year-old boy who presents to the emergency room with a possible broken left clavicle
2. A 76-year-old man with a fractured hip and dementia in a long-term care facility
3. A 25-year-old woman experiencing postoperative pain after a small bowel resection

It is important to remember that any child under stress or with anxiety will regress, and regression may make use of the verbal 0 to 10 scale in children under 8 to 10 years of age of questionable value.

### Older Clients

Pain may be manifested differently by older individuals. For example, pain may be referred (gallbladder pain is felt in the shoulder). Also, the intensity of pain in some older adults may not accurately reflect the severity of the underlying pathology (e.g., a myocardial infarction may be felt as a fluttering sensation, Eliopoulos, 1999).

Some of the outcomes of untreated pain in older adults include the following (Loeb, 1999):

- Sleep alterations
- Nutrition problems
- Impaired gait
- Cognitive impairments
- Decreased socialization
- Increased incidence of falls
- Decreasing ability to function independently

"Compared to race, site of pain, and intensity of pain, age is the most important variable influencing analgesic response" (Pasero, Reed, & McCaffery, 1998, p. 12.). The general guideline for administering analgesics to older clients is to *start low and go slow*.

Many older individuals receive health care in their homes. The accompanying display lists recommendations for a home health nurse to use with clients experiencing pain.

## Nursing Diagnosis

The two primary nursing diagnoses used to describe pain are *Acute Pain* and *Chronic Pain*. According to North American Nursing Diagnosis Association (NANDA) (2003), *Acute Pain* is defined as "an unpleasant sensory and emotional experience arising from actual or potential tissue damage or described in terms of such damage . . . (with) sudden or slow onset of any intensity from mild to severe, with an anticipated or predictable end and a duration of less than 6 months" (p. 72). *Chronic Pain* is defined as *Acute Pain*, with the last phrase replaced by "constant or recurring without an anticipated or predictable end and a duration of greater than 6 months." Presenting characteristics of *Acute Pain* and *Chronic Pain* are listed in Table 42-4.

If the client presents with problems in addition to pain, the nurse must be alert to the possibility that the pain may be the *cause* (not the effect) of another problem. For example, a client may be experiencing *Impaired Physical Mobility* or *Activity Intolerance* related to pain caused by a broken leg, as evidenced by verbal complaint, fatigue, and guarding of the affected leg.

# Outcome Identification and Planning

When planning care for the client experiencing pain, mutual goal setting is of utmost importance. After assessing the client's perception of the problem, work with the client in developing realistic outcomes. Be sure to use both nonpharmacological and pharmacological interventions

in planning strategies to help clients achieve desired levels of functioning and pain control.

When asking about the client's goal for pain relief, the nurse often has to state, "We can't usually get rid of all your pain, but if we could get it down to a place that it didn't bother you so much, what would that be?" Thus, the family, and health care professionals involved will all be aware of a realistic goal for pain relief. "Providing the best possible pain relief to patients requires regular and consistent communication among all members of the health care team, including the patient" (Collins, Sparger, Richardson, Schriver, & Bergenstock, 1999, p. 20). Treatment goals for CNP clients include the following (McCaffery & Pasero, 1999):

1. Reduce pain level whenever possible.
2. Improve functioning.
3. Develop self-help skills for coping.
4. Alleviate psychopathology, including anxiety and depression.
5. Improve relationships with family members and health care providers in order to meet individual needs.

Terminally ill clients pose a special challenge in the area of pain management. According to Bral (1998), approximately 15% of deaths occur in people receiving hospice care. Thus, pain management is the responsibility of nurses who have no specialization in palliative care. Joel (1999, p. 9) states "no death is a good or peaceful one if attended by suffering. Suffering can take the form of isolation, confusion, emotional deprivation, depersonalization, pain . . . All of this falls within the province of comfort and caring, and consequently becomes the work of nursing."

In its *Position Statement on Promotion of Comfort and Relief of Pain in Dying Patients*, the American Nurses Association (1991) states:

> One of the major concerns of dying patients and their families is the fear of intractable pain during the dying process. Indeed, overwhelming pain can cause sleeplessness, loss of morale, fatigue, irritability, restlessness, withdrawal, and other serious problems for the dying patient. (p. 1)

The American Nurses Association (1991) advises nurses to administer doses of pain medication that are effective enough to manage pain in the dying client.

Planning of care leads to the development of an individual treatment plan for each client. When nurses understand that the existence of pain and its intensity is best defined by the client, "they acknowledge that every person with pain has a complex, multidimensional, and unique experience" (Bral, 1998, p. 7).

# Implementation

"Assessing and managing pain has long been a core nursing responsibility. Now, The Joint Commission on the Accreditation of Healthcare Organizations (JCAHO) is

| TABLE 42-4 | NURSING DIAGNOSES |
| --- | --- |
| **Diagnosis** | **Selected Defining Characteristics** |
| *Acute Pain* | • Verbalization of severe discomfort<br>• Restlessness<br>• Variations in vital signs indicative of autonomic responses<br>• Guarding behavior<br>• Sleep disturbances<br>• Grimace<br>• Self-focus<br>• Distracted behavior<br>• Changes in appetite and eating |
| *Chronic Pain* | • Verbalization of pain over an extended period of time<br>• Impaired functional ability<br>• Sleep disturbances<br>• Guarding behavior<br>• Irritability<br>• Self-focus<br>• Restlessness<br>• Depression<br>• Muscle atrophy of affected area<br>• Weight changes<br>• Fatigue<br>• Fear of reinjury |

From NANDA. (2003). *Nursing diagnoses: Definitions and classifications: 2003-2004.* Philadelphia: Author.

requiring accredited facilities and organizations to develop policies and procedures that formalize this obligation" (Acello, 2000, p. 52). The JCAHO calls for health care providers to (Williams-Lee, 1999):

- Recognize each client's right to pain assessment and treatment
- Monitor client responses to pain management strategies
- Educate staff and clients about pain management

Some key concepts of JCAHO's standard on pain management include the following (Acello, 2000, p. 52):

- Clients have the right to appropriate pain assessment.
- Pain is to be assessed and regularly reassessed.
- Clients will be treated for pain or referred for treatment.
- Clients will be taught the importance of effective pain management.
- Clients will be taught that pain management is a part of treatment.
- Clients will be involved in making health care decisions.
- Analgesics are to be administered as needed.
- Discharge planning and teaching will include continuing needs for pain management.

## Nurse-Client Relationship

Establishment of a therapeutic relationship is the foundation for effective nursing care of the client experiencing pain. Clients who trust their nurses to be there, to listen, and to act, are the clients who are most likely to be comfortable. Clients also need to trust that the nurse believes their level and description of pain. See Chapter 4 for information on developing a therapeutic relationship.

## Client Education

Client education regarding pain management begins with defining pain, identifying the probable causes, introducing clients to pain assessment tools, and allowing them to choose the tool they would like to use. The importance of talking with health care providers about their pain and of using a preventive approach to pain management must also be emphasized. Provide written information to reinforce verbal explanations. Teach the importance of around-the-clock dosing instead of prn administration of analgesic medications.

When a client is to be discharged from a health care facility, discharge teaching should include pain management information with specific guidelines about the need for seeking follow-up advice/treatment. The Client Education box lists content for a comprehensive pain management teaching plan.

Both nonpharmacological and pharmacological interventions can be effective in caring for clients with pain. In some cases of mild pain, nonpharmacological techniques may be the primary intervention, with medication available as "backup." In cases of moderate to severe pain, nonpharmacological techniques can be an effective adjunctive, or complementary, treatment.

## Principles of Pharmacological Pain Management

Listed below are principles for the care of clients experiencing pain:

- Assess the pain.
- Treat the contributing factors (pathology).
- Individualize analgesic therapy to each client.
- Choose the least invasive route of administration.
- Administer analgesics at regularly scheduled intervals (around-the-clock dosing) rather than on an as-needed (prn) basis.
- Keep clients in control of their own analgesia as much as possible.
- Titrate doses to provide maximum pain relief and minimum side effects (Bral, 1998, p. 30). Know that the right dose is "whatever it takes to relieve the pain with the fewest side effects" (Newshan, 2000, p. 83).

Other general principles that guide practice are discussed below.

---

## CLIENT EDUCATION

### Pain Management Strategies

1. Instruct client on how to keep a pain diary, including functional abilities.
2. Have client identify barriers to pain management and ways to reduce these barriers.
3. Educate client about the need for intervention prior to pain becoming intolerable.
4. Discuss use of analgesic medications and the benefit of round-the-clock dosing versus prn use.
5. Discuss use of opioid analgesics and fears related to tolerance, dependence, and addiction.
6. Instruct client to call the health care provider if the pain is uncontrolled or interferes with ability to function.
7. Instruct client on how to control common side effects of medications, such as GI upset, nausea, lethargy, and constipation.
8. Instruct client on other health needs that facilitate pain management, such as stress reduction, rest and sleep, and support from family and friends.
9. Discuss the use of nonpharmacological interventions that can be effective in pain management, providing instruction on techniques of interest to the client.

Adapted from Ackley, B., & Ladwig, G. (2002). *Nursing diagnosis handbook* (5th ed.). St. Louis: Mosby.; Carpenito, L. (2002). *Handbook of nursing diagnosis* (8th ed.). Philadelphia: Lippincott.

## Combine Analgesics

Combining analgesics on the basis of the World Health Organization's (WHO) three-step analgesic ladder is imperative to provide effective pharmacological intervention for clients with all types of pain. The first step of the WHO analgesic ladder is to give nonopioid pain medications. Adjuvant medications may also be used at this first step. In the event of persistent or increasing pain, WHO recommends the addition of opioid analgesics at the second level of the analgesic ladder. Additional medications would be added at the third step of the WHO analgesic ladder if the pain persisted or continued to increase.

**Adjuvant medications** are those drugs used to enhance the analgesic efficacy of opioids, to treat concurrent symptoms that exacerbate pain, and to provide independent analgesia for specific types of pain. Adjuvant medication (medications without intrinsic analgesic properties) are often helpful in treating chronic pain. Adjuvant drugs include anticonvulsants, antidepressants, and sedatives. Gabapentin (Neurontin) is one anticonvulsant useful in treating older clients experiencing chronic pain

(Luggen, 2000) and in treatment of neuropathic pain. Education for clients taking adjuvant medication must explain the need to continue to take the analgesic drug with the adjuvant medication.

Table 42-5 lists some common adjuvant medications used in pain management.

## Maintain Therapeutic Serum Levels

Establishing and maintaining a therapeutic serum level is another important pharmacological pain management strategy. Peaks and valleys of drug serum levels often occur when analgesics are administered in the traditional prn manner. When the dose is administered on an intermittent schedule, a larger dose is often required, causing the client to have a peak serum drug level in the sedation range. The client must wait for the return of pain before requesting the next dose of analgesic. Depending on the length of time it takes to obtain the medication and, once taken, to reestablish an adequate blood level, there could be a period of up to an hour or so with inadequate pain control.

### TABLE 42-5    ADJUVANT MEDICATIONS FOR PAIN MANAGEMENT

| Medication | Type of Pain | Effects |
|---|---|---|
| *Tricyclic antidepressants* <br> Amitriptyline <br> Doxepin <br> Imipramine <br> Trazodone | Neuropathic pain frequently described as dull, aching, or throbbing | • Mood elevation, enhancement of opioid analgesia, direct analgesic effects <br> • Anticholinergic side effects: dry mouth, constipation, urinary retention |
| *Anticonvulsants* <br> Carbamazepine <br> Phenytoin <br> Clonazepam <br> Gabapentin | Neuropathic pain frequently described as sharp shooting, burning, or lancinating | • Suppresses the spontaneous neuronal firing as sharp, that causes this type of pain |
| *Corticosteroids* <br> Dexamethasone <br> Prednisone | Pain due to cerebral or spinal cord edema or that in peripheral nerves caused by perineural edema | • Mood elevation, strong anti-inflammatory activity, appetite stimulation |
| *Antihistamine* <br> Hydroxyzine | Pain or nausea in the anxious client | • Relief of complicating symptoms including anxiety, insomnia, nausea, and pruritus |
| *Neuroleptic* <br> Methotrimeprazine | Alternative analgesic for clients who are opioid-tolerant or have opioid-limiting side effects, especially constipation | • Antiemetic and anxiolytic. <br> • This is the one phenothiazine to date that has demonstrated analgesic properties: methotrimeprazine 15 mg IM was found to be equivalent to morphine 10 mg IM |
| *Psychostimulants* <br> Dextroamphetamine <br> Methylphenidate | Continued pain with opioid-induced sedation | • Improves opioid analgesia and decreases sedation |

Adapted from Acute Pain Management Guideline Panel. (1992). *Acute pain management: Operative or medical procedures and trauma. Clinical practice guideline.* (AHCPR Publication No. 92-0033). Rockville, MD: Agency for Health Care Policy and Research.

**Patient-controlled analgesia (PCA)** (client self-administration of intravenous pain medication via a programmable pump), with a loading dose when first started and a booster dose if needed, is a method to obtain a smooth analgesic level (Figure 42-5). PCA also allows the client to have control over pain management. The major advantage of PCA over the traditional, nurse-administered analgesia is that clients are enabled to seek pain relief whenever they feel it is necessary: "the best advice you can give your patients is to press the PCA button whenever they feel a need for pain medication" (Van-Couwenberghe & Pasero, 1998, p. 15). Requirements for the use of PCA are the cognitive ability to understand how to use the pump and the physical ability to push the button. The method is effective if the appropriate titrations are made on the basis of reassessment and client pain report.

Clients need to be taught that complete pain relief may be an unrealistic expectation. Instead, the goal of PCA is for the client to be comfortable and alert enough to participate in therapy. "The best time to teach patients about PCA is before it has started, when they're lucid enough to understand your instructions" (Van-Couwenberghe & Pasero, 1998, p. 14).

## Choose Appropriate Routes of Administration

Available routes of administration play an important role in choice of pain management technique. In general, the oral route (PO) of administration is preferred because it is the most convenient and cost-effective. When the oral route is not feasible, other routes (such as rectal or transdermal) can be used to administer analgesics.

The rectal route is effective when clients are nauseated and vomiting or when they are NPO. Suppositories of morphine, hydromorphone, and oxymorphone are available. Contraindications to rectal administration include diarrhea, lesions of the rectum or anus, or immunosuppressed status. The transdermal route bypasses gastrointestinal absorption but has a slow onset and a slow decline in blood level after the patch is removed.

With continuing documentation of unreliable absorption of intramuscular (IM) injections of opioids, the prudent approach is to switch to subcutaneous or intravascular administration. Continuous infusions are possible by either intravenous (IV) or subcutaneous methods.

Analgesia using epidural, intrathecal (intraspinal), or intraventricular routes are reserved for settings in which experience, expertise, extensive support systems, and sophisticated follow-up are available. See Table 42-6 for an overview of administration routes.

## Pain Medications
### Nonsteroidal Anti-Inflammatory Drugs

The nonopioid class of pharmacological agents consists of three groups of medications classified as nonsteroidal anti-inflammatory drugs (NSAIDs), acetaminophen, and

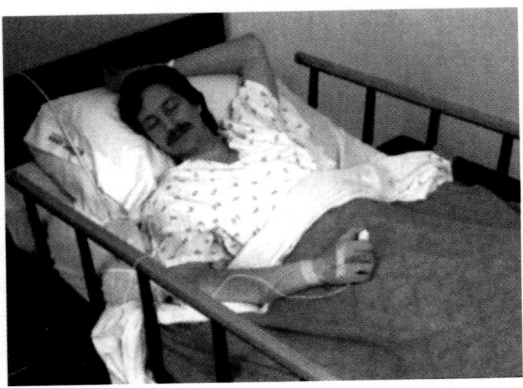

**Figure 42-5    Client is using patient-controlled analgesia (PCA).**

COX-2 inhibitors. NSAIDs work by inhibiting the synthesis of prostaglandin, a class of chemicals that:

- Can be found in almost every body tissue
- Cause allodynia even in low concentrations
- Are always released when cells are damaged
- Contribute to edema and erythema
- Sensitize afferent nerve endings to bradykinin (a pain substance) (McCaffery & Pasero, 1999)

NSAIDs are useful in treating mild to moderate pain, especially painful conditions involving inflammation. NSAIDs are used frequently because of the following (Cleland & Gebhart, 1997, p. 32):

- They can be administered orally.
- They do not cause CNS or respiration depression.
- Several are available over the counter.

The widespread use of NSAIDs makes them the culprit in many adverse drug effects. The use of some NSAIDs can result in adverse gastrointestinal, hematologic, liver, and renal effects. Aspirin is the standard NSAID against which the efficacy of all NSAIDs are measured, due to its long history of relative safe usage, low cost, and availability without a prescription (Jones, 1997). In fact, aspirin is so commonly used that many individuals fail to consider it as a drug. Clients must be taught about aspirin's adverse effects (see Table 42-7).

In addition to aspirin, other common NSAIDS are ibuprofen, ketorolac, and diclofenac. NSAIDs are also subject to the **ceiling effect** (as the dose of medication is increased above a certain level, the analgesic effect remains the same), and only the adverse effects continue to increase.

The remaining NSAIDs all have significant multisystem side effects and adverse effects, with the most worrisome being severe gastric irritation, gastric bleeding, and renal problems. NSAIDs must be used cautiously in older clients. The risk of gastrointestinal problems (such as peptic ulcer disease and gastrointestinal bleeding) increases with the use of NSAIDs in older clients (Pasero, Reed, & McCaffery, 1998). "Given the large number of NSAID

| TABLE 42-6 | ADVANTAGES AND DISADVANTAGES OF SELECTED MEDICATION ADMINISTRATION ROUTES | |
|---|---|---|
| **Intervention** | **Advantages** | **Disadvantages** |
| Oral NSAIDs | 1. Useful for a wide variety of mild to moderate pains.<br>2. Widely available, most over the counter.<br>3. Additive analgesia when combined with opioids and other modalities.<br>4. Can be administered by client or family.<br>5. Some are inexpensive. | 1. Ceiling effect to analgesia.<br>2. Side effects, especially gastritis, renal toxicity, and liver toxicity, can be serious.<br>3. May risk bleeding in severely thrombocytopenic patients.<br>4. Only one NSAID (ketorolac) is available now for parenteral administration.<br>5. Many are expensive. |
| Oral opioids | 1. Effective for both localized and generalized pain.<br>2. Ceiling to analgesic effectiveness imposed only by side effects.<br>3. Multiple drug choices in the class.<br>4. Sedative and anxiolytic properties useful in some acute treatment settings.<br>5. Can be administered by client or family.<br>6. Some are inexpensive.<br>7. Long-acting, controlled-release forms are available. | 1. Side effects may limit analgesic effectiveness.<br>2. Prescription of these substances is regulated.<br>3. Stigma or fears associated with use.<br>4. Dependency potential. |
| Transdermal opioids (fentanyl) | 1. Long duration of action (48–72 h) from single patch.<br>2. Allows use of a strong opioid (fentanyl) in outpatient settings for some clients who have not tolerated morphine and related drugs.<br>3. Many clients find them easy to use.<br>4. Provides continuous administration of an opioid without use of needles or pumps.<br>5. Can be administered by client or family. | 1. Side effects may not be as quickly reversible as in oral administration.<br>2. Difficult to modify dosage rapidly.<br>3. Relatively slow onset of action.<br>4. Requires additional short-acting medicine for breakthrough pain.<br>5. Expensive.<br>6. Dependency potential. |
| Rectal opioids | 1. Relatively easy-to-use alternative route when the oral route is unavailable.<br>2. Other opioid suppositories available for morphine-intolerant clients.<br>3. Can be administered by client or family.<br>4. Less expensive than subcutaneous or intravenous infusions. | 1. Not widely accepted by patients or families.<br>2. Side effects may limit analgesic effectiveness.<br>3. Relatively slow onset of action.<br>4. Contraindicated if low white blood cell or platelet count (risks of infection, bleeding). |

*(continues)*

## TABLE 42-6    ADVANTAGES AND DISADVANTAGES OF SELECTED MEDICATION ADMINISTRATION ROUTES (continued)

| Intervention | Advantages | Disadvantages |
|---|---|---|
| Subcutaneous infusion | 1. Can provide rapid pain relief without intravenous access.<br>2. Morphine and hydromorphone are the preferred drugs for this route when administered in the home.<br>3. When used in PCA mode, allows for rapid individual dose titration and provides sense of control for client. | 1. Only a limited volume of infusate can be administered (e.g., 2–4 ml/h).<br>2. Induration, irritation at infusion site may be a complication.<br>3. Requires skilled nursing and pharmacy support.<br>4. Often requires expensive drug infusion pump and recurring charges for disposables. |
| Intravenous infusion | 1. Can provide rapid pain relief.<br>2. Almost all opioids can be given by this route.<br>3. Not limited to infusate volumes.<br>4. When used in PCA mode, allows for rapid individual dose titration and provides sense of control for client. | 1. Infection and infiltration of intravenous lines are potential complications.<br>2. Requires skilled nursing and pharmacy support.<br>3. Often requires expensive drug infusion pump and recurring charges for disposables.<br>4. Client may not have easy venous access. |
| Epidural, intrathecal, and intracerebral ventricular routes | 1. Useful for pain that has not responded to less-invasive measures.<br>2. Local anesthetics may be added to spinal opioids and may produce additive analgesia. | 1. Tolerance may occur sooner than with oral or rectal administration.<br>2. Infection at catheter site can produce meningitis and/or epidural abscess.<br>3. Pruritus and urinary retention are more common than with oral or parenteral opioid administration.<br>4. Contraindicated in presence of acute spinal cord compression.<br>5. Requires special expertise.<br>6. Requires careful monitoring, especially when therapy begins and when doses are increased.<br>7. May require expensive drug infusion pump, intervention fees, and recurring charges for disposables.<br>8. Potential risk for paralysis. |
| Regional neurolytic blocks | 1. Effective for pain relief with certain diagnoses (e.g., pancreatic cancer).<br>2. May be useful for movement-related and abdominal visceral pain that is refractory to drug therapy.<br>3. Can allow dosage (and side effect) reduction of systemic drugs for localized pain. | 1. Risk of postural hypotension, bowel and bladder incontinence, and leg weakness.<br>2. Procedure is irreversible.<br>3. Requires special expertise.<br>4. Expenses for specialized care and operating room costs. |

Adapted from Management of Cancer Pain Guideline Panel. (1994). *Pain Assessment Methodology*. (AHCPR Publication No. 94-0592, pp. 42–43). Rockville, MD: Agency for Health Care Policy and Research.

| TABLE 42-7 | SYMPTOMS OF ASPIRIN TOXICITY | |
|---|---|---|
| Mild | Moderate | Severe |
| Tinnitus | Acne | Hallucinations |
| Vertigo | Diarrhea | Convulsions |
| Nausea and vomiting | Drowsiness | Coma |
| | Confusion | Cardiovascular collapse |
| | Hyperventilation | |
| | Hyperthermia | |
| | Electrolyte imbalances | |

Adapted from Jones, S. L. (1997). Pharmacology of pain management. In *Expert pain management* (p. 40). Springhouse, PA: Springhouse Corporation.

users, protection against GI complications is a priority" (Peloso, 2000, p. 36).

Cyclooxygenase-2 (COX-2) inhibitors are a relatively new classification of nonopioid analgesics (Kessenich, 2001). These drugs act by inhibiting the COX-2 enzyme, which prevents the arachidonic acid cascade. This cascade is believed to be responsible for inflammation, tissue edema, and pain. Thus, the COX-2 inhibitors are extremely useful in treatment of inflammatory pain, specifically arthritic conditions. The advantage of COX-2 inhibitors over NSAIDS is that they have little gastrointestinal (GI) side effects. The primary disadvantage is that they are much more costly than the NSAIDS.

Acetaminophen is a nonopioid analgesic and antipyretic, but it lacks an anti-inflammatory effect. The advantages of acetaminophen for use in pain relief is that it has fewer interactions with other drugs and less of an effect on bleeding tendencies. A major disadvantage of acetaminophen is the low ceiling effect and high risk of liver toxicity.

### Opioid Analgesics

The opioids and NSAIDs exert pain relief through different mechanisms. For example, the opioids act on several sites in the central nervous system (CNS) rather than on the peripheral nervous system as do the NSAIDs. Opioids alter the release of neurotransmitters, and, therefore, pain transmission is interrupted at several sites in the CNS. The result is an altered perception of and response to pain (Plaisance & Price, 1999).

The opioid analgesics fall into three classes: pure opioid agonists, partial agonists, and **mixed agonist-antagonists** (a compound that blocks opioid effects on one receptor type while producing opioid effects on a second receptor type). Pure agonists are those that produce a maximal response from cells when they bind to the cells' opioid receptor sites. Morphine (the gold standard against which all other opioids are measured), fentanyl, methadone,

hydromorphone, and codeine are pure agonists. Meperidine, although classified as a pure agonist, is not recommended except in clients with a true allergy to all other narcotics, because of its neurotoxicity. Meperidine creates a toxic metabolite, normeperidine, when it is metabolized in the liver. This metabolic has a half-life of 3 to 5 hours, much greater than the 1.5 to 2.0 hours of duration for meperidine's analgesic effects. Thus, frequent doses of meperidine are required to sustain an analgesic effect. The more frequent dosing, however, leads to high levels of metabolite normeperidine, which is neurotoxic. Meperidine used for more than short periods in treatment of acute pain has lead to seizures, coma, and death. Meperidine should never be used in chronic pain management and only sparingly in PCA (Reiss, Evans, & Broyles, 2002).

Meperidine should be reserved for very brief courses in otherwise healthy clients who have demonstrated an unusual reaction (e.g., local histamine release at the infusion site) or allergic response during treatment with other opioids such as morphine or hydromorphone. While technically meperidine does not have a ceiling effect, there is a ceiling effect in regard to the metabolite normeperidine.

Unlike the NSAIDs, pure agonist opioids are not subject to the ceiling effect. As the dosage is increased, there is increasing pain relief, with the only limiting factor being the degree of side effects, particularly respiratory depression and constipation. Many of the opioid analgesics can cause the unwanted effect of constipation. Because of the systemic effect of opioid analgesics on nerves to the GI tract, pharmacological treatment of constipation is indicated when a person has been on chronic or high-dose opioid use.

Other side effects that occur frequently in clients on opioid medications are pruritus and nausea, but the degree to which they are present from each medication varies among

### NURSING STRATEGY

#### OPIOID-INDUCED CONSTIPATION: PREVENTIVE APPROACHES

- Eat high-fiber foods.

- Drink 8 to 10 glasses of fluid per day.

- Eat foods that have helped relieve constipation previously.

- Increase physical activity, such as walking.

- Consume a hot beverage about 30 minutes prior to the planned time for a bowel movement.

- Use laxatives or stool softeners as prescribed by the health care provider.

individuals. Clients must be instructed regarding these *normal* responses to opioids and informed that it does not mean that they are allergic to them. A true allergy to opioids would be indicated by a rash or hives that starts after receiving the opioid, a local histamine release at the site of infusion, or anaphylaxis. Clients also need to know that the pruritus and nausea generally subside after 4 to 5 days of opioid therapy. In the meantime, an antihistamine such as diphenhydramine or hydroxyzine may be used for pruritus, and an antiemetic such as metoclopromide or trimethobenzamide can be used to treat the nausea. Almost all medications used to treat side effects have their own side effect of sedation. Thus, there is the possibility of a cumulative effect of severe sedation. Because of this additive sedative effect, the dosage of opioid analgesics may need to be decreased when antihistamines or antiemetics are also administered.

Mixed agonist-antagonist opioids are believed to be subject to the ceiling effect for pain relief, as well as a ceiling effect for respiratory depression. Mixed agonist-antagonist opioids activate one opioid receptor type while simultaneously blocking another type. Butorphanol, pentazocine, and nalbuphine are the most frequently used in pain management.

### Tolerance, Physical Dependence, and Addiction

Persons who have limited exposure to opioids or who are highly sensitive to opioids are known as being narcotic naïve. Narcotic-naïve clients often require low doses of narcotics for effective pain relief. **Tolerance** can occur after repeated administration of an opioid analgesic, when a specific dose loses its effectiveness and the client requires larger doses to produce the same level of analgesia. The first indication of tolerance is decreased duration of action, then decreased analgesia. If this pattern is noted in clients with continuing opioid needs, the analgesic dose needs to be titrated higher immediately. **Physical dependence** occurs when the body physiologically adapts to opioids. When the opioids are discontinued, withdrawal symptoms occur. McCaffery and Pasero (1999) define **addiction**, or psychological dependence, as behavior of overwhelming involvement with obtaining and using a drug for other than approved medical reasons. Therefore, a client taking opioids for an appropriate medical reason is not addicted. "The fear of addiction is perhaps the single most persistent barrier to achieving pain relief with opioid analgesics . . . it may be the most challenging aspect of educating patients, their families, and even health care professionals" (McCaffery & Pasero, 1998, p. 18).

**Respiratory Depression**   Titrating opioid analgesics to obtain optimal pain management with minimal side effects is a difficult task. See Table 42-8 for a list of risk factors predisposing to respiratory depression in clients receiving appropriate dosages of sedatives or opioid analgesics. This list should be used to identify clients of all ages who require increased vigilance, possible cardiac and pulse oximetry (determination of oxygen saturation of arterial blood) monitoring, and frequent assessment when taking opioid anal-

gesics. It is not to be construed as a reason for denying the client adequate pain management. When caring for clients receiving opioid analgesics, the nurse should periodically identify the presence and intensity of risk factors.

### Local Anesthesia

Local anesthetics are effective for pain management in a variety of settings. Topical anesthetics are available for teething, sore throats, denture pain, laceration repair, and intravenous catheter insertions. EMLA® cream is a mixture of local anesthetics, combining prilocaine and lidocaine. It produces complete anesthesia for at least 60 minutes when topically applied to intact skin.

Another topical anesthetic, TAC, is available for anesthesia during closure of lacerations. It is a combination of tetracaine 0.5%, adrenaline 1:2000, and cocaine 11.8% in a normal saline solution that can be applied directly to the open wound surface in place of local anesthetic infiltration with a needle. This allows pain-free cleansing of the laceration as well as suturing. Because both adrenaline (epinephrine) and cocaine cause vasoconstriction, TAC cannot be used in areas supplied by end-arteriolar blood supply such as digits, the ear, or the nose. It also is contraindicated on burned or abraded skin because this could lead to increased systemic absorption of cocaine and tetracaine, thus placing the client at risk for seizures.

## Treatment of Neuropathic Pain

Neuropathic pain is often refractory to treatment with NSAIDs and opioids. When increasing doses of opioids are ineffective in controlling postoperative pain, an immediate search for the underlying cause should begin, and the diagnosis of neuropathic pain should be considered. Once diagnosed, the focus of treatment is optimizing functional abilities.

Trial of a tricyclic antidepressant is frequently the first step in a client who describes dull, aching, or throbbing pain. Amitriptyline is often the drug of choice because it has been the most widely studied. This class of medications is useful in pain management as a result of:

- Mood elevation
- Potentiation of opioid analgesia
- Direct analgesic effects

### CLINICAL ALERT

#### Administering Opioid Medications

Health care workers often assume obese clients need more opioid pain medication because of their weight. This error can lead to overdose and respiratory depression. Opioids should be prescribed based on estimated lean body weight versus actual weight.

## TABLE 42-8   RISK FACTORS PREDISPOSING TO RESPIRATORY DEPRESSION WITH USE OF SEDATIVES OR OPIOID ANALGESICS

1. Neurologic impairment
   Cerebral palsy
   Altered level of consciousness

2. Respiratory compromise
   Thoracic skeletal deformities (e.g., scoliosis, kyphosis, contracture)
   Neurodegenerative disorders (e.g., muscular dystrophy, tuberous sclerosis, Werdnig-Hoffman disease, myasthenia gravis)
   Pulmonary disease (e.g., cystic fibrosis, reactive airway disease, bronchopulmonary dysplasia, chronic obstructive lung disease)
   Thoracic or high abdominal incision
   Abdominal distension

3. Metabolic alteration
   Liver dysfunction or failure
   Metabolic disease
   Sepsis

4. Renal compromise
   Kidney dysfunction or failure
   Single kidney
   Hypovolemia
   Urine output < 1 ml/kg/h in children, < 30 ml/h in adults, or elevated blood urea nitrogen (BUN) or creatinine

5. Other
   Obesity (when drug is ordered on actual weight rather than estimated lean body weight)
   Increasing sedation
   Agitation
   Preverbal or nonverbal client

6. Concurrent administration of other narcotics or sedatives
   Opioid analgesics
   Sedatives/hypnotics and tranquilizers
   Anticonvulsants
   Antihistamines
   Psychotropics

Adapted from Reiss, B., Evans, M., & Broyles, B. (2002). *Pharmacological aspects of nursing care.* Clifton Park, NY: Delmar Learning.

Clients with neuropathic pain often have significant sleep deprivation. Amitriptyline's action and the side effect of drowsiness improve the client's ability to fall asleep and to sleep for longer periods. Amitriptyline must be started at very low doses especially in children, the debilitated, or older clients, then increased slowly. It should be administered at bedtime to promote sleep and to minimize falls resulting from orthostatic hypotension. The onset of analgesic effects occurs within 1 to 2 weeks, and maximal effect can be seen in 4 to 6 weeks.

Anticonvulsants are often tried first for clients with burning, sharp, shocking, shooting, or **lancinating** (piercing or stabbing) pain. Carbamazepine is often the drug of choice, with other possibilities being clonazepam or phenytoin. These medications suppress spontaneous neuronal firing that leads to the lancinating pain of nerve injury. Carbamazepine may cause a transient bone marrow suppression and requires regular monitoring of serum drug levels, blood counts, and liver function. It should be avoided if possible in clients with any form of bone marrow suppression (e.g., those undergoing chemotherapy, radiation therapy, or taking immunosuppressants posttransplantation) (Reiss, Evans, & Broyles).

Corticosteroid effects include mood elevation, anti-inflammatory effects, and appetite stimulation. Corticosteriods are effective in reducing the neuropathic pain caused by pressure on nerves both centrally and peripherally. The two corticosteroids most frequently used in pain management are dexamethasone and prednisone.

If muscle spasms are a major contributor to the client's discomfort, baclofen can be tried for its antispasmodic effect. This is particularly effective for clients with spinal cord injury or upper motor neuron dysfunction, including cerebral palsy.

## Cognitive-Behavioral Interventions

Cognitive-behavioral interventions are designed to educate clients and to modify client attitudes and behaviors. These nonpharmacological approaches are an important part of the multimodal approach to pain management and can be used in conjunction with appropriate analgesics. A major goal of these interventions is to help the client gain a sense of control over the pain. The effectiveness of selected therapies is outlined in Table 42-9.

### Distraction

Distraction is a pain management strategy that focuses the client's attention on something other than the pain and associated negative emotions. Children and adolescents seem to be particularly adept at using distraction. As many parents know, interactive games or listening to music can be powerful distraction techniques for children; they can also be effective for adults experiencing pain.

## Reframing

**Reframing** is a technique that teaches clients to monitor their negative thoughts and replace them with ones that are more positive. Teaching a client to view pain by expressing not, "I can't stand this pain, it's never going away" but instead, "I've had similar pain before, and it's gotten better" is an example of effective reframing.

## Biofeedback

Biofeedback training is another method that may be helpful for the client in pain, especially one who has difficulty relaxing muscle tension. **Biofeedback** is a process through which individuals learn to influence their physiological responses. Through the use of biofeedback, clients can alter their pain experience.

---

**TABLE 42-9    ADVANTAGES AND DISADVANTAGES OF NONPHARMACOLOGICAL THERAPIES**

| Intervention | Advantages | Disadvantages |
|---|---|---|
| Relaxation, imagery, biofeedback, distraction, and reframing (Figure 42-6) | 1. May decrease pain and anxiety without drug-related side effects.<br>2. Can be used as adjuvant therapy with most other modalities.<br>3. Can increase client's sense of control.<br>4. Most are inexpensive, require no special equipment, and are easily administered. | 1. Client must be motivated to use self-management strategies.<br>2. Requires professional time to teach interventions. |
| Client education | 1. Effective in improving ability to follow medical regimen and in decreasing pain.<br>2. Multiple teaching aids available.<br>3. Promotes self-care in pain treatment and management of side effects. | 1. Requires professional time to teach pain management regimens. |
| Psychotherapy, structured support, and hypnosis | 1. May decrease pain and anxiety for clients who have pain that is difficult to manage.<br>2. May increase client's coping skills. | 1. Requires skilled therapist. |
| Cutaneous stimulation (superficial heat, cold, and massage) | 1. May reduce pain, inflammation, or muscle spasm.<br>2. Can be used as adjuvant therapy with most other modalities.<br>3. Relatively easy to use.<br>4. Can be administered by clients or families.<br>5. Relatively low cost. | 1. Heat may increase bleeding and edema after acute injury.<br>2. Cold is contraindicated for use over ischemic tissues. |
| Transcutaneous electrical nerve stimulation (TENS) | 1. May provide pain relief without drug-related side effects.<br>2. Can be used as adjuvant therapy with most other modalities.<br>3. Gives client sense of control over pain. | 1. Requires skilled therapist to initiate therapy.<br>2. Potential risk of infection, bleeding. |

Adapted from Acute Pain Management Guideline Panel. (1992). *Acute pain management: Operative or medical procedures and trauma. Clinical practice guideline.* (AHCPR Publication No. 92-0033). Rockville, MD: Agency for Health Care Policy and Research.

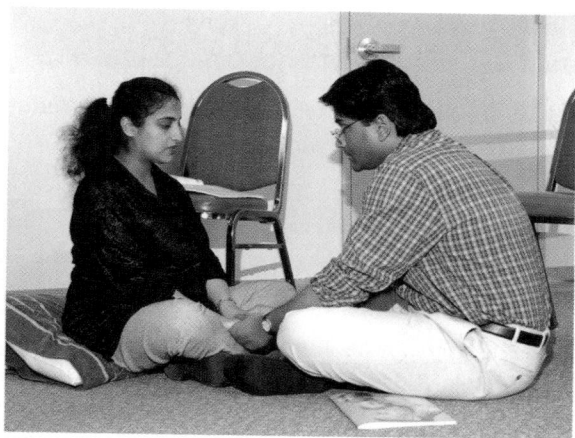

**Figure 42-6** A nonpharmacological therapy to reduce pain are childbirth preparation classes, which often include techniques wherein the partner helps the woman to relax, focus, and breathe deeply.

## Cutaneous Stimulation

**Counterstimulation** is the term used to identify techniques believed to activate the endogenous opioid and monoamine analgesia systems. These interventions are effective by decreasing swelling through cryotherapy (or cold applications), decreasing stiffness (heat applications), and increasing large-diameter nerve fiber input to block small-diameter pain fiber messages (cold, heat, pressure, vibration, or massage). Therapeutic heat and cold are effective pain management tools; they are readily available and easy to use. Both heat and cold can produce analgesia for pain. Heat therapy increases blood flow, increases tissue metabolism, decreases vasomotor tone, and increases the viscoelasticity of connective tissue, making it particularly effective in easing joint stiffness/pain (Bezkor & Lee, 1997). The use of heat as therapy should be closely monitored as it can produce increased inflammation and edema.

Cold therapy exerts many benefits, including the following:

- Alleviates edema by reducing vascular flow
- Counteracts inflammation
- Reduces fever
- Diminishes muscle spasms
- Elevates pain threshold as a result of decreasing the velocity of nerve conduction

Application of cold is inappropriate for clients with cold intolerance, vascular insufficiency, and conditions aggravated by cold (e.g., Reynaud's phenomenon).

## Transcutaneous Stimulation

Transcutaneous stimulation is achieved through use of transcutaneous electrical nerve stimulation, acupuncture, and acupressure. **Transcutaneous electrical nerve stimulation (TENS)** is a method of applying minute amounts of electrical stimulation to large-diameter nerve fibers via electrodes placed on the skin. Placement of the electrodes is deter-

### CLINICAL ALERT

Use heat therapy cautiously in clients with sensory impairment as they may experience burns. Bony prominences are especially vulnerable to the potential for burns.

mined by identifying which nerve innervates the painful area, then determining where that nerve is superficial, or where an anesthetic block would be placed to numb that nerve. Other modalities of pain management should *not* be abandoned while a trial of TENS occurs. Although TENS can be successful, there are two major contraindications:

1. No electrodes should be placed in the area over or surrounding demand cardiac pacemakers.
2. No electrodes can be placed over the uterus of a pregnant woman.

## Complementary/Alternative Therapies

Complementary/alternative methods are being used with increasing frequency to treat pain. The use of such strategies is often influenced by the client's culture. Box 42-2 lists some commonly used complementary therapies.

### Acupuncture and Acupressure

Acupuncture is an intervention from the field of traditional Chinese medicine (TCM). It involves the insertion of fine, solid needles into specific acupuncture points, enhancing the flow of qi (pronounced *chi*) through various meridians of the body (Kotani, Hashimoto, Sato, Sessler, Yoshioka, Kitayama, Yasuda, & Matsuki, 2001). Preoperative intradermal acupuncture reduces postoperative pain, nausea and vomiting, analgesic requirement, and sympathoadrenal responses. Acupuncture points are determined by the type of pain and corresponding TCM organ affected. It is believed that the enhanced qi flow decreases the pain response. Acupressure is the application of pressure to the same acupuncture points on the body. Figure 42-7 shows acupressure points specific to headache relief.

### Herbs

Many herbs are also useful in mediating pain; see Table 42-10. Howell (1997) reports treatment of mouth pain in cancer patients with candy that contains capsaicin.

### Nutrition

Dietary practices may affect pain by inhibiting biochemical events associated with inflammation. Some foods may actually trigger a painful episode; for example, red wine, cheese, citrus fruits, and cured meats often contribute to the onset of migraine headaches (Howell, 1997).

## BOX 42-2 COMPLEMENTARY THERAPIES AND PAIN MANAGEMENT

- Acupuncture and acupressure
  - Herbs
  - Nutrition
- Physical stimulation (passive and active)
  - Exercise
  - Massage
  - Tai chi
  - Yoga
- Relaxation techniques
  - Imagery
  - Progressive muscle relaxation
- Environment interventions
  - Music
  - Pet therapy
  - Horticulture therapy

See Chapter 31 for a complete discussion of complementary therapies.

## RESEARCH FOCUS

**Title of Study:** Relaxation and music reduce pain after gynecologic surgery

**Study Purpose:** The purpose of the study was to evaluate use of relaxation tapes, music, and a combination of relaxation tapes and music on pain management after gynecologic surgery.

**Methods:** Three hundred eleven clients were randomly assigned to three intervention groups or a control group. All clients received patient controlled analgesia (PCA). Three groups also received an intervention of music, relaxation tapes, or both music and relaxation tapes. Pain sensation was measured using a visual analogue scale.

**Findings:** The authors found that persons in the intervention groups had significantly less pain than those who received PCA alone. There was no difference among the three intervention groups in terms of pain reduction.

**Implications:** The findings reveal that music and relaxation tapes would improve pain management in post-gynecologic surgery clients. Nurses can add these interventions to the nonpharmacological methods of treating pain.

Good, M., Anderson, G., Stanton-Hicks, M., Grass, J., & Makii, M. (2002). Relaxation and music reduce pain after gynecologic surgery. *Pain Management Nursing, 3*(2), 21–26.

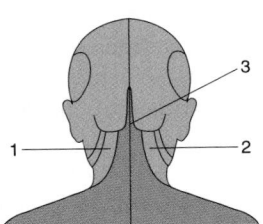

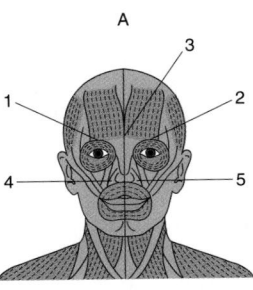

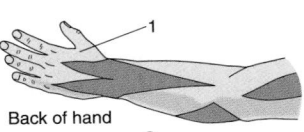

**Point Locations**

**A. Point Location: 1 and 2**
In the hollow, approximately 2 to 3 inches wide, between the two large vertical neck muscles below the base of the skull.

**A. Point Location: 3**
In the large hollow under the base of the skull in the center of the back of the head.

**B. Point Location: 1 and 2**
Where the bridge of the nose meets the inner ridge of the eyebrows, at the indentation of each inner eye socket.

**B. Point Location: 3**
Between the eyebrows where the bridge of the nose meets the forehead.

**B. Point Location: 4 and 5**
At the bottom of each cheekbone adjacent to the nose and in line with the pupil of each eye.

**C. Point Location: 1**
At the highest spot on the muscle in the webbing between the thumb and index finger. *(Do not press on pregnant individual.)*

**Figure 42-7 Acupressure points for headache relief**

Other foods may help alleviate the pain associated with chronic diseases. For example, cherries and berries with red, blue, or black skins have high amounts of bioflavonoids, substances with anti-inflammatory properties. Table 42-11 lists foods with properties that exert a pain-reducing effect.

## Physical Stimulation (Passive and Active)

Passive forms of physical stimulation include massage. There are various forms of massage, such as Swedish, tai, shiatsu, lymphatic, deep tissue, and myofacial release. The common result of massage is to promote muscle relaxation, and decreasing tension and stress. Additionally, it is believed that massage might stimulate release of endogenous endorphins, enhancing pain relief (Nurse Healers: Organization of Therapeutic Touch, 2003).

Active forms of physical stimulation can influence pain via two mechanisms. Tai chi and yoga both offer slow, deliberate movements that combine mental relaxation with physical movement and stretching. The resultant benefit is physical and mental stress reduction and thereby some pain relief.

## TABLE 42-10    HERBAL PAIN MANAGEMENT

| Name | Properties/Use | Contraindications/Side Effects |
|---|---|---|
| Bromelain (*Ananas comosus*) | Anti-inflammatory, smooth muscle relaxant Useful in pain related to oral surgery, sports injury, menstruation | Nontoxic Well tolerated in long-term usage |
| Cayenne pepper (*Capsicum frutescens*) | • Depletes substance P • Excites C fibers (repeated application to C fibers kills them) • For pain of osteoarthritis, neuropathy, postherpetic neuralgia, shingles, fibromyalgia | Avoid getting into eyes May cause brief burning or stinging sensation upon initial use Not for use in those allergic to ragweed |
| Chamomile (*Matricaria chamomilla*) | Antiinflammatory Antispasmodic Analgesic for intestinal spasms Infants' colic pain Stomachache Gastric ulcers | Not for use if allergic to ragweed, asters, or chrysanthemums |
| Feverfew (*Chrysanthemum parthenium*) | Prevention of migraines Rheumatoid arthritis | Not for use with prescription headache drugs Not for use by pregnant and lactating women Capsule preferred (chewing leaves may cause mouth ulcers and loss of taste) |
| Green tea (*Camellia sinensis*) | Produces antioxidant effects | Avoid large quantities during pregnancy Limit to 1 cup per day for those with anxiety disorders or cardiac arrhythmias |
| Kava | Produces relaxation Treatment of insomnia | Large amounts may be intoxicating Potential for abuse |
| Lavender oil (*Lavandula augustifolia*) | Analgesic Sedative Relaxant Useful in treating headaches, muscular sprains, arthritis, menstrual cramps | Warning: May cause extreme drowsiness |
| Licorice (*Glycyrrhiza glabra*) | Anti-inflammatory Inactivates herpes simplex (for treatment of oral and genital herpes lesions) Rheumatoid arthritis | Long-term use can cause hypertension |
| Valerian | Insomnia Muscle pain Menstrual cramps Intestinal cramps | Do not use with alcohol or other CNS depressants |

NOTE: This information is not intended to be a guide for self-medication or the treatment of others. Consult a health care practitioner with expertise in the use of herbs before using any herb for medicinal purposes.

Data from Cleland, C. L., & Gebhart, G. F. (1997). Principles of nociception and pain. In Springhouse Corporation. *Expert pain management* (p. 11). Springhouse, PA: Springhouse Corporation; Howell, S. (1997). Complementary therapies. In Springhouse Corporation. *Expert pain management* (p. 261). Springhouse, PA: Springhouse Corporation; Fontaine, K. (2000). *Healing practices: Alternative therapies for nursing* (pp. 121–123). Upper Saddle River, NJ: Prentice Hall; Tierra, M. (1998). *The way of herbs.* New York: Pocket Books; Walters, C. (1998). *Aromatherapy: A basic guide.* New York: Barnes & Noble.

## TABLE 42-11 NUTRITION AND THERAPEUTIC OUTCOMES

| Food | Therapeutic Effect |
|---|---|
| Cherries and berries with black or red-blue skins (raspberries, blackberries) | • Rich in bioflavonoids (anti-inflammatory substances)<br>• Used in pain associated with arthritis and gout |
| Calcium, magnesium, zinc, and Vitamins A, B-complex, C, D, and E (found in fruits, vegetables, legumes, whole grains, sunflower seeds, nuts) | |
| Fatty acid eicosapentaenoic acid (EPA), a component of certain fish oils (found in cold-water fish) | Inhibits formation of substances associated with inflammation |
| Amino acids (found in whole grains, starchy vegetables, dairy products, turkey) | Produces mild analgesia |

Data from Howell, S. (1997). Complementary therapies. In Springhouse Corporation. *Expert pain management* (pp. 258–259). Springhouse, PA: Springhouse Corporation.

## Relaxation Techniques

**Relaxation techniques** (a variety of methods used to decrease anxiety and muscle tension), **imagery** (a strategy that uses mental images to assist with relaxation), and **progressive muscle relaxation** (a strategy in which muscles are alternately tensed and relaxed) are used to achieve both mental and physical relaxation. Physical relaxation leads to reduction of skeletal muscle tension; mental relaxation is used to alleviate anxiety.

## Environment Manipulation

The environment can exert influence on the perception of pain; therefore, changes in one's environment may reduce pain levels. Pet therapy, consisting of interactive sessions between client and animals, is helpful for some people experiencing chronic pain.

Horticultural therapy (treatment that includes looking at, touching, and growing plants) has several therapeutic benefits, including pain reduction, relaxation, and improved energy level. Participation in gardening can provide distraction from chronic pain.

## LEGAL AND ETHICAL ISSUES

### The Use of Medicinal Marijuana

Currently six states (Alaska, California, Colorado, Maine, Oregon, and Washington) allow for the use of medical marijuana in treatment of anorexia and chronic pain. Several other states are in the process of having bills introduced that would allow for medical marijuana use. In 2001, the U.S. Supreme Court decided that federal law, which prohibits marijuana use, took precedence over state laws allowing for medical marijuana use. The result was numerous drug busts, mostly in California, by the Drug Enforcement Administration (DEA). Despite the Supreme Court ruling, medical marijuana continues to be an active program in states where it is allowed, creating tension between local and federal law enforcement agencies. It additionally puts clients and health care providers in legal limbo. Research has demonstrated that marijuana is useful in HIV and cancer pain management.

Marijuana Use. 2003. http://www.mayoclinic.com

## COMMUNITY/HOME CARE

### Pain Management Concepts

- On each visit, evaluate the client's pain.

- Assess factors influencing effective pain management (e.g., motor, cognitive, and functional alterations).

- Teach clients and family members adjunctive therapies to be used with analgesics to decrease pain.

- Identify barriers that hinder pain control.

- Encourage the homebound client to use around-the-clock dosing of analgesics.

Adapted from Luggen, A. S. (2000). Pain. In A. G. Lueckenotte, (Ed.), *Gerontologic nursing* (2nd ed., p. 300.). St. Louis: Mosby.

Music therapy may help ease pain by producing relaxation and providing distraction.

Another alternative therapy that has stimulated controversy is the potential use of marijuana for its medicinal purposes. Debate over the use of marijuana has been a state-by-state issue, with differences continuing to exist. Research has supported marijuana's positive effects in specific types of disorders.

## Evaluation

Evaluating the efficacy of the pain management interventions is ongoing, with client input throughout the process.

Evaluation focuses primarily on the client's subjective reports. Objective data used to evaluate pain management efficacy include:

- Client's facial expression and posture
- Presence (or absence) of restlessness
- Vital sign monitoring
- Ongoing use of pain assessment tools

Regular reassessment is an integral part of effective pain management. In addition to client self-report and nursing observation, family input is a valuable source of information for evaluating the effectiveness of care.

# CASE STUDY/NURSING CARE PLAN

Ms. Shandra Williams is a 22-year-old African American female with sickle cell disease, SS type. She comes to the emergency room in a sickling crisis, complaining of acute pain in her chest and extremities, especially her joints. Her vital signs are blood pressure 90/50, heart rate 110, respiration rate 24, and temperature 37.5°C. Her pulse oximetry is 80% on room air. She rates her pain a 10 and describes it as sharp, burning, and constant. The pain began 2 hours prior to coming to the emergency room. She took two analgesics at that time but came to the emergency room because the pain became worse and she experienced shortness of breath.

## Assessment

Ms. Williams is experiencing ischemic pain as a result of a sickling crisis, and her pain is 10 on a rating scale of 10. The client describes the pain as sharp and burning. In addition, Ms. Williams' pulse oximetry of 80% is indicative of a low oxygen state. Ms. Williams' is on MS Contin 100 mg BID for treatment of her chronic pain.

## Nursing Diagnosis

*Acute Pain* related to decreased oxygenation to tissues
**NOC:** Pain Level; Pain Control; Pain: Disruptive Effects; Comfort Level
**NIC:** Pain Management; Analgesic Administration; Patient-Controlled Analgesia Administration

## Expected Outcomes

The client will:

1. Rate her pain as < 3 on a 10-point rating scale within 48 hours.
2. Demonstrate a pulse oximetry at 95% or higher within 24 hours.

## Planning/Interventions/Rationales

1. Initiate patient-controlled analgesia (PCA) with morphine, titrated to control Ms. Williams' pain. *Continuous opioids are necessary for managing an acute pain episode, especially in a person who is narcotic tolerant. Use of the PCA allows the client to control pain medication without becoming over-sedated.*
2. Provide oxygen per nasal cannula. *Supplemental oxygen is necessary when treating ischemic pain to prevent infarction. In someone with sickle cell disease, it is necessary to prevent acute chest syndrome.*
3. Implement intravenous fluids. *Intravenous fluids are necessary to hydrate the person in an acute sickling crisis. Dehydration is a common contributor to sickling crises and hydration facilitates resolution of the crisis.*
4. Apply warm compresses to painful joints. *Warmth can help increase circulation to the joints and promote pain relief.*
5. Keep client on bed rest until acute crisis is over. *Bed rest decreases oxygen needs and promotes relaxation.*

## Evaluation

After 3 hours, Ms. Williams reports her pain as less: 5 on a scale of 1 to 10. Her oxygen saturation is 95% on 3 liters/minute (LPM) per nasal cannula. Her chest pain is gone, but the joint pain persists. Immediate pain interventions have been successful in decreasing her pain, but ongoing acute pain management is indicated. Ms. Williams is admitted to the hospital for ongoing treatment and evaluation.

# CARE MAP CASE STUDY

Arlene Johnson, age 52, has been diagnosed with ovarian cancer. For several months prior to her diagnosis she managed her abdominal discomfort and "gas" with over-the-counter (OTC) medications. Later on, she also noticed a vague pelvic aching, lower back pain, painful defecation, constipation, some urinary frequency, and painful intercourse (dyspareunia). She attributed these symptoms and changes in her menstrual cycle as signs of menopause. She delayed scheduling an appointment with her gynecologist because she was already scheduled for her annual physical in 3 months. Arlene is an elementary school teacher. She is married; the couple has no children. She likes to cook gourmet meals and they entertain friends frequently. They also enjoy their sailboat excursions on the weekends when weather permits. She is looking forward to her retirement in 3 years.

During her physical examination, Dr. Jamison notes that Arlene has gained 15 pounds (165 to 180 pounds) within the last year. Her height is 5 feet 3 inches; temperature, 98.6; pulse, 82; respirations, 20. The abdominal and pelvic exam revealed a large firm fixed mass on the left side. She is scheduled for a transvaginal ultrasound diagnostic test, an intravenous pyelogram, and a barium enema. Following these procedures, Dr. Jamison informs Arlene and her husband, John, of his tentative diagnosis, and that he would like to perform an exploratory laparotomy. He asks their permission to do a total abdominal hysterectomy if necessary. He also explains the potential treatment options.

You have selected Arlene as your client on the first postoperative day following the surgery, which included total hysterectomy and bilateral salpingo-oophorectomy. (The cancer had spread locally to the fallopian tubes and the broad ligament. She will be scheduled for systemic chemotherapy for at least 6 months). Arlene complains of pain in the incision area that interferes with her need to perform the exercises of coughing, deep breathing, and moving. A retention catheter is in place; however, the urinary drainage has been minimal in the last 2 hours. Palpation of her abdomen reveals a distended bladder. Arlene tells you she is very anxious about her condition and about what the future holds for her. Her husband tries to comfort her during her frequent crying spells. As he leaves, he tells you that he is devastated by the prognosis report given to him following his wife's surgery.

This scenario was designed to include an appropriate assessment of postoperative abdominal pain and the psychological discomfort associated with a life-threatening illness.

## Suggested References

1. Refer back to the discussion in this chapter and review content in a current medical-surgical text related to management of pain, ovarian cancer, postoperative care for abdominal hysterectomy, and the impact of psychological stress on the perception of pain.
2. Lasch, K. (2000). Culture, pain, and culturally sensitive pain care. *Pain Management Nursing*, *1*(3), 16–22.
3. Manz, B., Mosier, R., Nusser-Gerlach, M., Bergstrom, N., & Agrawal, S. (2000). Pain assessment in the cognitively impaired and unimpaired elderly. *Pain Management Nursing*, *1*(4), 106–115.
4. Vallerand, A., & Polomano, R. (2000). The relationship of gender to pain. *Pain Management Nursing*, *1*(3), 8–15.

Refer back to the care map example for areas to include in your map. Add concepts from the case study into the areas where you believe they belong. (Some concepts may belong in more than one area.)

1. Have you placed the couple as the client in the center of the map?
2. Cluster related concepts together. Draw connecting lines to indicate relationships.
3. What nursing actions would you do to determine why there has been no urinary drainage within the last 2 hours? Why would this problem contribute to Arlene's abdominal pain? What precautions would you take to eliminate this problem in the future?
4. What can you do to assist Arlene in following the instructions to cough and deep breathe and to minimize her discomfort when moving? Why are these exercises so important?
5. What independent nursing interventions can you use to help to minimize Arlene's pain and her perception of pain?

*(continues)*

## CARE MAP CASE STUDY (continued)

6.  Since thrombophlebitis is a common postoperative complication following a hysterectomy, what signs and symptoms will you assess?

7.  What additional information would you like to have to assist in planning Arlene's care? Consider the impact of the cancer diagnosis on her psychological and spiritual needs.

8.  Locate the cancer pain ladder tool originated by the World Health Organization (WHO) (usually found in nursing texts or on the WHO website.) Use the analgesia described in each of the three steps of the ladder for relief of persisting or increasing pain such as cancer pain.

9.  Arlene's postoperative pain is considered acute pain. How does acute pain management differ from chronic pain management or cancer pain management?

10. What would you include in your discharge plan for Arlene regarding pain management?

## Key Concepts

- Pain is a subjective and individualized experience.
- Pain is defined as whatever the client says it is.
- Pain is increased by anxiety and fatigue.
- Several factors influence the perception of pain, including developmental level, culture, and previous experience.
- Nonpharmacological interventions may be used in managing pain.
- Pharmacological agents can be therapeutic for clients experiencing pain
- Nonopioid analgesics, adjuvant medications, and opioid analgesics should all be used in pharmacological management of pain.
- Nonpharmacological interventions (e.g., herbs, biofeedback, distraction) are important in pain management.

## Review Questions and Activities

1.  How would you describe the different types of pain (somatic, cutaneous, visceral, referred, ischemic, acute, and chronic).

2.  What nonpharmacological interventions would be appropriate for a 50-year-old woman suffering from arthritis, a 9-year-old oncology client, a couple going through childbirth?

3.  What is the difference between nonopioid analgesics, adjuvant medications, and opioid analgesics?

4.  What are the principles that guide pharmacological pain management?

5.  What are the common side effects a nurse must watch for when giving opioid pain medications?

6.  What is the difference between tolerance, physical dependence, and addiction?

## Web Resources

Agency for Health Care Research and Quality
    http://www.ahrq.gov
American Pain Foundation
    http://www.painfoundation.org
American Pain Society
    http://www.ampainsoc.org
Marijuana Use
    http://www.mayoclinic.com
National Institutes of Health
    http://www.nih.gov
National Institutes of Health—Pain Guidelines Site
    http://www.nlm.nih.gov
Nurse Healers: Organization of Therapeutic Touch
    http://www.therapeutic-touch.org

## References

Acello, B. (2000). Meeting JCAHO standards for pain control. *Nursing2000, 30*(3), 52–54.

Ackley, B., & Ladwig, G. (2002). *Nursing diagnosis handbook* (5th ed.). St.Louis: Mosby.

Acute Pain Management Guideline Panel. (1992). *Acute pain management: Operative or medical procedures and trauma. Clinical practice guideline.* (AHCPR Publication No. 92-0033). Rockville, MD: Agency for Health Care Policy and Research.

American Nurses Association. (1991). *Position statement: Promotion of comfort and relief of pain in dying patients.* Washington, DC: Author.

American Pain Foundation. 2002. http://www.pain foundation.org

Anand, K. J. S., & McGrath, P. J. (1999). *Pain in neonates.* New York: Elsevier Science.

Bezkor, M. F., & Lee, M. H. M. (1997). Noninvasive techniques for managing pain. In Springhouse Corporation, *Expert pain management* (pp. 179–204). Springhouse, PA: Springhouse Corporation.

Bral, E. E. (1998). Caring for adults with chronic cancer pain. *American Journal of Nursing, 98*(4), 27–32.

Carpenito, L. J. (2002). *Handbook of nursing diagnosis* (8th ed.). Philadelphia: Lippincott.

Cheever, K. H. (1999). Control critically ill patients' active pain. *Nursing Management, 30*(8), 40–43.

Cleland, C. L., & Gebhart, G. F. (1997). Principles of nociception and pain. In Springhouse Corporation, *Expert pain management* (pp. 1–30). Springhouse, PA: Springhouse Corporation.

Collins, P. M., Sparger, K., Richardson, M., Schriver, T., & Bergenstock, D. (1999). Talking with physicians about pain. *American Journal of Nursing, 99*(10), 20.

Eliopoulos, C. (1999). *Manual of gerontologic nursing* (2nd ed.). St. Louis: Mosby.

Fontaine, K. (2000). *Healing practices: Alternative therapies for nursing* (pp. 113–133). Upper Saddle River, NJ: Prentice Hall.

Good, M., Anderson, G. C., Stanton-Hicks, M. Grass, J. A., & Makii, M. (2002). Relaxation and music reduce pain after gynecologic surgery. *Pain Management Nursing, 3*(2), 21–26.

Hockenberry, M., Wilson, D., Winkelstein, M., & Kline, N. (2003). *Wong's nursing care of infants and children* (7th ed.). St. Louis: Mosby.

Howell, S. (1997). Complementary therapies. In Springhouse Corporation, *Expert pain management* (pp. 224–282). Springhouse, PA: Springhouse Corporation.

Jacox, A., Carr, D. B., Payne, R., et al. (1994). *Pain Assessment Methodology* (Publication No. 94-0592). Rockville, MD: Agency for Health Care Policy and Research (AHCPR), U.S. Department of Health and Human Services, Public Health Service.

Joel, L. (1999). The fifth vital sign: Pain. *American Journal of Nursing, 99*(2), 9.

Jones, S. L. (1997). Pharmacology of pain management. In Springhouse Corporation, *Expert pain management* (pp. 31–65). Springhouse, PA: Springhouse Corporation.

Kessenich, C. R. (2001). Cyclo-oxygenase 2 inhibitors: An important new drug classification. *Pain Management Nursing, 2*(1), 13–18.

Kotani, N., Hashimoto, H., Sato, Y., Sessler, D. I., Yoshioka, H., Kitayama, M., Yasuda, T., & Matsuki, A. (2001). Preoperative intradermal acupuncture reduces postoperative pain, nausea and vomiting, analgesic requirement, and sympathoadrenal responses. *Anesthesiology, 95*(2), 349–356.

Loeb, J. L. (1999). Pain management in long-term care. *American Journal of Nursing, 99*(2), 48–52.

Luggen, A. S. (2000). Pain. In A. G. Lueckenotte (Ed.), *Gerontologic nursing* (2nd ed., pp. 281–301). St. Louis: Mosby.

Manz, B. D., Mosier, R., Nusser-Gerlach, M.A., Bergstrom, N., and Agrawal, S. (2000). Pain assessment in the cognitively impaired and unimpaired elderly. *Pain Management Nursing, 1*(4): 106-115.

Marijuana Use. 2003. http://www.mayoclinic.com

McCaffery, M., & Pasero, C. L. (1998). Pain control: Talking with patients and families about addiction. *American Journal of Nursing, 98*(3), 18–21.

McCaffery, M., & Pasero, C. (1999). *Pain: Clinical manual for nursing practice* (2nd ed.). St. Louis: Mosby.

Melzack, R., & Wall, D. W. (1965). Pain mechanisms: A new theory. *Science, 150*, 971–979.

Newshan, G. (2000). Pain management in the addicted patient: Practical considerations. *Nursing Outlook, 48*(2), 81–85.

North American Nursing Diagnosis Association. (2003). *Nursing diagnoses: Definitions and classification, 2003–2004*. Philadelphia: Author.

Nurse Healers: Organization of Therapeutic Touch. (2003). http://www.therapeutic-touch.org

Pasero, C. L., Reed, B., & McCaffery, M. (1998). How aging affects pain management. *American Journal of Nursing, 98*(6), 12–13.

Peloso, P. M. (2000). NSAIDs: A Faustian bargain. *American Journal of Nursing, 200*(6), 34–38.

Plaisance, L., & Price, T. F. (1999). A stepwise guide to cancer pain management in the home. *Home Healthcare Nurse, 17*(2), 96–104.

Porth, C. (2002). *Pathophysiology: Concepts in altered health states* (6th ed.). Philadelphia: J. B. Lippincott.

Purnell, L., & Paulanka, B. (1998). *Transcultural health care*. Philadelphia: F. A. Davis.

Reiss, B., Evans, M., & Broyles, B. (2002). *Pharmacological Aspects of Nursing Care*. Clifton Park: Delmar Learning.

Thomson, H. (2001). A new law to improve pain management and end-of-life care. *Western Journal of Medicine, 174*(3), 161–162.

Tierra, M. (1998). *The way of herbs*. New York: Pocket Books.

Travell, J., & Rinzler, S. H. (1952). The myofascial genesis of pain. *Postgraduate Medicine, 11*, 425.

Vallerand, A. H. & Polomano, R. C. (2000). The relationship of gender to pain. *Pain Management Nursing, 1*(3), 8–15.

Van-Couwenberghe, C., & Pasero, C. L. (1998). Teaching patients how to use PCA. *American Journal of Nursing, 98*(9), 14–15.

Walters, C. (1998). *Aromatherapy: A basic guide*. New York: Barnes & Noble.

Williams-Lee, P. (1999). Managing pain by the book. *Nursing Management, 30*(7), 9.

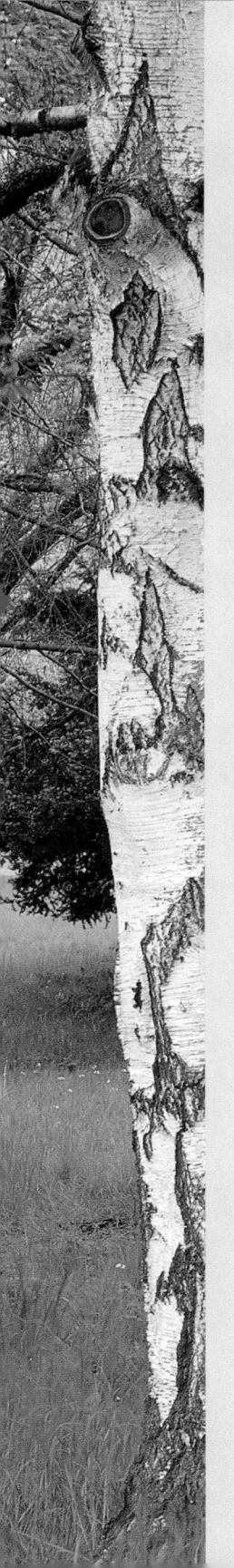

# XIII UNIT

# Self-Perception/ Self-Concept

Chapter 43  Self-Concept

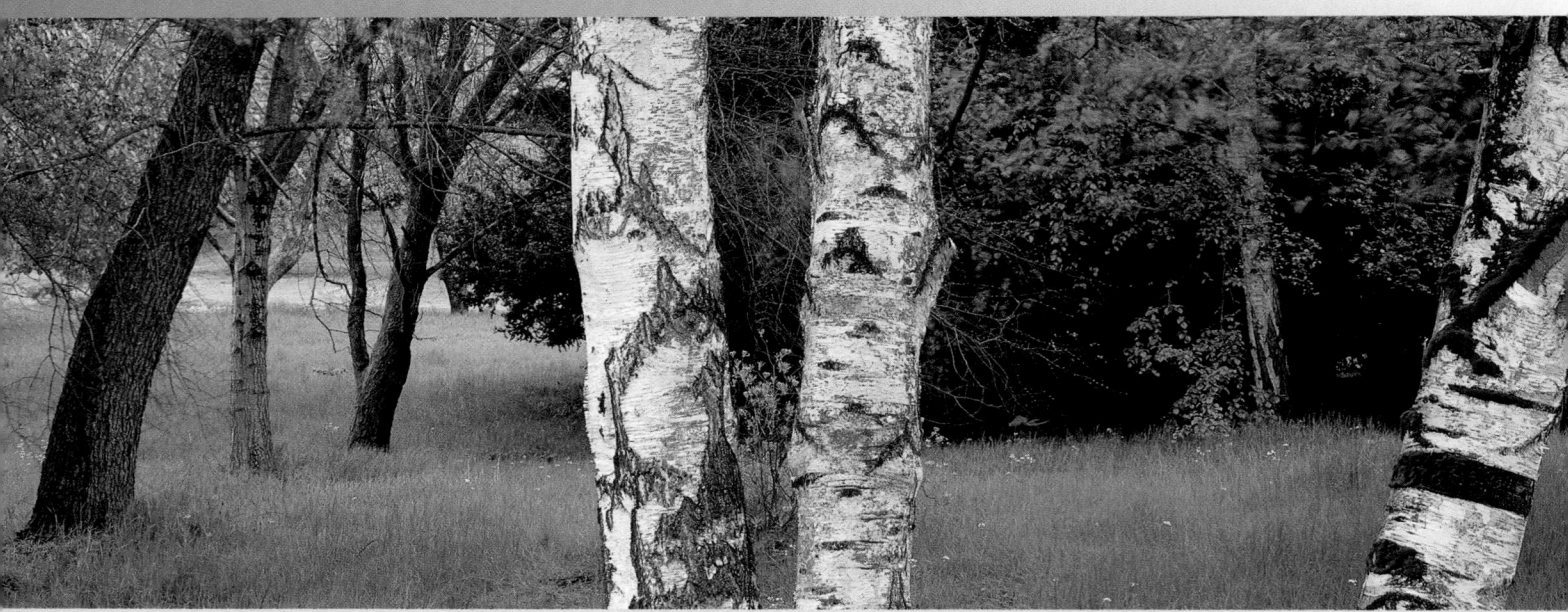

# Self-Concept

Ruth N. Grendell, DNSc, RN

*"If life is to have meaning, the extent to which you know your-self is the most important work you will ever do."*

(Gregory Crow, 2000)

# Chapter Competencies

*Upon completion of this chapter, the reader should be able to:*

1. Describe the different components of self-concept.
2. Explain the development of self-concept throughout the life span.
3. Discuss factors affecting self-concept.
4. Identify the variety of assessment skills necessary to evaluate for alterations of self-concept.
5. Identify nursing diagnoses that are common for clients with alterations of self-concept.
6. Create a plan to achieve the outcomes for client management.
7. Evaluate different nursing strategies for implementing interventions for clients with alterations in self-concept.
8. Synthesize methods for evaluating the nursing process in alterations of self-concept.
9. Identify strategies to promote positive self-esteem.

# Key Terms

body image
identity
role

role conflict
self-concept
self-esteem

self-ideal
sick role

**S**elf-concept (an individual's perception of self) affects every aspect of life, including relationships, functional abilities, and health status. No two people have an identical self-concept; self-concept is what helps make each individual unique. Everyone has both positive and negative self-assessments in the physical, emotional, intellectual, and functional dimensions, which change over time and according to the context of the situation. Because self-concept is an individual's frame of reference for perceiving and interacting with the world, it exerts a powerful influence on one's life. Though neither visible nor tangible, a positive self-concept is one of the greatest strengths a person can possess (Ball & Bindler, 2003; Stuart & Laraia, 2001).

One's view of self affects the ability to function. A person who sees self as a competent individual will behave competently and vice versa. Individuals with a positive self-concept approach new experiences and tasks with confidence; they expect to be accepted by others and to succeed. Conversely, the person with a negative self-concept tends to shy away from others and to avoid challenges. Self-concept greatly influences health status. For example, a person with a positive self-concept is more likely to care for one's self—physically, emotionally, and spiritually. The relationship of the components

of self-concept and mental health are discussed in Table 43-1.

| TABLE 43-1 | SELF-CONCEPT AND MENTAL HEALTH |
|---|---|
| **Component of Self-Concept** | **Relationship to Mental Health** |
| Strong sense of identity | Experiences self as a unique individual. |
| Accurate and positive | A healthy awareness of one's body image body is based on reality testing. |
| Positive self-esteem | A person with a high degree of self-esteem respects self and treats self with dignity. |
| Satisfying role performance | The person with healthy role performance relates well with others and receives gratification from fulfilling role expectations. |

# Components of Self-Concept

Self-concept is composed of four components: identity, body image, self-esteem, and role performance (Figure 43-1). By considering these four elements of self-concept, nurses can more effectively respond to a client. Several major theories have been introduced to explain human development, with each theory focusing on a particular aspect of development, including psychosexual, psychosocial, cognitive, moral, and learning development. These theories usually organize the developmental phases and their common characteristics into age-specific categories. A central theme among the different theories is the completion of tasks for a particular developmental phase before successfully moving on to the next phase (Ball & Binder, 2003).

The self-concept can be depicted as the central core surrounded by the overlapping circles of self-identity, body image, self-esteem, and role performance. These circles have broken lines signifying the influence of continual exchanges from inner and external forces. Changes in any of the components impact the others. The self-concept can be defined as the ideas, beliefs, and convictions that constitute an individual's self-knowledge. It includes the unique perspective of personal characteristics and abilities, and relationships with the surrounding world (Stuart & Laraia, 2001).

## Identity

A sense of personal **identity** is what sets one person apart as a unique individual (Figure 43-2). A well-formulated identity provides the answer to the question "Who am I?" Identity may include a person's name, gender, ethnic identity, family status, occupation, and various roles.

A person begins to develop identity during childhood and constantly reinforces and modifies it throughout life. First, parents or caretakers provide a child with elements of an emerging identity. Children may be told they are good or naughty, shy or outgoing, creative or dull, powerless or empowered. Children believe what they are told by others, and these beliefs influence the developing identi-

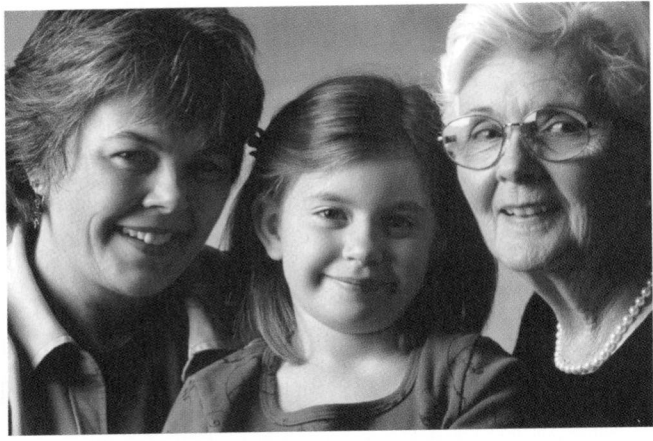

**Figure 43-2    Each of these three family members is a unique individual. *Courtesy of Photodisc***

ty. Erikson's psychosocial theory stressed the importance of the quality of parent-child interactions and facilitating the child's development (Orem, 2001; Stuart & Laraia, 2001; Erikson, 1963). During adolescence, the individual examines and redefines the self in relationship to the family, peer group, and community. Conflict often arises as the teenager struggles to become independent and to establish a unique identity. Those who have self-doubts regarding their place in society are at risk of role confusion, may lack self-confidence, and may be unsure of roles they must perform as adults. Self-identity is the integrating force of self-concept and is the combination of conscious and unconscious elements of self-respect, autonomy, and competency (Ball & Bindler, 2003; Berger, 1999; Stuart & Laraia, 2001). Eventually, people learn to observe themselves critically, as their social environment

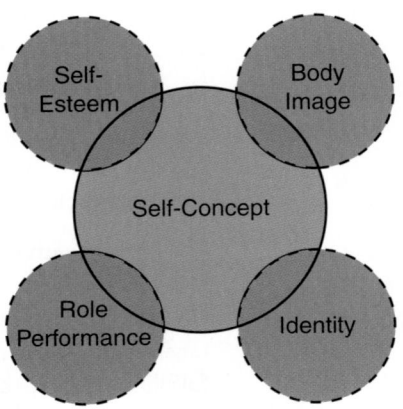

**Figure 43-1    The interrelationship of the components of self-concept**

## STOP AND THINK

### Sharing the Real Self with the Nurse

The private, or subjective, self is frequently not apparent to others. It is comprised of the ideas, attitudes, and feelings a person believes about who she *really* is. An individual may readily share some self-aspects, such as wishes, values, and problem-solving abilities.

- What comments could a client make that would cause you to think she is not sharing her private "self"?

- How would you encourage the client to share these elements of the self?

- What is the health value of a client being able to share her private self with the nurse?

expands. Feedback from others may support and strengthen an aspect of identity already implanted, or it may contradict an aspect and help change it (Oran, 2000; Berger, 1999).

## Body Image

**Body image** is an attitude about one's physical attributes and characteristics, appearance, and performance.

Body image is dynamic because any change in body structure or function, including the normal changes of growth and development, can affect body image. The adolescent years are a good example of the interplay between an individual's physical changes and a developing sense of body image. Many teenagers will have harmless body image distortions. It is not at all uncommon for adolescents to feel self-conscious because they think their noses are too big, their hips too wide, or their blemishes too prominent. Usually, these are normal concerns. Adolescents generally find that their perceptions continue to evolve as their physical development continues to mature.

Body image is continually modified throughout the life span. An individual's attitude toward physical appearance may reflect, or mirror, self-identity. An acceptance of one's body is most often related to higher levels of self-esteem and self-concept (Ball & Bindler, 2003; Berger, 1999).

## Self-Ideal

**Self-ideal** is the perception of behavior based on personal standards and self-expectations. Development begins in childhood and is continually influenced by culture, association with peers, and experiences. The ideal serves as an internal regulator to support self-respect and self-esteem. However, the perceptions may be unrealistic when goals are too demanding. Successful goal attainment is more feasible when there is congruence between expectations and abilities (Stuart & Laraia, 2001).

## Self-Esteem

**Self-esteem** is the judgment of personal performance compared with the self-ideal. It is derived from a sense of

### STOP AND THINK

### Developing Self-Esteem

- Why would a client with low self-esteem be vulnerable to depression?

- How would this perception affect your clients?

- How would you encourage clients to praise themselves for who they are and what they do?

giving and receiving love, and being respected by others. Self-esteem is most threatened during adolescence as the individual struggles with self-concept issues. It stabilizes as an adult when the individual is more self-accepting, less idealistic, and equipped with mature coping skills. Self-esteem of the aging individual is challenged again by negative stereotypes of older adults in a youth-oriented society, by role transitions, and by the losses associated with physical health problems and a diminished social support system.

Locus of control is closely associated with self-esteem. Individuals with an internal locus of control perceive themselves as actively controlling their destiny; individuals with external locus of control perceive themselves as incapable of control (Hollinger-Smith, 2000; Stuart & Laraia, 2001). The nurse can assist the client in developing control and increasing his self-esteem.

## Role Performance

**Role** refers to a set of expected behaviors that are determined by familial, cultural, and social norms Self-identity emerges from the self-concept and is expressed as role behavior. Individuals attempt to integrate self-identity within their various roles, such as a gender-identity, while simultaneously fulfilling the several roles of parent, sibling, friend, spouse, and student or worker. The level of self-esteem depends upon the self-perception of adequate role performance in these various social roles. Self-esteem also depends upon the similarity between cultural norms and the individual's own expectations for role behavior. The nurse gains a better understanding of individuals within the perspective of the performance patterns in their overlapping roles (Edminson, 2001; Pasquali, 1999; Stuart & Laraia, 2001).

The nurse theorist Peplau (1992) examined roles in the context of the nurse-client relationship. The nurse may assume several different roles, such as counselor, teacher, leader, or surrogate parent. As the relationship progresses, the client feels free to express deep feelings to the nurse because the nurse has assumed the roles of listener, counselor, and expert. As teacher, the nurse may provide information to the client or correct misconceptions. As counselor, the nurse responds to the client's feelings or behavior, helping the client to gain insight or self-care or a health-affirming outlook.

### Stressors Affecting Role

Roles have accompanying responsibilities that are affected by maturational and situational events. Whenever a person is unable to fulfill role responsibilities, self-concept is impaired. When an individual has too many roles to fulfill simultaneously, overload can occur. The person becomes overwhelmed by the many demands of several roles. The individual may complain of being stressed out and feeling unable to cope. In fact, the individual's coping skills are greatly taxed.

## STOP AND THINK

### Personal Roles

Consider the various roles you currently fulfill. What are some of the potential conflicts inherent in your multiple roles? For example, your role of student may at times conflict with your role of friend or parent (e.g., you need to be in class at the same time you need to attend a parent-teacher conference or be available to your friend who is undergoing a crisis). Or your need to study for an examination (student role) is superseded by your need to work (role of wage earner).

In addition to overload, another common problematic role experience is **role conflict**, which occurs when the expectations of one role compete with the expectations of other roles. The person may feel unable to establish priorities among competing role expectations. Table 43-2 describes the various types of role conflict.

The **sick role** is a set of social expectations met by an ill person, such as being exempt from the usual social role responsibilities, and being obligated to get well and to seek competent help. Individuals sometimes take on a deviant sick role, and use their illness to receive attention, to gain control over others, or as a means of avoiding responsibilities. The "invalid" role can also be a result of self-pity regarding a chronic illness or disability (Grendell, 2000). Depression and anxiety, preoccupation with illness symptoms, and dependency are common responses to acute illness that resolve as the person's health improves. However, perceptions of poor health, prolonged emotional distress, and interpersonal dependency for reassurance and attention can lead to "learned helplessness" and invalidism (Riegel, Dracup, & Glaser, 1998).

## STOP AND THINK

### Sick Role

● What happens when illness forces an individual to assume the "sick role"?

● What are the social expectations of a sick person?

● What effect does this new and often unexpected role have on all the other roles the individual performs?

### TABLE 43-2     TYPES OF ROLE CONFLICT

| Type | Description | Example |
|---|---|---|
| Interrole conflict | Expectations of one role oppose expectations of another role. | A woman's job requires travel at the same time her child's dance recital is scheduled. |
| Interpersonal role conflict | Incompatible role expectations are held by one or more people. | A husband and wife disagree on parental expectations (e.g., disciplinary methods). |
| Role overload | Excessive demands of numerous roles have conflicting priorities. | A nurse must decide which urgent task to do first. |
| Person-role conflict | The individual's values are violated by demands of a role. | A nurse who believes in always telling the truth is directed by the supervisor to withhold a diagnosis from a client. |

## Development of Self-Concept

Self-concept evolves throughout life and depends to an extent on an individual's developmental level. Self-concept changes during each developmental stage. According to Stuart and Laraia (2001), the ongoing process of self-concept development is facilitated by the following:

• Interpersonal and cultural experiences
• Self-perceived competence
• Self-actualization (living up to one's potential)

Self-concept is developed primarily in response to social interactions and experiences. Sullivan's classic theory (1953) states that self-concept is developed according to perceptions mirrored by others to the individual. A person's concept of self depends, to an extent, on what he thinks that others think about him.

As individuals mature, they can accept or reject the appraisals of others and change their behavior in a way that leads to a more positive self-concept (Stuart & Laraia, 2001).

# Childhood

Self-concept is not innate; rather, it develops throughout the life cycle as a result of social interactions. An infant whose basic needs are met in a warm, consistent manner develops positive feelings about self. Formation of self-concept occurs in the following manner: (1) during infancy, the child develops a self-perception of being separate from the environment (including parents); (2) as the child ages, perspectives (especially of the parents) are internalized; and (3) society's norms (e.g., expectations of appropriate behavior) are then internalized by the child.

A child's sense of self is shaped by interactions with parents and siblings, through shared experiences with extended family members, and in relationships with others. Children learn about their individual worth and their ability to be competent in the family unit, and their sense of self changes as they move through each developmental stage. Infants learn to trust based on the degree to which their needs are met, and begin to develop a sense of self as distinct from the primary caretaker and their surroundings. As new skills are mastered, toddlers begin to develop a sense of autonomy and self-image, yet they still remain very self-centered. Preschoolers have increasing initiative and self-awareness as their expanding language and motor skills broaden their horizons, and they begin to have an awareness of emotions and the values that their families embrace. When children reach school age, they will incorporate experiences and values of their new contacts and environments into their image of self and may start to have an understanding of their strengths as well as their shortcomings (Figure 43-3).

Positive experiences, role models, and family environment are all crucial to the healthy self-concept of the growing child. The impact of early parent-child experiences on the shaping of a child's self-concept was emphasized by Sullivan (1953), whose interpersonal theory of psychiatry has greatly influenced nursing. The child develops a sense of self according to the type of feedback received from significant others (parental figures). Positive feedback reinforces the development of a "Good-Me" sense of self. A negative self-concept ("Bad-Me") is reinforced by feedback that is consistently negative and anxiety-provoking (Ball & Binder, 2003; Berger, 1999; Stuart & Laraia, 2001).

# Adolescence

The numerous changes in physical, emotional, and psychosocial status that characterize the adolescent years bring about rapid and often continuous changes in self-concept. Impressions about self from childhood may be internalized or challenged. The primary benchmark for arriving at an overall perception of self can change from family or parental values to those held by peers and friends or embodied in desired role models. Teens typically invest tremendous energies in appearances and social status and often fail to see their positive traits if they feel deficient in these areas. Adolescents often cannot separate their opinion of their own body image, for instance, from their overall self-concept; the teen who views herself as fat, when in fact she is emaciated, is likely to have a disturbed self-concept based on her distorted body image, regardless of what other positive qualities she may possess (Ball & Bindler, 2003; Berger, 1999).

# Adulthood

Self-concept continues to develop and change as an individual progresses through the adult years. Periods of relative stability in self-image may be interspersed with realizations of physical changes in body size, proportion, characteristics, and energy levels, all of which will influence perception of self. Involvement in family, work, and

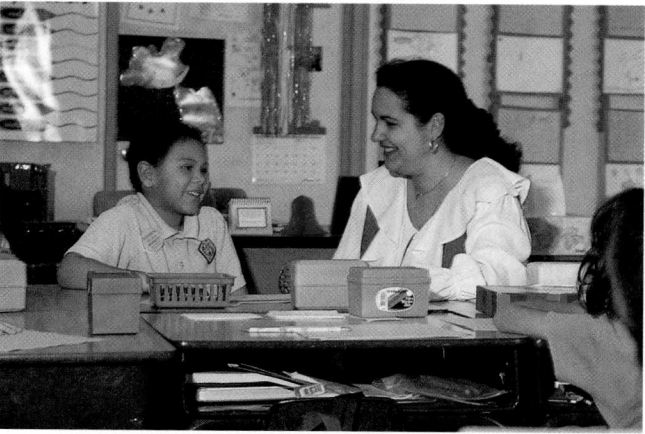

**Figure 43-3** For a school-age child, praise from teachers and a feeling of accomplishment in school can boost self-esteem.

## CLINICAL ALERT

### Teens and Self-Concept

Because of their emphasis on body image, teens are at particular risk for feelings of disturbed body image, which may lead to serious health concerns, such as anorexia nervosa and bulimia nervosa. The nurse needs to learn to distinguish between what might be a normal body image distortion ("I wish I were 3 inches taller.") and one that can have serious, even fatal, consequences ("Weighing 100 pounds is the most important thing in the world for me."). Determining a teen's self-concept and the importance she places on different aspects of self will help the nurse know which perceptions are normal reactions to the changes of adolescence and which are potentially harmful (Muscari, 1998).

## LEGAL AND ETHICAL ISSUES

### Confidentiality

Breeching confidentiality presents the potential problem of destroying adolescents' beginning trust in the health care system. Discuss the limits of confidentiality with adolescents regarding mandatory reporting of specific aspects of their behaviors and lives. Disclosure of information may cause psychological, social, and physical harm for some clients (Ball & Bindler, 2003).

community obligations and activities often contributes significantly to an individual's self-concept, as roles and responsibilities change and new roles are introduced. Healthy adjustment to these changes usually leads to a positive self-concept (Figure 43-4).

As the years pass, the older adult's perception of self continues to develop. Learning to adapt to the numerous physical changes that normally occur with aging, such as diminished eyesight and hearing, lower stamina levels, loss and change in color of hair, can be a true challenge for many individuals (Figure 43-5). Accompanying these changes is often the desire to look back on one's life and evaluate its overall success. Such reminiscence is usually a critical factor in an older adult's self-concept (Eliopoulos, 1999; Stuart and Laraia, 2001).

## Factors Affecting Self-Concept

There is a universal need for positive self-concept, which includes a high degree of self-esteem and self-acceptance. This need develops in childhood as a result of the approval

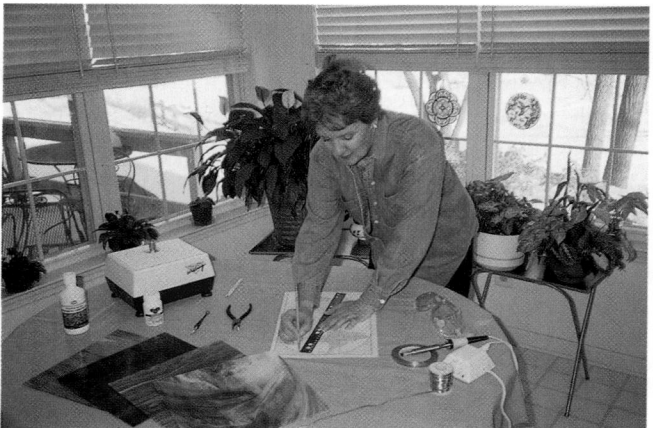

**Figure 43-4    The mature adult's self-concept can be enhanced by learning new skills and enjoying new activities.**

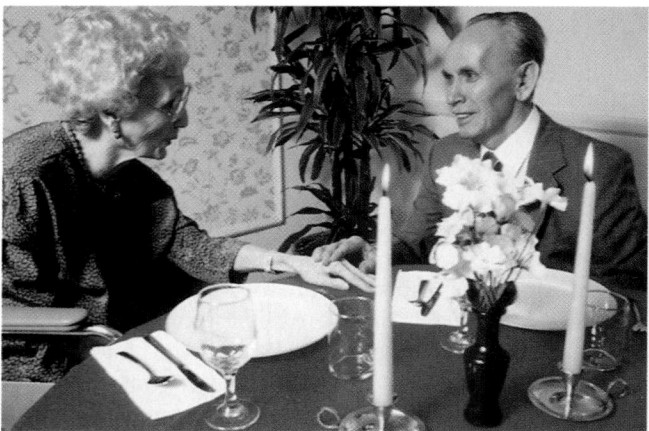

**Figure 43-5    Older adults need to adjust their self-concept, especially body image, in accordance with physical changes that affect appearance.**

the child receives from parents and other adults. Any type of threat (real or imagined, actual or anticipated) may challenge one's self-concept (Muscari, 1998).

## Altered Health Status

Illness evokes anxiety in most people; in turn, anxiety can result in illness. Every client will have some element of anxiety that influences behavioral and emotional responses. Most ill people are somewhat uneasy, especially if they are being treated in an unfamiliar environment. When anxiety level is heightened, recovery is compromised. Nurses, as professionals who focus on the human response to illness, must be aware of the anxiety level of clients to promote more effective adaptation. Table 43-3 shows common stressors experienced during illness.

By their very nature, some illnesses may impair self-concept. For example, there is a social stigma against mental illness; the reactions of other people to the mentally ill person affect the client's self-perceptions. Many people fear cancer and isolate those affected with the disease. A diagnosis of acquired immunodeficiency syndrome (AIDS) may also carry a stigma leading to low self-esteem. Society often shuns those with AIDS, which may make them feel embarrassed or ashamed about their illness. To improve clients' quality of life, the nurse caring for individuals with any of these disorders must intervene to promote positive self-concept.

Compromised health status that requires surgery can also lead to several psychological alterations, including an impaired body image. Altered body image may result from loss of a body part or function; surgical procedures often threaten body image. Some procedures (e.g., mastectomy, amputation, colostomy) may leave the individual feeling mutilated or flawed. Other common sequelae of surgery—decreased independence, loss of control, and disruption of routine—can also negatively affect self-concept. Self-esteem deficits related to surgery often include interference with

| TABLE 43-3 | STRESSORS ASSOCIATED WITH ILLNESS |
|---|---|
| Threat | Example |
| Threats to physical safety | Undergoing painful procedures (the thought of receiving an injection evokes anxiety in many) |
| | Fear of pain |
| | Fear of death |
| Threat to psychological integrity | One's image of self is threatened or challenged by new situations (such as moving to a nursing home) |
| Inability to exert control | Having little or no input into important decisions. Clients often feel as if they have no input into decision making regarding their treatment plan |
| | Loss of control may have a negative impact on self-concept and self-esteem, which in turn evokes anxiety |
| Unmet biologic needs | Hunger |
| | Thirst |
| | Urge to eliminate and lack of bathroom or privacy for toileting |
| | Physical pain, discomfort |

## STOP AND THINK

### Stigmatization of Illness

- Do you believe that there is a stigma against the mentally ill?

- What is your rationale for your answer?

- How do you feel about caring for someone infected with human immunodeficiency virus?

- Are there thoughts of blame directed toward the person with AIDS?

- What about the stigma against individuals with cancer?

role performance and interference with sexuality (Stuart & Laraia, 2001).

Bodily changes as a result of surgery have different meanings to different individuals. For example, consider a mastectomy. The woman whose feminine identity is symbolized by a voluptuous shape will likely be adversely affected by the surgery.

## Developmental Transitions

Developmental processes may also affect self-concept by introducing changes or challenges to an individual's identity, body image, self-esteem, and role expectations. For example, pregnancy is a process with resultant changes in all these factors of self-concept (Figure 43-6). In the early part of pregnancy, the woman incorporates the baby into her self-image. As the pregnancy progresses, the woman's body image adjusts to accommodate the idea that the baby is a separate individual (Kelly, 2001). After delivery, the woman who has positive self-esteem will accept and love the baby. One who feels unlovable or unattractive may make disparaging remarks about the infant and have difficulty bonding appropriately and adjusting to the life changes a new baby introduces. New roles of mother and parent need to be incorporated into a revised self-concept, and identity and self-esteem must be adjusted on the basis of new expectations.

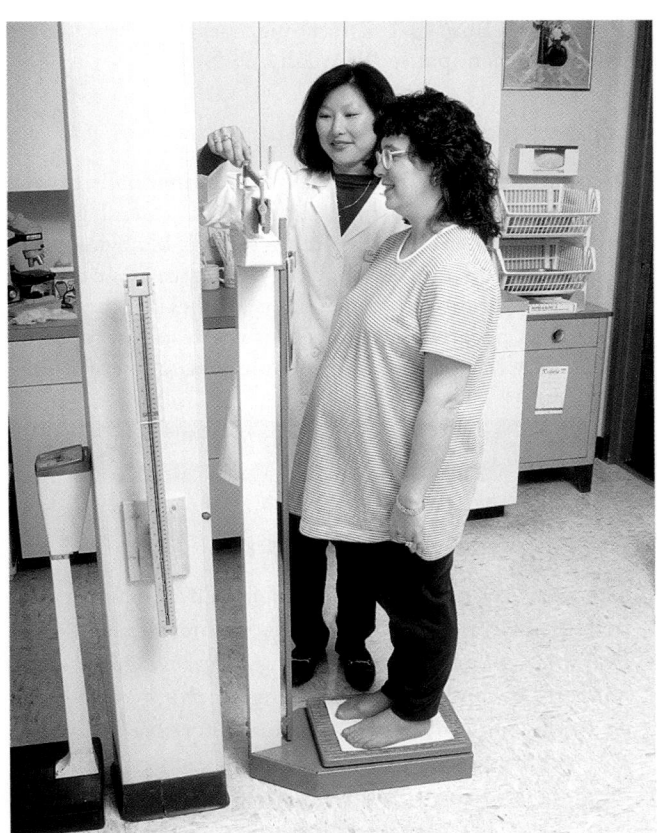

**Figure 43-6    Body image changes with developmental events such as pregnancy.**

Another example of a developmental issue that can affect the self-concept of an individual is menopause. The nurse must understand the meaning of this transitional period to the client and know that it varies with each individual. This normal developmental transition in a woman's life may have a negative psychological impact on some women. Some people view the female climacteric (menopausal phase) as an indication of loss of femininity with resultant decrease in value as a person. Other women view menopause as a sign of freedom from the risk of childbearing. Box 43-1 lists some common misconceptions about menopause (Pasquali, 1999).

## Experience

Self-concept is also influenced by an individual's experiences. Individuals who have experienced several failures begin to view themselves as failures; their behavior often becomes self-fulfilling in that they perform at an unsuccessful level because they feel that is all they are capable of achieving. A negative self-concept is the result of repeated failures. On the other hand, people who achieve a task

begin to see themselves in a positive manner, thus setting the foundation for a positive self-concept (Seigley, 1999; Stuart & Laraia, 2001).

## Assessment

When assessing a client's self-concept, the nurse must consider both the client's developmental level and chronological age. Clients need to be addressed at a level that reflects their current condition as well as their cognitive competence. For example, very young clients and those with low literacy skills may not be able to read; thus, the use of pictures would be helpful.

It is necessary to determine the client's perception of self-concept and the factors affecting it. For example, an adjustment to and recovery from an appendectomy may be uneventful for one person and difficult for another. The person who sees the surgery as a means to recovery will be healthier than the one who feels mutilated by a scarred abdomen.

Behavior, thoughts, and emotions are affected by self-concept. It is important to attend to the client's verbal and nonverbal clues. Self-concept is reflected in a person's behavior and conversation. Individuals who feel they are unable to accomplish goals will experience changes in eating, sleeping, and activity patterns (Barker, 2000).

The Nursing Strategy box offers some questions useful in assessing body image and self-esteem. Table 43-4 lists some indicators of high and low levels of self-esteem.

To provide quality care, the nurse must determine the client's strengths. Doing so enables assessment of characteristics that can be used for coping and problem solving. The client's strengths are a foundation on which to build therapeutic interventions. Some areas to assess include the client's ability to:

- Develop and maintain appropriate relationships
- Care for self in order to meet basic needs
- Adapt to stressors in a positive manner

The nurse should encourage clients to make a list of all the positive things they have done and then review the list. Also, the nurse can help clients identify how they have handled problems in the past: "When you were in a similar situation, what did you do? Was it helpful? Are you willing to try that now? If not, what else can you do?"

## NURSING STRATEGY

### Body Image and Self-Esteem

The nurse can ask the following questions when assessing body image and self-esteem:

#### Body Image

- What do you like best about your body?
- What do you like least about your body?
- If you could change how you look, what would you change?

#### Self-Esteem

- What do you like best about yourself?
- What do you like least about yourself?
- How do you describe yourself to others?
- How would others describe you?
- What are your strengths and weaknesses?

| TABLE 43-4 | INDICATORS OF HIGH AND LOW SELF-ESTEEM |
| --- | --- |
| **High Self-Esteem** | **Low Self-Esteem** |
| **Communication** | |
| Assertive | Passive or aggressive |
| Direct and honest | Indirect, dishonest |
| **Posture** | |
| Erect | Stooped |
| Moves briskly | Slow movement and activity |
| **General Appearance** | |
| Well-groomed | Unkempt and dirty |
| **Eye Contact** | |
| Frequent and appropriate to context of situation | Avoidance or intrusive staring |
| **Speech** | |
| Well modulated | Monotone |
| Speech flows smoothly | Mumbling |
| | Hesitant |
| **Self-Care** | |
| Attends to own needs | Neglects own needs by always caring for others first |
| | Denies or minimizes own needs |
| **Self-Talk** | |
| Praises self | Puts self down |
| | Highly self-critical |
| **Behavior** | |
| Appropriate to situation and context of interpersonal relationship | Socially inappropriate |
| | Violates social norms |
| | Counterproductive |
| **Measure of Worth** | |
| Values self | Has feelings of worthlessness |
| **Decision Making** | |
| Makes decisions appropriately for context of situation | Indecisive |
| | Hesitant |
| **Locus of Control** | |
| Internal | External |
| **Autonomy** | |
| Self-directed | Overly dependent on others |
| **Emotions** | |
| Able to experience a wide range of emotions | Wide range of emotions inappropriately expressed |
| Varies appropriately according to situation | Hostile |

Data from Stuart, G. W., & Laraia, M. T. (2001). *Principles and practices of psychiatric nursing* (7th ed.). St. Louis: Mosby.

The nurse should ask clients to describe their appearance and abilities. This information is an indicator of awareness of strengths as well as limitations; it is also important to assess the personal meaning of these assets and liabilities to clients.

## Nursing Diagnosis

Individuals experiencing self-concept disturbances usually have feelings of anxiety, hostility, guilt, and shame. Self-concept alterations affect every aspect of a person's life: emotions, relationships, and functional ability.

The nurse must conduct a thorough assessment to determine the nature and extent of problems to formulate accurate nursing diagnoses. Because of the extensive impact of self-concept problems, several diagnoses may be established by the nurse. Box 43-2 shows some primary nursing diagnoses associated with self-concept disturbances as defined by the North American Nursing Diagnosis Association (NANDA, 2003).

## Outcome Identification and Planning

For clients with an altered self-concept, a major nursing goal is to promote the client's sense of well-being and to facilitate growth. This involves teaching coping skills and the effective use of personal resources.

Together the nurse and client develop specific goals; mutually established goals encourage the client to assume an active role in recovery. Realistic planning involves examination of options and identification of available resources and methods to help a client regain responsibility for self-care. Realistic goals should be stated in terms of specific behavior that is measurable and should have an appropriate time frame for evaluation of outcome achievement.

## Implementation

Regardless of the setting in which they practice, nurses will inevitably encounter clients who are experiencing alterations in self-concept. Whether a client is experiencing optimal level of health or an alteration in health, a high degree of self-esteem is important to a positive outcome. The nurse needs to find ways to support positive self-esteem. High self-esteem can be associated with several different dimensions of the whole person, such as success in relationships, intelligence, or in being a member who is held in high regard of an ethnic or cultural group. In attempting to support the client's high self-esteem, the nurse should try to learn sources of self-esteem for the client and reinforce them (Edminson, 2001; Carnevale, 1999).

### Initiate Therapeutic Interaction

Self-concept, or lack of it, affects the nurse-client relationship. The nurse is a role model of an individual who has self-respect and also respects others. By using a nonjudgmental approach, the nurse encourages clients to feel more positive about themselves.

---

### BOX 43-2 NURSING DIAGNOSES

- *Disturbed Body Image*
- *Parental Role Conflict*
- *Disturbed Personal Identity*
- *Ineffective Role Performance*
- *Chronic Low Self-Esteem*
- *Situational Low Self-Esteem*
- *Disturbed Personal Identity*
- *Anxiety*
- *Social Isolation*
- *Hopelessness*
- *Powerlessness*

From NANDA. (2003). *Nursing diagnoses: Definitions and classification 2003–2004*. Philadelphia: Author.

---

### STOP AND THINK

### Defense Mechanisms Related to Body Image Changes

Individuals who have a disturbed body image protect themselves with a variety of ego-defense mechanisms. Behaviors include "acting-out," self-destructive behavior, anorexia, overeating, use of drugs, isolating themselves, and retreating to thoughts of fantasy.

- How should the nurse respond to clients with a disturbed body image from a surgery such as a mastectomy?

- What are potential cues of defense mechanisms the nurse might see with the client who has recently had a colostomy?

- Who could the nurse refer clients to for assistance with defense mechanisms related to body image disturbances?

The use of open-ended statements facilitates open, honest communication. Active listening is essential in working with clients experiencing self-concept alterations. By thoughtfully applying therapeutic communication skills, the nurse facilitates the development of trust and rapport (Figure 43-7).

## Support Healthy Defense Mechanisms

Use of defense mechanisms is a common reaction to anxiety or a perceived threat. When caring for a client with altered or threatened self-concept, it is wise to first identify the client's strengths and successful coping mechanisms before formulating and implementing a plan of care. It is important to not take away a client's defensive processes until another method of coping with anxiety has been developed. For example, breaking through a client's denial too soon can result in overwhelming anxiety. On the other hand, encouraging the use of denial beyond its helpful period will result in reality distortion (Stuart & Laraia, 2001).

## Ensure Satisfaction of Needs

The relationship between satisfaction of basic needs and psychological comfort is undeniable. When needs are unmet, anxiety increases.

### Physical Needs

Self-concept stems in part from the client's perception of personal appearance, competencies, and limitations. It includes the client's self-perception as well as perceptions of others. By assisting the client to maintain personal appearance, the nurse is also assisting the client to improve self-esteem. Being unable to meet one's basic needs usually results in self-concept impairment. Self-

esteem is generally decreased as a person becomes more dependent on others.

Providing for the client's well-being and comfort is the foundation of quality nursing care. When clients are treated in a caring, competent manner and their physical needs are met, self-concept is positively influenced (Hollinger-Smith, 2000; Stuart & Laraia, 2001).

### Psychosocial Needs

Uncertainty escalates anxiety. Explain procedures, telling the client what is expected and what is going to occur. All clients in every health care setting need clear statements of expected behavior. The following nursing actions promote the client's psychological safety:

- Respect a client's privacy. Loss of privacy triggers anxiety in most individuals. During treatment in any setting, personal probing questions must be asked; procedures often violate physical space and can be offensive; elimination processes often occur in the presence of others. Be sure to protect privacy as much as possible.
- Treat each client as an individual worthy of dignity. This means being sensitive to the feelings of others and recognizing that their feelings may differ from yours and those of other clients.
- Encourage the client to be as independent as possible, while providing assistance as needed.

## Promote Positive Self-Esteem Across the Life Span

### Childhood

The child's self-concept continues to develop over time and is greatly influenced by interactions and experiences with others. The nurse must consider that the child needs to feel successful and competent with tasks.

Some of the changes occurring with physical growth and maturation may be anxiety-provoking for the child; for instance, anxiety may result when the child loses baby teeth or experiences menstruation for the first time. The onset of physical changes of puberty can be frightening or unsettling to the child. The nurse is most effective by providing education and support and serving as a role model. The Client Education box provides information essential in helping parents promote positive self-concept development in children.

### Adolescence

Adolescents' sense of self is greatly influenced by how others, especially peers, view them. Acceptance and a sense of belonging to a peer group influence the adolescent's sense of worth and well-being (Figure 43-8). Feelings about one's self intensify during puberty. Adolescents may become very self-conscious because they often "feel that others are as concerned about them as they are themselves. Thus, they're overpowered by self-consciousness and the feeling that 'everyone is looking at them.' To blend in with peers,

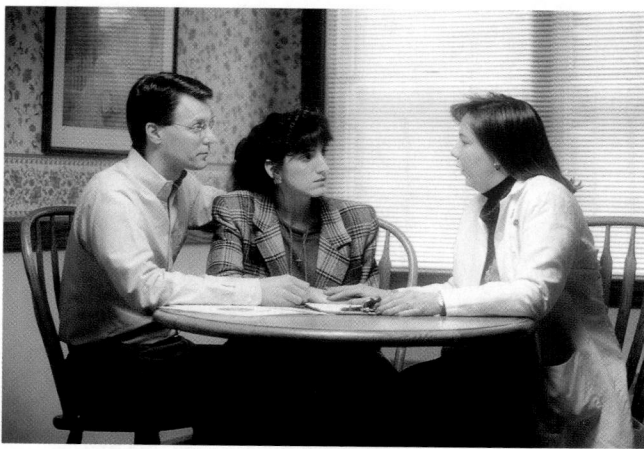

**Figure 43-7**    **A nurse uses therapeutic communication to establish trust and also to encourage a positive self-concept for this young couple.** *Photo courtesy of Bellevue, The Women's Hospital, Niskayuna, NY*

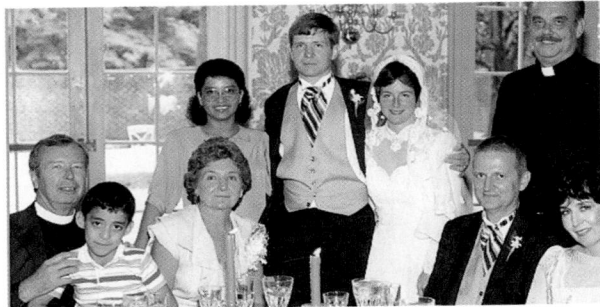

**Figure 43-9** Young adulthood often means assuming new roles. What role changes are this newly married couple likely to experience?

teenagers focus on complexion, hair, and clothing" (Muscari, 1998, p. 28).

As adolescents' bodies change, they must keep revising their body images. A severe or deep-rooted distortion of body image may be a manifestation of a mental illness, such as anorexia nervosa or bulimia nervosa, which occurs primarily during adolescence. The nurse needs to help the adolescent redirect energies and focus on positive traits and to view self as a compilation of many factors, not just one (e.g., weight, dieting).

### Adulthood

As adults continue to mature, self-concept changes in response to new self-perceptions and roles (Figure 43-9).

Young adults make a transition to independent living without parental assistance. The degree of ease or discomfort in making such a transition affects the young adult's self-concept by demonstrating a sense of competency.

The self-concept of an older person is the culmination of a variety of factors, including life experiences and interactions with others. Some life experiences that shape the older person's self-concept are adjusting to role loss and dealing with the loss of significant others. "Many of the realities of aging make the elderly vulnerable to self-perception problems. Older adults suffer numerous losses, have a decreased ability to protect themselves, and are confronted with many subtle messages that they are misplaced in a youth-oriented society" (Eliopoulos, 1999, pp. 362–363). Spending time with significant others may increase the older client's self-esteem by making him feel valued (Figure 43-10).

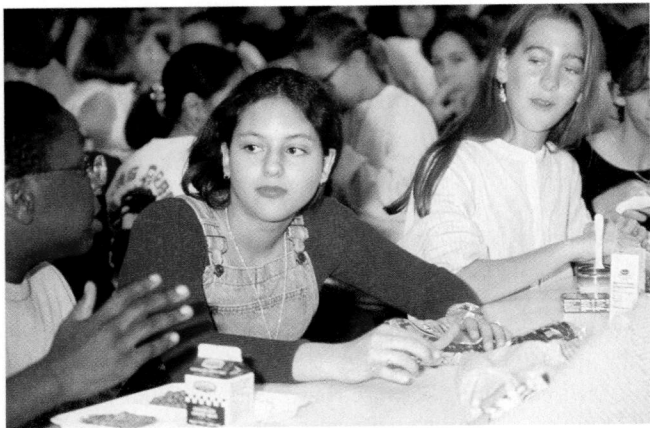

**Figure 43-8** Peers exert much influence on the adolescent's changing self-concept.

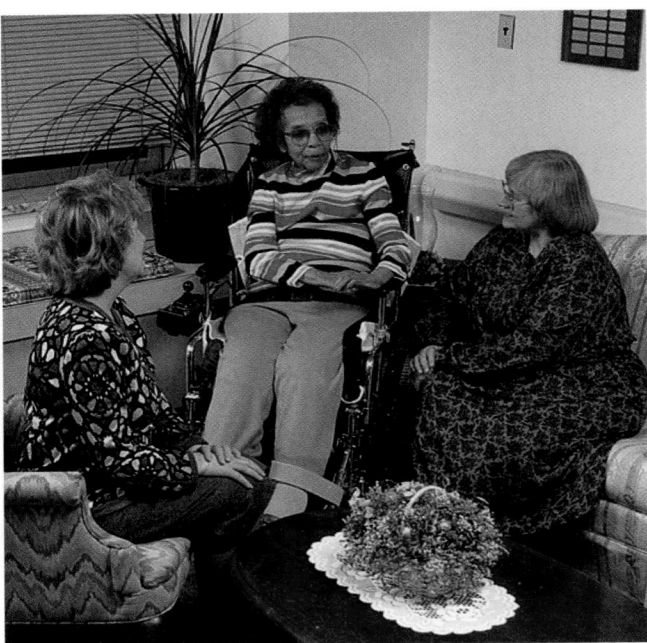

**Figure 43-10** Identify some factors that may contribute positively to this older client's self-esteem.

## RESEARCH FOCUS

**Title of Study:** Psychological aspects of breast reconstruction.

**Study Purpose:** To explore the rationale of women's decisions to have breast reconstruction following mastectomy for breast cancer

**Methods:** A retrospective study of published research articles was conducted to identify psychological outcomes for women following breast reconstruction.

**Findings:**

• More than one-third of the women reported anxiety and depression 1 year after a mastectomy. They perceived mastectomy as a blow to body-image, self-esteem, their femininity, and sense of wholeness. Wearing a prosthesis was a constant reminder of loss and disfigurement. The prosthesis was uncomfortable and inconvenient. Thirty percent opted for reconstructive surgery.

• Women who chose reconstruction were younger, married, and had higher social economic status than women who did not choose reconstruction.

• Following reconstruction, the women believed they made a better adjustment to cancer treatment and were confident of the outcome. Some women reported their decision to have reconstruction was a way to cope with their diagnosis. Many believed that the surgeon's willingness to do the surgery was an indication that the cancer would not return. A majority reported satisfaction with the results of reconstructive surgery as well as having increased self-esteem and self-confidence and a better quality of life.

• Women with unrealistic expectations expressed dissatisfaction with the results, stating the breast did not look normal. Some reported the reconstructive surgery as a traumatic experience.

• It was difficult for some women to make a decision soon after the cancer diagnosis.

**Implications:** Clients need psychological support and education throughout the decision-making process. Nurses can assist clients to set realistic expectations, provide support to clients, and serve as client advocates.

Harcourt, D., & Rumsey, N. (2001). Psychological aspects of breast reconstruction: A review of the literature. *Journal of Advanced Nursing, 35*(4), 477–487.

---

## BOX 43-3 FACTORS CONTRIBUTING TO SELF-CONCEPT ALTERATIONS IN THE OLDER CLIENT

• Changes in environment

• Ageism (social stigma against older adults)

• Loss of significant others (including pets)

• Social isolation

• Illness, acute or chronic

• Financial change

---

Throughout life, the individual has developed coping resources. Because self-concept is intertwined with competency, it is important for nurses to allow older clients the time to complete tasks that are meaningful to them (Zauszniewski & Martin, 1999). Some of the many factors that may negatively affect the older adult's self-esteem are shown in Box 43-3. The nurse can employ several interventions to boost the older client's self-concept. When caring for older clients, it is important to plan activities that promote a healthy self-concept (Grendell, 2000; Stuart & Laraia, 2001).

---

## CLIENT REFLECTIONS

### Living with Chronic Illness

Aging compounded by illness and pain brings about many role changes. Self-identity is threatened as a person takes on a new role or exits from a former role. Students, nurses, and older clients viewed master art pieces and explained how the art represented the effects of living with chronic illness. Responses of older persons with chronic illness included: "I try to smile and act like everything is OK. Even [when] taking medications, I have pain. You just learn to live with it. You try to be sociable, but it isn't easy."

"Of course I've lived with my poor eyesight for many years, and I do the best I can with it, and try not to be depressed. Now I'm getting cataracts, and my eyesight is getting worse. So I just make up my mind to do the best I can day by day."

How would you respond to these comments?

Hodges, H., Keeley, A., & Grier, E. (2001). Masterworks of art and chronic illness experiences in the elderly. *Journal of Advanced Nursing, 36*(3), 389–398.

## CLIENT EDUCATION

### Promoting Self-Concept in the Older Client

✓ Increase socialization.

✓ Encourage involvement and participation in care.

✓ For clients in the home setting, urge family members to allow client to be involved with household tasks and routines as much as possible.

✓ Elicit client feedback.

✓ Use touch to decrease feelings of isolation and to promote feelings of security and acceptance.

✓ Modesty is often important to the older client; therefore, maintain and promote privacy. For example, perform physical examinations or procedures without completely exposing the client.

✓ Do not remove all personal belongings because these are often invested with symbolic meaning (for example, let the older woman keep her purse at her bedside).

✓ Demonstrate patience; allow clients time to complete sentences and to finish one task before moving on to the next.

✓ Involve family or significant others as much as possible in the provision of care.

✓ Encourage the client to reminisce, especially focusing on individual strengths and accomplishments.

## Evaluation

A client's behavior and attitudes will reflect the degree of progress toward restoring an altered self-concept. The nurse must reconsider the alignment of the client's targeted self-concept with the plan of care to assess if the two are still congruent. Input from family members or significant others can be useful in seeing the client in a larger context of differing roles and expectations and may also highlight some of the similarities and differences between the client's perceived self-image and the impression of those closest to him.

Another crucial factor in evaluating success of attaining goals outlined in the care plan is the consideration of time. Because self-concept is based on personal attitudes, feelings, and impressions, it often requires months or even years to change. Nurses, clients, and their families all need to learn to be patient and to work together to improve or restore a client's self concept (Ackley & Ladwig, 2002).

##  CASE STUDY/NURSING CARE PLAN

Todd Lloyd is a 31-year-old civil engineer who has just left his job of 10 years to care full-time for his newborn daughter, Sarah. He and his wife decided that, after their child was born, she would return to work full-time outside the home, and he would be the primary caregiver for their daughter during the day. Mr. Lloyd arrives at the clinic, and states, "I am very eager and excited about being a full-time dad, but I'm also a little nervous because I really don't know what to expect." Mr. Lloyd is actually here for his newborn daughter's checkup, but asked that you check his blood pressure as he had not had it taken in several years. His blood pressure is 138/90, his pulse is 82/minute, and his respiratory rate = 18/minute. In the meantime, Sarah is "doing very well" and is without any problems for her 6-month checkup.

### Assessment

Your assessment finds that this is an open, communicating young family. The father is assuming a new role of "househusband and child-care provider." The child is developing without complications, and the father is somewhat stressed with his new role. In addition, the father has a lack of knowledge regarding the new parenting role.

### Nursing Diagnosis

*Ineffective Role Performance* related to change in roles and usual patterns of responsibility, as evidenced by verbalization of concern over lack of knowledge about new role.

**NOC:** Coping; Psychological Adjustment: Life change

**NIC:** Role Enhancement

*(continues)*

**CASE STUDY/NURSING CARE PLAN** *(continued)*

### Expected Outcomes

The client will:

1. Explain specific concerns about new roles by the end of his first appointment.
2. Identify realistic perception of role by the end of his first appointment.
3. State personal strengths by the end of his first appointment.
4. Verbalize acceptance and satisfaction with role performance after one month.

### Planning/Interventions/Rationales

1. Encourage the client to express his feelings about his new role. *Opens the door to communication and problem solving.*
2. Outline with client what aspects of his role(s) will be changing and what will be the same. *Helps client identify the ways in which his role is changing, so he can face the changes with a realistic frame of mind. Also highlights similarities, not just differences, between his past and present roles, thus helping client feel less overwhelmed.*
3. Assist the client in identifying specific concerns he has regarding the change in roles. *Helps the client determine exactly what his concerns are, so they can be addressed.*
4. Encourage client to discuss concerns with wife and to seek help together. *Support of spouse will be critical to client's success in overcoming concerns about changing roles.*
5. Help client gain confidence and competence with new role by demonstrating new role behaviors, offering literature and resources, and providing referral to parenting courses or counselors. *Assures client that resources are available to help him meet his needs and helps lessen his anxiety and his feeling of being overwhelmed.*
6. Have client return-demonstrate new behaviors and offer encouragement and additional teaching. *Allows client to try out new behaviors in a "safe" environment and provides a means for immediate feedback.*
7. Ask client for feedback on the new behaviors and information acquired. *Provides chance for client to evaluate progress in new role, which will increase client's confidence.*

### Evaluation

Mr. Lloyd is able to identify specific concerns about his new role as parent and has demonstrated a growing competence in some of the behaviors that will support this new role. He read the literature and has ordered a videotape designed for new parents. He is also planning to subscribe to a newsletter entitled "The Full-Time Father." Mr. Lloyd agrees that his wife's input would be very valuable to his gaining comfort and confidence in his new role, and he agrees to visit the clinic again with her in a week.

## Key Concepts

- Self-concept (an individual's perception of self) affects every aspect of a person's life.
- A person who sees oneself as a competent individual will behave competently and vice versa.
- Self-concept consists of interrelated components: identity, body image, self-ideal, self-esteem, and role performance.
- A well-formulated identity provides the answer to the question "Who am I?" and may consist of a person's name, family status, occupation, and various roles.
- Body image refers to a person's mental picture of and attitudes about her body. It includes physical attributes and characteristics, appearance, and performance.
- Self-esteem is the individual's generalized sense of worth and value.
- Role refers to a set of expected behaviors that are determined by social norms.

- The development of self-concept begins at birth and depends, to a degree, on interactions with others as the child grows and matures.
- The person's developmental level affects self-concept; with maturity comes a stronger self-concept.
- Illness evokes anxiety in most people; anxiety can cause illness. Any threat to self-concept arouses anxiety. When anxiety level is heightened, recovery is compromised.
- The sick role is a set of social expectations met by an ill person, such as being exempt from the usual social role responsibilities, and being obligated to get well and to seek competent help. Individuals sometimes take on a deviant sick role, and use their illness to receive attention, to gain control over others, or as a means of avoiding responsibilities.
- Surgery can result in body image disturbances. Altered body image results from loss of a body part or function, invasion of body space, and distortion of body image.

- Assessment of self-concept must consider both developmental level and chronological age.
- Identification of client strengths enables the nurse to determine the presence of factors the client can use for coping and problem solving.

## Review Questions and Activities

1. Consider self-concept and the factors that comprise it. How do these factors interface in contributing to overall self-concept?
2. Outline some of the specific factors that contribute to the development of self-concept throughout the life span.
3. What are some specific nursing strategies that you could use to promote the self-concept and comfort of a hospitalized client?
4. Refer to the chapter case study/nursing care plan. What other assessments might you expect to find in this client? How could the plan of care be modified to reflect these additional findings?

## Web Resources

American Holistic Nurses' Association
    http://www.ahna.org
American Nurses Association
    http://www.ana.org
American Psychiatric Nurses Association
    http://www.apna.org
American Psychological Association
    http://www.apa.org

## References

Ackley, B., & Ladwig, G. (2002). *Nursing diagnosis handbook: A guide to planning care.* St. Louis: Mosby.

Ball, J., & Bindler, R. (2003). *Pediatric nursing: Caring for children* (3rd ed.). Upper Saddle River, NJ: Prentice Hall.

Barker, M. (2000). Development of the adult. In K. Fortinash and P. Holoday-Worret (Eds.), *Psychiatric mental health nursing* (2nd ed.). St. Louis: Mosby.

Berger, K. S. (1999). *The developing person through childhood and adolescence* (4th ed.). New York: Worth.

Black, J., Hawks, J., & Keene, A. (2001). *Medical-surgical nursing: Clinical management for positive outcomes.* Philadelphia: W. B. Saunders.

Carnevale, F. A. (1999). Toward a cultural conception of the self. *Journal of Psychosocial Nursing, 37*(8), 26–31.

Crow, G. (2000). Knowing self. In F. Bower, *Nurses taking the lead: Personal qualities of effective leadership* (pp. 15–37). Philadelphia: W. B. Saunders.

Doenges, M., & Moorhouse, M. (1998). *Nurses pocket guide: Diagnoses, interventions, and rationales* (6th ed.) Philadelphia: F. A. Davis.

Edminson, K. (2001). Psychosocial dimensions of medical-surgical nursing. In J. Black, J. Hawks, & A. Keene (Eds.), *Medical-surgical nursing: Clinical management for positive outcomes.* Philadelphia: W. B. Saunders.

Eliopoulos, C. (1999). *Manual of gerontologic nursing* (2nd ed.). St. Louis: Mosby.

Erikson, E. (1963). *Childhood and society* (pp. 91–96). New York: W. W. Norton.

Grendell, R. (2000). Psychologic aspects of physiologic illness. In K. Fortinash & P. Holoday-Worret (Eds.), *Psychiatric mental health nursing* (2nd ed.). St. Louis: Mosby.

Harcourt, D., & Rumsey, N. (2001). Psychological aspects of breast reconstruction: A review of the literature. *Journal of Advances in Nursing, 35*(4), 477–487.

Hodges, H., Keeley, A. & Grier, E. (2001). Masterworks of art and chronic illness experiences in the elderly. *Journal of Advanced Nursing, 36*(3), 389–398.

Hollinger-Smith, L. (2000). The elderly. In K. Fortinash and P. Holoday-Worret (Eds.), *Psychiatric mental health nursing* (2nd ed. pp. 209–230). St. Louis: Mosby.

Kelly, G. (2001). *Sexuality today: The human perspective.* Boston: McGraw-Hill.

Muscari, M. E. (1998). Rebels with a cause: When adolescents won't follow medical advice. *American Journal of Nursing, 98*(12), 26–30.

North American Nursing Diagnosis Association (NANDA). (2003). *Nursing diagnoses: Definitions and classification 2003–2004.* Philadelphia: Author.

Oran, D. (2000). Children and adolescents. In K. Fortinash and P. Holoday-Worret (Eds.), *Psychiatric mental health nursing* (2nd ed., pp. 178–194) St. Louis: Mosby.

Orem, D. E. (2001). *Nursing: Concepts of practice* (6th ed.). St. Louis: Mosby.

Pasquali, E. A. (1999). The impact of premature menopause on women's experience of self. *Journal of Holistic Nursing, 17*(4), 346–364.

Peplau, H. (1992). Interpersonal relations: A theoretical framework for application in nursing practice. *Nursing Science Quarterly, 5,* 13–18.

Riegel, B., Dracup, K. & Glaser, D. (1998). A longitudinal causal model of cardiac invalidism following myocardial infarction. *Nursing Research, 47*(5), 285–292.

Seigley, L. A. (1999). Self-esteem and health behavior: Theoretic and empirical links. *Nursing Outlook, 47*(2), 74–77.

Stuart, G. W., & Laraia, M. T. (2001*). Principles and practices of psychiatric nursing* (7th ed.). St. Louis: Mosby.

Sullivan, H. S. (1953). *The interpersonal theory of psychiatry.* New York: Norton.

Zauszniewski, J. A., & Martin, M. H. (1999). Developmental task achievement and learned resourcefulness in healthy older adults. *Archives of Psychiatric Nursing, 13*(1), 41–47.

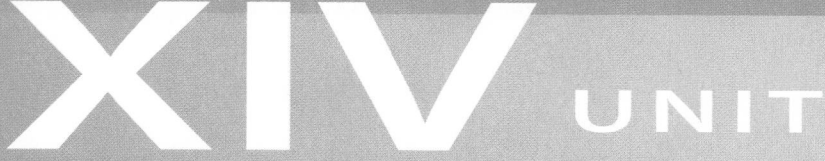

# XIV UNIT

# Role-Relationship

# 44 CHAPTER

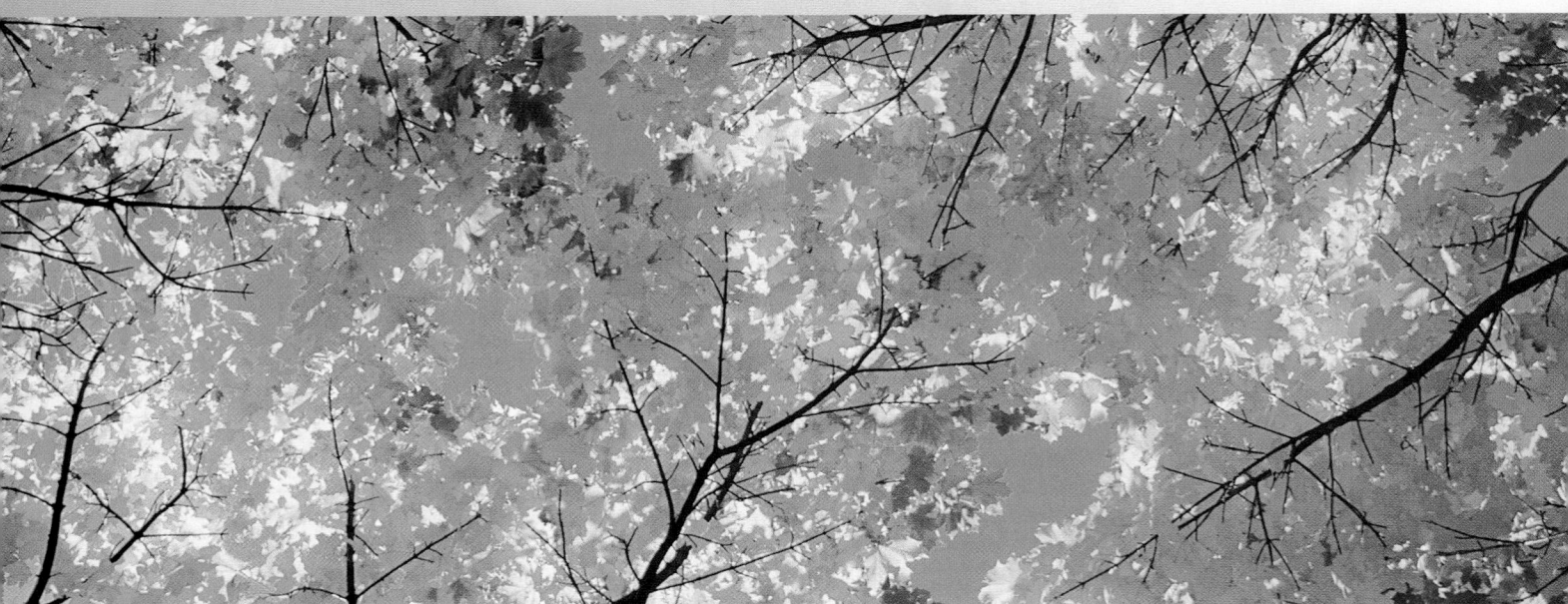

# Family, Roles, Relationships, and Social Support

Kathleen Lagana, RN, PhD

*"Don't try to be popular. Concentrate instead on competence, honesty, and fairness."*

*(Sharon LaDuke, 2000)*

# Chapter Competencies

## *Upon completion of this chapter, the reader should be able to:*

1. Describe the historical development of the concept of family.
2. Define structural-functional theory.
3. Discuss the roles evidenced in families.
4. Identify the concept of values as related to family.
5. Differentiate communication patterns present in families.
6. Evaluate the concept of power in the structure of the family.
7. Describe the processes of decision making and health in family.
8. Explain theories relevant to family processes.
9. Discuss family-based social support.
10. Describe mental health and family-based social support.
11. Identify the relationship between socioeconomic status and social support.
12. Discuss using the nursing process in supporting social support issues.

# Key Terms

| | | |
|---|---|---|
| actual social support | genogram | role overload |
| blended families | individualism | role strain |
| chaotic family power | locus of control | role stress |
| closed family system | nuclear dyads | role transition |
| cohabitate | nuclear family | situational role transitions |
| collectivism | open family system | social support |
| complementary family power | output | symmetrical (egalitarian) family power |
| ecomap | perceived social support | throughput |
| extended family | role competence | |
| family process | role conflict | |

Humans are social beings. As such, they congregate in small and usually biologically linked reciprocal groups. This social structure is particularly advantageous because of a relatively long pregnancy and the fact that

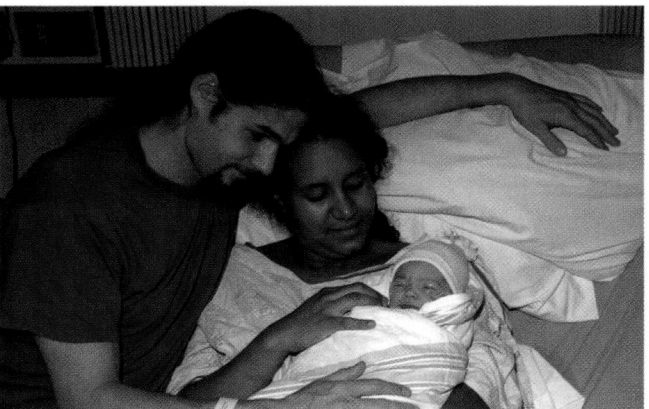

**Figure 44-1    Social support begins in infancy**

infants are born quite vulnerable and dependent. Human beings also have a relatively long maturation process to adulthood. Pregnant women, infants, and children require ongoing care from others to maintain health and safety. Providing for people in our social network is referred to as **social support** (Figure 44-1). The same need for caring relationships exists for adults in health and illness, as well as in old age. How social support is perceived or delivered varies across cultural groups and individual perceptions. The most common and long-term source of social support is the family, and the family is a key social institution that teaches social behavior to offspring. In addition, nursing can play a vital role in enhancing social support in individuals and families.

## Historical Trends of the Family as a Social Institution

Every society constructs specialized institutions to maintain and promote certain skills, values, or norms to be passed on between generations (Rokeach, 1973). Historically, the family has been recognized as a social institution that exists in some form in all cultures and societies (see Chapter 5 for cultural implications for the concept of family). As a social institution, the family has historically been responsible for socializing children with behaviors, knowledge, and skills they will need in the adult world (Hanson, 2001).

## The Family in Agrarian Times

Prior to the industrial revolution, agrarian economies predominated. Members of small groups worked together, and roles were clearly defined. Over time, genetic linkage was the inevitable outcome and the foundation was laid for the development of modern conjugal families. Family groups collected into small towns, increasing the complexity of society and social relationships. That complexity was the beginning of diversity in family structures (Hanson, 2001). The family, however, remained a stable economic unit and was responsible for socialization of the children. Patriarchal norms provided power to males as head of household and the legitimate voice for the family. Dependence on the family and other related small groups for basic needs led to the development of a cultural form known as **collectivism**. Collectivism called for loyalty and reciprocity to the group. Relationships formed slowly, tended to be genetically linked, and were long lasting. Collectivism was characterized by shared values and norms of behavior. Contemporary collectivism can be seen in rural settings and in developing countries with strong agrarian bases.

## Post-Industrial Revolution

Families have changed a great deal since the industrial revolution in the late 18th century. Following the industrial revolution, people moved away from their extended families on farms and in small towns to factory jobs in the cities. If the conjugal unit, including children, moved together, all were expected to work. Over time, socialization of children was increasingly delegated to institutions outside of the family. Urban lifestyles led to skill specializations and the need for unrelated individuals to provide for many basic needs, such as groceries, living quarters, or fictive (unrelated) kin. Relationships, while more superficial, were more readily established. Again, diversity increased and individual values began to gain favor over those of the original family unit.

### Individualism

**Individualism**, as this phenomenon is known, flourished in urban settings and has become the predominant cultural type in the United States and many other industrialized countries. In traditional societies, alienation from family, the source of most resources, could threaten survival. However, in urban settings where other supportive relationships are relatively easy to form, individuals are more likely to choose a more independent lifestyle and form nuclear families.

In contemporary society, where individualism still predominates, there is a growing recognition that closer family relations lead to increased care for children and older adults. This is especially apparent in light of the scarcity of government funding for family services. Collectivism is of value to health care providers looking for family-based resources for their clients. In fact, family-centered health care is not only advantageous from the perspective of resources; it also takes advantage of the health-promoting effect of family-based social support (Dracup, 2002).

## The Purposes of Family

The family serves two purposes. The first of these, as noted earlier, is as a social institution to socialize children. The second purpose is to serve the needs of the individual family members. As a cooperative system, the family shares food, shelter, property, values, social support, and activities, with the long-term goal of health maintenance and survival of the group. At a more fundamental level, cooperative social group behavior in human beings promotes the survival of the species (Ballard, 2001). Nurses working with families are usually guided by a theoretical model that helps to describe, explain, or predict dynamic family processes and needed nursing interventions. Theoretical models that are used frequently in working with families include structural-functional theory, family stress theory, family development theory, and family systems theory. These theoretical frameworks will be discussed in this chapter where appropriate. Structural-functional theory is especially useful for nurses to understand the processes that form shared family experiences.

## Structural-Functional Theory

Generally, the family meets the needs of individual members and the group by assigning certain roles and responsibilities to each family member. Structure helps family members meet personal and collective goals. Structural-functional theory is based on the assumptions that (1) the family functions to serve the needs of its members, and (2) that individual behavior is based on norms and values learned within the family (Artinian, 1999).

### Family Function

Membership in a healthy family is fundamental to the stabilization of adult personalities and the maintenance of health in individual family members. A healthy family demonstrates certain characteristics (Box 44-1). These characteristics include communication and time together, respect for individuality and trust among the members, play and leisure time, and reciprocal social support (Hanson, 2001).

Married people are generally happier than those who are not married (Friedman, 1998). In addition, married

| BOX 44-1 | CHARACTERISTICS OF THE HEALTHY FAMILY |
|---|---|

- Strong communication skills
- Time spent together
- Respect for individuality
- Trust among family members
- Adequate play and leisure time
- Reciprocal social support

Adapted from Hanson, S. M. (2001). *Family nursing and health care: Theory, practice, and research* (2nd ed.). Philadelphia: F. A. Davis Publishers.

individuals experience less mortality related to cardiovascular or immunological disease. While many factors contribute to family health, it appears that human beings generally fare better in small reciprocal groups than alone.

According to Friedman (1998), the family has specific benefits and functions (see Box 44-2). Specifically, families provide for the majority of health-promotion activities and the management of minor health problems (Spector, 2001).

How well a family functions depends on the structural organization of the family. Family functioning is greatly affected by cultural and social diversity and by the recognition of individuals' rights. Nurses must develop strong family assessment skills as well as cross-cultural competency. The way a family is organized to address functional needs is known as **family process**. By assessing family structure, the nurse gains insight about risks and strengths that may influence health status.

## Family Structure

Several aspects of family structure must be assessed. The first of these is the family form. Family forms can be tra-

| BOX 44-2 | FAMILY FUNCTIONS |
|---|---|

- Affective function
- Socialization
- Conjugal/reproductive function
- Family coping function
- Economic function
- Basic needs function
- Health-promotion function

Adapted from Friedman, M. (1998). *Family nursing: Theory and practice* (4th ed.). Norwalk, CT: Appleton & Lange.

ditional or nontraditional (see Box 44-3). The law sanctions some family forms, but not others. For example, the law in most societies ensures certain rights, responsibilities, and privileges to couples who are legally married. One of the most important of these is the right to make health care decisions for one's family member, if for some reason that family member cannot decide for himself.

A common family form in the world today is the traditional multigenerational **extended family** (family members from previous generations, such as grandparents, uncles, and aunts) (Friedman, 1998). Agrarian societies are more notable for this family form. As discussed earlier, the movement of families to urban centers promoted the emergence of the traditional **nuclear family**. The nuclear family consists of a married heterosexual man and woman and their biologic children, and accounts for only 36% of families in the United States (United States Bureau of the Census, 1998). **Nuclear dyads** are married heterosexual couples without children, either by choice or situation.

Nontraditional family forms include **blended families** in which children live with one birth parent and one stepparent. Other nontraditional family forms include single adults living communally or alone and single heterosexual or homosexual couples who **cohabitate** (live together without being married), with or without children (Ballard, 2001). Some of these nontraditional family forms are not legally sanctioned in some states and risk the loss of decision-making power. Some legal approaches can avoid such challenges, such as the medical durable power of attorney, which is an individual's legally binding written assignment of decision-making power. However, few people have a medical durable power of attorney, placing some nontraditional families in a less-than-empowered state. Nurses and

| BOX 44-3 | FAMILY FORMS |
|---|---|

*Traditional Family Forms*

Multigenerational extended family

Nuclear family

Nuclear dyads

*Nontraditional Family Forms*

Blended families

Single adults living alone

Single adults living communally

Cohabitating heterosexual couples

Cohabitating homosexual couples

Adapted from Ballard, N. (2001). Family structure, function, and process. In S. Hansen (Ed.), *Family nursing and health care: Theory, practice, and research* (2nd ed. pp. 79–99). Philadelphia: F. A. Davis; Friedman, M. (1998). *Family nursing: Theory and practice* (4th ed.). Norwalk, CT: Appleton & Lange.

## STOP AND THINK

### Constructing a Genogram

● What do you tell the client if she asks what good making a genogram serves?

● What could be the benefits of the client getting a copy of the genogram?

● What interventions can the nurse employ after reading a client's genogram?

other health care professionals can become entrenched in legal and ethical dilemmas regarding rights of the family and individuals. Clients must be informed of their rights at the time of accessing health care. A family-centered approach takes into consideration the unique challenges that nontraditional families may face (Farvis, 2002).

### Genogram

An easy-to-use tool to assess a family's structure is the **genogram**. The genogram is a graphic representation of the family form. Normally, nurses can gather data on three generations: the grandparents, the parents, and the children. Collection of multigenerational data assists the nurse in identifying family-linked health problems, as well as possible sources of support. It is important to remember that because of variations in family form, family members may not be genetically related. The genogram may also include extended family members if they are living in nearby or adjacent houses and are integral to the family functioning on a regular and ongoing basis (Figure 44-2). A genogram demonstrates how relationships between family members are indicated (Estes, 2002).

Members' ages, occupations, health status, and marital status as well as the nature of the relationships among family members, and the strength and quality of those bonds are graphically illustrated. Constructing a genogram with a client can assist in understanding the family dynamics that influence health.

## Family Role Structure

Families tend to develop roles for each member of the group. A variety of formal and informal roles are enumerated in Box 44-4. Having a determined role in the family contributes to a sense of belonging among its members. Family role-taking is best understood from the perspective of role theory (Biddle, 1979; Mead, 1934). Role theory is based on the sociological theory of structural-functionalism. According to role theory, formal roles are generally performed within a position in the social system. Some roles contribute to healthy family functioning, while others are associated with psychological or communication problems. For example, the informal role that requires one family member to be blamed for family problems (i.e., family scapegoat) is generally suggestive of family dysfunction. The so-called black sheep of the family is usually the person who tends to explore experiences outside of the family's norms and receives messages of invalidation or disapproval. At the same time, the black sheep who maintains contact with the family also brings diverse experiences to the family, contributing to its evolution over time.

## Formal Roles for Family

Formal roles for adult family members are shown in Box 44-4. Traditionally, formal roles were often assigned according to gender. Contemporary families, however,

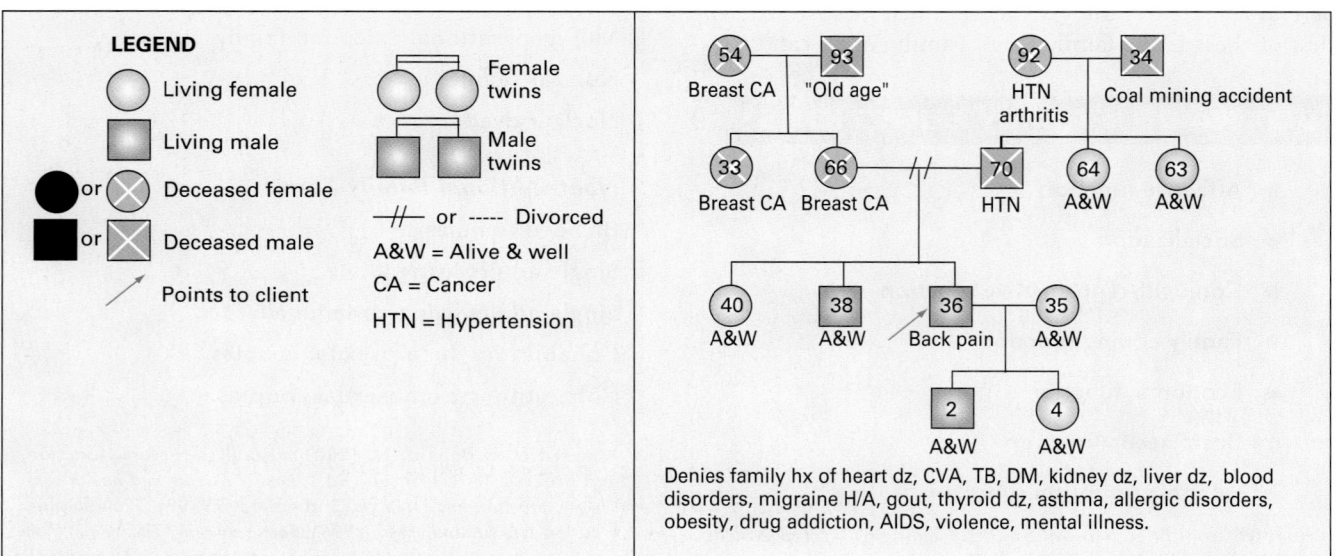

**Figure 44-2    Genogram**

## BOX 44-4 FORMAL AND INFORMAL FAMILY ROLES

- Provider
- Housekeeper
- Child-care provider
- Socializer
- Sexual partner
- Therapist
- Recreation organizer
- Kinship member

Adapted from Ballard, N. (2001). Family structure, function, and process. In S. Hansen (Ed.), *Family nursing and health care: Theory, practice, and research* (2nd ed., pp. 79–99). Philadelphia: F. A. Davis; Friedman, M. (1998). *Family nursing: Theory and practice* (4th ed.). Norwalk, CT: Appleton & Lange.

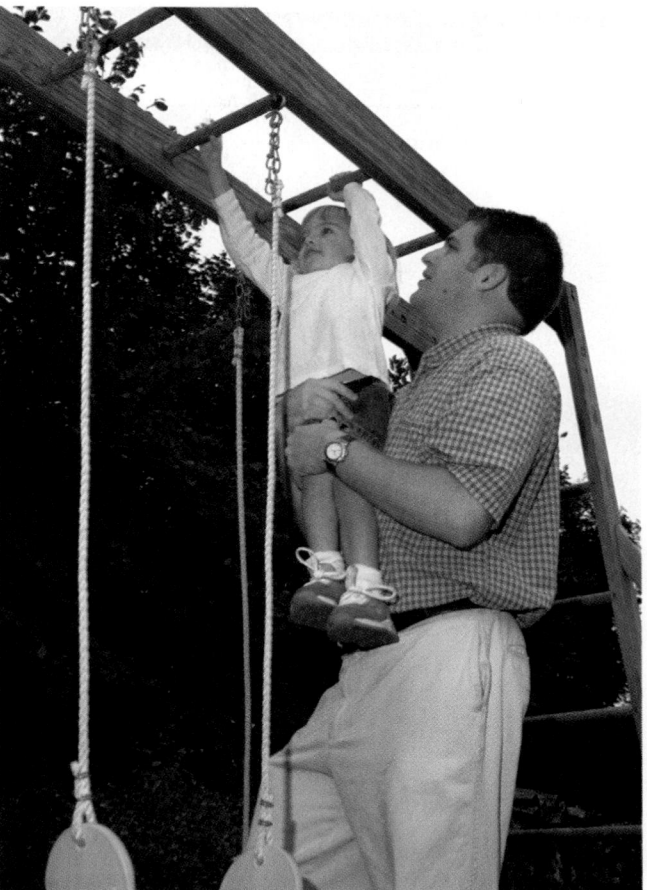

**Figure 44-3** **This stay-at-home father must balance the tug of war between home life, giving up a career for the time being, and finding time for himself.**

assign roles in a variety of ways. An example is the stay-at-home father, who performs many household and child-care responsibilities traditionally assigned to women (Figure 44-3). Multiple providers in the household also call for role flexibility, including perhaps greater shared responsibility for children. A gay couple may share parenthood with a biologically linked or adopted child and assign parental roles in nontraditional ways (Shears, 2002a).

While contemporary families have more freedom in negotiating roles, societal sanctions do exist when adult family members fail to ensure a minimal degree of family functioning. For example, in some societies, parental rights may be legally terminated if children are neglected or abused (Table 44-1). Family function and structure suggest how a given family function might be facilitated by various roles and positions within the families.

While parents and other adults are primarily responsible for ensuring family functioning, all family members, including older, more competent children, may perform formal roles. An older sibling may be responsible for escorting a younger sibling to school, teaching safe ways to cross the street, or correcting inappropriate social behavior.

### Position in the Family

The meaning of a person's position in the family is also socioculturally constructed. Family positions in traditional families, such as mother/wife, father/husband, daughter/sister, or son/brother are likely to come with shared social expectations for role performance. In nontraditional families, dysfunction in the family process can occur related to unclear consensus about what responsibilities are to be assigned to the positions. For example, there is great diversity in beliefs about the roles of the working mother/wife or the cohabiting "boyfriend" (Friedman, 1998).

### Role of Children in Family

The roles performed by children are limited by developmental stage, societal sanction, and in some cases, law. In the United States, children are generally not allowed to participate in the family provider role. Economic function is legally and socially held to be the responsibility of adults. However, teenagers are often encouraged to take jobs as part of socialization into the adult behavior of self-sufficiency. Theoretically, any income generated belongs to the child, not the family.

### CLIENT REFLECTIONS

#### Suspected Child Abuse

If the nurse suspects child abuse, the children's services agency must be contacted immediately. In addition, the nurse must document the "signs" that exist in the assessment of the child.

Martin, S. (2002). Children exposed to domestic violence: Psychiatric considerations for health care practitioners. *Holistic Nursing Practice, 16*(3), 7–15.

## TABLE 44-1    FAMILY FUNCTION AND STRUCTURE

| Family Function | Formal Role Structure | Responsible Family Member |
| --- | --- | --- |
| Affective function | Therapeutic role<br>Kinship role<br>Recreational role | All family members |
| Socialization function | Child-care role<br>Therapeutic role<br>Kinship role | Parent<br>Grandparent<br>Competent adult<br>Competent older child |
| Conjugal function | Sexual role | Husband<br>Wife<br>Partner |
| Economic function | Provider role | Parent<br>Grandparent<br>Competent adult |
| Basic needs function | Housekeeper role<br>Provider role | Husband/wife/partner<br>Parent<br>Grandparent<br>Other relative<br>Competent adult<br>Child (chores) |
| Health care function | Therapeutic role<br>Kinship role | Husband/wife/partner<br>Parent<br>Grandparent<br>Other relative<br>Competent adult |

Adapted from Ballard, N. (2001). Family structure, function, and process. In S. Hansen (Ed.), *Family nursing and health care: Theory, practice, and research* (2nd ed., pp. 79–99). Philadelphia: F. A. Davis; Hitchcock, J., Schubert, P., & Thomas, S. (2003). *Community health nursing: Caring in action.* Clifton Park, NY: Delmar Learning.

In many parts of the world, as well as within the United States, children continue to contribute to the economic functioning of the family. For example, agriculturally based cultures expect all family members to assist in labor-intensive activities such as harvest. Children may also contribute to daily chores. In most developed nations, law prohibits children from entering into the workforce outside of family enterprises. In developing countries, however, these protections are not always present, either through lack of law or lack of legal enforcement. Children may be assigned into servitude to satisfy family debt or sent out as vendors to pedal food or wares for the family's economic needs. Even in the United States, there is a current resurgence of child labor regardless of child labor laws. Landrigan and McCammon (1997) reported that poverty, large-scale immigration, and decreased enforcement of child labor laws have contributed

to 200,000 injuries in child workers and more than 70 deaths each year. Economic functioning based on child labor represents an emerging health problem in the United States.

## Performance of Roles in Family

How well a family member performs a role depends on several factors. First is the concept of **role competence**. Role competence refers to the family member's ability to perform a role. Role competency requires an individual to understand her roles. Role performance depends on established norms for how the role should be enacted (Fortinash & Holoday-Worret, 2000). For example, a mother needs to know what society expects of that role before she can address the functions of that role. However, as with any performance-based role, training and education are required.

## Gender

Traditionally, the responsibilities subsumed under certain family roles frequently have been defined by gender (Shears, 2002a). For example, Lagana (1996), in a study of motherhood in traditional Mexican culture, found that mothers were expected to role-model respectable social behavior to their children and to prioritize family needs over self-needs. In addition, the role of fathers in society has implications that are specific to their gender and are interrelated with the culture (see Chapter 5 for specific cultural expectations).

## Role Disorders

Four definite role disorders exist as persons take on different roles. Nurses must watch for these role disorders. The role disorders are role stress, role strain, role conflict, and role overload. They are described as follows.

## Role Stress

Without clear role consensus or agreement about expectations, role stress or role strain may occur. **Role stress** is a condition of role expectations that is likely to contribute to family or individual dysfunction. Lack of role competency or competing roles can be stressors on healthy family functioning. In contemporary families, each family member often performs multiple roles. For example, an older child may be expected to assist with housekeeping or child care, while also having responsibilities to school or friends. Stress results from the pressures of different persons' expectations of the older child (Roy, 2001).

## Role Strain

The inability to perform a role according to the expectations of others, or oneself, often leads to **role strain**. Role strain is a subjective personal response of psychological distress in which an individual anticipates or has an actual inability to satisfactorily perform a role. For example, Edwards, Zarit, Stephens, & Townsend (2002), in a study of caregivers for cognitively impaired older family members, found that working caregivers experienced greater role strain and depression when the work environment did not support their caregiving needs. For example, when employers were unable to allow the caregiver to have time off to make appointments or to meet crisis needs of the impaired family member, role strain resulted.

## Role Conflict

**Role conflict** occurs when the expectations for one role are incompatible with those of another role. A typical contemporary role conflict occurs for working mothers. When a child is ill, the provider role may conflict with the therapeutic role. The Family and Medical Leave Act (FMLA) of 1993 was a federal law passed to allow working family members to take time off to care for family members without losing their jobs. While the FMLA has limitations, it is an example of public health policy that recognized the impact of role conflict on family health (Grebowski, 2002).

## Role Overload

Finally, **role overload** is a form of role stress or strain that occurs when the family member lacks the time, resources, or energy to perform the role. Role overload may be related to unrealistic expectations of the amount of work the role entails. For example, the husband who works two jobs in his provider role for the family may not be able to contribute much to the child-care role without experiencing role overload. If role expectations are not renegotiated, role overload will interfere with some area of the family functioning (Pierce, Hong, Franks, & Ketterer, 2002). Nurses must realize that an important part of family assessment is the delineation of role expectations.

## Role Transition

Changes are often required in role assignment for developmental, situational, or illness-related reasons. **Role transition** may represent a stressor for the family, taxing family coping abilities. According to Meleis (1997), "Transition requires the person to incorporate new knowledge, to alter behavior, and therefore to change the definition of self in social context (p. 108)."

All families go through developmental role changes related to the aging of its members and to necessary changes in family functions. For example, when parents become older, adult children are often called upon to care for their parents. In this way, the adult children take on roles of provider and caregiver, formerly roles their parents held. There is inadequate research on the developmental role changes experienced by nontraditional families.

### Situational Role Transitions

**Situational role transitions** are changes that are made in roles when families experience the addition or loss of a family member. For example, a new baby requires increased child-care role performance; this may become the priority responsibility for the mother for a period of time. Housekeeping or provider role activities may need to be curtailed,

---

### CLIENT REFLECTIONS

#### A Working Mother and Role Conflict

Martha is the single parent of 7-year-old Stacy. Stacy requires chemotherapy every week and is hospitalized for 3 days during the treatments. Martha tells the nurse, "I have never felt so guilty as when I have to leave Stacy at the hospital while I go off to work. I have to work because we don't have much money. In fact, if I missed another day of work, I would lose my job. Then where would we be? And sometimes, Stacy gets sick and can't go to school. It is a real dilemma."

What options are available to Martha? What would you say to her?

## CLIENT REFLECTIONS

### A New Stepparent Role

The nurse can give the following suggestions to a new stepparent in regard to the parenting role of stepchildren:

- Provide "alone time" with the biologic parent and the biologic children.

- Be patient with the stepchild regarding the acceptance of the new parent.

- Avoid criticism of the child's estranged parent.

- Structure social events that allow the stepchildren and biologic children to get to know one another in nonthreatening settings.

Friedman, M. (1998). *Family nursing: Theory and practice* (4th ed.). Norwalk, CT: Appleton & Lange; Martin, S. (2002). Children exposed to domestic violence: Psychiatric considerations for health care practitioners. *Holistic Nursing Practice, 16*(3), 7–15.

requiring the assistance of other family members to assume these roles. Situational role transitions tend to be time limited and are characterized by flexibility, adaptation, and adjustment in the family or dysfunction. Newly blended families, or stepfamilies, often experience transition-related role conflict and role strain until role expectations can be negotiated between the stepparent and stepchildren (Friedman, 1998) (Figure 44-4). Professional guidance and open communication between family members can assist in making a smooth transition.

### Role Transition and Illness

Role transition related to illness can be temporary or long-term depending on the nature and duration of the illness. For example, when a family member requires surgery, role flexibility between family members allows for the temporary performance of that person's duties through the recovery

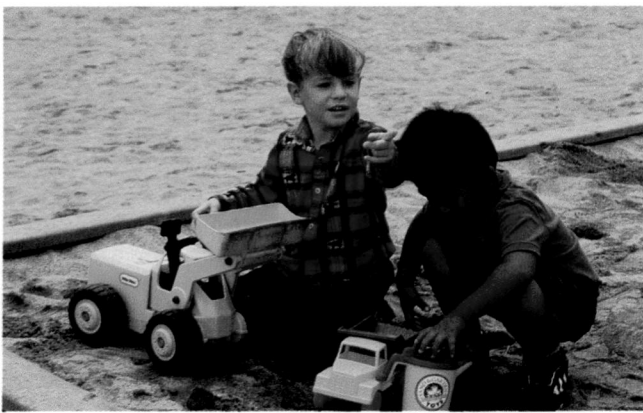

**Figure 44-4    Through remarriage, these boys became members of a blended family.**

period. If the illness is long-term or chronic, however, the family must make relatively permanent changes in role assignment and role expectations. If a wife must move from housekeeper to provider role following a disabling injury in her partner, performance expectations in her previous role(s) must be adjusted to take into account her new role as provider. Family nurses play an important part in family role transition through anticipatory guidance, family education, facilitation of open communication between family members, and sound discharge planning with referrals to helpful resources in the community (Parenthood, 2003).

## Values and Their Effect on Family Function

A family's functioning is strongly influenced by the values system learned during the socialization process. Established cultural norms in the surrounding community also have an influence on how the family interacts with the larger environment. Values and beliefs are associated with patterns of communication, ethnic norms, preferred language, religious affiliation, role expectations, availability of a supportive social network, and health practices. Strong family values are believed to have a beneficial effect on health (Dracup, 2002). When those values are markedly different than the surrounding community, however, conflict between the community and family members can exist. Value incongruence with the surrounding community can also lead to conflict within the family. The "generation gap" is a common phenomenon related to value changes in adolescents once they begin to interact more frequently with a diverse community and are exposed to a variety of values.

Health beliefs held by the family can also influence access to health care, as well as degree of agreement with recommended plans of care. Nurses must work with families to provide care that is congruent with the family's sociocultural values and belief system. Global migration and increasing societal diversity in the 21st century is leading to an increase in conflicting health beliefs and values. The term *noncompliance* was once used to describe a client's nonparticipation in a health care plan. Now, it is understood that the client has the right to decline to participate in a recommended plan of care. Nurses must assess the cultural and family-based health beliefs held by clients and advocate for a plan of care that is acceptable to the client (Chinn, 2000). Oftentimes, a thorough discussion of the rationale, risks, benefits, or alternatives for a recommended plan of care facilitates agreement.

If the client is a child, a family-based team approach is often successful in providing optimal care. All family members active in decision making for the family should be included in a family-based approach. Legal and ethical issues may arise for the health care team when health care decisions made by the parents are clearly not in the best interest of the child. Conflicting beliefs about health care needs create a complex situation that requires strong com-

## LEGAL AND ETHICAL ISSUES

### Parents Making Health Care Decisions for Their Children

Many ethical dilemmas are created by the "rights of the child" versus the "wishes of the parents" as related to the values and beliefs in family systems. Nurses must assess the situation carefully when health care decisions are made by the parents, particularly if the decisions are clearly not in the best interest of the child. For example, when a child has done something that is "embarrassing to their parents" (e.g., pregnancy out of wedlock), the parents might purport the child not telling anyone, having an abortion, and being "silent" about the entire incident. The child, however, needs to have the freedom to seek counseling, have other options (e.g., "adopting out") the infant, and pursuing interventions that are beneficial to the child.

Potts, N., & Mandleco, B. (2002). *Pediatric nursing: Caring for children and their families*. Clifton Park, NY: Delmar Learning.

## NURSING STRATEGY

### Communication with Culturally or Linguistically Diverse Clients

- For family nurses communicating with clients who are culturally or linguistically diverse, it is very important to use culturally informed medical interpreters to facilitate clear communication.

- Health care facilities need to keep records of medical persons with language skills who can be contacted whenever needed.

- For family members who are struggling with cross-cultural communication problems, simply pointing out the process of cross-cultural communication may be helpful.

- Adult family members are often unaware of differences in communication patterns until pointed out by a family nurse specialist or family therapist.

Chinn, J. L. (2000). Culturally competent health care. *Public Health Reports, 115*, 25–33.

munication skills and a multidisciplinary health care team approach. However, if a family lacks effective communication skills, such conflicts are very difficult to resolve.

## Communication Patterns in the Family

A family's communication pattern may be the most important factor in a healthy family process. Communication allows the family to share important information; conveys affection, support, and a sense of belonging; and aids in developing values needed to live in civilized society. Ultimately, how clearly and openly family members communicate with each other will be a strong determinant of how the family performs in any of the family functions. When assessing family communications, it is important to consider the principles of communication as depicted in Chapter 4.

Effective communication requires certain characteristics in the sender and receiver. The sender sends clear and congruent messages, makes sure the message is understood, invites feedback, and is open to that feedback. In effective communication, the receiver intently listens to the message and gives feedback, validating the importance of the message with phrases like "I hear what you are saying and can see how important of an issue this is to you." In this way, further discussion is invited.

Ineffective communication can be related to characteristics of the sender, the receiver, or both. Ineffective communication is a communication pattern that interferes with family processes. Oftentimes, communication prob-

lems impact the effective functioning in a family because of the inability to resolve conflict. However, ineffective communication impacts all areas of family process.

Communication patterns are learned in childhood during the socialization process. Native language patterns (related to the primary language learned and spoken as a child) and culturally sanctioned communication rules (e.g., rules about how children communicate with their elders) also influence communication patterns. As discussed in Chapter 4, the decoding and recoding process required for effective communication is very complex when attempted across languages and cultures. Misunderstanding of messages is common.

## Power Structure

Finally, power structure plays a critical role in family health functioning. Power has been defined as the ability to control, influence, or change another person's behavior (Friedman, 1998). Power is related to resources. Control over resources infers power. In most families, parents and other competent adults control the resources. It is important to assess family power bases when discussing health care issues.

### Family Power

There are three family power types, which are chaotic power, symmetrical power, and complementary power (Hanson,

2001). Each of these family power types are described in this section.

## Chaotic Family Power

**Chaotic family power** is an absence of power structure within a family structure. In a chaotic family, family process is dysfunctional because there is no clearly delineated group leadership, values are poorly defined, and socialization of children is unpredictable. In a chaotic family, there is no established plan for how primary family functions will be addressed. As a result, the health of the family members may suffer. Sociopathology is believed by some to be the result of growing up in a chaotic family (Hanson, 2001).

## Symmetrical (Egalitarian) Family Power

**Symmetrical (egalitarian) family power** is power shared between family members. This is an increasingly observed form of family power in the United States. With household adults working, it may be necessary for parents to share decision making and responsibilities for the family and household. However, it is important to remember that there are developmental constraints on how much younger members of the family can handle. A review of role theory suggests that parents or older, more mature adults must take a leadership role if a family is to function adequately. As children show increased competence and move toward adulthood, however, the egalitarian family does more power sharing (Hanson, 2001).

## Complementary Family Power

**Complementary family power** requires a dominion-submission dynamic within the family structure. In this family power type, healthy families are characterized by parents having a clear power advantage that their children recognize and accept. For example, in many cultures, the father has more power in the public sector, while the mother has more power in the private sector. Culturally appropriate health care recognizes established power structure and works within that structure to meet the health care needs of the individual client. However, it is also important to recognize family power structures that are coercive or abusive to members of the family and to assess the need for domestic violence intervention (Hanson, 2001).

# Decision-Making About Health Behaviors

Decision making about health behaviors or accessing health care services, while ultimately up to the individual, is often decided within the power structure of the family. It should be remembered that health care functioning is a major focus of the family, generally supported by the therapeutic role. In health care today, many health decisions are made by the family prior to accessing the health care system (Kaiser, Hays, Cho, & Agrawal, 2002). For example,

home remedies may have been tried. Perhaps a health problem did not seem like a problem until the family member could no longer function in his formal role. Health behaviors like nutritional intake, exercise patterns, dental hygiene, or the use of substances are all behaviors that may be learned within the family. How decisions are made varies. Egalitarian families usually make decisions by consensus. In consensus decision making, family members talk, often in consultation with health care providers, and arrive at a decision that the whole family can support.

Decision making by accommodation requires a change in one or more family members' first choice. One functional approach is to compromise. Compromise is a strategy for conflict resolution and requires that family members communicate effectively and come to a middle ground in a decision. Three other forms of the use of power in making health care decisions are bargaining, coercion, and de-facto decision making.

## Bargaining

In the bargaining form of power to make health care decisions, family members reach an agreement by give and take. A father and husband may say to family members: "OK, I will give up cigarettes, but do not ever bother me about my beer drinking again." In the father's statement, the family members are expected to "keep their end of the bargain" and to "never bother the father about his beer drinking."

## Coercion

Coercion or coercive power is considered unethical in the United States. In health care, a health care provider could theoretically coerce a client into agreeing to a plan of care that the provider supports by not informing the patient of risks or of viable alternative treatments. However, fully informed consent is the standard of care, and a health care professional's failure to provide it could result in civil or criminal legal challenges. When family members use coercion in health care decisions to maintain power, this behavior is often interpreted as abusive. Coercion is frequently observed in reproductive health. For example, in a recent study of contraceptive use among women living in a shelter for battered women, Davila and Brackley (1999) found that Hispanic women reported battering associated with asking the partner to use condoms. Among childbearing women, the decision to maintain or terminate a pregnancy is often coerced with threats of abandonment by the partner. In some cultures, pregnancy outside of marriage or marriage to a partner from a different religion, culture, or race can lead to social ostracism.

## De Facto

Finally, de-facto decision making is making no decision at all and allowing a condition to take its course (Friedman, 1998). De-facto decision making is commonly related to locus of control (Spector, 2001). A particular belief in

## FOCUS ON WELLNESS

### Locus of Control in Persons with Spinal Cord Injuries

In a study involving over 100 wheelchair athletes (persons with spinal cord injuries), there was a significant correlation among the concepts of locus of control, self-efficacy and self-esteem, and the healthy attitudes and behaviors of the athletes. The clients in this research with high levels of internal self-control, self-esteem, and self-efficacy were more likely to participate in wheelchair athletics and other health promotive attitudes and behaviors.

Daniels, R. (2000). Exploring the self-care variables that explain a wellness lifestyle in wheelchair basketball athletes with spinal cord injuries, *SCI Psychosocial Process, 13*(2), 50–58.

**locus of control** (a person's perception of the source of control over events and situations affecting the person's life) is strongly influenced by culture, religion, and family values. The Health Beliefs Model, originally developed by Becker (1974) and refined by Pender (1996), theorizes that the decision to take health-promoting actions is influenced by an individual's belief that her actions will be effective. If the individual believes that health is controlled by an external source (e.g., the health care professional, spiritual leader or deity, or destiny), there may be less self-motivation for action. This is also discussed in the literature as self-efficacy and is often influenced by the individual's level of self-esteem.

## Theories That Explain Family Processes

As the preceding discussion on family dynamics suggests, the family functions in multiple ways to contribute to the health of individual family members. Most important is the idea that healthy family functioning protects and supports its members in the face of many stressors and in so doing it facilitates health. Other theories that may help to explain family processes are family development theory, family systems theory, and family stress theory.

### Family Development Theory

Family development theory begins with the assumption that families are groups of long-term duration and an associated history that must be considered in a family assessment. There are several variations on family development theory, but all consider that human families move linearly and predictably through developmental stages in

time. This is often referred to as the family career or family life cycle. Family development stages are shown in Box 44-5. The challenge for families from a developmental perspective is to continue to function in a healthy way during times of transition when roles and values may change. Developmental transitions are characterized by stress that must be managed. Families often require assistance at this time (Rodgers & White, 1993).

Family development theory was constructed primarily on the observation of traditional nuclear families in the United States. For this reason, one concern about the application of family development theory today is that it does not adequately consider the broad variation in contemporary family forms. Many adults forego marriage or childbearing. It is also important to note that many families do not progress in a linear fashion through the stages of development. Clearly, further research is needed to examine the life careers of nontraditional families (Ballard, 2001).

### Family Systems Theory

Family systems theory is based in a very broad and abstract theory known as general systems theory. Systems theory defines the system as an enduring goal-directed unit. This is a concept that well describes the family unit. Systems are made up of interacting parts, are in some way distinct from the surrounding environment, and require input from the surrounding environment to maintain stability. Systems theory also recognizes that systems are holistic and greater than the sum of their parts. In other words, the integrity of a functioning system produces an energy output that its individual parts could not produce alone (Friedman, 1998).

Family systems theory applies these broad ideas to the family as a cohesive, goal-directed unit that, while interacting with the environment, maintains a distinct and

### BOX 44-5    STAGES OF FAMILY DEVELOPMENT BETWEEN FAMILIES

The following are the stages of family development that may occur between families:

Marriage

Childbearing

Child rearing

Launching of young adults

Middle-aged parents

Retirement and old age

Friedman, M. (1998). *Family nursing: Theory and practice* (4th ed.). Norwalk, CT: Appleton & Lange.

## LIFE SPAN CONSIDERATIONS

### Grandparents Raising Their Grandchildren

Parents who have launched their children may find themselves once again facing the task of parenting by raising their grandchildren. This is a known stressor for grandparents who had anticipated the end of child-rearing responsibilities. In addition, these grandparents who have become parents again may also face caring for their aging parents. Thus the term *sandwich generation* is used to label these middle adults who are "caught with child-rearing of their grandchildren and caregivers to their parents."

Hanson, S. (2001). *Family nursing and health care: Theory, practice, and research* (2nd ed., pp. 79–99). Philadelphia: F. A. Davis.

## RESEARCH FOCUS

**Title of Study:** Family survivorship and quality of life following a cancer diagnosis

**Study Purpose:** To test a model of family survivorship and its influence on quality of life for the family unit during the survivor phase of cancer illness

**Methods:** This exploratory, cross-sectional study interviewed a random, stratified sample of 123 families (N = 246 adult family members) for evidence to support the family survivorship model.

The family survivorship model assessed "Illness Survival Stressors," including (1) other concurrent family stressors, (2) fear of recurrence of the cancer, and (3) somatic concerns. It also assessed "Family Resources," including the family hardiness and family social support. Stressors and resources were then viewed through the lens of what meaning the family held for "Cancer Illness," resulting in the family's reported "Quality of Life."

After institutional review board approval, families with a member who had survived cancer for 1 to 5 years were recruited to the study by letters and follow-up phone calls. After informed consent, adult family members were interviewed in the home. Instruments used for data collection included the Family Pressures Index (FPI), Fear of Recurrence Questionnaire, the Functional Assessment of Cancer Therapy subscale for physical well-being, the Family Hardiness Index, the Social Support Index, the Constructed Meaning Scale, and the Quality of Life–Parent Form. Sociodemographic data, such as age, occupation, race and ethnicity, education level, and family income level, were also collected.

**Findings:** The research found that the strongest predictors of quality of life for families with cancer survivors were other concurrent family stressors, family social support, fear of recurrence, and the cancer survivor's employment status. Families in which the survivor was retired reported the highest quality of life. The family survivorship model explained 67% of the variance for quality of life. However, somatic concerns and meaning of the illness did not affect the quality of life. The authors attributed this to a possible lack of validity for patients who are no longer ill.

**Implications:** While the study showed that the family survivorship model did predict quality of life for the families of cancer survivors, it did not show a relationship with somatic concerts or the families' ideas about what it meant to have cancer. The model can be used by nurses in family-centered care to predict quality of life based on family hardiness, family social support, and illness-related and concurrent family stressors. Fear of recurrence of the cancer should be considered as a chronic stressor in families with cancer survivors.

Mellon, S., & Northouse, L. (2001). Family survivorship and quality of life following a cancer diagnosis. *Research in Nursing & Health, 24*, 446–459.

---

separate identity. An **open family system** is one that interacts with the environment and in so doing maintains growth and balance. A **closed family system** is a family system that is considered to be at risk for dysfunction because ideas and values may be out of sync with the broader community and because this isolation limits available resources to the family and its members.

In a family that is open to interaction with the community, input from the community is processed and labeled **throughput**. The resulting response from the family is labeled **output**. This response feeds back to the community, influencing future input from the community. The following example demonstrates this process. Six-year-old Jimmy is falling asleep in morning classes. The school nurse's nutritional assessment indicates that Jimmy's breakfast lacks adequate protein to last until lunchtime. The nurse calls Jimmy's parents with this information and suggests adding milk to his diet (input). This information is processed by the family unit (throughput) and results in a family decision to make nutritional changes (output). Jimmy is more alert in class (feedback). The responsiveness of open family systems to environmental resources helps the family unit meet individual family members' needs and often leads to healthier family functioning. Closed family systems tend to resist interaction with the community and have fewer opportunities for growth and adaptation to change. Situations that challenge a family's ability to cope may present as crisis and dysfunction (Hanson, 2001).

## Family-Based Social Support

Human beings are by nature social animals that live in organized groups that provide mutual or reciprocal support to group members. As discussed earlier, the family is the most frequent source of social support. An **ecomap** is a graphic representation of the family within the social network (Figure 44-5).

## Concept of Social Support

Social support can be defined as the perception that one has emotional and tangible resources to call on when needed. It is associated with a sense of belonging as a valued and respected member of the group. Also, social support is involved in mitigating the human stress response and associated illness. It meets a fundamental human need for social ties, making life less stressful, and social support buffers the negative effects of stress, thus indirectly contributing to good health outcomes (Friedman, 1998; Smith, 1998).

Components of the social network may include people at school, church, or work, as well as neighbors and other members of the community. During illness, one role of the nurse is to assist the individual to identify and mobilize the social network. Research indicates that network variables have direct effects on health outcomes, whereas perceived social support interacts with or buffers the impact of stress on health (Family Social Support, 2003).

In the case of inadequate social support from family, integration in this broader social network can help to meet a person's social support needs. Empirical evidence shows that social ties have a protective effect on mortality risks and mental health (Farvis, 2002). For example, post-myocardial infarction clients who are integrated in a social network demonstrate higher level functioning and longevity. Integration in a social network also appears to have a generalized protective effect on physiological processes (immune response, cardiovascular activity, neuroendocrine response).

## Social Isolation

Social isolation may be experienced as a stressor due to the unavailability of social support or network resources. Social isolation in sociological terms can be broadly conceived as the converse of social integration or a deficit in social integration. Individuals who are married, hold group memberships, live with others, share social norms

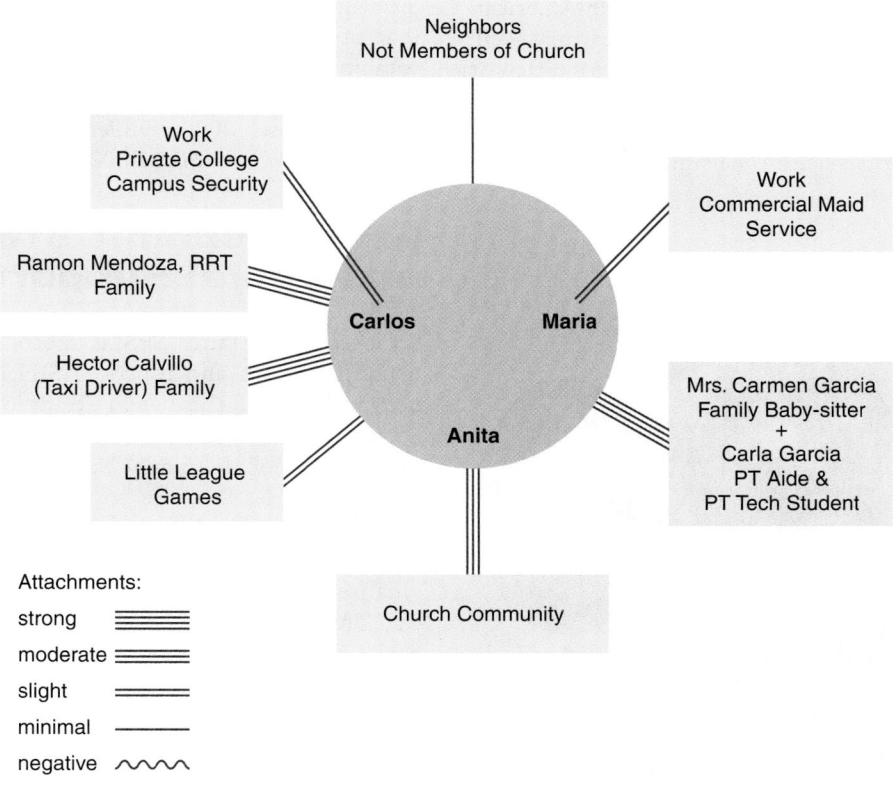

**Figure 44-5    An ecomap**

and values, have multiple network members, and long-standing relationships with frequent contact are less likely to experience social isolation (MacKinlay, 2001). A loss of social network and the associated support can represent a health crisis in physical and psychological terms.

The Lagana Model of Social Isolation (2001) represents the possible effect of social isolation on health outcomes (Figure 44-6). Based on the idea that social support buffers life stressors, thus promoting health and minimizing illness, the model identifies social isolation as a complex, multidimensional phenomenon. Numerous variables gleaned from the literature are conceptualized as interacting and contributing to a state of social isolation in the individual. For example, suppose an older male who has chronic congestive heart failure becomes widowed when his wife dies of cancer. The new situation of social isolation adds to the stressor of the congestive heart failure, and the widower begins to have a variety of cardiovascular system problems and subsequent illness.

## Social Support from Others

An individual may receive different types of social support from different individuals. On the one hand, social support is identified as **perceived social support** (social support that is perceived by the recipient of the support). And on the other hand, **actual social support** is identified as social support that is given by others regardless of the recipient's perception of the support. In either case, social support can be provided from others. For example, in a qualitative study of social support in Mexican-American childbearing women in Southern Colorado, Lagana, Weil, and Saiz (2001) found that women reported different types of social support from their male partners than from women in their families. But social support was provided by both the male partners and the women.

## Conflict and Negative Social Support

A supportive social climate is required for social support to occur. A network that is composed of conflicted relationships may not be perceived as supportive. Therefore, it is necessary to assess not only the structure of the network that exists, but the quality of the social relationships that are present within the network. Conflicted relationships, also referred to as negative support, have been shown to contribute to poor health outcomes (e.g., immune, neuroendocrine, or cardiovascular disorders) (Kaiser, Hays, Cho, & Agrawal, 2002).

## Mental Health and Family-Based Social Support

Lonely people are more often depressed. This is related to the notion that human beings are social animals with fundamental needs for social interaction. Whereas poor health is related to both social isolation and loneliness, mental health is more related to only social isolation. There is inadequate understanding of the role social support plays in other more serious mental health problems, such as schizophrenia. Medical focus on the known physiological aspects of severe mental illness may overlook the complex multidimensional social backgrounds of the mentally ill. Mental illness is the frequently seen response to overwhelming stressors related to major family transitions and health problems. Management of the client's mental health and that of the family requires a multidisciplinary approach combining pharmacological intervention, family and individual counseling, and social support (Carlson, McNutt, Choi, & Rose, 2002; DuPertuis, Aldwin, Bosse, 2001; Katerndahl & Parchman, 2002; Saunders & Byrne, 2002).

## Socioeconomic Status and Social Support

Socioeconomic status (SES) is another factor contributing to family health and function. SES is influenced by the occupation(s) of the parent (traditionally the husband's occupation), the education level of the parents, and the income level of the family. Social class is associated with social inequities in access to resources and related power, social privilege, and social prestige (Hanson, 2001). The health status and longevity of socially and culturally marginalized groups is less optimal. Furthermore, the trend in the United States for social and cultural disparities in health is growing. Immigrants who may have held prestigious social positions in their home countries often find it very difficult to establish themselves in the same social class in the United States. It often takes generations to overcome the barriers related to SES and social class. Stress-related illness such as heart disease, diabetes, substance use, and depression are common among families of lower SES.

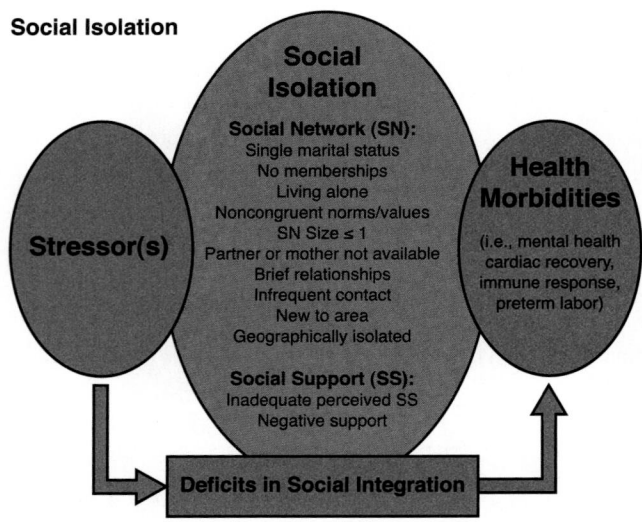

**Figure 44-6** Lagana Model of Social Isolation (Lagana, 2002)

Unlike many countries, social class in the United States depends on income rather than birthright. With the promise of higher paying jobs, education appears to be an important factor in social mobility in the United States.

## Social Support and the Nursing Process

The concept of social support is interrelated with family theory and the roles and relationships that exist among persons. As shown throughout this chapter, persons with alterations in social support often require assistance from the health care provider. Specifically, nursing can have a vital position in working with clients who have problems with social support. The following section displays the elements of the nursing process as affiliated with problems that clients can have in their social support.

### Assessment

Family-based social support is a naturally occurring resource for promoting individual health. However, family dysfunction can undermine the effectiveness of social support efforts. The nurse must assess the family and network structures using assessment tools (see the genogram in Figure 44-2 and ecomap in Figure 44-5). The nurse must also assess the family's ability to function in a supportive way to individual family members. Individual and family interviews help to identify sources of support. The impact of negative (conflicted) relationships on human health must be considered. The nurse must assess if any observed affective dysfunction is acute, related to the crisis of illness or chronic dysfunction. Chronic dysfunction often requires the assessment skills of an advanced practice nurse.

### Nursing Diagnosis

Nursing diagnoses are developed after assessing clients with disturbances in their social support—for example, "*Compromised Family Coping* related to an unexpected alteration in the health state of a family member, as evidenced by emotional distress and communication dysfunction in the family members." Relatedly, another nursing diagnosis involving social support dysfunction is "*Interrupted Family Processes* related to recent divorce between parents, as evidenced by a lack of demonstrated family cohesiveness and nurturing behaviors." Both of these diagnoses can be addressed by the nurse in effectively caring for clients with problems in social support.

### Outcome Identification and Planning

Education, referral, and developing therapeutic relationships with clients who are experiencing social support alterations are valuable functions of the nurse. In addition, nurses can encourage family members to assist in setting realistic goals for their loved ones as related to social support problems. Family members can be taught to practice effective communication skills with the client and report their progress to the nurse and other health care providers. The nurse can also instruct family members to demonstrate evidence of family cohesiveness, including emotional and instrumental social support. The client's social support problems can often be changed with their family members demonstrating nurturing behaviors toward each other.

### Implementation

Nurses can implement a wide variety of strategies in meeting the needs of their clients with alterations in social support. A focus of nurses' care can be on the position of the families as a primary means of addressing the needs of the client (Figure 44-7). For example, nurses can provide information to the client and family regarding the alteration in health state, its cause, and the recommended multidisciplinary plan of care. The nurse can encourage family members to verbalize their concerns in working with the client and suggest supportive behaviors. In addition, the nurse can assist family members in identifying social network resources that can assist in role performance and social support. During this time, the family may require nursing support as well. Nurses can suggest that family members provide rest and respite for exhaustion and encourage interaction between individual family members. In addition, other members of the health care team can be sought for assistance, such as obtaining a social worker consultation for long-term planning.

### Evaluation

As the client begins to improve in problems related to social support, the nurse's assessment with the client will reveal affirmations of increased self-esteem, self-efficacy, and lessened symptomatology from the client. Also, the family members will begin to cope, and the nurse should observe calmer emotions and improved communication

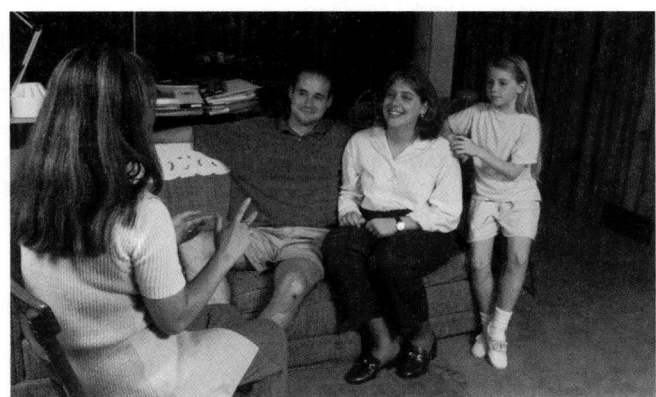

**Figure 44-7 A nurse meets with a family to work with them concerning their recent social support issues with grandparents who are struggling with having moved into a convalescent care facility.**

among family members, the clients, and the health care providers. In addition, in effective care, the family members should (1) congregate and communicate functionally, (2) report adequate rest and nutrition, and (3) display effective functioning demonstrated in the form of nurturing interactions. Also, a broader social network of resources will be engaged in assisting the family in the client's time-altered social support problems.

# CASE STUDY/NURSING CARE PLAN

Carter Tierny is a 29-year-old single woman who has recently been divorced and moved to "take a new job to take her mind off the divorce." She came to your medical clinic because she has been having "panic attacks" and is "fighting depression." Upon questioning, you find that Ms. Tierny does not have any family or friends within 200 miles of her recent location. She chose the city because it has one of the branch offices of the bank she works for and it had an opening in her area of expertise. Her history reveals 5 years of infrequent panic attacks and an isolated bout of depression 4 years ago when her father died. At that time, she had difficulty sleeping and the depression was resolved within a matter of 2 months. Otherwise, the only medications she takes is an occasional mild sedative for sleeplessness.

## Assessment
Client is a 29-year-old with social isolation, slight depression, and occasional panic attacks. She does not have social contacts in her area and is not currently affiliated with any social groups. She does not have suicidal ideation and states that the depression only causes her to not sleep well and to have panic attacks. Her panic attacks occur at least 1 to 2 times a day, and they last for about 15 minutes with her "feeling nervous, jittery, and a little short of breath." Her blood pressure is 132/86 and her pulse is 78/minute.

## Nursing Diagnosis
*Social Isolation* related to recent change of employment and move away from family and friends.
**NOC:** Loneliness; Mood Equilibrium; Social Interaction Skills; Social Involvement; Social Support
**NIC:** Socialization Enhancement

## Expected Outcomes
The client will:
1. Describe strategies to promote effective socialization by her second appointment.
2. Make constructive use of her "free time" and specify the activities in which she plans to participate by her second appointment.
3. Experience less than three panic attacks within the next week.

## Planning/Interventions/Rationales
1. Refer client to social groups (e.g., church, professional organization, fitness center) in which she could participate. *Increases social contacts and decreases social isolation.*
2. Work with client to develop recreational activities throughout the times that she is home alone. *Diversional activities decrease tendencies to depression.*
3. Educate client in biofeedback, imaging, and deep breathing techniques. *Decreases anxiety and stress.*

## Evaluation
Client worked out at a local fitness center three times per week. She also began cooking gourmet meals and practicing her piano by the second appointment. In addition, Ms. Tierny had only two panic attacks per week.

## Key Concepts
- Families changed in their focus after the industrial revolution.
- The family's purposes are to socialize children and serve individual family members.
- Common family forms are nuclear families and nuclear dyads.
- There are both formal and informal roles for the family.
- Role disorders are role stress, role strain, role conflict, and role overload.
- The value system of a family strongly influences the socialization process.

- Communication is a strong determinant of how a family functions.
- The three family power types are chaotic power, symmetrical power, and complementary power.
- De-facto decision making allows a condition to take its course and is correlated with locus of control.
- Family development theory was constructed primarily on the observation of nuclear families in the United States.
- The family is the most frequent source of social support.
- An ecomap graphically represents the family within its social network.
- Social isolation exists when there are no network resources or social support structures.
- Mental health influences family-based support.
- Socioeconomic status is an important variable influencing social support.
- Nurses can work with families to develop strategies of care for clients with social support alterations.

## Review Questions and Activities

1. What are the historical differences between the agrarian and postindustrial times as related to family development trends?
2. What are the main assumptions of structural-functional theory applied to families?
3. Construct a genogram of your family.
4. Describe the roles for each member in your family. Are there any role disorders in your family? What are they?
5. What are the values to which your family ascribes? How are they different from your closest friend's family?
6. Which of the six communication patterns does your family practice the best? Worst?
7. What are examples of complementary power in two cultures other than in the United States?
8. How would you describe family development theory as related to most of the families in your home area?
9. Draw an ecomap of your family, and evaluate how a family member activates the social network during illness.
10. Who are the persons that provide social support for your family?
11. How does socioeconomic status affect social support?
12. What can nurses do with families to increase the social support of the client?

## Web Resources

Family Social Support
   http://www.carlow.edu
Health and Social Support
   http://stauffer.queensu.ca
Parenthood
   http://www.parenthood.com

Social Support in Midwifery Practice
   http://www.efn.org
United States Bureau of the Census
   http://www.census.gov

## References

Artinian, N. T. (1999). Selecting a model to guide family assessment. In G. Wegner & R. Alexander (Eds.), *Readings in family nursing* (2nd ed., pp. 447–459), Philadelphia: Lippincott.

Ballard, N. (2001). Family structure, function, and process. In S. Hansen (Ed.), *Family nursing and health care: Theory, practice, and research* (2nd ed., pp. 79–99). Philadelphia: F. A. Davis.

Becker, M. H.(1974). *The health beliefs model and personal health behavior.* Thorofare, NJ: Charles B. Slack.

Biddle, B. J. (1979). *Role theory: Expectations, identities, and behaviors.* New York: Academic Press.

Carlson, B., McNutt, L., Choi, D. Y., & Rose, I. M. (2002). Intimate partner abuse and mental health: The role of social support and other protective factors. *Violence Against Women, 8*(6), 720–745.

Chinn, J. L. (2000). Culturally competent health care. *Public Health Reports, 115*, 25–33.

Daniels, R. (2000). Exploring the self-care variables that explain a wellness lifestyle in wheelchair basketball athletes with spinal cord injuries. *SCI Psychosocial Process, 13*(2), 50–58.

Davila, Y., & Brackley, M. (1999). Mexican and Mexican-American women in a battered women's shelter: Barriers to condom negotiation for HIV/AIDS. *Issues in Mental Health Nursing, 20*(4), 333–355.

Dracup, K. (2002). Beyond the patient: Caring for families. *Communicating Nursing Research, 35*, 53–61.

DuPertuis, L. L., Aldwin, C.M., & Bosse, R. (2001). Does the source of support matter for different health outcomes? Findings from the normative aging study. *Journal of Aging and Health, 13*(4), 494–510.

Edwards, A. B., Zarit, S. H., Stephens, M., & Townsend, A. (2002). Employed family caregivers of cognitively impaired elderly: An examination of role strain and depressive symptoms. *Aging and Mental Health, 6*(1), 55–61.

Estes, M. (2002). *Health assessment & physical examination* (2nd ed.). Clifton Park, NY: Delmar Learning.

Family Social Support. (2003). http://www.carlow.edu

Farvis, M. (2002). The family: An important nursing resource for holistic client care. *Australian Nursing Journal, 10*(5), 1–3.

Fortinash, K., & Holoday-Worret, P. (2000). *Psychiatric mental health nursing* (2nd ed.). St. Louis: Mosby.

Friedman, M. (1998). *Family nursing: Theory and practice* (4th ed.). Norwalk, CT: Appleton & Lange.

Grebowski, L. S. (2002). Managing overlapping federal FMLA and state leave regulations. *Employee Benefits Journal, 27*(1), 41–44.

Hanson, S. (2001). *Family nursing and health care: Theory, practice, and research* (2nd ed., pp. 79-99). Philadelphia: F. A. Davis.

Hitchcock, J., Schubert, P., & Thomas, S. (2003). *Community health nursing: Caring in action.* Clifton Park, NY: Delmar Learning.

Kaiser, K. L., Hays B. J., Cho, W. J., & Agrawal, S. (2002). Examining health problems and intensity of need for care in family-focused community and public health nursing. *Journal of Community Health Nursing, 19*(1), 17-32.

Katerndahl, D. A., & Parchman, M. (2002). The ability of the stress process model to explain mental health outcomes. *Comprehensive Psychiatry, 43*(5), 351-360.

LaDuke, S. (2000). NIC puts musing into words. *Nursing Management, 31(2),* 43-44.

Lagana, K. L. (1996). *Preventing low birthweight: Cultural influences on Mexican immigrant and Mexican-American prenatal care. A community study.* (Doctoral dissertation, research, University of California, San Francisco).

Lagana, K., Weil, B., & Saiz, J. (2001). Acculturation and social support among childbearing women in a U.S. Mexican-American community. *International Nursing Perspectives, 1*(1), 23-31.

Landrigan, P.J., & McCammon, J.B. (1997). Child labor: Still with us after all these years. *Public Health Reports, 112*(6), 466-473.

MacKinlay, E. (2001). Aging and isolation: Is the issue social isolation or is it a lack of meaning in life? *Journal of Religious Gerontology, 12*(3-4), 89-99.

Martin, S. (2002). Children exposed to domestic violence: Psychiatric considerations for health care practitioners. *Holistic Nursing Practice, 16*(3), 7-15.

Mead, G. H. (1934). *Mind, self, and society.* Chicago: University of Chicago Press.

Meleis, A. I. (1997). *Theoretical nursing: Development and progress* (3rd ed.). Philadelphia: Lippincott.

Mellon, S., & Northouse, L. (2001). Family survivorship and quality of life following a cancer diagnosis. *Research in Nursing & Health, 24,* 446-459.

Parenthood. (2003). http://www.parenthoodweb.com

Pender, N. J. (1996). *Health promotion in nursing* (3rd ed.). Stamford, CT: Appleton & Lange.

Pierce, L. S., Hong, T. B., Franks, M. M., & Ketterer, M. W. (2002). Health-related interactions and the self in marriage. *Journal of Women & Aging, 14*(3-4), 149-164.

Potts, N., & Mandleco, B. (2002). *Pediatric nursing: Caring for children and their families.* Clifton Park, NY: Delmar Learning.

Rodgers, R. H., & White, J. M. (1993). Family development theory. In Pauline G. Boss & William J. Doherty, (Eds.), *Sourcebook of family theories and methods: A contextual approach* (pp. 225-257).

Rokeach, M. (1973). *The nature of human values.* New York: The Free Press.

Roy, C. (2001). Roy adaptation model and perspectives on the family. *Nursing science quarterly, 14*(1), 9-13.

Saunders, J. C., & Byrne, M. M. (2002). A thematic analysis of families living with schizophrenia. *Archives of Psychiatric Nursing, 16*(5), 217-223.

Shears, K. H. (2002a). Gender stereotypes compromise sexual health. *Network, 21*(4), 12-13, 15-18.

Shears, K. H. (2002b). Youth programs challenge stereotypes. *Network, 21*(4), 16-17.

Smith, R. D. (1998). Social structures and chaos theory. *Sociological research, 3*(1), 12-16.

Spector, R. (2001). *Cultural diversity in health and illness* (5th ed.). Upper Saddle River, NJ: Prentice Hall.

United States Bureau of the Census. (1998). http://www.census.gov

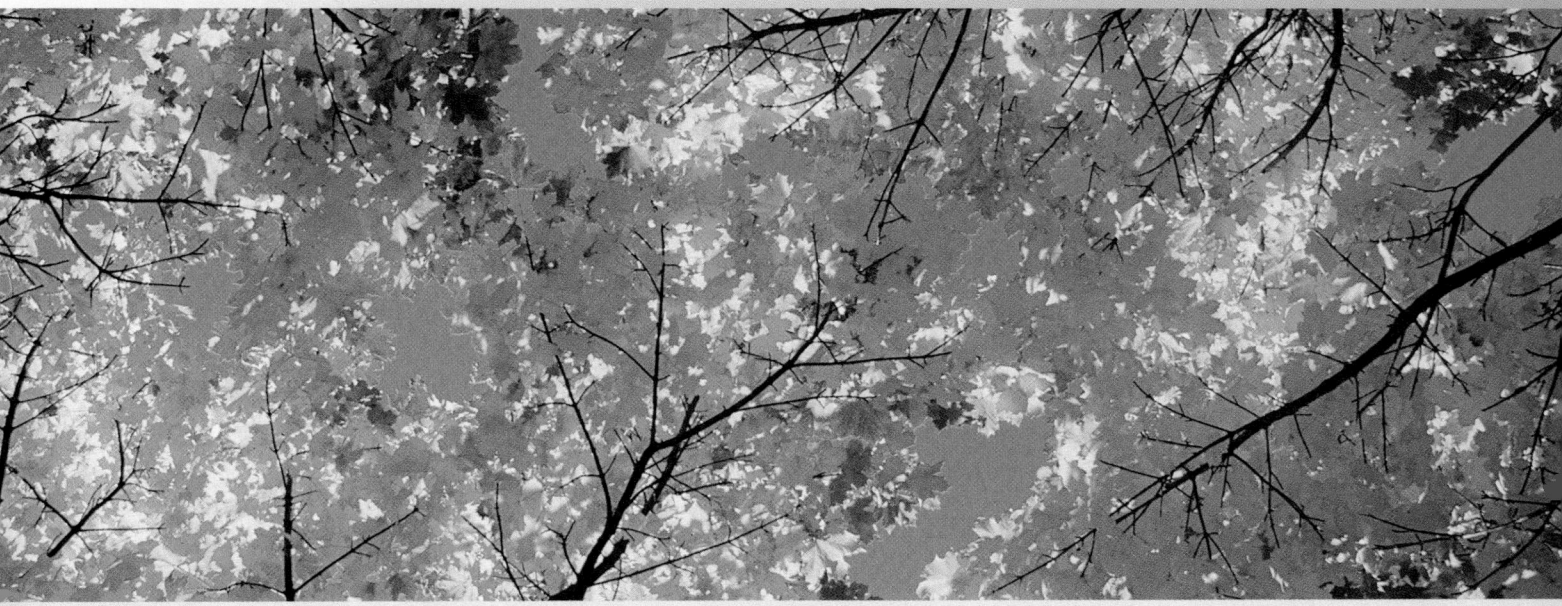

# CHAPTER 45

# Loss and Grief

Debra L. Topham, PhD, RN, CNS, ACRN

*"Death has always been and always will be with us. It is an integral part of human existence."*

(Elizabeth Kübler-Ross, 1975)

# Chapter Competencies

*Upon completion of this chapter, the reader should be able to:*

1. Discuss the concept of loss and theories around grief and death.
2. Describe various losses that affect individuals at different stages of the life cycle.
3. Explain the relationship between loss and grief.
4. Describe the characteristics of an individual experiencing grief.
5. Differentiate between uncomplicated and dysfunctional grief.
6. Discuss use of the nursing process with a grieving individual.
7. Discuss the holistic needs of the dying person and family.
8. Define the purpose of hospice care.
9. Develop a plan for end-of-life (EOL) care.
10. Discuss nursing responsibilities when a client dies.
11. Identify ethical and legal issues related to the end of life.
12. Describe ways in which nurses can cope with their own grief.

# Key Terms

| | | |
|---|---|---|
| algor mortis | dysfunctional grief | maturational loss |
| anticipatory grief | grief | mourning |
| autopsy | grief work | palliative care |
| bereavement | hospice | rigor mortis |
| complicated grief | liver mortis | situational loss |
| disenfranchised grief | loss | uncomplicated grief |

In contemporary society, individuals constantly experience loss. Frequent episodes of terrorism, natural disaster, and personal crises result in the universal experience of loss. Throughout the life cycle, people are faced with loss, without which growth would not continue. Many people consider loss only in terms of death and dying; however, loss of every type occurs daily. Nurses must be aware of the potential for loss in today's world, as well as the processes by which individuals adapt.

Every day nurses encounter clients who experience grief associated with losses. Thus, nurses must have an understanding of the major concepts related to loss and grieving. Grief is a response to losses of all types, especially death. Nurses also care for dying clients. This chapter provides information on meeting the special needs of dying clients and their families.

## Loss

**Loss** is any situation in which a valued object is changed or is no longer accessible to the individual. Because change is a major constant in life, everyone experiences losses. Loss can be actual (e.g., a spouse is lost through divorce) or anticipated (a person is diagnosed with a terminal illness and has only a short time to live). A loss can be tangible or intangible. For example, when a person is fired from a job, the tangible loss is income, whereas the loss of self-esteem is intangible.

Losses occur as a result of moving from one developmental stage to another. An example of such a **maturational loss** is the adolescent who loses the younger child's freedom from responsibility. Other examples of losses associated with growth and development are discussed later in this chapter. A **situational loss** occurs in response to external events, usually beyond the individual's control (such as the death of a significant other) (Figure 45-1).

Loss can also be experienced as a collective. On September 11, 2001, all Americans experienced significant loss as a result of a terrorist attack on the World Trade Center in New York City and the Pentagon in Washington, D.C. Individuals directly experienced loss of people, jobs, and material objectives. The collective of Americans has experienced the loss of security and invulnerability to foreign threats of violence on American soil.

## Types of Loss

Loss occurs when a valued object is changed or is no longer available. Not everyone responds to loss in the same

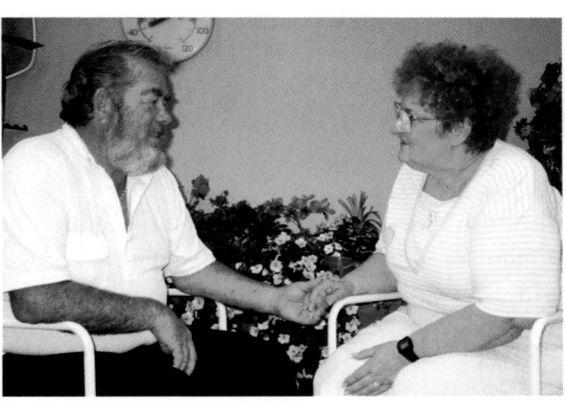

**Figure 45-1    An example of situational loss is the death of a spouse. These two friends have lost their spouses and are comforting one another.**

way, because the significance of the lost object or person is determined by individual perceptions. There are many types of loss, including:

- *Actual loss:* Loss that is perceived by others, such as death of a loved one, theft of one's property
- *Perceived loss:* Occurs when a sense of loss is felt by an individual but is not tangible to others, such as the loss of youth or stamina
- *Physical loss:* Loss of an extremity in an accident, scarring from burns, permanent injury
- *Psychological loss:* Such as a woman feeling inadequate after menopause and resultant infertility

There are four major categories of loss: loss of external objects, loss of familiar environment, loss of aspects of self, and loss of significant other (Antai-Otong, 2003).

### Loss of an External Object

When an object that a person highly values is damaged, changed, or disappears, loss occurs. The significance of the lost object to the individual determines the type and amount of grieving that occurs. The valued object may be a person, pet, prized possession, or one's home. The loss of

---

## STOP AND THINK

### Loss and September 11, 2001

Think about where you were and what you were doing on September 11, 2001:

1. What losses did you experience that day?
2. What emotions did you feel?
3. How did your behavior change for the days and weeks after September 11, 2001?

---

a pet, especially for those who live alone, can be a devastating loss (Figure 45-2).

### Loss of Familiar Environment

The loss of a familiar environment occurs when a person moves to another home or a different community, changes schools, or starts a new job. A client who is hospitalized or institutionalized experiences loss when faced with new surroundings. This type of loss may evoke anxiety.

### Loss of Aspect of Self

Loss of an aspect of self can be physiological or psychological. A psychological aspect of self that may be lost is ambition, a sense of humor, or enjoyment of life. An example of physiological loss includes loss of physical function as a result of illness or injury. Loss also occurs when there is disfigurement or disappearance of a body part, such as having an amputation or mastectomy. Loss of an aspect of self can result from illness, trauma, or treatment methodologies (such as surgery).

### Loss of Significant Other

The loss of a loved one is a significant loss. Such a loss can be the result of separation, divorce, running away, moving to a different area, or death. Responses to loss are highly individualized as each person perceives the meaning of loss differently. For example, the death of a spouse is different for men and women.

## Loss as Crisis

Loss precipitates anxiety and a feeling of vulnerability—which may lead to crisis. For example, when a significant

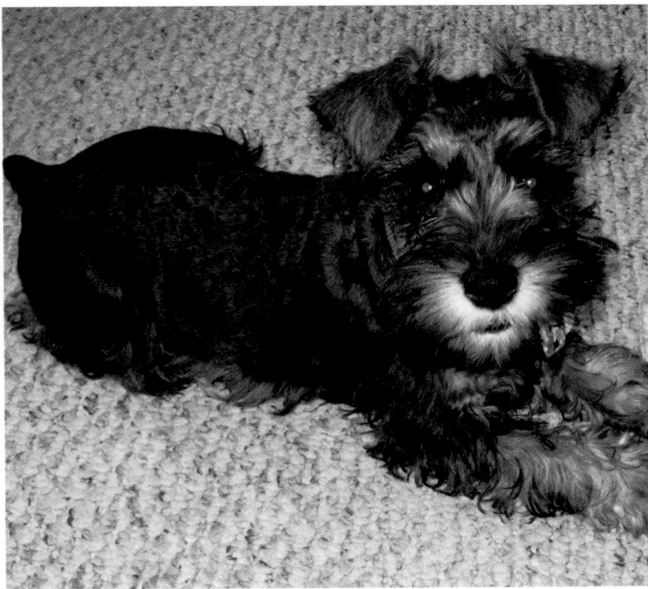

**Figure 45-2    Loss of a pet can lead to a grief response.**

other dies, one's sense of safety and security is disrupted. Grieving is a mechanism for coping with loss. When an individual feels overwhelmed by stress and the usual coping mechanisms are no longer effective, crisis occurs. Crisis intervention may be necessary to help the person grieve successfully.

# Grief

**Grief** is a series of responses that occur following a loss. It is a normal, natural, necessary, and adaptive response to a loss. **Bereavement** is the period of grief following a significant loss, especially the death of a person or pet. Bereavement may be a time when people may neglect their own health or are unable to continue day-to-day functioning. **Mourning** is the period of time during which the grief is expressed. Resolution and integration of the loss occur during mourning, and people are able to maintain their day-to-day activities. Mourning is an adaptive response to loss (Hospice Foundation of America, 2003).

## Theories of the Grieving Process

No one comprehensive theory explains the grief process, which may consist of a series of phases. Several theories have allowed delineation of predictable symptoms and grief states. When reviewing the following theories, remember that people do not experience each phase in the order described. The theories of Erich Lindemann, George L. Engle, and J. William Worden are discussed in the following section.

### Lindemann

In 1944, after the Coconut Grove fire in Boston in which over 400 people died, Lindemann studied survivors of the disaster and their families. Lindemann coined the phrase **grief work**, which is still used today to describe the process experienced by the bereaved. During grief work, the person experiences freedom from attachment to the deceased, becomes reoriented to the environment in which the deceased is no longer present, and establishes new relationships (Lindemann, 1944). Lindemann's classic work is the foundation for current crisis and grief resolution theories. Box 45-1 provides a description of Lindemann's concepts.

### Engle

Engle (1961) describes three stages of mourning, and progression through each stage is necessary for healing. The grieving process, which may take several years for completion, is experienced differently by each person. The goal of the grieving process is for the mourner to accept the loss and let go of the deceased. Box 45-2 provides an overview of Engle's theory of grief.

---

## BOX 45-1   LINDEMANN'S THEORY: REACTIONS TO NORMAL GRIEF

**Somatic Distress**
Episodic waves of discomfort in duration of 10 to 60 minutes; multiple somatic complaints, fatigue, and extreme physical or emotional pain.

**Preoccupation with the Image of the Deceased**
The bereaved experience a sense of unreality, emotional detachment from others, and an overwhelming pre-occupation with visualizing the deceased.

**Guilt**
The bereaved consider the death to be a result of their own negligence or lack of attentiveness; they look for evidence of how they could have contributed to the death.

**Hostile Reactions**
Relationships with others become impaired owing to the bereaved's desire to be left alone, irritability, and anger.

**Loss of Patterns of Conduct**
The bereaved exhibit an inability to sit still, generalized restlessness, and continual search for something to do.

Adapted from Lindemann, E. (1944). Symptomatology and management of acute grief. *American Journal of Psychiatry, 101,* 141–148; Roach, S. S., & Nieto, B. C. (1997). *Healing and the grief process* (pp. 1–24). Clifton Park, NY: Delmar Learning.

---

### Worden

Worden (1982) has identified four tasks that an individual must perform in order to successfully deal with a loss:

- Accept the fact that the loss is real.
- Experience the emotional pain of grief.
- Adjust to an environment without the deceased.
- Reinvest the emotional energy once directed at the deceased into another relationship (Worden, 1982).

Worden categorized the behavioral responses that grieving individuals experienced (Table 45-1).

Elizabeth Kübler-Ross (1975) has done extensive research around dying clients and their families. Her theory on death and dying is similar to some of the grief theories and is presented later in this chapter. It is important to remember that while there are many theories around

## BOX 45-2   ENGLE'S THEORY OF GRIEF: THREE STAGES OF MOURNING

### Stage I: Shock and Disbelief

- Disorientation
- Feeling of helplessness
- Denial gives protection until person is able to face reality

Stage I can last from minutes to days.

### Stage II: Developing Awareness

- Emotional pain occurs with increased reality of loss
- Recognition that one is powerless to change the situation
- Feelings of helplessness
- Anger and hostility may be directed at others
- Guilt
- Sadness
- Isolation
- Loneliness

Stage II may last from 6 to 12 months.

### Stage III: Restitution and Resolution

- Emergence of bodily symptoms
- May idealize the deceased
- Mourner starts to come to terms with the loss
- Establishment of new social patterns and relationships

Stage III marks the beginning of the healing process and may take up to several years.

Adapted from Engle, G. L. (1961). Is grief a disease? *Psychosomatic Medicine, 23,* 18–22; Engle, G. L. (1964). Grief and grieving. *American Journal of Nursing, 64*(9), 93-98; Roach, S. S., & Nieto, B. C. (1997). *Healing and the grief process* (pp. 1–24). Clifton Park, NY: Delmar Learning.

grief and loss, each person experiences loss and grief in her own unique way.

## Types of Grief

Grief is a universal, normal response to loss. Grief drains people, both emotionally and physically. Because grief consumes so much emotional energy, relationships may be impaired and health status may become altered. There are different types of grief, including uncomplicated (normal), dysfunctional, and anticipatory.

## Uncomplicated Grief

Many individuals use the term *normal grief.* Engle (1961) proposed use of the term **uncomplicated grief** to describe a grief reaction that normally follows a significant loss. Uncomplicated grief runs a fairly predictable course that ends with the relinquishing of the lost object and resumption of the previous life. Of course, the bereaved person's life is changed forever, but the person is able to regain the ability to function.

Some of the common responses experienced by grieving individuals are shown in Table 45-2. Not every mourner will experience all the reactions, but the reactions most often experienced in response to a recent loss are listed.

Many grieving people experience feelings of anger or blame; these feelings may be directed toward those perceived to have caused or contributed to the death. Often the anger associated with grief is directed at one's self, that is, expressed as guilt or depression. Some survivors have a strong need to assign blame. If someone else can be blamed, then the survivors can rid themselves of any responsibility. Those who are experiencing grief must be provided an opportunity to express feelings—both positive and negative—in order to alleviate guilt.

## Dysfunctional Grief

Persons experiencing **dysfunctional grief** do not progress through the stages of overwhelming emotions associated with grief, or they may fail to demonstrate any behaviors commonly associated with grief. The person experiencing dysfunctional grief continues to have strong emotional reactions, does not return to a normal sleep pattern or work routine, usually remains isolated, and has altered eating habits. The bereaved may have the need to endlessly tell and retell the story of loss but without subsequent healing. The pathologically grieving person is unable to reestablish a routine. Visits to the gravesite or mausoleum may be made often or not at all. Schattner (2000) refers to a type of dysfunctional grief as unspoken grief that "can lead to a variety of unresolved grief symptoms . . . and isolation from support of friends, family, and activities" (p. 11).

Dysfunctional grief is a demonstration of a persistent pattern of intense grief that does not result in reconciliation of feelings. A person experiencing chronic grief continues to focus on the deceased, may overvalue objects that belonged to the deceased, and may engage in depressive brooding. Several factors predispose a person to experience dysfunctional grieving, including:

- Uncertain, sudden, or overcomplicated circumstance surrounding the loss
- A loss that is socially unspeakable or socially negated (e.g., suicide)
- A relationship with the deceased characterized by ambivalence or excessive dependency (Worden, 1991)

## TABLE 45-1    MANIFESTATIONS OF NORMAL GRIEF (WORDEN)

| Emotions | Physical Settings | Behaviors | Thought Processes |
|---|---|---|---|
| • Sadness<br>• Anxiety<br>• Guilt<br>• Relief<br>• Emancipation<br>• Self-blame<br>• Fatigue<br>• Numbness<br>• Shock<br>• Helplessness<br>• Yearning<br>• Loneliness | • Increased sensitivity to noise<br>• Constricted feeling in throat and chest<br>• Shortness of breath<br>• Hollow feeling in stomach<br>• Dry mouth<br>• Muscular weakness<br>• Lethargy | • Disrupted sleep patterns<br>• Dreaming about the deceased<br>• Forgetfulness<br>• Crying<br>• Avoiding reminders of the deceased<br>• Treasuring objects belonging to the deceased<br>• Social withdrawal | • Disbelief<br>• Preoccupation<br>• Confusion<br>• Sense of presence of the deceased<br>• Hallucinations (such as seeing or hearing the deceased) |

## TABLE 45-2    REACTIONS COMMONLY EXPERIENCED DURING GRIEF

| Physical Reactions | Psychosocial Reactions | Cognitive Reactions | Behavioral Reactions |
|---|---|---|---|
| • Loss of appetite<br>• Weight loss<br>• Insomnia<br>• Fatigue<br>• Decreased libido<br>• Decreased immune functioning (increased susceptibility to illness)<br>• Multiple somatic complaints (e.g., headache, backache)<br>• Restlessness | • Profound sadness<br>• Helplessness<br>• Hopelessness<br>• Denial<br>• Anger<br>• Hostility<br>• Guilt<br>• Nightmares<br>• Ennui (overwhelming sense of emptiness)<br>• Preoccupation with lost object<br>• Loneliness | • Inability to concentrate<br>• Forgetfulness<br>• Impaired judgment<br>• Decreased problem-solving ability | • Impulsivity<br>• Indecisiveness<br>• Social withdrawal<br>• Distancing |

## Disenfranchised Grief

Disenfranchised grief is a type of grief that is a major contributor to dysfunctional grief. It has not received a lot of attention, especially as a focus of research. **Disenfranchised grief** is grief experienced in situations where grief is discouraged and social supports are absent (Doka, 1989). Such situations include, but are not limited to, death of partners of gays and lesbians, close friends, opposite-gender non-married partners, lovers of married persons, and clients of health care workers.

## Anticipatory Grief

**Anticipatory grief** is the occurrence of grief work before an expected loss. Anticipatory grief may be experienced by the terminally ill person as well as family. This phenomenon promotes adaptive grieving by freeing up the mourn-

er's emotional energy. Although anticipatory grieving may be helpful in adjusting to the loss, it may also result in some disadvantages. For example, for the dying client, anticipatory grieving may lead to family members' distancing themselves and not being available to provide support. Also, if the family members have separated themselves emotionally from the dying client, they may seem cold and distant, thus, not meeting society's expectations of mourning behavior. This response can prevent the mourners from receiving their own much needed support from others.

Nurses play an important role in assisting mourners to develop and understand the normal grieving process and the complex feelings exhibited when grief becomes more complicated. Nurses with a sound knowledge base of both normal grief and dysfunctional grief will be better pre-

## CLINICAL ALERT

### Severe Depression

Nurses must know the clinical manifestations of severe depression associated with grief in order to initiate treatment measures. Examples of symptomatology are flat affect, depressed mood most of the day, markedly diminished interest or pleasure in activities of the day, significant weight loss, insomnia, psychomotor agitation, and fatigue.

Hogstel, M. (2001). *Gerontology: Nursing care of the older adult.* Clifton Park, NY: Delmar Learning.

## CLIENT REFLECTIONS

### Support Groups During Grief

Vicki is a 24-year-old woman who has been married the last 2 years to her husband, Mark. While showering one day, Mark noticed a small lump in his left testicle. After examination and several tests, his doctor determined that he had advanced testicular cancer with metastasis. Despite treatment, Mark died within 4 weeks. When Mark died, Vicki was 6 weeks pregnant. Vicki's minister referred her to a support group for widows, as she was extremely distraught and thought her life had ended when her husband's did. Vicki makes the following statements to her nurse: "I am only 24 years old, and I am the youngest person in the group. In fact, the next youngest person is 67 years old and had been married for 45 years. I can't relate to any of the women in the group."

1. What factors could have predicted Vicki's difficulty in coping with her husband's death?
2. Would you anticipate any grief response problems when Vicki's baby is born? Why or why not?

pared to assist the survivors than nurses who believe that all grief is the same.

## Factors Affecting Grief

The experience of grief is individual and is influenced by various factors. Factors that influence grief include the person's developmental level, religious and cultural beliefs, relationship to the lost object, and the cause of death.

### Developmental Considerations

Depending on a client's development level, the grief response to a loss will be experienced differently. Nurses practice in many settings in which children, adolescents, and adults, as a result of growth and development, experience changes that result in loss. For example, a pregnant woman will, to some degree, experience loss after delivery, even delivery of a normal healthy infant. This might be the loss of freedom and identity as a nonparent. See Table 45-3 for other examples of developmental losses that may precipitate grieving. Certain kinds of loss at key developmental points may have a profound effect on a person's ability to work through grief, as well as possible inadequate achievement of the developmental task.

### Childhood

The many losses associated with childhood are often not appreciated unless the loss is the death of a person or pet. Children vary in their ability to comprehend the meaning of death. It is important to understand how a child's concept of death evolves, because it varies with developmental level and may affect mastery of developmental tasks (Table 45-4, Figure 45-3).

Well-meaning adults often try to protect children from the realities of death by excluding them from mourning rituals. However, children need to be included as appropriate to their developmental level. Children who are grieving need explanations about death that are honest and in language that can be comprehended. See Table 45-5 for suggestions on talking to children about death.

### Adolescence

Most adolescents value physical attractiveness and athletic abilities. Grief may occur when the adolescent suffers the loss of a body part or function. Because of the strong influence of peer groups, adolescents seek approval of their friends and fear being rejected if a loss affects their acceptance by others (e.g., grief after a disfiguring accident is usually intense in adolescents). Even though they have an intellectual understanding of death, adolescents feel they are immune to death and therefore do not accept the possibility of their own mortality. This perception is caused by the sense of invulnerability that normally occurs during adolescence. Adolescents perceive themselves as being invulnerable and death as something that will not happen to them. The loss of a parent may seriously disrupt developmental tasks at this level. The adolescent loses a very important role model, as well as has to take on more of the burden of supporting the household and younger siblings (Potts & Mandleco, 2002).

### Early Adulthood

In the young adult, grief is usually precipitated by loss of role or status. For example, unemployment or breakup of a relationship causes significant grief for the young adult. Similar to adolescents, young adults often view themselves

## CLIENT REFLECTIONS

### A Widower's Grief

Jerry was a 76-year-old widower whose wife died after a long, terminal illness. While she was dying, Jerry was supportive of his wife, constantly at her side. After her death, he held an elaborate "Celebration of Life" service that was well attended by family and friends. Nine months after his wife's death, Jerry attended a health screening for older people. When asked about his marital status, Jerry began sobbing and stated, "My wife died and I just don't know what to do without her." The nurse was able to find out that Jerry cried almost every day, had difficulty sleeping, had lost 20 pounds in the last 3 months, and often thought about dying himself. The nurse suggested that Jerry talk with his primary care provider about getting some antidepressant medication. Jerry burst into more tears and stated he was sad and grieving but didn't think that was abnormal. The nurse explained that sadness and grief was normal, but that his response was longer and affecting his health. She also explained that the medication would help him through this rough time while he received some grief counseling and support. Jerry saw his primary care provider and started on Celexa®, an antidepressant. He also attended some grief support groups and began going to senior lunches during the week. After 6 months, Jerry felt like he was a "new man." He had gained his weight back, was sleeping at night, and found that while he missed his wife and remembered her, he didn't cry every day or every time he thought of her. He had also developed a small network of friends and was considering dating one of the women he eats lunch with.

1. To what community resources could the nurse have referred Jerry?
2. Is Jerry's grief reaction typical?

and their lives as invulnerable to the impact of death. In addition to loss of a parent, loss of a partner or child during this developmental stage can be extremely disruptive and often leaves the young adult at risk for dysfunctional grief. An example is the couple who experiences the birth of a stillborn child. Over 50% of these couples divorce within 2 years of the stillbirth, secondary to dysfunctional grief responses.

### Middle Adulthood

During middle adulthood the potential for experiencing loss increases. The death of parents begins to occur. Because loss of parents is an anticipated task during middle adulthood, dysfunctional grief is less likely than in young adulthood. Dysfunctional grief is more of a risk if a peer dies. As an individual ages, it can be especially threatening for peers to die because their death forces acknowledgment of one's own vulnerability to death. Other losses frequently experienced during middle age are those associated with changes in employment and relationships (e.g., divorce), children leaving home, and decreasing functional abilities.

### Older Adulthood

During late adulthood, most individuals recognize the inevitability of death. Most older adults experience numerous losses as they age. Losses commonly experienced by older adults include loss of (Bowlby, 1982):

- Loved ones and friends
- Occupational role as a result of retirement
- Material possessions
- Dreams and hopes
- Physical and cognitive function

In the United States, women are more likely than men to experience the death of a spouse or partner. Regardless of gender, the bereaved may need to develop new skills in order to adapt. For example, a man who was married for 50 years may have to learn meal preparation after his wife dies (Callahan, 1999).

### Religious and Cultural Beliefs

Religious and cultural beliefs can have a significant effect on an individual's grief. Every culture has certain religious beliefs about the significance of death, as well as rituals for care of the dying. See Chapters 5 and 48 for discussion of the impact of religious and cultural beliefs. Beliefs about an after-life, faith in God, redemption of the soul, and reincarnation are important aspects that often assist one in grief work.

### Relationship with the Lost Entity

It is usually more difficult to cope with the loss of an ambivalent relationship, as such relationships are characterized by many "if only" and "I should have" thoughts. "Unfinished business" and regrets about the deceased make coping with their loss more problematic. When individuals of stormy relationships have time to work on issues prior to the death, grieving is usually facilitated.

In general, the more intimate the relationship with the deceased, the more intense the grief experienced by the bereaved. The death of a child poses a particular risk for dysfunctional grieving to occur.

The death of a parent or a sibling can pose a major challenge for children. The child's feelings may often go

## TABLE 45-3 LOSSES ASSOCIATED WITH DEVELOPMENTAL STAGE

| Developmental Stage | Related Loss | Developmental Stage | Related Loss |
|---|---|---|---|
| Infants | • Intrauterine environment (warmth and protection) <br> • Comfort of sucking breast or bottle | Young adults | • Friends through leaving school, moving, changing jobs <br> • Financial support from parents when leaving home <br> • Freedom when assuming more adult responsibilities <br> • Sexual activity |
| Toddlers/ Preschoolers | • Security object <br> • Immediate gratification of needs as child gains independence <br> • Familiar environment as child attends day care or nursery school | Middle adults | • Spouse, through separation, divorce, or death <br> • Children as they leave home <br> • Friends through job changes, moving, or death <br> • Parents through death <br> • "Youth" (as related to physical appearance, decreased libido, physical stamina) <br> • Women experiencing loss of fertility through menopause |
| School-aged children | • Periodic loss of body function caused by normal childhood illnesses and injuries <br> • Friends and significant others (teachers, coaches) as they progress through school | | |
| Adolescents | • Changing schools <br> • Familiarity of body with onset of puberty <br> • Childhood freedoms in response to social expectation to act mature <br> • First love (as adolescent "crushes" end) <br> • Familiar environment when leaving home for work or education | Older adults | • Spouse and friends through death <br> • Sensory perceptual acuity <br> • Job, as a result of retirement <br> • Body image changes related to decline in some physiological functions <br> • Independence <br> • Cognitive abilities |

unrecognized by adults who fail to understand the child's need to mourn (Mallow & Bechtel, 1999).

Individuals experiencing parental grief usually have intense reactions and responses. In the United States today, it is expected that children outlive their parents. When a child dies, the parent loses not only the child, but also experiences losses of the parental role. Bowlby (1961) describes parents who talk about losing a part of themselves as a result of their child's death. "The death of a child disrupts family homeostasis and the psychological and physiologic equilibrium of family members" (Levin, 1998, p. 70). The uniqueness of parental grief for a deceased child may be the loss of the perceived potential for that child who has died. It is the loss of the parents'

hopes for the child, for "the things that could have been." Table 45-6 provides a listing of characteristics of parents of infants and children who have died (see Box 45-3).

### Cause of Death
#### Anticipated Death

Anticipated death, such as death after a lengthy terminal illness, often results in an uncomplicated grief response. Other types of death may affect the intensity of the grief response, especially unexpected death or death from trauma or suicide.

#### Unexpected Death

The loss occurring with an unexpected death poses particular difficulty for the bereaved in achieving closure. As

## TABLE 45-4 PERCEPTION OF DEATH BY CHILDREN AND ADOLESCENTS

| Developmental Stage | Perception | Potential Developmental Disruptions |
|---|---|---|
| Infancy, toddler | • Not aware of death<br>• Is aware of disruptions in normal routine<br>• Can react to family's expressions of grief | • If the mother or surrogate dies during the first 2 years of life, may have significant long-lasting psychosocial problems |
| Preschool | • Views death as a temporary separation<br>• Able to react to the gravity of death in accordance with the reactions of parents or other adults | • May have significant psychosocial problems if either parent is lost at this stage, especially between ages 4 and 6 (owing to *magical thinking,* in which children may believe death is their fault) |
| School-age | • Appreciates that death is final and inevitable<br>• Fantasizes about and tends to personify death ("the boogie-man") | • May have nightmares<br>• May engage in death-avoidance behaviors (e.g., hiding under the covers, leaving the lights on, closing closet doors)<br>• May experience intense guilt and a sense of responsibility for the death |
| Preadolescent and adolescent | • Recognizes that death is final<br>• Understands that death is inevitable<br>• Preadolescents: tend to worry about dying<br>• Adolescents: tend to deny that death could happen to them | • Loss of a parent may interfere with mastery of the young adulthood task of forming an intimate relationship with members of opposite sex |

Roach and Nieto (1997) stated, any death, even anticipated death, is a traumatic experience to the surviving loved ones. Unexpected death, such as a death from complications after a successful surgery, leaves survivors shocked and bereaved. Often, the inability to say good-bye compounds the trauma of the death and may be a factor contributing to complicated grieving.

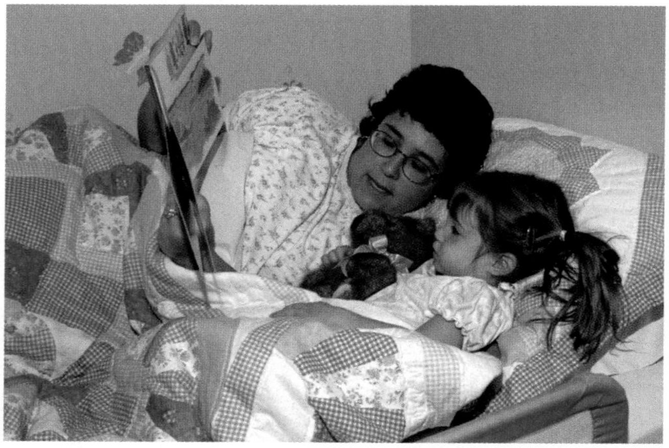

**Figure 45-3** **This child has lost her father to cancer. Her mother is providing extra care and attention during this time of loss.**

### Traumatic Death

**Complicated grief** is also associated with traumatic death such as death by homicide, suicide, or an accident. Although traumatic death does not necessarily predispose the survivor to complications in mourning, survivors may suffer emotions of greater intensity than those associated with normal grief (James & Friedman, 1998).

When loved ones die violently, the grievers may suffer from traumatic imagery—that is, reliving the terror of the incident or imagining the feelings of horror felt by the victim. Traumatic imagery is a common occurrence with traumatic death. Such thoughts, coupled with intense grief, can lead to *post-traumatic stress disorder* (PTSD). Nurses must be aware of the possibility of PTSD and be alert for the presence of symptoms, which may include:

• Sleep disturbances, such as recurrent, terror-filled nightmares

## TABLE 45-5 COMMUNICATING WITH CHILDREN ABOUT DEATH

| Therapeutic | Nontherapeutic |
|---|---|
| • Use simple, concrete language. | • Use of euphemisms (e.g., "he's gone to sleep" or "she passed away") |
| • Involve the child in mourning rituals (take to funeral home and/or cemetery); explain what is going to happen. | • Overexplanations |
| • Encourage the child to express feelings. | • Minimizing child's experience |
| • Reassure children that they will not be abandoned. | • Judgmental statements |
| • Answer all questions truthfully. | • Hiding/sheltering child |

## TABLE 45-6 CHARACTERISTICS OF PARENTS WHOSE INFANT OR UNBORN CHILD DIES

| Death | Characteristics |
|---|---|
| Spontaneous abortion (miscarriage) and stillbirth | Parents, especially the mother, may have feelings of intense sadness, anger, or guilt. The death is often inadequately recognized by others, especially if the loss occurs in early weeks of pregnancy. The death may be considered a personal failure. Parents may dwell on details, designating blame to themselves or others. Grief from previous miscarriages may be relived. Anticipatory grief may occur if the condition of the infant is known early. Ambivalence experienced in early pregnancy may increase grief. Hopes for the future must be modified or changed. Despair may peak when the parents must leave the hospital without the baby. |
| Neonatal death | Feelings are similar to stillbirth. Parents have had the time to form a bond with the infant, intensifying the grief. Grief may be intense by both parents. |
| Sudden infant death syndrome (SIDS) | Death is unexplainable and totally unexpected. Pain is increased by lack of knowledge and misinformation. Parental bonding is complete. Death is silent, no signs of distress. Guilt may be present. Police may investigate, adding to the guilt. Grief is acute because there is no time to prepare. Parents, especially the mother, may be preoccupied with the details of the death. |
| Abortion | Shame, secrecy, and guilt may accompany grief. Highly ambivalent feelings may be present. Little support or comfort is offered by others. Feelings of relief are expected, but despair and depression may surface. No guilt may be felt, especially if the woman did not want a child. |

## BOX 45-3    GRIEF IN BRAZIL

Parkes (2002) related the story of researcher Nancy Sheper-Hughes, who studied poor people of northeast Brazil and the high infant mortality rate. She found mothers did not grieve at the death of children, because they were "just babies."

- Psychological distress
- Chronic anxiety

Unless this problem is recognized and the survivors are encouraged to express the intense feelings, they will not be able to progress through the normal, adaptive grieving process.

### Suicide

The loss of a loved one to suicide is frequently compounded by feelings of blame in the survivors. They feel guilty for failing to recognize clues that may have enabled the victim to receive help. These feelings of guilt and self-blame can be transformed into anger at the victim for inflicting such pain, at themselves and at caregivers. Feelings of shame for having a suicide in the family may also be present. Because of the social unacceptability of suicide, grief related to suicide is one form of disenfranchised grief.

## Nursing Care of the Grieving Person

Resolution of a loss is a painful process and must be done by clients in their own way. Nurses can assist by providing support as the client moves through the process of mourning. Grief changes people by affecting self-esteem, triggering the development of new ways of coping, and precipitating a change in lifestyle without the deceased.

Nurses can play an active role in assisting people to grieve. Encourage clients to do their grief work, that is, to experience their feelings to the fullest in order to work through them. Provide support and explain to the bereaved that it will take time to grieve the loss and to

## RESEARCH FOCUS

**Title of Study:** Chronic sorrow: The experience of parents with children who are developmentally disabled

**Study Purpose:** To compare chronic sorrow experiences of mothers with those of fathers of developmentally disabled children.

**Methods:** A qualitative survey design was used to identify patterns of feelings and emotions among parents residing in the same household with a developmentally disabled child.

**Findings:** Different patterns of chronic sorrow among mothers and fathers of developmentally disabled children were identified. Adaptation mechanisms differ between mothers and fathers. Mothers' emotions evolve into chronic sorrow, while fathers' reactions move toward resignation.

**Implications:** This study points out the need for continued support to parents; involvement in community support groups may be helpful in coping with chronic sorrow and resignation.

Mallow, G. E., & Bechtel, G. A. (1999). Chronic sorrow: The experience of parents with children who are developmentally disabled. *Journal of Psychosocial Nursing, 37*(7), 31–35.

## CLIENT EDUCATION

### Risk Factors for Complicated Grief

Clients can be informed of the following risk factors for complicated grief:

***Mode of Loss***
- ✓ Loss is sudden or unexpected, leaving the survivor little time for preparation
- ✓ Multiple losses
- ✓ Violent or horrific loss
- ✓ Loss for which the person is responsible or feels responsible
- ✓ Loss for which others are seen as responsible
- ✓ Disenfranchised losses (cannot be acknowledged or mourned)

***Personal Vulnerability***
- ✓ Dependent on deceased person (or deceased person dependent on survivor)
- ✓ Ambivalence toward the deceased person
- ✓ Survivor lacks self-esteem and/or trust in others
- ✓ Survivor is psychologically vulnerable (or has history of psychological vulnerability)

***Lack of Social Support***
- ✓ Absent or nonsupportive family
- ✓ Social isolation

Adapted from Parkes, C. M. (2002). Grief: Lessons from the past, visions for the future. *Death Studies, 26*, 367–385.

## NURSING STRATEGY

### Questions to Ask a Grieving Client

1. How have your hygiene habits been affected? (Cues of complicated grief include wearing dirty clothes, not showering or bathing, not brushing hair or teeth, not shaving, etc.)

2. How has your diet changed? (Cues of complicated grief include eating more or less than usual; eating more sugar, fast foods, and high-fat foods; and eating less of healthy foods.)

3. How has your sleep changed? (Cues of complicated grief include more or less sleep than usual, difficulty falling asleep, and interrupted sleep.)

4. Are you socializing less than previously? (Cues of complicated grief include less socialization and more solitary activities.)

5. Are you able to work normal hours? (Cues of complicated grief include missing more work than usual, habitual tardiness to work, and lack of interest in work.)

Levin, B. (1998). Grief Counseling. *American Journal of Nursing,* 98(5), 69–72.

gain some closure to the relationship (Ferrell, Grant, & Virani, 1999).

## Assessment

A thorough assessment of the grieving client and family begins with a determination of the personal meaning of the loss. Another key assessment area is deciding where the person is in terms of the grieving process. The nurse understands that the stages of grieving are not necessarily mastered sequentially, but that instead individuals may vacillate in progression through the stages of grief. Levin (1998) recommends that assessment be done to differentiate the signs of healthy grieving from complicated grieving. The key to distinguishing between uncomplicated and complicated grieving is in assessing the person's self-care behavior and ability to continue her normal day-to-day routines.

## Nursing Diagnosis

The North American Nursing Diagnosis Association (NANDA) defines *Dysfunctional Grieving* as "extended, unsuccessful use of intellectual and emotional responses by which individuals (families, communities) attempt to work through the process of modifying self-concept based upon the perception of potential loss" (NANDA, 2003). Another diagnosis that may be applicable is *Anticipatory*

*Grieving*, defined as "intellectual and emotional responses and behavior by which individuals (families, communities) work through the process of modifying self-concept based on the perception of potential loss" (NANDA, 2003). See Box 45-4 for a discussion of the two NANDA diagnoses specifically developed to address grieving individuals.

### Outcome Identification and Planning

It is important to clarify the expected outcomes when planning care for the grieving client. Listed below are some expected outcome criteria for the person experiencing grief:

- Verbalize feelings of grief.
- Share grief with significant others.
- Accept the loss.
- Renew activities and relationships.

Some of these expected outcomes will take a long period of time to achieve, and some must be achieved before others are mastered. For example, to accept the loss, the person must begin to share grief with others by verbalizing feelings. Two expected outcomes for the bereaved are discussed.

### Acceptance of the Loss

Only by going through grief work are individuals able to reach some acceptance and, ultimately, resolution of feelings about the loss. Often, people try to find some meaning in their situations. This search involves introspection in which spiritual support is of therapeutic value.

### Renewal of Activities and Relationships

The very core of grief work revolves around acceptance of the fact that the needs met by key people in clients' lives can be met in other ways and by other people or the clients themselves. The deceased cannot be replaced; however, enough healing must occur so that new relationships can be initiated.

How long does the process of adaptive grieving take? The length of time for grief to be resolved is as individual as the person experiencing it and its intensity. Grief work takes time. There are no definite time frames in which grief should occur. Each person grieves in his own way and at his own pace.

### Implementation

Therapeutic nursing care is based on an understanding of the significance of the loss to the client. To understand the client's perspective, the nurse must spend time listening. As the client expresses feelings, the nurse must demonstrate acceptance, even if the client is not responding according to the nurse's expectations or belief system. The nurse's non-judgmental, accepting attitude is essential while the bereaved expresses anger and other emotions. The nurse communicates an understanding of the client's emotions—and avoids personalizing and using defensive behaviors.

Grieving people need reassurance, counseling, and support (Figure 45-4). One mechanism of providing support

## BOX 45-4    NURSING DIAGNOSES FOR GRIEF

### Diagnosis: Dysfunctional Grieving
**Defining Characteristics**
*Major*

- Unsuccessful adaptation to loss
- Prolonged denial or depression
- Inability to resume normal living patterns
- Delayed emotional response

*Minor*

- Failure to restructure life after the loss
- Social isolation or withdrawal from others
- Failure to develop new interests or relationships

*Related Factors*

- Loss of physiological function related to disease or trauma
- Surgery (colostomy, hysterectomy, mastectomy, amputation)
- Terminal illness
- Chronic pain
- Death
- Developmental life changes
- Loss of a relationship

### Diagnosis: Anticipatory Grieving
**Defining Characteristics**
*Major*

- Expressed emotional pain over a potential loss

*Minor*

- Sorrow
- Anger
- Guilt
- Altered sleep patterns
- Changes in eating patterns
- Decreased libido
- Communication alterations

*Related Factors*

- Diagnosis of terminal illness (self or significant other)
- Upcoming lifestyle change (divorce, child leaving home)
- Potential job loss
- Loss associated with aging

Data from North American Nursing Diagnosis Association. (NANDA). (2003). *Nursing diagnoses: Definitions & classification, 2003–2004.* Philadelphia: Author.

---

 **STOP AND THINK**

### Allowing Time to Grieve

Your coworker, who is also your friend, has just lost a loved one whose funeral was today. Tomorrow your friend must return to work because his 3-day bereavement leave is over. He is dealing with many intense emotions as well as a lack of energy. Society dictates that he return to work.

- How would you feel if you were in his place?
- How do you deal with his lack of productivity at work?
- How do you provide support to him?

---

on a long-term basis is support groups. Thus, the nurse needs to be aware of the availability of such groups within the community to make appropriate referrals. When bereaved people join support groups, they will be with others who have experienced the same situation. This sharing decreases the feelings of loneliness and social isolation that are so common in grief. The accompanying Nursing Strategy box lists steps for working through loss.

### Evaluation

People follow their own time schedule for grief work. In general, it takes months or years for resolution of grief. It is important to teach grieving individuals that resolution of the loss is generally a process of lifelong adjustment. Therefore, nurses usually do not have an opportunity to be with the bereaved family when grief work is completed. However, the nurse has a unique opportunity to lay the foundation for adaptive grieving

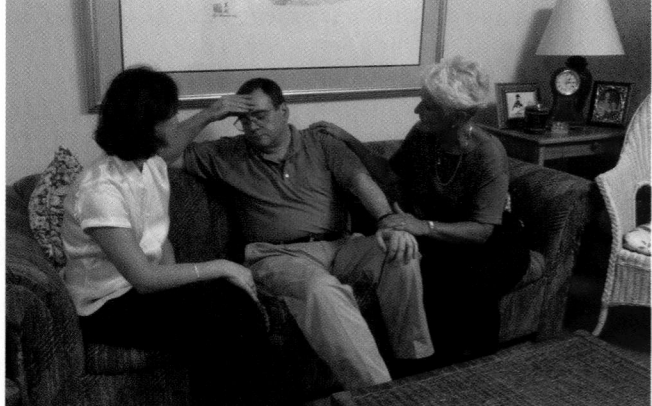

**Figure 45-4    A home health nurse and spouse are comforting this husband in his grieving over the loss of his father.**

## NURSING STRATEGY

### Assisting Clients to Grieve Successfully

When working with bereaved clients, encourage them to:

- Recognize the loss by acknowledging the loss.

- Express feelings related to the loss.

- Remember the deceased in a realistic (versus idealistic) manner.

- Relinquish old attachments of the deceased (e.g., give away some of the deceased's possessions).

- Readjust to the community without the deceased.

- Reinvest the emotional energy into something else (e.g., begin to socialize).

Data modified from Schattner, J. (2000). A ritual to help participants grieve the loss of another member in their cardiac rehabilitation program. *Journal of Psychosocial Nursing, 38*(1), 13.

| TABLE 45-7 | KÜBLER-ROSS'S STAGES OF DYING AND DEATH |
|---|---|
| **Stage** | **Example** |
| First stage: **Denial** | *Verbal:* "This can't be happening to me!" *Behavioral:* Client is diagnosed with terminal lung cancer; client continues to smoke two packs of cigarettes daily. |
| Second stage: **Anger** | *Verbal:* "Why me?" *Behavioral:* Client strikes out at caregivers. |
| Third stage: **Bargaining** | *Verbal:* Client prays, "Please, God, just let me live long enough to see my grandchild graduate." *Behavioral:* Client promises to change behaviors if God will let client live. |
| Fourth stage: **Depression** | *Verbal:* "Go away. I just want to lie here in bed. What's the use?" *Behavioral:* Client withdraws and isolates self. |
| Fifth stage: **Acceptance** | *Verbal:* "I feel ready. At least, I'm more at peace now." *Behavioral:* Client gets financial or legal affairs in order. Client says goodbye to significant others. |

Data from Kübler-Ross, E. (1969). *On death and dying.* New York: Macmillan.

by encouraging the bereaved to share their feelings and continue to verbalize their experience with significant others. Goals mutually established with client and family are the foundation for evaluation.

## Death

Historically, while death has been viewed as a normal part of life, many have often sought illusive immortality. As Western medicine and science have developed, the technology to prolong life has allowed health care workers to save the lives of people who previously would have died. Death became viewed as something to be avoided at all costs. Despite this perspective, everyone does die.

## Stages of Death and Dying

In her classic works, Elizabeth Kübler-Ross (1969, 1974) identified five possible stages of dying experienced by clients and their families (Table 45-7). Every person does not move sequentially through each stage. These stages are experienced in varying degrees and for varying lengths of time. The client may express anger, a few minutes later express acceptance of death, and then express anger again. The value in Kübler-Ross's work is that it helps increase sensitivity to the needs of the dying client and her family.

### Denial

In the first stage of dying, the initial shock can be overwhelming. Denial, which is an immediate response to loss experienced by most people, is a useful tool for coping. It is an essential and protective mechanism that may last for only a few minutes or may manifest itself for months.

### Anger

The initial stage of denial is followed by anger. The client's security is being threatened by the unknown. All the normal daily routines have become disrupted. The client has no control over the situation and thus becomes angry in response to this powerlessness. The anger may be directed at self, God, and others. Often the nurse is the recipient of the anger when the client lashes out (Figure 45-5).

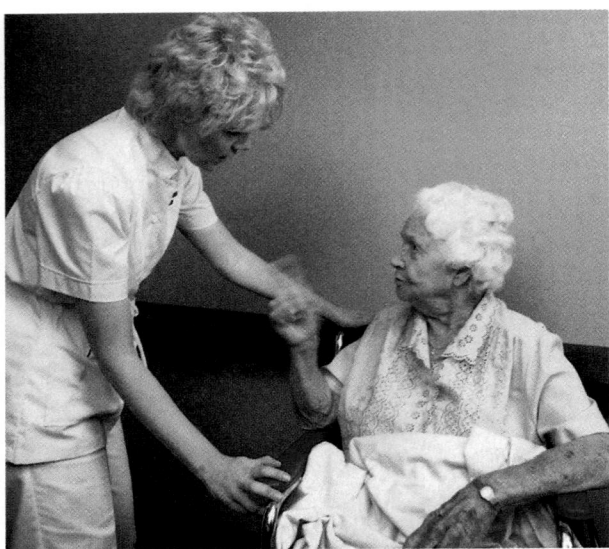

**Figure 45-5** Anger is a common response of grieving individuals. What is the nurse's priority action in the situation depicted with this angry client?

### Bargaining

The anticipation of the loss through death brings about bargaining through which the client attempts to postpone or reverse the inevitable. The client promises to do something (such as be a better person, change lifestyle) in exchange for a longer life. Significant others may try to bargain with God, offering their own life so that their loved one can live.

### Depression

When the realization comes that the loss can no longer be delayed, the client moves to the stage of depression. This depression can be different from dysfunctional depression in that it helps the client detach from life to be able to accept death. This type of depression can become dysfunctional and immobilizing. Too often this depression is not treated because people are expected to experience depression when they are dying or when a loved one has died. Depression should be treated as any other symptom associated with end-of-life care, such as pain or fatigue (Antai-Otong, 2003).

### Acceptance

The final stage of acceptance may not be reached by every dying client. However, "most dying persons eventually accept the inevitability of death. Many want to talk about their feelings with family members" (Ward, 1999, p. 1). Verbalization of emotions facilitates acceptance. With acceptance comes growing awareness of peace and contentment. The feeling that all that could be done has been done is often expressed during this stage. Reinforcement of the client's feelings and sense of personal worth are important during this stage. In addition, the concept of death is very different in children and requires nurses to have knowledge specific to pediatric clients.

## Ethical and Legal Issues Related to End of Life

The meaning of death and the role of medicine in addressing the needs of terminal clients have entered into great debate in the past decade. At the beginning of the 20th century, death was more readily accepted as a part of life. With advances in allopathic medical science, such as the perfection of anesthesia and surgery and the development of thousands of medications, death became viewed as something to be avoided at all costs. Any and every medical intervention was used to try and sustain life.

Moving into the 21st century, however, great ethical debates have arisen as technology has outpaced ethical science. People are beginning to question medical intervention at all costs, especially when death is inevitable. The struggle between intervening to prolong life and allowing for a peaceful death has given rise to end-of-life care, palliative care, hospice, and physician-assisted suicide. End-of-life (EOL) care and physician-assisted suicide will be discussed here.

## LIFE SPAN CONSIDERATIONS

### Children and Death

Children react to the death of a family member differently than adults. Preschoolers view death as temporary or reversible. Children between ages 5 and 9 view death as permanent, but don't believe it will happen to them or someone they know. Things to know about grief and children:

1. Upon the death of a family member, children may have an immediate grief reaction or believe that the family member is still alive.
2. Children should be allowed to attend funerals, but never forced to. If the child asks to go, then he is ready, although an adult may need to explain to the child what is happening. If the child doesn't want to go, he should not be forced to, no matter what the age. If the child doesn't go to a funeral, it is helpful to have him honor or remember the person through a prayer or lighting a candle.
3. Children may display feelings of sadness off and on over a long period of time and at unexpected moments.
4. Children often respond to death through anger, especially if the person was a part of the child's stability. Anger is directed toward surviving family members and is displayed in a variety of ways, often by the child acting out.
5. Children often regress, or act younger than they are, when a parent dies.
6. Children may feel guilty if someone whom they wished were dead actually dies. The child may believe that his wish has come true.
7. Children with the following symptoms are having serious problems with grief and need professional help: inability to sleep, loss of appetite, fear of being alone, loss of interest in daily activities, repeating desire to join the dead person, withdrawal from friends, sharp drop in school performance, or refusal to attend school.

Potts, N., & Mandleco, B. (2002). *Pediatric nursing: Caring for children and their families.* Clifton Park, NY: Delmar Learning.

## End-of-Life (EOL) Care

Death is one of two life events that all humans share, the other being birth. Dying is a normal part of the life cycle. Technological advances in medicine have caused care of those who are dying to become depersonalized and mechanical.

In an attempt to humanize care of the dying, proponents of improved EOL care are looking to nurses. "Nurses spend more time with patients who are facing the end of life than any other member of the health care team" (Ferrell, Grant, & Virani, 1999, p. 252). In 1997, the Institute of Medicine (IOM) made six recommendations for improving EOL care (see Box 45-5).

## Physician-Assisted Suicide

The legal grounds for physician-assisted suicide is currently under debate in the United States (Emanuel, 2002). Emanuel found that pain was not the primary deciding factor for clients who chose to commit suicide and that clients with cancer were most likely to use euthanasia. At least seven states have passed laws that prohibit euthanasia. The state of Oregon, however, did pass a physician-assisted

---

### BOX 45-5   IMPROVING END-OF-LIFE CARE: IOM RECOMMENDATIONS

1. Create and facilitate client and family expectations for reliable, skillful, and supportive care.
2. Ask health care professionals to commit themselves to improving care for dying clients and using existing knowledge to prevent and relieve pain and other symptoms.
3. Address deficiencies in the health care system through improved methods for measuring quality, tools for provider accountability, revised financial systems to encourage better coordination of care, and reformed drug prescribing laws.
4. Develop medical education to ensure practitioners have relevant attitudes, knowledge, and skills to provide excellent EOL care.
5. Make palliative care a defined area of expertise, education, and research.
6. Pursue public discussion about the modern experience of dying, options available to dying clients and families, and community obligations to those nearing death.

Data from Field, M. J., & Cassel, C. K. (Eds.). (1997). *Approaching death: Improving care at the end of life (report of the Institute of Medicine Task Force).* Washington, DC: National Academy Press.

suicide law that allows physicians to prescribe medications that could be used by clients to facilitate their death. These clients must have an irreversible, terminal illness; have extensive psychiatric evaluations on at least two occasions; undergo counseling; and meet certain other conditions.

In 2001, U.S. Attorney General John Ashcroft sought to have states' physician-suicide laws negated. He had a federal law passed that makes it a federal crime for a physician to prescribe controlled substances to assist suicide of clients (Dispensing of, 2001). Ashcroft has threatened prosecution of physicians who prescribe any controlled substance to be used for the purpose of assisted suicide. There continues to be great ethical and legal debate around this very sensitive issue.

# Nursing Care of the Dying Client

## Assessment

Nursing interventions are based on a thorough assessment of the client's holistic needs. While the end of life can be a difficult time, it is an important time for the nurse to confidently assess a client's death readiness. Most clients are relieved when they are asked about their death readiness and have someone who is willing to listen and assist them in this last of life's processes. Assessment areas in the dying client are shown in Box 45-6.

## Nursing Diagnosis

Because death is a natural part of life processes, no nursing diagnoses are specific to dying. Nursing diagnoses related to grieving, which were previously discussed in this chapter, are most appropriately used with the dying client and family. Numerous other nursing diagnoses may be applicable to the dying client. These would include nursing diagnoses related to any physical and

# LEGAL AND ETHICAL ISSUES

### Dilemma Around Dying

In March 2002, Ms. Bartlett, paralyzed from the neck down, was allowed to have her ventilator shut off, ending her life. Mrs. Peters petitioned the court to be allowed to have her physician assist her in a peaceful death. Mrs. Peters had a degenerative disease, was on a feeding tube, was unable to speak, and was unable to move from the neck down. With disease progression, she would soon end up on a ventilator. The courts upheld the decision to not support assisted suicide, but they allowed for Ms. Bartlett's refusal of medical treatment, even as termination of such treatment resulted in her immediate death. Singer (2002) notes that legally the decisions were both correct. Refusal of medical treatment is a legal right, even if it means death. Assisted suicide is not legal, even in a similar situation in which the person has not yet become dependent upon a medical intervention that could be removed and thus facilitate death. Singer argues that while the legal line is clear, the ethical issue remains unclear. Morally, Singer asks, why is there a difference between the case where a doctor turns off a ventilator and the other case where he gives a drug, if both result in the ending of a life?

Singer, P. (2002). Ms. B and Diane Pretty: A commentary. *Journal of Medical Ethics, 28,* 234–235.

emotional conditions present. Diagnoses that may be directly related to the dying client include *Powerlessness, Helplessness, High Risk for Spiritual Distress,* and *Altered Family Processes.* The reader is referred to NANDA's (2003) book for more detailed information about these nursing diagnoses.

## Outcome Identification and Planning

Nursing care promotes the optimal quality of life, which means treating the client and family in a respectful manner and providing a safe environment for the expression of feelings. Sensitive nursing care recognizes and respects the cultural, ethnic, spiritual, and religious beliefs of clients and families. Planning focuses on meeting the holistic needs and goals of the client and family. Essential elements to consider when planning care of the dying person, include:

- Schedule time to be available to client.
- Offer to contact clergy or spiritual guide.

# STOP AND THINK

### Communicating with the Family

Relief from pain, constipation, nausea, dry mouth, and reactions to treatments are basic needs of dying people. Being able to take nourishment, to be active, and to occupy oneself are also needs.

- What should the nurse tell the family as physiological changes occur?

- How can nurses help both the client and the family deal with these changes?

## BOX 45-6  ASSESSING THE DYING CLIENT

- Client and family's knowledge about the nature of terminal illness and its trajectory

- Availability of support systems for client and family

- Physical condition and symptoms, such as pain, anxiety, and fatigue

- Emotional status including assessment for depression

- Presence of advanced directives for health care decisions

- Concern about unfinished business

- Client priorities and preparation needs before death

Hospice Foundation of America. (2003). http://www.hospice foundation.org

- Balance the client's need for independence and need for assistance.
- Respect the client's confidentiality.
- Answer all questions and provide factual information to client and family.

## Implementation

Proficient nursing care during the final stage of life requires a unique knowledge base and skills. The American Association of Colleges of Nursing (1999) has developed a list of competencies necessary to provide quality EOL care (see Box 45-7).

The nurse's first priority is to communicate a caring attitude to the client. Establishment of rapport facilitates the client's verbalization of feelings. The nurse establishes a safe environment in which the client does not feel chided or chastised for experiencing those feelings. Nonverbal communication can be used very effectively with dying individuals. Sitting with the client, touching the client, and being physically present are often the most effective methods of communicating a caring, compassionate, and accepting attitude.

## Palliative Care

With the movement to provide compassionate EOL care, the concept of palliative care has arisen. **Palliative care** is care provided for the sole purpose of providing comfort to the client rather than curing any problems. The focus is on symptom management. The most common symptoms of priority for palliative care are pain, dyspnea, anxiety, and fatigue.

## BOX 45-7  COMPETENCIES NECESSARY FOR NURSES TO PROVIDE HIGH-QUALITY CARE TO CLIENTS AND FAMILIES DURING THE TRANSITION TO THE END OF LIFE: AACN

1. Recognize changes (social, demographic, economic) necessitating improved EOL care.
2. Promote provision of comfort care to the dying.
3. Communicate with client, family, and colleagues about EOL issues.
4. Recognize one's own attitudes, feelings, values, and expectations about death; acknowledge diversity (individual, cultural, and spiritual) in beliefs and customs.
5. Demonstrate respect for the client's view and wishes during EOL care.
6. Collaborate with interdisciplinary team members during EOL care.
7. Use scientifically based standardized tools to assess symptoms experienced by client at the end of life.
8. Use assessment data to plan and intervene using traditional and complementary approaches.
9. Evaluate the impact of traditional, complementary, and technological therapies on client-centered outcomes.
10. Assess and treat multiple dimensions (physical, psychological, social, and spiritual needs) to improve quality at the end of life.
11. Assist client, family, colleagues, and one's self in coping with suffering, grief, loss, and bereavement in EOL care.
12. Apply legal and ethical principles in the analysis of complex EOL issues.
13. Identify barriers and facilitators to clients' and caregivers' effective use of resources.
14. Demonstrate skill at implementing a plan for improved EOL care.
15. Apply knowledge gained from palliative care research to EOL education and care.

Adapted from American Association of Colleges of Nursing. (1999). *Peaceful death: Recommended competencies and curricular guidelines for end-of-life nursing care.* Washington, DC: Author.

## NURSING STRATEGY

### Meeting the Comfort Needs of the Terminally Ill Client

1. Encourage client to verbalize presence of pain.
2. Discuss pain relief options with client and family.
3. Administer medication on a regular schedule instead of prn to ensure maximum pain relief.
4. Assist client and family to identify the stressors that influence pain.
5. Teach noninvasive pain relief measures:
   - Relaxation techniques such as deep breathing, imagery
   - Use of heat and cold
   - Massage
   - Topical ointments, such as soothing salves, deep-heating rubs, herbal-scented lotions

## COMMUNITY/HOME CARE

### Do Not Resuscitate Orders

Clients in home hospice should have a "Do Not Resuscitate Order" on a prescription, which is kept at home. Sometimes as death becomes imminent, family members call 911 and these responders are required to resuscitate unless there is a written order. With a written order, these responders can then just transport the client without initiating unnecessary interventions.

National Hospice and Palliative Care Organization. (2003). http://www.nhpco.org

## Physiological Needs

According to Maslow's hierarchy of needs, physiological needs must be met before others because they are essential for existence. Areas that are often problematic for the terminally ill client are nutrition, breathing, elimination, comfort, and mobility. Table 45-8 provides information on meeting the client's physiological needs.

## Promoting Comfort

The primary activities directed at promoting physical comfort include pain relief, keeping the client clean and dry, and providing a safe, nonthreatening environment. Many, though certainly not all, dying clients experience pain. Comfort should be maximized by management of pain and other discomforting factors. The American Society of Pain Management Nurses (ASPMN) advocates "for a healthcare environment that fosters humane and dignified care. ASPMN promotes ethical and effective pain and symptom management as an integral part of palliative care" (ASPMN, 1999, p. 2). The Nursing Strategy box provides a list of interventions to promote comfort. See Chapter 42 for further discussion of pain management.

## Hospice Care

**Hospice**, a type of care for the terminally ill, is founded on the concept of allowing individuals to die with dignity and be surrounded by those who love them. Hospice care is one of the fastest growing segments of the health care industry. There are currently over 1,800 hospice programs in the United States (Roach & Nieto, 1997). Clients enter hospice care when aggressive medical treatment is no longer an option or when the client refuses further aggressive medical treatment.

Managing the care of a dying person requires many skills. Because of the complexity of care required by the hospice client, an interdisciplinary team is essential for delivering quality, compassionate care. The interdisciplinary team consists of nurses, physicians, social workers, psychologists, clergy, ancillary personnel, and volunteers. The health care team members meet regularly to solve problems, make decisions, and assure that care is coordinated (Beyers, 2000).

Traditionally hospices have been a part of hospital-based units or freestanding institutions. Because of rising health care costs and the desire to be at home, home hospices have grown rapidly in the past 10 years. The advantages of home hospices are that the dying person can stay in a familiar and safe environment, family and friends can be present and participate in client care, and costs are generally less for home hospice care. Hospice team members, especially nurses, make frequent visits to the dying client and continue to provide care to family members after the client's death.

## Psychosocial Needs

Death presents a threat not only to a person's physical existence but also to the person's psychological integrity. The nurse who demonstrates a respectful, caring attitude promotes the client's psychological comfort.

Clients may experience many fears related to death. They may fear helplessness, dependence on others, loss of abilities, mutilation, or uncontrollable pain. See Table 45-9 for a discussion of ways to meet the psychosocial needs of the dying client.

## Spiritual Needs

In times of crisis, such as death, spirituality may be a source of comfort and support for the client and family. Dying can also be a time of spiritual crisis for many clients. Clients who may not have been very spiritual can become distressed when faced with death. Nurses respect

## TABLE 45-8    MEETING THE PHYSIOLOGICAL NEEDS OF THE DYING CLIENT

| Area of Need | Discussion | Nursing Implications |
| --- | --- | --- |
| Nutrition | Anorexia, nausea, and vomiting are common. | • Give antiemetic medications and avoid spicy foods.<br>• Give foods that are easy to swallow.<br>• Small, frequent feedings of favorite foods is most successful in maintaining food intake. |
| Breathing | Respirations at end of life may become labored, irregular, and difficult; clients often breathe through the mouth, leading to dryness of oral mucosa. | • Keep client's head of bed elevated.<br>• Give medications that decrease respiratory secretions.<br>• Provide oxygen as necessary to ease respiratory effort.<br>• Suction client as needed to remove secretions.<br>• Perform oral care to keep mouth moist. |
| Elimination | Clients who are close to dying often become incontinent (or have constipation if on high doses of narcotics). | • Keep client clean and dry, performing pericare as necessary.<br>• Keep linens clean and dry.<br>• Monitor bowel status if on high doses of narcotics. |
| Comfort | Some clients, especially those with cancer, have a great deal of pain at end of life. | • Aggressive pain relief is necessary at end of life.<br>• Administer narcotics and adjuvant medications as necessary to keep the client comfortable.<br>• Position client to promote comfort.<br>• Use noninvasive pain-management techniques in addition to pain medications. |
| Mobility | Clients close to dying will have decreased mobility and become stiff. | • Positioning and turning clients every two hours is important to prevent unnecessary skin and tissue destruction, which would lead to more client discomfort. |
| Fatigue | Clients have decreased energy and stamina and experience increased fatigue toward end of life. | • Schedule care activities to ensure uninterrupted rest times for energy conservation.<br>• Monitor hemoglobin and hematocrit levels; in some cases, transfusions can be used in palliative care to combat extreme fatigue. |

Adapted from Beyers, M. (2000). About how to implement a palliative-care program. *Nursing Management, 31*(1), 56; Hospice Foundation of America. (2003). http://www.hospicefoundation.org

clients' reliance on spiritual support by listening and contacting clergy or spiritual guides if requested.

Nurses play a major role in promoting the dying client's spiritual comfort. Dying is a personal process, but it need not be a lonely one. The presence of a spiritual guide can assist in making dying a less lonely process. The nurse can serve as a sounding board for the client who expresses values and beliefs related to death. The following are therapeutic nursing interventions that address the spiritual needs of the dying:

• Listening to the client and reinforcing the normalcy of the client's dying process
• Communicating empathy
• Using touch
• Praying with the client
• Contacting clergy if requested by the client
• Reading religious literature aloud at the client's request

See Chapter 31 for a discussion of complementary and alternative modalities that are therapeutic to the dying client.

## TABLE 45-9 MEETING THE PSYCHOSOCIAL NEEDS OF THE DYING CLIENT

| Problem | Discussion | Nursing Implications |
|---|---|---|
| Anxiety | A combination of factors contribute to anxiety of the dying client and family:<br><br>• Client's fear of death (and the loss of the known world)<br>• Caregiver's fear of loss of the loved one<br>• Client's sense of abandonment by the family, friends, and health care providers<br><br>Loss of independence and social isolation increase anxiety. | • Spend as much time as possible with the dying client.<br>• Encourage verbalization of feelings.<br>• Listen in a nonjudgmental manner.<br>• Answer all questions in an honest, factual manner.<br>• Provide explanation of all procedures.<br>• Encourage family and friends to spend time with client. |
| Decreased independence | Independence is threatened by powerlessness.<br>Independence is promoted by having control over one's life. | • Seek client's opinion on treatment issues.<br>• Involve client in developing plan of care.<br>• Encourage continued interaction of client with family and friends.<br>• Assist the client to develop goals that are realistic within the limitations of the illness (realistic hope).<br>• Avoid always emphasizing limitations.<br>• Allow client and family to ventilate feelings about not being able to change the course of events.<br>• Help the client to identify those things over which he does have power. |
| Social interaction | Loneliness is increased when others detach themselves in order to disengage from the dying person's pain.<br><br>Health care providers tend to avoid interacting with the dying.<br><br>Sensory deprivation (dimly lit rooms and out-of-the-way rooms) can increase feelings of abandonment. | • Encourage family to remain with the dying person.<br>• Stay with the dying person as much as possible.<br>• Provide support through your presence and active listening.<br>• Be available to discuss the client's situation.<br>• Use touch to communicate caring.<br>• Provide meaningful sensory stimuli. |

Adapted from Antai-Otong, D. (2003). *Psychiatric Nursing*. Clifton Park, NY: Delmar Learning.

## Support for the Family

Family members need to be involved in the care of their dying loved one. Unrealistic guilt is increased by feelings of powerlessness; thus it is important to involve family members in the caregiving. It is equally important to give family permission to not participate in care if it is too difficult. The amount of care asked of family members should be determined by the family members. Families facing the impending death of a loved one require much support and reassurance from nurses and other caregivers.

### Learning Needs of Client and Family

Bereaved families need much support and information. The nurse's role is to support and educate family members. Knowledge about the client's physical condition and treatment regimen, and ways to support the dying client are commonly needed. For families with little or no experience in dealing with dying, a great deal of education might be needed. Family members will also need to be educated about how to handle medical crises and what to do for emergency care, especially if the client is at home.

The accompanying Client Education box provides guidelines for educating families of dying clients.

## Evaluation

Evaluation primarily focuses on evaluating the death experience for the client's family and friends. The nurse needs to determine the goals for a peaceful death and provide a supportive environment for the client and the family members. After the client's death, nursing staff often need to discuss the death experience with others not only for debriefing, but also for evaluating so that key learning can assist in providing care for future dying clients.

## Care After Death

Caring for the deceased body and meeting the needs of the grieving family are important nursing responsibilities. This section discusses care of the body and responding to the needs of bereaved family and friends.

## Care of the Body

The body of the deceased needs to be treated in a way that respects the sanctity of the human body. Nursing care includes maintaining privacy and preventing damage to the body.

### Physiological Changes

Several physiological changes occur after death. The body temperature decreases with a resultant lack of skin elasticity (**algor mortis**). Therefore, the nurse must use caution to avoid skin breakdown when removing tape from the body. Another physiological change, **liver mortis**, is the bluish purple discoloration that is a by-product of red blood cell destruction. This discoloration occurs in dependent areas of the body; therefore, the nurse should elevate the head to prevent discoloration from the pooling of blood. Approximately 2 to 4 hours after death, **rigor mortis** occurs; this is stiffening of the body caused by contraction of skeletal and smooth muscles. To prevent disfiguring effects of rigor mortis, as soon as possible after death the nurse should close the eyelids, insert dentures (if applicable), close the mouth, and position the body in a natural position (Figure 45-6).

In preparing the body for family viewing, the nurse seeks to make the body look comfortable and natural. This means removing all tubes and positioning the body in a supine position covered with a clean sheet and hands on top of the sheet (to allow the family to touch the body). After the family has viewed the body, the nurse places identification tags on the body's toe and wrist. The body is then placed in a plastic or fabric shroud and the shroud is tagged. Then the body is transported to the institution's morgue. In some cases, the body stays in the room and the mortuary responsible for funeral services picks the body up from the room. In the case of organ donation or autopsy, the body is always taken to the institution's morgue. During this time, a legal pronouncement of death has been made. The nurse is also responsible for returning the deceased's possessions to

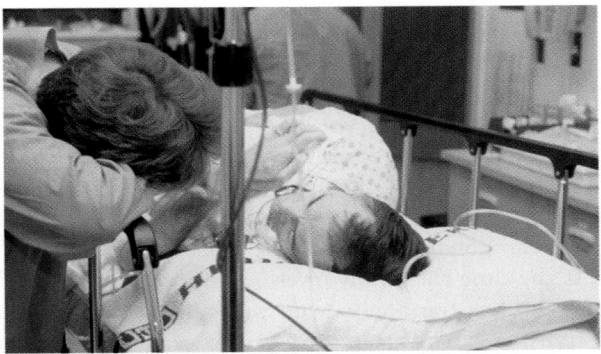

**Figure 45-6    Allow family and friends time to view the deceased.**

## LEGAL AND ETHICAL ISSUES

### Death Certificates

In most states, the physician is legally responsible for determining the cause of death and signing the death certificate. The nurse may, in certain situations, be the person responsible for certifying the death. It is important for nurses to know their legal responsibilities, which are defined by their state or provincial board of nursing.

the family. Jewelry, eyeglasses, clothing, and all other personal items are returned to the family.

## Autopsy

An **autopsy** (postmortem examination to determine the cause of death) is mandated in situations in which an unusual death has occurred. For example, an unexpected death, a suspicious death, and a violent death are circumstances that would necessitate an autopsy. Families must give consent for an autopsy to be performed. In the case of a violent death, the legal system may seek a court order to obtain an autopsy.

## Organ Donation

The donation of organs for transplantation is a matter that requires compassion and sensitivity from the caregivers. Health care institutions are required to have policies related to the referral of potential donors to organ procurement agencies. It is important that families of the deceased know the importance of and process for organ donation. There is an inadequate supply of organs and tissues to meet the demand for transplants. The following organs and tissues can be used for transplantation:

- Kidneys
- Heart
- Lungs
- Liver
- Pancreas
- Skin
- Corneas
- Bones (long bones and middle ear bones)

Some of these tissues or organs must be harvested prior to physiological death. Others may be harvested immediately after death. All hospitals are to inquire as to the possibility of organ donation prior to the death of a person.

At the time the family gives consent for donation, the nurse notifies the donor team that an organ is available for transplant. Time is of the essence because the organ or tissue must be harvested and transplanted quickly to maintain viability.

## STOP AND THINK

### Nurses and the Vulnerability of Grieving

Nurses need to feel as free to ask for help in dealing with feelings about a dying client as they would in asking for assistance in lifting and repositioning a client in bed. Asking for help means taking a risk to being vulnerable; some nurses fear appearing emotionally vulnerable or overwhelmed.

- What are some ways for nurses to support each other in dealing with the grief of caring for dying people?

- Who can a nurse be referred to for grief counseling?

## Care of the Family

At the time of death, the nurse provides invaluable support to the family of the deceased. When an individual dies, family members' anxiety is commonly increased due to their uncertainties about what to do. Informing the family of the type and circumstances surrounding the death is extremely important. The nurse provides information about viewing the body and offers to contact support people (e.g., other relatives, clergy). Sometimes, the nurse needs to help the family with decision making regarding a funeral home, transportation, and removal of the deceased's belongings. Using sensitive and compassionate interpersonal skills is essential in providing information and support to families.

## Nurse's Self-Care

Working with dying clients can evoke both a personal and a professional threat in the nurse. "Death, and the process of dying, represent a personal crisis not only for the dying person but for the caregivers who share life's most profound moment" (Ward, 1999, p. 3). Because many nurses are confronted with death and loss daily, grief is a common experience for nurses. Frequent exposure to death can interfere in the nurse's effectiveness unless the nurse has support and effectively processes the multiple losses she has experienced.

Whether working in a hospice, hospital, long-term care facility, or the home, nurses are at particular risk for experiencing complicated grief.

To cope with their own grief, nurses need support, education, and assistance in coping with the death of clients. Nurses who have had a client die should have

## STOP AND THINK

### Responses to Death

How might you respond to the death of the following clients? What would influence the difference in your responses?

- A 6-year-old with leukemia

- A client 1 year younger than you with end-stage liver disease

- A client the age of your parents killed in a car accident

- A client the age of your grandparents dying because of heart disease

## NURSING STRATEGY

### Nurse's Grief and Self-Care

- Set aside some time for your own grieving.

- Ask for help.

- Use support from within your agency—counselors, clergy, support groups.

- Find a way to say good-bye to the deceased client—rituals bring closure, which is a necessary part of grieving.

immediate support of peers. Care of other assigned clients should be covered by peers while the nurse takes some time to process the loss. This is in addition to the time to care for the family and dispose of the body. Even if the time is short, it is very important to have this. Staff education should focus on how to seek support and how to provide support to coworkers. An institution's pastoral care department should be offered to support the nurse whose client has died. Additionally, coworkers may need to share stories and experiences about the dead person and the dying process. This sharing is important in working through the grief process. If a nurse is faced with an overwhelming number of deaths in a short period of time, the nurse may need to take some vacation

time or a short leave of absence to be able to process all of the losses (Herrman, 2001).

Other ways that nurses can cope with the death of a client is through self-care. This includes a healthy, balanced diet; adequate sleep; regular aerobic exercise; and stress management techniques. Such stress management techniques include meditation, yoga, progressive relaxation, or tai chi. Spiritual practices have also been found to be effective in helping nurses cope with the death of clients.

Some nurses may struggle with the death of a client, especially if it is unexpected—for instance, during labor and delivery. The death of a client may also cause nurses to feel their own mortality. The death of a client may also raise feelings of the nurse's own mortality. Nurses need to be reassured that these feelings are normal and to be reminded to seek care for themselves.

## CASE STUDY/NURSING CARE PLAN

Mrs. Jane Schmidt is a 56-year-old African American female who is in the hospital completing her first round of chemotherapy, after having been diagnosed with stage IV ovarian cancer and metastasis to the liver. She and her husband of 37 years have three grown children and six grandchildren. She has recently retired from teaching physics at the local high school. Her husband, John, also has recently retired from teaching drama at the same high school. They were looking forward to traveling around the country and overseas. Mrs. Schmidt has been very involved in the Unitarian Church, having taught Sunday school classes for the past 10 years. She was found to have an abdominal mass during a routine physical examination. After extensive testing, it was determined that she had inoperable ovarian cancer with metastasis to the liver. At this point, she has been told that chemotherapy would only be palliative and there was no cure for her condition. She decided to complete one round of chemotherapy. Physically, she is experiencing fatigue, constipation, dyspnea, nausea, and fevers. Emotionally, she feels well supported by her family and church, but has decided not to continue with chemotherapy. She is concerned about her husband's well-being after she dies.

*(continues)*

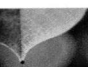

## CASE STUDY/NURSING CARE PLAN (*continued*)

### Assessment

Mrs. Schmidt has a terminal diagnosis of stage IV ovarian cancer with metastasis to the liver and has accepted her diagnosis and prognosis. She has not talked with her husband about her feelings and is concerned for his ability to care for himself after she dies. Mr. Schmidt refuses to believe his wife is dying and wants her to continue chemotherapy.

### Nursing Diagnosis

*Interrupted Family Process* related to husband's nonacceptance of wife's impending death.
**NOC:** Family Coping; Family Environment: Internal; Psychosocial Adjustment: Life Changes
**NIC:**  Family Integrity Promotion; Family Process Maintenance

### Expected Outcomes

The client will:

1. Discuss her feelings and her decision to stop chemotherapy with her husband, within one week.
2. Listen to her husband verbalize his acceptance of her decision to stop chemotherapy, within 2 weeks.
3. Communicate with her husband regarding his plans after her death, within 2 to 4 weeks.

### Planning/Interventions/Rationales

1. Talk with Mr. and Mrs. Schmidt individually about each other's perceptions of Mrs. Schmidt's prognosis. *Individual discussion will facilitate support of each person and allow for open discussion without fear of offending the other spouse.*
2. Practice role-play with Mrs. Schmidt on how to discuss her feelings with Mr. Schmidt. Inquire as to her fears concerning telling Mr. Schmidt and exploring what Mr. Schmidt will do after her death. *Having the client focus on fears often leads to the realization that the fears are unrealistic. Role-playing allows for the client to practice sharing her feelings and often leads to greater courage to talk with spouse.*
3. In talking with Mr. Schmidt, be honest and clear about Mrs. Schmidt's health and prognosis. *Client's families need factual information to prevent creating false hope and to facilitate movement through the stages of grief.*
4. Offer to be present or have a spiritually trained counselor present when Mrs. Schmidt talks with Mr. Schmidt about her feelings. *A third person present may facilitate this conversation as the third person can provide support to both people and factually answer questions that either may have.*
5. Provide reassurance to both Mr. and Mrs. Schmidt that palliative care will be provided and that she will be treated respectfully and with dignity. *A common fear of stopping curative treatment is that palliative care will also be stopped. Reassuring clients and families that this is not true can facilitate acceptance of stopping curative treatment.*

### Evaluation

Mr. and Mrs. Schmidt did talk within 1 week. Mr. Schmidt's biggest fear was that his wife would suffer severe pain if she stopped the chemotherapy. While he was reluctant to have her stop therapy, he also wanted to respect her wishes. Mr. Schmidt assured his wife that he would miss her, but would take care of himself after she died. Mrs. Schmidt verbalized her acceptance of the plans that Mr. Schmidt had after her death.

## Key Concepts

- Loss is a universal response experienced by an individual when someone (or something) of value is no longer available.

- Grief is a psychological adaptive response to loss. Grieving people experience various stages of grief differently.
- The difference between normal and complicated grief is the inability of the individual to adapt to life without the loved one.

- There are five psychological stages involved in the dying process: denial, anger, bargaining, depression, and acceptance.
- Legal and ethical dilemmas are created in the struggle between intervening to prolong life and allowing for a client to have a peaceful death.
- Complicated grief is associated with traumatic death such as death by accident, homicide, or suicide.
- Hospice care offers clients an alternative to hospitalization when aggressive medical treatment is no longer an option.
- After death, the nurse focuses on supporting the family and caring for the deceased body.
- Nurses must care for themselves in order to continue to provide quality, compassionate care to dying persons.

## Review Questions and Activities

1. What are Engle's three stages of mourning, and what feelings are related to each stage?
2. What is the difference between complicated grief and uncomplicated grief?
3. Does everyone advance through all the stages of grief?
4. What are some of the identifying behaviors that would indicate that the survivors and family have not progressed through the grief process?
5. What are some normal responses to grief?
6. What are some factors that affect the grief response?
7. What is the focus of palliative care?
8. What are common physiological needs of a dying client?

## Web Resources

American Society of Pain Management Nurses
http://www.aspmn.org
Association for Pet Loss and Bereavement
http://www.aplb.org
Hospice and Palliative Nurses Association
http://www.hpna.org
Hospice Foundation of America
http://www.hospicefoundation.org
National Hospice and Palliative Care Organization
http://www.nhpco.org
Organ Donor Information
http://www.organdonor.gov

## References

American Association of Colleges of Nursing (1999). *Peaceful death: Recommended competencies and curricular guidelines for end-of-life nursing care*. Washington, DC: Author.

American Society of Pain Management Nurses (ASPMN). (1999). *ASPMN position statement on end-of-life care*. Pensacola, FL: Author.

Antai-Otong, D. (2003). *Psychiatric nursing*. Clifton Park, NY: Delmar Learning.

Beyers, M. (2000). About how to implement a palliative-care program. *Nursing Management, 31*(1), 56.

Bowlby, J. (1982). *Attachment and loss: Vol. 2, Separation anxiety and anger*. New York: Basic Books.

Callahan, D. (1999). Aging, death, and population. *Journal of the American Medical Association, 282*(21), 2077.

Dispensing of controlled substances to assist suicide. (2001, November). *Federal Register, 66*(218). Retrieved from http://fr.cos.com.

Doka, K. (1989). *Disenfranchised grief*. Lexington, MA: Lexington Books.

Emanuel, E. J. (2002). Euthanasia and physician-assisted suicide: A review of the empirical data from the United States. *Archives of Internal Medicine, 162*(2), 142–152.

Engle, G. L. (1961). Is grief a disease? *Psychosomatic Medicine, 23,* 18–22.

Engle, G. L. (1964). Grief and grieving. *American Journal of Nursing, 64*(9), 93–98.

Ferrell, B. R., Grant, M., & Virani, R. (1999). Strengthening nursing education to improve end-of-life care. *Nursing Outlook, 47*(6), 252–256.

Field, M. J., & Cassel, C. K. (Eds.). (1997). Approaching death: Improving care at the end of life (report of the Institute of Medicine Task Force). Washington, DC: National Academy Press.

Herrman, C. P. (2001). Spiritual needs of dying patients: A qualitative study. *Oncology Nursing Forum, 28*(1), 67–72.

Hogstel, M. (2001). *Gerontology: Nursing care of the older adult*. Clifton Park, NY: Delmar Learning.

Hospice Foundation of America. (2003). Retrieved from http://www.hospicefoundation.org

James, J. W., & Friedman, R. (1998). *The grief recovery handbook*. New York: HarperPerennial.

Kübler-Ross, E. (1969). *On death and dying*. New York: Macmillan.

Kübler-Ross, E. (1974). *Questions and answers on death and dying*. New York: Macmillan.

Kübler-Ross, E. (1975). *Death: The final stage of growth*. Englewood Cliffs, NJ: Prentice Hall.

Levin, B. (1998). Grief counseling. *American Journal of Nursing, 98*(5), 69–72.

Lindemann, E. (1944). Symptomatology and management of acute grief. *American Journal of Psychiatry, 101,* 141–148.

Mallow, G. E., & Bechtel, G. A. (1999). Chronic sorrow: The experience of parents with children who are developmentally disabled. *Journal of Psychosocial Nursing, 37*(7), 31–35.

National Hospice and Palliative Care Organization. (2003). Retrieved from http://www.nhpco.org

North American Nursing Diagnosis Association (NANDA). (2003). *Nursing diagnoses: Definitions and classification, 2003–2004.* Philadelphia: Author.

Parkes, C. M. (2002). Grief: Lessons from the past, visions for the future. *Death Studies, 26,* 367–385.

Potts, N., & Mandleco, B. (2002). *Pediatric nursing: Caring for children and their families.* Clifton Park, NY: Delmar Learning.

Roach, S. S., & Nieto, B. C. (1997). *Healing and the grief process.* Clifton Park, NY: Delmar Learning.

Schattner, J. (2000). A ritual to help participants grieve the loss of another member in their cardiac rehabilitation program. *Journal of Psychosocial Nursing, 38*(1), 9–14.

Singer, P. (2002). Ms. B and Diane Pretty: A commentary. *Journal of Medical Ethics, 28,* 234–235.

Ward, G. G. (1999). Saying goodbye. *Dialogue, 14*(4), 1–3.

Worden, J. W. (1982). *Grief counseling and grief therapy: A handbook for the mental health practitioner.* New York: Springer.

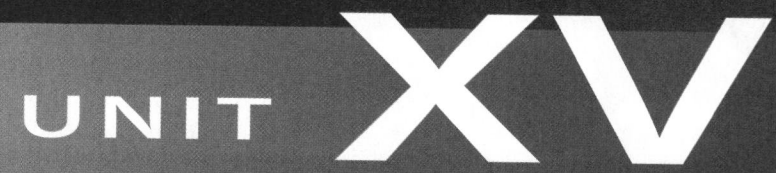
# Sexuality-Reproductive

Chapter 46  Sexuality

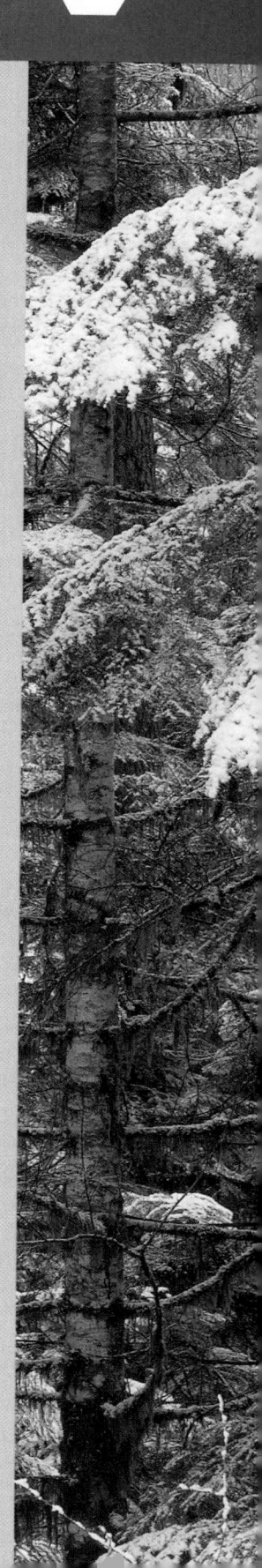

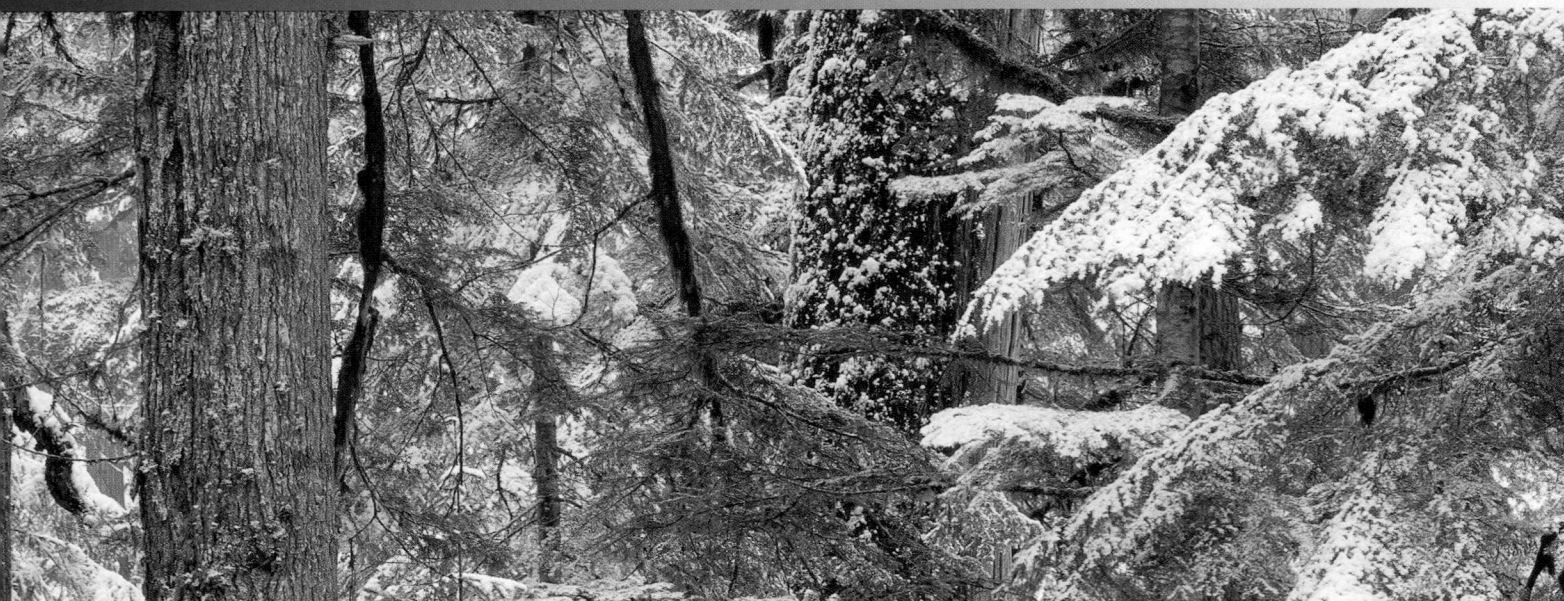

# Sexuality

## Debra L. Topham, PhD, RN, CNS, ACRN

*"The organ that appears to be critical to psychosexual development and adaptation is not the external genitalia, but the brain."*

*(William Reiner [Graff, 2001])*

# Chapter Competencies

*Upon completion of this chapter, the reader should be able to:*

1. Describe sexual health and sexuality and its components.
2. Discuss factors that influence sexual health.
3. Explain sexual development across the life span.
4. Describe the nurse's role related to applying the nursing process with clients having sexual alterations.
5. Evaluate wellness practices as related to sexual health.
6. Describe the anatomy and physiology of the male and female reproductive systems.
7. Explain the process and importance of performing the breast self-exam (BSE) and the testicular self-exam (TSE).

# Key Terms

anhedonia
bisexual
breast clinical exam (BCE)
breast self-exam (BSE)
coitus
erectile dysfunction
female genital mutilation (FGM)
frigidity
gay
gender
gender bender

gender identity
gender role
heterosexism
heterosexual
high-risk sexual behavior
homosexual
impotence
infertility
intersexed
lesbian
libido
pansexual

Papanicolaou (PAP) test
sexual dysfunction
sexual health
sexuality
sexually transmitted infections (STIs)
sexual orientation
straight
testicular self-exam (TSE)
transgender
transsexual
transvestite

Sexuality can be a difficult topic to discuss, despite it being an integral part of human life. Sex, sexual images, sexual behavior, and sexuality are prevalent in U.S. culture through the media. Sexual content is implicitly and explicitly present in advertising, books, magazines, movies, and videos, as well as on television. Yet there tends to be a taboo on open and explicit discussion about sexuality, which often leads to misconceptions and misunderstandings.

As health care providers, nurses need to know about basic sexuality and the range of sexual behaviors they will encounter from their clients. Research has demonstrated that while nurses and physicians fail to ask about sexuality, most clients expect them to (Rosenthal, Lewis, Succop, Burklow, Nelson, Shedd, Heyman, & Biro, 1999). Clients' reluctance to bring up sexual issues varies in form, but may include embarrassment, the social taboo against talking openly about sex, and feelings that they should already know about sex.

The purpose of this chapter is to introduce basic terminology about sexuality and sexual health. Additionally, provided scenarios will offer ways to assist clients with issues around sexuality. The nurse is not intended to be qualified to treat clients for complex sexual dysfunctions; that is the role of certified sex therapists. Finally, societal and cultural influences on sexuality and sexual behaviors will be discussed.

## Sexual Health

Because of the many social and cultural influences, sexual health can be difficult to define. Two beliefs are clear. First, sexual health goes beyond prevention of sexually transmitted infections (STIs) and prevention of the reproductive function. Second, discussion of sexuality fosters sexual health (Smith, 2002). The World Health Organization (WHO) in 1987 concluded that there could be no single definition of a sexually healthy person. However, in 1986, WHO did define sexual health as having three components: (1) a capacity to enjoy and control sexual and reproductive behavior in accordance with social and personal ethic; (2) freedom from fear, shame, guilt, false beliefs, and other psychological factors inhibiting sexual response and impairing sexual relationships; and (3) freedom from disease and deficiencies that interfere with sexual and reproductive function. For the purposes of this text, **sexual health** is defined as ability to form developmentally appropriate sexual relationships that are safe and respectful of one's self and others.

Most authors agree that sexual health includes the physical ability to engage in sexual activity. Too often the focus on sexual health is translated into the ability to have an orgasm or to engage in vaginal/penile intercourse, also known as **coitus**. Limiting sexual health to prescribed physical acts can seriously affect a person's emotional health when physical illness or injury inhibits physiological sexual functioning. While physical performance is important, it is the emotional, developmental, and psychological components that honor all aspects of sexual health.

It is important to note that WHO's definition encompasses both personal and social ethics. This is consistent with acknowledging the variations in what is considered acceptable sexual behaviors. This also assists the nurse in moving away from the idea that coitus between a married man and woman is the only acceptable form of sexual behavior. Prior to 1973, the American Psychiatric Association (APA) listed homosexuality as a mental illness. After much research, homosexuality was removed from the APA list and is now considered natural sexual behavior for some people.

## Sexuality

**Sexuality** is a major part of being human. Byer and Shainberg (1994) define sexuality as the aspect of the self that deals with reproduction, pursuit of sexual pleasure, love, and personal fulfillment. Gender identity, gender role, and sexual orientation are all components of sexuality (Table 46-1).

## Gender Identity

**Gender identity**, also known as **gender**, refers to the biologic sex of male, female, or intersexed. **Intersexed** people, formerly known as hermaphrodites, are people who are born with both sets or ambiguous genitalia. More than 2,000 infants are born as intersexed people each year in the United States (Graff, 2001). These infants are usually surgically assigned gender by physicians who perform the most expedient surgery (Fausto-Sterling, 2001) (see Box 46-1). Unfortunately, an increasing number of these infants grow up and find, when their hormones of puberty are fully functioning, they had been assigned the wrong gender.

## Gender Role

**Gender role** is the masculine or feminine role adopted by a person, which is often culturally and socially determined. While masculine and feminine roles vary among cultures around the world, the gender stereotypes of the submissive female and dominant male are most prevalent and most harmful to sexual health. According to Shears (2002), traditional gender roles hinder communications, which often leads to violence, sexual exploitation, unplanned pregnancy, and STIs.

In addition, as research in the area of psychosexual development has progressed, the area of gender role has been expanded to include transgendered persons. The term

## STOP AND THINK

### Sexual Understanding

- How comfortable are you with discussing sexual health issues?

- How often do you assume your client is heterosexual?

- What do you think are the differences between gender role, gender identity, and sexual orientation?

- How often do you assume that older adults (married and single) are celibate?

| TABLE 46-1 | COMPONENTS OF SEXUALITY |
| --- | --- |
| Component of Sexuality | Manifestation |
| Gender identity | Male |
| | Female |
| | Intersexed |
| Gender role | Masculine |
| | Feminine |
| | Transgendered |
| Sexual orientation | Straight (heterosexual) |
| | Gay or lesbian (homosexual) |
| | Pansexual (bisexual) |

Adapted from Byer, C. O., & Shainberg, L. W. (1994). *Dimensions of human sexuality* (4th ed.). Madison, WI: Brown & Benchmark Publishers.

societal beliefs about sexual behavior. David Satcher, the 16th surgeon general of the United States, left his office in February 2002. One major reason for his leaving was President George W. Bush's disagreement with his report, which found that abstinence was not an effective strategy for decreasing the teen pregnancy rate (Recer, 2001). Satcher advocated teaching abstinence as one option, along with birth control techniques. Previous surgeon generals who have been dismissed for views on open discussion about sexuality and sexual behavior include Jocelyn Elders, who advocated teaching masturbation to youth as a form of healthy sexual expression to prevent STI transmission and teenage pregnancy.

## Religious Factors

According to Byer and Shainberg (1994), early religious ceremonies, predominantly pagan religions, often involved sexual activity. With the beginning of patriarchal religions, sexual behavior became more proscribed and separated from spiritual practice. The Hebrew influence introduced a focus on procreation and protecting the family lineage, thus nonreproductive sex and sex between nonmarried partners were discouraged. The early Christian influence also emphasized the value of sex to marriage for the purpose of procreation. Celibacy was advocated for any unmarried persons, and sex for any other purpose than procreation was inappropriate. Sexual norms varied throughout Christian history, but most consistent was the idea that sex was only considered normal when engaged in by married couples. The sexual revolution of the 1960s brought about a resistance to the influence of religious teachings on sexual activity. Religion has been less influential on sexual activity, but still continues to influence many peoples' beliefs about what is acceptable sexual behavior.

In addition to the above factors, sexuality is also heavily influenced by a person's developmental stage. There are many theories related to psychosexual development. The following discussion is based upon commonly accepted precepts about sexual development throughout the life span.

## Sexual Development Across the Life Span

It is important to note that from birth, sexuality is a large part of being human. At each stage in life, certain stages of sexual development occur. For instance, puberty is a time of enormous physical, emotional, and sexual growth. This is when male and female hormones transform young children into young adults who are physiologically inclined to greater sexual activity. During adolescence, a time of rapid sex organ development, the focus tends to be on physical sexual activity. It is a time of great sexual experimentation. Research has shown that most adolescents have had more than one sexual partner by the time they graduate from high school.

Sexual development continues beyond adolescence as it takes on a more emotional and psychological dimension.

Although adolescence is a publicly accepted time of sexual development, sexual development begins much closer to birth. As young as 6 months old, infants begin an awareness of their sexual self. This is generally manifested as genital touching. Through this time to around age 5, young children move from indiscriminate genital touching to intentional genital touching. Parental responses during this time will have a major impact on children's sexual development. If treated with shame, children may feel embarrassment and guilt when engaging in sexual activity later in life. If treated as a normal part of children's growth and development, children may have a better chance of developing into sexually healthy adults. Parental guidance at this time should focus on teaching children

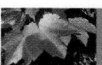

## RESEARCH FOCUS

**Title of Study:** Lessons learned: European approaches to adolescent sexual behavior and responsibility

**Study Purpose:** The purpose of the study was to compare sexual health indicators in the United States and European nations.

**Methods:** A team of 40 adolescent health specialists conducted a qualitative, critical analyses of factors that determined adolescent reproductive and sexual health attitudes, behaviors, and outcomes.

**Findings:** The research team found that adolescents in France, Germany, and the Netherlands have lower teen pregnancy and sexually transmitted diseases than in the United States. They also found more reproductive health services, sexuality education in schools, and reproductive and sexual health policies.

**Implications:** Recommendations are made for approaches to adolescent sexual health in the United States. This includes adding protective sexual behavior to abstinence-only education, expanding sexual health resources for adolescents, providing age and developmentally appropriate sexuality education in schools, providing ongoing media campaigns promoting protective behaviors in sexually active adolescents, providing resources to communities and families to support sexual education programs, and developing a nationwide agenda that is proactive for sexual health.

Berne, L. A., & Huberman, B. K. (2000). Lessons learned: European approaches to adolescent sexual behavior and responsibility. *Journal of Sex Education and Therapy, 25*(2, 3), 189–199.

## LIFE SPAN CONSIDERATIONS

### Changes in Sexuality with Aging

- Women will notice a decrease in elasticity of the vaginal wall and decrease in natural lubrication, which may affect sexual pleasure. A significant percentage of postmenopausal women tend to have decreased libido.

- Men take longer to achieve an erection, have a less firm erection, and notice a shortened ejaculation time. Impotence increases with men as they age, especially if they have a history of cardiovascular disease.

Leiblum, S. R. (1999). Sexual problems and dysfunction: Epidemiology, classification, and risk factors. *Journal of Gender-Specific Medicine, 2*(5), 41–45.

---

about privacy by directing children to engage in genital touching in private.

From age 5 to puberty, children begin to engage in genital touching, but more often begin hiding it. This is also the time they are generally beginning exploration of other children. In adolescence, when sex hormones are triggered, children become much more focused upon the corresponding sexual response to genital stimulation. This is a time when breasts change, pubic hair grows, and sex organs mature. Girls begin their menses at the end of puberty. During this time, boys begin to ejaculate and have nocturnal emissions (Potts & Mandleco, 2002).

It is during this time that sexual experimentation with others occurs. It is important to note that sexual experimentation often occurs with people of both genders. This is not indicative of an adolescent's sexual orientation. Thus, it is important not to label adolescents who engage in such sexual experimentation as being pansexual, gay, lesbian, or straight. In addition to the physical sexual experimentation, adolescents engage in sexual fantasy and tend to have a preoccupation with physical sex. Most sexual relationships at this time are superficial and the needs of the self are most dominant. Adolescence is a very important developmental time for sexuality and has special considerations for education.

As adolescents enter into adulthood, sexual development moves to psychosexual mutuality, where the needs of both partners become more equal. The focus of the relationship moves from sexual gratification to becoming inclusive of needs related to intimacy and connection. The stage of pregnancy has specific sexuality implications. As adults mature, they enter into a phase of psychosexual integration. This integration happens when sexual behavior becomes embedded within the context of a mutually satisfying intimate relationship.

## CLIENT EDUCATION

### Pregnancy and Sexual Functioning

Pregnancy can affect a woman's sexual functioning with varying degrees of increase or decrease in sexual desire. The client and her partner need to be reassured that this fluctuation is normal. Additionally, the client should be educated about the following:

✓ In the absence of other health problems, like bleeding, the client may have sexual intercourse up until labor begins.

✓ Orgasm may stimulate a contraction, but this is not a harmful contraction.

✓ A change in coital position may be necessary in later pregnancy to decrease abdominal discomfort for the woman.

✓ The first 6 weeks after birth can be difficult for the couple as the postpartum woman may have many feelings of self-doubt and mood alterations. The partner may feel displaced by the newborn.

Littleton, L., & Engebretson, J. (2002). *Maternal, neonatal, and women's health nursing.* Clifton Park, NY: Delmar Learning.

---

## Sexual Dysfunction

**Sexual dysfunction** is defined as the inability to engage in sexual activity. Leiblum (1999) found that as many as 43% of women and 31% of men have sexual dysfunction. Sexual dysfunction can be a result of physical illness, psychological illness, interpersonal factors, or medication side effects. Physical illness such as diabetes mellitus and cardiovascular disease can have a direct effect on sexual functioning. Table 46-3 discusses common physical illnesses and related sexual dysfunction. Psychological illness, such as depression, mania, and borderline personality disorders, can also have a direct effect on sexual functioning. Table 46-4 discusses common psychological problems and relat-

## CLINICAL ALERT

### Administering Viagra

Clients who use Viagra™ should be assessed for use of cardiac medications. Drug interactions have been known to cause death.

Reiss, B., Evans, M., & Broyles, B. (2002). *Pharmacological aspects of nursing care.* Clifton Park, NY: Delmar Learning.

## TABLE 46-3　PHYSICAL ILLNESSES CONTRIBUTING TO SEXUAL DYSFUNCTION

| Disease | Possible Causes of Dysfunction | Treatment |
|---|---|---|
| Arthritis, Fibromyalgia | Pain decreases libido, medications decrease sexual response; fear of hurting partner inhibits sexual activity | Timing of activity, change of activity, change of position, prophylactic use of pain relievers |
| Cancer | Loss of breast, genital, or parts of genitalia | Explore alternate forms of sexual expression and stimulation |
| Cardiovascular Disease | Fear of performance, chest pain, and death; decreased desire and arousal | Explore client's fears; teach about timing of sexual activity and alternate forms of sexual expression |
| Chronic Obstructive Pulmonary Disease (COPD) | Interferes with ability to oxygenate during sexual activity and leads to decreased stamina | Alter activity, timing, and use of oxygen; plan for sexual activity |
| Chronic Renal Failure (CRF) | Untreated uremia causes cessation of ovulation, decreased spermatogenesis, decreased libido, and erectile dysfunction | Dialysis to remove uremic buildup |
| Colostomy/Ileostomy | Changes in body image and self-concept; decreased libido; anxiety over spillage and odor | Explore client's fears and anxieties; have client meet another ostomite; empty ostomy bag prior to sexual activity |
| Diabetes Mellitus | Microvascular changes decrease ability to have erection or orgasm | Penile implants; no current treatment to address women's sexual needs |
| Spinal Cord Injury | Decreased nerve stimulation of genitals | Altered position, altered forms of sexual stimulation |

Adapted from Centers for Disease Control and Prevention. (2002). http://www.cdc.org; Leiblum, S. R. (1999). Sexual problems and dysfunction: Epidemiology, classification, and risk factors. *Journal of Gender-Specific Medicine, 2*(5), 41–45.

## TABLE 46-4　PSYCHOLOGICAL AND INTERPERSONAL FACTORS CONTRIBUTING TO SEXUAL DYSFUNCTION

| Psychological Factors | Interpersonal Factors |
|---|---|
| Anxiety | Communications |
| Depression | Interpersonal stress |
| Mania | Privacy |
| Personality disorders | Time |
| Self-esteem issues | |

Adapted from Andrews, W. C. (2000). Approaches to taking a sexual history. *Journal of Women's Health & Gender-Based Medicine, 9*, S1, S21–S24; Bruess, C. E., Haffner, D. W., & Greenberg, J. S. (2002). *Exploring the dimensions of human sexuality.* Sudbury, MA: Jones and Bartlett Publishers.

ed sexual dysfunctions. Finally, numerous medications, such as beta-blockers and antidepressants, may affect sexual function. Table 46-5 discusses common medications with their corresponding sexual dysfunctions.

# Common Risks to Sexual Health

The greatest risk to sexuality is being a childhood survivor of sexual abuse. Research has shown that some people who were sexually abused as children may tend to act out sexually, either through multiple partners or engaging in high-risk sexual behaviors (Maltz & Holman, 1987). The abuse during childhood often erodes self-esteem, which fosters the tendency of abuse survivors to acquiesce to their partners' sexual desires. Some survivors of childhood sexual abuse may do the opposite and avoid any form of sexual activity.

Sexually transmitted infections (STIs) are a major threat to sexuality and reproductive function. Many untreated STIs can lead to pelvic inflammatory disease, infertility, and cancers. The most common STIs are chlamydia, genital herpes,

## TABLE 46-5    MEDICATIONS THAT ALTER SEXUAL FUNCTION

| Drug or Medication | Effect on Sexuality |
|---|---|
| Alcohol | Small amounts increase libido and decrease inhibitions; large amounts impair neural reflexes involved in erection; chronic use causes impotence and sterility |
| Antidepressants | Blocks nerve innervation of sex organs; decreases libido |
| Antihistamines | Blocks nerve innervation of sex organs |
| Antihypertensives | Decreases libido; decreases blood flow during sexual excitement, leading to impotence and ejaculatory dysfunction |
| Antispasmodics | Blocks parasympathetic nerve innervation of sex organs; may cause impotence |
| Central nervous system (CNS) depressants | Decreases libido and may cause orgasmic dysfunction and impotence |
| Chemotherapy | Decreases libido; may lead to ovarian dysfunction and erectile dysfunction; may lead to sterility; decreases vaginal lubrication |
| Oral contraceptives | May decrease libido |

Adapted from Reiss, B., Evans, M., & Broyles, B. (2002). *Pharmacological aspects of nursing care.* Clifton Park, NY: Delmar Learning.

and gonorrhea. Human immunodeficiency virus (HIV) infections are also considered to be an STI. More than half of recorded STIs occur in persons under the age of 25. Sexual abuse and molestation should be considered when children under the age of 10 are diagnosed with having an STI (Potts & Mandleco, 2002).

Persons with sexuality risks can be diagnosed with altered sexuality patterns. Specifically altered patterns include erectile dysfunction or impotence, frigidity, and infertility. **Erectile dysfunction**, also known as **impotence**, is the inability for a man to achieve or maintain an erection. **Frigidity** is the lack of sexual desire in a woman. **Infertility** is the inability of a man to produce adequate sperm counts, or a woman to produce ova and/or implant fertilized ova.

## Nursing's Role in Clients with Sexual Alterations

When the nurse suspects or knows that a client has alterations in sexual health, she should take the initiative in performing a full sexual assessment. Prior to doing this assessment, the nurse must first work through her own level of comfort and knowledge about sexuality. As a nurse learns how to perform a sexual assessment, she will become more comfortable with the assessment. Additionally, the nurse must also be aware of resources available to the client, specifically the names of sexual counselors or therapists if the need is indicated.

## Assessment

Prior to beginning a sexual assessment, the nurse must first ensure client privacy. This includes conducting the assessment when the partner is not present. The first part of a sexual assessment includes taking a complete health history and medication history. This also includes asking about over-the-counter medications, hormonal influences on sexual libido, and any herbal remedies the client may be taking. Once the history is completed, the

### LEGAL AND ETHICAL ISSUES

#### Sexual Abuse

Sexual abuse or suspected sexual abuse in children under the age of 18 is reportable in all states in the United States. One of five girls ages 14 to 18 is sexually abused by dates. Those who have been sexually abused have higher incidences of drug use or other risky behavior, which makes them more susceptible to engaging in high-risk sexual behaviors. This puts them at greater risk for acquiring an STI.

Leiblum, S. R. (1999). Sexual problems and dysfunction: Epidemiology, classification, and risk factors. *Journal of Gender-Specific Medicine, 2*(5), 41–45.

## NURSING STRATEGY

### Performing a Sexual Assessment

When performing a sexual assessment:

- Make client feel comfortable by talking with ease and being natural in conversation.

- Reassure the client that information will remain confidential.

- Choose appropriate terminology.

- Use open-ended questions.

- A sexual history includes a social history, medical history, medication history, and recreational drug use history.

Andrews, W. C. (2000). Approaches to taking a sexual history. *Journal of Women's Health & Gender-Based Medicine, 9,* S1, S21–S24.

nurse should inform the client that he will be asking some questions related to sex, which may be embarrassing but will assist the nurse in providing the best care for the client. Additionally, the nurse should explain to the client why a sexual history is relevant and necessary. During the sexual assessment, the nurse should inform the client why individual questions may be relevant (Estes, 2002).

All clients should have a sexual health assessment. For those with more than one sexual partner, high-risk behavior, or indications of sexual dysfunction, a more detailed sexual assessment is necessary. The short form sexual history should include the following questions:

- Are you currently sexually active? If not, would you like to be and is something stopping you?
- If yes, with one or more than one partner? Men, women, or both?
- Is sex satisfying to you? For your partner?
- Do you have difficulty achieving erection or orgasm?
- Do you ever experience pain or bleeding with sexual activity? If so, what kind and under what circumstances?
- Do you have any questions or concerns about your sexual functioning? About your partner's sexual functioning?

For a comprehensive sexual assessment, see Chapter 11 and Andrews (2000), "Approaches to taking a sexual history."

## Nursing Diagnosis

The North America Nursing Diagnosis Association (NANDA, 2003) has identified two nursing diagnoses specifically related to sexual health: *Altered Sexuality Patterns* and *Sexual Dysfunction*. Etiologies for these diag-

noses are many, but common ones include deficient knowledge, pain, anxiety, fear, body image disturbance, emotional stress, and medication side effects.

## Planning

After assessment and identification of a nursing diagnosis, the nurse plans for care related to sexual health. The key behavior here is including the client in goal setting. Without including the client in goal setting, the nurse runs the risk of imposing her values on the client. It is important to establish a time frame for intervention and evaluation that fits the client's need, not the nurse's need. Because most clients engage in sexual activity with a partner or partners, it is also important to include the partner in goal setting.

## Intervention

Interventions should be timed appropriately. For instance, 2 days after a motor vehicle accident while a client is still in the intensive care unit is not the best time to discuss sexual function of a person with a spinal cord injury. Interventions should occur when partners are present and in an environment that ensures privacy.

One intervention strategy in working with clients with sexual dysfunction or altered sexuality patterns is use of the PLISSIT model, which guides the practitioner from the level of least intervention to the most intensive intervention. The acronym is described as follows:

*P* stands for permission. The nurse gives the client permission to discuss any sexual concerns he may have. This is done by providing privacy and bringing up the subject of sexuality. For example, the nurse may ask if the client has any concerns about sexual function after he has had a myocardial infarction (MI). *LI* stands for limited information. This means the nurse may share with the client some limited knowledge about the subject. For example, if the client states he has no concerns about sexual function, the nurse may state, "It is common for people who have had a myocardial infarction to wonder when it is appropriate to resume sexual activity. Do you have any concerns about this?" *SS* stands for specific suggestion. The nurse might offer specific suggestions about how to deal with a sexual problem. For example, if the client is unable to use problem solving to find different times for sexual activity, the nurse might state, "Clients with arthritis often find it more enjoyable and less painful if they engage in sexual activity after a warm shower, first thing in the morning." *IT* stands for intensive therapy, which should be performed by a certified sex therapist. This would be appropriate for a person who has suffered a spinal cord injury and needs intensive therapy and education to explore new options for sexual expression (Bruess, et al., 2002; Estes, 2002).

# Evaluation

The evaluation process is directed by the goals set by the client and nurse. Of most importance is the satisfaction of the client and her partner or partners.

# Wellness Practices and Sexual Health

The most important wellness practice to ensure sexual health is knowing oneself and one's partner. As a result of the sexual revolution in the 1960s and the AIDS epidemic, which began in the 1980s, knowledge about sexual behaviors has expanded greatly. In separate studies, Kinsey, and the team of Masters and Johnson both found human sexuality falls along a continuum. While it was once thought that "normal" people were heterosexual and had sex only within the confines of marriage, this perspective has been challenged. Over time, some authors ascribe to the notion that people fall along a continuum from 100% homosexuality to 100% heterosexuality, with bisexuality in the middle. What has been discovered is that "normal" behavior is culturally and socially defined, and the definition of "normal" has changed over the years (Masters, Johnson, & Kolodyny, 1995; Neal, 2002).

Physical wellness practices include keeping oneself free from STIs, including HIV. The most effective way to prevent an STI is to have one lifetime, mutually monogamous sexual partner. For those people who have multiple sexual partners, it is recommended that various barriers be used to provide protection from transmission of STIs. It is important to note that these barriers are not 100% effective, but are more effective than no barriers in preventing transmission of STIs. These barriers include using a condom during vaginal-penile intercourse, rectal-penile intercourse, or oral-penile stimulation. A dental dam or other barrier is recommended for oral-vulva stimulation or oral-rectal stimulation. Gloves are recommended for insertion of fingers or fists into the vagina or rectum. For persons with multiple sexual partners who do not use barriers, it is recommended that STI screening be done at least annually. This would include testing for HIV (Bruess, Haffner, & Greenberg, 2002).

Emotional and psychological wellness practices focus on open communication between sexual partners. It is important that partners talk about what is comfortable and not comfortable for them. Best (2002) found that enhanced partner communication not only prevents sexual dysfunction, but also enhances satisfaction with sexual health. Communication is the key to exploring sexual activity with partners, which then promotes physical and psychological safety. With open communication, partners will be better able to adjust when confronted by sexual health problems. In addition to these general wellness practices for sexual health, specific wellness practices are relevant to each dominant gender.

# Female Reproductive Anatomy and Wellness Practices

The female reproductive system includes the breasts, vulva, labia majora and minora, clitoris, vagina, cervix, uterus, fallopian tubes, and ovaries (Figure 46-1).

The reproductive role of the breasts is predominantly for feeding infants and young children. The role of the vulva and labias are to protect the vaginal opening. The vagina is a muscular organ where the penis is inserted for delivery of sperm. Sperm travels from the vagina, through the cervix, and into the uterus. Sperm travels up the uterus where it meets the ovum, secreted from the ovary. The ovum travels down the fallopian tube. When sperm fertilizes an ovum, it is implanted in the uterine wall until the fetus is fully developed and the baby is ready to be born (Littleton & Engebretson, 2002).

While it is not known to have a role in reproduction, it is important to note the role of the clitoris in the sexual pleasure of women. While it is possible to have an orgasm through vaginal intercourse or digital-vaginal stimulation, many women find orgasms from clitoral stimulation more intense, more easily attained, and more pleasurable. Clitoral stimulation occurs more frequently through oral contact, digital stimulation, or when the woman is engaged in vaginal-penile intercourse while on top of the man.

Prevention of STIs is an important component of female sexual health. Many common STIs, such as gonorrhea, may result in female sterility if left untreated. Additionally, human papilloma virus (HPV) is thought to be an indicator for high risk of developing cervical cancer. Besides freedom from STIs, other sexual health concerns for women include breast, ovarian, uterine, and cervical cancers. Breast cancer is the leading cancer in women, with 1 in 9 women getting breast cancer in her lifetime. However, breast cancer is not the leading cause of death in women. Lung cancer, from the increasing number of women smok-

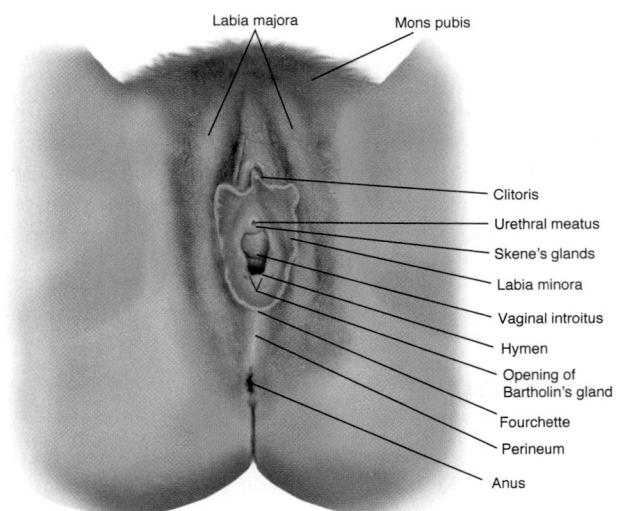

**Figure 46-1    Female genitalia**

ing, is the number one cause of cancer death in women. Breast cancer used to be the number one cause of cancer death in women, but due to intensive prevention efforts, it is being detected early enough for successful cures (Bruess, Haffner, & Greenberg, 2002). One of the key screening tools for breast cancer is the breast self-examination (BSE).

## Breast Self-Examination

All women should perform a **breast self-exam(BSE)** monthly once they begin menstruation (Figure 46-2). It is recommended to perform BSE 2 to 3 days after the end of a menstrual cycle, as breasts tend to be less tender then. Although the incidence of breast cancer increases with age, women in their early 20s have died from breast cancer.

Beginning BSE with menstruation teaches young women about breast health and preventive measures to ensure breast health. When women learn to do the breast exam monthly, it becomes a lifelong habit for them. It also accustoms women to their breasts so that any changes can be detected early. In addition to BSE, a yearly **breast clinical exam (BCE)** should be performed by women's health care practitioners. The BCE is most often performed when women receive their annual vaginal exams (Littleton & Engebretson, 2002).

## Vaginal/Cervical Exam

The vaginal/cervical examination involves inspection of the outer genitals (labia majora, labia minor, vulva, clitoris),

---

## FOCUS ON WELLNESS

### How to Do a Breast Self-Exam

1. Lie down. Flatten your right breast by placing a pillow under your right shoulder. Place your right arm behind your head.
2. Use the sensitive fingerpads (where your fingerprints are, not the tips) of the middle three fingers on your left hand. Feel for lumps using a circular, rubbing motion in small, dime-sized circles without lifting the fingers. Powder, oil, or lotion can be applied to the breast to make it easier for the fingers to glide over the surface and feel changes.
3. Press firmly enough to feel different breast tissues, using three different pressures. First, use light pressure to just move the skin without jostling the tissue beneath, then medium pressure pressing midway into the tissue, and finally deep pressure to probe more deeply down to the ribs or to the point just short of discomfort.
4. Completely feel all of the breast and chest area up under your armpit, up to the collarbone, and all the way over to your shoulder to cover breast tissue that extends toward the shoulder.
5. Use the same pattern to feel every part of the breast tissue. Choose the method easiest for you:
   - *Lines:* Start in the underarm area and move your fingers downward little by little until they are below the breast. Then move your fingers slightly toward the middle, and slowly move back up. Go up and down until you cover the whole area.
   - *Circles:* Beginning at the outer edge of your breast, move your fingers slowly around the breast in a circle. Move around the breast in smaller and smaller circles, gradually working toward the nipple. Don't forget to check the underarm and upper chest areas, too.
   - *Wedges:* Starting at the outer edge of the breast, move your fingers toward the nipple and back to the edge. Check your whole breast, covering one small wedge-shaped section at a time. Be sure to check the underarm area and the upper chest.
6. After you have completely examined your right breast, examine your left breast using the same method and your right hand, with a pillow under your left shoulder.
7. You will want to examine your breasts or do an extra exam while showering. It's easy to slide soapy hands over your skin and to feel anything unusual.
8. You should also check your breasts in a mirror, looking for any change in size or contour, dimpling of the skin, or spontaneous nipple discharge.

American Cancer Society. (2003). http://www.cancer.org

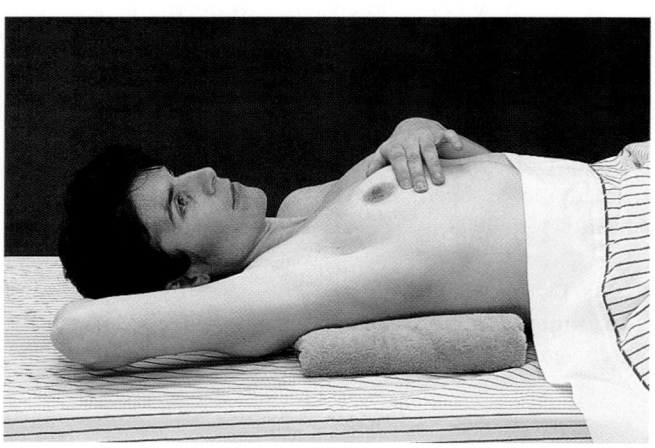

**A. In bed**

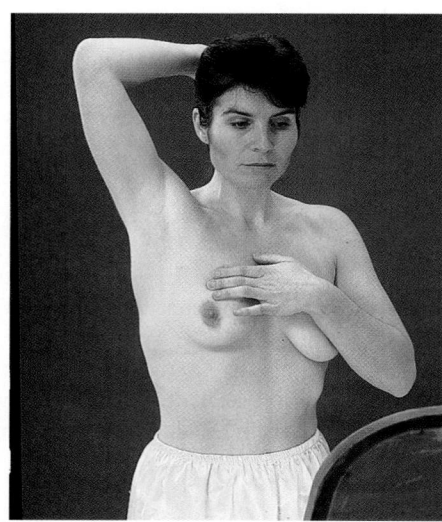

**B. Standing**

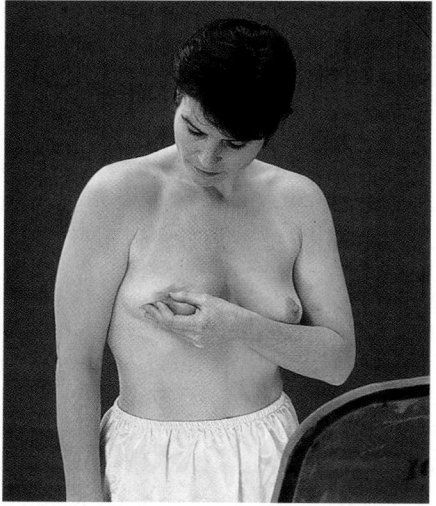

**C. Compression of the nipple**

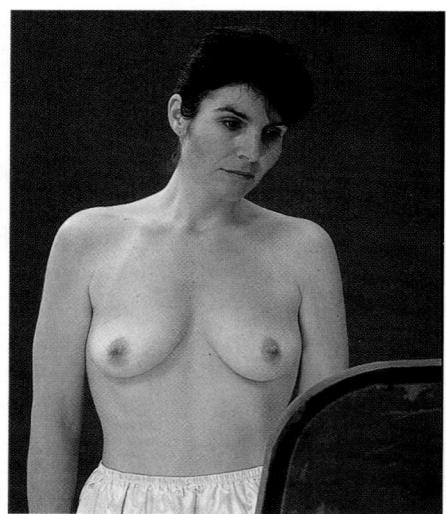

**D. Before a mirror: arms at side**

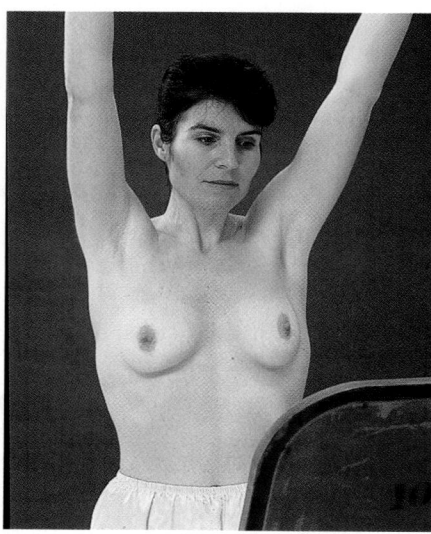

**E. Before a mirror: arms overhead**

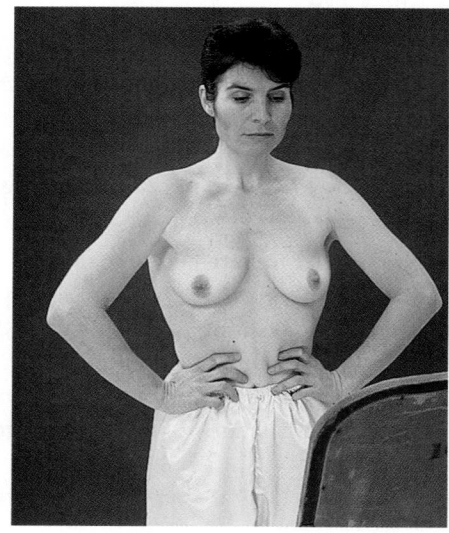

**F. Before a mirror: hands pressed into hips**

**Figure 46-2    Breast self-exam**

## STOP AND THINK

### Papanicolaou Test and Pain

During a routine PAP test, 31-year-old Cathy begins to cry and tells the practitioner to not insert the speculum. She states that PAP smears have always been painful for her.

- As the nurse assisting with the gynecological exam, what would your response be?

- What might be behind Cathy's pain and fear of PAP smears?

inspection of the vaginal wall and cervix through insertion of a speculum, manual palpation of the vagina and ovaries, and rectal examination. During inspection of the cervix and vaginal wall, specimens are taken for laboratory testing for cell changes that may indicate precancerous or cancerous conditions. This is known as a **Papanicolaou (PAP) test.** The incidence of cervical cancers has decreased significantly after the initiation of routine annual PAP tests.

### Mammograms

Mammograms are recommended to be done annually for women beginning at age 40. With breast cancer being a risk for women of any age, there is controversy in excluding women under the age of 40 from mammography screenings. The American Cancer Society recommends a baseline mammogram and bilateral breast ultrasound at ages 35 to 40 to establish a baseline. After that, annual mammograms should begin at age 40. For women with a significant family history or women with palpable masses (breast cancer increases with age), mammography should be performed as needed, regardless of age.

## Male Reproductive Anatomy and Physiology and Wellness Practices

The male reproductive system consists of the penis, scrotum, seminal vesicles, prostate gland, and testes (Figure 46-3). During sexual activity, the penis enlarges in width and length, and becomes hard from increased blood flow to the shaft. The testes produce sperm that is stored in the seminal vesicles as semen. During sexual activity at the point of ejaculation, the seminal vesicles contract and the semen moves along the urethra and out the penis. If the penis is in the vagina, the semen moves into the uterus to fertilize an ovum (White & Duncan, 2002).

Prevention of STIs in men is equally important as with women. Men tend to have more symptoms when infected with an STI—most notably discharge from the urinary

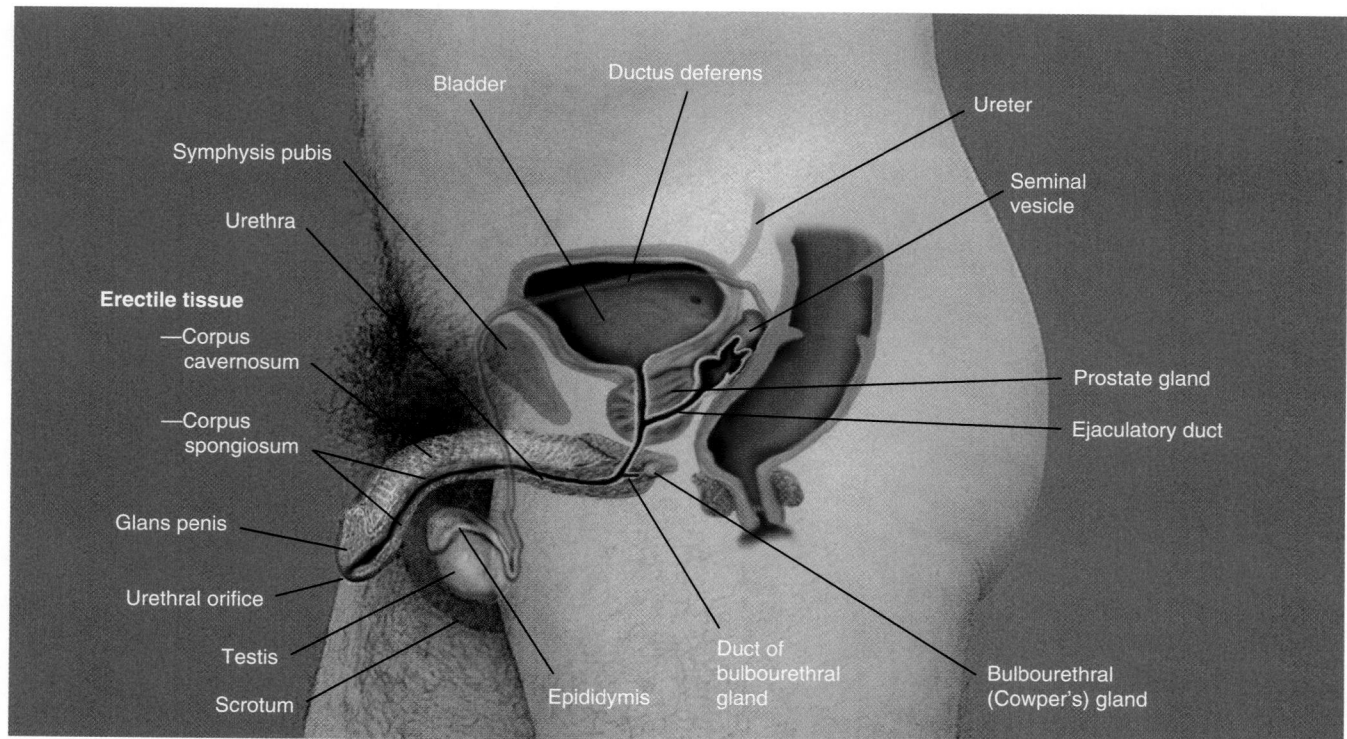

**Figure 46-3    Male genitalia**

meatus or lesions on the penis or scrotum. Condoms are effective in prevention of some STIs, but they only protect the shaft and head of the penis. As with women, cancer prevention is as important as STI prevention. The most common cancers to affect men's reproductive organs are prostate and testicular cancers. While more rare, there is a significant incidence of penile cancers in older men.

## Prostate Exams

Health care practitioners perform prostate exams, or screenings. This is usually done by urologists because of the influence of an enlarged prostate gland on urinary and sexual function. Because the risk of prostate cancer rises as men age, annual prostate exams should begin around age 50. Prostate cancer is one of the top five cancers in men. As with other cancers, if it is detected early, treatment can be curative. Testicular cancer, which mostly affects younger men, is a type of cancer that can be screened for thorough self-examination (Estes, 2002).

## Testicular Self-Examination

**Testicular self-exam(TSE)** is the male's self-examination of the testes for suspicious lumps (Figure 46-4). The incidence of testicular cancer is on the increase and is especially high in the African American population. As with breast cancer, early screening and intervention can significantly increase the survival rate of men treated for testicular cancer. TSE should begin with the onset of puberty and be performed on a monthly basis. As with BSE for women, this is to accustom men to the texture of the testes so that changes may be detected early. Performing TSE monthly during puberty helps it to become a lifelong habit. Unlike prostate cancer, most men with testicular cancer are diagnosed in their 20s and early 30s (Estes, 2002).

## FOCUS ON WELLNESS

### How to Do a Testicular Self-Exam

1. Stand in front of a mirror. Check for any swelling on the scrotal skin.
2. Examine each testicle with both hands. Place the index and middle fingers under the testicle with the thumbs placed on top. Roll the testicle gently between the thumbs and fingers; you shouldn't feel any pain when doing the exam. Don't be alarmed if one testicle seems slightly larger than the other—that's normal.
3. Find the epididymis, the soft, tubelike structure behind the testicle that collects and carries sperm. If you are familiar with this structure, you won't mistake it for a suspicious lump. Cancerous lumps usually are found on the sides of the testicle but can also show up on the front. Lumps on the epididymis are not cancerous.
4. If you find a lump, see a doctor, preferably a urologist, right away. The abnormality may not be cancer; it may just be an infection. But if it is testicular cancer, it will spread if it is not stopped by treatment. Waiting and hoping will not fix anything. Please note that free-floating lumps in the scrotum that are not attached in any way to a testicle are not testicular cancer.

Testicular self-exam. (2002). http://www.acor.org

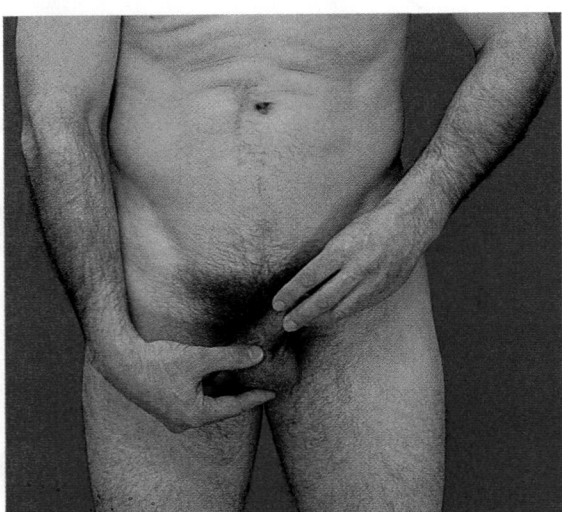

**A. Palpating the testis**

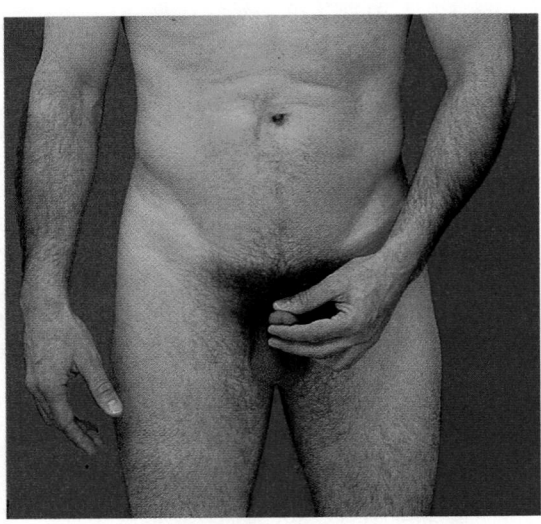

**B. Assessing for penile discharge**

**Figure 46-4    Testicular self-examination**

# CASE STUDY/NURSING CARE PLAN

John and Carol, both 58, have been married for 36 years. For the past several years, Carol has suffered from increasingly painful osteoarthritis. She is in the hospital after receiving a right knee replacement. As you are reviewing her discharge plans, John comments that now he hopes they can be intimate again. When you ask him to clarify what he means, Carol blushes and states that she avoids sex because it is so painful for her.

### Assessment

A married couple are having difficulty in their sexual activities for a variety of reasons. They do not communicate well and are not open in their expressions regarding their sexual activities. In addition, the wife has osteoarthritis, which causes her to have pain; consequently, this interrupts her outlook on sexual behaviors.

### Nursing Diagnosis

*Ineffective Sexual Patterns* related to painful and swollen joints.
**NOC:** Risk Control: Role Performance; Self-Esteem; Sexual Functioning
**NIC:** Sexual Counseling

### Expected Outcomes

The client will:

1. Verbalize a sexually satisfying relationship with spouse by second counseling appointment.
2. Acknowledge strategies to decrease pain by end of first counseling appointment.

### Planning/Interventions/Rationales

1. Explore with client current methods used to enhance sexual function, including open communication. *Increases knowledge level.*
2. Encourage client to take a hot bath or shower prior to sexual activity. *Potentially increases libido.*
3. Apply anti-inflammatory creams over joints prior to sexual activity. *Decreases pain during sexual activities and increases satisfaction during sexual intercourse.*
4. Explore alternative positions for sexual activity. *Decreases the amount of strain on arthritic joints.*
5. Explore the best time of day for sexual activity. *Pain may be lowest in the morning or after gentle physical activity.*

### Evaluation

After 2 months, Carol and John both verbalize satisfaction with sexual function. Morning is the best time for Carol to participate in sexual intercourse, after taking ibuprofen followed by a hot shower and gentle range-of-motion exercises. The couple is most satisfied with a side-lying position for sex. They have also incorporated more massage and touch in sexual activity, lengthening the amount of foreplay and leading to more satisfactory sexual activity for both Carol and John. Both also acknowledge that improved communications has led to fewer misunderstandings and frustrations.

## Key Concepts

- Sexual health involves physiological as well as psychological components.
- Sexuality is comprised of gender identity (biologic sex), gender role, and sexual orientation.
- Sexuality is influenced by physiological, emotional and psychological, cultural, social, and religious factors throughout the life span.
- Self-knowledge and interpersonal communications skills are key for nurses working with clients with alterations in sexual health.
- The PLISSIT model is useful in intervening with clients with sexual health problems.

- A detailed sexual health assessment needs to be taken when a client has more than one sexual partner, high-risk behavior, or indications of sexual dysfunction.
- BSE and TSE are two health-screening activities that clients should perform on a monthly basis.

## Review Questions and Activities

1. What are the three components of sexuality?
2. What factors influence sexuality?
3. What factors influence sexual health and functioning?

**4.** Give an example of medications and diseases that affect sexual functioning.

**5.** Describe how to do a breast self-exam.

**6.** Describe how to do a testicular self-exam.

## Multimedia Links

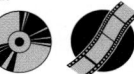

Altman *Basic Care DVD: Breast Examination*

## Web Resources

American Cancer Society
   http://www.cancer.org
Centers for Disease Control and Prevention
   http: //www.cdc.gov
Intersex Society
   http://www.isna.org
Sexual Health for Adolescents
   http://www.coolnurse.com
Testicular Self-Exam
   http://www.acor.org

## References

American Cancer Society. 2003. http://www.cancer.org

American Psychological Association (2001). *Publication Manual of the American Psychological Association* (5th ed.). Washington, DC: American Psychological Association.

Andrews, W. C. (2000). Approaches to taking a sexual history. *Journal of Women's Health & Gender-Based Medicine, 9*, S1, S21–S24.

Berne, L. A., & Huberman, B. K. (2000). Lessons learned: European approaches to adolescent sexual behavior and responsibility. *Journal of Sex Education and Therapy, 25*(2–3), 189–199.

Best, K. (2002). When partners talk, behavior may change. *Network, 21*(4), 19–24.

Bruess, C. E., Haffner, D. W., & Greenberg, J. S. (2002). *Exploring the dimensions of human sexuality.* Sudbury, MA: Jones and Bartlett Publishers.

Byer, C. O., & Shainberg, L. W. (1994). *Dimensions of human sexuality* (4th ed.). Madison, WI: Brown & Benchmark Publishers.

Centers for Disease Control and Prevention. (2002). http://www.cdc.gov

Estes, M. (2002). *Health assessment & physical examination* (2nd ed.). Clifton Park, NY: Delmar Learning.

Fausto-Sterling, A. (2001). *Sexing the Body: Gender Politics and the Construction of Sexuality.* New York: Basic Books.

Feinberg, L. (2001). Trans health crisis: For us it's life or death. *American Journal of Public Health, 92*(6), 897–900.

Graff, E. J. (2001, December 17). The M/F boxes. *The Nation*, pp. 20–23.

Intersex Society. (2003). http://www.isna.org

Leiblum, S. R. (1999). Sexual problems and dysfunction: Epidemiology, classification, and risk factors. *Journal of Gender-Specific Medicine, 2*(5), 41–45.

Littleton, L., & Engebretson, J. (2002). *Maternal, neonatal, and women's health nursing.* Clifton Park, NY: Delmar Learning.

Maltz, W., & Holman, B. (1987). *Incest and sexuality: A guide to understanding and healing.* Lexington, MA: Lexington Books.

Masters, W. H., Johnson, V. E., & Kolodyny, R. C. (1995). *Human sexuality* (5th ed.). Little, Brown, & Co.

Neal, G. (2002). *St. James encyclopedia of popular culture.* Detroit: Gale Group.

North American Nursing Diagnosis Association (NANDA). (2003). *Nursing diagnoses: Definitions and classification, 2003–2004* (4th ed.). Philadelphia: Author.

Potts, N., & Mandleco, B. (2002). *Pediatric nursing: Caring for children and their families.* Clifton Park, NY: Delmar Learning.

Recer, P. (2001). *Surgeon general will leave when his 4-year term ends.* Associated Press Release.

Reiss, B., Evans, M., & Broyles, B. (2002). *Pharmacological aspects of nursing care.* Clifton Park, NY: Delmar Learning.

Rosenthal, S. L., Lewis, L. M., Succop, P. A., Burklow, K. A., Nelson, P. R., Shedd, K. D., Heyman, R. B., & Biro, F. M. (1999). *Clinical Pediatrics, 38*(4), 227.

Shears, K. H. (2002). Gender stereotypes compromise sexual health. *Network, 21*(4), 12–13, 15–18.

Smith, E. F. (2002). Discussing sexuality fosters sexual health. *Network, 21*(4), 5–6, 8.

Testicular self-exam. (2002). http://www.acor.org

White, L., & Duncan, G. (2002). *Medical-surgical nursing: An integrated approach* (2nd ed.). Clifton Park, NY: Delmar Learning.

WHO. (1986). *Concepts for sexual health.* Copenhagen: WHO.

WHO. (1987). *Concepts of sexual health, report of a working group convened by the World Health Organization (EURO).* Copenhagen: WHO.

# Coping-Stress Tolerance

Chapter 47  Stress, Anxiety, Coping, and Adaptation

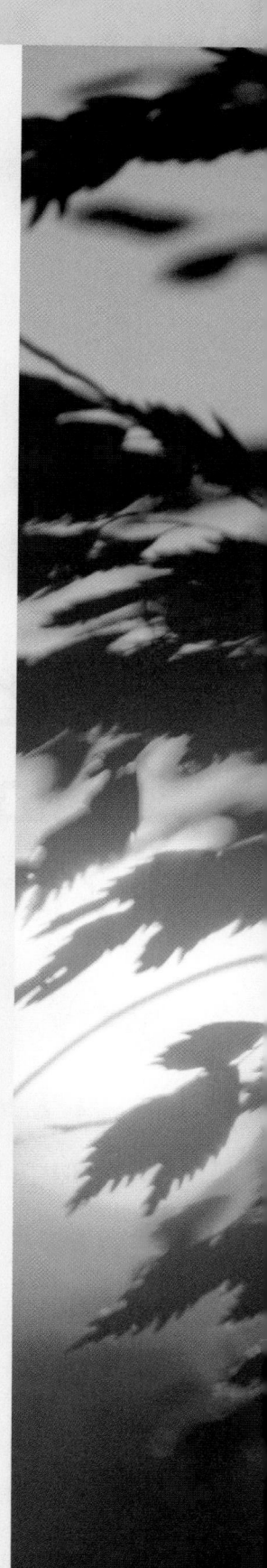

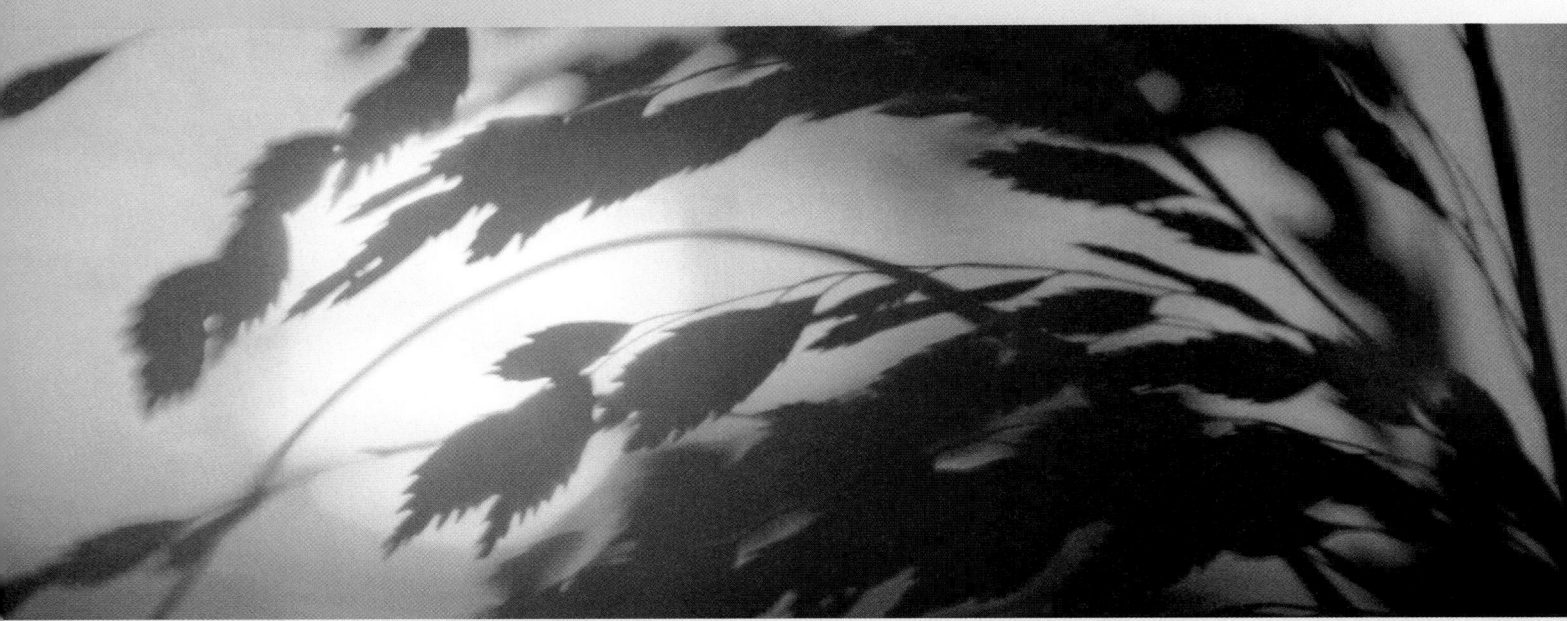

# Stress, Anxiety, Coping, and Adaptation

Ruth N. Grendell, DNSc, RN

*"What lies behind us and what lies before us are tiny matters compared to what lies within us."*

*(Ralph Waldo Emerson, 1862/2000)*

# Chapter Competencies

## Upon completion of this chapter, the reader should be able to:

1. Discuss stress, anxiety, coping, and adaptation as they affect health.
2. Identify factors contributing to the stress response.
3. Evaluate the role of stress in illness.
4. Explain stressors inherent in the change process.
5. Discuss the role of the nurse as a change agent.
6. Explain nursing interventions that promote positive adaptation to stress.
7. Develop an individualized stress management plan for use as a nurse.

# Key Terms

| | | |
|---|---|---|
| adaptation | depersonalization | maladaptation |
| anxiety | distress | paradigm |
| catharsis | eustress | proactive |
| change | fight-or-flight response | progressive muscle relaxation |
| change agent | general adaptation syndrome | rapid relaxation response |
| cognitive reframing | (GAS) | (RRR) |
| coping | guided imagery | stress |
| crisis | homeostasis | stressor |
| crisis intervention | local adaptation syndrome | suppression |
| defense mechanisms | (LAS) | |

Stress, a universal experience, can be the catalyst for positive change or it can be the source of discomfort and pain. Stress can be contagious. Caring for clients who are experiencing high levels of anxiety can be stress-provoking for nurses. Nurses are involved with stress management from a teaching perspective, helping clients learn to cope with the stress imposed by illness, injury, disability, or treatment approaches. Nurses also encounter stress as a personal experience. Successful stress management is necessary for wellness of both clients and nurses. This chapter discusses the major concepts related to stress and anxiety and presents strategies for coping with stress and change.

## Stress, Anxiety, Coping, and Adaptation

**Stress** is the body's physiological reaction to any stimulus that evokes a change. "A certain amount of stress is necessary for survival" (Stuart & Laraia, 2002, p. 34). Any situation, event, or agent that threatens a person's security is a **stressor**. A stressor is a stimulus that evokes the need to adapt and can be internal or external. For example, a headache is an internal stressor, whereas a difficult assignment is an external stressor. A stressor can be physical (such as a laceration), physiological (e.g., hypertension), or psychosocial (e.g., graduation from school). Even pleasant events can be stressful in that they evoke the need to adapt. Stressors in themselves are neutral; in other words, a stressor is neither good nor bad. The individual's *perception* of the stressor greatly determines whether the outcome is positive or negative. Any event can be stressful, depending on the person's interpretation of that event.

**Anxiety** is a vague, nonspecific, uncomfortable, subjective response as the result of a perceived or actual threat to one's biologic, psychological, or social integrity. It is a pervasive feeling of dread or apprehension (Molloy, 2000). Some authors refer to stress as the person's physiological response to a stimulus, and others define anxiety as the psychological response to a threat. People respond to the same situation in different ways. There is a close relationship between stress and anxiety. Anxiety can be both an activator of stress and a response to stress. It is usually activated by stress and may, in and of itself, lead to more stress.

**Coping** is a complex of behavioral, cognitive, and physiological responses that aim to prevent or minimize unpleasant or harmful experiences that challenge one's personal resources. Persons use their coping strengths in specific ways depending on whether the situation is "normal" or difficult. Some researchers suggest that one's reactions to stressful events will vary between active coping (e.g., assertiveness, imagery, self-statements) and restful coping (e.g., progressive relaxation, meditation). Both of these aspects are necessary, separately and in combination with one another. Coping strategies are vital to clients in their adapting to disorders and in maintaining their health.

**Adaptation** is an ongoing process by which individuals adjust to stressors in order to achieve **homeostasis** (equilibrium between physiological, psychological, sociocultural, intellectual, and spiritual needs). Adaptation is a holistic response that involves all dimensions of an individual. Individuals, as holistic beings, seek to maintain a *steady state* (another term for homeostasis) in all dimensions of life: physiological, psychological, cognitive, social, and spiritual. Wellness is an adaptive state; that is, the well person is one who is coping effectively with stressors to maintain a high level of well-being. The nurse's goal is to identify and support the client's positive adaptive responses (Armstrong, 2000; Molloy, 2000).

## Sources of Stress

Individuals experience stress from multiple sources, primarily their bodies, their thoughts, and the environment. A situation or event that evokes stress in one person may not affect another. Loss is a primary theme that permeates all life changes. It is a series of overlapping experiences that requires recognition of the loss, adjustment to the changes that result, and resolution of the loss. The process of mourning a loss and continuing with one's life is influenced by personality, culture, and socialization (Armstrong, 2000). Examples of factors contributing to stress are shown in Table 47-1.

## Responses to Stress

Every individual has unique responses to stress. A person's response to stress is influenced by several variables: mental attitude, lifestyle, perception, and heredity.

## Physiological Response to Stress

The physiological stress response, which can be adaptive or maladaptive, is the nonspecific response of the body to any demand (Selye, 1974). When the response is adaptive, the individual achieves and is able to maintain homeostasis. If the stress response is maladaptive, health status is altered.

### General Adaptation Syndrome

Hans Selye (1976), a Canadian physiologist, introduced the concept of the **general adaptation syndrome (GAS),**

the physiological response to stress. The GAS is the same whether the stressor is actual or imagined, present or potential. In other words, the physiological reactions of the body are essentially the same regardless of the source of the stress. For example, the mind can imagine a stressor, and the physiological response (GAS) will be the same as if the body had actually experienced the stressor. According to Selye (1976), all stress reactions involve similar physiological reactions. The three stages of the GAS are described in Figure 47-1.

### Fight-or-Flight Response

During the resistance stage of the GAS, an individual attempts to defend against the stressor through the **fight-or-flight response**. The body becomes physiologically ready to defend itself by either fighting or running away from the danger (stressor). Hormones, such as adrenaline

| TABLE 47-1 | COMMON STRESSORS |
|---|---|
| **Type of Stressor** | **Examples** |
| Physiological | • Maturation (moving from one developmental stage to another)<br>• Trauma<br>• Illness<br>• Poor nutrition<br>• Sleep disturbances<br>• Hunger<br>• Discomfort<br>• Pain |
| Psychological | • Worry<br>• Fear<br>• Anger<br>• Happiness |
| Cognitive | • Thoughts<br>• Perceptions<br>• Interpretation of events |
| Environmental | • Temperature (weather)<br>• Air pollution<br>• Noise pollution<br>• Crowding<br>• Time pressures |
| Sociocultural | • Job loss or promotion<br>• Changes in interpersonal relationships<br>• Interpersonal conflict<br>• Living conditions<br>• Loss of loved one |

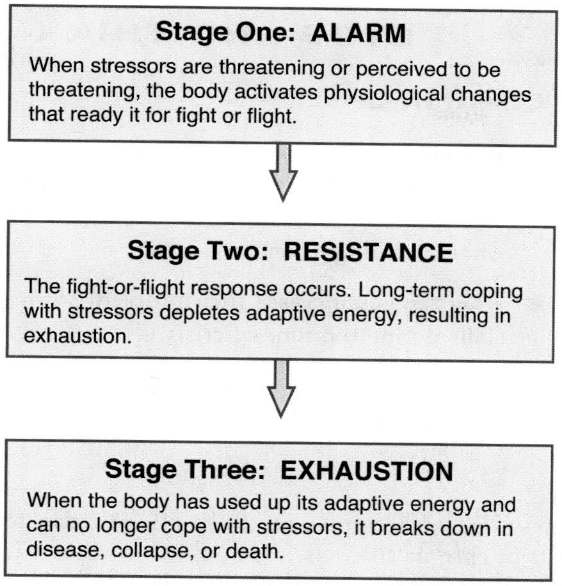

## Stage One: ALARM

When stressors are threatening or perceived to be threatening, the body activates physiological changes that ready it for fight or flight.

## Stage Two: RESISTANCE

The fight-or-flight response occurs. Long-term coping with stressors depletes adaptive energy, resulting in exhaustion.

## Stage Three: EXHAUSTION

When the body has used up its adaptive energy and can no longer cope with stressors, it breaks down in disease, collapse, or death.

**Figure 47-1** Stages of the general adaptation syndrome

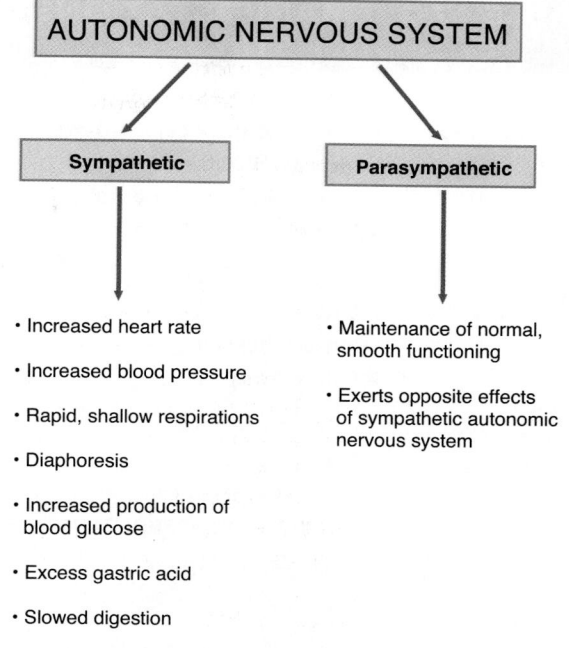

**Figure 47-2** Physiology of autonomic nervous system: arousal and homeostasis *Adapted from Delaune, S.C. (1996). Applying the nursing process for clients with anxiety, somatoform, and dissociative disorders. In H. S. Wilson & C. R. Kneisl (Eds.), Psychiatric nursing (5th ed., p. 368). Menlo Park, CA: Addison-Wesley.*

and norepinephrine, are secreted that cause various biologic changes. Arousal of the autonomic nervous system (ANS) (particularly the sympathetic branch) characterizes the fight-or-flight phenomenon (Figure 47-2). The endocrine system is also involved in maintaining physiological homeostasis.

### Local Adaptation Syndrome

The **local adaptation syndrome (LAS)** is the physiological response to a stressor (e.g., trauma, illness) affecting a specific part of the body. For example, if a person experiences a puncture wound on the foot, the LAS is initiated and leads to localized inflammation. The classic symptoms of inflammation (redness, warmth, and swelling) occur at the injured site. The LAS is usually a temporary process that is resolved when the traumatic area is restored to its steady state. However, if the inflammation is not resolved with the LAS, the individual will then experience the GAS as the entire body becomes affected.

## Psychoneurologic Regulation, Neuroendocrine Regulation, and the Stress Response

Psychoneuroimmunology is the study of the interaction of consciousness, the nervous system (i.e., brain, central nervous system), and immunology. Psychoneuroimmunology explains the connection between immune-related diseases and the implications of psychosocial factors as they combine with the endocrine system and changes in the nervous system. Immune-related illnesses are associated with stress, albeit the mechanisms of causation are not clearly established. Current research focuses on the pathways for stress-related immune disorders, including cancer, autoimmune diseases, and allergies.

The stress response is interconnected to psychoneuroimmunology because stress is initiated by the nervous system and the endocrine system. The sympathetic nervous system stimulates the adrenal glands to release catecholamines (via the adrenal medulla), cortisol (via the adrenal cortex), and a variety of other hormones (e.g., endorphins, enkephalins, somatotropin). Overall, the stress response is interwoven among the nervous, endocrine, and immune systems.

## Manifestations of Stress

The manifestations of stress are numerous and affect every dimension of a person. Common manifestations of stress are described in Table 47-2.

## Outcomes of Stress

Stress is an experience that provides the individual with two possibilities: (1) an opportunity for personal growth or (2) the risk of disorganization and distress. When stressors are responded to appropriately, adaptation is successful and the body returns to its normal steady state.

When stress is not handled within a short period of time, however, problems may occur. Individuals who experience chronic periods of stress are the ones who have the

## TABLE 47-2    MANIFESTATIONS OF STRESS

| Physiological | • Cardiovascular/respiratory effects<br>—Increased pulse<br>—Increased blood pressure<br>—Rapid, shallow breathing |
|---|---|
| | • Neurologic effects<br>—Dizziness<br>—Headaches<br>—Dilated pupils |
| | • Gastrointestinal effects<br>—Nausea<br>—Altered appetite<br>—Diarrhea or constipation |
| | • Genitourinary effects<br>—Polyuria |
| | • Musculoskeletal effects<br>—Tension<br>—Twitching |
| | • Endocrine effects<br>—Increased levels of blood glucose and cortisol |
| Psychological | • Irritability<br>• Increased sensitivity (feelings are easily hurt)<br>• Sadness, depression<br>• Feeling "on edge" |
| Cognitive | • Impaired memory<br>• Confusion<br>• Impaired judgment<br>• Poor decision making<br>• Delayed response time<br>• Altered perceptions<br>• Inability to concentrate |
| Behavioral | • Pacing<br>• Sweaty palms<br>• Rapid speech<br>• Insomnia<br>• Withdrawal<br>• Exaggerated startle reflex |
| Spiritual | • Alienation<br>• Social isolation<br>• Feeling of emptiness |

Adapted from Molloy, M. (2000). Anxiety and related disorders. In K. Fortinash & P. Holoday-Worret (Eds.), *Psychiatric mental health nursing* (2nd ed., pp. 233–256); Stuart, G. W., & Laraia, M. T. (2000). *Principles and practice of psychiatric nursing* (7th ed.). St. Louis: Mosby.

### STOP AND THINK

#### Client in Crisis

● What are some ways to encourage your clients to use their adaptive energy in a productive manner when they are "spinning their wheels" during a time of stress?

● How can you increase their problem-solving skills during the time of crisis?

● What coping mechanisms can you assess with the client in crisis?

greatest risk of becoming ill. Selye (1976) refers to the effects of chronic stress as "dis-ease," which occurs in the third stage of the GAS, exhaustion. The person becomes dis-eased when coping mechanisms are ineffective. This process of coping ineffectively with stressors is referred to as **maladaptation**. The inability to adapt to continued demands of stress can have harmful results, such as illness.

The term **eustress** is used to describe a type of stress that results in positive outcomes. Consider, for example, students who have an examination scheduled the following week. The stress over the impending test motivates them to study early. As a result, they pass the examination.

When stressors evoke an ineffective response, **distress** is experienced. For example, consider students who have an examination scheduled for the next day. They had plenty of time to study, but because they put it off until the last minute, they take the examination unprepared. As a result of "cramming" all night, they are not alert, do not know the material, and fail the examination; they are experiencing distress. In general, when people say *stress* they are referring to distress, the negative outcomes of an ineffectual stress response.

### STOP AND THINK

#### Eustressors

● What are several eustressors in your life?

● How do they help "balance" the difficult things when you are in a crisis?

● How does your body normally respond during times of stress?

● What do you feel emotionally during the stressful times?

● How do you respond behaviorally during these stressful times?

## Crisis

When stressors exceed the person's ability to cope, a crisis develops. A **crisis** (an acute state of disorganization) occurs when the individual's usual coping mechanisms are no longer effective. Crisis is characterized by extreme anxiety, inability to function, and disorganized behavior. A crisis is time-limited; that is, no one can remain in acute disequilibrium for a long period of time because of the degree of discomfort that is experienced. Owing to the time-limited nature of crisis, a client experiencing a crisis needs immediate intervention to reach a successful resolution. For example, when the client with diabetes mellitus has a hypoglycemic reaction, it is a crisis that is often resolved with a form of glucose.

The source of the stressful event may not always be defined clearly or determined immediately for every individual. Certain events may cause a severe emotional response in one person, but have no detrimental effect for another person. The three types of crises, developmental or maturational, situational, and adventitious are depicted in Table 47-3. Crisis intervention is discussed later in this chapter.

A crisis can be a negative experience, but it also has the potential to be an opportunity for growth and learning. The outcome is unique according to each individual's perception and coping abilities. Nurses are challenged to help clients discover the opportunity in their crises to adapt in a positive, healthy manner (Figure 47-3).

Not every person will experience a crisis as a result of stressful events. Each crisis is unique according to the individual and circumstances. However, some characteristics are common to all crises, including the following:

- A crisis is experienced as a sudden event.
- A crisis has an identifiable precipitating event.

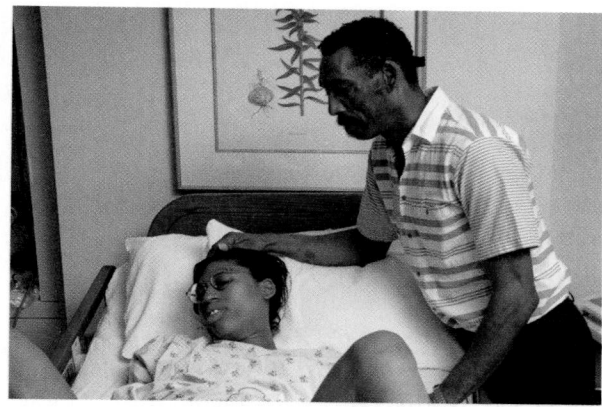

**Figure 47-3    The process of labor and delivery can be a time of crisis, which requires the support of family and significant others.**

- The situation is perceived as overwhelming or life-threatening.
- The situation cannot be resolved with usual coping skills.
- Intervention is required for equilibrium to be achieved.

A crisis is *not* a mental illness even though it is not uncommon for a person experiencing the acute discomfort and anxiety to fear "I'm losing my mind." There are three types of crises, which are shown in Table 47-3 (Aguilera, 2000).

### Balancing Factors

Three factors that influence a person's resolution of a crisis (Aguilera, 1997) are perception, coping mechanisms, and situational support. During a crisis, one (or sometimes more) of these factors is out of balance. When the factors return to a balanced state, the individual is able to resolve the crisis effectively. Nursing interventions focus on reestablishing equilibrium among these factors.

## TABLE 47-3    TYPES OF CRISES

| Type | Definition | Examples |
|------|-----------|----------|
| Developmental or maturational | • Occur as a person ages and moves from one developmental stage to another<br>• Are universal | • An adolescent attempting to gain independence from parents<br>• A middle-aged woman experiencing menopause |
| Situational | • Can occur at any time and are not predictable<br>• Are not experienced by everyone<br>• Occur when there is change in role or function | • Illness<br>• Loss (death, divorce)<br>• Graduation<br>• Job promotion<br>• Retirement |
| Adventitious | • Are unpredictable events that rarely occur | • Being in an airplane crash<br>• Losing one's home in a tornado<br>• Being a victim of a school shooting<br>• Winning a $10 million lottery |

## LIFE SPAN CONSIDERATIONS

### Crises in Older Adults

Generally speaking, crises in the older population are of greater consequence than in the younger population. Older adults often have a more compromised general body system, including the immune system capabilities. In addition, aged individuals often have several "diseases" that exist in their person, and the ability to "deal with the crisis" is affected by their condition. Nurses must recognize that the older client may require special interventions and strategies for care during a time of crisis.

## Anxiety

"Anxiety is an integral part of the universal human experience" (Molloy, 2000). A mild level of anxiety that is associated with the tensions of daily life helps increase a person's awareness of surroundings, and can actually promote growth and creativity. A severe level of anxiety, such as a motor vehicle accident, triggers the fight-or-flight response—the perception is narrowed, problem solving is difficult, activity may increase or decrease, and the person may even freeze in position (Stuart & Laraia, 2000).

Behavioral responses observed in the anxious person are personal and interpersonal. Higher levels of anxiety affect psychomotor functions such as muscle tension, lack of coordination, and tremors. The person who startles easily is at higher risk for accidents. Withdrawal from the situation and disruption of interpersonal relationships are typical responses. Common cognitive responses to anxiety are poor concentration, forgetfulness, errors in judgment, and preoccupation. For example, the adult child who is anxious about an older parent living alone may find himself preoccupied with worry about the parent and not be able to remember appointments. In addition, the anxious person may be hypervigilant or confused, and have loss of objectivity. Affective responses are the individual's description of feeling tense, jittery, worried, restless, or anticipating something dreadful will happen. Refer to Tables 47-2 and 47-4.

Anxiety is usually accompanied by other emotions such as anger, guilt, hostility, or depression. These emotions are closely connected and reciprocal, resulting in an increased cycle of destructive responses (Molloy, 2000; Reed & Pettigrew, 1999; Stuart & Laraia, 2000).

### Coping Behaviors

Coping has been used interchangeably with similar concepts of adaptation, defense, mastery, and adjustment reactions. People use a variety of conscious and unconscious, overt or covert strategies to cope with stress and anxiety. Coping is a process of attempting to solve threats to ego integrity (Aguilera, 2000). Conscious protective measures include exercising, seeking social or spiritual support, crying, laughing, journaling and reading, practicing relaxation techniques, and becoming involved in purposeful work (Holoday-Worret, 2000). The three main types of coping mechanisms are:

1. Problem-focused mechanisms—Involve tasks or direct efforts to cope with stress. For example, the person worrying about coordinating a large dinner might choose to have the meal catered.
2. Cognitively focused mechanisms—Attempt to control the meaning of a problem and thus neutralize it. For example, the adult experiencing uncontrolled depres-

## TABLE 47-4     LEVELS OF ANXIETY

| Anxiety Level | Characteristics of Anxious Person | Nursing Implications |
|---|---|---|
| Mild | • Increased degree of alertness<br>• Increased vigilance | • Optimal time for client teaching because of heightened awareness and increased perceptual field |
| Moderate | • Subjective distress<br>• Decreased perception and attention | • Help the client to determine a cause-and-effect relationship between stressor and anxiety |
| Severe | • Increased subjective distress<br>• Selective attention<br>• Distorted perception | • Encourage verbalization<br>• Engage in motor activity<br>• Give specific directions |
| Panic | • Major perceptual distortion<br>• Immobilization; inability to function<br>• Impaired communication | • Provide limits and structure<br>• Maintain client safety (both physical and psychological) |

From Peplau, H. E. (1952). *Interpersonal relations in nursing.* New York: Putnam; Sullivan, H. S. (1953). *The interpersonal theory of psychiatry.* New York: Norton.

sion might choose to attend counseling sessions to uncover the root of the depression.

3. Emotion-focused—Use of ego-defense mechanisms such as denial or projection. For example, the spouse who has lost her husband to illness might worry needlessly about the children's health.

The disciplines of nursing, social work, psychology, and psychiatry are examining the protective (problem-focused and cognitively focused) defenses as potential useful strategies that can be learned.

### Defense Mechanisms

"**Defense mechanisms** are mental processes the ego (person) uses as attempts to control or cope with anxi-

ety" (Molloy, 2000, p. 56). They are protective measures against the feelings of inadequacy and unworthiness; they also decrease the awareness of anxiety (Stuart & Laraia, 2000). Some of the methods are automatic responses, whereas other responses are purposeful and planned techniques used by individuals to manage conflicts and other negative events (Table 47-5). Denial is probably the simplest and most primitive of all unconscious defense mechanisms. Repression, the unconscious exclusion of a painful thought or memory, begins early in life and underlies all other defense mechanisms. **Suppression**, the counterpart to repression, is the conscious inhibition of a thought or perceived threat. Continued use of suppression can result in repression

### TABLE 47-5  COMMON DEFENSE MECHANISMS

| Mechanism | Description | Example |
|---|---|---|
| Denial | Negation of reality of threatening situations, despite factual evidence | The client refuses to admit to anger, even though the situation warrants it and the client's voice indicates anger. |
| Projection | Attribution of one's own thoughts, feelings, or impulses to others | "I'm not attracted to him. My best friend is." |
| Repression | Unconscious blocking from awareness any material that is threatening or painful | "I never got angry at my father; our family lived in harmony and love" (when such descriptions of the family life would not fit with anyone else's interpretation of the events). |
| Rationalization | Intellectual explaining away of threatening circumstances | "The test had too many trick questions; I really know all the material; our instructor was out to get me." |
| Introjection | Incorporating, without examination or thought, the qualities or attitudes of others | The adolescent who takes on all the values and styles of an admired teacher. |
| Displacement | Transfer of feelings or reactions evoked by one topic or event to another that is less threatening | The husband who is angry at his wife and yells at the family dog rather than dealing directly with his anger. |
| Reaction formation | Expression of a feeling that is the opposite of one's authentic feeling or of feelings that would be appropriate in the situation | A client who brings gifts to the nurse at whom he is really angry. |
| Regression | Retreat to a previous developmental level | A child starts to suck his thumb (after 2 years of no thumb sucking) when admitted to the hospital. |
| Suppression | Conscious attempt to keep threatening material out of consciousness | A student nurse decides not to think about a family problem at the moment so he can study for an upcoming examination. |
| Sublimation | Channeling of socially unacceptable impulses into socially acceptable activities | A young man who is dealing with aggression by playing football. |
| Symbolization | Use of an object, idea, or act to express emotion that is not expressed directly | The client who leaves the nurse a flower rather than directly saying she cares about the nurse. |

(Stuart & Laraia, 2000). See the Client Reflections box for an example of the use of suppression.

Defense mechanisms are universal. Their use does not indicate psychosocial imbalance or mental illness; however, defense mechanisms are pathological when they become a stereotyped pattern—that is, the only way that an individual responds to a threat. Defense mechanisms are also considered to be pathological when they limit the individual's ability to function. Physiological and psychological problems may occur when an individual's perception of an obstacle, or stress is insurmountable, when internal and external stressors exceed the individual's capacity to deal with them, or when one or more defenses are exclusively used, especially those that distort reality (Holoday-Worret, 2000).

The nurse who is unfamiliar with defense mechanisms is likely to be judgmental about clients who do not respond according to the nurse's expectations. If, for example, the nurse tries to break through a client's denial too quickly by presenting reality, the client will likely be overwhelmed by anxiety and will panic.

## Stress and Illness

Everyone experiences stress and accompanying anxiety; this anxiety is increased during illness and the recovery process. Illness and stress are interwoven to such a degree that it is difficult to determine which precedes the other. When a person's adaptive attempts are unsuccessful, illness occurs. Also, a person who is ill has fewer adaptive resources available to cope with stressors. Even though some stressors may not directly cause illness, stress is a sig-

nificant component in the onset and progression of many diseases. Table 47-6 lists some disorders commonly associated with stress.

One of the major outcomes of prolonged periods of stress is impairment of the immune system. As the body continues to fight off the threat (actual or perceived), steroid production is increased. Increased steroid production is helpful on a short-term basis because steroids speed up the healing process. However, increased steroid production over a period of time will impair the immune system. Thus, the body is less able to protect itself from disease.

| TABLE 47-6 | STRESS-RELATED DISORDERS |
|---|---|
| Respiratory disorders | • Emphysema<br>• Chronic bronchitis<br>• Asthma |
| Cardiovascular disorders | • Hypertension<br>• Cardiac arrhythmias<br>• Migraine headaches |
| Endocrine disorders | • Thyroid problems<br>• Amenorrhea, anovulation<br>• Diabetes<br>• Excessive weight gain or weight loss |
| Musculoskeletal disorders | • Chronic back pain<br>• Arthritis |
| Genitourinary disorders | • Enuresis<br>• Urinary frequency |
| Sexual and reproductive disorders | • Low libido<br>• Impotence (erectile dysfunction, or ED)<br>• Menstrual irregularities |
| Gastrointestinal disorders | • Colitis<br>• Chronic constipation<br>• Ulcers<br>• Gastritis |
| Integumentary disorders | • Eczema<br>• Hives<br>• Psoriasis |

## CLIENT REFLECTIONS

### Suppression

Mrs. James, a 34-year-old mother of two small children, has just been informed by her physician that she has cervical cancer. She is also told that her prognosis is dire; she has about 3 months left to live. Mrs. James asks questions and appears to be very calm. Later, the nurse asks Mrs. James if she wants to talk. Mrs. James replies, "I can't deal with this right now. I'll wait until my family is here and then I'll want to talk to you." Mrs. James's use of suppression allows her to postpone attempting to deal with the threatening diagnosis until she has members of her support system available to help her cope.

## CLINICAL ALERT

### To Prevent Panic

To prevent panic, never attempt to take away a defense mechanism until the client has learned another method of coping. Denying a client the use of a defense mechanism will cause more anxiety.

## Impact of Illness and Treatment

Everyone entering the health care system experiences a change in the usual routine. For example, hospitalization, surgery, and admission to a long-term care facility are major disruptions in one's routine. Such changes evoke the stress response.

Being in an unfamiliar environment, losing control over one's schedule, and being dependent on others for care are all issues with which hospitalized clients must cope. Each of these issues is a stressor that requires adaptation in order to maintain a steady state. Most clients do not have the energy to cope with numerous changes simultaneously, particularly young persons. Some cues that a person may be reacting adversely to hospitalization include:

- Increased stress response
- Higher levels of anxiety
- Increased or impaired use of coping mechanisms
- Inability to function
- Disorganized behavior

## COMMUNITY/HOME CARE

### Stress in the Home Setting

Clients who have home health care nursing needs are automatically more at risk for stress and anxiety simply because they require outside assistance. Regardless of the primary needs of these clients, the home health nurse must recognize that the client is likely to experience increased stress. This requires the nurse to carefully assess the client for the effects of stress on the body system and to incorporate stress management into the client's care plan in their home setting. The nurse must be aware of the variety of clinical manifestations of stress and design the interventions accordingly.

## LIFE SPAN CONSIDERATIONS

### Stress and the Hospitalized Child

Hospitalization of a child produces an intense form of stress for both the child and family. Parents are often highly impacted when their children experience acute illnesses, and stress is expected. The nurse must remember to exercise extremely caring attitudes and behaviors toward the client and family. Also, the nurse needs to use sound judgment in deciding what the parents will be able to tolerate in terms of caregiving or their involvement during medical procedures. For example, the nurse may notice that a mother is turning somewhat pale when her child's wound care is being performed. The nurse may want to ask the mother to wait outside the child's hospital room during the procedure.

Individuals do not have to be hospitalized to experience stressors associated with the client role. Consider, for example, the person having "minor" surgery at an outpatient center, the employee being treated at the industrial clinic for a work-related injury, or the adolescent being treated by the school nurse. Even clients who are treated by home health agencies experience stressors associated with having a health care provider enter their personal environment.

The greater the threat (or perceived threat), the greater the level of the client's anxiety. The nurse must be sensitive to stress and anxiety stemming from the multiple changes imposed by illness on the client, family, and/or significant others. The nurse's sensitivity to clients' stress reduces the risk of depersonalizing the client.

## STOP AND THINK

### Stressors Associated with Hospitalization

Think of some major changes that people experience when they are hospitalized. Can you identify at least three changes? What can you do to significantly reduce threats (real or perceived) in acute care settings? In long-term care settings?

# Stress and Change

**Change** (a dynamic process in which an individual's behavior is altered in response to a stressor) is an inherent part of life. It is the process that causes individuals to adapt. Whether it is planned or unplanned, change is both inevitable and constant. Change can be constructive or destructive and is stressful to individuals because it activates the GAS. Box 47-1 lists characteristics of change.

Nurses must be able to initiate and cope with change. Proficiency in critical-thinking and problem-solving skills is necessary to initiate positive change.

The pace of change is rapidly increasing in health care agencies, which have been changing and continue to change in response to consumer demands. "Change is inevitable and nurses have the qualities and a strategic position to participate actively" (Joel, 1998, p. 7). Some changes that have evolved from consumer demands and needs include:

## NURSING STRATEGY

### Actions to Promote Client Control

- *Communicate clearly.* Use terms easily understood by clients and families. Avoid using medical jargon with clients.

- *Answer questions thoroughly.* Validate client's and family's level of understanding.

- *Teach the use of relaxation techniques,* such as progressive muscle relaxation (a stress management technique involving the tensing and relaxing of muscles) and guided imagery (a relaxation technique in which the individual uses the imagination to experience a pleasant, soothing image).

- *Instruct clients on the use of* cognitive reframing (a technique in which the individual changes her negative perception of a situation or event to a more positive, less-threatening perspective).

- *Provide support and reassurance.* The nurse's presence ("being with" the client) can alleviate anxiety levels. The most therapeutic tool in alleviating client anxiety is the nurse's therapeutic use of self.

- *Break down the information shared with clients.* Too much information at once can make the client feel overwhelmed and less likely to listen. When clients have adequate information, they can make informed decisions and maintain some degree of control over their lives.

## BOX 47-1    CHARACTERISTICS OF CHANGE

- Is an inevitable part of life.
- May be eustressful or distressful.
- Can be self-initiated or externally imposed.
- Can occur abruptly or have a gradual onset with insidious progression.
- Energy is required to effect change, as well as to resist change.

- Sports medicine clinics
- Substance abuse treatment programs
- Day treatment programs for geriatric and psychiatric clients
- Weight control programs
- Exercise programs

## Types of Change

Change is either planned or unplanned. Unplanned change is the change that "just happens"; it is unpredictable and may be imposed by others or by uncontrollable natural events (e.g., losing one's home in a flood). On the other hand, planned change results from a deliberate effort to improve a situation. In addition to planned and unplanned change, there are other types of changes (Table 47-7).

## TABLE 47-7    TYPES OF CHANGE

| Type of Change | Description |
| --- | --- |
| Developmental | • Physical and emotional changes that occur at different stages of the life cycle |
| | • Generally predictable |
| | • Usually occur gradually |
| Reactive | • Adaptive responses to external stimuli |
| | • Efforts to cope with change imposed by others |
| Covert | • Occur without person's conscious awareness |
| Overt | • Person is aware of the change |
| | • Usually not under individual's direct control |

## Theories of Change

Nurses must have a thorough understanding of the change process in order to effectively implement change with clients and within the health care delivery system. Planned change theories are most useful for low-level and low-complex change situations in stable environments. These linear theories propose that change occurs in sequential or incremental stages, and is most effective in improving a situation when guided by change leaders. An example would be assisting a client with lifestyle changes that promote a better quality of life. Strategies of planned change can also be used in coping with the resulting stress from unpredictable or uncontrollable changes (Manix, 1999).

Nonlinear change theories suggest that organizations exist in rapidly changing and chaotic environments where times of stability are interrupted by intense periods of varying forms of change. An example would be a health care system's attempts to control long-term outcomes in a rapidly changing and unpredictable social environment. Such changes are stressors to the organization and all persons involved. Yet, if a status quo is maintained, there would be no individual growth, and the organization's survival would be threatened (Grossman & Valiga, 2000). Nurses must be able to strategize creatively and visualize several alternative outcomes in more complex situations as well as in less complex situations related to the change process. Proficiency in critical-thinking and problem-solving skills is necessary to initiate positive change. (Manix, 1999). Two major theories of planned change are discussed below.

### Lewin's Theory of Change

A classic theory of change was developed by Lewin (1951), who stated that the change process occurs in three stages: unfreezing, moving, and refreezing (Figure 47-4). In the unfreezing stage, the person recognizes a need for change and becomes motivated to move in a new direction. Stage two, moving, is the actual implementation of the change. In the third stage, refreezing, new changes are incorporated into behavior and these new behaviors stabilize. Because the change process is dynamic, these stages are not rigid. The process of change may quickly move through all stages, or it may become "stuck" in one stage.

### Lippitt's Theory of Change

Lippitt (Lippitt, Watson, & Westley, 1958) proposed a theory of change that consists of seven phases:

1. Diagnose the problem (need for change).
2. Assess the change target's motivation and capacity for change.
3. Assess the change agent's motivation and capacity for change.
4. Establish objectives for change.
5. Determine the role of the change agent.
6. After change has occurred, maintain it.
7. Terminate the role of the change agent.

## Resistance to Change

Many people tend to resist change because of the energy required to adapt. Conversely, energy is also required to resist change, or to maintain the *status quo*. Individuals differ in their ability to tolerate (or even thrive on) change.

There are many reasons why people tend to resist change (Table 47-8). There are no absolute guarantees that the change activity will lead to positive outcomes; this uncertainty about outcomes is a major barrier to change.

## Changing Paradigms

Changing involves questioning and frequently results in the development of a new **paradigm** (a pattern, model, or mindset that strongly influences one's decisions and behaviors). One's paradigm greatly colors one's perceptions and behaviors. By changing paradigms, an individual can determine what is positive in the old system and use it to create a newer, better system (Alfaro-LeFevre, 1998).

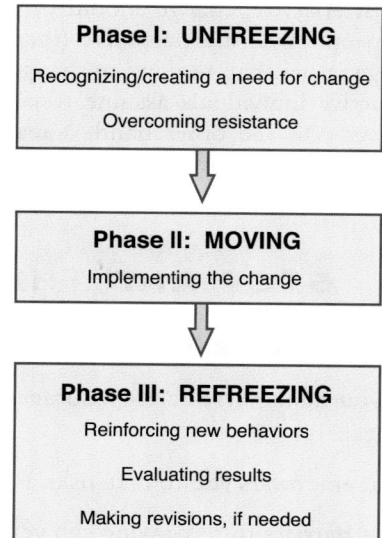

**Figure 47-4  Lewin's Theory of Change.** *From Lewin, K. (1951). Field theory in social science, New York: Harper.*

### STOP AND THINK

#### Responses to Change

What is your typical response when first learning that a change is imminent? Do you feel threatened, afraid, anxious? Do you feel excited and optimistic? Perhaps you feel something in between resistance and excitement. It is important for you to be aware of your automatic thoughts that influence your response to change.

## TABLE 47-8     REASONS PEOPLE RESIST CHANGE

| | |
|---|---|
| Conformity | Often referred to as "groupthink"; complying with the group's expectations; going along with others to avoid conflict. |
| Dissimilar beliefs and values | Differences in attitudes and expectations regarding health and illness behaviors; differences between client and nurse that can impede positive change. |
| Habits | Routine, "set" behaviors are often hard to change. |
| Satisfaction with *status quo* | Seeing only advantages to the present system can blind one to the possible need for change. Satisfaction with the way things are now reinforces resistance to change. |
| **Secondary gains** (outcomes other than alleviation of anxiety) | Benefits or pay-offs of the sick role (such as gaining attention and sympathy, avoiding responsibilities, and getting financial compensation or reward) often are so desirable that the client has little incentive to change. |
| Threats to satisfying basic needs | Change may be perceived as a threat to self-esteem, security, or survival. |
| Fear | Fear of failure and fear of the unknown especially block change. |
| Unrealistic goals | Set up the individual for failure in change efforts. |

It is risky to initiate change, to challenge one's own paradigms and those of others. One of the first signs of the need for change is questioning. The nurse who wonders Why? or Why not? or What if? is the nurse who will likely take the risk to initiate change activity. The effective risk taker is neither reckless nor overly cautious. Successful risk takers consider possible outcomes before initiating action. "Accepting change as inevitable and taking personal control and responsibility for it needs to be acknowledged by all in the health service industry today" (Bonalumi & Fisher, 1999, p. 70).

## Overcoming Barriers to Change

Because change is inevitable, learning how to deal with it is crucial for nurses. Resistance occurs when the individual rejects proposed new ideas without critically thinking about the proposal.

> Overcoming this barrier doesn't mean embracing every new idea uncritically. It means being willing to suspend judgment long enough to make an informed decision on whether the change is worthwhile. (Alfaro-LeFevre, 1998, p. 25)

Coping with change of any type calls for flexibility, adaptability, and resilience.

## Nurse as Change Agent

Initiating change is an expectation for professional nurses. The American Nurses Association (1991) calls for nurses to bring about changes in practice as well as changes in the system of delivering health care. Nurses experience stress daily as a result of changes within their immediate work environment as well as changes in the entire health care delivery system. The uncertainty over health care reform is very distressful to some nurses. Others see opportunity for positive change in the future. "Nursing staff members need to realize that change is not something that happens to them, but something that they can influence" (Bonalumi & Fisher, 1999, p. 72).

In bringing about change to promote positive adaptation, the nurse serves as a **change agent** (a person who intentionally initiates and creates change). True change agents constantly seek ways to make improvements. They use critical-thinking skills to develop creative, innovative solutions. Critical thinking is also required to determine the outcome of initiating change. Evaluating the effects of change is key to bringing about positive change.

To be most effective, change should be planned and directed by people who are **proactive** (individuals who initiate change rather than respond to change imposed by others). Proactive individuals assume responsibility for their own lives. On the other hand, a reactive person responds only to externally imposed change. Proactive

 ## STOP AND THINK

### Nurses As Risk Takers

- Do you think nurses are encouraged to be risk takers?

- What empowers you to take risks as a student?

- What barriers to risk-taking can you identify in academic and health care settings?

## LEGAL AND ETHICAL ISSUES

### Changes That Result in Legal Implications

When nurses make a change in an intervention policy, they must remember to examine the change in regard to any potential legal implications. For example, if a different acuity system for categorizing clients is developed, the nurses must remember to evaluate the quality of care that is the outcome of the new staffing measures. If the new acuity changes do not leave a safe staff-to-client ratio, then the system would need further refining. Otherwise, there would be obvious legal implications of a changed, unsafe system of care.

## STOP AND THINK

### Stress and You

Some questions to ask your client are:

● What aspects of your life are stressful?

● What have you tried before to cope with a stressful problem?

● How well did your methods work?

● Can you tell me about your current problem?

● Has this particular problem occurred before?

nurses are change agents who affect the entire health care system as well as individual clients. However, when nurses makes changes in policy, there may be resulting legal implications.

Change agents keep the change process moving toward a positive outcome. As an advocate for change, the nurse empowers the client to initiate change in order to adapt more successfully; client education is a powerful tool for initiating change. Teaching a client about a disease process, a treatment modality, or a lifestyle alteration provides the client with an opportunity to change. In fact, learning results in behavioral changes (Reed & Pettigrew, 1999).

## Assessment

Many times, clients with anxiety symptoms may seek treatment for other reasons. "It is important for all nurses to identify dysfunctional manifestations of anxiety so that treatment can be implemented promptly" (Molloy, 2000, p. 18). When caring for an anxious client, the nurse must first determine the client's perception of the situation. This determination is done by directly asking for the client's input and carefully listening to the client's response. Because the nurse's nonverbal behavior can affect the client's anxiety level, nurses must be aware of their own body language. Anxiety is a subjective experience, thus, it cannot be directly observed. Therefore, the nurse must look for the signs indicative of anxiety (previously discussed in Table 47-2).

A thorough assessment of stress and anxiety levels includes eliciting client input to evaluate the following factors:

• Patterns of stressors
• Typical responses to stressful situations

• Cause-and-effect relationships between stressors and thoughts, feelings, and behaviors
• Past history of successful coping mechanisms

Assessing the client's coping abilities can be done in various ways. For example, use open-ended questions to determine previously used coping mechanisms.

Identification of the client's coping abilities assists in establishing appropriate nursing diagnoses and developing an effective plan of care. Assessment, which relies heavily on the nurse's observation and listening skills, provides the data necessary for formulating nursing diagnoses.

## Nursing Diagnosis

Several nursing diagnoses may apply to clients experiencing anxiety. See Table 47-9 for selected diagnoses and their defining characteristics and related factors. In addition to the four diagnoses listed in Table 47-9, the following NANDA (2003) diagnoses may also be appropriate for anxious clients.

• *Impaired Adjustment*
• *Ineffective Role Performance*
• *Disturbed Thought Processes*
• *Defensive Coping*
• *Fear*
• *Post-Trauma Syndrome*
• *Impaired Social Interaction*
• *Spiritual Distress*

## Outcome Identification and Planning

Client involvement in planning care is essential because helping clients learn to cope successfully is part of the empowerment process. Planning means exploring self-responsibility issues with the client.

## TABLE 47-9 NURSING DIAGNOSIS: CLIENTS EXPERIENCING ANXIETY

| Nursing Diagnosis: Definition | Defining Characteristics | Related Factors |
|---|---|---|
| **Anxiety:** Feelings of apprehension and arousal of the autonomic nervous system in response to a threat (which may be specific or vague) | Note: Manifestations will vary according to the level of anxiety.<br>• Physiological<br> –Changes in vital signs (increased pulse, respirations, blood pressure)<br> –Diaphoresis (increased sweating)<br> –Restlessness, tremors<br> –Frequent urination<br>• Emotional<br> –Verbalization of feelings of helplessness, losing control, nervousness, fear<br> –Inability to relax<br> –Increased irritability<br> –Withdrawal or angry outbursts<br>• Cognitive<br> –Forgetfulness<br> –Impaired ability to concentrate<br> –Inability to remember | • Any threat, real or perceived<br>• Unmet needs (biologic, safety and security, belonging, self-esteem)<br>• A loss (e.g., of a relationship as a result of death or divorce; a job; functional ability)<br>• Loss of control (over one's situation or events)<br>• Conflict (interpersonal or intrapersonal)<br>• Environmental changes |
| **Ineffective Coping:** The inability to manage stressors because problem-solving behaviors are no longer effective | • Inability to meet basic needs<br>• Inability to solve problems<br>• Altered patterns of communication<br>• Inappropriate use of defense mechanisms<br>• Verbalization of inability to ask for help<br>• Destructive behavior toward self or others | • Low self-esteem<br>• Alterations in body integrity (e.g., disfigurement secondary to trauma or surgery; loss of body part)<br>• Disruption of emotional ties<br>• Unsatisfactory support system<br>• Separation from home and family<br>• Sensory overload |
| **Ineffective Denial:** Occurrence in which the person minimizes or negates symptoms to the point of being injurious to his health status | • Refusal of health care treatment<br>• Delay in seeking treatment<br>• Resistance to treatment program<br>• Failure to perceive danger of presence of symptoms<br>• Relinquishing of self-responsibility (frequent verbalizations of "I can't")<br>• Blaming other people or circumstances ("It's not my fault")<br>• Inability or unwillingness to admit impact of illness or trauma on self | • Presence of chronic and/or terminal disease<br>• Loss (e.g., of job, significant other, income)<br>• Personal vulnerability<br>• Fear<br>• Difficulty handling new situations<br>• Learned response<br>• Cultural factors<br>• Personal and/or family value system |
| **Powerlessness:** Situation in which the person perceives a lack of control over situations or events | • Verbalization of dissatisfaction over inability to control the situation<br>• Passive, "giving-up" behavior or aggressive, hostile behavior<br>• Difficulty in expressing self directly<br>• Anxiety<br>• Resignation<br>• Depression | • Illness (both acute and chronic)<br>• Hospitalization or institutionalization<br>• Expressed feelings of insecurity and/or resentment<br>• Multiple life changes and/or losses |

From Carpenito, L. J. (2002). *Handbook of nursing diagnosis* (9th ed.). Philadelphia: Lippincott; Doenges, M. E., Townsend, M. C., & Moorhouse, M. F. (2002). *Psychiatric care plans: Guidelines for planning and documenting client care* (4th ed.). Philadelphia: F. A. Davis; North American Nursing Diagnosis Association (NANDA). (2003). *Nursing Diagnoses: Definitions and classifications, 2003–2004*. Philadelphia: Author.

The Nursing Strategy box shows expected outcomes appropriate for many anxious clients.

## Implementation

Teaching, a major nursing intervention for managing stress, is inherent in holistic nursing practice. Stress management approaches can be taught to clients of every age and developmental stage in all health care settings: acute care (inpatient and outpatient), long-term care, and the home.

Teaching clients to reduce their own levels of stress is a major step in promoting self-care. Client education provides clients with options. Clients who have a thorough understanding of their options can make informed decisions about necessary lifestyle changes (Figure 47-5). Following is a discussion of some of the many interventions that can be used with anxious clients.

### Meeting Basic Needs

There is a close relationship between basic physiological needs and stress. Anything that interferes with the satisfaction of basic needs evokes the stress response and attendant anxiety. Clients who are cold, hungry, or in pain have higher anxiety levels than those who are comfortable. When anxiety levels increase, so does the perception of pain. Nurses who empower clients to meet basic needs are laying the foundation for a less stressful, more caring treatment process. By reducing anxiety, the nurse is improving the client's healing potential.

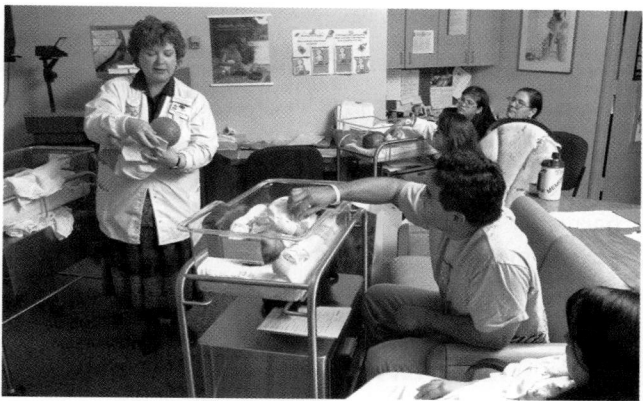

**Figure 47-5**    By discussing options for infant care with this father, the nurse is providing him with the information he needs to plan effective lifestyle changes. What methods can the nurse use to assess whether the client fully understands the information?

### Environmental Strategies

Because an individual's immediate environment can influence stress levels, it is important for the nurse to decrease environmental stimuli that may contribute to anxiety. Some specific ways to limit environmental stimuli are listed in the Nursing Strategy box.

## NURSING STRATEGY

### Client Coping

The nurse should work with clients in coping with their crises by establishing outcomes such as the following:

- Verbalizes absence of or decrease in subjective distress

- Has vital signs that reflect baseline or decreased sympathetic stimulation

- Has posture, facial expressions, gestures, and activity levels that reflect decreased distress

- Demonstrates return of basic problem-solving skills

- Demonstrates increased interest in social interactions

- Demonstrates some ability to reassure self

From Ackley, B., & Ladwig, G. (2002). *Nursing diagnosis handbook: A guide to planning care.* St. Louis: Mosby.

## NURSING STRATEGY

### Reducing Environmental Distressors

To decrease environmental stimulants that increase client's anxiety:

- Provide private room if possible.

- Dim the lights or close window blinds.

- Maintain an environment in which the client feels free to express emotions.

- Limit contacts with other clients to minimize contagious aspects of anxiety.

- Limit the length of stay and number of visitors at any one time.

- Limit visits with family and visitors that may contribute to client's anxiety.

- Assist anxious family members to relax.

- Introduce supportive measures such as massage, warm baths, and relaxation techniques.

- Use soft background music if it soothes client.

- Personalize the environment with client's familiar objects.

## Verbalization

Encouraging clients to express their feelings is especially valuable in stress reduction. Freud (1959) used the term **catharsis** to describe the process of talking out one's feelings. People instinctively know the value of "getting things off their chest" through verbalization. Verbalization promotes relaxation primarily in two ways. First, when a feeling is described it becomes *real*. Once the problem is identified, the person can begin to deal effectively with it. Also, the actual activity of talking uses energy and, therefore, reduces anxiety.

## Involvement of Family and Significant Others

The client's developmental stage influences the type of intervention for stress management. Children and adolescents have varying coping skills; children of all ages rely on their parents to a varying degree for security and support. It is important to include the entire family in the care of the client whenever possible (Figure 47-6). Such an approach is useful in decreasing the stress levels of everyone involved, because families provide essential support for clients.

Family members who are extremely anxious often have a negative impact on the client's health status. Therefore, nurses often need to help family members relax; one way to accomplish this is by providing explanations and information. Thus, it is often necessary for nurses to teach stress management techniques to the client's family.

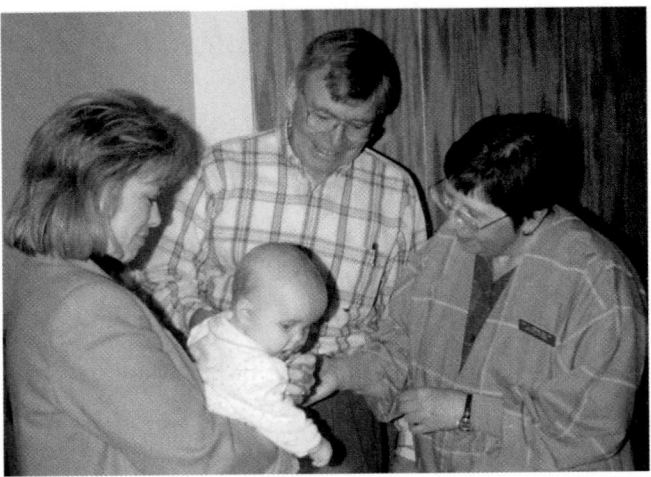

**Figure 47-6**    Nurses can encourage the interaction of clients with family members and significant others in various health care settings. This involvement is helpful in easing the client's anxiety and can also serve as a method through which the family member is kept informed about the client's care.

## Stress Management Techniques

A variety of stress management techniques can easily be taught to clients, families, and significant others. Many of these techniques are considered to be complementary modalities, as they are used in conjunction with traditional medical treatment methods (i.e., medication, radiation therapy). Some of the most common approaches for managing stress are discussed below.

### Exercise

Physical exercise is a powerful way to reduce anxiety and can be used by clients of all ages and with varying physical abilities (Figure 47-7). Client teaching should emphasize

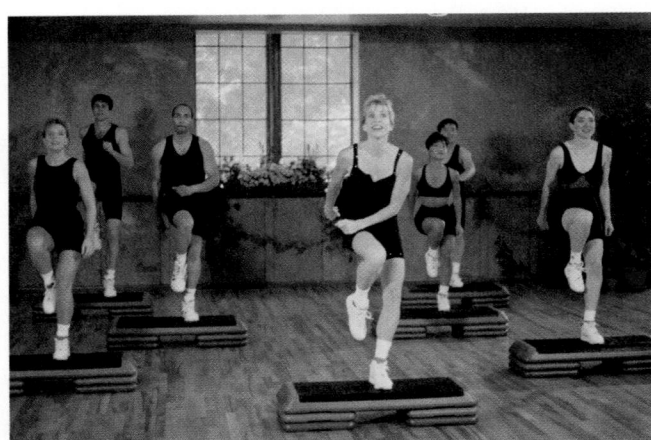

**Figure 47-7**    Exercise provides physiological and psychological benefits to individuals. Fitness centers are common places for persons to participate in organized aerobic activities. *Courtesy of Photodisc*

### Guidelines for Establishing an Exercise Program

- Explore the availability of different exercise programs.

- Consult with a health care provider about the safety of a specific exercise program.

- Set realistic goals.

- Plan a routine, allow for a warm-up and cool-down period using stretch exercises.

- Engage in activity that increases heart rate for a period of time and is followed by a cool-down period.

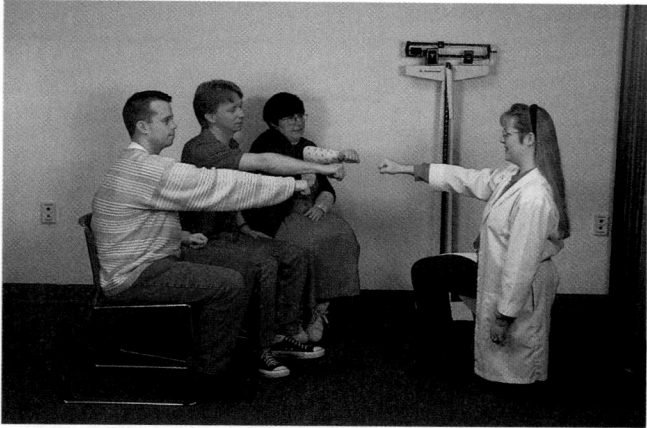

**Figure 47-8**   This nurse is demonstrating the technique of progressive muscle relaxation in a client education program. How does instruction in this method enhance the self-responsibility that clients need to develop in order to manage their stress?

the need for incorporating exercise into one's lifestyle. In other words, if exercise is to reduce anxiety, it must be done on an ongoing and regular basis.

"Exercise can bring a general sense of well-being and vitality, increase respiratory and cardiovascular efficiency, and promote a longer life. Exercise is now considered a major factor in self-care. Exercise can also enhance the self-image and general health" (Grendell, 2000, p. 714). Additional psychological benefits include decreased stress, improved concentration and memory, reduced depression, and less dependence on external stimulants or relaxants. A good exercise program includes aerobic activities such as walking, jogging, swimming, bicycling, and dancing (Michaels, 1999).

### Relaxation Techniques

There are several approaches that help individuals relax. See Chapter 31 for a discussion of complementary/alternative modalities (such as aromatherapy, herbals, music, and humor) that promote relaxation. The following discussion describes some specific relaxation techniques that are easily learned and can be effective in a variety of stressors.

### Progressive Muscle Relaxation

**Progressive muscle relaxation (PMR)** is a method of inducing relaxation by tensing and releasing various muscle groups. For example, the individual tightens her hands into a fist, holds the tension for a few seconds, then slowly relaxes her fingers and hands, paying particular attention to the different sensations of tension and relaxation (Figure 47-8). This tense-release action is applied to all muscle groups of the body. PMR is especially helpful in promoting sleep. PMR is a technique that can successfully be taught to clients for use in any health care setting, including the home.

### Progressive Muscle Relaxation

After explaining the purpose and process of progressive muscle relaxation, instruct the client to:

1. Assume a comfortable position in a quiet environment.
2. Close eyes and keep them closed until the exercise is completed.
3. Inhale deeply to a count of 4.
4. Hold breath for a count of 4.
5. Exhale to a count of 4.
6. Continue to breathe slowly and deeply.
7. Tense both feet until muscle tension is felt. Caution the client to tighten the muscles only until the muscles are tensed, not to the point of pain. Hold a gentle state of tension in both feet for a count of 3.

   *NOTE*: If muscle cramps occur, stop the procedure and gently massage the affected area. Then begin the cycle of slight muscle tension and relaxation again.

8. Slowly release the tension from the feet.
9. Fully experience the difference between tension and relaxation.
10. Repeat steps 3 to 6.

Repeat the above sequence with all the muscle groups to experience relaxation throughout your body. To be effective, this procedure requires approximately 20 to 30 minutes. Like all other relaxation exercises, progressive muscle relaxation is most effective with repetition.

## Guided Imagery

Another technique for helping clients manage stress successfully is **guided imagery**, a process in which the person uses all the senses to experience the sensation of relaxation. During guided imagery, the client is directed to concentrate on a pleasant scene or image in order to become more relaxed. In many situations, music is a helpful adjunct to guided imagery (Figure 47-9). The Client Education box describes the steps involved in using this technique. See Chapter 31 for further discussion of guided imagery. Note that imagery is not recommended for individuals experiencing emotional instability.

## Cognitive Reframing or Thought Stopping

**Cognitive reframing** is a technique based on a theory proposed by Aaron Beck (1976), who stated that a person's emotional response is determined by the meaning attached to an event. For example, if an event is perceived to be threatening, the client is likely to feel anxious. If the interpretation of the event can be modified, the client will be less anxious. Reframing is a technique used to alter one's perceptions and interpretations by changing one's thoughts. Box 47-2 describes the thought-stopping process, a cognitive reframing technique.

## Rapid Relaxation Response

The **rapid relaxation response (RRR)** is a useful method that is similar to transcendental meditation. The person selects a mantra, a word or phrase (e.g., "ocean waves") that can be used repetitively to help manage symptoms or unwanted emotions. The mantra becomes a rapid focus tool that can be used at any time and any place to block the mind/body interactive effects of anxiety and other disturbing emotions. Individuals who have practiced RRR have reported decrease in anger, anxiety, feelings of hopelessness, and insomnia; they have been able to manage their moods more effectively and believe they have better

coping skills. Their concentration also has improved (Borman, 2002).

## Crisis Intervention

Some clients will be in an acute crisis state and require **crisis intervention**, a specific technique that helps clients regain equilibrium. Clients are viewed as having the abili-

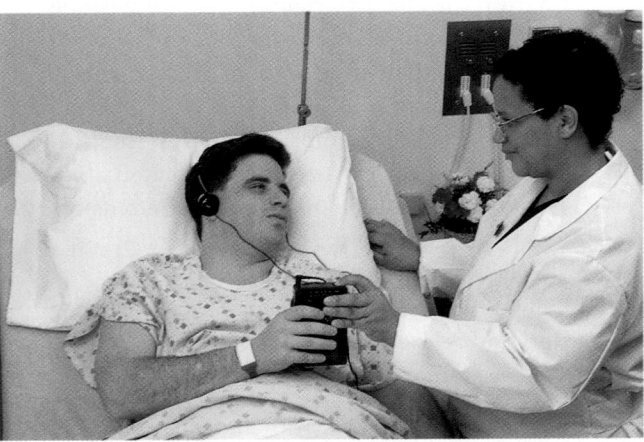

**Figure 47-9** To help relieve this client's stress, the nurse is giving him a tape recorder and a relaxation tape. In your opinion, are there any situations where this type of intervention may be inappropriate?

---

## CLIENT EDUCATION

### Guided Imagery

After explaining the purpose and process of guided imagery, instruct the client to:

✓ Assume a comfortable position in a quiet environment.

✓ Close your eyes and keep them closed until the exercise is completed.

✓ Inhale deeply to a count of 4.

✓ Hold breath for a count of 4.

✓ Exhale to a count of 4.

✓ Continue to breathe slowly and deeply.

✓ Think of a favorite place and prepare to take an imaginary journey there. Select a place in which you are relaxed and at peace.

✓ Picture in your mind's eye your favorite place. Look around you. See all the colors, the light and shadows. Look at all the pleasant sights.

✓ Listen to all the sounds. Pay attention to what you hear.

✓ Feel all the physical sensations . . . the temperature . . . the textures . . . the movement of the air.

✓ As you take in a deep breath, smell the aromas of your favorite place.

✓ Taste the foods and drinks you usually consume in your favorite place. Savor each taste fully.

✓ Focus all your attention totally on your favorite place.

✓ Inhale deeply to a count of 4.

✓ Hold breath for a count of 4.

✓ Exhale to a count of 4.

✓ Resume your usual breathing pattern.

✓ Slowly open your eyes and stretch, if desired.

This procedure works best when all five senses are used. Like all other relaxation exercises, guided imagery becomes more effective with repetition. This technique (as all imagery exercises) is not recommended for individuals with emotional instability.

## BOX 47-2    THOUGHT STOPPING: A COGNITIVE REFRAMING TECHNIQUE

- Listen to self-talk (thoughts).

- Recognize when the self-talk is negative.

- When a negative thought is detected, do something physical to stop the train of thought. For example, clap your hands or snap a rubber band on your wrist. Tell yourself, "Stop!"

- Replace the negative thought with one that is both positive and realistic.

Like all other relaxation exercises, thought stopping becomes more effective with repetition

---

ty to control their own lives. The five steps of crisis intervention are illustrated in Figure 47-10.

The client is an active participant in the process of resolving the crisis in order to restore equilibrium. If the client is unable to participate in problem solving (e.g., because of delayed developmental stage or altered mental status), then crisis intervention should not be attempted. However, the family can be approached with the crisis intervention method.

Sometimes clients need more assistance than the nurse can provide. Recognition of such situations calls for prompt consultation with and, sometimes, referral to other health care providers, such as:

- Psychiatric clinical nurse specialists
- Nurse psychotherapists
- Psychologists
- Social workers
- Psychiatrists
- Clergy and other counselors

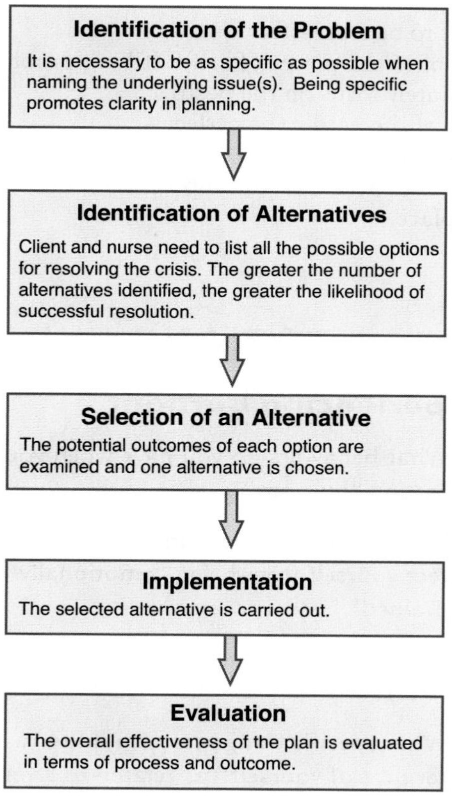

## Evaluation

Evaluating the effectiveness of clients' coping abilities is an ongoing comprehensive process that must include client input. It is imperative that the nurse evaluate client outcomes as well as the process of delivering nursing care.

In addition to eliciting verbal input from the client and significant others, nurses also collect evaluation data by observation of client behavior. See the Nursing Strategy box for some questions that the nurse may consider in evaluating the effectiveness of interventions to reduce anxiety.

## Personal Stress Management Approaches for the Nurse

"Before nurses can care for clients, they must first learn to value and care for themselves" (Fontaine, 2000, p. 18). There are many stressors inherent in nursing. Learning to cope successfully with stressors is essential for nurses.

---

**Identification of the Problem**
It is necessary to be as specific as possible when naming the underlying issue(s). Being specific promotes clarity in planning.

↓

**Identification of Alternatives**
Client and nurse need to list all the possible options for resolving the crisis. The greater the number of alternatives identified, the greater the likelihood of successful resolution.

↓

**Selection of an Alternative**
The potential outcomes of each option are examined and one alternative is chosen.

↓

**Implementation**
The selected alternative is carried out.

↓

**Evaluation**
The overall effectiveness of the plan is evaluated in terms of process and outcome.

**Figure 47-10    Steps of crisis intervention.** *Aguilera, D., 1998; 2000.*

---

## NURSING STRATEGY

### Evaluation

Consider these questions when evaluating the effectiveness of your anxiety-reducing interventions:

- Does the client exhibit decreased fidgeting and pacing?

- Is the client's tone of voice calm?

- Is the client's problem-solving ability unimpaired?

- Is ability to concentrate intact?

- Are the vital signs within normal limits (client's baseline)?

Two major reasons nurses must cope successfully with stress are to maintain their own wellness and to model health-promoting behaviors to others. In order to help clients learn to manage stress, nurses must first be able to manage their own stress.

Exercise, relaxation techniques, and environmental changes are beneficial for nurses as well as for their clients. In addition to relaxation techniques mentioned previously, and complementary/alternative modalities discussed in Chapter 31, the nurse may choose journaling, writing poetry, and hobbies as health promoting strategies. Kulbe's (2001) study of coping measures used by hospice nurses revealed that exercise and recreational activities were perceived as the greatest stress-reduction methods. Additional supportive measures were a professional team spirit, a personal spiritual practice, use of humor, working part time, and taking "time out to rest and for reflection."

## Burnout and Nurses

The burnout phenomenon is evident in occupations where individuals spend a significant amount of time in close personal interaction with others. Nurses are particularly vulnerable to burnout due to their daily involvement with people in crisis, and being in stressful work situations (see Box 47-3). The defining characteristics include tension and irritability, mental and physical fatigue, appetite changes, and sleep deprivation associated with rotating work schedules. Additional hazards are work-related injuries, exposure to chemicals, potential infection from human blood or body fluids, and communicable diseases. The current emphasis on managed care and cost-containment, shorter hospital stays, and time constraints is in conflict with the nurses' expectations for providing quality care. Nurses cope with these situations by depersonalizing clients and removing themselves from the close nurse-client relationship. **Depersonalization** describes the process in which an individual is treated as an object rather than as a person with unique characteristics. Absenteeism and job turnover are common occurrences, and the potential for drug and alcohol abuse increases (Kilfedder, Power, & Wells, 2001; Michaels, 2000; Reed & Pettigrew, 1999).

Many new graduates quickly realize that accomplishing their own role expectations depends upon many factors other than their own perceptions of how nursing should be performed. The realities of the clinical setting may not allow sufficient time or resources to meet the total needs of clients. Such situations result in cognitive dissonance, where there is knowledge of what should be done but circumstances do not permit fulfilling expectations. The end results are disappointment, lack of personal accomplishment, and increased anxiety (Catalano, 2000).

---

### BOX 47-3    PHASES OF BURNOUT

Phase 1: Initial feeling of enthusiasm for the job

Phase 2: Loss of enthusiasm

Phase 3: Continuous deterioration

Phase 4: Crisis

Phase 5: Inability to work effectively

From Michaels, B. (2000). Self-care strategies. In J. Zerwekh & J. Claborn (Eds.), *Nursing today: Transitions and trends* (pp. 517–535). Philadelphia: W. B. Saunders.

---

There are numerous and varied strategies to combat burnout. "Learning about self-care is really about empowerment. With empowerment comes a feeling of well-being and effectiveness" (Michaels, 2000, p. 52). In finding an "inner balance," the nurse is more effective in caring for others (Folsom, 1999, p. 80).

Nurses can use many strategies to help manage professional and personal stress. In addition to the techniques listed in Box 47-4, the following Client Education box provides strategies that are also helpful in managing professional stress. Helpful guidelines for changing from a negative to a positive outlook include:

- Expect to be successful.
- Remember the power of self-fulfilling prophecies and deliberately focus on the positive.
- Let go of the need to be perfect.
- Listen to your self-talk.
- Encourage the use of appropriate humor in the workplace.

---

    **STOP AND THINK**

### Experiencing Burnout

- What behaviors do you have when you are getting "burnout"?

- What coping mechanisms do you use to protect yourself from being "emotionally drained" by your clients?

- Who do you "connect with" when you are stressed?

- What specific things can you do to take "better care of yourself" as related to stress and potential issues of burnout?

## BOX 47-4   STRATEGIES FOR SELF-MANAGEMENT AND COPING WITH STRESS

- Use your high-priority goals as guides in making decisions.

- Make your personal health a priority.

- Know your personal response to stress.

- Self-evaluate your responses frequently.

- Use strategies that help you maintain balance and self-control.

- Refocus on your priorities whenever you begin to feel overwhelmed.

- Network with colleagues and members of interdisciplinary team.

- Maintain an attitude of openness to new ideas.

- Avoid overcommitment. Learn to say no!

- Manage time effectively.

- Recognize your own limitations.

- Affirm self-esteem and accomplishments.

Michaels, B. (2000). Self-care strategies. In J. Zerwekh & J. Claborn (Eds.), *Nursing today: Transitions and trends* (pp. 517–535). Philadelphia: W. B. Saunders; Reed, F., & Pettigrew, A. (1999). Self-management: Stress and time. In P. Yoder-Wise (Ed.), *Leading and managing in nursing* (pp. 186–204). St. Louis: Mosby.

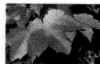

## RESEARCH FOCUS

**Title of Study:** Hardiness, help-seeking behavior, and social support of baccalaureate nursing students

**Study Purpose:** To (1) examine the effects of hardiness, social support, and help-seeking behavior on academic performance, and (2) determine the relationship among hardiness, social support, and help-seeking behavior.

**Methods:** This descriptive correlational study used a questionnaire with a self-selected sample. Surveys were administered to students who remained after class.

**Findings:** (1) Students indicated that they sometimes seek help, with more students seeking help for academic than personal situations. (2) General students were more likely to seek help than nursing students. (3) As hardiness increases, academic performance increases slightly.

**Implications:** The study results reinforce the importance of social support to success in any challenging life situation. Faculty should build on students' perseverance, persistence, and hardiness.

Hegge, M., Melcher, P., & Williams, S. (1999). Hardiness, help-seeking behavior, and social support of baccalaureate nursing students. *Journal of Nursing Education, 38*(4), 178–182.

Nurses who cultivate the hardiness factor will likely be resilient to stress. Kobasa (1979) originated the concept of hardiness in the late 1970s. Hardiness consists of a set of attitudes, beliefs, and behaviors that result in individuals being more resilient (or hardy) to the negative effects of stress. There are three components to stress hardiness:

1. *Commitment.* Becoming involved in what one is doing
2. *Challenge.* Perceiving change as an opportunity for growth rather than an obstacle or threat
3. *Control.* Believing that one is influential in directing what happens to oneself rather than feeling helpless and victimized

According to studies (Kobasa, 1979; Kobasa, Maddi, & Kahn, 1982), individuals who have higher degrees of har-

diness are healthier than individuals with low degrees of hardiness. Such people develop fewer illnesses when they experience multiple stressors.

Lambert & Lambert (1999) surveyed more than 50 journal articles on hardiness published since 1987. The themes indicated that individuals with psychological hardiness have a sense of purpose, are involved in life events, have a sense of control, and use more positive coping behaviors. These individuals view change as normal and as a stimulus for growth. Hardiness may be an ascribed (innate) trait, a learned socialized trait, or a trait derived from a strong social support system. Hardiness is a multifaceted concept.

Resilience theory has evolved from the studies conducted on hardiness. The ability to respond quickly and "bounce back" from traumatic experiences are hallmarks of resilience. Humphreys' (2001) study of resilient daughters of battered women identified the use of perseverance and optimism as coping mechanisms throughout the critical life events. They learned to seek help as a means of

## CLIENT EDUCATION

### Managing Professional Stress

✓ *Develop and maintain active support systems,* both at work and away from work. Having friends who are not health care providers helps maintain a sense of balance and separateness between personal and professional domains.

✓ *Develop decision-making skills.* For example, break large tasks down into small, realistic, achievable objectives. This strategy avoids your becoming overwhelmed by the seemingly "impossible" task before you.

✓ *Avoid consumption of noxious substances.* Practice a substance-free lifestyle to manage stress well. Do not depend on these unhealthy behaviors as avenues to relaxation: smoking, overeating, drinking alcohol and caffeine.

✓ *Nourish your body* with a healthy diet and adequate amounts of sleep and rest balanced with activity and exercise. Care for yourself as you would for clients.

✓ *Maintain a sense of humor while you work.* Humor helps a person maintain a positive outlook; therefore, it can be used to reframe situations to reduce distress (Figure 47-11).

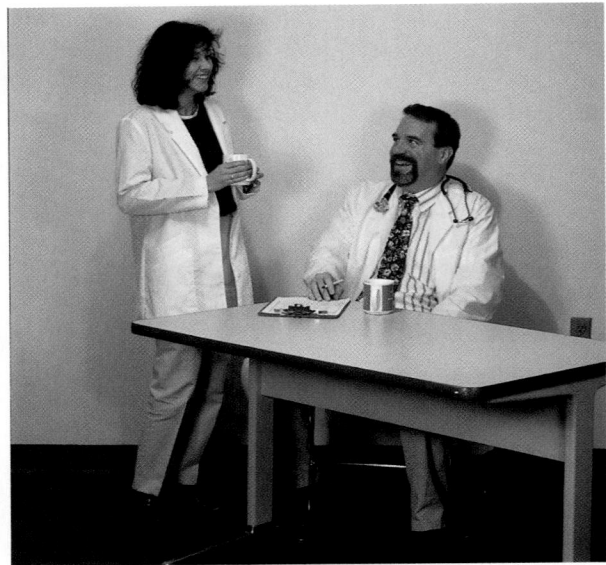

**Figure 47-11**    Humor helps nurses manage the stress created by the nature and intensity of their work. What can you do to help your fellow nursing students cope with the inherent anxiety in this stage of your academic experience?

healing. "As these women grew into adults, they consciously sought to heal themselves. They described battling back against their circumstances by asserting themselves and their goals," and they used self-reflection to uncover the past and its effect on them. Hardiness and resilience are not static characteristics. Individuals who sometimes are able to adapt effectively to stressful events at times may still require interventions to assist them at other times.

Nurses must learn to care for themselves in order to care for others. Primary responsibilities include the use of supportive coping mechanisms in reducing stress, making personal health a priority, taking time for relaxation and socialization, and avoiding overcommitment. An example of an effective strategy is journaling. When under stress, nurses can write down their thoughts and feelings. Writing down emotions and thoughts may help clarify issues related to anxiety. Journaling is also an effective method for venting feelings that have not been released.

 ## CASE STUDY/NURSING CARE PLAN

Weston Ramsey is a 42-year-old man seeking treatment in the emergency department of a regional teaching hospital. He is very anxious, and is pacing and wringing his hands. He is also complaining of severe chest pain, a pounding headache, and back pain. He is sweating profusely and exhibits fine hand tremors. His blood pressure and pulse are elevated, and his respirations are rapid and shallow. He states that he hasn't slept well since his wife left him 3 months ago. He says, "I'm afraid that I'm losing my mind! My heart is racing and I can't seem to sit still. Please help me! I'm afraid that I'm going to die." The nurse continues the client assessment and provides nursing measures aimed at decreasing his stress and evaluating his condition.

*(continues)*

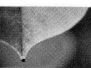 **CASE STUDY/NURSING CARE PLAN** (continued)

## Assessment

The assessment reveals an anxious 42-year-old male who has a variety of clinical manifestations that necessitate further investigation. The client is experiencing chest pain, headache, back pain, and profuse sweating; has elevated pulse, blood pressure, and respirations; and has fine hand tremors. In addition, he is stressed over his spouse leaving him recently. He appears very anxious and is obviously stressed.

## Nursing Diagnosis #1

*Anxiety* related to feelings of powerlessness and lifestyle change.
**NOC:** Anxiety Control; Coping
**NIC:** Anxiety Reduction; Presence; Calming Technique; Emotional Support

### Expected Outcomes

The client will:
1. Identify effective coping mechanisms to decrease anxiety after first nurse intervention counseling session.
2. Report that anxiety is reduced to a manageable level within 24 hours.
3. Demonstrate relaxation skills at completion of first nurse intervention setting.

### Planning/Interventions/Rationales

1. Establish a trusting relationship. *The client may perceive the nurse or emergency department as a threat and thus anxiety will increase.*
2. Have the client identify and describe physical and emotional feelings. *The first step in coping with anxiety is to recognize the anxiety and become aware of feelings in order to link emotions with maladaptive coping responses.*
3. Help the client to relate cause-and-effect relationships between stressors and anxiety. *Increases the client's sense of control and power over the situation.*
4. Teach the client relaxation techniques (such as imagery and meditation). *The relaxation response is the opposite of the stress response and, therefore, counters the physiological effects of the stress response. The relaxation response leads to lowered blood pressure, decreased heart rate, deeper and slower respirations.*
5. Administer antianxiety medication as indicated. *Antianxiety agents provide relief from the immobilizing effects of anxiety.* **NOTE:** *This is a collaborative-dependent nursing action.*

## Evaluation

The client is visibly relaxed. Vital signs are within normal limits. The client verbalizes that he is calmer and no longer afraid.

## Nursing Diagnosis #2

*Ineffective Coping* related to inappropriate use of defense mechanisms.
**NOC:** Coping; Decision-Making; Information Processing
**NIC:** Coping Enhancement

### Expected Outcomes

The client will:
1. Verbalize feelings related to his emotional state in the first counseling session.
2. Identify coping patterns and the consequences of the behavior by the second counseling session.
3. Identify personal strengths and accept support throughout the nurse-client relationship.
4. Make decisions and follow through with appropriate actions to change situations after each nurse-client interaction.

### Planning/Interventions/Rationales

1. Encourage client to use coping mechanisms that have been previously successful. *Increases confidence in own abilities to cope.*

*(continues)*

## CASE STUDY/NURSING CARE PLAN (continued)

2. Offer support and encourage expression of feelings. Offer matter-of-fact appraisals in a realistic manner. *Provides caring support.*
3. Convey honesty and empathy. *Develops a trusting relationship.*

**Evaluation**

The client is verbally able to identify his condition and provide a realistic appraisal of his coping mechanisms.

## Key Concepts

- Stress is an individual's physiological response to stimuli.
- Individuals who experience prolonged periods of stress are at risk for developing stress-related diseases.
- Anxiety is the psychological response to a threat to the health and well-being of an individual and activates the stress response.
- Coping mechanisms are valuable strategies in which individuals can deal with their stressful circumstances.
- An individual seeks equilibrium through the process of adaptation. When adaptation is effective, homeostasis (the body's self-regulation of physiological processes) is maintained.
- Many factors, such as physiological, psychological, cognitive, or environmental changes, contribute to stress.
- The general adaptation syndrome (GAS), the physiological response to stress, consists of three stages: alarm, resistance, and exhaustion. The GAS is the same whether the stressor is actual or imagined, present or potential.
- Illness and hospitalization are major stressors for individuals and their families. To alleviate the stress of hospitalization, nursing interventions should reduce the client's feelings of unfamiliarity and loss of control.
- Change can be perceived as stressful because of a fear of failure, a threat to security, a potential for loss of self-esteem, and the need to develop new paradigms.
- Nurses act as change agents by consciously empowering the client through education to initiate change in order to successfully adapt to perceived stressful situations.
- Nursing interventions that promote positive adaptation to stress are the empowerment of clients to meet basic needs; the minimization of environmental stimuli; the encouragement of verbalization of feelings; the inclusion of family members and significant others into client care; and the use of various relaxation techniques, such as progressive muscle relaxation (PMR) and guided imagery.
- Rapid relaxation response (RRR) is a useful stress management intervention that is similar to transcendental meditation.
- Stress management techniques can be used by both clients and nurses to facilitate effective coping.

- The thought-stopping technique, a cognitive approach to stress management, involves removing or reducing anxiety by changing negative thoughts to positive and realistic thoughts.
- Burnout occurs when the nurse is overwhelmed by stress. As a result, the nurse experiences physical, emotional, and behavioral dysfunction, including decreased productivity.
- Elements of a stress management plan for professional nurses consist of maintaining support systems, developing time-management and decision-making skills, identifying and changing stressors that can be managed, and knowing personal limits.

## Review Questions and Activities

1. Identify positive and negative outcomes of an upcoming change in your life.
2. Reflect on the past 4 months. List some of the changes that you experienced during that time. What were the outcomes of the changes? Would you now respond differently in similar situations? If so, what would be altered?
3. Explain the fight-or-flight response.
4. Describe how you would explain to a client the relationship between stress and illness.
5. List some ways in which your life has changed since becoming a nursing student.
6. How can you act as a change agent in your school?
7. Identify some ways you can become a change agent for clients.
8. Select one stress management exercise described in this chapter and practice it three times a week for 4 weeks. Keep a journal reflecting your experience, including your emotions, physical responses, and behaviors.
9. What are some changes you can begin now to improve your ability to handle personal and professional stress in your life?

10. Answer the following as true or false to determine how well you care for yourself.

|  | TRUE | FALSE |
|---|---|---|
| **a.** I exercise regularly. | _____ | _____ |
| **b.** I eat a well-balanced diet. | _____ | _____ |
| **c.** I get enough sleep and rest. | _____ | _____ |
| **d.** I have specific techniques for managing stress. | _____ | _____ |
| **e.** I'm healthier now than I was 5 years ago. | _____ | _____ |

11. Which of the following are physiological indicators of anxiety?
    a. Decreased pulse rate
    b. Constricted pupils
    c. Increased blood pressure
    d. Warm, dry skin

12. Keep a dietary journal for 2 weeks to monitor food and fluid intake. Note the time of day when your appetite is greatest, as well as situations that trigger snacking or overeating. Identify times when skipped meals occur. Identify what you do to contribute to your good nutrition.

## Web Resources

American Holistic Nurses Association
   http://www.ahna.org
American Psychiatric Nurses Association
   http://www.apna.org
National Institute of Mental Health
   http://www.nimh.nih.gov

## References

Ackley, B., & Ladwig, G. (2002). *Nursing diagnosis handbook: A guide to planning care.* St. Louis: Mosby.

Aguilera, D. C. (1997). *Crisis intervention: Theory and methodology* (8th ed.). St. Louis: Mosby.

Aguilera, D. (2000). Crisis intervention. In K. Fortinash & P. Holoday-Worret (Eds.), *Psychiatric mental health nursing* (2nd ed., pp. 591–602). St. Louis: Mosby.

Alfaro-LeFevre, R. (1998). *Critical thinking in nursing: A practical approach.* (2nd ed.) Philadelphia: Saunders.

American Nurses Association. (1991). *Standards of clinical nursing practice.* Washington, DC: Author.

Armstrong, M. (2000). Adjustment disorders. In K. Fortinash & P. Holoday-Worret (Eds.), *Psychiatric mental health nursing* (2nd ed., pp. 493–504).

Beck, A. (1976). *Cognitive therapy and emotional disorders.* New York: International Universities Press.

Bonalumi, N., & Fisher, K. (1999). Health care change: Challenge for nurse administrators. *Nursing Administration Quarterly, 23*(2), 69–73.

Borman, J. (2002, March 20). *Rapid relaxation response for clear-mindedness and symptom management.* Research presentation, Zeta-Mu Chapter of Sigma Theta Tau, San Diego, CA.

Carpenito, L. J. (2002). *Handbook of nursing diagnosis* (9th ed.). Philadelphia: Lippincott.

Catalano, J. (2000). Reality shock in the workplace. In *Nursing now! Today's issues, tomorrow's trends* (pp. 231–260). (Author) Philadelphia: F. A. Davis.

Clark, M.J. *Nursing in the community.* (1999). Stamford, CT: Appleton & Lange.

DeLaune, S. C. (1996). Applying the nursing process for clients with anxiety, somatoform, and dissociative disorders. In H. S. Wilson, & C. R. Kneisl (Eds.), *Psychiatric nursing* (5th ed., p. 368). Menlo Park, CA: Addison-Wesley.

Doenges, M. E., Townsend, M. C., & Moorhouse, M. F. (2002). *Psychiatric care plans: Guidelines for planning and documenting care* (4th ed.). Philadelphia: Davis.

Emerson, R., Atkinson, B., & Oliver, M. (2000). *Essential Writings of Ralph Waldo Emerson.* New York: Random House.

Folsom, D. (1999). Nursing the patient within. *American Journal of Nursing, 99*(3), 80.

Fontaine, K. L. (2000). *Healing practices: Alternative therapies for nursing.* Upper Saddle River, NJ: Prentice Hall.

Fortinash, K. (2000). The nursing process. In K. Fortinash & P. Holoday-Worret (Eds.), *Psychiatric mental health nursing* (2nd ed., pp. 123–147).

Freud, S. (1959). Inhibitions, symptoms and anxiety. In J. Strachey (Trans.), *The standard edition of the complete psychological works of Sigmund Freud* (Vol. 20). London: The Hogarth Press.

Grendell, R. (2000). Psychologic aspects of physiologic illness. In K. Fortinash & P. Holoday-Worret (Eds.), *Psychiatric mental health nursing* (2nd ed., pp. 709–725).

Grossman, S. & Valiga, T. (2000). Chaos and disequilibrium: Invigorating, challenging and growth-producing. In *The new leadership challenge: Creating the future of nursing* (Authors). Philadelphia: F. A. Davis.

Hegge, M., Melcher, P., & Williams, S. (1999). Hardiness, help-seeking behavior, and social support of baccalaureate nursing students. *Journal of Nursing Education, 38*(4), 178–183.

Holoday-Worret, P. (2000). Foundations of psychiatric mental health nursing. In K. Fortinash & P. Holoday-Worret (Eds.), *Psychiatric mental health nursing* (2nd ed., pp. 3–25).

Humphreys, J. (2001). Turnings and adaptation in resilient daughters of battered women. *Image: Journal of Nursing Scholarship, 33*(3). 245–251.

Joel, L. A. (1998). Absolutes and indefinites. *American Journal of Nursing, 90*(2), 7.

Kilfedder, C., Power, K., & Wells, T. (2001). Burnout in psychiatric nursing. *Journal of Advanced Nursing, 34*(3), 383–396.

Kobasa, S. C. (1979). Stressful life events, personality and health. An inquiry into hardiness. *Journal of Personality and Social Psychology, 37*(1), 1–11.

Kobasa, S. C., Maddi, S. R., & Kahn, S. (1982). Hardiness and health: A prospective study. *Journal of Personality and Social Psychology, 45*(4), 839–850.

Kulbe, J. (2001). Stressors and coping measures of hospice nurses. *Home Health Care Nurse, 19*(11), 707–711.

Lambert, C., & Lambert, V. (1999). Psychological hardiness: State of the science. *Holistic Nursing Practice, 13*(3), 11–19.

Lewin, K. (1951). *Field theory in social science.* New York: Harper.

Lippitt, R., Watson, J., & Westley, B. (1958). *The dynamics of planned change.* New York: Harcourt Brace.

Manix, K. (1999). Leading change. In P. Yoder-Wise (Ed.), *Leading and managing in nursing* (pp. 73–89). St. Louis: Mosby.

Michaels, B. (2000). Self-care strategies. In J. Zerwekh & J. Claborn (Eds.), *Nursing today: Transitions and trends* (pp. 517–535). Philadelphia: W. B. Saunders.

Molloy, M. (2000). Anxiety and related disorders. In K. Fortinash & P. Holoday-Worret (Eds.), *Psychiatric mental health nursing* (2nd ed., pp. 233–256).

North American Nursing Diagnosis Association. (NANDA). (2003*). Nursing diagnoses: Definitions and classification, 2003–2004.* Philadelphia: Author.

Peplau, H. E. (1952). *Interpersonal relations in nursing.* New York: Putnam.

Reed, F., & Pettigrew, A. (1999). Self-management: Stress and time. In P. Yoder-Wise (Ed.), *Leading and managing in nursing* (pp. 186–204). St. Louis: Mosby.

Selye, H. (1974). *Stress without distress.* New York: New American Library.

Selye, H. (1976). *Stress in health and disease* (Rev. ed.). Boston: Butterworths.

Stuart, G. W., & Laraia, M. T. (2002). *Principles and practice of psychiatric nursing* (7th ed.). St. Louis: Mosby.

Sullivan, H. S. (1953). *The interpersonal theory of psychiatry.* New York: Norton.

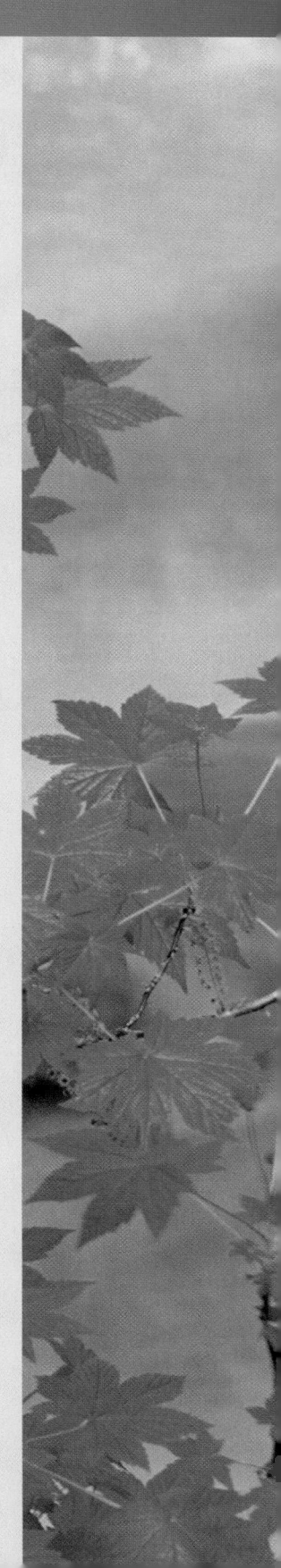

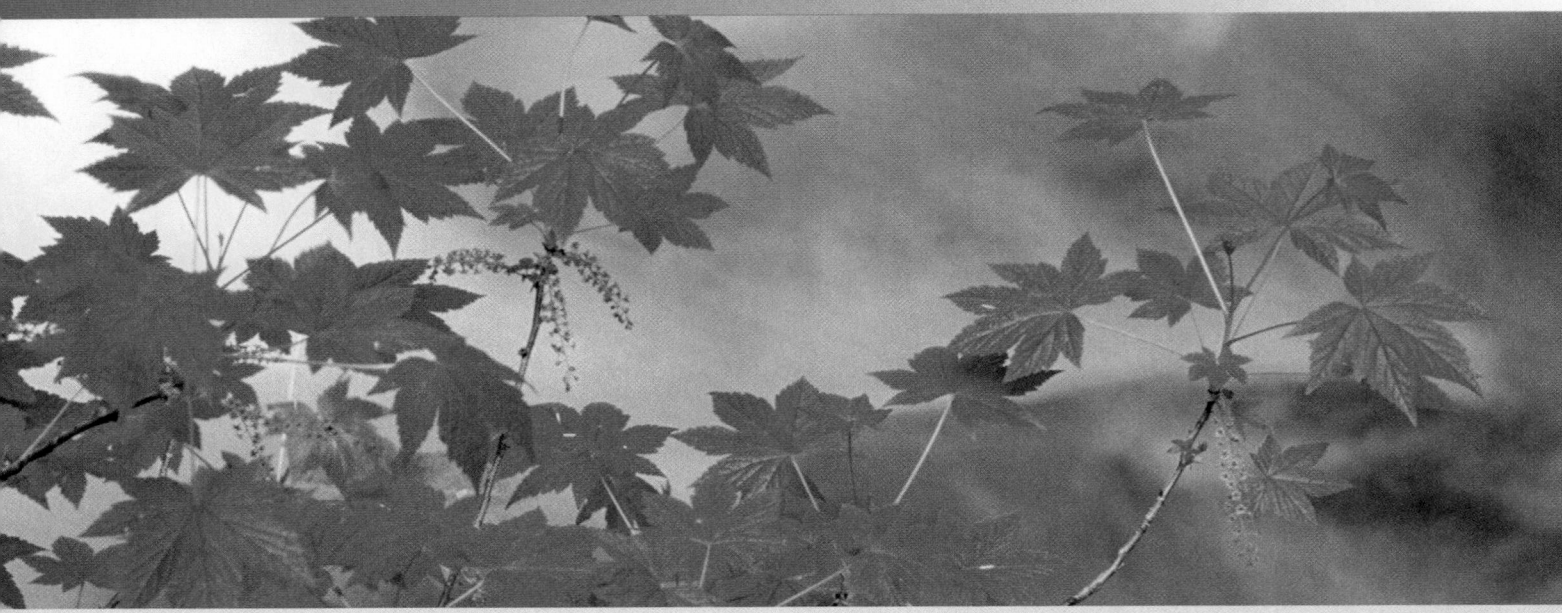

# 48 CHAPTER

# Spiritual Health

## Carol Craig, PhD, FNP-C, RN

*"The infrequency with which nurses identify spiritual needs and provide spiritual care is inconsistent with the prominent place allocated to spirituality by nursing tradition, nurse theorists, codes of professional conduct, and professional organizations."*

(Stranahan, 2001)

# Chapter Competencies

*Upon completion of this chapter, the reader should be able to:*

1. Compare and contrast the concepts of spirituality and religion.
2. Describe beliefs and practices of the world religions, including their relationships to health care.
3. Identify the spiritual development of individuals across the life span and the interrelationship between nursing and health care.
4. Synthesize the components necessary for performing a spiritual assessment.
5. Compare the characteristics of the nursing diagnoses: spiritual well-being and spiritual distress.
6. Analyze the nurse's role in the nursing process as related to spiritual health (strategies of assessment, care, etc.)

# Key Terms

agnostics
atheists
balance
connection

Fowler's stages of spiritual development
generalized spiritual assessment
New Age spirituality
purpose

religion
reincarnation
spirituality
transcendence

Nurses have been committed to the alleviation of sufferingfor many years. Florence Nightingale started modern nursing's involvement in spiritual concerns through her interest in mysticism and her belief that attention to a person's spiritual life would promote healing (Macrae, 1995). Nurses are concerned with the relief of pain, the promotion of healing, and the prevention of disease. Experienced nurses are aware that people suffer from far more than just physical pain, and that physical pain frequently is the least part of the distress that illness brings. One person can be dying of a painful condition and yet be at peace, while another can have a minor physical problem but be deeply distressed. The recognition that people are holistic beings with interconnected minds, bodies, and spirits is an acknowledgment that physical pain is only one part of the pain that nurses must address to provide client care. Furthermore, spiritual issues are apt to be very prominent at critical junctures in clients' lives. Birth, serious illness, and death are times at which nurses are often present. Learning to work with people who have spiritual concerns is therefore a crucial part of nursing care.

This chapter will discuss spirituality as a part of holistic nursing care. Since religion is often intertwined with spirituality in people's daily lives, definitions of the two concepts and how they differ is provided. Spiritual development across the life span and expression of spiritual beliefs are also considered. Finally, the nursing process will be used as a framework for how nurses can assist people with spiritual concerns.

## Spirituality

Of the two concepts, spirituality and religion, spirituality is the broadest and incorporates religion. **Spirituality** has many different definitions, but common threads in most definitions include transcendence, connection, balance, and purpose. **Transcendence** involves finding meaning larger than the person's individual self and life. Spirituality entails a search for meaning in events that may be either joyous or tragic, as in the birth of a child or the death of a spouse. Finding meaning can be so powerful that assigning meaning to the injurious condition often reduces or even resolves the suffering associated with it. In addition, transcendence allows a person to love unconditionally. Such unconditional love encourages people to work for "larger than the self" issues such as universal justice and acceptance.

**Connection** is integration of all of the aspects of being human. Those connections would include the self, other people (Figure 48-1), the surrounding world, and for some people, a supreme being. To be connected is to feel part of the universe and in relationship with all creation. **Balance** is often defined as "harmony." Many cultures place high value on living in harmony with self, others, and nature.

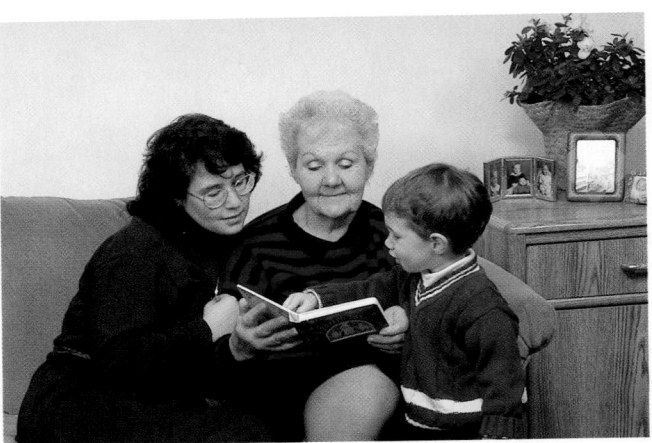

**Figure 48-1    Connections are vital, as shown in this grandmother reading to her daughter and grandson.**

Illness is described as imbalance within the self, or being out of harmony with others, or violating the balance of the self with nature. Healing involves restoring a person's balance on any or all of these levels. Purpose is a person's understanding of the impact of her life and includes the understanding of life events. **Purpose** involves answering questions such as "Why am I here?", "Why did this happen to me?", "What should I be doing?", and "What should I do because I have experienced these things?"

In summary, spirituality is an overreaching human need to understand and develop connections with a larger world. Spirituality is an integrating force that allows people to be most fully human. Feelings of love, forgiveness, despair, self-esteem, hope, and relationship involve people's spiritual selves. Everyone has spiritual needs and concerns, but the language that each person uses will differ according to cultural values and personal beliefs. Significant events in a

## FOCUS ON WELLNESS

### Spiritual Wellness

When there are religious symbols in the client's sleeping area (whether they are in their own home or not), be sure to use therapeutic communication techniques in ascertaining the intrinsic value of these items to the client. Also, ask clients if there are other items that they would like to obtain from their home or have a family member bring them. In addition, explore the possibility of a referral from a religious leader of their faith or from the clergy or chaplain member of the health care facility. Spiritual wellness is invaluable regardless of the client's current illness and condition.

person's life lead to spiritual questioning. The practice of spiritual care occurs when a nurse helps a client to strengthen hope and relationship, enables a client to find meaning and purpose, and assists a client in overcoming despair and finding forgiveness.

## Religion

Many people confuse spirituality and religion. People with strong spiritual beliefs and lives may not belong to any organized religion. Religion is a system of beliefs and practices that usually involves a community of like-minded people. Religion has also taken on more individual aspects in recent years, with some people taking pieces of many religions and weaving them into a personal philosophy and practice.

A compelling reason to address spiritual concerns is the amount of faith, both religious and nonreligious, professed by Americans. Americans, on the whole, place tremendous value in faith. Gallup studies over the past 6 decades indicate both a religious nation and a predominant belief in God that has remained surprisingly constant through the years. A synopsis by Gallup indicated five constant variables in American beliefs: belief in God or a universal spirit (consistently about 95%); importance of religion in people's lives (about 85%); membership in a religious organization (about 66%); religious preference (about 90%); and weekly worship attendance (about 41%) (Gallup, 2003). These data underscore an important point. While the vast majority of Americans believe in God or a universal spirit, organized religion, although important, may not be the avenue through which people address their spiritual beliefs. "Americans tend to view their faith as a matter between them and God, to be aided, but not necessarily influenced, by religious institutions" (Gallup, 2003). Given the high percentage of people with spiritual beliefs, it isn't surprising that many people would like a care provider to discuss spiritual concerns with them, or even to pray with them. Two-thirds of respondents in a recent study strongly agreed that if they become gravely ill, their physicians should ask them about their religious beliefs (Ehman, 1999). A similar figure was found in a *USA Today* poll using spiritual, rather than religious, beliefs. Many people claim to have had spiritual experiences whether or not they have formal religious beliefs (Sherwood, 2000). A number of people use prayer as an alternative or complementary therapy. With a large number of people who would like to be asked about their spiritual selves, few health care providers actually explore this issue. About 15% of people state a health care provider ever asked them about their spiritual beliefs. Other studies indicated that 20% or fewer physicians ask clients about spiritual concerns, with the exception of fear of death and dying. In 1994, the Joint Commission for Accreditation of Healthcare Organizations stated that a client has a right to care that respects spiritual values, but those values remain largely unexplored in the world of health care.

# Overview of Major World Religions

Religions and religious expression in the United States are increasingly diverse and difficult to place into categories. New religions are evolving, including new branches of older religions and entirely new religions, and increasing numbers of new immigrants bring their religions with them. A few definitions can be helpful when thinking about the wide variety of religious groups.

- Prophetic religions are those that believe in a personal God who rules the universe. This God is concerned with human existence and behavior, and is present in human affairs. Prophetic religions try to save the soul from evil. Examples of major prophetic religions are Judaism, Christianity, and Islam.
- Mystic religions are those in which God is a principle rather than a being. This principle is the source of all life, is unchanging, and is a path to the liberation of the soul from human existence. Major mystical religions are Hinduism, Buddhism, Sikhism, and Shintoism.
- **Atheists** are those who do not believe in the existence of a God in any form. Atheists may have ethical principles that are important to them, or they may not have any particular ethical code.
- **Agnostics** are those who do not know if a God exists or not. They generally state that the existence of a God is unknowable.

As Table 48-1 indicates, the extent of membership in religions around the world is very large (Adherents, 2001).

| TABLE 48-1 | MEMBERSHIP OF MAJOR WORLD RELIGIONS | |
|---|---|
| Group | Approximate Number Worldwide |
| Christianity | 2.0 billion |
| Islam | 1.3 billion |
| Hinduism | 900 million |
| Buddhism | 360 million |
| Sikhism | 23 million |
| Judaism | 14 million |

Adherents. (2001, July 16). Major religions of the world ranked by number of adherents. http://www.adherents.com

The religion with the greatest number of members is Christianity, and within that group Catholics are the majority. A close second, and the fastest-growing religion in the world, is Islam. Hindus and Buddhists are the next largest, followed by a number of smaller groups. Jews are the smallest group on this list, but their influence on theological and philosophical thinking has far exceeded their rank.

## Christianity

Christianity is probably the most familiar faith to nurses in the Western world. It is one of the prophetic religions. The religion began with its founder, Jesus Christ. "Christ" is not a name, but a title that means "the one chosen and anointed by God." Jesus was a Jew, and many Jewish concepts were incorporated into Christianity. The moral code that Christians follow is essentially Jewish, and Christians believe that Jesus was the Jewish Messiah, the Savior. Jesus was an itinerant teacher who ignored class distinctions and taught that faith in God was superior to outward religious acts. The central tenet of Christianity is that after Jesus' death he rose from the dead, thus giving all people the opportunity for eternal life. Christians have formed many groups that typically attend churches and have varying beliefs, but all Christians take Jesus as their founder and follow an interpretation of his teachings.

## Islam

Islam also began with a single founder and is a prophetic religion. The prophet Muhammed is not considered to be God, but a man to whom God's word was revealed. This word was recorded by Muhammed in the Qur'an. The basic creed that all Muslims follow is "There is only one God, and Muhammed is his prophet." The duty of human beings is to worship and obey God. A faithful Muslim is expected to believe in the basic creed, pray five times during the day, be charitable, fast at appropriate times, and make a pilgrimage to Mecca at least once during his lifetime.

## Hinduism

Hinduism is a very broad term that encompasses a wide variety of religious beliefs. The term "Hindu" simply means "Indian" in the Persian language. These religions are very old and have no known founder. Although they differ enough to cover a wide range of beliefs from many gods to no God, basic Hindu thought is mystic. Hindus do not support missions, so the religion has remained basically an Indian phenomenon. A central tenet of Hinduism is a belief in **reincarnation**. The soul is an eternal entity that is reborn in many physical bodies. The behavior of a person in a particular life determines the position the soul will have in the next life: a person who leads a good life will have his soul reborn in a higher status in the next life and vice versa. The ultimate goal of life is to escape the cycle of rebirth and live forever in nirvana. Principle gods in Hindu belief include Vishnu, Siva, Krishna, and Brahma.

## Buddhism

Buddhism developed as a splinter group from Hinduism, and the religion remains in the mystic tradition. Classic Buddhism has no belief in any God. Buddhism was started by Siddartha Gautama, who became known as the "Buddha," or "enlightened one." The goal of Buddhism is to free the self from craving both material goods and pleasures in order to achieve nirvana, which is an eternal life without further reincarnation. Meditation is used as a means to learn to overcome desires and free the self from worldly entanglements. The Path to Enlightenment is founded on morality, meditation, and wisdom.

## Sikhism

The founder of the Sikhs was a Hindu who traveled widely and came into contact with Muslims and Buddhists. He was a monotheist who disapproved of polytheism but believed in reincarnation. Sikhism may have been an attempt to reconcile a belief in one God with a belief in rebirth. Sikhs do not believe in prophets, and Sikhism is a mystic religion. Sikhs have strong beliefs about care of the body, and both sexes do not cut their hair, as the body should remain intact as given by God. The goal of the religion is to form a close relationship with God. Sikhs rejected the Hindu caste system, and equality of all people is a central tenet of their religious faith.

## Judaism

The Jewish religion is unusual because this small group has been so influential in the development of other religious traditions, especially Christianity and Islam. Judaism is considered both a religion and an ethnicity. Judaism is a prophetic religion concerned with belief in one God and appropriate behavior in relationship to God. The Jewish declaration of faith is "Hear, O Israel; the Lord is our God, the Lord is One God." The moral code of the Jews is the foundation for the morality of the Western world in the form of the Ten Commandments.

## Comparing Common Concepts Among Religions

Taking religious beliefs into account for holistic nursing practice (Figure 48-2) is far different from promoting religion as a means of healing. Respect for particular religious beliefs and remembering how religious beliefs may impact a client's choices and comfort are important aspects of nursing care. Recommending that people use religion as the sole form of care can be dangerous, however, for both

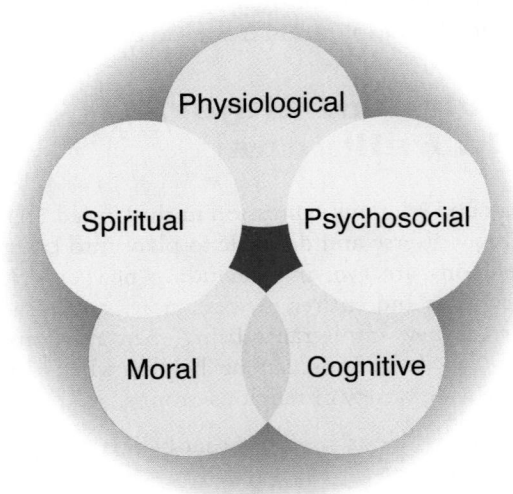

**Figure 48-2** **Holistic nature of human beings**

nurse and client. While some interesting studies have indicated a link between religious activities, spirituality, and health or healing (Aldridge, 1993; Cerranto, 1998; Oxman, Freeman, & Manheimer, 1995), these studies have not been definitive enough to allow nurses to recommend religious activities as a means of healing.

Table 48-2 considers a number of religions in the context of some common beliefs about healing, which can assist a nurse in recognizing religious practices that may be important to a client. Religion is an important element in how people approach health and illness. Religions usually play especially prominent roles in conceptualizations of birth, death, illness, and diet, all of which will influence

### LEGAL AND ETHICAL ISSUES

#### Spiritual Conflicts

Occasionally the client's religious practices conflict with typical ideology of treatment in Western health care practices (refusing blood transfusions, wearing ritual undergarments at all times, declining medical treatments). The nurse must learn both to accept these practices and to encourage alternate methods of treatment without being aggressive or coercive in the process. For example, the client may not realize that it would be helpful to find practitioners of their own faith who may have specific interventions that keep the client's beliefs in consideration. In addition, providing accurate information about the health regimen, treatments, and medications may alleviate some of the misunderstandings that are causing "spiritual conflicts."

personal preference and comfort in a specific health or illness event. Schisms and individualization of religious tenets may conflict with individual health practices, however, and it is important not to make assumptions about a person's beliefs.

## Birth

Birth is an important event in all cultures and religions. Many religions have specific ceremonies that mark the birth of a child and define the child as a member of a specific religious group. Traditional Jews have male children circumcised on the 8th day of life as a sign that the child is dedicated to a covenant between God and the Jewish people. A number of Christian groups perform the ceremony of baptism into the Christian faith early in life, and the parents of a seriously ill newborn may request that baptism be done in the hospital. Related to birth are issues around birth control and abortion. Abortion is prohibited by some religions, sometimes even to save the mother's life. Birth control methods may be acceptable or unacceptable. Traditional Roman Catholics may practice rhythm methods of birth control, but find other methods unacceptable.

## Death

Death is another important event that is noted in all cultures and religions. Some Christian groups want last rites to be said before death. People from some faith traditions will want to confess their sins before death. Hindus, many of whom believe in reincarnation, may want to be alert and focused at their death to help guide the soul to a new life. Muslims may wish to face Mecca at the moment of death. After death, many religious groups have important rituals for preparing the body for burial or cremation. These rituals may include prayers, and the anointing, positioning, or cleansing of the body. Some religions will discourage cremation while others will promote it. Some

### COMMUNITY/HOME CARE

#### A Church's Role in Home Care

Mrs. Jackson is a member of the Church of Jesus Christ of Latter-Day Saints (i.e., Mormon) and is immobilized at home after a recent motor vehicle accident. She lives alone. When her home health nurse visits her initially, she finds that Mrs. Jackson has not notified her ward of her condition. The nurse should assist Mrs. Jackson in contacting her church for help with shopping for groceries or with other needs. This particular faith strongly supports their members and is exceptional in assisting members during times of need.

religious groups will want to have all limbs and organs buried with the body.

## Illness

Religious beliefs may impact illness in a number of ways. Some religions, such as the Church of Christ, Scientist, believe that illness should be treated entirely by prayer. Jehovah's Witnesses may refuse blood transfusions and, in some cases, organ transplants and vaccinations. Shaving and cutting hair may be unacceptable to men of some religions. While prayer is common to all religious traditions, prayers for healing are not appropriate for some religions, including the Unitarian Church.

## Cultural Practices and Religion

Religious and spiritual practices are frequently rooted in culture, although a nurse should never assume that a person of a specific culture is a member of a specific religion. Culture and religion, often working in tandem, help to define what is health, illness, and the cause of an illness; how to cure a specific illness; who is the appropriate person to treat an illness; and how to maintain health (White, 2000). Knowing that a person is from Vietnam, however, does not tell a nurse how closely he maintains ties to traditional Vietnamese cultural values and beliefs, nor what specific spiritual and religious practices he maintains. A common problem in spiritual assessment is to assume that a person's culture determines religious orientation. A person from India may or may not be a Hindu; someone from Mexico may or may not be Catholic. Cultural variations of religious beliefs are also important. Muslims from India, Africa, the Philippines, and the United States will differ in their practice of Islam.

### LIFE SPAN CONSIDERATIONS

#### Last Rites Ritual

In the Roman Catholic faith, it is important to have last rites performed at the end of life. This ritual ideally is performed by a Roman Catholic priest, but other persons familiar with the statements of belief can also perform this ritual. Nurses providing care for Roman Catholic clients who are older or of terminal disease conditions should advocate for clergy members or chaplains to be prepared for this event.

## TABLE 48-2    OVERVIEW OF RELIGIOUS BELIEFS AND PRACTICES

| Religion | Birth | Death | Illness | Diet | Sacred Texts | Nursing Implications |
|---|---|---|---|---|---|---|
| **Baha'i** | No special birth ceremony takes place. Abortion is not permissible. Birth control is allowed. | Cremation is discouraged. Embalming is not practiced. The dead should be buried within 1 hour's travel from where the death took place. | The Baha'i religion has no clergy. Spiritual comfort is provided by the Baha'i community. | Alcohol is not consumed. | Writings of Baha'u'llah | Giving information and client education about birth control would be acceptable. When providing after-death care, let the mortuary know that embalming and cremation are not acceptable. |
| **Buddhism (Buddhist Churches of America)** | No formal ceremonies take place. Abortion depends on the mother's condition. No restrictions are placed on birth control. | No formal ceremonies take place. Autopsy is permitted. | Healing through prayer is not practiced. Illness is tolerated as a part of life. | Frequently vegetarian diet—check for egg/ milk product restrictions. Alcohol is not consumed. | *Visuddhi-magga (The Path of Purification)* Sutras Other texts depending on particular sect | Giving information and client education about birth control would be acceptable. Discuss dietary preferences. Do not offer to pray for healing with client. |
| **Christian Scientists (Church of Christ, Scientist)** | Baptism does not take place. Abortion is prohibited. Birth control is acceptable. | No last rites are practiced. | Illness is believed to be an illusion; all forms of medicine and medication are prohibited. Healing is accomplished by prayer. Special practitioners pray for the sick. Only legally required immunizations are permitted. Prayers for healing are appropriate. Illness may be seen as a punishment from God. | Coffee, alcohol, and tobacco are not consumed. | *Science and Health with Key to the Scriptures* Miscellaneous Writings *Manual of the Mother Church* | People who choose to enter the health care system despite their Christian Scientist beliefs may feel very guilty and anxious; assess their comfort level. |

*(continues)*

## TABLE 48-2    OVERVIEW OF RELIGIOUS BELIEFS AND PRACTICES (continued)

| Religion | Birth | Death | Illness | Diet | Sacred Texts | Nursing Implications |
|---|---|---|---|---|---|---|
| Evangelical Protestants (e.g., Baptist/ Churches of God/ Assemblies of God/ Pentecostal/ Churches of Christ) | No infant baptism takes place. Abortion is generally not approved. Birth control is generally acceptable. | No last rites are practiced. | Some practice healing through "laying on of hands." Some may want the sacrament of communion. | Most avoid alcohol. Some avoid coffee and tea. Some may wish to fast on certain days. Some avoid tobacco, pork, and strangled animals. | Bible | Do a careful dietary assessment to ensure client gets acceptable foods. Assess the meaning of the illness to the client. |
| Hinduism | Abortion is allowed. Birth control is permitted. | Belief in life after death is upheld; most believe in reincarnation. Cremation is preferred. Some may wish to be alert at the time of death. | Illness may be a result of actions in a past life. | Most Hindus are vegetarians and do not eat meat. Alcohol is not consumed. | *Bhagavad Gita* (*Song of the Lord*) Many other texts depending on sect | Do a careful dietary assessment to ensure client gets acceptable foods. Assess the meaning of the illness to the client. |
| Jehovah's Witnesses | No infant baptism takes place. Abortion is not permitted. Birth control is acceptable except for sterilization. | No last rites are practiced. | No transfusions or organ transplants are permitted; some may refuse vaccination. Surgery is permitted except when blood products are used. Prayers for healing are appropriate. | No foods to which blood has been added (such as sausage) and no tobacco are consumed. | Bible | Do a careful dietary assessment to ensure client gets acceptable foods. Check with client that procedures are acceptable. |

(continues)

## TABLE 48-2 OVERVIEW OF RELIGIOUS BELIEFS AND PRACTICES (continued)

| Religion | Birth | Death | Illness | Diet | Sacred Texts | Nursing Implications |
|---|---|---|---|---|---|---|
| Judaism | Ritual circumcision 8 days after birth takes place. Abortion is often permitted. Birth control is acceptable for most. | Burial must be as soon as possible. Some oppose cremation. Most do not believe in life after death; immortality lies in memories of those who loved you. Most do not believe in prolonging life. Body parts should be buried together. | Some may request visit from Rabbi. Prayers for healing are appropriate. Organ donation and transplant need prior consultation with Rabbi. Men may wish to keep head and feet covered. Women may wish to keep hair covered. Shaving may be forbidden except as medically necessary. | Most do not eat pork or shellfish. Some do not eat meat and dairy at the same meal. Meat may need to be kosher (slaughtered in a particular way). | Torah | Do a careful dietary assessment to ensure client gets acceptable foods. Check with client for acceptable exposure of body. Ask family if they require assistance with burial plans. |
| Lutherans, Episcopals | Infant baptism is usual. Abortion is not encouraged, but it is a matter of private conscience. Birth control is acceptable. | Last rites are often requested but are optional. Cremation is not practiced. No last rites are practiced. | Some may request communion. Prayers for healing are appropriate. | Some may wish to fast on certain days. | Bible Prayer book | Check with family members about baptism of critically ill neonate. Check with client and family about last rites for dying client. |
| Mormons (Church of Jesus Christ of Latter-Day Saints) | No infant baptism takes place. Abortion is prohibited. Birth control is up to the individual. | | Prayers for healing are appropriate. Some may request visit from healing minister within the congregation. | No coffee, tea, alcohol, or tobacco are consumed. Eat sparingly. | Book of Mormon Doctrine & Covenants Pearl of Great Price | Do a careful dietary assessment to ensure client gets acceptable foods. Do not remove undergarment worn next to skin except in emergency. |

(continues)

## TABLE 48-2  OVERVIEW OF RELIGIOUS BELIEFS AND PRACTICES (continued)

| Religion | Birth | Death | Illness | Diet | Sacred Texts | Nursing Implications |
|---|---|---|---|---|---|---|
| **Muslims** | Circumcision is a routine practice.<br><br>Abortion is permitted.<br><br>Birth control is permitted. | Cremation is not practiced.<br><br>Confession before death is practiced.<br><br>Some may wish to face Mecca.<br><br>Belief in life after death is upheld. | Prayers for healing are acceptable.<br><br>Many pray 5 times a day facing Mecca. | Some may wish to fast from sunrise to sunset during Ramadan.<br><br>No pork or alcohol is consumed. | Qur'an | Do a careful dietary assessment to ensure client gets acceptable foods<br><br>Ask dying client if he wishes to face Mecca.<br><br>Help client to maintain prayers if client wishes |
| **Native American/ American Indian Religions** | The more than 700 tribes or groups of Native Americans have a wide variety of spiritual beliefs and practices. Most Native Americans would consider their traditional religion to be an integrated part of life and not a separate practice. Therefore, cultural and religious practices are very close to one another and may be considered one entity. As the U.S. Congress banned traditional religion until the Indian Freedom of Religion Act in 1979, people may be very reluctant to discuss traditional religious beliefs. Traditional healing practices may not be discussed with non-tribal members, so contact with the person's designated healer may be best. The following is a broad generalization to help guide individual assessment. | | | | | |
| | Abortion is often not acceptable.<br><br>Birth control is often a matter of individual choice. | Some cultures avoid contact with the dead; others will want to prepare the body in a ritual way after death.<br><br>Many will want to maintain a positive attitude in the face of impending death.<br><br>Autopsy is usually avoided.<br><br>Some cultures may avoid discussion of impending death and planning for death. | See above; bring person in contact with spiritual healer if requested. | Diet is highly varied.<br><br>Traditional foods are consumed for health and healing. | Most traditions were passed down orally; therefore, a written text does not exist.<br><br>Songs, stories, and dances may be used to relate spiritual concepts. | Ask client about particular spiritual comfort measures. |

*(continues)*

# TABLE 48-2  OVERVIEW OF RELIGIOUS BELIEFS AND PRACTICES (continued)

| Religion | Birth | Death | Illness | Diet | Sacred Texts | Nursing Implications |
|---|---|---|---|---|---|---|
| New Age Spiritualists | New Age spirituality is not one particular spiritual philosophy but rather an approach in which individuals take pieces from various religions and weave them into a personal spiritual ethic. People may also add ideas from New Age thinking to a traditional religious foundation. The "New Age" is a reference to an astrological concept in which the Earth is moving from one astrological configuration to another, a process that occurs over thousands of years. The Earth moved into a new astrological age in the early 1980s. Many New Age believers use beliefs from Eastern religions, particularly karma, reincarnation, astrology, and pantheism. New Age concepts include the idea that everything is God, and therefore God is within the self; religion is universal; people should live in a balance with nature; and caring for the spirit is part of holistic health. New Age health care practices may include meditation, yoga, crystals, gestalt therapy, primal scream therapy, massage, and homeopathy, among others. Eastern medical practices that involve energy manipulation such as acupuncture and acupressure may also be used. Most people who identify with New Age ideas would be comfortable with prayers for healing and faith healing. Specific practices involving birth, death, illness, and diet cannot be provided in this table, as New Age practices are too diverse. The nurse must make an individual assessment for the specific influences of New Age beliefs. | | | | | |
| Orthodox Catholic | Infant baptism is usual; parents may desire immediate baptism for seriously ill newborn. | Cremation and embalming are discouraged. Last rites are given by a priest before death. | Anointing for healing is common during illness. Prayers for healing are appropriate. Confession of sins may be important for some. Some may want communion during hospitalization. Men may not wish to be shaved except as required for surgery. Many will want every effort to preserve life. | Some may wish to fast from meat, olive oil, and dairy on holy days. Some may wish to fast before taking communion. | Bible Prayer book | Check with family members about baptism of critically ill neonate. Check with client and family about last rites for dying client. |

*(continues)*

**TABLE 48-2 OVERVIEW OF RELIGIOUS BELIEFS AND PRACTICES (continued)**

| Religion | Birth | Death | Illness | Diet | Sacred Texts | Nursing Implications |
|---|---|---|---|---|---|---|
| **Protestant Non-Evangelicals (e.g., Presbyterians, Methodists)** | No infant baptism takes place.<br><br>Abortion is not encouraged but is a matter of private conscience.<br><br>Birth control is acceptable. | Last rites are optional. | Some may request communion.<br><br>Prayers for healing are appropriate. | Diet is not restricted. | Bible | Ask client about particular spiritual comfort measures. |
| **Quakers (Society of Friends)** | Birth control is a matter of private conscience.<br><br>Most oppose abortion.<br><br>Baptism is not practiced.<br><br>No rituals take place around the birth of a child. | No rituals take place at death.<br><br>Many do not believe in life after death. | No ordained clergy | Many abstain from alcohol. | Bible | Ask client about particular spiritual comfort measures. |
| **Roman Catholics** | Infant baptism is usual; parents may desire immediate baptism for seriously ill newborn.<br><br>Abortion and sterilization are forbidden.<br><br>Rhythm birth control is permitted. | Last rites are given by a priest before death.<br><br>Cremation is not common.<br><br>Burial of surgically removed limbs may be requested. | Anointing for healing is common during illness.<br><br>Prayers for healing are appropriate.<br><br>Confession of sins may be important for some.<br><br>Some may want communion during hospitalization. | Traditional Catholics may prefer not to eat meat on days of fasting.<br><br>Some may wish to fast before taking communion. | Bible<br><br>Prayer book | Check with family members about baptism of critically ill neonate.<br><br>Check with client and family about last rites for dying client. |

*(continues)*

## TABLE 48-2 OVERVIEW OF RELIGIOUS BELIEFS AND PRACTICES (continued)

| Religion | Birth | Death | Illness | Diet | Sacred Texts | Nursing Implications |
|---|---|---|---|---|---|---|
| **Seventh Day Adventists** | Therapeutic abortions are permitted. Birth control is allowed. No infant baptism takes place. | The dead "sleep" until the second coming of Christ; they do not enter heaven at the time of death. | Prayers for healing are appropriate. Pastors offer prayers for the sick and anointing with oil for healing. | No alcohol, caffeine, narcotics, or stimulants are consumed. Some follow vegetarian diets. | Bible | Do a careful dietary assessment to ensure client gets acceptable foods. Do not comfort newly bereaved with idea that loved one is in heaven. |
| **Sikhs** | No special birth ritual takes place. | Belief in life after death is upheld; most believe in reincarnation. Some may wish to be alert at the time of death. | Illness may be seen as a result of actions in a past life. | No alcohol is consumed. Many prefer to follow a vegetarian diet. | Siri Guru Granth Sahib | Sikhs are expected to pray multiple times each day; assist the person to accomplish this if possible. Check for dietary preferences. |
| **Tao** | Abortion is left for the individual to decide the greater good. Birth control is acceptable. | Being kept alive at all costs is opposed. | Prayers for healing not appropriate. Stress the achievement of harmony; illness is due to an imbalance. Extremes of behavior that result in imbalance are avoided. | Food and drink should be in moderation. | *Tao Te Ching (The Way and Its Power)* | Ask client about particular spiritual comfort measures. |

*(continues)*

## TABLE 48-2  OVERVIEW OF RELIGIOUS BELIEFS AND PRACTICES (continued)

| Religion | Birth | Death | Illness | Diet | Sacred Texts | Nursing Implications |
|---|---|---|---|---|---|---|
| Unitarian/ Universalist | No infant baptism takes place.<br><br>Abortion is acceptable.<br><br>Birth control is acceptable. | Cremation is usual. | Some may prefer not to see clergy, as individual connection with God is emphasized.<br><br>Prayers for healing are often not accepted; they may be seen as superstitious.<br><br>Science is preferred to faith healing. | Diet is not restricted. | Some may use Bible (very diverse theological beliefs). | Ask client about particular spiritual comfort measures. |

Davidhizar, R., Bechtel, G. A., & Cosey, E. J. (2000). The spiritual needs of hospitalized patients. *American Journal of Nursing, 100*(7), 24C–D; Marty, M. E. (1998). Revising the map of American religion. In W. C. Roof (Ed.), *The Annals of the American Academy of Political and Social Science: Religion in the Nineties,* Volume 558 (pp. 13–27). Newbury Park, CA: Sage; Sloan, R. P., Bagiella, E., & Powell, T. (1999). Religion, spirituality, and medicine. *The Lancet, 353*(9153), 664–667; Sherwood, G. D. (2000). The power of nurse-client encounters: Interpreting spiritual themes. *Journal of Holistic Nursing, 18*(2), 159–175; Wright, K. B. (1998). Professional, ethical and legal implications for spiritual care in nursing. *Image: The Journal of Nursing Scholarship, 30*(1), pp. 81–83.

## CLINICAL ALERT

### Respect for Rituals

Some Native Americans have specific rituals which may be performed as end-of-life customs or routines. These rituals may include having specific tribal members present with the family during the last stages of physical life. In addition, these persons may perform specific verbalizations, dances, or singing at this time. The nurse must recognize the ethnic variance of this situation and must be prepared to make allowances for this type of ritual. The nurse must advocate for continued nursing care that respects the faith and belief practices of the dying Native American client.

Table 48-2 lists some of the important scriptures for a number of religions. It includes a section on sacred writings, as they may provide comfort and strength during stressful times. The table is meant to be a starting guideline and to give a very broad overview of religious traditions.

## Spirituality in Nursing Theory

The concern for spirituality that Florence Nightingale brought to nursing slowly eroded as nursing fought to become a science as well as an art. Science as interpreted in this century has dealt with five-sense data: if a phenomenon cannot be seen, heard, touched, smelled, or tasted, then it is not the business of science. It may be that the lack of "scientific objectivity" that is inherent in spirituality accounts for the absence of spirituality in nursing theory. A review of 26 nursing theories in relationship to spirituality revealed only two theorists who acknowledged the development of spirituality in their respective theories. The two theorists who explicitly included spirituality were Jean Watson and Margaret Newman. Only their two metatheories in nursing have explicit content addressing theoretical aspects of spiritual nursing care. Of the two, Jean Watson has most directly dealt with the human soul, or spirit, as part of her theory.

## Watson's Theory of Nursing and Spirituality

Watson's Theory of Human Science and Human Care (Watson, 1985), states that the human soul is an essential part of each human being. In Watson's theory, the human soul is the "spirit, inner self, or essence of the person" (p. 46) and is "tied to a greater sense of self-awareness, a higher degree of consciousness, an inner strength, and a power that can expand human capacities and allow a person to transcend his or her usual self" (p. 46). The nurse promotes healing through assisting a person to find meaning and autonomy.

Assisting clients to find meaning in life provides guidelines for how a nurse might act when a person is in spiritual distress or when spiritual well-being is threatened. According to Watson, when an illness experience causes people to be confronted with concerns about existence and meaning, clients need to examine the meaning of the illness and to have that meaning become part of the nurse's response to the client. This is part of what Watson calls the "transpersonal caring relationship," in which both nurse and client develop a shared experience that leads to healing. The nurse, therefore, must develop a relationship with the client that encourages exploration of meaning, listen carefully, and assist the client to use this new insight in the healing process. Watson's theory thus encompasses the definition of spirituality used in this chapter: transcendence, connection, balance, and purpose.

An application of Watson's theory (1985) in clinical care was the use of a "Laughing Spirit Listening Circle" with a group of older women living in a retirement care center. The Listening Circle was designed to have the women speak freely about whatever they chose to share, without formal leadership or direction. The participants told one another stories about important events in their lives, and discussed how they coped with obstacles and managed difficulties. Through this experience, the women felt cared for and created an environment of healing. The "transpersonal caring relationship" allowed for relationships to develop, the exploration of meaning, and new insights.

## Connection Between Spirituality and Health

A number of studies indicate a relationship between spiritual well-being and mental and physical health. A typical example is the positive relationship between religious strength and survival following cardiac surgery (Oxman, Freeman, & Manheimer, 1995). Studies have indicated the same positive relationship between spiritual well-being and stress, depression, AIDS complications, and myocardial infarction (Sicher, Targ, Moore, & Smith, 1998; Tuck, McCain, & Elswick, 2001). More surprising are the number of studies that indicate improved outcomes for people who receive remote, intercessory prayer for their well-being. O'Laoire (1997) conducted a randomized, double-blind study of people who suffered from anxiety and depression. Those subjects who were prayed for improved significantly more than controls, even though the subjects were unaware of the prayers. While studies such as these are controversial, both spiritual support and prayer appear to support mental and physical health. Another research example is seen in the Research Focus box.

## RESEARCH FOCUS

**Title of Study:** Spiritual activities as a resistance resource for women with human immunodeficiency virus

**Study Purpose:** This study examined the role of spiritual activities as a resource that might reduce the negative effects of the impact of the HIV disease process on 184 HIV positive women.

**Methods:** Initially, 54 women participated in focus groups to provide measurement scales for the analysis of the interviews for the larger sample. Then demographic characteristics and the variables of interest (developed from the focus groups) were collected in interview settings. The larger sample (n = 184) consisted primarily of African American women who were single, urban residing, and made less than $10,000 annually. This was a longitudinal study that used 1.5–2-hour interview techniques with trained research assistants. Data collected from focus groups and open-ended questions were developed into analysis scales. These scales provided cultural and contextual relevant measurements for women with HIV disease.

**Findings:** The results revealed that as spiritual activities increased, emotional distress decreased when adjustments were made for HIV-related stressors. A positive relationship between spiritual activities and quality of life was found. The identified spiritual activities (e.g., praying, taking problems to God) were consistent with the practice of Judeo-Christianity in the southeastern United States, which was typical for the type of population from which the sample in this study was derived. In addition, HIV-related stressors were found to have a significant negative effect on both emotional distress and quality of life. Overall, the findings in this research support the notion that spiritual activities are an important psychological resource that accounts for individual variability in adjustment to the stressors associated with HIV disease.

**Implications:** The future implications indicate a need for health care providers to implement spiritual interventions in persons with serious illnesses such as HIV disease.

Sowell, R., Moneyham, L., Hennessy, M., Buillory, J., Demi, A., & Seals, B. (2000). Spiritual activities as a resistance resource for women with human immunodeficiency virus. *Nursing Research, 49*(2), 73–82.

## Nursing Care

Nurses and other health caregivers are frequently uncomfortable in exploring spiritual concerns with clients. Some of this discomfort may reflect personal confusion or rejection of religion. As discussed above, everyone has spiritual concerns when spirituality is defined as finding meaning, connection, and purpose in their lives. The logical conclusion is that every nurse, along with every client, is a spiritual being with spiritual concerns. Nurses are likely to work within their own system of spiritual values and beliefs. A first step in assisting others with spiritual concerns is to assess your own personal spiritual beliefs. This assessment provides the nurse with a chance to develop skills in spiritual assessment as well as a means of self-discovery. Asking the same questions of yourself as you would ask others about spiritual concerns is an important first step. Nurses with strong religious and/or spiritual beliefs can also use this exercise as a way of "setting aside" their own convictions when dealing with a client from a different spiritual background. It is also important for those with antireligious feelings to recognize their antagonism toward particular beliefs. Discomfort toward spirituality may stem from not knowing how to intervene with spiritual problems. Nursing education frequently does not provide much information about working with a client's spiritual needs, despite the commitment to holistic nursing care. The next section will use the nursing process as a framework to assess, plan, diagnose, and evaluate a client's spiritual dimension.

## Assessment

Spiritual assessment begins with the consideration of how spirituality develops across the life span. Many people have noted that spirituality is an important aspect for children who are seriously ill or dying, but their spirituality is quite different from adult spirituality. Adolescents are often spiritual seekers, and their spiritual development affects how a nurse will assess their needs. Adults, and in particular older adults, may have very deep spiritual concerns that influence their approach to illness and dying.

### Spiritual Development Across the Life Span

James Fowler did the seminal work on spiritual development through the life span, and his categories are still widely used today (Fowler, 1981). He based his stages of spiritual development on the works of Piaget, Erickson, and Kohlberg. While physical and cognitive development are important in moving from one stage to the next, people may never move beyond an early stage. **Fowler's stages of spiritual development** (Table 48-3) point out that spiritual needs and understanding will change as a person

## TABLE 48-3     FOWLER'S STAGES OF SPIRITUAL DEVELOPMENT

| Stage | Age | Description |
|---|---|---|
| 0. Undifferentiated | 0 to 3 years | Infant has no concepts about self or the environment. |
| 1. Intuitive-Projective | 4 to 6 years | Spiritual beliefs imitate those of influential adults; child uses fantasy; first understanding of death and morality. |
| 2. Mythic-Literal | 7 to 12 years | Stories and myths are used to communicate spiritual meanings and to create understanding of experience. |
| 3. Synthetic-Conventional | Adolescence | Relationships are key to understanding of self and others; spiritual concepts tend to be relational. |
| 4. Individuating-Reflective | After 18 | Spiritual identity no longer defined by others; creation of unique identity is involved. |
| 5. Paradoxical-Consolidative | After 30 | Person moves beyond dichotomy into an awareness of truth from a multifaceted viewpoint. |
| 6. Universalizing | Older adult | This stage is reached by very few, some of whom may be spiritual leaders who work against hate and injustice in the world. |

Fowler, J. (1981). *Stages of faith: The psychology of human development and the quest for meaning.* San Francisco: Harper.

ages. At every age, however, spiritual concerns may be extremely important.

Stage 1 is the first stage in which spiritual understanding can be identified. Children from about ages 2 to 7 are influenced by the important adults in their lives. A child in this stage can be powerfully influenced by adult actions. The first awareness of death occurs in stage 1. Stage 2 is characterized by spiritual understanding through the use of stories. God or goodness tends to be a person with human characteristics, as is Satan or evil. Stories are used to make sense of experience and to create meaning. Stage 3 often occurs during adolescence and involves reflection on the contradictions in spiritual myths and stories. Contradictions lead the person to build a more personal relationship with the world and with spiritual beliefs. This new identity is predicated on relationships to God and others. Stage 4 is where the individual claims an identity no longer defined by relationships to others. Young adulthood is the typical time to move into stage 4, and the spiritual task is to take the symbols that were adopted from childhood and put them into conceptual meaning. Stage 5 is a complex stage in which a person moves beyond stage 4's "either-or" and sees spiritual issues as multifaceted. Stage 5 is unusual before midlife, as it involves an in-depth examination and recognition of one's "deeper self." The last stage is stage 6, which few people accomplish. Those who do achieve stage 6 tend to be spiritual leaders who break down barriers between classes and social conditions to promote justice and understanding. A synopsis of Fowler's stages of spiritual development is depicted in Table 48-3.

## STOP AND THINK

### Assessing Spirituality

- What specific clues can the nurse identify in "detecting" the need for spiritual interventions?

- What preparatory questions or conversations can the nurse use to engage the client in discussions of spirituality?

- What physiological clinical manifestations can a client exhibit that indicate a need for spiritual interventions?

## General Spiritual Assessment

A **generalized spiritual assessment** should include the four elements of spirituality: transcendence, connection, balance, and purpose. Box 48-1 lists questions that would elicit each of these four components. A spiritual assessment can be performed either by using a standardized form or by asking general questions. Standardized forms have the advantage of systematic data collection that can be used for evaluation. A disadvantage of using a standard form is that it may not be appropriate for people of different age groups or cultural backgrounds. In addition, spir-

## BOX 48-1    QUESTIONS TO ASK IN A SPIRITUAL ASSESSMENT

### Transcendence

- What gives your life meaning and hope?

- Has this illness/event made you wonder why this happened to you?

### Connection

- Are spiritual relationships important to you?

- Do you have a spiritual or religious leader who you would like me to contact?

- Has this illness/event caused you to question your relationship to God or a higher being?

- What are the important relationships in your life?

### Balance

- Are there any spiritual guidelines that you follow that relate to your health or illness?

- Has this illness/event interfered with your spiritual practices?

- How can I help you make your spiritual practice easier in this situation?

- Have you had feelings of doubt, anger, or hopelessness since this happened?

### Purpose

- Has this illness/event caused you to question your understanding of what's important in your life?

- Has this illness/event changed your ideas about what you should do in life?

ment should include the person's concept of God or a supreme being, spiritual belief and practice, any spiritual questioning or doubts, and source of spiritual strength.

Spiritual concerns may be "invisible" to the nurse, especially if observations are concentrated on physical and psychological responses to illness. Observations about a person's spiritual life include noting objects in the client's environment and a client's comments about God, religious activities, and spiritual practices. Verbal expressions of spiritual concern are comments such as, "Why did God do this to me?", "I feel useless.", "Nothing can help me now.", "I have no reason to go on.", and "No one cares what happens to me." General expressions of

## TABLE 48-4    SPIRITUALITY ASSESSMENT INSTRUMENTS

| Name of Instrument | Characteristics |
|---|---|
| Spiritual Well-Being Scale | Measures relationship with God (vertical dimension) and purpose and satisfaction with life (horizontal dimension) (20 items) |
| Spiritual Health Inventory | Measures spiritual need for self-acceptance, relationships, and hope (31 items) |
| Index of Core Spiritual Experiences | Measures spiritual experience, sense of well-being, and response to stress (68 items) |
| Spiritual Perspective Scale | Measures spiritual depth and engagement in spiritual activities (10 items) |
| COOP Charts of Spirituality | Visual analogue scale with three questions that ask about closeness to God, spiritual practices, and spiritual experiences (3 items) |
| Spiritual Coping Interview | Measures relationship with God, use of spiritual behaviors or resources, expressions of spiritual needs and perception of the nurse's role (30 items) |

Ellerhorst-Ryan, J. M. (1997). Instruments to measure aspects of spirituality. In M. Frank-Stromberg & S. J. Olsen (Eds.), *Instruments for clinical health-care research* (2nd ed., pp. 202–212). Boston: Jones and Bartlett.

itual assessment questionnaires may measure only some of the spiritual questions (see Box 48-1) that are important for an individual. Some of the questionnaires were developed for clinical purposes, while some reflect research concerns. A number of standardized forms have been developed; see Table 48-4 for a list of some of the forms and their general characteristics. For nurses who work in agencies that have not adopted a specific spiritual assessment tool, an assessment can be focused around several general areas, including the importance of spirituality in the person's life, connection to self and others, and meaning and purpose in the person's life. Basic areas of assess-

spiritual distress include feelings of loss, alienation, anger, and grieving.

## Spiritual Assessment for Children

Fowler's stages of spiritual development (Table 48-3) can be used as a framework for assessing the spiritual concerns of children. Children below age 3 do not have an understanding or conception of the spiritual aspects of being. Toddlers may have spiritual rituals such as prayer, but they do not have an understanding yet of the meaning of prayer. Preschool and young school-age children, on the other hand, have many spiritual questions and concerns. Young children do not make distinctions between religion and spirituality, however; and religious traditions within their families may be very important to them. Therefore, it is important to assess the family's religious values and practices to help children cope with chronic illness or a terminal diagnosis. Morality is conceptualized during stage 1, and some children may feel that their illness is a punishment for being "bad." Since children at this age have a concept of death, a child with a serious or terminal illness may have many fears about death and what will happen after death. Older children in stage 2 make sense of pain and illness through stories; having a child tell a story about the illness will help the nurse assess the child's concept of the illness and what it means to the child.

Adolescents question their parents' spiritual beliefs and their family's religious and spiritual practices. Adolescents may not have the same beliefs and practices as their parents, so it is important to ask them directly rather than relying on a parent's report. Relationships with others form the foundation of spiritual belief for stage 3, so asking about relationships in conjunction with their illness will be important.

## Spiritual Assessment for Adults

Adults in stages 3, 4, and 5 are consolidating their beliefs and values in light of their experience as adults. Adults are busy with work, life partners, and raising children; all of these experiences will challenge and refine spiritual beliefs. Values that may have been important in adolescence may change radically as a person matures. The nurse may find that opening a discussion of spiritual beliefs will assist a person to clarify and redefine what is important.

## Spiritual Assessment for Older Adults

Older adults may have a well-developed sense of their spirituality (Figure 48-3), or they may have never confronted their spiritual concerns until diagnosed with a serious or terminal illness. Adults in stage 4 will view spir-

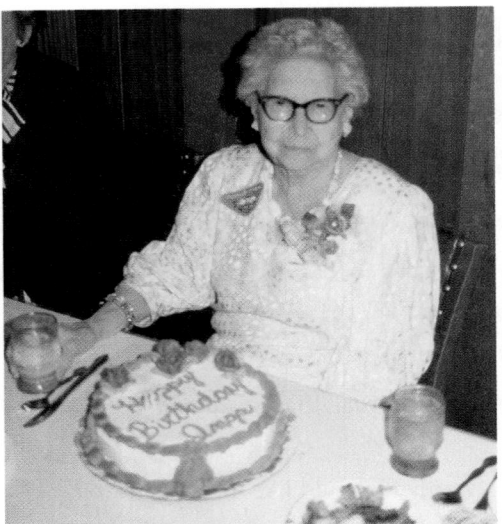

**Figure 48-3    The elderly often have a well-developed sense of their spirituality.**

itual problems in more black-and-white terms than will an adult in stage 5, who will have a very multifaceted understanding of spiritual questions. In either case, spiritual questions are likely to be important. Furthermore, older adults tend to be more involved in religious activities and to state that religion is very important in their daily lives (Ehmann, 1999).

## Nursing Diagnoses

Common nursing diagnoses that result from a spiritual assessment are *Risk for Spiritual Distress* and *Readiness for Enhanced Spiritual Well-Being*. The North American Nursing Diagnosis Association (NANDA) (2003) guidelines define spiritual distress as "altered sense of harmonious connectedness with all of life and the universe in which dimensions that transcend and enforce the self may be disrupted"

---

### NURSING STRATEGY

#### Assessing Spirituality in Older Adults

To assess spirituality, consider asking the following questions:

- Is religion or God significant to you?

- Do you feel your faith (or religion) is helpful to you?

- Are religious practices meaningful to you?

- Has your current illness affected your spiritual perspective?

(NANDA, 2003, p. 179). Spiritual well-being has been defined as "personal expressions of connectedness with self, others, higher power, all life, nature and the universe that transcend and empower the self" (Johnson & Maas, 1997). Outcomes for these two diagnoses are complex, since these diagnoses involve so much of a person's integrated being. In general, good outcomes are that the person maintains feelings of connectedness and peace while continuing activities that promote meaning in the person's life.

## Spiritual Distress

Related factors that might create spiritual distress are separation from religious ties and supports, and when beliefs or values are challenged by medical treatment. An example would be when a person who is a Christian Scientist agrees to accept treatment for an illness rather than relying entirely on prayer for healing. Circumstances that bring a person to spiritual distress may also create problems for an individual with coping, anxiety, or grieving. Spiritual distress is distinguished by anger with God or a higher power, inability to find meaning in an illness or event, or feeling that purpose in life has been lost. Ineffective coping occurs when a person is unable to use usual mechanisms to manage life's stressors. When a person has lost a spiritual support, the appropriate diagnosis is spiritual distress rather than ineffective coping. Anxiety is distinguished by globalized, vague feelings, worry, or threat from an unidentified source. While people may feel worried about their spiritual beliefs or relationship to God, a specific spiritual concern should be called spiritual distress. Only vague, unidentified worry is diagnosed as anxiety. Grieving can be for the loss of an individual, role, or cherished object in a person's life. Grieving may also involve a perceived rather than an actual loss. If the loss involves spiritual support, beliefs, or values, the appropriate diagnosis is spiritual distress.

Many of the interventions for a client with spiritual distress are the same as for any distress that a person may feel. Some examples of these interventions are providing support and encouragement, conveying a caring presence, and listening. Interventions for a client experiencing spiritual distress may also include calling for the person's spiritual counselor (e.g., minister, priest, rabbi), but every nurse can assist a person who is in spiritual distress. The nurse can pray with the client if the client is comfortable with prayer. In addition, touching the person, if the person is comfortable with being touched, can provide support (Figure 48-4). The nurse's role in spiritual care may not be to provide specific religious actions, but rather to assist the person in finding connection, meaning, and hope.

## Spiritual Well-Being

Spiritual well-being may be seen in any type of individual in any position on the health-illness continuum. Several concepts important to spiritual well-being are transcen-

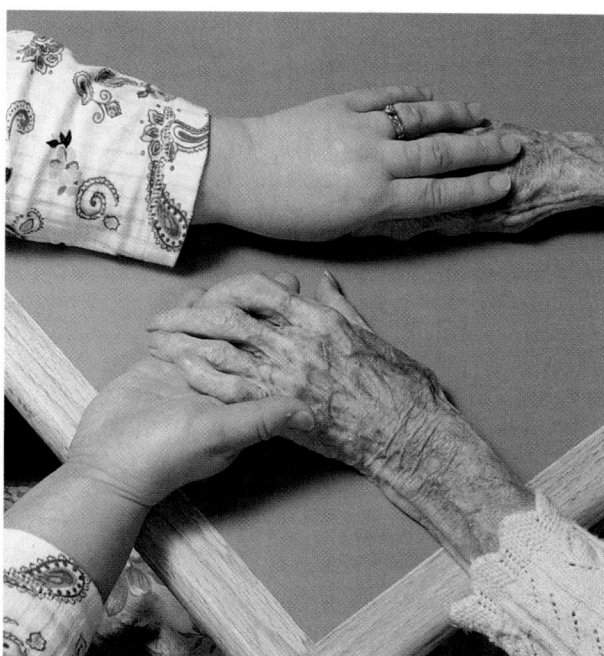

**Figure 48-4    Touching can be an important spiritual intervention.**

dence, connection, **balance** (a sense of inner peace), and **purpose** (a sense of meaning and purpose in life). Defining characteristics of spiritual well-being related to transcendence are compassion for others, working toward universal justice and acceptance, a capacity for unconditional love, and expressing an understanding of the illness/event that helps them find meaning. Characteristics of well-being as related to connection are feeling loved and cared for, being connected to God or a Higher Being in a meaningful way, and having a capacity for love and acceptance of self and others' needs. A client with balance in life

---

## CLIENT EDUCATION

### Nursing Interventions for Spiritual Distress

✓ Discuss with the client in spiritual distress that it is normal to doubt one's quality or strength of faith during a time of crisis or illness.

✓ Offer to contact spiritual leaders consistent with the client's beliefs (but the nurse should be cautioned against establishing a practice pattern that only includes this intervention).

✓ Give "permission" for the client to discuss spiritual concerns with you by broaching the subject of spiritual welfare in a "natural manner."

✓ Provide uninterrupted quiet time for prayer, reading, or meditation on spiritual concerns.

will exhibit such behaviors as having inner peace, and feeling hopeful, integrated, and whole.

There are many potential nursing interventions for spiritual well-being. The following are examples of these actions of care: helping the client find a reason to live and to discover meaning in life, encouraging the exploration of the meaning of the illness/event in the client's life, and assisting the client to identify beliefs and values. The nurse should also provide assistance with enabling spiritual and religious rituals and actions, and encourage family and friends to provide meaningful religious objects. In addition, when a spiritual counselor comes to visit, provide a quiet place for them to talk and pray. The nurse must learn to adapt nursing therapeutics to the client's specific spiritual requirements as much as possible.

## Intervention

Nursing interventions for spirituality may be very intrinsic to the client and somewhat complicated to design. In addition, each developmental stage must be looked at individually as depicted in Fowler's stages of development (Fowler, 1981). The nurse must remember that one nursing diagnosis may have very different interventions for the different ages of clients. For example, an intervention that might have positive results with an adolescent might not be effective for a younger child. The nurse must strive to intervene with strategies that have been well planned.

### Interventions with Children

Young children find meaning and comfort in ritual. Helping a child to maintain religious practice will ease fear and confusion. Telling stories and listening to stories may help an older child come to terms with an illness experience. Ask the child to tell you a story about being sick, and use stories to explain how people may feel lost, alone, or confused by an illness. Adolescents may need help with discovering values and actions that are important for them. Encouraging exploration of meaning and purpose in life within a framework of relationship may be helpful. Spiritual intervention with an adolescent may have far-

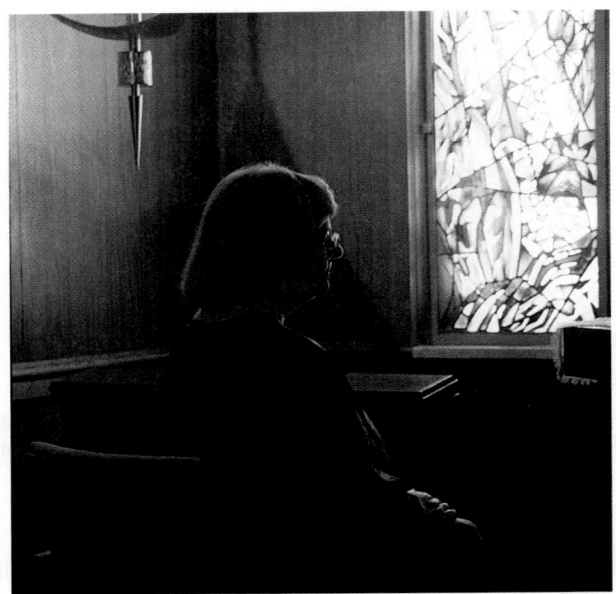

**Figure 48-5 Frequency of praying increases with age.**

reaching consequences. Adolescents who maintain or adopt spiritual practice during their adolescent years are less likely to engage in self-destructive behavior, and in general feel happier and better adjusted late in life (Pfund, 2000).

### Interventions with Older Adults

While prayer appears to be practiced by all age groups, frequency of prayer increases with age (Figure 48-5). With an older adult, ask if prayers would be welcomed. Helping an older person to maintain usual religious and spiritual observances is important. Older adults who have an active religious or spiritual life appear to be healthier and more likely to heal than those who do not. Several studies have indicated that people who do not have the comfort and support of spirituality or religion are at increased risk for poor outcomes following surgery, myocardial infarction, or other life stressors.

Those who are dying have extraordinary spiritual needs. These needs may or may not include a need for religion, but are likely to include needs for companionship and connection with important others. People frequently express a need to finish important "business" in their lives, whether it be physical or emotional tasks. Many people welcome a chance to do a "life review" in which the meaning and accomplishments of their lives are examined.

## Evaluation

The suggested Nursing Outcomes Classification (NOC) for spiritual distress is dignified dying, hope, and spiritual well-being (Johnson & Maas, 1997). The client outcomes

### CLIENT REFLECTIONS

#### A Terminal Client

Mr. Stypinski is 83 years old and has nonoperable, terminal cancer of the brain. He states to the nurse, "I am not afraid of dying, because I believe I will go to heaven—but I am worried for my wife. She will have to live alone, and I know that will be hard for her." How would you respond to his statements as Mr. Stypinski's nurse?

that would support the NOC are that a client discusses conflicts or disturbances in relation to spiritual beliefs, states feeling of trust in the self or in a higher being, continues spiritual practices, discusses feelings about death, and expresses a mood that is appropriate for the situation. More specifically, a spiritual evaluation can take the format of asking open-ended questions to obtain the more internal aspects of how the client is spiritually. For example, two questions to evaluate the nursing intervention outcomes for a person with spiritual distress are (1) does the client state that he feels more comfortable spiritually?, and (2) can the client describe at least *x* number of support systems to use when spiritual conflict arises? In addition, the evaluation questions that Cox and her colleagues suggest for spiritual well-being are (1) is the client expressing satisfaction with spirituality?, and (2) does the client exhibit a stated percentage of defining characteristics of spiritual well-being?

Overall, achieving spiritual health requires creativity and a variety of communication and assessment skills of the nurse. Obtaining a spiritual evaluation is fundamental to evaluating the nursing interventions for spiritual problems and the effectiveness of the nursing care provided for the client.

# CASE STUDY/NURSING CARE PLAN

Mrs. Snodgrass is in her 80s and slowly dying of cancer. She has been in the hospital for several weeks and when the nurse heard of the extent of her disease, the nurse was certain that she must be suffering terribly. It surprised the nurse to hear that Mrs. Snodgrass hadn't had any pain medication on the previous shift, and the nurse wondered if her colleagues had given Mrs. Snodgrass enough attention. As the nurse made her assessment rounds, she was startled to find Mrs. Snodgrass sitting up in bed, watching out her window with a quiet expression. When the nurse offered her morphine, Mrs. Snodgrass just smiled. "Oh, no, honey," she said, and patted the nurse's hand. "I don't need much and I'm fine just now," stated Mrs.Snodgrass. "I really would like to be left alone to pray." As the nurse got to know Mrs. Snodgrass better in the 2 weeks before she died, the nurse discovered that Mrs. Snodgrass was often able to control her pain through her prayer time. Mrs. Snodgrass even comforted the nurse when the nurse was stressed by her first full-time nursing position. "I've had a good life, and I've made my peace with God," Mrs. Snodgrass said just before she died. "I'm ready to go."

## Assessment

Client is physically dying of cancer and is experiencing intermittent pain at a level of 8 (scale 1 to 10), which is sometimes controlled with prayer. She places great importance on her spirituality and is self-actualized through the inner qualities of her faith, which is so important to her.

## Nursing Diagnosis #1

*Acute Pain* related to terminal cancer.
**NOC:** Comfort Level; Medication Response; Pain Control
**NIC:** Analgesic Administration; Conscious Sedation; Pain Management

## Expected Outcome

The client will:
1. Maintain a prayer time throughout hospitalization to allow time to cope with pain level.

## Planning/Interventions/Rationales

1. Provide privacy and quiet two to four times a day or as requested for daily prayer times. *Encourages individual practice of prayer time.*
2. Inform nursing station area to hold client calls during this time. *Provides privacy for client and creates environment conducive to prayer.*
3. Note spiritual intervention of prayer on Kardex and include in care plan. *Provides continuity for nurses related to client's praying.*
4. Assess level of pain; determine the intensity of the pain with rating scale from 1 to 10. *Provides ongoing assessment of pain level and quantifies the amount of pain client is experiencing.*

*(continues)*

# CASE STUDY/NURSING CARE PLAN (continued)

## Evaluation
Client was provided times of prayer every 4 hours and privacy was maintained for each prayer time. Pain level was assessed every 2 hours and level was between 5 and 8.

## Nursing Diagnosis #2
*Spiritual Distress* related to coping with terminal cancer.
**NOC:** Hope; Spiritual Well-Being
**NIC:** Spiritual Support; Coping Enhancement; Emotional Support

## Expected Outcome
The client will:
1. Maintain spiritual practices throughout hospitalization.

## Planning/Interventions/Rationales
1. Provide privacy at prearranged intervals for spiritual practices (e.g., praying, reading, meditating). *Promotes an environment conducive to participating in spiritual observances.*
2. Explore whether client needs assistance in selected positions for praying or meditating and provide assistance as necessary. *Provides aid as related to physical limitations during times of spiritual practices.*
3. Contact spiritual leader recommended by client. *Provides holistic management by trained personnel in arena of spirituality.*
4. Express understanding and acceptance of the importance of client's religious or spiritual beliefs and practices. *Validates the nurse's awareness and support of the client's spirituality.*

## Evaluation
Privacy maintained each time client expressed desire to pray, read the Bible, or talk with her pastor. Client did not need physical assistance during these times of spiritual interventions. The pastor was contacted by the nurse and came to visit client each day in the afternoon. The nurse verbalized support of the client's spiritual health regularly during the hospitalization.

## Key Concepts

- Spirituality may or may not involve religious beliefs. While most Americans express a belief in God or a higher power, religious practice varies widely.
- Religious beliefs will vary globally and within the individual, even for those who affiliate with a particular congregation or religious philosophy.
- Spiritual development occurs throughout the life span. Spiritual assessment and intervention need to take spiritual development into consideration to provide appropriate nursing care.
- Spiritual assessment includes the four elements of transcendence, connection, balance, and purpose.
- Two common nursing diagnoses are spiritual distress and spiritual well-being.
- The nurse's role is instrumental in the client's spiritual health.

## Review Questions and Activities

1. What measures can a nurse take to increase her comfort level in approaching clients' spiritual needs?
2. Compare and contrast the concepts of spirituality and religion.
3. How do three to five prominent religions view birth?
4. What are some critical beliefs of several religions as related to health care practices?
5. Describe two specific religions in regard to creating ethical dilemmas for health care practices.
6. How should the nurse approach a client who chooses dietary restrictions, based on spiritual beliefs, that are contraindicated by the client's physical condition?
7. Why is it valuable for the nurse to be familiar with Fowler's spiritual stages when providing care for pediatric clients with terminal disorders?

**8.** What are several questions the nurse could ask the client to assess the client's spiritual condition?

**9.** What are several specific nursing interventions a nurse could develop for a client with a nursing diagnosis of spiritual distress?

## Web Resources

America and Religion
   http://www.gallup.com
New Age Spirituality
   http://www.religioustolerance.org
Taoism
   http://www.religioustolerance.org

## References

Ackley, B. J. (1999). *Nursing diagnosis handbook: A guide to planning care* (4th ed.). St. Louis: Mosby.

Adherents, (2001, July 16). Major religions of the world ranked by number of adherents (94 paragraphs). Retrieved from http://www.adherents.com

Albert, M. L. (1999). Spirituality and healing in medicine. *HealthInform: Essential Information on Alternative Health Care, 4*(10), 7–9.

Aldridge, D. (1993). Is there evidence for spiritual healing? *Advances: The Journal of Mind-Body Health, 9*(4), 4–21.

Carpenito, L. J. (2000). *Nursing diagnosis: An application to clinical practice* (8th ed.). Philadelphia: Lippincott.

Cerranto, P. L. (1998). *Spirituality and healing. RN, 61*(2), 49–51.

Davidhizar, R., Bechtel, G. A., & Cosey, E. J. (2000). The spiritual needs of hospitalized patients. *American Journal of Nursing, 100*(7), 24C–D.

Ehman, C. (1999). *The age factor in religious attitudes and behavior* (9 paragraphs). http://www.gallup.com

Ellerhorst-Ryan, J. M. (1997). Instruments to measure aspects of spirituality. In M. Frank-Stromberg & S. J. Olsen (Eds.), *Instruments for clinical health-care research* (2nd ed., pp. 202–212). Boston: Jones and Bartlett.

Ellis, M. R., Vinson, D. C., & Ewigman, B. (1999). Addressing spiritual concerns of patients: Family physicians' attitudes and practices. *The Journal of Family Practice, 48*(2), 105–109.

Fowler, J. (1981). *Stages of Faith: The Psychology of Human Development and the Quest for Meaning.* San Francisco: Harper.

Gallup. (2003). http://www.gallup.com.

Hatch, R. L., Burg, M. A., Naberhaus, D. S., & Hellmich, L. K. (1998). The spiritual involvement and beliefs scale: Development and testing of a new instrument. *The Journal of Family Practice, 46*(6), 476–483.

Herrman, C. P. (2001). Spiritual needs of dying patients: A qualitative study. *Oncology Nursing Forum, 28*(1), 67–72.

Johnson, M., & Maas, M. (1997). Nursing outcomes classification (NOC). St. Louis: Mosby.

Kendrick, D. D., & Robinson, S. (2000). Spirituality: Its relevance and purpose for clinical nursing in a new millennium. *Journal of Clinical Nursing, 9*(5), 701–705.

Kozier, B., Erb, G., Berman, A. J., & Burke, K. (2000). Spirituality. In B. Kozier, G. Erb, A. J. Berman, & K. Burke (Eds.), *Fundamentals of nursing: Concepts, process and practice* (6th ed., pp 219–233). Upper Saddle River, NJ: Prentice Hall.

Levin, J. S., & Taylor, R. J. (1997). Age differences in patterns and correlates of the frequency of prayer. *Gerontologist, 37*(1), 75–88.

Magida, A. J., & Matlins, S. M. (1999a). *How to be the perfect stranger: A guide to etiquette in other people's religious ceremonies,* Volume 1. Woodstock, VT: Skylight Paths.

Magida, A. J., & Matlins, S. M. (1999b). *How to be the perfect stranger: A guide to etiquette in other people's religious ceremonies,* Volume 2. Woodstock, VT: Skylight Paths.

Marty, M. E. (1998). Revising the map of American religion. In W. C. Roof (Ed.), *The annals of the American Academy of Political and Social Science: Religion in the nineties,* Volume 558 (pp. 13–27). Newbury Park, CA: Sage.

McBride, J. L., Pilkington, L., & Arthur, G. (1998). Development of brief pictorial instruments for assessing spirituality in primary care. *Journal of Ambulatory Care Management, 21*(4), 53–61.

Mccrae, J. (1995). Nightingale's spiritual philosophy and its significance for modern nursing. *Image: Journal of Nursing Scholarship, 27*(1), 8–10.

Meraviglia, M. G. (1999). Critical analysis of spirituality and its empirical indicators. Prayer and meaning in life. *Journal of Holistic Nursing, 17*(1), 18–33.

Moberg, D. O. (1999). Spiritual well-being questionnaire. In P. C. Hill & R. W. Hood, Jr. (Eds.), *Measures of religiosity.* Birmingham, AL: Religious Education Press.

North American Nursing Diagnosis Association (NANDA). (2003). *Nursing diagnoses: Definitions and classification, 2003–2004.* Philadelphia: Author.

O'Laoire, S. (1997). An experimental study of the effects of distant, intercessory prayer on self-esteem, anxiety, and depression. *Alternative Therapies in Health & Medicine, 3*(6), 38–53.

Oxman, T. E., Freeman, D. H., Jr., & Manheimer, E. D. (1995). Lack of social participation or religious strength and comfort as risk factors for death after cardiac surgery in the elderly. *Psychosomatic Medicine, 57,* 5–15.

Perrin, J. M., Barnes, L. L., Plotnikoff, G. A., Fox, K., & Pendleton, S. (2000). Spirituality, religion and pediatrics: Intersecting worlds of healing. *Pediatrics, 106* (suppl.), 899–908.

Pfund, R. (2000). Nurturing a child's spirituality. *Journal of Child Health Care, 4*(4), 143–148.

Sherwood, G. D. (2000). The power of nurse-client encounters: Interpreting spiritual themes. *Journal of Holistic Nursing, 18*(2), 159–175.

Sicher, F., Targ, E., Moore, D., & Smith, H. (1998, December). A randomized double-blind study of the effect of distant healing in a population with advanced AIDS. *Western Journal of Medicine,* pp. 356–363.

Sloan, R. P., Bagiella, E., & Powell, T. (1999). Religion, spirituality, and medicine. *The Lancet, 353*(9153), 664–667.

Smucker, C. J. (1998). Nursing, healing and spirituality. *Complementary Therapies in Nursing and Midwifery, 4*(4), 95–97.

Sowell, R., Moneyham, L., Hennessy, M., Buillory, J., Demi, A., & Seals, B. (2000). Spiritual activities as a resistance resource for women with human immuno-deficiency virus. *Nursing Research, 49*(2), 73–82.

Stranahan, S. (2001). Spiritual perception, attitudes about spiritual care, and spiritual care practices among nurse practitioners. *Western Journal of Nursing Research, 23(1)*, 90–104.

Sumner, C. H. (1998). Recognizing and responding to spiritual concerns. *American Journal of Nursing, 98*(1), 26–30.

Tuck, I., McCain, N., & Elswick, R. (2001). Spirituality and psychosocial factors in persons living with HIV. *Journal of Advanced Nursing, 33*(6), pp. 776–783.

Watson, J. (1985). *Nursing science and human care.* Norwalk: CT: Appleton-Century-Crofts.

White, G. (2000). An inquiry into the concepts of spirituality and spiritual care. *International Journal of Palliative Nursing, 6*(10), 479–484.

Wright, K. B. (1998). Professional, ethical and legal implications for spiritual care in nursing. *Image: The Journal of Nursing Scholarship, 30*(1), pp. 81–83.

Zentner, J. P., Murray, R. B., Samiezade-Yazd, C., Adams, S., Talley, P., Atkins, F., & Cox, E. (2001). Spiritual and religious influences on the person and family. In R. B. Murray and J. P. Zentner (Eds.), *Health promotion strategies through the life span* (7th ed., pp. 115–153). Upper Saddle River, NJ: Prentice Hall.

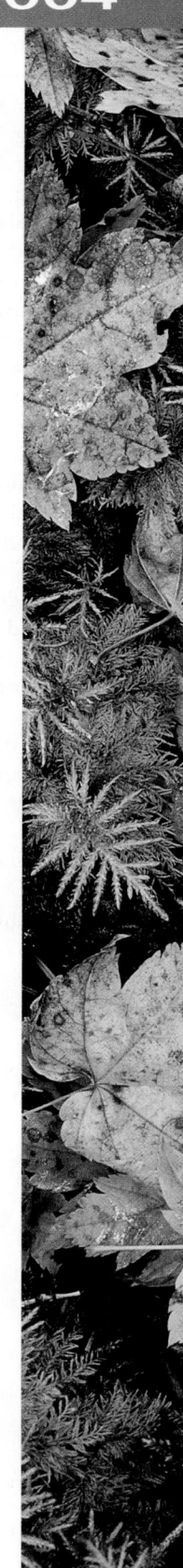

Activity intolerance
Activity intolerance, Risk for
Adjustment, Impaired
Airway clearance, Ineffective
Allergy response, Risk for latex
Anxiety
Anxiety, Death
Aspiration, Risk for
Body image, Disturbed
Body temperature, Risk for imbalanced
Bowel incontinence
Breastfeeding, Effective
Breastfeeding, Ineffective
Breastfeeding, Interrupted
Breathing pattern, Ineffective
Cardiac output, Decreased
Caregiver role strain
Caregiver role strain, Risk for
Communication, Impaired verbal
Communication, Readiness for enhanced
Confusion, Acute
Confusion, Chronic
Constipation
Constipation, Perceived
Constipation, Risk for
Coping, Community, Ineffective
Coping, Community, Readiness for enhanced
Coping, Defensive
Coping, Family, Compromised
Coping, Family, Disabled
Coping, Family, Readiness for enhanced
Coping, Ineffective
Coping, Readiness for enhanced
Conflict, Decisional (specify)
Conflict, Parental role
Denial, Ineffective
Dentition, Impaired
Development, Risk for delayed
Diarrhea
Disuse syndrome, Risk for
Diversional activity, Deficient
Dysreflexia, Autonomic
Energy field, Disturbed
Environmental interpretation syndrome, Impaired
Failure to thrive, Adult
Falls, Risk for
Family processes, Dysfunctional: Alcoholism

Family processes, Interrupted
Family processes, Readiness for enhanced
Fatigue
Fear
Fluid balance, Readiness for enhanced
Fluid volume, Deficient
Fluid volume, Excess
Fluid volume, Risk for deficient
Fluid volume, Risk for imbalanced
Gas exchange, Impaired
Grieving, Anticipatory
Grieving, Dysfunctional
Growth and development, Delayed
Growth, Risk for disproportionate
Health maintenance, Ineffective
Health-seeking behaviors (specify)
Home maintenance, Impaired
Hopelessness
Hyperthermia
Hypothermia
Identity, Disturbed personal
Incontinence, Functional urinary
Incontinence, Reflex urinary
Incontinence, Stress urinary
Incontinence, Total urinary
Incontinence, Urge urinary
Incontinence, Urge urinary, Risk for
Infant behavior, Disorganized
Infant behavior, Readiness for enhanced organized
Infant behavior, Risk for disorganized
Infant feeding pattern, Ineffective
Infection, Risk for
Injury, Perioperative positioning, Risk for
Injury, Risk for
Intracranial adaptive capacity, Decreased
Knowledge, Deficient
Knowledge, Readiness for enhanced (specify)
Loneliness, Risk for
Memory, Impaired
Mobility, Impaired bed
Mobility, Impaired physical
Mobility, Impaired wheelchair
Nausea
Noncompliance (specify)
Nutrition, Imbalanced:
    Less than body requirements

Nutrition, Imbalanced: More than body requirements

Nutrition, Imbalance: More than body requirements, Risk for

Nutrition, Readiness for enhanced

Oral mucous membrane, Impaired

Pain, Acute

Pain, Chronic

Parent/infant/child attachment, Risk for impaired

Parenting, Impaired

Parenting, Impaired, Risk for

Parenting, Readiness for enhanced

Peripheral neurovascular dysfunction, Risk for

Poisoning, Risk for

Post-trauma syndrome

Post-trauma syndrome, Risk for

Powerlessness

Powerlessness, Risk for

Protection, Ineffective

Rape-trauma syndrome

Rape-trauma syndrome, Compound reaction

Rape-trauma syndrome, Silent reaction

Relocation stress syndrome

Relocation stress syndrome, Risk for

Role performance, Ineffective

Self-care deficit, Bathing/hygiene

Self-care deficit, Dressing/grooming

Self-care deficit, Feeding

Self-care deficit, Toileting

Self-concept, Readiness for enhanced

Self-esteem, Low, Chronic

Self-esteem, Low, Situational

Self-esteem, Low, Situational, Risk for

Self-mutilation

Self-mutilation, Risk for

Sensory perception, Disturbed (specify: visual, auditory, kinesthetic, gustatory, tactile, olfactory)

Sexual dysfunction

Sexuality patterns, Ineffective

Skin integrity, Impaired

Skin integrity, Impaired, Risk for

Sleep deprivation

Sleep pattern, Disturbed

Sleep, Readiness for enhanced

Social interaction, Impaired

Social isolation

Sorrow, Chronic

Spiritual distress

Spiritual distress, Risk for

Spiritual well-being, Readiness for enhanced

Sudden infant death syndrome, Risk for

Suffocation, Risk for

Suicide, Risk for

Surgical recovery, Delayed

Swallowing, Impaired

Therapeutic regimen management, Effective

Therapeutic regimen management, Ineffective

Therapeutic regimen management, Ineffective community

Therapeutic regimen management, Ineffective family

Therapeutic regimen management, Readiness for enhanced

Thermoregulation, Ineffective

Thought process, Disturbed

Tissue integrity, Impaired

Tissue perfusion, Ineffective (specify type: renal, cerebral, cardiopulmonary, gastrointestinal, peripheral)

Transfer ability, Impaired

Trauma, Risk for

Neglect, unilateral

Urinary elimination, Impaired

Urinary elimination, Readiness for enhanced

Urinary retention

Ventilation, Impaired spontaneous

Ventilatory weaning response, Dysfunctional

Violence, Risk for other-directed

Violence, Risk for self-directed

Walking, Impaired

Wandering

Source: North American Nursing Diagnosis Association. (2003). *Nursing Diagnoses: Definitions and Classifications, 2003–2004.* Philadelphia: Author.

### Symbols

| | | | |
|---|---|---|---|
| ~ | similar | > | greater than |
| ≅ | approximately | < | less than |
| @ | at | % | percent |
| √ | check | + | positive |
| Δ | change | − | negative |
| ↑ | increased | ♀ | female |
| ↓ | decreased | ♂ | male |
| = | equals | △₁△₂△₃ | trimester of pregnancy (one |
| # | pounds | | triangle for each trimester) |

### Abbreviations

| | | | |
|---|---|---|---|
| 2,3-DPG | 2,3-diphosphoglycerate | APN | advanced practice nurse |
| AACN | American Association of Colleges of Nursing | APRN | advanced practice registered nurse |
| AAOHN | American Association of Occupational Health Nurses | APTT | activated partial thromboplastin time |
| AARP | American Association of Retired Persons | AST | aspartate aminotransferase |
| | | AT | axillary temperature |
| ABG | arterial blood gases | ATP | adenosine triphosphate |
| A/C | alternative/complementary | ATSDR | Agency for Toxic Substances and Disease Registry |
| Acetyl-CoA | acetyl coenzyme A | | |
| ADA | Americans with Disabilities Act | BCR | bulbocavernosus reflex |
| ADAMHA | Alcohol, Drug Abuse, and Mental Health Administration | BMI | body mass index |
| | | BMR | basal metabolic rate |
| ADH | antidiuretic hormone | BN | bachelor's degree in nursing |
| ADL | activities of daily living | BP | blood pressure |
| ADP | adenosine diphosphate | BScN | bachelor of science in nursing (in Canada) |
| ADR | adverse drug reactions | | |
| AEB | as evidenced by | BSE | breast self-examination |
| AGF | angiogenesis factor | BSN | bachelor of science in nursing |
| AHA | American Hospital Association | BUN | blood urea nitrogen |
| AHNA | American Holistic Nurses Association | C | Celsius; also called centigrade |
| | | CAT | computerized adaptive testing |
| AHRQ | Agency for Health Care Research and Policy | CAUSN | Canadian Association of University Schools of Nursing |
| AIDS | acquired immunodeficiency syndrome | CBC | complete blood count |
| | | CBE | charting by exception |
| AJN | *American Journal of Nursing* | CDC | Centers for Disease Control and Prevention |
| AMB | as manifested by | | |
| ANA | American Nurses Association | CEUs | continuing education units |
| ANS | autonomic nervous system | CHD | coronary heart disease |
| AONE | Association of Nurse Executives | CLIA | Clinical Laboratory Improvement Act |
| AORN | Association for Operating Room Nurses | | |
| | | cm | centimeter |

| | | | |
|---|---|---|---|
| CMS | Centers for Medicare & Medicaid Services | GNP | gross national product |
| CNA | Canadian Nurses Association | HBD | alpha-hydroxybutyrate dehydrogenase |
| CNATS | Canadian Nurses Association Testing Service | HBV | hepatitis B virus |
| | | HCFA | Health Care Financing Administration |
| CNM | certified nurse midwife | | |
| CNO | community nursing organization | Hct | hematocrit |
| CNS | central nervous system | HDL | high-density lipoprotein |
| CNS | clinical nurse specialist | HEPA | high-efficiency particulate air |
| $CO_2$ | carbon dioxide | Hgb | hemoglobin |
| COBRA | Consolidated Omnibus Budget Reconciliation Act | HIS | hospital information system |
| | | HIV | human immunodeficiency virus |
| COPD | chronic obstructive pulmonary disease | HMO | health maintenance organization |
| | | HPN | home parenteral nutrition |
| CPK | creatine phosphokinase | HQIA | Healthcare Quality Improvement Act |
| CPM | continuous passive motion | | |
| CPN | central parenteral nutrition | HRSA | Health Resources and Services Administration |
| CPR | cardiopulmonary resuscitation | | |
| CPT | chest physiotherapy | HSV-2 | herpes simplex virus 2 |
| CQI | continuous quality improvement | HT | healing touch |
| CRNA | certified registered nurse anesthetist | IHS | Indian Health Service |
| | | IM | intramuscular |
| CSF | cerebrospinal fluid | in | inch |
| CST | computerized clinical simulation testing | I&O | intake and output |
| | | IOM | Institute on Medicine |
| CT | computed tomography | IPPB | intermittent positive-pressure breathing |
| CVA | cerebral vascular accident | | |
| DDS | doctor of dental science | IRA | individual retirement account |
| DHHS | Department of Health and Human Services | IV | intravenous |
| | | IVP | intravenous pyelogram |
| dl | deciliter | JCAHO | Joint Commission on Accreditation of Healthcare Organizations |
| DNR | do not resuscitate | | |
| DNSc | doctorate of nursing in science | kcal | kilocalorie |
| DRGs | diagnosis-related groups | kg | kilogram |
| DSN | doctorate of science in nursing | LAS | localized adaptation syndrome |
| DUS | Doppler ultrasound stethoscope | lb | pound |
| DVT | deep vein thrombosis | LDH | lactic dehydrogenase |
| ECG | electrocardiogram (also known as an EKG) | LDL | low-density lipoprotein |
| | | LLQ | left lower quadrant |
| EEG | electroencephalogram | LOC | level of consciousness |
| EN | enteral nutrition | LPN | licensed practical nurse |
| EPA | Environmental Protection Agency | LUQ | left upper quadrant |
| EPO | exclusive provider organization | LVN | licensed vocational nurse |
| ESR | erythrocyte sedimentation rate | m | meter |
| ET | ear canal temperature | MA | master of arts degree |
| F | Fahrenheit | MAC | mid-upper-arm circumference |
| FAF | fibroblase activating factor | MAR | medication administration record |
| FAS | fetal alcohol syndrome | MD | doctor of medicine |
| FDA | Food and Drug Administration | MDR | multi-drug-resistant |
| $FiO_2$ | fraction of inspired oxygen | mEq | milliequivalent |
| ft | feet | mEq/L | milliequivalent per liter |
| g | gram | mg | milligram |
| GAS | general adaptation syndrome | MH | malignant hyperthermia |
| GCS | Glasgow Coma Scale | MI | myocardial infarction |
| gH | drop | ml | milliliter; also abbreviated mL |
| GI | gastrointestinal tract | mm | millimeter |

| | | | |
|---|---|---|---|
| mm Hg | millimeters of mercury | PC | potential complication |
| MN | master's degree in nursing | PCA | patient-controlled analgesia |
| mOsm | milliosmole; also spelled milliosmol | $PCO_2$ | partial pressure of carbon dioxide dissolved in arterial blood plasma |
| mOsm/L | milliosmole per liter | PCP | primary care provider |
| MRI | magnetic resonance imaging | PEG | percutaneous endoscopic gastrostomy |
| MRSA | methicillin-resistant *Staphylococcus aureus* | PERRLA | pupils equal, round, reactive to light, and accommodation |
| MSN | master of science in nursing | | |
| NACGN | National Association of Colored Graduate Nurses | pH | hydrogen ion concentration of a solution |
| NANDA | North American Nursing Diagnosis Association | PID | pelvic inflammatory disease |
| | | PIE | problem, intervention, evaluation |
| NCEP | National Cholesterol Education Program | PIEE | pulsed irrigation enhanced evacuation |
| NCLEX | National Council Licensing Examination | PKU | phenylketonuria |
| | | PMR | progressive muscle relaxation |
| NCLEX-PN | National Council Licensure Examination for Practical Nurses | PMS | premenstrual syndrome |
| | | PN | parenteral nutrition |
| NCLEX-RN | National Council Licensure Examination for Registered Nurses | PNI | psychoneuroimmunology |
| | | PNS | peripheral nervous system |
| NCNR | National Center for Nursing Research | PO | *per os* (by mouth) |
| | | POMR | problem-oriented medical record |
| NCSBN | National Council of State Boards of Nursing | POR | problem-oriented record |
| | | PPN | peripheral parenteral nutrition |
| NIC | Nursing Interventions Classification | PPO | preferred provider organization |
| | | PPS | prospective payment system |
| NIH | National Institutes of Health | prn | *pro re nata* (as needed) |
| NINR | National Institute of Nursing Research | PRO | peer review organization |
| | | PSRO | professional standards review organization |
| NLN | National League for Nursing | | |
| NMDS | Nursing Minimum Data Set | PT | physical therapist |
| NP | nurse practitioner | PT | prothrombin |
| NPO | *non per os* (nothing by mouth— to eat or drink) | PT | prothrombin time |
| | | PTSD | post-traumatic stress disorder |
| NS | nutrition support | PTT | partial thromboplastin |
| NST | nutritional support team | PURT | prompted urge response toileting |
| OAM | Office of Alternative Medicine | q | every |
| OBRA | Omnibus Budget Reconciliation Act | QA | quality assurance |
| | | R | respiration |
| OR | operative room | RAS | reticular activating system |
| OSHA | Occupational Safety and Health Administration | RBC | red blood cell |
| | | RD | registered dietitian |
| OT | occupational therapist | RDA | recommended dietary allowance |
| OT | oral temperature | RDDA | recommended daily dietary allowances |
| OTC | over-the-counter drugs | | |
| oz | ounce | RHC | Rural Health Clinic |
| P | pulse | RLQ | right lower quadrant |
| $PO_2$ | partial pressure of oxygen in a mixture of gasses, or in solution | RN | registered nurse |
| | | RNA | registered nurse's assistant |
| $PO_2$ | partial pressures of oxygen | ROM | range-of-motion |
| PA | physician's assistant | RPCH | rural primary care hospital |
| $PaO_2$ ($PAO_2$) | partial pressure of oxygen dissolved in arterial blood plasma | RPh | registered pharmacist |
| | | RT | rectal temperature |
| PAP | Papanicolaou test | RT | related to |
| PAT | pulmonary artery temperature | RT | respiratory therapist |

| | | | |
|---|---|---|---|
| RUQ | right upper quadrant | SUI | stress urinary incontinence |
| S-CDTN | Self-Care Deficit Theory of Nursing | SW | social worker |
| | | T | temperature |
| SA | sinoatrial node | TEFRA | Tax Equity Fiscal Responsibility Act |
| SAECG | signal-averaged electrocardiography | TENS | transcutaneous electrical nerve stimulation |
| SaO$_2$ | percent saturation of arterial blood (hemoglobin) with oxygen | TMJ | temporomandibular joint |
| SBC | school-based clinic | TNA | total nutrient admixture |
| SI | le Système International d'Unités (the international system of units) | TPN | total parenteral nutrition |
| | | TQM | total quality management |
| SL | sublingual | TSE | testicular self-examination |
| SLT | social learning theory | TT | therapeutic touch |
| SMDA | Safe Medical Devices Act | UAP | unlicensed assistive personnel |
| SMI | sustained maximum inspiration | UHDDS | uniform hospital discharge data set |
| SO | source-oriented charting | USPHS | United States Public Health Service |
| SOAP | Subjective data, Objective data, Assessment, Plan | VA | Veterans Affairs |
| | | VLDL | very low density lipoprotein |
| SOAPIE | Subjective data, Objective data, Assessment, Plan, Implementation, Evaluation | V/Q | ventilation/perfusion mismatch |
| | | VRE | vancomycin-resistant enterococci |
| | | WBC | white blood cell |
| STD | sexually transmitted disease | WIC | Women, Infants, and Children |

| Category | Age (yr) or Condition | Weight[b] (kg) | (lb) | Height[b] (cm) | (in) | KCal per Day | Protein (g) | Fat-Soluble Vitamins Vitamin A (µg RE)[c] | Vitamin D (µg)[d] | Vitamin E (µg α-TE)[e] | Vitamin K (µc) |
|---|---|---|---|---|---|---|---|---|---|---|---|
| Infants | 0.0–0.5 | 6 | 13 | 60 | 24 | 650 | 13 | 375 | 7.5 | 3 | 5 |
| | 0.5–1.0 | 9 | 20 | 71 | 28 | 850 | 14 | 375 | 10 | 4 | 10 |
| Children | 1–3 | 13 | 29 | 90 | 35 | 1300 | 16 | 400 | 10 | 6 | 15 |
| | 4–6 | 20 | 44 | 112 | 44 | 1800 | 24 | 500 | 10 | 7 | 20 |
| | 7–10 | 28 | 62 | 132 | 52 | 2000 | 28 | 700 | 10 | 7 | 30 |
| Men | 11–14 | 45 | 99 | 157 | 62 | 2500 | 45 | 1000 | 10 | 10 | 45 |
| | 15–18 | 66 | 145 | 176 | 69 | 3000 | 59 | 1000 | 10 | 10 | 65 |
| | 19–24 | 72 | 160 | 177 | 70 | 2900 | 58 | 1000 | 10 | 10 | 70 |
| | 25–50 | 79 | 174 | 176 | 70 | 2900 | 63 | 1000 | 5 | 10 | 80 |
| | Over 51 | 77 | 170 | 173 | 68 | 2300 | 63 | 1000 | 5 | 10 | 80 |
| Women | 11–14 | 46 | 101 | 157 | 62 | 2200 | 46 | 800 | 10 | 8 | 45 |
| | 15–18 | 55 | 120 | 163 | 64 | 2200 | 44 | 800 | 10 | 8 | 55 |
| | 19–24 | 58 | 128 | 164 | 65 | 2200 | 46 | 800 | 10 | 8 | 60 |
| | 25–50 | 63 | 138 | 163 | 64 | 2200 | 50 | 800 | 5 | 8 | 65 |
| | Over 51 | 65 | 143 | 160 | 63 | 1900 | 50 | 800 | 5 | 8 | 65 |
| Pregnant/ Lactating: | | | | | | 2200 | 60 | 800 | 10 | 10 | 65 |
| | 1st 6 mo | | | | | 2700 | 65 | 1300 | 10 | 12 | 65 |
| | 2nd 6 mo | | | | | 2700 | 62 | 1200 | 10 | 11 | 65 |

*(continues)*

| Water-Soluble Vitamins | | | | | | | Minerals | | | | | | |
|---|---|---|---|---|---|---|---|---|---|---|---|---|---|
| Vita-<br>min C<br>(mg) | Thia-<br>min<br>(mg) | Ribo-<br>flavin<br>(mg) | Niacin<br>(mg<br>NE)[f] | Vita-<br>min B$_6$<br>(mg) | Fo-<br>late<br>(µg) | Vita-<br>min B$_{12}$<br>(µg) | Cal-<br>cium<br>(mg) | Phos-<br>phorus<br>(mg) | Mag-<br>nesium<br>(mg) | Iron<br>(mg) | Zinc<br>(mg) | Iodine<br>(µg) | Sele-<br>nium<br>(µg) |
| 30 | 0.3 | 0.4 | 5 | 0.3 | 25 | 0.3 | 400 | 300 | 40 | 6 | 5 | 40 | 10 |
| 35 | 0.4 | 0.5 | 6 | 0.6 | 35 | 0.5 | 600 | 500 | 60 | 10 | 5 | 50 | 15 |
| 40 | 0.7 | 0.8 | 9 | 1.0 | 50 | 0.7 | 800 | 800 | 80 | 10 | 10 | 70 | 20 |
| 45 | 0.9 | 1.1 | 12 | 1.1 | 75 | 1.0 | 800 | 800 | 120 | 10 | 10 | 90 | 20 |
| 45 | 1.0 | 1.2 | 13 | 1.4 | 100 | 1.4 | 800 | 800 | 170 | 10 | 10 | 120 | 20 |
| 50 | 1.3 | 1.5 | 17 | 1.7 | 150 | 2.0 | 1200 | 1200 | 270 | 12 | 15 | 150 | 40 |
| 60 | 1.5 | 1.8 | 20 | 2.0 | 200 | 2.0 | 1200 | 1200 | 400 | 12 | 15 | 150 | 50 |
| 60 | 1.5 | 1.7 | 29 | 2.0 | 200 | 2.0 | 1200 | 1200 | 350 | 10 | 15 | 150 | 70 |
| 60 | 1.5 | 1.7 | 19 | 2.0 | 200 | 2.0 | 800 | 800 | 350 | 10 | 15 | 150 | 70 |
| 60 | 1.2 | 1.4 | 15 | 2.0 | 200 | 2.0 | 800 | 800 | 350 | 10 | 15 | 150 | 70 |
| 50 | 1.1 | 1.3 | 15 | 1.4 | 150 | 2.0 | 1200 | 1200 | 280 | 15 | 12 | 150 | 45 |
| 60 | 1.1 | 1.3 | 15 | 1.5 | 180 | 2.0 | 1200 | 1200 | 300 | 15 | 12 | 150 | 50 |
| 60 | 1.1 | 1.3 | 15 | 1.6 | 180 | 2.0 | 1200 | 1200 | 280 | 15 | 12 | 150 | 55 |
| 60 | 1.1 | 1.3 | 15 | 1.6 | 180 | 2.0 | 800 | 800 | 280 | 15 | 12 | 150 | 55 |
| 60 | 1.0 | 1.3 | 13 | 1.6 | 180 | 2.0 | 800 | 800 | 280 | 10 | 12 | 150 | 55 |
| 70 | 1.5 | 1.6 | 17 | 2.2 | 400 | 2.2 | 1200 | 1200 | 320 | 30 | 15 | 175 | 65 |
| 95 | 1.6 | 1.8 | 20 | 2.1 | 280 | 2.6 | 1200 | 1200 | 355 | 15 | 19 | 200 | 75 |
| 90 | 1.6 | 1.7 | 20 | 2.1 | 260 | 2.6 | 1200 | 1200 | 340 | 15 | 16 | 200 | 75 |

[a] The allowances, expressed as average daily intakes over time, are intended to provide for individual variations among most normal persons as they live in the United States under usual environmental stresses. Diets should be based on a variety of common foods to provide other nutrients for which human requirements have been less well defined.

[b] Weights and heights of Reference Adults are actual medians for the U.S. population of the designated age.

[c] Retinol equivalents. 1 RE = 1 µg retinol or 6 µg b-carotene.

[d] As cholecalciferol. 10 mg cholecalciferol = 400 U of vitamin D.

[e] Tocopherol equivalents. 1 mg d-a-tocopherol = 1 α-TE.

[f] Ne Niacin equivalent = 1 mg of niacin or 60 mg of dietary tryptophan.

Source: Reprinted with permission from *Recommended Dietary Allowances*, 10th edition. Copyright 1989 by the National Academy of Sciences. Courtesy of the National Academy Press, Washington, DC.

| Laboratory Tests | Conventional Units | SI Units |
|---|---|---|
| Acid hemolysis | No hemolysis | No hemolysis |
| Alkaline phosphatase | 14–100 | 14–100 |
| Cell counts | | |
|   Erythrocytes | | |
|     Male | 4.6–6.2 million/mm$^3$ | 4.6–6.2 $\times$ 10$^{12}$/L |
|     Female | 4.2–5.4 million/mm$^3$ | 4.2–5.4 $\times$ 10$^{12}$/L |
|     Children (varies with age) | 4.5–5.1 million/mm$^3$ | 4.5–5.1 $\times$ 10$^{12}$/L |
| Leukocytes, total | 4,500–11,000 /mm$^3$ | |
| Leukocytes, differential counts | | |
|   Myelocytes | 0% | 0/L |
|   Band neutrophils | 3–5% | 150–400 $\times$ 10$^6$/L |
|   Segmented neutrophils | 54–62% | 3,000–5.800 $\times$ 10$^6$/L |
|   Lymphocytes | 25–33% | 1,500–3,000 $\times$ 10$^6$/L |
|   Monocytes | 3–7% | 300–500 $\times$ 10$^6$/L |
|   Eosinophils | 1–3% | 50–250 $\times$ 10$^6$/L |
|   Basophils | 0–1% | 15–50 $\times$ 10$^6$/L |
| Platelets | 150,000–400,000/mm$^3$ | 150–400 $\times$ 10$^9$/L |
| Reticulocytes | 25,000–75,000/mm$^3$ | 25–75 $\times$ 10$^9$/L |
| Coagulation tests | | |
|   Bleeding time | 2.75–8.0 min | 2.75–8.0 min |
|   Coagulation time | 5–15 min | 5–15 min |
|   D-dimer | < 0.5 µg/mL | < 0.5 mg/L |
|   Factor VIII and other coagulation factors | 50–150 of normal | 0.5–1.5 of normal |
|   Fibrin split products | < 10 µg/mL | < 10 mg/L |
|   Fibrinogen | 200–400 mg/dL | 2.0–4.0 g/L |
|   Partial thromboplastin time (PTT) | 20–35 sec | 20–35 sec |
|   Prothrombin time (PT) | 12.0–14.0 sec | 12.0–14.0 sec |
| Coombs' test | | |
|   Direct | Negative | |
|   Indirect | Negative | |

*(continues)*

| Laboratory Tests | Conventional Units | SI Units |
| --- | --- | --- |
| Corpuscular values of erythrocytes | | |
| Mean corpuscular hemoglobin | 26–34 pg/cell | 26–34 pg/cell |
| Mean corpuscular volume | 80–96 $\mu m^3$ | 80–96 fL |
| Mean corpuscular hemoglobin concentration (MCHC) | 32–36 g/dL | 320–360 g/L |
| Haptoglobin | 20–165 mg/dL | 0.20–1.65 g/L |
| Hematocrit | | |
| Male | 40–54 mL/dL | 0.40–0.54 |
| Female | 37–47 mL/dL | 0.37–0.47 |
| Newborn | 49–54 mL/dL | 0.49–0.54 |
| Children (varies with age) | 35–49 mL/dL | 0.35–0.49 |
| Hemoglobin | | |
| Male | 13.0–18.0 g/dL | 8.1–11.2 mmol/L |
| Female | 12.0–16.0 g/dL | 7.4–9.9 mmol/L |
| Newborn | 16.5–19.5 g/dL | 10.2–12.1 mmol/L |
| Children (varies with age) | 11.2–16.5 g/dL | 7.0–10.2 mmol/L |
| Hemoglobin, fetal | < 1.0% of total | < 0.01 of total |
| Hemoglobin A1C | 3–5% of total | 0.03–0.05 of total |
| Hemoglobin A2 | 1.5–3.0% of total | 0.015–0.03 of total |
| Hemoglobin, plasma | 0.0–5.0 mg/dL | 0.0–3.2 $\mu$mol/L |
| Methemoglobin | 30–130 mg/dL | 19–80 $\mu$mol/L |
| Erythrocyte sedimentation rate (ESR) | | |
| Wintrobe | | |
| Male | 0–5 mm/hr | 0–5 mm/h |
| Female | 0–55 mm/hr | 0–15 mm/h |
| Westergren | | |
| Male | 0–15 mm/hr | 0–15 mm/h |
| Female | 0–20 mm/hr | 0–20 mm/h |

Being able to say a few words or phrases in the client's language is one way to show that you care. It lets the client know that you as a nurse are interested in the individual. There are three rules to keep in mind regarding the pronunciation of Spanish words.

- If a word ends in a vowel, or in *n* or *s,* the accent is on the next to the last syllable.
- If the word ends in a consonant other than *n* or *s,* the accent is on the last syllable.
- If the word does not follow these rules, it has a written accent over the vowel of the accented syllable.

Courtesy phrases, names of body parts, and expressions of time and numbers are included in this section for quick reference. The English version will appear first, followed by the Spanish translation and Spanish pronunciation.

## Courtesy Phrases

| | | |
|---|---|---|
| Please | Por favor | Por-fah-**vor** |
| Thank you | Grácias | **Grah**-the-as |
| Good morning | Buénos dias | Boo-**ay**-nos **dee**-as |
| Good afternoon | Buénas tardes | Boo-**ay**-nas **tar**-days |
| Good evening | Buénas noches | Boo-**ay**-nas **no**-chays |
| Yes/No | Si/No | See/No |
| Good | Bien | Be-en |
| Bad | Mal | Mahl |
| How many? | Cuántos? | Coo-**ahn**-tos? |
| Where? | Dónde? | **Don**-day? |
| When? | Cuándo? | Coo-**ahn**-do? |

## Body Parts

| | | |
|---|---|---|
| abdomen | el abdomen | el ab-doh-men |
| ankle | el tobillo | el to-**beel**-lyo |
| anus | el ano | el **ah**-no |
| anvil (incus) | el yunque | el **yoon**-kay |
| appendix | el apéndice | el ah-**pen**-de-thay |
| aqueous humor | el humor acuoso | el oo-**mor** ah-coo-**o**-so |
| bladder | la vejiga | lah vah-**nee**-gah |
| brain | el cerebro | el thay-**ray**-bro |
| breast | el pecho | el **pay**-cho |
| buttock | la nalga | lah **nahl**-gah |
| calf | la pantorrilla | lah pan-tor-**reel**-lyah |
| cervix | la cerviz | lah ther-**veth** |
| cheek | la mejilla | lah mah-**heel**-lyah |
| chin | la barbilla | lah bar-**beel**-lyah |
| choroid | la coroidea | lah co-ro-e-**day**-ah |
| ciliary body | el cuerpo ciliar | el coo-**err**-po the-le-**ar** |
| clitoris | el clitoris | el **clee**-to-ris |
| coccyx | el coxis | el **coc**-sees |
| conjunctiva | la conjuntiva | lah con-hoon-**tee**-vah |

| cornea | la córnea | lah **cor**-nay-ah |
|---|---|---|
| penis | el pene | el **pay**-nay |
| prostate gland | la próstata | lah **pros**-ta-tah |
| pupil | la pupila | lah poo-**pee**-lah |
| rectum | el recto | el **rec**-to |
| retina | la retina | lah ray-**tee**-nah |
| sclera | la esclerótica | lah es-clay-**ro**-te-cah |
| scrotum | el escroto | el es-**cro**-to |
| seminal vesicle | la vesícula seminal | lah vay-**see**-coo-lah say-me-**nahl** |
| shoulder | el hombro | el **om**-bro |
| small intestine | el intestino delgado | el in-tes-**tee**-no del-**gah**-do |
| spinal cord | la médula espinal | lah **may**-doo-lah es-pe-**nahl** |
| spleen | el bazo | el **bah**-tho |
| stirrup (stapes) | el estribo | el es-**tree**-bo |
| stomach | el estómago | el es-**toh**-mah-go |
| temple | la sien | lah se-**ayn** |
| testis | el testículo | el tes-**tee**-coo-lo |
| thigh | el muslo | el **moos**-lo |
| thorax | el tórax | el **to**-rax |
| tongue | la lengua | lah **len**-goo-ah |
| trachea | la tráquea | lah **trah**-kay-ah |
| upper extremities | las extremidades superiores | las ex-tray-me-**dahd**-es soo-pay-re-**or**-es |
| ureter | el uréter | el oo-**ray**-ter |
| uterus | el útero | el **oo**-tay-ro |
| vagina | el vagina | lah vah-**hee**-nah |
| vitreous humor | el humor vítreo | el oo-**mor vee**-tray-o |
| wrist | la muñeca | lah moo-**nyay**-cah |

## Expressions of Time, Calendar, and Numbers

| after meals | después de comer | des-poo-**es** day co-**merr** |
|---|---|---|
| at bedtime | al acostarse | al ah-cos-**tar**-say |
| before meals | antes de comer | **ahn**-tes day co-**merr** |
| daily | el diario | el de-**ah**-re-o |
| date | la fecha | lah **fay**-chah |
| day | el dia | el **dee**-ah |
| every hour | a cada hora | ah **cah**-dah **o**-rah |
| hour (time) | la hora | lah **o**-rah |
| how often | cada cuánto tiempo | **cah**-dah coo-**ahn**-to te-**em**-po |
| noon | el mediodia | el may-de-o-**dee**-ah |
| now | ahora | ah-**o**-rah |
| once | una vez | **oo**-nah veth |
| today | hoy | **oh**-e |
| tomorrow | mañana | mah-**nyah**-nah |
| tonight | esta noche | **es**-tah **no**-chay |
| week | la semana | lah say-**mah**-nah |
| year | año | **a**-nyo |
| Sunday | el domingo | el do-**meen**-go |
| Monday | el lunes | el **loo**-nes |
| Tuesday | el martes | el **mar**-tes |
| Wednesday | el miércoles | el me-**err**-co-les |
| Thursday | el jueves | el hoo-**ay**-ves |
| Friday | el viernes | el ve-**err**-nes |
| Saturday | el sábado | el **sah**-bah-do |
| zero | cero | **thay**-ro |
| one | uno | **oo**-no |

| | | |
|---|---|---|
| two | dos | dose |
| three | tres | trays |
| four | cuatro | coo-**ah**-tro |
| five | cinco | **theen**-co |
| six | seis | **say**-ees |
| seven | siete | se-**ay**-tay |
| eight | ocho | **o**-cho |
| nine | nueve | noo-**ay**-vay |
| ten | diez | de-**eth** |

## Nursing Care Sentences and Questions

What is your name?
¿Como se llama usted?
¿**Co**-mo say **lyah**-mah oos-**ted?**

I am a student nurse.
Soy estudiente enfermera(o).
Soy es-too-de-**ahn**-tay en-fer-**may**-ra(o).

My name is . . .
Mi nombre es . . .
Mee **nom**-bray es . . .

Do you need a wheelchair?
¿Necesita usted una silla de rueda?
¿Nay-thay-**se**-ta oos-**ted oo**-nah **seel**-lyah day roo-**ay**-dah?

How do you feel?
¿Como se siente?
¿**Co**-mo say se-**ayn**-tah?

When is your family coming?
¿Cuándo viene su familia?
¿Coo-**ahn**-do vee-**en**-nah soo fah-**mee**-le-ah?

This is the call light.
Esta es la luz para llamar a la enfermera.
**Es**-tah es lah looth **pay**-ra lyah-**mar** a lah en-fer-**may**-ra.

If you need anything, press the button.
Si usted necesita algo, oprima el botón.
See oos-**ted** nay-thay-**se**-ta **ahl**go o-pre-**ma** el bo-**tone.**

Do not turn without calling the nurse.
No se voltee sin llamar a la enfermera.
No say **vol**-tay seen lyah-**mar** a lah en-fer-**may**-ra.

The side rails on your bed are for your protection.
Los rieles del costado están para su protección.
Los re-**el**-es del cos-**tah**-do es-**tahn pah**-ra soo pro-tec-the-**on.**

Please do not try to lower or climb over the side rail.
Por favor no pretenda bajarlos (barjarlas) o treparse sobre ellos.
Por fah-**vor** no pray-**ten**-dah ba-**har**-los o tray-**par**-say **so**-bray **ayl**-lyos.

The head nurse is . . .
La jefa de enfermeras es . . .
La **hay**-fay day en-fer-**may**-ras es . . .

Do you need more blankets or another pillow?
¿Necesita usted más frazadas u orta almohada?
¿Nay-thay-**si**-ta oos-**ted** mahs frah-**thad**-dahs oo **o**-trah al-mo-**ah**-dah?

You may not smoke in the room.
No se puede fumar en el cuarto.
No say poo-**ay**-day foo-**mar** en el coo-**ar**-to.

Do you want me to turn on (turn off) the lights?
¿Quiere usted que encienda (apague) la luz?
¿Ke-**ay**-ray oos-**ted** day en-the-**en**-dah (a-**pah**-gay) lah looth?

Are you thirsty?
¿Tiene usted sed?
¿Tee-**en**-nah oos-**ted** sayd?

Are you allergic to any medication?
¿Es usted alérgico(a) a alguna medicina?
¿Es oos-**ted** ah-**lehr**-hee-co(a) ah ah-**goo**-nah nay-de-**thee**-nah?

You may take a bath.
Usted puede bañarse.
Oos-**ted** poo-**ay**-day bah-**nyar**-say.

Do not lock the door, please.
No cierre usted la puerta con llave, por favor.
No the-**err**-ray oos-**ted** lah poo-**err**-tah con **lyah**-vay por-fah-**vor.**

Call if you feel faint or in need of help.
Llame si usted se siente débil o si necesita ayuda.
**Lyah**-mah see oos-**ted** say se-**ayn**-tah **day**-bil o see nay-thay-**se**-ta ah-**yoo**-dah.

Call when you have to go to the toilet.
Llame cuando tenga que ir al inodoro.
**Lyah**-mah coo-**ahn**-do **ten**-gah kay eer al in-o-**do**-ro.

I will give you an enema.
Le pondré una enema.
Lay pon-**dray oo**-nah ay-**nay**-mah.

Turn on your left (right) side.
Voltese a su lado izquierdo (derecho).
Vol-**tay**-say ah soo **lah**-do ith-ke-**er**-do(dah)
    (day-**ray**-cho[cha]).

Here is an appointment card.
Aqui tiene usted una tarjeta con la información escrito.
Ah-**kee** tee-**en**-nah oos-**ted oo**-nah tar-**hay**-tah con lah
    in-for-mah-the-**on** es-**cree**-to.

You are going to be discharged (released) today.
A usted le van a dar de alta hoy.
Ah oos-**ted** lay vahn ah dar day **ahl**-tah **oh**-e.

How did this illness begin?
¿Como empezó esta enfermedad?
¿**Co**-mo em-pa-**tho es**-tah en-fer-may-**dahd**?

Is the pain better after the medicine?
Siente usted alivio depués de tomar la medicina?
¿Se-**ayn**-tah oos-**ted** al-lee-ve-o des-poo-**es** day to-**mar**
    lah may-de-**thee**-nah?

Where is the pain?
¿Que la duele? (or) Dónde le duele?
¿Kay lah doo-**ay**-le? (or) **Don**-day lay doo-**ay**-le?

Do you have pains in your chest?
¿Tiene usted dolores in el pecho?
¿Tee-**en**-nah oos-**ted** do-**lor**-es en el **pay**-cho?

Are you in pain now?
¿Tiene usted dolores ahora?
¿Tee-**en**-nah oos-**ted** do-**lor**-es ah-**o**-rah?

Is it constant pain or does it come and go?
¿Es un dolor constante or va y vuelve?
¿Es oon do-**lor** cons-**tahn**-tay o vah ee voo-**el**-vah?

Is there anything that makes the pain better?
¿Hay algo que lo alivie?
¿**Ah**-ee **ahl**-go kay lo al-**le**-ve?

Is there anything that makes the pain worse?
¿Hay algo que lo aumente?
¿**Ah**-ee **ahl**-go kay lo ah-oo-**men**-tay?

Where do you feel the pain?
¿Dónde siente usted el dolor?
¿**Don**-day se-**ayn**-tah oos-**ted** el do-**lor**?

Point to where it hurts.
Apunte usted por favor, adonde le duele.
Ah-**poon**-tay oos-**ted** por fah-**vor** ah-**don**-day lay doo-**ay**-le.

Show me where it hurts.
Enséñeme usted donde l duele.
En-**say**-nah-may oos-**ted don**-day lay doo-**ay**-le.

Is the pain sharp or dull?
¿Es agudo o sordo el dolor?
¿Es ah-**goo**-do o **sor**-do el do-**lor**?

Do you know where you are?
¿Sabe usted donde esta?
¿Sah-**bay** oos-**ted don**-day es-**tah**?

You are in a hospital.
Usted está en el hospital.
Oos-**ted** es-**tah** en el os-pee-**tahl**.

You will be okay.
Usted va a estar bien.
Oos-**ted** vah a es-**tar be**-en.

Do you have any drug reactions?
¿Tiene usted alguna sensibilidad a productos químicos?
¿Te-**en** nah oos-**ted** al-**goo**-nah sen-se-be-le-**dahd** a
    pro-**dooc**-tos **kee**-me-cos?

Have you seen another doctor or native healer for this
    problem?
¿Ha visto usted a otro médico o curandero tocante a este
    problema?
¿Ah **vees**-to oos-**ted** a **o**-tro **may**-de-co o coo-ran-**day**-ro
    to-**cahn**-tay a **es**-ah pro-**blay**-mah?

Have you vomited?
¿Ha vomitado usted?
¿Ah vo-me-**tah**-do oos-**ted**?

Do you have any difficulty in breathing?
¿Tiene usted alguna dificultad para respirar?
Te-**en**-nah oos-**ted** ah-**goo**-nah de-fe-cool-**tahd pah**-ra
    res-pe-**rar**?

Do you smoke?
¿Fuma usted?
¿Foo-**mar** oos-**ted**?

How many per day?
¿Cuántos al dia?
¿Coo-**ahn**-tos al **dee**-ah?

For how many years?
¿Por cuántos años?
¿Por coo-**ahn**-tos **a**-nos?

Do you awaken in the night because of shortness of breath?
¿Se despierta usted por la noche por falta de respiración?
¿Say des-pee-**err**-tah oos-**ted** por lah **no**-chay por
  **fahl**-tah day res-pe-rah-the-**on**?

Is any part of your body swollen?
¿Tiene usted alguna parte del cuerpo hinchada?
¿Te-**en**-nah oos-**ted** ah-**goo**-nah **par**-tay del coo-**err**-po
  in-**chah**-da?

How much water do you drink daily?
Cuántos vasos de agua bebe usted diariamente?
¿Coo-**ahn**-tos **vah**-sos day **ah**-goo-ah **bay**-be oos-**ted**
  de-ah-re-ah-**men**-tay?

Are you nauseated?
¿Tiene náusea?
¿Te-**en**-nah **nah**-oo-say-ah?

Are you going to vomit?
¿Va a vomitar?
¿Vah a vo-me-**tar**?

When was your last bowel movement?
¿Cuánto tiempo hace que evacúa usted?
¿Coo-**ahn**-to te-**em**-po **ah**-the kay ay-vah-**coo**-ah oos-**ted**?

Do you have diarrhea?
¿Tiene usted diarrea?
¿Te-**en**-nah oos-**ted** der-ar-**ray**-ah?

How much do you urinate?
¿Cuánto orina usted?
¿Coo-**ahn**-to o-**re**-nah oos-**ted**?

Did you urinate?
¿Orino usted?
¿O-re-**no** oos-**ted**?

What color is your urine?
¿De qué color es la orina?
¿Day kay co-**lor** es lah o-**re**-nah?

Call when you have to go to the toilet.
Llame usted cuando tenga que ir al inodoro.
**Lyah**-mah oos-**ted** coo-**ahn**-do **ten**-gah kay eer al
  in-o-**do**-ro.

I need a urine specimen from you.
Necesito una muestra de orina de usted.
Nay-thay-**se**-to **oo**-nah moo-**ays**-trah day o-**re**-nah day
  oos-**ted**.

We will put a tube in your bladder so that you can urinate.
Le pondremos un tubo en la vejiga para que puede orinar.
Lay pon-**dray**-mos un **too**-be en lah vay-**hee**-gah **pah**-rah
  kay poo-**ay**-day o-re **nar**.

When was your last menstrual period?
¿Cuándo fue se última menstruación?
¿Coo-**ahn**-do foo-**ay** soo **ool**-te-mah mens-troo-ah-the-**on**?

Are you bleeding heavily?
¿Está sangrando mucho?
¿Es-tah san-**grahn**-do **moo**-cho?

Take off your clothes, please.
Desvístase usted, por favor.
Des-**ves**-tah-say oos-**ted** por-fah-**vor**.

Just relax.
Relaje usted el cuerpo.
Ray-**lah**-he oos-**ted** el coo-**err**-po.

I am going to listen to your chest.
Voy a escucharle el pecho.
Voye a es-coo-**char**-lay el **pay**-cho.

Let me feel your pulse.
Déjeme tomarle el pulso.
**Day**-ha-me to-**mar**-lay el **pool**-so.

I am going to take your temperature.
Voy a tomarle la temperatura.
Voye a to-**mar**-lay lah tem-pay-rah-**too**-rah.

Lie down, please.
Acuéstese, por favor.
Ah-coo-**es**-tah-say por fah-**vor**.

Do you understand?
¿Me comprende usted?
¿May com-**pren**-day oos-**ted**?

That's right.
Así. Bien.
Ah-**see. Be**-en.

You are doing very well.
Usted va muy bien.
Oos-**ted** vah **moo**-e be-en.

Do not take any medicine from home.
No tome usted ninguna medicina traída de su casa.
No **to**-may oos-**ted** nin-**goon**-ay may-de-**thee**-nah trah-**ee**
  dah day soo **cah**-sah.

I am going to give you an injection.
Voy a ponerle ana inyección.
Voye a po-**nerr**-lay **oo**-nah in-yec-the-**on**.

Take a sip of water.
Tome usted un traguito de agua.
**To**-may oos-**ted** un trah-**gee**-to day **ah**-goo-ah.

Very good. That was fine.
Muy bien. Excelente.
**Moo**-e **be**-en. Ex-thay-**len**-tay.

Don't be nervous.
No se ponga nervioso(a).
No say **pon**-gah ner-ve-**o**-so(ah).

Do you feel dizzy?
¿Se siente vertigo?
¿Say see-**ayn**-tah **verr**-to-go?

Please lie still.
Quédese inmóvil, por favor.
**Kay**-day-say in-**mo**-veel por fah-**vor.**

You must drink lots of liquids.
Usted debe tomar muchos liquidos.
Oos-**ted day**-bay to-**mar moo**-chos **lee**-ke-dos.

## References

Kelz, R. K. (1997). *Conversational Spanish for Health Professionals* (3rd ed.). Clifton Park, NY: Delmar Learning.

Velazquez de la Cadena, M., Gray, E., and Iribas, J. (1985). *New Revised Velazquez Spanish and English Dictionary.* Clinton, N.J.: New Win Publishing, Inc., 1985.

# STANDARD PRECAUTIONS

## FOR INFECTION CONTROL

**Wash Hands** (Plain soap)
Wash after touching **blood, body fluids, secretions, excretions**, and **contaminated items**.
Wash immediately **after gloves are removed** and **between patient contacts**.
Avoid transfer of microorganisms to other patients or environments.

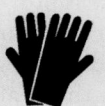

**Wear Gloves**
Wear when touching **blood, body fluids, secretions, excretions**, and **contaminated items**.
Put on **clean** gloves just **before touching mucous membranes** and **nonintact skin**.
Change gloves between tasks and procedures on the same patient after contact with material that may contain high concentrations of microorganisms. Remove gloves promptly after use, before touching noncontaminated items and environmental surfaces, and before going to another patient, and wash hands immediately to avoid transfer of microorganisms to other patients or environments.

**Wear Mask and Eye Protection or Face Shield**
Protect mucous membranes of the eyes, nose and mouth during procedures and patient–care activities that are likely to generate **splashes** or **sprays** of **blood, body fluids, secretions**, or **excretions**.

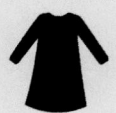

**Wear Gown**
Protect skin and prevent soiling of clothing during procedures that are likely to generate **splashes** or **sprays** of **blood, body fluids, secretions**, or **excretions**. Remove a soiled gown as promptly as possible and wash hands to avoid transfer of microorganisms to other patients or environments.

**Patient-Care Equipment**
Handle used patient–care equipment soiled with **blood, body fluids, secretions**, or **excretions** in a manner that prevents skin and mucous membrane exposures, contamination of clothing, and transfer of microorganisms to other patients and environments. Ensure that reusable equipment is not used for the care of another patient until it has been appropriately cleaned and reprocessed and single use items are properly discarded.

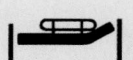

**Environmental Control**
Follow hospital procedures for routine care, cleaning, and disinfection of environmental surfaces, beds, bedrails, bedside equipment and other frequently touched surfaces.

**Linen**
Handle, transport, and process used linen soiled with **blood, body fluids, secretions**, or **excretions** in a manner that prevents exposures and contamination of clothing, and avoids transfer of microorganisms to other patients and environments.

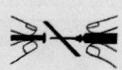

**Occupational Health and Bloodborne Pathogens**
Prevent injuries when using needles, scalpels, and other sharp instruments or devices; when handling sharp instruments after procedures; when cleaning used instruments; and when disposing of used needles.

**Never recap used needles using both hands** or any other technique that involves directing the point of a needle toward any part of the body; rather, use either a one-handed "scoop" technique or a mechanical device designed for holding the needle sheath.

Do not remove used needles from disposable syringes by hand, and do not bend, break, or otherwise manipulate used needles by hand. Place disposable syringes and needles, scalpel blades, and other sharp items in puncture–resistant sharps containers located as close as practical to the area in which the items were used, and place reusable syringes and needles in a puncture–resistant container for transport to the reprocessing area.

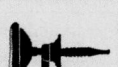

Use **resuscitation devices** as an alternative to mouth–to–mouth resuscitation.

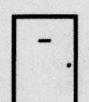

**Patient Placement**
Use a **private room** for a patient who contaminates the environment or who does not (or cannot be expected to) assist in maintaining appropriate hygiene or environmental control. Consult Infection Control if a private room is not available.

The information on this sign is abbreviated from the HICPAC Recommendations for Isolation Precautions in Hospitals.

Form No. **SPR**    BREVIS CORP, 3310 S 2700 E, SLC, UT 84109    © 1996 Brevis Corp.

*Courtesy of the Brevis Corporation*

# APPENDIX G
## Concept Mapping

**C**oncept mapping is the process of analyzing the meaning of interrelationships among several concepts. Concept mapping has many synonyms including cognitive mapping, mind mapping, concept trees, and semantic networking (Beitz, 1998). A **concept map** is a graphic design that provides a visual picture of the analytical thinking process and interpretation of the information (Kathol, Geiger, & Hartig, 1998). The major concept is usually placed in the center of the map. Concepts or words related to the major concept are situated around it in categories or clusters. The concept clusters are linked to the major concept by lines, arrows, or significant words similar to the connecting roads and topographical areas between cities on a geographic map. Concept maps have three characteristics: hierarchical structure, chains or links, and clustering (Bietz, 1998).

The mapping process is associated with problem-solving learning. Educators have found concept mapping to be an innovative teaching method that promotes critical thinking, communication, categorization of information, and self-directed learning. The tool is relatively new to nursing; however, it has been used for several years in a variety of disciplines including education and education psychology, business, medicine, the social sciences, and research (Beitz, 1998; Kathol et al., 1998).

In nursing education, the concept map is primarily used as an alternative to the traditional linear care plan. Visual learners particularly value the map design because it provides a visuo-spatial illustration of patient/client information. Creating the map assists students to gain a holistic perspective of the client, the health problem and all the contributing factors, as well as realizing the implications for each phase of the nursing process (Alexander, McDaniel, Baldwin, & Money, 2002; Mueller, Johnston, & Bligh, 2001; Schuster, 2000; Beitz, 1998; Kathol et al., 1998).

## Creating a Concept Map

Concept maps can be very simple or elaborate and creatively designed, and either handwritten or computer generated. An entire page is used, usually in landscape form. The client's name and the

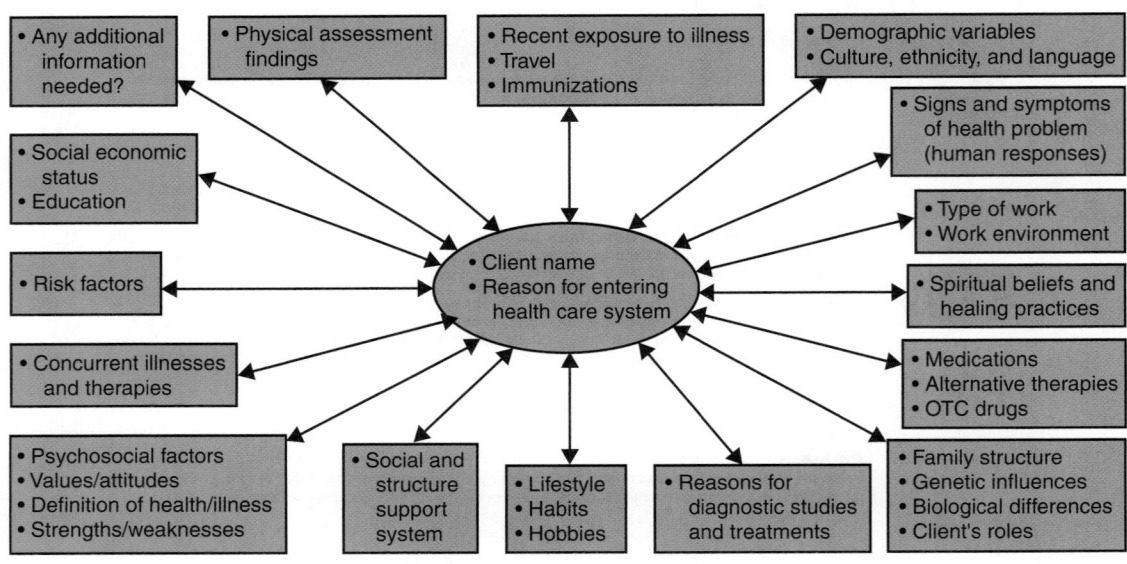

**Figure G-1   Concept Mapping Client Information**

reason for entering the health care system are placed in the center of the diagram. Client information is gathered through assessment, interviews with the client or others, and review of the client's record. The information can be clarified by reviewing texts, professional journal articles, and other literature. All concepts are analyzed for a possible connection to each other. Clusters of similar or related client information are linked to the client according to the best fit envisioned by the mapmaker. As concepts are added, the relationships and links may change (see Figure G-1). Color-coding is often used to sort and categorize the information and to signify priority needs and nursing actions. Arrows identify the direction of the connecting links among the various concepts and the relationship of the client's responses to the health problem (Heinrich, Karner, Gagline, & Lambert, 2002; King & Shell, 2002; Kathol et al., 1998).

Concept mapping also includes the organization of client information within the phases of the nursing process to demonstrate the connections to the plan of care (Figure G-2 is an example). The end product is a unique representation "of an individual's health status as well as those concepts that affect the individual, such as social, cultural, ethnicity, and psychosocial state" (King & Shell, 2002, p. 36). Each map is considered a unique representation of the learner's ability to link theory to clinical practice.

## Preparation for Concept Mapping

Students must have an understanding of the concepts and principles of the life sciences and a working knowledge of the nursing process prior to creating concept maps.

Concept mapping can be introduced by mapping one's plan to visit a specific area or by creating a map of one's personal experiences and their effects on learning. These activities facilitate the transition to using nursing concepts in planning care. Case studies aid students in designing a map that illustrates the connections between clusters of information and selecting appropriate nursing diagnoses, client outcomes, and nursing activities. Other helpful activities are mapping the effects of nursing concepts, such as immobility, oxygenation, pain, or anxiety on a client's systems, and correlating the effects of a medication or therapy to a nursing diagnosis (King & Shell, 2002; Mueller et al., 2001).

## Clinical Application

Students learn the practice of clinical nursing by relating concepts, drawing on past learning and experience, and organizing conceptual meanings that make sense to them (Kathol et al., 1998). A simple, or "micro," map is often used as a worksheet for a clinical day. Throughout the day, the instructor and student can evaluate where new information should be added and where changes need to be made. An updated version of the map is completed following the clinical experience.

## Advantages of Concept Mapping

Concept mapping enhances motivation and facilitates the learning process (Beitz, 1998). Critical thinking skills can be used for developing creative pictorial designs, such as

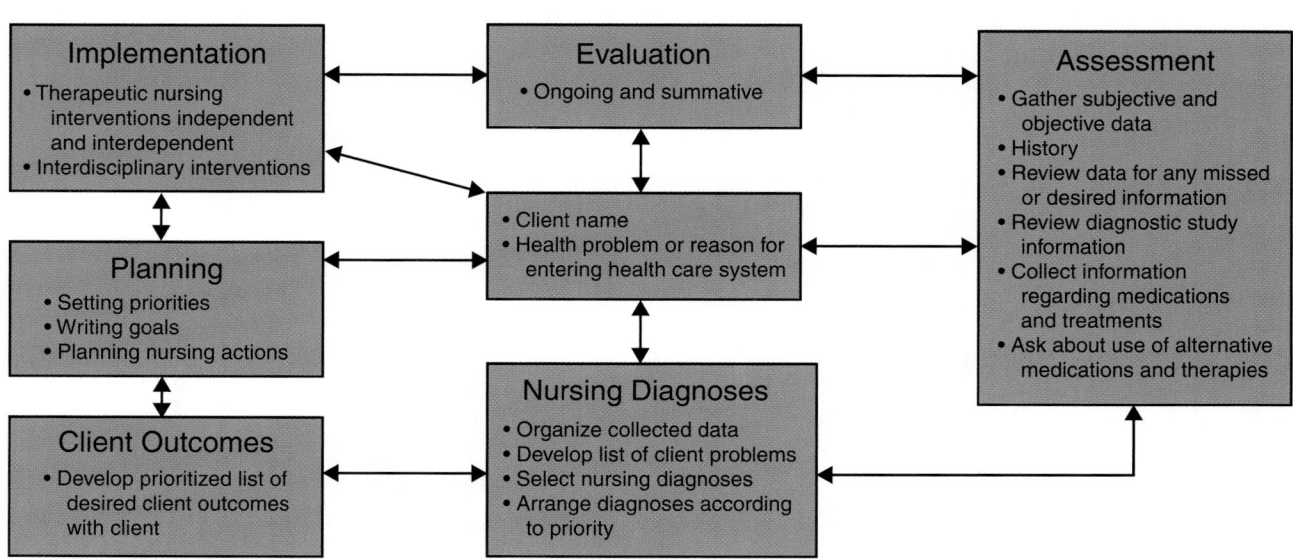

**Figure G-2    Concept Mapping**

placing concepts related to a respiratory problem in a lung-shaped map, inserting client information related to a urinary problem within a kidney shape, or drawing a map of the country of origin for content related to a client from a different culture. Concept mapping can be an individual or group activity in the classroom or clinical settings for short-term or long-term assignments. Simple maps can be expanded throughout the curriculum to include more complex ideas, such as ethical/legal and leadership/management issues. They can also be used as study guides and for evaluation purposes. Concept mapping can be used as a curriculum matrix to track major concepts and themes, thus illustrating to faculty and students how the concepts and subject matter of the various courses are related to each other (Heinrich et al., 2002; Beitz, 1998). It also correlates well with the current emphasis on research and Evidence-Based Practice (King & Shell, 2002; Burns & Grove, 2001).

## Disadvantages of Concept Mapping

Since there are many ways to demonstrate connections between concepts, concept mapping may be difficult for individuals who believe there is only one way. The mapping process may also be challenging for persons who think in a linear manner. Mapping may not be appropriate for all areas of learning. Concept mapping is time consuming; however, computer graphics facilitate the development process. Educators must value its importance and take time to prepare students to use the mapping process.

## Application

Five case studies are included in Chapters 5, 17, 19, 34, and 42 to assist in learning the process of concept mapping. Statements and questions are listed as prompts for developing a concept map. However, the mapmaker is encouraged to be creative!

## References

Alexander, J., McDaniel, G., Baldwin, M., & Money, B. (2002). Promoting, applying, and evaluating problem-based learning in the undergraduate nursing curriculum. *NLN Perspectives, 23*(5), 248–254.

Beitz, J. (1998). Concept mapping: Navigating the learning process. *Nurse Educator, 23*(5), 35–41.

Burns, N., & Grove, S. (2001). Cognitive mapping. In *The practice of nursing research, conduct, critique and utilization* (4th ed.). Philadelphia: W. B. Saunders.

Heinrich, C., Karner, K., Gaglione, B., & Lambert, L. (2002). Order out of chaos: The use of a matrix to validate curriculum integrity. *Nurse Educator, 27*(3), 136–140.

Kathol, D., Geiger, M., & Hartig, J. (1998). Clinical correlation map: A tool for linking theory and practice. *Nurse Educator, 23*(4), 31–34.

King, M., & Shell, R. (2002). Teaching and evaluating critical thinking with concept maps. *Nurse Educator, 27*(5), 214–216.

Mueller, A., Johnston, M., & Bligh, D. (2001). Mind-mapped care plans: A remarkable alternative to traditional nursing care plans. *Nurse Educator, 26*(2), 75–80.

Schuster, P. (2000). Concept mapping: Reducing clinical care plan paperwork and increasing learning. *Nurse Educator, 25*(2), 78–91.

**Abduction**   To move a body part away from the midline.

**Abrasion**   Surface wounds involving loss of the epidermis and possibly part of the dermis that are caused by "dragging" of epidermal surface against another surface such as pavement, dirt, or gravel.

**Absorption**   Process by which the end products of digestion pass through the epithelial membranes in the small and large intestines into the blood or lymph system; passage of a drug from the site of administration into the bloodstream.

**Abstract**   Summary statement of a research article that identifies the purpose, methodology, findings, and conclusions.

**Accommodation**   Component of cognitive development that allows for readjustment of the cognitive structure (mind-set) in order to take in new information.

**Accountability**   Process that mandates that individuals are answerable for their actions and have an obligation (or duty) to act.

**Accreditation**   Process by which a voluntary, nongovernmental agency or organization appraises and grants accredited status to institutions, programs, and services that meet predetermined structure, process, and outcome criteria.

**Acculturation**   Process that consists of learning norms, beliefs, and behavioral expectations of a group through which people of a subculture assume the characteristics of the dominant culture.

**Acid**   A molecule or an ion that can function as a hydrogen ion donor.

**Acid-Base Balance**   Regulation of hydrogen ion concentration.

**Acid-Base Buffer System**   A solution containing two or more chemical compounds that prevent marked changes in the hydrogen ion concentration when either an acid or a base is added to the solution.

**Acidosis**   A condition that occurs when there is an excessive number of hydrogen ions in a solution.

**Acquired Immunity**   Formation of antibodies (memory B cells) to protect against future invasions of an already experienced antigen.

**Active-Assistive Range of Motion**   Range-of-motion exercises performed by the client with the assistance of the nurse.

**Active Euthanasia**   Process of taking deliberate action that will hasten the client's death.

**Active Immunity**   The development within the body of antibodies that neutralize or destroy the infective agent.

**Active Listening**   Listening that focuses on the feelings of the individual who is speaking.

**Active Range-of-Motion**   Range-of-motion exercises performed independently by the client.

**Activities of Daily Living**   Activities of self-care related to bathing, hygiene, dressing, grooming, toileting, and eating.

**Actual Nursing Diagnosis**   Nursing diagnosis that indicates that a problem exists; composed of the diagnostic label, related factors, and signs and symptoms.

**Actual Social Support**   Social support that is given by others regardless of the recipient's perception of the support.

**Acuity**   A patient classification based on amount of skilled nursing care needed; amount of independence versus dependence in self-care activities.

**Acupressure**   The use of finger pressure applied to specific points (energy pathways) on the body to promote healing.

**Acupuncture**   The use of needles inserted at specific points on the body (energy pathways) to promote healing.

**Acute Care**   Short-term hospital care provided to patients with conditions of short duration requiring stays of, on average, less than 30 days.

**Acute Illness**   Disruption (usually reversible) in functional ability characterized by a rapid onset, intense manifestations, and a relatively short duration.

**Acute Pain**   Discomfort identified by sudden onset and relatively short duration, mild to severe intensity, and a steady decrease in intensity over several days or weeks.

**Acute Wound**   Wound that is incurred suddenly and that heals in an orderly and predictable cascade of overlapping events.

**Adaptation**   Component of cognitive development that refers to the changes that occur as a result of assimilation and accommodation; ongoing process by which an individual adjusts to stressors in order to achieve homeostasis.

**Addiction**   Physiological and psychological dependence upon a substance.

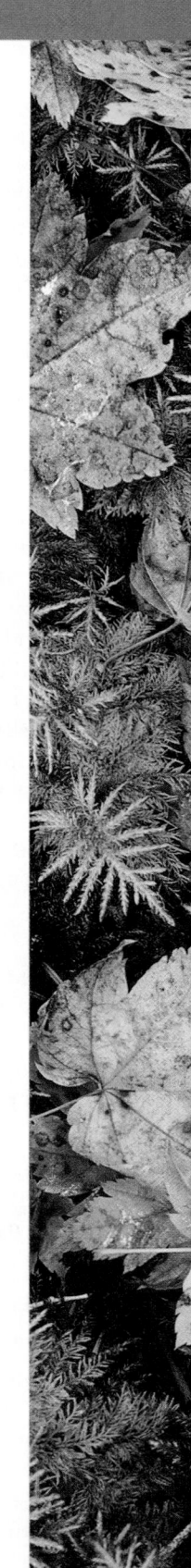

**Adduction**   To move a body part toward the midline.

**Adherence**   Remaining faithful to a program of instruction or activity.

**Adjuvant Medication**   Drugs used to enhance the analgesic efficacy of opioids, treat concurrent symptoms that exacerbate pain, and provide independent analgesia for specific types of pain.

**Administrative Controls**   Strategies that minimize hazard exposure by altering work practices, such as training and policies and procedures.

**Administrative Law**   Laws developed by groups who are appointed to governmental administrative agencies and who are entrusted with enforcing the statutory laws passed by the legislature.

**Adolescence**   Developmental stage from the ages of 12 to 20 years that begins with the appearance of the secondary sex characteristics (puberty).

**Advance Care Medical Directive**   Document in which a client, in consultation with the physician, relatives, or other personal advisers, provides precise instructions for the type of health care the client wants or does not want in a number of scenarios (e.g., end-of-life decisions).

**Advance Directive**   Written instruction for health care that is recognized under state law and is related to the provision of such care when the individual is incapacitated.

**Advanced Practice Nursing**   Practice of nursing at a level requiring an expanded knowledge base and clinical expertise in a specialty area.

**Adventitious Breath Sounds**   Superimposed sounds on the normal vesicular, bronchovesicular, and bronchial breath sounds.

**Adverse Reaction**   Any drug effect other than what is therapeutically intended.

**Advocate**   Taking action to achieve a goal on behalf of another.

**Aerobic Metabolism**   Metabolism of nutrients in the presence of oxygen; a metabolic pathway that uses oxygen to convert glucose into cellular energy.

**Affect**   Mood or feeling.

**Affective Domain**   Area of learning that involves attitudes, beliefs, and emotions.

**Afferent Nerve Pathway**   Ascending pathways that transmit sensory impulses to the brain.

**Afferent Pain Pathway**   Ascending spinal cord.

**Ageism**   Imposition of age stereotypes and discrimination.

**Agent**   Entity capable of causing disease.

**Agglutination**   Clumping together of red blood cells.

**Agglutinin**   A specific kind of antibody whose interaction with antigens is manifested as agglutination.

**Agglutinogen**   Any antigenic substance that causes agglutination by the production of agglutinin.

**Agnostics**   Those who do not know if God exists or not. They generally state that the existence of God is unknowable.

**Airborne Controls**   Protective actions taken to minimize disease exposure risk when disease is transmitted via an airborne route.

**Airborne Precautions**   Caregiving measures used to prevent the spread of airborne contaminants.

**Airborne Transmission**   Mode of transfer of disease through contact with droplet, nuclei, or dust particles suspended in the air.

**Algorithm**   Graphical representation or flowchart describing a set of steps used in a particular clinical decision-making process.

**Algor Mortis**   Lack of skin elasticity as a result of death.

**Alkalosis**   Excessive removal of hydrogen ions from a solution.

**Allen Test**   Assessment procedure that measures the collateral circulation to the radial artery.

**Allodynia**   Pain caused by a stimulus that does not normally evoke pain.

**Allopathic**   That which is recognized by a specific culture as being traditional, conventional, or mainstream (e.g., Western medicine).

**Alternative Therapies**   Treatment approaches that are not accepted by mainstream medical practice.

**Ambulation**   Assisted or unassisted walking.

**Ambulatory Care**   Care that is delivered to individuals whose institutional episodes of care are less than 24 hours.

**Amniocentesis**   Withdrawal of amniotic fluid to obtain a sample for specimen examination.

**Anabolism**   Constructive phase of metabolism.

**Anaerobic Metabolism**   Metabolism of nutrients in the absence of oxygen; a metabolic pathway that converts glucose into energy in the absence of oxygen.

**Analysis**   Breaking the whole down into parts that can be examined.

**Analyte**   A substance dissolved in a solution; also called solute.

**Anemia**   Reduction in the amount of hemoglobin in the blood, thus decreasing the oxygen-carrying capacity of the blood.

**Anesthesia**   Absence of pain.

**Aneurysm**   Localized (aortic) abnormal dilation or weakness of a wall of a blood vessel.

**Angina**   Pain in the chest, neck, or arm resulting from myocardial ischemia.

**Angina Pectoris**   Pain caused by tissue ischemia in the heart.

**Angiocatheter**   An intracatheter with a metal stylet.

**Angiogenesis**   Formation of new blood vessels.

**Angiography**   Visualization of the vascular structures through the use of fluoroscopy with contrast medium.

**Anhedonia**   Loss of pleasure from previously pleasurable activities.

**Anions**   Ions with a negative charge.

**Anorexia Nervosa**   Self-imposed starvation that results in a 15% or more loss of body weight.

**Anthropogenic**   Descriptor for transmission of microorganisms resulting from changes in the relationship between humans and the environment.

**Anthropometric Measurements**   Measurement of the size, weight, and proportions of the body.

**Antibody**   An immunoglobulin produced by the body in response to bacteria, viruses, or other antigenetic substances; counteracts and neutralizes the effects of antigens, and destroys bacteria and other cells. Agglutinin is one type of antibody.

**Anticipatory Grief**   Occurrence of grief work before an expected loss.

**Antigen**   A substance, usually a protein, that causes the formation of an antibody and reacts specifically with that antibody (e.g., agglutinogen).

**Antioxidant**   An agent that prevents or inhibits oxidation.

**Anxiety**   Subjective response that occurs when a person experiences a threat to well-being; it is a diverse feeling of dread or apprehension.

**Aphasia**   Impairment or absence of language function that can result from an injury to the cortex.

**Apnea**   Temporary cessation of breathing.

**Apnea Monitor**   Machine with chest leads that monitors the movement of the chest.

**Appetite**   Desire for specific foods instead of food in general (hunger); involves a psychological desire or craving.

**Aromatherapy**   Therapeutic use of concentrated essences or essential oils that have been extracted from plants and flowers.

**Arousal**   A component linked closely to the appearance of wakefulness and alertness.

**Arterial Blood Gases (ABGs)**   Measurement of levels of oxygen and carbon dioxide, as well as pH and bicarbonate ion in arterial blood.

**Arterial Ulcer**   Lower extremity ulcers caused by chronic arterial insufficiency, which in turn causes chronic ischemia and marked tissue vulnerability.

**Arteriography**   Radiographic study of the vascular system following the injection of a radiopaque dye through a catheter.

**Arthritis**   An inflammation of the joints that causes pain and swelling.

**Arthroplasty**   Total hip replacement.

**Artifact**   Specific type of nonverbal message that includes items in the client's environment, manner of grooming, or use of clothing and jewelry.

**Artificial Immunity**   Immunity produced following a vaccine, which may not last a lifetime.

**Ascites**   Accumulation of fluid in the abdomen.

**Asepsis**   Absence of microorganisms.

**Aseptic Technique**   Infection control practice used to prevent the transmission of pathogens.

**Aspiration**   Procedure performed to withdraw fluid that has abnormally collected or to obtain a specimen.

**Assault**   Intentional and unlawful offer to touch a person in an offensive, insulting, or physically intimidating manner.

**Assessment**   First step in the nursing process; includes collection, verification, organization, interpretation, and documentation of data.

**Assessment Model**   Framework that provides a systematic method for organizing data.

**Assimilation**   Component of cognitive development that involves taking in new experiences or information.

**Assisted Suicide**   Situation in which a health care professional provides a client with the means to end his own life.

**Atelectasis**   Collapsed alveoli.

**Atheists**   Those who do not believe in the existence of God in any form.

**Atherosclerosis**   Disease characterized by narrowing and eventual occlusion of the lumen (opening of the arteries) by deposits of lipids, fibrin, and calcium on the interior walls of the arteries.

**Atherosclerotic Plaque**   A thick, hard deposit on the walls of the inner arteries that can clog the arteries in the heart and the brain.

**Atrophy**   Reduction in muscle size and shape, resulting in thin, flabby muscles.

**Attending Behaviors**   A set of nonverbal listening skills that conveys interest in what the other person is saying.

**Auditory Channel**   Transmission of messages through spoken words and by cues.

**Auditory Learner**   An individual who learns by hearing.

**Auscultation**   Physical examination technique that involves listening to sounds in the body that are created by movement of air or fluid.

**Auscultatory Gap**   The temporary disappearance of sounds at the end of Korotkoff phase I and beginning of phase II.

**Autoantigen**   Antigen that originates from the body's own proteins.

**Autocratic Leadership Style**   Style of leadership in which the leader maintains strong control, makes the decisions, and solves all the problems.

**Autoimmune Disorder**   Condition in which the specific immune defense inappropriately reacts to the host's own tissue.

**Autonomy**   Being self-directed, taking initiative instead of waiting for direction from others; ethical principle that refers to the individual's right to choose for oneself and the ability to act on that choice.

**Autopsy**   Postmortem examination to determine the cause of death.

**Autoregulation**   Redistribution of blood flow to areas of greatest need.

**Avoidance**    A method of conflict management where the difficult situation is avoided with the assumption that given enough time, the issue will resolve itself and just go away.

**Awareness**    The capacity to perceive sensory impressions and react appropriately through thoughts and actions.

**Ayurveda**    A healing system based on Hindu philosophy and Indian philosophy that embraces the concept of an energy force in the body that seeks to maintain balance or harmony.

**Bacteremia**    Bacteria in the blood.

**Bacteriuria**    Bacteria in the urine.

**Balance**    Coordination and stability of the body in space; having a sense of inner peace.

**Barium**    Chalky-white contrast medium.

**Barium Enema**    Rectal infusion of barium sulfate used to visualize the colon.

**Barium Swallow**    Fluoroscopic visualization of the esophagus following the ingestion of barium sulfate.

**Barrier Precautions**    Physical precautions used to minimize the risk of exposure to blood and body fluids.

**Barthel Index**    A formal tool that evaluates an individual's ability to safely and independently perform activities of daily living in 10 areas of functioning.

**Basal Metabolic Rate (BMR)**    Energy needed to maintain essential physiological functions when a person is at complete rest both physically and mentally.

**Base**    A molecule or an ion that will combine with hydrogen ions.

**Baseline Values**    The norms against which subsequent vital sign measurements can be compared.

**Base of Support**    Foundation on which a person or object rests.

**Basic Human Need**    Need that must be met for survival.

**Battery**    Touching another person without consent.

**Behavior**    Observable response of an individual to external stimuli.

**Benchmarking**    Process that evaluates products, services, and priorities against the performance of others.

**Beneficence**    Ethical principle regarding the duty to promote good and prevent harm.

**Bereavement**    Period of grieving following the death of a loved one.

**Bioavailability**    Readiness to produce a drug effect.

**Bioethics**    Application of general ethical principles to health care.

**Biofeedback**    Measurement of physiological responses that yields information about the relationship between the mind and body and helps clients learn how to manipulate these responses through mental activity.

**Biographical Method**    A form of qualitative research in which research is performed on a specific person's life.

**Biological Agent**    Living organism that invades a host, causing disease.

**Biological Clock**    Endogenous mechanism capable of measuring time in a living organism.

**Biopsy**    Excision of a small amount of tissue.

**Biotransformation**    The chemical alteration of a medication in the body, usually by enzymes, into a form that can be excreted; also known as metabolism of a medication.

**Bisexual**    Having an equal or almost equal preference for sexual partners of either gender.

**Black Wound**    Wound containing necrotic tissue.

**Bladder Training**    A program with the goal of teaching the client to suppress the urge to void and thereby gradually increasing the intervals between voiding.

**Blanching**    White color of the skin when pressure is applied.

**Blended Families**    Families in which children live with one birth parent and one stepparent.

**Blood Pressure**    Measurement of pressure pulsations exerted against the blood vessel walls during systole and diastole.

**Body Alignment**    Position of body parts in relation to each other.

**Body Image**    Individual's perception of physical self, including appearance, function, and ability.

**Body Mass Index (BMI)**    Determines whether a person's weight is appropriate for height by dividing the weight in kilograms by the height in meters squared.

**Body Mechanics**    Purposeful and coordinated use of body parts and positions during activity.

**Bodymind**    Inseparable connection and operation of thoughts, feelings, and physiological functions.

**Bonding**    Formation of attachment between parent and child.

**Bradycardia**    A heart rate less than 60 beats per minute in an adult.

**Bradypnea**    Respiratory rate of 10 or fewer breaths per minute.

**Breast Clinical Exam (BCE)**    Systematic palpation of the breasts by health care practitioner trained to do breast examination for the purpose of finding potentially cancerous lumps; performed annually.

**Breast Self-Exam (BSE)**    Systematic palpation of the breasts by a woman on herself for the purpose of finding potentially cancerous lumps; performed monthly.

**Bronchial Sounds**    Loud and high-pitched sounds with a hollow quality heard longer on expiration than inspiration from air moving through the trachea.

**Bronchography**    Radiographic study of the trachea and bronchi following the injection of a contrast agent through a catheter.

**Bronchovesicular Sounds**    Medium-pitched and blowing sounds heard equally on inspiration and expiration from air moving through the large airways, posteriorly between the scapula and anteriorly over bronchioles lateral to the sternum and second intercostal spaces.

**Bruits** Blowing sounds that are heard when the blood flow becomes turbulent as it rushes past an obstruction.

**Bruxism** Teeth grinding during sleep.

**Buccal** Pertaining to the inside cheek.

**Budget** A plan that provides formal quantitative expression for acquiring and distributing funds over the ensuing time period.

**Bulimia** Insatiable appetite.

**Bulimia Nervosa** An eating disorder characterized by episodic binge eating followed by purging.

**Burnout** State of physical and emotional exhaustion that occurs when caregivers deplete their adaptive energy; characterized by fatigue, depersonalization, and decreased feelings of personal accomplishment.

**Burns** Tissue injuries resulting from thermal, chemical, or electrical trauma.

**Butterfly Needles** Winged-tipped needle.

**Cachexia** Weight loss marked by weakness and emaciation that usually occurs with a chronic illness such as tuberculosis or cancer.

**Calorie** Quantity of heat required to raise the temperature of 1 gram of water 1°C.

**Capitated Rate** Preset fees based on membership, not services provided; payment system used in managed care.

**Carbohydrate** Organic compound composed of carbon, hydrogen, and oxygen.

**Carcinogens** Chemicals that cause cancer.

**Cardiac Catheterization** Radiographic study with the use of a contrast medium injected into a vascular catheter that is threaded into the heart, coronary, and/or pulmonary vessels.

**Cardiac Conduction System** Specialized cells in the heart that generate and conduct electrical impulses; consists of the sinoatrial node, internodal pathways, atrioventricular node, bundle of His, right and left bundle branches, and Purkinje fibers.

**Cardiac Cycle** Series of electrical and mechanical events resulting in a cycle of atrial and ventricular contraction and relaxation.

**Cardiac Output** Measurement of blood pumped by the heart in 1 minute; measured by multiplying the heart rate by the ventricle's stroke volume.

**Cardiopulmonary Resuscitation (CPR)** Technique of applying respiration and chest compressions to support oxygenation in the event of cardiac and respiratory arrest.

**Care Map** A plan of care that is based on standards, reflects optimal timing of sequential steps provided by all members of the health care team, and identifies expected outcomes of this care.

**Case Management** Methodology for organizing client care through an episode of illnesses to achieve specific clinical and financial outcomes within an allotted time frame.

**Case Study Method** A type of qualitative research in which research is performed on a specific individual (case), a group, or an institution.

**Catabolism** Destructive phase of metabolism.

**Categorical Imperative** Concept that states that one should act only if the action is based on a principle that is universal.

**Catharsis** Process of talking out one's feelings; "getting things off the chest" through verbalization.

**Cations** Ions with a positive charge.

**Causation** Breach of duty that must be legally proved to have caused an injury.

**Cavities** Dental caries.

**Ceiling Effect** Phenomenon in which increasing doses of a medication above a certain level does not result in increased analgesic effect.

**Cell-Mediated Immunity (Cellular Immunity)** An immune process initiated when the antigen stimulates the release of activated T cells.

**Centering** Process of bringing oneself to an inward focus of serenity that is done before beginning an energetic touch therapy treatment.

**Central Line** Venous catheter inserted into the superior vena cava through the subclavian, internal, or external jugular vein.

**Certification** Process by which a nongovernmental agency or association certifies that an individual licensed to practice a profession has met predetermined standards specified by that profession for specialty practice.

**Certified Nurse Midwife** Advanced practice nurse who is prepared in nursing and midwifery.

**Certified Registered Nurse Anesthetist** Advanced practice nurse who is prepared in the science of anesthesiology.

**Chain of Infection** Phenomena of developing an infectious process.

**Chakra** A concentrated area of energy that influences the physical body, emotions, mental patterns, and spiritual awareness.

**Change** Dynamic process in which an individual's response to a stressor leads to an alteration in behavior.

**Change Agent** Individual who intentionally creates and implements change.

**Channel** Medium through which a message is transmitted.

**Chaotic Family Power** An absence of power structure within a family structure.

**Charting by Exception (CBE)** Charting method that requires the nurse to document only deviations from preestablished norms.

**Chemical Agent** Substance that interacts with a host, causing disease.

**Chemical Restraints** Medications used to control the client's behavior.

**Chest Physiotherapy (CPT)**    Technique of percussing or vibrating the chest wall in an effort to mobilize pulmonary secretions; usually accompanies postural drainage.

**Chiropractic**    Promotion of healing through manipulation of the spinal column.

**Cholangiography**    Roentgenographic visualization of the integrity of the biliary system by a radiopaque contrast medium.

**Cholesterol**    Lipid that is produced by the body and used in the synthesis of steroid hormones. Cholesterol is excreted in bile.

**Cholinesterase**    Enzyme manufactured in the liver that is responsible for the breakdown of acetylcholine and other choline esters.

**Chronemics**    Study of the effects of time on the communication process.

**Chronic Acute Pain**    Discomfort that occurs almost daily over a long period (months or years) and that has a high probability of ending; also known as progressive pain.

**Chronic Illness**    Disruption in functional ability usually characterized by a gradual, insidious onset with lifelong changes that are usually irreversible.

**Chronic Malignant Pain**    Chronic pain as a result of progressive tissue injury.

**Chronic Nonmalignant Pain**    Discomfort that occurs almost daily, has been present for at least 6 months, and ranges in intensity from mild to severe; also known as chronic benign pain.

**Chronic Obstructive Pulmonary Disease (COPD)**    Category of alterations in ventilation including emphysema, asthma, and chronic bronchitis.

**Chronic Pain**    Discomfort that is persistent, nearly constant, and long-lasting (6 months or longer); or recurrent pain that produces significant negative changes in a person's life.

**Chronic Wound**    Wound that is caused by a chronic condition or that fails to heal in an orderly manner.

**Chronobiology**    Science of studying biorhythms.

**Chronological Age**    Exact age of a person from birth.

**Chylomicrons**    Lipoproteins synthesized in the intestines that transport triglycerides to the liver.

**Circadian Rhythm**    Biorhythm that cycles on a daily basis.

**Civil Law**    Law that deals with relations between individuals.

**Clean-Contaminated Wound**    Intentional wound created by entry into the alimentary, respiratory, or genitourinary tract under controlled conditions.

**Clean Object**    Object on which there are microorganisms that are not usually pathogenic.

**Cleansing**    Removal of soil or organic material from instruments and equipment used in providing client care.

**Clean Wound**    Intentional wound in which no inflammation was encountered and the respiratory, alimentary, and oropharyngeal tracts were not entered.

**Client Advocate**    Person who speaks up or acts on behalf of the client.

**Client Behavior Incidents**    Mishaps that occur when the client's behavior or actions precipitate the incident.

**Clinical Guidelines**    Consensus statements that are systematically developed to assist practitioners in making patient management decisions related to special clinical circumstances.

**Clinical Nurse Specialist**    Advanced practice nurse who is educated in a recognized nursing specialty area and is authorized to provide direct nursing care to a select population.

**Clinical Practice Guidelines**    Evidence-based standards of nursing and medical care for clients with the same clinical problem.

**Closed-Ended Question**    Interviewing technique that consists of questions that can be answered briefly with one-word responses.

**Closed Family System**    Family system that is considered to be at risk for dysfunction because its ideas and values may be out of sync with the broader community and because its isolation limits available resources to the family and its members.

**Closed Suction Drainage System**    Drain with a reservoir that when compressed creates negative pressure, or a vacuum, which draws exudate away from a wound.

**Cluster**    Set of data cues in which relationships between and among cues are established to identify a specific health state or condition.

**Cognition**    The intellectual ability to think.

**Cognitive Domain**    Area of learning that involves intellectual understanding.

**Cognitive Reframing**    Stress management technique in which the individual changes her own negative perception of a situation or event to a more positive, less threatening perspective.

**Cohabitate**    To live together without being married.

**Cohesiveness**    The bonding among members of a group.

**Coitus**    Vaginal/penile intercourse.

**Colic**    Acute abdominal pain.

**Collaboration**    A partnership in which all parties are valued for their contribution.

**Collaborative Problems**    Certain physiological complications that nurses monitor to detect onset of changes in status.

**Collagen**    Protein responsible for tissue repair.

**Collagen Synthesis**    The production of collagen, which is a strong, fibrous, insoluble protein found in connective tissue.

**Collectivism**    A cultural form where there is dependence on the family and other related small groups for basic needs.

**Colloid**    Nondiffusible substances.

**Colonization**    Multiplication of microorganisms on or within a host that does not result in cellular injury.

**Communicable Agent**    Infectious agent transmitted to a client by direct or indirect contact, vehicle or vector, or airborne route.

**Communicable Disease**    Disease caused by a communicable agent.

**Communication**   Dynamic, continuous, and multidimensional process for sharing information as determined by standards or policies.

**Community**   A group of people engaged in multifaceted relationships, sharing a common culture with the capacity to act collectively over a period of time.

**Community Development Society (CDS)**   An organization that identifies communities as the building blocks for society.

**Community Health Information Networks (CHINs)**   A computer-connecting network between a variety of agencies (e.g., hospitals, suppliers, physicians, laboratories) that facilitates coordinating client care.

**Community Health Nursing (CHN)**   The field of nursing that provides health care to a wide variety of populations (e.g., communities, groups).

**Community Partnerships**   Health care providers that bring together a large number of community-based agencies, health care clinicians, educational institutions, and public organizations to address the health needs of a specific community.

**Comorbidity**   Existence of simultaneous disease processes within an individual.

**Competency**   Ability, qualities, and capacity to function in a particular way.

**Complementary Family Power**   A dominion-submission dynamic process existing within the family structure.

**Complementary Therapies**   Treatment approaches that can be used in conjunction with conventional medical therapies.

**Compliance**   A client's agreement with and ability to follow through with a health care practitioner's therapeutic recommendations.

**Complicated Grief**   Associated with traumatic death such as death by homicide, suicide, or an accident.

**Comprehensive Assessment**   Type of assessment that provides baseline client data, including a complete health history and current needs assessment.

**Compromised Host**   Person whose normal defense mechanisms are impaired.

**Computed Tomography**   Radiologic scanning of the body with x-ray beams and radiation detectors that transmit data to a computer, which transcribes the data into quantitative measurement and multidimensional images of the internal structures.

**Concept**   Vehicle of thought.

**Conceptual Framework (Model)**   Structure that links global concepts together to form a unified whole.

**Conceptualization**   Process of developing and refining abstract ideas.

**Conditions of Participation (COPs)**   Medicare requirements for services and reimbursement that are based on the client being homebound and requiring skilled services on an intermittent basis.

**Conduction**   Loss of heat to an object in contact with the body.

**Connection**   The integration of all of the aspects of being human; these connections include the self, other people, the world around us, and for some people, a supreme being.

**Conscious Sedation**   Minimally depressed level of consciousness during which the client retains the ability to maintain a continuously patent airway and to respond appropriately to physical stimulation or verbal commands.

**Consciousness**   State of awareness of self, others, and the surrounding environment.

**Consent**   Voluntary act by which a person agrees to allow someone else to do something.

**Constipation**   Infrequent and difficult passage of hard stool.

**Constitution**   Set of basic laws that defines and limits the powers of government.

**Construct**   Abstraction or mental representation inferred from situations, events, or behaviors.

**Consultation**   Method of soliciting help from a specialist in order to resolve diagnoses.

**Consultative Leadership Style**   Leadership style that is based on the concepts of consultation. The leader carefully explains the rationale for a decision and its effect on followers so as to allow greater understanding and acceptance of the decision.

**Contact Precautions**   Caregiving measures used to prevent the direct transmission of a communicable disease from the host.

**Contact Transmission**   Mode of transfer of disease through direct contact.

**Contaminated Wound**   Open, traumatic wound or intentional wound with acute nonpurulent inflammation.

**Continuous Passive Motion Device (CPM)**   Device that increases range of motion and stimulates healing of the articular cartilage by decreasing swelling and the formation of adhesions.

**Continuous Quality Improvement**   Approach to quality management in which scientific, data-driven approaches are used to study work processes that lead to long-term system improvements.

**Contraction**   Mobilization of wound edges to reduce the size of the tissue defect.

**Contract Law**   Enforcement of agreements among private individuals.

**Contrast Medium**   Radiopaque substance that facilitates roentgen imaging of the body's internal structures.

**Controlled Substance**   The Comprehensive Drug Abuse Prevention and Control Act of 1971 established five classes (called schedules) of drugs that require detailed records of distribution and use (most of these drugs are CNS stimulants or depressants, which have high risk for abuse or addiction).

**Contusion**    Disruption of blood vessels in the soft tissue caused by blunt trauma and resulting in bruising with no disruption of the skin surface.

**Convalescent Stage**    Period of time in which acute symptoms of an infection begin to disappear until the client returns to the previous state of health.

**Convection**    Movement of heat away from the body's surface.

**Coping**    A complex of behavioral, cognitive, and physiological responses that aim to prevent or minimize unpleasant or harmful experiences that challenge one's personal resources.

**Correlational Designs**    Methods of data analysis that investigate the correlation (relationship) of one variable with another variable or multiple variables.

**Corrosives**    Health hazard classification; substances that will erode or damage skin on contact.

**Costal (Thoracic) Breathing**    Occurs when the external intercostal muscles are used to move the chest upward and outward.

**Counterstimulation**    Technique used to achieve relaxation by activating the endogenous opioid and monoamine analgesia systems.

**Crackle**    An audible breath sound heard on inspiration over the base of the lungs. May be either a dry, high-pitched popping of short duration or a moist, low-pitched gurgling of long duration.

**Creative Problem Solving**    Goal-directed thinking that leads to achievement by using a new idea or method.

**Credibility**    The quality or power of inspiring beliefs.

**Crepitus**    Grating or crackling sensation caused by two rough surfaces rubbing together, as in subcutaneous emphysema.

**Criminal Law**    Acts or offenses against the welfare or safety of the public.

**Crisis**    Acute state of disorganization that occurs when the individual's usual coping mechanisms are no longer effective.

**Crisis Intervention**    Specific technique used to assist clients in regaining equilibrium.

**Criteria**    Standards that are used to evaluate whether the behavior demonstrated indicates accomplishment of the goal.

**Critical Pathway**    Abbreviated summary of key elements from the case management plan.

**Critical Period**    Time of the most rapid growth or development in a particular stage of the life cycle in which an individual is most vulnerable to stressors of any type.

**Critical Social Theory**    A theory that is directed toward making social changes to alter health-damaging conditions.

**Critical Thinking**    Disciplined, deliberate method of thinking used to search for meaning; employs strategies such as asking questions, evaluating evidence, identifying assumptions, examining alternatives, and seeking to understand various points of view.

**Cross-Functional Team**    Interdepartmental, multidisciplinary group that is assigned to study an organization-wide process.

**Cross-Section Studies**    Studies involving data collection at one specific measurement point in time.

**Crystallized Intelligence**    The application of life experiences and learned skills to solve problems.

**Crystalloid**    Electrolyte solution with the potential to form crystals.

**Cues**    Small amounts of data that are applied to the decision-making process.

**Cullen's Sign**    Bluish discoloration around the umbilicus in postoperative clients; can indicate intra-abdominal or perineal bleeding.

**Cultural Assimilation**    Process by which individuals from a minority group are absorbed by the dominant culture and take on the characteristics of the dominant culture.

**Cultural Competence**    Process through which the nurse provides care that is appropriate to the client's cultural context.

**Cultural Diversity**    Individual differences among people that result from racial, ethnic, and cultural variables.

**Culture**    Dynamic and integrated structures of knowledge, beliefs, behaviors, ideas, attitudes, values, habits, customs, languages, symbols, rituals, ceremonies, and practices that are unique to a particular group of people; growing microorganisms to identify a pathogen.

**Customer**    Anyone who uses the products, services, or processes provided by an organization.

**Cutaneous Pain**    Discomfort caused by stimulation of the cutaneous nerve endings in the skin.

**Cyanosis**    Blue or gray discoloration of the skin, resulting from reduced oxygen levels in the arterial blood.

**Cystocele**    Bladder hernia that protrudes through the vagina.

**Cystography**    Radiographic study used to visualize the excretory function by instilling an aqueous iodine contrast agent into the bladder through a urinary catheter.

**Cytology**    Study of cells.

**Cytomegalovirus (CMV)**    DNA virus that causes intranuclear and intracytoplasmic changes in infected cells.

**Data Clustering**    Process of grouping significant cues together according to a specific assessment model to establish a nursing diagnosis.

**Data Interpretation**    Recognition of patterns in data to determine nursing diagnoses.

**Data Verification**    Process through which data are validated as being complete and accurate.

**Deadspace**    Condition in which lung tissue is well ventilated but poorly perfused.

**Deamination**    Removal of the amino groups from the amino acids.

**Debridement**    Removal of necrotic tissue.

**Decision Making**    The consideration and selection of interventions that facilitate the achievement of a desired outcome.

**Declarative Knowledge**    Specific facts or information and an understanding of the nature of that knowledge.

**Defamation**   Act that occurs when information that damages an individual's reputation is communicated to a third party either in writing (libel) or verbally (slander).

**Defecation**   Evacuation of feces from the rectum.

**Defendant**   Person being sued in a lawsuit.

**Defense Mechanisms**   Unconscious operations that protect the mind from anxiety.

**Defining Characteristics**   Collected data that are also known as signs and symptoms, subjective and objective data, or clinical manifestations.

**Deglutition**   Swallowing of food.

**Degree**   Unit that measures the heat of the body.

**Dehiscence**   Partial or complete separation of the wound edges and the layers below the skin.

**Delegation**   Process of transferring a selected nursing task in a situation to an individual who is competent to perform that task.

**Democratic Leadership Style**   Style of leadership (also called participative leadership) that is based on the belief that every group member should have input into the development of goals and problem solving.

**Deontology**   Ethical theory that considers the intrinsic moral significance of an act itself as the criterion for determination of good.

**Dependence**   Reliance on or need to take a drug.

**Dependent Nursing Intervention**   Nursing action that requires an order from a physician or other health care professional.

**Dependent Variable**   Outcome variable of interest.

**Depersonalization**   Treating an individual as an object rather than as a person.

**Dermal-Epidermal Junction**   Anatomical point at which epidermis connects with dermis, characterized by interdigitating connections.

**Dermatome Map**   Cutaneous area whose sensory receptors and axons feed into a single dorsal root of the spinal cord.

**Dermis**   Innermost layer of skin.

**Descriptive Studies**   Those studies that describe a phenomenon of interest.

**Detrusor Muscle**   Smooth muscle of the bladder wall.

**Development**   Behavioral changes in functional abilities and skills.

**Developmental Tasks**   Certain goals that must be achieved during each developmental stage of the life cycle.

**Diabetes Mellitus**   A disease in which the pancreas fails to secrete adequate levels of insulin to accommodate blood glucose levels.

**Diagnosis**   Science and art of identifying problems or conditions.

**Dialectic Process**   Process involving a transaction that the changing person has with the changing world.

**Diaphoresis**   Profuse perspiration.

**Diaphragmatic (Abdominal) Breathing**   Occurs when the diaphragm contracts and relaxes as observed by the movement of the abdomen.

**Diarrhea**   Passage of liquified stool (increased frequency and consistency of stool sufficient to represent a change in bowel habits).

**Diastole**   Process of cardiac chamber filling.

**Dietary Fiber**   The part of food that body enzymes cannot digest and absorb.

**Diffusion**   Movement of molecules in a solution or a gas from an area of high concentration to one of low concentration.

**Diffusion Defect**   Decrease in efficiency of gas diffusion from the alveolar space into the pulmonary capillary blood.

**Digestion**   Mechanical and chemical processes that convert nutrients into a physically absorbable state.

**Digital Subtraction Angiography**   Computerized imaging of the vasculature with visualization on a monitor screen following the intravenous injection of iodine through a catheter.

**Direct Contact**   Transmission of a communicable disease from the host.

**Direct Expenses**   Those expenditures that are directly attributable to the department and will include both labor and nonlabor components.

**Dirty and Infected Wound**   Traumatic wound with retained dead tissue, or intentional wound created when purulent drainage was present.

**Dirty Object**   Object on which there is a high number of microorganisms, including some that are potentially pathogenic.

**Disability**   A lack of ability to perform an activity a normal person can perform.

**Disaccharide**   Double sugar.

**Discharge Planning**   Planning that involves critical anticipation and consideration for the client's needs after discharge; the client begins to resume self-care activities before leaving the health care environment.

**Discipline**   Field of study.

**Disease Prevention/Health Protection**   Behavior motivated by a desire to actively avoid illness, detect it early, or maintain functioning within the constraints of an illness.

**Disenfranchised Grief**   Grief experienced in situations where grief is discouraged and social supports are absent.

**Disinfectant**   Chemical solution used to clean inanimate objects.

**Disinfection**   Elimination of pathogens, with the exception of spores, from inanimate objects.

**Disorientation**   A mentally confused state in which the person's awareness of time, place, self, and/or situation is impaired.

**Disseminated Intravascular Coagulation (DIC)**   An acquired hemorrhagic syndrome characterized by uncontrollable formation and deposition of thrombi.

**Dissolution**   Rate at which a drug becomes a solution.

**Distance Learning**   Educational courses designed in formats that allow the educators and the students to be in different geographic locations.

**Distraction**   Technique of focusing attention on stimuli other than pain.

**Distress**   Experienced when stressors evoke an ineffective response.

**Distribution**   Movement of drugs from the blood into various body fluids and tissues.

**Documentation**   Written evidence of the interactions between and among health care professionals, clients and their families, and health care organizations; the administration of tests, procedures, treatments, and client education; the result or client's response to these diagnostic tests and interventions.

**Dominant Culture**   Group whose values prevail within a society.

**Doppler**   Handheld transducer.

**Droplet Precautions**   Methods of care used for suspected or confirmed diagnosis of infectious disease transmitted via attachment to large droplets of moisture during exhalation.

**Drug**   Any substance that, when taken into a living organism, may modify one or more of its functions.

**Drug Allergy**   Hypersensitivity to a drug.

**Drug Incompatibility**   Undesired chemical or physical reaction between a drug and a solution, between two drugs, or between a drug and the container or tubing.

**Drug Tolerance**   Reaction that occurs when the body becomes accustomed to a specific drug and requires larger doses of the drug to produce the desired therapeutic effect.

**Dullness**   A high-pitched sound of short duration.

**Durable Power of Attorney**   Document or legal status that enables any competent individual to name someone to exercise health-related decision-making authority, under specific circumstances, on the client's behalf when the client is incapable of making own decisions.

**Duration**   The time period that a medication has its action.

**Duty**   Obligation created either by law or contract, or by any voluntary action.

**Dysfunctional Grief**   Failure to progress through the stages of overwhelming emotions associated with grief; or failure to demonstrate any behaviors commonly associated with grief.

**Dyspnea**   Difficulty in breathing as observed by labored or forced respirations through the use of accessory muscles in the chest and neck to breathe.

**Dysrhythmia**   Irregular heartbeat.

**Dysuria**   Painful urination.

**Echocardiography**   Ultrasonic procedure used to reveal abnormal structure or motion of the heart wall and thrombi.

**Ecomap**   A graphic representation of the family within the social network.

**Edema**   Detectable accumulation of increased interstitial fluid.

**Efferent Nerve Pathway**   Descending pathways that send sensory impulses from the brain.

**Efferent Pain Pathway**   Descending spinal cord.

**Effleurage**   Massage technique consisting of long, smooth strokes used at the beginning and end of treatment and between other movements.

**Electrocardiogram (ECG or EKG)**   Graphic recording of the heart's electrical activity.

**Electrochemical Gradient**   Sum of all the diffusion forces acting on the membrane.

**Electroencephalogram (EEG)**   Graphic recording of the brain's electrical activity.

**Electrolyte**   Element or compound that when dissolved in water or another solvent dissociates (separates) into ions (electrically charged particles) and provides for cellular reactions.

**Electronic Health Record (EHR)**   Method of documentation where all information related to the client is recorded electronically rather than on a traditional paper record. It is sometimes referred to as a computerized patient/client record.

**Electronic Mail (e-mail)**   Method of transmitting data or text files from one computer to another over an intranet or the Internet.

**Embryonic Stage**   Developmental stage that occurs during the first 2 to 8 weeks after fertilization of a human egg.

**Emergency Assessment**   A rapid assessment of a client who is experiencing a life-threatening problem or crisis.

**Emollients**   Products that penetrate the epidermis to restore lost skin oils that keep the skin soft and supple.

**Emotional Intelligence (EI)**   Leadership effectiveness that focuses on emotional considerations of the persons in the group.

**Empathy**   Understanding another person's perception of a situation.

**Empowerment**   Process of enabling others to do for themselves.

**Encoding**   Use of language and other specific signs and symbols for sending messages.

**Endorphins**   Group of opiate-like substances produced naturally by the brain; these substances raise the pain threshold, produce sedation and euphoria, and promote a sense of well-being.

**Endoscopy**   Visualization of a body organ or cavity through a scope.

**Energetic-Touch Therapies**   Techniques in which the hands are used to direct or redirect the flow of the body's energy fields to enhance balance within the fields.

**Engineering Controls**   Strategies that eliminate or minimize the hazard exposure through substitution, mechanical devices, or a process change.

**Enteral Instillation**   Administration of drugs through a gastrointestinal tube.

**Enteral Nutrition**  The nonvolitional delivery of nutrients through a gastrointestinal tube.

**Environment**  Place or community where care is provided.

**Environment of Care**  The organizational safety program as defined by JCAHO, developed to provide a safe environment for clients, visitors, and staff; encompasses management of seven specific areas: safety, security, utilities, medical equipment, emergency, hazardous materials and waste, and fire prevention.

**Enzyme**  Protein produced in the body that catalyzes chemical reactions in organic matter.

**Epidemiology**  The study of the cause and distribution of diseases, disability, and death among populations.

**Epidermis**  Outermost layer of skin.

**Epithelialization**  Growth of epithelial tissue.

**Equipment Incidents**  Accidents resulting from the malfunction or improper use of medical equipment.

**Equity**  Process that acts in accordance with the spirit, not the letter, of the law.

**Erectile Dysfunction**  Inability of a man to achieve or maintain an erection.

**Ergonomic Stressors**  Working conditions such as repetitive tasks and manual client lifting that have the potential to lead to work-related injury.

**Erythema**  Increased blood flow to an inflamed area.

**Erythrocytes**  Red blood cells.

**Erythrocyte Sedimentation Rate (ESR)**  The rate with which the RBCs settle in saline or plasma over a specified time period.

**Eschar**  Necrotic (dead) tissue that is brown or black and usually dry.

**Essential Amino Acids**  Amino acids that are required for growth and development and must be obtained from food.

**Ethical Dilemma**  Situation that occurs when there is a conflict between two or more ethical principles.

**Ethical Principles**  Tenets that direct or govern actions.

**Ethical Reasoning**  Process of thinking through what one ought to do in an orderly, systematic manner in order to provide justification of actions based on principles.

**Ethics**  Branch of philosophy concerned with determining right from wrong on the basis of a body of knowledge.

**Ethnicity**  Cultural group's perception of themselves (group identity) and others' perception of them.

**Ethnocentrism**  Assumption of cultural superiority and an inability to accept other cultures' ways of organizing reality.

**Ethnography**  A type of qualitative research whose approach involves anthropology, in which a person's culture is examined by studying the meanings of the actions and events of the culture's members.

**Ethnomethodology**  A type of qualitative methodology in which interpretations of ethnography are made in a particular social world.

**Etiology**  Related cause of or contributor to a problem.

**Eupnea**  Easy respirations with a normal breath rate of breaths per minute that are age-specific.

**Eustress**  Type of stress that results in positive outcomes.

**Euthanasia**  Intentional action or lack of action causing the merciful death of someone suffering from a terminal illness or incurable condition; derived from the Greek word *euthanatos*, which literally means "good or gentle death."

**Evaluation**  Fifth step in the nursing process; involves determining whether client goals have been met, partially met, or not met.

**Evaporation**  Continuous insensible heat loss from the skin and lungs when water is converted from a liquid to a gas.

**Evidenced-Based Nursing**  A decision-making approach based on integrating clinical expertise with the best available evidence from systematic research.

**Evidenced-Based (Nursing) Practice**  The application of the best available empirical evidence, including recent research findings, to clinical practice in order to aid clinical decision making.

**Evisceration**  Protrusion of the internal viscera through a disrupted wound.

**Exclusive Provider Organization**  Organization in which care must be delivered by the plan in order for clients to receive reimbursement for health care services.

**Excretion**  Elimination of drugs from the body.

**Existentialism**  Movement that is centered on individual existence in an incomprehensible world and the role that free will plays in it.

**Expected Outcome**  Detailed, specific statement that describes the methods through which a goal will be achieved and includes aspects such as direct nursing care, client teaching, and continuity of care.

**Experimental Design**  A method of statistical analysis in which an independent variable is tested against a dependent variable.

**Expert Systems**  Decision-making support systems.

**Expert Witness**  Person called by parties in a malpractice suit who is a member of the same profession as the party being sued and who is qualified to testify to the expected behaviors usually employed by members of the profession when in a similar situation.

**Expiration (Exhalation)**  Movement of gases from the lungs to the atmosphere.

**Exploratory Studies**  Those studies that describe in detail the nature of phenomena and try to identify contributing factors.

**Expressed Contract**  Conditions and terms of a contract given in writing by the concerned parties.

**Expressive Aphasia**  The ability to understand communication, but inability to speak clearly back to the sender of a message.

**Extended Family**  Family members from previous generations, such as grandparents, uncles, and aunts.

**Extension**     Straightening of a joint.

**External Customer**     An individual who is not employed by the organization, and who uses the services the organization provides.

**External Respiration**     See *Oxygen Uptake*.

**External Stimuli**     Elements that generate messages from outside the person in the environment and include sensations, sights, sounds, touch, taste, and smells.

**Extinction**     Ability to discriminate the points of distance when two body parts are simultaneously touched.

**Extraurethral Incontinence**     Uncontrolled loss of urine caused when the sphincter mechanism has been bypassed.

**Extubation**     Removal of an endotracheal tube.

**Exudate**     Material and cells discharged from blood vessels.

**Facilitator**     A person who assists others in making decisions or developing a plan of action.

**False Imprisonment**     Situation that occurs when clients are made to wrongfully believe they cannot leave a place.

**Family Process**     The way a family is organized to address functional needs.

**Fascia**     Thin layer of connective tissue covering the muscle.

**Fat-Soluble Vitamins**     Vitamins that require the presence of fats for their absorption from the gastrointestinal tract and for cellular metabolism.

**Fatty Acids**     Basic structural units of most lipids that contain carbon chains and hydrogen.

**Fecal Incontinence**     Involuntary loss of stool of sufficient duration and volume to create a social or hygienic problem.

**Feedback**     Information the sender receives about the receiver's reaction to a message.

**Fee-for-Service**     Where health care recipient directly pays the provider for services as they are provided.

**Felony**     Crime of a serious nature usually punishable by imprisonment in a state penitentiary or by death.

**Female Genital Mutilation (FGM)**     Ritualistic removal of clitoris; often culturally based to control female sexual drive.

**Fetal Alcohol Syndrome**     Condition in which fetal development is impaired by maternal consumption of alcohol.

**Fetal Stage**     Intrauterine developmental period from 8 weeks to birth.

**Fibroblast**     Any cell from which connective tissue is developed.

**Fidelity**     Ethical concept that means faithfulness and keeping promises.

**Fight-or-Flight Response**     State in which the body becomes physiologically ready to respond to a stressor by either fighting or running away from the danger (which may be actual or perceived).

**Firewall**     A protective mechanism that establishes limited access into a computer system.

**Fixation**     Inadequate mastery or failure to achieve a developmental task that inhibits healthy progression through subsequent stages.

**Flashback**     Rush of blood back into intravenous tubing when a negative pressure is created on the tubing.

**Flatulence**     Discharge of gas from the rectum.

**Flexion**     To bend a joint.

**Flora**     Vegetation of microorganisms on the human body.

**Flow Rate**     Volume of fluid to infuse over a set period of time.

**Fluency**     Ability to talk in a steady manner.

**Fluid Intelligence**     Ability to acquire new concepts and adapt to unfamiliar situations; mental activities based on organizing information.

**Fluoroscopy**     Immediate, serial images of the body's structure or function.

**Focus Charting**     Documentation method using a columnar format to chart data, action, and response.

**Focused Assessment**     Type of assessment that is limited in scope in order to focus on a particular need or health care problem or potential health care risks.

**Focused Questions**     Questions asked to obtain information that is more specific about a problem or condition.

**FOCUS PDCA**     An acronym describing the Shewhart/Deming model for quality improvement.

**Fomite**     Object that has become contaminated with a microorganism.

**Formal Contract**     Written contract that cannot be changed legally by an oral agreement.

**Fowler's Stages of Spiritual Development**     Six categories of spiritual development across the life span purported by James Fowler in 1981.

**Fraud**     Wrong that results from a deliberate deception intended to produce unlawful gain.

**Free Radicals**     A molecule containing an odd number of electrons; free radicals are released during times of ischemic injury.

**Friction**     Force of two surfaces moving against one another; massage technique whereby the heels of the hands or the thumb pads are used to apply deep, penetrating pressure on knotted muscles.

**Frigidity**     A women's lack of desire for sex or inability to achieve orgasm.

**Full Disclosure**     Communication of complete information to potential research subjects regarding the nature of the study, the subjects' right to refuse participation, and the likely risks and benefits that will be incurred.

**Full-Thickness Wound**     Wound involving the entire epidermis and dermis.

**Functional Ability**     Physical, cognitive, and psychological skills needed to carry out activities of daily living, mobility, work, and family roles.

**Functional Assessment**    Assessment of the client's ability to perform activities of daily living.

**Functional Health Patterns**    A systematic holistic approach to evaluate all areas of human needs, recognizing that the needs are interdependent.

**Functional Incontinence**    Loss of urine caused by altered mobility or dexterity, access to the toilet, or changes in mentation.

**Functional Independence Measurement (FIM)**    A formal tool that evaluates an individual's ability to safely and independently perform activities of daily living specific to self-care, sphincter control, transfers, locomotion, communication, and social cognition.

**Functional Team**    Departmental or unit-specific group whose scope is limited to departmental or work area processes.

**Gait or Transfer Belt**    Two-inch-wide webbed belt worn by the client for the purpose of stabilization during transfers and ambulation.

**Gallop**    Extra heart sounds.

**Gate Control Pain Theory**    Theory proposing that the cognitive, sensory, emotional, and physiological components of the body can act together to block an individual's perception of pain.

**Gay**    Male who has affectional and sexual tendencies for males; more holistic term than *homosexual* when it includes women who have affectional tendencies for females.

**Gender (Biologic Sex)**    Biologic structure of a person's genitals that designate them as male, female, or intersexed.

**Gender Bender**    A person who dresses as opposite gender or androgynously, challenging societally prescribed gender behaviors, especially dress.

**Gender Identity**    View of one's self as male or female in relationship to others.

**Gender Role**    Masculine or feminine role adopted by a person; often culturally and socially determined.

**General Adaptation Syndrome**    Physiological response that occurs when a person experiences a stressor.

**General Anesthesia**    Anesthesia that causes the client to lose all sensation and consciousness; used for major surgical procedures.

**Generalized Spiritual Assessment**    An assessment that includes the four elements of spirituality: transcendence, connection, balance, and purpose.

**Generativity**    A sense that one is making a contribution to society.

**Genogram**    A graphic representation of the family form.

**Genome**    The DNA contained in an organism or a cell, which includes both the chromosomes within the nucleus and the DNA in the mitochondria.

**Germicide**    Chemical that can be applied to both animate and inanimate objects to kill pathogens.

**Germinal Stage**    Developmental stage that begins with conception and lasts approximately 10 to 14 days.

**Gingivitis**    Inflammation of the gums.

**Glasgow Coma Scale (GCS)**    An international scale used in grading neurologic responses to determine the client's level of consciousness.

**Global Migration**    An ongoing trend of people crossing regions, countries, and international boundaries to reside and maintain themselves in new and unfamiliar places.

**Gluconeogenesis**    Conversion of amino acids into glucose or glycogen.

**Glucose 6-Phosphate Dehydrogenace (G6PD)**    An enzyme in RBCs that metabolizes glucose.

**Glycolysis**    Breakdown of glucose by enzymes located inside the cell's cytoplasm.

**Glycosylated Hemoglobin A$_1$ (Hb A$_1$)**    A form of hemoglobin (hemoglobin A$_1$) in the red blood cells; it combines strongly with glucose in the process called glycosylation.

**Goal**    Aim, intent, or end.

**Goniometer**    A protractor with two movable arms used to measure the angles of skeletal joint during range of motion.

**Good Samaritan Acts**    Laws that provide protection to health care providers by ensuring immunity from civil liability when the caregiver provides assistance at the scene of an emergency and does not intentionally or recklessly cause the client injury.

**Grand Theory**    Theory composed of concepts representing global and complex phenomena.

**Granulation Tissue**    Tissue consisting of newly formed blood vessels and newly synthesized connective tissue.

**Graphesthesia**    Ability to identify numbers, letters, or shapes when drawn on the skin.

**Grief**    Series of intense physical and psychological responses that occur following a loss.

**Grief Work**    Phrase coined from Lindemann, it describes the process experienced by the bereaved. It consists of freedom from attachment to the deceased, becoming reoriented to the environment in which the deceased is no longer present, and establishing new relationships.

**Grounded Theory**    A type of qualitative research in which field research seeks to explore and describe the phenomena in naturalistic settings.

**Group Communication**    A complex level of communication that occurs when three or more people meet in face-to-face encounters or through another communication medium, such as a conference call.

**Group Dynamics**    Study of the events that take place during small-group interaction and the development of subgroups.

**Groupthink**    Going along with the majority opinion while personally having another viewpoint.

**Growth**    Quantitative (measurable) changes in the physical size of the body and its parts.

**Growth Factors**    Polypeptides released during clot breakdown and synthesized by a number of cells that serve as primary regulators of wound repair.

**Guided Imagery**    A process in which the person uses all the senses to experience the sensation of relaxation.

**Half-Life**    Time it takes the body to eliminate half of the blood concentration level of the original drug dose.

**Halitosis**    Bad breath.

**Hallucination**    A sensory perception that occurs in the absence of external stimuli and is not based on reality.

**Handicap**    Inability to perform one's roles in society.

**Handwashing**    Rubbing together of all surfaces and crevices of the hands using a soap or chemical and water.

**Hardiness**    The ability to survive stress.

**Hazardous Condition**    A situation (aside from the disease for which treatment is provided) that increases the risk of a serious adverse outcome.

**Healing**    Process of recovery from illness, accident, or disability.

**Healing Touch**    Energy-based therapeutic modality that alters the energy fields through the use of touch, thereby affecting physical, mental, emotional, and spiritual health.

**Health**    Process through which the person seeks to maintain an equilibrium that promotes stability and comfort; includes physiological, psychological, sociocultural, intellectual, and spiritual well-being.

**Health Care Delivery System**    Mechanism for providing services that meet the health-related needs of individuals.

**Health History**    Review of the client's functional health patterns prior to the current contact with a health care agency.

**Health Maintenance**    Behavior directed toward maintaining a current level of health.

**Health Maintenance Activities**    The activities and behaviors an individual performs to maintain or improve a current level of health.

**Health Maintenance Organization (HMO)**    Prepaid health plan that provides primary health care services for a preset fee and focuses on cost-effective treatment methods.

**Health Policies**    Written decisions directing or influencing the actions or decisions of others.

**Health-Promoting Behaviors**    Actions that increase well-being or quality of life.

**Health Promotion**    Process undertaken to increase levels of wellness in individuals, families, and communities.

**Health-Seeking Behaviors**    Activities that are directed toward attaining and maintaining a state of well-being.

**Heart Failure**    Inability of the heart to pump enough blood to meet the metabolic needs of the body; often accompanied by a backup of blood in the venous circuits (congestive heart failure).

**Heaves**    Lifting of the cardiac area secondary to an increased workload and force of left ventricular contraction.

**Heimlich Maneuver**    Application of sharp, upward thrusts to the abdomen in order to remove an airway obstruction.

**Hematoma**    Localized collection of blood underneath the tissue.

**Hematuria**    Blood in the urine; *microscopic hematuria* is the presence of blood noted on microscopic examination of the urine; *gross hematuria* is the presence of blood visible to the naked eye.

**Hemoconcentration**    Reduced volume of plasma water and the increased concentration of blood cells, plasma proteins, and protein-bound constituents; occurs with increased capillary hydrostatic pressure, which causes water to shift from the intravascular into the interstitial space.

**Hemodynamic Regulation**    Physiological function of blood circulating to maintain an appropriate environment in tissue fluids.

**Hemoglobin Electrophoresis**    A laboratory test that uses an electromagnetic field to identify various types of hemolytic anemia.

**Hemolysis**    A breakdown of red cells and the release of hemoglobin.

**Hemorrhage**    Persistent bleeding.

**Hemorrhagic Exudate**    Discharge with a large component of red blood cells; present with severe inflammation.

**Hemorrhoids**    Perianal varicosity of the hemorrhoidal veins.

**Hemostasis**    Cessation of bleeding.

**Heterosexism**    Perspective of assumption that people are heterosexual.

**Heterosexual**    Describes sexual activity between a man and a woman.

**High-Biological-Value Proteins (Complete Proteins)**    Proteins that contain all of the essential amino acids.

**High-Level Wellness**    State in which individuals function at their maximum health potential while remaining in balance with the environment.

**High-Risk Sexual Behavior**    Behavior that leads to increased risk of contracting STIs (e.g., unprotected sex, multiple sexual partners, sexual activity that involves blood or exposure to blood).

**Historical Research**    A type of research in which data relating to past events is systematically collected.

**History**    Study of the past, including events, situations, and individuals.

**Holism**    The belief that individuals function as complete units that cannot be reduced to the sum of their parts.

**Home Health Agencies**    Organizations that provide services using health professionals in an individual's place of residence.

**Home Health Care**    An organized, nonphysician health service provided by professionals to clients in their homes.

**Home Health Care Nursing**    A subspecialty of community health nursing and can be offered to a variety of clients throughout the age spectrum.

**Homeopathy**    The treatment of disease with minute drug dosages.

**Homeostasis**    Equilibrium (balance) between physiological, psychological, sociocultural, intellectual, and spiritual needs.

**Homosexuality** Sexual activity between two members of the same sex.

**Hospice** Type of care for the terminally ill founded on the concept of allowing individuals to die with dignity and surrounded by those who love them.

**Host** Simple or complex organism that can be affected by an agent.

**Human Genome Project** An international research project to map each human gene and to completely sequence human DNA.

**Humectants** Products that attract and hold water in the epidermal layer.

**Humoral Immune Response** An immune response initiated when an antigen is recognized and B lymphocytes are activated.

**Humoral Immunity** Stimulation of B cells and antibody production.

**Hydrostatic Pressure** Pressure that a liquid exerts on the sides of the container that holds it; also called filtration force.

**Hygiene** Science of health.

**Hyperalgesia** Extreme sensitivity to pain.

**Hypercalcemia** Excess in the extracellular level of calcium.

**Hypercapnia** Elevation of carbon dioxide levels in the blood indicating inadequate alveolar ventilation.

**Hyperchloremia** Excess in the extracellular level of chloride.

**Hyperglycemia** Condition characterized by a blood glucose level greater than 110 mg/dl.

**Hyperkalemia** Excess in the extracellular level of potassium.

**Hypermagnesemia** Excess in the extracellular level of magnesium.

**Hypernatremia** Excess in the extracellular level of sodium.

**Hyperphosphatemia** Excess in the extracellular level of phosphorus.

**Hypersomnia** Alteration in sleep pattern characterized by excessive sleep, especially in the daytime.

**Hypertension** Refers to a persistent systolic pressure greater than 135–140 mm Hg and a diastolic pressure greater than 90 mm Hg.

**Hyperthyroidism** Increased secretion of thyroid hormones, which increases the rate of metabolism.

**Hypertonic** Solution with more solutes in proportion to the volume of body water; also called a hyperosmolar solution.

**Hypertonicity** Increased muscle tone.

**Hypertrophy** Refers to an increase in muscle size and shape due to an increase in muscle fiber.

**Hyperventilation** Characterized by deep, rapid ventilations.

**Hypervolemia** Increased circulating fluid volume.

**Hypnagogic Hallucinations** Lifelike dreams and hallucinations that often incorporate elements of the environment and are experienced during the hypnagogic state.

**Hypnagogic State** Condition experienced when one is between sleep and wake.

**Hypnosis** State of heightened awareness and focused concentration.

**Hypocalcemia** Deficit in the extracellular level of calcium.

**Hypochloremia** Deficit in the extracellular level of chloride.

**Hypodermis** Tissue layer underlying the dermis, composed of adipose tissue and connective tissue (also known as subcutaneous tissue).

**Hypoglycemia** Condition characterized by a blood glucose level less than 80 mg/dl.

**Hypokalemia** Deficit in the extracellular level of potassium.

**Hypomagnesemia** Deficit in the extracellular level of magnesium.

**Hyponatremia** Deficit in the extracellular level of sodium.

**Hypophosphatemia** Deficit in the extracellular level of phosphorus.

**Hypotension** A systolic blood pressure less than 90 mm Hg or 20–30 mm Hg below the client's normal blood pressure.

**Hypothesis** Statement of an asserted relationship between dependent variables.

**Hypothyroidism** Decreased secretion of thyroid hormones, which decreases the metabolic rate.

**Hypotonic** Solution with less solute in proportion to the volume of water; also called a hypo-osmolar solution.

**Hypotonicity** A flabby muscle with poor tone.

**Hypoventilation** Characterized by shallow respirations.

**Hypoxemia** Decreased oxygen level in the blood.

**Hypoxia** Oxygen deprivation of the body's cells.

**Identity** What sets one person apart as a unique individual; it may include a person's name, gender, ethnic identity, family status, occupation, and various roles.

**Idiopathic Insomnia** Sleeplessness with an unknown origin.

**Idiosyncratic Reaction** Reaction of overresponse, underresponse, or an atypical response.

**Illness** Inability of an individual's adaptive responses to maintain physical and emotional balance that subsequently results in an impairment in functional abilities.

**Illness Stage** Time interval when client is presenting or manifesting specific signs and symptoms of an infectious agent.

**Illusion** An inaccurate perception or misinterpretation of sensory stimuli.

**Imagery** Relaxation technique in which the individual uses the imagination to visualize a pleasant, soothing image.

**Immediate Memory**   The retention of information for a specified and usually short period of time.

**Immunity**   A specific defense mechanism used to combat infection.

**Immunoglobulins**   Plasma protein cells that produce large amounts of antibodies in five different classes (IgM, IgG, IgA, IgD, and IgE).

**Impaction**   Hard bolus of stool that obstructs the fecal stream.

**Impaired Nurse**   Nurse who is habitually intemperate or is addicted to the use of alcohol or habit-forming drugs.

**Impairment**   Loss of function at the organ level.

**Implantable Port**   Device with a radiopaque silicone catheter and a plastic or stainless steel injection port with a self-sealing silicone-rubber septum.

**Implementation**   Fourth step in the nursing process; involves the execution of the nursing plan of care formulated during the planning phase of the nursing process.

**Implied Contract**   Contract that recognizes a relationship between parties for services.

**Impotence**   Male's inability to have or sustain an erection.

**Incentive Spirometers**   Breathing devices that measure the client's ventilatory volumes.

**Incidence**   Refers to the prevalence of a disease in a population or community. The predictive value of the same test can be different when applied to people of differing ages, genders, and geographic locations.

**Incident Report**   Documentation of an unusual occurrence or an accident in delivery of client care.

**Incontinence**   Loss of the ability to initiate, control, or inhibit elimination.

**Incubation Period**   Time interval between the entry of an infectious agent in the host and the onset of symptoms.

**Independent Nursing Intervention**   Nursing action initiated by the nurse that does not require direction or an order from another health care professional.

**Independent Variable**   Variable that is believed to cause or influence the dependent variable.

**Indirect Contact**   Transmission of a communicable disease by any medium.

**Indirect Expenses**   Those costs that are allocated from the operation of the larger organization to the various service units.

**Individualism**   A predominant cultural type that focuses on an independent lifestyle that flourishes in urban settings.

**Infancy**   Developmental stage from the first month to the first year of life.

**Infarction**   Death (necrosis) of an area of tissue caused by oxygen deprivation.

**Infection**   Actual invasion and multiplication of microorganisms in body tissue with cellular injury.

**Infection Chain**   A process of elements that when linked together result in an infection.

**Infectious Agent**   Microorganism that causes infections.

**Infertility**   Inability to conceive.

**Infiltration**   See page of foreign substances into the interstitial tissue.

**Inflammation**   Nonspecific cellular response to tissue injury or infection; involves increased blood flow in the affected area.

**Inflammatory Phase**   Initial phase of wound repair, characterized by vessel dilatation, migration of white blood cells to wound bed, and clinical signs of erythema, edema, and exudate production.

**Information Technology**   The use of computers to gather, organize, process, and communicate information.

**Informed Consent**   Client understands the reason for the proposed intervention, its benefits, and risks, and agrees to the treatment by signing a consent form.

**Ingestion**   Route of exposure whereby exposure to chemical or microorganism is via gastrointestinal tract.

**Inhalation**   Route of exposure whereby exposure to chemical or microorganism is via respiratory tract.

**Initial Planning**   Planning that involves development of an initial plan of care by the nurse who performs the admission assessment and gathers the comprehensive admission assessment data.

**Injection**   Route of exposure whereby exposure to chemical or microorganism is via percutaneous exposure or compromised skin.

**Injury**   Physical, financial, or emotional harm.

**Insensible Heat Loss**   Heat that is lost through the continuous, unnoticed water loss that occurs with vaporation.

**Insomnia**   Chronic inability to sleep, or inadequate quality of sleep.

**Inspection**   Physical examination technique that involves careful visual observation.

**Inspiration (Inhalation)**   Intake of air into the lungs.

**Insulin**   Pancreatic hormone that aids in the diffusion of glucose into the liver and muscle cells and the synthesis of glycogen.

**Integrative Therapy**   A clinical approach that combines Western technological medicine with techniques from Eastern medicine.

**Integumentary System**   Skin, hair, scalp, and nails; provides the body with external protection, regulates temperature, and is a sensory organ for pain, temperature, and touch.

**Intentional Wound**   Wound acquired during treatment (such as surgery) or therapy (such as venipuncture).

**Interdependent Nursing Intervention**   Nursing action that is implemented in a collaborative manner with other health care professionals.

**Intermittent Claudication**   Ischemia to the extremities usually brought on by activity and relieved by rest.

**Internal Customer**   An individual employed by the organization who must depend on the efficiency and productivity of other employees to do his work.

**Internal Respiration**   Process of gas exchange between capillary blood and the body's cells, in which the cells receive oxygen and carbon dioxide is removed.

**Internal Stimuli**   Those elements that generate messages and are found within the person, including such things as hunger, fatigue, and myriad cognitive experiences (e.g., thoughts, fantasies).

**Interpersonal Communication**   Process that occurs between two people in face-to-face encounters, over the telephone, or through other communication media.

**Intersexed**   Person born with both sets or ambiguous genitalia.

**Interstate Nursing Practice**   An agreement among states to mutually recognize each other's licenses.

**Interview**   Therapeutic interaction that has a specific purpose.

**Intracath**   Plastic tube for insertion into a vein.

**Intractable Pain**   Pain that is resistant to all pain-relieving therapies.

**Intradermal (ID)**   Injection into the dermis.

**Intramuscular (IM)**   Injection into the muscle.

**Intraoperative** (during surgery)   Phase that begins when the client is transferred to the operating room and ends when the client is transferred to a postanesthesia care unit.

**Intrapersonal Communication**   Messages one sends to oneself, including "self-talk," or communication with oneself.

**Intrapsychic Theory**   Theory that focuses on an individual's unconscious processes. Feelings, needs, conflicts, and drives are considered to be motivators of behavior.

**Intravenous (IV)**   Injection into a vein.

**Intravenous Pyelogram**   A series of x-rays of the kidneys, ureters, and bladder following the administration of an intravenous iodine preparation.

**Intravenous (IV) Therapy**   Administration of nutrients, fluids, electrolytes, or medications by the venous route.

**Intubation**   Insertion of an endotracheal tube into the bronchus through the nose or mouth to ensure an airway.

**Invasive**   Accessing the body tissues, organs, or cavities through some type of instrumentation procedure.

**Ischemia**   Oxygen deprivation, usually caused by poor perfusion, that is usually temporary and localized.

**Ischemic Pain**   Discomfort resulting when the blood supply of an area is restricted or obstructed.

**Isotonic**   Solution with body water and solutes (sodium) in equal amounts; also called an isosmolar solution.

**Jargon**   Technical language that is often specific to a discipline.

**Joint Commission on Accreditation of Healthcare Organizations (JCAHO)**   An independent, non-profit health care accrediting body, charged with setting health care quality standards.

**Judgment**   The ability to compare or evaluate alternatives to life situations and arrive at an appropriate course of action.

**Judicial Decisions**   Authoritative decisions based on the interpretation of laws; made by a judge.

**Jurisprudence**   Body of judge-made law.

**Justice**   Ethical principle based on the concept of fairness that is extended to each individual.

**Kardex**   Summary worksheet reference of basic client care information.

**Keloid**   Scar tissue that extends beyond the boundaries of the original wound.

**Ketogenesis**   Conversion of amino acids into keto acids or fatty acids.

**Ketones**   Products of incomplete fat metabolism.

**Ketonuria**   Abnormally high concentration of ketones in the urine.

**Kilocalorie**   Equivalent to 1,000 calories.

**Kinesthetic Channel**   Transmission of messages through sensation of touch.

**Kinesthetic Learner**   A person who processes information by experiencing the information or by touching and feeling.

**Laceration**   Cuts to skin and soft tissues.

**Laissez-Faire Leadership Style**   Style of leadership in which the leader assumes a passive, nondirective, and inactive style.

**Lancinating**   Type of pain that is typically described as piercing or stabbing.

**Laser Plume**   Product of combustion when laser is applied to living human tissue; may contain pathogens.

**Late Potentials**   Electrical activity that occurs after normal depolarization of the ventricles.

**Law**   That which is laid down or fixed.

**Leadership**   Interpersonal process that involves motivating and guiding others to achieve goals.

**Leadership Theory**   Conceptual support framework for leadership.

**Learning**   Process of assimilating information with a resultant change in behavior.

**Learning Plateau**   Peak in effectiveness of teaching and depth of learning.

**Learning Style**   Way in which an individual incorporates new information.

**Legal Regulation**   Process by which the state attests to the public that the individual licensed to practice is competent to do so.

**Lentigo Senilis**   Benign, brown pigmented areas on the face, hands, and arms of older people.

**Lesbian**   Female who has affectional and sexual tendencies toward females.

**Leukocytes**   White blood cells.

**Level of Evidence**   A categorization of research support (with four levels) generated to support a particular strategy of care.

**Liability**   Obligation one has incurred or might incur through any act or failure to act.

**Libido**   Level of desire for sexual activity.

**Licensure**   Method by which a state holds the nurse accountable for safe practice to citizens of that state.

**Licensure by Endorsement**   Process by which an individual who is duly licensed as a registered nurse under the laws of one state or country has her credentials accepted and approved by another state or country.

**Licensure by Examination**   Process by which an individual who has completed an approved program of studies leading to registered nurse licensure seeks initial licensure by successfully passing a standardized competency examination.

**Line of Gravity**   Vertical line passing through the center of gravity.

**Lipids**   Organic compounds that are insoluble in water but soluble in organic solvents such as ether and alcohol; also known as fats.

**Lipoproteins**   Blood lipids bound to protein.

**Literature Review**   The part of the research process that involves reviewing the published and unpublished sources of information used in a given study.

**Liver Mortis**   Bluish purple discoloration that is a by-product of red blood cell destruction.

**Living Will**   Document prepared by a competent adult that provides direction regarding medical care should the person become incapacitated or otherwise unable to make decisions personally.

**Local Adaptation Syndrome**   Physiological response to a stressor (e.g., trauma, illness) affecting a specific part of the body.

**Local Anesthesia**   Anesthesia that causes the client to lose sensation to a localized body part (e.g., spraying the back of the throat with lidocaine decreases the gag reflex).

**Localized Infection**   Infection limited to a defined area or single organ.

**Lock-Out Interval**   Minimum time allowed between doses for the client to self-medicate; feature found in infusion pumps used for patient-controlled analgesia.

**Locus of Control**   A person's perception of the source of control over events and situations affecting the person's life.

**Logrolling**   A technique for moving a client whose body must remain in straight alignment.

**Longitudinal Studies**   Studies that involve data collection over time in a particular research sample.

**Long-Term Acute Care**   Care arenas provided in acute facilities to clients with conditions of longer duration than acute care clients.

**Long-Term Outcome**   Statement written in objective format demonstrating an expectation to be achieved in resolution of the nursing diagnosis over a long period of time, usually over weeks or months.

**Loss**   Any situation in which a valued object is changed or is no longer accessible to an individual.

**Low-Biological-Value Proteins (Incomplete Proteins)**   Proteins lacking in one or more of the essential amino acids.

**Lumbar Puncture**   Aspiration of cerebrospinal fluid from the subarachnoid space.

**Lymphangiography**   Radiographic study of the lymphatic system following a catheter injection of an oil-based dye.

**Lymphokine**   Mediator substance released by lymphocytes.

**Maceration**   Overhydration of skin secondary to diaphoresis or to prolonged exposure to exogenous moisture.

**Macrophages**   Immunologically active cells that phagocytize pathogens and break down necrotic tissue; they also secrete growth factors to regulate wound repair.

**Magnetic Resonance Imaging (MRI)**   An imaging technique that uses radiowaves and a strong magnetic field to make continuous cross-sectional images of the body.

**Maladaptation**   Process of ineffective coping with stressors.

**Malignant Hyperthermia (MH)**   A potentially lethal syndrome caused by a hypermetabolic state that is precipitated by the administration of certain anesthetic agents.

**Malnutrition**   Nutritional alterations related to inadequate intake, disorders of digestion or absorption, or overeating.

**Malpractice**   Professional person's wrongful conduct, improper discharge of professional duties, or failure to meet the standards of acceptable care that results in harm to another person.

**Mammography**   A low-dose radiographic study of the breast tissue.

**Managed Care**   System of providing and monitoring care in which access, cost, and quality are controlled before or during delivery of services. These networks "manage" or control costs in many ways (e.g., by limiting referrals to costly specialists). HMOs are a common form of managed care.

**Management**   Accomplishment of tasks either by oneself or by directing others.

**Mandatory Licensure Laws**   Legislation that prohibits any individual from practicing as a registered nurse without a current license.

**Mandatory Overtime**   Work hours imposed on a nurse over an agreed-upon, predetermined work schedule.

**Mastication**   Chewing into fine particles and then mixing the food with enzymes in saliva.

**Material Principle of Justice**   Rationale for determining when there can be unequal allocation of scarce resources.

**Material Safety Data Sheet (MSDS)**   Reference sheet supplied by the manufacturer and kept on file by the employer; contains safety information on hazardous chemicals in the workplace.

**Maturation**   Process of becoming fully grown and developed; involves physiological and behavioral aspects.

**Maturation Phase**   Third phase of full-thickness wound repair, during which the scar tissue is remodeled via the simultaneous processes of collagen lysis and collagen synthesis.

**Maturational Loss**   Adolescent that loses the younger child's freedom from responsibility.

**Medical Asepsis**   Practices that reduce the number, growth, and spread of microorganisms.

**Medical Diagnosis**   Clinical judgment by the physician that identifies or determines a specific disease, condition, or pathological state.

**Medical Model**   Traditional approach to health care in which the focus is on treatment and cure of disease.

**Medicare Certified**   A process that requires an agency to have inspections (e.g., reviews of charts, policies/procedures, billing practices, qualifications of care providers) from Medicare representatives in order to receive funding from the Medicare program.

**Medication**   A medicinal substance.

**Medication Interaction**   The effects caused when multiple medications are administered together.

**Medicine**   A drug or remedy.

**Meditation**   Quieting the mind by focusing one's attention.

**Melanocyte**   A melanin-forming cell.

**Menarche**   Onset of the first menstrual period.

**Message**   Stimulus produced by a sender and responded to by a receiver.

**Metabolic Rate**   Rate of heat liberated during chemical reactions.

**Metabolism**   Aggregate of all chemical reactions in every body cell.

**Metacommunication**   Relationship aspect of communication, which refers to the message about the message.

**Metaparadigm**   Unifying force in a discipline that names the phenomena of concern to that discipline.

**Micro-Range Theory**   Theory that explains a specific phenomenon of concern to a discipline.

**Middle Adulthood**   Developmental stage from the ages of 40 to 65 years.

**Middle-Range Theory**   Theory that addresses more concrete and more narrowly defined phenomena than a grand theory but does not cover the full range of phenomena of concern to a discipline.

**Mid-Upper-Arm Circumference**   Measures skeletal muscle mass and serves as an indicator of protein reserve.

**Migrants**   Laborers who move from one location to another in pursuit of work.

**Minerals**   Inorganic elements.

**Minority Group**   Group of people who constitute less than a numerical majority of the population and who, because of their cultural or physical characteristics, are labeled and treated differently from others in the society.

**Misdemeanor**   Offense less serious than a felony that may be punished by a fine or sentence to a local prison for less than 1 year.

**Mixed Agonist-Antagonist**   Compound that blocks opioid effects on one receptor type while producing opioid effects on a second receptor type.

**Mobility**   Ability to engage in activity and free movement.

**Modeling**   The process the nurse uses in developing an image and understanding within the client's framework and from the client's perspective.

**Mode of Transmission**   Process that bridges the gap between the portal of exit of the biological agent from the reservoir and the portal of entry of the susceptible "new" host.

**Monosaccharides**   Simple sugars.

**Monounsaturated Fatty Acids**   Fatty acids with one double or triple bond.

**Morality**   Behavior in accordance with custom or tradition that usually reflects personal or religious beliefs.

**Moral Maturity**   Ability to decide for oneself what is right.

**Motivation**   The internal drive or externally arising stimulus to action or thought.

**Mourning**   Period of time during which grief is expressed and resolution and integration of the loss occur.

**Moxibustion**   Type of acupuncture that involves the application of heat from certain burning substances, such as herbs, at acupuncture points on the body.

**Murmur**   Swishing or blowing sounds of long duration heard in the heart during the systolic and diastolic phases, created by turbulent blood flow through a valve.

**Muscle**   Tissue composed of contractile fibers that control position and movement.

**Muscle Layer**   A type of tissue layer composed of contractile cells or fibers that affects the movement of an organ or a part of the body.

**Muscle Tone**   Normal state of balanced tension present in the body that allows muscles to respond quickly to stimuli.

**Musculoskeletal Disorders**   Soft tissue injuries related to repeated trauma or other ergonomic stressors.

**Music-Thanatology**   Holistic and palliative method for use of music with dying clients; solely concerned with dissipating any obstacle to a peaceful passage.

**Myelography**   Study of the spinal cord and its surrounding subarachnoid spaces through the use of radiography and pantopaque, a contrast agent.

**Myocardial Infarction**   Necrosis of the heart muscle.

**Myofascial Pain Syndromes**   Group of muscle disorders characterized by pain, muscle spasm, tenderness, stiffness, and limited motion.

**Myoneuronal Junction**   Point at which nerve endings come in contact with muscle cells.

**N-95 Particulate Filtering Respirator**   A filter device commonly used in health care for protection against diseases transmitted by tiny particles of virus or bacteria remaining suspended in the air for long periods of time.

**Narcolepsy**   Sleep alteration characterized by sudden uncontrollable urges to fall asleep.

**Narrative Charting**    A story format of documentation that describes the client's status, interventions and treatments, and the response to treatments.

**Natural Immunity**    The genetically determined response of protection within a specific species.

**Near Miss**    A deviation from a process that does not actually harm the client, but could place the client at risk if it were to occur again.

**Necrosis**    Tissue death as the result of disease or injury.

**Necrotizing Fasciitis**    Severe and rapidly progressing infectious process caused by beta-hemolytic strep; spreads along fascial planes.

**Need**    Anything that is absolutely essential for existence.

**Negative Nitrogen Balance**    Condition that exists when nitrogen output exceeds intake or protein catabolism exceeds anabolism.

**Negligence**    Failure of an individual to provide the care in a situation that a reasonable person would ordinarily provide in a similar circumstance.

**Negotiation**    A method of conflict management whereby the parties decide what they must retain and what they are willing to give up in order to reach a compromise position.

**Neonatal Period**    First 28 days of life following birth.

**Networking**    Process of building connections with others.

**Neuralgia**    Paroxysmal pain that extends along the course of one or more nerves.

**Neuropathic Pain**    Discomfort from damage to portions of the peripheral or central nervous system.

**Neuropathic Ulcer**    Ulcers caused by painless repetitive trauma in clients with reduced sensory awareness due to neurologic lesions or disease processes.

**Neuropeptides**    Amino acids produced in the brain and other sites in the body that act as chemical communicators.

**Neurotransmitters**    Chemical substances produced by the body that facilitate nerve impulse transmission.

**New Age Spirituality**    A spiritual philosophy that incorporates various religions into a personal spiritual ethic; these concepts include such ideas as everything is God, and therefore God is within the self; religion is universal; and people should live in balance with nature.

**Nitrogen Balance**    Net result of intake and loss of nitrogen that measures protein anabolism and catabolism.

**Nociception**    Process by which an individual becomes aware of pain.

**Nociceptor**    Receptive neuron for painful sensations.

**Nocturia**    Awakening from sleep to urinate.

**Nonblanching Erythema**    Redness of the skin that cannot be dissipated with direct pressure; usually reflects vascular injury and extravasation of blood out into the tissues.

**Nonessential Amino Acids**    Amino acids that can be synthesized in the adult body.

**Noninvasive**    Body is *not* entered with any type of instrument.

**Nonmaleficence**    Ethical principle that means the duty to cause no harm to others.

**Nonprofit Agencies**    Those agencies that have a tax-exempt status.

**Nonverbal Message**    Message communicated without words.

**Nosocomial Infection**    Infection acquired in the hospital that was not present or incubating at the time of the client's admission.

**Nuclear Dyads**    Married heterosexual couples without children, either by choice or situation.

**Nuclear Family**    A married heterosexual man and woman and their biologic children.

**Nurse-Client Relationship**    One-to-one interactive process between client and nurse that is directed at improving the client's health status or assisting in problem solving.

**Nurse Epidemiologist**    A direct care provider role in which the nurse studies illnesses, their causes, and the illnesses distribution in groups of people.

**Nurse Practice Act**    Law determined by each state governing the practice of nursing.

**Nurse Practitioner**    Advanced practice nurse educated in a specified area of care who is authorized to provide primary care to individuals, families, and other groups in a variety of settings.

**Nursing**    An art and a science that assists individuals to learn to care for themselves whenever possible; it also involves caring for others when they are unable to meet their own needs.

**Nursing Audit**    Process of collecting and analyzing data to evaluate the effectiveness of nursing interventions.

**Nursing Diagnosis**    Second step in the nursing process; a clinical judgment about individual, family, or community (aggregate) responses to actual, possible, or risk (potential) health problems, wellness states, or syndromes.

**Nursing Informatics**    The use of information technologies by nurses.

**Nursing Intervention**    Action performed by a nurse that helps the client achieve the results specified by the expected outcomes.

**Nursing Intervention Classification (NIC)**
Standardized language for nursing interventions.

**Nursing Leadership**    Interpersonal process in nursing that involves motivating and guiding others to achieve goals.

**Nursing Minimum Data Set (NMDS)**    Elements contained in clinical records and abstracted for studies on the effectiveness and costs of nursing care.

**Nursing Order**    Statement written by the nurse that is within the scope of nursing practice to plan and initiate.

**Nursing Process**    Systematic method of providing care to clients; consists of five steps: (1) assessment, (2) diagnosis, (3) outcome identification and planning, (4) implementation, and (5) evaluation.

**Nursing Research**    Systematic application of formalized methods for generating valid and dependable information about the phenomena of concern to the discipline of nursing.

**Nursing Sensitive Outcome**    Changes in client health status that reflect direct influence of nursing interventions.

**Nutraceuticals**    Natural substances found in plant or animal foods that act as protective or healing agents.

**Nutrition**    Process by which the body metabolizes and uses nutrients.

**Nystagmus**    Involuntary, rhythmical oscillation of the eyes.

**Obesity**    Weight that is 20% or more above the ideal body weight.

**Objective Data**    Observable and measurable data that are obtained through both standard assessment techniques performed during the physical examination, and laboratory and diagnostic tests.

**Obligatory Loss of Proteins**    Degradation of the body's own proteins into amino acids in response to inadequate protein intake.

**Observation**    Skill of watching carefully and attentively.

**Obstructive Pulmonary Disease**    Category of lung diseases characterized by obstruction of the airways and trapping of air distal to the obstruction.

**Occult**    Blood in the stool that can be detected only through a microscope or by chemical means.

**Older Adulthood**    Developmental stage occurring from the age of 65 and beyond.

**Oliguria**    Diminished production of urine (typically less than 400 ml/24 hours).

**Ongoing Assessment**    Type of assessment that includes systematic monitoring and observation related to specific problems.

**Ongoing Planning**    Planning that entails continuous updating of the client's plan of care.

**Onset of Action**    Time it takes the body to respond to a drug after administration.

**Open-Ended Questions**    Interview technique that encourages the client to elaborate about a particular concern or problem.

**Open Family System**    A family system that interacts with the environment and in doing so maintains growth and balance.

**Operational Decisions**    Similar to rules and regulations, having the same authority, but less permanent.

**Operative Knowledge**    An understanding of the nature of knowledge (knowing the "how" or "why").

**Opposition**    One body part being across from another part at nearly 180 degrees.

**Oppression**    Condition in which the rules, modes, and ideals of one group are imposed on another group.

**Oral Cholecystography**    Visualization of the gallbladder and presence of stones through the administration of radiopaque iodine tablets.

**Organization**    Means by which members of a profession join together to promote and protect the profession as a valuable service to society.

**Organizational Culture**    Commonly held beliefs, values, norms, and expectations that drive the workforce.

**Orientation**    Perception of self in relation to the surrounding environment.

**Orientation Phase**    First stage of the therapeutic relationship in which the nurse and client become acquainted, establish trust, and determine the expectations of each other.

**Orthostatic Hypotension (Postural Hypotension)**    Refers to a sudden drop of 25 mm Hg in systolic pressure and 10 mm Hg in diastolic pressure when the client moves from a lying to a sitting or a sitting to a standing position.

**Osmolality**    Measurement of the total concentration of dissolved particles (solutes) per kilogram of water.

**Osmolarity**    Concentration of solutes per liter of cellular fluid.

**Osmole**    Unit of measure of osmotic pressure.

**Osmosis**    Process caused by a concentration difference of water.

**Osmotic Pressure**    Force that develops when two solutions of different strengths are separated by a selectively permeable membrane.

**Osteoarthritis**    The most common type of degenerative arthritis in which the joints become stiff and tender to touch.

**Osteoporosis**    Process in which reabsorption exceeds accretion of bone.

**Outcome**    A domain in Donabedian's quality assurance model, which evaluates health and disability consequences, positive and negative, related to health care delivery.

**Outcome and Assessment Information Set (OASIS)**    A method to collect needed information on all Medicare home health beneficiaries. Data is collected electronically from all Medicare-certified agencies and is used to provide a foundation for OBQI.

**Outcome Based Quality Improvement (OBQI)**    A process to increase quality care and determine those services that are contributing (or not contributing) to the outcomes of care.

**Outcome Evaluation**    Process of comparing the client's current status with the expected outcomes.

**Output**    The response from the family to throughput.

**Oxygen Uptake**    Process of oxygen diffusing from the alveolar space into the pulmonary capillary blood; also called external respiration.

**Oxyhemoglobin Dissociation Curve**    Graphic representation of the relationship between partial pressure of oxygen and oxygen saturation.

**Pain**    State in which an individual experiences and reports the presence of physical discomfort; may range in intensity from uncomfortable sensation to severe discomfort.

**Pain Threshold**    Level of intensity at which pain becomes appreciable or perceptible.

**Pain Tolerance**　Level of intensity or duration of pain that a person is willing to endure.

**Palliative Care**　Control of the symptoms rather than cure.

**Palpation**　Physical examination technique that uses the sense of touch to assess texture, temperature, moisture, organ location and size, vibrations and pulsations, swelling, masses, and tenderness.

**Pansexual**　Crosses all sexual proclivities.

**Papanicolaou Test**　Smear method of examining stained exfoliative cells.

**Paracentesis**　Aspiration of fluid from the abdominal cavity.

**Paradigm**　Pattern, model, or mind-set that strongly influences one's decisions and behaviors.

**Paradigm Revolution**　Turmoil experienced by a discipline when a competing paradigm gains acceptance over the dominant, prevailing paradigm.

**Paradigm Shift**　Acceptance of a competing paradigm over the prevailing paradigm.

**Parasomnia**　Sleep alteration resulting from activation of physiological systems at inappropriate times during the sleep-wake cycle.

**Paraverbal Communication**　The way in which a person speaks, including voice tone, pitch, and inflection.

**Paraverbal Cue**　Verbal message accompanied by cues, such as tone and pitch of voice, speed, inflection, volume, and other nonlanguage vocalizations.

**Parenteral**　Denoting any medication route other than the alimentary canal (e.g., intravenous, subcutaneous, intramuscular).

**Parenteral Nutrition**　Nutrients bypass the small intestine and enter the blood directly.

**Paresthesia**　Abnormal sensation such as burning, prickling, or tingling.

**Parish Nursing**　An organization whereby a religious or health care system coordinates registered nurses in providing nursing care to members of a church congregation.

**Paroxysmal Nocturnal Dyspnea**　Episode of sudden shortness of breath occurring during sleep.

**Partial Thickness Wound**　Wound involving the epidermis and part of the dermis.

**Participative Leadership Style**　Leadership style where every person's viewpoints are considered as valuable and have equal voice in making decisions.

**Passive Euthanasia**　Process of cooperating with the client's dying process.

**Passive Immunity**　Immunity that is acquired by the introduction of preformed antibodies.

**Passive Range of Motion**　Range-of-motion exercises performed by the nurse for the dependent client.

**Patency**　Openness of tube lock or bodily passageway.

**Paternalism**　Practice by which health care providers decide what is "best" for clients and then attempt to coerce clients to act against their own choices.

**Pathogen**　Microorganism that causes disease.

**Pathogenicity**　Ability of a microorganism to cause disease.

**Patient-Controlled Analgesia (PCA)**　Device that allows the client to control the delivery of intravenous or subcutaneous pain medication in a safe, effective manner through a programmable pump.

**Patient-Focused Care**　Specific approach to care delivery that involves the decentralization of services, physical redesign of units, and cross-training of employees to bring client care and services to the client in order to minimize contacts with large numbers of staff and to increase overall client satisfaction.

**Peak Plasma Level**　Achievement of the highest blood concentration of a single drug dose until the elimination rate equals the rate of absorption.

**Peer Evaluation**　Process by which professionals provide critical performance appraisal and feedback that is geared toward corrective action.

**Peer Review**　Chart review by a peer to assess appropriateness of physician treatment and interventions.

**Penrose Drain**　Flexible drain that functions by gravity.

**Perceived Social Support**　Social support that is perceived by the recipient of the support.

**Perception**　Person's sense and understanding of the world.

**Percussion**　Physical examination technique that uses short, tapping strokes on the surface of the skin to create vibrations of underlying organs.

**Percutaneous**　When an action is effected through the layers of the skin.

**Performance Improvement**　Activities and behaviors that each individual does to meet customers' expectations.

**Perineal Care**　Cleansing of the external genitalia, perineum, and surrounding area.

**Perioperative**　Refers to the management and treatment of the surgical client during the three phases of surgery: preoperative, intraoperative, and postoperative.

**Peripherally Inserted Central Catheters (PICC)**　Large-bore catheters inserted into large vessels and are used for (1) specific types of prolonged IV therapy or (2) to administer fluids that are damaging to the vessels (e.g., chemotherapy).

**Peristalsis**　Coordinated, rhythmic, serial contraction of the smooth muscles of the gastrointestinal tract.

**Permeability**　Capability of a substance, molecule, or ion to diffuse through a membrane.

**Person**　One of the four metaparadigm concepts in nursing that refers to the individual, family, or group who are the interest of nursing.

**Personal Digital Assistants (PDA)**　Handheld wireless computer devices.

**Personal Protective Equipment**　Clothing and equipment worn to provide a barrier between the hazard and an individual.

**Petrissage**   Massage technique using squeezing, kneading, and rolling movements to release muscle tension and stimulate circulation.

**Phagocytosis**   Process by which certain cells engulf and dispose of foreign bodies.

**Phantom Limb Pain**   Neuropathic pain in which pain sensations are referred to an area from which an extremity has been amputated.

**Pharmacodynamics**   Effects that the medication causes at the site of action in the body; includes biochemical changes, functional changes, and therapeutic and nontherapeutic effects.

**Pharmacokinetics**   Study of the absorption, distribution, metabolism, and excretion of drugs.

**Phenomenon**   Observable fact or event that can be perceived through the senses and is susceptible to description and explanation.

**Phenomenology**   A type of philosophy used in qualitative research whereby the approach (methods) to research is considered.

**Phenylketonuria (PKU)**   Genetic disorder that can lead to impaired intellectual functioning if untreated.

**Philosophy**   Statement of beliefs that is the foundation for one's thoughts and actions.

**Phlebitis**   Inflammation of a vein.

**Phlebotomist**   Individual who performs venipuncture.

**Phospholipids**   Composed of one or more fatty acid molecules and one phosphoric acid radical, and usually contain a nitrogenous base.

**Physical Agent**   Factor in the environment capable of causing disease in a host.

**Physical Dependence**   Reaction of the body to abrupt discontinuation of a medication; also known as withdrawal syndrome.

**Physical Restraints**   Manual methods or physical equipment attached to the client to reduce the client's movement.

**Phytonutrients**   Chemical found in plants.

**PIE Charting**   Documentation method using problem, intervention, evaluation (PIE) format.

**Piggybacked**   Addition of an intravenous solution to infuse concurrently with another infusion.

**Piloerection**   Hairs standing on end as a result of the body's decrease in body temperature.

**Plaintiff**   Party who initiates a lawsuit that seeks damages or other relief.

**Planning**   Third step of the nursing process; includes the formulation of guidelines that establish the proposed course of nursing action in the resolution of nursing diagnoses and the development of the client's plan of care.

**Plan of Care**   Written guide that organizes data about a client's care into a formal statement of the strategies that will be implemented to help the client achieve optimal health.

**Plateau**   Level at which a drug's blood concentration is maintained.

**Pleura**   Lining of the chest cavity.

**Pleural Friction Rub**   Heard on either inspiration or expiration over anterior lateral lungs as a continuous creaking, grating sound.

**Pneumatic Compression Device**   Device that provides intermittent compression cycles to the veins of the extremities to promote circulation.

**Pneumothorax**   Collection of air or gas in the pleural space, causing the lungs to collapse.

**Point-of-Care Charting**   Documentation system that allows health care providers to gain immediate access to client information at the bedside.

**Poison**   Any substance that causes an alteration such as injury or death in the client's health when inhaled, injected, ingested, or absorbed by the body.

**Political Action Teams**   Often developed within professional organizations to analyze or address a particular policy issue of concern.

**Politics**   Way in which people try to influence decision making, especially decisions about the use of resources.

**Polyp**   A small, abnormal growth of tissue.

**Polypharmacy**   Concurrent use of several different medications.

**Polysaccharide**   Complex sugar.

**Polyunsaturated Fatty Acids**   Fatty acids that have many carbons unbonded to hydrogen atoms.

**Port-a-Cath**   A port that has been implanted under the skin with a catheter inserted into the superior vena cava or right atrium through the subclavian or internal jugular vein.

**Portal of Entry**   Pathway by which infectious agents gain access to the body.

**Portal of Exit**   Pathway by which pathogens leave the body of a host.

**Positive Nitrogen Balance**   Condition that exists when nitrogen intake exceeds output and protein anabolism exceeds catabolism.

**Possible Nursing Diagnosis**   Nursing diagnosis that indicates a situation exists in which a problem could arise unless preventive action is taken; or a "hunch" or intuition by the nurse that cannot be confirmed or eliminated until more data have been collected. It is composed of the diagnostic label and related factors.

**Postoperative** (after surgery)   Begins when the client leaves the operating room and is taken to a postanesthesia care unit; this phase continues until the client is discharged from the care of the surgeon.

**Postural Drainage**   A technique of positioning that promotes gravity drainage of specific lung lobes.

**Power**   Ability to do or act, resulting in the achievement of desired results.

**Prana**   The flow of life energy referred to in the practice of yoga.

**Preadolescence**   Developmental stage from the ages of approximately 10 to 12 years.

**Pre-Albumin**   Precursor of albumin.

**Precapillary Sphincters**   Smooth muscles surrounding the smallest arterioles that control blood flow through the capillary beds.

**Predictive Value**   The ability of screening test results to correctly identify the disease state, such as a true-positive correctly identifies persons who actually have the disease, whereas a true-negative correctly identifies persons who do not actually have the disease.

**Preferred Provider Organization (PPO)**   Type of managed care model in which member choice is limited to providers within the system.

**Prenatal Period**   Developmental stage beginning with conception and ending with birth.

**Preoperative**   (Before surgery) Refers to the time interval that begins when the decision is made for surgery until the client is transferred to the operating room.

**Presbycusis**   Hearing loss associated with old age.

**Presbyopia**   The inability of the lens to change shape causing the farsightedness of the middle years.

**Preschool Stage**   Developmental stage from the ages of 3 to 6 years.

**Prescriptive Authority**   Legal recognition of the ability to prescribe medications.

**Presence**   The process of "just being" with another; a therapeutic nursing intervention.

**Pressing**   A conflict resolution approach where there is an exchange for support or acquiescence relative to the decision in question.

**Pressure/Shear Force**   Deep wounds caused by prolonged pressure and exposure to sliding force.

**Pressure Ulcer**   Localized area of tissue necrosis that develops when soft tissue is compressed between a bony prominence and an external surface for a prolonged period of time; also known as bedsore or decubitus ulcer.

**Primary Care Provider**   Health care provider whom a client sees first for health care; typically, a family practitioner (physician/nurse), internist, or pediatrician.

**Primary Health Care**   Client's point of entry into the health care system; includes assessment, diagnosis, treatment, coordination of care, education, preventive services, and surveillance.

**Primary Intention Healing**   Healing process of a wound with minimal tissue loss and well-approximated edges; occurs with minimal granulation tissue and scarring.

**Primary Source**   Major provider of information about client; research article written by one or more researchers.

**prn (As Necessary) Orders**   Prescribed actions that are implemented according to circumstances.

**Proactive**   Initiating change rather than responding to change imposed by others.

**Problem-Oriented Medical Record (POMR)**   Documentation focused on the client's problem with a structured, logical format to narrative charting called SOAP (subjective and objective data, assessment, plan).

**Procedures**   Specific step-by-step evidence-based directions on how to perform a specific clinical activity or technical skill.

**Process**   Series of steps or acts that lead to accomplishment of a goal or purpose.

**Process Evaluation**   Measurement of nursing actions by examination of each phase of the nursing process.

**Process Improvement**   Process that examines the flow of client care between departments in order to ensure that the processes work as they were designed and that acceptable levels of performance are achieved.

**Prodromal Stage**   Time interval from the onset of non-specific symptoms until specific symptoms of the infectious agent begin to manifest themselves.

**Profession**   Group (vocational or occupational) that requires specialized education and intellectual knowledge.

**Professional Organizations**   Members engaged in the same professional pursuit, often with similar goals and concerns.

**Professional Regulation**   Process by which nursing ensures that its members act in the public interest by providing a unique service that society has entrusted to them.

**Professional Standards**   Authoritative statements developed by the profession by which quality of practice, service, and/or education can be judged.

**Progressive Muscle Relaxation**   Stress management technique involving tensing and relaxing muscles.

**Proliferative Phase**   Second phase of wound healing in which there is rapid regeneration of new tissue cells.

**Proposition**   Statement that proposes a relationship between concepts.

**Proprietary Agencies**   Private organizations that were not tax-exempt, and their profits did not have to be reinvested into the agency but could be used to reward investors.

**Proprioception**   Awareness of posture, movement, and changes in equilibrium and the knowledge of position, weight, and resistance of objects in relation to the body.

**Prosody**   Melody of speech that conveys meaning through changes in the tempo, rhythm, and intonation.

**Prospective Payment System (PPS)**   Reimbursement for client care according to the client's diagnosis.

**Prospective Study**   A study that actively follows subjects over the period of the study and does not rely on data collected retrospectively, except as background information.

**Proteins**   Organic compounds of amino acid polymers connected by peptide bonds that contain carbon, hydrogen, oxygen, and nitrogen.

**Protocol**   Series of standing orders or procedures that should be followed under certain specific conditions.

**Proxemics**   Study of the distance between people and objects.

**Psychomotor Domain**   Area of learning that involves performance of motor skills.

**Psychoneuroimmunology**   Study of the complex relationship between the cognitive, affective, and physical aspects of humans.

**Puberty**   Appearance of secondary sex characteristics that signals the beginning of adolescence.

**Public Law**   Law that deals with an individual's relationship to the state.

**Pulse**   Bounding of blood flow in an artery that is palpable at various points on the body.

**Pulse Deficit**   Condition in which the apical pulse rate is greater than the radial pulse rate.

**Pulse Oximeter**   Sensor device used to measure the oxygen saturation level of blood.

**Pulse Oximetry**   The use of an oximeter to determine the oxygen saturation of blood.

**Pulse Pressure**   Measurement of the ratio of stroke volume to compliance (total distensibility) of the arterial system.

**Pulse Quality**   Refers to the "feel" of the pulse, its rhythm and forcefulness.

**Pulse Rate**   Indirect measurement of cardiac output obtained by counting the number of apical or peripheral pulse waves over a pulse point.

**Pulse Rhythm**   Regularity of the heartbeat.

**Pulse Volume**   Measurement of the strength or amplitude of the force exerted by the ejected blood against the arterial wall with each contraction.

**Purpose**   Having a sense of meaning and purpose in life.

**Purulent Exudate**   Thick discharge composed of leukocytes, liquefied dead tissue debris, and dead and living bacteria; also known as pus.

**Pyogenic Bacteria**   Bacteria that produce pus.

**Pyorrhea**   Periodontal disease.

**Pyrexia**   When heat production exceeds heat loss and body temperature rises above the normal range.

**Pyrogens**   Bacteria, viruses, fungi, and some antigens.

**Pyuria**   Pus (white blood cells) in the urine.

**Qualitative Analysis**   Integration and synthesis of narrative, nonnumerical data.

**Qualitative Research**   Systematic collection and analysis of subjective narrative materials, using procedures for which there tends to be a minimum of research-imposed control.

**Quality**   Meeting or exceeding requirements of the client.

**Quality Assurance Framework**   Traditional approach to quality management in which monitoring and evaluation focus on individual performance, deviation from standards, and problem solving.

**Quality Improvement**   A process for change using a multidisciplinary approach to problem identification and resolution.

**Quantitative Research**   Systematic collection of numerical information, often under conditions of considerable control.

**Quasi-Experimental Design**   A method of statistical analysis that is a modified experiment where control or randomization is not possible, so that all subjects have some exposure to the independent variable.

**Race**   Grouping of people based on biologic similarities such as physical characteristics.

**Racism**   Discrimination directed toward individuals who are misperceived to be inferior because of biologic factors.

**Radiation**   Loss of heat in the form of infrared rays.

**Radiofrequency Ablation**   The delivery of low-voltage, high-frequency, alternating electrical current to cauterize the abnormal myocardial tissue.

**Radiography**   Study of x-rays or gamma-ray-exposed film through the action of ionizing radiation.

**Range of Motion (ROM)**   Extent to which a joint can move.

**Rapid Relaxation Response (RRR)**   A useful coping method that is similar to transcendental meditation. The person selects a mantra, a word or phrase that can be used repetitively to help manage symptoms or unwanted emotions.

**Rapport**   Bond or connection between two people that is based on mutual trust.

**Rationale**   Explanation based on the theories and scientific principles of natural and behavioral sciences and the humanities.

**Readiness for Learning**   Evidence of willingness to learn.

**Receiver**   Person who intercepts the sender's message.

**Recent Memory**   The result of events that have occurred over the past 24 hours.

**Receptive Aphasia**   The ability to speak well, but the inability to understand the message that is spoken.

**Recommended Dietary Allowances (RDA)**   Recommended allowances of essential nutrients established by the Food and Nutritional Academy of Sciences–National Research Council.

**Recurrent Acute Pain**   Discomfort marked by cycles of repetitive pain episodes that alternate with pain-free intervals; this pain may recur over a prolonged period or throughout a person's lifetime.

**Red Cell Indices**   Laboratory measurement of the size and hemoglobin content of the red cells.

**Red Wound**   Wound in the proliferative phase of repair.

**Referred Pain**   Discomfort from the internal organs that is felt in another area of the body.

**Reflexology**   A system of massage in which the feet and hands are massaged in an attempt to favorably influence other body functions.

**Reframing**   Technique of monitoring negative thoughts and replacing them with positive ones.

**Regeneration**   Method of tissue repair in which lost tissue is replaced with no cosmetic or functional deficit.

**Regional Anesthesia**   Anesthesia that causes the client to lose sensation in a particular area of the body (e.g., laparoscope for a tubal sterilization).

**Regurgitation**    Backward flow of blood through a diseased heart valve, also known as insuffiency.

**Rehabilitate**    To restore to a normal, healthy, or highest level of functioning possible.

**Reiki**    A form of energy work that was founded in the 1800s when Mikao Usui studied a tradition of using hands for healing by Buddhist monks.

**Reincarnation**    A belief that one will be reborn in another form of life after own physical death.

**Relaxation Response**    State of increased arousal of the parasympathetic nervous system that leads to a relaxed physiological state.

**Relaxation Techniques**    Methods used to decrease anxiety and muscle tension.

**Religion**    A system of beliefs and practices that usually involves a community of like-minded people.

**Relocation Stress Syndrome**    A nursing diagnosis that applies when a client experiences physiological and psychological symptoms when moved to a different environment.

**Remote Memory**    The retention of experiences that occurred during earlier periods of life.

**Research**    Systematic method of exploring, describing, explaining, relating, or establishing the existence of a phenomenon, the factors that cause changes in the phenomenon, and how the phenomenon influences other phenomena.

**Research Design**    Overall plan used to conduct research.

**Reservoir (or Source)**    A place for an organism to live while awaiting a host.

**Resident Flora**    Microorganisms that are always present, usually without altering the client's health.

**Resident Infectious Agents**    Microorganisms that are always present on skin and can be reduced through handwashing, but not totally removed.

**Residual**    The amount of substance left during and after the organ's normal functioning (e.g., the amount of fluids remaining in the stomach during and after tube feeding).

**Respiration**    The act of breathing.

**Respirator**    Protective devices worn to protect the respiratory tract from exposure to inhalation hazards.

**Rest**    State of relaxation and calmness, both mental and physical.

**Restorative Nursing Care**    Nursing care provided to clients who have residual impairment as a result of disease or injury; seeks to increase the client's independence and ability to perform self-care.

**Restraints**    Protective devices used to limit the physical activity of a client or to immobilize a client or extremity.

**Restrictive Pulmonary Disease**    A category of lung diseases characterized by impaired mobility or elasticity of the lungs or chest wall.

**Retrospective Studies**    Studies involving existing data usually found in medical records or client care records.

**Review of Systems**    A brief account of any recent signs or symptoms related to any body system.

**Rhonchi**    Heard predominantly on expiration over the trachea and bronchi as a continuous, low-pitched musical sound.

**Rigor Mortis**    Stiffening of the body after death caused by contraction of the skeletal and smooth muscles.

**Risk for Infection**    State in which an individual is at increased risk for being invaded by pathogenic organisms.

**Risk Nursing Diagnosis**    Nursing diagnosis that indicates that a problem does not yet exist but specific risk factors are present; composed of the diagnostic label preceded by the phrase "Risk for" with the specific risk factors listed.

**Role**    Set of expected behaviors associated with a person's status or position.

**Role Competence**    The family member's ability to perform a role.

**Role Conflict**    When the expectations of one role compete with the expectations of other roles.

**Role Overload**    A form of role stress or strain that occurs when the family member lacks the time, resources, or energy to perform the role.

**Role Strain**    A subjective personal response of psychological distress in which an individual anticipates or has an actual inability to satisfactorily perform a role.

**Role Stress**    A condition of role expectations that is likely to contribute to family or individual dysfunction.

**Role Transition**    Changes in role assignment for developmental, situational, or illness-related reasons.

**Rolfing**    A form of deep tissue massage and manipulation to correct body posture.

**Rounds**    Reporting method; care team members walk to clients' rooms and discuss care and progress with each other and with the clients.

**Routes of Exposure**    Methods by which chemicals and other potentially hazardous substances are assimilated into the body (e.g., inhalation, ingestion, injection).

**Rules and Regulations**    Provide specific guidance for implementation of a law.

**Saccharides**    Sugar units.

**Satiety**    Feeling of fulfillment from food.

**Saturated Fatty Acids**    Glycerol esters of organic acids whose atoms are joined by a single-valence bond.

**Scar Formation**    Method of repair involving replacement of lost tissue with connective tissue and an epithelial cover.

**School-Age Period**    Developmental stage from the ages of 6 to 12 years.

**Scope of Practice**    Legal boundaries of practice for health care providers as defined in state statutes.

**Sebum**    Substance produced by the skin to kill bacteria.

**Secondary Gain**    Outcomes of the sick role other than alleviation of anxiety (primary gain); examples include gaining attention and sympathy, avoiding responsibilities, and receiving financial compensation or reward.

**Secondary Intention Healing** Healing process of a wound that has extensive tissue loss and poorly approximated edges; occurs with gradual tissue replacement and scarring.

**Secondary Source** Source of data other than the client, family members, other health care providers, or medical records; article in which an author addresses the research of someone else.

**Self-Care** Learned behavior and a deliberate action in response to a need.

**Self-Care Deficit** State in which an individual is not able to perform one or more activities of daily living.

**Self-Concept** Individual's perception of self; includes self-esteem, body image, and ideal self.

**Self-Efficacy** Belief in one's ability to succeed; according to social cognitive theory of learning, this serves as an internal motivator for change.

**Self-Esteem** Individual's perception of self-worth; includes judgments about one's self and one's capabilities.

**Self-Ideal** The perception of behavior based on personal standards and self-expectations.

**Semipermeable** Selective permeability of membranes.

**Sender** Person who generates a message.

**Sensation** The ability to receive and process stimuli received through the sensory organs.

**Sensitivity** Determines the susceptibility of a pathogen to an antibiotic; the ability of a test to correctly identify those individuals who have the disease.

**Sensitizer** Chemical or substance that causes allergy in susceptible individuals.

**Sensory Deficit** A change in the perception of sensory stimuli.

**Sensory Deprivation** A state of reduced sensory input from the internal or external environment, manifested by alterations in sensory perceptions.

**Sensory Overload** Increased perception of the intensity of auditory and visual stimuli.

**Sensory Perception** The ability to receive sensory impressions and, through cortical association, relate the stimuli to past experiences to form an impression of the nature of the stimulus.

**Sentinel Event** Unexpected event involving client death or serious injury; includes near misses.

**Serous Exudate** Watery discharge composed primarily of serum, with a low protein count.

**Servant Leadership** Leadership that is based on the needs of others and on helping those served.

**Sex Roles** Culturally determined patterns associated with being male or female.

**Sexual Dysfunction** Physical inability to perform sexually, but can also be a psychological inability to perform sexually.

**Sexual Health** Ability to form mutually consensual, developmental-appropriate sexual relationships that are safe and respectful of self and others; includes emotional, physical, and psychological components.

**Sexuality** Human characteristic that refers not just to gender but to all the aspects of being male or female, including feelings, attitudes, beliefs, and behavior.

**Sexually Transmitted Infections (STIs)** Formerly known as sexually transmitted diseases (STDs); infections most notably transmitted via sexual activity, including any oral, anal, vaginal, or penile activity.

**Sexual Orientation** Individual's preference for ways of expressing sexual feelings.

**Shaman** Folk healer-priest who uses natural and supernatural forces to help others.

**Shamanism** Practice of entering altered states of consciousness with the intent of helping others.

**Shear Force** Forces exerted against the skin by movement or repositioning.

**Shiatsu** A combination of acupressure, massage, and joint manipulation.

**Short-Term Outcome** Statement written in objective format demonstrating an expectation to be achieved in resolution of the nursing diagnosis in a short period of time, usually a few hours or days.

**Shunting** Condition in which alveolar regions are well-perfused but not adequately ventilated.

**Sick Role** A set of social expectations met by an ill person, such as being exempt from the usual social role responsibilities and being obligated to get well and to seek competent help.

**Side Effects** Mild nontherapeutic drug effect.

**Signal-Averaged Electrocardiography (SAECG)** Surface ECG that amplifies late potentials.

**Simultaneity Paradigm** Nursing viewpoint that focuses on the quality of life from the client's perspective and conceptualizes the interaction between person and environment as mutual and simultaneous.

**Single-Payer System** Health care delivery model in which the government is the only entity to reimburse.

**Single Point of Entry** Entry into the health care system is required through a point designated by the plan.

**Situational Leadership** Style of leadership in which there is a blending of styles based on current circumstances and events.

**Situational Loss** Occurs in response to external events, usually beyond the individual's control (such as the death of a significant other).

**Situational Role Transitions** Changes that are made in role when families experience the addition or loss of a family member.

**Skin Absorption** Route of exposure whereby exposure to chemical or biologic substances occurs via passage through the skin barrier.

**Skin Contact** Route of exposure whereby exposure to chemical or biologic substances occurs via contact with skin.

**Skinfold Measurement**   Measures the amount of body fat.

**Skin Shear**   Result of dragging skin across a hard surface.

**Skin Tear**   Superficial skin lesion that occurs when the superficial layers of the skin separate from the underlying tissues.

**Skin Turgor**   Normal resiliency of the skin.

**Sleep**   State of altered consciousness during which an individual experiences fluctuations in level of consciousness, minimal physical activity, and a general slowdown of the body's physiological processes.

**Sleep Apnea**   A syndrome in which breathing periodically ceases during sleep, often associated with heavy snoring.

**Sleep Cycle**   Sequence of sleep that begins with the four stages of no rapid eye movement (NREM) sleep, a return to stage 3, then stage 2, and then passage into the first rapid eye movement (REM) stage.

**Sleep Deprivation**   Prolonged inadequate quality and quantity of sleep.

**Sleep Paralysis**   Experience of waking from sleep and being unable to move, speak, or cry out.

**Slough**   Necrotic (dead) tissue that is gray, yellow, or white and usually soft.

**Small-Group Ecology**   Study of proxemics in small-group situations.

**Smart Card**   A computerized disk that stores client information.

**Snellen Chart**   A chart of graduating black letters that test visual acuity.

**SOAP Charting**   Documentation method using subjective data, objective data, assessment, and plan.

**Social Marketer**   A role that uses marketing techniques and skills to promote healthy living as well as health promotion programs.

**Social Support**   Providing for people in a social network.

**Solute**   A substance dissolved in a solution; also called analyte.

**Solvent**   A liquid with a substance in solution.

**Somatic Pain**   Nonlocalized discomfort originating in tendons, ligaments, and nerves.

**Somnambulism**   Sleepwalking.

**Source-Oriented (SO) Charting**   Narrative recording by each member (source) of the health care team on a separate record.

**Spasticity**   Increase in muscle tension.

**Specific Gravity**   Weight of urine compared with weight of distilled water; a specific gravity greater than 1.000 indicates solutes in the urine.

**Specificity**   The ability of a test to correctly identify those individuals who do not have the disease.

**Spherocytes**   Small, thick red cells.

**Spiritual Distress**   The client's perception that his belief system, or his place within it, is threatened.

**Spirituality**   Relationship with one's self, a sense of connection with others, and a relationship with a higher power or divine source.

**Spores**   Single-celled microorganisms or microorganisms in the resting or inactive stage.

**Sprain**   Trauma to ligaments, tendons, or bones around joint caused by twisting or pulling.

**Stagnation**   A sense of nonmeaning in one's life.

**Standard of Care**   Delineates the extent and character of the nurse's duty to the client; defined by organizational policy or professional standards of practice.

**Standard Precautions**   Guidelines recommended by the Centers for Disease Control and Prevention to reduce the risk of infection.

**Standing Order**   Standardized intervention written, approved, and signed by a physician that is kept on file within health care agencies to be used in predictable situations or in circumstances requiring immediate attention.

**Stat Order**   An order for a single dose of medication to be given immediately.

**Statutory Law**   Laws enacted by legislative bodies.

**Stenosis**   Narrowing or constriction of a blood vessel or valve.

**Stereognosis**   Ability to identify objects by manipulation and touch.

**Stereotyping**   Belief that all people within the same racial, ethnic, or cultural group act alike and share the same beliefs and attitudes.

**Sterilization**   Total elimination of all microorganisms including spores.

**Stock Supplied**   Medications dispensed and labeled in large quantities for storage in the medication room or nursing unit.

**Stoma**   Surgically created opening.

**Stomatitis**   Inflammation of the oral mucosa.

**Stool**   Fecal material.

**Straight**   Holistic term for a person who has sexual contact and engages in intimate relationships with people of the opposite gender.

**Strain**   Stretch injury of muscles, tendons, or ligaments.

**Stress**   Body's reaction to any stimulus.

**Stressor**   Any stimulus encountered by an individual; leads to the need to adapt.

**Stress Test**   Measures the client's cardiovascular response to exercise tolerance.

**Stress Urinary Incontinence**   Uncontrolled loss of urine caused by physical exertion in the absence of a bladder contraction.

**Striae**   Red or silver-white streaks over the breasts or axillae.

**Stridor**   Heard predominantly on inspiration as a continuous crowing sound.

**Stroke Volume**   Measurement of blood that enters the aorta with each ventricular contraction.

**Structure**   A domain in Donabedian's quality assurance model encompassing the integrity of the infrastructure within the health care organization (e.g., physical environment, human resources).

**Structure Evaluation**   Determination of the health care agency's ability to provide the services offered to its client population.

**Subacute Care**   Short-term aggressive care that emphasizes restorative interventions before the client's reentry into the community.

**Subculture**   Group of people with characteristic patterns of behavior that distinguish it from the larger culture or society.

**Subcutaneous (SC/SQ)**   Injection into the subcutaneous tissue.

**Subjective Data**   Data from the client's point of view, including feelings, perceptions, and concerns.

**Sublingual**   Under the tongue.

**Substitution**   Replacing a particular substance with a less hazardous alternative.

**Superficial Wound**   Wound confined to the epidermis layer.

**Supination**   Turning a body part upward.

**Supplemental Recommendation**   Area of noncompliance is identified during a JCAHO survey, not as serious as a Type I; must be resolved in a timely fashion.

**Suppository**   A substance specifically designed to insert into a bodily orifice other than the mouth (anus, vagina, urethra). The suppository is typically composed of a vehicle containing a medication.

**Suppression**   Conscious defense mechanism whereby a person decides to avoid dealing with a stressor at the present time.

**Suppuration**   Formation of pus, or purulent exudate.

**Surfactant**   Phospholipid secreted by Type II alveolar cells that reduces the alveolar surface tension and thus helps prevent alveolar collapse.

**Surgical Asepsis**   Practices that eliminate all microorganisms from an object or area.

**Survey Method**   Those studies that involve surveying the subjects in a research study for responses to given questions or statements.

**Susceptible Host**   Person who lacks resistance to an agent and is therefore vulnerable to disease.

**Sustained Release**   Specially coated medication that allows for slow, controlled absorption over an extended period of time.

**Suture**   Surgical means of closing a wound by sewing, wiring, or stapling.

**Symmetrical (Egalitarian) Family Power**   Power that is shared between family members.

**Synergy**   Combined power of many people.

**Synthesis**   Putting data together in a new way.

**Systemic Infection**   Infection that affects the entire body with involvement of multiple organs.

**Systole**   Process of cardiac chamber emptying or ejecting blood.

**Tachycardia**   A heart rate in excess of 100 beats per minute in an adult.

**Tachypnea**   Respiratory rate greater than 24 breaths per minute.

**Tactile Fremitus**   Vibrations created by sound waves.

**Tao**   A spiritual belief system (with its roots in China) that is ascribed to the oneness of all things in nature.

**Tapotement**   Massage technique using a light tapping of the fingers that stimulates movement in tired muscles.

**Target Organ Chemicals**   Chemicals that have health effects on a particular organ.

**Taxonomy of Nursing Diagnoses**   Type of classification where the diagnostic label is grouped according to which human response the client demonstrates to the actual or perceived stressor.

**Teaching**   Active process in which one individual shares information with another as a means to facilitate behavioral changes.

**Teaching-Learning Process**   Planned interaction promoting a behavioral change that is not a result of maturation or coincidence.

**Teaching Strategies**   Techniques employed by the teacher to promote learning.

**Team**   Group of individuals who work together to achieve a common goal.

**Telecare**   Nursing care and community support to clients at a distance.

**Telehealth**   Using telecommunication and information technology to provide health care at a distance from the care setting.

**Telemedicine**   The delivery of medical care via computerized equipment.

**Telenursing**   The delivery of nursing care via computerized equipment.

**Teleology**   Ethical theory that states that the moral value of a situation is determined by its consequences.

**Teratogen**   Anything that adversely affects normal cellular development in the embryo or fetus.

**Teratogenic Substance**   Substance that can cross the placental barrier and impair normal growth and development.

**Termination Phase**   Third and final stage of the therapeutic relationship; focuses on evaluation of goal achievement and effectiveness of treatment.

**Tertiary Intention Healing**   Healing process of a wound in which primary closure of a wound is undesirable; occurs when circulation is poor or when infection is present.

**Testicular Self-Exam (TSE)**   Systematic palpation of the testicles by a man on himself for the purpose of finding lumps that potentially may be cancerous; should be done monthly after a hot shower.

**Testimony**   Written or verbal evidence given by a qualified expert in an area.

**Thallium**   Radionuclide that is the physiological analogue of potassium.

**Theory**   Set of concepts and propositions that provide an orderly way to view phenomena.

**Therapeutic**   Describes actions that are beneficial to the client.

**Therapeutic Communication**   Use of communication for the purpose of creating a beneficial outcome for the client.

**Therapeutic Massage**   Application of pressure and motion by the hands with the intent of improving the recipient's well-being.

**Therapeutic Procedure Incidents**   Accidents that occur during the delivery of medical or nursing interventions.

**Therapeutic Range**   Achievement of a constant therapeutic blood level of a medication within a safe range.

**Therapeutic Relationship**   Relationship that benefits the client's health status.

**Therapeutic Touch**   Holistic technique that consists of assessing alterations in a person's energy fields and using the hands to direct energy to achieve a balanced state.

**Therapeutic Use of Self**   Process in which nurses deliberately plan their actions and approach the relationship with a specific goal in mind before interacting with the client.

**Thermoregulation**   Body's physiological function of heat regulation to maintain a constant internal body temperature.

**Thoracentesis**   The aspiration of fluids from the pleural cavity.

**Thrills**   Vibrations that feel similar to a purring cat.

**Thrombus**   Blood clot.

**Throughput**   Input from the community that is processed.

**Toddler**   Developmental stage beginning at approximately 12 to 18 months of age, when a child begins to walk, and ending at approximately age 3.

**Tolerance**   Phenomenon of requiring larger and larger doses of an analgesic to achieve the same level of pain relief.

**Tort**   Civil wrong committed upon a person or property stemming from a direct invasion of some legal right of the person, the infraction of some public duty, or the violation of some private obligation by which damages accrue to the person.

**Tort Law**   Enforcement of duties and rights among individuals independent of contractual agreements.

**Totality Paradigm**   Nursing viewpoint that conceptualizes the interaction between person and environment as constant in order to accomplish goals and maintain balance.

**Total Parenteral Nutrition**   Intravenous infusion of a solution containing dextrose, amino acids, fats, essential fatty acids, vitamins, and minerals.

**Total Quality Management**   Method of management and system operation that is used to achieve continuous quality improvement.

**Touch**   Means of perceiving or experiencing through tactile sensation.

**Toxic Effect**   Reaction that occurs when the body cannot metabolize a drug, causing the drug to accumulate in the blood.

**Tracheotomy**   A surgical procedure in which an opening (stoma) is made through the anterior neck into the trachea; an artificial airway (tracheostomy tube) is placed into the stoma.

**Transcendence**   Finding meaning larger than the person's individual self and life.

**Transcultural Nursing**   Formal area of study and practice focused on comparative analysis of different cultures and subcultures with respect to cultural care, health and illness beliefs, and values and practices, with the goal of providing health care within the context of the client's culture.

**Transcutaneous Electrical Nerve Stimulation (TENS)**   Method of applying minute amounts of electrical stimulation to large-diameter nerve fibers via electrodes placed on the skin to block the passage of pain to the dorsal spinal root.

**Transdermal**   Absorption through the skin into the systemic circulation.

**Transducer**   Instrument that converts electrical energy to sound waves.

**Transferrin** (nonheme iron)   Combination of a blood protein and iron.

**Transformational Leadership**   Leadership that promotes the end values of justice, equality, and human rights, as well as endorses the modal values of honesty, loyalty, and fairness.

**Transgender**   Person who dresses and engages in roles of the person of the opposite gender.

**Transient Flora**   Microorganisms that attach to the skin for a brief period of time but do not continuously live on the skin.

**Transient Infectious Agents**   Those microorganisms that are picked up by the skin from another person or object.

**Transmission-Based Precautions**   Precautions designed for clients documented or suspected to be infected with highly transmissible pathogens for which additional precautions beyond Standard Precautions are needed.

**Transsexual**   Belief that one is psychologically of the sex opposite own anatomical gender.

**Transvestite**   Person who dresses as the opposite gender than birth gender.

**Trigger Point**   Hypersensitive point in a muscle, ligament, fascia, or joint capsule that when stimulated causes a local twitch or jump response.

**Triglycerides**   Lipid compounds consisting of three fatty acids and a glycerol molecule.

**Trocar**   Large-bored abdominal paracentesis needle.

**Troponin**  Cardiac-specific proteins involved in muscle contraction.

**Trough**  A groove or channel in which substances may travel through.

**T-Tube**  Artificial drain placed in the common bile duct during surgery.

**Tunneling**  Areas of soft tissue destruction underlying intact skin that extend in one direction (usually at right angles) from the primary ulcer bed.

**Tympany**  A low-pitched sound of long duration.

**Type and Crossmatch**  Laboratory test that identifies the client's blood type (e.g., A or B) and determines the compatibility of the blood between potential donor and recipient.

**Type I Recommendation**  Typically the most serious finding during JCAHO survey process; requires resolution of deficiency within a specified time frame.

**Ultrasound**  Use of high-frequency sound waves instead of x-ray film to visualize deep body structures; also called an echogram.

**Uncomplicated Grief**  A fairly predictable grief reaction following a significant loss, ending with the relinquishing of the lost object and resumption of the previous life.

**Understaffing**  Failure of a facility to provide a sufficient number of professional staff to meet the needs of their clients.

**Unified Nursing Language System (UNLS)** A language system developed by the American Nurses Association in 1991 that encompasses common nursing terms from a variety of vocabularies that can be used interchangeably as synonyms for the same concept.

**Unintentional Wound**  Wound resulting from trauma or accident.

**Unit Dose Form**  System of packaging and labeling each dose of medication, usually for a 24-hour period.

**Unprofessional Conduct**  Conduct that could adversely affect the health and welfare of the public.

**Unsaturated Fatty Acids**  Glycerol esters of organic acids whose atoms are joined by double or triple valence bonds.

**Urgency**  Timely intervention of surgery.

**Urge Urinary Incontinence**  Uncontrolled discharge of urine caused by hyperactive (unstable) contractions of the detrusor muscle.

**Urinalysis**  Laboratory analysis of the urine.

**Urinary Incontinence**  Uncontrolled loss of urine of sufficient duration and volume to create a social or hygienic problem.

**Urinary Retention**  Inability to completely evacuate the bladder.

**Urobilinogen**  Derived from the normal bacterial action of intestinal flora on bilirubin.

**Urodynamics**  A set of tests that measure bladder and surrounding abdominal pressures.

**Utility**  Ethical principle that states that an act must result in the greatest amount of good for the greatest number of people involved in a situation.

**Vaccination**  Inoculation with a vaccine to produce immunity against specific diseases.

**Value**  Variation of the variable.

**Values**  Principles that influence the development of beliefs and attitudes.

**Values Clarification**  Process of analyzing one's own values to better understand what is truly important to oneself.

**Variable**  Anything that may differ from the norm.

**Variations**  Goals not met or interventions not performed according to the time frame; also called variance.

**Vasoconstriction**  The narrowing of the vessels, usually leading to reduced blood flow.

**Vasodilation**  The widening of the vessels, usually leads to increased blood flow.

**Vector-Borne Transmission**  Mode of transmission of disease through animate objects.

**Vehicle Transmission**  Mode of transmission of disease through inanimate objects.

**Venipuncture**  Puncturing of a vein with a needle to aspirate blood.

**Venography**  Radiographic study of the venous system of the lower extremities following the injection of an iodine contrast agent.

**Venous Access Devices (VAD)**  Venous catheters made of different types of materials and available in single, double, triple, or even quadruple lumens.

**Venous Ulcers**  Lower extremity ulcers caused by chronic venous insufficiency and the resultant fragility of the tissues.

**Ventilation**  Movement of air into and out of the lungs for the purpose of delivering fresh air to the alveoli.

**Ventilation–Perfusion (V/Q) Mismatching**  Condition in which perfusion and ventilation of the lung areas are not adequately balanced.

**Veracity**  Ethical principle that means that one should be truthful, neither lying nor deceiving others.

**Verbal Message**  Message communicated through words or language, both spoken and written.

**Vesicant**  Medication that causes blisters and tissue injury when it escapes into surrounding tissue.

**Vesicular Sounds**  Soft, breezy, and low-pitched sounds heard longer on inspiration than expiration that result from air moving through the smaller airways over the lung's periphery, with the exception of the scapular area.

**Vibration**  Massage technique using rapid movements that stimulate or relax muscles.

**Virulence**  Degree of pathogenicity of an infectious microorganism (pathogen).

**Visceral Pain**  Discomfort felt in the internal organs.

**Visual Channel**  Transmission of messages through sight, observation, and perception.

**Visual Learner**  A person who learns by processing information by seeing.

**Vital Capacity**    Amount of air exhaled from the lungs after a minimal full inspiration.

**Vital Signs**    Measurement of the client's body temperature (T), pulse (P) rate, respiratory (R) rate, and blood pressure (BP).

**Vitamins**    Organic compounds.

**Voiding**    Process of urine evacuation.

**Walking Rounds**    Reporting method used when the members of the care team walk to each client's room and discuss care and progress with each other and the client.

**Water-Soluble Vitamins**    Vitamins that require daily ingestion in normal quantities because they are not stored in the body.

**Wellness**    Condition in which an individual functions at optimal levels.

**Wellness Nursing Diagnosis**    Nursing diagnosis that indicates the client's expression of a desire to obtain a higher level of wellness in some area of function. It is composed of the diagnostic label preceded by the phrase "potential for enhanced."

**Wheezes**    Heard predominantly on expiration all over the lungs as a continuous sonorous wheeze or sibilant wheeze.

**Whistle-blowing**    Calling attention to the unethical, illegal, or incompetant actions of others.

**Withdrawal Syndrome**    State in which symptoms occur after abrupt discontinuation of a narcotic.

**Work of Breathing**    Amount of muscular energy (work) required to accomplish ventilation.

**Working Phase**    Second stage of the therapeutic relationship in which problems are identified, goals are established, and problem-solving methods are selected.

**Wound**    Disruption in the integrity of a body tissue.

**Yellow Wound**    Wound with fibrinous slough or purulent exudate from bacteria.

**Young Adulthood**    Developmental stage from the ages of 21 to approximately 40 years.

**Z-Track Technique**    Method of intramuscular (IM) injection to seal the medication in the muscle, preventing the drug from irritating the subcutaneous tissue.